Ackley and Ladwig's

NURSING DIAGNOSIS HANDBOOK

An Evidence-Based Guide to Planning Care

NANDA-I Diagnoses

Mary Beth Flynn Makic PhD, RN, CCNS, CCRN-K, FAAN, FNAP, FCNS
Professor
Program Director, Adult-Gerontology Clinical Nurse Specialist Program
College of Nursing
University of Colorado
Aurora, Colorado

Marina Reyna Martinez-Kratz MS, RN, CNE
Professor
Department of Nursing
Jackson College
Jackson, Michigan

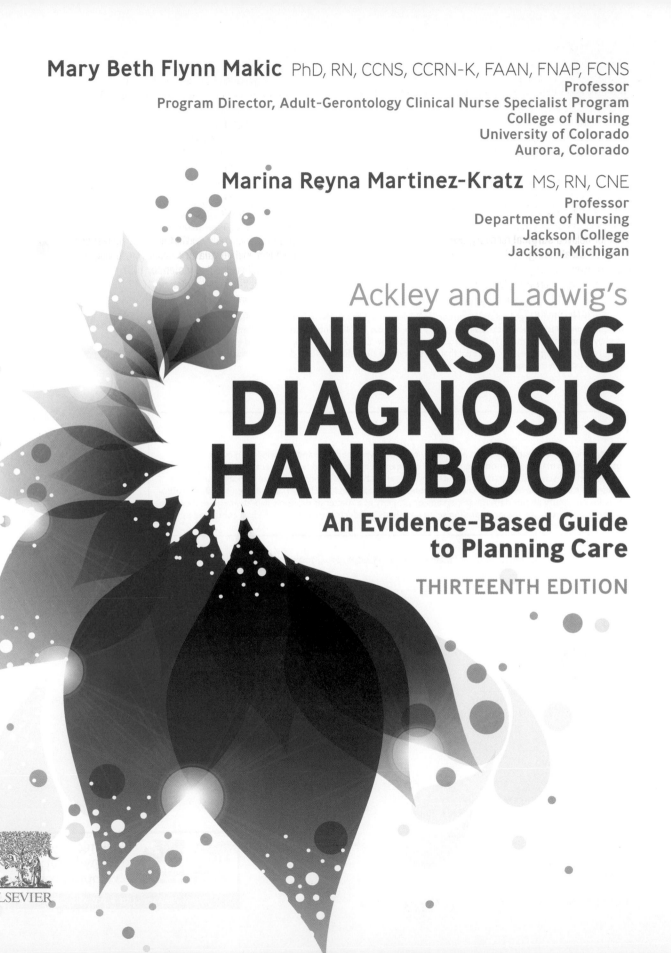

Ackley and Ladwig's

NURSING DIAGNOSIS HANDBOOK

An Evidence-Based Guide to Planning Care

THIRTEENTH EDITION

ELSEVIER

3251 Riverport Lane
St. Louis, Missouri 63043

ACKLEY AND LADWIG'S NURSING DIAGNOSIS HANDBOOK, THIRTEENTH EDITION

ISBN: 978-0-323-77683-7

Notice

Practitioners and researchers must always rely on their own experience and knowledge in evaluating and using any information, methods, compounds or experiments described herein. Because of rapid advances in the medical sciences, in particular, independent verification of diagnoses and drug dosages should be made. To the fullest extent of the law, no responsibility is assumed by Elsevier, authors, editors or contributors for any injury and/or damage to persons or property as a matter of products liability, negligence or otherwise, or from any use or operation of any methods, products, instructions, or ideas contained in the material herein.

Previous editions copyrighted 2020, 2017, 2014, 2011, 2008, 2006, 2004, 2002, 1999, 1997, 1995, and 1993.

Senior Content Strategist: Sandra Clark
Senior Content Development Specialist: Rae L. Robertson
Publishing Services Manager: Julie Eddy
Book Production Specialist: Clay S. Broeker
Design Direction: Amy Buxton

Printed in Canada

Last digit is the print number: 9 8 7 6 5 4 3 2 1

To nursing colleagues throughout the world who continue to demonstrate unwavering commitment to providing exceptional care, physical, emotional, and spiritual care. Special thanks to my family. To my husband and children, whose unconditional love and support are ever present in my life. To my parents and sisters for always encouraging me to follow my passion. Finally, to Betty Ackley and Gail Ladwig for their steadfast commitment to the profession of nursing as expert teachers and prolific authors. Your leadership and spirit continue to inform nursing practice excellence.
Mary Beth Flynn Makic

To all the nurses who are working on the front lines. To my best friend and the love of my life, Kent Martinez-Kratz. To my children, Maxwell, Jesse, and Sierra, whose love, inspiration, and wit make my life complete. To my first fans, my parents Angel and Eva, and siblings, Debra and Jason. To Gail Ladwig for being the absolute best nursing professor, mentor, colleague, and comadre. And finally, to Betty Ackley's memory, for inspiring excellence in nursing education and practice.
Marina Reyna Martinez-Kratz

About the Authors

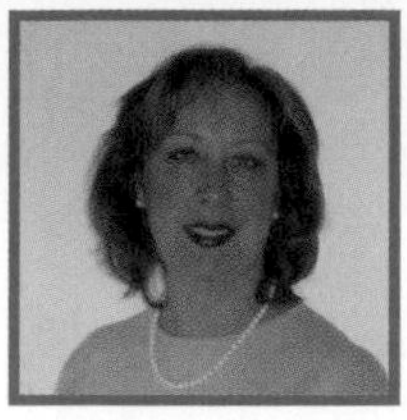

Mary Beth Flynn Makic is a Professor at the University of Colorado College of Nursing in Aurora, Colorado, where she teaches in the undergraduate, graduate, and doctoral programs. She is the director of the Adult-Gerontology Clinical Nurse Specialist Program at the College of Nursing. She has worked predominately in critical care for 33 years. Mary Beth is best known for her publications and presentations, regionally and nationally, as an expert on evidence-based practice in nursing. Her practice expertise and research focus are trauma, general surgical, and burn-injured client populations; acute wound healing; pressure ulcer prevention; and hospital-acquired conditions (HACs). She is passionate about nurses' understanding and translating current best evidence into practice to optimize client and family outcomes. She is coeditor of *Trauma Nursing: from Resuscitation through Rehabilitation,* fifth edition, and *Introduction to Critical Care Nursing,* eighth edition. She is actively involved in several professional nursing and interprofessional organizations.

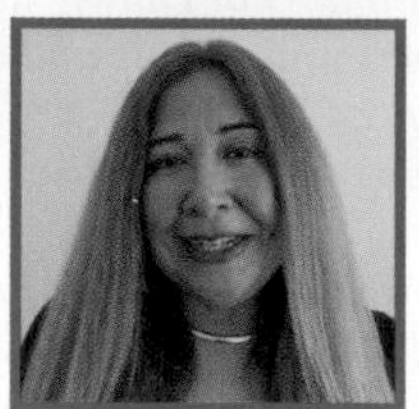

Marina Reyna Martinez-Kratz is a Professor of Nursing at Jackson College in Jackson, Michigan. She is a registered nurse with 33 years of experience and is a Certified Nurse Educator. She received her nursing degrees from Jackson Community College and the University of Michigan. Her expertise in nursing practice has focused on psychiatric nursing, professional issues, and nutrition. In 1998 Marina joined the faculty at Jackson Community College and currently teaches nursing courses in Behavioral Health, Capstone Nursing, and Nutrition. In addition, Marina serves on the Nursing Outcomes and Professional Development Committees and is a Mandated Reporter Trainer. She has served as a behavioral health consultant for several health care facilities, contributes to and reviews many academic publications, and has presented at the state and national level. Marina belongs to many professional organizations and serves as the National League for Nursing Ambassador for Jackson College. Marina's passion is helping students learn to think like nurses! Marina is the proud mother of three children and has been married to her partner and best friend Kent for 32 years.

Contributors

Keith A. Anderson, PhD, MSW
Associate Professor
School of Social Work
University of Montana
Missoula, Montana

Amanda Andrews, BSc (Hons), MA
Senior Teaching Fellow
Birmingham City University
Birmingham, United Kingdom

Carla Aresco, MSL, CRNP
Clinical Program Manager
Department of Neurosurgery
University of Maryland Medical Center
Baltimore, Maryland

Suzanne C. Ashworth, MSN, APRN, CCRN, CCNS
Clinical Nurse Specialist
Center for Nursing Research
ORMC/Orlando Health
Orlando, Florida

Kathaleen C. Bloom, PhD, CNM
Professor Emeritus
School of Nursing
University of North Florida
Jacksonville, Florida

Susan Bonini, EdD, MSN, RN
Assistant Professor
Division of Adult and Senior Health
College of Nursing
University of Colorado
Aurora, Colorado

Monica Brock, MSN, RN, CCRN, CNEcl
Clinical Scholar
Professional Development
UCHealth/University of Colorado Hospital
Aurora, Colorado

Elyse Bueno, MS, ACCNS-AG, CCRN, NE-BC
Nurse Manager
Surgical Trauma Intensive Care Unit
UCHealth/University of Colorado Hospital
Aurora, Colorado

Stacey M. Carroll, PhD, APRN-BC
Assistant Professor
College of Nursing
Rush University
Chicago, Illinois

Nadia Ali Muhammad Ali Charania, PhD, RN
Clinical Assistant Professor
School of Nursing
University of Michigan
Ann Arbor, Michigan

Nichol Chesser, RN, CNM, DNP
Assistant Professor
OB/GYN
School of Medicine
University of Colorado
Aurora, Colorado

Lorraine Chiappetta, MSN, RN, CNE
Emeritus Professional Faculty, Nursing
Washtenaw Community College
Ann Arbor, Michigan

JoAnn Coar, MSN, RN-BC, A-GNP-C, CWOCN
Nursing Education Department
Chilton Medical Center
Pompton Plains, New Jersey

Maureen F. Cooney, DNP, FNP-BC, ACHPN, AP-PMN
Nurse Practitioner
Department of Pain Management
Westchester Medical Center
Instructor of Anesthesiology
New York Medical College
Valhalla, New York
Adjunct Associate Professor
Lienhard School of Nursing, College of Health Professions
Pace University
New York, New York

Mary Rose Day, DN, MA, PGDip PHN, BSc, RPHN, RM, RGN
School of Nursing and Midwifery
University College Cork
Cork, Ireland

Helen I. de Graaf-Waar, MSc, RN
Consultant
Dutch Association for Nursing Diagnoses, Interventions, Outcomes
Groningen, The Netherlands

Mary E. Desmond, PhD, RN, MA, MSN, AHN-BC
Assistant Professor and Associate Director of Master's Entry to Nursing Practice (MENP) Program
College of Science and Health
DePaul University
Chicago, Illinois
Research Health Scientist
Center of Innovation for Complex Chronic Healthcare (CINCCH) Research
Hines VA Medical Center
Hines, Illinois
Faculty Associate
Caritas Leader Faculty
Watson Caring Science Institute
Boulder, Colorado

Julianne E. Doubet, BSN, RN, EMT-B
Certified Emergency Nurse (Retired)
Bethesda North Hospital
Mason, Ohio

Margaret M. Egan-Touw, DNP, RN, CNE
Assistant Professor
University of Texas Medical Branch School of Nursing
Galveston, Texas

Dawn Fairlie, PhD, NP
Assistant Professor
Department of Nursing
School of Health Sciences
College of Staten Island
City University of New York
Staten Island, New York

Arlene T. Farren, PhD, RN, AOCN, CTN-A
Associate Professor Emerita and Adjunct Associate Professor
Department of Nursing
College of Staten Island
Staten Island, New York
Associate Professor Emerita
Department of Nursing
City University of New York Graduate Center
New York, New York

Judith Ann Floyd, PhD, RN, FNAP, FAAN
Professor Emerita
College of Nursing
Wayne State University
Detroit, Michigan

Meredith Ford, MSN, RN, CNE
Assistant Professor
University of Texas Medical Branch School of Nursing
Galveston, Texas

Katherine Foss, MSN, RN
Instructor, Clinical Teaching
Assistant Director, Experiential Learning Team
College of Nursing
University of Colorado
Supervisor, Clinical Entry Programs
Department of Professional Development
UCHealth/University of Colorado Hospital
Aurora, Colorado

Maria Galletto, MSN, RN, CNL, CPHQ
Lead Quality Nurse Consultant
Kaiser Foundation Hospital
Oakland, California

Tracy P. George, DNP, APRN-BC, CNE
Assistant Professor of Nursing
Francis Marion University
Florence, South Carolina

Susanne W. Gibbons, PhD, C-ANP/GNP
Clinical Nurse Practitioner, Adult and Geriatric
Greater Baltimore Medical Center
Towson, Maryland

Barbara A. Given, PhD, RN, FAAN
University Distinguished Professor
College of Nursing
Michigan State University
East Lansing, Michigan

Pauline McKinney Green, PhD, RN, CNE
Professor Emerita
College of Nursing and Allied Health Sciences
Howard University
Washington, District of Columbia

Sherry A. Greenberg, PhD, RN, GNP-BC, FGSA, FAANP, FAAN
Associate Professor
College of Nursing
Seton Hall University
South Orange, New Jersey

Linda J. Hassler, DNP, RN, GCNS-BC, FGNLA
Assistant Professor
Rutgers School of Nursing
Newark, New Jersey

Dianne F. Hayward, RN, MSN, WHNP
Adjunct Faculty
Department of Nursing
Oakland Community College
Waterford, Michigan

Kelly Henrichs, DNP, RN, GNP-BC
Assistant Professor
College of Nursing
University of Colorado
Aurora, Colorado

Dina M. Hewett, PhD, RN, NEA-BC
Associate Dean of Nursing Operations
Department of Nursing
Herzing University
Menomonee Falls, Wisconsin

Patricia Hindin, PhD, CNM
Associate Professor
Advanced Nursing Practice
Rutgers University School of Nursing
Newark, New Jersey

Paula D. Hopper, MSN, RN, CNE
Professor Emeritus
Department of Nursing
Jackson College
Jackson, Michigan

Wendie A. Howland, MN, RN-BC, CRRN, CCM, CNLCP, LNCC
Principal
Legal Nurse Consulting and Life Care Planning
Howland Health Consulting
Cape Cod, Massachusetts

Teri Hulett, RN, BSN, CIC, FAPIC
Infection Prevention Consultant
Infection Prevention Strategies, LLC
Thornton, Colorado

Nicole Huntley, MS, RN, APN, ACCNS-AG
Clinical Nurse Specialist
Department of Professional Development
UCHealth/University of Colorado Hospital
Aurora, Colorado

Olga F. Jarrín, PhD, RN
Assistant Professor
School of Nursing
Assistant Professor
Institute for Health, Health Care Policy, and Aging Research
Rutgers, The State University of New Jersey
New Brunswick, New Jersey
Adjunct Assistant Professor
School of Nursing
University of Pennsylvania
Philadelphia, Pennsylvania

Laura King, DNP, RN, MSN, CNE
Assistant Professor and BSN Program Director, Junior Level
University of Texas Medical Branch School of Nursing
Galveston, Texas

Rachel Klompmaker, BScN, NP-PHC, MScN
Nurse Practitioner
Durham Christian Homes
Newcastle, Ontario, Canada

Gail B. Ladwig, MSN, RN
Professor Emeritus
Jackson Community College
Jackson, Michigan
Consultant in Guided Imagery, Healing Touch, and Nursing Diagnosis
Hilton Head, South Carolina

Patrick Luna, MSN, RN, CEN, NRP
Senior Instructor of Clinical Teaching
Experiential Learning Team
College of Nursing
University of Colorado
Aurora, Colorado

Mary Beth Flynn Makic, PhD, RN, CCNS, CCRN-K, FAAN, FNAP, FCNS
Professor
Program Director, Adult-Gerontology Clinical Nurse Specialist Program
College of Nursing
University of Colorado
Aurora, Colorado

Mary Patricia Mancuso, MA
Professional Research Assistant
General Internal Medicine
School of Medicine
University of Colorado
Aurora, Colorado

Marina Reyna Martinez-Kratz, MS, RN, CNE
Professor
Department of Nursing
Jackson College
Jackson, Michigan

Lauren McAlister, MSN, FNP-BC, DNP
School of Nursing
University of North Florida
Jacksonville, Florida

Kimberly S. Meyer, PhD, ACNP-BC, CNRN
Neurotrauma/Cerebrovascular Nurse Practitioner
Department of Neurological Surgery
AGACNP Track Instructor
School of Nursing
University of Louisville
Louisville, Kentucky

Daniela Moscarella, DNP, APN, CPNP-PC, CCRN-K
Clinical Instructor
Entry to Baccalaureate Nursing Practice
Rutgers, The State University of New Jersey
Newark, New Jersey

Morgan Nestingen, MSN, APRN, AGCNS-BC, OCN, ONN-CG
Director of Nursing, Intake and Navigation Services
Department of Nursing
Miami Cancer Institute
Miami, Florida
PhD Student
College of Nursing
University of Colorado
Aurora, Colorado

Katherina A. Nikzad-Terhune, PhD, MSW
Assistant Professor
School of Social Work
Northern Kentucky University
Highland Heights, Kentucky

Darcy O'Banion, RN, MS, ACCNS-AG
Senior Instructor
Department of Neurology
School of Medicine
University of Colorado
Aurora, Colorado

Kenneth J. Oja, PhD, RN
Nurse Scientist
Nursing Education and Research
Denver Health
Denver, Colorado
Assistant Professor Adjunct
College of Nursing
University of Colorado
Aurora, Colorado

Kristen A. Oster, DNP, APRN, ACNS-BC, CNOR, CNS-CP
Assistant Nurse Manager, Operating Room
Parker Adventist Hospital
Parker, Colorado

Kathleen L. Patusky, PhD, MA, RN, CNS
Associate Professor
School of Nursing
Rutgers, The State University of New Jersey
Newark, New Jersey

Kim L. Paxton, DNP, APRN, ANP-BC, LHIT-C
Assistant Professor
College of Nursing
University of Colorado
Aurora, Colorado

Nishat S. Poppy, BSN, RN
Registered Nurse
Post ICU
Jersey City Medical Center
Jersey City, New Jersey

Ann Will Poteet, MS, RN, CNS, AGNP-C
Nurse Practitioner
Division of Cardiology
School of Medicine
University of Colorado
Aurora, Colorado

Margaret Quinn, DNP, CPNP, CNE
Clinical Associate Professor, Advanced Practice Division
Specialty Director, Pediatric Nurse Practitioner Program
Rutgers, The State University of New Jersey
Newark, New Jersey

Friso Raemaekers, B Health, RN, CEN
Health Informatics Nurse
R&D Department
Nursing Quality Concept
The Hague, The Netherlands

Barbara A. Reyna, PhD, RN, NNP-BC
Associate Professor
School of Nursing, University of Virginia
Charlottesville, Virginia
Neonatal Nurse Practitioner
Children's Hospital of Richmond
VCU Health System
Richmond, Virginia

Mamilda Robinson, DNP, APN, PMHNP-BC
Clinical Instructor
Division of Advanced Nursing Practice
Rutgers, The State University of New Jersey
Newark, New Jersey

Kimberly Anne Rumsey, MSN, RN, CNE
Assistant Professor
University of Texas Medical Branch School of Nursing
Galveston, Texas

Debra Siela, PhD, RN, ACNS-BC, CCRN-K, CNE, RRT
Associate Professor
School of Nursing
Ball State University
Muncie, Indiana

Tammy Spencer, DNP, RN, CNE, AGCNS-BC, CCNS
Assistant Professor
College of Nursing
University of Colorado
Aurora, Colorado

Bernie St Aubyn, BSc (Hons), MSc
Senior Lecturer
Dame Edith Cavell Department of Adult Nursing
Birmingham City University
Birmingham, United Kingdom

Denise Sullivan, MSN, ANP-BC, ACHPN, AP-PMN
Nurse Practitioner
Department of Pain Management
NYC Health + Hospitals/Jacobi
Bronx, New York

Jacquelyn Svoboda, DNP, RN, WHNP-C
Assistant Professor and Advanced Practice Nurse
University of Texas Medical Branch School of Nursing
Galveston, Texas

Philemon Tedros, BSN, RN
BSN Student
Rutgers, The State University of New Jersey
Newark, New Jersey

Krystal Chamberlain Tenure, MS, RN, CCRN, SCRN
Clinical Nurse Educator
Neurosurgical ICU
UCHealth/University of Colorado Hospital
Aurora, Colorado

Rosemary Timmerman, DNP, APRN, CCNS, CCRN-CSC-CMC
Clinical Nurse Specialist
Intensive Care Unit
Providence Alaska Medical Center
Anchorage, Alaska
Adjunct Faculty
University of Providence School of Nursing
Great Falls, Montana

Janelle M. Tipton, DNP, APRN-CNS, AOCN
Clinical Assistant Professor
School of Nursing
Purdue University
West Lafayette, Indiana

Mary Velahos, BSN
Traditional BSN Honors Student
School of Nursing
Rutgers, The State University of New Jersey
Newark, New Jersey

Barbara Baele Vincensi, PhD, RN, FNP-BC
Associate Professor
Department of Nursing
Hope College
Holland, Michigan

Jody L. Vogelzang, PhD, RDN, CHES, FAND
Associate Professor
Allied Health Sciences
Grand Valley State University
Grand Rapids, Michigan

Suzanne White, MSN, RN, PHCNS-BC
Associate Professor
Department of Nursing
Morehead State University
Morehead, Kentucky

David M. Wikstrom, BSN, RN, CMSRN
Graduate Student, Nursing Research
Michigan State University
Lansing, Michigan

Ruth A. Wittmann-Price, PhD, RN, CNS, CNE, CNEcl, CHSE, ANEF, FAAN
Dean and Professor of Nursing
School of Health Sciences
Francis Marion University
Florence, South Carolina

Wendy R. Worden, MS, APRN, CNS, CRRN, CWCN
Clinical Nurse Specialist
Departments of Nursing and Physical Medicine and Rehabilitation
Mayo Clinic
Rochester, Minnesota

Reviewers

Valerie Beshears, MSN, RN, NCSN
Nursing Instructor
College of Health Sciences
University of Arkansas-Fort Smith
Fort Smith, Arkansas

Amelia D. Davis, PhD, RN
Coordinator of Simulation and Clinical Learning
School of Nursing
North Carolina Agricultural and Technical State University
Greensboro, North Carolina

Lorraine C. Haertel, PhD, RN, CS, APRN
Assistant Professor of Clinical Nursing
School of Nursing
The University of Texas at Austin
Austin, Texas

Kathleen Hughes, DNP, RN, CNE
Undergraduate Nursing Program Director
Nursing Department
Marian University Wisconsin
Fond du Lac, Wisconsin

Silvia Imanda, PhD, RN
Department of Nursing
University of Arkansas-Fort Smith
Fort Smith, Arkansas

Alisha H. Johnson, MSN, RN
Clinical Assistant Professor
Department of Nursing
St. David's School of Nursing at Texas State University
Round Rock, Texas

Paula Julian, PhD, APRN, FNP-C, CPN
Interim Executive Director of Nursing
Department of Nursing
University of Arkansas-Fort Smith
Fort Smith, Arkansas

Susan Wynn, MSN, RN
Nurse Educator
Nursing Faculty
University of Arkansas-Fort Smith
Fort Smith, Arkansas

Preface

Ackley and Ladwig's Nursing Diagnosis Handbook: An Evidence-Based Guide to Planning Care is a convenient reference to help the practicing nurse or nursing student make a nursing diagnosis and write a care plan with ease and confidence. This handbook helps nurses correlate nursing diagnoses with known information about clients on the basis of assessment findings; established medical, surgical, or psychiatric diagnoses; and the current treatment plan.

Making a nursing diagnosis and planning care are complex processes that involve diagnostic reasoning and critical thinking skills. Nursing students and practicing nurses cannot possibly memorize the extensive list of defining characteristics, related factors, and risk factors for the 267 diagnoses approved by NANDA-International (NANDA-I). There are also two additional diagnoses that the authors think are significant: Hearing Loss and Vision Loss. These diagnoses are contained in Appendix E (on the Evolve website). This book correlates suggested nursing diagnoses with what nurses know about clients and offers a care plan for each nursing diagnosis.

Section I, Nursing Process, Clinical Reasoning, Nursing Diagnosis, and Evidence-Based Nursing, is divided into two parts. Part A includes an overview of the nursing process. This section provides information on how to make a nursing diagnosis and directions on how to plan nursing care. It also includes information on using clinical reasoning and judgment skills, eliciting the "client's story," recognizing patterns in client responses, and synthesizing information to form decisions that will guide care based on analyzing and understanding the client's concerns. Part B includes advanced nursing concepts: concept mapping, QSEN (Quality and Safety Education for Nurses), evidence-based nursing care, quality nursing care, person-centered care, safety, informatics in nursing, and team/collaborative work with a multiprofessional team.

In **Section II, Guide to Nursing Diagnosis,** the nurse can look up symptoms and problems and their suggested nursing diagnoses for more than 1450 client symptoms; medical, surgical, and psychiatric diagnoses; diagnostic procedures; surgical interventions; and clinical states.

In **Section III, Guide to Planning Care,** the nurse can find care plans for all nursing diagnoses suggested in Section II. We have included the suggested nursing outcomes from the Nursing Outcomes Classification (NOC) and interventions from the Nursing Interventions Classification (NIC) by the Iowa Intervention Project. We believe this work is a significant addition to the nursing process to further define nursing practice with standardized language.

Scientific rationales based on research are included for most of the interventions. This is done to make the evidence basis for the specific nursing practice apparent to the nursing student and practicing nurse.

Special features of the 13th edition of *Ackley and Ladwig's Nursing Diagnosis Handbook: An Evidence-Based Guide to Planning Care* include the following:

- Labeling of classic older research studies that are still relevant as Classic Evidence-Based (CEB)
- Sixty-seven revised nursing diagnoses approved by NANDA-I
- Use of the terms *At-Risk Populations* and *Associated Conditions* with the diagnostic indicators as approved by NANDA-I.
- Twenty-nine new nursing diagnoses recently approved by NANDA-I, along with the retirement of four nursing diagnoses: Reflex Urinary Incontinence, Grieving, Decreased Intracranial Adaptive Capacity, and Latex Allergy Reaction.
- Seventeen revisions of nursing diagnoses made by NANDA-I in existing nursing diagnoses:
    - **Old diagnosis:** Ineffective Health Maintenance
      Revised diagnosis: Ineffective Health Maintenance Behaviors
    - **Old diagnosis:** Ineffective Health Management
      Revised diagnosis: Ineffective Health Self-Management
    - **Old diagnosis:** Readiness for Enhanced Health Management
      Revised diagnosis: Readiness for Enhanced Health Self-Management
    - **Old diagnosis:** Ineffective Family Health Management
      Revised diagnosis: Ineffective Family Health Self-Management
    - **Old diagnosis:** Impaired Home Maintenance
      Revised diagnosis: Ineffective Home Maintenance Behaviors
        - **Old domain:** 4 Activity/Rest
        - **New domain:** 1 Health Promotion
    - **Old diagnosis:** Ineffective Infant Feeding Pattern
      Revised diagnosis: Ineffective Infant Suck-Swallow Response
    - **Old diagnosis:** Risk for Metabolic Imbalance Syndrome
      Revised diagnosis: Risk for Metabolic Syndrome
    - **Old diagnosis:** Functional Urinary Incontinence
      Revised diagnosis: Disability-Associated Urinary Incontinence
    - **Old diagnosis:** Bowel Incontinence
      Revised diagnosis: Impaired Bowel Continence

    - **Old diagnosis:** Activity Intolerance
      Revised diagnosis: Decreased Activity Tolerance
    - **Old diagnosis:** Risk for Activity Intolerance
      Revised diagnosis: Risk for Decreased Activity Tolerance
    - **Old diagnosis:** Complicated Grieving
      Revised diagnosis: Maladaptive Grieving
    - **Old diagnosis:** Risk for Complicated Grieving
      Revised diagnosis: Risk for Maladaptive Grieving
    - **Old diagnosis:** Risk for Falls
      Revised diagnosis: Risk for Adult Falls
    - **Old diagnosis:** Risk for Pressure Ulcer
      Revised diagnosis: Risk for Adult Pressure Injury
    - **Old diagnosis:** Risk for Suicide
      Revised diagnosis: Risk for Suicidal Behavior
    - **Old diagnosis:** Risk for Delayed Development
      Revised diagnosis: Risk for Delayed Child Development
- Further addition of pediatric and critical care interventions to appropriate care plans
- An associated Evolve Online Course Management System that includes a Care Plan Template, critical thinking case studies, NIC and NOC labels, PowerPoint slides, review questions for the NCLEX-RN® exam, and appendixes for Nursing Diagnoses Arranged by Maslow's Hierarchy of Needs, Nursing Diagnoses Arranged by Gordon's Functional Health Patterns, Motivational Interviewing for Nurses, Wellness-Oriented Diagnostic Categories, and Nursing Care Plans for Hearing Loss and Vision Loss

The following features of *Ackley and Ladwig's Nursing Diagnosis Handbook: A Guide to Planning Care* are also available:

- Suggested nursing diagnoses for more than 1450 clinical entities, including signs and symptoms, medical diagnoses, surgeries, maternal-child disorders, mental health disorders, and geriatric disorders
- Labeling of nursing research as EBN (Evidence-Based Nursing) and clinical research as EB (Evidence-Based) to identify the source of evidence-based rationales
- An Evolve Online Courseware System with a Care Plan Template that helps the student or nurse write a nursing care plan
- Rationales for nursing interventions that are based on nursing research and best practices
- Nursing references identified for each care plan
- A complete list of NOC Outcomes on the Evolve website
- A complete list of NIC Interventions on the Evolve website
- Nursing care plans that contain many holistic interventions
- Care plans written by leading national nursing experts from throughout the United States, along with international contributors, who together represent all of the major nursing specialties and have extensive experience with nursing diagnoses, the nursing process, and evidence-based practice. Several contributors are the original submitters/authors of the nursing diagnoses established by NANDA-I
- A format that facilitates analyzing signs and symptoms by the process already known by nurses, which involves using defining characteristics of nursing diagnoses to make a diagnosis
- Use of NANDA-I terminology and approved diagnoses
- An alphabetical format for Sections II and III, which allows rapid access to information
- Nursing care plans also listed by domains and class, consistent with NANDA-I
- Nursing care plans for all nursing diagnoses listed in Section II
- Specific geriatric interventions in appropriate plans of care
- Specific client/family teaching interventions in each plan of care
- Information on culturally competent nursing care included where appropriate
- Inclusion of commonly used abbreviations (e.g., AIDS, MI, HF) and cross-references to complete terms in Section II

We acknowledge the work of NANDA-I, which is used extensively throughout this text. The original NANDA-I work can be found in *NANDA-I Nursing Diagnoses: Definitions & Classification 2021–2023*, 12th edition.

We and the consultants and contributors trust that nurses will find this 13th edition of *Ackley and Ladwig's Nursing Diagnosis Handbook: An Evidence-Based Guide to Planning Care* a valuable tool that simplifies the process of identifying appropriate nursing diagnoses for clients and planning for their care, thus allowing nurses more time to provide evidence-based care that promote each client's recovery.

Mary Beth Flynn Makic
Marina Reyna Martinez-Kratz

Acknowledgments

We would like to thank the following people at Elsevier: Sandy Clark, Senior Content Strategist, who supported us with the 13th edition of the text with intelligence and kindness; Jennifer Wade and Rae Robertson, Senior Content Development Specialists, who were a continual source of support; and a special thank you to Clay Broeker for the project management of this edition.

With gratitude, we acknowledge nurses and student nurses, who are always an inspiration for us to provide fresh and accurate material. We are honored that they continue to value this text and to use it in their studies and practice.

We would like to thank all of the dedicated contributors who are experts in their fields of nursing. We appreciate all of their hard work.

Care has been taken to confirm the accuracy of the information presented in this book. However, the authors, editors, and publisher cannot accept any responsibility for consequences resulting from errors or omissions of the information in this book and make no warranty, expressed or implied, with respect to its contents. The reader should use practices suggested in this book in accordance with agency policies and professional standards. Every effort has been made to ensure the accuracy of the information presented in this text.

We hope you find this text a useful resource for your nursing practice.

Mary Beth Flynn Makic
Marina Reyna Martinez-Kratz

How to Use *Nursing Diagnosis Handbook: An Evidence-Based Guide to Planning Care*

STEP 1: ASSESS

Following the guidelines in Section I (Nursing Process, Clinical Reasoning, Nursing Diagnosis, and Evidence-Based Nursing), begin to formulate your nursing diagnosis by gathering and documenting the objective and subjective information about the client.

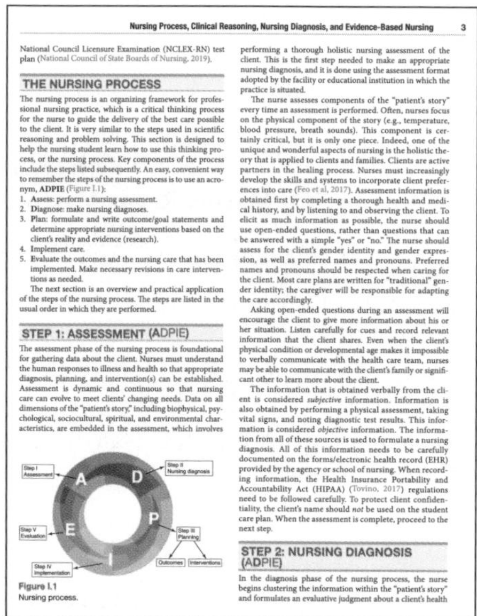

Nursing Process, Clinical Reasoning, Nursing Diagnosis, and Evidence-Based Nursing 3

National Council Licensure Examination (NCLEX-RN) test plan (National Council of State Boards of Nursing, 2019).

THE NURSING PROCESS

The nursing process is an organizing framework for professional nursing practice, which is a critical thinking process for the nurse to guide the delivery of the best care possible to the client. It is very similar to the steps used in scientific reasoning and problem solving. This section is designed to help the nursing student learn how to use this thinking process, or the nursing process. Key components of the process include the steps listed subsequently. An easy, convenient way to remember the steps of the nursing process is to use an acronym, **ADPIE** (Figure I.1):

1. **Assess:** perform a nursing assessment.
2. **Diagnose:** make nursing diagnoses.
3. **Plan:** formulate and write outcome/goal statements and determine appropriate nursing interventions based on the client's reality and evidence (research).
4. Implement care.
5. Evaluate the outcomes and the nursing care that has been implemented. Make necessary revisions in care interventions as needed.

The next section is an overview and practical application of the steps of the nursing process. The steps are listed in the usual order in which they are performed.

STEP 1: ASSESSMENT (ADPIE)

The assessment phase of the nursing process is foundational for gathering data about the client. Nurses must understand the human responses to illness and health so that appropriate diagnosis, planning, and intervention(s) can be established. Assessment is dynamic and continuous so that nursing care can evolve to meet clients' changing needs. Data on all dimensions of the "patient's story," including biophysical, psychological, sociocultural, spiritual, and environmental characteristics, are embedded in the assessment, which involves performing a thorough holistic nursing assessment of the client. This is the first step needed to make an appropriate nursing diagnosis, and it is done using the assessment format adopted by the facility or educational institution in which the practice is situated.

The nurse assesses components of the "patient's story" every time an assessment is performed. Often, nurses focus on the physical component of the story (e.g., temperature, blood pressure, breath sounds). This component is certainly critical, but it is only one piece. Indeed, one of the unique and wonderful aspects of nursing is the holistic theory that is applied to clients and families. Clients are active partners in the healing process. Nurses must increasingly develop the skills and systems to incorporate client preferences into care (Feo et al, 2017). Assessment information is obtained first by completing a thorough health and medical history, and by listening to and observing the client. To elicit as much information as possible, the nurse should use open-ended questions, rather than questions that can be answered with a simple "yes" or "no." The nurse should assess for the client's gender identity and gender expression, as well as preferred names and pronouns. Preferred names and pronouns should be respected when caring for the client. Most care plans are written for "traditional" gender identity; the caregiver will be responsible for adapting the care accordingly.

Asking open-ended questions during an assessment will encourage the client to give more information about his or her situation. Listen carefully for cues and record relevant information that the client shares. Even when the client's physical condition or developmental age makes it impossible to verbally communicate with the health care team, nurses may be able to communicate with the client's family or significant other to learn more about the client.

The information that is obtained verbally from the client is considered *subjective* information. Information is also obtained by performing a physical assessment, taking vital signs, and noting diagnostic test results. This information is considered *objective* information. The information from all of these sources is used to formulate a nursing diagnosis. All of this information needs to be carefully documented on the forms/electronic health record (EHR) provided by the agency or school of nursing. When recording information, the Health Insurance Portability and Accountability Act (HIPAA) (Tovino, 2017) regulations need to be followed carefully. To protect client confidentiality, the client's name should *not* be used on the student care plan. When the assessment is complete, proceed to the next step.

Figure I.1
Nursing process.

STEP 2: NURSING DIAGNOSIS (ADPIE)

In the diagnosis phase of the nursing process, the nurse begins clustering the information within the "patient's story" and formulates an evaluative judgment about a client's health

STEP 2: DIAGNOSE

Turn to Section II, Guide to Nursing Diagnosis, and locate the client's symptoms, clinical state, medical or psychiatric diagnoses, and anticipated or prescribed diagnostic studies or surgical interventions (listed in alphabetical order). Note suggestions for appropriate nursing diagnoses.

Then use Section III, Guide to Planning Care, to evaluate each suggested nursing diagnosis and "related to" (r/t) etiology statement. Section III is a listing of care plans according to NANDA-I, arranged alphabetically by diagnostic concept, for each nursing diagnosis referred to in Section II. Determine the appropriateness of each nursing diagnosis by comparing the Defining Characteristics and/or Risk Factors to the client data collected.

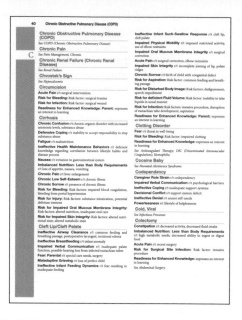

40 Chronic Obstructive Pulmonary Disease (COPD)

C

Chronic Obstructive Pulmonary Disease (COPD)

See COPD (Chronic Obstructive Pulmonary Disease)

Chronic Pain

See Pain Management, Chronic

Chronic Renal Failure (Chronic Renal Disease)

See Renal Failure

Chvostek's Sign

See Hypocalcemia

Circumcision

Acute Pain r/t surgical intervention

Risk for Bleeding: Risk factor: surgical trauma

Risk for Infection: Risk factor: surgical wound

Readiness for Enhanced Knowledge: Parent: expresses an interest in learning

Cirrhosis

Chronic Confusion r/t chronic organic disorder with increased ammonia levels, substance abuse

Defensive Coping r/t inability to accept responsibility to stop substance abuse

Fatigue r/t malnutrition

Ineffective Health Maintenance Behaviors r/t deficient knowledge regarding correlation between lifestyle habits and disease process

Nausea r/t irritation to gastrointestinal system

Imbalanced Nutrition: Less than Body Requirements r/t loss of appetite, nausea, vomiting

Chronic Pain r/t liver enlargement

Chronic Low Self-Esteem r/t chronic illness

Chronic Sorrow r/t presence of chronic illness

Risk for Bleeding: Risk factors: impaired blood coagulation, bleeding from portal hypertension

Risk for Injury: Risk factors: substance intoxication, potential delirium tremens

Risk for Impaired Oral Mucous Membrane Integrity: Risk factors: altered nutrition, inadequate oral care

Risk for Impaired Skin Integrity: Risk factors: altered nutritional state, altered metabolic state

Cleft Lip/Cleft Palate

Ineffective Airway Clearance r/t common feeding and breathing passage, postoperative laryngeal, incisional edema

Ineffective Breastfeeding r/t infant anomaly

Impaired Verbal Communication r/t inadequate palate function, possible hearing loss from infected eustachian tubes

Fear: Parental r/t special care needs, surgery

Maladaptive Grieving r/t loss of perfect child

Ineffective Infant Feeding Dynamics r/t fear resulting in inadequate feeding

Ineffective Infant Suck-Swallow Response r/t cleft lip, cleft palate

Impaired Physical Mobility r/t imposed restricted activity, use of elbow restraints

Impaired Oral Mucous Membrane Integrity r/t surgical correction

Acute Pain r/t surgical correction, elbow restraints

Impaired Skin Integrity r/t incomplete joining of lip, palate ridges

Chronic Sorrow r/t birth of child with congenital defect

Risk for Aspiration: Risk factor: common feeding and breathing passage

Risk for Disturbed Body Image: Risk factors: disfigurement, speech impediment

Risk for deficient Fluid Volume: Risk factor: inability to take liquids in usual manner

Risk for Infection: Risk factors: invasive procedure, disruption of eustachian tube development, aspiration

Readiness for Enhanced Knowledge: Parent: expresses an interest in learning

Clotting Disorder

Fear r/t threat to well-being

Risk for Bleeding: Risk factor: impaired clotting

Readiness for Enhanced Knowledge: expresses an interest in learning

See Anticoagulant Therapy; DIC (Disseminated Intravascular Coagulation); Hemophilia

Cocaine Baby

See Neonatal Abstinence Syndrome

Codependency

Caregiver Role Strain r/t codependency

Impaired Verbal Communication r/t psychological barriers

Ineffective Coping r/t inadequate support systems

Decisional Conflict r/t support system deficit

Ineffective Denial r/t unmet self-needs

Powerlessness r/t lifestyle of helplessness

Cold, Viral

See Infectious Processes

Colectomy

Constipation r/t decreased activity, decreased fluid intake

Imbalanced Nutrition: Less than Body Requirements r/t high metabolic needs, decreased ability to ingest or digest food

Acute Pain r/t recent surgery

Risk for Surgical Site Infection: Risk factor: invasive procedure

Readiness for Enhanced Knowledge: expresses an interest in learning

See Abdominal Surgery

STEP 3: DETERMINE OUTCOMES

Use Section III, Guide to Planning Care, to find appropriate outcomes for the client. Use either the NOC Outcomes with the associated rating scales or Client Outcomes as desired.

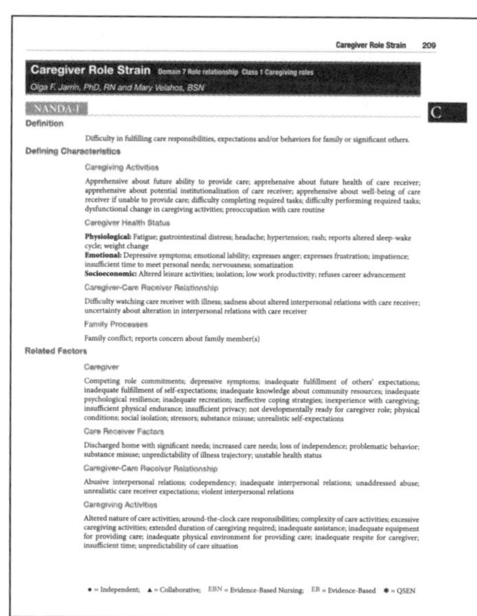

Caregiver Role Strain 209

Caregiver Role Strain Domain 7 Role relationship Class 1 Caregiving roles

Olga F. Jarrin, PhD, RN and Mary Velahos, BSN

C

NANDA-I

Definition

Difficulty in fulfilling care responsibilities, expectations and/or behaviors for family or significant others.

Defining Characteristics

Caregiving Activities

Apprehensive about future ability to provide care; apprehensive about future health of care receiver; apprehensive about potential institutionalization of care receiver; apprehensive about well-being of care receiver if unable to provide care; difficulty completing required tasks; difficulty performing required tasks; dysfunctional change in caregiving activities; preoccupation with care routine

Caregiver Health Status

Physiological: Fatigue; gastrointestinal distress; headache; hypertension; rash; reports altered sleep-wake cycle; weight change
Emotional: Depressive symptoms; emotional lability; expresses anger; expresses frustration; impatience; insufficient time to meet personal needs; nervousness; somatization
Socioeconomic: Altered leisure activities; isolation; low work productivity; refuses career advancement

Caregiver-Care Receiver Relationship

Difficulty watching care receiver with illness; sadness about altered interpersonal relations with care receiver; uncertainty about alteration in interpersonal relations with care receiver

Family Processes

Family conflict; reports concern about family member(s)

Related Factors

Caregiver

Competing role commitments; depressive symptoms; inadequate fulfillment of others' expectations; inadequate fulfillment of self-expectations; inadequate knowledge about community resources; inadequate psychological resilience; inadequate recreation; ineffective coping strategies; inexperience with caregiving; insufficient physical endurance; insufficient privacy; not developmentally ready for caregiver role; physical conditions; social isolation; stressors; substance misuse; unrealistic self-expectations

Care Receiver Factors

Discharged home with significant needs; increased care needs; loss of independence; problematic behavior; substance misuse; unpredictability of illness trajectory; unstable health status

Caregiver-Care Receiver Relationship

Abusive interpersonal relations; codependency; inadequate interpersonal relations; unaddressed abuse; unrealistic care receiver expectations; violent interpersonal relations

Caregiving Activities

Altered nature of care activities; around-the-clock care responsibilities; complexity of care activities; excessive caregiving activities; extended duration of caregiving required; inadequate assistance; inadequate equipment for providing care; inadequate physical environment for providing care; inadequate respite for caregiver; insufficient time; unpredictability of care situation

● = Independent; ▲ = Collaborative; EBN = Evidence-Based Nursing; EB = Evidence-Based ✱ = QSEN

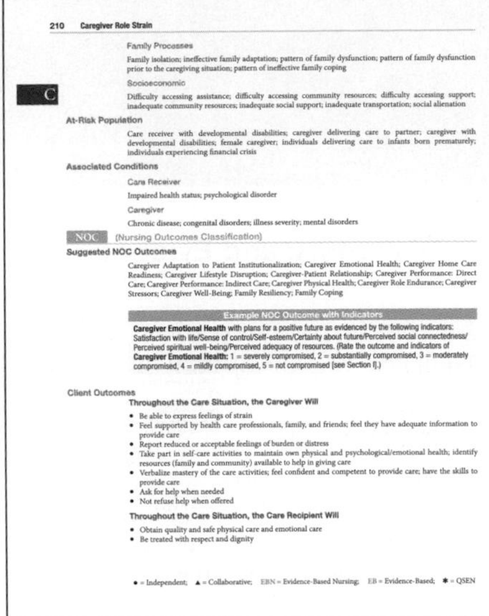

210 **Caregiver Role Strain**

C

Family Processes

Family isolation; ineffective family adaptation; pattern of family dysfunction; pattern of family dysfunction prior to the caregiving situation; pattern of ineffective family coping

Socioeconomic

Difficulty accessing assistance; difficulty accessing community resources; difficulty accessing support; inadequate community resources; inadequate social support; inadequate transportation; social alienation

At-Risk Population

Care receiver with developmental disabilities; caregiver delivering care to partner; caregiver with developmental disabilities; female caregiver; individuals delivering care to infants born prematurely; individuals experiencing financial crisis

Associated Conditions

Care Receiver

Impaired health status; psychological disorder

Caregiver

Chronic disease; congenital disorders; illness severity; mental disorders

NOC (Nursing Outcomes Classification)

Suggested NOC Outcomes

Caregiver Adaptation to Patient Institutionalization; Caregiver Emotional Health; Caregiver Home Care Readiness; Caregiver Lifestyle Disruption; Caregiver-Patient Relationship; Caregiver Performance: Direct Care; Caregiver Performance: Indirect Care; Caregiver Physical Health; Caregiver Role Endurance; Caregiver Stressors; Caregiver Well-Being; Family Resiliency; Family Coping

Example NOC Outcome with Indicators

Caregiver Emotional Health with plans for a positive future as evidenced by the following indicators: Satisfaction with life/Sense of control/Self-esteem/Certainty about future/Perceived social connectedness/Perceived spiritual well-being/Perceived adequacy of resources. (Rate the outcome and indicators of **Caregiver Emotional Health:** 1 = severely compromised, 2 = substantially compromised, 3 = moderately compromised, 4 = mildly compromised, 5 = not compromised [see Section I].)

Client Outcomes

Throughout the Care Situation, the Caregiver Will

- Be able to express feelings of strain
- Feel supported by health care professionals, family, and friends; feel they have adequate information to provide care
- Report reduced or acceptable feelings of burden or distress
- Take part in self-care activities to maintain own physical and psychological/emotional health; identify resources (family and community) available to help in giving care
- Verbalize mastery of the care activities; feel confident and competent to provide care; have the skills to provide care
- Ask for help when needed
- Not refuse help when offered

Throughout the Care Situation, the Care Recipient Will

- Obtain quality and safe physical care and emotional care
- Be treated with respect and dignity

● = Independent; ▲ = Collaborative; EBN = Evidence-Based Nursing; EB = Evidence-Based; ✱ = QSEN

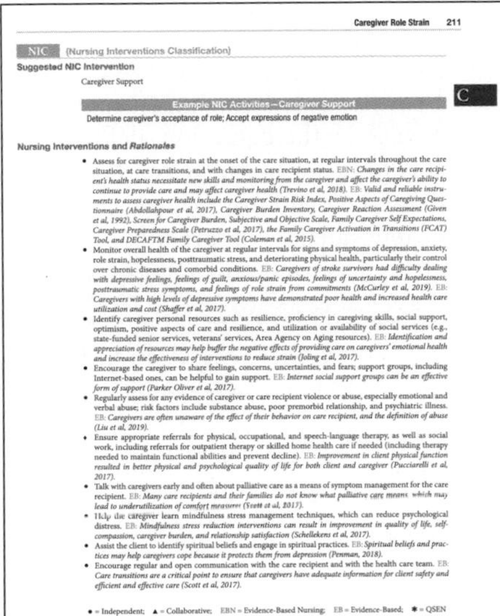

Caregiver Role Strain 211

NIC (Nursing Interventions Classification)

Suggested NIC Intervention

Caregiver Support

C

Example NIC Activities—Caregiver Support

Determine caregiver's acceptance of role; Accept expressions of negative emotion

Nursing Interventions and *Rationales*

- Assess for caregiver role strain at the onset of the care situation, at regular intervals throughout the care situation, at care transitions, and with changes in care recipient status. EBN: *Changes in the care recipient's health status necessitate new skills and monitoring from the caregiver and affect the caregiver's ability to continue to provide care and may affect caregiver health (Trevino et al, 2018).* EB: *Valid and reliable instruments to assess caregiver health include the Caregiver Strain Risk Index, Positive Aspects of Caregiving Questionnaire (Abdollahpour et al, 2017), Caregiver Burden Inventory, Caregiver Reaction Assessment (Given et al, 1992), Screen for Caregiver Burden, Subjective and Objective Scale, Family Caregiver Self Expectations, Caregiver Preparedness Scale (Petruzzo et al, 2017), the Family Caregiver Activation in Transitions (FCAT) Tool, and DECAFTM Family Caregiver Tool (Coleman et al, 2015).*
- Monitor overall health of the caregiver at regular intervals for signs and symptoms of depression, anxiety, role strain, hopelessness, posttraumatic stress, and deteriorating physical health, particularly their control over chronic diseases and comorbid conditions. EB: *Caregivers of stroke survivors had difficulty dealing with depressive feelings, feelings of guilt, anxious/panic episodes, feelings of uncertainty and hopelessness, posttraumatic stress symptoms, and feelings of role strain from commitments (McCurley et al, 2019).* EB: *Caregivers with high levels of depressive symptoms have demonstrated poor health and increased health care utilization and cost (Shaffer et al, 2017).*
- Identify caregiver personal resources such as resilience, proficiency in caregiving skills, social support, optimism, positive aspects of care and resilience, and utilization or availability of social services (e.g., state-funded senior services, veterans' services, Area Agency on Aging resources). EB: *Identification and appreciation of resources may help buffer the negative effects of providing care on caregivers' emotional health and increase the effectiveness of interventions to reduce strain (Joling et al, 2017).*
- Encourage the caregiver to share feelings, concerns, uncertainties, and fears; support groups, including Internet-based ones, can be helpful to gain support. EB: *Internet social support groups can be an effective form of support (Parker Oliver et al, 2017).*
- Regularly assess for any evidence of caregiver or care recipient violence or abuse, especially emotional and verbal abuse; risk factors include substance abuse, poor premorbid relationship, and psychiatric illness. EB: *Caregivers are often unaware of the effect of their behavior on care recipient, and the definition of abuse (Liu et al, 2019).*
- Ensure appropriate referrals for physical, occupational, and speech-language therapy, as well as social work, including referrals for outpatient therapy or skilled home health care if needed (including therapy needed to maintain functional abilities and prevent decline). EB: *Improvement in client physical function resulted in better physical and psychological quality of life for both client and caregiver (Pucciarelli et al, 2017).*
- Talk with caregivers early and often about palliative care as a means of symptom management for the care recipient. EB: *Many care recipients and their families do not know what palliative care means, which may lead to underutilization of comfort measures (Scott et al, 2017).*
- Help the caregiver learn mindfulness stress management techniques, which can reduce psychological distress. EB: *Mindfulness stress reduction interventions can result in improvement in quality of life, self-compassion, caregiver burden, and relationship satisfaction (Schellekens et al, 2017).*
- Assist the client to identify spiritual beliefs and engage in spiritual practices. EB: *Spiritual beliefs and practices may help caregivers cope because it protects them from depression (Penman, 2018).*
- Encourage regular and open communication with the care recipient and with the health care team. EB: *Care transitions are a critical point to ensure that caregivers have adequate information for client safety and efficient and effective care (Scott et al, 2017).*

● = Independent; ▲ = Collaborative; EBN = Evidence-Based Nursing; EB = Evidence-Based; ✱ = QSEN

PLAN INTERVENTIONS

Use Section III, Guide to Planning Care, to find appropriate interventions for the client. Use the Nursing Interventions as found in that section.

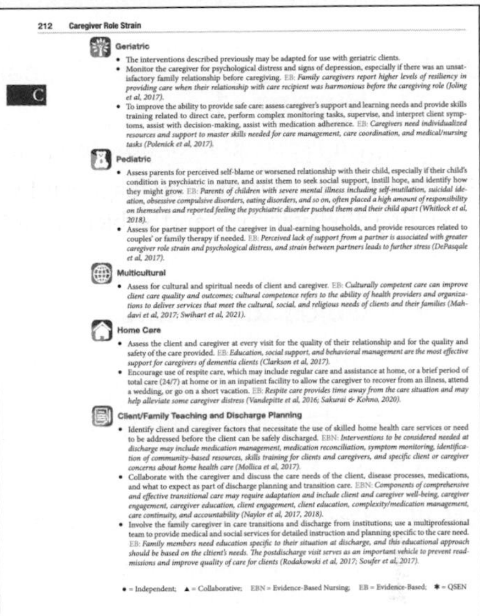

212 **Caregiver Role Strain**

C

Geriatric

- The interventions described previously may be adapted for use with geriatric clients.
- Monitor the caregiver for psychological distress and signs of depression, especially if there was an unsatisfactory family relationship before caregiving. EB: *Family caregivers report higher levels of resiliency in providing care when their relationship with care recipient was harmonious before the caregiving role (Joling et al, 2017).*
- To improve the ability to provide safe care: assess caregiver's support and learning needs and provide skills training related to direct care, perform complex monitoring tasks, supervise, and interpret client symptoms, assist with decision-making, assist with medication adherence. EB: *Caregivers need individualized resources and support to master skills needed for care management, care coordination, and medical/nursing tasks (Polenick et al, 2017).*

Pediatric

- Assess parents for perceived self-blame or worsened relationship with their child, especially if their child's condition is psychiatric in nature, and assist them to seek social support, instill hope, and identify how they might grow. EB: *Parents of children with severe mental illness including self-mutilation, suicidal ideation, obsessive compulsive disorders, eating disorders, and so on, often placed a high amount of responsibility on themselves and reported feeling the psychiatric disorder pushed them and their child apart (Whitlock et al, 2018).*
- Assess for partner support of the caregiver in dual-earning households, and provide resources related to couples' or family therapy if needed. EB: *Perceived lack of support from a partner is associated with greater caregiver role strain and psychological distress, and strain between partners leads to further stress (DePasqale et al, 2017).*

Multicultural

- Assess for cultural and spiritual needs of client and caregiver. EB: *Culturally competent care can improve client care quality and outcomes; cultural competence refers to the ability of health providers and organizations to deliver services that meet the cultural, social, and religious needs of clients and their families (Mahdavi et al, 2017; Swihart et al, 2021).*

Home Care

- Assess the client and caregiver at every visit for the quality of their relationship and for the quality and safety of the care provided. EB: *Education, social support, and behavioral management are the most effective support for caregivers of dementia clients (Clarkson et al, 2017).*
- Encourage use of respite care, which may include regular care and assistance at home, or a brief period of total care (24/7) at home or in an inpatient facility to allow the caregiver to recover from an illness, attend a wedding, or go on a short vacation. EB: *Respite care provides time away from the care situation and may help alleviate some caregiver distress (Vandepitte et al, 2016; Sakurai & Kohno, 2020).*

Client/Family Teaching and Discharge Planning

- Identify client and caregiver factors that necessitate the use of skilled home health care services or need to be addressed before the client can be safely discharged. EBN: *Interventions to be considered needed at discharge may include medication management, medication reconciliation, symptom monitoring, identification of community-based resources, skills training for clients and caregivers, and specific client or caregiver concerns about home health care (Mollica et al, 2017).*
- Collaborate with the caregiver and discuss the care needs of the client, disease processes, medications, and what to expect as part of discharge planning and transition care. EBN: *Components of comprehensive and effective transitional care may require adaptation and include client and caregiver well-being, caregiver engagement, caregiver education, client engagement, client education, complexity/medication management, care continuity, and accountability (Naylor et al, 2017, 2018).*
- Involve the family caregiver in care transitions and discharge from institutions; use a multiprofessional team to provide medical and social services for detailed instruction and planning specific to the care need. EB: *Family members need education specific to their situation at discharge, and this educational approach should be based on the cltient's needs. The postdischarge visit serves as an important vehicle to prevent readmissions and improve quality of care for clients (Rodakowski et al, 2017; Soufer et al, 2017).*

● = Independent; ▲ = Collaborative; EBN = Evidence-Based Nursing; EB = Evidence-Based; ✱ = QSEN

GIVE NURSING CARE

Administer nursing care following the plan of care based on the interventions.

EVALUATE NURSING CARE

Evaluate nursing care administered using either the NOC Outcomes or Client Outcomes. If the outcomes were not met and the nursing interventions were not effective, reassess the client and determine if the appropriate nursing diagnoses were made.

DOCUMENT

Document all of the previous steps using the format provided in the clinical setting. A Care Plan Template is available in the Evolve online resources to assist with documentation.

Contents

SECTION I

Nursing Process, Clinical Reasoning, Nursing Diagnosis, and Evidence-Based Nursing

Mary Beth Flynn Makic, PhD, RN, CCNS, CCRN-K, FAAN, FNAP, FCNS, and
Marina Martinez-Kratz, MS, RN, CNE

Section I is divided into two parts. Part A includes an overview of the nursing process. This section provides information on how to make a nursing diagnosis and directions on how to plan nursing care. It also includes information on using clinical reasoning skills and eliciting the "patient's story." Part B includes advanced nursing concepts.

Part A: The Nursing Process: Using Clinical Reasoning Skills to Determine Nursing Diagnoses and Plan Care

1. **A**ssessing: performing a nursing assessment by gathering subjective and objective data.
2. **D**iagnosing: identifying and making nursing diagnoses.
3. **P**lanning: formulating and writing outcome statements and determining appropriate nursing interventions based on appropriate best evidence (e.g., research, practice guidelines, practice standards).
4. **I**mplementing: applying nursing care interventions to achieve client outcomes.
5. **E**valuating: appraising the outcomes and the nursing care that has been implemented. Make necessary revisions in care interventions as needed to achieve client-centered goals.

Part B: Advanced Nursing Process Concepts

- Concept mapping
- Evidence-based nursing care
- Person-centered care
- Quality and Safety Education for Nurses (QSEN)

PART A The Nursing Process: Using Clinical Reasoning Skills to Determine Nursing Diagnoses and Plan Care

The primary goals of nursing care are to (1) determine client/family responses to human problems, level of wellness, and need for assistance; (2) provide physical care, emotional care, teaching, guidance, and counseling; and (3) implement interventions aimed at prevention and assisting the client in meeting his or her own needs and health-related goals. The nurse must always focus on assisting clients and families to their highest level of functioning and self-care. The nursing care that is provided should be structured in a way that allows clients the ability to influence their health care and accomplish their self-efficacy goals.

The nursing process, which is a problem-solving approach to the identification and treatment of client problems, provides a framework for assisting clients and families to their optimal level of functioning. The nursing process involves five dynamic and fluid phases: **assessment, diagnosis, planning, implementation,** and **evaluation.** Clinical reasoning is inherent within the nursing process and is an iterative process by which the nurse makes clinical judgments to analyze and understand clients' concerns and form decisions to guide care (Tanner, 2006; Koharchik et al, 2015). It is a process by which the nurse gathers data, recognizes patterns in client responses, and synthesizes information to guide nursing care decisions. Although clinical reasoning skills evolve with experience, it is a logical process by which nurses gather cues (assessment and outcome data), process the information to understand the client's needs and goals (diagnosis), initiate a plan of care (planning and implementation), observe and evaluate outcomes (evaluation), and finally reflect on what was learned from this client–nurse interaction (Levett-Jones et al, 2010; Cappelletti et al, 2014). Clinical judgment is the prioritization of decisions based on the assessment data to guide nursing care (Thompson et al, 2013; Cappelletti et al, 2014). The nurse employs complex cognitive processes that require gathering and analyzing client data and understanding the significance of the information to determine interventions, weigh alternative actions, and adjust the plan of care as deemed necessary based on the nurse's clinical judgment (Cappelletti et al, 2014; Wright & Scardaville, 2021). Identifying priority nursing diagnoses can facilitate clinical judgment based on the understanding of client priorities for care and desired health outcomes.

Within each phase of the nursing process, the client and family story is embedded and is used as a foundation for knowledge, judgment, and actions brought to the client care experience. A description of the "patient's story" and each aspect of the nursing process follows.

THE "PATIENT'S STORY"

The "patient's story" is a term used to describe objective and subjective information about the client that describes who the client is as a person in addition to their medical history. Specific aspects of the story include physiological, psychological, family, and social characteristics; available resources; environmental context; knowledge; and motivation. Care is influenced, and often driven, by what the client states—verbally, nonverbally, and through their physiological state. The "patient's story" is fluid and must be explored and understood throughout the client's health care experience.

There are multiple sources for obtaining the "patient's story." The primary source for eliciting this story is through communicating directly with the client and the client's family. It is important to understand how the illness (or wellness) state has affected the client physiologically, psychologically, and spiritually. The client's perception of his or her health state is important to understand and may have an impact on subsequent interventions and the established goals for care. At times, clients will be unable to tell their story verbally, but there is still much they can communicate through their physical state. The client's family (as the client defines them) is a valuable source of information and can provide a rich perspective on the client. Other valuable sources of the "patient's story" include the client's health record. Every time a piece of information is added to the health record, it becomes a part of the "patient's story."

Understanding the "patient's story" is critically important, in that psychological, socioeconomic, and spiritual characteristics play a significant role in the client's ability and desire to access health care. Also, knowing and understanding the "patient's story" is an integral first step in giving person-centered care. In today's health care world, the focus is on the client, which leads to increased satisfaction with care. Improving the client's health care experience is tied to reimbursement through value-based purchasing of care to reward providers for the quality of care they provide (Centers for Medicare and Medicaid Services, 2019).

All nursing care is driven by the client's story. The nurse must have a clear understanding of the story to effectively complete the nursing process. Understanding the full story also provides an avenue for identifying mutual goals with the client and family aimed at improving client outcomes and goals. The "patient's story" is terminology that is used to describe a holistic assessment of information about the client, including the client's and the family's input as much as possible. In this text, we use the term "patient's story" in quotes whenever we refer to the specific process. In all other places, we use the term *client* in place of the word *patient*. The term *patient* aligns with the understanding of an individual awaiting medical care (Merriam-Webster, 2021). Use of the word *client,* on the other hand, represents engagement in service, which we believe is more respectful and empowering for the person. *Client* is also the term that is used in the National

Council Licensure Examination (NCLEX-RN) test plan (National Council of State Boards of Nursing, 2019).

THE NURSING PROCESS

The nursing process is an organizing framework for professional nursing practice, which is a critical thinking process for the nurse to guide the delivery of the best care possible to the client. It is very similar to the steps used in scientific reasoning and problem solving. This section is designed to help the nursing student learn how to use this thinking process, or the nursing process. Key components of the process include the steps listed subsequently. An easy, convenient way to remember the steps of the nursing process is to use an acronym, **ADPIE** (Figure I.1):

1. **A**ssess: perform a nursing assessment.
2. **D**iagnose: make nursing diagnoses.
3. **P**lan: formulate and write outcome/goal statements and determine appropriate nursing interventions based on the client's reality and evidence (research).
4. **I**mplement care.
5. **E**valuate the outcomes and the nursing care that has been implemented. Make necessary revisions in care interventions as needed.

The next section is an overview and practical application of the steps of the nursing process. The steps are listed in the usual order in which they are performed.

STEP 1: ASSESSMENT (ADPIE)

The assessment phase of the nursing process is foundational for gathering data about the client. Nurses must understand the human responses to illness and health so that appropriate diagnosis, planning, and intervention(s) can be established. Assessment is dynamic and continuous so that nursing care can evolve to meet clients' changing needs. Data on all dimensions of the "patient's story," including biophysical, psychological, sociocultural, spiritual, and environmental characteristics, are embedded in the assessment, which involves performing a thorough holistic nursing assessment of the client. This is the first step needed to make an appropriate nursing diagnosis, and it is done using the assessment format adopted by the facility or educational institution in which the practice is situated.

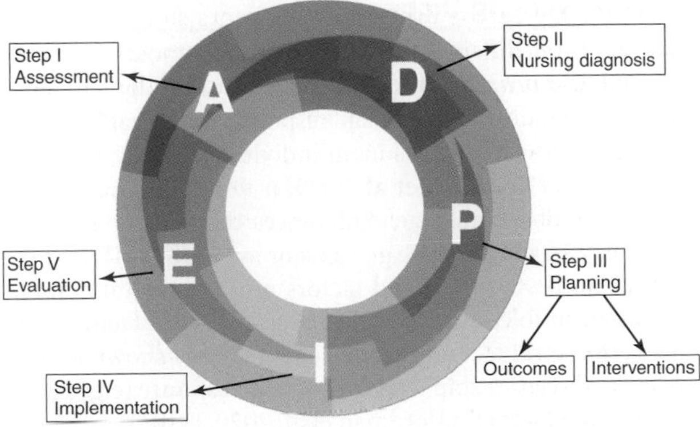

Figure I.1
Nursing process.

The nurse assesses components of the "patient's story" every time an assessment is performed. Often, nurses focus on the physical component of the story (e.g., temperature, blood pressure, breath sounds). This component is certainly critical, but it is only one piece. Indeed, one of the unique and wonderful aspects of nursing is the holistic theory that is applied to clients and families. Clients are active partners in the healing process. Nurses must increasingly develop the skills and systems to incorporate client preferences into care (Feo et al, 2017). Assessment information is obtained first by completing a thorough health and medical history and by listening to and observing the client. To elicit as much information as possible, the nurse should use open-ended questions rather than questions that can be answered with a simple "yes" or "no." The nurse should assess for the client's gender identity and gender expression, as well as preferred names and pronouns. Preferred names and pronouns should be respected when caring for the client. Most care plans are written for "traditional" gender identity; the caregiver will be responsible for adapting the care accordingly.

Asking open-ended questions during an assessment will encourage the client to give more information about his or her situation. Listen carefully for cues and record relevant information that the client shares. Even when the client's physical condition or developmental age makes it impossible to verbally communicate with the health care team, nurses may be able to communicate with the client's family or significant other to learn more about the client.

The information that is obtained verbally from the client is considered *subjective* information. Information is also obtained by performing a physical assessment, taking vital signs, and noting diagnostic test results. This information is considered *objective* information. The information from all of these sources is used to formulate a nursing diagnosis. All of this information needs to be carefully documented on the forms/electronic health record (EHR) provided by the agency or school of nursing. When recording information, Health Insurance Portability and Accountability Act (HIPAA) (Tovino, 2017) regulations need to be followed carefully. To protect client confidentiality, the client's name should *not* be used on the student care plan. When the assessment is complete, proceed to the next step.

STEP 2: NURSING DIAGNOSIS (ADPIE)

In the diagnosis phase of the nursing process, the nurse begins clustering the information within the "patient's story" and formulates an evaluative judgment about a client's health status. Only after a thorough analysis—which includes recognizing cues, sorting through and organizing or clustering the information, and determining client strengths and unmet needs—can an appropriate diagnosis be made. This process of thinking is called *clinical reasoning*. Clinical reasoning is a cognitive process that uses formal and informal thinking strategies to gather and analyze client information, evaluate the significance of this information, and determine the value of alternative actions (Benner, 2010). Benner (2010) described this cognitive process as "thinking like a nurse." Watson and Rebair (2014) referred to "noticing" as a precursor to clinical reasoning. By noticing, the nurse can preempt possible risks or support subtle changes toward recovery. Noticing can be the activity that stimulates nursing action before words are exchanged, preempting need. The nurse synthesizes the evidence while also knowing the client as part of clinical reasoning that informs client-specific diagnoses (Cappelletti et al, 2014; Koharchik et al, 2015).

The nursing diagnoses that are used throughout this book are taken from NANDA International, Inc. (NANDA-I) (Herdman et al, 2020). The complete nursing diagnosis list is on the inside front cover of this text, and it can also be found on the Evolve website that accompanies this text. The diagnoses used throughout this text are listed in alphabetical order by the **diagnostic concept.** For example, *impaired wheelchair mobility* is found under *mobility,* not under *wheelchair* or *impaired* (Herdman et al, 2020). There are 13 domains for nursing diagnosis and these are listed below the nursing diagnosis along with the class.

The holistic assessment of the client helps determine the type of diagnosis that should be used to guide nursing interventions. For example, if during the assessment a client is noted to have unsteady gait and balance disturbance and states, "I'm concerned I will fall while walking down my stairs," but has not fallen previously, the client would be identified as having a "risk" nursing diagnosis. However, if a client states, "I am having increasing problems with leaking urine when I sneeze or cough," this is an actual problem for the client.

Once the diagnosis is determined, the next step is to determine defining characteristics and related factors. A client may have many nursing and medical diagnoses, and determining the priority with which each should be addressed requires clinical reasoning and application of knowledge.

Formulating a Nursing Diagnosis With Defining Characteristics and Related Factors

A working nursing diagnosis may have two or three parts. The two-part system consists of the nursing diagnosis and the "related to" (r/t) statement: "Related factors are etiologies, circumstances, facts, or influences that have some type of relationship with the nursing diagnosis (e.g., cause, contributed factor)" (Herdman et al, 2020). The two-part system is often used when the defining characteristics, or signs and symptoms identified in the assessment, may be obvious to those caring for the client.

The three-part system consists of the nursing diagnosis, the r/t statement, and the defining characteristics, which are "observable cues/inferences that cluster as manifestations of an actual or wellness nursing diagnosis" (Herdman et al, 2020).

Some nurses refer to the three-part diagnostic statement as the **PES system:**

P (problem)—The nursing diagnosis label: a concise term or phrase that represents a pattern of related cues. The nursing diagnosis is taken from the official NANDA-I list.
E (etiology)—"Related to" (r/t) phrase or etiology: related cause or contributor to the problem.
S (symptoms)—Defining characteristics phrase: symptoms that the nurse identified in the assessment.

Here we use the example of a beginning nursing student who is attempting to understand the nursing process and how to make a nursing diagnosis:

Problem: Use the nursing diagnosis label deficient **Knowledge** from the NANDA-I list. Remember to check the definition: "Absence or deficiency of cognitive information related to a specific topic" (Herdman et al, 2020).
Etiology: r/t unfamiliarity with information about the nursing process and nursing diagnosis. At this point, the beginning nurse would not be familiar with available resources regarding the nursing process.
Symptoms: Defining characteristics, as evidenced by (aeb) verbalization of lack of understanding: "I don't understand this, and I really don't know how to make a nursing diagnosis."

When using the **PES** system, look at the **S** first and then formulate the three-part statement. (You would have gotten the **S,** symptoms, which are defining characteristics, from your assessment.)

Therefore, the three-part nursing diagnosis is: Deficient **Knowledge** r/t unfamiliarity with information about the nursing process and nursing diagnosis aeb verbalization of lack of understanding.

Types of Nursing Diagnoses

There are three different types of nursing diagnoses.

Problem-Focused Diagnosis. "A clinical judgment concerning an undesirable human response to a health condition/life process that exists in an individual, family, group or community" (Herdman et al, 2020, p 98). Defining characteristics are observable cues/inferences that cluster as manifestations of a diagnosis (e.g., signs or symptoms) (Herdman et al, 2020, p 103). "Related factors are an integral component of all problem-focused diagnoses. Related factors, also called etiological factors are antecedent factors shown to have a patterned relationship with the human response (e.g., cause, contributing factor)" (Herdman et al, 2020, p 103).

Example of a Problem-Focused Nursing Diagnosis. **Overweight** related to excessive intake in relation to metabolic needs, concentrating food intake at the end of the day aeb weight 25% over ideal for height and frame. Note: This is a three-part nursing diagnosis.

Risk Diagnosis. Risk nursing diagnosis is a "clinical judgment concerning the susceptibility of an individual, caregiver, family, group, or community for developing an undesirable human response to health conditions/life processes" (Herdman et al, 2020, p 98). "Risk factors are antecedent factors that increase the susceptibility of an individual, caregiver, family, group, or community to an undesirable human response (e.g. environmental, psychological)" (Herdman et al, 2020, p 103).

Example of a Risk Nursing Diagnosis. Risk for **Overweight:** Risk factor: abnormal eating behavior pattern, concentrating food at the end of the day. Note: This is a two-part nursing diagnosis.

Health Promotion Nursing Diagnosis. A clinical judgment concerning motivation and desire to increase well-being and to actualize health potential. These responses are expressed by a readiness to enhance specific health behaviors and can be used in any health state. Health promotion responses may exist in an individual, caregiver, family, group, or community (Herdman et al, 2020). Health promotion is different from prevention in that health promotion focuses on being as healthy as possible, as opposed to preventing a disease or problem. The difference between health promotion and disease prevention is that the reason for the health behavior should always be a positive one. *With a health promotion diagnosis, the outcomes and interventions should be focused on enhancing health.*

Example of a Health Promotion Nursing Diagnosis. Readiness for Enhanced **Nutrition** aeb willingness to change eating pattern and eat healthier foods. Note: This is a two-part nursing diagnosis.

Application and Examples of Making a Nursing Diagnosis

When the assessment is complete, identify common patterns/symptoms of response *to actual or potential health problems from the assessment* and select an appropriate nursing diagnosis label using clinical reasoning skills. Use the steps with Case Study 1. (The same steps can be followed using an actual client assessment in the clinical setting or in a student assessment.)

A. Highlight or underline the relevant symptoms (defining characteristics). As you review your assessment information, ask the following questions: Is this normal? Is this an ideal situation? Is this a problem for the client? You may go back and validate information with the client.
B. Make a list of the symptoms (underlined or highlighted information).
C. Cluster similar symptoms.
D. Analyze/interpret the symptoms. (What do these symptoms mean or represent when they are together?)
E. Select a nursing diagnosis label from the NANDA-I list that fits the appropriate defining characteristics and nursing diagnosis definition.

Case Study 1—Older Client with Breathing Problems

A. Underline the Symptoms (Defining Characteristics)

A 73-year-old man has been admitted to the unit with a diagnosis of chronic obstructive pulmonary disease (COPD). He states that he has "difficulty breathing when walking short distances." He also states that his "heart feels like it is racing" (heart rate is 110 beats per minute) at the same time. He states that he is "tired all the time," and while talking to you about his story, he is continually wringing his hands and looking out the window.

B. List the Symptoms (Subjective and Objective)

"Difficulty breathing when walking short distances"; "heart feels like it is racing"; heart rate is 110 beats per minute; "tired all the time"; continually wringing his hands and looking out the window.

C. Cluster Similar Symptoms

"Difficulty breathing when walking short distances"
"Heart feels like it is racing"; heart rate = 110 beats per minute
"Tired all the time"
Continually wringing his hands
Looking out the window

D. Analyze

Interpret the Subjective Symptoms (What the Client Has Stated)

"Difficulty breathing when walking short distances" = exertional discomfort: a defining characteristic of Decreased **Activity** Tolerance
"Heart feels like it is racing" = abnormal heart rate response to activity: a defining characteristic of Decreased **Activity** Tolerance
"Tired all the time" = verbal report of weakness: a defining characteristic of Decreased **Activity** Tolerance

Interpret the Objective Symptoms (Observable Information)

Continually wringing his hands = extraneous movement, hand/arm movements: a defining characteristic of **Anxiety**
Looking out the window = poor eye contact, glancing about: a defining characteristic of **Anxiety**
Heart rate = 110 beats per minute

E. Select the Nursing Diagnosis Label

In Section II look up *dyspnea (difficulty breathing)* or *dysrhythmia (abnormal heart rate or rhythm),* which are chosen because they are high priority, and you will find the nursing diagnosis Decreased **Activity** Tolerance listed with these symptoms. Is this diagnosis appropriate for this client?

To validate that the diagnosis Decreased **Activity** Tolerance is appropriate for the client, turn to Section III and read the NANDA-I definition of the nursing diagnosis Decreased **Activity** Tolerance: "Insufficient endurance to complete required or desired daily activities" (Herdman et al, 2020, p 307). When reading the definition, ask, "Does this definition describe the symptoms demonstrated by the client?" "Is any more assessment information needed?" "Should I take his blood pressure or take an apical pulse rate?" If the appropriate nursing diagnosis has been selected, the definition should describe the condition that has been observed.

The client may also have defining characteristics for this particular diagnosis. Are the client's symptoms that you identified in the list of defining characteristics (e.g., verbal report of fatigue, abnormal heart rate response to activity, exertional dyspnea)?

Another way to use this text and to help validate the diagnosis is to look up the client's medical diagnosis in Section II. This client has a medical diagnosis of COPD. Is Decreased **Activity** Tolerance listed with this medical diagnosis? Consider whether the nursing diagnosis makes sense given the client's medical diagnosis (in this case, COPD). There may be times when a nursing diagnosis is not directly linked to a medical diagnosis (e.g., Ineffective **Coping**) but is nevertheless appropriate given nursing's holistic approach to the client/family.

The process of identifying significant symptoms, clustering or grouping them into logical patterns, and then choosing an appropriate nursing diagnosis involves diagnostic reasoning (critical thinking) skills that must be learned in the process of becoming a nurse. This text serves as a tool to help the learner in this process.

"Related to" Phrase or Etiology

The second part of the nursing diagnosis is the "related to" (r/t) phrase. Related factors (etiological factors) are those that appear to show some type of patterned relationship with the human response that supports the nursing diagnosis. Such factors may be described as antecedent to, associated with, related to, contributing to, or abetting. Pathophysiological and psychosocial changes, such as developmental age and cultural and environmental situations, may be causative or contributing factors.

Often, a nursing diagnosis is complementary to a medical diagnosis and vice versa. Ideally, the etiology (r/t statement), or cause, of the nursing diagnosis is something that can be treated independently by a nurse. When this is the case, the diagnosis is identified as an independent nursing diagnosis.

If medical intervention is also necessary, it might be identified as a collaborative nursing diagnosis. A carefully written, individualized r/t statement enables the nurse to plan nursing interventions and refer for diagnostic procedures, medical treatments, pharmaceutical interventions, and other interventions that will assist the client/family in accomplishing goals and return to a state of optimum health. Diagnoses and treatments provided by the multiprofessional team all contribute to the client/family outcome. The coordinated effort of the team can only improve outcomes for the client/family and decrease duplication of effort and frustration among the health care team and the client/family.

The etiology is *not* the medical diagnosis. It may be the underlying issue contributing to the nursing diagnosis, but a medical diagnosis is *not* something the nurse can treat independently, without provider orders. In the case of the client with COPD, think about what happens when someone has COPD. How does this condition affect the client? What is happening to him because of this diagnosis?

For each suggested nursing diagnosis, the nurse should refer to the statements listed under the heading Related Factors (r/t) in Section III. These r/t factors may or may not be appropriate for the individual client. If they are not appropriate, the nurse should develop and write an r/t statement that is appropriate for the client. For the client from Case Study 1, a two-part statement could be made here:

Problem = Decreased **Activity** Tolerance
Etiology = r/t imbalance between oxygen supply and demand

It was already determined that the client had Decreased **Activity** Tolerance. With the respiratory symptoms identified from the assessment, the imbalance between oxygen supply and demand is appropriate.

Defining Characteristics Phrase

The defining characteristics phrase is the third part of the three-part diagnostic system, and it consists of the signs and symptoms that have been gathered during the assessment phase. The phrase "as evidenced by" (aeb) may be used to connect the etiology (r/t) with the defining characteristics. The use of identifying defining characteristics is similar to the process that the health care provider uses when making a medical diagnosis. For example, the health care provider who observes the following signs and symptoms—diminished inspiratory and expiratory capacity of the lungs, complaints of dyspnea on exertion, difficulty in inhaling and exhaling deeply, and sometimes chronic cough—may make the medical diagnosis of COPD. This same process is used to identify the nursing diagnosis of Decreased **Activity** Tolerance.

Put It All Together: Writing the Three-Part Nursing Diagnosis Statement

Problem—Choose the label (nursing diagnosis) using the guidelines explained previously. A list of nursing diagnosis labels can be found in Section II.

Etiology—Write an r/t phrase (etiology). These can be found in Section II.

Symptoms—Write the defining characteristics (signs and symptoms) or the "as evidenced by" (aeb) list. A list of the signs and symptoms associated with each nursing diagnosis can be found in Section III.

Case Study 1—73-Year-Old Male Client With Chronic Obstructive Pulmonary Disease (Continued)

Using the information from the earlier case study/example, the nursing diagnostic statement would be as follows:

Problem—Decreased **Activity** Tolerance.
Etiology—r/t imbalance between oxygen supply and demand.

Symptoms—Verbal reports of fatigue, exertional dyspnea ("difficulty breathing when walking"), and abnormal heart rate response to activity ("racing heart"); heart rate 110 beats per minute.

Therefore, the nursing diagnostic statement for the client with COPD is Decreased **Activity** Tolerance r/t imbalance between oxygen supply and demand aeb verbal reports of fatigue, exertional dyspnea, and abnormal heart rate in response to activity.

Consider a second case study:

Case Study 2—Woman with Insomnia

As before, the nurse always begins with an assessment. To make the nursing diagnosis, the nurse follows the steps below.

A. Underline the Symptoms

A 45-year-old woman comes to the clinic and asks for medication to help her sleep. She states that she is worrying too much and adds, "It takes me about an hour to get to sleep, and it is very hard to fall asleep. I feel like I can't do anything because I am so tired. My job has become very stressful because of a new boss and too much work."

B. List the Symptoms (Subjective and Objective)

Asks for medication to help her sleep; states she is worrying about too much; "It takes me about an hour to get to sleep"; "it is very hard to fall asleep"; "I feel like I can't do anything because I am so tired"; "My job has become very stressful because of a new boss and too much work."

C. Cluster Similar Symptoms

Asks for medication to help her sleep.
"It takes me about an hour to get to sleep."
"It is very hard to fall asleep."
"I feel like I can't do anything because I am so tired."
"I am worrying too much."
"My job is stressful."
"Too much work."

D. Analyze/Interpret the Symptoms
Subjective Symptoms

Asks for medication to help her sleep; "It takes me about an hour to get to sleep"; "it is very hard to fall asleep"; "I feel like I can't do anything because I am so tired." (All defining characteristics = verbal complaints of difficulty with sleeping.)

States she is worrying too much (anxiety): "My job is stressful."

Objective Symptoms

None

E. Select a Nursing Diagnosis with Related Factors and Defining Characteristics

Look up "sleep" in Section II. Listed under the heading "Disturbed **Sleep** Pattern" in Section II is the following information:

Insomnia (nursing diagnosis) r/t anxiety and stressors

This client states she is worrying too much, which may indicate anxiety; she also recently has increased job stress.

Look up **Insomnia** in Section III. Check the definition: "Inability to initiate or maintain sleep, which impairs functioning" (Herdman et al, 2020, p 301). Does this describe the client in the case study? What are the related factors? What are the symptoms? Write the diagnostic statement:

Problem—**Insomnia**
Etiology—r/t anxiety, stressors
Symptoms—Difficulty falling asleep; "I am so tired, I can't do anything."

The nursing diagnostic statement is written in this format: **Insomnia** r/t anxiety and stressors aeb difficulty falling asleep.

Note: There are additional case studies available for both student and faculty use on the Evolve website that accompanies this text.

After the diagnostic statement is written, proceed to the next step: planning.

STEP 3: PLANNING (ADPIE)

The planning phase of the nursing process includes the identification of priorities and the determination of appropriate client-specific outcomes and interventions. The nurse, in collaboration with the client and family (as applicable) and the rest of the health care team, must determine the urgency of the identified problems and prioritize client needs. *Mutual goal setting,* along with *symptom pattern recognition* and *triggers,* helps prioritize interventions and determine which interventions are going to provide the greatest impact. *Symptom pattern recognition* and/or *triggers* is a process of identifying symptoms that clients have related to their illness, understanding which symptom patterns require intervention, and identifying the associated time frame to intervene effectively. For example, a client with heart failure is noted to gain 5 pounds overnight. Coupling this symptom with other symptoms of edema and shortness of breath while walking can be referred to as "symptom pattern recognition"; in this case, that the client is retaining fluid. The nurse, and often the client/family, recognize these symptoms as an immediate *cause* and that more action/intervention is needed to avoid a potential adverse outcome.

Nursing diagnoses should be prioritized based on urgent needs, diagnoses with a high level of congruence with defining characteristics, related factors, or risk factors (Herdman et al, 2020, p 105). The use of ABC (airway, breathing, and circulation) and safety is a method to rank threats to the client's immediate survival or safety. The highest priority can also be determined by using Maslow's hierarchy of needs. In this hierarchy, priority is given to immediate problems that may be life-threatening (thus ABC). For example, Ineffective **Airway** Clearance, aeb the symptoms of increased secretions and increased use of inhaler related to asthma, creates an immediate cause compared with the nursing diagnosis of **Anxiety,** a love and belonging or security need, which makes it a lesser priority than Ineffective **Airway** Clearance. Refer to Appendix A on Evolve for assistance in prioritizing nursing diagnoses.

The planning phase should be done, whenever possible, with the client/family and the multidisciplinary team to maximize efforts and understanding and increase compliance with the proposed plan and outcomes. For a successful plan of care, measurable goals and outcomes, including nursing interventions, must be identified.

SMART Outcomes

When writing outcome statements, it can be helpful to use the acronym SMART, which means the outcome must be:

Specific
Measurable
Attainable
Realistic
Timed

The SMART acronym is used in business, education, and health care settings. This method assists the nurse in identifying client outcomes more effectively.

Once priorities are established, outcomes for the client can be easily identified. Client-specific outcomes are determined based on the mutually set goals. Outcomes refer to the measurable degree of the client's response. The client's response/outcome may be intentional and favorable, such as leaving the hospital 2 days after surgery without any complications. The client's outcome can be negative and unintentional, such as demonstrating a surgical site infection. Generally, outcomes are described in relation to the client's response to interventions; for example, the client's cough becomes more productive after the client begins using the controlled coughing technique.

Based on the "patient's story"; the nursing assessment; the mutual goals and outcomes identified by the caregiving team and the client, caregiver, and family; and the clinical reasoning that the nurse uses to prioritize his or her work, the nurse then decides what interventions to use. Based on the nurse's clinical judgment and knowledge, nursing interventions are defined as *all treatments that a nurse performs to enhance client outcomes.*

The selection of appropriate, effective interventions can be individualized to meet the mutual goals established by the client/family. It is then the nurses' education, experiences, and skills that allow them to select and carry out interventions to meet that mutual goal.

Outcomes

After the appropriate priority setting of the nursing diagnoses and interventions are determined, outcomes are developed and decided on. This text includes standardized Nursing Outcomes Classification (NOC) measurement of health outcomes written by a large team of University of Iowa College of Nursing faculty and students in conjunction with clinicians from a variety of settings (Moorhead et al, 2018). NOC was developed to be used with nursing diagnosis and provides a standard language by which nurse-sensitive outcomes can be measured along a continuum in response to a nursing intervention or interventions. The outcomes are stated as concepts that reflect a client, caregiver, family, or community state, as a perception of behavior rather than as expected goals (Moorhead et al, 2018).

It is very important for the nurse to *involve* the client and/or family in determining appropriate outcomes. The use of outcomes information creates a continuous feedback loop that is essential to improve nursing quality, ensure client safety, and secure the best possible client outcomes (Sim et al, 2018). The minimum requirements for rating an outcome are when the outcome is selected (i.e., the baseline measure) and when care is completed (i.e., the discharge summary). Depending on how rapidly the client's condition is expected to change, some settings (e.g., acute care hospitals, rehabilitation centers, community care settings) may evaluate once a week, once a day, or once a shift. A five-point Likert-type scale is used with all outcomes and indications used to evaluate progress toward achieving the outcome; however, because measurement times are not standardized, they can be individualized for the client and the setting (Moorhead et al, 2018).

Development of appropriate outcomes can be completed one of two ways: using the NOC list or developing an appropriate outcome statement, both of which are included in Section III with each nursing diagnosis. The suggested outcome statements for each nursing diagnosis in this text can be used as written or modified as necessary to meet the needs of the client. The Evolve website includes a list of additional NOC outcomes. For more information about NOC, refer to the NOC text (Moorhead et al, 2018).

Because the NOC outcomes are specific, they enhance nursing professional practice by helping the nurse measure and record the nurse sensitive outcomes before and after interventions have been performed. The nurse can also choose to have clients rate their own progress using the Likert-type rating scale. This involvement can help increase client motivation to progress *toward* outcomes.

After client outcomes are selected or written and *discussed* with a client, the nurse plans nursing care with the client and establishes a means that will help the client achieve the selected outcomes. The usual means are through nursing interventions.

Interventions

Interventions are like road maps directing the best ways to provide nursing care. The more clearly a nurse writes an intervention, the easier it will be to complete the journey and arrive at the destination of desired client outcomes. Nursing interventions are treatments based on clinical judgment and knowledge, supported by evidence, that a nurse performs to enhance client outcomes (Butcher et al, 2018). Section

III includes suggested interventions and rationales for each nursing diagnosis. The interventions are identified as independent (autonomous actions that are initiated by the nurse in response to a nursing diagnosis) or collaborative (actions that the nurse performs in collaboration with other health care professionals and that may require a health care provider's order and may be in response to both medical and nursing diagnoses). The nurse may choose the interventions appropriate for the client and individualize them accordingly or determine additional interventions.

This text also contains several suggested interventions from the Nursing Interventions Classification (NIC), which is a comprehensive standardized classification of interventions that nurses perform (Butcher et al, 2018). NIC is used along with NOC and nursing diagnoses as client-specific care plans are developed. NIC includes both physiological and psychosocial interventions and covers all nursing specialties. A list of NIC interventions is included on the Evolve website. For more information about NIC interventions, refer to the NIC text (Butcher et al, 2018).

Putting It All Together—Recording the Care Plan

The nurse must document the actual care plan, including prioritized nursing diagnostic statements, outcomes, and interventions. This may be done electronically or in writing. To ensure continuity of care, the plan must be documented and shared with all health care personnel caring for the client. This text provides rationales, most of which are research based, to validate that the interventions are appropriate and workable.

The Evolve website includes an electronic care plan constructor that can be easily accessed, updated, and individualized. Many agencies are using electronic records, and this is an ideal resource. See the inside front cover of this text for information regarding access to the Evolve website, or go to http://evolve.elsevier.com/Ackley/NDH.

STEP 4: IMPLEMENTATION (ADPIE)

The implementation phase includes the "carrying out" of the specific, individualized, jointly agreed-on interventions in the plan of care. Often, the interventions implemented are focused on *symptom management,* which is alleviating symptoms. Typically, nursing care does not involve "curing" the medical condition causing the symptom; rather, nursing care focuses on caring for the client, caregiver, and family so that they can function at their highest level.

The implementation phase of the nursing process is the point at which you actually give nursing care. You perform the interventions that have been individualized to the client. All the hard work you put into the previous steps (ADP) can now be actualized to assist the client. As the interventions are performed, make sure that they are appropriate for the client. Consider that the client who was having difficulty breathing was also older. He may need extra time to carry out any activity. Check the rationale and research that are provided to determine why the intervention is being used. The evidence should support the individualized actions that you are implementing.

Client outcomes are achieved by the performance of the nursing interventions in collaboration with other disciplines and the client, caregiver, or family. During this phase, the nurse continues to assess the client to determine whether the interventions are effective and the desired outcomes are met.

STEP 5: EVALUATION (ADPIE)

The final phase of the nursing process is evaluation. This step occurs not only at the end of the nursing process but also throughout the process. Evaluation of an intervention is, in essence, another nursing assessment; hence, the dynamic feature of the nursing process. The nurse reassesses the client, taking into consideration where the client was before the intervention (i.e., baseline) and where the client is after the intervention. Nurses are also in a great place (at the bedside) to evaluate how clients respond to other, multiprofessional interventions, and their assessment of the client's response is valuable to determine whether the client's plan of care needs to be altered or not. For example, the client may receive 2 mg of morphine intravenously for pain (a pharmaceutical intervention to treat pain), and the nurse is the member of the health care team who can best assess how the client responded to that medication. Did the client receive relief from pain? Did the client develop any side effects? The nurse's documented evaluation of the client's response will be very helpful to the entire health care team.

The client/family can often tell the nurse how the intervention helped or did not help. This reassessment requires the nurse to revisit the mutual outcomes and goals set earlier and ask, "Are we moving toward that goal, or does the goal seem unreachable after the intervention?" If the outcomes were not met, the nurse begins again with assessment and determines the reason they were not met. Consider the SMART acronym and Case Study 1. Were the outcomes **S**pecific? Were the outcomes **M**easurable? Did the client's heart rate decrease? Did the client indicate that it was easier to breathe when walking from his bed to the bathroom? Were the outcomes **A**ttainable and **R**ealistic? Did he still report "being tired"? Did you allow adequate **T**ime for a positive outcome? Also ask yourself whether you identified the correct nursing diagnosis. Should the interventions be changed? At this point, the nurse can look up any new symptoms or conditions that have been identified and adjust the care plan as needed. Decisions about implementing additional interventions may be necessary; if so, they should be made in collaboration with the client, caregiver, and family, if possible. In some instances, the client/caregiver-family/nurse triad will establish new, achievable goals and continue to cycle through the nursing process until the mutual goals are achieved.

Another important part of the evaluation phase is documentation. The nurse should use the facility's tool for documentation and record the nursing activity that was performed, as well as the results of the nursing interventions. Many facilities use problem-oriented charting, in which the nurse evaluates the care and client outcomes as part of charting. Documentation is also necessary for legal reasons, because in a legal dispute, *if it wasn't charted or recorded, it wasn't done.*

Many health care providers use critical pathways or care maps to plan nursing care. The use of nursing diagnoses should be an integral part of any critical pathway/care map to ensure that nursing care needs are being assessed and appropriate nursing interventions are planned and implemented.

PART B Advanced Nursing Process Concepts

Conceptual Mapping and the Nursing Process

Conceptual mapping is an active learning strategy that promotes critical thinking and clinical judgment by providing a schematic representation of concepts and meaning within a framework that helps increase clinical understanding and competency (George et al, 2014; Daley et al, 2016; Kaddoura et al, 2016). Nurses identify complex client problems that require critical thinking to identify priority interventions based on current best evidence to affect client outcomes (Kaddoura et al, 2016). Concept mapping facilitates critical thinking and encourages a deeper understanding of the complexity of concepts that influence nursing practice interventions (George et al, 2014; Daley et al, 2016). The process involves developing a diagram or pictorial representation of newly generated ideas. A concept map begins with a central theme or concept, and then related information is diagrammed radiating from the central theme. A concept map can be used to diagram the critical thinking strategy involved in applying the nursing process in practice.

Start with a blank sheet of paper; the client should be at the center of the paper. The next step involves linking to the person, via lines, the symptoms (defining characteristics, related factors, and risk factors) from the assessment to help determine the appropriate nursing diagnosis.

Figure I.2 is an example of how a concept map can be used to begin the nursing diagnostic process.

After the symptoms are visualized, similar ones can be put together to formulate a nursing diagnosis using another concept map (Figure I.3).

The central theme in this concept map is the nursing diagnosis: Decreased **Activity** Tolerance, with the defining characteristics/client symptoms as concepts that lead to and support the nursing diagnosis. The conceptual map can then be used as a method for determining outcomes and interventions as desired. The nursing process is a thinking process. Using conceptual mapping is a method to help the nurse or nursing student think more effectively about the client.

Quality and Safety Education for Nurses

The Quality and Safety Education for Nurses (QSEN; https://qsen.org/) project represents the nursing profession's response to the five health care competencies articulated by the Institute of Medicine (now called the National Academy of Medicine) (Institute of Medicine, 2003). These competencies were adopted by nursing leaders to guide nursing education to better meet the evolving needs of clients and the health care system (Cronenwett et al, 2007). The QSEN project defined the six competencies for nursing: person-centered care, teamwork and collaboration, evidence-based practice (EBP), quality improvement, safety, and informatics (Cronenwett et al, 2007). The objective of the QSEN project is to provide nurses with the knowledge, skills, and attitudes critical for improving the quality and safety of health care systems. Initially, QSEN was developed to enhance nursing education, but it has since been incorporated into practice settings (Lyle-Edrosolo & Waxman, 2016). Additionally, the core elements of the QSEN map to key practice initiatives identified by The Joint Commission (TJC) and the American Nurses Credentialing Center Magnet (Magnet) recognition program (The Joint Commission, 2021). A crosswalk of the similarities of the QSEN competencies to TJC and Magnet demonstrates the alignment of the QSEN competencies to guide nursing practice excellence to improve the quality and safety of health care (Lyle-Edrosolo & Waxman, 2016; QSEN, 2020). The following are the competencies that were identified.

Person-Centered Care

Person-centered care is the ability to "recognize the patient or designee as the source of control and full partner in providing compassionate and coordinated care based on respect

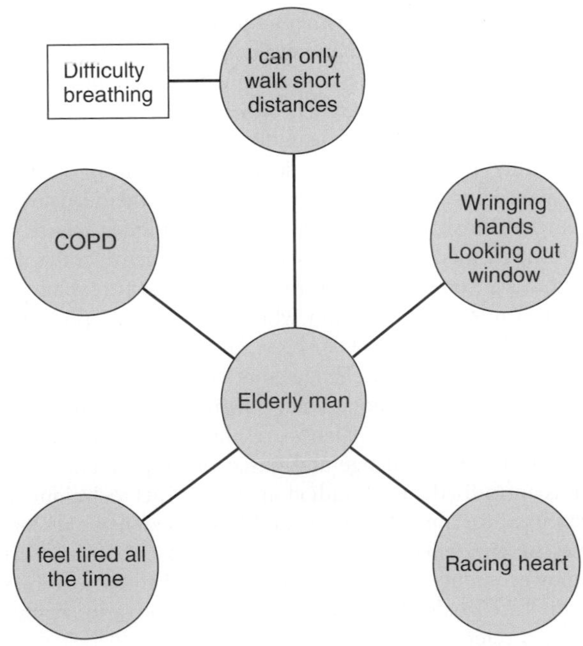

Figure I.2
Example of a concept map.

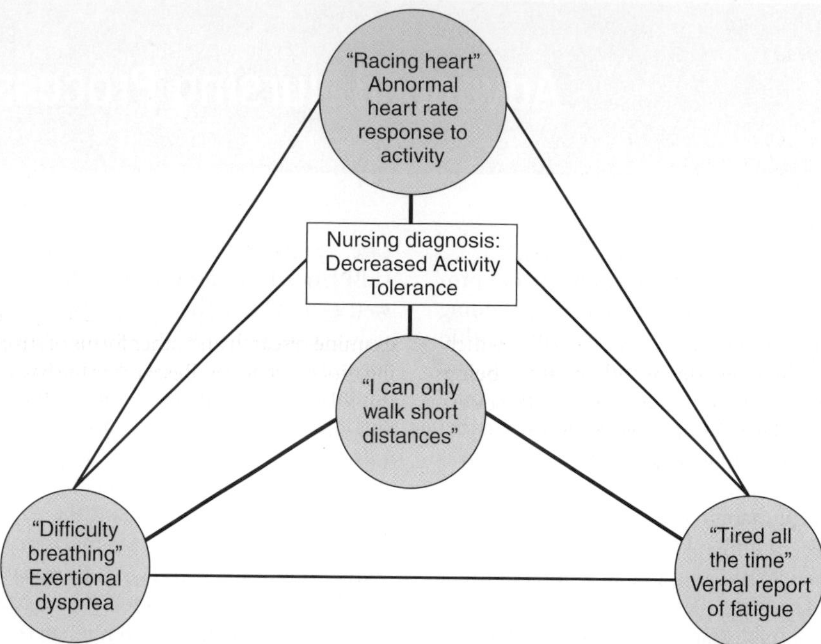

Figure I.3
Formulating a nursing diagnosis using a concept map.

for patient's preferences, values, and needs" (QSEN, 2020). Person-centered care begins with the nurse learning as much as possible about the client, including their "patient's story," as explained in Part A of this text. The nursing process, using nursing diagnosis, is intrinsically all about person-centered care when the nurse engages the client/family as a full partner in the entire process: assessment, nursing diagnosis selection, outcomes, interventions, and evaluation. This competency is about providing care in partnership with the client and family. The client, family, nurse, health care provider, and other health care workers form a team to collaborate with the client and family in every way possible to achieve health.

Client education needs to be centered on the needs of the client, addressing behavior-changing techniques to accomplish the defined goals. At present, too often new health information is given to clients in the form of a lecture, handout, admonishment, or direction where the client is powerless. Conversations need to occur between the client and nurse to understand behavioral changes that can be implemented to achieve goals. Motivational interviewing is a technique based on reinforcement of the client's present thoughts and motivations on behavior change and based on respect for the client as an individual (Moradi et al, 2016). This technique has been used for almost 30 years and has an extensive research base showing effectiveness by engaging in conversations to empower clients to identify strategies and tools to achieve health care goals. To learn more about motivational interviewing, refer to Appendix C on Evolve.

Addressing the unique cultural needs of clients is another example of person-centered care. Culturally competent care planning is based on cultural awareness and assessments, which enables integration of client values, beliefs, and preferences linked to culture(s). Cultural awareness encompasses the nurse's assessment of personal knowledge, sensitivity, humility, and organizational support to deliver culturally focused care (Sharifi et al, 2019). This text provides the addition of multicultural interventions that reflect the client's cultural preferences, values, and needs.

Person-centered care can help nurses change attitudes toward clients, especially when caring for older clients (Flagg, 2015). Caring for the retired school teacher who raised four children can be different from just caring for the client woman in Room 234 who has her call light on frequently and is incontinent of urine at too-frequent intervals. Including the client and family in the bedside report and care decisions is key to client satisfaction and enhances the overall quality of care (Flagg, 2015).

Teamwork and Collaboration

Teamwork and collaboration are defined as the ability to "function effectively within nursing and interprofessional teams, fostering open communication, mutual respect, and shared decision-making to achieve quality client care" (QSEN, 2020). Multiprofessional collaboration and practice has the ability to embrace care interventions that improve quality and safety initiatives across clients' lifespans and all health care settings (Stalter et al, 2017). The need for collaboration by health care professionals is a reality of contemporary health care practice and is identified within each nursing diagnosis in this text. Many nursing interventions are referrals to other health care personnel to best meet the client's needs; thus collaborative interventions are designated with a triangular symbol ▲.

Evidence-Based Practice

QSEN defines evidence-based practice (EBP) as the integration of best current evidence with clinical expertise and client, caregiver, and family preferences and values for delivery of optimal health care (QSEN, 2020). It is well established that EBP results in higher quality care for clients than care that is based on traditional nursing knowledge (Buccheri & Sharifi, 2017; Makic & Granger, 2019). It is imperative that each nurse and nursing student develop clinical inquiry skills, which means the nurse continually questions whether care is being given in the best way possible based on a review of the quality and strength of the evidence (Buccheri & Sharifi, 2017). Basing nursing practice on evidence, inclusive of research and other forms of evidence, is a concept that is incorporated throughout this text. EBP is a systematic process that uses current evidence in making decisions about the care of clients, including evaluation of quality and applicability of existing research, client preferences, clinical expertise, and available health care resources (Melnyk & Fineout-Overholt, 2019). To determine the best way of giving care, the use of EBP is needed. To make this happen, nurses need to access the evidence, critically appraise the evidence, and then apply the evidence in practice (Makic & Granger, 2019).

This text includes evidence-based rationales whenever possible. An effort is made to provide research-based rationales. The evidence ranges along a continuum from a case study about a single client to a systematic review performed by experts to quality improvement reports that provide information to guide nursing care. Every attempt has been made to supply the most current evidence for the nursing interventions. In Section III, the abbreviation **EBN** is used when interventions have a scientific rationale supported by nursing research. The abbreviation **EB** is used when interventions have a scientific rationale supported by research that has been obtained from disciplines other than nursing. **CEB** is used as a heading for classic research that has not been replicated or is older. It may be either nursing research or research from other disciplines. Many times the **CEB**-labeled research will be the seminal studies that were conducted addressing client concern or nursing care intervention.

When using **EBP**, it is vitally important that the client's concerns and individual situations be taken into consideration. The nurse must always use critical thinking when applying evidence-based guidelines to any particular nursing situation. Each client is unique in his or her needs and capabilities. To improve outcomes, clinicians and clients should collaborate to formulate a treatment plan that incorporates both evidence-based data and client preferences within the context of each client's specific clinical situation (Mackey & Bassendowski, 2017). This text integrates current best evidence and the nursing process, and it assists the nurse in increasing the use of evidence-based interventions in the clinical setting.

Quality Improvement

Quality improvement has been used for many years, with processes in place to ensure that the client receives appropriate care. The QSEN quality improvement competency is defined as the ability of the nurse to use data to monitor the outcomes of care processes and use improvement methods to design and test changes to continuously improve the quality and safety of health care systems (QSEN, 2020). QSEN resources supporting quality improvement initiatives are available at the QSEN website (http://qsen.org/competencies/quality-improvement-resources-2/). As with EBP, quality improvement initiatives need to critically examine research and other forms of strong evidence in supporting process changes. Research is the basis on which best practices should be supported (Makic, 2020). Research and other forms of evidence, such as quality improvement studies, provide a growing body of evidence to guide practice.

It is essential for nurses to participate in the work of quality and performance improvement to attain and sustain excellence in nursing care. As nurses are educated about performance and quality measures, they are more likely to value these activities and make quality improvement part of their nursing practice (Trent et al, 2017). Although there is a potential overlap of work in quality departments and EBP/research departments, the hope is that quality departments collaborate closely with EBP/research departments to improve the practice of nursing. Best evidence should be used to guide nursing practice interventions, and quality improvement critically evaluates and enhances the process of care to ensure effective delivery of high-quality, evidence-based care to clients.

Safety

Safety is defined as minimizing risk of harm to clients and providers through both system effectiveness and individual performance (QSEN, 2020). Client safety is a priority when health care is delivered. Nurses are required to adhere to established standards of care as a guideline for providing safe client care. Internal organizational policies and procedures established by health care institutions should be based on the most relevant and current evidence to guide safe practice standards. External standards of care are established by regulatory agencies (e.g., TJC), professional organizations (e.g., the American Nurses Association), and health care organizations. QSEN competencies align well with external agencies guiding safe practice expectations (Lyle-Edrosolo & Waxman, 2016).

Client safety was identified as a priority of care by TJC through the launch of the National Patient Safety Goals in 2002. TJC continually reviews and establishes standards for improving client safety that include the need for increased handwashing, better client identification before receiving medications or treatments, and protection of suicidal clients from self-harm. Many of the safety standards have been incorporated into the care plans in this text.

Informatics

QSEN defines informatics as the nurse's ability to use information and technology to communicate, manage knowledge, mitigate error, and support decision-making (QSEN, 2020). The use of information technology is a critical part of the nurse's professional role, and every nurse must be computer literate (Technology Informatics Guiding Education Reform [TIGER], 2018). Key technology and computer proficiencies for nursing practice should include basic computer system and desktop skills; the ability to search for client information; communication using email; ability to search electronic health care databases; and use of technology for client education, client documentation, and client monitoring (Hubner et al, 2017; TIGER, 2018).

In addition to computer literacy, nurses must also acquire informatic knowledge that addresses client privacy and the security of health care information as it applies to the use of technology (Hubner et al, 2017; TIGER, 2018). Because nurses document on the EHR and use smartphones for access to information on medications, diagnoses, and treatments, there are constant threats to client confidentiality, which needs to be maintained through secure-access systems. Nurses also use clinical decision support systems in many facilities that contain order sets tailored for conditions or types of clients. These systems include information vital to nurses and also may provide alerts about potentially dangerous situations when giving client care.

Nurses need access to technology to effectively bring evidence to the client's bedside because evidence is constantly evolving. The use of informatics is integral in the use of EBP. As evidence changes, practice should also change. Moving best evidence consistently into practice requires behavior changes by the clinician and system to effectively implement best evidence into practice. Similarly, habits in practice that result in unnecessary care need to be deimplemented (van Bodegrom-Vos et al, 2017). The Choosing Wisely campaign primarily focused on deimplementing unnecessary medical tests or treatments that were found to not provide benefit to clients (Levinson et al, 2015). Similarly, there are interventions that nurses should question because these interventions may not be beneficial for clients. The American Academy of Nursing maintains a list of nursing interventions that should be questioned as to client benefit. Continually reviewing the evidence to implement best practices while deimplementing interventions that are no longer supported by evidence or may no longer be truly necessary requires the nurses to remain actively engaged in EBP as a practice norm (Makic & Granger, 2019; American Academy of Nursing, 2021).

EBP, safety initiatives, informatics, person-centered care, teamwork, and quality work together in a synergistic manner, leading to excellence in nursing care. Quality care needs to be more than safe; the care should result in the best outcome possible for the client. For this to happen, the client should receive care that is based on evidence of the effectiveness of the nursing care interventions.

The nursing process is continually evolving. This text is all about *thinking* for the nurse to help the client in any way possible. Our goal is to present state-of-the-art information to help the nurse and nursing student provide the best care possible.

REFERENCES

American Academy of Nursing. (2021). *Choosing wisely: Twenty-five things nurses and patients should question.* Retrieved from https://www.aannet.org/initiatives/choosing-wisely. (Accessed 11 January 2021).

Benner, P. (2010). *Educating nurses: A call for radical transformation.* San Francisco: Jossey-Bass.

Buccheri, R. K., & Sharifi, C. (2017). Critical appraisal of tools and reporting guidelines for evidence-based practice. *World Views on Evidence-Based Nursing, 14*(6), 463–472.

Butcher, H., Bulechek, G., et al. (2018). *Nursing interventions classification (NIC) e-book* (7th ed.). St Louis: Mosby/Elsevier.

Cappelletti, A., Engel, J. E., & Prentice, D. (2014). Systematic review of clinical judgment and reasoning in nursing. *The Journal of Nursing Education, 53*(8), 453–458.

Centers for Medicare and Medicaid Services. (2019). *Hospital value-based purchasing.* Retrieved from https://www.cms.gov/Medicare/Quality-Initiatives-Patient-Assessment-Instruments/HospitalQualityInits/Hospital-Value-Based-Purchasing-.html. (Accessed 10 January 2021).

Cronenwett, L., Sherwood, G., Barnsteiner, J., et al. (2007). Quality and safety education for nurses. *Nursing Outlook, 55*, 121–131.

Daley, B. J., Morgan, S., & Black, S. B. (2016). Concept maps in nursing education: A historical literature review and research directions. *The Journal of Nursing Education, 55*(11), 631–639. https://doi.org/10.3928/01484834-20161011-05.

Feo, R., et al. (2017). Using holistic interpretive synthesis to create practice-relevant guidance for person-centred fundamental care delivered by nurses. *Nursing Inquiry, 24*(2), 1–11. https://doi.org/10.1111/nin.12152.

Flagg, A. J. (2015). The role of patient centered care in nursing. *The Nursing Clinics of North America, 50*(1), 75–86.

George, A., Geethakrishnan, R., & D'Souza, P. (2014). Concept mapping. *Holistic Nursing Practice, 28*(1), 43–47.

Herdman, T. H., Kamitsuru, S., & Lopes, C. T. (Eds.). (2020). *NANDA International, Inc. Nursing diagnoses. Definitions and classification. 2021-2023.* New York: Thieme Medical Publishers, Inc.

Hubner, U., Shaw, T., Thye, J., et al. (2017). *Towards an international framework for recommendations of core competencies in nursing and interprofessional informatics: The TIGER competency synthesis project.* Retrieved from http://www.himss.org/library/towards-international-framework-recommendations-core-competencies-nursing-and-interprofessional. (Accessed 1 January 2021).

Institute of Medicine (IOM). (2003). *Health professions education: a bridge to quality.* Washington, DC: National Academies Press. Retrieved from https://www.ncbi.nlm.nih.gov/books/NBK221528/pdf/Bookshelf_NBK221528.pdf. (Accessed 11 January 2021).

Levett-Jones, T., Hoffman, K., Dempsey, J., Jeong, S. Y., Noble, D., Norton, C. A., et al. (2010). The "five rights" of clinical reasoning: An educational model to enhance nursing students' ability to identify and manage clinically "at risk" patients. *Nurse Education Today, 30*(6), 515–520. https://doi.org/10.1016/j.nedt.2009.10.020.

The Joint Commission. (2021). *2018 National patient safety goals.* Retrieved from https://www.jointcommission.org/standards_information/npsgs.aspx. (Accessed 11 January 2021).

Kaddoura, M., Van-Dyke, O., & Yang, Q. (2016). Impact of a concept map teaching approach on nursing students' critical thinking skills. *Nursing and Health Sciences, 18*(3), 350–354.

Koharchik, L., Caputi, L., Robb, M., & Culleiton, A. L. (2015). Fostering clinical reasoning in nursing students. *The American Journal of Nursing*, *115*(1), 58–61. https://doi.org/10.1097/01.NAJ.0000459638.68657.9b.

Levinson, W., Kallewaard, M., Bhatia, S. R., et al. (2015). Choosing wisely: A growing international campaign. *BMJ Quality and Safety*, *24*(12), 167–174.

Lyle-Edrosolo, G., & Waxman, K. T. (2016). Aligning healthcare safety and quality competencies: Quality and safety education for nurses, the Joint Commissions, and American Nurses Credentialing Center, Magnet Standards Crosswalk. *Nurse Leader*, *7*(2), 70–75.

Mackey, A., & Bassendowski, S. (2017). The history of evidence-based practice in nursing education and practice. *Journal of Professional Nursing*, *33*(1), 51–55.

Makic, M., & Granger, B. B. (2019). Deimplementation in clinical practice: What are we waiting for? *AACN Advanced Critical Care*, *30*(3), 282–286. https://doi.org/10.4037/aacnacc2019607.

Makic, M. (2020). Providing evidence-based practice during the COVID-19 Pandemic. *Critical Care Nurse*, *40*(5), 72–74. https://doi.org/10.4037/ccn2020908.

Melnyk, B., & Fineout-Overholt, E. (2019). *Evidence-based practice in nursing & healthcare: A guide to best practice* (4th ed.). Philadelphia: Wolters Kluwer Health.

Merriam-Webster Dictionary. (2021). https://www.merriam-webster.com/dictionary/patient?utm_campaign=sd&utm_medium=serp&utm_source=jsonld (Accessed 10 January 2021)

Moorhead, S., Johnson, M., Maas, M. L., et al. (Eds.). (2018). *Nursing outcomes classification (NOC): Measurement of health outcomes* (6th ed.) St Louis: Elsevier.

Moradi, K., Najarkolai, A. R., & Keshmiri, F. (2016). Interprofessional Teamwork Education: Moving toward the patient-centered approach. *Journal of Continuing Education in Nursing*, *47*(10), 449–460. https://doi.org/10.3928/00220124-20160920-06.

National Council of State Boards of Nursing. (2019). *NCLEX-RN examination, detailed test plan*. Retrieved from https://www.ncsbn.org/2019_RN_TestPlan-English.pdf. (Accessed 11 January 2021).

Quality and Safety Education for Nurses (QSEN). (2020). Retrieved from http://qsen.org/competencies/pre-licensure-ksas/. (Accessed 11 January 2021).

Sharifi, N., Adib-Hajbaghery, M., & Najafi, M. (2019). Cultural competence in nursing: A concept analysis. *International Journal of Nursing Studies*, *99*, 103386. https://doi.org/10.1016/j.ijnurstu.2019.103386.

Sim, J., et al. (2018). Measuring the outcomes of nursing practice: A Delphi study. *Journal of Clinical Nursing*, *27*(1–2), e368–e378. https://doi.org/10.1111/jocn.13971.

Stalter, A. M., Phillips, J. M., Ruggiero, J. S., Scardaville, D. L., Merriam, D., Dolansky, M. A., et al. (2017). A concept analysis of systems thinking. *Nursing Forum*, *52*(4), 323–330. https://doi.org/10.1111/nuf.12196.

Tanner, C. A. (2006). Thinking like a nurse: a research-based model of clinical judgment in nursing. *The Journal of Nursing Education*, *45*(6), 204–211. https://doi.org/10.3928/01484834-20060601-04.

Technology Informatics Guiding Education Reform (TIGER). (2018). *The TIGER initiative: Informatics competencies for every practicing nurse: Recommendations from the TIGER Collaborative*. Retrieved from http://www.himss.org/professionaldevelopment/tiger-initiative. (Accessed 1 January 2021).

Thompson, C., Aiken, L., Doran, D., et al. (2013). An agenda for clinical decision making and judgement in nursing research and education. *International Journal of Nursing Studies*, *50*, 1720–1726.

Tovino, S. A. (2017). Teaching the HIPAA privacy rule. *Saint Louis University Law Journal*, *61*(3), 469–494.

Trent, P., Dolansky, M. A., DeBrew, J. K., & Petty, G. M. (2017). RN-to-BSN Students' quality improvement knowledge, skills, confidence, and systems thinking. *The Journal of Nursing Education*, *56*(12), 737–740. https://doi.org/10.3928/01484834-20171120-06.

van Bodegrom-Vos, L., Davidoff, F., & Marang-van de Mheen, P. (2017). Implementation and de-implementation: Two sides of the same coin? *BMJ Quality & Safety*, *26*(8), 495–501.

Watson, F., & Rebair, A. (2014). The art of noticing: Essential to nursing practice. *The British Journal of Nursing*, *23*(10), 514–517.

Wright, J., & Scardaville, D. (2021). A nursing residency program: A window into clinical judgement and clinical decision making. *Nurse Education in Practice*, *50*, 102931. https://doi.org/10.1016/j.nepr.2020.102931.

SECTION

II Guide to Nursing Diagnosis

Mary Beth Flynn Makic, PhD, RN, CCNS, CCRN-K, FAAN, FNAP, FCNS and
Marina Martinez-Kratz, MS, RN, CNE

Section II is an alphabetical listing of client symptoms, client problems, medical diagnoses, psychosocial diagnoses, and clinical states. Each of these will have a list of possible nursing diagnoses. You may use this section to find suggestions for nursing diagnoses for your client.

- Assess the client using the format provided by the clinical setting.
- Locate the client's symptoms, problems, clinical state, diagnoses, surgeries, and diagnostic testing in the alphabetical listing contained in this section.
- Note suggestions given for appropriate nursing diagnoses.
- Evaluate the suggested nursing diagnoses to determine whether they are appropriate for the client and are supported by the information that was found in the assessment.
- Use Section III (which contains an alphabetized list of all NANDA-I approved nursing diagnoses) to validate this information and check the definition, defining characteristics (if appropriate), risk factors, related factors, at-risk populations, and associated conditions. Determine whether the nursing diagnosis you have selected is appropriate for the client.

A

A

Abdominal Distention

Chronic Functional Constipation r/t habitually suppresses urge to defecate, impaired physical mobility, inadequate dietary intake, insufficient fiber intake, insufficient fluid intake

Constipation r/t decreased activity, decreased fluid intake, decreased fiber intake, pathological process

Dysfunctional Gastrointestinal Motility r/t decreased perfusion of intestines, medication effect

Nausea r/t irritation of gastrointestinal tract

Imbalanced Nutrition: Less Than Body Requirements r/t nausea, vomiting

Acute Pain r/t retention of air, gastrointestinal secretions

Delayed Surgical Recovery r/t retention of gas, secretions

Abdominal Hysterectomy

See Hysterectomy

Abdominal Pain

Dysfunctional Gastrointestinal Motility r/t decreased perfusion, medication effect

Acute Pain r/t injury, pathological process

Abdominal Surgery

Constipation r/t decreased activity, decreased fluid intake, anesthesia, opioids

Dysfunctional Gastrointestinal Motility r/t medication or anesthesia effect, trauma from surgery

Imbalanced Nutrition: Less Than Body Requirements r/t high metabolic needs, decreased ability to ingest or digest food

Acute Pain r/t surgical procedure

Ineffective Peripheral Tissue Perfusion r/t immobility, abdominal surgery

Risk for Delayed Surgical Recovery: Risk factor: extensive surgical procedure

Risk for Surgical Site Infection: Risk factor: invasive procedure

Risk for Thrombosis: Risk factor: impaired physical mobility, smoking

Readiness for Enhanced Knowledge: expresses an interest in learning

See Surgery, Perioperative Care; Surgery, Postoperative Care; Surgery, Preoperative Care

Abdominal Trauma

Disturbed Body Image r/t scarring, change in body function, need for temporary colostomy

Ineffective Breathing Pattern r/t abdominal distention, pain

Deficient Fluid Volume r/t hemorrhage, active fluid volume loss

Dysfunctional Gastrointestinal Motility r/t decreased perfusion

Acute Pain r/t abdominal trauma

Risk for Bleeding: Risk factor: trauma and possible contusion/rupture of abdominal organs

Risk for Infection: Risk factor: possible perforation of abdominal structures

Ablation, Radiofrequency Catheter

Fear r/t invasive procedure

Risk for Decreased Cardiac Tissue Perfusion: Risk factor: catheterization of heart

Abortion, Induced

Compromised Family Coping r/t unresolved feelings about decision

Acute Pain r/t surgical intervention

Chronic Low Self-Esteem r/t feelings of guilt

Chronic Sorrow r/t loss of potential child

Risk for Bleeding: Risk factor: trauma from abortion

Risk for Infection: Risk factors: open uterine blood vessels, dilated cervix

Risk for Post-Trauma Syndrome: Risk factor: psychological trauma of abortion

Risk for Spiritual Distress: Risk factor: perceived moral implications of decision

Readiness for Enhanced Health Literacy: expresses desire to enhance personal health care decisions

Readiness for Enhanced Knowledge: expresses an interest in learning

Abortion, Spontaneous

Disturbed Body Image r/t perceived inability to carry pregnancy, produce child

Disabled Family Coping r/t unresolved feelings about loss

Ineffective Coping r/t personal vulnerability

Interrupted Family Processes r/t unmet expectations for pregnancy and childbirth

Fear r/t implications for future pregnancies

Risk for Maladaptive Grieving r/t loss of fetus

Acute Pain r/t uterine contractions, surgical intervention

Situational Low Self-Esteem r/t feelings about loss of fetus

Chronic Sorrow r/t loss of potential child

Risk for Bleeding: Risk factor: trauma from abortion

Risk for Infection: Risk factors: septic or incomplete abortion of products of conception, open uterine blood vessels, dilated cervix

Risk for Post-Trauma Syndrome: Risk factor: psychological trauma of abortion

Risk for Spiritual Distress: Risk factor: loss of fetus

Readiness for Enhanced Knowledge: expresses an interest in learning

Abruptio Placentae <36 Weeks

Anxiety r/t unknown outcome, change in birth plans

Death Anxiety r/t unknown outcome, hemorrhage, or pain

Interrupted Family Processes r/t unmet expectations for pregnancy and childbirth

Fear r/t threat to well-being of self and fetus

Impaired Gas Exchange: Placental r/t decreased uteroplacental area

Acute Pain r/t irritable uterus, hypertonic uterus

Impaired Tissue Integrity: Maternal r/t possible uterine rupture

Risk for Bleeding: Risk factor: separation of placenta from uterus causing bleeding

Risk for Infection: Risk factor: partial separation of placenta

Risk for Disturbed Maternal–Fetal Dyad: Risk factors: trauma of process, lack of energy of mother

Risk for Shock: Risk factor: separation of placenta from uterus

Readiness for Enhanced Knowledge: expresses an interest in learning

Abscess Formation

Acute Pain r/t inflammation

Ineffective Protection r/t inadequate nutrition, abnormal blood profile, drug therapy, depressed immune function

Impaired Tissue Integrity r/t altered circulation, nutritional deficit or excess

Readiness for Enhanced Knowledge: expresses an interest in learning

Abuse, Child

See Child Abuse

Abuse, Spouse, Parent, or Significant Other

Anxiety r/t threat to self-concept, situational crisis of abuse

Caregiver Role Strain r/t chronic illness, self-care deficits, lack of respite care, extent of caregiving required

Impaired Verbal Communication r/t psychological barriers of fear

Compromised Family Coping r/t abusive patterns

Defensive Coping r/t low self-esteem

Disturbed Family Identity Syndrome r/t unaddressed domestic violence

Dysfunctional Family Processes r/t inadequate coping skills

Insomnia r/t psychological stress

Post-Trauma Syndrome r/t history of abuse

Powerlessness r/t lifestyle of helplessness

Chronic Low Self-Esteem r/t negative family interactions

Risk for Impaired Emancipated Decision-Making: Risk factor: inability to verbalize needs and wants

Risk for Female Genital Mutilation: Risk factor: lack of family knowledge about impact of practice on physical health

Risk for Self-Directed Violence: Risk factor: history of abuse

Accessory Muscle Use (to Breathe)

Ineffective Breathing Pattern (See **Breathing Pattern, Ineffective,** Section III)

See Asthma; Bronchitis; COPD (Chronic Obstructive Pulmonary Disease); Respiratory Infections, Acute Childhood (Croup, Epiglottis, Pertussis, Pneumonia, Respiratory Syncytial Virus)

Accident Prone

Frail Elderly Syndrome r/t history of falls

Acute Confusion r/t altered level of consciousness

Ineffective Coping r/t personal vulnerability, situational crises

Ineffective Impulse Control (See **Impulse Control, Ineffective,** Section III)

Risk for Injury: Risk factor: history of accidents

Wandering r/t overstimulating environment

Achalasia

Ineffective Coping r/t chronic disease

Acute Pain r/t stasis of food in esophagus

Impaired Swallowing r/t neuromuscular impairment

Risk for Aspiration: Risk factor: nocturnal regurgitation

Acid-Base Imbalances

Risk for Electrolyte Imbalance: Risk factors: renal dysfunction, diarrhea, treatment-related side effects (e.g., medications, drains)

Acidosis, Metabolic

Acute Confusion r/t acid-base imbalance, associated electrolyte imbalance

Impaired Memory r/t effect of metabolic acidosis on brain function

Imbalanced Nutrition: Less Than Body Requirements r/t inability to ingest, absorb nutrients

Risk for Electrolyte Imbalance: Risk factor: effect of metabolic acidosis on renal function

Risk for Injury: Risk factors: disorientation, weakness, stupor

Risk for Decreased Cardiac Tissue Perfusion: Risk factor: dysrhythmias from hyperkalemia

Risk for Shock: Risk factors: abnormal metabolic state, presence of acid state impairing function, decreased tissue perfusion

Acidosis, Respiratory

Decreased Activity Tolerance r/t imbalance between oxygen supply and demand

Impaired Gas Exchange r/t ventilation-perfusion imbalance

Impaired Memory r/t hypoxia

Risk for Decreased Cardiac Tissue Perfusion: Risk factor: dysrhythmias associated with respiratory acidosis

Acne

Disturbed Body Image r/t biophysical changes associated with skin disorder

Ineffective Health Self-Management r/t insufficient knowledge of therapeutic regimen

Impaired Skin Integrity r/t hormonal changes (adolescence, menstrual cycle)

Acromegaly

Decreased Activity Tolerance

Ineffective Airway Clearance r/t airway obstruction by enlarged tongue

Disturbed Body Image r/t changes in body function and appearance

A

Impaired Physical Mobility r/t joint pain

Risk for Decreased Cardiac Tissue Perfusion: Risk factor: increased atherosclerosis from abnormal health status

Risk for Unstable Blood Glucose Level: Risk factor: abnormal physical health status

Sexual Dysfunction r/t changes in hormonal secretions

Risk for Overweight: Risk factor: energy expenditure less than energy intake

Activity Intolerance, Potential to Develop

Decreased Activity Tolerance r/t sedentary behavior, deconditioning

Acute Abdominal Pain

Deficient Fluid Volume r/t air and fluids trapped in bowel, inability to drink

Acute Pain r/t pathological process

Risk for Dysfunctional Gastrointestinal Motility: Risk factor: ineffective gastrointestinal tissue perfusion

See Abdominal Pain

Acute Alcohol Intoxication

Ineffective Breathing Pattern r/t depression of the respiratory center from excessive alcohol intake

Acute Confusion r/t central nervous system depression

Dysfunctional Family Processes r/t abuse of alcohol

Risk for Aspiration: Risk factor: depressed reflexes with acute vomiting

Risk for Infection: Risk factor: impaired immune system from malnutrition associated with chronic excessive alcohol intake

Risk for Injury: Risk factor: chemical (alcohol)

Acute Back Pain

Anxiety r/t situational crisis, back injury

Constipation r/t decreased activity, effect of pain medication

Ineffective Coping r/t situational crisis, back injury

Impaired Physical Mobility r/t pain

Acute Pain r/t back injury

Readiness for Enhanced Knowledge: expresses an interest in learning

Acute Confusion

See Confusion, Acute

Acute Coronary Syndrome

Decreased Cardiac Output r/t cardiac disorder

Risk for Decreased Cardiac Tissue Perfusion (See **Cardiac Tissue Perfusion, Risk for Decreased,** Section III)

See Angina; Myocardial Infarction (MI)

Acute Lymphocytic Leukemia (ALL)

See Cancer; Chemotherapy; Child with Chronic Condition; Leukemia

Acute Renal Failure

See Renal Failure

Acute Respiratory Distress Syndrome

See ARDS (Acute Respiratory Distress Syndrome)

Acute Substance Withdrawal

Acute Substance Withdrawal Syndrome: Risk factor: developed dependence to alcohol or other addictive substances

Anxiety r/t unknown outcome of withdrawal sequence, physiological effects

Imbalanced Energy Field r/t hyperactivity of energy flow

Impaired Comfort r/t restlessness and agitation

Acute Confusion r/t effects of substance withdrawal

Ineffective Coping r/t situational crisis, withdrawal

Labile Emotional Control r/t lack of control over the progression of withdrawal process

Fear r/t threat to well-being of self

Insomnia r/t physical and psychological effects of substance withdrawal

Imbalanced Nutrition: Less than Body Requirements r/t nausea, anxiety

Powerlessness r/t loss of ability to control withdrawal process

Risk for Acute Confusion: Risk factor: possible alteration in level of consciousness

Risk for Injury: Risk factor: alteration in sensory perceptual functioning

Risk for Suicidal Behavior: Risk factor: psychic pain

Risk for Other-Directed Violence: Risk factors: poor impulse control, hallucinations

Risk for Self-Directed Violence: Risk factors: poor impulse control, hallucinations

Adams–Stokes Syndrome

See Dysrhythmia

Addiction

See Alcoholism; Substance Abuse

Addison's Disease

Decreased Activity Tolerance r/t weakness, fatigue

Disturbed Body Image r/t increased skin pigmentation

Deficient Fluid Volume r/t failure of regulatory mechanisms

Imbalanced Nutrition: Less than Body Requirements r/t chronic illness

Risk for Injury: Risk factor: weakness

Readiness for Enhanced Knowledge: expresses an interest in learning

Adenoidectomy

Acute Pain r/t surgical incision

Ineffective Airway Clearance r/t hesitation or reluctance to cough as a result of pain, fear

Nausea r/t anesthesia effects, drainage from surgery

Risk for Aspiration: Risk factors: postoperative drainage, impaired swallowing

Risk for Bleeding: Risk factor: surgical incision

Risk for Deficient Fluid Volume: Risk factors: decreased intake as a result of painful swallowing, effects of anesthesia

Risk for Dry Mouth: Risk factor: mouth breathing due to nasal congestion

Risk for Imbalanced Nutrition: Less than Body Requirements: Risk factor: reluctance to swallow

Readiness for Enhanced Knowledge: expresses an interest in learning

Adhesions, Lysis of

See Abdominal Surgery

Adjustment Disorder

Anxiety r/t inability to cope with psychosocial stressor

Ineffective Coping r/t stressors

Impaired Mood Regulation r/t emotional instability

Labile Emotional Control r/t emotional disturbance

Risk-Prone Health Behavior r/t assault to self-esteem

Disturbed Personal Identity r/t psychosocial stressor (specific to individual)

Situational Low Self-Esteem r/t change in role function

Impaired Social Interaction r/t absence of significant others or peers

Adjustment Impairment

Risk-Prone Health Behavior (See **Health Behavior, Risk-Prone,** Section III)

Adolescent, Pregnant

Anxiety r/t situational and maturational crisis, pregnancy

Disturbed Body Image r/t pregnancy superimposed on developing body

Decisional Conflict: Keeping Child Versus Giving up Child Versus Abortion r/t lack of experience with decision-making, interference with decision-making, multiple or divergent sources of information, lack of support system

Disabled Family Coping r/t highly ambivalent family relationships, chronically unresolved feelings of guilt, anger, despair

Ineffective Coping r/t situational and maturational crisis, personal vulnerability

Ineffective Denial r/t fear of consequences of pregnancy becoming known

Ineffective Adolescent Eating Dynamics r/t lack of knowledge of nutritional needs during pregnancy

Interrupted Family Processes r/t unmet expectations for adolescent, situational crisis

Fear r/t labor and delivery

Deficient Knowledge r/t pregnancy, infant growth and development, parenting

Imbalanced Nutrition: Less than Body Requirements r/t lack of knowledge of nutritional needs during pregnancy and as growing adolescent

Ineffective Role Performance r/t pregnancy

Situational Low Self-Esteem r/t feelings of shame and guilt about becoming or being pregnant

Impaired Social Interaction r/t self-concept disturbance

Social Isolation r/t absence of supportive significant others

Risk for Impaired Attachment: Risk factor: anxiety associated with the parent role

Risk for Disturbed Family Identity Syndrome: Risk Factor: excessive stress

Risk for Urge Urinary Incontinence: Risk factor: pressure on bladder by growing uterus

Risk for Disturbed Maternal–Fetal Dyad: Risk factors: immaturity, substance use

Risk for Impaired Parenting: Risk factors: adolescent parent, unplanned or unwanted pregnancy, single parent

Readiness for Enhanced Childbearing Process: reports appropriate prenatal lifestyle

Readiness for Enhanced Health Literacy: expresses desire to enhance social support for health

Readiness for Enhanced Knowledge: expresses an interest in learning

Adoption, Giving Child up for

Decisional Conflict r/t unclear personal values or beliefs, perceived threat to value system, support system deficit

Ineffective Coping r/t stress of loss of child

Interrupted Family Processes r/t conflict within family regarding relinquishment of child

Maladaptive Grieving r/t loss of child, loss of role of parent

Insomnia r/t depression or trauma of relinquishment of child

Social Isolation r/t making choice that goes against values of significant others

Chronic Sorrow r/t loss of relationship with child

Risk for Spiritual Distress: Risk factor: perceived moral implications of decision

Readiness for Enhanced Spiritual Well-Being: harmony with self-regarding final decision

Adrenocortical Insufficiency

Deficient Fluid Volume r/t insufficient ability to reabsorb water

Ineffective Protection r/t inability to tolerate stress

Delayed Surgical Recovery r/t inability to respond to stress

Risk for Shock: Risk factors: deficient fluid volume, decreased cortisol to initiate stress response to insult to body

See Addison's Disease; Shock, Hypovolemic

Advance Directives

Death Anxiety r/t planning for end-of-life health decisions

Decisional Conflict r/t unclear personal values or beliefs, perceived threat to value system, support system deficit

Maladaptive Grieving r/t possible loss of self, significant other

Readiness for Enhanced Spiritual Well-Being: harmonious interconnectedness with self, others, higher power, God

Affective Disorders

See Depression (Major Depressive Disorder); Dysthymic Disorder; Manic Disorder, Bipolar I; SAD (Seasonal Affective Disorder)

A

Age-Related Macular Degeneration

See Macular Degeneration

Aggressive Behavior

Fear r/t real or imagined threat to own well-being

Risk for Other-Directed Violence (See **Violence, Other-Directed, Risk for,** Section III)

Aging

Death Anxiety r/t fear of unknown, loss of self, impact on significant others

Impaired Dentition r/t ineffective oral hygiene

Risk for Frail Elderly Syndrome: Risk factors: >70 years, activity intolerance, impaired vision

Maladaptive Grieving r/t multiple losses, impending death

Ineffective Health Maintenance Behaviors r/t powerlessness

Hearing Loss r/t exposure to loud noises, aging

Impaired Urinary Elimination r/t impaired vision, impaired cognition, neuromuscular limitations, altered environmental factors

Impaired Resilience r/t aging, multiple losses

Sleep Deprivation r/t aging-related sleep-stage shifts

Risk for Caregiver Role Strain: Risk factor: inability to handle increasing needs of significant other

Risk for Impaired Emancipated Decision-Making: Risk factor: inability to process information regarding health care decisions

Risk for Injury: Risk factors: vision loss, hearing loss, decreased balance, decreased sensation in feet

Risk for Loneliness: Risk factors: inadequate support system, role transition, health alterations, depression, fatigue

Risk for Ineffective Thermoregulation: Risk factor: aging

Readiness for Enhanced Community Coping: providing social support and other resources identified as needed for elderly client

Readiness for Enhanced Family Coping: ability to gratify needs, address adaptive tasks

Readiness for Enhanced Health Self-Management: knowledge about medication, nutrition, exercise, coping strategies

Readiness for Enhanced Knowledge: specify need to improve health

Readiness for Enhanced Nutrition: need to improve health

Readiness for Enhanced Relationship: demonstrates understanding of partner's insufficient function

Readiness for Enhanced Sleep: need to improve sleep

Readiness for Enhanced Spiritual Well-Being: one's experience of life's meaning, harmony with self, others, higher power, God, environment

Agitation

Acute Confusion r/t side effects of medication, hypoxia, decreased cerebral perfusion, alcohol abuse or withdrawal, substance abuse or withdrawal, sensory deprivation or overload

Sleep Deprivation r/t sustained inadequate sleep hygiene, sundown syndrome

Agoraphobia

Anxiety r/t real or perceived threat to physical integrity

Ineffective Coping r/t inadequate support systems

Fear r/t leaving home, going out in public places

Impaired Social Interaction r/t disturbance in self-concept

Social Isolation r/t altered thought process

Agranulocytosis

Delayed Surgical Recovery r/t abnormal blood profile

Risk for Infection: Risk factor: abnormal blood profile

Readiness for Enhanced Knowledge: expresses an interest in learning

AIDS (Acquired Immunodeficiency Syndrome)

Death Anxiety r/t fear of premature death

Disturbed Body Image r/t chronic contagious illness, cachexia

Caregiver Role Strain r/t unpredictable illness course, presence of situation stressors

Diarrhea r/t inflammatory bowel changes

Interrupted Family Processes r/t distress about diagnosis of human immunodeficiency virus (HIV) infection

Fatigue r/t disease process, stress, decreased nutritional intake

Fear r/t powerlessness, threat to well-being

Maladaptive Grieving: Family/Parental r/t potential or impending death of loved one

Maladaptive Grieving: Individual r/t loss of physical and psychosocial well-being

Hopelessness r/t deteriorating physical condition

Imbalanced Nutrition: Less than Body Requirements r/t decreased ability to eat and absorb nutrients as a result of anorexia, nausea, diarrhea; oral candidiasis

Chronic Pain r/t tissue inflammation and destruction

Impaired Resilience r/t chronic illness

Situational Low Self-Esteem r/t crisis of chronic contagious illness

Ineffective Sexuality Pattern r/t possible transmission of disease

Social Isolation r/t self-concept disturbance, therapeutic isolation

Chronic Sorrow r/t chronic illness

Spiritual Distress r/t challenged beliefs or moral system

Risk for Deficient Fluid Volume: Risk factors: diarrhea, vomiting, fever, bleeding

Risk for Infection: Risk factor: inadequate immune system

Risk for Loneliness: Risk factor: social isolation

Risk for Impaired Oral Mucous Membrane Integrity: Risk factor: immunological deficit

Risk for Impaired Skin Integrity: Risk factors: immunological deficit, diarrhea

Risk for Spiritual Distress: Risk factor: physical illness

Readiness for Enhanced Health Literacy: expresses desire to enhance understanding of health information to make health care choices

Readiness for Enhanced Knowledge: expresses an interest in learning

See AIDS, Child; Cancer; Pneumonia

AIDS, Child

Impaired Parenting r/t congenital acquisition of infection secondary to intravenous (IV) drug use, multiple sexual partners, history of contaminated blood transfusion

Risk for Disturbed Family Identity Syndrome: Risk factor: excessive stress

See AIDS (Acquired Immunodeficiency Syndrome); Child with Chronic Condition; Hospitalized Child; Terminally Ill Child, Adolescent; Terminally Ill Child, Infant/Toddler; Terminally Ill Child, Preschool Child; Terminally Ill Child, School-Age Child/Preadolescent; Terminally Ill Child/Death of Child, Parent

AIDS Dementia

Chronic Confusion r/t viral invasion of nervous system

See Dementia

Airway Obstruction/Secretions

Ineffective Airway Clearance (See **Airway Clearance, Ineffective,** Section III)

Alcohol Withdrawal

Anxiety r/t situational crisis, withdrawal

Acute Confusion r/t effects of alcohol withdrawal

Ineffective Coping r/t personal vulnerability

Dysfunctional Family Processes r/t abuse of alcohol

Insomnia r/t effect of alcohol withdrawal, anxiety

Imbalanced Nutrition: Less than Body Requirements r/t poor dietary habits

Chronic Low Self-Esteem r/t repeated unmet expectations

Acute Substance Withdrawal Syndrome: Risk factor: developed dependence to alcohol

Risk for Deficient Fluid Volume: Risk factors: excessive diaphoresis, agitation, decreased fluid intake

Risk for Other-Directed Violence: Risk factor: substance withdrawal

Risk for Self-Directed Violence: Risk factor: substance withdrawal

Readiness for Enhanced Knowledge: expresses an interest in learning

Alcoholism

Anxiety r/t loss of control

Risk-Prone Health Behavior r/t lack of motivation to change behaviors, addiction

Acute Confusion r/t alcohol abuse

Chronic Confusion r/t neurological effects of chronic alcohol intake

Defensive Coping r/t denial of reality of addiction

Disabled Family Coping r/t codependency issues due to alcoholism

Ineffective Coping r/t use of alcohol to cope with life events

Labile Emotional Control r/t substance abuse

Ineffective Denial r/t refusal to acknowledge addiction

Dysfunctional Family Processes r/t alcohol abuse

Ineffective Home Maintenance Behaviors r/t memory deficits, fatigue

Insomnia r/t irritability, nightmares, tremors

Impaired Memory r/t alcohol abuse

Self-Neglect r/t effects of alcohol abuse

Imbalanced Nutrition: Less than Body Requirements r/t anorexia, inappropriate diet with increased carbohydrates

Powerlessness r/t alcohol addiction

Ineffective Protection r/t malnutrition, sleep deprivation

Chronic Low Self-Esteem r/t failure at life events

Social Isolation r/t unacceptable social behavior, values

Acute Substance Withdrawal Syndrome: Risk factor: developed dependence to alcohol

Risk for Injury: Risk factor: alteration in sensory or perceptual function

Risk for Loneliness: Risk factor: unacceptable social behavior

Risk for Acute Substance Withdrawal Syndrome: Risk factor: developed dependence to alcohol

Risk for Other-Directed Violence: Risk factors: reactions to substances used, impulsive behavior, disorientation, impaired judgment

Risk for Self-Directed Violence: Risk factors: reactions to substances used, impulsive behavior, disorientation, impaired judgment

Alcoholism, Dysfunctional Family Processes

Dysfunctional Family Processes (See **Family Processes, Dysfunctional,** Section III)

Disturbed Family Identity Syndrome: Risk factor: excessive stress

Alkalosis

See Metabolic Alkalosis

ALL (Acute Lymphocytic Leukemia)

See Cancer; Chemotherapy; Child with Chronic Condition; Leukemia

Allergies

Risk for Allergy Reaction: Risk factors: chemical factors, dander, environmental substances, foods, insect stings, medications

Risk for Latex Allergic Reaction: Risk factor: repeated exposure to products containing latex

Readiness for Enhanced Knowledge: expresses an interest in learning

Alopecia

Disturbed Body Image r/t loss of hair, change in appearance

A

Readiness for Enhanced Knowledge: expresses an interest in learning

ALS (Amyotrophic Lateral Sclerosis)

See Amyotrophic Lateral Sclerosis (ALS)

Altered Mental Status

See Confusion, Acute; Confusion, Chronic; Memory Deficit

Alzheimer's Disease

Caregiver Role Strain r/t duration and extent of caregiving required

Chronic Confusion r/t loss of cognitive function

Compromised Family Coping r/t interrupted family processes

Frail Elderly Syndrome r/t alteration in cognitive functioning

Ineffective Home Maintenance Behaviors r/t impaired cognitive function, inadequate support systems

Hopelessness r/t deteriorating condition

Insomnia r/t neurological impairment, daytime naps

Impaired Memory r/t neurological disturbance

Impaired Physical Mobility r/t severe neurological dysfunction

Self-Neglect r/t loss of cognitive function

Powerlessness r/t deteriorating condition

Self-Care Deficit: Specify r/t loss of cognitive function, psychological impairment

Social Isolation r/t fear of disclosure of memory loss

Wandering r/t cognitive impairment, frustration, physiological state

Risk for Chronic Functional Constipation: Risk factor: impaired cognitive functioning

Risk for Injury: Risk factor: confusion

Risk for Loneliness: Risk factor: potential social isolation

Risk for Relocation Stress Syndrome: Risk factors: impaired psychosocial health, decreased health status

Risk for Other-Directed Violence: Risk factors: frustration, fear, anger, loss of cognitive function

Readiness for Enhanced Knowledge: Caregiver: expresses an interest in learning

See Dementia

AMD (Age-Related Macular Degeneration)

See Macular Degeneration

Amenorrhea

Imbalanced Nutrition: Less than Body Requirements r/t inadequate food intake

See Sexuality, Adolescent

AMI (Acute Myocardial Infarction)

See MI (Myocardial Infarction)

Amnesia

Acute Confusion r/t alcohol abuse, delirium, dementia, drug abuse

Dysfunctional Family Processes r/t alcohol abuse, inadequate coping skills

Impaired Memory r/t excessive environmental disturbance, neurological disturbance

Post-Trauma Syndrome r/t history of abuse, catastrophic illness, disaster, accident

Amniocentesis

Anxiety r/t threat to self and fetus, unknown future

Decisional Conflict r/t choice of treatment pending results of test

Risk for Infection: Risk factor: invasive procedure

Amnionitis

See Chorioamnionitis

Amniotic Membrane Rupture

See Premature Rupture of Membranes

Amputation

Disturbed Body Image r/t negative effects of amputation, response from others

Maladaptive Grieving r/t loss of body part, future lifestyle changes

Impaired Physical Mobility r/t musculoskeletal impairment, limited movement

Acute Pain r/t surgery, phantom limb sensation

Chronic Pain r/t surgery, phantom limb sensation

Ineffective Peripheral Tissue Perfusion r/t impaired arterial circulation

Impaired Skin Integrity r/t poor healing, prosthesis rubbing

Risk for Bleeding: Risk factor: vulnerable surgical site

Risk for Impaired Tissue Integrity: Risk factor: mechanical factors impacting site

Readiness for Enhanced Knowledge: expresses an interest in learning

Amyotrophic Lateral Sclerosis (ALS)

Death Anxiety r/t impending progressive loss of function leading to death

Ineffective Breathing Pattern r/t compromised muscles of respiration

Impaired Verbal Communication r/t weakness of muscles of speech, deficient knowledge of ways to compensate and alternative communication devices

Decisional Conflict: Ventilator Therapy r/t unclear personal values or beliefs, lack of relevant information

Impaired Resilience r/t perceived vulnerability

Chronic Sorrow r/t chronic illness

Impaired Swallowing r/t weakness of muscles involved in swallowing

Impaired Spontaneous Ventilation r/t weakness of muscles of respiration

Risk for Aspiration: Risk factor: impaired swallowing

Risk for Spiritual Distress: Risk factor: chronic debilitating condition

See Neurological Disorders

Anal Fistula

See Hemorrhoidectomy

Anaphylactic Shock

Deficient Fluid Volume r/t compromised regulatory mechanism

Ineffective Airway Clearance r/t laryngeal edema, bronchospasm

Risk for Latex Allergic Reaction r/t abnormal immune mechanism response

Impaired Spontaneous Ventilation r/t acute airway obstruction from anaphylaxis process

Anaphylaxis Prevention

Risk for Allergy Reaction (See **Allergy Reaction, Risk for,** Section III)

Anasarca

Excess Fluid Volume r/t excessive fluid intake, cardiac/renal dysfunction, loss of plasma proteins

Risk for Decreased Cardiac Output: Risk factor: imbalanced fluid volume

Risk for Impaired Skin Integrity: Risk factor: impaired circulation to skin from edema

Anemia

Anxiety r/t cause of disease

Impaired Comfort r/t feelings of always being cold from decreased hemoglobin and decreased metabolism

Fatigue r/t decreased oxygen supply to the body, increased cardiac workload

Impaired Memory r/t change in cognition from decreased oxygen supply to the body

Delayed Surgical Recovery r/t decreased oxygen supply to body, increased cardiac workload

Risk for Bleeding (See **Bleeding, Risk for,** Section III)

Risk for Injury: Risk factor: alteration in peripheral sensory perception

Readiness for Enhanced Knowledge: expresses an interest in learning

Anemia, in Pregnancy

Anxiety r/t concerns about health of self and fetus

Fatigue r/t decreased oxygen supply to the body, increased cardiac workload

Risk for Infection: Risk factor: reduction in oxygen-carrying capacity of blood

Risk for Disturbed Maternal–Fetal Dyad: Risk factor: compromised oxygen transport

Readiness for Enhanced Knowledge: expresses an interest in learning

Anemia, Sickle Cell

See Anemia; Sickle Cell Anemia/Crisis

Anencephaly

See Neural Tube Defects (Meningocele, Myelomeningocele, Spina Bifida, Anencephaly)

Aneurysm, Abdominal Aortic Repair Surgery

Risk for Deficient Fluid Volume: Risk factor: hemorrhage r/t potential abnormal blood loss

Risk for Surgical Site Infection: Risk factor: invasive procedure

See Abdominal Surgery

Aneurysm, Cerebral

See Craniectomy/Craniotomy; Subarachnoid Hemorrhage

Anger

Anxiety r/t situational crisis

Defensive Coping r/t inability to acknowledge responsibility for actions and results of actions

Labile Emotional Control r/t stressors

Fear r/t environmental stressor, hospitalization

Maladaptive Grieving r/t significant loss

Risk-Prone Health Behavior r/t assault to self-esteem, disability requiring change in lifestyle, inadequate support system

Powerlessness r/t health care environment

Risk for Compromised Human Dignity: Risk factors: inadequate participation in decision-making, perceived dehumanizing treatment, perceived humiliation, exposure of the body, cultural incongruity

Risk for Post-Trauma Syndrome: Risk factor: inadequate social support

Risk for Other-Directed Violence: Risk factors: history of violence, rage reaction

Risk for Self-Directed Violence: Risk factors: history of violence, history of abuse, rage reaction

Angina

Decreased Activity Tolerance r/t acute pain, dysrhythmias

Anxiety r/t situational crisis

Decreased Cardiac Output r/t myocardial ischemia, medication effect, dysrhythmia

Ineffective Coping r/t personal vulnerability to situational crisis of new diagnosis, deteriorating health

Ineffective Denial r/t deficient knowledge of need to seek help with symptoms

Maladaptive Grieving r/t pain, loss of health

Acute Pain r/t myocardial ischemia

Ineffective Sexuality Pattern r/t disease process, medications, loss of libido

Readiness for Enhanced Knowledge: expresses an interest in learning

See MI (Myocardial Infarction)

Angiocardiography (Cardiac Catheterization)

See Cardiac Catheterization

Angioplasty, Coronary

Fear r/t possible outcome of interventional procedure

Ineffective Peripheral Tissue Perfusion r/t vasospasm, hematoma formation

Risk for Bleeding: Risk factors: possible damage to coronary artery, hematoma formation

Risk for Decreased Cardiac Tissue Perfusion: Risk factors: ventricular ischemia, dysrhythmias

Readiness for Enhanced Knowledge: expresses an interest in learning

Anomaly, Fetal/Newborn (Parent Dealing with)

Anxiety r/t threat to role functioning, situational crisis

Decisional Conflict: Interventions for Fetus or Newborn r/t lack of relevant information, spiritual distress, threat to value system

Disabled Family Coping r/t chronically unresolved feelings about loss of perfect baby

Ineffective Coping r/t personal vulnerability in situational crisis

Interrupted Family Processes r/t unmet expectations for perfect baby, lack of adequate support systems

Fear r/t real or imagined threat to baby, implications for future pregnancies, powerlessness

Maladaptive Grieving r/t loss of ideal child

Hopelessness r/t long-term stress, deteriorating physical condition of child, lost spiritual belief

Deficient Knowledge r/t limited exposure to situation

Impaired Parenting r/t interruption of bonding process

Powerlessness r/t complication threatening fetus or newborn

Parental Role Conflict r/t separation from newborn, intimidation with invasive or restrictive modalities, specialized care center policies

Situational Low Self-Esteem r/t perceived inability to produce a perfect child

Social Isolation r/t alterations in child's physical appearance, altered state of wellness

Chronic Sorrow r/t loss of ideal child, inadequate bereavement support

Spiritual Distress r/t test of spiritual beliefs

Risk for Impaired Attachment: Risk factor: ill infant unable to effectively initiate parental contact as result of altered behavioral organization

Risk for Disorganized Infant Behavior: Risk factor: congenital disorder

Risk for Impaired Parenting: Risk factors: interruption of bonding process; unrealistic expectations for self, infant, or partner; perceived threat to own emotional survival; severe stress; lack of knowledge

Risk for Spiritual Distress: Risk factor: lack of normal child to raise and carry on family name

Anorectal Abscess

Disturbed Body Image r/t odor and drainage from rectal area

Acute Pain r/t inflammation of perirectal area

Risk for Constipation: Risk factor: fear of painful elimination

Readiness for Enhanced Knowledge: expresses an interest in learning

Anorexia

Deficient Fluid Volume r/t inability to drink

Imbalanced Nutrition: Less than Body Requirements r/t loss of appetite, nausea, vomiting, laxative abuse

Delayed Surgical Recovery r/t inadequate nutritional intake

Risk for Delayed Surgical Recovery: Risk factor: inadequate nutritional intake

Anorexia Nervosa

Decreased Activity Tolerance r/t fatigue, weakness

Disturbed Body Image r/t misconception of actual body appearance

Constipation r/t lack of adequate food, fiber, and fluid intake

Defensive Coping r/t psychological impairment, eating disorder

Disabled Family Coping r/t highly ambivalent family relationships

Ineffective Denial r/t fear of consequences of therapy, possible weight gain

Diarrhea r/t laxative abuse

Interrupted Family Processes r/t situational crisis

Ineffective Adolescent Eating Dynamics r/t food refusal

Ineffective Family Health Self-Management r/t family conflict, excessive demands on family associated with complexity of condition and treatment

Imbalanced Nutrition: Less than Body Requirements r/t inadequate food intake, excessive exercise

Chronic Low Self-Esteem r/t repeated unmet expectations

Ineffective Sexuality Pattern r/t loss of libido from malnutrition

Risk for Infection: Risk factor: malnutrition resulting in depressed immune system

Risk for Spiritual Distress: Risk factor: low self-esteem

See Maturational Issues, Adolescent

Anosmia (Smell, Loss of Ability to)

Imbalanced Nutrition: Less than Body Requirements r/t loss of appetite associated with loss of smell

Antepartum Period

See Pregnancy, Normal; Prenatal Care, Normal

Anterior Repair, Anterior Colporrhaphy

Urinary Retention r/t edema of urinary structures

Risk for Urge Urinary Incontinence: Risk factor: trauma to bladder

Readiness for Enhanced Knowledge: expresses an interest in learning

See Vaginal Hysterectomy

Anticoagulant Therapy

Risk for Bleeding: Risk factor: altered clotting function from anticoagulant

Risk for Deficient Fluid Volume: Hemorrhage: Risk factor: altered clotting mechanism

Readiness for Enhanced Knowledge: expresses an interest in learning

Antisocial Personality Disorder

Defensive Coping r/t excessive use of projection

Ineffective Coping r/t frequently violating the norms and rules of society

Labile Emotional Control r/t psychiatric disorder

Hopelessness r/t abandonment

Impaired Social Interaction r/t sociocultural conflict, chemical dependence, inability to form relationships

Spiritual Distress r/t separation from religious or cultural ties

Ineffective Health Self-Management r/t excessive demands on family

Risk for Loneliness: Risk factor: inability to interact appropriately with others

Risk for Impaired Parenting: Risk factors: inability to function as parent or guardian, emotional instability

Risk for Self-Mutilation: Risk factors: self-hatred, depersonalization

Risk for Other-Directed Violence: Risk factor: history of violence, altered thought patterns

Anuria

See Renal Failure

Anxiety

See **Anxiety,** Section III

Anxiety Disorder

Ineffective Activity Planning r/t unrealistic perception of events

Anxiety r/t unmet security and safety needs

Death Anxiety r/t fears of unknown, powerlessness

Decisional Conflict r/t low self-esteem, fear of making a mistake

Defensive Coping r/t overwhelming feelings of dread

Disabled Family Coping r/t ritualistic behavior, actions

Imbalanced Energy Field r/t feelings of restlessness and apprehension

Impaired Mood Regulation r/t functional impairment, impaired social functioning, alteration in sleep pattern

Ineffective Coping r/t inability to express feelings appropriately

Ineffective Denial r/t overwhelming feelings of hopelessness, fear, threat to self

Insomnia r/t psychological impairment, emotional instability

Labile Emotional Control r/t emotional instability

Powerlessness r/t lifestyle of helplessness

Self-Care Deficit r/t ritualistic behavior, activities

Sleep Deprivation r/t prolonged psychological discomfort

Risk for Spiritual Distress: Risk factor: psychological distress

Readiness for Enhanced Knowledge: expresses an interest in learning

Aortic Valvular Stenosis

See Congenital Heart Disease/Cardiac Anomalies

Aphasia

Anxiety r/t situational crisis of aphasia

Impaired Verbal Communication r/t decrease in circulation to brain

Ineffective Coping r/t loss of speech

Ineffective Health Maintenance Behaviors r/t deficient knowledge regarding information on aphasia and alternative communication techniques

Aplastic Anemia

Decreased Activity Tolerance r/t imbalance between oxygen supply and demand

Fear r/t ability to live with serious disease

Risk for Bleeding: Risk factor: inadequate clotting factors

Risk for Infection: Risk factor: inadequate immune function

Readiness for Enhanced Knowledge: expresses an interest in learning

Apnea in Infancy

See Premature Infant (Child); Premature Infant (Parent); SIDS (Sudden Infant Death Syndrome)

Apneustic Respirations

Ineffective Breathing Pattern r/t perception or cognitive impairment, neurological impairment

Appendectomy

Deficient Fluid Volume r/t fluid restriction, hypermetabolic state, nausea, vomiting

Acute Pain r/t surgical incision

Delayed Surgical Recovery r/t rupture of appendix

Risk for Infection: Risk factors: perforation or rupture of appendix, peritonitis

Risk for Surgical Site Infection: Risk factor: surgical incision

Readiness for Enhanced Knowledge: expresses an interest in learning

See Hospitalized Child; Surgery, Postoperative Care

Appendicitis

Deficient Fluid Volume r/t anorexia, nausea, vomiting

Acute Pain r/t inflammation

Risk for Infection: Risk factor: possible perforation of appendix

Readiness for Enhanced Knowledge: expresses an interest in learning

Apprehension

Anxiety r/t threat to self-concept, threat to health status, situational crisis

Death Anxiety r/t apprehension over loss of self, consequences to significant others

A

ARDS (Acute Respiratory Distress Syndrome)

Ineffective Airway Clearance r/t excessive tracheobronchial secretions

Death Anxiety r/t seriousness of physical disease

Impaired Gas Exchange r/t damage to alveolar-capillary membrane, change in lung compliance

Impaired Spontaneous Ventilation r/t damage to alveolar-capillary membrane

See Ventilated Client, Mechanically

Arrhythmia

See Dysrhythmia

Arterial Insufficiency

Ineffective Peripheral Tissue Perfusion r/t interruption of arterial flow

Delayed Surgical Recovery r/t ineffective tissue perfusion

Arthritis

Decreased Activity Tolerance r/t chronic pain, fatigue, weakness

Disturbed Body Image r/t ineffective coping with joint abnormalities

Impaired Physical Mobility r/t joint impairment

Chronic Pain r/t progression of joint deterioration

Self-Care Deficit: Specify r/t pain with movement, damage to joints

Readiness for Enhanced Knowledge: expresses an interest in learning

See JRA (Juvenile Rheumatoid Arthritis)

Arthrocentesis

Acute Pain r/t invasive procedure

Arthroplasty (Total Hip Replacement)

See Total Joint Replacement (Total Hip/Total Knee/Shoulder); Surgery, Perioperative Care; Surgery, Postoperative Care; Surgery, Preoperative Care

Arthroscopy

Impaired Physical Mobility r/t surgical trauma of knee

Readiness for Enhanced Knowledge: expresses an interest in learning

Ascites

Ineffective Breathing Pattern r/t increased abdominal girth

Imbalanced Nutrition: Less than Body Requirements r/t loss of appetite

Chronic Pain r/t altered body function

Readiness for Enhanced Knowledge: expresses an interest in learning

See Ascites; Cancer; Cirrhosis

Asperger's Syndrome

Ineffective Relationship r/t poor communication skills, lack of empathy

See Autism

Asphyxia, Birth

Ineffective Breathing Pattern r/t depression of breathing reflex secondary to anoxia

Ineffective Coping r/t uncertainty of child outcome

Fear (Parental) r/t concern over safety of infant

Impaired Gas Exchange r/t poor placental perfusion, lack of initiation of breathing by newborn

Maladaptive Grieving r/t loss of perfect child, concern of loss of future abilities

Impaired Spontaneous Ventilation r/t brain injury

Risk for Impaired Attachment: Risk factors: ill infant who is unable to initiate parental contact, hospitalization in critical care environment

Risk for Delayed Child Development: Risk factors: lack of oxygen to brain

Risk for Disorganized Infant Behavior: Risk factor: lack of oxygen to brain

Risk for Injury: Risk factor: lack of oxygen to brain

Risk for Ineffective Cerebral Tissue Perfusion: Risk factor: poor placental perfusion or cord compression resulting in lack of oxygen to brain

Aspiration, Danger of

Risk for Aspiration (See **Aspiration, Risk for,** Section III)

Assault Victim

Post-Trauma Syndrome r/t assault

Rape-Trauma Syndrome r/t rape

Impaired Resilience r/t frightening experience, post-trauma stress response

Risk for Post-Trauma Syndrome: Risk factors: perception of event, inadequate social support, unsupportive environment, diminished ego strength, duration of event

Risk for Spiritual Distress: Risk factors: physical, psychological stress

Assaultive Client

Risk for Injury: Risk factors: confused thought process, impaired judgment

Risk for Other-Directed Violence: Risk factors: paranoid ideation, anger

Asthma

Decreased Activity Tolerance r/t fatigue, energy shift to meet muscle needs for breathing to overcome airway obstruction

Ineffective Airway Clearance r/t tracheobronchial narrowing, excessive secretions

Anxiety r/t inability to breathe effectively, fear of suffocation

Disturbed Body Image r/t decreased participation in physical activities

Ineffective Breathing Pattern r/t anxiety

Ineffective Coping r/t personal vulnerability to situational crisis

Ineffective Health Self-Management (See **Health Management, Ineffective,** Section III)

Ineffective Home Maintenance Behaviors r/t deficient knowledge regarding control of environmental triggers

Sleep Deprivation r/t ineffective breathing pattern, cough

Readiness for Enhanced Health Self-Management (See **Health Self-Management, Readiness for Enhanced,** Section III)

Readiness for Enhanced Knowledge: expresses an interest in learning

See Child with Chronic Condition; Hospitalized Child

Ataxia

Anxiety r/t change in health status

Disturbed Body Image r/t staggering gait

Impaired Physical Mobility r/t neuromuscular impairment

Risk for Falls: Risk factors: gait alteration, instability

Atelectasis

Ineffective Breathing Pattern r/t loss of functional lung tissue, depression of respiratory function or hypoventilation because of pain

Impaired Gas Exchange r/t decreased alveolar-capillary surface

Anxiety r/t alteration in respiratory pattern

See Atelectasis

Atherosclerosis

See MI (Myocardial Infarction); CVA (Cerebrovascular Accident); Peripheral Vascular Disease (PVD)

Athlete's Foot

Impaired Skin Integrity r/t effects of fungal agent

Readiness for Enhanced Knowledge: expresses an interest in learning

See Pruritus

ATN (Acute Tubular Necrosis)

See Renal Failure

Atrial Fibrillation

See Dysrhythmia

Atrial Septal Defect

See Congenital Heart Disease/Cardiac Anomalies

Attention Deficit Disorder

Risk-Prone Health Behavior r/t intense emotional state

Disabled Family Coping r/t significant person with chronically unexpressed feelings of guilt, anxiety, hostility, and despair

Ineffective Impulse Control (See **Impulse Control, Ineffective,** Section III)

Chronic Low Self-Esteem r/t difficulty in participating in expected activities, poor school performance

Social Isolation r/t unacceptable social behavior

Risk for Delayed Child Development: Risk factor: behavior disorders

Risk for Falls: Risk factor: rapid non-thinking behavior

Risk for Loneliness: Risk factor: social isolation

Risk for Impaired Parenting: Risk factor: lack of knowledge of factors contributing to child's behavior

Risk for Spiritual Distress: Risk factor: poor relationships

Autism

Impaired Verbal Communication r/t speech and language delays

Compromised Family Coping r/t parental guilt over etiology of disease, inability to accept or adapt to child's condition, inability to help child and other family members seek treatment

Disturbed Personal Identity r/t inability to distinguish between self and environment, inability to identify own body as separate from those of other people, inability to integrate concept of self

Self-Neglect r/t impaired socialization

Impaired Social Interaction r/t communication barriers, inability to relate to others, failure to develop peer relationships

Risk for Delayed Child Development: Risk factor: autism

Risk for Disturbed Family Identity Syndrome: Risk factor: excessive stress

Risk for Loneliness: Risk factor: difficulty developing relationships with other people

Risk for Self-Mutilation: Risk factor: autistic state

Risk for Other-Directed Violence: Risk factors: frequent destructive rages toward others secondary to extreme response to changes in routine, fear of harmless things

Risk for Self-Directed Violence: Risk factors: frequent destructive rages toward self, secondary to extreme response to changes in routine, fear of harmless things

See Child with Chronic Condition

Autonomic Dysreflexia

Autonomic Dysreflexia r/t bladder distention, bowel distention, noxious stimuli

Risk for Autonomic Dysreflexia: Risk factors: bladder distention, bowel distention, noxious stimuli

Autonomic Hyperreflexia

See Autonomic Dysreflexia

B

Baby Care

Readiness for Enhanced Childbearing Process: demonstrates appropriate feeding and baby care techniques, along with attachment to infant and providing a safe environment

Anxiety r/t situational crisis, back injury

Ineffective Coping r/t situational crisis, back injury

Impaired Physical Mobility r/t pain

Acute Pain r/t back injury

Chronic Pain r/t back injury

Risk for Constipation: Risk factors: decreased activity, side effect of pain medication

Risk for Disuse Syndrome: Risk factor: severe pain

Readiness for Enhanced Knowledge: expresses an interest in learning

Bacteremia

Risk for Infection: Risk factor: compromised immune system

Risk for Shock: Risk factor: development of systemic inflammatory response from presence of bacteria in bloodstream

B

Balanced Energy Field

Imbalanced Energy Field (See **Energy Field, Imbalanced,** Section III)

Barrel Chest

See Aging (if appropriate); COPD (Chronic Obstructive Pulmonary Disease)

Bathing/Hygiene Problems

Impaired Mobility r/t chronic physically limiting condition

Self-Neglect (See **Self-Neglect,** Section III)

Bathing Self-Care Deficit (See **Self-Care Deficit, bathing,** Section III)

Battered Child Syndrome

Dysfunctional Family Processes r/t inadequate coping skills

Sleep Deprivation r/t prolonged psychological discomfort

Chronic Sorrow r/t situational crises

Risk for Post-Trauma Syndrome: Risk factors: physical abuse, incest, rape, molestation

Risk for Self-Mutilation: Risk factors: feelings of rejection, dysfunctional family

Risk for Suicidal Behavior: Risk factor: childhood abuse

See Child Abuse

Battered Person

See Abuse, Spouse, Parent, or Significant Other

Bedbugs, Infestation

Ineffective Home Maintenance Behaviors r/t deficient knowledge regarding prevention of bedbug infestation

Impaired Skin Integrity r/t bites of bedbugs

See Pruritus

Bed Mobility, Impaired

Impaired Bed Mobility (See **Mobility, Bed, Impaired,** Section III)

Bed Rest, Prolonged

Decreased Diversional Activity Engagement r/t prolonged bed rest

Impaired Bed Mobility r/t neuromuscular impairment

Social Isolation r/t prolonged bed rest

Risk for Chronic Functional Constipation: Risk factor: insufficient physical activity

Risk for Disuse Syndrome: Risk factor: prolonged immobility

Risk for Frail Elderly Syndrome: Risk factor: prolonged immobility

Risk for Loneliness: Risk factor: prolonged bed rest

Risk for Overweight: Risk factor: energy expenditure below energy intake

Risk for Pressure Ulcer: Risk factor: prolonged immobility

Risk for Thrombosis: Risk factor: prolonged immobility

Bedsores

See Pressure Ulcer

Bedwetting

Ineffective Health Maintenance Behaviors r/t unachieved developmental level, neuromuscular immaturity, diseases of the urinary system

Bell's Palsy

Disturbed Body Image r/t loss of motor control on one side of face

Imbalanced Nutrition: Less than Body Requirements r/t difficulty with chewing

Acute Pain r/t inflammation of facial nerve

Risk for Injury (Eye): Risk factors: decreased tears, decreased blinking of eye

Readiness for Enhanced Knowledge: expresses an interest in learning

Benign Prostatic Hypertrophy

See BPH (Benign Prostatic Hypertrophy); Prostatic Hypertrophy

Bereavement

Maladaptive Grieving r/t loss of significant person

Insomnia r/t grief

Risk for Maladaptive Grieving: Risk factor: emotional instability, lack of social support

Risk for Spiritual Distress: Risk factor: death of a loved one

Biliary Atresia

Anxiety r/t surgical intervention, possible liver transplantation

Impaired Comfort r/t inflammation of skin, itching

Imbalanced Nutrition: Less than Body Requirements r/t decreased absorption of fat and fat-soluble vitamins, poor feeding

Risk for Bleeding: Risk factors: vitamin K deficiency, altered clotting mechanisms

Ineffective Breathing Pattern r/t enlarged liver, development of ascites

Risk for Impaired Skin Integrity: Risk factor: pruritus

See Child with Chronic Condition; Cirrhosis; Hospitalized Child

Biliary Calculus

See Cholelithiasis

Biliary Obstruction

See Jaundice

Bilirubin Elevation in Neonate

See Hyperbilirubinemia, Neonatal

Biopsy

Fear r/t outcome of biopsy

Readiness for Enhanced Knowledge: expresses an interest in learning

Bioterrorism

Contamination r/t exposure to bioterrorism

Risk for Infection: Risk factor: exposure to harmful biological agent

Risk for Post-Trauma Syndrome: Risk factor: perception of event of bioterrorism

Bipolar Disorder I (Most Recent Episode, Depressed or Manic)

Ineffective Activity Planning r/t unrealistic perception of events

Fatigue r/t psychological demands

Risk-Prone Health Behavior: Risk factor: low state of optimism

Ineffective Health Maintenance Behaviors r/t lack of ability to make good judgments regarding ways to obtain help

Self-Care Deficit: Specify r/t depression, cognitive impairment

Chronic Low Self-Esteem r/t repeated unmet expectations

Social Isolation r/t ineffective coping

Risk for Maladaptive Grieving: Risk factor: lack of previous resolution of former grieving response

Risk for Loneliness: Risk factors: stress, conflict

Risk for Spiritual Distress: Risk factor: mental illness

Risk for Suicidal Behavior: Risk factors: psychiatric disorder, poor support system

See Depression (Major Depressive Disorder); Manic Disorder, Bipolar I

Birth Asphyxia

See Asphyxia, Birth

Birth Control

See Contraceptive Method

Bladder Cancer

Urinary Retention r/t clots obstructing urethra

See Cancer; TURP (Transurethral Resection of the Prostate)

Bladder Distention

Urinary Retention r/t high urethral pressure caused by weak detrusor, inhibition of reflex arc, blockage, strong sphincter

Bladder Training

Disturbed Body Image r/t difficulty maintaining control of urinary elimination

Disability-Associated Urinary Incontinence r/t altered environment; sensory, cognitive, mobility deficit

Stress Urinary Incontinence r/t degenerative change in pelvic muscles and structural supports

Urge Urinary Incontinence r/t decreased bladder capacity, increased urine concentration, overdistention of bladder

Readiness for Enhanced Knowledge: expresses an interest in learning

Bladder Training, Child

See Toilet Training

Bleeding Tendency

Risk for Bleeding (See **Bleeding, Risk for,** Section III)

Risk for Delayed Surgical Recovery: Risk factor: bleeding tendency

Blepharoplasty

Disturbed Body Image r/t effects of surgery

Readiness for Enhanced Knowledge: expresses an interest in learning

Blindness

Interrupted Family Processes r/t shift in health status of family member (change in visual acuity)

Ineffective Home Maintenance Behaviors r/t decreased vision

Ineffective Role Performance r/t alteration in health status (change in visual acuity)

Self-Care Deficit: Specify r/t inability to see to be able to perform activities of daily living

Risk for Injury: Risk factor: sensory dysfunction

Readiness for Enhanced Knowledge: expresses an interest in learning

Blood Disorder

Ineffective Protection r/t abnormal blood profile

Risk for Bleeding: Risk factor: abnormal blood profile

See ITP (Idiopathic Thrombocytopenic Purpura); Hemophilia; Lacerations; Shock, Hypovolemic

Blood Glucose Control

Risk for Unstable Blood Glucose Level (See **Glucose Level, Blood, Unstable, Risk for,** Section III)

Blood Pressure Alteration

See Hypotension; HTN (Hypertension)

(See **Unstable Blood Pressure, Risk for,** Section III)

Blood Transfusion

Anxiety r/t possibility of harm from transfusion

See Anemia

Body Dysmorphic Disorder

Anxiety r/t perceived defect of body

Disturbed Body Image r/t over-involvement in physical appearance

Chronic Low Self-Esteem r/t lack of self-valuing because of perceived body defects

Social Isolation r/t distancing self from others because of perceived self-body defects

Risk for Suicidal Behavior: Risk factor: perceived defects of body affecting self-valuing and hopes

Body Image Change

Disturbed Body Image (See **Body Image, Disturbed,** Section III)

Body Temperature, Altered

Ineffective Thermoregulation (See **Thermoregulation, Ineffective,** Section III)

Bone Marrow Biopsy

Fear r/t unknown outcome of results of biopsy

Acute Pain r/t bone marrow aspiration

Readiness for Enhanced Knowledge: expresses an interest in learning

See Disease Necessitating Bone Marrow Biopsy (e.g., Leukemia)

B

Borderline Personality Disorder

Ineffective Activity Planning r/t unrealistic perception of events

Anxiety r/t perceived threat to self-concept

Defensive Coping r/t difficulty with relationships, inability to accept blame for own behavior

Ineffective Coping r/t use of maladjusted defense mechanisms (e.g., projection, denial)

Powerlessness r/t lifestyle of helplessness

Social Isolation r/t immature interests

Ineffective Family Health Self-Management r/t manipulative behavior of client

Risk for Caregiver Role Strain: Risk factors: inability of care receiver to accept criticism, care receiver taking advantage of others to meet own needs or having unreasonable expectations

Risk for Self-Mutilation: Risk factors: ineffective coping, feelings of self-hatred

Risk for Spiritual Distress: Risk factor: poor relationships associated with abnormal behaviors

Risk for Self-Directed Violence: Risk factors: feelings of need to punish self, manipulative behavior

Boredom

Decreased Diversional Activity Engagement r/t environmental lack of diversional activity

Impaired Mood Regulation r/t emotional instability

Social Isolation r/t altered state of wellness

Botulism

Deficient Fluid Volume r/t profuse diarrhea

Readiness for Enhanced Knowledge: expresses an interest in learning

Bowel Incontinence

Impaired Bowel Continence r/t decreased awareness of need to defecate, loss of sphincter control, fecal impaction

Readiness for Enhanced Knowledge: expresses an interest in learning

Bowel Obstruction

Constipation r/t decreased motility, intestinal obstruction

Deficient Fluid Volume r/t inadequate fluid volume intake, fluid loss in bowel

Imbalanced Nutrition: Less than Body Requirements r/t nausea, vomiting

Acute Pain r/t pressure from distended abdomen

Bowel Resection

See Abdominal Surgery

Bowel Sounds, Absent or Diminished

Constipation r/t decreased or absent peristalsis

Deficient Fluid Volume r/t inability to ingest fluids, loss of fluids in bowel

Delayed Surgical Recovery r/t inability to obtain adequate nutritional status

Risk for Dysfunctional Gastrointestinal Motility (See **Gastrointestinal Motility, Dysfunctional, Risk for,** Section III)

Bowel Sounds, Hyperactive

Diarrhea r/t increased gastrointestinal motility

Bowel Training

Impaired Bowel Continence r/t loss of control of rectal sphincter

Readiness for Enhanced Knowledge: expresses an interest in learning

Bowel Training, Child

See Toilet Training

BPH (Benign Prostatic Hypertrophy)

Ineffective Health Maintenance Behaviors r/t deficient knowledge regarding self-care with prostatic hypertrophy

Insomnia r/t nocturia

Urinary Retention r/t obstruction of urethra

Risk for Urge Urinary Incontinence: Risk factors: detrusor muscle instability with impaired contractility, involuntary sphincter relaxation

Risk for Infection: Risk factors: urinary residual after voiding, bacterial invasion of bladder

Readiness for Enhanced Knowledge: expresses an interest in learning

See Prostatic Hypertrophy

Bradycardia

Decreased Cardiac Output r/t slow heart rate supplying inadequate amount of blood for body function

Risk for Ineffective Cerebral Tissue Perfusion: Risk factors: decreased cardiac output secondary to bradycardia, vagal response

Readiness for Enhanced Knowledge: expresses an interest in learning

Bradypnea

Ineffective Breathing Pattern r/t neuromuscular impairment, pain, musculoskeletal impairment, perception or cognitive impairment, anxiety, fatigue or decreased energy, effects of drugs

See Sleep Apnea (See **Airway Clearance, Ineffective,** Section III)

Brain Injury

Risk for Ineffective Thermoregulation: Risk factor: posttraumatic inflammation or infection

See Intracranial Pressure, Increased

Brain Surgery

See Craniectomy/Craniotomy

Brain Tumor

Acute Confusion r/t pressure from tumor

Fear r/t threat to well-being

Maladaptive Grieving r/t potential loss of physiological-psychosocial well-being

Acute Pain r/t pressure from tumor

Vision Loss r/t tumor growth compressing optic nerve and/or brain tissue

Risk for Injury: Risk factors: sensory-perceptual alterations, weakness

Risk for Ineffective Thermoregulation: Risk factor: changes in metabolic activity of the brain

See Cancer; Chemotherapy; Child with Chronic Condition; Craniectomy/Craniotomy; Hospitalized Child; Radiation Therapy; Terminally Ill Child, Adolescent; Terminally Ill Child, Infant/Toddler; Terminally Ill Child, Preschool Child; Terminally Ill Child, School-Age Child/Preadolescent; Terminally Ill Child/Death of Child, Parent

Braxton Hicks Contractions

Decreased Activity Tolerance r/t increased contractions with increased gestation

Anxiety r/t uncertainty about beginning labor

Fatigue r/t lack of sleep

Stress Urinary Incontinence r/t increased pressure on bladder with contractions

Insomnia r/t contractions when lying down

Ineffective Sexuality Pattern r/t fear of contractions associated with loss of infant

Breast Biopsy

Fear r/t potential for diagnosis of cancer

Risk for Spiritual Distress: Risk factor: fear of diagnosis of cancer

Readiness for Enhanced Knowledge: expresses an interest in learning

Breast Cancer

Death Anxiety r/t diagnosis of cancer

Ineffective Coping r/t treatment, prognosis

Fear r/t diagnosis of cancer

Sexual Dysfunction r/t loss of body part, partner's reaction to loss

Chronic Sorrow r/t diagnosis of cancer, loss of body integrity

Risk for Spiritual Distress: Risk factor: fear of diagnosis of cancer

Readiness for Enhanced Health Literacy: expresses desire to enhance understanding of health information to make health care choices

Readiness for Enhanced Knowledge: expresses an interest in learning

See Cancer; Chemotherapy; Mastectomy; Radiation Therapy

Breast Examination, Self

See SBE (Self-Breast Examination)

Breast Lumps

Fear r/t potential for diagnosis of cancer

Readiness for Enhanced Knowledge: expresses an interest in learning

Breast Pumping

Risk for Infection: Risk factors: possible contaminated breast pump, incomplete emptying of breast

Risk for Impaired Skin Integrity: Risk factor: high suction

Readiness for Enhanced Knowledge: expresses an interest in learning

Breastfeeding, Effective

Readiness for Enhanced Breastfeeding (See **Breastfeeding, Readiness for Enhanced,** Section III)

Breastfeeding, Ineffective

Ineffective Breastfeeding (See **Breastfeeding, Ineffective,** Section III)

See Ineffective Infant Suck-Swallow Response; Painful Breasts, Engorgement; Painful Breasts, Sore Nipples

Breastfeeding, Interrupted

Interrupted Breastfeeding (See **Breastfeeding, Interrupted,** Section III)

Breast Milk Production, Insufficient

Insufficient Breast Milk Production (See **Breast Milk Production, Insufficient,** Section III)

Breath Sounds, Decreased or Absent

See Atelectasis; Pneumothorax

Breathing Pattern Alteration

Ineffective Breathing Pattern r/t neuromuscular impairment, pain, musculoskeletal impairment, perception or cognitive impairment, anxiety, decreased energy or fatigue

Breech Birth

Fear: Maternal r/t danger to infant, self

Impaired Gas Exchange: Fetal r/t compressed umbilical cord

Risk for Aspiration: Fetal: Risk factor: birth of body before head

Risk for Impaired Tissue Integrity: Fetal: Risk factor: difficult birth

Risk for Impaired Tissue Integrity: Maternal: Risk factor: difficult birth

Bronchitis

Ineffective Airway Clearance r/t excessive thickened mucus secretion

Readiness for Enhanced Health Self-Management: wishes to stop smoking

Readiness for Enhanced Knowledge: expresses an interest in learning

Bronchopulmonary Dysplasia

Decreased Activity Tolerance r/t imbalance between oxygen supply and demand

Excess Fluid volume r/t sodium and water retention

Imbalanced Nutrition: Less than Body Requirements r/t poor feeding, increased caloric needs as a result of increased work of breathing

See Child with Chronic Condition; Hospitalized Child; Respiratory Conditions of the Neonate

Bronchoscopy

Risk for Aspiration: Risk factor: temporary loss of gag reflex

Risk for Injury: Risk factors: complication of pneumothorax, laryngeal edema, hemorrhage (if biopsy done)

B

Bruits, Carotid

Risk for Ineffective Cerebral Tissue Perfusion: Risk factors: interruption of carotid blood flow to brain

Bryant's Traction

See Traction and Casts

Buck's Traction

See Traction and Casts

Buerger's Disease

See Peripheral Vascular Disease (PVD)

Bulimia

Disturbed Body Image r/t misperception about actual appearance, body weight

Compromised Family Coping r/t chronically unresolved feelings of guilt, anger, hostility

Defensive Coping r/t eating disorder

Diarrhea r/t laxative abuse

Fear r/t food ingestion, weight gain

Imbalanced Nutrition: Less than Body Requirements r/t induced vomiting, excessive exercise, laxative abuse

Ineffective Adolescent Eating Dynamics r/t overeating, leading to purge

Powerlessness r/t urge to purge self after eating

Chronic Low Self-Esteem r/t lack of positive feedback

See Maturational Issues, Adolescent

Bullying

Anxiety r/t specific or nonspecific threat to self

Impaired Social Interaction r/t dysfunctional interactions with others

Fear r/t perceived threat to self

Risk for Compromised Human Dignity: Risk factors: dehumanizing treatment, humiliation

Risk for Other-Directed Violence: Risk factors: social isolation, unresolved interpersonal conflicts

Risk for Powerlessness: Risk factor: ineffective coping strategies

Risk for Impaired Resilience: Risk factor: insufficient familial and social support

Risk for Self-Directed violence: Risk factors: unresolved interpersonal conflicts, social isolation

Risk for Chronic Low Self-Esteem: Risk factors: ineffective coping strategies, absence of sense of belonging, inadequate respect from others

Bunion

Readiness for Enhanced Knowledge: expresses an interest in learning

Bunionectomy

Impaired physical Mobility r/t sore foot

Impaired Walking r/t pain associated with surgery

Risk for Surgical Site Infection: Risk factors: surgical incision

Readiness for Enhanced Knowledge: expresses an interest in learning

Burn Risk

Risk for Thermal Injury (See **Thermal Injury, Risk for,** Section III)

Burns

Anxiety r/t burn injury, treatments

Disturbed Body Image r/t altered physical appearance

Decreased Diversional Activity Engagement r/t long-term hospitalization

Fear r/t pain from treatments, possible permanent disfigurement

Deficient Fluid Volume r/t loss of protective skin

Maladaptive Grieving r/t loss of bodily function, loss of future hopes and plans

Hypothermia r/t impaired skin integrity

Impaired Physical Mobility r/t pain, musculoskeletal impairment, contracture formation

Imbalanced Nutrition: Less than Body Requirements r/t increased metabolic needs, anorexia, protein and fluid loss

Acute Pain r/t burn injury, treatments

Chronic Pain r/t burn injury, treatments

Ineffective Peripheral Tissue Perfusion r/t circumferential burns, impaired arterial/venous circulation

Post-Trauma Syndrome r/t life-threatening event

Impaired Skin Integrity r/t injury of skin

Delayed Surgical Recovery r/t ineffective tissue perfusion

Risk for Ineffective Airway Clearance: Risk factors: potential tracheobronchial obstruction, edema

Risk for Deficient Fluid Volume: Risk factors: loss from skin surface, fluid shift

Risk for Infection: Risk factors: loss of intact skin, trauma, invasive sites

Risk for Peripheral Neurovascular Dysfunction: Risk factor: eschar formation with circumferential burn

Risk for Post-Trauma Syndrome: Risk factors: perception, duration of event that caused burns

Risk for Ineffective Thermoregulation: Risk factor: disruption of skin integrity

Readiness for Enhanced Knowledge: expresses an interest in learning

See Hospitalized Child; Safety, Childhood

Bursitis

Impaired Physical Mobility r/t inflammation in joint

Acute Pain r/t inflammation in joint

Bypass Graft

See Coronary Artery Bypass Grafting (CABG)

C

CABG (Coronary Artery Bypass Grafting)

See Coronary Artery Bypass Grafting (CABG)

Cachexia

Frail Elderly Syndrome r/t fatigue, feeding self-care deficit

Imbalanced Nutrition: Less than Body Requirements r/t inability to ingest food because of physiological factors

Risk for Infection: Risk factor: inadequate nutrition

Calcium Alteration

See Hypercalcemia; Hypocalcemia

Cancer

Decreased Activity Tolerance r/t side effects of treatment, weakness from cancer

Death Anxiety r/t unresolved issues regarding dying

Disturbed Body Image r/t side effects of treatment, cachexia

Decisional Conflict r/t selection of treatment choices, continuation or discontinuation of treatment, "do not resuscitate" decision

Constipation r/t side effects of medication, altered nutrition, decreased activity

Compromised Family Coping r/t prolonged disease or disability progression that exhausts supportive ability of significant others

Ineffective Coping r/t personal vulnerability in situational crisis, terminal illness

Ineffective Denial r/t complicated grieving process

Fear r/t serious threat to well-being

Maladaptive Grieving r/t potential loss of significant others, high risk for infertility

Ineffective Health Maintenance Behaviors r/t deficient knowledge regarding prescribed treatment

Hopelessness r/t loss of control, terminal illness

Insomnia r/t anxiety, pain

Impaired Physical Mobility r/t weakness, neuromusculoskeletal impairment, pain

Imbalanced Nutrition: Less than Body Requirements r/t loss of appetite, difficulty swallowing, side effects of chemotherapy, obstruction by tumor

Impaired Oral Mucous Membrane Integrity r/t chemotherapy, effects of radiation, oral pH changes, decreased oral secretions

Chronic Pain r/t metastatic cancer

Powerlessness r/t treatment, progression of disease

Ineffective Protection r/t cancer suppressing immune system

Ineffective Role Performance r/t change in physical capacity, inability to resume prior role

Self-Care Deficit: Specify r/t pain, intolerance to activity, decreased strength

Impaired Skin Integrity r/t immunological deficit, immobility

Social Isolation r/t hospitalization, lifestyle changes

Chronic Sorrow r/t chronic illness of cancer

Spiritual Distress r/t test of spiritual beliefs

Risk for Bleeding: Risk factor: bone marrow depression from chemotherapy

Risk for Disuse Syndrome: Risk factors: immobility, fatigue

Risk for Ineffective Home Maintenance Behaviors: Risk factor: lack of familiarity with community resources

Risk for Infection: Risk factor: inadequate immune system

Risk for Impaired Resilience: Risk factors: multiple stressors, pain, chronic illness

Risk for Spiritual Distress: Risk factor: physical illness of cancer

Readiness for Enhanced Knowledge: expresses an interest in learning

Readiness for enhanced spiritual well-being: desire for harmony with self, others, higher power, God, when faced with serious illness

See Chemotherapy; Child with Chronic Condition; Hospitalized Child; Leukemia; Radiation Therapy; Terminally Ill Child, Adolescent; Terminally Ill Child, Infant/Toddler; Terminally Ill Child, Preschool Child; Terminally Ill Child, School-Age Child/Preadolescent; Terminally Ill Child/Death of Child, Parent

Candidiasis, Oral

Readiness for Enhanced Knowledge: expresses an interest in learning

Impaired Oral Mucous Membrane Integrity r/t overgrowth of infectious agent, depressed immune function

Acute Pain r/t oral condition

Capillary Refill Time, Prolonged

Impaired Gas Exchange r/t ventilation perfusion imbalance

Ineffective Peripheral Tissue Perfusion r/t interruption of arterial flow

See Shock, Hypovolemic

Carbon Monoxide Poisoning

See Smoke Inhalation

Cardiac Arrest

Post-Trauma Syndrome r/t experiencing serious life event

See Dysrhythmia; MI (Myocardial Infarction)

Cardiac Catheterization

Fear r/t invasive procedure, uncertainty of outcome of procedure

Risk for Injury: Hematoma: Risk factor: invasive procedure

Risk for Decreased Cardiac Tissue Perfusion: Risk factors: ventricular ischemia, dysrhythmia

Risk for Peripheral Neurovascular Dysfunction: Risk factor: vascular obstruction

Risk for Impaired Tissue Integrity: Risk factor: invasive procedure

Readiness for Enhanced Knowledge: expresses an interest in learning postprocedure care, treatment, and prevention of coronary artery disease

C

Cardiac Disorders in Pregnancy

Decreased Activity Tolerance r/t cardiac pathophysiology, increased demand for cardiac output because of pregnancy, weakness, fatigue

Death Anxiety r/t potential danger of condition

Compromised Family Coping r/t prolonged hospitalization or maternal incapacitation that exhausts supportive capacity of significant others

Ineffective Coping r/t personal vulnerability

Interrupted Family Processes r/t hospitalization, maternal incapacitation, changes in roles

Fatigue r/t physiological, psychological, and emotional demands

Fear r/t potential maternal effects, potential poor fetal or maternal outcome

Powerlessness r/t illness-related regimen

Ineffective Role Performance r/t changes in lifestyle, expectations from disease process with superimposed pregnancy

Situational Low Self-Esteem r/t situational crisis, pregnancy

Social Isolation r/t limitations of activity, bed rest or hospitalization, separation from family and friends

Risk for Decreased Cardiac Tissue Perfusion: Risk factor: strain on compromised heart from work of pregnancy, delivery

Risk for Imbalanced Fluid Volume: Risk factor: sudden changes in circulation after delivery of placenta, compromised regulatory mechanism with increased afterload, preload, circulating blood volume

Risk for Impaired Gas Exchange: Risk factor: pulmonary edema

Risk for Disturbed Maternal–Fetal Dyad: Risk factor: compromised oxygen transport

Risk for impaired Resilience: Risk factors: multiple stressors, fear

Risk for Spiritual Distress: Risk factor: fear of diagnosis for self and infant

Readiness for Enhanced Knowledge: expresses an interest in learning

Cardiac Dysrhythmia

See Dysrhythmia

Cardiac Output, Decreased

Decreased Cardiac Output r/t cardiac dysfunction

Decreased Cardiac Output (See **Cardiac Output, Decreased,** Section III)

Risk for Decreased Cardiac Output (See **Cardiac Output, Risk for Decreased,** Section III)

Cardiac Tamponade

Decreased Cardiac Output r/t fluid in pericardial sac

See Pericarditis

Cardiogenic Shock

See Shock, Cardiogenic

Caregiver Role Strain

Caregiver Role Strain (See **Caregiver Role Strain,** Section III)

Risk for Impaired Resilience: Risk factor: stress of prolonged caregiving

Carious Teeth

See Cavities in Teeth

Carotid Endarterectomy

Fear r/t surgery in vital area

Risk for Ineffective Airway Clearance: Risk factor: hematoma compressing trachea

Risk for Bleeding: Risk factor: possible hematoma formation, trauma to region

Risk for Ineffective Cerebral Tissue Perfusion: Risk factors: hemorrhage, clot formation

Readiness for Enhanced Knowledge: expresses an interest in learning

Carpal Tunnel Syndrome

Impaired Physical Mobility r/t neuromuscular impairment

Chronic Pain r/t unrelieved pressure on median nerve

Self-Care Deficit: Bathing, Dressing, Feeding r/t pain

Carpopedal Spasm

See Hypocalcemia

Casts

Decreased Diversional Activity Engagement r/t physical limitations from cast

Impaired Physical Mobility r/t limb immobilization

Self-Care Deficit: Bathing, Dressing, Feeding r/t presence of cast(s) on upper extremities

Self-Care Deficit: Toileting r/t presence of cast(s) on lower extremities

Impaired Walking r/t cast(s) on lower extremities, fracture of bones

Risk for Peripheral Neurovascular Dysfunction: Risk factors: mechanical compression from cast, trauma from fracture

Risk for Impaired Skin Integrity: Risk factor: unrelieved pressure on skin from cast

Readiness for Enhanced Knowledge: expresses an interest in learning

See Traction and Casts

Cataract Extraction

Anxiety r/t threat of permanent vision loss, surgical procedure

Vision Loss r/t edema from surgery (see Appendix E on Evolve)

Risk for Injury: Risk factors: increased intraocular pressure, accommodation to new visual field

Readiness for Enhanced Knowledge: expresses an interest in learning

Catatonic Schizophrenia

Impaired Verbal Communication r/t cognitive impairment

Impaired Memory r/t cognitive impairment

Impaired Physical Mobility r/t cognitive impairment, maintenance of rigid posture, inappropriate or bizarre postures

Imbalanced Nutrition: Less than Body Requirements r/t decrease in outside stimulation, loss of perception of hunger, resistance to instructions to eat

Social Isolation r/t inability to communicate, immobility

See Schizophrenia

Catheterization, Urinary

Risk for Infection: Risk factor: invasive procedure

Readiness for Enhanced Knowledge: expresses an interest in learning

Cavities in Teeth

Impaired Dentition r/t ineffective oral hygiene, barriers to self-care, economic barriers to professional care, nutritional deficits, dietary habits

Celiac Disease

Diarrhea r/t malabsorption of food, immune effects of gluten on gastrointestinal system

Imbalanced Nutrition: Less than Body Requirements r/t malabsorption caused by immune effects of gluten

Readiness for Enhanced Knowledge: expresses an interest in learning

Cellulitis

Acute Pain r/t inflammatory changes in tissues from infection

Impaired Tissue Integrity r/t inflammatory process damaging skin and underlying tissue

Ineffective Peripheral Tissue Perfusion r/t edema of extremities

Risk for Vascular Trauma: Risk factor: infusion of antibiotics

Readiness for Enhanced Knowledge: expresses an interest in learning

Cellulitis, Periorbital

Acute Pain r/t edema and inflammation of skin/tissues

Impaired Skin Integrity r/t inflammation or infection of skin, tissues

Vision Loss r/t decreased visual field secondary to edema of eyelids (see Appendix E on Evolve)

Readiness for Enhanced Knowledge: expresses an interest in learning

See Hospitalized Child

Central Line Insertion

Risk for Infection: Risk factor: invasive procedure

Risk for Vascular Trauma (See **Vascular Trauma, Risk for,** Section III)

Readiness for Enhanced Knowledge: expresses an interest in learning

Cerebral Aneurysm

See Craniectomy/Craniotomy; Intracranial Pressure, Increased; Subarachnoid Hemorrhage

Cerebral Palsy

Impaired Verbal Communication r/t impaired ability to articulate or speak words because of facial muscle involvement

Decreased Diversional Activity Engagement r/t physical impairments, limitations on ability to participate in recreational activities

Impaired Physical Mobility r/t spasticity, neuromuscular impairment or weakness

Imbalanced Nutrition: Less than Body Requirements r/t spasticity, feeding or swallowing difficulties

Self-Care Deficit: Specify r/t neuromuscular impairments, sensory deficits

Impaired Social Interaction r/t impaired communication skills, limited physical activity, perceived differences from peers

Chronic Sorrow r/t presence of chronic disability

Risk for Adult Falls: Risk factor: impaired physical mobility

Risk for Child Falls: Risk factor: impaired physical mobility

Risk for Injury: Risk factors: muscle weakness, inability to control spasticity

Risk for Impaired Parenting: Risk factor: caring for child with overwhelming needs resulting from chronic change in health status

Risk for Spiritual Distress: Risk factor: psychological stress associated with chronic illness

See Child with Chronic Condition

Cerebral Perfusion

Risk for Ineffective Cerebral Tissue Perfusion (See **Cerebral Tissue Perfusion, Ineffective, Risk for,** Section III)

Cerebrovascular Accident (CVA)

See CVA (Cerebrovascular Accident)

Cervicitis

Ineffective Health Maintenance Behaviors r/t deficient knowledge regarding care and prevention of condition

Ineffective Sexuality Pattern r/t abstinence during acute stage

Risk for Infection: Risk factors: spread of infection, recurrence of infection

Cesarean Delivery

Disturbed Body Image r/t surgery, unmet expectations for childbirth

Interrupted Family Processes r/t unmet expectations for childbirth

Fear r/t perceived threat to own well-being, outcome of birth

Impaired Physical Mobility r/t pain

Acute Pain r/t surgical incision

Ineffective Role Performance r/t unmet expectations for childbirth

Situational Low Self-Esteem r/t inability to deliver child vaginally

Risk for Bleeding: Risk factor: surgery

Risk for Imbalanced Fluid Volume: Risk factors: loss of blood, fluid shifts

Risk for Surgical Site Infection: Risk factor: surgical incision

Risk for Urinary Retention: Risk factor: regional anesthesia

Readiness for Enhanced Childbearing Process: a pattern of preparing for, maintaining, and strengthening care of newborn

Readiness for Enhanced Knowledge: expresses an interest in learning

Chemical Dependence

See Alcoholism; Substance Abuse

Chemotherapy

Death Anxiety r/t chemotherapy not accomplishing desired results

Disturbed Body Image r/t loss of weight, loss of hair

Fatigue r/t disease process, anemia, drug effects

Nausea r/t effects of chemotherapy

Imbalanced Nutrition: Less than Body Requirements r/t side effects of chemotherapy

Impaired Oral Mucous Membrane Integrity r/t effects of chemotherapy

Ineffective Protection r/t suppressed immune system, decreased platelets

Risk for Bleeding: Risk factors: tumor eroding blood vessel, stress effects on gastrointestinal system

Risk for Infection: Risk factor: immunosuppression

Risk for Vascular Trauma: Risk factor: infusion of irritating medications

Readiness for Enhanced Knowledge: expresses an interest in learning

See Cancer

Chest Pain

Fear r/t potential threat of death

Acute Pain r/t myocardial injury, ischemia

Risk for Decreased Cardiac Tissue Perfusion: Risk factor: ventricular ischemia

See Angina; MI (Myocardial Infarction)

Chest Tubes

Ineffective Breathing Pattern r/t asymmetrical lung expansion secondary to pain

Impaired Gas Exchange r/t decreased functional lung tissue

Acute Pain r/t presence of chest tubes, injury

Risk for Injury: Risk factor: presence of invasive chest tube

Cheyne-Stokes Respiration

Ineffective Breathing pattern r/t critical illness

Chickenpox

See Communicable Diseases, Childhood

Child Abuse

Interrupted Family Processes r/t inadequate coping skills

Fear r/t threat of punishment for perceived wrongdoing

Insomnia r/t hypervigilance, fear

Imbalanced Nutrition: Less than Body Requirements r/t inadequate caretaking

Acute Pain r/t physical injuries

Impaired Parenting r/t psychological impairment, physical or emotional abuse of parent, substance abuse, unrealistic expectations of child

Ineffective Child Eating Dynamics r/t hostile parental relationship

Post-Trauma Syndrome r/t physical abuse, incest, rape, molestation

Chronic Low Self-Esteem r/t lack of positive feedback, excessive negative feedback

Impaired Skin Integrity r/t altered nutritional state, physical abuse

Social Isolation: Family Imposed r/t fear of disclosure of family dysfunction and abuse

Risk for Poisoning: Risk factors: inadequate safeguards, lack of proper safety precautions, accessibility of illicit substances because of impaired home maintenance

Risk for Suffocation: Risk factors: unattended child, unsafe environment

Risk for Physical Trauma: Risk factors: inadequate precautions, cognitive or emotional difficulties

Childbearing Problems

Ineffective Childbearing Process (See **Childbearing Process, Ineffective,** Section III)

Risk for Ineffective Childbearing Process (See **Childbearing Process, Risk for Ineffective,** Section III)

Child Neglect

See Child Abuse; Failure to Thrive

Child with Chronic Condition

Decreased Activity Tolerance r/t fatigue associated with chronic illness

Compromised Family Coping r/t prolonged overconcern for child; distortion of reality regarding child's health problem, including extreme denial about its existence or severity

Disabled Family Coping r/t prolonged disease or disability progression that exhausts supportive capacity of significant others

Ineffective Coping: Child r/t situational or maturational crises

Decisional Conflict r/t treatment options, conflicting values

Decreased Diversional Activity Engagement r/t immobility, monotonous environment, frequent or lengthy treatments, reluctance to participate, self-imposed social isolation

Interrupted Family Processes r/t intermittent situational crisis of illness, disease, hospitalization

Ineffective Health Maintenance Behaviors r/t exhausting family resources (finances, physical energy, support systems)

Ineffective Home Maintenance Behaviors r/t overtaxed family members (e.g., exhausted, anxious)

Hopelessness: Child r/t prolonged activity restriction, long-term stress, lack of involvement in or passively allowing care as a result of parental overprotection

Insomnia: Child or Parent r/t time-intensive treatments, exacerbation of condition, 24-hour care needs

Deficient Knowledge r/t knowledge or skill acquisition regarding health practices, acceptance of limitations, promotion of maximal potential of child, self-actualization of rest of family

Imbalanced Nutrition: Less than Body Requirements r/t anorexia, fatigue from physical exertion

Risk for Overweight r/t effects of steroid medications on appetite

Chronic Pain r/t physical, biological, chemical, or psychological factors

Powerlessness: Child r/t health care environment, illness-related regimen, lifestyle of learned helplessness

Parental Role Conflict r/t separation from child as a result of chronic illness, home care of child with special needs, interruptions of family life resulting from home care regimen

Chronic Low Self-Esteem r/t actual or perceived differences; peer acceptance; decreased ability to participate in physical, school, and social activities

Ineffective Sexuality Pattern: Parental r/t disrupted relationship with sexual partner

Impaired Social Interaction r/t developmental lag or delay, perceived differences

Social Isolation: Family r/t actual or perceived social stigmatization, complex care requirements

Chronic Sorrow r/t developmental stages and missed opportunities or milestones that bring comparisons with social or personal norms, unending caregiving as reminder of loss

Risk for Delayed Child Development: Risk factor: chronic illness

Risk for Infection: Risk factor: debilitating physical condition

Risk for Impaired Parenting: Risk factors: impaired or disrupted bonding, caring for child with perceived overwhelming care needs

Readiness for Enhanced Family Coping: impact of crisis on family values, priorities, goals, or relationships; changes in family choices to optimize wellness

Childbirth

Readiness for Enhanced Childbearing Process (See **Childbearing Process, Readiness for Enhanced,** Section III)

See Labor, Normal; Postpartum, Normal Care

Childhood Obesity

Obesity r/t disordered eating behaviors

Risk for Unstable Blood Glucose Level: Risk factor: excessive weight gain

Risk for Metabolic Syndrome: Risk factors: obesity, sedentary lifestyle

Readiness for Enhanced Exercise Engagement: expresses desire to engage in regular exercise

Readiness for Enhanced Knowledge: expresses desire to make healthier nutrition choices

Chills

Hyperthermia r/t infectious process

Chlamydia Infection

See STD (Sexually Transmitted Disease)

Chloasma

Disturbed Body Image r/t change in skin color

Choking or Coughing with Eating

Impaired Swallowing r/t neuromuscular impairment

Risk for Aspiration: Risk factors: depressed cough and gag reflexes

Cholecystectomy

Imbalanced Nutrition: Less than Body Requirements r/t high metabolic needs, decreased ability to digest fatty foods

Acute Pain r/t trauma from surgery

Risk for Deficient Fluid Volume: Risk factors: restricted intake, nausea, vomiting

Risk for Surgical Site Infection: Risk factor: invasive procedure

Readiness for Enhanced Knowledge: expresses an interest in learning

See Abdominal Surgery

Cholelithiasis

Nausea r/t obstruction of bile

Imbalanced Nutrition: Less than Body Requirements r/t anorexia, nausea, vomiting

Acute Pain r/t obstruction of bile flow, inflammation in gallbladder

Readiness for Enhanced Knowledge: expresses an interest in learning

Chorioamnionitis

Anxiety r/t threat to self and infant

Maladaptive Grieving r/t guilt about potential loss of ideal pregnancy and birth

Hyperthermia r/t infectious process

Situational Low Self-Esteem r/t guilt about threat to infant's health

Risk for Infection: Risk factors: infection transmission from mother to fetus; infection in fetal environment

Chronic Confusion

See Confusion, Chronic

Chronic Functional Constipation

(See **Constipation, Chronic Functional,** Section III)

(See **Constipation, Chronic Functional, Risk for,** Section III)

Chronic Lymphocytic Leukemia

See Cancer; Chemotherapy; Leukemia

C

Chronic Obstructive Pulmonary Disease (COPD)

See COPD (Chronic Obstructive Pulmonary Disease)

Chronic Pain

See Pain Management, Chronic

Chronic Renal Failure (Chronic Renal Disease)

See Renal Failure

Chvostek's Sign

See Hypocalcemia

Circumcision

Acute Pain r/t surgical intervention

Risk for Bleeding: Risk factor: surgical trauma

Risk for Infection: Risk factor: surgical wound

Readiness for Enhanced Knowledge: Parent: expresses an interest in learning

Cirrhosis

Chronic Confusion r/t chronic organic disorder with increased ammonia levels, substance abuse

Defensive Coping r/t inability to accept responsibility to stop substance abuse

Fatigue r/t malnutrition

Ineffective Health Maintenance Behaviors r/t deficient knowledge regarding correlation between lifestyle habits and disease process

Nausea r/t irritation to gastrointestinal system

Imbalanced Nutrition: Less than Body Requirements r/t loss of appetite, nausea, vomiting

Chronic Pain r/t liver enlargement

Chronic Low Self-Esteem r/t chronic illness

Chronic Sorrow r/t presence of chronic illness

Risk for Bleeding: Risk factors: impaired blood coagulation, bleeding from portal hypertension

Risk for Injury: Risk factors: substance intoxication, potential delirium tremens

Risk for Impaired Oral Mucous Membrane Integrity: Risk factors: altered nutrition, inadequate oral care

Risk for Impaired Skin Integrity: Risk factors: altered nutritional state, altered metabolic state

Cleft Lip/Cleft Palate

Ineffective Airway Clearance r/t common feeding and breathing passage, postoperative laryngeal, incisional edema

Ineffective Breastfeeding r/t infant anomaly

Impaired Verbal Communication r/t inadequate palate function, possible hearing loss from infected eustachian tubes

Fear: Parental r/t special care needs, surgery

Maladaptive Grieving r/t loss of perfect child

Ineffective Infant Feeding Dynamics r/t fear resulting in inadequate feeding

Ineffective Infant Suck-Swallow Response r/t cleft lip, cleft palate

Impaired Physical Mobility r/t imposed restricted activity, use of elbow restraints

Impaired Oral Mucous Membrane Integrity r/t surgical correction

Acute Pain r/t surgical correction, elbow restraints

Impaired Skin Integrity r/t incomplete joining of lip, palate ridges

Chronic Sorrow r/t birth of child with congenital defect

Risk for Aspiration: Risk factor: common feeding and breathing passage

Risk for Disturbed Body Image: Risk factors: disfigurement, speech impediment

Risk for Deficient Fluid Volume: Risk factor: inability to take liquids in usual manner

Risk for Infection: Risk factors: invasive procedure, disruption of eustachian tube development, aspiration

Readiness for Enhanced Knowledge: Parent: expresses an interest in learning

Clotting Disorder

Fear r/t threat to well-being

Risk for Bleeding: Risk factor: impaired clotting

Readiness for Enhanced Knowledge: expresses an interest in learning

See Anticoagulant Therapy; DIC (Disseminated Intravascular Coagulation); Hemophilia

Cocaine Baby

See Neonatal Abstinence Syndrome

Codependency

Caregiver Role Strain r/t codependency

Impaired Verbal Communication r/t psychological barriers

Ineffective Coping r/t inadequate support systems

Decisional Conflict r/t support system deficit

Ineffective Denial r/t unmet self-needs

Powerlessness r/t lifestyle of helplessness

Cold, Viral

See Infectious Processes

Colectomy

Constipation r/t decreased activity, decreased fluid intake

Imbalanced Nutrition: Less than Body Requirements r/t high metabolic needs, decreased ability to ingest or digest food

Acute Pain r/t recent surgery

Risk for Surgical Site Infection: Risk factor: invasive procedure

Readiness for Enhanced Knowledge: expresses an interest in learning

See Abdominal Surgery

Colitis

Diarrhea r/t inflammation in colon

Deficient Fluid Volume r/t frequent stools

Acute Pain r/t inflammation in colon

Readiness for Enhanced Knowledge: expresses an interest in learning

See Crohn's Disease; Inflammatory Bowel Disease (Child and Adult)

Collagen Disease

See specific disease (e.g., Lupus Erythematosus; JRA [Juvenile Rheumatoid Arthritis]); Congenital Heart Disease/Cardiac Anomalies

Colostomy

Disturbed Body Image r/t presence of stoma, daily care of fecal material

Ineffective Sexuality Pattern r/t altered body image, self-concept

Social Isolation r/t anxiety about appearance of stoma and possible leakage of stool

Risk for Constipation: Risk factor: inappropriate diet

Risk for Diarrhea: Risk factor: inappropriate diet

Risk for Impaired Skin Integrity: Risk factor: irritation from bowel contents

Readiness for Enhanced Knowledge: expresses an interest in learning

Colporrhaphy, Anterior

See Vaginal Hysterectomy

Coma

Death Anxiety: Significant Others r/t unknown outcome of coma state

Interrupted Family Processes r/t illness or disability of family member

Disability-Associated Urinary Incontinence r/t presence of comatose state

Self-Care Deficit r/t neuromuscular impairment

Ineffective Family Health Self-Management r/t complexity of therapeutic regimen

Risk for Aspiration: Risk factors: impaired swallowing, loss of cough or gag reflex

Risk for Disuse Syndrome: Risk factor: altered level of consciousness impairing mobility

Risk for Dry Mouth: Risk factor: inability to perform own oral care

Risk for Hypothermia: Risk factors: inactivity, possible pharmaceutical agents, possible hypothalamic injury

Risk for Injury: Risk factor: potential seizure activity

Risk for Corneal Injury: Risk factor: suppressed corneal reflex

Risk for Urinary Tract Injury: Risk factor: long-term use of urinary catheter

Risk for Impaired Oral Mucous Membrane Integrity: Risk factors: dry mouth, inability to do own mouth care

Risk for Pressure Ulcer: Risk factor: prolonged immobility

Risk for Impaired Skin Integrity: Risk factor: immobility

Risk for Spiritual Distress: Significant Others: Risk factors: loss of ability to relate to loved one, unknown outcome of coma

Risk for Impaired Tissue Integrity: Risk factor: impaired physical mobility

See Head Injury; Subarachnoid Hemorrhage; Intracranial Pressure, Increased

Comfort, Loss of

Impaired Comfort (See **Comfort, Impaired,** Section III)

Readiness for Enhanced Comfort (See **Comfort, Readiness for Enhanced,** Section III)

Communicable Diseases, Childhood (e.g., Measles, Mumps, Rubella, Chickenpox, Scabies, Lice, Impetigo)

Impaired Comfort r/t pruritus, inflammation or infection of skin, subdermal organisms

Decreased Diversional Activity Engagement r/t imposed isolation from peers, disruption in usual play activities, fatigue, activity intolerance

Ineffective Health Maintenance Behaviors r/t nonadherence to appropriate immunization schedules, lack of prevention of transmission of infection

Acute Pain r/t impaired skin integrity, edema

Risk for Infection: Transmission to Others: Risk factor: contagious organisms

See Meningitis/Encephalitis; Respiratory Infections, Acute Childhood

Communication

Readiness for Enhanced Communication (See **Communication, Readiness for Enhanced,** Section III)

Communication Problems

Impaired Verbal Communication (See **Communication, Verbal, Impaired,** Section III)

Community Coping

Ineffective Community Coping (See **Coping, Community, Ineffective,** Section III)

Readiness for Enhanced Community Coping: community sense of power to manage stressors, social supports available, resources available for problem solving

Community Health Problems

Deficient community Health (See **Health, Deficient, Community,** Section III)

Companion Animal

Anxiety r/t environmental and personal stressors

Impaired Comfort r/t insufficient environmental control

Compartment Syndrome

Fear r/t possible loss of limb, damage to limb

Acute Pain r/t pressure in compromised body part

Ineffective Peripheral Tissue Perfusion r/t increased pressure within compartment

Compulsion

See OCD (Obsessive-Compulsive Disorder)

Conduction Disorders (Cardiac)

See Dysrhythmia

C

Confusion, Acute

Acute Confusion r/t older than 70 years of age with hospitalization, alcohol abuse, delirium, dementia, substance abuse

Frail Elderly Syndrome r/t impaired memory

Risk for Acute Confusion: Risk factor: alteration in level of consciousness

Confusion, Chronic

Chronic Confusion r/t dementia, Korsakoff's psychosis, multi-infarct dementia, cerebrovascular accident, head injury

Frail Elderly Syndrome r/t impaired memory

Impaired Memory r/t fluid and electrolyte imbalance, neurological disturbances, excessive environmental disturbances, anemia, acute or chronic hypoxia, decreased cardiac output

Impaired Mood Regulation r/t emotional instability

See Alzheimer's Disease; Dementia

Congenital Heart Disease/Cardiac Anomalies

Decreased Activity Tolerance r/t fatigue, generalized weakness, lack of adequate oxygenation

Ineffective Breathing Pattern r/t pulmonary vascular disease

Decreased Cardiac Output r/t cardiac dysfunction

Excess Fluid Volume r/t cardiac dysfunction, side effects of medication

Impaired Gas Exchange r/t cardiac dysfunction, pulmonary congestion

Imbalanced Nutrition: Less than Body Requirements r/t fatigue, generalized weakness, inability of infant to suck and feed, increased caloric requirements

Risk for Deficient Fluid Volume: Risk factor: side effects of diuretics

Risk for Disorganized Infant Behavior: Risk factor: invasive procedures

Risk for Poisoning: Risk factor: potential toxicity of cardiac medications

Risk for Ineffective Thermoregulation: Risk factor: neonatal age

See Child with Chronic Condition; Hospitalized Child

Congestive Heart Failure (CHF)

See Heart Failure

Conjunctivitis

Acute Pain r/t inflammatory process

Vision Loss r/t change in visual acuity resulting from inflammation

Consciousness, Altered Level of

Acute Confusion r/t alcohol abuse, delirium, dementia, drug abuse, head injury

Chronic Confusion r/t multi-infarct dementia, Korsakoff's psychosis, head injury, cerebrovascular accident, neurological deficit

Disability-Associated Urinary Incontinence r/t neurological dysfunction

Impaired Memory r/t neurological disturbances

Self-Care Deficit: Specify r/t neuromuscular impairment

Risk for Aspiration: Risk factors: impaired swallowing, loss of cough or gag reflex

Risk for Disuse Syndrome: Risk factor: impaired mobility resulting from altered level of consciousness

Risk for Dry Mouth: Risk factor: inability to perform own oral care

Risk for Falls: Risk factor: diminished mental status

Risk for Impaired Oral Mucous Membrane Integrity: Risk factors: dry mouth, interrupted oral care

Risk for Ineffective Cerebral Tissue Perfusion: Risk factors: increased intracranial pressure, altered cerebral perfusion

Risk for Impaired Skin Integrity: Risk factor: immobility

See Coma; Head Injury; Subarachnoid Hemorrhage; Intracranial Pressure, Increased

Constipation

Constipation (See **Constipation,** Section III)

Constipation, Chronic Functional

Constipation (See **Constipation, Chronic Functional,** Section III)

Constipation, Perceived

Perceived Constipation (See **Perceived Constipation,** Section III)

Constipation, Risk for

Risk for Constipation (See **Constipation, Risk for,** Section III)

Risk for chronic functional Constipation (See **Constipation, Chronic Functional, Risk for,** Section III)

Contamination

Contamination (See **Contamination,** Section III)

Risk for Contamination (See **Contamination, Risk for,** Section III)

Continent Ileostomy (Kock Pouch)

Ineffective Coping r/t stress of disease, exacerbations caused by stress

Imbalanced Nutrition: Less than Body Requirements r/t malabsorption from disease process

Risk for Injury: Risk factors: failure of valve, stomal cyanosis, intestinal obstruction

Readiness for Enhanced Knowledge: expresses an interest in learning

See Abdominal Surgery; Crohn's Disease

Contraceptive Method

Decisional Conflict: Method of Contraception r/t unclear personal values or beliefs, lack of experience or interference with decision-making, lack of relevant information, support system deficit

Ineffective Sexuality Pattern r/t fear of pregnancy

Readiness for Enhanced Health Self-Management: requesting information about available and appropriate birth control methods

Convulsions

Anxiety r/t concern over controlling convulsions

Impaired Memory r/t neurological disturbance

Risk for Aspiration: Risk factor: impaired swallowing

Risk for Injury: Risk factor: seizure activity

Readiness for Enhanced Knowledge: expresses an interest in learning

See Seizure Disorders, Adult; Seizure Disorders, Childhood

COPD (Chronic Obstructive Pulmonary Disease)

Decreased Activity Tolerance r/t imbalance between oxygen supply and demand

Ineffective Airway Clearance r/t bronchoconstriction, increased mucus, ineffective cough, infection

Anxiety r/t breathlessness, change in health status

Death Anxiety r/t seriousness of medical condition, difficulty being able to "catch breath," feeling of suffocation

Interrupted Family Processes r/t role changes

Impaired Gas Exchange r/t ventilation-perfusion inequality

Ineffective Health Self-Management (See **Health Management, Ineffective,** Section III)

Imbalanced Nutrition: Less than Body Requirements r/t decreased intake because of dyspnea, unpleasant taste in mouth left by medications, increased need for calories from work of breathing

Powerlessness r/t progressive nature of disease

Self-Care Deficit r/t fatigue from the increased work of breathing

Chronic Low Self-Esteem r/t chronic illness

Sleep Deprivation r/t breathing difficulties when lying down

Impaired Social Interaction r/t social isolation because of oxygen use, activity intolerance

Chronic Sorrow r/t presence of chronic illness

Risk for Infection: Risk factor: stasis of respiratory secretions

Readiness for Enhanced Health Self-Management (See **Health Management, Readiness for Enhanced,** Section III)

Coping

Readiness for Enhanced Coping (See **Coping, Readiness for Enhanced,** Section III)

Risk for Complicated Immigration Transition: Risk factors: insufficient knowledge about the process to access resources in the host country, insufficient social support in the host country, overt discrimination

Coping Problems

Compromised Family Coping (See **Coping, Compromised Family,** Section III)

Defensive Coping (See **Coping, Defensive,** Section III)

Disabled Family Coping (See **Coping, Disabled Family,** Section III)

Ineffective Coping (See **Coping, Ineffective,** Section III)

Ineffective Community Coping (See **Coping, Ineffective Community,** Section III)

Corneal Injury

Risk for Corneal Injury (See **Corneal Injury, Risk for,** Section III)

Corneal Reflex, Absent

Risk for Injury: Risk factors: accidental corneal abrasion, drying of cornea

Corneal Transplant

Risk for Surgical Site Infection: Risk factors: invasive procedure, surgery

Readiness for Enhanced Health Self-Management: describes need to rest and avoid strenuous activities during healing phase

Coronary Artery Bypass Grafting (CABG)

Decreased Cardiac Output r/t dysrhythmia, depressed cardiac function, change in preload, contractility or afterload

Fear r/t outcome of surgical procedure

Deficient Fluid Volume r/t intraoperative blood loss, use of diuretics in surgery

Acute Pain r/t traumatic surgery

Risk for Perioperative Positioning Injury: Risk factors: hypothermia, extended supine position

Risk for Surgical Site Infection: Risk factor: surgical incision

Risk for Impaired Tissue Integrity: Risk factor: surgical procedure

Readiness for Enhanced Knowledge: expresses an interest in learning

Costovertebral Angle Tenderness

See Kidney Stone; Pyelonephritis

Cough, Ineffective

Ineffective Airway Clearance r/t decreased energy, fatigue, normal aging changes

See Bronchitis; COPD (Chronic Obstructive Pulmonary Disease); Pulmonary Edema

Crackles in Lungs, Coarse

Ineffective Airway Clearance r/t excessive secretions in airways, ineffective cough

See Heart Failure; Pneumonia; Pulmonary Edema

Crackles in Lungs, Fine

Ineffective Breathing Pattern r/t fatigue, surgery, decreased energy

See Bronchitis or Pneumonia (if from pulmonary infection); Congestive Heart Failure (CHF) (if cardiac in origin); Infection, Potential for

Craniectomy/Craniotomy

Frail Elderly Syndrome r/t alteration in cognition

C

Fear r/t threat to well-being

Impaired Memory r/t neurological surgery

Acute Pain r/t recent brain surgery, increased intracranial pressure

Risk for Ineffective Cerebral Tissue Perfusion: Risk factors: cerebral edema, increased intracranial pressure

Risk for Injury: Risk factor: potential confusion

See Coma (if relevant)

Crepitation, Subcutaneous

See Pneumothorax

Crisis

Anxiety r/t threat to or change in environment, health status, interaction patterns, situation, self-concept, or role functioning; threat of death of self or significant other

Death Anxiety r/t feelings of hopelessness associated with crisis

Compromised Family Coping r/t situational or developmental crisis

Ineffective Coping r/t situational or maturational crisis

Fear r/t crisis situation

Maladaptive Grieving r/t potential significant loss

Impaired Resilience r/t onset of crisis

Situational Low Self-Esteem r/t perception of inability to handle crisis

Stress Overload (See **Stress Overload,** Section III)

Risk for Spiritual Distress: Risk factors: physical or psychological stress, natural disasters, situational losses, maturational losses

Crohn's Disease

Anxiety r/t change in health status

Ineffective Coping r/t repeated episodes of diarrhea

Diarrhea r/t inflammatory process

Ineffective Health Maintenance Behaviors r/t deficient knowledge regarding management of disease

Imbalanced Nutrition: Less than Body Requirements r/t diarrhea, altered ability to digest and absorb food

Acute Pain r/t increased peristalsis

Powerlessness r/t chronic disease

Risk for Deficient Fluid Volume: Risk factor: abnormal fluid loss with diarrhea

Croup

See Respiratory Infections, Acute Childhood (Croup, Epiglottitis, Pertussis, Pneumonia, Respiratory)

Cryosurgery for Retinal Detachment

See Retinal Detachment

Cushing's Syndrome

Decreased Activity Tolerance r/t fatigue, weakness

Disturbed Body Image r/t change in appearance from disease process

Excess Fluid Volume r/t failure of regulatory mechanisms

Sexual Dysfunction r/t loss of libido

Impaired Skin Integrity r/t thin vulnerable skin from effects of increased cortisol

Risk for Infection: Risk factor: suppression of immune system caused by increased cortisol levels

Risk for Injury: Risk factors: decreased muscle strength, brittle bones

Readiness for Enhanced Knowledge: expresses an interest in learning

Cuts (Wounds)

See Lacerations

CVA (Cerebrovascular Accident)

Anxiety r/t situational crisis, change in physical or emotional condition

Disturbed Body Image r/t chronic illness, paralysis

Caregiver Role Strain r/t cognitive problems of care receiver, need for significant home care

Impaired Verbal Communication r/t pressure damage, decreased circulation to brain in speech center informational sources

Chronic Confusion r/t neurological changes

Constipation r/t decreased activity

Ineffective Coping r/t disability

Interrupted Family Processes r/t illness, disability of family member

Frail Elderly Syndrome r/t alteration in cognitive functioning

Maladaptive Grieving r/t loss of health

Ineffective Home Maintenance Behaviors r/t neurological disease affecting ability to perform activities of daily living

Disability-Associated Urinary Incontinence r/t neurological dysfunction

Impaired Memory r/t neurological disturbances

Impaired Physical Mobility r/t loss of balance and coordination

Unilateral Neglect r/t disturbed perception from neurological damage

Self-Care Deficit: Specify r/t decreased strength and endurance, paralysis

Impaired Social interaction r/t limited physical mobility, limited ability to communicate

Impaired Swallowing r/t neuromuscular dysfunction

Impaired Transfer Ability r/t limited physical mobility

Vision Loss r/t pressure damage to visual centers in the brain (*see Appendix E on Evolve*)

Impaired Walking r/t loss of balance and coordination

Risk for Aspiration: Risk factors: impaired swallowing, loss of gag reflex

Risk for Chronic Functional Constipation: Risk factor: immobility

Risk for Disuse Syndrome: Risk factor: paralysis

Risk for Adult Falls: Risk factor: paralysis, decreased balance

Risk for Injury: Risk factors: vision loss, decreased tissue perfusion with loss of sensation

Risk for Ineffective Cerebral Tissue Perfusion: Risk factor: clot, emboli, or hemorrhage from cerebral vessel

Risk for Impaired Skin Integrity: Risk factor: immobility

Readiness for Enhanced Knowledge: expresses an interest in learning

Cyanosis, Central with Cyanosis of Oral Mucous Membranes

Impaired Gas Exchange r/t alveolar-capillary membrane changes

Cyanosis, Peripheral with Cyanosis of Nail Beds

Ineffective Peripheral Tissue Perfusion r/t interruption of arterial flow, severe vasoconstriction, cold temperatures

Cystic Fibrosis

Decreased Activity Tolerance r/t imbalance between oxygen supply and demand

Ineffective Airway Clearance r/t increased production of thick mucus

Anxiety r/t dyspnea, oxygen deprivation

Disturbed Body Image r/t changes in physical appearance, treatment of chronic lung disease (clubbing, barrel chest, home oxygen therapy)

Impaired Gas Exchange r/t ventilation-perfusion imbalance

Ineffective Home Maintenance Behaviors r/t extensive daily treatment, medications necessary for health

Imbalanced Nutrition: Less than Body Requirements r/t anorexia; decreased absorption of nutrients, fat; increased work of breathing

Chronic Sorrow r/t presence of chronic disease

Risk for Caregiver Role Strain: Risk factors: illness severity of care receiver, unpredictable course of illness

Risk for Deficient Fluid Volume: Risk factors: decreased fluid intake, increased work of breathing

Risk for Infection: Risk factors: thick, tenacious mucus; harboring of bacterial organisms; immunocompromised state

Risk for Spiritual Distress: Risk factor: presence of chronic disease

See Child with Chronic Condition; Hospitalized Child; Terminally Ill Child, Adolescent; Terminally Ill Child, Infant/Toddler; Terminally Ill Child, Preschool Child; Terminally Ill Child, School-Age Child/Preadolescent; Terminally Ill Child/Death of Child, Parent

Cystitis

Acute Pain: Dysuria r/t inflammatory process in bladder and urethra

Impaired Urinary Elimination: Frequency r/t urinary tract infection

Urge Urinary Incontinence: Risk factor: infection in bladder

Readiness for Enhanced Knowledge: expresses an interest in learning

Cystocele

Stress Urinary Incontinence r/t prolapsed bladder

Readiness for Enhanced Knowledge: expresses an interest in learning

Cystoscopy

Urinary Retention r/t edema in urethra obstructing flow of urine

Risk for Infection: Risk factor: invasive procedure

Readiness for Enhanced Knowledge: expresses an interest in learning

D

Deafness

Impaired Verbal Communication r/t impaired hearing

Hearing Loss r/t alteration in sensory reception, transmission, integration

Risk for Injury: Risk factor: alteration in sensory perception

Death

Risk for Sudden Infant Death (See **Sudden Infant Death, Risk for,** Section III)

Death, Oncoming

Death Anxiety r/t unresolved issues surrounding dying

Compromised Family Coping r/t client's inability to provide support to family

Ineffective Coping r/t personal vulnerability

Fear r/t threat of death

Maladaptive Grieving r/t loss of significant other

Powerlessness r/t effects of illness, oncoming death

Social Isolation r/t altered state of wellness

Spiritual Distress r/t intense suffering

Readiness for Enhanced Spiritual Well-Being: desire of client and family to be in harmony with each other, higher power, God

See Terminally Ill Child, Adolescent; Terminally Ill Child, Infant/Toddler; Terminally Ill Child, Preschool Child; Terminally Ill Child, School-Age Child/Preadolescent; Terminally Ill Child/Death of Child, Parent

Decisions, Difficulty Making

Decisional Conflict r/t support system deficit, perceived threat to value system, multiple or divergent sources of information, lack of relevant information, unclear personal values or beliefs

Risk for Impaired Emancipated Decision-Making: Risk factor: insufficient self-confidence in decision-making

Readiness for Enhanced Decision-Making (See **Decision-Making, Readiness for Enhanced,** Section III)

Decubitus Ulcer

See Pressure Ulcer; Pressure Injury

D

Deep Vein Thrombosis (DVT)

See DVT (Deep Vein Thrombosis); Venous Thromboembolism

Defensive Behavior

Defensive Coping r/t nonacceptance of blame, denial of problems or weakness

Ineffective Denial r/t inability to face situation realistically

Dehiscence, Abdominal

Fear r/t threat of death, severe dysfunction

Acute Pain r/t stretching of abdominal wall

Impaired Skin Integrity r/t altered circulation, malnutrition, opening in incision

Delayed Surgical Recovery r/t altered circulation, malnutrition, opening in incision

Impaired Tissue Integrity r/t exposure of abdominal contents to external environment

Risk for Deficient Fluid Volume: Risk factor: altered circulation associated with opening of wound and exposure of abdominal contents

Risk for Surgical Site Infection: Risk factors: loss of skin integrity, open surgical wound

Dehydration

Deficient Fluid Volume r/t active fluid volume loss

Impaired Oral Mucous Membrane Integrity r/t decreased salivation, fluid deficit

Risk for Chronic Functional Constipation: Risk factor: decreased fluid volume

Risk for Dry Mouth: Risk factor: decreased fluid volume

Risk for Ineffective Thermoregulation: Risk factor: decreased fluid volume

Risk for Unstable Blood Pressure: Risk factor: hypotension caused by insufficient fluid volume

See Burns; Heat Stroke; Vomiting; Diarrhea

Delirium

Acute Confusion r/t effects of medication, response to hospitalization, alcohol abuse, substance abuse, sensory deprivation or overload, infection, polypharmacy

Impaired Memory r/t delirium

Sleep Deprivation r/t sustained inadequate sleep hygiene

Risk for Injury: Risk factor: altered level of consciousness

Delirium Tremens (DT)

See Alcohol Withdrawal

Delivery

See Labor, Normal

Delusions

Impaired Verbal Communication r/t psychological impairment, delusional thinking

Acute Confusion r/t alcohol abuse, delirium, dementia, substance abuse

Ineffective Coping r/t distortion and insecurity of life events

Fear r/t content of intrusive thoughts

Risk for Other-Directed Violence: Risk factor: delusional thinking

Risk for Self-Directed Violence: Risk factor: delusional thinking

Dementia

Chronic Confusion r/t neurological dysfunction

Interrupted Family Processes r/t disability of family member

Frail Elderly Syndrome r/t alteration in cognitive functioning

Ineffective Home Maintenance Behaviors r/t inadequate support system, neurological dysfunction

Imbalanced Nutrition: Less than Body Requirements r/t neurological impairment

Disability-Associated Urinary Incontinence r/t neurological dysfunction

Insomnia r/t neurological impairment, naps during the day

Impaired Physical Mobility r/t alteration in cognitive function

Self-Neglect r/t cognitive impairment

Self-Care Deficit: Specify r/t psychological or neuromuscular impairment

Chronic Sorrow: Significant Other r/t chronic long-standing disability, loss of mental function

Impaired Swallowing r/t neuromuscular changes associated with long-standing dementia

Risk for Caregiver Role Strain: Risk factors: number of caregiving tasks, duration of caregiving required

Risk for Chronic Functional Constipation: Risk factor: decreased fluid intake

Risk for Adult Falls: Risk factor: diminished mental status

Risk for Frail Elderly Syndrome: Risk factors: cognitive impairment

Risk for Injury: Risk factors: confusion, decreased muscle coordination

Risk for Impaired Skin Integrity: Risk factors: altered nutritional status, immobility

Denial of Health Status

Ineffective Denial r/t lack of perception about the health status effects of illness

Ineffective Health Self-Management r/t denial of seriousness of health situation

Dental Caries

Impaired Dentition r/t ineffective oral hygiene, barriers to self-care, economic barriers to professional care, nutritional deficits, dietary habits

Ineffective Health Maintenance Behaviors r/t lack of knowledge regarding prevention of dental disease

Depression (Major Depressive Disorder)

Death Anxiety r/t feelings of lack of self-worth

Constipation r/t inactivity, decreased fluid intake

Fatigue r/t psychological demands

Ineffective Health Maintenance Behaviors r/t lack of ability to make good judgments regarding ways to obtain help

Hopelessness r/t feeling of abandonment, long-term stress

Impaired Mood Regulation r/t emotional instability

Insomnia r/t inactivity

Self-Neglect r/t depression, cognitive impairment

Powerlessness r/t pattern of helplessness

Chronic Low Self-Esteem r/t repeated unmet expectations

Sexual Dysfunction r/t loss of sexual desire

Social Isolation r/t ineffective coping

Chronic Sorrow r/t unresolved grief

Risk for Maladaptive Grieving: Risk factor: lack of previous resolution of former grieving response

Risk for Suicidal Behavior: Risk factor: grieving, hopelessness

Dermatitis

Anxiety r/t situational crisis imposed by illness

Impaired Comfort r/t itching

Impaired Skin Integrity r/t side effect of medication, allergic reaction

Readiness for Enhanced Knowledge: expresses an interest in learning

See Itching

Despondency

Hopelessness r/t long-term stress

See Depression (Major Depressive Disorder)

Destructive Behavior Toward Others

Risk-Prone Health Behavior r/t intense emotional state

Ineffective Coping r/t situational crises, maturational crises, disturbance in pattern of appraisal of threat

Risk for Other-Directed Violence (See **Violence, Other-Directed, Risk for,** Section III)

Developmental Concerns

Risk for Delayed Child Development: Risk factor: growth and development lag

Risk for Delayed Infant Motor Development: Risk factor: growth and development lag

Diabetes in Pregnancy

See Gestational Diabetes (Diabetes in Pregnancy)

Diabetes Insipidus

Deficient Fluid Volume r/t inability to conserve fluid

Ineffective Health Maintenance Behaviors r/t deficient knowledge regarding care of disease, importance of medications

Diabetes Mellitus

Ineffective Health Maintenance Behaviors r/t complexity of therapeutic regimen

Ineffective Health Self-Management (See **Health Management, Ineffective,** Section III)

Imbalanced Nutrition: Less than Body Requirements r/t inability to use glucose (type 1 [insulin-dependent] diabetes)

Risk for Overweight: Risk factor: excessive intake of nutrients (type 2 diabetes)

Ineffective Peripheral Tissue Perfusion r/t impaired arterial circulation

Powerlessness r/t perceived lack of personal control

Sexual Dysfunction r/t neuropathy associated with disease

Vision Loss r/t ineffective tissue perfusion of retina

Risk for Unstable Blood Glucose Level (See **Glucose Level, Blood, Unstable, Risk for,** Section III)

Risk for Infection: Risk factors: hyperglycemia, impaired healing, circulatory changes

Risk for Injury: Risk factors: hypoglycemia or hyperglycemia from failure to consume adequate calories, failure to take insulin

Risk for Dysfunctional Gastrointestinal Motility: Risk factor: complication of diabetes

Risk for Metabolic Syndrome: Risk factor: complication of diabetes

Risk for Impaired Skin Integrity: Risk factor: loss of pain perception in extremities

Risk for Delayed Surgical Recovery: Risk factor: impaired healing due to circulatory changes

Readiness for Enhanced Health Literacy: expresses desire to enhance understanding of health information to make health care choices

Readiness for Enhanced Health Self-Management (See **Health Self-Management, Readiness for Enhanced,** Section III)

Readiness for Enhanced Knowledge: expresses an interest in learning

See Hyperglycemia; Hypoglycemia

Diabetes Mellitus, Juvenile (Insulin-Dependent Diabetes Mellitus Type 1)

Risk-Prone Health Behavior r/t inadequate comprehension, inadequate social support, low self-efficacy, impaired adjustment attributable to adolescent maturational crises

Disturbed Body Image r/t imposed deviations from biophysical and psychosocial norm, perceived differences from peers

Impaired Comfort r/t insulin injections, peripheral blood glucose testing

Ineffective Health Maintenance Behaviors r/t inadequate trust in health care professional, ineffective communication skills, ineffective coping strategies, ineffective family coping

Imbalanced Nutrition: Less than Body Requirements r/t inability of body to adequately metabolize and use glucose and nutrients, increased caloric needs of child to promote growth and physical activity participation with peers

Risk for Metabolic Syndrome: Risk factor: complication of diabetes

Readiness for Enhanced Knowledge: expresses an interest in learning

See Diabetes Mellitus; Child with Chronic Condition; Hospitalized Child

Diabetic Coma

Acute Confusion r/t hyperglycemia, presence of excessive metabolic acids

D

Deficient Fluid Volume r/t hyperglycemia resulting in polyuria

Ineffective Health Self-Management r/t lack of understanding of preventive measures, adequate blood glucose control

Risk for Unstable Blood Glucose Level (See **Glucose Level, Blood, Unstable, Risk for,** Section III)

Risk for Infection: Risk factors: hyperglycemia, changes in vascular system

See Diabetes Mellitus

Diabetic Ketoacidosis

See Ketoacidosis, Diabetic

Diabetic Neuropathy

See Neuropathy, Peripheral

Diabetic Retinopathy

Maladaptive Grieving r/t loss of vision

Ineffective Health Maintenance Behaviors r/t deficient knowledge regarding preserving vision with treatment if possible, use of low-vision aids

See Vision Impairment; Blindness

Dialysis

See Hemodialysis; Peritoneal Dialysis

Diaphragmatic Hernia

See Hiatal Hernia

Diarrhea

Diarrhea r/t infection, change in diet, gastrointestinal disorders, stress, medication effect, impaction

Deficient Fluid Volume r/t excessive loss of fluids in liquid stools

Risk for Electrolyte Imbalance: Risk factor: effect of loss of electrolytes from frequent stools

DIC (Disseminated Intravascular Coagulation)

Fear r/t threat to well-being

Deficient Fluid Volume: Hemorrhage r/t depletion of clotting factors

Risk for Bleeding: Risk factors: microclotting within vascular system, depleted clotting factors

Digitalis Toxicity

Decreased Cardiac Output r/t drug toxicity affecting cardiac rhythm, rate

Ineffective Health Self-Management r/t deficient knowledge regarding action, appropriate method of administration of digitalis

Dignity, Loss of

Risk for Compromised Human Dignity (See **Human Dignity, Compromised, Risk for,** Section III)

Dilation and Curettage (D&C)

Acute Pain r/t uterine contractions

Risk for Bleeding: Risk factor: surgical procedure

Risk for Surgical Site Infection: Risk factor: surgical procedure

Ineffective Sexuality Pattern r/t painful coitus, fear associated with surgery on genital area

Readiness for Enhanced Knowledge: expresses an interest in learning

Dirty Body (for Prolonged Period)

Self-Neglect r/t mental illness, substance abuse, cognitive impairment

Discharge Planning

Ineffective Home Maintenance Behaviors r/t family member's disease or injury interfering with home maintenance

Deficient Knowledge r/t lack of exposure to information for home care

Relocation Stress Syndrome: Risk factors: insufficient predeparture counseling, insufficient support system, unpredictability of experience

Readiness for Enhanced Health Literacy: expresses desire to enhance understanding of health information to make health care choices

Readiness for Enhanced Knowledge: expresses an interest in learning

Discomforts of Pregnancy

Disturbed Body Image r/t pregnancy-induced body changes

Impaired Comfort r/t enlarged abdomen, swollen feet

Fatigue r/t hormonal, metabolic, body changes

Stress Urinary Incontinence r/t enlarged uterus, fetal movement

Insomnia r/t psychological stress, fetal movement, muscular cramping, urinary frequency, shortness of breath

Nausea r/t hormone effect

Acute Pain: Headache r/t hormonal changes of pregnancy

Acute Pain: Leg Cramps r/t nerve compression, calcium/phosphorus/potassium imbalance

Risk for Constipation: Risk factors: decreased intestinal motility, inadequate fiber in diet

Risk for Injury: Risk factors: faintness and/or syncope caused by vasomotor lability or postural hypotension, venous stasis in lower extremities

Dislocation of Joint

Acute Pain r/t dislocation of a joint

Self-Care Deficit r/t inability to use a joint

Risk for Injury: Risk factor: unstable joint

Dissecting Aneurysm

Fear r/t threat to well-being

See Abdominal Surgery; Aneurysm, Abdominal Aortic Repair

Disseminated Intravascular Coagulation (DIC)

See DIC (Disseminated Intravascular Coagulation)

Dissociative Identity Disorder (Not Otherwise Specified)

Anxiety r/t psychosocial stress

Ineffective Coping r/t personal vulnerability in crisis of accurate self-perception

Disturbed Personal Identity r/t inability to distinguish self-caused by multiple personality disorder, depersonalization, disturbance in memory

Impaired Memory r/t altered state of consciousness

See Multiple Personality Disorder (Dissociative Identity Disorder)

Distress

Anxiety r/t situational crises, maturational crises

Death Anxiety r/t denial of one's own mortality or impending death

Disuse Syndrome, Potential to Develop

Risk for Disuse Syndrome: Risk factors: paralysis, mechanical immobilization, prescribed immobilization, severe pain, altered level of consciousness

Diversional Activity Engagement, Lack of

Decreased Diversional Activity Engagement r/t environmental lack of diversional activity as in frequent hospitalizations, lengthy treatments

Diverticulitis

Constipation r/t dietary deficiency of fiber and roughage

Diarrhea r/t increased intestinal motility caused by inflammation

Deficient Knowledge r/t diet needed to control disease, medication regimen

Imbalanced Nutrition: Less than Body Requirements r/t loss of appetite

Acute Pain r/t inflammation of bowel

Risk for Deficient Fluid Volume: Risk factor: diarrhea

Dizziness

Decreased Cardiac Output r/t alteration in heart rate and rhythm, altered stroke volume

Deficient Knowledge r/t actions to take to prevent or modify dizziness and prevent falls

Impaired Physical Mobility r/t dizziness

Risk for Adult Falls: Risk factor: difficulty maintaining balance

Risk for Ineffective Cerebral Tissue Perfusion: Risk factor: interruption of cerebral arterial blood flow

Domestic Violence

Impaired Verbal Communication r/t psychological barriers of fear

Compromised Family Coping r/t abusive patterns

Defensive Coping r/t low self-esteem

Disturbed Family Identity Syndrome r/t domestic violence

Dysfunctional Family Processes r/t inadequate coping skills

Fear r/t threat to self-concept, situational crisis of abuse

Insomnia r/t psychological stress

Post-Trauma Syndrome r/t history of abuse

Powerlessness r/t lifestyle of helplessness

Situational Low Self-Esteem r/t negative family interactions

Risk for Compromised Resilience: Risk factor: effects of abuse

Risk for Other-Directed Violence: Risk factor: history of abuse

Down Syndrome

See Child with Chronic Condition; Intellectual Disability

Dress Self (Inability to)

Dressing Self-Care Deficit r/t intolerance to activity, decreased strength and endurance, pain, discomfort, perceptual or cognitive impairment, neuromuscular impairment, musculoskeletal impairment, depression, severe anxiety

Dribbling of Urine

Urinary Retention r/t degenerative changes in pelvic muscles and urinary structures

Stress Urinary Incontinence r/t degenerative changes in pelvic muscles and urinary structures

Drooling

Impaired Swallowing r/t neuromuscular impairment, mechanical obstruction

Risk for Aspiration: Risk factor: impaired swallowing

Dropout from School

Impaired Resilience (See **Resilience, Individual, Impaired,** Section III)

Anxiety r/t conflict about life goals

Ineffective Coping r/t inadequate resources

Drug Abuse

See Substance Abuse

Drug Withdrawal

See Acute Substance Withdrawal Syndrome

Dry Eye

Risk for Dry Eye: Risk factors (See **Dry Eye, Risk for,** Section III)

Risk for Corneal Injury: Risk factor: suppressed corneal reflex

Readiness for Enhanced Knowledge: expresses an interest in learning

See Conjunctivitis; Keratoconjunctivitis Sicca (Dry Eye Syndrome)

Dry Mouth

Risk for Dry Mouth: Risk factors (See **Dry Mouth, Risk for,** Section III)

Risk for Impaired Oral Mucous Membrane Integrity: Risk factor: reduced quality or quantity of saliva caused by decreased fluid volume

DT (Delirium Tremens)

See Alcohol Withdrawal

DVT (Deep Vein Thrombosis)

Constipation r/t inactivity, bed rest

Impaired Physical Mobility r/t pain in extremity

Acute Pain r/t vascular inflammation, edema

Ineffective Peripheral Tissue Perfusion r/t deficient knowledge of aggravating factors

Delayed Surgical Recovery r/t impaired physical mobility

Readiness for Enhanced Knowledge: expresses an interest in learning

Risk for Ineffective Thermoregulation: Risk factor: inactivity

See Anticoagulant Therapy; Venous Thromboembolism, Risk for (See Section III)

D

Dying Client

See Terminally Ill Adult; Terminally Ill Adolescent; Terminally Ill Child, Infant/Toddler; Terminally Ill Child, Preschool Child; Terminally Ill Child, School-Age Child/Preadolescent; Terminally Ill Child/Death of Child, Parent

Dysfunctional Eating Pattern

Imbalanced Nutrition: Less than Body Requirements r/t psychological factors

Risk for Overweight: Risk factor: psychological factors

See Anorexia Nervosa; Bulimia; Maturational Issues, Adolescent; Obesity

Dysfunctional Family Unit

See Family Problems

Dysfunctional Ventilatory Weaning

Dysfunctional Ventilatory Weaning Response r/t physical, psychological, situational factors

Dysmenorrhea

Nausea r/t prostaglandin effect

Acute Pain r/t cramping from hormonal effects

Readiness for Enhanced Knowledge: expresses an interest in learning

Dyspareunia

Sexual Dysfunction r/t lack of lubrication during intercourse, alteration in reproductive organ function

Dyspepsia

Anxiety r/t pressures of personal role

Acute Pain r/t gastrointestinal disease, consumption of irritating foods

Readiness for Enhanced Knowledge: expresses an interest in learning

Dysphagia

Impaired Swallowing r/t neuromuscular impairment

Risk for Aspiration: Risk factor: loss of gag or cough reflex

Dysphasia

Impaired Verbal Communication r/t decrease in circulation to brain

Impaired Social Interaction r/t difficulty in communicating

Dyspnea

Decreased Activity Tolerance r/t imbalance between oxygen supply and demand

Ineffective Breathing Pattern r/t compromised cardiac or pulmonary function, decreased lung expansion, neurological impairment affecting respiratory center, extreme anxiety

Fear r/t threat to state of well-being, potential death

Impaired Gas Exchange r/t alveolar-capillary damage

Insomnia r/t difficulty breathing, positioning required for effective breathing

Sleep Deprivation r/t ineffective breathing pattern

Dysrhythmia

Decreased Activity Tolerance r/t decreased cardiac output

Decreased Cardiac Output r/t alteration in heart rate, rhythm

Fear r/t threat of death, change in health status

Risk for Ineffective Cerebral Tissue Perfusion: Risk factor: decreased blood supply to the brain from dysrhythmia

Risk for Unstable Blood Pressure r/t cardiac arrhythmia and electrolyte imbalance

Readiness for Enhanced Knowledge: expresses an interest in learning

Dysthymic Disorder

Ineffective Coping r/t impaired social interaction

Ineffective Health Maintenance Behaviors r/t inability to make good judgments regarding ways to obtain help

Insomnia r/t anxious thoughts

Chronic Low Self-Esteem r/t repeated unmet expectations

Ineffective Sexuality Pattern r/t loss of sexual desire

Social Isolation r/t ineffective coping

See Depression (Major Depressive Disorder)

Dystocia

Anxiety r/t difficult labor, deficient knowledge regarding normal labor pattern

Ineffective Coping r/t situational crisis

Fatigue r/t prolonged labor

Maladaptive Grieving r/t loss of ideal labor experience

Acute Pain r/t difficult labor, medical interventions

Powerlessness r/t perceived inability to control outcome of labor

Risk for Bleeding: Risk factor: hemorrhage secondary to uterine atony

Risk for Ineffective Cerebral Tissue Perfusion (Fetal): Risk factor: difficult labor and birth

Risk for Infection: Risk factor: prolonged rupture of membranes

Risk for Impaired Tissue Integrity (Maternal and Fetal): Risk factor: difficult labor

Dysuria

Impaired Urinary Elimination r/t infection/inflammation of the urinary tract

Risk for Urge Urinary Incontinence: Risk factor: detrusor hyperreflexia from infection in the urinary tract

Acute Pain r/t infection/inflammation of the urinary tract

E

Ear Surgery

Acute Pain r/t edema in ears from surgery

Hearing Loss r/t invasive surgery of ears, dressings

Risk for Delayed Child Development: Risk factor: hearing impairment

Risk for Adult Falls: Risk factor: dizziness from excessive stimuli to vestibular apparatus

Readiness for Enhanced Knowledge: expresses an interest in learning

See Hospitalized Child

Earache

Acute Pain r/t trauma, edema, infection

Hearing Loss r/t altered sensory reception, transmission

Eating Dynamics, Adolescent

Imbalanced Nutrition: Less than Body Requirements r/t negative perception of one's body

Ineffective Adolescent Eating Dynamics r/t altered family dynamics, eating disorder, excessive stress

Risk for Overweight: Risk factor: media influence resulting in unhealthy choices, insufficient interest in physical activity

Readiness for Enhanced Health Literacy: expresses desire to learn to make healthy food choices

Eating Dynamics, Child

Imbalanced Nutrition: Less than Body Requirements r/t excessive of parental control over quantity and choices of foods

Ineffective Child Eating Dynamics r/t bribing child to eat, forcing child to eat

Risk for Delayed Child Development: Risk factor: inadequate nutrition to meet metabolic needs for normal development

Risk for Overweight: Risk factors: unhealthy choices, frequent snacking, low physical activity

Eating Dynamics, Infant

See Feeding Dynamics, Infant

Eclampsia

Interrupted Family Processes r/t unmet expectations for pregnancy and childbirth

Fear r/t threat of well-being to self and fetus

Risk for Aspiration: Risk factor: seizure activity

Risk for Ineffective Cerebral Tissue Perfusion: Fetal: Risk factor: uteroplacental insufficiency

Risk for Imbalanced Fluid Volume: Risk factor: decreased urine output as a result of renal dysfunction

Risk for unstable Blood Pressure: Risk factor: hypertension caused by excess fluid volume

ECMO (Extracorporeal Membrane Oxygenator)

Death Anxiety r/t emergency condition, hemorrhage

Decreased Cardiac Output r/t altered contractility of the heart

Impaired Gas Exchange (See **Gas Exchange, Impaired,** Section III)

See Respiratory Conditions of the Neonate

ECT (Electroconvulsive Therapy)

Decisional Conflict r/t lack of relevant information

Fear r/t real or imagined threat to well-being

Impaired Memory r/t effects of treatment

See Depression (Major Depressive Disorder)

Ectopic Pregnancy

Death Anxiety r/t emergency condition, hemorrhage

Disturbed Body Image r/t negative feelings about body and reproductive functioning

Fear r/t threat to self, surgery, implications for future pregnancy

Acute Pain r/t stretching or rupture of implantation site

Ineffective Role Performance r/t loss of pregnancy

Situational Low Self-Esteem r/t loss of pregnancy, inability to carry pregnancy to term

Chronic Sorrow r/t loss of pregnancy, potential loss of fertility

Risk for Bleeding: Risk factor: possible rupture of implantation site, surgical trauma

Risk for Ineffective Coping: Risk factor: loss of pregnancy

Risk for Interrupted Family Processes: Risk factor: situational crisis

Risk for Infection: Risk factors: traumatized tissue, surgical procedure

Risk for Spiritual Distress: Risk factor: grief process

Eczema

Disturbed Body Image r/t change in appearance from inflamed skin

Impaired Comfort: Pruritus r/t inflammation of skin

Impaired Skin Integrity r/t side effect of medication, allergic reaction

Readiness for Enhanced Knowledge: expresses an interest in learning

ED (Erectile Dysfunction)

See Erectile Dysfunction (ED); Impotence

Edema

Excess Fluid Volume r/t excessive fluid intake, cardiac dysfunction, renal dysfunction, loss of plasma proteins

Ineffective Health Maintenance Behaviors r/t deficient knowledge regarding treatment of edema

Risk for Impaired Skin Integrity: Risk factors: impaired circulation, fragility of skin

See Heart Failure; Renal Failure

Elder Abuse

See Abuse, Spouse, Parent, or Significant Other

E

Elderly

See Aging; Frail Elderly Syndrome

Electroconvulsive Therapy

See ECT (Electroconvulsive Therapy)

Electrolyte Imbalance

Risk for Electrolyte Imbalance (See **Electrolyte Imbalance, Risk for,** Section III)

Risk for Unstable Blood Pressure: Risk factor: fluid volume changes

Emaciated Person

Frail Elderly Syndrome r/t living alone, malnutrition, alteration in cognitive functioning

Imbalanced Nutrition: Less than Body Requirements r/t inability to ingest food, digest food, absorb nutrients because of biological, psychological, economic factors

Emancipated Decision-Making, Impaired

Risk for Impaired Emancipated Decision-Making: Risk factor: inability or unwillingness to verbalize needs and wants

Readiness for Enhanced Emancipated Decision-Making: expresses desire to enhance decision-making process

Embolectomy

Fear r/t threat of great bodily harm from embolus

Ineffective Peripheral Tissue Perfusion r/t presence of embolus

Risk for Bleeding: Risk factors: postoperative complication, surgical area

See Surgery, Postoperative Care

Emboli

See Pulmonary Embolism (PE)

Embolism in Leg or Arm

Ineffective Peripheral Tissue Perfusion r/t arterial/venous obstruction from clot

See DVT (Deep Vein Thrombosis); Risk for Thrombosis

Emesis

Nausea (See **Nausea,** Section III)

See Vomiting

Emotional Problems

See Coping Problems

Empathy

Readiness for Enhanced Community Coping: social supports, being available for problem solving

Readiness for Enhanced Family Coping: basic needs met, desire to move to higher level of health

Readiness for Enhanced Spiritual Well-Being: desire to establish interconnectedness through spirituality

Emphysema

See COPD (Chronic Obstructive Pulmonary Disease)

Emptiness

Social Isolation r/t inability to engage in satisfying personal relationships

Chronic Sorrow r/t unresolved grief

Spiritual Distress r/t separation from religious or cultural ties

Encephalitis

See Meningitis/Encephalitis

Endocardial Cushion Defect

See Congenital Heart Disease/Cardiac Anomalies

Endocarditis

Decreased Activity Tolerance r/t reduced cardiac reserve, prescribed bed rest

Decreased Cardiac Output r/t inflammation of lining of heart and change in structure of valve leaflets, increased myocardial workload

Risk for Imbalanced Nutrition: Less than Body Requirements: Risk factors: fever, hypermetabolic state associated with fever

Risk for Ineffective Cerebral Tissue Perfusion: Risk factor: possible presence of emboli in cerebral circulation

Risk for Ineffective Peripheral Tissue Perfusion: Risk factor: possible presence of emboli in peripheral circulation

Readiness for Enhanced Knowledge: expresses an interest in learning

Endometriosis

Maladaptive Grieving r/t possible infertility

Nausea r/t prostaglandin effect

Acute Pain r/t onset of menses with distention of endometrial tissue

Sexual Dysfunction r/t painful intercourse

Readiness for Enhanced Knowledge: expresses an interest in learning

Endometritis

Anxiety r/t, fear of unknown

Ineffective Thermoregulation r/t infectious process

Acute Pain r/t infectious process in reproductive tract

Readiness for Enhanced Knowledge: expresses an interest in learning

Enuresis

Ineffective Health Maintenance Behaviors r/t unachieved developmental task, neuromuscular immaturity, diseases of urinary system

See Toilet Training

Environmental Interpretation Problems

See Chronic Confusion

Epididymitis

Anxiety r/t situational crisis, pain, threat to future fertility

Acute Pain r/t inflammation in scrotal sac

Ineffective Sexuality Pattern r/t edema of epididymis and testes

Readiness for Enhanced Knowledge: expresses an interest in learning

Epiglottitis

See Respiratory Infections, Acute Childhood (Croup, Epiglottitis, Pertussis, Pneumonia, Respiratory Syncytial Virus)

Epilepsy

Anxiety r/t threat to role functioning

Ineffective Health Self-Management r/t deficient knowledge regarding seizure control

Impaired Memory r/t seizure activity

Risk for Aspiration: Risk factors: impaired swallowing, excessive secretions

Risk for Injury: Risk factor: environmental factors during seizure

Readiness for Enhanced Knowledge: expresses an interest in learning

See Seizure Disorders, Adult; Seizure Disorders, Childhood (Epilepsy, Febrile Seizures, Infantile Spasms)

Episiotomy

Anxiety r/t fear of pain

Disturbed Body Image r/t fear of resuming sexual relations

Impaired Physical Mobility r/t pain, swelling, tissue trauma

Acute Pain r/t tissue trauma

Sexual Dysfunction r/t altered body structure, tissue trauma

Impaired Skin Integrity r/t perineal incision

Risk for Infection: Risk factor: tissue trauma

Epistaxis

Fear r/t large amount of blood loss

Risk for Deficient Fluid Volume: Risk factor: excessive blood loss

Epstein-Barr Virus

See Mononucleosis

Erectile Dysfunction (ED)

Situational Low Self-Esteem r/t physiological crisis, inability to practice usual sexual activity

Sexual Dysfunction r/t altered body function

Readiness for Enhanced Knowledge: information regarding treatment for erectile dysfunction

See Impotence

Escherichia coli Infection

Fear r/t serious illness, unknown outcome

Deficient Knowledge r/t how to prevent disease; care of self with serious illness

See Gastroenteritis; Gastroenteritis, Child; Hospitalized Child

Esophageal Varices

Fear r/t threat of death from hematemesis

Risk for Bleeding: Risk factors: portal hypertension, distended variceal vessels that can easily rupture

See Cirrhosis

Esophagitis

Acute Pain r/t inflammation of esophagus

Readiness for Enhanced Knowledge: expresses an interest in learning

Evisceration

See Dehiscence, Abdominal

Exhaustion

Impaired Resilience (See **Resilience, Individual, Impaired,** Section III)

Disturbed Sleep Pattern (See **Sleep Pattern, Disturbed,** Section III)

Exposure to Hot or Cold Environment

Hyperthermia r/t exposure to hot environment, abnormal reaction to anesthetics

Hypothermia r/t exposure to cold environment

Risk for Ineffective Thermoregulation: Risk factors: extremes of environmental temperature, inappropriate clothing for environmental temperature

External Fixation

Disturbed Body Image r/t trauma, change to affected part

Risk for Infection: Risk factor: presence of pins inserted into bone

See Fracture

Extracorporeal Membrane Oxygenator (ECMO)

See ECMO (Extracorporeal Membrane Oxygenator)

Eye Discomfort

Risk for Dry Eye (See **Eye, Dry, Risk for,** Section III)

Risk for Corneal Injury: Risk factors: exposure of the eyeball, blinking less than five times per minute

Eye Surgery

Anxiety r/t possible loss of vision

Self-Care Deficit: Specify r/t impaired vision

Vision Loss r/t surgical procedure, eye pathology

Risk for Injury: Risk factor: impaired vision

Readiness for Enhanced Knowledge: expresses an interest in learning

See Hospitalized Child

F

F

Failure to Thrive, Child

Disorganized Infant Behavior (See **Infant Behavior, Disorganized,** Section III)

Ineffective Child Eating Dynamics r/t lack of knowledge or resources regarding nutritional needs of child

Ineffective Infant Feeding Dynamics r/t lack of knowledge regarding nutritional needs of infant

Ineffective Infant Suck-Swallow Response r/t unsatisfactory sucking behavior

Insomnia r/t inconsistency of caretaker; lack of quiet, consistent environment

Imbalanced Nutrition: Less than Body Requirements r/t inadequate type or amounts of food for infant or child, inappropriate feeding techniques

Impaired Parenting r/t lack of parenting skills, inadequate role modeling

Chronic Low Self-Esteem: Parental r/t feelings of inadequacy, support system deficiencies, inadequate role model

Social Isolation r/t limited support systems, self-imposed situation

Risk for Impaired Attachment: Risk factor: inability of parents to meet infant's needs

Readiness for Enhanced Knowledge: parent expresses willingness to learn how to meet infant/child nutritional needs

Falls, Risk for

Risk for Adult Falls (See **Adult Falls, Risk for,** Section III)

Risk for Child Falls (See **Child Falls, Risk for,** Section III)

Family Problems

Compromised Family Coping (See **Coping, Family, Compromised,** Section III)

Disabled Family Coping (See **Coping, Family, Disabled,** Section III)

Interrupted Family Processes r/t situation transition and/or crises, developmental transition and/or crises

Ineffective Family Health Self-Management (See **Family Health Management, Ineffective,** Section III)

Readiness for Enhanced Family Coping: needs sufficiently gratified, adaptive tasks effectively addressed to enable goals of self-actualization to surface

Family Process

Dysfunctional Family Processes (See **Family Processes, Dysfunctional,** Section III)

Interrupted Family Processes (See **Family Processes, Interrupted,** Section III)

Readiness for Enhanced Family Processes (See **Family Processes, Readiness for Enhanced,** Section III)

Readiness for Enhanced Relationship (See **Relationship, Readiness for Enhanced,** Section III)

Fatigue

Fatigue (See **Fatigue,** Section III)

Fear

Death Anxiety r/t fear of death

Fear r/t identifiable physical or psychological threat to person

Febrile Seizures

See Seizure Disorders, Childhood (Epilepsy, Febrile Seizures, Infantile Spasms)

Fecal Impaction

See Impaction of Stool

(See **Constipation,** Section III)

(See **Constipation, Chronic Functional,** Section III)

Fecal Incontinence

Impaired Bowel Continence r/t neurological impairment, gastrointestinal disorders, anorectal trauma, weakened perineal muscles

Feeding Dynamics, Infant

Ineffective Infant Eating Dynamics r/t inappropriate transition to sold foods

Ineffective Infant Suck-Swallow Response r/t unsatisfactory sucking behavior

Risk for Caregiver Role Strain: Risk factor: fatigue leading to ineffective or insufficient feeding

Risk for Impaired Attachment: Risk factor: inability physically or psychologically to meet nutritional needs of newborn

Risk for Impaired Parenting: Risk factors: stress, sleep deprivation, insufficient knowledge, and/or social isolation

Readiness for Enhanced Health Literacy: expresses a desire to enhance knowledge of appropriate feeding dynamics for each developmental stage (See **Ineffective Feeding Dynamics, Infant,** Section III)

Feeding Problems, Newborn

Ineffective Breastfeeding (See **Breastfeeding, Ineffective,** Section III)

Ineffective Infant Feeding Dynamics r/t attachment issues, lack of knowledge of appropriate methods of feeding infant for each stage of development

Ineffective Infant Suck-Swallow Response r/t unsatisfactory sucking behavior

Insufficient Breast Milk Production (See **Breast Milk Production, Insufficient,** Section III)

Disorganized Infant Behavior r/t prematurity, immature neurological system

Ineffective Infant Feeding Dynamics r/t parental lack of knowledge of appropriate feeding methods for each stage of development

Ineffective Infant Feeding Pattern r/t prematurity, neurological impairment or delay, oral hypersensitivity, prolonged nothing-by-mouth status

Impaired Swallowing r/t prematurity

Neonatal Abstinence Syndrome: At-risk population: in utero substance exposure secondary to maternal substance use

Nipple-Areolar Complex Injury r/t maternal impatience with breastfeeding process

Risk for Deficient Fluid Volume: Risk factor: inability to take in adequate amount of fluids

Female Genital Mutilation

Acute Pain r/t traumatic surgical procedure

Anxiety r/t situational crisis

Disturbed Body Image r/t scarring, changes in body function

Fear r/t threat to well-being

Powerlessness r/t absence of control of decision-making

Impaired Skin Integrity r/t traumatic surgical procedure

Impaired Tissue Integrity r/t wound, potential for infection

Risk for Compromised Human Dignity: Risk factor: dehumanizing treatment

Risk for Infection: Risk factor: invasive procedure

Risk for Post-Trauma Syndrome: Risk factor: experiencing traumatic surgery

Risk for Chronic Low Self-Esteem: Risk factor: cultural incongruence (See **Female Genital Mutilation, Risk for,** Section III)

Femoral Popliteal Bypass

Anxiety r/t threat to or change in health status

Acute Pain r/t surgical trauma, edema in surgical area

Ineffective Peripheral Tissue Perfusion r/t impaired arterial circulation

Risk for Bleeding: Risk factor: surgery on arteries

Risk for Surgical Site Infection: Risk factor: invasive procedure

Fetal Alcohol Syndrome

See Neonatal Abstinence Syndrome

Fetal Distress/Nonreassuring Fetal Heart Rate Pattern

Fear r/t threat to fetus

Ineffective Peripheral Tissue Perfusion: fetal r/t interruption of umbilical cord blood flow

Fever

Ineffective Thermoregulation r/t infectious process

Fibrocystic Breast Disease

See Breast Lumps

Filthy Home Environment

Ineffective Home Maintenance Behaviors (See **Home Maintenance Behaviors, Ineffective,** Section III)

Self-Neglect r/t mental illness, substance abuse, cognitive impairment

Financial Crisis in the Home Environment

Ineffective Home Maintenance Behaviors r/t insufficient finances

Fistulectomy

See Hemorrhoidectomy

Flail Chest

Ineffective Breathing Pattern r/t chest trauma

Fear r/t difficulty breathing

Impaired Gas Exchange r/t loss of effective lung function

Impaired Spontaneous Ventilation r/t paradoxical respirations

Flashbacks

Post-Trauma Syndrome r/t catastrophic event

Flat Affect

Hopelessness r/t prolonged activity restriction creating isolation, failing or deteriorating physiological condition, long-term stress, abandonment, lost belief in transcendent values or higher power or God

Risk for Loneliness: Risk factors: social isolation, lack of interest in surroundings

See Depression (Major Depressive Disorder); Dysthymic Disorder

Fluid Volume Deficit

Deficient Fluid Volume r/t active fluid loss, vomiting, diarrhea, failure of regulatory mechanisms

Risk for Shock: Risk factors: hypovolemia, sepsis, systemic inflammatory response syndrome (SIRS)

Risk for Unstable Blood Pressure: Risk factor: hypotension, excessive loss or insufficient intake of fluid

Fluid Volume Excess

Excess Fluid Volume r/t compromised regulatory mechanism, excess sodium intake

Risk for Unstable Blood Pressure: Risk factor: hypertension, excessive intake or retention of fluid

Fluid Volume Imbalance, Risk for

Risk for Imbalanced Fluid Volume: Risk factor: major invasive surgeries

Food Allergies

Diarrhea r/t immune effects of offending food on gastrointestinal system

Risk for Allergy Reaction: Risk factor: specific foods

Readiness for Enhanced Knowledge: expresses an interest in learning

See Anaphylactic Shock

F

F

Foodborne Illness

Diarrhea r/t infectious material in gastrointestinal tract

Deficient Fluid Volume r/t active fluid loss from vomiting and diarrhea

Deficient Knowledge r/t care of self with serious illness, prevention of further incidences of foodborne illness

Nausea r/t contamination irritating stomach

Risk for Dysfunctional Gastrointestinal Motility: Risk factor: contaminated food

See Gastroenteritis; Gastroenteritis, Child; Hospitalized Child; Escherichia coli *Infection*

Food Intolerance

Risk for Dysfunctional Gastrointestinal Motility: Risk factor: food intolerance

Foreign Body Aspiration

Ineffective Airway Clearance r/t obstruction of airway

Ineffective Health Maintenance Behaviors r/t parental deficient knowledge regarding high-risk items

Risk for Suffocation: Risk factor: inhalation of small objects

See Safety, Childhood

Formula Feeding of Infant

Maladaptive Grieving: Maternal r/t loss of desired breastfeeding experience

Ineffective Infant Feeding Dynamics r/t lack of knowledge of appropriate methods of feeding infant for each stage of development

Ineffective Infant Suck-Swallow Response r/t unsatisfactory sucking behavior

Risk for Constipation: Infant: Risk factor: iron-fortified formula

Risk for Infection: Infant: Risk factors: lack of passive maternal immunity, supine feeding position, contamination of formula

Readiness for Enhanced Knowledge: expresses an interest in learning

Fracture

Decreased Diversional Activity Engagement r/t immobility

Impaired Physical Mobility r/t limb immobilization

Acute Pain r/t muscle spasm, edema, trauma

Post-Trauma Syndrome r/t catastrophic event

Impaired Walking r/t limb immobility

Risk for Ineffective Peripheral Tissue Perfusion: Risk factors: immobility, presence of cast

Risk for Peripheral Neurovascular Dysfunction: Risk factors: mechanical compression, treatment of fracture

Risk for Impaired Skin Integrity: Risk factors: immobility, presence of cast

Risk for Thrombosis: Risk factors: trauma, immobility

Readiness for Enhanced Knowledge: expresses an interest in learning

Fractured Hip

See Hip Fracture

Frail Elderly Syndrome

Decreased Activity Tolerance r/t sensory changes

Risk for Frail Elderly Syndrome (See **Frail Elderly Syndrome, Risk for,** Section III)

Risk for Injury: Risk factors: impaired vision, impaired gait

Risk for Powerlessness: Risk factor: inability to maintain independence

Frequency of Urination

Stress Urinary Incontinence r/t degenerative change in pelvic muscles and structural support

Urge Urinary Incontinence r/t decreased bladder capacity, irritation of bladder stretch receptors causing spasm, alcohol, caffeine, increased fluids, increased urine concentration, overdistended bladder

Impaired Urinary Elimination r/t urinary tract infection

Urinary Retention r/t high urethral pressure caused by weak detrusor, inhibition of reflex arc, strong sphincter, blockage

Friendship

Readiness for Enhanced Relationship: expresses desire to enhance communication between partners

Frostbite

Acute Pain r/t decreased circulation from prolonged exposure to cold

Ineffective Peripheral Tissue Perfusion r/t damage to extremities from prolonged exposure to cold

Impaired Tissue Integrity r/t freezing of skin and tissues

Risk for Ineffective Thermoregulation: Risk factor: prolonged exposure to cold

See Hypothermia

Frothy Sputum

See CHF (Congestive Heart Failure); Pulmonary Edema; Seizure Disorders, Adult; Seizure Disorders, Childhood (Epilepsy, Febrile Seizures, Infantile Spasms)

Fusion, Lumbar

Anxiety r/t fear of surgical procedure, possible recurring problems

Impaired Physical Mobility r/t limitations from surgical procedure, presence of brace

Acute Pain r/t discomfort at bone donor site, surgical operation

Risk for Injury: Risk factor: improper body mechanics

Risk for Perioperative Positioning Injury: Risk factor: immobilization during surgery

Readiness for Enhanced Knowledge: expresses an interest in learning

G

Gag Reflex, Depressed or Absent

Impaired Swallowing r/t neuromuscular impairment

Risk for Aspiration: Risk factors: depressed cough or gag reflex

Gallop Rhythm

Decreased Cardiac Output r/t decreased contractility of heart

Gallstones

See Cholelithiasis

Gang Member

Impaired Resilience (See **Resilience, Individual, Impaired,** Section III)

Gangrene

Fear r/t possible loss of extremity

Ineffective Peripheral Tissue Perfusion r/t obstruction of arterial flow

See Diabetes Mellitus; Peripheral Vascular Disease

Gas Exchange, Impaired

Impaired Gas Exchange r/t ventilation-perfusion imbalance

Dysfunctional Ventilatory Weaning Response r/t psychomotor agitation

Gastric Ulcer

See GI Bleed (Gastrointestinal Bleeding); Ulcer, Peptic (Duodenal or Gastric)

Gastritis

Imbalanced Nutrition: Less than Body Requirements r/t vomiting, inadequate intestinal absorption of nutrients, restricted dietary regimen

Acute Pain r/t inflammation of gastric mucosa

Risk for Deficient Fluid Volume: Risk factors: excessive loss from gastrointestinal tract from vomiting, decreased intake

Gastroenteritis

Diarrhea r/t infectious process involving intestinal tract

Deficient Fluid Volume r/t excessive loss from gastrointestinal tract from diarrhea, vomiting

Nausea r/t irritation to gastrointestinal system

Imbalanced Nutrition: Less than Body Requirements r/t vomiting, inadequate intestinal absorption of nutrients, restricted dietary intake

Acute Pain r/t increased peristalsis causing cramping

Risk for Electrolyte Imbalance: Risk factor: loss of gastrointestinal fluids high in electrolytes

Readiness for Enhanced Knowledge: expresses an interest in learning

See Gastroenteritis, Child

Gastroenteritis, Child

Impaired Skin Integrity: Diaper Rash r/t acidic excretions on perineal tissues

Readiness for Enhanced Knowledge: expresses an interest in learning

Acute Pain r/t increased peristalsis causing cramping

See Gastroenteritis; Hospitalized Child

Gastroesophageal Reflux Disease (GERD)

Ineffective Airway Clearance r/t reflux of gastric contents into esophagus and tracheal or bronchial tree

Ineffective Health Maintenance Behaviors r/t deficient knowledge regarding antireflux regimen (e.g., positioning, change in diet)

Acute Pain r/t irritation of esophagus from gastric acids

Risk for Aspiration: Risk factor: entry of gastric contents in tracheal or bronchial tree

Gastroesophageal Reflux, Child

Ineffective Airway Clearance r/t reflux of gastric contents into esophagus and tracheal or bronchial tree

Anxiety: Parental r/t possible need for surgical intervention

Deficient Fluid Volume r/t persistent vomiting

Imbalanced Nutrition: Less than Body Requirements r/t poor feeding, vomiting

Risk for Aspiration: Risk factor: entry of gastric contents in tracheal or bronchial tree

Risk for Impaired Parenting: Risk factors: disruption in bonding as a result of irritable or inconsolable infant; lack of sleep for parents

Readiness for Enhanced Knowledge: expresses an interest in learning

See Child with Chronic Condition; Hospitalized Child

Gastrointestinal Bleeding (GI Bleed)

See GI Bleed (Gastrointestinal Bleeding)

Gastrointestinal Hemorrhage

See GI Bleed (Gastrointestinal Bleeding)

Gastrointestinal Surgery

Risk for Injury: Risk factor: inadvertent insertion of nasogastric tube through gastric incision line

See Abdominal Surgery

Gastroschisis/Omphalocele

Ineffective Airway Clearance r/t complications of anesthetic effects

Impaired Gas Exchange r/t effects of anesthesia, subsequent atelectasis

Maladaptive Grieving r/t threatened loss of infant, loss of perfect birth or infant because of serious medical condition

Risk for Deficient Fluid Volume: Risk factors: inability to feed because of condition, subsequent electrolyte imbalance

Risk for Infection: Risk factor: disrupted skin integrity with exposure of abdominal contents

Risk for Injury: Risk factors: disrupted skin integrity, ineffective protection

Gastrostomy

Risk for Impaired Skin Integrity: Risk factor: presence of gastric contents on skin

See Tube Feeding

Gender Dysphoria

Anxiety r/t conflict between physical (assigned) gender and gender they identify with

Decisional Conflict r/t uncertainty about choices regarding gender reassignment

Disturbed Body Image r/t alteration in self-perception, inability to identify with own body

Ineffective Denial r/t insufficient emotional support

Fear r/t victimization

Disturbed Personal Identity r/t gender confusion

Ineffective Sexuality Pattern r/t conflict surrounding gender identity

Risk for Compromised Human Dignity: Risk factor: cultural incongruence, humiliation

Readiness for Enhanced Decision-Making: expresses desire to enhance understanding of choices for decision-making

Genital Herpes

See Herpes Simplex II

Genital Warts

See STD (Sexually Transmitted Disease)

GERD

See Gastroesophageal Reflux Disease (GERD)

Gestational Diabetes (Diabetes in Pregnancy)

Anxiety r/t threat to self and/or fetus

Impaired Nutrition: Less than Body Requirements r/t decreased insulin production and glucose uptake in cells

Risk for Overweight: Fetal r/t excessive glucose uptake

Impaired Nutrition: More than Body Requirements: Fetal r/t excessive glucose uptake

Risk for Unstable Blood Glucose: Risk factor: excessive intake of carbohydrates

Risk for Disturbed Maternal–Fetal Dyad: Risk factor: impaired glucose metabolism

Risk for Impaired Tissue Integrity: Fetal: Risk factors: large infant, congenital defects, birth injury

Risk for Impaired Tissue Integrity: Maternal: Risk factor: delivery of large infant

Readiness for Enhanced Knowledge: expresses an interest in learning

See Diabetes Mellitus

GI Bleed (Gastrointestinal Bleeding)

Fatigue r/t loss of circulating blood volume, decreased ability to transport oxygen

Fear r/t threat to well-being, potential death

Deficient Fluid Volume r/t gastrointestinal bleeding, hemorrhage

Imbalanced Nutrition: Less than Body Requirements r/t nausea, vomiting

Acute Pain r/t irritated mucosa from acid secretion

Risk for Ineffective Coping: Risk factors: personal vulnerability in crisis, bleeding, hospitalization

Readiness for Enhanced Knowledge: expresses an interest in learning

Gingivitis

Impaired Oral Mucous Membrane Integrity r/t ineffective oral hygiene

Glaucoma

Deficient Knowledge r/t treatment and self-care for disease

See Vision Impairment

Glomerulonephritis

Excess Fluid Volume r/t renal impairment

Imbalanced Nutrition: Less than Body Requirements r/t anorexia, restrictive diet

Acute Pain r/t edema of kidney

Readiness for Enhanced Knowledge: expresses an interest in learning

Gluten Allergy

See Celiac Disease

Gonorrhea

Acute Pain r/t inflammation of reproductive organs

Risk for Infection: Risk factor: spread of organism throughout reproductive organs

Readiness for Enhanced Knowledge: expresses an interest in learning

See STD (Sexually Transmitted Disease)

Gout

Impaired Physical Mobility r/t musculoskeletal impairment

Chronic Pain r/t inflammation of affected joint

Readiness for Enhanced Knowledge: expresses an interest in learning

Grandiosity

Defensive Coping r/t inaccurate perception of self and abilities

Grand Mal Seizure

See Seizure Disorders, Adult; Seizure Disorders, Childhood (Epilepsy, Febrile Seizures, Infantile Spasms)

Grandparents Raising Grandchildren

Anxiety r/t change in role status

Decisional Conflict r/t support system deficit

Parental Role Conflict r/t change in parental role

Compromised Family Coping r/t family role changes

Interrupted Family Processes r/t family roles shift

Ineffective Role Performance r/t role transition, aging

Ineffective Family Health Self-Management r/t excessive demands on individual or family

Risk for Impaired Parenting: Risk factor: role strain

Risk for Powerlessness: Risk factors: role strain, situational crisis, aging

Risk for Spiritual Distress: Risk factor: life change

Readiness for Enhanced Parenting: physical and emotional needs of children are met

Graves' Disease

See Hyperthyroidism

Grieving, Maladaptive

Complicated Grieving r/t expected or sudden death of a significant other with whom there was a volatile relationship, emotional instability, lack of social support

Risk for Maladaptive Grieving: Risk factors: death of a significant other with whom there was a volatile relationship, emotional instability, lack of social support

Groom Self (Inability to)

Bathing Self-Care Deficit (See **Self-Care Deficit, Bathing,** Section III)

Dressing Self-Care Deficit (See **Self-Care Deficit, Dressing,** Section III)

Growth and Development Lag

See Failure to Thrive, Child

Guillain-Barré Syndrome

Dysfunctional Ventilatory Weaning Response r/t fatigue

Impaired Spontaneous Ventilation r/t weak respiratory muscles

Risk for Aspiration: Risk factors: ineffective cough; depressed gag reflex

See Neurological Disorders

Guilt

Maladaptive Grieving r/t potential loss of significant person, animal, prized material possession, change in life role

Impaired Resilience (See **Resilience, Individual, Impaired,** Section III)

Situational Low Self-Esteem r/t unmet expectations of self

Risk for Maladaptive Grieving: Risk factors: actual loss of significant person, animal, prized material possession, change in life role

Risk for Post-Trauma Syndrome: Risk factor: exaggerated sense of responsibility for traumatic event

Readiness for Enhanced Spiritual Well-Being: desire to be in harmony with self, others, higher power or God

H

Hair Loss

Disturbed Body Image r/t psychological reaction to loss of hair

Imbalanced Nutrition: Less than Body Requirements r/t inability to ingest food because of biological, psychological, economic factors

Halitosis

Impaired Dentition r/t ineffective oral hygiene

Impaired Oral Mucous Membrane Integrity r/t ineffective oral hygiene

Hallucinations

Anxiety r/t threat to self-concept

Acute Confusion r/t alcohol abuse, delirium, dementia, mental illness, substance abuse

Ineffective Coping r/t distortion and insecurity of life events

Risk for Self-Mutilation: Risk factor: command hallucinations

Risk for Other-Directed Violence: Risk factors: catatonic excitement, manic excitement, rage or panic reactions, response to violent internal stimuli

Risk for Self-Directed Violence: Risk factors: catatonic excitement, manic excitement, rage or panic reactions, response to violent internal stimuli

Headache

Acute Pain r/t lack of knowledge of pain control techniques or methods to prevent headaches

Ineffective Health Self-Management r/t lack of knowledge, identification, elimination of aggravating factors

Head Injury

Ineffective Breathing Pattern r/t pressure damage to breathing center in brainstem

Acute Confusion r/t increased intracranial pressure

Risk for Ineffective Cerebral Tissue Perfusion: Risk factors: effects of increased intracranial pressure, trauma to brain

See Neurological Disorders

Health Behavior, Risk-Prone

Risk-Prone Health Behavior: Risk factors (See **Health Behavior, Risk-Prone,** Section III)

Risk for Metabolic Syndrome r/t obesity

Health Maintenance Problems

Ineffective Health Maintenance Behaviors (See **Health Maintenance Behaviors, Ineffective,** Section III)

Ineffective Health Self-Management (See **Health Self-Management, Ineffective,** Section III)

Health-Seeking Person

Readiness for Enhanced Health literacy (See **Health Literacy, Readiness for Enhanced,** Section III)

Readiness for Enhanced Health Self-Management (See **Health Self-Management, Readiness for Enhanced,** Section III)

Hearing Impairment

Impaired Verbal Communication r/t inability to hear own voice

Hearing Loss (see Appendix E on Evolve)

Social Isolation r/t difficulty with communication

Heart Attack

See MI (Myocardial Infarction)

Heartburn

Nausea r/t gastrointestinal irritation

Acute Pain: Heartburn r/t inflammation of stomach and esophagus

Risk for Imbalanced Nutrition: Less than Body Requirements: Risk factor: pain after eating

Readiness for Enhanced Knowledge: expresses an interest in learning

See Gastroesophageal Reflux Disease (GERD)

Heart Failure

Decreased Activity Tolerance r/t weakness, fatigue, shortness of breath

Decreased Cardiac Output r/t impaired cardiac function, increased preload, decreased contractility, increased afterload

Constipation r/t activity intolerance

Fatigue r/t disease process with decreased cardiac output

Fear r/t threat to one's own well-being

Excess Fluid Volume r/t impaired excretion of sodium and water

Impaired Gas Exchange r/t excessive fluid in interstitial space of lungs

Powerlessness r/t illness-related regimen

Risk for Shock (Cardiogenic): Risk factors: decreased contractility of heart, increased afterload

Readiness for Enhanced Health Management (See **Health Management, Readiness for Enhanced,** Section III)

See Child with Chronic Condition; Congenital Heart Disease/Cardiac Anomalies; Hospitalized Child

Heart Surgery

See Coronary Artery Bypass Grafting (CABG)

Heat Stroke

Deficient Fluid Volume r/t profuse diaphoresis from high environmental temperature

Hyperthermia r/t vigorous activity, high environmental temperature, inappropriate clothing

Hematemesis

See GI Bleed (Gastrointestinal Bleeding)

Hematuria

See Kidney Stone; UTI (Urinary Tract Infection)

Hemianopia

Anxiety r/t change in vision

Unilateral Neglect r/t effects of disturbed perceptual abilities

Risk for Injury: Risk factor: disturbed sensory perception

Hemiplegia

Anxiety r/t change in health status

Disturbed Body Image r/t functional loss of one side of body

Impaired Physical Mobility r/t loss of neurological control of involved extremities

Self-Care Deficit: Specify r/t neuromuscular impairment

Impaired Sitting r/t partial paralysis

Impaired Standing r/t partial paralysis

Impaired Transfer Ability r/t partial paralysis

Unilateral Neglect r/t effects of disturbed perceptual abilities

Impaired Walking r/t loss of neurological control of involved extremities

Risk for Adult Falls: Risk factor: impaired mobility

Risk for Impaired Skin Integrity: Risk factors: alteration in sensation, immobility; pressure over bony prominence

See CVA (Cerebrovascular Accident)

Hemodialysis

Ineffective Coping r/t situational crisis

Interrupted Family Processes r/t changes in role responsibilities as a result of therapy regimen

Excess Fluid Volume r/t renal disease with minimal urine output

Powerlessness r/t treatment regimen

Risk for Caregiver Role Strain: Risk factor: complexity of care receiver treatment

Risk for Electrolyte Imbalance: Risk factor: effect of metabolic state on renal function

Risk for deficient Fluid Volume: Risk factor: excessive removal of fluid during dialysis

Risk for Infection: Risk factors: exposure to blood products, risk for developing hepatitis B or C, impaired immune system

Risk for Injury: Risk factors: clotting of blood access, abnormal surface for blood flow

Risk for Impaired Tissue Integrity: Risk factor: mechanical factor associated with fistula formation

Readiness for Enhanced Knowledge: expresses an interest in learning

See Renal Failure; Renal Failure, Child with Chronic Condition

Hemodynamic Monitoring

Risk for Infection: Risk factor: invasive procedure

Risk for Injury: Risk factors: inadvertent wedging of catheter, dislodgment of catheter, disconnection of catheter

Risk for Impaired Tissue Integrity: Risk factor: invasive procedure

See Shock, Cardiogenic; Shock, Hypovolemic; Shock, Septic

Hemolytic Uremic Syndrome

Fatigue r/t decreased red blood cells

Fear r/t serious condition with unknown outcome

Deficient Fluid Volume r/t vomiting, diarrhea

Nausea r/t effects of uremia

Risk for Injury: Risk factors: decreased platelet count, seizure activity

Risk for Impaired Skin Integrity: Risk factor: diarrhea

See Hospitalized Child; Renal Failure, Acute/Chronic, Child

Hemophilia

Fear r/t high risk for AIDS infection from contaminated blood products

Impaired Physical Mobility r/t pain from acute bleeds, imposed activity restrictions, joint pain

Acute Pain r/t bleeding into body tissues

Risk for Bleeding: Risk factors: deficient clotting factors, child's developmental level, age-appropriate play, inappropriate use of toys or sports equipment

Readiness for Enhanced Knowledge: expresses an interest in learning

See Child with Chronic Condition; Hospitalized Child; Maturational Issues, Adolescent

Hemoptysis

Fear r/t serious threat to well-being

Risk for Ineffective Airway Clearance: Risk factor: obstruction of airway with blood and mucus

Risk for Deficient Fluid Volume: Risk factor: excessive loss of blood

Hemorrhage

Fear r/t threat to well-being

Deficient Fluid Volume r/t massive blood loss

See Hypovolemic Shock

Hemorrhoidectomy

Anxiety r/t embarrassment, need for privacy

Constipation r/t fear of pain with defecation

Acute Pain r/t surgical procedure

Urinary Retention r/t pain, anesthetic effect

Risk for Bleeding: Risk factors: inadequate clotting, trauma from surgery

Readiness for Enhanced Knowledge: expresses an interest in learning

Hemorrhoids

Impaired Comfort r/t itching in rectal area

Constipation r/t painful defecation, poor bowel habits

Impaired Sitting r/t pain and pressure

Readiness for Enhanced Knowledge: expresses an interest in learning

Hemothorax

Deficient Fluid Volume r/t blood in pleural space

See Pneumothorax

Hepatitis

Decreased Activity Tolerance r/t weakness or fatigue caused by infection

Decreased Diversional Activity Engagement r/t isolation

Fatigue r/t infectious process, altered body chemistry

Imbalanced Nutrition: Less than Body Requirements r/t anorexia, impaired use of proteins and carbohydrates

Acute Pain r/t edema of liver, bile irritating skin

Social Isolation r/t treatment-imposed isolation

Risk for Imbalanced Fluid Volume: Risk factor: excessive loss of fluids from vomiting and diarrhea

Readiness for Enhanced Knowledge: expresses an interest in learning

Hernia

See Hiatal Hernia; Inguinal Hernia Repair

Herniated Disk

See Low Back Pain

Herniorrhaphy

See Inguinal Hernia Repair

Herpes in Pregnancy

Fear r/t threat to fetus, impending surgery

Situational Low Self-Esteem r/t threat to fetus as a result of disease process

Risk for Infection: Infant: Risk factors: transplacental transfer during primary herpes, exposure to active herpes during birth process

See Herpes Simplex II

Herpes Simplex I

Impaired Oral Mucous Membrane Integrity r/t inflammatory changes in mouth

Herpes Simplex II

Ineffective Health Maintenance Behaviors r/t deficient knowledge regarding treatment, prevention, spread of disease

Acute Pain r/t active herpes lesion

Situational Low Self-Esteem r/t expressions of shame or guilt

Sexual Dysfunction r/t disease process

Impaired Tissue Integrity r/t active herpes lesion

Impaired Urinary Elimination r/t pain with urination

Herpes Zoster

See Shingles

HHNS (Hyperosmolar Hyperglycemic Nonketotic Syndrome)

See Hyperosmolar Hyperglycemic Nonketotic Syndrome (HHNS)

Hiatal Hernia

Ineffective Health Maintenance Behaviors r/t deficient knowledge regarding care of disease

Nausea r/t effects of gastric contents in esophagus

Imbalanced Nutrition: Less than Body Requirements r/t pain after eating

Acute Pain r/t gastroesophageal reflux

Hip Fracture

Acute Confusion r/t sensory overload, sensory deprivation, medication side effects, advanced age, pain

Constipation r/t immobility, opioids, anesthesia

Fear r/t outcome of treatment, future mobility, present helplessness

Impaired Physical Mobility r/t surgical incision, temporary absence of weight bearing, pain when walking

Acute Pain r/t injury, surgical procedure, movement

Powerlessness r/t health care environment

Self-Care Deficit: Specify r/t musculoskeletal impairment

Impaired Transfer Ability r/t immobilization of hip

Impaired Walking r/t temporary absence of weight bearing

Risk for Bleeding: Risk factors: postoperative complication, surgical blood loss

Risk for Surgical Site Infection: Risk factor: invasive procedure

Risk for Injury: Risk factors: activities such as greater than 90-degree flexion of hips that can result in dislodged prosthesis, unsteadiness when ambulating

Risk for Perioperative Positioning Injury: Risk factors: immobilization, muscle weakness, emaciation

Risk for Peripheral Neurovascular Dysfunction: Risk factors: trauma, vascular obstruction, fracture

Risk for Impaired Skin Integrity: Risk factor: immobility

Risk for Thrombosis: Risk factors: immobility, trauma

Hip Replacement

See Total Joint Replacement (Total Hip/Total Knee/Shoulder)

Hirschsprung's Disease

Constipation: Bowel Obstruction r/t inhibited peristalsis as a result of congenital absence of parasympathetic ganglion cells in distal colon

Maladaptive Grieving r/t loss of perfect child, birth of child with congenital defect even though child expected to be normal within 2 years

Imbalanced Nutrition: Less than Body Requirements r/t anorexia, pain from distended colon

Acute Pain r/t distended colon, incisional postoperative pain

Impaired Skin Integrity r/t stoma, potential skin care problems associated with stoma

Readiness for Enhanced Knowledge: expresses an interest in learning

See Hospitalized Child

Hirsutism

Disturbed Body Image r/t excessive hair

Hitting Behavior

Acute Confusion r/t dementia, alcohol abuse, drug abuse, delirium

Risk for Other-Directed Violence (See **Violence, Other-Directed, Risk for,** Section III)

HIV (Human Immunodeficiency Virus)

Fear r/t possible death

Ineffective Protection r/t depressed immune system

Readiness for Enhanced Health Literacy: expresses desire to enhance understanding of health information to make health care choices

See AIDS (Acquired Immunodeficiency Syndrome)

Hodgkin's Disease

See Anemia; Cancer; Chemotherapy

Homelessness

Ineffective Home Maintenance Behaviors r/t impaired cognitive or emotional functioning, inadequate support system, insufficient finances

Home Maintenance Problems

Ineffective Home Maintenance Behaviors (See **Home Maintenance, Impaired,** Section III)

Self-Neglect r/t mental illness, substance abuse, cognitive impairment

Powerlessness r/t interpersonal interactions

Risk for Physical Trauma: Risk factor: being in high-crime neighborhood

Hope

Readiness for Enhanced Hope (See **Hope, Readiness for Enhanced,** Section III)

Hopelessness

Hopelessness (See **Hopelessness,** Section III)

Hospitalized Child

Decreased Activity Tolerance r/t fatigue associated with acute illness

Anxiety: Separation: Child r/t familiar surroundings and separation from family and friends

Compromised Family Coping r/t possible prolonged hospitalization that exhausts supportive capacity of significant people

Ineffective Coping: Parent r/t possible guilt regarding hospitalization of child, parental inadequacies

Decreased Diversional Activity Engagement r/t immobility, monotonous environment, frequent or lengthy treatments, reluctance to participate, therapeutic isolation, separation from peers

Interrupted Family Processes r/t situational crisis of illness, disease, hospitalization

Fear r/t deficient knowledge or maturational level with fear of unknown, mutilation, painful procedures, surgery

Hopelessness: Child r/t prolonged activity restriction, uncertain prognosis

Insomnia: Child or Parent r/t 24-hour care needs of hospitalization

Acute Pain r/t treatments, diagnostic or therapeutic procedures, disease process

Powerlessness: Child r/t health care environment, illness-related regimen

Risk for Impaired Attachment: Risk factor: separation

Risk for Injury: Risk factors: unfamiliar environment, developmental age, lack of parental knowledge regarding safety (e.g., side rails, IV site/pole)

Risk for Imbalanced Nutrition: Less than Body Requirements: Risk factors: anorexia, absence of familiar foods, cultural preferences

Readiness for Enhanced Family Coping: impact of crisis on family values, priorities, goals, relationships in family

See Child with Chronic Condition

Hostile Behavior

Risk for Other-Directed Violence: Risk factor: antisocial personality disorder

HTN (Hypertension)

Ineffective Health Self-Management (See **Health Management, Ineffective,** Section III)

Readiness for Enhanced Health Self-Management (See **Health Management, Readiness for Enhanced,** Section III)

Risk for Overweight: Risk factor: lack of knowledge of relationship between diet and disease process

Human Energy Field

Energy Field, Imbalanced (See **Imbalanced Energy Field,** Section III)

Humiliating Experience

Risk for Compromised Human Dignity (See **Human Dignity, Compromised, Risk for,** Section III)

Huntington's Disease

Decisional Conflict r/t whether to have children

See Neurological Disorders

Hydrocele

Acute Pain r/t severely enlarged hydrocele

Ineffective Sexuality Pattern r/t recent surgery on area of scrotum

Hydrocephalus

Decisional Conflict r/t unclear or conflicting values regarding selection of treatment modality

Interrupted Family processes r/t situational crisis

Imbalanced Nutrition: Less than Body Requirements r/t inadequate intake as a result of anorexia, nausea, vomiting, feeding difficulties

Risk for Infection: Risk factor: sequelae of invasive procedure (shunt placement)

Risk for Ineffective Cerebral Tissue Perfusion: Risk factors: interrupted flow, hypervolemia of cerebral ventricles

Risk for Adult Falls: Risk factors: acute illness, alteration in cognitive functioning

See Normal Pressure Hydrocephalus (NPH); Child with Chronic Condition; Hospitalized Child; Premature Infant (Child); Premature Infant (Parent)

Hygiene, Inability to Provide Own

Frail Elderly Syndrome r/t living alone

Self-Neglect (See **Self-Neglect,** Section III)

Bathing Self-Care Deficit (See **Self-Care Deficit, Bathing,** Section III)

Hyperactive Syndrome

Decisional Conflict r/t multiple or divergent sources of information regarding education, nutrition, medication regimens; willingness to change own food habits; limited resources

Parental Role Conflict: When Siblings Present r/t increased attention toward hyperactive child

Compromised Family Coping r/t unsuccessful strategies to control excessive activity, behaviors, frustration, anger

Ineffective Impulse Control r/t disorder of development, environment that might cause frustration or irritation

Ineffective Role Performance: Parent r/t stressors associated with dealing with hyperactive child, perceived or projected blame for causes of child's behavior, unmet needs for support or care, lack of energy to provide for those needs

Chronic Low Self-Esteem r/t inability to achieve socially acceptable behaviors; frustration; frequent reprimands, punishment, or scolding for uncontrolled activity and behaviors; mood fluctuations and restlessness; inability to succeed academically; lack of peer support

Impaired Social Interaction r/t impulsive and overactive behaviors, concomitant emotional difficulties, distractibility and excitability

Risk for Impaired Parenting: Risk factor: disruptive or uncontrollable behaviors of child

Risk for Other-Directed Violence: Parent or Child: Risk factors: frustration with disruptive behavior, anger, unsuccessful relationships

Hyperbilirubinemia, Neonatal

Anxiety: Parent r/t threat to infant, unknown future

Parental Role Conflict r/t interruption of family life because of care regimen

Neonatal Hyperbilirubinemia r/t abnormal breakdown of red blood cells following birth

Imbalanced Nutrition: Less than Body Requirements: Infant r/t disinterest in feeding because of jaundice-related lethargy

Risk for Injury: Infant: Risk factors: kernicterus, phototherapy lights

Risk for Ineffective Thermoregulation: Risk factor: phototherapy

Readiness for Enhanced Health Self-Management: Parent: expresses desire to manage treatment: assessment of jaundice when infant is discharged from the hospital, when to call the physician, and possible preventive measures such as frequent breastfeeding (See **Neonatal Hyperbilirubinemia, Risk for,** Section III)

Hypercalcemia

Decreased Cardiac Output r/t bradydysrhythmia

Impaired Physical Mobility r/t decreased muscle tone

Imbalanced Nutrition: Less than Body Requirements r/t gastrointestinal manifestations of hypercalcemia (nausea, anorexia, ileus)

Risk for Disuse Syndrome: Risk factor: comatose state impairing mobility

Hypercapnia

Fear r/t difficulty breathing

Impaired Gas Exchange r/t ventilation-perfusion imbalance, retention of carbon dioxide

See ARDS (Adult Respiratory Distress Syndrome); COPD (Chronic Obstructive Pulmonary Disorder); Sleep Apnea

Hyperemesis Gravidarum

Anxiety r/t threat to self and infant, hospitalization

Deficient Fluid Volume r/t excessive vomiting

Ineffective Home Maintenance Behaviors r/t chronic nausea, inability to function

Nausea r/t hormonal changes of pregnancy

Imbalanced Nutrition: Less than Body Requirements r/t excessive vomiting

Powerlessness r/t health care regimen

Social Isolation r/t hospitalization

Risk for Electrolyte Imbalance: Risk factor: vomiting

Hyperglycemia

Ineffective Health Self-Management r/t complexity of therapeutic regimen, decisional conflicts, economic difficulties, unsupportive family, insufficient cues to action, deficient knowledge, mistrust, lack of acknowledgment of seriousness of condition

Risk for Unstable Blood Glucose Level (See **Glucose Level, Blood, Unstable, Risk for,** Section III)

See Diabetes Mellitus

Hyperkalemia

Risk for Decreased Activity Tolerance: Risk factor: muscle weakness

Risk for Decreased Cardiac Tissue Perfusion: Risk factor: abnormal electrolyte level affecting heart rate and rhythm

Risk for Excess Fluid Volume: Risk factor: untreated renal failure

Hypernatremia

Risk for Imbalanced Fluid Volume: Risk factors: abnormal water loss, inadequate water intake

Hyperosmolar Hyperglycemic Nonketotic Syndrome (HHNS)

Acute Confusion r/t dehydration, electrolyte imbalance

Deficient Fluid Volume r/t polyuria, hyperglycemia, inadequate fluid intake

Risk for Electrolyte Imbalance: Risk factor: effect of metabolic state on kidney function

Risk for Injury: Seizures: Risk factors: hyperosmolar state, electrolyte imbalance

See Diabetes Mellitus; Diabetes Mellitus, Juvenile (Insulin-Dependent Diabetes Mellitus Type 1)

Hyperphosphatemia

Deficient Knowledge r/t dietary changes needed to control phosphate levels

See Renal Failure

Hypersensitivity to Slight Criticism

Defensive Coping r/t situational crisis, psychological impairment, substance abuse

Hypertension (HTN)

See HTN (Hypertension)

Risk for Decreased Cardiac Output: Risk factors: decreased contractility and altered conductivity associated with myocardial damage

Risk for Unstable Blood Pressure (See **Unstable Blood Pressure, Risk for,** Section III)

Hyperthermia

Hyperthermia (See **Hyperthermia,** Section III)

Hyperthyroidism

Anxiety r/t increased stimulation, loss of control

Diarrhea r/t increased gastric motility

Insomnia r/t anxiety, excessive sympathetic discharge

Imbalanced Nutrition: Less than Body Requirements r/t increased metabolic rate, increased gastrointestinal activity

Risk for Injury: Eye Damage: Risk factor: protruding eyes without sufficient lubrication

Risk for Unstable Blood Pressure r/t hyperthyroidism

Readiness for Enhanced Knowledge: expresses an interest in learning

Hyperventilation

Ineffective Breathing Pattern r/t anxiety, acid-base imbalance

See Anxiety Disorder; Dyspnea; Heart Failure

Hypocalcemia

Decreased Activity Tolerance r/t neuromuscular irritability

Ineffective Breathing Pattern r/t laryngospasm

Imbalanced Nutrition: Less than Body Requirements r/t effects of vitamin D deficiency, renal failure, malabsorption, laxative use

Hypoglycemia

Acute Confusion r/t insufficient blood glucose to brain

Ineffective Health Self-Management r/t deficient knowledge regarding disease process, self-care

Imbalanced Nutrition: Less than Body Requirements r/t imbalance of glucose and insulin level

Risk for Unstable Blood Glucose Level (See **Glucose Level, Blood, Unstable, Risk for,** Section III)

See Diabetes Mellitus; Diabetes Mellitus, Juvenile (IDDM Type 1)

Hypokalemia

Decreased Activity Tolerance r/t muscle weakness

Risk for Decreased Cardiac Tissue Perfusion: Risk factor: possible dysrhythmia from electrolyte imbalance

Hypomagnesemia

Imbalanced Nutrition: Less than Body Requirements r/t deficient knowledge of nutrition, alcoholism

See Alcoholism

Hypomania

Insomnia r/t psychological stimulus

See Manic Disorder, Bipolar I

Hyponatremia

Acute Confusion r/t electrolyte imbalance

Excess Fluid Volume r/t excessive intake of hypotonic fluids

Risk for Injury: Risk factors: seizures, new onset of confusion

Hypoplastic Left Lung

See Congenital Heart Disease/Cardiac Anomalies

Hypotension

Decreased Cardiac Output r/t decreased preload, decreased contractility

Risk for Deficient Fluid Volume: Risk factor: excessive fluid loss

Risk for Ineffective Cerebral Tissue Perfusion: Risk factors: hypovolemia, decreased contractility, decreased afterload

Risk for Shock (See **Shock, Risk for,** Section III)

Risk for Unstable Blood Pressure (See **Unstable Blood Pressure, Risk for,** Section III)

See Dehydration; Heart Failure; MI (Myocardial Infarction)

Hypothermia

Hypothermia (See **Hypothermia,** Section III)

Risk for Hypothermia (See **Hypothermia, Risk for,** Section III)

Hypothyroidism

Decreased Activity Tolerance r/t muscular stiffness, shortness of breath on exertion

Constipation r/t decreased gastric motility

Impaired Gas Exchange r/t respiratory depression

Impaired Skin Integrity r/t edema, dry or scaly skin

Risk for Overweight: Risk factor: decreased metabolic process

Hypovolemic Shock

See Shock, Hypovolemic

Hypoxia

Acute Confusion r/t decreased oxygen supply to brain

Fear r/t breathlessness

Impaired Gas Exchange r/t altered oxygen supply, inability to transport oxygen

Risk for Shock (See **Shock, Risk for,** Section III)

Hysterectomy

Constipation r/t opioids, anesthesia, bowel manipulation during surgery

Ineffective Coping r/t situational crisis of surgery

Maladaptive Grieving r/t change in body image, loss of reproductive status

Acute Pain r/t surgical injury

Sexual Dysfunction r/t disturbance in self-concept

Urinary Retention r/t edema in area, anesthesia, opioids, pain

Risk for Bleeding: Risk factor: surgical procedure

Risk for Constipation: Risk factors: opioids, anesthesia, bowel manipulation during surgery

Risk for Ineffective Peripheral Tissue Perfusion: Risk factor: deficient knowledge of aggravating factors

Risk for Surgical Site Infection: Risk factor: invasive procedure

Readiness for Enhanced Knowledge: Expresses an interest in learning

See Surgery, Perioperative Care; Surgery, Preoperative Care; Surgery, Postoperative Care

I

IBS (Irritable Bowel Syndrome)

Constipation r/t low-residue diet, stress

Diarrhea r/t increased motility of intestines associated with disease process, stress

Ineffective Health Self-Management r/t deficient knowledge, powerlessness

Chronic Pain r/t spasms, increased motility of bowel

Risk for Electrolyte Imbalance: Risk factor: diarrhea

Readiness for Enhanced Health Self-Management: expresses desire to manage illness and prevent onset of symptoms

ICD (Implantable Cardioverter/Defibrillator)

Anxiety r/t possible dysrhythmia, threat of death

Decreased Cardiac Output r/t possible dysrhythmia

Readiness for Enhanced Knowledge: expresses an interest in learning

IDDM (Insulin-Dependent Diabetes Mellitus)

See Diabetes Mellitus

Identity Disturbance/Problems

Disturbed Personal Identity r/t situational crisis, psychological impairment, chronic illness, pain

Risk for Disturbed Personal Identity (See **Identity, Personal, Risk for Disturbed,** Section III)

Idiopathic Thrombocytopenic Purpura (ITP)

See ITP (Idiopathic Thrombocytopenic Purpura)

Ileal Conduit

Disturbed Body Image r/t presence of stoma

Ineffective Health Self-Management r/t new skills required to care for appliance and self

Ineffective Sexuality Pattern r/t altered body function and structure

Social Isolation r/t alteration in physical appearance, fear of accidental spill of urine

Risk for Latex Allergy Reaction: Risk factor: repeated exposures to latex associated with treatment and management of disease

Risk for Impaired Skin Integrity: Risk factor: difficulty obtaining tight seal of appliance

Readiness for Enhanced Knowledge: expresses an interest in learning

Ileostomy

Disturbed Body Image r/t presence of stoma

Diarrhea r/t dietary changes, alteration in intestinal motility

Deficient Knowledge r/t limited practice of stoma care, dietary modifications

Ineffective Sexuality Pattern r/t altered body function and structure

Social Isolation r/t alteration in physical appearance, fear of accidental spill of ostomy contents

Risk for Impaired Skin Integrity: Risk factors: difficulty obtaining tight seal of appliance, caustic drainage

Readiness for Enhanced Knowledge: expresses an interest in learning

Ileus

Deficient Fluid Volume r/t loss of fluids from vomiting, fluids trapped in bowel

Dysfunctional Gastrointestinal Motility r/t effects of surgery, decreased perfusion of intestines, medication effect, immobility

Nausea r/t gastrointestinal irritation

Acute Pain r/t pressure, abdominal distention

Readiness for Enhanced Knowledge: expresses an interest in learning

Immigration Transition, Risk for Complicated

Anxiety r/t changes in safety and security needs

Fear r/t unfamiliar environment, separation from support system, possible language barrier

Impaired Social Interaction r/t possible communication or sociocultural barriers

Risk for Loneliness: Risk factor: separation from support system

Risk for Powerlessness: Risk factor: insufficient social support

Risk for Relocation Stress Syndrome: Risk factors: insufficient support system, social isolation, and potential communication barriers

Risk for Impaired Resilience: Risk factor: decreased ability to adapt to adverse or changing situations

Readiness for Enhanced Coping: expresses desire to enhance social support

Readiness for Enhanced Knowledge: expresses a desire to become familiar with resources within their environment

Immobility

Ineffective Breathing Pattern r/t inability to deep breathe in supine position

Acute Confusion: Elderly r/t sensory deprivation from immobility

Constipation r/t immobility

Risk for Frail Elderly Syndrome: Risk factors: low physical activity, bed rest

Impaired Physical Mobility r/t medically imposed bed rest

Ineffective Peripheral Tissue Perfusion r/t interruption of venous flow

Powerlessness r/t forced immobility from health care environment

Impaired Walking r/t limited physical mobility, deconditioning of body

Risk for Disuse Syndrome: Risk factor: immobilization

Risk for Impaired Skin Integrity: Risk factors: pressure over bony prominences, shearing forces when moved; pressure from devices

Risk for Impaired Tissue Integrity: Risk factors: mechanical factors from pressure over bony prominences, shearing forces when moved; pressure from devices

Risk for Overweight: Risk factor: energy expenditure less than energy intake

Risk for Thrombosis: Risk factor: lack of physical activity

Readiness for Enhanced Knowledge: expresses an interest in learning

Immunization

(See **Readiness for Enhanced Health Literacy,** Section III)

(See **Readiness for Enhanced Health Self-Management,** Section III)

Immunosuppression

Risk for Infection: Risk factors: immunosuppression; exposure to disease outbreak

Impaired Social Interaction r/t therapeutic isolation

Impaction of Stool

Constipation r/t decreased fluid intake, less than adequate amounts of fiber and bulk-forming foods in diet, medication effect, or immobility

Impaired Sitting

Impaired Physical Mobility r/t musculoskeletal, cognitive, or neuromuscular disorder

Impaired Standing

Decreased Activity Tolerance r/t insufficient physiological or psychological energy

Powerlessness r/t loss of function

Imperforate Anus

Anxiety r/t ability to care for newborn

Deficient Knowledge r/t home care for newborn

Impaired Skin Integrity r/t pruritus

Impetigo

Impaired Skin Integrity r/t infectious disease

Readiness for Enhanced Knowledge: expresses an interest in learning

See Communicable Diseases, Childhood (e.g., Measles, Mumps, Rubella, Chickenpox, Scabies, Lice)

Implantable Cardioverter/Defibrillator (ICD)

See ICD (Implantable Cardioverter/Defibrillator)

Impotence

Situational Low Self-Esteem r/t physiological crisis, inability to practice usual sexual activity

Sexual Dysfunction r/t altered body function

Readiness for Enhanced Knowledge: treatment information for erectile dysfunction

See Erectile Dysfunction (ED)

Impulsiveness

Ineffective Impulse Control (See **Impulse Control, Ineffective,** Section III)

Inactivity

Decreased Activity Tolerance r/t imbalance between oxygen supply and demand, sedentary lifestyle, weakness, immobility

Hopelessness r/t deteriorating physiological condition, long-term stress, social isolation

Impaired Physical Mobility r/t intolerance to activity, decreased strength and endurance, depression, severe anxiety, musculoskeletal impairment, perceptual or cognitive impairment, neuromuscular impairment, pain, discomfort

Risk for Constipation: Risk factor: insufficient physical activity

Incompetent Cervix

See Premature Dilation of the Cervix (Incompetent Cervix)

Incontinence of Stool

Disturbed Body Image r/t inability to control elimination of stool

Impaired Bowel Continence r/t decreased awareness of need to defecate, loss of sphincter control

Toileting Self-Care Deficit r/t cognitive impairment, neuromuscular impairment, perceptual impairment, weakness

Situational Low Self-Esteem r/t inability to control elimination of stool

Risk for Impaired Skin Integrity: Risk factor: presence of stool

Incontinence of Urine

Disability-Associated Urinary Incontinence r/t altered environment; sensory, cognitive, or mobility deficits

Stress Urinary Incontinence (See **Incontinence, Urinary, Stress,** Section III)

Urge Urinary Incontinence (See **Incontinence, Urinary, Urge,** Section III)

Toileting Self-Care Deficit r/t cognitive impairment

Situational Low Self-Esteem r/t inability to control passage of urine

Risk for Impaired Skin Integrity: Risk factor: presence of urine on perineal skin

Indigestion

Nausea r/t gastrointestinal irritation

Imbalanced Nutrition: Less than Body Requirements r/t discomfort when eating

Induction of Labor

Anxiety r/t medical interventions, powerlessness

Decisional Conflict r/t perceived threat to idealized birth

Ineffective Coping r/t situational crisis of medical intervention in birthing process

Acute Pain r/t contractions

Situational Low Self-Esteem r/t inability to carry out normal labor

Risk for Injury: Maternal and Fetal: Risk factors: hypertonic uterus, potential prematurity of newborn

Readiness for Enhanced Family Processes: family support during induction of labor

Infant Apnea

See Premature Infant (Child); Respiratory Conditions of the Neonate; Sudden Infant Death Syndrome (SIDS)

Infant Behavior

Disorganized Infant Behavior r/t pain, oral/motor problems, feeding intolerance, environmental overstimulation, lack of containment or boundaries, prematurity, invasive or painful procedures

Risk for Disorganized Infant Behavior: Risk factors: pain, oral/motor problems, environmental overstimulation, lack of containment or boundaries

Readiness for Enhanced Organized Infant behavior: stable physiologic measures, use of some self-regulatory measures

Infant Care

Readiness for Enhanced Childbearing Process: a pattern of preparing for, maintaining, and strengthening care of newborn infant

Infant Feeding Dynamic, Ineffective

Ineffective Infant Feeding Dynamic r/t prematurity, neurological impairment or delay, oral hypersensitivity, prolonged nothing-by-mouth order

Infant of Diabetic Mother

Decreased Cardiac Output r/t cardiomegaly

Deficient Fluid Volume r/t increased urinary excretion and osmotic diuresis

Imbalanced Nutrition: Less than Body Requirements r/t hypotonia, lethargy, poor sucking, postnatal metabolic changes from hyperglycemia to hypoglycemia and hyperinsulinism

Risk for Impaired Gas Exchange: Risk factors: increased incidence of cardiomegaly, prematurity

Risk for Unstable Blood Glucose Level: Risk factor: metabolic change from hyperglycemia to hypoglycemia and hyperinsulinism

Risk for Disturbed Maternal–Fetal Dyad: Risk factor: impaired glucose metabolism

See Premature Infant (Child); Respiratory Conditions of the Neonate

Infant of Substance-Abusing Mother

See Neonatal Abstinence Syndrome

Infantile Polyarteritis

See Kawasaki Disease

Infection, Potential for

Risk for Infection (See **Infection, Risk for,** Section III)

Infectious Processes

I

Impaired Comfort r/t distressing symptoms

Diarrhea r/t gastrointestinal inflammation

Ineffective Health Maintenance Behaviors r/t knowledge deficit regarding transmission, symptoms, and treatment

Ineffective Health Self-Management r/t lack of knowledge regarding preventive immunizations

Ineffective Protection r/t inadequate nutrition, abnormal blood profiles, drug therapies, treatments

Impaired Social Interaction r/t therapeutic isolation

Risk for Electrolyte Imbalance: Risk factors: vomiting, diarrhea

Risk for Deficient Fluid Volume: Risk factors: vomiting, diarrhea, inadequate fluid intake

Risk for Infection: Risk factor: increased environmental exposure when in close proximity to infected persons

Risk for Surgical Site Infection r/t immunosuppression

Risk for Ineffective Thermoregulation: Risk factor: infectious process

Readiness for Enhanced Knowledge: expresses desire for information regarding prevention and treatment

Infertility

Ineffective Health Self-Management r/t deficient knowledge about infertility

Powerlessness r/t infertility

Chronic Sorrow r/t inability to conceive a child

Spiritual Distress r/t inability to conceive a child

Inflammatory Bowel Disease (Child and Adult)

Ineffective Coping r/t repeated episodes of diarrhea

Diarrhea r/t effects of inflammatory changes of the bowel

Deficient Fluid Volume r/t frequent and loose stools

Imbalanced Nutrition: Less than Body Requirements r/t anorexia, decreased absorption of nutrients from gastrointestinal tract

Acute Pain r/t abdominal cramping and anal irritation

Impaired Skin Integrity r/t frequent stools, development of anal fissures

Social Isolation r/t diarrhea

See Child with Chronic Condition; Crohn's Disease; Hospitalized Child; Maturational Issues, Adolescent

Influenza

See Infectious Processes

Inguinal Hernia Repair

Impaired Physical Mobility r/t pain at surgical site and fear of causing hernia to rupture

Acute Pain r/t surgical procedure

Urinary Retention r/t possible edema at surgical site

Risk for Surgical Site Infection: Risk factor: surgical procedure

Injury

Risk for Adult Falls: Risk factors: orthostatic hypotension, impaired physical mobility, diminished mental status

Risk for Child Falls: Risk factors: impaired physical mobility, diminished mental status

Risk for Injury: Risk factor: environmental conditions interacting with client's adaptive and defensive resources

Risk for Corneal Injury: Risk factors: blinking less than five times per minute, mechanical ventilation, pharmaceutical agent, prolonged hospitalization

Risk for Thermal Injury: Risk factors: cognitive impairment, inadequate supervision, developmental level

Risk for Urinary Tract Injury: Risk factor: inflammation and/or infection from long-term use of urinary catheter

Insomnia

(See **Insomnia,** Section III)

Insulin Shock

See Hypoglycemia

Intellectual Disability

Impaired Verbal Communication r/t developmental delay

Interrupted Family Processes r/t crisis of diagnosis and situational transition

Maladaptive Grieving r/t loss of perfect child, birth of child with congenital defect or subsequent head injury

Deficient Community Health r/t lack of programs to address developmental deficiencies

Ineffective Home Maintenance Behaviors r/t insufficient support systems

Self-Neglect r/t learning disability

Self-Care Deficit: Bathing, Dressing, Feeding, Toileting r/t perceptual or cognitive impairment

Self-Mutilation r/t inability to express tension verbally

Social Isolation r/t delay in accomplishing developmental tasks

Spiritual Distress r/t chronic condition of child with special needs

Stress Overload r/t intense, repeated stressor (chronic condition)

Impaired Swallowing r/t neuromuscular impairment

Risk for Ineffective Activity Planning r/t inability to process information

Risk for Impaired Religiosity: Risk factor: social isolation

Risk for Self-Mutilation: Risk factors: separation anxiety, depersonalization

Readiness for Enhanced Family Coping: adaptation and acceptance of child's condition and needs

See Child with Chronic Condition; Safety, Childhood

Intermittent Claudication

Deficient Knowledge r/t lack of knowledge of cause and treatment of peripheral vascular diseases

Acute Pain r/t decreased circulation to extremities with activity

Ineffective Peripheral Tissue Perfusion r/t interruption of arterial flow

Risk for Injury: Risk factor: tissue hypoxia

Readiness for Enhanced Knowledge: prevention of pain and impaired circulation

See Peripheral Vascular Disease (PVD)

Internal Cardioverter/Defibrillator (ICD)

See ICD (Implantable Cardioverter/Defibrillator)

Internal Fixation

Impaired Walking r/t repair of fracture

Risk for Infection: Risk factors: traumatized tissue, broken skin

See Fracture

Interstitial Cystitis

Acute Pain r/t inflammatory process

Impaired Urinary Elimination r/t inflammation of bladder

Risk for Infection: Risk factor: suppressed inflammatory response

Readiness for Enhanced Knowledge: expresses an interest in learning

Intervertebral Disk Excision

See Laminectomy

Intestinal Obstruction

See Ileus; Bowel Obstruction

Intestinal Perforation

See Peritonitis

Intoxication

Anxiety r/t loss of control of actions

Acute Confusion r/t alcohol abuse

Ineffective Coping r/t use of mind-altering substances as a means of coping

Impaired Memory r/t effects of alcohol on mind

Risk for Aspiration: Risk factors: diminished mental status, vomiting

Risk for Adult Falls: Risk factor: diminished mental status

Risk for Other-Directed Violence: Risk factor: inability to control thoughts and actions

Intraaortic Balloon Counterpulsation

Anxiety r/t device providing cardiovascular assistance

Decreased Cardiac Output r/t heart dysfunction needing counterpulsation

Compromised Family Coping r/t seriousness of significant other's medical condition

Impaired Physical Mobility r/t restriction of movement because of mechanical device

Risk for Peripheral Neurovascular Dysfunction: Risk factors: vascular obstruction of balloon catheter, thrombus formation, emboli, edema

Risk for Infection: Risk factor: invasive procedure

Risk for Impaired Tissue Integrity: Risk factor: invasive procedure

Intracranial Pressure, Increased

Ineffective Breathing Pattern r/t pressure damage to breathing center in brainstem

Acute Confusion r/t increased intracranial pressure

Impaired Memory r/t neurological disturbance

Vision Loss r/t pressure damage to sensory centers in brain

Risk for Ineffective Cerebral Tissue Perfusion: Risk factors: body position, cerebral vessel circulation deficits

See Head Injury; Subarachnoid Hemorrhage

Intrauterine Growth Retardation

Anxiety: Maternal r/t threat to fetus

Ineffective Coping: Maternal r/t situational crisis, threat to fetus

Impaired Gas Exchange r/t insufficient placental perfusion

Imbalanced Nutrition: Less than Body Requirements r/t insufficient placenta

Situational Low Self-Esteem: Maternal r/t guilt about threat to fetus

Spiritual Distress r/t unknown outcome of fetus

Risk for Powerlessness: Risk factor: unknown outcome of fetus

Intravenous Therapy

Risk for Vascular Trauma: Risk factor: infusion of irritating chemicals

Intubation, Endotracheal or Nasogastric

Disturbed Body Image r/t altered appearance with mechanical devices

Impaired Verbal Communication r/t endotracheal tube

Imbalanced Nutrition: Less than Body Requirements r/t inability to ingest food because of the presence of tubes

Impaired Oral Mucous Membrane r/t presence of tubes

Acute Pain r/t presence of tube

Iodine Reaction with Diagnostic Testing

Risk for Adverse Reaction to Iodinated Contrast Media (See **Reaction to Iodinated Contrast Media, Risk for Adverse,** Section III)

Irregular Pulse

See Dysrhythmia

Irritable Bowel Syndrome (IBS)

See IBS (Irritable Bowel Syndrome)

Isolation

Impaired Resilience (See **Resilience, Individual, Impaired,** Section III)

Social Isolation (See **Social Isolation,** Section III)

Itching

See Pruritus

ITP (Idiopathic Thrombocytopenic Purpura)

Decreased Diversional Activity Engagement r/t activity restrictions, safety precautions

Ineffective Protection r/t decreased platelet count

Risk for Bleeding: Risk factors: decreased platelet count, developmental level, age-appropriate play

J

Jaundice

Imbalanced Nutrition: Less than Body Requirements r/t decreased appetite with liver disorder

Risk for Bleeding: Risk factor: impaired liver function

Risk for Impaired Liver Function: Risk factors: possible viral infection, medication effect

Risk for Impaired Skin Integrity: Risk factors: pruritus, itching

See Cirrhosis; Hepatitis

Jaundice, Neonatal

See Hyperbilirubinemia, Neonatal

Jaw Pain and Heart Attacks

See Angina; Chest Pain; MI (Myocardial Infarction)

Jaw Surgery

Deficient Knowledge r/t emergency care for wired jaws (e.g., cutting bands and wires), oral care

Imbalanced Nutrition: Less than Body Requirements r/t jaws wired closed, difficulty eating

Acute Pain r/t surgical procedure

Impaired Swallowing r/t edema from surgery

Risk for Aspiration: Risk factor: wired jaws

Jittery

Anxiety r/t unconscious conflict about essential values and goals, threat to or change in health status

Death Anxiety r/t unresolved issues relating to end of life

Risk for Post-Trauma Syndrome: Risk factors: occupation, survivor's role in event, inadequate social support

Jock Itch

Ineffective Health Self-Management r/t prevention and treatment of disorder

Impaired Skin Integrity r/t moisture and irritating or tight-fitting clothing

See Pruritus

Joint Dislocation

See Dislocation of Joint

Joint Pain

See Arthritis; Bursitis; JRA (Juvenile Rheumatoid Arthritis); Osteoarthritis; Rheumatoid Arthritis (RA)

Joint Replacement

Risk for Peripheral Neurovascular Dysfunction: Risk factor: orthopedic surgery

Risk for Impaired Tissue Integrity: Risk factor: invasive procedure

See Total Joint Replacement (Total Hip/Total Knee/Shoulder)

JRA (Juvenile Rheumatoid Arthritis)

Impaired Comfort r/t altered health status

Fatigue r/t chronic inflammatory disease

Impaired Physical Mobility r/t pain, restricted joint movement

Acute Pain r/t swollen or inflamed joints, restricted movement, physical therapy

Self-Care Deficit: feeding, bathing, dressing, toileting r/t restricted joint movement, pain

Risk for Compromised Human Dignity: Risk factors: perceived intrusion by clinicians, invasion of privacy

Risk for Injury: Risk factors: impaired physical mobility, splints, adaptive devices, increased bleeding potential from anti-inflammatory medications

Risk for Impaired Resilience: Risk factor: chronic condition

Risk for Situational Low Self-Esteem: Risk factor: disturbed body image

Risk for Impaired Skin Integrity: Risk factors: splints, adaptive devices

See Child with Chronic Condition; Hospitalized Child

K

Kaposi's Sarcoma

Risk for Maladaptive Grieving: Risk factor: loss of social support

Risk for Impaired Religiosity: Risk factors: illness/hospitalization, ineffective coping

Risk for Impaired Resilience: Risk factor: serious illness

See AIDS (Acquired Immunodeficiency Syndrome)

Kawasaki Disease

Anxiety: Parental r/t progression of disease, complications of arthritis, and cardiac involvement

Impaired Comfort r/t altered health status

Hyperthermia r/t inflammatory disease process

Imbalanced Nutrition: Less than Body Requirements r/t impaired oral mucous membrane integrity

Impaired Oral Mucous Membrane Integrity r/t inflamed mouth and pharynx; swollen lips that become dry, cracked, fissured

Acute Pain r/t enlarged lymph nodes; erythematous skin rash that progresses to desquamation, peeling, denuding of skin

Impaired Skin integrity r/t inflammatory skin changes

Risk for Imbalanced Fluid Volume: Risk factor: hypovolemia

Risk for Decreased Cardiac Tissue Perfusion: Risk factor: cardiac involvement

Risk for Dry Mouth: Risk factor: decreased fluid intake

See Hospitalized Child

Keloids

Disturbed Body Image r/t presence of scar tissue at site of a healed skin injury

Readiness for Enhanced Health Self-Management: desire to have information to manage condition

Keratoconjunctivitis Sicca (Dry Eye Syndrome)

Risk for Dry Eye: Risk factors: aging, staring at a computer screen for long intervals

Risk for Infection: Risk factor: dry eyes that are more vulnerable to infection

Risk for Corneal Injury: Risk factors: dry eye, exposure of the eyeball

See Conjunctivitis

Keratoplasty

See Corneal Transplant

Ketoacidosis, Alcoholic

See Alcohol Withdrawal; Alcoholism

Ketoacidosis, Diabetic

Deficient Fluid Volume r/t excess excretion of urine, nausea, vomiting, increased respiration

Impaired Memory r/t fluid and electrolyte imbalance

Imbalanced Nutrition: Less than Body Requirements r/t body's inability to use nutrients

Risk for Unstable Blood Glucose Level: Risk factor: deficient knowledge of diabetes management (e.g., action plan)

Risk for Powerlessness: Risk factor: illness-related regimen

Risk for Impaired Resilience: Risk factor: complications of disease

See Diabetes Mellitus

Keyhole Heart Surgery

See MIDCAB (Minimally Invasive Direct Coronary Artery Bypass)

Kidney Disease Screening

Readiness for Enhanced Health Self-Management: seeks information for screening

Risk for Electrolyte Imbalance r/t renal dysfunction

Kidney Failure

See Renal Failure

Kidney Failure Acute/Chronic, Child

See Renal Failure, Acute/Chronic, Child

Kidney Failure, Nonoliguric

See Renal Failure, Nonoliguric

Kidney Stone

Acute Pain r/t obstruction from kidney calculi

Impaired Urinary Elimination: Urgency and Frequency r/t anatomical obstruction, irritation caused by stone

Risk for Infection: Risk factor: obstruction of urinary tract with stasis of urine

Readiness for Enhanced Knowledge: expresses an interest in learning about prevention of stones

Kidney Transplant

Ineffective Protection r/t immunosuppressive therapy

Readiness for Enhanced Decision-Making: expresses desire to enhance understanding of choices

Readiness for Enhanced Family Processes: adapting to life without dialysis

Readiness for Enhanced Health Self-Management: desire to manage the treatment and prevention of complications after transplantation

Readiness for Enhanced Spiritual Well-Being: heightened coping, living without dialysis

See Renal Failure, Kidney Transplantation, Donor; Kidney Transplantation, Recipient; Nephrectomy; Surgery, Perioperative Care; Surgery, Postoperative Care; Surgery, Preoperative Care

Kidney Transplantation, Donor

Impaired Emancipated Decision-Making r/t harvesting of kidney from traumatized donor

Moral Distress r/t conflict among decision makers, end-of-life decisions, time constraints for decision-making

Spiritual Distress r/t grieving from loss of significant person

Risk for Surgical Site Infection: Risk factor: surgical procedure

Readiness for Enhanced Communication: expressing thoughts and feelings about situation

Readiness for Enhanced Family Coping: decision to allow organ donation

Readiness for Enhanced Emancipated Decision-Making: expresses desire to enhance understanding and meaning of choices

Readiness for Enhanced Resilience: decision to donate organs

Readiness for Enhanced Spirituality: inner peace resulting from allowance of organ donation

See Nephrectomy

Kidney Transplantation, Recipient

Anxiety r/t possible rejection, procedure

Ineffective Health Maintenance Behaviors r/t long-term home treatment after transplantation, diet, signs of rejection, use of medications

Deficient Knowledge r/t specific nutritional needs, possible paralytic ileus, fluid or sodium restrictions

Impaired Urinary Elimination r/t possible impaired renal function

Risk for Bleeding: Risk factor: surgical procedure

Risk for Infection: Risk factor: use of immunosuppressive therapy to control rejection

Risk for Surgical Site Infection: Risk factor: surgical procedure

Risk for Shock: Risk factor: possible hypovolemia

Risk for Spiritual Distress: Risk factor: obtaining transplanted kidney from someone's traumatic loss

Readiness for Enhanced Spiritual Well-Being: acceptance of situation

Kidney Tumor

See Wilms' Tumor

Kissing Disease

See Mononucleosis

Knee Replacement

See Total Joint Replacement (Total Hip/Total Knee/Shoulder)

Knowledge

Readiness for Enhanced Knowledge (See **Knowledge, Readiness for Enhanced,** Section III)

Knowledge, Deficient

Ineffective Health maintenance behaviors r/t lack of or significant alteration in communication skills (written, verbal, and/or gestural)

Deficient Knowledge (See **Knowledge, Deficient,** Section III)

Readiness for Enhanced Knowledge (See **Knowledge, Readiness for Enhanced,** Section III)

Kock Pouch

See Continent Ileostomy (Kock Pouch)

Korsakoff's Syndrome

Acute Confusion r/t alcohol abuse

Dysfunctional Family Processes r/t alcoholism as possible cause of syndrome

Impaired Memory r/t neurological changes associated with excessive alcohol intake

Self-Neglect r/t cognitive impairment from chronic alcohol abuse

Risk for Adult Falls: Risk factor: cognitive impairment from chronic alcohol abuse

Risk for Injury: Risk factors: sensory dysfunction, lack of coordination when ambulating from chronic alcohol abuse

Risk for Impaired Liver function: Risk factor: substance abuse (alcohol)

Risk for Imbalanced Nutrition: Less than Body Requirements: Risk factor: lack of adequate balanced intake from chronic alcohol abuse

L

Labor, Induction of

See Induction of Labor

Labor, Normal

Anxiety r/t fear of the unknown, situational crisis

Impaired Comfort r/t labor

Fatigue r/t childbirth

Deficient Knowledge r/t lack of preparation for labor

Labor Pain r/t uterine contractions, stretching of cervix and birth canal

Impaired Tissue Integrity r/t passage of infant through birth canal, episiotomy

Risk for Ineffective Childbearing Process (See **Childbearing Process,** Section III)

Risk for Adult Falls: Risk factors: excessive loss or shift in intravascular fluid volume, orthostatic hypotension

Risk for Deficient Fluid Volume: Risk factor: excessive loss of blood

Risk for Infection: Risk factors: multiple vaginal examinations, tissue trauma, prolonged rupture of membranes

Risk for Injury: Fetal: Risk factor: hypoxia

Risk for Post-Trauma Syndrome: Risk factors: trauma or violence associated with labor pains, medical or surgical interventions, history of sexual abuse

Readiness for Enhanced Childbearing Process: responds appropriately, is proactive, bonds with infant, uses support systems

Risk for Nipple-Areolar Complex Injury: breast engorgement; inappropriate positioning of the mother during breastfeeding

Readiness for Enhanced Family Coping: significant other provides support during labor

Readiness for Enhanced Health Management: prenatal care and childbirth education birth process

Readiness for Enhanced Power: expresses readiness to enhance participation in choices regarding treatment during labor

Labor Pain

Labor Pain r/t uterine contractions, stretching of cervix and birth canal

Labyrinthitis

Ineffective Health Self-Management r/t delay in seeking treatment for respiratory and ear infections

Risk for Injury r/t dizziness

Readiness for Enhanced Health Management: management of episodes

See Ménière's Disease

Lacerations

Readiness for Enhanced Health Management: appropriate care of injury

Risk for Infection: Risk factor: broken skin

Risk for Physical Trauma: Risk factor: children playing with dangerous objects

Lactation

See Breastfeeding, Ineffective; Breastfeeding, Interrupted

Lactic Acidosis

Decreased Cardiac Output r/t altered heart rate/rhythm, preload, and contractility

Risk for Electrolyte Imbalance: Risk factor: impaired regulatory mechanism

Risk for Decreased Cardiac Tissue Perfusion: Risk factor: hypoxia

Impaired Gas Exchange r/t ineffective breathing pattern, pain, ineffective airway clearance

See Ketoacidosis, Diabetic

Lactose Intolerance

Readiness for Enhanced Knowledge: interest in identifying lactose intolerance, treatment, and substitutes for milk products

See Abdominal Distention; Diarrhea

Laminectomy

Anxiety r/t change in health status, surgical procedure

Impaired Comfort r/t surgical procedure

Deficient Knowledge r/t appropriate postoperative and post-discharge activities

Impaired Physical Mobility r/t neuromuscular impairment

Acute Pain r/t localized inflammation and edema

Urinary Retention r/t competing sensory impulses, effects of opioids or anesthesia

Risk for Bleeding: Risk factor: surgery

Risk for Surgical Site Infection: Risk factor: invasive procedure, surgery

Risk for Perioperative Positioning Injury: Risk factor: prone position

See Surgery, Perioperative Care; Surgery, Postoperative Care; Surgery, Preoperative Care

Language Impairment

See Speech Disorders

Laparoscopic Laser Cholecystectomy

See Cholecystectomy; Laser Surgery

Laparoscopy

Urge Urinary Incontinence r/t pressure on the bladder from gas

Acute Pain: Shoulder r/t gas irritating the diaphragm

Laparotomy

See Abdominal Surgery

Large Bowel Resection

See Abdominal Surgery

Laryngectomy

Ineffective Airway Clearance r/t surgical removal of glottis, decreased humidification

Death Anxiety r/t unknown results of surgery

Disturbed Body Image r/t change in body structure and function

Impaired Comfort r/t surgery

Impaired Verbal Communication r/t removal of larynx

Interrupted Family Processes r/t surgery, serious condition of family member, difficulty communicating

Grieving r/t loss of voice, fear of death

Ineffective Health Self-Management r/t deficient knowledge regarding self-care with laryngectomy

Imbalanced Nutrition: Less than Body Requirements r/t absence of oral feeding, difficulty swallowing, increased need for fluids

Impaired Oral Mucous Membrane r/t absence of oral feeding

Chronic Sorrow r/t change in body image

Impaired Swallowing r/t edema, laryngectomy tube

Risk for Electrolyte Imbalance: Risk factor: fluid imbalance

Risk for Maladaptive Grieving: Risk factors: loss, major life event

Risk for Compromised Human Dignity: Risk factor: inability to communicate

Risk for Surgical Site Infection: Risk factors: invasive procedure, surgery

Risk for Powerlessness: Risk factors: chronic illness, change in communication

Risk for Impaired Resilience: Risk factor: change in health status

Risk for Situational Low Self-Esteem: Risk factor: disturbed body image

Laser Surgery

Impaired Comfort r/t surgery

Constipation r/t laser intervention in vulval and perianal areas

Deficient Knowledge r/t preoperative and postoperative care associated with laser procedure

Acute Pain r/t heat from laser

Risk for Bleeding: Risk factor: surgery

Risk for Infection: Risk factor: delayed heating reaction of tissue exposed to laser

Risk for Injury: Risk factor: accidental exposure to laser beam

LASIK Eye Surgery (Laser-Assisted in Situ Keratomileusis)

Impaired Comfort r/t surgery

Decisional Conflict r/t decision to have surgery

Risk for Infection: Risk factor: invasive procedure/surgery

Readiness for Enhanced Health Management: surgical procedure preoperative and postoperative teaching and expectations

L

Latex Allergic Reaction

Latex Allergic Reaction (See **Latex Allergic Reaction,** Section III)

Risk for Latex Allergic Reaction (See **Latex Allergic Reaction, Risk for,** Section III)

Readiness for Enhanced Knowledge: prevention and treatment of exposure to latex products

Laxative Abuse

Perceived Constipation r/t health belief, faulty appraisal, impaired thought processes

Lead Poisoning

Contamination r/t flaking, peeling paint in presence of young children

Ineffective Home Maintenance Behaviors r/t presence of lead paint

Risk for Delayed Child Development: Risk factor: lead poisoning

Left Heart Catheterization

See Cardiac Catheterization

Legionnaires' Disease

Contamination r/t contaminated water in air-conditioning systems

See Pneumonia

Lens Implant

See Cataract Extraction; Vision Impairment

Lethargy/Listlessness

Frail Elderly Syndrome r/t alteration in cognitive function

Fatigue r/t decreased metabolic energy production

Insomnia r/t internal or external stressors

Risk for Ineffective Cerebral Tissue Perfusion: Risk factor: carbon dioxide retention and/or lack of oxygen supply to brain

Leukemia

Ineffective Protection r/t abnormal blood profile

Fatigue r/t abnormal blood profile and/or side effects of chemotherapy treatment

Risk for Imbalanced Fluid Volume: Risk factors: nausea, vomiting, bleeding, side effects of treatment

Risk for Infection: Risk factor: ineffective immune system

Risk for Impaired Resilience: Risk factor: serious illness

See Cancer; Chemotherapy

Leukopenia

Ineffective Protection r/t leukopenia

Risk for Infection: Risk factor: low white blood cell count

Level of Consciousness, Decreased

See Confusion, Acute; Confusion, Chronic

Lice

Impaired Comfort r/t inflammation, pruritus

Readiness for Enhanced Health Management: preventing and treating infestation

Ineffective Home Maintenance Behaviors r/t close unsanitary, overcrowded conditions

Self-Neglect r/t lifestyle

See Communicable Diseases, Childhood (e.g., Measles, Mumps, Rubella, Chickenpox, Scabies, Lice)

Lifestyle, Sedentary

Sedentary Lifestyle (See **Sedentary Lifestyle,** Section III)

Risk for Ineffective Peripheral Tissue Perfusion: Risk factor: lack of movement

Decreased Activity Tolerance: Related factor: impaired physical mobility

Lightheadedness

See Dizziness; Vertigo; Falls

Limb Reattachment Procedures

Anxiety r/t unknown outcome of reattachment procedure, use and appearance of limb

Disturbed Body Image r/t unpredictability of function and appearance of reattached body part

Grieving r/t unknown outcome of reattachment procedure

Spiritual Distress r/t anxiety about condition

Stress Overload r/t multiple coexisting stressors, physical demands

Risk for Bleeding: Risk factor: severed vessels

Risk for Perioperative Positioning Injury: Risk factor: immobilization

Risk for Peripheral Neurovascular Dysfunction: Risk factors: trauma, orthopedic and neurovascular surgery, compression of nerves and blood vessels

Risk for Powerlessness: Risk factor: unknown outcome of procedure

Risk for Impaired Religiosity: Risk factors: suffering, hospitalization

See Surgery, Postoperative Care

Liposuction

Disturbed Body Image r/t dissatisfaction with unwanted fat deposits in body

Risk for Impaired Resilience: Risk factor: body image disturbance

Readiness for Enhanced Decision-Making: expresses desire to make decision regarding liposuction

Readiness for Enhanced Self-Concept: satisfaction with new body image

See Surgery, Perioperative Care; Surgery, Postoperative Care; Surgery, Preoperative Care

Lithotripsy

Readiness for Enhanced Health Management: expresses desire for information related to procedure and aftercare and prevention of stones

See Kidney Stone

Liver Biopsy

Anxiety r/t procedure and results

Risk for Deficient Fluid Volume: Risk factor: hemorrhage from biopsy site

Risk for Infection: Risk factor: invasive procedure

Risk for Powerlessness: Risk factor: inability to control outcome of procedure

Liver Cancer

Risk for Bleeding: Risk factor: liver dysfunction

Risk for Adult Falls: Risk factor: confusion associated with liver dysfunction

Risk for Impaired Liver Function: Risk factor: disease process

Risk for Impaired Resilience: Risk factor: serious illness

See Cancer; Chemotherapy; Radiation Therapy

Liver Disease

See Cirrhosis; Hepatitis

Liver Function

Risk for Impaired Liver Function (See **Liver Function, Impaired, Risk for,** Section III)

Liver Transplant

Impaired Comfort r/t surgical pain

Decisional Conflict r/t acceptance of donor liver

Ineffective Protection r/t immunosuppressive therapy

Risk for Impaired Liver Function: Risk factors: possible rejection, infection

Readiness for Enhanced Family Processes: change in physical needs of family member

Readiness for Enhanced Health Management: desire to manage the treatment and prevention of complications after transplantation

Readiness for Enhanced Spiritual Well-Being: heightened coping

See Surgery, Perioperative Care; Surgery, Postoperative Care; Surgery, Preoperative Care

Living Will

Moral Distress r/t end-of-life decisions

Readiness for Enhanced Decision-Making: expresses desire to enhance understanding of choices for decision-making

Readiness for Enhanced Relationship: shares information with others

Readiness for Enhanced Religiosity: request to meet with religious leaders or facilitators

Readiness for Enhanced Resilience: uses effective communication

Readiness for Enhanced Spiritual Well-Being: acceptance of and preparation for end of life

See Advance Directives

Lobectomy

See Thoracotomy

Loneliness

Spiritual Distress r/t loneliness, social alienation

Risk for Loneliness (See **Loneliness, Risk for,** Section III)

Risk for Impaired Religiosity: Risk factor: lack of social interaction

Readiness for Enhanced Hope: expresses desire to enhance interconnectedness with others

Readiness for Enhanced Relationship: expresses satisfaction with complementary relationship between partners

Loose Stools (Bowel Movements)

Diarrhea r/t increased gastric motility

Risk for Dysfunctional Gastrointestinal Motility (See **Gastrointestinal Motility, Dysfunctional, Risk for,** Section III)

See Diarrhea

Loss of Bladder Control

See Incontinence of Urine

Loss of Bowel Control

See Incontinence of Stool

Lou Gehrig's Disease

See Amyotrophic Lateral Sclerosis (ALS)

Low Back Pain

Impaired Comfort r/t back pain

Ineffective Health Maintenance Behaviors r/t deficient knowledge regarding self-care with back pain

Impaired Physical Mobility r/t back pain

Chronic Pain r/t degenerative processes, musculotendinous strain, injury, inflammation, congenital deformities

Urinary Retention r/t possible spinal cord compression

Risk for Powerlessness: Risk factor: living with chronic pain

Readiness for Enhanced Health Management: expresses desire for information to manage pain

Low Blood Glucose

See Hypoglycemia

Low Blood Pressure

See Hypotension

Lower GI Bleeding

See GI Bleed (Gastrointestinal Bleeding)

Lumbar Puncture

Anxiety r/t invasive procedure and unknown results

Deficient Knowledge r/t information about procedure

Acute Pain r/t possible loss of cerebrospinal fluid

Risk for Ineffective Cerebral Tissue Perfusion: Risk factor: treatment-related side effects

Risk for Infection: Risk factor: invasive procedure

Lumpectomy

Decisional Conflict r/t treatment choices

Readiness for Enhanced Knowledge: preoperative and postoperative care

Readiness for Enhanced Spiritual Well-Being: hope of benign diagnosis

See Cancer

Lung Cancer

See Cancer; Chemotherapy; Radiation Therapy; Thoracotomy

Lung Surgery

See Thoracotomy

Lupus Erythematosus

Disturbed Body Image r/t change in skin, rash, lesions, ulcers, mottled erythema

Fatigue r/t increased metabolic requirements

Ineffective Health Maintenance Behaviors r/t deficient knowledge regarding medication, diet, activity

Acute Pain r/t inflammatory process

Powerlessness r/t unpredictability of course of disease

Impaired Religiosity r/t ineffective coping with disease

Chronic Sorrow r/t presence of chronic illness

Spiritual Distress r/t chronicity of disease, unknown etiology

Risk for Decreased Cardiac Tissue Perfusion: Risk factor: altered circulation

Risk for Impaired Resilience: Risk factor: chronic disease

Risk for Impaired Skin Integrity: Risk factors: chronic inflammation, edema, altered circulation

Lyme Disease

Impaired Comfort r/t inflammation

Fatigue r/t increased energy requirements

Deficient Knowledge r/t lack of information concerning disease, prevention, treatment

Acute Pain r/t inflammation of joints, urticaria, rash

Chronic Pain r/t chronic inflammation

Risk for Decreased Cardiac Output: Risk factor: dysrhythmia

Risk for Powerlessness: Risk factor: possible chronic condition

Lymphedema

Disturbed Body Image r/t change in appearance of body part with edema

Excess Fluid Volume r/t compromised regulatory system; inflammation, obstruction, or removal of lymph glands

Deficient Knowledge r/t management of condition

Risk for Infection: Risk factors: abnormal lymphatic system allowing stasis of fluids with decreased resistance to infection

Risk for Situational Low Self-Esteem: Risk factor: disturbed body image

Ineffective Lymphedema Self-Management r/t difficulty managing complex treatment regimen

Risk for Ineffective Lymphedema Self-Management: Risk factors: decreased perceived quality of life; inadequate commitment to a plan of action; unrealistic perception of susceptibility to sequelae

Lymphoma

See Cancer

M

Macular Degeneration

Anxiety r/t expressed insecurity with visual loss

Ineffective Coping r/t visual loss

Compromised Family Coping r/t deteriorating vision of family member

Risk-Prone Health Behavior r/t deteriorating vision while trying to maintain usual lifestyle

Hopelessness r/t deteriorating vision

Sedentary Lifestyle r/t visual loss

Self-Neglect r/t change in vision

Social Isolation r/t inability to drive because of visual changes

Risk for Falls: Risk factor: visual difficulties

Risk for Injury: Risk factor: inability to distinguish traffic lights and safety signs

Risk for Powerlessness: Risk factor: deteriorating vision

Risk for Impaired Religiosity: Risk factor: possible lack of transportation to church

Risk for Impaired Resilience: Risk factor: changing vision

Readiness for Enhanced Health Management: appropriate choices of daily activities for meeting the goals of a treatment program

Magnetic Resonance Imaging (MRI)

See MRI (Magnetic Resonance Imaging)

Major Depressive Disorder

See Depression (Major Depressive Disorder)

Malabsorption Syndrome

Diarrhea r/t lactose intolerance, gluten sensitivity, resection of small bowel

Dysfunctional Gastrointestinal Motility r/t disease state

Deficient Knowledge r/t lack of information about diet and nutrition

Imbalanced Nutrition: Less than Body Requirements r/t inability of body to absorb nutrients because of physiological factors

Risk for Electrolyte Imbalance: Risk factors: hypovolemia, hyponatremia, hypokalemia

Risk for Imbalanced Fluid Volume: Risk factors: diarrhea, hypovolemia

See Abdominal Distention

Maladaptive Behavior

See Crisis; Post-Trauma Syndrome; Suicide Attempt

Malaise

See Fatigue

Malaria

Contamination r/t geographic area

Risk for Contamination: Risk factors: increased environmental exposure (not wearing protective clothing, not using insecticide or repellant on skin, clothing, and in room in areas in which infected mosquitoes are present); inadequate defense mechanisms (inappropriate use of prophylactic regimen)

Risk for Impaired Liver Function: Risk factor: complications of disease

Readiness for Enhanced Community Coping: uses resources available for problem-solving

Readiness for Enhanced Health Management: expresses desire to enhance immunization status/vaccination status

Readiness for Enhanced Resilience: immunization status

See Anemia

Male Infertility

See Erectile Dysfunction (ED); Infertility

Malignancy

See Cancer

Malignant Hypertension (Arteriolar Nephrosclerosis)

Decreased Cardiac Output r/t altered afterload, altered contractility

Fatigue r/t disease state, increased blood pressure

Excess Fluid Volume r/t decreased kidney function

Risk for Ineffective Cerebral Tissue Perfusion: Risk factor: elevated blood pressure damaging cerebral vessels

Risk for Acute Confusion: Risk factors: increased blood urea nitrogen or creatinine levels

Risk for Imbalanced Fluid Volume: Risk factors: hypertension, altered kidney function

Risk for Unstable Blood Pressure: Risk factor: damaged vessels due to disease process

Readiness for Enhanced Health Management: expresses desire to manage the illness, high blood pressure

Malignant Hyperthermia

Hyperthermia r/t anesthesia reaction associated with inherited condition

Readiness for Enhanced Health Management: knowledge of risk factors

Risk for Shock r/t deficient fluid volume

Malnutrition

Insufficient Breast Milk Production (See **Breast Milk, Insufficient Production,** Section III)

Frail Elderly Syndrome r/t undetected malnutrition

Deficient Knowledge r/t misinformation about normal nutrition, social isolation, lack of food preparation facilities

Imbalanced Nutrition: Less than Body Requirements r/t inability to ingest food, digest food, or absorb nutrients because of biological, psychological, or economic factors; institutionalization (i.e., lack of menu choices)

Ineffective Protection r/t inadequate nutrition

Ineffective Health Management r/t inadequate nutrition

Self-Neglect r/t inadequate nutrition

Risk for Powerlessness: Risk factor: possible inability to provide adequate nutrition

Mammography

Readiness for Enhanced Health Management: follows guidelines for screening

Readiness for Enhanced Resilience: responsibility for self-care

Manic Disorder, Bipolar I

Anxiety r/t change in role function

Ineffective Coping r/t situational crisis

Ineffective Denial r/t fear of inability to control behavior

Interrupted Family Processes r/t family member's illness

Risk-Prone Health Behavior r/t low self-efficacy

Ineffective Health Management r/t unpredictability of client, excessive demands on family, chronic illness, social support deficit

Ineffective Home Maintenance Behaviors r/t altered psychological state, inability to concentrate

Disturbed Personal Identity r/t manic state

Insomnia r/t constant anxious thoughts

Imbalanced Nutrition: Less than Body Requirements r/t lack of time and motivation to eat, constant movement

Impaired individual Resilience r/t psychological disorder

Ineffective Role Performance r/t impaired social interactions

Self-Neglect r/t manic state

Sleep Deprivation r/t hyperagitated state

Risk for Ineffective Activity Planning r/t inability to process information

Risk for Caregiver Role Strain: Risk factor: unpredictability of condition

Risk for Imbalanced Fluid Volume: Risk factor: hypovolemia

Risk for Powerlessness: Risk factor: inability to control changes in mood

Risk for Spiritual Distress: Risk factor: depression

Risk for Suicidal Behavior: Risk factor: bipolar disorder

Risk for Self-Directed Violence: Risk factors: hallucinations, delusions

Risk for Other-Directed Violence: Risk factor: pathologic intoxication

Readiness for Enhanced Hope: expresses desire to enhance problem-solving goals

Manipulative Behavior

Defensive Coping r/t superior attitude toward others

Ineffective Coping r/t inappropriate use of defense mechanisms

M

Self-Mutilation r/t use of manipulation to obtain nurturing relationship with others

Self-Neglect r/t maintaining control

Impaired Social Interaction r/t self-concept disturbance

Risk for Loneliness: Risk factor: inability to interact appropriately with others

Risk for Situational Low Self-Esteem: Risk factor: history of learned helplessness

Risk for Self-Mutilation: Risk factor: inability to cope with increased psychological or physiological tension in healthy manner

Marfan Syndrome

Decreased Cardiac Output r/t dilation of the aortic root, dissection or rupture of the aorta

Risk for Decreased Cardiac Tissue Perfusion: Risk factor: heart-related complications from Marfan syndrome

Risk for Impaired Cardiovascular Function: Risk factor: heart-related valve disorders form Marfan syndrome

Readiness for Enhanced Health Management: describes reduction of risk factors

See Mitral Valve Prolapse; Scoliosis

Mastectomy

Disturbed Body Image r/t loss of sexually significant body part

Impaired Comfort r/t altered body image; difficult diagnosis

Death Anxiety r/t threat of mortality associated with breast cancer

Fatigue r/t increased metabolic requirements

Fear r/t change in body image, prognosis

Deficient Knowledge r/t self-care activities

Insomnia r/t impaired health status

Nausea r/t chemotherapy

Acute Pain r/t surgical procedure

Sexual Dysfunction r/t change in body image, fear of loss of femininity

Chronic Sorrow r/t disturbed body image, unknown long-term health status

Spiritual Distress r/t change in body image

Risk for Surgical Site Infection: Risk factors: surgical procedure, broken skin

Risk for Impaired Physical Mobility: Risk factors: nerve or muscle damage, pain

Risk for Post-Trauma Syndrome: Risk factors: loss of body part, surgical wounds

Risk for Powerlessness: Risk factor: fear of unknown outcome of procedure

Risk for Impaired Resilience: Risk factor: altered body image

See Cancer; Modified Radical Mastectomy; Surgery, Perioperative Care; Surgery, Postoperative Care; Surgery, Preoperative Care

Mastitis

Anxiety r/t threat to self, concern over safety of milk for infant

Ineffective Breastfeeding r/t breast pain, conflicting advice from health care providers

Deficient Knowledge r/t antibiotic regimen, comfort measures

Acute Pain r/t infectious disease process, swelling of breast tissue

Ineffective Role Performance r/t change in capacity to function in expected role

Maternal Infection

Ineffective Protection r/t invasive procedures, traumatized tissue

See Postpartum, Normal Care

Maturational Issues, Adolescent

Ineffective Coping r/t maturational crises

Risk-Prone Health Behavior r/t inadequate comprehension, negative attitude toward health care

Interrupted Family Processes r/t developmental crises of adolescence resulting from challenge of parental authority and values, situational crises from change in parental marital status

Deficient Knowledge: Potential for Enhanced Health Maintenance r/t information misinterpretation, lack of education regarding age-related factors

Impaired Social Interaction r/t ineffective, unsuccessful, or dysfunctional interaction with peers

Social Isolation r/t perceived alteration in physical appearance, social values not accepted by dominant peer group

Risk for Ineffective Activity Planning: Risk factor: unrealistic perception of personal competencies

Risk for Disturbed Personal Identity: Risk factor: maturational issues

Risk for Injury: Risk factor: thrill-seeking behaviors

Risk for Chronic Low Self-Esteem: Risk factor: lack of sense of belonging in peer group

Risk for Situational Low Self-Esteem: Risk factor: developmental changes

Readiness for Enhanced Communication: expressing willingness to communicate with parental figures

Readiness for Enhanced Relationship: expresses desire to enhance communication with parental figures

See Sexuality, Adolescent; Substance Misuse (if relevant)

Maze III Procedure

See Dysrhythmia; Open Heart Surgery

MD (Muscular Dystrophy)

See Muscular Dystrophy (MD)

Measles (Rubeola)

See Communicable Diseases, Childhood (e.g., Measles, Mumps, Rubella, Chickenpox, Scabies, Lice)

Meconium Aspiration

See Respiratory Conditions of the Neonate

Meconium Delayed

Risk for Neonatal Hyperbilirubinemia: Risk factor: delayed meconium

Medical Marijuana

Imbalanced Nutrition: Less than Body Requirements r/t eating disorder, appetite loss, effects of chemotherapy

Chronic Pain Syndrome r/t persistence of pain as a result of physical injury or condition

Nausea r/t effects of chemotherapy

Melanoma

Disturbed Body Image r/t altered pigmentation, surgical incision

Death Anxiety r/t threat of mortality associated with cancer

Fear r/t threat to well-being

Ineffective Health Maintenance Behaviors r/t deficient knowledge regarding self-care and treatment of melanoma

Acute Pain r/t surgical incision

Chronic Sorrow r/t disturbed body image, unknown long-term health status

Readiness for Enhanced Health Management: describes reduction of risk factors; protection from sunlight's ultraviolet rays

See Cancer

Melena

Fear r/t presence of blood in feces

Risk for Imbalanced Fluid volume: Risk factor: hemorrhage

See GI Bleed (Gastrointestinal Bleeding)

Memory Deficit

Impaired Memory (See **Memory, Impaired,** Section III)

Ménière's Disease

Risk for Injury: Risk factor: symptoms of disease

Readiness for Enhanced Health Management: expresses desire to manage illness

See Dizziness; Nausea; Vertigo

Meningitis/Encephalitis

Ineffective Airway Clearance r/t seizure activity

Impaired Comfort r/t altered health status

Excess Fluid Volume r/t increased intracranial pressure, syndrome of inappropriate secretion of antidiuretic hormone

Impaired Mobility r/t neuromuscular or central nervous system insult

Acute Pain r/t biological injury

Risk for Aspiration: Risk factor: seizure activity

Risk for Acute Confusion: Risk factor: infection of brain

Risk for Falls: Risk factors: neuromuscular dysfunction and confusion

Risk for Injury: Risk factor: seizure activity

Risk for Impaired Resilience: Risk factor: illness

Risk for Shock: Risk factor: infectious process

Risk for Ineffective Cerebral Tissue Perfusion: Risk factors: cerebral tissue edema and inflammation of meninges, increased intracranial pressure; infection

Risk for Ineffective Thermoregulation: Risk factor: infectious process

Risk for Unstable Blood Pressure r/t fluid shifts

See Hospitalized Child

Meningocele

See Neural Tube Defects

Menopause

Impaired Comfort r/t symptoms associated with menopause

Insomnia r/t hormonal shifts

Impaired Memory r/t change in hormonal levels

Sexual Dysfunction r/t menopausal changes

Ineffective Sexuality Pattern r/t altered body structure, lack of lubrication, lack of knowledge of artificial lubrication

Ineffective Thermoregulation r/t changes in hormonal levels

Risk for Urge Urinary Incontinence: Risk factor: changes in hormonal levels affecting bladder function

Risk for Overweight: Risk factor: change in metabolic rate caused by fluctuating hormone levels

Risk for Powerlessness: Risk factor: changes associated with menopause

Risk for Impaired Resilience: Risk factor: menopause

Risk for Situational Low Self-Esteem: Risk factors: developmental changes, menopause

Readiness for Enhanced Health Management: verbalized desire to manage menopause

Readiness for Enhanced Self-Care: expresses satisfaction with body image

Readiness for Enhanced Spiritual Well-Being: desire for harmony of mind, body, and spirit

Menorrhagia

Fear r/t loss of large amounts of blood

Risk for Deficient Fluid Volume: Risk factor: excessive loss of menstrual blood

Mental Illness

Defensive Coping r/t psychological impairment, substance misuse

Ineffective Coping r/t situational crisis, coping with mental illness

Compromised Family Coping r/t lack of available support from client

Disabled Family Coping r/t chronically unexpressed feelings of guilt, anxiety, hostility, or despair

Ineffective Denial r/t refusal to acknowledge abuse problem, fear of the social stigma of disease

Risk-Prone Health Behavior r/t low self-efficacy

Disturbed Personal Identity r/t psychoses

Ineffective Relationship r/t effects of mental illness in partner relationship

Chronic Sorrow r/t presence of mental illness

Stress Overload r/t multiple coexisting stressors

Ineffective Family Health Self-Management r/t chronicity of condition, unpredictability of client, unknown prognosis

Risk for Loneliness: Risk factor: social isolation

Risk for Powerlessness: Risk factor: lifestyle of helplessness

Risk for Impaired Resilience: Risk factor: chronic illness

Risk for Chronic Low Self-Esteem: Risk factor: presence of mental illness/repeated negative reinforcement

Metabolic Acidosis

See Ketoacidosis, Alcoholic; Ketoacidosis, Diabetic

Metabolic Alkalosis

Deficient Fluid Volume r/t fluid volume loss, vomiting, gastric suctioning, failure of regulatory mechanisms

Metabolic Imbalance Syndrome

Ineffective Health Maintenance Behaviors r/t deficient knowledge regarding basic health practice

Obesity r/t energy expenditure below energy intake

Risk for Unstable Blood Glucose Level: Risk factor: variations in serum glucose levels

Metastasis

See Cancer

Methicillin-Resistant *Staphylococcus aureus* (MRSA)

See MRSA (Methicillin-Resistant Staphylococcus aureus*)*

MI (Myocardial Infarction)

Decreased Activity Tolerance r/t imbalance between oxygen supply and demand

Anxiety r/t threat of death, possible change in role status

Death Anxiety r/t seriousness of medical condition

Constipation r/t decreased peristalsis from decreased physical activity, medication effect, change in diet

Ineffective Family Coping r/t spouse or significant other's fear of partner loss

Ineffective Denial r/t fear, deficient knowledge about heart disease

Interrupted Family Processes r/t crisis, role change

Fear r/t threat to well-being

Ineffective Health Maintenance Behaviors r/t deficient knowledge regarding self-care and treatment

Acute Pain r/t myocardial tissue damage from inadequate blood supply

Situational Low Self-Esteem r/t crisis of MI

Ineffective Sexuality Pattern r/t fear of chest pain, possibility of heart damage

Risk for Powerlessness: Risk factor: acute illness

Risk for Shock: Risk factors: hypotension, myocardial dysfunction, hypoxia

Risk for Spiritual Distress: Risk factor: physical illness

Risk for Decreased Cardiac Output: Risk factors: alteration in heart rate, rhythm, and contractility

Risk for Decreased Cardiac Tissue Perfusion: Risk factors: coronary artery spasm, hypertension, hypotension, hypoxia

Risk for Unstable Blood Pressure r/t cardiac dysrhythmia

Readiness for Enhanced Knowledge: expresses an interest in learning about condition

See Angioplasty, Coronary; Coronary Artery Bypass Grafting (CABG)

MIDCAB (Minimally Invasive Direct Coronary Artery Bypass)

Risk for Bleeding: Risk factor: surgery

Readiness for Enhanced Health Management: preoperative and postoperative care associated with surgery

Risk for Surgical Site Infection: Risk factor: surgical procedure

See Angioplasty, Coronary; Coronary Artery Bypass Grafting (CABG)

Midlife Crisis

Ineffective Coping r/t inability to deal with changes associated with aging

Powerlessness r/t lack of control over life situation

Spiritual Distress r/t questioning beliefs or value system

Risk for Disturbed Personal Identity: Risk factor: alteration in social roles

Risk for Chronic Low Self-Esteem: Risk factor: ineffective coping with loss

M

Readiness for Enhanced Relationship: meets goals for lifestyle change

Readiness for Enhanced Spiritual Well-Being: desire to find purpose and meaning to life

Migraine Headache

Ineffective Health Maintenance Behaviors r/t deficient knowledge regarding prevention and treatment of headaches

Readiness for Enhanced Health Management: expresses desire to manage illness

Acute Pain: Headache r/t vasodilation of cerebral and extracerebral vessels

Risk for Impaired Resilience: Risk factors: chronic illness, disabling pain

Military Families, Personnel

Anxiety r/t apprehension and helplessness caused by uncertainty of family members' situation

Interrupted Family Processes r/t possible change in family roles, decrease in available emotional support

Relocation Stress Syndrome r/t unpredictability of experience, powerlessness, significant environmental change

Milk Intolerance

See Lactose Intolerance

Minimally Invasive Direct Coronary Artery Bypass (MIDCAB)

See MIDCAB (Minimally Invasive Direct Coronary Artery Bypass)

Miscarriage

See Pregnancy Loss

Mitral Stenosis

Decreased Activity Tolerance r/t imbalance between oxygen supply and demand

Anxiety r/t possible worsening of symptoms, activity intolerance, fatigue

Decreased Cardiac Output r/t incompetent heart valves, abnormal forward or backward blood flow, flow into a dilated chamber, flow through an abnormal passage between chambers

Fatigue r/t reduced cardiac output

Ineffective Health Maintenance Behaviors r/t deficient knowledge regarding self-care with disorder

Risk for Decreased Cardiac Tissue Perfusion: Risk factor: incompetent heart valve

Risk for Infection: Risk factors: invasive procedure, risk for endocarditis

Mitral Valve Prolapse

Anxiety r/t symptoms of condition: palpitations, chest pain

Fatigue r/t abnormal catecholamine regulation, decreased intravascular volume

Fear r/t lack of knowledge about mitral valve prolapse, feelings of having heart attack

Ineffective Health Maintenance Behaviors r/t deficient knowledge regarding methods to relieve pain and treat dysrhythmia and shortness of breath, need for prophylactic antibiotics before invasive procedures

Acute Pain r/t mitral valve regurgitation

Risk for Ineffective Cerebral Tissue Perfusion: Risk factor: postural hypotension

Risk for Infection: Risk factor: invasive procedures

Risk for Powerlessness: Risk factor: unpredictability of onset of symptoms

Readiness for Enhanced Knowledge: expresses interest in learning about condition

Mobility, Impaired Bed

Impaired Bed Mobility (See **Mobility, Bed, Impaired,** Section III)

Mobility, Impaired Physical

Impaired Physical Mobility (See **Mobility, Physical, Impaired,** Section III)

Risk for Falls: Risk factor: impaired physical mobility

Mobility, Impaired Wheelchair

Impaired Wheelchair Mobility (See **Mobility, Wheelchair, Impaired,** Section III)

Modified Radical Mastectomy

Readiness for Enhanced Communication: willingness to enhance communication

See Mastectomy

Mononucleosis

Decreased Activity Tolerance r/t generalized weakness

Impaired Comfort r/t sore throat, muscle aches

Fatigue r/t disease state, stress

Ineffective Health Maintenance Behaviors r/t deficient knowledge concerning transmission and treatment of disease

Acute Pain r/t enlargement of lymph nodes, oropharyngeal edema

Impaired Swallowing r/t enlargement of lymph nodes, oropharyngeal edema

Risk for Injury: Risk factor: possible rupture of spleen

Risk for Loneliness: Risk factor: social isolation

Mood Disorders

Caregiver Role Strain r/t overwhelming needs of care receiver, unpredictability of mood alterations

Labile Emotional Control (See **Labile Emotional Control,** Section III)

Risk-Prone Health Behavior r/t hopelessness, altered locus of control

Impaired Mood Regulation (See **Mood Regulation, Impaired,** Section III)

Self-Neglect r/t inability to care for self

Social Isolation r/t alterations in mental status

Risk for Situational Low Self-Esteem: Risk factor: unpredictable changes in mood

Readiness for Enhanced Communication: expresses feelings

See specific disorder: Depression (Major Depressive Disorder); Dysthymic Disorder; Hypomania; Manic Disorder, Bipolar I

Moon Face

Disturbed Body Image r/t change in appearance from disease and medication(s)

Risk for Situational Low Self-Esteem: Risk factor: change in body image

See Cushing's Syndrome

Moral/Ethical Dilemmas

Impaired Emancipated Decision-Making r/t questioning personal values and belief, which alter decision

Moral Distress r/t conflicting information guiding moral or ethical decision-making

Risk for Powerlessness: Risk factor: lack of knowledge to make a decision

Risk for Spiritual Distress: Risk factor: moral or ethical crisis

Readiness for Enhanced Emancipated Decision-Making: expresses desire to enhance congruency of decisions with personal values and goals

Readiness for Enhanced Religiosity: requests assistance in expanding religious options

Readiness for Enhanced Resilience: vulnerable state

Readiness for Enhanced Spiritual Well-Being: request for interaction with others regarding difficult decisions

M

Morning Sickness

See Hyperemesis Gravidarum; Pregnancy, Normal

Motion Sickness

See Labyrinthitis

Mottling of Peripheral Skin

Ineffective Peripheral Tissue Perfusion r/t interruption of arterial flow, decreased circulating blood volume

Risk for Shock: Risk factor: inadequate circulation to perfuse body

Mourning

See Grieving

Mouth Lesions

See Mucous Membrane Integrity, Impaired Oral

MRI (Magnetic Resonance Imaging)

Anxiety r/t fear of being in closed spaces

Readiness for Enhanced Health Management: describes reduction of risk factors associated with exam

Deficient Knowledge r/t unfamiliarity with information resources; exam information

Readiness for Enhanced Knowledge: expresses interest in learning about exam

MRSA (Methicillin-Resistant *Staphylococcus aureus*)

Impaired Skin Integrity r/t infection

Delayed Surgical Recovery r/t infection

Ineffective Thermoregulation r/t severe infection stimulating immune system

Impaired Tissue Integrity r/t wound, infection

Risk for Loneliness: Risk factor: physical isolation

Risk for Impaired Resilience: Risk factor: illness

Risk for Shock: Risk factor: sepsis

MS (Multiple Sclerosis)

See Multiple Sclerosis

Mucocutaneous Lymph Node Syndrome

See Kawasaki Disease

Mucous Membrane Integrity, Impaired Oral

Impaired Oral Mucous Membrane Integrity (See **Oral Mucous Membrane Integrity, Impaired,** Section III)

Multi-Infarct Dementia

See Dementia

Multiple Gestations

Anxiety r/t uncertain outcome of pregnancy

Death Anxiety r/t maternal complications associated with multiple gestations

Insufficient Breast Milk Production r/t multiple births

Ineffective Childbearing Process r/t unavailable support system

Fatigue r/t physiological demands of a multifetal pregnancy and/or care of more than one infant

Ineffective Home Maintenance Behaviors r/t fatigue

Stress Urinary Incontinence r/t increased pelvic pressure

Insomnia r/t impairment of normal sleep pattern; parental responsibilities

Deficient Knowledge r/t caring for more than one infant

Neonatal Hyperbilirubinemia r/t feeding pattern not well established

Deficient Knowledge r/t caring for more than one infant

Imbalanced Nutrition: Less than Body Requirements r/t physiological demands of a multifetal pregnancy

Stress Overload r/t multiple coexisting stressors, family demands

Impaired Walking r/t increased uterine size

Risk for Ineffective Breastfeeding: Risk factors: lack of support, physical demands of feeding more than one infant

Risk for Delayed Child Development: Fetus: Risk factor: multiple gestations

Risk for Neonatal Hyperbilirubinemia: Risk factors: abnormal weight loss, prematurity, feeding pattern not well established

Readiness for Enhanced Childbearing Process: demonstrates appropriate care for infants and mother

Readiness for Enhanced Family Processes: family adapting to change with more than one infant

Multiple Personality Disorder (Dissociative Identity Disorder)

Anxiety r/t loss of control of behavior and feelings

Disturbed Body Image r/t psychosocial changes

Defensive Coping r/t unresolved past traumatic events, severe anxiety

Ineffective Coping r/t history of abuse

Hopelessness r/t long-term stress

Disturbed Personal Identity r/t severe child abuse

Chronic Low Self-Esteem r/t rejection, failure

Risk for Self-Mutilation: Risk factor: need to act out to relieve stress

Readiness for Enhanced Communication: willingness to discuss problems associated with condition

See Dissociative Identity Disorder (Not Otherwise Specified)

Multiple Sclerosis (MS)

Ineffective Activity Planning r/t unrealistic perception of personal competence

Ineffective Airway Clearance r/t decreased energy or fatigue

Impaired Physical Mobility r/t neuromuscular impairment

Self-Neglect r/t functional impairment

Powerlessness r/t progressive nature of disease

Self-Care Deficit: Specify r/t neuromuscular impairment

Sexual Dysfunction r/t biopsychosocial alteration of sexuality

Chronic Sorrow r/t loss of physical ability

Spiritual Distress r/t perceived hopelessness of diagnosis

Urinary Retention r/t inhibition of the reflex arc

Risk for Disuse Syndrome: Risk factor: physical immobility

Risk for Injury: Risk factors: altered mobility, sensory dysfunction

Risk for Imbalanced Nutrition: Less than Body Requirements: Risk factors: impaired swallowing, depression

Risk for Powerlessness: Risk factor: chronic illness

Risk for Impaired Religiosity: Risk factor: illness

Risk for Thermal Injury: Risk factor: neuromuscular impairment

Readiness for Enhanced Health Management: expresses a desire to manage condition

Readiness for Enhanced Self-Care: expresses desire to enhance knowledge of strategies and responsibility for self-care

Readiness for Enhanced Spiritual Well-Being: struggling with chronic debilitating condition

See Neurological Disorders

Mumps

See Communicable Diseases, Childhood (e.g., Measles, Mumps, Rubella, Chickenpox, Scabies, Lice)

Murmurs

Decreased Cardiac Output r/t altered preload/afterload

Risk for Decreased Cardiac Tissue Perfusion: Risk factor: incompetent valve

Risk for Fatigue: Risk factor: decreased cardiac output

Muscular Atrophy/Weakness

Risk for Disuse Syndrome: Risk factor: impaired physical mobility

Risk for Adult Falls: Risk factor: impaired physical mobility

Risk for Child Falls: Risk factor: impaired physical mobility

Muscular Dystrophy (MD)

Decreased Activity Tolerance r/t fatigue, muscle weakness

Ineffective Activity Planning r/t unrealistic perception of personal competence

Ineffective Airway Clearance r/t muscle weakness and decreased ability to cough

Constipation r/t immobility

Fatigue r/t increased energy requirements to perform activities of daily living

Impaired Physical Mobility r/t muscle weakness and development of contractures

Imbalanced Nutrition: Less than Body Requirements r/t impaired swallowing or chewing

Self-Care Deficit: Feeding, Bathing, Dressing, Toileting r/t muscle weakness and fatigue

Self-Neglect r/t functional impairment

Impaired Transfer Ability r/t muscle weakness

Impaired Swallowing r/t neuromuscular impairment

Impaired Walking r/t muscle weakness

Risk for Aspiration: Risk factor: impaired swallowing

Risk for Decreased Cardiac Tissue Perfusion: Risk factor: hypoxia associated with cardiomyopathy

Risk for Disuse Syndrome: Risk factor: complications of immobility

Risk for Falls: Risk factor: muscle weakness

Risk for Infection: Risk factor: pooling of pulmonary secretions as a result of immobility and muscle weakness

Risk for Injury: Risk factors: muscle weakness and unsteady gait

Risk for Overweight: Risk factor: inactivity

Risk for Powerlessness: Risk factor: chronic condition

Risk for Impaired Religiosity: Risk factor: illness

Risk for Impaired Resilience: Risk factor: chronic illness

Risk for Situational Low Self-Esteem: Risk factor: presence of chronic condition

Risk for Impaired Skin Integrity: Risk factors: immobility, braces, or adaptive devices

Readiness for Enhanced Self-Concept: acceptance of strength and abilities

See Child with Chronic Condition; Hospitalized Child

MVC (Motor Vehicle Crash)

See Fracture; Head Injury; Injury; Pneumothorax

Myasthenia Gravis

Ineffective Airway Clearance r/t decreased ability to cough and swallow

Interrupted Family Processes r/t crisis of dealing with diagnosis

Fatigue r/t paresthesia, aching muscles, weakness of muscles

Impaired Physical Mobility r/t defective transmission of nerve impulses at the neuromuscular junction

Imbalanced Nutrition: Less than Body Requirements r/t difficulty eating and swallowing

Impaired Swallowing r/t neuromuscular impairment

Risk for Caregiver Role Strain: Risk factors: severity of illness of client, overwhelming needs of client

Risk for Impaired Religiosity: Risk factor: illness

Risk for Impaired Resilience: Risk factor: new diagnosis of chronic, serious illness

Readiness for Enhanced Spiritual Well-Being: heightened coping with serious illness

See Neurological Disorders

Mycoplasma Pneumonia

See Pneumonia

Myelocele

See Neural Tube Defects

Myelomeningocele

See Neural Tube Defects

N

Myocardial Infarction (MI)

See MI (Myocardial Infarction)

Myocarditis

Decreased Activity Tolerance r/t reduced cardiac reserve and prescribed bed rest

Decreased Cardiac Output r/t altered preload/afterload

Fear r/t dyspnea and reduced cardiac reserve

Deficient Knowledge r/t treatment of disease

Risk for Decreased Cardiac Tissue Perfusion: Risk factors: hypoxia, hypovolemia, cardiac tamponade

Readiness for Enhanced Knowledge: treatment of disease

See Heart Failure, if appropriate

Myringotomy

Fear r/t hospitalization, surgical procedure

Ineffective Health Maintenance r/t deficient knowledge regarding care after surgery

Acute Pain r/t surgical procedure

Risk for Surgical Site Infection: Risk factor: invasive procedure

See Ear Surgery

Myxedema

See Hypothyroidism

N

Narcissistic Personality Disorder

Defensive Coping r/t grandiose sense of self

Impaired Emancipated Decision-Making r/t lack of realistic problem-solving skills

Interrupted Family Processes r/t taking advantage of others to achieve own goals

Risk-Prone Health Behavior r/t low self-efficacy

Disturbed Personal Identity r/t psychological impairment

Ineffective Relationship r/t lack of mutual support/respect between partners

Impaired Individual Resilience r/t psychological disorders

Impaired Social Interaction r/t self-concept disturbance

Risk for Loneliness: Risk factors: emotional deprivation, social isolation

Narcolepsy

Anxiety r/t fear of lack of control over falling asleep

Disturbed Sleep Pattern r/t uncontrollable desire to sleep

Risk for Physical Trauma: Risk factor: falling asleep during potentially dangerous activity

Readiness for Enhanced Sleep: expresses willingness to enhance sleep

Narcotic Use

See Opioid Use (preferred terminology)

Nasogastric Suction

Impaired Oral Mucous Membrane Integrity r/t presence of nasogastric tube

Risk for Electrolyte Imbalance: Risk factor: loss of gastrointestinal fluids that contain electrolytes

Risk for Imbalanced Fluid Volume: Risk factor: loss of gastrointestinal fluids without adequate replacement

Risk for Dysfunctional Gastrointestinal Motility: Risk factor: decreased intestinal motility

Nausea

Nausea (See **Nausea,** Section III)

Near-Drowning

Ineffective Airway Clearance r/t aspiration of fluid

Aspiration r/t aspiration of fluid into lungs

Fear: Parental r/t possible death of child, possible permanent and debilitating sequelae

Impaired Gas Exchange r/t laryngospasm, holding breath, aspiration, inflammation

Maladaptive Grieving r/t potential death of child, unknown sequelae, guilt about accident

Ineffective Health Maintenance Behaviors r/t parental deficient knowledge regarding safety measures appropriate for age

Hypothermia r/t central nervous system injury, prolonged submersion in cold water

Risk for Delayed Child Development: Risk factors: hypoxemia, cerebral anoxia

Risk for Maladaptive Grieving: Risk factors: potential death of child, unknown sequelae, guilt about accident

Risk for Infection: Risk factors: aspiration, invasive monitoring

Risk for Ineffective Cerebral Tissue Perfusion: Risk factor: hypoxia

Readiness for Enhanced Spiritual Well-Being: struggle with survival of life-threatening situation

See Child with Chronic Condition; Hospitalized Child; Safety, Childhood; Terminally Ill Child/Death of Child, Parent

Nearsightedness

Readiness for Enhanced Health Management: need for correction of myopia

Nearsightedness; Corneal Surgery

See LASIK Eye Surgery (Laser-Assisted in Situ Keratomileusis)

Neck Vein Distention

Decreased Cardiac Output r/t decreased contractility of heart resulting in increased preload

Excess Fluid Volume r/t excess fluid intake, compromised regulatory mechanisms

Risk for Thrombosis r/t blood coagulation disorders

See Congestive Heart Failure (CHF); Heart Failure

Necrosis, Kidney Tubular; Necrosis, Acute Tubular

See Renal Failure

Necrotizing Enterocolitis

Ineffective Breathing Pattern r/t abdominal distention, hypoxia

Diarrhea r/t infection

Impaired Bowel Continence r/t infection

Deficient Fluid Volume r/t vomiting, gastrointestinal bleeding

Neonatal Hyperbilirubinemia r/t feeding pattern not well established

Imbalanced Nutrition: Less than Body Requirements r/t decreased ability to absorb nutrients, decreased perfusion to gastrointestinal tract

Risk for Dysfunctional Gastrointestinal Motility: Risk factor: infection

Risk for Infection: Risk factors: bacterial invasion of gastrointestinal tract, invasive procedures

See Hospitalized Child; Premature Infant (Child)

Negative Feelings About Self

Chronic Low Self-Esteem r/t long-standing negative self-evaluation

Self-Neglect r/t negative feelings

Readiness for Enhanced Self-Concept: expresses willingness to enhance self-concept

Neglect, Unilateral

Unilateral Neglect (See **Unilateral Neglect,** Section III)

Neglectful Care of Family Member

Caregiver Role Strain r/t overwhelming care demands of family member, lack of social or financial support

Disabled Family Coping r/t highly ambivalent family relationships, lack of respite care

Interrupted Family Processes r/t situational transition or crisis

Deficient Knowledge r/t care needs

Impaired Individual Resilience r/t vulnerability from neglect

Risk for Compromised Human Dignity: Risk factor: inadequate participation in decision-making

Neonatal Abstinence Syndrome

Ineffective Airway Clearance r/t pooling of secretions from lack of adequate cough reflex, effects of viral or bacterial lower airway infection as a result of altered protective state

Interrupted Breastfeeding r/t use of drugs or alcohol by mother

Ineffective Childbearing Process r/t inconsistent prenatal health visits, suboptimal maternal nutrition, substance abuse

Impaired Comfort r/t irritability and inability to relax

Diarrhea r/t effects of withdrawal, increased peristalsis from hyperirritability

Disorganized Infant Behavior r/t exposure and/or withdrawal from toxic substances (alcohol or drugs), lack of attachment

Imbalanced Nutrition: Less than Body Requirements r/t feeding problems; uncoordinated or ineffective suck and swallow; effects of diarrhea, vomiting, or colic associated with maternal substance abuse

Impaired Parenting r/t impaired or absent attachment behaviors, inadequate support systems

Ineffective Infant Suck-Swallow Response r/t uncoordinated or ineffective sucking reflex, neurological delay

Disturbed Sleep Pattern r/t hyperirritability or hypersensitivity to environmental stimuli

Risk for Impaired Attachment: Risk factor: (parent) substance misuse, inability to meet infant's needs

Risk for Delayed Child Development: Risk factor: effects of prenatal substance abuse

Risk for Infection: Risk factor: stress effects of withdrawal

Risk for Disturbed Maternal–Fetal Dyad: Risk factor: substance abuse

Risk for Sudden Infant Death: Risk factor: prenatal illicit drug exposure

Risk for Ineffective Thermoregulation: Risk factor: immature nervous system

See Anomaly, Fetal/Newborn (Parent Dealing with); Cerebral Palsy; Child with Chronic Condition; Failure to Thrive; Hospitalized Child; Hyperactive Syndrome; Premature Infant/Child; Sudden Infant Death, Risk for

Neonatal Hyperbilirubinemia

Neonatal Hyperbilirubinemia (See **Neonatal Hyperbilirubinemia,** Section III)

Neonate

Readiness for Enhanced Childbearing Process: appropriate care of newborn

See Newborn, Normal; Newborn, Postmature; Newborn, Small for Gestational Age (SGA)

Neoplasm

Fear r/t possible malignancy

See Cancer

Nephrectomy

Anxiety r/t surgical recovery, prognosis

Ineffective Breathing Pattern r/t location of surgical incision

Constipation r/t lack of return of peristalsis

Acute Pain r/t incisional discomfort

Spiritual Distress r/t chronic illness

Risk for Bleeding: Risk factor: surgery

Risk for Imbalanced Fluid Volume: Risk factors: vascular losses, decreased intake

Risk for Surgical Site Infection: Risk factor: surgical procedure

Nephrostomy, Percutaneous

Acute Pain r/t invasive procedure

Impaired Urinary Elimination r/t nephrostomy tube

Risk for Infection: Risk factor: invasive procedure

Nephrotic Syndrome

Decreased Activity Tolerance r/t generalized edema

Disturbed Body Image r/t edematous appearance and side effects of steroid therapy

Excess Fluid Volume r/t edema resulting from oncotic fluid shift caused by serum protein loss and kidney retention of salt and water

Imbalanced Nutrition: Less than Body Requirements r/t anorexia, protein loss

Imbalanced Nutrition: More than Body Requirements r/t increased appetite attributable to steroid therapy

Social Isolation r/t edematous appearance

Risk for Infection: Risk factor: altered immune mechanisms caused by disease and effects of steroids

Risk for Impaired Skin Integrity: Risk factor: edema

See Child with Chronic Condition; Hospitalized Child

Neural Tube Defects (Meningocele, Myelomeningocele, Spina Bifida, Anencephaly)

Chronic Functional Constipation r/t immobility or less than adequate mobility

Maladaptive Grieving r/t loss of perfect child, birth of child with congenital defect

Mixed Urinary Incontinence r/t neurogenic impairment

Urge Urinary Incontinence r/t neurogenic impairment

Impaired Mobility r/t neuromuscular impairment

Chronic Low Self-Esteem r/t perceived differences, decreased ability to participate in physical and social activities at school

Impaired Skin Integrity r/t incontinence

Risk for Delayed Child Development: Risk factor: inadequate nutrition

Risk for Latex Allergic Reaction: Risk factor: multiple exposures to latex products

Risk for Imbalanced Nutrition: More than Body Requirements: Risk factors: diminished, limited, or impaired physical activity

Risk for Powerlessness: Risk factor: debilitating disease

Risk for Impaired Skin Integrity: Lower Extremities: Risk factor: decreased sensory perception

Readiness for Enhanced Family Coping: effective adaptive response by family members

Readiness for Enhanced Family Processes: family supports each other

See Child with Chronic Condition; Premature Infant (Child)

Neuralgia

See Trigeminal Neuralgia

Neuritis (Peripheral Neuropathy)

Decreased Activity Tolerance r/t pain with movement

Ineffective Health Maintenance Behaviors r/t deficient knowledge regarding self-care with neuritis

Acute Pain r/t stimulation of affected nerve endings, inflammation of sensory nerves

See Neuropathy, Peripheral

Neurogenic Bladder

Mixed Urinary Incontinence r/t neurological impairment

Urinary Retention r/t interruption in the lateral spinal tracts

Neurological Disorders

Ineffective Airway Clearance r/t perceptual or cognitive impairment, decreased energy, fatigue

Acute Confusion r/t dementia, alcohol abuse, drug abuse, delirium

Ineffective Coping r/t disability requiring change in lifestyle

Interrupted Family Processes r/t situational crisis, illness, or disability of family member

Maladaptive Grieving r/t loss of usual body functioning

Ineffective Home Maintenance Behaviors r/t client's or family member's disease

Risk for Corneal Injury: Risk factor: lack of spontaneous blink reflex

Impaired Memory r/t neurological disturbance

Impaired Physical Mobility r/t neuromuscular impairment

Imbalanced Nutrition: Less than Body Requirements r/t impaired swallowing, depression, difficulty feeding self

Powerlessness r/t progressive nature of disease

Self-Care Deficit: Specify r/t neuromuscular dysfunction

Sexual Dysfunction r/t biopsychosocial alteration of sexuality

Social Isolation r/t altered state of wellness

Impaired Swallowing r/t neuromuscular dysfunction

Risk for Disuse Syndrome: Risk factors: physical immobility, neuromuscular dysfunction

Risk for Injury: Risk factors: altered mobility, sensory dysfunction, cognitive impairment

Risk for Ineffective Cerebral Tissue Perfusion: Risk factor: cerebral disease/injury

Risk for Impaired Religiosity: Risk factor: life transition

Risk for Impaired Skin Integrity: Risk factors: altered sensation, altered mental status, paralysis

See specific condition: Alcohol Withdrawal; Amyotrophic Lateral Sclerosis (ALS); CVA (Cerebrovascular Accident); Delirium; Dementia; Guillain-Barré Syndrome; Head Injury; Huntington's Disease; Spinal Cord Injury; Myasthenia Gravis; Muscular Dystrophy (MD); Parkinson's Disease

Neuropathy, Peripheral

Chronic Pain r/t damage to nerves in the peripheral nervous system as a result of medication side effects, vitamin deficiency, or diabetes

Ineffective Thermoregulation r/t decreased ability to regulate body temperature

Risk for Injury: Risk factors: lack of muscle control, decreased sensation

Risk for Impaired Skin Integrity: Risk factor: poor perfusion

Risk for Thermal Injury: Risk factor: nerve damage

See Peripheral Vascular Disease (PVD)

Neurosurgery

See Craniectomy/Craniotomy

Newborn, Normal

Breastfeeding r/t normal oral structure and gestational age greater than 34 weeks

Ineffective Thermoregulation r/t immaturity of neuroendocrine system

Risk for Sudden Infant Death: Risk factors: lack of knowledge regarding infant sleeping in prone or side-lying position, prenatal or postnatal infant smoke exposure, infant overheating or overwrapping, loose articles in the sleep environment

Risk for Infection: Risk factors: open umbilical stump, immature immune system

Risk for Injury: Risk factors: immaturity, need for caretaking

Readiness for Enhanced Childbearing Process: appropriate care of newborn

Readiness for Enhanced Organized Infant Behavior: demonstrates adaptive response to pain

Readiness for Enhanced Parenting: providing emotional and physical needs of infant

Newborn, Postmature

Hypothermia r/t depleted stores of subcutaneous fat

Impaired Skin Integrity r/t cracked and peeling skin as a result of decreased vernix

Risk for Ineffective Airway Clearance: Risk factor: meconium aspiration

Risk for Unstable Blood Glucose Level: Risk factor: depleted glycogen stores

Newborn, Small for Gestational Age (SGA)

Neonatal Hyperbilirubinemia r/t neonate age and difficulty feeding

Imbalanced Nutrition: Less than Body Requirements r/t history of placental insufficiency

Ineffective Thermoregulation r/t decreased brown fat, subcutaneous fat

Risk for Delayed Child Development: Risk factor: history of placental insufficiency

Risk for Injury: Risk factors: hypoglycemia, perinatal asphyxia, meconium aspiration

Risk for Sudden Infant Death: Risk factor: low birth weight

Nicotine Addiction

Risk-Prone Health behavior r/t smoking

Ineffective Health Maintenance Behaviors r/t lack of ability to make a judgment about smoking cessation

Risk for Impaired Skin Integrity: Risk factor: poor tissue perfusion associated with nicotine

Powerlessness r/t perceived lack of control over ability to give up nicotine

Readiness for Enhanced Emancipated Decision-Making: expresses desire to enhance understanding and meaning of choices

Readiness for Enhanced Health Literacy: expresses desire to enhance understanding of health information to make health care choices

Readiness for Enhanced Health Management: expresses desire to learn measures to stop smoking

NIDDM (Non–Insulin-Dependent Diabetes Mellitus)

Readiness for Enhanced Health Management: expresses desire for information on exercise and diet to manage diabetes

See Diabetes Mellitus

Nightmares

Post-Trauma Syndrome r/t disaster, war, epidemic, rape, assault, torture, catastrophic illness, or accident

Nipple Soreness

Impaired Comfort r/t physical condition

See Painful Breasts, Sore Nipples; Sore Nipples, Breastfeeding

Nocturia

Urge Urinary Incontinence r/t decreased bladder capacity, irritation of bladder stretch receptors causing spasm, alcohol, caffeine, increased fluids, increased urine concentration, overdistention of bladder

Impaired Urinary Elimination r/t sensory motor impairment, urinary tract infection

Risk for Powerlessness: Risk factor: inability to control nighttime voiding

Nocturnal Myoclonus

See Restless Leg Syndrome; Stress

Nocturnal Paroxysmal Dyspnea

See PND (Paroxysmal Nocturnal Dyspnea)

Non–Insulin-Dependent Diabetes Mellitus (NIDDM)

See Diabetes Mellitus

Normal Pressure Hydrocephalus (NPH)

Impaired Verbal Communication r/t obstruction of flow of cerebrospinal fluid affecting speech

Acute Confusion r/t increased intracranial pressure caused by obstruction to flow of cerebrospinal fluid

Impaired Memory r/t neurological disturbance

Risk for Ineffective Cerebral Tissue Perfusion: Risk factor: fluid pressing on the brain

Risk for Adult Falls: Risk factor: unsteady gait as a result of obstruction of cerebrospinal fluid

Risk for Child Falls: Risk factor: unsteady gait as a result of obstruction of cerebrospinal fluid

NSTEMI (Non–ST-Elevation Myocardial Infarction)

See MI (Myocardial Infarction)

Nursing

See Breastfeeding, Effective; Breastfeeding, Ineffective; Breastfeeding, Interrupted, Nipple-Areolar Complex Injury

Nutrition

Readiness for Enhanced Nutrition (See **Nutrition, Readiness for Enhanced,** Section III)

Nutrition, Imbalanced

Imbalanced Nutrition: Less than Body Requirements (See **Nutrition: Less than Body Requirements, Imbalanced,** Section III)

Obesity (See **Obesity,** Section III)

Overweight (See **Overweight,** Section III)

Risk for Dry Mouth r/t depression

Risk for Overweight (See **Overweight, Risk for,** Section III)

Risk for Metabolic Syndrome r/t inadequate dietary habits

Obesity

Disturbed Body Image r/t eating disorder, excess weight

Risk-Prone Health Behavior r/t negative attitude toward health care

Obesity (See **Obesity,** Section III)

Chronic Low Self-Esteem r/t ineffective coping, overeating

Risk for Metabolic Syndrome: Risk factor: obesity

Risk for ineffective Peripheral Tissue Perfusion: Risk factor: sedentary lifestyle

Readiness for Enhanced Nutrition: expresses willingness to enhance nutrition

OBS (Organic Brain Syndrome)

See Organic Mental Disorders; Dementia

Obsessive-Compulsive Disorder (OCD)

See OCD (Obsessive-Compulsive Disorder)

Obstruction, Bowel

See Bowel Obstruction

Obstructive Sleep Apnea

Insomnia r/t blocked airway

Obesity r/t excessive intake related to metabolic need

See PND (Paroxysmal Nocturnal Dyspnea)

OCD (Obsessive-Compulsive Disorder)

Ineffective Activity Planning r/t unrealistic perception of events

Anxiety r/t threat to self-concept, unmet needs

Impaired Emancipated Decision-Making r/t inability to make a decision for fear of reprisal

Disabled Family Coping r/t family process being disrupted by client's ritualistic activities

Ineffective Coping r/t expression of feelings in an unacceptable way, ritualistic behavior

Risk-Prone Health behavior r/t inadequate comprehension associated with repetitive thoughts

Powerlessness r/t unrelenting repetitive thoughts to perform irrational activities

Impaired Individual Resilience r/t psychological disorder

Risk for Situational Low Self-Esteem: Risk factor: inability to control repetitive thoughts and actions

Occupational Injury

Fatigue r/t lack of sleep

Deficient Knowledge r/t inadequate training, improper use of equipment

Stress Overload r/t feelings of pressure

Risk for Occupational Injury (See **Risk for Occupational Injury,** Section III)

ODD (Oppositional Defiant Disorder)

Anxiety r/t feelings of anger and hostility toward authority figures

Ineffective Coping r/t lack of self-control or perceived lack of self-control

Disabled Family Coping r/t feelings of anger, hostility; defiant behavior toward authority figures

Risk-Prone Health Behavior r/t multiple stressors associated with condition

Ineffective Impulse Control r/t anger/compunction to engage in disruptive behaviors

Chronic or Situational Low Self-Esteem r/t poor self-control and disruptive behaviors

Impaired Social Interaction r/t being touchy or easily annoyed, blaming others for own mistakes, constant trouble in school

Social Isolation r/t unaccepted social behavior

Ineffective Family Health Self-Management r/t difficulty in limit setting and managing oppositional behaviors

Risk for Ineffective Activity Planning: Risk factors: unrealistic perception of events, hedonism, insufficient social support

Risk for Impaired Parenting: Risk factors: children's difficult behaviors and inability to set limits

Risk for Powerlessness: Risk factor: inability to deal with difficult behaviors

Risk for Spiritual Distress: Risk factors: anxiety and stress in dealing with difficult behaviors

Risk for Other-Directed Violence: Risk factors: history of violence, threats of violence against others, history of antisocial behavior, history of indirect violence

Older Adult

See Aging

Oliguria

Deficient Fluid Volume r/t active fluid loss, failure of regulatory mechanism, inadequate intake

Risk for Electrolyte Imbalance r/t inadequate knowledge of modifiable factors

See Cardiac Output, Decreased; Renal Failure; Shock, Hypovolemic

Omphalocele

See Gastroschisis/Omphalocele

Oophorectomy

Risk for Ineffective Sexuality Pattern: Risk factor: altered body function

See Surgery, Perioperative Care; Surgery, Postoperative Care; Surgery, Preoperative Care

OPCAB (Off-Pump Coronary Artery Bypass)

See Angioplasty, Coronary; Coronary Artery Bypass Grafting (CABG)

Open Heart Surgery

Risk for Decreased Cardiac Tissue Perfusion: Risk factor: cardiac surgery

See Coronary Artery Bypass Grafting (CABG); Dysrhythmia

Open Reduction of Fracture with Internal Fixation (Femur)

Anxiety r/t outcome of corrective procedure

Impaired Physical Mobility r/t postoperative position, abduction of leg, avoidance of acute flexion

Powerlessness r/t loss of control, unanticipated change in lifestyle

Risk for Surgical Site Infection: Risk factor: surgical procedure

Risk for Perioperative Positioning injury: Risk factor: immobilization

Risk for Peripheral Neurovascular Dysfunction: Risk factors: mechanical compression, orthopedic surgery, immobilization

Risk for Thrombosis: Risk factor: impaired mobility

See Surgery, Postoperative Care

Opioid Addiction

See Substance Abuse

Opioid Use

Acute Pain r/t physical injury or surgical procedure

Chronic Pain Syndrome r/t prolonged use of opioids

Risk for Constipation: Risk factor: effects of opioids on peristalsis

See Substance Abuse; Substance Withdrawal; Pain Management, Acute; Pain Management, Chronic

Opportunistic Infection

Delayed Surgical Recovery r/t abnormal blood profiles, impaired healing

Risk for Infection: Risk factor: abnormal blood profiles

See AIDS (Acquired Immunodeficiency Syndrome); HIV (Human Immunodeficiency Virus)

Oppositional Defiant Disorder (ODD)

See ODD (Oppositional Defiant Disorder)

Oral Mucous Membrane Integrity, Impaired

Impaired Oral Mucous Membrane Integrity (See **Oral Mucous Membrane Integrity, Impaired,** Section III)

Oral Thrush

Impaired Oral Mucous Membrane Integrity: Risk factors: effects of chemotherapy, radiotherapy, oral trauma, immune system disease

See Candidiasis, Oral

Orchitis

Readiness for Enhanced Health Self-Management: follows recommendations for mumps vaccination

See Epididymitis

Organic Mental Disorders

Chronic Confusion r/t progressive impairment in cognitive functioning

Frail Elderly Syndrome r/t alteration in cognitive function

Impaired Social Interaction r/t disturbed thought processes

Risk for Disturbed Personal Identity: Risk factor: delusions/fluctuating perceptions of stimuli

See Dementia

Orthopedic Traction

Ineffective Role Performance r/t limited physical mobility

Impaired Social Interaction r/t limited physical mobility

Impaired Transfer Ability r/t limited physical mobility

Risk for Impaired Religiosity: Risk factor: immobility

See Traction and Casts

Orthopnea

Ineffective Breathing Pattern r/t inability to breathe with head of bed flat

Decreased Cardiac Output r/t inability of heart to meet demands of body

Orthostatic Hypotension

See Dizziness

Osteoarthritis

Acute Pain r/t movement

Impaired Walking r/t inflammation and damage to joints

See Arthritis

Osteomyelitis

Decreased Diversional Activity Engagement r/t prolonged immobilization, hospitalization

Fear: Parental r/t concern regarding possible growth plate damage caused by infection, concern that infection may become chronic

Ineffective Health Maintenance Behaviors r/t continued immobility at home, possible extensive casts, continued antibiotics

Impaired Physical Mobility r/t imposed immobility as a result of infected area

Acute Pain r/t inflammation in affected extremity

Ineffective Thermoregulation r/t infectious process

Risk for Constipation: Risk factor: immobility

Risk for Infection: Risk factor: inadequate primary and secondary defenses

Risk for Impaired Skin Integrity: Risk factor: irritation from splint or cast

See Hospitalized Child

Osteoporosis

Deficient Knowledge r/t diet, exercise, need to abstain from alcohol and nicotine

Impaired Physical Mobility r/t pain, skeletal changes

Imbalanced Nutrition: Less than Body Requirements r/t inadequate intake of calcium and vitamin D

Acute Pain r/t fracture, muscle spasms

Risk for Injury: Fracture: Risk factors: lack of activity, risk of falling resulting from environmental hazards, neuromuscular disorders, diminished senses, cardiovascular responses to drugs

Risk for Adult Falls r/t decreased lower extremity strength

Risk for Powerlessness: Risk factor: debilitating disease

Readiness for Enhanced Health Self-Management: expresses desire to manage the treatment of illness and prevent complications

Ostomy

See Child with Chronic Condition; Colostomy; Ileal Conduit; Ileostomy

Otitis Media

Acute Pain r/t inflammation, infectious process

Risk for Delayed Child Development: Speech and Language: Risk factor: frequent otitis media

Anxiety r/t pain

Risk for Infection: Risk factors: eustachian tube obstruction, traumatic eardrum perforation, infectious process

Readiness for Enhanced Knowledge: information on treatment and prevention of disease

Ovarian Carcinoma

Death Anxiety r/t unknown outcome, possible poor prognosis

Fear r/t unknown outcome, possible poor prognosis

Ineffective Health Maintenance Behaviors r/t deficient knowledge regarding self-care, treatment of condition

Readiness for Enhanced Family Processes: family functioning meets needs of client

Readiness for Enhanced Resilience: participates in support groups

See Chemotherapy; Hysterectomy; Radiation Therapy

P

Pacemaker

Anxiety r/t change in health status, presence of pacemaker

Death Anxiety r/t worry over possible malfunction of pacemaker

Deficient Knowledge r/t self-care program, when to seek medical attention

Acute Pain r/t surgical procedure

Risk for Bleeding: Risk factor: surgery

Risk for Decreased Cardiac Tissue Perfusion: Risk factor: pacemaker malfunction

Risk for Impaired Cardiovascular Function: Risk factor: cardiac dysrhythmias

Risk for Infection: Risk factors: invasive procedure, presence of foreign body (catheter and generator)

Risk for Powerlessness: Risk factor: presence of electronic device to stimulate heart

Readiness for Enhanced Health Management: appropriate health care management of pacemaker

Paget's Disease

Disturbed Body Image r/t possible enlarged head, bowed tibias, kyphosis

Deficient Knowledge r/t appropriate diet high in protein and calcium, mild exercise

Chronic Sorrow r/t chronic condition with altered body image

Risk for Physical Trauma: Fracture: Risk factor: excessive bone destruction

Pain Management, Acute

Acute Pain r/t injury or surgical procedure

Imbalanced Energy Field r/t unpleasant sensory and emotional feelings

Pain Management, Chronic

Chronic Pain (See **Pain, Chronic,** Section III)

Chronic Pain Syndrome r/t persistent pain affecting daily living

Risk for Constipation: Risk factor: effects of medications on peristalsis

Readiness for Enhanced Knowledge: expresses a desire to learn alternative methods of nonpharmaceutical pain control

See Substance Misuse

Painful Breasts, Engorgement

Acute Pain r/t distention of breast tissue

Ineffective Role Performance r/t change in physical capacity to assume role of breastfeeding mother

Impaired Tissue Integrity r/t excessive fluid in breast tissues

Risk for Ineffective Breastfeeding: Risk factors: pain, infant's inability to latch on to engorged breast

Risk for Infection: Risk factor: milk stasis

Risk for Nipple-Areolar Complex Injury r/t breast engorgement

Painful Breasts, Sore Nipples

Insufficient Breast Milk Production r/t long breastfeeding time/pain response

Ineffective Breastfeeding r/t pain

Acute Pain r/t cracked nipples

Ineffective Role Performance r/t change in physical capacity to assume role of breastfeeding mother

Impaired Skin Integrity r/t mechanical factors involved in suckling, breastfeeding management

Nipple-Areolar Complex Injury r/t Maternal impatience with the breastfeeding process

Risk for Infection: Risk factor: break in skin

Pallor of Extremities

Ineffective Peripheral Tissue Perfusion r/t interruption of vascular flow

See Shock; Peripheral Vascular disease (PVD)

Palpitations (Heart Palpitations)

See Dysrhythmia

Pancreatic Cancer

Death Anxiety r/t possible poor prognosis of disease process

Ineffective Family Coping r/t poor prognosis

Fear r/t poor prognosis of the disease

Maladaptive Grieving r/t shortened lifespan

Deficient Knowledge r/t disease-induced diabetes, home management

Spiritual Distress r/t poor prognosis

Risk for impaired Liver Function: Risk factor: complications from underlying disease

See Cancer; Chemotherapy; Radiation Therapy; Surgery, Perioperative Care; Surgery, Postoperative Care; Surgery, Preoperative Care

Pancreatitis

Ineffective Breathing Pattern r/t splinting from severe pain, disease process, and inflammation

Ineffective Denial r/t ineffective coping, alcohol use

Diarrhea r/t decrease in pancreatic secretions resulting in steatorrhea

Deficient Fluid Volume r/t vomiting, decreased fluid intake, fever, diaphoresis, fluid shifts

Ineffective Health Maintenance Behaviors r/t deficient knowledge concerning diet, alcohol use, medication

Nausea r/t irritation of gastrointestinal system

Imbalanced Nutrition: Less than Body Requirements r/t inadequate dietary intake, increased nutritional needs as a result of acute illness, increased metabolic needs caused by increased body temperature, disease process

Acute Pain r/t irritation and edema of the inflamed pancreas

Chronic Sorrow r/t chronic illness

Readiness for Enhanced Comfort: expresses desire to enhance comfort

Panic Disorder (Panic Attacks)

Ineffective Activity Planning r/t unrealistic perception of events

Anxiety r/t situational crisis

Ineffective Coping r/t personal vulnerability

Risk-Prone Health Behavior r/t low self-efficacy

Disturbed Personal Identity r/t situational crisis

Post-Trauma Syndrome r/t previous catastrophic event

Social Isolation r/t fear of lack of control

Risk for Loneliness: Risk factor: inability to socially interact because of fear of losing control

Risk for Post-Trauma Syndrome: Risk factors: perception of the event, diminished ego strength

Risk for Powerlessness: Risk factor: ineffective coping skills

Readiness for Enhanced Coping: seeks problem-oriented and emotion-oriented strategies to manage condition

See Anxiety; Anxiety Disorder

Paralysis

Disturbed Body Image r/t biophysical changes, loss of movement, immobility

Impaired Comfort r/t prolonged immobility

Constipation r/t effects of spinal cord disruption, inadequate fiber in diet

Ineffective Health Maintenance Behaviors r/t deficient knowledge regarding self-care with paralysis

Ineffective Home Maintenance Behaviors r/t physical disability

Mixed Urinary Incontinence r/t neurological impairment

Impaired Physical Mobility r/t neuromuscular impairment

Impaired Wheelchair Mobility r/t neuromuscular impairment

Self-Neglect r/t functional impairment

Powerlessness r/t illness-related regimen

Self-Care Deficit: Specify r/t neuromuscular impairment

Sexual Dysfunction r/t loss of sensation, biopsychosocial alteration

Chronic Sorrow r/t loss of physical mobility

Impaired Transfer Ability r/t paralysis

Risk for Autonomic Dysreflexia: Risk factor: cause of paralysis

Risk for Disuse Syndrome: Risk factor: paralysis

Risk for Adult Falls: Risk factor: paralysis

Risk for Injury: Risk factors: altered mobility, sensory dysfunction

Risk for Post-Trauma Syndrome: Risk factor: event causing paralysis

Risk for Impaired Religiosity: Risk factors: immobility, possible lack of transportation

Risk for Impaired Resilience: Risk factor: chronic disability

Risk for Situational Low Self-Esteem: Risk factor: change in body image and function

Risk for Impaired Skin integrity: Risk factors: altered circulation, altered sensation, immobility

Risk for Thrombosis: Risk factor: prolonged immobility

Readiness for Enhanced Self-Care: expresses desire to enhance knowledge and responsibility for strategies for self-care

See Child with Chronic Condition; Hemiplegia; Hospitalized Child; Neural Tube Defects (Meningocele, Myelomeningocele, Spina Bifida, Anencephaly); Spinal Cord Injury

P

Paralytic Ileus

Constipation r/t decreased gastrointestinal motility

Deficient Fluid Volume r/t loss of fluids from vomiting, retention of fluid in bowel

Dysfunctional Gastrointestinal Motility r/t recent abdominal surgery, electrolyte imbalance

Nausea r/t gastrointestinal irritation

Acute Pain r/t pressure, abdominal distention, presence of nasogastric tube

See Bowel Obstruction

Paranoid Personality Disorder

Ineffective Activity Planning r/t unrealistic perception of events

Anxiety r/t uncontrollable intrusive, suspicious thoughts

Risk-Prone Health Behavior r/t intense emotional state

Disturbed Personal Identity r/t difficulty with reality testing

Impaired Individual Resilience r/t psychological disorder

Chronic Low Self-Esteem r/t inability to trust others

Social Isolation r/t inappropriate social skills

Risk for Loneliness: Risk factor: social isolation

Risk for Other-Directed Violence: Risk factor: being suspicious of others and their actions

Paraplegia

See Spinal Cord Injury

Parathyroidectomy

Anxiety r/t surgery

Risk for Ineffective Airway Clearance: Risk factors: edema or hematoma formation, airway obstruction

Risk for Bleeding: Risk factor: surgery

Risk for Impaired Verbal Communication: Risk factors: possible laryngeal damage, edema

Risk for Infection: Risk factor: surgical procedure

See Hypocalcemia

Parent Attachment

Risk for Impaired Attachment (See **Attachment, Impaired, Risk for,** Section III)

Readiness for Enhanced Childbearing Process: demonstrates appropriate care of newborn

See Parental Role Conflict

Parental Role Conflict

Parental Role Conflict (See **Role Conflict, Parental,** Section III)

Ineffective Relationship r/t unrealistic expectations

Chronic Sorrow r/t difficult parent–child relationship

Risk for Spiritual Distress: Risk factor: altered relationships

Readiness for Enhanced Parenting: willingness to enhance parenting

Parenting

Readiness for Enhanced Parenting (See **Parenting, Readiness for Enhanced,** Section III)

Parenting, Impaired

Impaired Parenting (See **Parenting, Impaired,** Section III)

Chronic Sorrow r/t difficult parent–child relationship

Risk for Spiritual Distress: Risk factor: altered relationships

Parenting, Risk for Impaired

Risk for Impaired Parenting (See **Parenting, Impaired, Risk for,** Section III)

See Parenting, Impaired

Paresthesia

Risk for Injury: Risk factors: inability to feel temperature changes, pain

Risk for Impaired Skin Integrity: Risk factor: impaired sensation

Risk for Thermal Injury: Risk factor: neuromuscular impairment

Parkinson's Disease

Impaired Verbal Communication r/t decreased speech volume, slowness of speech, impaired facial muscles

Constipation r/t weakness of muscles, lack of exercise, inadequate fluid intake, decreased autonomic nervous system activity

Frail Elderly Syndrome r/t chronic illness

Imbalanced Nutrition: Less than Body Requirements r/t tremor, slowness in eating, difficulty in chewing and swallowing

Chronic Sorrow r/t loss of physical capacity

Risk for Injury: Risk factors: tremors, slow reactions, altered gait

See Neurologic Disorders

Paroxysmal Nocturnal Dyspnea (PND)

See PND (Paroxysmal Nocturnal Dyspnea)

Patent Ductus Arteriosus (PDA)

See Congenital Heart Disease/Cardiac Anomalies

Patient-Controlled Analgesia (PCA)

See PCA (Patient-Controlled Analgesia)

Patient Education

Deficient Knowledge r/t lack of exposure to information misinterpretation, unfamiliarity with information resources to manage illness

Readiness for Enhanced Emancipated Decision-Making: expresses desire to enhance understanding of choices for decision-making

Readiness for Enhanced Knowledge (Specify): interest in learning

Readiness for Enhanced Health Management: expresses desire for information to manage the illness

PCA (Patient-Controlled Analgesia)

Deficient Knowledge r/t self-care of pain control

Nausea r/t side effects of medication

Risk for Injury: Risk factors: possible complications associated with PCA

Risk for Vascular Trauma: Risk factors: insertion site and length of insertion time

Readiness for Enhanced Knowledge: appropriate management of PCA

Acute Pain: guarding behaviors

Pectus Excavatum

See Marfan Syndrome

Pediculosis

See Lice

PEG (Percutaneous Endoscopic Gastrostomy)

See Tube Feeding

Pelvic Inflammatory Disease (PID)

See PID (Pelvic Inflammatory Disease)

Penile Prosthesis

Ineffective Sexuality Pattern r/t use of penile prosthesis

Risk for Surgical Site Infection: Risk factor: invasive surgical procedure

Risk for Situational Low Self-Esteem: Risk factor: ineffective sexuality pattern

Readiness for Enhanced Health Management: seeks information regarding care and use of prosthesis

See Erectile Dysfunction (ED); Impotence

Peptic Ulcer

See Ulcer, Peptic (Duodenal or Gastric)

Percutaneous Transluminal Coronary Angioplasty (PTCA)

See Angioplasty, Coronary

Pericardial Friction Rub

Decreased Cardiac Output r/t inflammation

Acute Pain r/t inflammation, effusion

Risk for Decreased Cardiac Tissue Perfusion: Risk factors: inflammation in pericardial sac, fluid accumulation compressing heart

Pericarditis

Decreased Activity Tolerance r/t reduced cardiac reserve, prescribed bed rest

Decreased Cardiac Output r/t impaired cardiac function from inflammation of pericardial sac

Risk for Decreased Cardiac Tissue Perfusion: Risk factor: inflammation in pericardial sac

Deficient Knowledge r/t unfamiliarity with information sources

Risk for Imbalanced Nutrition: Less than Body Requirements: Risk factors: fever, hypermetabolic state associated with fever

Acute Pain r/t biological injury, inflammation

Periodontal Disease

Risk for Impaired Oral Mucous Membrane Integrity (See **Oral Mucous Membrane Integrity, Impaired, Risk for,** Section III)

Perioperative Hypothermia

Risk for Perioperative Hypothermia (See **Perioperative Hypothermia, Risk for,** Section III)

Perioperative Positioning

Risk for Perioperative Positioning Injury (See **Perioperative Positioning injury, Risk for,** Section III)

Peripheral Neuropathy

See Neuropathy, Peripheral

Peripheral Neurovascular Dysfunction

Risk for Peripheral Neurovascular Dysfunction (See **Peripheral Neurovascular Dysfunction, Risk for,** Section III)

See Neuropathy, Peripheral; Peripheral Vascular Disease (PVD)

Peripheral Vascular Disease (PVD)

Ineffective Health Maintenance Behaviors r/t deficient knowledge regarding self-care and treatment of disease

Chronic Pain: Intermittent Claudication r/t ischemia

Ineffective Peripheral Tissue Perfusion r/t disease process

Risk for Adult Falls: Risk factor: altered mobility

Risk for Injury: Risk factors: tissue hypoxia, altered mobility, altered sensation

Risk for Peripheral Neurovascular Dysfunction: Risk factor: possible vascular obstruction

Risk for Impaired Tissue Integrity: Risk factor: altered circulation or sensation

Readiness for Enhanced Health Management: self-care and treatment of disease

See Neuropathy, Peripheral; Peripheral Neurovascular Dysfunction

Peritoneal Dialysis

Ineffective Breathing Pattern r/t pressure from dialysate

Impaired Comfort r/t instillation of dialysate, temperature of dialysate

Ineffective Home Maintenance Behaviors r/t complex home treatment of client

Deficient Knowledge r/t treatment procedure, self-care with peritoneal dialysis

Chronic Sorrow r/t chronic disability

Risk for Ineffective Coping: Risk factor: disability requiring change in lifestyle

Risk for Unstable Blood Glucose Level: Risk factors: increased concentrations of glucose in dialysate, ineffective medication management

Risk for Imbalanced Fluid Volume: Risk factor: medical procedure

P

Risk for Infection: Peritoneal: Risk factors: invasive procedure, presence of catheter, dialysate

Risk for Powerlessness: Risk factors: chronic condition and care involved

See Child with Chronic Condition; Hemodialysis; Hospitalized Child; Renal Failure; Renal Failure, Acute/Chronic, Child

Peritonitis

Ineffective Breathing Pattern r/t pain, increased abdominal pressure

Constipation r/t decreased oral intake, decrease of peristalsis

Deficient Fluid Volume r/t retention of fluid in bowel with loss of circulating blood volume

Nausea r/t gastrointestinal irritation

Imbalanced Nutrition: Less than Body Requirements r/t nausea, vomiting

Acute Pain r/t inflammation and infection of gastrointestinal system

Risk for Dysfunctional Gastrointestinal Motility: Risk factor: gastrointestinal disease

Risk for Infection r/t inadequate knowledge to avoid exposure to pathogens

Pernicious Anemia

Diarrhea r/t malabsorption of nutrients

Fatigue r/t imbalanced nutrition: less than body requirements

Impaired Memory r/t lack of adequate red blood cells

Nausea r/t altered oral mucous membrane; sore tongue, bleeding gums

Imbalanced Nutrition: Less than Body Requirements r/t lack of appetite associated with nausea and altered oral mucous membrane

Impaired Oral Mucous Membrane Integrity r/t vitamin deficiency; inability to absorb vitamin B_{12} associated with lack of intrinsic factor

Risk for Adult Falls: Risk factors: dizziness, lightheadedness

Risk for Peripheral Neurovascular Dysfunction: Risk factor: anemia

Persistent Fetal Circulation

See Congenital Heart Disease/Cardiac Anomalies

Personal Identity Problems

Disturbed Personal Identity (See **Identity, Personal, Disturbed,** Section III)

Risk for Disturbed Personal Identity (See **Disturbed Personal Identity, Risk for,** Section III)

Personality Disorder

Ineffective Activity Planning r/t unrealistic perception of events

Impaired Individual Resilience r/t psychological disorder

See specific disorder: Antisocial Personality Disorder; Borderline Personality Disorder; OCD (Obsessive-Compulsive Disorder); Paranoid Personality Disorder

Pertussis (Whooping Cough)

Risk for Impaired Emancipated Decision-Making: Risk factor: indecision regarding administration of usual childhood vaccinations

See Respiratory Infections, Acute Childhood

Pesticide Contamination

Contamination r/t use of environmental contaminants; pesticides

Risk for Allergic Reaction: Risk factor: repeated exposure to pesticides

Petechiae

See Anticoagulant Therapy; Clotting Disorder; DIC (Disseminated Intravascular Coagulation); Hemophilia

Petit Mal Seizure

Readiness for Enhanced Health Management: wears medical alert bracelet; limits hazardous activities such as driving, swimming, working at heights, operating equipment

See Epilepsy

Pharyngitis

See Sore Throat

Phenylketonuria (PKU)

See PKU (Phenylketonuria)

Pheochromocytoma

Anxiety r/t symptoms from increased catecholamines—headache, palpitations, sweating, nervousness, nausea, vomiting, syncope

Ineffective Health Maintenance Behaviors r/t deficient knowledge regarding treatment and self-care

Insomnia r/t high levels of catecholamines

Nausea r/t increased catecholamines

Risk for Decreased Cardiac Tissue Perfusion: Risk factor: hypertension

See Surgery, Perioperative Care; Surgery, Postoperative Care; Surgery, Preoperative Care

Phlebitis

See Thrombophlebitis

Phobia (Specific)

Fear r/t presence or anticipation of specific object or situation

Powerlessness r/t anxiety about encountering unknown or known entity

Impaired Individual Resilience r/t psychological disorder

Readiness for Enhanced Power: expresses readiness to enhance identification of choices that can be made for change

See Anxiety; Anxiety Disorder; Panic Disorder (Panic Attacks)

Photosensitivity

Ineffective Health Maintenance Behaviors r/t deficient knowledge regarding medications inducing photosensitivity

Risk for Dry Eye: Risk factors: pharmaceutical agents, sunlight exposure

Risk for Impaired Skin Integrity: Risk factor: exposure to sun

Physical Abuse

See Abuse, Child; Abuse, Spouse, Parent, or Significant Other

Pica

Anxiety r/t stress

Imbalanced Nutrition: Less than Body Requirements r/t eating nonnutritive substances

Impaired Parenting r/t lack of supervision, food deprivation

Risk for Constipation: Risk factor: presence of undigestible materials in gastrointestinal tract

Risk for Dysfunctional Gastrointestinal Motility: Risk factor: abnormal eating behavior

Risk for Infection: Risk factor: ingestion of infectious agents via contaminated substances

Risk for Poisoning: Risk factor: ingestion of substances containing lead

See Anemia

PID (Pelvic Inflammatory Disease)

Ineffective Health Maintenance Behaviors r/t deficient knowledge regarding self-care, treatment of disease

Acute Pain r/t biological injury; inflammation, edema, congestion of pelvic tissues

Ineffective Sexuality Pattern r/t medically imposed abstinence from sexual activities until acute infection subsides, change in reproductive potential

Risk for Infection: Risk factors: insufficient knowledge to avoid exposure to pathogens; proper hygiene, nutrition, other health habits

See Maturational Issues, Adolescent; STD (Sexually Transmitted Disease)

PIH (Pregnancy-Induced Hypertension/ Preeclampsia)

Anxiety r/t fear of the unknown, threat to self and infant, change in role functioning

Death Anxiety r/t threat of preeclampsia

Decreased Diversional Activity Engagement r/t bed rest

Interrupted Family Processes r/t situational crisis

Ineffective Home Maintenance Behaviors r/t bed rest

Deficient Knowledge r/t lack of experience with situation

Impaired Physical Mobility r/t medically prescribed limitations

Impaired Parenting r/t prescribed bed rest

Powerlessness r/t complication threatening pregnancy, medically prescribed limitations

Ineffective Role Performance r/t change in physical capacity to assume role of pregnant woman or resume other roles

Situational Low Self-Esteem r/t loss of idealized pregnancy

Impaired Social Interaction r/t imposed bed rest

Risk for Imbalanced Fluid Volume: Risk factors: hypertension, altered kidney function

Risk for Injury: Fetal: Risk factors: decreased uteroplacental perfusion, seizures

Risk for Injury: Maternal: Risk factors: vasospasm, high blood pressure

Risk for Unstable Blood Pressure: Risk factor: hypertension, imbalanced fluid volume

Readiness for Enhanced Knowledge: exhibits desire for information on managing condition

Piloerection

Hypothermia r/t exposure to cold environment

Pink Eye

See Conjunctivitis

Pinworms

Impaired Comfort r/t itching

Ineffective Home Maintenance Behaviors r/t inadequate cleaning of bed linen and toilet seats

Insomnia r/t discomfort

Readiness for Enhanced Health Management: proper handwashing; short, clean fingernails; avoiding hand, mouth, nose contact with unwashed hands; appropriate cleaning of bed linen and toilet seats

Pituitary Tumor, Benign

See Cushing's Disease

PKU (Phenylketonuria)

Risk for Delayed Child Development: Risk factors: not following strict dietary program; eating foods extremely low in phenylalanine; avoiding eggs, milk, any foods containing aspartame (e.g., NutraSweet)

Readiness for Enhanced Health Management: testing for PKU and following prescribed dietary regimen

Placenta Abruptio

Death Anxiety r/t threat of mortality associated with bleeding

Fear r/t threat to self and fetus

Ineffective Health Maintenance Behaviors r/t deficient knowledge regarding treatment and control of hypertension associated with placenta abruptio

Acute Pain: Abdominal/Back r/t premature separation of placenta before delivery

Risk for Bleeding: Risk factor: placenta abruptio

Risk for Deficient Fluid Volume: Risk factor: maternal blood loss

Risk for Powerlessness: Risk factors: complications of pregnancy and unknown outcome

Risk for Shock: Risk factor: hypovolemia

Risk for Spiritual Distress: Risk factor: fear from unknown outcome of pregnancy

Placenta Previa

Death Anxiety r/t threat of mortality associated with bleeding

Disturbed Body Image r/t negative feelings about body and reproductive ability, feelings of helplessness

Ineffective Coping r/t threat to self and fetus

Decreased Diversional Activity Engagement r/t long-term hospitalization

Interrupted Family Processes r/t maternal bed rest, hospitalization

Fear r/t threat to self and fetus, unknown future

Ineffective Home Maintenance Behaviors r/t maternal bed rest, hospitalization

Impaired Physical Mobility r/t medical protocol, maternal bed rest

Ineffective Role Performance r/t maternal bed rest, hospitalization

Situational Low Self-Esteem r/t situational crisis

Spiritual Distress r/t inability to participate in usual religious rituals, situational crisis

Risk for Bleeding: Risk factor: placenta previa

Risk for Constipation: Risk factors: bed rest, pregnancy

Risk for Deficient Fluid Volume: Risk factor: maternal blood loss

Risk for Imbalanced Fluid Volume: Risk factor: maternal blood loss

Risk for Injury: Fetal and Maternal: Risk factors: threat to uteroplacental perfusion, hemorrhage

Risk for Disturbed Maternal–Fetal Dyad: Risk factor: complication of pregnancy

Risk for Impaired Parenting: Risk factors: maternal bed rest, hospitalization

Risk for Ineffective Peripheral Tissue Perfusion: Placental: Risk factors: dilation of cervix, loss of placental implantation site

Risk for Powerlessness: Risk factors: complications of pregnancy, unknown outcome

Risk for Shock: Risk factor: hypovolemia

Plantar Fasciitis

Impaired Comfort r/t inflamed structures of feet

Impaired Physical Mobility r/t discomfort

Acute Pain r/t inflammation

Chronic Pain r/t inflammation

Pleural Effusion

Ineffective Breathing Pattern r/t pain

Excess Fluid Volume r/t compromised regulatory mechanisms; heart, liver, or kidney failure

Acute Pain r/t inflammation, fluid accumulation

Pleural Friction Rub

Ineffective Breathing Pattern r/t pain

Acute Pain r/t inflammation, fluid accumulation

Pleural Tap

See Pleural Effusion

Pleurisy

Ineffective Breathing Pattern r/t pain

Impaired Gas Exchange r/t ventilation perfusion imbalance

Acute Pain r/t pressure on pleural nerve endings associated with fluid accumulation or inflammation

Impaired Walking r/t activity intolerance, inability to "catch breath"

Risk for Ineffective Airway Clearance: Risk factors: increased secretions, ineffective cough because of pain

Risk for Infection: Risk factor: exposure to pathogens

PMS (Premenstrual Syndrome)

Fatigue r/t hormonal changes

Excess Fluid Volume r/t alterations of hormonal levels inducing fluid retention

Deficient Knowledge r/t methods to deal with and prevent syndrome

Acute Pain r/t hormonal stimulation of gastrointestinal structures

Risk for Powerlessness: Risk factors: lack of knowledge and ability to deal with symptoms

Risk for Impaired Resilience: Risk factor: PMS symptoms

Readiness for Enhanced Communication: willingness to express thoughts and feelings about PMS

Readiness for Enhanced Health Management: desire for information to manage and prevent symptoms

PND (Paroxysmal Nocturnal Dyspnea)

Anxiety r/t inability to breathe during sleep

Ineffective Breathing Pattern r/t increase in carbon dioxide levels, decrease in oxygen levels

Insomnia r/t suffocating feeling from fluid in lungs on awakening from sleep

Sleep Deprivation r/t inability to breathe during sleep

Risk for Decreased Cardiac Tissue Perfusion: Risk factor: hypoxia

Risk for Powerlessness: Risk factor: inability to control nocturnal dyspnea

Readiness for Enhanced Sleep: expresses willingness to learn measures to enhance sleep

Pneumonectomy

See Thoracotomy

Pneumonia

Decreased Activity Tolerance r/t imbalance between oxygen supply and demand

Ineffective Airway Clearance r/t inflammation and presence of secretions

Impaired Gas Exchange r/t decreased functional lung tissue

Dysfunctional Adult Ventilatory Weaning Response r/t fatigue

Ineffective Health Management r/t deficient knowledge regarding self-care and treatment of disease

Imbalanced Nutrition: Less than Body Requirements r/t loss of appetite

Impaired Oral Mucous Membrane Integrity r/t dry mouth from mouth breathing, decreased fluid intake

Ineffective Thermoregulation r/t infectious process

Risk for Acute Confusion: Risk factors: underlying illness, hypoxia

Risk for Deficient Fluid Volume: Risk factor: inadequate intake of fluids

Risk for Vascular Trauma: Risk factor: irritation from intravenous antibiotics

See Respiratory Infections, Acute Childhood

Pneumothorax

Fear r/t threat to own well-being, difficulty breathing

Impaired Gas Exchange r/t ventilation-perfusion imbalance, decreased functional lung tissue

Impaired Spontaneous Ventilation r/t respiratory muscle fatigue with difficulty breathing

Acute Pain r/t recent injury, coughing, deep breathing

Risk for Injury: Risk factor: possible complications associated with closed chest drainage system

See Chest Tubes

Poisoning, Risk for

Risk for Poisoning (See **Poisoning, Risk for,** Section III)

Poliomyelitis

See Paralysis

Polydipsia

See Diabetes Mellitus

Polyphagia

Readiness for Enhanced Nutrition: knowledge of appropriate diet for diabetes

See Diabetes Mellitus

Polyuria

See Diabetes Mellitus

Postoperative Care

See Surgery, Postoperative Care

Postpartum Depression

Anxiety r/t new responsibilities of parenting

Disturbed Body Image r/t normal postpartum recovery

Ineffective Childbearing Process r/t depression/lack of support system

Ineffective Coping r/t hormonal changes

Fatigue r/t childbirth, postpartum state, crying child

Risk-Prone Health Behavior r/t lack of support systems

Ineffective Home Maintenance Behaviors r/t fatigue, care of newborn

Hopelessness r/t stress, exhaustion

Deficient Knowledge r/t lifestyle changes

Impaired Parenting r/t hormone-induced depression

Ineffective Role Performance r/t new responsibilities of parenting

Sexual Dysfunction r/t fear of another pregnancy, postpartum pain, lochia flow

Sleep Deprivation r/t environmental stimulation of newborn

Impaired Social Interaction r/t change in role functioning

Risk for Disturbed Personal Identity: Risk factor: role change/depression/inability to cope

Risk for Situational Low Self-Esteem: Risk factor: decreased power over feelings of sadness

Risk for Spiritual Distress: Risk factors: altered relationships, social isolation

Readiness for Enhanced Hope: expresses desire to enhance hope and interconnectedness with others

See Depression (Major Depressive Disorder)

Postpartum Hemorrhage

Decreased Activity Tolerance r/t anemia from loss of blood

Death Anxiety r/t threat of mortality associated with bleeding

Disturbed Body Image r/t loss of ideal childbirth

Insufficient Breast Milk Production r/t fluid volume depletion

Interrupted Breastfeeding r/t separation from infant for medical treatment

Decreased Cardiac Output r/t hypovolemia

Fear r/t threat to self, unknown future

Deficient Fluid Volume r/t uterine atony, loss of blood

Ineffective Home Maintenance Behaviors r/t lack of stamina

Deficient Knowledge r/t lack of exposure to situation

Acute Pain r/t nursing and medical interventions to control bleeding

Ineffective Peripheral Tissue Perfusion r/t hypovolemia

Risk for Bleeding: Risk factor: postpartum complications

Risk for Impaired Childbearing: Risk factor: postpartum complication

Risk for Imbalanced Fluid Volume: Risk factor: maternal blood loss

Risk for Infection: Risk factors: loss of blood, depressed immunity

Risk for Impaired Parenting: Risk factor: weakened maternal condition

Risk for Powerlessness: Risk factor: acute illness

Risk for Shock: Risk factor: hypovolemia

Postpartum, Normal Care

Anxiety r/t change in role functioning, parenting

Effective Breastfeeding r/t basic breastfeeding knowledge, support of partner and health care provider

Fatigue r/t childbirth, new responsibilities of parenting, body changes

Acute Pain r/t episiotomy, lacerations, bruising, breast engorgement, headache, sore nipples, epidural or intravenous site, hemorrhoids

Sexual Dysfunction r/t recent childbirth

Impaired Tissue Integrity r/t episiotomy, lacerations

Sleep Deprivation r/t care of infant

Impaired Urinary Elimination r/t effects of anesthesia, tissue trauma

Risk for Constipation: Risk factors: hormonal effects on smooth muscles, fear of straining with defecation, effects of anesthesia

Risk for Infection: Risk factors: tissue trauma, blood loss

Readiness for Enhanced family Coping: adaptation to new family member

Readiness for Enhanced Hope: desire to increase hope

Readiness for Enhanced Parenting: expresses willingness to enhance parenting skills

Post-Trauma Syndrome

Post-Trauma Syndrome (See **Post-Trauma Syndrome,** Section III)

Post-Trauma Syndrome, Risk for

Risk for Post-Trauma Syndrome (See **Post-Trauma Syndrome, Risk for,** Section III)

Posttraumatic Stress Disorder (PTSD)

See PTSD (Post-Traumatic Stress Disorder)

Potassium, Increase/Decrease

See Hyperkalemia; Hypokalemia

Power/Powerlessness

Powerlessness (See **Powerlessness,** Section III)

Risk for Powerlessness (See **Powerlessness, Risk for,** Section III)

Readiness for Enhanced Power (See **Power, Readiness for Enhanced,** Section III)

Preeclampsia

See PIH (Pregnancy-Induced Hypertension/Preeclampsia)

Pregnancy, Cardiac Disorders

See Cardiac Disorders in Pregnancy

Pregnancy-Induced Hypertension/ Preeclampsia (PIH)

See PIH (Pregnancy-Induced Hypertension/Preeclampsia)

Pregnancy Loss

Anxiety r/t threat to role functioning, health status, situational crisis

Compromised Family Coping r/t lack of support by significant other because of personal suffering

Ineffective Coping r/t situational crisis

Maladaptive Grieving r/t loss of pregnancy, fetus, or child

Acute Pain r/t surgical intervention

Ineffective Role Performance r/t inability to assume parenting role

Ineffective Sexuality Pattern r/t self-esteem disturbance resulting from pregnancy loss and anxiety about future pregnancies

Chronic Sorrow r/t loss of a fetus or child

Spiritual Distress r/t intense suffering from loss of child

Risk for Deficient Fluid Volume: Risk factor: blood loss

Risk for Maladaptive Grieving: Risk factor: loss of pregnancy

Risk for Infection: Risk factor: retained products of conception

Risk for Powerlessness: Risk factor: situational crisis

Risk for Ineffective Relationship: Risk factor: poor communication skills in dealing with the loss

Risk for Spiritual Distress: Risk factor: intense suffering

Readiness for Enhanced Communication: willingness to express feelings and thoughts about loss

Readiness for Enhanced Hope: expresses desire to enhance hope

Readiness for Enhanced Spiritual Well-Being: desire for acceptance of loss

Pregnancy, Normal

Anxiety r/t unknown future, threat to self secondary to pain of labor

Disturbed Body Image r/t altered body function and appearance

Interrupted Family Processes r/t developmental transition of pregnancy

Fatigue r/t increased energy demands

Fear r/t labor and delivery

Deficient Knowledge r/t primiparity

Nausea r/t hormonal changes of pregnancy

Imbalanced Nutrition: Less than Body Requirements r/t growing fetus, nausea

Imbalanced Nutrition: More than Body Requirements r/t deficient knowledge regarding nutritional needs of pregnancy

Sleep Deprivation r/t uncomfortable pregnancy state

Impaired Urinary Elimination r/t frequency caused by increased pelvic pressure and hormonal stimulation

Risk for Constipation: Risk factor: pregnancy

Risk for Sexual Dysfunction: Risk factors: altered body function, self-concept, body image with pregnancy

Readiness for Enhanced Childbearing Process: appropriate prenatal care

Readiness for Enhanced Family Coping: satisfying partner relationship, attention to gratification of needs, effective adaptation to developmental tasks of pregnancy

Readiness for Enhanced Family Processes: family adapts to change

Readiness for Enhanced Health Management: seeks information for prenatal self-care

Readiness for Enhanced Nutrition: desire for knowledge of appropriate nutrition during pregnancy

Readiness for Enhanced Parenting: expresses willingness to enhance parenting skills

Readiness for Enhanced Relationship: meeting developmental goals associated with pregnancy

Readiness for Enhanced Spiritual Well-Being: new role as parent

See Discomforts of Pregnancy

Premature Dilation of the Cervix (Incompetent Cervix)

Ineffective Activity Planning r/t unrealistic perception of events

Ineffective Coping r/t bed rest, threat to fetus

Decreased Diversional Activity Engagement r/t bed rest

Fear r/t potential loss of infant

Maladaptive Grieving r/t potential loss of infant

Deficient Knowledge r/t treatment regimen, prognosis for pregnancy

Impaired Physical Mobility r/t imposed bed rest to prevent preterm birth

Powerlessness r/t inability to control outcome of pregnancy

Ineffective Role Performance r/t inability to continue usual patterns of responsibility

Situational Low Self-Esteem r/t inability to complete normal pregnancy

Sexual Dysfunction r/t fear of harm to fetus

Impaired Social Interaction r/t bed rest

Risk for Infection: Risk factor: invasive procedures to prevent preterm birth

Risk for Injury: Fetal: Risk factors: preterm birth, use of anesthetics

Risk for Injury: Maternal: Risk factor: surgical procedures to prevent preterm birth (e.g., cerclage)

Risk for Impaired Resilience: Risk factor: complication of pregnancy

Risk for Spiritual Distress: Risk factors: physical/psychological stress

Premature Infant (Child)

Insufficient Breast Milk Production r/t ineffective sucking, latching on of the infant

Impaired Gas Exchange r/t effects of cardiopulmonary insufficiency

Disorganized Infant Behavior r/t prematurity

Insomnia r/t noisy and noxious intensive care environment

Neonatal Hyperbilirubinemia r/t infant experiences difficulty making transition to extrauterine life

Imbalanced Nutrition: Less than Body Requirements r/t delayed or understimulated rooting reflex, easy fatigue during feeding, diminished endurance

Impaired Swallowing r/t decreased or absent gag reflex, fatigue

Ineffective Thermoregulation r/t large body surface/weight ratio, immaturity of thermal regulation, state of prematurity

Risk for Delayed Child Development: Risk factor: prematurity

Risk for Infection: Risk factors: inadequate, immature, or undeveloped acquired immune response

Risk for Injury: Risk factor: prolonged mechanical ventilation, retinopathy of prematurity (ROP) secondary to 100% oxygen environment

P

Risk for Neonatal Hyperbilirubinemia: Risk factor: late preterm birth

Readiness for Enhanced Organized Infant Behavior: use of some self-regulatory measures

Premature Infant (Parent)

Ineffective Breastfeeding r/t disrupted establishment of effective pattern secondary to prematurity or insufficient opportunities

Decisional Conflict r/t support system deficit, multiple sources of information

Compromised Family Coping r/t disrupted family roles and disorganization, prolonged condition exhausting supportive capacity of significant persons

Ineffective Infant Feeding Dynamics r/t insufficient knowledge of nutritional needs

Maladaptive Grieving r/t loss of perfect child possibly leading to complicated grieving

Risk for Maladaptive Grieving (Prolonged) r/t unresolved conflicts

Parental Role Conflict r/t expressed concerns, expressed inability to care for child's physical, emotional, or developmental needs

Chronic Sorrow r/t threat of loss of a child, prolonged hospitalization

Spiritual Distress r/t challenged belief or value systems regarding moral or ethical implications of treatment plans

Risk for Impaired Attachment: Risk factors: separation, physical barriers, lack of privacy

Risk for Disturbed Maternal–Fetal Dyad: Risk factor: complication of pregnancy

Risk for Powerlessness: Risk factor: inability to control situation

Risk for Impaired Resilience: Risk factor: premature infant

Risk for Spiritual Distress: Risk factor: challenged belief or value systems regarding moral or ethical implications of treatment plans

Readiness for Enhanced Family Process: adaptation to change associated with premature infant

See Child with Chronic Condition; Hospitalized Child

Premature Rupture of Membranes

Anxiety r/t threat to infant's health status

Disturbed Body Image r/t inability to carry pregnancy to term

Ineffective Coping r/t situational crisis

Maladaptive Grieving r/t potential loss of infant

Situational Low Self-Esteem r/t inability to carry pregnancy to term

Risk for Ineffective Childbearing Process: Risk factor: complication of pregnancy

Risk for Infection: Risk factor: rupture of membranes

Risk for Injury: Fetal: Risk factor: risk of premature birth

Premenstrual Tension Syndrome (PMS)

See PMS (Premenstrual Tension Syndrome)

Prenatal Care, Normal

Readiness for Enhanced Childbearing Process: appropriate prenatal lifestyle

Readiness for Enhanced Knowledge: appropriate prenatal care

Readiness for Enhanced Spiritual Well-Being: new role as parent

See Pregnancy, Normal

Prenatal Testing

Anxiety r/t unknown outcome, delayed test results

Acute Pain r/t invasive procedures

Risk for Infection: Risk factor: invasive procedures during amniocentesis or chorionic villus sampling

Risk for Injury: Risk factor: invasive procedures

Preoperative Teaching

See Surgery, Preoperative Care

Pressure Injury

Impaired Bed Mobility r/t intolerance to activity, pain, cognitive impairment, depression, severe anxiety, severity of illness

Imbalanced Nutrition: Less than Body Requirements r/t limited access to food, inability to absorb nutrients because of biological factors, anorexia

Acute Pain r/t tissue destruction, exposure of nerves

Impaired Skin Integrity: Stage I or II Pressure Injury r/t physical immobility, mechanical factors, altered circulation, skin irritants, excessive moisture

Impaired Tissue Integrity: Stage III or IV Pressure Injury r/t altered circulation, impaired physical mobility, excessive moisture

Risk for Infection: Risk factors: physical immobility, mechanical factors (shearing forces, pressure, restraint, altered circulation, skin irritants, excessive moisture, open wound)

Risk for Adult Pressure Injury (See **Adult Pressure Injury,** Section III)

Risk for Child Pressure Injury (See **Child Pressure Injury,** Section III)

Risk for Neonate Pressure Injury (See **Neonate Pressure Injury,** Section III)

Preterm Labor

Anxiety r/t threat to fetus, change in role functioning, change in environment and interaction patterns, use of tocolytic drugs

Ineffective Coping r/t situational crisis, preterm labor

Decreased Diversional Activity Engagement r/t long-term hospitalization

Risk for Maladaptive Grieving r/t loss of idealized pregnancy, potential loss of fetus

Ineffective Home Maintenance Behaviors r/t medical restrictions

Impaired Physical Mobility r/t medically imposed restrictions

Ineffective Role Performance r/t inability to carry out normal roles secondary to bed rest or hospitalization, change in expected course of pregnancy

Situational Low Self-Esteem r/t threatened ability to carry pregnancy to term

Sexual Dysfunction r/t actual or perceived limitation imposed by preterm labor and/or prescribed treatment, separation from partner because of hospitalization

Sleep Deprivation r/t change in usual pattern secondary to contractions, hospitalization, treatment regimen

Impaired Social Interaction r/t prolonged bed rest or hospitalization

Risk for Injury: Fetal: Risk factors: premature birth, immature body systems

Risk for Injury: Maternal: Risk factor: use of tocolytic drugs

Risk for Powerlessness: Risk factor: lack of control over preterm labor

Risk for Vascular Trauma: Risk factor: intravenous medication

Readiness for Enhanced Childbearing Process: appropriate prenatal lifestyle

Readiness for Enhanced Comfort: expresses desire to enhance relaxation

Readiness for Enhanced Communication: willingness to discuss thoughts and feelings about situation

Problem-Solving Dysfunction

Defensive Coping r/t situational crisis

Impaired Emancipated Decision-Making r/t problem-solving dysfunction

Risk for Chronic Low Self-Esteem: Risk factor: repeated failures

Readiness for Enhanced Communication: willing to share ideas with others

Readiness for Enhanced Relationship: shares information and ideas between partners

Readiness for Enhanced Resilience: identifies available resources

Readiness for Enhanced Spiritual Well-Being: desires to draw on inner strength and find meaning and purpose to life

Projection

Anxiety r/t threat to self-concept

Defensive Coping r/t inability to acknowledge that own behavior may be a problem, blaming others

Chronic Low Self-Esteem r/t failure

Impaired Social Interaction r/t self-concept disturbance, confrontational communication style

Risk for Loneliness: Risk factor: blaming others for problems

See Paranoid Personality Disorder

Prolapsed Umbilical Cord

Fear r/t threat to fetus, impending surgery

Ineffective Peripheral Tissue Perfusion: Fetal r/t interruption in umbilical blood flow

Risk for Ineffective Cerebral Tissue Perfusion: Fetal: Risk factor: cord compression

Risk for Injury: Risk factor (maternal): emergency surgery

See TURP (Transurethral Resection of the Prostate)

Prostatic Hypertrophy

Ineffective Health Maintenance Behaviors r/t deficient knowledge regarding self-care and prevention of complications

Sleep Deprivation r/t nocturia

Urinary Retention r/t obstruction

Risk for Infection: Risk factors: urinary residual after voiding, bacterial invasion of bladder

See BPH (Benign Prostatic Hypertrophy)

Prostatitis

Impaired Comfort r/t inflammation

Ineffective Health Maintenance Behaviors r/t deficient knowledge regarding treatment

Urge Urinary Incontinence r/t irritation of bladder

Ineffective Protection r/t depressed immune system

Pruritus

Impaired Comfort r/t inflammation of skin causing itching

Deficient Knowledge r/t methods to treat and prevent itching

Risk for Impaired Skin Integrity: Risk factors: scratching, dry skin

Psoriasis

Disturbed Body Image r/t lesions on body

Impaired Comfort r/t irritated skin

Ineffective Health Maintenance Behaviors r/t deficient knowledge regarding treatment modalities

Powerlessness r/t lack of control over condition with frequent exacerbations and remissions

Impaired Skin Integrity r/t lesions on body

Psychosis

Ineffective Activity Planning r/t compromised ability to process information

Ineffective Health Maintenance Behaviors r/t cognitive impairment, ineffective individual and family coping

Self-Neglect r/t mental disorder

Impaired Individual Resilience r/t psychological disorder

Situational Low Self-Esteem r/t excessive use of defense mechanisms (e.g., projection, denial, rationalization)

Risk for Disturbed Personal Identity: Risk factor: psychosis

Impaired Mood Regulation r/t psychosis

Risk for Post-Trauma Syndrome: Risk factor: diminished ego strength

See Schizophrenia

PTCA (Percutaneous Transluminal Coronary Angioplasty)

See Angioplasty, Coronary

P

PTSD (Posttraumatic Stress Disorder)

Anxiety r/t exposure to internal or external cues that symbolize or resemble an aspect of the traumatic event

Chronic Sorrow r/t chronic disability (e.g., physical, mental)

Death Anxiety r/t psychological stress associated with traumatic event

Ineffective Breathing Pattern r/t hyperventilation associated with anxiety

Ineffective Coping r/t extreme anxiety

Ineffective Impulse Control r/t thinking of initial trauma experience

Ineffective Relationship r/t stressors

Insomnia r/t recurring nightmares

Post-Trauma Syndrome r/t exposure to a traumatic event

Sleep Deprivation r/t nightmares interrupting sleep associated with traumatic event

Spiritual Distress r/t feelings of detachment or estrangement from others

Risk for Impaired Resilience: Risk factor: chronicity of existing crisis

Risk for Powerlessness: Risk factors: flashbacks, reliving event

Risk for Ineffective Relationship: Risk factor: stressful life events

Risk for Self- or Other-Directed Violence: Risk factors: fear of self or others

Readiness for Enhanced Comfort: expresses desire to enhance relaxation

Readiness for Enhanced Communication: willingness to express feelings and thoughts

Readiness for Enhanced Spiritual Well-Being: desire for harmony after stressful event

Pulmonary Edema

Anxiety r/t fear of suffocation

Ineffective Airway Clearance r/t presence of tracheobronchial secretions

Decreased Cardiac Output r/t increased preload, infective forward perfusion

Impaired Gas Exchange r/t extravasation of extravascular fluid in lung tissues and alveoli

Ineffective Health Maintenance Behaviors r/t deficient knowledge regarding treatment regimen

Sleep Deprivation r/t inability to breathe

Risk for Acute Confusion: Risk factor: hypoxia

See Heart Failure

Pulmonary Embolism (PE)

Anxiety r/t fear of suffocation

Decreased Cardiac Output r/t right ventricular failure secondary to obstructed pulmonary artery

Fear r/t severe pain, possible death

Impaired Gas Exchange r/t altered blood flow to alveoli secondary to embolus

Deficient Knowledge r/t activities to prevent embolism, self-care after diagnosis of embolism

Acute Pain r/t biological injury, lack of oxygen to cells

Ineffective Peripheral Tissue Perfusion r/t deep vein thrombus formation

Risk for Thrombosis r/t sedentary lifestyle

See Anticoagulant Therapy

Pulmonary Stenosis

See Congenital Heart Disease/Cardiac Anomalies

Pulse Deficit

Risk for Decreased Cardiac Output r/t dysrhythmia

See Dysrhythmia

Pulse Oximetry

Readiness for Enhanced Knowledge: information about treatment regimen

See Hypoxia

Pulse Pressure, Increased

See Intracranial Pressure, Increased

Pulse Pressure, Narrowed

See Shock, Hypovolemic

Pulses, Absent or Diminished Peripheral

Ineffective Peripheral Tissue Perfusion r/t interruption of arterial flow

Risk for Peripheral Neurovascular Dysfunction: Risk factors: fractures, mechanical compression, orthopedic surgery trauma, immobilization, burns, vascular obstruction

Purpura

See Clotting Disorder

Pyelonephritis

Ineffective Health Maintenance Behaviors r/t deficient knowledge regarding self-care, treatment of disease, prevention of further urinary tract infections

Acute Pain r/t inflammation and irritation of urinary tract

Disturbed Sleep Pattern r/t urinary frequency

Impaired Urinary Elimination r/t irritation of urinary tract

Pyloric Stenosis

Imbalanced Nutrition: Less than Body Requirements r/t vomiting secondary to pyloric sphincter obstruction

Acute Pain r/t abdominal fullness

Risk for Decreased Fluid Volume: Risk factors: vomiting, dehydration

See Hospitalized Child

Pyloromyotomy (Pyloric Stenosis Repair)

See Surgery Preoperative Care, Perioperative Care, Postoperative Care

R

RA (Rheumatoid Arthritis)

See Rheumatoid Arthritis (RA)

Rabies

Ineffective Health Maintenance Behaviors r/t deficient knowledge regarding care of wound, isolation, and observation of infected animal

Acute Pain r/t multiple immunization injections

Risk for Ineffective Cerebral Tissue Perfusion: Risk factor: rabies virus

Radial Nerve Dysfunction

Acute Pain r/t trauma to hand or arm

Chronic Pain r/t trauma hand or arm

See Neuropathy, Peripheral

Radiation Therapy (Radiotherapy)

Decreased Activity Tolerance r/t fatigue from possible anemia

Disturbed Body Image r/t change in appearance, hair loss

Diarrhea r/t irradiation effects

Fatigue r/t malnutrition from lack of appetite, nausea, and vomiting; side effect of radiation

Deficient Knowledge r/t what to expect with radiation therapy, how to do self-care

Nausea r/t side effects of radiation

Imbalanced Nutrition: Less than Body Requirements r/t anorexia, nausea, vomiting, irradiation of areas of pharynx and esophagus

Impaired Oral Mucous Membrane Integrity r/t irradiation effects

Ineffective Protection r/t suppression of bone marrow

Risk for Dry Mouth: Risk factor: possible side effect of radiation treatments

Risk for Impaired Oral Mucous Membrane Integrity: Risk factor: radiation treatments

Risk for Powerlessness: Risk factors: medical treatment and possible side effects

Risk for Impaired Resilience: Risk factor: radiation treatment

Risk for Impaired Skin Integrity: Risk factor: irradiation effects

Risk for Spiritual Distress: Risk factors: radiation treatment, prognosis

Ineffective Dry Eye Self-Management inattentive to dry eye symptoms from radiotherapy treatment regimen

Radical Neck Dissection

See Laryngectomy

Rage

Risk-Prone Health Behavior r/t multiple stressors

Labile Emotional Control r/t psychiatric disorders and mood disorders

Impaired Individual Resilience r/t poor impulse control

Stress Overload r/t multiple coexisting stressors

Risk for Self-Mutilation: Risk factor: command hallucinations

Risk for Suicidal Behavior: Risk factor: desire to kill self

Risk for Other-Directed Violence: Risk factors: panic state, manic excitement, organic brain syndrome

Rape-Trauma Syndrome

Rape-Trauma Syndrome (See **Rape-Trauma Syndrome,** Section III)

Chronic Sorrow r/t forced loss of virginity

Risk for Ineffective Childbearing Process r/t to trauma and violence

Risk for Post-Trauma Syndrome: Risk factor: trauma or violence associated with rape

Risk for Powerlessness: Risk factor: inability to control thoughts about incident

Risk for Ineffective Relationship: Risk factor: trauma and violence

Risk for Chronic Low Self-Esteem: Risk factors: perceived lack of respect from others, feeling violated

Risk for Spiritual Distress: Risk factor: forced loss of virginity

Rash

Impaired Comfort r/t pruritus

Impaired Skin Integrity r/t mechanical trauma

Risk for Infection: Risk factors: traumatized tissue, broken skin

Rationalization

Defensive Coping r/t situational crisis, inability to accept blame for consequences of own behavior

Ineffective Denial r/t fear of consequences, actual or perceived loss

Impaired Individual Resilience r/t psychological disturbance

Risk for Post-Trauma Syndrome: Risk factor: survivor's role in event

Readiness for Enhanced Communication: expresses desire to share thoughts and feelings

Readiness for Enhanced Spiritual Well-Being: possibility of seeking harmony with self, others, higher power, God

Rats, Rodents in Home

Ineffective Home Maintenance Behaviors r/t lack of knowledge, insufficient finances

Risk for Allergic Reaction: Risk factor: repeated exposure to environmental contamination

See Filthy Home Environment

Raynaud's Disease

Deficient Knowledge r/t lack of information about disease process, possible complications, self-care needs regarding disease process and medication

Ineffective Peripheral Tissue Perfusion r/t transient reduction of blood flow

Acute Pain r/t transient reduction in blood flow

RDS (Respiratory Distress Syndrome)

See Respiratory Conditions of the Neonate

Rectal Fullness

Chronic Functional Constipation r/t decreased activity level, decreased fluid intake, inadequate fiber in diet, decreased peristalsis, side effects of antidepressant or antipsychotic therapy

Risk for Chronic Functional Constipation: Risk factor: habitual denial of or ignoring urge to defecate

Rectal Lump

See Hemorrhoids

Rectal Pain/Bleeding

Chronic Functional Constipation r/t pain on defecation

Deficient Knowledge r/t possible causes of rectal bleeding, pain, treatment modalities

Acute Pain r/t pressure of defecation

Risk for Bleeding: Risk factor: rectal disease

Rectal Surgery

See Hemorrhoidectomy

Rectocele Repair

Chronic Functional Constipation r/t painful defecation

Ineffective Health Maintenance Behaviors r/t deficient knowledge of postoperative care of surgical site, dietary measures, exercise to prevent constipation

Acute Pain r/t surgical procedure

Urinary Retention r/t edema from surgery

Risk for Bleeding: Risk factor: surgery

Risk for Surgical Site Infection: Risk factors: surgical procedure, possible contamination of area with feces

Reflex Incontinence

Mixed Urinary Incontinence (See **Incontinence, Urinary, Reflex**, Section III)

Regression

Anxiety r/t threat to or change in health status

Defensive Coping r/t denial of obvious problems, weaknesses

Self-Neglect r/t functional impairment

Powerlessness r/t health care environment

Impaired Individual Resilience r/t psychological disturbance

Ineffective Role Performance r/t powerlessness over health status

See Hospitalized Child; Separation Anxiety

Regretful

Anxiety r/t situational or maturational crises

Death Anxiety r/t feelings of not having accomplished goals in life

Risk for Spiritual Distress: Risk factor: inability to forgive

Rehabilitation

Ineffective Coping r/t loss of normal function

Impaired Physical Mobility r/t injury, surgery, psychosocial condition warranting rehabilitation

Self-Care Deficit: Specify r/t impaired physical mobility

Risk for Adult Falls: Risk factor: physical deconditioning

Risk for Child Falls: Risk factor: Decreased lower extremity strength

Readiness for Enhanced Comfort: expresses desire to enhance feeling of comfort

Readiness for Enhanced Self-Concept: accepts strengths and limitations

Readiness for Enhanced Health Self-Management: expresses desire to manage rehabilitation

Relationship

Ineffective Relationship (See **Ineffective Relationship,** Section III)

Readiness for Enhanced Relationship (See **Risk for Enhanced Relationship,** Section III)

Relaxation Techniques

Anxiety r/t situational crisis

Readiness for Enhanced Comfort: expresses desire to enhance relaxation

Readiness for Enhanced Health Self-Management: desire to manage illness

Readiness for Enhanced Religiosity: requests religious materials or experiences

Readiness for Enhanced Resilience: desire to enhance resilience

Readiness for Enhanced Self-Concept: willingness to enhance self-concept

Readiness for Enhanced Spiritual Well-Being: seeking comfort from higher power

Religiosity

Impaired Religiosity (See **Religiosity, Impaired,** Section III)

Risk for Impaired Religiosity (See **Religiosity, Impaired, Risk for,** Section III)

Readiness for Enhanced Religiosity (See **Religiosity, Readiness for Enhanced,** Section III)

Religious Concerns

Spiritual Distress r/t separation from religious or cultural ties

Risk for Impaired Religiosity: Risk factors: ineffective support, coping, caregiving

Risk for Spiritual Distress: Risk factors: physical or psychological stress

Readiness for Enhanced Spiritual Well-Being: desire for increased spirituality

Relocation Stress Syndrome

Relocation Stress Syndrome (See **Relocation Stress Syndrome,** Section III)

Risk for Relocation Stress Syndrome (See **Relocation Stress Syndrome, Risk for,** Section III)

Renal Failure

Decreased Activity Tolerance r/t effects of anemia, heart failure

Death Anxiety r/t unknown outcome of disease

Decreased Cardiac Output r/t effects of heart failure, elevated potassium levels interfering with conduction system

Impaired Comfort r/t pruritus

Ineffective Coping r/t depression resulting from chronic disease

Fatigue r/t effects of chronic uremia and anemia

Excessive Fluid Volume r/t decreased urine output, sodium retention, inappropriate fluid intake

Ineffective Health Self-Management r/t complexity of health care regimen, inadequate number of cues to action, perceived barriers, powerlessness

Imbalanced Nutrition: Less than Body Requirements r/t anorexia, nausea, vomiting, altered taste sensation, dietary restrictions

Impaired Oral Mucous Membrane Integrity r/t irritation from nitrogenous waste products

Chronic Sorrow r/t chronic illness

Spiritual Distress r/t dealing with chronic illness

Impaired Urinary Elimination r/t effects of disease, need for dialysis

Risk for Electrolyte Imbalance: Risk factor: renal dysfunction

Risk for Infection: Risk factor: altered immune functioning

Risk for Injury: Risk factors: bone changes, neuropathy, muscle weakness

Risk for Impaired Oral Mucous Membrane Integrity: Risk factors: dehydration, effects of uremia

Risk for Powerlessness: Risk factor: chronic illness

Risk for Sepsis: Risk factor: infection

Renal Failure Acute/Chronic, Child

Disturbed Body Image r/t growth retardation, bone changes, visibility of dialysis access devices (shunt, fistula), edema

Decreased Diversional Activity Engagement r/t immobility during dialysis

See Child with Chronic Condition; Hospitalized Child

Renal Failure, Nonoliguric

Anxiety r/t change in health status

Risk for Deficient Fluid Volume: Risk factor: loss of large volumes of urine

See Renal Failure

Respiratory Acidosis

See Acidosis, Respiratory

Respiratory Conditions of the Neonate (Respiratory Distress Syndrome [RDS], Meconium Aspiration, Diaphragmatic Hernia)

Ineffective Airway Clearance r/t sequelae of attempts to breathe in utero resulting in meconium aspiration

Fatigue r/t increased energy requirements and metabolic demands

Impaired Gas Exchange r/t decreased surfactant, immature lung tissue

Dysfunctional Ventilator Weaning Response r/t immature respiratory system

Risk for Infection: Risk factors: tissue destruction or irritation as a result of aspiration of meconium fluid

See Bronchopulmonary Dysplasia; Hospitalized Child; Premature Infant, Child

Respiratory Distress

See Dyspnea

Respiratory Distress Syndrome (RDS)

See Respiratory Conditions of the Neonate

Respiratory Infections, Acute Childhood (Croup, Epiglottitis, Pertussis, Pneumonia, Respiratory Syncytial Virus)

Decreased Activity Tolerance r/t generalized weakness, dyspnea, fatigue, poor oxygenation

Ineffective Airway Clearance r/t excess tracheobronchial secretions

Ineffective Breathing Pattern r/t inflamed bronchial passages, coughing

Fear r/t oxygen deprivation, difficulty breathing

Deficient Fluid Volume r/t insensible losses (fever, diaphoresis), inadequate oral fluid intake

Impaired Gas Exchange r/t insufficient oxygenation as a result of inflammation or edema of epiglottis, larynx, bronchial passages

Imbalanced Nutrition: Less than Body Requirements r/t anorexia, fatigue, generalized weakness, poor sucking and breathing coordination, dyspnea

Ineffective Thermoregulation r/t infectious process

Risk for Aspiration: Risk factors: inability to coordinate breathing, coughing, sucking

Risk for Infection: Transmission to Others: Risk factor: virulent infectious organisms

Risk for Injury (to Pregnant Others): Risk factors: exposure to aerosolized medications (e.g., ribavirin, pentamidine), resultant potential fetal toxicity

Risk for Suffocation: Risk factors: inflammation of larynx, epiglottis

See Hospitalized Child

Respiratory Syncytial Virus

See Respiratory Infections, Acute Childhood

Restless Leg Syndrome

Disturbed Sleep Pattern r/t leg discomfort during sleep relieved by frequent leg movement

Chronic Pain r/t leg discomfort

See Stress

Retinal Detachment

Anxiety r/t change in vision, threat of loss of vision

Deficient Knowledge r/t symptoms, need for early intervention to prevent permanent damage

Vision Loss r/t impaired visual acuity

Risk for Ineffective Home Maintenance Behaviors: Risk factors: postoperative care, activity limitations, care of affected eye

Risk for Impaired Resilience: Risk factor: possible loss of vision

See Vision Impairment

Retinopathy, Diabetic

See Diabetic Retinopathy

Retinopathy of Prematurity (ROP)

Risk for Injury: Risk factors: prolonged mechanical ventilation, ROP secondary to 100% oxygen environment

See Retinal Detachment

Rh Factor Incompatibility

Anxiety r/t unknown outcome of pregnancy

Neonatal Hyperbilirubinemia r/t Rh factor incompatibility

Deficient Knowledge r/t treatment regimen from lack of experience with situation

Powerlessness r/t perceived lack of control over outcome of pregnancy

Risk for Injury: Fetal: Risk factors: intrauterine destruction of red blood cells, transfusions

Risk for Neonatal Hyperbilirubinemia: Risk factor: Rh factor incompatibility

Readiness for Enhanced Health Management: prenatal care, compliance with diagnostic and treatment regimen

Rhabdomyolysis

Ineffective Coping r/t seriousness of condition

Impaired Physical Mobility r/t myalgia and muscle weakness

Risk for Deficient Fluid Volume: Risk factor: reduced blood flow to kidneys

Risk for Shock: Risk factor: hypovolemia

Readiness for Enhanced Health Management: seeks information to avoid condition

See Kidney Failure

Rheumatic Fever

See Endocarditis

Rheumatoid Arthritis (RA)

Imbalanced Nutrition: Less than Body Requirements r/t loss of appetite

Chronic Pain r/t joint inflammation

Disturbed Body Image r/t joint deformity and muscle atrophy

Impaired Physical Mobility r/t pain, impaired joints

Risk for Impaired Resilience: Risk factor: chronic, painful, progressive disease

See Arthritis; JRA (Juvenile Rheumatoid Arthritis)

Rib Fracture

Ineffective Breathing Pattern r/t fractured ribs

Acute Pain r/t movement, deep breathing

Impaired Gas Exchange r/t ventilation-perfusion imbalance, decreased depth of ventilation

Ridicule of Others

Defensive Coping r/t situational crisis, psychological impairment, substance abuse

Risk for Post-Trauma Syndrome: Risk factor: perception of event

Ringworm of Body

Impaired Comfort r/t pruritus

Impaired Skin Integrity r/t presence of macules associated with fungus

See Itching; Pruritus

Ringworm of Nails

Disturbed Body Image r/t appearance of nails, removed nails

Ringworm of Scalp

Disturbed Body Image r/t possible hair loss (alopecia)

See Itching; Pruritus

Roaches, Invasion of Home with

Ineffective Home maintenance Behaviors r/t lack of knowledge, insufficient finances

See Filthy Home Environment

Role Performance, Altered

Ineffective Role Performance (See **Role Performance, Ineffective,** Section III)

ROP (Retinopathy of Prematurity)

See Retinopathy of Prematurity (ROP)

RSV (Respiratory Syncytial Virus)

See Respiratory Infection, Acute Childhood

Rubella

See Communicable Diseases, Childhood (e.g., Measles, Mumps, Rubella, Chickenpox, Scabies, Lice, Impetigo)

Rubor of Extremities

Ineffective Peripheral Tissue Perfusion r/t interruption of arterial flow

See Peripheral Vascular Disease (PVD)

Ruptured Disk

See Low Back Pain

S

SAD (Seasonal Affective Disorder)

Readiness for Enhanced Resilience: uses SAD lights during winter months

See Depression (Major Depressive Disorder)

Sadness

Risk for Maladaptive Grieving r/t actual or perceived loss

Impaired Mood Regulation r/t chronic illness (See **Mood Regulation, Impaired,** Section III)

Spiritual Distress r/t intense suffering

Risk for Powerlessness: Risk factor: actual or perceived loss

Risk for Spiritual Distress: Risk factor: loss of loved one

Readiness for Enhanced Communication: willingness to share feelings and thoughts

Readiness for Enhanced Spiritual Well-Being: desire for harmony after actual or perceived loss

See Depression (Major Depressive Disorder); Major Depressive Disorder

Safe Sex

Readiness for Enhanced Health Self-Management: takes appropriate precautions during sexual activity to keep from contracting sexually transmitted disease

See Sexuality, Adolescent; STD (Sexually Transmitted Disease)

Safety, Childhood

Deficient Knowledge: Potential for Enhanced Health Self-Maintenance r/t parental knowledge and skill acquisition regarding appropriate safety measures

Risk for Aspiration (See **Aspiration, Risk for,** Section III)

Risk for Injury: Risk factors: developmental age, altered home maintenance

Risk for Impaired Parenting: Risk factors: lack of available and effective role model, lack of knowledge, misinformation from other family members (old wives' tales)

Risk for Poisoning: Risk factors: use of lead-based paint; presence of asbestos or radon gas; drugs not locked in cabinet; household products left in accessible area (bleach, detergent, drain cleaners, household cleaners); alcohol and perfume within reach of child; presence of poisonous plants; atmospheric pollutants

Risk for Thermal injury: Risk factor: inadequate supervision

Readiness for Enhanced Childbearing Process: expresses appropriate knowledge for care of child

Salmonella

Impaired Home Maintenance r/t improper preparation or storage of food, lack of safety measures when caring for pet reptile

Risk for Shock: Risk factors: hypovolemia, diarrhea, sepsis

Readiness for Enhanced Health Self-Management: avoiding improperly prepared or stored food, wearing gloves when handling pet reptiles or their feces

See Gastroenteritis; Gastroenteritis, Child

Salpingectomy

Decisional Conflict r/t sterilization procedure

Maladaptive Grieving r/t possible loss from tubal pregnancy

Risk for Impaired Urinary Elimination: Risk factor: trauma to ureter during surgery

See Hysterectomy; Surgery, Perioperative Care; Surgery, Postoperative Care; Surgery, Preoperative Care

Sarcoidosis

Anxiety r/t change in health status

Impaired Gas Exchange r/t ventilation-perfusion imbalance

Ineffective Health Maintenance Behaviors r/t deficient knowledge regarding home care and medication regimen

Acute Pain r/t possible disease affecting joints

Ineffective Protection r/t immune disorder

Risk for Decreased Cardiac Tissue Perfusion: Risk factor: dysrhythmias

Risk for Impaired Skin integrity: Risk factor: immunological disorder

SBE (Self–Breast Examination)

Readiness for Enhanced Health Self-Management: desires to have information about SBE

Readiness for Enhanced Knowledge: SBE

Scabies

See Communicable Diseases, Childhood (e.g., Measles, Mumps, Rubella, Chickenpox, Scabies, Lice, Impetigo)

Scared

Anxiety r/t threat of death, threat to or change in health status

Death Anxiety r/t unresolved issues surrounding end-of-life decisions

Fear r/t hospitalization, real or imagined threat to own well-being

Impaired Individual Resilience r/t violence

Readiness for Enhanced Communication: willingness to share thoughts and feelings

Schizophrenia

Ineffective Activity Planning r/t compromised ability to process information

Anxiety r/t unconscious conflict with reality

Impaired Verbal Communication r/t psychosis, disorientation, inaccurate perception, hallucinations, delusions

Ineffective Coping r/t inadequate support systems, unrealistic perceptions, inadequate coping skills, disturbed thought processes, impaired communication

Decreased Diversional Activity Engagement r/t social isolation, possible regression

Interrupted Family Processes r/t inability to express feelings, impaired communication

Fear r/t altered contact with reality

Ineffective Health Maintenance Behaviors r/t cognitive impairment, ineffective individual and family coping, lack of material resources

Ineffective Family Health Self-Management r/t chronicity and unpredictability of condition

Ineffective Home Maintenance Behaviors r/t impaired cognitive or emotional functioning, insufficient finances, inadequate support systems

Hopelessness r/t long-term stress from chronic mental illness

Disturbed Personal Identity r/t psychiatric disorder

Impaired Memory r/t psychosocial condition

Imbalanced Nutrition: Less than Body Requirements r/t fear of eating, lack of awareness of hunger, disinterest toward food

Impaired Individual Resilience r/t psychological disorder

Self-Care Deficit: Specify r/t loss of contact with reality, impairment of perception

Self-Neglect r/t psychosis

Sleep Deprivation r/t intrusive thoughts, nightmares

Impaired Social Interaction r/t impaired communication patterns, self-concept disturbance, disturbed thought processes

Social Isolation r/t lack of trust, regression, delusional thinking, repressed fears

Chronic Sorrow r/t chronic mental illness

Spiritual Distress r/t loneliness, social alienation

Risk for Caregiver Role Strain: Risk factors: bizarre behavior of client, chronicity of condition

Risk for Compromised Human Dignity: Risk factor: stigmatizing label

Risk for Loneliness: Risk factor: inability to interact socially

Risk for Post-Trauma Syndrome: Risk factor: diminished ego strength

Risk for Powerlessness: Risk factor: intrusive, distorted thinking

Risk for Impaired Religiosity: Risk factors: ineffective coping, lack of security

Risk for Suicidal Behavior: Risk factor: psychiatric illness

Risk for Self-Directed Violence: Risk factors: lack of trust, panic, hallucinations, delusional thinking

Risk for Other-Directed Violence: Risk factor: psychotic disorder

Readiness for Enhanced Hope: expresses desire to enhance interconnectedness with others and problem-solve to meet goals

Readiness for Enhanced Power: expresses willingness to enhance participation in choices for daily living and health and enhance knowledge for participation in change

Sciatica

See Neuropathy, Peripheral

Scoliosis

Risk-Prone Health Behavior r/t lack of developmental maturity to comprehend long-term consequences of noncompliance with treatment procedures

Disturbed Body Image r/t use of therapeutic braces, postsurgery scars, restricted physical activity

Impaired Comfort r/t altered health status and body image

Impaired Gas Exchange r/t restricted lung expansion as a result of severe presurgery curvature of spine, immobilization

Ineffective Health Maintenance Behaviors r/t deficient knowledge regarding treatment modalities, restrictions, home care, postoperative activities

Impaired Physical Mobility r/t restricted movement, dyspnea caused by severe curvature of spine

Acute Pain r/t musculoskeletal restrictions, surgery, reambulation with cast or spinal rod

Impaired Skin Integrity r/t braces, casts, surgical correction

Chronic Sorrow r/t chronic disability

Risk for Perioperative Positioning Injury: Risk factor: prone position

Risk for Impaired Resilience: Risk factor: chronic condition

Readiness for Enhanced Health Self-Management: desires knowledge regarding treatment for condition

See Hospitalized Child; Maturational Issues, Adolescent

S

Sedentary Lifestyle

Decreased Activity Tolerance r/t sedentary lifestyle

Sedentary Lifestyle (See **Sedentary Lifestyle,** Section III)

Obesity (See **Obesity,** Section III)

Overweight (See **Overweight,** Section III)

Risk for Overweight (See **Overweight,** Section III)

Risk for Ineffective Peripheral Tissue Perfusion: Risk factor: insufficient knowledge of aggravating factors (e.g., immobility, obesity)

Readiness for Enhanced Coping: seeking knowledge of new strategies to adjust to sedentary lifestyle

Seizure Disorders, Adult

Acute Confusion r/t postseizure state

Social Isolation r/t unpredictability of seizures, community-imposed stigma

Risk for Ineffective Airway Clearance: Risk factor: accumulation of secretions during seizure

Risk for Child Falls: Risk factor: uncontrolled seizure activity

Risk for Powerlessness: Risk factor: possible seizure

Risk for Impaired Resilience: Risk factor: chronic illness

Readiness for Enhanced Knowledge: anticonvulsive therapy

Readiness for Enhanced Self-Care: expresses desire to enhance knowledge and responsibility for self-care

See Epilepsy

Seizure Disorders, Childhood (Epilepsy, Febrile Seizures, Infantile Spasms)

Ineffective Health Maintenance Behaviors r/t lack of knowledge regarding anticonvulsive therapy, fever reduction (febrile seizures)

Social Isolation r/t unpredictability of seizures, community-imposed stigma

Risk for Ineffective Airway Clearance: Risk factor: accumulation of secretions during seizure

Risk for Delayed Child Development: Risk factors: effects of seizure disorder, parental overprotection

Risk for Child Falls: Risk factor: possible seizure

Risk for Injury: Risk factors: uncontrolled movements during seizure, falls, drowsiness caused by anticonvulsants

See Epilepsy

Self–Breast Examination (SBE)

See SBE (Self–Breast Examination)

Self-Care

Readiness for Enhanced Self-Care (See **Self-Care, Readiness for Enhanced,** Section III)

Self-Care Deficit, Bathing

Bathing Self-Care Deficit (See **Self-Care Deficit, Bathing,** Section III)

Self-Care Deficit, Dressing

Dressing Self-Care Deficit (See **Self-Care Deficit, Dressing,** Section III)

Self-Care Deficit, Feeding

Feeding Self-Care Deficit (See **Self-Care Deficit, Feeding,** Section III)

Self-Care Deficit, Toileting

Toileting Self-Care Deficit (See **Self-Care Deficit, Toileting,** Section III)

Self-Concept

Readiness for Enhanced Self-Concept (See **Self-Concept, Readiness for Enhanced,** Section III)

Self-Destructive Behavior

Post-Trauma Syndrome r/t unresolved feelings from traumatic event

Risk for Self-Mutilation: Risk factors: feelings of depression, rejection, self-hatred, depersonalization; command hallucinations

Risk for Suicidal Behavior: Risk factor: history of self-destructive behavior

Risk for Self-Directed Violence: Risk factors: panic state, history of child abuse, toxic reaction to medication

Self-Esteem, Chronic Low

Chronic Low Self-Esteem (See **Self-Esteem, Low, Chronic,** Section III)

Risk for Disturbed Personal Identity: Risk factor: chronic low self-esteem

Self-Esteem, Situational Low

Situational Low Self-Esteem (See **Self-Esteem, Low, Situational,** Section III)

Risk for Situational Low Self-Esteem (See **Self-Esteem, Low, Situational, Risk For,** Section III)

Self-Mutilation

Ineffective Impulse Control r/t ineffective management of anxiety

Self-Mutilation (See **Self-Mutilation,** Section III)

Risk for Self-Mutilation (See **Self-Mutilation, Risk for,** Section III)

Senile Dementia

Ineffective Relationship r/t cognitive changes in one partner

Sedentary Lifestyle r/t lack of interest in movement

See Dementia

Separation Anxiety

Ineffective Coping r/t maturational and situational crises, vulnerability related to developmental age, hospitalization, separation from family and familiar surroundings, multiple caregivers

Insomnia r/t separation for significant others

Risk for Impaired Attachment: Risk factor: separation

See Hospitalized Child

Sepsis, Child

Impaired Gas Exchange r/t pulmonary inflammation associated with disease process

Imbalanced Nutrition: Less than Body Requirements r/t anorexia, generalized weakness, poor sucking reflex

Delayed Surgical Recovery r/t presence of infection

Ineffective Thermoregulation r/t infectious process, septic shock

Ineffective Peripheral Tissue Perfusion r/t arterial or venous blood flow exchange problems, septic shock

Risk for Deficient Fluid Volume: Risk factor: inflammation leading to decreased systemic vascular resistance

Risk for Impaired Skin Integrity: Risk factor: desquamation caused by disseminated intravascular coagulation

See Hospitalized Child; Premature Infant, Child

Septicemia

Imbalanced Nutrition: Less than Body Requirements r/t anorexia, generalized weakness

Ineffective Peripheral Tissue Perfusion r/t decreased systemic vascular resistance

Risk for Deficient Fluid Volume: Risk factors: vasodilation of peripheral vessels, leaking of capillaries

Risk for Shock: Risk factors: hypotension, hypovolemia

Risk for Unstable Blood Pressure: Risk factor: hypovolemia

See Sepsis, Child; Shock, Septic

Service Animal

Readiness for Enhanced Power: expresses desire to enhance independence with actions for change

Readiness for Enhanced Resilience: expresses desire to enhance involvement in activities, desire to enhance environmental safety

Severe Acute Respiratory Syndrome (SARS)

See Pneumonia

Sexual Dysfunction

Sexual Dysfunction r/t insufficient knowledge about sexual function

Ineffective Relationship r/t reported sexual dissatisfaction between partners

Chronic Sorrow r/t loss of ideal sexual experience, altered relationships

Risk for Situational Low Self-Esteem: Risk factor: alteration in body function

See Erectile Dysfunction (ED)

Sexual Harassment Victim

Anxiety r/t situational crisis

Risk for Compromised Human Dignity: Risk factors: humiliation, dehumanizing treatment

Risk for Post-Trauma Syndrome: Risk factors: perceived traumatic event, insufficient social support

Risk for Spiritual Distress: Risk factors: physical, psychological stress

See Assault Victim

Sexuality, Adolescent

Disturbed Body Image r/t anxiety caused by unachieved developmental milestone (puberty) or deficient knowledge regarding reproductive maturation with expressed concerns regarding lack of growth of secondary sex characteristics

Impaired Emancipated Decision-Making: Sexual Activity r/t undefined personal values or beliefs, multiple or divergent sources of information, lack of relevant information

Ineffective Impulse control r/t denial of consequences of actions

Deficient Knowledge: Potential for Enhanced Health Self-Maintenance r/t multiple or divergent sources of information or lack of relevant information regarding sexual transmission of disease, contraception, prevention of toxic shock syndrome

See Maturational Issues, Adolescent

Sexuality Pattern, Ineffective

Ineffective Sexuality Pattern (See **Sexuality Pattern, Ineffective,** Section III)

Sexually Transmitted Disease (STD)

See STD (Sexually Transmitted Disease)

Shaken Baby Syndrome

Impaired Parenting r/t stress, history of being abusive

Impaired Individual Resilience r/t poor impulse control

Stress Overload r/t intense repeated family stressors, family violence

Risk for Other-Directed Violence: Risk factors: history of violence against others, perinatal complications

See Child Abuse; Suspected Child Abuse and Neglect (SCAN), Child; Suspected Child Abuse and Neglect (SCAN), Parent

Shakiness

Anxiety r/t situational or maturational crisis, threat of death

Shame

S

Situational Low Self-Esteem r/t inability to deal with past traumatic events, blaming of self for events not in one's control

Shingles

Acute Pain r/t vesicular eruption along the nerves

Ineffective Protection r/t abnormal blood profiles

Social Isolation r/t altered state of wellness, contagiousness of disease

Risk for Infection: Risk factor: tissue destruction

See Itching

Shivering

Impaired Comfort r/t altered health status

Fear r/t serious threat to health status

Hypothermia r/t exposure to cool environment

Ineffective Thermoregulation r/t serious infectious process resulting in immune response of fever

See Shock, Septic

Shock, Cardiogenic

Decreased Cardiac Output r/t decreased myocardial contractility, dysrhythmia

Shock, Hypovolemic

Deficient Fluid Volume r/t abnormal loss of fluid, trauma, third spacing

Shock, Septic

Deficient Fluid Volume r/t abnormal loss of intravascular fluid, pooling of blood in peripheral circulation, overwhelming inflammatory response

Ineffective Protection r/t inadequately functioning immune system

See Sepsis, Child; Septicemia

Shoulder Repair

Self-Care Deficit: Bathing, Dressing, Feeding r/t immobilization of affected shoulder

Risk for Perioperative Positioning Injury: Risk factor: immobility

See Surgery, Preoperative Care; Surgery, Perioperative Care; Surgery, Postoperative Care; Total Joint Replacement (Total Hip/Total Knee/Shoulder)

Sickle Cell Anemia/Crisis

Decreased Activity Tolerance r/t fatigue, effects of chronic anemia

Deficient Fluid Volume r/t decreased intake, increased fluid requirements during sickle cell crisis, decreased ability of kidneys to concentrate urine

Impaired Physical Mobility r/t pain, fatigue

Acute Pain r/t viscous blood, tissue hypoxia

Ineffective Peripheral Tissue Perfusion r/t effects of red cell sickling, infarction of tissues

Risk for Decreased Cardiac Tissue Perfusion: Risk factors: effects of red cell sickling, infarction of tissues

Risk for Infection: Risk factor: alterations in splenic function

Risk for Impaired Resilience: Risk factor: chronic illness

Risk for Ineffective Cerebral Tissue Perfusion: Risk factors: effects of red cell sickling, infarction of tissues

See Child with Chronic Condition; Hospitalized Child

SIDS (Sudden Infant Death Syndrome)

Anxiety: Parental Worry r/t life-threatening event

Interrupted Family Processes r/t stress as a result of special care needs of infant with apnea

Maladaptive Grieving r/t potential loss of infant

Insomnia: Parental/Infant r/t home apnea monitoring

Deficient Knowledge: Potential For Enhanced Health Self-Maintenance r/t knowledge or skill acquisition of cardiopulmonary resuscitation and home apnea monitoring

Impaired Resilience r/t sudden loss

Risk for Sudden Infant Death (See **Sudden Infant Death, Risk for,** Section III)

Risk for Powerlessness: Risk factor: unanticipated life-threatening event

See Terminally Ill Child/Death of Child, Parent

Sitting Problems

Impaired Sitting (See **Sitting, Impaired,** Section III)

Situational Crisis

Imbalanced Energy Field r/t hyperactivity of the energy flow

Ineffective Coping r/t situational crisis

Interrupted Family Processes r/t situational crisis

Risk for Ineffective Activity Planning: Risk factor: inability to process information

Risk for Disturbed Personal Identity: Risk factor: situational crisis

Readiness for Enhanced Communication: willingness to share feelings and thoughts

Readiness for Enhanced Religiosity: requests religious material and/or experiences

Readiness for Enhanced Resilience: desire to enhance resilience

Readiness for Enhanced Spiritual Well-Being: desire for harmony following crisis

SJS (Stevens-Johnson Syndrome)

See Stevens-Johnson Syndrome (SJS)

Skin Cancer

Ineffective Health Maintenance Behaviors r/t deficient knowledge regarding self-care with skin cancer

Ineffective Protection r/t weakened immune system

Impaired Tissue Integrity r/t abnormal cell growth in skin, treatment of skin cancer

Readiness for Enhanced Health Self-Management: follows preventive measures

Readiness for Enhanced Knowledge: self-care to prevent and treat skin cancer

Skin Disorders

Impaired Skin Integrity (See **Skin Integrity, Impaired,** Section III)

Skin Turgor, Change in Elasticity

Deficient Fluid Volume r/t active fluid loss

Sleep

Readiness for Enhanced Sleep (See **Sleep, Readiness for Enhanced,** Section III)

Sleep Apnea

Ineffective Breathing Pattern r/t obesity, substance misuse, enlarged tonsils, smoking, or neurological pathology such as a brain tumor

Impaired Comfort r/t use of bilevel positive airway pressure (BiPAP)/continuous positive airway pressure (CPAP) machine

Sleep Deprivation

Fatigue r/t lack of sleep

Sleep Deprivation (See **Sleep Deprivation,** Section III)

Insomnia (See **Insomnia,** Section III)

Sleep Problems

Insomnia (See **Insomnia,** Section III)

Sleep Pattern, Disturbed, Parent/Child

Insomnia: Child r/t anxiety or fear

Insomnia: Parent r/t parental responsibilities, stress

See Suspected Child Abuse and Neglect (SCAN), Child; Suspected Child Abuse and Neglect (SCAN), Parent

Slurring of Speech

Impaired Verbal Communication r/t decrease in circulation to brain, brain tumor, anatomical defect, cleft palate

Situational Low Self-Esteem r/t speech impairment

See Communication Problems

Small Bowel Resection

See Abdominal Surgery

Smell, Loss of Ability to

Risk for Injury: Risk factors: inability to detect gas fumes, smoke smells

See Anosmia (Smell, Loss of Ability to)

Smoke Inhalation

Ineffective Airway Clearance r/t smoke inhalation

Impaired Gas Exchange r/t ventilation-perfusion imbalance

Risk for Acute Confusion: Risk factor: decreased oxygen supply

Risk for Infection: Risk factors: inflammation, ineffective airway clearance, pneumonia

Risk for Poisoning: Risk factor: exposure to carbon monoxide

Readiness for Enhanced Health Self-Management: functioning smoke detectors and carbon monoxide detectors in home and work, escape route planned and reviewed

See Atelectasis; Burns; Pneumonia

Smoking Behavior

Insufficient Breast Milk Production r/t smoking

Risk-Prone Health Behavior Risk factor: smoking

Ineffective Health Maintenance Behaviors r/t denial of effects of smoking, lack of effective support for smoking withdrawal

Readiness for Enhanced Knowledge: expresses interest in smoking cessation

Risk for Dry Eye: Risk factor: smoking

Risk for Ineffective Peripheral Tissue Perfusion: Risk factor: effect of nicotine

Risk for Thermal Injury: Risk factor: unsafe smoking behavior

Readiness for Enhanced Health Literacy: verbalizes desire to enhance understanding of health information to make health care choices

Social Interaction, Impaired

Impaired Social Interaction (See **Social Interaction, Impaired,** Section III)

Social Isolation

Social Isolation (See **Social Isolation,** Section III)

Sociopathic Personality

See Antisocial Personality Disorder

Sodium, Decrease/Increase

See Hyponatremia; Hypernatremia

Somatization Disorder

Anxiety r/t unresolved conflicts channeled into physical complaints or conditions

Ineffective Coping r/t lack of insight into underlying conflicts

Ineffective Denial r/t displaced psychological stress to physical symptoms

Nausea r/t anxiety

Chronic Pain r/t unexpressed anger, multiple physical disorders, depression

Impaired Individual Resilience r/t possible psychological disorders

Sore Nipples, Breastfeeding

Ineffective Breastfeeding r/t deficient knowledge regarding correct feeding procedure

Nipple-Areolar Complex Injury r/t breast engorgement

See Painful Breasts, Sore Nipples

Sore Throat

Impaired Comfort r/t sore throat

Deficient Knowledge r/t treatment, relief of discomfort

Impaired Oral Mucous Membrane Integrity r/t inflammation or infection of oral cavity

Impaired Swallowing r/t irritation of oropharyngeal cavity

Risk for Dry Mouth: Risk factor: painful swallowing

Sorrow

Maladaptive Grieving r/t loss of significant person, object, or role

Chronic Sorrow (See **Sorrow, Chronic,** Section III)

Readiness for Enhanced Communication: expresses thoughts and feelings

Readiness for Enhanced Spiritual Well-Being: desire to find purpose and meaning of loss

Spastic Colon

See IBS (Irritable Bowel Syndrome)

Speech Disorders

Anxiety r/t difficulty with communication

Impaired Verbal Communication r/t anatomical defect, cleft palate, psychological barriers, decrease in circulation to brain

Spina Bifida

See Neural Tube Defects (Meningocele, Myelomeningocele, Spina Bifida, Anencephaly)

Spinal Cord Injury

Decreased Diversional Activity Engagement r/t long-term hospitalization, frequent lengthy treatments

Fear r/t powerlessness over loss of body function

Disturbed Body Image r/t alteration in body function

Chronic Functional Constipation r/t inhibition of reflex arc

Maladaptive Grieving r/t loss of usual body function

Ineffective Coping r/t inability to meet basic needs and insufficient sense of control

Sedentary Lifestyle r/t lack of resources or interest

Impaired Physical Mobility r/t neuromuscular impairment

Impaired Wheelchair Mobility r/t neuromuscular impairment

Impaired Standing r/t spinal cord injury

Urinary Retention r/t inhibition of reflex arc

Risk for Autonomic Dysreflexia: Risk factors: bladder or bowel distention, skin irritation, deficient knowledge of client and caregiver

Risk for Ineffective Breathing Pattern: Risk factor: neuromuscular impairment

Risk for Infection: Risk factors: chronic disease, stasis of body fluids

Risk for Loneliness: Risk factor: physical immobility

Risk for Powerlessness: Risk factor: loss of function

Risk for Adult Pressure Injury: Risk factor: immobility and decreased sensation

Risk for Child Pressure Injury: Risk factor: immobility and decreased sensation

Risk for Thermal Injury: Risk factor: physical immobility

Risk for Thrombosis: Risk factor: physical immobility

See Child with Chronic Condition; Hospitalized Child; Neural Tube Defects (Meningocele, Myelomeningocele, Spina Bifida, Anencephaly); Paralysis

Spinal Fusion

Impaired Bed Mobility r/t impaired ability to turn side to side while keeping spine in proper alignment

Impaired Physical Mobility r/t musculoskeletal impairment associated with surgery, possible back brace

Readiness for Enhanced Knowledge: expresses interest in information associated with surgery

Risk for Adult Pressure Injury: Risk factor: immobility

Risk for Child Pressure Injury: Risk factor: immobility

See Acute Back Pain; Scoliosis; Surgery, Preoperative Care; Surgery, Perioperative Care; Surgery, Postoperative Care

Spiritual Distress

Spiritual Distress (See **Spiritual Distress,** Section III)

Risk for Chronic Low Self-Esteem: Risk factor: unresolved spiritual issues

Risk for Spiritual Distress (See **Spiritual Distress, Risk for,** Section III)

Spiritual Well-Being

Readiness for Enhanced Spiritual Well-Being (See **Spiritual Well-Being, Readiness for Enhanced,** Section III)

Splenectomy

See Abdominal Surgery

Sprains

Acute Pain r/t physical injury

Impaired Physical Mobility r/t injury

Impaired Walking r/t injury

Stable Blood Pressure, Risk for Unstable

Deficient Knowledge r/t inconsistency with medication regiment (See **Unstable Blood Pressure, Risk for,** Section III)

Standing Problems

Impaired Standing (See **Impaired Standing,** Section III)

Stapedectomy

Hearing Loss r/t edema from surgery

Acute Pain r/t headache

Risk for Adult Falls: Risk factor: dizziness

Risk for Infection: Risk factor: invasive procedure

Stasis Ulcer

Impaired Tissue Integrity r/t chronic venous congestion

Risk for Infection: Risk factor: open wound

See CHF (Congestive Heart Failure); Varicose Veins

STD (Sexually Transmitted Disease)

Impaired Comfort r/t infection

Fear r/t altered body function, risk for social isolation, fear of incurable illness

Ineffective Health Maintenance Behaviors r/t deficient knowledge regarding transmission, symptoms, treatment of STD

Ineffective Sexuality Pattern r/t illness, altered body function, need for abstinence to heal

Social Isolation r/t fear of contracting or spreading disease

Risk for Infection: Spread of Infection: Risk factor: lack of knowledge concerning transmission of disease

Readiness for Enhanced Knowledge: seeks information regarding prevention and treatment of STDs

See Maturational Issues, Adolescent; PID (Pelvic Inflammatory Disease)

STEMI (ST-Elevation Myocardial Infarction)

See MI (Myocardial Infarction)

Stent (Coronary Artery Stent)

Risk for Injury: Risk factor: complications associated with stent placement

Risk for Decreased Cardiac Tissue Perfusion: Risk factor: possible restenosis

Risk for Vascular Trauma: Risk factors: insertion site, catheter width

Readiness for Enhanced Decision-Making: expresses desire to enhance risk-benefit analysis, understanding and meaning of choices, and decisions regarding treatment

See Angioplasty, Coronary; Cardiac Catheterization

Sterilization Surgery

Decisional Conflict r/t multiple or divergent sources of information, unclear personal values or beliefs

See Surgery, Preoperative Care; Surgery, Perioperative Care; Surgery, Postoperative Care; Tubal Ligation; Vasectomy

Stertorous Respirations

Ineffective Airway Clearance r/t pharyngeal obstruction

Stevens-Johnson Syndrome (SJS)

Impaired Oral Mucous Membrane Integrity r/t immunocompromised condition associated with allergic medication reaction

Acute Pain r/t painful skin lesions and painful mucosa lesions

Impaired Skin Integrity r/t allergic medication reaction

Risk for Deficient Fluid Volume: Risk factors: factors affecting fluid needs (hypermetabolic state, fever), excessive losses through normal routes (vomiting and diarrhea)

Risk for Infection: Risk factor: sloughing skin

Risk for Impaired Liver Function: Risk factor: impaired immune response

Stillbirth

See Pregnancy Loss

Stoma

See Colostomy; Ileostomy

Stomatitis

Impaired Oral Mucous Membrane Integrity r/t pathological conditions of oral cavity; side effects of chemotherapy

Risk for Impaired Oral Mucous Membrane Integrity (See **Impaired Oral Mucous Membrane Integrity, Risk for,** Section III)

Stool, Hard/Dry

Chronic Functional Constipation r/t inadequate fluid intake, inadequate fiber intake, decreased activity level, decreased gastric motility

Straining with Defecation

Chronic Functional Constipation r/t less than adequate fluid intake, less than adequate dietary intake

Risk for Decreased Cardiac Output: Risk factor: vagal stimulation with dysrhythmia resulting from Valsalva maneuver

Strep Throat

Risk for Infection: Risk factor: exposure to pathogen

See Sore Throat

Stress

Anxiety r/t feelings of helplessness, feelings of being threatened

Ineffective Coping r/t ineffective use of problem-solving process, feelings of apprehension or helplessness

Fear r/t powerlessness over feelings

Stress Overload r/t intense or multiple stressors

Readiness for Enhanced Communication: shows willingness to share thoughts and feelings

Readiness for Enhanced Spiritual Well-Being: expresses desire for harmony and peace in stressful situation

See Anxiety

Stress Urinary Incontinence

Stress Urinary Incontinence r/t degenerative change in pelvic muscles

Stridor

Ineffective Airway Clearance r/t obstruction, tracheobronchial infection, trauma

Stroke

See CVA (Cerebrovascular Accident)

Stuttering

Anxiety r/t impaired verbal communication

Impaired Verbal Communication r/t anxiety, psychological problems

Subarachnoid Hemorrhage

Acute Pain: Headache r/t irritation of meninges from blood, increased intracranial pressure

Risk for Ineffective Cerebral Tissue Perfusion: Risk factor: bleeding from cerebral vessel

See Intracranial Pressure, Increased

Substance Misuse

Acute Substance Withdrawal Syndrome: Risk factor: developed dependence to alcohol or other addictive substances

Anxiety r/t threat to self-concept, lack of control of drug use

Compromised Family Coping r/t codependency issues

Defensive Coping r/t substance misuse

Disabled Family Coping r/t differing coping styles between support persons

Ineffective Coping r/t use of substances to cope with life events

S

Ineffective Denial r/t refusal to acknowledge substance misuse problem

Dysfunctional Family Processes r/t substance misuse

Risk-Prone Health behavior r/t addiction

Deficient Community Health r/t prevention and control of illegal substances in community

Ineffective Impulse Control r/t addictive process

Insomnia r/t irritability, nightmares, tremors

Imbalanced Nutrition: Less than Body Requirements r/t poor eating habits

Powerlessness r/t feeling unable to change patterns of drug abuse

Ineffective Relationship r/t inability for well-balanced collaboration between partners

Sexual Dysfunction r/t actions and side effects of drugs

Sleep Deprivation r/t prolonged psychological discomfort

Impaired Social Interaction r/t disturbed thought processes from drug abuse

Risk for Acute Substance Withdrawal Syndrome: Risk factor: developed dependence to alcohol or other addictive substances

Risk for Impaired Attachment: Risk factor: substance misuse

Risk for Injury: Risk factors: hallucinations, drug effects

Risk for Disturbed Personal Identity: Risk factor: ingestion/inhalation of toxic chemicals

Risk for Chronic Low Self-Esteem: Risk factors: perceived lack of respect from others, repeated failures, repeated negative reinforcement

Risk for Thermal Injury: Risk factor: intoxication with drugs or alcohol

Risk for Unstable Blood Pressure: Risk factor: vasoconstriction of cardiac arteries

Risk for Vascular Trauma: Risk factor: chemical irritant self injected into veins

Risk for Self-Directed Violence: Risk factors: reactions to substances used, impulsive behavior, disorientation, impaired judgment

Risk for Other-Directed Violence: Risk factor: poor impulse control

Readiness for Enhanced Coping: seeking social support and knowledge of new strategies

Readiness for Enhanced Self-Concept: accepting strengths and limitations

See Alcoholism

Substance Misuse, Adolescent

See Alcoholism; Maturational Issues, Adolescent; Substance Misuse

Substance Misuse in Pregnancy

Ineffective Childbearing Process r/t substance misuse

Defensive Coping r/t denial of situation, differing value system

Ineffective Health Self-Management r/t addiction

Deficient Knowledge r/t lack of exposure to information regarding effects of substance misuse in pregnancy

Neonatal Abstinence Syndrome r/t in utero substance exposure secondary to maternal substance use

Risk for Impaired Attachment: Risk factors: substance misuse, inability of parent to meet infant's or own personal needs

Risk for Infection: Risk factors: intravenous drug use, lifestyle

Risk for Injury: Fetal: Risk factor: effects of drugs on fetal growth and development

Risk for Injury: Maternal: Risk factor: drug or alcohol misuse

Risk for Impaired Parenting: Risk factor: lack of ability to meet infant's needs due to addiction with use of alcohol or drugs

See Alcoholism; Substance Misuse

Substance Withdrawal

See Acute Substance Withdrawal Syndrome

Sucking Reflex

Effective Breastfeeding r/t regular and sustained sucking and swallowing at breast

Sudden Infant Death Syndrome (SIDS)

See SIDS (Sudden Infant Death Syndrome)

Suffocation, Risk for

Risk for Suffocation (See **Suffocation, Risk for,** Section III)

Suicide Attempt

Risk-Prone Health Behavior r/t low self-efficacy

Ineffective Coping r/t anger, complicated grieving

Hopelessness r/t perceived or actual loss, substance misuse, low self-concept, inadequate support systems

Ineffective Impulse Control r/t inability to modulate stress, anxiety

Post-Trauma Syndrome r/t history of traumatic events, abuse, rape, incest, war, torture

Impaired Individual Resilience r/t poor impulse control

Situational Low Self-Esteem r/t guilt, inability to trust, feelings of worthlessness or rejection

Social Isolation r/t inability to engage in satisfying personal relationships

Spiritual Distress r/t hopelessness, despair

Risk for Post-Trauma Syndrome: Risk factor: survivor's role in suicide attempt

Risk for Suicidal Behavior (See **Suicide, Risk for,** Section III)

Readiness for Enhanced Communication: willingness to share thoughts and feelings

Readiness for Enhanced Spiritual Well-Being: desire for harmony and inner strength to help redefine purpose for life

See Violent Behavior

Support System, Inadequate

Readiness for Enhanced Family Coping: ability to adapt to tasks associated with care, support of significant other during health crisis

Readiness for Enhanced Family Processes: activities support the growth of family members

Readiness for Enhanced Parenting: children or other dependent person(s) expressing satisfaction with home environment

Suppression of Labor

See Preterm Labor

Surgery, Perioperative Care

Risk for Imbalanced Fluid Volume: Risk factor: surgery

Risk for Perioperative Hypothermia: Risk factors: inadequate covering of client, cold surgical room

Risk for Perioperative Positioning Injury: Risk factors: predisposing condition, prolonged surgery

Surgery, Postoperative Care

Decreased Activity Tolerance r/t pain, surgical procedure

Anxiety r/t change in health status, hospital environment

Deficient Knowledge r/t postoperative expectations, lifestyle changes

Nausea r/t manipulation of gastrointestinal tract, postsurgical anesthesia

Imbalanced Nutrition: Less than Body Requirements r/t anorexia, nausea, vomiting, decreased peristalsis

Ineffective Peripheral Tissue Perfusion r/t hypovolemia, circulatory stasis, obesity, prolonged immobility, decreased coughing, decreased deep breathing

Acute Pain r/t inflammation or injury in surgical area

Delayed Surgical Recovery r/t extensive surgical procedure, postoperative surgical infection

Urinary Retention r/t anesthesia, pain, fear, unfamiliar surroundings, client's position

Risk for Bleeding: Risk factor: surgical procedure

Risk for Ineffective Breathing Pattern: Risk factors: pain, location of incision, effects of anesthesia or opioids

Risk for Constipation: Risk factors: decreased activity, decreased food or fluid intake, anesthesia, pain medication

Risk for Imbalanced Fluid Volume: Risk factors: hypermetabolic state, fluid loss during surgery, presence of indwelling tubes, fluids used to distend organ structures being absorbed into body

Risk for Surgical Site Infection: Risk factors: invasive procedure, pain, anesthesia, location of incision, weakened cough as a result of aging

Surgery, Preoperative Care

Anxiety r/t threat to or change in health status, situational crisis, fear of the unknown

Insomnia r/t anxiety about upcoming surgery

Deficient Knowledge r/t preoperative procedures, postoperative expectations

Readiness for Enhanced Knowledge: shows understanding of preoperative and postoperative expectations for self-care

Surgical Recovery, Delayed

Delayed Surgical Recovery (See **Surgical Recovery, Delayed,** Section III)

Risk for Delayed Surgical Recovery (See **Surgical Recovery, Delayed, Risk for,** Section III)

Surgical Site Infection

Anxiety r/t unforeseen result of surgery

Impaired Comfort r/t surgical site pain

Risk for Ineffective Thermoregulation: Risk factor: infectious process

Risk for Delayed Surgical Recovery: Risk factor: interrupted healing of surgical site

Readiness for Enhanced Knowledge: expresses desire for knowledge of prevention and symptoms of infection

Suspected Child Abuse and Neglect (SCAN), Child

Ineffective Activity Planning r/t lack of family support

Anxiety: Child r/t threat of punishment for perceived wrongdoing

Deficient Community Health r/t inadequate reporting and follow-up of SCAN

Disturbed Personal Identity r/t dysfunctional family processes

Rape-Trauma Syndrome r/t altered lifestyle because of abuse, changes in residence

Risk for Impaired Resilience: Risk factor: adverse situation

Readiness for Enhanced Community Coping: obtaining resources to prevent child abuse, neglect

See Child Abuse; Hospitalized Child; Maturational Issues, Adolescent

Suspected Child Abuse and Neglect (SCAN), Parent

Disabled Family Coping r/t dysfunctional family, underdeveloped nurturing parental role, lack of parental support systems or role models

Dysfunctional Family Processes r/t inadequate coping skills

Ineffective Health Maintenance Behaviors r/t deficient knowledge of parenting skills as result of unachieved developmental tasks

Impaired Home Maintenance r/t disorganization, parental dysfunction, neglect of safe and nurturing environment

Ineffective Impulse Control r/t projection of anger, frustration onto child

Impaired Parenting r/t unrealistic expectations of child; lack of effective role model; unmet social, emotional, or maturational needs of parents; interruption in bonding process

Impaired Individual Resilience r/t poor impulse control

Chronic Low Self-Esteem r/t lack of successful parenting experiences

Risk for Other-Directed Violence: Parent to Child: Risk factors: inadequate coping mechanisms, unresolved stressors, unachieved maturational level by parent

Suspicion

Disturbed Personal Identity r/t psychiatric disorder

Powerlessness r/t repetitive paranoid thinking

Impaired Social Interaction r/t disturbed thought processes, paranoid delusions, hallucinations

Disturbed Thought Process r/t psychiatric disorder

Risk for Self-Directed Violence: Risk factor: inability to trust

Risk for Other-Directed Violence: Risk factor: impulsiveness

Swallowing Difficulties

Impaired Swallowing (See **Swallowing, Impaired,** Section III)

Risk for Aspiration r/t difficulty swallowing

Syncope

Anxiety r/t fear of falling

Impaired Physical Mobility r/t fear of falling

Ineffective Health Management Behaviors r/t lack of knowledge in how to prevent syncope

Social Isolation r/t fear of falling

Risk for Decreased Cardiac Output: Risk factor: dysrhythmia

Risk for Adult Falls: Risk factor: syncope

Risk for Injury: Risk factors: altered sensory perception, transient loss of consciousness, risk for falls

Risk for Ineffective Cerebral Tissue Perfusion: Risk factor: interruption of blood flow

Syphilis

See STD (Sexually Transmitted Disease)

Systemic Lupus Erythematosus

See Lupus Erythematosus

T

T & A (Tonsillectomy and Adenoidectomy)

Ineffective Airway Clearance r/t hesitation or reluctance to cough because of pain

Deficient Knowledge: Potential for Enhanced Health Maintenance Behaviors r/t insufficient knowledge regarding postoperative nutritional and rest requirements, signs and symptoms of complications, positioning

Nausea r/t gastric irritation, pharmaceuticals, anesthesia

Acute Pain r/t surgical incision

Risk for Aspiration: Risk factors: postoperative drainage and impaired swallowing

Risk for Deficient Fluid Volume: Risk factors: decreased intake because of painful swallowing, effects of anesthesia (nausea, vomiting), hemorrhage

Risk for Imbalanced Nutrition: Less than Body Requirements: Risk factors: hesitation or reluctance to swallow

Tachycardia

See Dysrhythmia

Tachypnea

Ineffective Breathing Pattern r/t pain, anxiety, hypoxia

See cause of Tachypnea

Tardive Dyskinesia

Ineffective Health Self-Management r/t complexity of therapeutic regimen or medication

Deficient Knowledge r/t cognitive limitation in assimilating information relating to side effects associated with neuroleptic medications

Risk for Injury: Risk factor: drug-induced abnormal body movements

Taste Abnormality

Frail Elderly Syndrome r/t chronic illness

TB (Pulmonary Tuberculosis)

Ineffective Airway Clearance r/t increased secretions, excessive mucus

Ineffective Breathing Pattern r/t decreased energy, fatigue

Fatigue r/t disease state

Impaired Gas Exchange r/t disease process

Ineffective Health Self-Management r/t deficient knowledge of prevention and treatment regimen

Ineffective Home Maintenance Behaviors r/t client or family member with disease

Ineffective Thermoregulation r/t presence of infection

Risk for Infection: Risk factor: insufficient knowledge regarding avoidance of exposure to pathogens

Readiness for Enhanced Health Self-Management: takes medications according to prescribed protocol for prevention and treatment

TBI (Traumatic Brain Injury)

Interrupted Family Processes r/t traumatic injury to family member

Chronic Sorrow r/t change in health status and functional ability

Risk for Post-Trauma Syndrome: Risk factor: perception of event causing TBI

Risk for Impaired Religiosity: Risk factor: impaired physical mobility

Risk for Impaired Resilience: Risk factor: crisis of injury

See Head Injury; Neurologic Disorders

TD (Traveler's Diarrhea)

See Traveler's Diarrhea (TD)

Technology Addiction

Decreased Diversional Activity Engagement r/t insufficient motivation to separate from electronic devices

Impaired Social Interaction r/t lack of desire to engage in personal face-to-face contact with others

Risk for Impaired Attachment: Risk factor: preoccupation with electronic devices

Risk for Impaired Parenting: Risk factor: insufficient uninterrupted meaningful interaction between parent and child as the result of preoccupation with electronic devices

Risk for Ineffective Relationship: Risk factor: ineffective face-to-face communication skills

Temperature, Decreased

Hypothermia r/t exposure to cold environment

Temperature, High

Hyperthermia r/t neurological damage, disease condition with high temperature, excessive heat, inflammatory response

Temperature Regulation, Impaired

Ineffective Thermoregulation r/t trauma, illness, cerebral injury

TEN (Toxic Epidermal Necrolysis)

See Toxic Epidermal Necrolysis (TEN)

TENS Unit (Transcutaneous Electrical Nerve Stimulation)

Risk for Unstable Blood Pressure: Risk factor: improper use of TENS unit (front of neck)

Readiness for Enhanced Comfort: expresses desire to enhance resolution of complaints

Tension

Anxiety r/t threat to or change in health status, situational crisis

Readiness for Enhanced Communication: expresses willingness to share feelings and thoughts

See Stress

Terminally Ill Adult

Death Anxiety r/t unresolved issues relating to death and dying

Imbalanced Energy Field r/t weak energy field patterns

Risk for Spiritual Distress: Risk factor: impending death

Readiness for Enhanced Religiosity: requests religious material and/or experiences

Readiness for Enhanced Spiritual Well-Being: desire to achieve harmony of mind, body, spirit

See Terminally Ill Child/Death of Child, Parent

Terminally Ill Child, Adolescent

Disturbed Body Image r/t effects of terminal disease, already critical feelings of group identity and self-image

Ineffective Coping r/t inability to establish personal and peer identity because of the threat of being different or not being healthy, inability to achieve maturational tasks

Impaired Social Interaction r/t forced separation from peers

See Child with Chronic Condition; Hospitalized Child, Terminally Ill Child/Death of Child, Parent

Terminally Ill Child, Infant/Toddler

Ineffective Coping r/t separation from parents and familiar environment from inability to understand dying process

See Child with Chronic Condition, Terminally Ill Child/Death of Child, Parent

Terminally Ill Child, Preschool Child

Fear r/t perceived punishment, bodily harm, feelings of guilt caused by magical thinking (i.e., believing that thoughts cause events)

See Child with Chronic Condition, Terminally Ill Child/Death of Child, Parent

Terminally Ill Child, School-Age Child/Preadolescent

Fear r/t perceived punishment, body mutilation, feelings of guilt

Maladaptive Grieving r/t difficulty dealing with concurrent crises

See Child with Chronic Condition, Terminally Ill Child/Death of Child, Parent

Terminally Ill Child/Death of Child, Parent

Compromised Family Coping r/t inability or unwillingness to discuss impending death and feelings with child or support child through terminal stages of illness

Decisional Conflict r/t continuation or discontinuation of treatment, do-not-resuscitate decision, ethical issues regarding organ donation

Ineffective Denial r/t complicated grieving

Interrupted Family Processes r/t situational crisis

Maladaptive Grieving r/t death of child

Hopelessness r/t overwhelming stresses caused by terminal illness

Insomnia r/t grieving process

Impaired Parenting r/t risk for overprotection of surviving siblings

Powerlessness r/t inability to alter course of events

Impaired Social Interaction r/t complicated grieving

Social Isolation: Imposed by Others r/t feelings of inadequacy in providing support to grieving parents

Social Isolation: Self-Imposed r/t unresolved grief, perceived inadequate parenting skills

Spiritual Distress r/t sudden and unexpected death, prolonged suffering before death, questioning the death of youth, questioning the meaning of one's own existence

Risk for Maladaptive Grieving: Risk factors: prolonged, unresolved, obstructed progression through stages of grief and mourning

Risk for Impaired Resilience: Risk factor: impending death

Readiness for Enhanced Family Coping: impact of crisis on family values, priorities, goals, or relationships; expressed interest or desire to attach meaning to child's life and death

Tetralogy of Fallot

See Congenital Heart Disease/Cardiac Anomalies

Tetraplegia

Autonomic Dysreflexia r/t bladder or bowel distention, skin irritation, infection, deficient knowledge of client and caregiver

Maladaptive Grieving r/t loss of previous functioning

Powerlessness r/t inability to perform previous activities

Impaired Sitting r/t paralysis of extremities

Impaired Spontaneous Ventilation r/t loss of innervation of respiratory muscles, respiratory muscle fatigue

Risk for Aspiration: Risk factor: inadequate ability to protect airway from neurological damage

Risk for Infection: Risk factor: urinary stasis

Risk for Impaired Skin Integrity: Risk factor: physical immobilization and decreased sensation

Risk for Adult Pressure Injury: Risk factor: immobility and sensory loss

Risk for Child Pressure Injury: Risk factor: immobility and sensory loss

Risk for Ineffective Thermoregulation: Risk factors: inability to move to increase temperature, possible presence of infection to increase temperature

Thermoregulation, Ineffective

Ineffective Thermoregulation (See **Thermoregulation, Ineffective,** Section III)

Risk for Ineffective Thermoregulation (See **Ineffective Thermoregulation, Risk for,** Section III)

Thoracentesis

See Pleural Effusion

Thoracotomy

Decreased Activity Tolerance r/t pain, imbalance between oxygen supply and demand, presence of chest tubes

Ineffective Airway Clearance r/t drowsiness, pain with breathing and coughing

Ineffective Breathing Pattern r/t decreased energy, fatigue, pain

Deficient Knowledge r/t self-care, effective breathing exercises, pain relief

Acute Pain r/t surgical procedure, coughing, deep breathing

Risk for Bleeding: Risk factor: surgery

Risk for Surgical Site Infection: Risk factor: invasive procedure

Risk for Injury: Risk factor: disruption of closed-chest drainage system

Risk for Perioperative Positioning Injury: Risk factors: lateral positioning, immobility

Risk for Vascular Trauma: Risk factors: chemical irritant; antibiotics

Thought Disorders

See Schizophrenia

Thrombocytopenic Purpura

See ITP (Idiopathic Thrombocytopenic Purpura)

Thrombophlebitis

See Deep Vein Thrombosis (DVT)

Thyroidectomy

Risk for Ineffective Airway Clearance: Risk factor: edema or hematoma formation, airway obstruction

Risk for Impaired Verbal Communication: Risk factors: edema, pain, vocal cord or laryngeal nerve damage

Risk for Injury: Risk factor: possible parathyroid damage or removal

See Surgery, Preoperative Care; Surgery, Perioperative Care; Surgery, Postoperative Care

TIA (Transient Ischemic Attack)

Acute Confusion r/t hypoxia

Readiness for Enhanced Health Self-Management: obtains knowledge regarding treatment prevention of inadequate oxygenation

See Syncope

Tic Disorder

See Tourette's Syndrome (TS)

Tinea Capitis

Impaired Comfort r/t inflammation from skin irritation

See Ringworm of Scalp

Tinea Corporis

See Ringworm of Body

Tinea Cruris

See Jock Itch; Itching; Pruritus

Tinea Pedis

See Athlete's Foot; Itching; Pruritus

Tinea Unguium (Onychomycosis)

See Ringworm of Nails

Tinnitus

Ineffective Health Maintenance Behaviors r/t deficient knowledge regarding self-care with tinnitus

Hearing Loss r/t ringing in ears obscuring hearing

Tissue Damage, Integumentary

Impaired Tissue Integrity (See **Tissue Integrity, Impaired,** Section III)

Risk for Impaired Tissue Integrity (See **Tissue Integrity, Impaired, Risk for,** Section III)

Tissue Perfusion, Peripheral

Ineffective Peripheral Tissue Perfusion (See **Tissue Perfusion, Peripheral, Ineffective,** Section III)

Risk for Ineffective Peripheral Tissue Perfusion (See **Tissue Perfusion, Peripheral, Ineffective, Risk for,** Section III)

Toileting Problems

Toileting Self-Care Deficit r/t impaired transfer ability, impaired mobility status, intolerance of activity, neuromuscular impairment, cognitive impairment

Impaired Transfer Ability r/t neuromuscular deficits

Toilet Training

Deficient Knowledge: Parent r/t signs of child's readiness for training

Risk for Constipation: Risk factor: withholding stool

Risk for Infection: Risk factor: withholding urination

Tonsillectomy and Adenoidectomy (T & A)

See T & A (Tonsillectomy and Adenoidectomy)

Toothache

Impaired Dentition r/t ineffective oral hygiene, barriers to self-care, economic barriers to professional care, nutritional deficits, lack of knowledge regarding dental health

Acute Pain r/t inflammation, infection

Total Anomalous Pulmonary Venous Return

See Congenital Heart Disease/Cardiac Anomalies

Total Joint Replacement (Total Hip/Total Knee/Shoulder)

Disturbed Body Image r/t large scar, presence of prosthesis

Impaired Physical Mobility r/t musculoskeletal impairment, surgery, prosthesis

Risk for Injury: Neurovascular: Risk factors: altered peripheral tissue perfusion, impaired mobility, prosthesis

Risk for Peripheral Neurovascular Dysfunction: Risk factors: immobilization, surgical procedure

Ineffective Peripheral Tissue Perfusion r/t surgery

See Surgery, Preoperative Care; Surgery, Perioperative Care; Surgery, Postoperative Care

Total Parenteral Nutrition (TPN)

See TPN (Total Parenteral Nutrition)

Tourette's Syndrome (TS)

Hopelessness r/t inability to control behavior

Impaired Individual Resilience r/t uncontrollable behavior

Risk for Situational Low Self-Esteem: Risk factors: uncontrollable behavior, motor and phonic tics

See Attention Deficit Disorder

Toxemia

See PIH (Pregnancy-Induced Hypertension/Preeclampsia)

Toxic Epidermal Necrolysis (TEN) (Erythema Multiforme)

Death Anxiety r/t uncertainty of prognosis

Risk for Shock r/t deficient fluid volume

TPN (Total Parenteral Nutrition)

Imbalanced Nutrition: Less than Body Requirements r/t inability to digest food or absorb nutrients as a result of biological or psychological factors

Risk for Electrolyte Imbalance: Risk factor: need for regulation of electrolytes in TPN fluids

Risk for Excess Fluid Volume: Risk factor: rapid administration of TPN

Risk for Unstable Blood Glucose Level: Risk factor: high glucose levels in TPN to be regulated according to blood glucose levels

Risk for Infection: Risk factors: concentrated glucose solution, invasive administration of fluids

Risk for Vascular Trauma: Risk factors: insertion site, length of treatment time

Tracheoesophageal Fistula

Ineffective Airway Clearance r/t aspiration of feeding because of inability to swallow

Imbalanced Nutrition: Less than Body Requirements r/t difficulties swallowing

Risk for Aspiration: Risk factor: common passage of air and food

Risk for Vascular Trauma: Risk factors: venous medications and site

See Respiratory Conditions of the Neonate; Hospitalized Child

Tracheostomy

Ineffective Airway Clearance r/t increased secretions, mucous plugs

Anxiety r/t impaired verbal communication, ineffective airway clearance

Disturbed Body Image r/t abnormal opening in neck

Impaired Verbal Communication r/t presence of mechanical airway

Deficient Knowledge r/t self-care, home maintenance management

Acute Pain r/t edema, surgical procedure

Risk for Aspiration: Risk factor: presence of tracheostomy

Risk for Bleeding: Risk factor: surgical incision

Risk for Surgical Site Infection: Risk factors: invasive procedure, pooling of secretions

Traction and Casts

Constipation r/t immobility

Decreased Diversional Activity Engagement r/t immobility

Impaired Physical Mobility r/t imposed restrictions on activity because of bone or joint disease injury

Acute Pain r/t immobility, injury, or disease

Self-Care Deficit: Feeding, Dressing, Bathing, Toileting r/t degree of impaired physical mobility, body area affected by traction or cast

Impaired Transfer Ability r/t presence of traction, casts

Risk for Disuse Syndrome: Risk factor: mechanical immobilization

Risk for Child Pressure Injury: Risk factor: immobility and pressure over bony prominence

See Casts

Transfer Ability

Impaired Transfer Ability (See **Transfer Ability, Impaired,** Section III)

Transient Ischemic Attack (TIA)

See TIA (Transient Ischemic Attack)

Transposition of Great Vessels

See Congenital Heart Disease/Cardiac Anomalies

Transurethral Resection of the Prostate (TURP)

See TURP (Transurethral Resection of the Prostate)

T

Trauma in Pregnancy

Anxiety r/t threat to self or fetus, unknown outcome

Deficient Knowledge r/t lack of exposure to situation

Acute Pain r/t trauma

Impaired Skin Integrity r/t trauma

Risk for Bleeding: Risk factor: trauma

Risk for Deficient Fluid Volume: Risk factor: fluid loss

Risk for Infection: Risk factor: traumatized tissue

Risk for Injury: Fetal: Risk factor: premature separation of placenta

Risk for Disturbed Maternal–Fetal Dyad: Risk factor: complication of pregnancy

Trauma, Physical, Risk for

Risk for Physical Trauma (See **Physical Trauma, Risk for,** Section III)

Traumatic Brain Injury (TBI)

See TBI (Traumatic Brain Injury); Intracranial Pressure, Increased

Traumatic Event

Post-Trauma Syndrome r/t previously experienced trauma

Traveler's Diarrhea (TD)

Diarrhea r/t travel with exposure to different bacteria, viruses

Risk for Deficient Fluid Volume: Risk factor: excessive loss of fluids

Risk for Infection: Risk factors: insufficient knowledge regarding avoidance of exposure to pathogens (water supply, iced drinks, local cheese, ice cream, undercooked meat, fish and shellfish, uncooked vegetables, unclean eating utensils, improper handwashing)

Trembling of Hands

Fear r/t threat to or change in health status, threat of death, situational crisis

Tricuspid Atresia

See Congenital Heart Disease/Cardiac Anomalies

Trigeminal Neuralgia

Ineffective Health Self-Management r/t deficient knowledge regarding prevention of stimuli that trigger pain

Imbalanced Nutrition: Less than Body Requirements r/t pain when chewing

Acute Pain r/t irritation of trigeminal nerve

Risk for Corneal Injury: Risk factor: possible decreased corneal sensation

Truncus Arteriosus

See Congenital Heart Disease/Cardiac Anomalies

TS (Tourette's Syndrome)

See Tourette's Syndrome (TS)

TSE (Testicular Self-Examination)

Readiness for Enhanced Health Self-Management: seeks information regarding self-examination

Tubal Ligation

Decisional Conflict r/t tubal sterilization

See Laparoscopy

Tube Feeding

Risk for Aspiration: Risk factors: improper placement of feeding tube, improper positioning of client during and after feeding, excessive residual feeding or lack of digestion, altered gag reflex

Risk for Deficient Fluid Volume: Risk factor: inadequate water administration with concentrated feeding

Risk for Imbalanced Nutrition: Less than Body Requirements: Risk factors: intolerance to tube feeding, inadequate calorie replacement to meet metabolic needs

Impaired Bowel Continence: Risk factor: tube feeding osmolality too high for proper nutrient absorption

Tuberculosis (TB)

See TB (Pulmonary Tuberculosis)

TURP (Transurethral Resection of the Prostate)

Deficient Knowledge r/t postoperative self-care, home maintenance management

Acute Pain r/t incision, irritation from catheter, bladder spasms, kidney infection

Urinary Retention r/t obstruction of urethra or catheter with clots

Risk for Bleeding: Risk factor: surgery

Risk for Deficient Fluid Volume: Risk factors: fluid loss, possible bleeding

Risk for Urge Urinary Incontinence: Risk factor: edema from surgical procedure

Risk for Infection: Risk factors: invasive procedure, route for bacteria entry

Risk for Urinary Tract Injury: Risk factor: invasive procedure

U

Ulcer, Peptic (Duodenal or Gastric)

Fatigue r/t loss of blood, chronic illness

Ineffective Health Maintenance Behaviors r/t lack of knowledge regarding health practices to prevent ulcer formation

Nausea r/t gastrointestinal irritation

Acute Pain r/t irritated mucosa from acid secretion

See GI Bleed (Gastrointestinal Bleeding)

Ulcerative Colitis

See Inflammatory Bowel Disease (Child and Adult)

Ulcers, Stasis

See Stasis Ulcer

Unilateral Neglect of One Side of Body

Unilateral Neglect (See **Unilateral Neglect,** Section III)

Unsanitary Living Conditions

Impaired Home Maintenance r/t impaired cognitive or emotional functioning, lack of knowledge, insufficient finances, addiction

Risk for Allergic Reaction: Risk factor: exposure to environmental contaminants

Upper Respiratory Infection

See Cold, Viral

Urgency to Urinate

Urge Urinary Incontinence (See **Incontinence, Urinary, Urge,** Section III)

Risk for Urge Urinary Incontinence (See **Incontinence, Urinary, Urge, Risk for,** Section III)

Urinary Catheter

Risk for Urinary Tract Injury: Risk factors: confused client, long-term use of catheter, large retention balloon or catheter, perirectal burn injured client

Risk for Infection: Risk factors: difficulty managing long-term invasive urinary catheter devices

Urinary Diversion

See Ileal Conduit

Urinary Elimination, Impaired

Impaired Urinary Elimination (See **Urinary Elimination, Impaired,** Section III)

Urinary Incontinence

See Incontinence of Urine

Urinary Retention

Urinary Retention (See **Urinary Retention,** Section III)

Urinary Tract Infection (UTI)

See UTI (Urinary Tract Infection)

Urolithiasis

See Kidney Stone

Uterine Atony in Labor

See Dystocia

Uterine Atony in Postpartum

See Postpartum Hemorrhage

Uterine Bleeding

See Hemorrhage; Postpartum Hemorrhage; Shock, Hypovolemic

UTI (Urinary Tract Infection)

Ineffective Health Maintenance Behaviors r/t deficient knowledge regarding methods to treat and prevent UTIs, prolonged use of indwelling urinary catheter

Acute Pain: Dysuria r/t inflammatory process in bladder

Impaired Urinary Elimination: Frequency r/t urinary tract infection

Risk for Acute Confusion: Risk factor: infectious process

Risk for Urge Urinary Incontinence: Risk factor: hyperreflexia from cystitis

Risk for Urinary Tract Injury: Risk factors: confused client, long-term use of catheter, large retention balloon or catheter

V

VAD (Ventricular Assist Device)

See Ventricular Assist Device (VAD)

Vaginal Hysterectomy

Urinary Retention r/t edema at surgical site

Risk for Urge Urinary Incontinence: Risk factors: edema, congestion of pelvic tissues

Risk for Infection: Risk factor: surgical site

Risk for Perioperative Positioning Injury: Risk factor: lithotomy position

Vaginitis

Impaired Comfort r/t pruritus, itching

Ineffective Health Maintenance Behaviors r/t deficient knowledge regarding self-care with vaginitis

Ineffective Sexuality Pattern r/t abstinence during acute stage, pain

Vagotomy

See Abdominal Surgery

Value System Conflict

Decisional Conflict r/t unclear personal values or beliefs

Spiritual Distress r/t challenged value system

Readiness for Enhanced Spiritual Well-Being: desire for harmony with self, others, higher power, God

Varicose Veins

Ineffective Health Maintenance Behaviors r/t deficient knowledge regarding health care practices, prevention, treatment regimen

Chronic Pain r/t impaired circulation

Ineffective Peripheral Tissue Perfusion r/t venous stasis

Risk for Impaired Tissue Integrity: Risk factor: altered peripheral tissue perfusion

Vascular Dementia (Formerly Called Multi-Infarct Dementia)

See Dementia

Vasectomy

Decisional Conflict r/t surgery as method of permanent sterilization

Venereal Disease

See STD (Sexually Transmitted Disease)

Venous Thromboembolism (VTE)

Anxiety r/t lack of circulation to body part

Acute Pain r/t vascular obstruction

Ineffective Peripheral Tissue Perfusion r/t interruption of circulatory flow

Risk for Peripheral Neurovascular Dysfunction: Risk factor: vascular obstruction

Ventilated Client, Mechanically

V

Ineffective Airway Clearance r/t increased secretions, decreased cough and gag reflex

Ineffective Breathing Pattern r/t decreased energy and fatigue as a result of possible altered nutrition: less than body requirements, neurological disease or damage

Impaired Verbal Communication r/t presence of endotracheal tube, inability to phonate

Fear r/t inability to breathe on own, difficulty communicating

Impaired Gas Exchange r/t ventilation-perfusion imbalance

Powerlessness r/t health treatment regimen

Social Isolation r/t impaired mobility, ventilator dependence

Impaired Spontaneous Ventilation r/t metabolic factors, respiratory muscle fatigue

Dysfunctional Ventilatory Weaning Response r/t psychological, situational, physiological factors

Risk for Adult Falls: Risk factors: impaired mobility, decreased muscle strength

Risk for Child Falls: Risk factors: impaired mobility, decreased lower extremity strength

Risk for Infection: Risk factors: presence of endotracheal tube, pooled secretions

Risk for Pressure Ulcer: Risk factor: decreased mobility

Risk for Impaired Resilience: Risk factor: illness

See Child With Chronic Condition; Hospitalized Child; Respiratory Conditions of the Neonate

Ventricular Assist Device (VAD)

Anxiety r/t possible failure of device

Risk for Infection: Risk factor: device insertion site

Risk for Vascular Trauma: Risk factor: insertion site

Readiness for Enhanced Decision-Making: expresses desire to enhance the understanding of the meaning of choices regarding implanting a VAD

See Open Heart Surgery

Ventricular Fibrillation

See Dysrhythmia

Veterans

Anxiety r/t possible unmet needs, both physical and psychological

Risk for Post-Trauma Syndrome: Risk factors: witnessing death, survivor role, guilt, environment not conducive to needs

Risk for Suicide: Risk factors: substance abuse, insufficient social support, physical injury, psychiatric disorder

Vertigo

See Syncope

Violent Behavior

Risk for Other-Directed Violence (See **Violence, Other-Directed, Risk for,** Section III)

Risk for Self-Directed Violence (See **Violence, Self-Directed, Risk for,** Section III)

Viral Gastroenteritis

Diarrhea r/t infectious process, Norovirus

Deficient Fluid Volume r/t vomiting, diarrhea

Ineffective Health Self-Management r/t inadequate handwashing

See Gastroenteritis, Child

Vision Impairment

Fear r/t loss of sight

Social Isolation r/t altered state of wellness, inability to see

Risk for Impaired Resilience: Risk factor: presence of new crisis

See Blindness; Cataracts; Glaucoma

Vomiting

Nausea r/t infectious processes, chemotherapy, postsurgical anesthesia, irritation to the gastrointestinal system, stimulation of neuropharmacological mechanisms

Imbalanced Nutrition: Less than Body Requirements r/t inability to ingest food

Risk for Electrolyte Imbalance: Risk factor: vomiting

VTE (Venous Thromboembolism)

Risk for Thrombosis r/t ineffective management of preventive measures, immobility, dehydration

(See **Venous Thromboembolism, Risk for,** Section III)

W

Walking Impairment

Impaired Walking (See **Walking, Impaired,** Section III)

Wandering

Wandering (See **Wandering,** Section III)

Weakness

Fatigue r/t decreased or increased metabolic energy production

Risk for Adult Falls: Risk factor: weakness

Weight Gain

Overweight (See **Overweight,** Section III)

Risk for Metabolic Syndrome r/t absence of interest in improving health behaviors

Weight Loss

Imbalanced Nutrition: Less than Body Requirements r/t inability to ingest food because of biological, psychological, economic factors

Wellness-Seeking Behavior

Readiness for Enhanced Health Self-Management: Expresses desire for increased control of health practice

Wernicke-Korsakoff Syndrome

See Korsakoff's Syndrome

West Nile Virus

See Meningitis/Encephalitis

Wheelchair Use Problems

Impaired Wheelchair Mobility (See **Mobility, Wheelchair, Impaired,** Section III)

Wheezing

Ineffective Airway Clearance r/t tracheobronchial obstructions, secretions

Ineffective Breathing Pattern r/t tracheobronchial obstructions and fatigue

Wilms' Tumor

Chronic Functional Constipation r/t obstruction associated with presence of tumor

Acute Pain r/t pressure from tumor

See Chemotherapy; Hospitalized Child; Radiation Therapy; Surgery, Preoperative Care; Surgery, Perioperative Care; Surgery, Postoperative Care

Withdrawal from Alcohol

See Alcohol Withdrawal

Withdrawal from Drugs

See Acute Substance Withdrawal Syndrome; Substance Misuse

Wound Debridement

Acute Pain r/t debridement of wound

Impaired Tissue Integrity r/t debridement, open wound

Risk for Infection: Risk factors: open wound, presence of bacteria

Wound Dehiscence, Evisceration

Fear r/t client fear of body parts "falling out," surgical procedure not going as planned

Disturbed Body Image r/t change in body structure and wound appearance

Imbalanced Nutrition: Less than Body Requirements r/t inability to digest nutrients, need for increased protein for healing

Risk for Deficient Fluid Volume: Risk factors: inability to ingest nutrients, obstruction, fluid loss

Risk for Injury: Risk factor: exposed abdominal contents

Risk for Delayed Surgical Recovery: Risk factors: separation of wound, exposure of abdominal contents

Risk for Surgical Site Infection: Risk factor: open wound after surgical procedure

Wound Infection

Disturbed Body Image r/t open wound

Imbalanced Nutrition: Less than Body Requirements r/t biological factors, infection, fever

Ineffective Thermoregulation r/t infection in wound resulting in fever

Impaired Tissue Integrity r/t wound, presence of infection

Risk for Imbalanced Fluid Volume: Risk factor: increased metabolic rate

Risk for Infection: Spread of: Risk factor: imbalanced nutrition: less than body requirements

Risk for Delayed Surgical Recovery: Risk factor: presence of infection

Wounds, Open

See Lacerations

SECTION

III Guide to Planning Care

Section III is a collection of NANDA-I nursing diagnosis care plans. The care plans are arranged alphabetically by diagnostic concept. Each care plan includes the diagnosis label, domain and class, definition, defining characteristics and if appropriate risk factors, related factors, at-risk populations, and associated conditions. Risk diagnoses, however, only contain definition and risk factors. Care plans include suggested outcomes and interventions for all nursing diagnoses.

MAKING AN ACCURATE NURSING DIAGNOSIS

Verify the accuracy of the previously suggested nursing diagnoses (from Section II) or from the alphabetized list (front of the book) for the client.

STEPS

- Read the definition for the suggested nursing diagnosis and determine if it is appropriate.
- Compare the Defining Characteristics with the symptoms that were identified from the client data collected.

or

- Compare the Risk Factors with the factors that were identified from the client data collected.

WRITING OUTCOMES STATEMENTS AND NURSING INTERVENTIONS

After selecting the appropriate nursing diagnosis, use this section to identify appropriate client outcomes and interventions.

STEPS

- Use the Client Outcomes/Nursing Interventions as written by the authors and contributors (select ones that are appropriate for your client).

or

- Use the NOC/NIC outcomes and interventions (as appropriate for your client).
- Read the rationales; the majority of rationales are based on evidence supported by nursing research (EBN), clinical research, or clinical practice guidelines (EB) that validate the efficacy of the interventions. Every attempt has been made to use current references. Important research studies that are older than 5 years are included because they are either seminal research or the current best evidence available. They are designated as CEB (Classic Evidence-Based).

Following these steps, you will be able to write an evidence-based nursing care plan.

- Follow this care plan to administer evidence-based nursing care to the client.
- Document all steps and evaluate and update the care plan as needed.

A

Decreased Activity Tolerance

Domain 4 Activity/rest Class 2 Activity/exercise

Kelly Henrichs, DNP, RN, GNP-BC

NANDA-I

Definition

Insufficient endurance to complete required or desired daily activities.

Defining Characteristics

Abnormal blood pressure response to activity; abnormal heart rate response to activity; anxious when activity is required; electrocardiogram change; exertional discomfort; exertional dyspnea; expresses fatigue; generalized weakness

Related Factors

Decreased muscle strength; depressive symptoms; fear of pain; imbalance between oxygen supply/demand; impaired physical mobility; inexperience with an activity; insufficient muscle mass; malnutrition; pain; physical deconditioning; sedentary lifestyle

At-Risk Population

Individuals with history of decreased activity tolerance; older adults

Associated Conditions

Neoplasms; neurodegenerative diseases; respiration disorders; traumatic brain injuries; vitamin D deficiency

NOC (Nursing Outcomes Classification)

Suggested NOC Outcomes

Activity Tolerance; Endurance; Energy Conservation; Self-Care: Instrumental Activities of Daily Living (IADLs)

Example NOC Outcome with Indicators

Activity Tolerance as evidenced by the following indicators: Oxygen saturation with activity/Pulse rate with activity/Respiratory rate with activity/Blood pressure with activity/Electrocardiogram findings/Skin color/Walking distance. (Rate the outcome and indicators of **Activity Tolerance:** 1 = severely compromised, 2 = substantially compromised, 3 = moderately compromised, 4 = mildly compromised, 5 = not compromised [see Section I].)

Client Outcomes

Client Will (Specify Time Frame)

- Participate in prescribed physical activity with appropriate changes in heart rate, blood pressure, and breathing rate; maintain monitor patterns (rhythm and ST segment) within normal limits
- State symptoms of adverse effects of exercise and report onset of symptoms immediately
- Maintain normal skin color; skin is warm and dry with activity
- Verbalize an understanding of the need to gradually increase activity based on testing, tolerance, and symptoms
- Demonstrate increased tolerance to activity

NIC (Nursing Interventions Classification)

Suggested NIC Interventions

Activity Therapy; Energy Management; Exercise Therapy: Ambulation

Example NIC Activities—Energy Management

Monitor cardiorespiratory response to activity; Monitor location and nature of discomfort or pain during movement/activity

Nursing Interventions and *Rationales*

- ✱ Determine cause of Decreased Activity Tolerance (see Related Factors) and decide whether cause is physical, psychological, or motivational. EB: *As nurses, we are called on to ensure higher levels of safety and quality for our clients by our governments, professional organizations, and hospital administrations. It is essential that we implement evidence-based nursing care strategies to reduce avoidable errors in care so that clinical outcomes improve (Chu, 2017).*
- ● If mainly on bed rest, minimize cardiovascular, neuromuscular, and skeletal deconditioning by positioning the client in an upright position several times daily as tolerated and perform simple range-of-motion (ROM) techniques (passive or active). EB: *Physical inactivity leads to a deconditioning of the skeletal, neuromuscular, and cardiovascular systems. It can lead to impaired quality of life, loss of autonomy, falls, and fractures (Kramer et al, 2017).*
- ● Assess the client daily for appropriateness of activity and bed rest orders. Mobilize the client as soon as possible. EB: Mobilization is a simple method of maintaining stable cardiovascular parameters (i.e., blood pressure, heart rate), countering orthostatic intolerance, and reducing the risk of secondary problems in clients during long-term immobilization (Constantin & Dahlke, 2018).
- ● If the client is mostly immobile, consider use of a transfer chair or a chair that becomes a stretcher. EB: The use of simple shifting aids can optimize the client transfer by avoiding heavy lifting situations and possible back injury to the caregivers. It reduces the effort of the caregivers and makes sure that the client is not hurt during the process of conversion (Ahmed et al, 2015).
- ● When appropriate, gradually increase activity, allowing the client to assist with positioning, transferring, and self-care as able. Progress the client from sitting in bed to dangling, to standing, to ambulation. Always have the client dangle at the bedside before standing to evaluate for postural hypotension. EB: *A reduction in plasma volume associated with bed rest impacts the physiological responses of autonomic control of circulation (Goswami et al, 2017)*
- ▲ When getting a client up, observe for symptoms of intolerance such as nausea, pallor, dizziness, visual dimming, and impaired consciousness, as well as changes in vital signs; manual blood pressure monitoring is more accurate than use of an automated blood pressure device. When an adult rises to the standing position, blood pools in the lower extremities; symptoms of central nervous system hypoperfusion may occur, including feelings of weakness, nausea, headache, lightheadedness, dizziness, blurred vision, fatigue, tremulousness, palpitations, and impaired cognition. EB: *Impaired orthostatic blood pressure recovery, delayed recovery, and/or sustained orthostatic hypotension are independent risk factors for falls, unexplained falls, and falls with injury (Ciaren et al, 2017).*
- ● If the client has symptoms of postural hypotension, such as dizziness, lightheadedness, or pallor, take precautions, such as dangling the client and applying leg compression stockings, before the client stands. EB: *Put graduated compression stockings on the client or use lower limb compression bandaging, if ordered, to return blood to the heart and brain. Have the client dangle at the side of the bed with legs hanging over the edge of the bed, flexing and extending the feet several times after sitting up, then standing slowly with someone holding the client. If the client becomes lightheaded or dizzy, return him or her to bed immediately (Crawford & Harris, 2016).*
- ● Perform ROM exercises if the client is unable to tolerate activity or is mostly immobile. See care plan for Risk for **Disuse Syndrome**.
- ● Monitor and record the client's ability to tolerate activity: changes in mentation, pulse rate, blood pressure, respiratory pattern, dyspnea, use of accessory muscles, and skin color before, during, and after the activity. If the following signs and symptoms of cardiac decompensation develop, activity should be stopped immediately:
  - Lightheadedness, confusion, ataxia, pallor, cyanosis, nausea, or any peripheral circulatory insufficiency
  - Onset of chest discomfort or pain
  - Changes in heart rate: increased, decreased, palpitations, dysrhythmia
  - Drop in blood pressure or hypotension
  - Rise in blood pressure or hypertension
  - Dyspnea
  - Decreased oxygen saturation
  - Excessive fatigue
- ▲ Instruct the client to stop the activity immediately and report to the health care provider if the client is experiencing the following symptoms: new or worsened intensity or increased frequency of discomfort; tightness or pressure in chest, back, neck, jaw, shoulders, and/or arms; palpitations; dizziness; weakness; unusual and extreme fatigue; or excessive air hunger. EB: *Cardiovascular deconditioning has long been*

recognized as a characteristic of the physiological adaptation to long-term bed rest in clients. The process is thought to contribute to orthostatic intolerance and enhance secondary complications in a significant way (Kehler et al, 2019).

- ● Observe and document skin integrity several times a day. Decreased **Activity Tolerance** if resulting in immobility, may lead to pressure ulcers. Mechanical pressure, moisture, friction, and shearing forces all predispose to their development. Refer to the care plan Risk for Impaired **Skin** Integrity.
- ● Assess for constipation. If present, refer to care plan for **Constipation.** Decreased **Activity** Tolerance is associated with increased risk of **Constipation.**
- ▲ Refer the client to physical therapy to help increase activity levels and strength.
- ▲ Consider a dietitian referral to assess nutritional needs related to Decreased **Activity** Tolerance and provide nutrition as indicated. If the client is unable to eat food, use enteral or parenteral feedings as needed.
- ● Recognize that malnutrition causes significant morbidity because of the loss of lean body mass.
- ● Provide emotional support and encouragement to the client to gradually increase activity. Work with the client to set mutual goals that increase activity levels. *Fear of breathlessness, pain, or falling may decrease willingness to increase activity.*
- ▲ Observe for pain before activity. If possible, treat pain before activity and ensure that the client is not heavily sedated. *Pain restricts the client from achieving a maximal activity level and is often exacerbated by movement.*
- ▲ Obtain any necessary assistive devices or equipment needed before ambulating the client (e.g., walkers, canes, crutches, portable oxygen).
- ▲ Use a gait-walking belt when ambulating the client. **EBN:** *Use of gait belts is a nurse-driven intervention and encouraged to be used to assist in ambulation and transfer (King et al, 2018).*
- ▲ *Use evidence-based practices for safe client handling to reduce the risk of injury for both clients and health care workers (King et al, 2018).*

Decreased Activity Tolerance Due to Respiratory Disease

- ● If the client is able to walk and has chronic obstructive pulmonary disease (COPD), use the traditional 6-minute walk distance to evaluate activity tolerance with ambulation.
- ▲ Ensure that the client with pulmonary diseases has oxygen saturation testing with exercise. Use supplemental oxygen to keep oxygen saturation 90% or above or as prescribed with activity. **EB:** *Oxygen therapy can prolong life (Apps et al, 2016).*
- ● Monitor a respiratory client's response to activity by observing for symptoms of respiratory intolerance, such as increased dyspnea, loss of ability to control breathing rhythmically, use of accessory muscles, nasal flaring, appearance of facial distress, and skin tone changes such as pallor and cyanosis, changes in mentation, or inability to talk during activity.
- ● Instruct and assist the client in using conscious, controlled breathing techniques during exercise, including pursed-lip breathing, and inspiratory muscle use.
- ▲ Evaluate the client's nutritional status. Use nutritional supplements to increase nutritional level if needed. Refer to a dietitian if indicated.
- ▲ For the client in the intensive care unit, consider mobilizing the client with passive exercise. **EBN:** *Nurses should consider incorporating at least 20 minutes of passive exercise early in the plan of care for critically ill clients treated with mechanical ventilation so that opportunities to improve client outcomes are not missed (Sommers et al, 2015).*
- ▲ Refer the COPD client to a pulmonary rehabilitation program. **EB:** *Pulmonary rehabilitation improves client's functionality and decreases hospital admissions (Apps et al, 2016).*

Decreased Activity Tolerance Due to Cardiovascular Disease

- ● If the client is able to walk and has heart failure, consider use of the 6-minute walk test to determine physical ability.
- ● Allow for periods of rest before and after planned exertion periods such as meals, baths, treatments, and physical activity.
- ▲ Refer to a heart failure program or cardiac rehabilitation program for education, evaluation, and guided support to increase activity and rebuild life. **EB:** *Exercise training improves functional capacity, the ability to perform activities of daily living (ADLs), and quality of life, and it reduces the risk for subsequent cardiovascular events (Simon et al, 2018).*

▲ Refer to a community support program that includes support of significant others. EB: *Contemporary studies now suggest that behavior change and multifactorial risk factor modification—especially smoking cessation and more intensive measures to control hyperlipidemia with diet, drugs, and exercise—may slow, halt, or even reverse (albeit modestly) the otherwise inexorable progression of atherosclerotic coronary artery disease (CAD) (Feigin et al, 2016).*

● See care plan for **Decreased Cardiac Output** for further interventions.

Pediatric

● Focus interview questions toward exercise tolerance, specifically including any history of asthma exacerbations. EB: *Cardiopulmonary deconditioning should be considered as an important differential diagnosis for breathlessness among obese adolescents. Some of these children may need pulmonary rehabilitation if difficulty breathing is the perceived reason for not exercising (Carpaji & van den Berge, 2018).*

Geriatric

✱ Slow the pace of care. Allow the client extra time to perform physical activities. Slow gait in older adults may be related to fear of falling, decreased strength in muscles, reduced balance or visual acuity, knee flexion contractures, and foot pain. EB: *Older clients with chronic cardiac conditions are more vulnerable to falls and injuries. Cardiovascular conditions, prevalent in older people, are also the frequent cause of potentially harmful fall injuries in this group. The need to identify the fall risk–related factors that cluster with arrhythmia and syncope is relevant, in that it will potentially reduce clients' risk for falls and fall injuries (Goswami et al, 2017).*

● Encourage families to help/allow an older client to be independent in whatever activities possible. EB: *Older adults can engage in a variety of physical activities to advance health ranging from walking and gardening to household chores and/or planned group exercise (World Health Organization, 2020).*

▲ Assess for swaying, poor balance, weakness, and fear of falling while older clients stand/walk. Refer to physical therapy if appropriate. EB: *A home exercise program was beneficial to improve the balance of community-dwelling frail older adults (Light et al, 2016).*

● Refer to the care plan for Risk for Adult **Falls** and Impaired **Walking**.

▲ Initiate ambulation by simply ambulating a client a few steps from bed to chair, once a health care provider's out-of-bed order is obtained. EBN: *Lack of ambulation and deconditioning effects of bed rest are some of the most predictable causes of loss of independent ambulation in hospitalized older persons. Nurses have been identified as the professionals most capable of promoting walking independence in the hospital setting (King et al, 2016).*

▲ Evaluate medications the client is taking to see if they could be causing Decreased **Activity** Tolerance. EB: *Polypharmacy and potentially inappropriate medications are associated with an increased risk of falls. The potential harms versus benefits of medications should be weighed in deciding to continue treatment in older adults with multiple chronic conditions (Masumoto et al, 2018).*

▲ Refer the disabled older client to physical therapy for functional training including gait training, stepping, and sit-to-stand exercises, or for strength training. EBN: *Older adults often experience functional losses during hospitalization. Clinical care activities have been increasingly promoted as a way to help older hospitalized clients offset these losses and recover from acute illness (Casey et al, 2016).*

Home Care

▲ Begin discharge planning as soon as possible with the case manager or social worker to assess the need for home support systems and the need for community or home health services. EB: *Discharging clients from acute care hospitals is complex and requires effective collaboration between multiprofessional teams and clients. Miscommunication around discharge instructions and/or follow-up care can lead to posthospital adverse events, client dissatisfaction, and increased 30-day readmissions (Patel et al, 2019).*

▲ Assess the home environment for factors that contribute to decreased activity tolerance such as stairs or distance to the bathroom. Refer the client for occupational therapy, if needed, and to assist the client in restructuring the home and ADL patterns. *During hospitalization, clients and families often estimate energy requirements at home inaccurately because the hospital's availability of staff support distorts the level of care that will be needed.*

▲ Refer the client for physical therapy for strength training and possible weight training to regain strength, increase endurance, and improve balance. If the client is homebound, the physical therapist can also initiate cardiac rehabilitation. EB: *The older and frailer the individual, the greater the rationale for the addition*

A

of progressive resistance and balance training to aerobic exercise programs, given the prevalence of sarcopenia, mobility impairment, and functional dependency in this group. Frailty is not a contraindication to exercise, but conversely, one of the most important reasons to prescribe it (Bauman et al, 2016).

- ● Encourage progress with positive feedback. The client's experience should be validated within expected norms. Recognition of progress enhances motivation.
- ● Teach the client/family the importance of and methods for setting priorities for activities, especially those having a high energy demand (e.g., home/family events). Instruct on realistic expectations.
- ● Encourage routine low-level exercise periods such as a daily short walk or chair exercises.
- ● Provide the client/family with resources such as senior centers, exercise classes, educational and recreational programs, and volunteer opportunities that can aid in promoting socialization and appropriate activity. Social isolation can be an outcome of and contribute to Decreased **Activity** Tolerance.
- ● Instruct the client and family on the importance of maintaining proper nutrition and use of dietary supplements as indicated. Illness may suppress appetite, leading to inadequate nutrition.
- ▲ Refer to medical social services as necessary to assist the family in adjusting to major changes in patterns of living because of Decreased **Activity** Tolerance.
- ▲ Assess the need for long-term supports for optimal activity tolerance of priority activities (e.g., assistive devices, oxygen, medication, catheters, massage), especially for a hospice client. Evaluate intermittently.
- ▲ Refer to home health aide services to support the client and family through changing levels of activity tolerance. Introduce aide support early. Instruct the aide to promote independence in activity as tolerated.
- ● Allow terminally ill clients and their families to guide care. Control by the client or family respects their autonomy and promotes effective coping.
- ● Provide increased attention to comfort and dignity of the terminally ill client in care planning. *Interventions should be provided as much for psychological effect as for physiological support. For example, oxygen may be more valuable as a support to the client's psychological comfort than as a booster of oxygen saturation.*
- ▲ Institute case management of frail elderly to support continued independent living.

Client/Family Teaching and Discharge Planning

- ● Instruct the client on techniques for avoiding Decreased **Activity** Tolerance, such as controlled breathing techniques.
- ● Teach the client techniques to decrease dizziness from postural hypotension when changing positions, especially when standing up.
- ● Help client with energy conservation and work simplification techniques in ADLs.
- ● Describe to the client the symptoms of Decreased **Activity** Tolerance, including which symptoms to report to the health care provider.
- ● Explain to the client how to use assistive devices, oxygen, or medications before or during activity.
- ● Help the client set up an activity log to record exercise and exercise tolerance.

REFERENCES

Ahmed, R., Razack, S., Salam, S., et al. (2015). Design and fabrication of pneumatically powered wheel chair-stretcher device. *International Journal of Innovative Research in Science, Engineering and Technology, 4*(10).

Apps, M., Mukherjee, D., Abbas, S., et al. (2016). A chronic obstructive pulmonary disease service integrating community and hospital services can improve patient care and reduce hospital stays. *American Journal of Respiratory and Critical Care Medicine, 193*, A1523.

Bauman, A., Merom, D., Bull, F., et al. (2016). Updating the evidence for physical activity: Summative reviews of the epidemiological evidence, prevalence, and interventions to promote active aging. *The Gerontologist, 56*(S2), S268–S280.

Carpaji, O. A., & van den Berge, M. (2018). The asthma-obesity relationship: Underlying mechanisms and treatment implications. *Current Opinion in Pulmonary Medicine, 24*(1), 42–49.

Casey, C., Bennett, J., Winters-Stone, K., et al. (2016). Measuring activity levels associated with rehabilitative care in hospitalized older adults. *Geriatric Nursing, 35*(2), S3–S10.

Chu, R. (2017). Preventing in-patient falls: The nurse's pivotal role. *Nursing 2020, 47*(3), 24–30.

Ciaren, F., O'Connell, M., Donogjue, O., et al. (2017). Impaired orthostatic blood pressure recovery is associated with unexplained and injurious falls. *Journal of the American Geriatrics Society, 65*(3), 474–482.

Constantin, S., & Dahlke, S. (2018). How nurses restore and maintain mobility in hospitalised older people: An integrative literature review. *International Journal of Older People Nursing, 13*(3). https://doi.org/10.1111/opn.12200.

Crawford, A., & Harris, H. (2016). Caring for adults with impaired physical mobility. *Nursing 2020, 46*(12), 36–41.

Feigin, V., Norrving, B., George, M., Foltz, J., Roth, G., & Mensah, G. A. (2016). Prevention of stroke: A strategic global imperative. *Nature Reviews Neurology, 12*(9), 501–512.

Goswami, N., Blaber, A. P., Hinghofer-Szalkay, H., & Montani, J. (2017). Orthostatic intolerance in older persons: Etiology and countermeasures. *Frontiers in Physiology, 8*(803). https://doi.org/10.3389/fphys.2017.00803.

Kehler, D. S., Theou, O., & Rockwood, K. (2019). Bed rest and accelerated aging in relation to the musculoskeletal and cardiovascular systems and frailty biomarkers: A review. *Experimental Gerontology, 124*. https://doi.org/10.1016/j.exger.2019.110643.

King, B. J., Pecanac, K., Krupp, A., Liebzeit, D., & Mahoney, J. (2018). Impact of fall prevention on nurses and care of fall risk patients. *The Gerontologist*, *58*(2), 331–340.

King, B. J., Steege, L. M., Winsor, K., VanDenbergh, S., & Brown, C. J. (2016). Getting patients walking: A pilot study of mobilizing older adult patients via a nurse-driven intervention. *Journal of the American Geriatrics Society*, *64*(10), 2088–2094.

Kramer, A., Gollhofer, A., Armbrecht, G., et al. (2017). How to prevent the detrimental effects of two months of bed-rest on muscle, bone and cardiovascular system: An RCT. *Scientific Reports*, *7*, 13177.

Light, K., Bishop, M., & Wright, T. (2016). Telephone calls make a difference in home balance training outcomes: A randomized trial. *Journal of Geriatric Physical Therapy*, *39*(3), 97–101.

Masumoto, S., Sato, M., Maeno, T., Ichinohe, Y., & Maeno, T. (2018). Potentially inappropriate medications with polypharmacy increase the risk of falls in older Japanese patients: 1 year prospective cohort study. *Geriatrics & Gerontology International*, *18*(7), 1064–1070.

Patel, H., Yirdaw, E., Yu, A., Slater, L., Perica, K., Pierce, R., et al. (2019). Improving early discharge using a team-based structure for discharge multidisciplinary rounds. *Professional Case Management*, *24*(2), 83–89.

Simon, M., Korn, K., Cho, L., Blackburn, G., & Raymond, C. (2018). Cardiac rehabilitation: A class 1 recommendation. *Cleveland Clinic Journal of Medicine*, *85*(7), 551–558.

Sommers, J., Engelbert, R., & Dettling-Ihnenfeldt, D. (2015). Physiotherapy in the intensive care unit: An evidence-based, expert driven, practical statement and rehabilitation recommendations. *Clinical Rehabilitation*, *29*(11). https://doi.org/10.1177/0269215514567156.

World Health Organization. (2020). *Physical activity and older adults*. Retrieved from http://www.who.int/dietphysicalactivity/factsheet_olderadults/en/.

A

Risk for Decreased Activity Tolerance Domain 4 Activity/rest Class 2 activity/exercise

Mary Beth Flynn Makic, PhD, RN, CCNS, CCRN-K, FAAN, FNAP, FCNS

NANDA-I

Definition

Susceptible to experiencing insufficient endurance to complete required or desired daily activities.

Risk Factors

Decreased muscle strength; depressive symptoms; fear of pain; imbalance between oxygen supply/demand; impaired physical mobility; inexperience with an activity; insufficient muscle mass; malnutrition; pain; physical deconditioning; sedentary lifestyle

At-Risk Population

Individuals with history of decreased activity tolerance; older adults

Associated Conditions

Neoplasms; neurodegenerative diseases; respiration disorders; traumatic brain injuries; vitamin D deficiency

NOC, NIC, Client Outcomes, Nursing Interventions and *Rationales,* and References

Refer to care plan for Decreased **Activity** Tolerance

Ineffective Activity Planning Domain 9 Coping/stress tolerance Class 2 Coping responses

Jacquelyn Svoboda, DNP, RN, WHNP-C

NANDA-I

Definition

Inability to prepare for a set of actions fixed in time and under certain conditions.

Defining Characteristics

Absence of plan; excessive anxiety about a task; inadequate health resources; inadequate organizational skills; pattern of failure; reports fear of performing a task; unmet goals for chosen activity

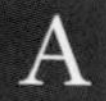

Related Factors

Flight behavior when faced with proposed solution; hedonism; inadequate information processing ability; inadequate social support; unrealistic perception of event; unrealistic perception of personal abilities

At-Risk Population

Individuals with history of procrastination

NOC (Nursing Outcomes Classification)

Suggested NOC Outcomes

Cognition; Cognition; Orientation; Concentration; Decision-Making; Information Processing; Memory

Example NOC Outcome with Indicators

Cognition as evidenced by the following indicators: Communication clear and appropriate for age/ Comprehension of the meaning of situations/Information processing/Alternatives weighed when making decisions. (Rate the outcome and indicators of **Cognition:** 1 = severely compromised, 2 = substantially compromised, 3 = moderately compromised, 4 = mildly compromised, 5 = not compromised [see Section I].)

Client Outcomes

Client Will (Specify Time Frame)

- Verbalize need for self-directed activity
- Choose the health care option that fits his or her lifestyle within an appropriate amount of time that allows enactment of the choice
- Describe how the chosen option fits into current lifestyle before or after the decision has been made
- Verbalize the need for a behavioral change to improve physical activity
- Offer alternative options to those with barriers to participating in physical activity

NIC (Nursing Interventions Classification)

Suggested NIC Interventions

Activity Therapy; Anxiety Reduction; Behavior Management; Behavior Modification; Calming Technique; Coping Enhancement; Cognitive Restructuring; Decision-Making Support; Life Skills Enhancement

Example NIC Activities—Coping Enhancement

Assist client in developing an objective appraisal of the event; Explore with client previous methods of dealing with life problems

Nursing Interventions and *Rationales*

- Identify the client's perception of the problem and how they envision their participation to improve goal setting. EB: *Clients prioritize planning based on experiences with their specific illness, while caregivers prioritize future consequences of the illness* (*Sathanapally et al, 2020*).
- Identify the informational needs of the client such as client's understanding of health condition, treatment options, health system processes, diet, exercise, and access to important telephone numbers. EB: *This study of clients with breast cancer and lymphedema validated the need for an individual assessment to determine the unique informational needs, preference in delivery method, and timing of receipt of information for each client (Dorri et al, 2020).*
- Address the client's fears and anxieties and encourage him or her to modify their cognitive approach to planning. EB: *A systematic review and meta-analysis supports the concept that improvements can be made for addictive behaviors through the assessment of desired thinking and modifying those responses (Mansueto et al, 2019).*
- Client verbalizes need for behavioral change for improved physical activity. EB: *This study reports that clear direction and encouragement from health care providers on the benefits that exercise can have on the symptom progression and on exercise opportunities can promote client participation and engagement* (*Hurley et al, 2018*).

- Encourage clients to verbalize the need for physical activity to help reduce role overload. EB: *This study demonstrated that the importance of integrating physical activity and exercise into life planning benefited the individuals affected by role overload, as well as benefited the family of the individuals* (Shelton, 2018).
- ▲ Determine factors that will increase opportunities to successfully plan activities and increase the success of the project: financial resources; family situation; prior medical, psychiatric, and psychosocial conditions; material resources; and the ability to manage stress. EB: *Discussions related to client lived experiences, cultural concepts, family dynamics, the etiology of health condition, and the barriers to physical activity are important in modifying and supporting healthy planning for diet and exercise (Lappan et al, 2020).*
- ▲ Encourage physical actively. Collaborate with occupational and/or physical therapy to establish activity opportunities and limitations. EB: *Cognitive impairment is correlated with higher mortality rates in the elderly clients who are inactive (Esteban-Cornejo et al, 2019).*

Pediatric

- Begin activity planning in preschool-age children of working parents. EB: *This study focused on preschool-age children and noted that sports participation resulted in better rule comprehension, improved memory, goal setting, and improved cognitive flexibility* (Bryant et al, 2020).
- Establish a contract. EB: *This study of adolescents with type 1 diabetes indicated that positive psychology intervention and behavioral contracts may be an important intervention to improve coping and glycemic control* (Jaser et al, 2020).
- Provide support to the schools for physical activities in all school venues. EB: *Urban schools are more successful in implementing physical activities when educators are allowed to formulate engaging and community-specific physical education curriculum that meets the needs of the students within the community and also when schools identify collaborating partnerships in the community to assist in funding needs* (Sliwa et al, 2017).
- Support safe neighborhood activity programs. EB: *Children of low-income households have a lower level of physical activity than average and the contributing factors that affect this activity were identified as working parents, dangerous activities in the neighborhood, lack of physical activity planning information, and lack of community input* (Finkelstein et al, 2017).

Geriatric

- Plan activities for older clients. EB: *In a study of elderly clients, it was found that physical activity may preserve cognitive function and the quality of memory* (Kurdi & Flora, 2019).
- Plan activities for older clients with impaired mental function. EB: *In this study, it was found that clients with impaired mental function have greater success in participating in a physical activity program that is formulated to address individual needs when there is ongoing supervision from the team to ensure adherence* (Eckert et al, 2020).
- Community-based activities for older adults. EB: *A study of certified nursing homes (CNH) identified that women clients who resided at higher star rated CNH had higher attendance in physical and social activity programs compared to lower star rated CNH and their male counterparts* (Neils-Strunjas et al, 2020).

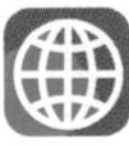

Multicultural

- ✱ Provide literature and information in the appropriate language for the client who speaks little to no English. EB: *This study reinforces the importance of addressing cultural and language needs of underserved populations to increased participation in physical activity (Bantham et al, 2020).*
- Preplanning educational programs for the culturally diverse population needs to be developed. EB: *By providing activities close in proximity and utilizing native linguistics instructions, along with culturally applicable activities, there is improved participation in the activity programming* (Montayre et al, 2020).
- ▲ Support and education by the physician and family on how exercise can help reduce and/or prevent falls of older adults improves adherence to physical activity. EB: *A study done on factors that affect the older client's belief on fall risk and prevention noted that providers can influence how clients perceive fall prevention and how they adopt fall risk prevention activities such as exercise through engagement and encouragement (Stevens et al, 2018).*

Home Care

- Have a preplanned activity exercise for the home client with a debilitating musculoskeletal disease to help improve functional status. EB: *This study showed that for Parkinson's disease clients, an individualized home exercise and walking program prevented the anticipated physical decline over 12 months (Ellis et al, 2019).*

A

- Assess the home environment for barriers that can impact the client's motivation to be a participant in the activity planned. EB: *This study on homebound heart failure clients showed that facilitators to client participation in physical activity programming include an individualized intervention created by the health care team, which considers individual barriers as well as the participation of the family in planning sessions (Okwose et al, 2020).*
- Home care for the cardiac rehabilitation client. EB: *Providing a home exercise plan with telemonitoring guidance for the home care cardiac rehabilitation client resulted in improvement of the health status for the client and resulted in being as efficacious as rehabbing in a care center (Avila et al, 2018).*
- For additional interventions, refer to care plans for **Anxiety,** Readiness for Enhanced Family **Coping,** Readiness for Enhanced **Decision-Making, Fear,** Readiness for Enhanced **Hope,** Readiness for Enhanced **Power,** Readiness for Enhanced **Spiritual** Well-Being, and Readiness for Enhanced **Health** Self-Management

REFERENCES

Avila, A., Claes, J., Goetschalckx, K., et al. (2018). Home-based rehabilitation with telemonitoring guidance for patients with coronary artery disease (short-term results of the TRiCH study): Randomized controlled trial. *Journal of Medical Internet Research*, *20*(6), e225.

Bantham, A., Ross, S. E. T., Sebastião, E., & Hall, G. (2020). Overcoming barriers to physical activity in underserved populations. *Progress in Cardiovascular Diseases, 64,* 64.

Bryant, L. M., Duncan, R. J., & Schmitt, S. A. (2020). The cognitive benefits of participating in structured sports for preschoolers. *Early Education & Development*, 1–12.

Dorri, S., Olfatbakhsh, A., & Asadi, F. (2020). Informational needs in patients with breast cancer with lymphedema: Is it important? *Breast Cancer: Basic and Clinical Research*, *14*, 1178223420911033.

Eckert, T., Bongartz, M., Ullrich, P., et al. (2020). Promoting physical activity in geriatric patients with cognitive impairment after discharge from ward-rehabilitation: A feasibility study. *European Journal of Ageing*, 1–12.

Ellis, T. D., Cavanaugh, J. T., DeAngelis, T., et al. (2019). Comparative effectiveness of mHealth-supported exercise compared with exercise alone for people with Parkinson disease: Randomized controlled pilot study. *Physical Therapy*, *99*(2), 203–216.

Esteban-Cornejo, I., Cabanas-Sánchez, V., Higueras-Fresnillo, S., et al. (2019). Cognitive frailty and mortality in a national cohort of older adults: The role of physical activity. *Mayo Clinic Proceedings*, *94*(7), 1180–1189.

Finkelstein, D. M., Petersen, D. M., & Schottenfeld, L. S. (2017). Peer reviewed: Promoting children's physical activity in low-income communities in Colorado: What are the barriers and opportunities? *Preventing Chronic Disease, 14.*

Hurley, M., Dickson, K., Hallett, R., et al. (2018). Exercise interventions and patient beliefs for people with hip, knee or hip and knee osteoarthritis: A mixed methods review. *Cochrane Database of Systematic Reviews*, 4.

Jaser, S. S., Datye, K., Morrow, T., et al. (2020). THR1VE! Positive psychology intervention to treat diabetes distress in teens with type 1 diabetes: Rationale and trial design. *Contemporary Clinical Trials*, *96*, 106086.

Kurdi, F. N., & Flora, R. (2019). The impact of physical exercise on Brain-Derived Neurotrophic Factor (BDNF) level in elderly population. *Open Access Macedonian Journal of Medical Sciences*, *7*(10), 1618.

Lappan, S. N., Carolan, M., Parra-Cardona, J. R., & Weatherspoon, L. (2020). Promoting healthy eating and regular physical activity in low-income families through family-centered programs: Implications for practice. *Journal of Primary Prevention*, 1–26.

Mansueto, G., Martino, F., Palmieri, S., et al. (2019). Desire thinking across addictive behaviours: A systematic review and meta-analysis. *Addictive Behaviors*, *98*, 106018.

Montayre, J., Neville, S., Dunn, I., Shrestha-Ranjit, J., Wright, S., & Clair, V. (2020). What makes community-based physical activity programs for culturally and linguistically diverse older adults effective? A systematic review. *Australasian Journal on Ageing, 39,* 331.

Neils-Strunjas, J., Crandall, K. J., Ding, X., Gabbard, A., Rassi, S., & Otto, S. (2020). Facilitators and barriers to attendance in a nursing home exercise program. *Journal of the American Medical Directors Association, 22,* 803.

Okwose, N. C., O'brien, N., Charman, S., et al. (2020). Overcoming barriers to engagement and adherence to a home-based physical activity intervention for patients with heart failure: A qualitative focus group study. *BMJ Open*, *10*(9), e036382.

Sathanapally, H., Sidhu, M., Fahami, R., Gillies, C., et al. (2020). Priorities of patients with multimorbidity and of clinicians regarding treatment and health outcomes: A systematic mixed studies review. *BMJ Open*, *10*(2), e033445. https://doi.org/10.1136/bmjopen-2019-033445.

Shelton, S. L. (2018). Women's self-reported factors that influence their postpartum exercise levels. *Nursing for Womens Health*, *22*(2), 148–157.

Sliwa, S., Nihiser, A., Lee, S., McCaughtry, N., Culp, B., & Michael, S. (2017). Engaging students in physical education: Key challenges and opportunities for physical educators in urban settings. *Journal of Physical Education, Recreation & Dance*, *88*(3), 43–48.

Stevens, J. A., Sleet, D. A., & Rubenstein, L. Z. (2018). The influence of older adults' beliefs and attitudes on adopting fall prevention behaviors. *American Journal of Lifestyle Medicine*, *12*(4), 324–330.

Risk for Ineffective Activity Planning

Domain 9 Coping/stress tolerance Class 2 Coping responses

Mary Beth Flynn Makic, PhD, RN, CCNS, CCRN-K, FAAN, FNAP, FCNS

NANDA-I

Definition

Susceptible to an inability to prepare for a set of actions fixed in time and under certain conditions, which may compromise health.

Risk Factors

Flight behavior when faced with proposed solution; hedonism; inadequate information processing ability; inadequate social support; unrealistic perception of event; unrealistic perception of personal abilities

At-Risk Population

Individuals with history of procrastination

NOC, NIC, Client Outcomes, Nursing Interventions and *Rationales,* Client/Family Teaching and Discharge Planning, and References

Refer to care plan for Ineffective **Activity** Planning.

Ineffective Airway Clearance Domain 11 Safety/protection Class 2 Physical injury

Debra Siela, PhD, RN, ACNS-BC, CCRN-K, CNE, RRT

Definition

Reduced ability to clear secretions or obstructions from the respiratory tract to maintain a clear airway.

Defining Characteristics

Absence of cough; adventitious breath sounds; altered respiratory rhythm; altered thoracic percussion; altered thoraco-vocal fremitus; bradypnea; cyanosis; difficulty verbalizing; diminished breath sounds; excessive sputum; hypoxemia; ineffective cough; ineffective sputum elimination; nasal flaring; orthopnea; psychomotor agitation; subcostal retraction; tachypnea; use of accessory muscles of respiration

Related Factors

Dehydration; excessive mucus; exposure to harmful substance; fear of pain; foreign body in airway; inattentive to second-hand smoke; mucus plug; retained secretions; smoking

At-Risk Population

Children; infants

Associated Conditions

Airway spasm; allergic airway; asthma; chronic obstructive pulmonary disease; congenital heart disease; critical illness; exudate in the alveoli; general anesthesia; hyperplasia of the bronchial walls; neuromuscular diseases; respiratory tract infection

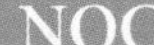

NOC (Nursing Outcomes Classification)

Suggested NOC Outcomes

Aspiration Prevention; Respiratory Status: Airway Patency, Gas Exchange, Ventilation

Example NOC Outcome with Indicators

Respiratory Status: Ventilation as evidenced by the following indicators: Respiratory rate/Respiratory rhythm/Depth of inspiration/Chest expansion symmetrical/Ease of breathing/Tidal volume/Vital capacity. (Rate each indicator of **Respiratory Status: Ventilation:** 1 = severe deviation from normal range, 2 = substantial deviation from normal range, 3 = moderate deviation from normal range, 4 = mild deviation from normal range, 5 = no deviation from normal range [see Section I].)

Client Outcomes

Client Will (Specify Time Frame)

- Demonstrate effective coughing and clear breath sounds
- Maintain a patent airway at all times
- Explain methods useful to enhance secretion removal

- Explain the significance of changes in sputum to include color, character, amount, and odor
- Identify and avoid specific factors that inhibit effective airway clearance

NIC (Nursing Interventions Classification)

Suggested NIC Interventions

Airway Management; Airway Suctioning; Cough Enhancement

Example NIC Activities—Airway Management

Instruct how to cough effectively; Auscultate breath sounds, noting areas of decreased or absent ventilation and presence of adventitious sounds

Nursing Interventions and *Rationales*

- ● Auscultate breath sounds every 1 to 4 hours. The presence of crackles and wheezes may alert the nurse to airway obstruction, which may lead to or exacerbate existing hypoxia. EB: *In severe exacerbations of chronic obstructive pulmonary disease (COPD), lung sounds may be diminished or distant with air trapping (Bickley et al, 2020).*
- ● Monitor respiratory patterns, including rate, depth, and effort. EB: *A normal respiratory rate for an adult without dyspnea is 12 to 16 breaths per minute (Bickley et al, 2020). With secretions in the airway, the respiratory rate will increase.*
- ● Monitor blood gas values and pulse oxygen saturation levels as available. An oxygen saturation of less than 90% (normal: 95%–100%) or a partial pressure of oxygen of less than 80 mm Hg (normal: 80–100 mm Hg) indicates significant oxygenation problems (Bickley et al, 2020).
- ▲ Administer oxygen as ordered. Oxygen administration has been shown to correct hypoxemia (Sauls, 2021). EB: *Administer humidified oxygen through an appropriate device (e.g., nasal cannula or Venturi mask per the health care provider's order); aim for an oxygen (O_2) saturation level of 90% or above. Oxygen should be titrated to target an SpO_2 of 94% to 98%, except with carbon monoxide poisoning (100% oxygen), acute respiratory distress syndrome (ARDS) (88%–95%), those at risk for hypercapnia (88%–92%), and premature infants (88%–94%) (Siela & Kidd, 2017; Sauls, 2021).*
- ● Position the client in a semirecumbent position with the head of the bed at a 30- to 45-degree angle to decrease the aspiration of gastric, oral, and nasal secretions (Siela, 2010; Vollman et al, 2017; Sauls, 2021). CEB/EB: *In a mechanically ventilated client, there is a decreased incidence of ventilator-associated pneumonia (VAP) if the client is positioned at a 30- to 45-degree semirecumbent position rather than a supine position (Siela, 2010; American Association of Critical Care Nurses, 2017)*
- ● Help the client deep breathe and perform controlled coughing. Have the client inhale deeply, hold breath for several seconds, and cough two or three times with mouth open while tightening the upper abdominal muscles. CEB/EB: *Controlled coughing uses the diaphragmatic muscles, making the cough more forceful and effective (Gosselink et al, 2008; Sommers et al, 2015; Bickley et al, 2020).*
- ● If the client has obstructive lung disease, such as chronic obstructive pulmonary disease (COPD), cystic fibrosis, or bronchiectasis, consider helping the client use the forced expiratory technique, the "huff cough." The client does a series of coughs while saying the word "huff." EB: *This technique prevents the glottis from closing during the cough and is effective in clearing secretions (Chalmers et al, 2015; Sommers et al, 2015).*
- ▲ Encourage the client to use an incentive spirometer. Recognize that controlled coughing and deep breathing may be just as effective as incentive spirometry (Chalmers et al, 2015).
- ● Encourage activity and ambulation as tolerated. If the client cannot be ambulated, turn the client from side to side at least every 2 hours. *Body movement helps mobilize secretions.*
- ● Encourage fluid intake of up to 2500 mL/day within cardiac or renal reserve. *Fluids help minimize mucosal drying and maximize ciliary action to move secretions.*
- ▲ Administer medications such as bronchodilators or inhaled steroids as ordered. Watch for side effects such as tachycardia or anxiety with bronchodilators or inflamed pharynx with inhaled steroids. EB: *Bronchodilators decrease airway resistance, improve the efficiency of respiratory movements, improve exercise tolerance, and can reduce symptoms of dyspnea on exertion (Anzueto & Miravitlles, 2017). Pharmacologic therapy in COPD is used to reduce symptoms, reduce the frequency and severity of exacerbation, and improve health strategies and exercise tolerance (GOLD, 2020).*
- ▲ Provide percussion, vibration, and oscillation as appropriate for individual client needs. EB: *Airway clearance techniques for clients with acute exacerbations of COPD may have a small but important positive effect*

on the need for and duration of ventilatory assistance and may reduce hospital length of stay (Chalmers, Aliberti, & Blasi, 2015; Sommers et al, 2015). Mucoregulators such as N-acetylcysteine and carbocysteine are recommended to reduce the frequency of COPD acute exacerbations (GOLD, 2020). High-frequency chest wall oscillation (HFCWO) significantly improves aeration of the dorsal lung region in hypersecretive clients with acute respiratory failure (Longhini et al, 2020).

- Use of positive expiratory pressure (PEP) with a mask for airway clearance shows a significant reduction in pulmonary exacerbations in people with cystic fibrosis (McIlwaine, Button, & Nevitt, 2019).
- Observe sputum, noting color, odor, and volume. EB: *Normal sputum is clear or gray and minimal; abnormal sputum is green, yellow, or bloody; malodorous; and often copious. The presence of purulent sputum during a COPD exacerbation can be sufficient indication for starting empirical antibiotic treatment. Notify health care provider of purulent sputum (GOLD, 2020).*

Critical Care

▲ In intubated clients, body positioning and mobilization may optimize airway secretion clearance. Lateral rotational movement provides continuous postural drainage and mobilization of secretions (St. Clair & MacDermott, 2017).

- Reposition the client as needed. Use rotational or kinetic bed therapy in clients for whom side-to-side turning is contraindicated or difficult. EBN: *Changing position frequently decreases the incidence of atelectasis, pooling of secretions, and resultant pneumonia. Continuous, lateral rotational therapy has been shown to improve oxygenation and decrease the incidence of VAP (St. Clair & MacDermott, 2017).*
- If the client is intubated, consider use of kinetic therapy, using a kinetic bed that slowly moves the client with 40-degree turns. EB: *Rotational therapy may decrease the incidence of pulmonary complications in high-risk clients with increasing ventilator support requirements, who are at risk for VAP, and with clinical indications for acute lung injury or ARDS with worsening PaO_2:FiO_2 ratio, presence of fluffy infiltrates via chest radiograph concomitant with pulmonary edema, and refractory hypoxemia (Case, 2021).*
- Assess for the presence or absence of a gag reflex. EB: *In individuals with prolonged ventilation, the presence of one or both gag reflexes could predict a reduction in extubation failure related to aspiration or excessive upper airway secretions (Howes et al, 2020).*

▲ Early mobility and physical rehabilitation can reduce muscle weakness, mechanical ventilation duration, intensive care unit stay, delirium, and hospitalization. CEB/EB: *The Awakening and Breathing Coordination, Delirium Monitoring and Management, and Early Mobility (ABCDEF) bundle has criteria to determine when clients are candidates for early mobility. An early mobility and walking program can promote weaning from ventilator support as a client's overall strength and endurance (Balas et al, 2012; Devlin et al, 2018).*

- If the client is intubated and is stable, consider getting the client up to sit at the edge of the bed, transfer to a chair, or walk as appropriate, if an effective interdisciplinary team is developed to keep the client safe *(Dirkes & Kozlowski, 2019).* CEB: *A study found that for every week of bed rest, muscle strength can decrease 20%; early ambulation also helped clients develop a positive outlook (Perme & Chandrashekar, 2009).* EB: *A systematic review and meta-analysis found that while early mobility programs did not influence overall morbidity, clients did demonstrate improvement in mobility status, muscle strength, and days alive out of hospital up to 180 days (Tipping et al, 2017).*
- When suctioning an endotracheal tube or tracheostomy tube for a client on a ventilator, do the following:
  - Explain the process of suctioning beforehand and ensure the client is not in pain or overly anxious. Suctioning can be a frightening experience; an explanation along with adequate pain relief or needed sedation can reduce stress, anxiety, and pain (Seckel, 2017).
  - Hyperoxygenate before and between endotracheal suction sessions. Studies have demonstrated that hyperoxygenation may help prevent oxygen desaturation in a suctioned client (Pedersen et al, 2009; Siela, 2010; Seckel, 2017; Vollman, Sole, & Quinn, 2017).
  - Suction for less than 15 seconds. Studies demonstrated that because of a drop in the partial pressure of oxygen with suctioning, preferably no more than 10 seconds should be used actually suctioning, with the entire procedure taking 15 seconds (Pedersen et al, 2009; Seckel, 2017).
  - Use a closed, in-line suction system. Closed in-line suctioning has minimal effects on heart rate, respiratory rate, tidal volume, and oxygen saturation and may reduce contamination (Seckel, 2017).
  - Avoid saline instillation during suctioning. CEB/EBN: Repeated studies have demonstrated that saline instillation before suctioning has an adverse effect on oxygen saturation in both adults and children (Pederson et al, 2009; Siela, 2010; Caparros, 2014; Seckel, 2017).

A

- ○ Use of a subglottic suctioning endotracheal tube reduces the incidence of VAP or ventilator-associated complications (Vollman, Sole, & Quinn, 2017; Pozuelo-Carrascosa et al, 2020). A decrease in mortality occurs with use of subglottic secretion drainage (Pozuelo-Carrascosa et al, 2020).
- ○ Document results of coughing and suctioning, particularly client tolerance and secretion characteristics such as color, odor, and volume (Seckel, 2017).

Pediatric

- ● Educate parents about the risk factors for ineffective airway clearance such as foreign body ingestion and passive smoke exposure.
- ● Educate children and parents on the importance of adherence to peak expiratory flow monitoring for asthma self-management.
- ● Educate parents and other caregivers that cough and cold medications bought over the counter are not safe for a child younger than 2 unless specifically ordered by a health care provider.
- ● See the care plan for Risk for **Suffocation**

Geriatric

- ● Encourage ambulation as tolerated without causing exhaustion. *Immobility is often harmful to older adults because it decreases ventilation and increases stasis of secretions, leading to atelectasis or pneumonia.*
- ● Actively encourage older adults to deep breathe and cough. *Cough reflexes are blunted, and coughing is decreased in older adults.*
- ● Ensure adequate hydration within cardiac and renal reserves. *Older adults are prone to dehydration and therefore more viscous secretions, because they frequently use diuretics or laxatives and forget to drink adequate amounts of water.*

Home Care

- ● Some of the above interventions may be adapted for home care use.
- ▲ Begin discharge planning as soon as possible with case manager or social worker to assess need for home support systems, assistive devices, and community or home health services.
- ● Assess home environment for factors that exacerbate airway clearance problems (e.g., presence of allergens, lack of adequate humidity in air, poor air flow, stressful family relationships).
- ● Assess affective climate within family and family support system. EB: *Problems with respiratory function and resulting anxiety can provoke anger and frustration in the client. Feelings may be displaced onto caregiver and require intervention to ensure continued caregiver support.* Refer to care plan for **Caregiver Role Strain.**
- ● Refer to GOLD guidelines for management of home care and indications of hospital admission criteria. http://www.goldcopd.org/.
- ● When respiratory procedures are being implemented, explain equipment and procedures to family members and caregivers, and provide needed emotional support. *Family members assuming responsibility for respiratory monitoring often find this stressful. They may not have been able to assimilate fully any instructions provided by hospital staff.*
- ● When electrically based equipment for respiratory support is being implemented, evaluate home environment for electrical safety, proper grounding, and so on. Ensure that notification is sent to the local utility company, the emergency medical team, and police and fire departments.
- ● Provide family with support for care of a client with chronic or terminal illness. *Breathing difficulty can provoke extreme anxiety, which can interfere with the client's ability or willingness to adhere to the treatment plan.*
- ● Witnessing breathing difficulties and facing concerns of dealing with chronic or terminal illness can create fear in caregiver. Fear inhibits effective coping. Refer to care plans for **Anxiety** and **Powerlessness.**
- ● Instruct the client to avoid exposure to persons with upper respiratory infections, avoid crowds of people, and wash hands after each exposure to groups of people or public places.
- ▲ Determine client adherence to medical regimen. Instruct the client and family on importance of reporting effectiveness of current medications to health care provider. *Inappropriate use of medications (too much or too little) can influence amount of respiratory secretions.*
- ● Teach the client when and how to use inhalant or nebulizer treatments at home.
- ● Teach the client/family importance of maintaining regimen and having "as-needed" drugs easily accessible at all times. *Success in avoiding emergency or institutional care may rest solely on medication compliance or availability.*

- Instruct the client and family on the importance of maintaining proper nutrition, adequate fluids, rest, and behavioral pacing for energy conservation and rehabilitation.
- Instruct in use of dietary supplements as indicated. *Illness may suppress appetite, leading to inadequate nutrition. Supplements will allow clients to eat with minimal energy consumption.*
- Identify an emergency plan, including criteria for use. *Ineffective airway clearance can be life-threatening.*
- ▲ Refer for home health aide services for assistance with activities of daily living (ADLs). Clients with decreased oxygenation and copious respiratory secretions are often unable to maintain energy for ADLs.
- ▲ Assess family for role changes and coping skills. Refer to medical social services as necessary. *Clients with decreased oxygenation are unable to maintain role activities and therefore experience frustration and anger, which may pose a threat to family integrity. Family counseling to adapt to role changes may be needed.*
- ▲ For the client dying at home with a terminal illness, if the "death rattle" is present with gurgling, rattling, or crackling sounds in the airway with each breath, recognize that anticholinergic medications can often help control symptoms, if given early in the process. *Anticholinergic medications can help decrease the accumulation of secretions but do not decrease existing secretions. This medication must be administered early in the process to be effective.*
- ▲ For the client with a death rattle, nursing care includes turning to mobilize secretions, keeping the head of the bed elevated for postural drainage of secretions, and avoiding suctioning. EB: *Suctioning is a distressing and painful event for clients and families and is rarely effective in decreasing the death rattle (Kolb, Snowden, & Stevens, 2018).*

Client/Family Teaching and Discharge Planning

- ▲ Teach the importance of not smoking. Refer to a smoking cessation program, and encourage clients who relapse to keep trying to quit. Ensure that the client receives appropriate medications to support smoking cessation from the primary health care provider. EB: *A Cochrane review found that use of the antidepressant medications increased the rate of smoking withdrawal two to three times more than smoking withdrawal without use of medications (Howes et al, 2020).*
- ▲ Teach the client how to use a flutter clearance device if ordered, which vibrates to loosen mucus and gives positive pressure to keep airways open. CEB: *Studies have demonstrated that use of the mucus clearance device had improved exercise performance compared with COPD clients who use a sham device (Osadnik, McDonald, & Holland, 2013).*
- ▲ Teach the client how to use peak expiratory flow rate (PEFR) meter if ordered and when to seek medical attention if PEFR reading drops. Also teach how to use metered dose inhalers and self-administer inhaled corticosteroids as ordered following precautions to decrease side effects.
- Teach the client how to deep breathe and cough effectively. Controlled coughing uses the diaphragmatic muscles, making the cough more forceful and effective (Sommers et al, 2015).
- Teach the client/family to identify and avoid specific factors that exacerbate ineffective airway clearance, including known allergens and especially smoking (if relevant) or exposure to secondhand smoke (SHS).
- Educate the client and family about the significance of changes in sputum characteristics, including color, character, amount, and odor. With this knowledge, the client and family can identify early the signs of infection and seek treatment before acute illness occurs.
- Teach the client/family the importance of taking antibiotics as prescribed, consuming all tablets until the prescription has run out. Taking the entire course of antibiotics helps eradicate bacterial infection, which decreases lingering, chronic infection.
- Teach the family of the dying client in hospice with a death rattle that rarely are clients aware of the fluid that has accumulated, and help them find evidence of comfort in the client's nonverbal behavior (Kolb et al, 2018).

REFERENCES

American Association of Critical Care Nurses. (2017). *AACN Practice Alert-Prevention of ventilator-associated pneumonia in adults.* American Association of Critical Care Nurses. Retrieved from https://www.aacn.org/~/media/aacn-website/clinical-resources/practice-alerts/preventingvapinadults2017.pdf.

Anzueto, A., & Miravitlles, M. (2017). Pathophysiology of dyspnea in COPD. *Postgraduate Medicine, 129*(3), 366–374. https://doi.org/10.1080/00325481.2017.1301190.

Balas, M. C., Vasilevskis, E. E., Burke, W. J., et al. (2012). Critical care nurses' role in implementing the "ABCDE Bundle" into practice. *Critical Care Nurse, 32*(2), 40–48, 35–38.

Bickley, L. S., Szilagyi, P., Hoffman, R. M., & Soriano, R. P. (2020). Foundations of health assessment. In *Bate's guide to physical examination* (13th ed.). Philadelphia: Lippincott, Williams and Wilkins.

A

Caparros, A. (2014). Mechanical ventilation and the role of saline instillation in suctioning adult intensive care patients. *Dimensions of Critical Care Nursing, 33*, 246–253.

Case, G. (2021). *Procedure for initiating continuous lateral rotation therapy (CLRT)*. London Health Sciences Center. Retrieved from https://www.lhsc.on.ca/critical-care-trauma-centre/procedure-for-initiating-continuous-lateral-rotation-therapy-clrt.

Chalmers, J. D., Aliberti, S., & Blasi, F. (2015). Management of bronchiectasis in adults. *The European Respiratory Journal, 45*(5), 1446–1462. https://doi.org/10.1183/09031936.00119114.

Devlin, J. W., Skrobik, Y., Gélinas, C., et al. (2018). Clinical practice guidelines for the prevention and management of pain, agitation/sedation, delirium, immobility, and sleep disruption in adult patients in the ICU. *Critical Care Medicine, 46*(9), e825–e873. doi:10.1097/CCM.0000000000003299.

Dirkes, S. M., & Kozlowski, C. (2019). Early mobility in the intensive care unit: evidence, barriers, and future directions. *Critical Care Nurse, 39*(3), 33–42. https://doi.org/10.4037/ccn2019654.

Global Initiative for Chronic Obstructive Lung Disease (GOLD). (2020). *Global strategy for the diagnosis, management, and prevention of COPD (2020 report)*. Global Initiative for Chronic Obstructive Lung Disease. Retrieved from ht tps://goldcopd.org/wp-content/uploads/2019/12/GOLD-2020-FINAL-ver1.2-03Dec19_WMV.pdf.

Gosselink, R., Bott, J., Johnson, M., et al. (2008). Physiotherapy for adult patients with critical illness: Recommendations of the European Respiratory Society and European Society of Critical Care Medicine task force on physiotherapy for critically ill patients. *Intensive Care Medicine, 34*(7), 1188–1199.

Howes, S., Hartmann-Boyce, J., Livingstone–Banks, J., Hong, B., & Lindson, N. (2020). Antidepressants for smoking cessation. *The Cochrane Database of Systematic Reviews, 4*, CD000031. doi:10.1002/14651858.CD000031.pub5.

Kolb, H., Snowden, A., & Stevens, E. (2018). Systematic review and narrative summary: Treatments for and risk factors associated with respiratory tract secretions (death rattle) in the dying adult. *Journal of Advanced Nursing, 74*(7), 1446–1462. https://doi.org/10.1111/jan.13557.

Longhini, F., Bruni, A., Garofalo, E., et al. (2020). Chest physiotherapy improves lung aeration in hypersecretive critically ill patients: A pilot randomized physiological study. *Critical Care, 24*(1), 479. doi:10.1186/s13054-020-03198-6.

McIlwaine, M., Button, B., & Nevitt, S. J. (2019). Positive expiratory pressure physiotherapy for airway clearance in people with cystic fibrosis. *Cochrane Database of Systematic Reviews, 11*, CD003147. doi:10.1002/14651858.CD003147.pub5.

Osadnik, C., McDonald, C., & Holland, A. (2013). Advances in airway clearance technologies for chronic obstructive pulmonary disease. *Expert Review in Respiratory Medicine, 7*(6), 673–685.

Pedersen, C. M., Rosendahl-Nielsen, M., Hjermind, J., et al. (2009). Endotracheal suctioning of the adult intubated patient—what is the evidence? *Intensive and Critical Care Nursing, 25*(1), 21–30.

Perme, C., & Chandrashekar, R. (2009). Early mobility and walking program for patients in intensive care units: Creating a standard of care. *American Journal of Critical Care, 18*(3), 212–220.

Pozuelo-Carrascosa, D. P., Herráiz-Adillo, Á., Alvarez-Bueno, C., Añón, J. M., Martínez-Vizcaíno, V., & Cavero-Redondo, I. (2020). Subglottic secretion drainage for preventing ventilator-associated pneumonia: An overview of systematic reviews and an updated meta-analysis. *European Respiratory Review, 29*(155), 190107. doi:10.1183/16000617.0107-2019.

Sauls, J. L. (2021). Acute respiratory failure. In M. Sole, D. Klein, M. Moseley, et al. (Eds.), *Introduction to critical care nursing* (pp. 375–403). St. Louis: Elsevier. https://doi.org/10.4037/ccn2017627.

Seckel, M. (2017). Suctioning: Endotracheal tube or tracheostomy tube. In D. L. Wiegland (Ed.), *AACN procedure manual for critical care* (7th ed.). Philadelphia: Elsevier.

Siela, D. (2010). Evaluation standards for management of artificial airways. *Critical Care Nurse, 30*(4), 76–78.

Siela, D., & Kidd, M. (2017). Oxygen requirements for acutely and critically ill patients. *Critical Care Nurse, 37*(4), 58–70.

Sommers, J., Engelbert, R. H., Dettling-Ihnenfeldt, D., et al. (2015). Physiotherapy in the intensive care unit: An evidence-based, expert driven, practical statement and rehabilitation recommendations. *Clinical Rehabilitation, 29*(11), 1051–1063. https://doi.org/10.1177/0269215514567156.

St. Clair, J., & MacDermott, J. (2017). Continuous lateral rotation therapy. In D. L. Wiegand (Ed.), *AACN procedure manual for critical care* (7th ed.). Philadelphia: Elsevier.

Tipping, C. J., Harrold, M., Holland, A., et al. (2017). The effects of active mobilisation and rehabilitation in ICU on mortality and function: A systematic review. *Intensive Care Medicine, 43*(2), 171–183. https://doi.org/10.1007/s00134-016-4612-0.

Vollman, K., Sole, M., & Quinn, B. (2017). Endotracheal tube care and oral care practices for ventilated and non-ventilated patients. In D. L. Wiegand (Ed.), *AACN procedure manual for high acuity, progressive, and critical care* (7th ed.). Philadelphia: Elsevier.

Risk for Allergy Reaction Domain 11 Safety/protection Class 5 Defensive processes

Julianne E. Doubet, BSN, RN, EMT-B

NANDA-I

Definition

Susceptible to an exaggerated immune response or reaction to substances, which may compromise health.

Risk Factors

Exposure to allergen; exposure to environmental allergen; exposure to toxic chemicals; inadequate knowledge about avoidance of relevant allergens; inattentive to potential allergen exposure

At-Risk Population

Individuals with history of food allergy; individuals with history of insect sting allergy; individuals with repeated exposure to allergen-producing environmental substance

NOC (Nursing Outcomes Classification)

Suggested NOC Outcomes

Allergic Response: Systemic; Immune Hypersensitivity Response; Knowledge: Health Behavior, Risk Control, Risk Detection; Tissue Integrity: Skin and Mucous Membranes

Example NOC Outcome with Indicators

Immune Hypersensitivity Response as evidenced by the following indicators: Respiratory, cardiac, gastrointestinal, renal and neurological function status IER/Free of allergic reactions. (Rate each indicator of **Immune Hypersensitivity Response:** 1 = not controlled, 2 = slightly controlled, 3 = moderately controlled, 4 = well controlled, 5 = very well controlled [see Section I].)

IER, In expected range.

Client Outcomes

Client Will (Specify Time Frame)

- State risk factors for allergies
- Demonstrate knowledge of plan to treat allergic reaction

NIC (Nursing Interventions Classification)

Suggested NIC Interventions

Allergy Management; Environmental Risk Protection

Example NIC Activity

Place an allergy band on client

Nursing Interventions and *Rationales*

- ● A careful history is important in detecting allergens and avoidance of these allergens. EB: *In a review of the National Institute for Health and Care Excellence (NICE) recommendations, Walsh (2017) agreed that food allergies may be identified by using an "allergy-focused clinical history."*
- ● Obtain a precise history of allergies, as well as medications taken and foods ingested before surgery. EB: *In their study of perioperative anaphylaxis, Meng et al (2017) confirmed that antibiotics and neuromuscular blocking agents are common producers of anaphylaxis.*
- ▲ Teach the client about the correct use of the injectable epinephrine and have the client do a return demonstration. EB: *Research on the correct use of the injectable epinephrine showed that 84% of the clients were unable to do it correctly (Bonds, Asawa, & Ghazi, 2015).*
- ▲ Carefully assess the client for allergies. *Below is information that is important for clients with allergies. Refer for immediate treatment if anaphylaxis is suspected.*

Causes

Common allergens include animal dander; bee stings or stings from other insects; foods, especially nuts, fish, and shellfish; insect bites; medications; plants; pollens

Symptoms

Common symptoms of a mild allergic reaction include hives (especially over the neck and face); itching; nasal congestion; rashes; watery, red eyes

Symptoms of a moderate or severe reaction include cramps or pain in the abdomen; chest discomfort or tightness; diarrhea; difficulty breathing; difficulty swallowing; dizziness or lightheadedness; fear or feeling of apprehension or anxiety; flushing or redness of the face; nausea and vomiting; palpitations; swelling of the face, eyes, or tongue; weakness; wheezing; unconsciousness

First Aid

For a mild to moderate reaction: calm and reassure the person having the reaction because anxiety can worsen symptoms.

1. Try to identify the allergen and have the person avoid further contact with it. If the allergic reaction is from a bee sting, scrape the stinger off the skin with something firm (e.g., fingernail or plastic credit card). Do not use tweezers; squeezing the stinger will release more venom.
2. Apply cool compresses and over-the-counter hydrocortisone cream for itchy rash.
3. Watch for signs of increasing distress.
4. Get medical help. For a mild reaction, a health care provider may recommend over-the-counter medications (e.g., antihistamines).

For a Severe Allergic Reaction (Anaphylaxis)

1. Check the person's airway, breathing, and circulation (the ABCs of Basic Life Support). A warning sign of dangerous throat swelling is a very hoarse or whispered voice or coarse sounds when the person is breathing in air. If necessary, begin rescue breathing and cardiopulmonary resuscitation.
2. Call 911.
3. Calm and reassure the person.
4. If the allergic reaction is from a bee sting, scrape the stinger off the skin with something firm (e.g., fingernail or plastic credit card). Do not use tweezers; squeezing the stinger will release more venom.
5. If the person has emergency allergy medication on hand, help the person take or inject the medication as soon as possible. Avoid oral medication if the person is having difficulty breathing. EB: *Delaying the administration of epinephrine for anaphylaxis may be associated with higher morbidity and mortality (Shaker et al, 2020).*
6. Take steps to prevent shock. Have the person lie flat, raise the person's feet about 12 inches, and cover him or her with a coat or blanket. Do NOT place the person in this position if a head, neck, back, or leg injury is suspected or if it causes discomfort.

Do NOT

- Do NOT assume that any allergy shots the person has already received will provide complete protection.
- Do NOT place a pillow under the person's head if he or she is having trouble breathing. This can block the airways.
- Do NOT give the person anything by mouth if the person is having trouble breathing.

When to Contact a Medical Professional

Call for immediate medical emergency assistance if:

- The person is having a severe allergic reaction—always call 911. Do not wait to see if the reaction is getting worse.
- The person has a history of severe allergic reactions (check for a medical ID tag).

Prevention

- Avoid triggers such as foods and medications that have caused an allergic reaction (even a mild one) in the past. Ask detailed questions about ingredients when you are eating away from home. Carefully examine ingredient labels. EB: *Education concerning allergen vulnerability will help clients to prevent most accidental exposures to known allergic triggers (Mahr & Hernandez-Trujillo, 2017).*
- If you have a child who is allergic to certain foods, introduce one new food at a time in limited amounts so you can recognize an allergic reaction. EB: *There is a decrease in the threat for the evolution of food allergies in clients who are at risk with the early introduction of known allergy-producing foods: abstaining from these types of foods, without a clear history of allergic reactions, may increase the chances of developing an allergy (Schroer, Bjelac, & Leonard, 2017).*
- People who know that they have had serious allergic reactions should wear a medical ID tag. EBN: *Anaphylaxis is a dangerous, unpredictable, and usually rapid hypersensitivity response to an allergen and is generally caused by a known irritant; it is advised, then, that those who have had a severe allergic reaction wear medical alert jewelry (Hunt, 2016).*
- Preoperative clients should be closely assessed for allergies. EB: *According to Kuric et al (2017), general anesthesia may mask the classic, initial signs of allergy, which would be seen in the conscious client.*
- For clients with a history of serious allergic reactions, counsel to carry emergency medications (e.g., a chewable form of diphenhydramine and injectable epinephrine or a bee sting kit) according to their health care provider's instructions. EB: *The initial intervention for anaphylaxis should be epinephrine; medical providers across the board agree that its quick administration is vital to prevent progression of the reaction and improve client outcomes and that epinephrine use will contribute to a decrease in hospitalizations and fatalities (Fromer, 2016).*
- Instruct clients to not give their injectable epinephrine (or any other personal medication) to anyone else as they may have a condition (e.g., a heart problem) that could be negatively affected by this drug. EB:

Those who "borrow" medications may defer primary treatment and delay professional assistance for their illness, plus the borrowed medication could mask serious symptoms of severe disease (Markotic et al, 2017).

- ▲ Refer the client for skin testing to confirm IgE-mediated allergic response. EB: *Stylianou et al (2016) stated that allergen-specific immunotherapy (SIT) is thought to be the most effective remedy for immunoglobulin E (IgE)–mediated allergies.*
- ● Provide all clients with a history of anaphylaxis with education about anaphylaxis, risk of recurrence, trigger avoidance, self-injectable epinephrine, and thresholds for further care. EB: *Evidence related to client education for anaphylaxis is associated with optimal outcomes (Shaker et al, 2020).*
- ▲ Refer all clients with a history of anaphylaxis to an allergist for follow-up evaluation. EB: *Evidence related to allergist referral for anaphylaxis is associated with optimal outcomes (Shaker et al, 2020).*
- ● See care plan for Risk for **Latex Allergy** Reaction.

Pediatric

- ● Teach parents and children with allergies to peanuts and tree nuts to avoid them and to identify them. EBN: *Nut allergies can have an undesirable impact on both the individual and their family; the key responsibilities of the nurse is ongoing support of those affected and aiding in creating a management plan to control allergen response (Proudfoot & Saul, 2016).*
- ● Teach parents and children with asthma about modifiable risk factors, which include allergy triggers. EBN: *Proudfoot & Saul (2016) recommended that those who care for asthmatic children have a "Risk Assessment Management Plan" that includes avoidance of the allergen (e.g., nuts), rescue medication, diabetic referral as needed, and continued support for both child and family.*
- ● Counsel parents to limit infant exposure to traffic and cigarette carbon monoxide pollution. EBN: *Children exposed to secondhand smoke (SHS) have an elevated rate of respiratory infections, ear infections, SHS-triggered asthma attacks, and sudden infant death syndrome (Kleier, Mites-Campbell, & Henson-Evertz, 2017).*
- ▲ Refer clients for food protein–induced enterocolitis syndrome (FPIES) in formula-fed infants with repetitive emesis, diarrhea, dehydration, and lethargy 1 to 5 hours after ingesting the offending food (the most common are cow's milk, soy, and rice). Remove the offending food. EB: *If FPIES becomes chronic, it may lead to an infant's failure to thrive (Nowak-Wegrzyn et al, 2015).*
- ▲ Children should be screened for seafood allergies and if an allergy is detected, avoid seafood and any foods containing seafood. EB: *According to a study by Presler (2016), fish and shellfish are powerful allergens that cause grave IgE antibody–mediated untoward reactions in those who are sensitive.*

REFERENCES

Bonds, R. S., Asawa, A., & Ghazi, A. I. (2015). Misuse of medical devices: A persistent problem in self-management of asthma and allergic disease. *Annals of Allergy, Asthma and Immunology, 114*(1), 74–76.e2. https://doi.org/10.1016/j.anai.2014.10.016.

Fromer, L. (2016). Prevention of anaphylaxis: The role of epinephrine auto injectors. *Journal of Medicine, 129*(12), 1244–1250. https//doi.org/10.1016/j.amjmed.2016.07.018.

Hunt, K. (2016). Anaphylaxis. *Practice Nurse, 46*(12), 13–18.

Kleier, J., Mites-Campbell, M., & Henson-Evertz, K. (2017). Children's exposure secondhand smoke and parental nicotine dependence and motivation to quit smoking. *Pediatric Nursing, 43*(1), 35–39. PMID:29406665.

Kuric, V., ZaZa, K., & Algazian, S. (2017). Atypical presentation to rocuronium allergy in a 19-year-old patient. *Journal of Clinical Anesthesia, 37*, 163–165. https://doi.org/10.1016/j.jclinane.2016.11.007.

Mahr, T., & Hernandez-Trujillo, V. (2017). First-ever action plan for epinephrine and anaphylaxis. *Contemporary Pediatrics, 34*(8), 16–42.

Markotic, F., Vrdoljak, D., Puljiz, M., & Puljak, L. (2017). Risk perception about medication sharing among patients: A focus group qualitative study on borrowing and lending of prescription analgesics. *Journal of Pain Research, 10*, 365–374. doi:10.2147/JPR.5123554.

Meng, J., Rotiroti, G., Burdett, E., et al. (2017). Anaphylaxis during general anesthesia: Experiences from a drug allergy centre in the UK. *ACTA Anaesthesiologica Scandinavica, 61*(3), 281–289. https://doi.org/10.1111/aas.12858.

Nowak-Wegrzyn, A., Yitzhak, K., Mehr, S., et al. (2015). Non-IgE-mediated gastrointestinal food allergy. *Journal of Allergy and Clinical Immunology, 135*(5), 1114–1124. https://doi.org/10.1016/j.jaci.2015.03.025.

Presler, L. (2016). Seafood allergy, toxicity and occupational health, Zagreb, Croatia. *Journal of American College of Nutrition, 35*(3), 271–283. https://doi.org/10.1080/07315724.2015.1014120.

Proudfoot, C., & Saul, P. (2016). Nut allergy in children: A growing concern. *Practice Nurse, 46*(12), 30–36.

Schroer, B., Bjelac, J., & Leonard, M. (2017). What is new in managing patients with food allergy? Almost everything. *Current Opinion in Pediatrics, 29*(5), 578–583. https://doi.org/10.1097/mop.0000000000000534.

Shaker, M. S., Wallace, D. V., Golden, D. B. K., et al. (2020). Anaphylaxis—a 2020 practice parameter update, systematic review, and Grading of Recommendations, Assessment, Development and Evaluation (GRADE) analysis. *Journal of Allergy and Clinical Immunology, 145*(4), 1082–1123. https://doi.org/10.1016/j.jaci.2020.01.017.

Stylianou, E., Ueland, T., Borchsenius, F., et al. (2016). Specific allergen immunotherapy: Effects on IgE, IgG4 and chemokines in patients with allergic rhinitis. *Scandinavian Journal of Clinical & Laboratory Investigations, 76*(2), 118–127. https://doi.org/10.3109/00365513.2015.1110856.

Walsh, J. (2017). NICE food allergy and anaphylaxis quality standards: A review of the 2016 quality standards. *British Journal of General Practice, 67*(656), 138–139. https://doi.org/10.3399/bjgp17x689833.

A

Anxiety Domain 9 Coping/stress tolerance Class 2 Coping responses

Lorraine Chiappetta, MSN, RN, CNE

NANDA-I

Definition

An emotional response to a diffuse threat in which the individual anticipates nonspecific impending danger, catastrophe, or misfortune.

Defining Characteristics

Behavioral/Emotional

Crying; decrease in productivity; expresses anguish; expresses anxiety about life event changes; expresses distress; expresses insecurity; expresses intense dread; helplessness; hypervigilance; increased wariness; insomnia; irritable mood; nervousness; psychomotor agitation; reduced eye contact; scanning behavior; self-focused

Physiological Factors

Altered respiratory pattern; anorexia; brisk reflexes; chest tightness; cold extremities; diarrhea; dry mouth; expresses abdominal pain; expresses feeling faint; expresses muscle weakness; expresses tension; facial flushing; increased blood pressure; increased heart rate; increased sweating; nausea; pupil dilation; quivering voice; reports altered sleep-wake cycle; reports heart palpitations; reports tingling in extremities; superficial vasoconstriction; tremors; urinary frequency; urinary hesitancy

Cognitive Factors

Altered attention; confusion; decreased perceptual field; expresses forgetfulness; expresses preoccupation; reports blocking of thoughts; rumination

Related Factors

Conflict about life goals; interpersonal transmission; pain; stressors; substance misuse; unfamiliar situation; unmet needs; value conflict

At-Risk Population

Individuals experiencing developmental crisis; individuals experiencing situational crisis; individuals exposed to toxins; individuals in the perioperative period; individuals with family history of anxiety; individuals with hereditary predisposition

Associated Conditions

Mental disorders

NOC (Nursing Outcomes Classification)

Suggested NOC Outcomes

Anxiety Level; Anxiety Self-Control; Coping; Impulse Self-Control Fear Level; Fear Self-Control; Mood Equilibrium

Example NOC Outcome with Indicators

Anxiety Self-Control as evidenced by the following indicators: Eliminates precursors of anxiety/Monitors physical manifestations of anxiety/Controls anxiety response. (Rate the outcome and indicators of **Anxiety Self-Control:** 1 = never demonstrated, 2 = rarely demonstrated, 3 = sometimes demonstrated, 4 = often demonstrated, 5 = consistently demonstrated [see Section I].)

A

Client Outcomes

Client Will (Specify Time Frame)

- Identify and verbalize symptoms of anxiety
- Identify, verbalize, and demonstrate techniques to manage anxiety
- Verbalize absence of or decrease in subjective distress
- Have vital signs that reflect baseline or decreased sympathetic stimulation
- Have posture, facial expressions, gestures, and activity levels that reflect decreased distress or a more tolerable level of anxiety
- Demonstrate improved concentration and accuracy of thoughts
- Demonstrate return of basic problem-solving skills
- Demonstrate increased external focus
- Demonstrate some ability to reassure self

NIC (Nursing Interventions Classification)

Suggested NIC Interventions

Anxiety Reduction; Calming Technique; Coping Enhancement; Impulse Control Training; Relaxation Therapy

Example NIC Activities—Anxiety Reduction

Use calm, reassuring approach; Explain all procedures, including sensations likely to be experienced during the procedure

Nursing Interventions and *Rationales*

- ● Assess the client's level of anxiety by noticing the physiologic, emotional, cognitive, and behavioral symptoms associated with the feeling state of anxiety. EBN: *Understanding the different levels of anxiety determines the most effective interventions. Assessing anxiety level on admission may help nurses develop plans of care that improve the client experience (Baldwin & Spears, 2019).*
- ● Introduce yourself and your role, explain what you will be doing and why, and explain usual hospital procedures. EBN: *Nurses can attempt to reduce any anxiety that clients experience by explaining the planned medical intervention and providing accurate information at the optimum time (Price, 2017).*
- ● Intervene when possible to remove sources of anxiety. EBN: *Aiding in the reduction of anxiety is an essential nursing intervention in client care state (Elham et al, 2015).*
- ● Explain all activities, procedures, and issues that involve the client; use nonmedical terms and calm, slow speech; and then validate the client's understanding. EBN: *In a study of the needs of anxious and/or depressed clients, Kim (2016) found that nursing care must include person-centered undertakings to form a bond between client and nurse, therefore reassuring and empowering these clients.*
- ▲ Use massage therapy to reduce anxiety. EBN: The use of massage therapy has been shown to markedly reduce psychological stress and anxiety (Kim et al, 2016).
- ▲ Consider massage therapy for preoperative clients. EBN: Complementary therapies, including massage, have been shown to aid client relaxation before surgery (Hansen, 2015).
- ● Use guided imagery to decrease anxiety. EBN: *Guided imagery can be used to aid clients in handling undesirable emotions connected with the symptoms of their illness* (Nooner et al, 2016).
- ● Suggest yoga to the client. EBN: *In a study by Centrella-Negro (2017), it was noted that the practice of yoga was beneficial to the welfare and comfort of cardiac clients.*
- ● Provide clients with a means to listen to music of their choice or audiotapes. EBN: *According to Quach (2017), nurses and other providers should recognize the value of music therapies and use them in client care when appropriate.*
- ▲ Refer to cognitive behavioral therapy (CBT). EB: *A systematic review found that Internet-delivered CBT was a cost-effective treatment for anxiety when compared with control treatments (Ophuis et al, 2017).*

Pediatric

- ● The previously mentioned interventions may be adapted for the pediatric client.

Geriatric

▲ Monitor the client for depression. Use appropriate interventions and referrals. EBN/EB: *Gould et al (2016) stated that "Anxiety disorders are common and debilitating in older individuals" and further noted that simple tests used to recognize anxiety symptoms in the older client are beneficial because they can begin discussions about current treatments.*

- Limit the use of benzodiazepines and nonbenzodiazepine agents for anxiety in the older adult. If these drugs must be used, give the lowest dose possible for short-term use only. EB: *Use of these medications increases the risk of development of delirium and increases fall risk in the elderly population (Subramanyam et al, 2018).*

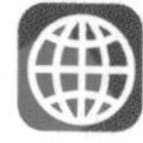

Multicultural

- Identify how anxiety is manifested in the culturally diverse client. EB: *People of non-Western ethnocultural origins many times have diverse ideas and contrasting perceptions of mental health and illness as opposed to those from Western societies (Neftçi & Barnow, 2016).*

▲ Refer to culturally adapted CBT. EB: *A systematic review found that CBT was an effective anxiety treatment for Latinos and that cultural adaptations addressed some treatment barriers (Casas, Benuto, & González, 2020).*

Home Care

- The previously mentioned interventions may be adapted for home care use.
- Encourage effective communication between family members. EB: *Family can be a key site of support for individuals who are diagnosed with a health issue, as long as the health condition is known within the family unit (Hays, Maliski, & Warner, 2017).*
- Assist family in being supportive of the client in the face of anxiety symptoms. EBN: *Vieira et al (2015) surmised in a study that both client and caregiver/family must realize and accept that medical conditions will bring a change of lifestyle for each and they should adapt as best they can.*

▲ Consider referral for the prescription of antianxiety or antidepressant medications for clients who have panic disorder or other anxiety-related psychiatric disorders. EBN: *Pharmacotherapy is an effective intervention for anxiety disorders because it decreases symptoms and enhances a sense of well-being for the client (da Cruz et al, 2016).*

▲ Assist the client/family to institute the medication regimen appropriately. Instruct in side effects and the importance of taking medications as ordered. EBN: *Instruct the client and/or caregivers concerning possible drug side effects and interactions that could have detrimental results (e.g., sleepiness, nausea) on the client and be certain the client/caregiver understands how the medication is to be given (Creed, 2017).*

Client/Family Teaching and Discharge Planning

- Provide basic teaching information about anxiety and anxiety disorders that includes signs and symptoms, risk factors, treatments, and therapies. EB: *The results of this study indicate that higher stress perception scores are significantly correlated with the need for more client and caregiver education on health-related issues (Abuatiq et al, 2020).*
- Provide client education about medications that includes side effects, ways to manage side effects, special administration issues (e.g., take with food, take at night), including which medications to avoid using concurrently. Education should also include a list of adverse effects that should be reported to the health care practitioner. EBN: *For safe and effective therapy, clients need to understand their medications, especially at discharge (Talbot, 2018).*

▲ Teach use of appropriate community resources in emergency situations (e.g., suicidal thoughts), such as hotlines, emergency departments, law enforcement, and judicial systems. EB: *Boudreaux et al (2016) suggested that community mental health services, delivered in conjunction with community emergency departments, may improve client commitment to aftercare and, as a result, reduce future behavioral health crises as well as decrease return visits to the emergency department.*

- Teach the client to visualize or fantasize about the absence of anxiety or pain, successful experience of the situation, resolution of conflict, or outcome of procedure. EB: *Guided imagery has been shown to augment comfort and can be used as a psychosupportive intervention (Satija & Bhatnagar, 2017).*
- Teach the relationship between a healthy physical and emotional lifestyle and a realistic mental attitude. EBN: *Jiwani (2016) stated that "anxiety leads to physiological and psychological changes in the human body" and can be controlled with various learned self-help techniques.*

A

REFERENCES

Abuatiq, A., Brown, R., Wolles, B., & Randall, R. (2020). Perceptions of stress. *Clinical Journal of Oncology Nursing*, *5*(24), 51–57. https://doi.org/10.1188/20.CJON.51-57.

Baldwin, K. M., & Spears, M. J. (2019). Improving the patient experience and decreasing patient anxiety with nursing bedside report. *Clinical Nurse Specialist CNS*, *33*(2), 82–89. https://doi.org/10.1097/NUR.0000000000000428.

Boudreaux, J., Crapanzano, K., Jones, G., et al. (2016). Using mental health outreach teams in the emergency department to improve engagement in treatment. *Community Mental Health Journal*, *52*(18), 1009–1014. https://doi.org/10.1007/s10597-015-9935-8.

Casas, J. B., Benuto, L. T., & González, F. (2020). Latinos, anxiety, and cognitive behavioral therapy: A systematic review. *International Journal of Psychology & Psychological Therapy*, *20*(1), 91–104.

Centrella-Negro, A. (2017). Evaluating the edition of hatha yoga in cardiac rehabilitation. *Medsurg Nursing*, *26*(1), 39–43.

Creed, S. (2017). Avoiding medication errors in general practice. *Practice Nurse*, *47*(2), 24–26.

da Cruz, A., Giacchero, K., do Carmo, M., et al. (2016). Difficulties related to medication therapies for anxiety disorder. *Revista Eletronica de Enfermagem*, *18*, 1–10. http://dx.doi.org/10.5216/rec.v18.32741.

Elham, H., Hazrat, M., Mommennasab, M., et al. (2015). The effect of need-based spiritual/religious intervention on spiritual well-being and anxiety of elderly. *Holistic Nursing Practice*, *29*(3), 136–143. https://doi.org/10.1097/HNP.0000000000000083.

Gould, C., Beaudreau, S., Gullickson, G., et al. (2016). Implementation of brief anxiety assessment and evaluation in a Department of Veterans Affairs geriatric pulmonary clinic. *Journal of Rehabilitation Research Development*, *53*(3), 335–344. https://doi.org/10.1682/JRRD.2014.10.0258.

Hansen, M. (2015). A feasibility pilot study on the use of complimentary therapies delivered via mobile technologies on Icelandic surgical patients reports of anxiety, pain and self-efficacy in healing. *BMC Complementary Alternative Medicine*, *15*(1), 11–12. https://doi.org/10.1186/s12906-015-0613-8.

Hays, A., Maliski, R., & Warner, B. (2017). Analyzing the effects of family communication patterns on the decision to disclose a health issue to a parent: The benefits of conversation and dangers of conformity. *Health Communication*, *32*(7), 837–844. https://doi.org/10.1080/10410236.2016.1177898.

Jiwani, K. (2016). Handling challenging emotions in nursing care. *Journal of Nursing*, *6*(2), 13–15. https://doi.org/10.26634/jnur.6.2.6042.

Kim, D., Lee, D., Schreiber, J., et al. (2016). Integrative evaluation of automatic massage combined with thermotherapy: Physical, physiological and psychological viewpoints. *BioMed Research International*, *2016*, 1–8. https://doi.org/10.1155/2016/2826905.

Kim, J. (2016). Phase II cardiac rehabilitation participants' perception of nurse caring correlated with participants' depression, anxiety, and adherence. *International Journal for Human Caring*, *20*(4), 213–219. https://doi.org/10.20467/1091-5710-20.4.213.

Neftçi, N. B., & Barnow, S. (2016). One size does not fit all in psychotherapy: Understanding depression among patients of Turkish behavior origin in Europe. *Archives of Neuropsychiatry*, *53*(1), 72–79.

Nooner, A., Dwyer, K., DeShea, L., et al. (2016). Using relaxation and guided imagery to address pain, fatigue, and sleep disturbances: A pilot study. *Clinical Journal of Oncology Nursing*, *20*(5), 547–552. https://doi.org/10.1188/16.CJON.547-552.

Ophuis, R. H., Lokkerbol, J., Heemskerk, S. C. M., et al. (2017). Cost-effectiveness of interventions for treating anxiety disorders: A systematic review. *Journal of Affective Disorders*, *210*(1), 1–13. https://doi.org/10.1016/j.jad.2016.12.005.

Price, B. (2017). Managing patients' anxiety about planned medical interventions. *Nursing Standard*, *31*(47), 53–63. https://doi.org/10.7748/ns.2017.e10544.

Quach, J. (2017). Do music therapies reduce depressive symptoms and improve QOL in older adults with chronic disease? *Nursing*, *47*(6), 58–63. https://doi.org/10.1097/01.NURSE.0000513604.41152.0c.

Satija, A., & Bhatnagar, S. (2017). Complimentary therapies for symptom management in cancer patients. *Indian Journal of Palliative Care*, *23*(4), 468–479. https://doi.org/10.4103/IJPC.IJPC_100_17.

Subramanyam, A. A., Kedare, J., Singh, O. P., & Pinto, C. (2018). Clinical practice guidelines for geriatric anxiety disorders. *Indian Journal of Psychiatry*, *60*(Suppl. 3), S371–S382. https://doi.org/10.4103/0019-5545.224476.

Talbot, B. (2018). Improving patient medication education. *Nursing*, *48*(5), 58–60. https://doi.org/10.1097/01.NURSE.0000531909.68714.85.

Vieira, G., Cavalcanti, A., da Silva, S., et al. (2015). Quality of life of caregivers to patients with heart failure: Integrative review. *Journal of Nursing UFPE*, *9*(2), 750–758. https://doi.org/10.5205/reuol.7028-60723-1-SM.0902201533.

Death Anxiety Domain 9 Coping/stress tolerance Class 2 Coping responses

Lorraine Chiappetta, MSN, RN, CNE

NANDA-I

Definition

Emotional distress and insecurity, generated by anticipation of death and the process of dying of oneself or significant others, which negatively effects one's quality of life.

Defining Characteristics

Dysphoria; expresses concern about caregiver strain; expresses concern about the impact of one's death on significant other; expresses deep sadness; expresses fear of developing terminal illness; expresses fear of loneliness; expresses fear of loss of mental abilities when dying; expresses fear of pain related to dying; expresses fear of premature death; expresses fear of prolonged dying process; expresses fear of separation from loved ones; expresses fear of suffering related to dying; expresses fear of the dying process; expresses fear of the unknown; expresses powerlessness; reports negative thoughts related to death and dying

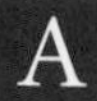

Related Factors

Anticipation of adverse consequences of anesthesia; anticipation of impact of death on others; anticipation of pain; anticipation of suffering; awareness of imminent death; depressive symptoms; discussions on the topic of death; impaired religiosity; loneliness; low self-esteem; nonacceptance of own mortality; spiritual distress; uncertainty about encountering a higher power; uncertainty about life after death; uncertainty about the existence of a higher power; uncertainty of prognosis; unpleasant physical symptoms

At-Risk Population

Individuals experiencing terminal care of significant others; individuals receiving terminal care; individuals with history of adverse experiences with death of significant others; individuals with history of near-death experience; older adults; women; young adults

Associated Conditions

Depression; stigmatized illnesses with high fear of death; terminal illness

NOC (Nursing Outcomes Classification)

Suggested NOC Outcomes

Acceptance: Health Status; Anxiety Self-Control; Comfort Status: Psychospiritual; Comfortable Death; Coping; Dignified Life Closure; Family Coping; Fear Self-Control; Grief Resolution; Health Beliefs: Perceived Threat: Hope; Personal Resiliency; Psychosocial Adjustment; Life Change; Quality of Life

Example NOC Outcome with Indicators

Dignified Life Closure as evidenced by the following indicators: Expresses readiness for death/Resolves important issues/Shares feelings about dying/Discusses spiritual concerns. (Rate the outcome and indicators of **Dignified Life Closure:** 1 = never demonstrated, 2 = rarely demonstrated, 3 = sometimes demonstrated, 4 = often demonstrated, 5 = consistently demonstrated [see Section I].)

Client Outcomes

Client Will (Specify Time Frame)

- Express feelings associated with death and the process of dying
- State concerns about impact of death on others
- Seek help in dealing with feelings
- Discuss realistic goals
- State concerns about the impact of death on significant others
- Use strategies to lessen anxiety surrounding death and dying including spiritual intelligence and finding meaning in one's life
- Use spiritual support for comfort

NIC (Nursing Interventions Classification)

Suggested NIC Interventions

Active Listening; Animal Assisted Therapy; Anticipatory Guidance; Anxiety Reduction; Aromatherapy; Coping Enhancement; Dying Care; Emotional Support; Grief Work Facilitation; Journaling; Respite Care; Spiritual Support; Support System Enhancement

Example NIC Activities—Dying Care

Communicate willingness to discuss death; Support client and family through stages of grief

Nursing Interventions and *Rationales*

- Complete a comprehensive nursing assessment on individuals with life-limiting illnesses. EB: The National Consensus Project Clinical Practice Guidelines for Quality Palliative Care includes the following content domains of palliative care assessment and interventions: Structures and processes of care; physical aspects of care; psychological and psychiatric aspects of care; social aspects of care; spiritual, religious, and existential aspects of care; cultural aspects of care; care of the imminently dying client; ethical and legal aspects of care (*Ahluwalia et al, 2018*). EB: A thorough assessment paves the way to the most effective treatments of death anxiety, tailored to the individual's unique needs (*Menzies & Menzies, 2020*).

- Assess family and caregivers' responses to death and dying, looking for symptoms of death anxiety. EB: *Despite a high prevalence of death anxiety among family caregivers, it is frequently undiagnosed and can lead to denial of the client's death, a worse quality of life, greater risk of depression, and caregiver overwork (Abreu-Figueiredo et al, 2019).*
- Assess for the development of new maladaptive coping in response to the powerful sense of fear or meaninglessness that is associated with awareness of death. EB: *Awareness of death may also produce a powerful sense of fear or meaninglessness and may drive a number of maladaptive coping behaviors (Menzies & Menzies, 2020).*
- Develop a trusting therapeutic relationship with the client and family. EB: *A trusting relationship is important for the delivery of client-focused care and the development of trust is an essential component of that relationship (Polansky, 2019).*
- Continue to remain available and to use empathetic communication skills so that the client and family will continue to feel comfortable discussing ongoing concerns. EB: *In a study in which caregivers were interviewed, participation in the study was viewed as a positive experience because it gave participants the opportunity to express certain fears and concerns and because they felt that they were understood (Abreu-Figueiredo et al, 2019).*
- Assess clients for pain and provide pain relief measures. EB: *Pain can be a significant problem that has important ramifications on clients' quality of life and the management of pain can be obstructed by poor client–provider communication (Johnsen et al, 2016).*
- Assess client for fears related to death. EB: *In their study of chronic obstructive pulmonary disease (COPD) clients with end-of-life issues, Stenzel et al (2015) found that client care should not be limited to managing just the physical manifestation of the disease but also the need to address psychological anxiety and disease-specific concerns.*
- Use psychosocial techniques to decrease distress. EB: *Meta-analysis showed life review and meaning-based techniques/interventions such as dignity therapy (a therapy that gives clients the opportunity to speak about their life accomplishments and roles), mindfulness, and creative arts–based therapy to be effective in improving quality of life and in reducing emotional distress and existential suffering in clients receiving palliative care (Warth et al, 2019).*
- Assist clients with life planning: consider and redefine main life goals, focus on areas of strength and/or goals that will provide satisfaction, adopt realistic goals, and recognize those that are impossible to achieve. EBN: *Nurses have an obligation to communicate with those under their care, which should include the discussion of life preferences and relating pertinent, personal information (Coyle et al, 2015).*
- Assist clients with life review and reminiscence. EBN: *Chen et al (2017) found in their studies of life review, for those suffering life-threatening illnesses, that this practice aided in diminishing depression and augmenting self-esteem.*
- Provide music of the client's choosing. EB: *There is convincing evidence that music effectively assists those facing end-of-life concerns (Clement-Cortis, 2016).*
- Provide social support for families: understanding what is most important to families who are caring for clients at the end of life. EBN: *Nurses, who deal not only with technical and resuscitative aspects of critical client care, are now developing their expertise to include "advocating for, communicating with, teaching, and guiding clients and families through end-of-life issues" (Banjar, 2017).*
- Encourage clients to use spiritual supports. EBN: *The Society of Critical Care Medicine recommends that the spiritual needs of clients facing a critical end-of-life illness should be recognized and managed by the health care team (Fournier, 2017).*
- Explore ways to provide spiritual support by asking clients what is important to them and what you can do to help and refer as needed. EB: *Specific interventions, such as spiritual support and logotherapy (finding meaning in life), can reduce death anxiety (Abreu-Figueiredo et al, 2019).*
- As a nurse, be aware of your own increased risk of experiencing symptoms of death anxiety and the negative impact this may have on your well-being. Seek support as needed. EB: *Death anxiety is commonly experienced (by nurses) and is associated with more negative consequences for self and clients (Sharif Nia et al, 2016).*

Geriatric

- Carefully assess older adults for issues regarding death anxiety. EB: *This study by Bonnewyn et al (2016) proposed that the way older adults perceive dying, in part, affects whether they have a desire to die: it could be advantageous to explore the subject of death with your client.*
- Assess the individual's resolution of Erikson's developmental stage of integrity versus despair. In this stage those age 65 and older reflect on their life and either move into feeling satisfied and happy with one's life or feel a deep sense of regret. EB: *Successful resolution of integrity versus despair developmental crisis in old age is associated with decreased death anxiety (Taghiabadi et al, 2017).*
- Teach components of spiritual intelligence (the adaptive use of spiritual information to facilitate everyday problem solving and goal attainment). EB: *Learning the components of spiritual intelligence reduces the extent of death anxiety in the elderly (Majidi & Moradi, 2018).*
- Use strategies to strengthen the individual's spiritual health and support use of religion as a coping strategy when applicable. EB: *There is a positive relationship between spiritual health, religious coping, and reduced death anxiety in the elderly (Solaimanizadeh et al, 2020).*
- Refer to care plan for Maladaptive **Grieving.**

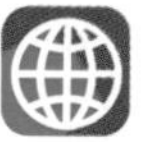

Multicultural

- Assist clients to identify with their culture and its values. EBN: *Cultures stand apart in their approach to how death is framed, viewed, and accepted (MacCloud et al, 2016).*
- Refer to care plans for **Anxiety** and Maladaptive **Grieving.**

Home Care

- The previously mentioned interventions may be adapted for home care.
- ▲ Support and facilitate a discussion of advance care plans/advanced directives as another strategy to lessen verbalized fears and concerns about death and the dying process. Document decisions. EB: *Residents with end-of-life care instructions in place were three times less likely to experience fear and anxiety in their last days than those who did not (Carr & Luth, 2017).*
- ▲ Make referrals to mental health professionals for CBT or logotherapy. EB: *Logotherapy is an existential psychotherapy that can help a person find meaning in life (Abreu-Figueiredo et al, 2019).* EB: *Meta-analysis revealed that psychosocial interventions produced significant reductions in death anxiety relative to control conditions (Menzies & Menzies, 2020).*
- ▲ Refer to appropriate medical services, social services, and/or mental health services, as needed. EBN: *The union between physical health and mental health needs requires added awareness and acknowledgment in the contemporary nursing care of palliative clients (Hayes, 2017).*
- ▲ Identify the client's preferences for end-of-life care; aid in honoring preferences as much as practicable. EBN: *To engage in person-centered care at end of life requires the entire health care team to enlist clients and families in communication and decision-making, especially about the clients' preferences and decisions concerning the use of life-extending technologies (Nouvet et al, 2016).*
- Refer to care plan for **Powerlessness.**

Client/Family Teaching and Discharge Planning

- Give information and reassurance to clients and families that distressing symptoms can often be anticipated and prevented and, when present, can be treated by health care professionals. EB: *A significant factor in the development of death anxiety was identified as fear of loneliness and abandonment (Abreu-Figueiredo et al, 2019).*
- Keep client and families informed about current health status and what to expect in the future. EB: *The findings of this study showed that the use of a health literacy might decrease levels of death anxiety in breast cancer clients (Bahrami & Behbahani, 2019).*
- Promote more effective communication to family members engaged in the caregiving role. EB: *Nurses can support family caregivers by fostering client–caregiver teamwork, family communication, and self-care; providing information; and referring to appropriate resources (Wittenberg et al, 2017).*

REFERENCES

Abreu-Figueiredo, R. M. S., de Sá, L. O., Lourenço, T. M. G., & de Almeida, S. S. B. P. (2019). Death anxiety in palliative care: Validation of the nursing diagnosis. *Acta Paulista de Enfermagem*, *32*(2), 178–185. https://doi.org/10.1590/1982-0194201900025.

Ahluwalia, S. C., Chen, C., Raaen, L., et al. (2018). A systematic review in support of the National Consensus Project Clinical Practice Guidelines for Quality Palliative Care, fourth edition. *Journal of Pain and Symptom Management*, *56*(6), 831–870. https://doi.org/10.1016/j.jpainsymman.2018.09.008.

Bahrami, M., & Behbahani, M. A. (2019). The effect of a health literacy promotion program on the level of health literacy and death anxiety in women with breast cancer. *Iranian Journal of Nursing and Midwifery Research*, *24*(4), 286–290. https://doi.org/10.4103/ijnmr.IJNMR_178_18.

Banjar, A. (2017). Till death do us part: The evolution of end-of-life and death attitudes. *Canadian Journal of Critical Care*, *28*(3), 34–40.

Bonnewyn, A., Shah, A., Bruffaerts, R., & Demyttenaere, K. (2016). Are religiousness and death attitudes associated with the wish to die in older people? *International Psychogeriatrics*, *28*(3), 397–404. https://doi.org/10.1017/S1041610215001192.

Carr, D., & Luth, E. A. (2017). Advance care planning: contemporary issues and future directions. *Innovation in Aging*, *1*(1), igx012. https://doi.org/10.1093/geroni/igx012.

Chen, Y., Xiao, H., Yang, Y., & Lan, X. (2017). The effects of life review on psycho-spiritual well-being among patients with life-threatening illness: A systematic review and meta-analysis. *Journal of Advanced Nursing*, *73*(7), 1539–1554. https://doi.org/10.1111/jan.13208.

Clement-Cortis, A. (2016). Development and efficacy of music therapy techniques with palliative care. *Complimentary Therapies in Clinical Practice*, *23*, 125–129. https://doi.org/10.1016/j.ctcp.2015.04.004.

Coyle, N., Manna, R., Shen, M., et al. (2015). Discussing death, dying and end-of-life care: A communications skills training module for oncology nurses. *Clinical Journal of Oncology Nursing*, *19*(6), 697–702. https://doi.org/10.1188/15.CJON.697-702.

Fournier, A. (2017). Creating a sacred place in the intensive care unit at the end-of-life. *Dimensions of Critical Care Nursing*, *36*(2), 110–115. https://doi.org/10.1097/DCC.0000000000000231.

Hayes, J. (2017). Specialist palliative care nurses' management of the needs of patients with depression. *International Journal of Palliative Medicine*, *23*(6), 298–305. https://doi.org/10.12968/ijpn.2017.23.6.298.

Johnsen, A. T., Petersen, M. A., Snyder, C. F., Pederson, L., & Groenvold, M. (2016). How does pain experience relate to the need for pain relief? A secondary exploratory analysis in a larger sample of cancer patients. *Supportive Care in Cancer*, *24*(10), 4187–4195. https://doi.org/10.1007/s00520-016-3246-7.

MacCloud, R., Crandall, J., Wilson, D., & Austin, P. (2016). Death anxiety among New Zealanders: The predictive role of gender and marital status. *Mental Health, Religion & Culture*, *19*(4), 339–349. https://doi.org/10.1080/13674676.2016.1187590.

Majidi, A., & Moradi, O. (2018). Effect of teaching the components of spiritual intelligence on death anxiety in the elderly. *Salmand: Iranian Journal of Ageing*, *13*(1), 110–123. https://doi.org/10.21859/sija.13.1.110.

Menzies, R. E., & Menzies, R. G. (2020). Death anxiety in the time of COVID-19: theoretical explanations and clinical implications. *Cognitive Behaviour Therapist*, *13*, e19. https://doi.org/10.1017/S1754470X20000215.

Nouvet, E., Strachan, P., Kryworuchko, J., & Downar, J. (2016). Waiting for the body to fail: Limits to end-of-life communication in Canadian hospitals. *Mortality*, *21*(4), 340–346. https://doi.org/10.1080/13576275.2016.1140133.

Polansky, M. (2019). Building trust in home healthcare. *Nursing2020*, *49*(10), 16–17. https://doi.org/10.1097/01.NURSE.0000580700.09898.05.

Sharif Nia, H., Lehto, R. H., Ebadi, A., & Peyrovi, H. (2016). Death anxiety among nurses and health care professionals: A review article. *International Journal of Community Based Nursing and Midwifery*, *4*, 2–10. PMID:26793726.

Solaimanizadeh, F., Mohammadinia, N., & Solaimanizadeh, L. (2020). The relationship between spiritual health and religious coping with death anxiety in the elderly. *Journal of Religious Health*, *59*, 1925–1932. https://doi.org/10.1007/s10943-019-00906-7.

Stenzel, N. M., Vaske, I., Kühl, K., Kenn, K., & Rief, W. (2015). Prediction of end-of-life fears in COPD—Hoping for the best but preparing for the worst. *Psychology & Health*, *30*(9), 1017–1034. https://doi.org/10.1080/08870446.2015.1014816.

Taghiabadi, M., Kavosi, A., Mirhafez, S. R., Keshvari, M., & Mehrabi, T. (2017). The association between death anxiety with spiritual experiences and life satisfaction in elderly people. *Electronic Physician*, *9*(3), 3980–3985. https://doi.org/10.19082/3980.

Warth, M., Kessler, J., Koehler, F., Aguilar-Raab, C., Bardenheuer, H. J., & Ditzen, B. (2019). Brief psychosocial interventions improve quality of life of patients receiving palliative care: A systematic review and meta-analysis. *Palliative Medicine*, *33*(3), 332–345. https://doi.org/10.1177/0269216318818011.

Wittenberg, E., Buller, H., Ferrell, B., Koczywas, M., & Borneman, T. (2017). Understanding family caregiver communication to provide family-centered cancer care. *Seminars in Oncology Nursing*, *33*(5), 507–516. https://doi.org/10.1016/j.soncn.2017.09.001.

Risk for Aspiration

Domain 11 Safety/protection Class 2 Physical injury

Debra Siela, PhD, RN, ACNS-BC, CCRN-K, CNE, RRT

NANDA-I

Definition

Susceptible to entry of gastrointestinal secretions, oropharyngeal secretions, solids, or fluids to the tracheobronchial passages, which may compromise health.

Risk Factors

Barrier to elevating upper body; decreased gastrointestinal motility; difficulty swallowing; enteral nutrition tube displacement; inadequate knowledge of modifiable factors; increased gastric residue; ineffective airway clearance

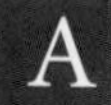

At-Risk Population

Older adults; premature infants

Associated Conditions

Chronic obstructive pulmonary disease; critical illness; decreased level of consciousness; delayed gastric emptying; depressed gag reflex; enteral nutrition; facial surgery; facial trauma; head and neck neoplasms; incompetent lower esophageal sphincter; increased intragastric pressure; jaw fixation techniques; medical devices; neck surgery; neck trauma; neurological diseases; oral surgical procedures; oral trauma; pharmaceutical preparations; pneumonia; stroke; treatment regimen

NOC (Nursing Outcomes Classification)

Suggested NOC Outcomes

Aspiration Prevention; Respiratory Status: Ventilation; Swallowing Status

Example NOC Outcome with Indicators

Aspiration Prevention as evidenced by the following indicators: Avoids risk factors/Maintains oral hygiene/Positions self upright for eating and drinking/Selects foods according to swallowing ability/Selects foods and fluid of proper consistency/Remains upright for 30 minutes after eating. (Rate the outcome and indicators of **Aspiration Prevention:** 1 = never demonstrated, 2 = rarely demonstrated, 3 = sometimes demonstrated, 4 = often demonstrated, 5 = continually demonstrated [see Section I].)

Client Outcomes

Client Will (Specify Time Frame)

- Maintain patent airway and clear lung sounds
- Swallow and digest oral, nasogastric, or gastric feeding without aspiration

NIC (Nursing Interventions Classification)

Suggested NIC Interventions

Aspiration Precautions

Example NIC Activities—Airway Management

Monitor level of consciousness, cough reflex, gag reflex, and swallowing ability; Check nasogastric or gastrostomy residual before feeding

Nursing Interventions and *Rationales*

- Monitor respiratory rate, depth, and effort. Note any signs of aspiration such as dyspnea, cough, cyanosis, wheezing, hoarseness, foul-smelling sputum, or fever. If there is a new onset of symptoms, perform oral suction and notify provider immediately. EB: *Signs of aspiration should be detected as soon as possible to prevent further aspiration and to initiate treatment that can be lifesaving (Gamache & Kamangar, 2018). Because of laryngeal pooling and residue in clients with dysphagia, silent aspiration may occur (Metheny, 2011b; Velayutham et al, 2018).*
- Auscultate lung sounds frequently and before and after feedings; note any new onset of crackles or wheezing. EB: *With decreased symptoms of pneumonia, an increased respiratory rate and/or crackles may be the first sign of pneumonia (Velayutham et al, 2018).*
- Take vital signs frequently, noting onset of a fever, increased respiratory rate, and increased heart rate. EB: *Implementation of an adapted aspiration risk assessment screening tool to document risk of hospital-acquired aspiration pneumonia and aspiration precautions protocol was associated with a decrease in aspiration pneumonia rates (Cipra, 2019).*
- Use of a bedside-aspiration risk screening process along with dysphagia therapists for acutely ill clients is a factor in decreasing client mortality from acquired aspiration. EB: *A systematic review and meta-analysis found that bedside aspiration risk screening with water offers sufficient information concerning aspiration risk, especially when other symptoms such as cough and choking with or without voice change occurs during the introduction of sips of water (Brodsky et al, 2016).*

- Before initiating oral feeding, check client's gag reflex and ability to swallow by feeling the laryngeal prominence as the client attempts to swallow (American Association of Critical Care Nurses, 2016a; Wangen, et al., 2019). If client is having problems swallowing, see nursing interventions for Impaired **Swallowing.**
- If client needs to be fed, feed slowly and allow adequate time for chewing and swallowing. EB: *Slowed feeding and fully chewing food allows time for more deliberate swallowing, reducing aspiration (Lee & Huang, 2019).* EB: *When feeding client, watch for signs of impaired swallowing or aspiration, including coughing, choking, change in voice, and spitting food (Brodsky et al, 2016).*
- Have suction machine available when feeding high-risk clients. If aspiration does occur, suction immediately. EB: *A client with aspiration needs immediate suctioning and may need further lifesaving interventions such as intubation and mechanical ventilation (Morata & Walsh, 2021).*
- Keep the head of the bed (HOB) elevated at 30 to 45 degrees, preferably with the client sitting up in a chair at 90 degrees when feeding. Keep head elevated for an hour after eating. CEB/EB: *Decreased gastric reflux occurs at both 30- and 45-degree HOB elevation. Thus, gastric-fed clients should be maintained at the highest HOB elevation that is comfortable to prevent aspiration (Metheny & Frantz, 2013; Morata & Walsh, 2021).*
- Note presence of nausea, vomiting, or diarrhea. Treat nausea promptly with antiemetics.
- If the client shows symptoms of nausea and vomiting, position on side. EB: *The side-lying position can help the client expel the vomitus and decrease the risk for aspiration (Morata & Walsh, 2021).*
- Assess the abdomen and listen to bowel sounds frequently, noting if they are decreased, absent, or hyperactive. EB: *Decreased or absent bowel sounds can indicate an ileus with possible vomiting and aspiration; increased high-pitched bowel sounds can indicate a mechanical bowel obstruction with possible vomiting and aspiration (Hasler & Owyang, 2018).*
- Note new onset of abdominal distention or increased rigidity of abdomen. EB: *Abdominal distention or rigidity can be associated with paralytic or mechanical obstruction and an increased likelihood of vomiting and aspiration (Hasler & Owyang, 2018).*
- If client has a tracheostomy, ask for referral to speech pathologist for swallowing studies before attempting to feed. EB: *There is an increased risk for aspiration when tracheostomy tubes are in place, and inflating the cuff does not prevent aspiration (Morata & Walsh, 2021).*
- Provide meticulous oral care including brushing of teeth at least two times per day. EB: *Good oral care can prevent bacterial or fungal contamination of the mouth, which can be aspirated (American Association of Critical Care Nurses, 2017a).* CEB: *Research has shown that excellent dental care/oral care can be effective in preventing hospital-acquired (or extended care–acquired) pneumonia (Munro, 2014).* EB: *Chlorhexidine mouthwash or gel reduces the incidence of developing ventilator-associated pneumonia in critically ill clients compared to placebo or usual care (Veitz-Keenan & Ferraiolo, 2017; Zhao et al, 2020).*
- Sedation agents can reduce cough and gag reflexes as well as interfere with the client's ability to manage oropharyngeal secretions. EB: *Using the smallest effective level of sedation may help reduce risk of aspiration (American Association of Critical Care Nurses, 2016a; Devlin et al, 2018).*

Enteral Feedings

- Insert nasogastric feeding tube using the internal nares to distal-lower esophageal-sphincter distance, an updated version of the Hanson method. The ear-to-nose-to-xiphoid process is often inaccurate. CEB: *A study demonstrated that the revised Hanson's method was more accurate in predicting the correct distance than the traditional method (Ellett et al, 2011).*
- Before instilling medication or enteral feeding, ensure proper gastric/duodenal tube placement. CEB/EB: *Verification of gastric tube placement should initially be obtained by radiography. Other methods of assessing proper gastric tube placement include capnography, aspirate assessment, tube markings, and pH tests. Auscultation should not be used to assess gastric tube placement (Metheny, Stewart, & McClave, 2011; Amirlak et al, 2012; Williams et al, 2014; American Association of Critical Care Nurses, 2016b).* EB: *If technology is present for confirmation by electromagnetic placement device, an x-ray confirmation of proper placement may not be* required *(Carter, Roberts, & Carson, 2018; Powers et al, 2018).*
- After radiographic verification of correct placement of the tube or the intestines, mark the tube's exit site clearly with tape or a permanent marker. EB: *Marking the tube's exit point can enable the nurse to identify possible migration or dislodgement of the tube (McGinnis, 2017).*
- Secure the nasogastric tube securely to the nose using a skin protectant under the tape or commercially available securement device. CEBN: *A research study found that insertion of the feeding tube into the small intestine and keeping the HOB position elevated to at least 30 degrees reduced the incidence of aspiration and aspiration-related pneumonia drastically in critically ill clients (Metheny, Davis-Jackson, & Stewart, 2010). Another study found that aspiration and pneumonia were reduced by feeding the clients in the mid-duodenum or farther in the*

A

small intestine (Metheny, Stewart, & McClave, 2011). **EBN:** *A study conducted in a critical care unit found that the nurse placement of a nasal bridal resulted in an 80% reduction in tube dislodgement (Taylor et al, 2018).*

- Measure and record the length of the tube that is outside of the body at defined intervals to help ensure correct placement. **EB:** *Note the length of the tube outside of the body; it is possible for a tube to slide out and be in the esophagus, without obvious disruption of the tape (American Association of Critical Care Nurses, 2016b).*
- Note the placement of the tube on any chest or abdominal radiographs that are obtained for the client. *Acutely ill clients receive frequent x-ray examinations. These are available for the nurse to determine continued correct placement of the nasogastric tube (American Association of Critical Care Nurses, 2016b; Boullata et al, 2017).*
- Check the pH of the aspirate. **EB:** *If the pH reading is 4 or less, the tube is probably in the stomach. Recognize that the pH may not indicate correct placement if the client is receiving continuous tube feedings, is receiving a hydrogen ion blocker or proton pump inhibitor, has blood in the aspirate, or is receiving antacids (American Association of Critical Care Nurses, 2016b). Enteral feeding tube pH can be recommended to evaluate gastric placement in neonates (Metheny et al, 2017; Kemper et al, 2019).*
- Do not rely on the air insufflation method to assess correct tube placement. **CEB/EBN:** *The auscultatory air insufflation method is not reliable for differentiating between gastric or respiratory placement; the "whooshing" sound can be heard even if the tube is incorrectly placed in the lung (Williams et al, 2014; American Association of Critical Care Nurses, 2016b; Boullata et al, 2017).*
- Follow unit policy regarding checking for gastric residual volume during continuous feedings or before feedings and holding feedings if increased residual is present. **CEB/EBN:** *There is little evidence to support the use of measurement of gastric residual volume, and the practice may or may not be effective in preventing aspiration (Boullata et al, 2017). It is still done at intervals if there is a question of tube feeding intolerance (Metheny et al, 2012; American Association of Critical Care Nurses, 2016b).*
- The practice of holding tube feedings if there is increased residual reduces the amount of calories given to the client. **EB:** *If the client has a small-bore feeding tube, it is difficult to check gastric residual volume and may be inaccurate. It is unclear if aspiration for residual volumes helps reduce the risk of aspiration (Metheny et al, 2012). Practice guidelines suggest continuing to feed the client until the residual is greater than 500 mL (Elke, Felbinger, & Heyland, 2015; Boullata et al, 2017; Yasuda et al, 2019).*
- Follow unit protocol regarding returning or discarding gastric residual volume. At this time there is not a definitive research base to guide practice. **EB:** *A recent systematic review and meta-analysis did not find compelling evidence that confirms that returning residual gastric aspirates provides more benefits than discarding them without increasing potential complications (Wen et al, 2019).*
- Do not use blue dye to tint enteral feedings. **CEB:** *The presence of blue and green skin and urine and serum discoloration from use of blue dye has been associated with the death of clients. The U.S. Food and Drug Administration (2003) has reported at least 12 deaths from the use of blue dye in enteral feedings.*
- During enteral feedings, position client with HOB elevated 30 to 45 degrees *(Schallom et al, 2015; American Association of Critical Care Nurses, 2016a).* **EB:** *HOB elevation greater than 30 degrees is feasible and preferred to 30 degrees for reducing oral secretion volume, reflux, and aspiration without pressure ulcer development in gastric-fed clients receiving mechanical ventilation (Schallom et al, 2015; American Association of Critical Care Nurses, 2017b).* **CEBN:** *A seminal study of mechanically ventilated clients receiving tube feedings demonstrated that there was an increase of the presence of pepsin (from gastric contents) in pulmonary secretions if the client was in a flat position versus being positioned with head elevated (Metheny & Frantz, 2013).* **EBN:** *Generally, do not turn off the tube feeding when repositioning clients. Stopping the tube feeding during repositioning is counterproductive because the client receives less nutrition and the rate of emptying of the stomach is slow. If it is imperative to keep the HOB elevated, consider use of reverse Trendelenburg (head higher than feet) when repositioning (Metheny, 2011a). Precautionary withholding of enteral feedings during repositioning does not reduce the incidence of aspiration in critically ill clients (DiLibero et al, 2015).*
- Nursing ventilated premature infants in right lateral position is associated with decreased aspiration of gastric secretions (Imam et al, 2019).
- Take actions to prevent inadvertent misconnections with enteral feeding tubes into intravenous (IV) lines or other harmful connections. Safety actions that should be taken to prevent misconnections include the following:
  - Trace tubing back to origin. Recheck connections at time of client transfer and at change of shift.
  - Label all tubing.
  - Use oral syringes for medications through the enteral feeding; do not use IV syringes.
  - Teach nonprofessional personnel "Do Not Reconnect" if a line becomes dislodged; rather, find the nurse instead of taking the chance of plugging the tube into the wrong place.

A

Critical Care

- Recognize that critically ill clients are at an increased risk for aspiration because of severe illness and interventions that compromise the gag reflex. EB: *Predisposing causes of aspiration include sedation, endotracheal intubation and mechanical ventilation, neurological disorders, altered level of consciousness, hemodynamic instability, sepsis, and client transport (American Association of Critical Care Nurses, 2016a; Talbert et al, 2020).*
- Recognize that intolerance to feeding as defined by increased gastric residual is more common early in the feeding process. EB: *For clients receiving gastric tube feedings, assess for gastrointestinal intolerance to the feedings at 4-hour intervals (American Association of Critical Care Nurses, 2016a).*
- Avoid bolus feedings in tube-fed clients who are at high risk for aspiration (American Association of Critical Care Nurses, 2016a).
- Maintain endotracheal cuff pressures at an appropriate level to prevent leakage of secretions around the cuff (American Association of Critical Care Nurses, 2016a).

Geriatric

- Carefully check older client's gag reflex and ability to swallow before feeding. *A slowed rate of swallowing is common in older adults (Morata & Walsh, 2021).*
- Watch for signs of aspiration pneumonia in older adults with cerebrovascular accidents, even if there are no apparent signs of difficulty swallowing or of aspiration. EB: *Bedside evaluation for swallow and aspiration can be inaccurate.* CEB/EB: *Silent aspiration can occur in the older population (Metheny, 2011b; Lee & Huang, 2019).*
- Recognize that older adults with aspiration pneumonia have fewer symptoms than younger people; repeat cases of pneumonia in older adults are generally associated with aspiration. EB: *Aspiration pneumonia can be undiagnosed in older adults because of decreased symptoms; sometimes the only obvious symptom may be new onset of delirium (Rodriguez & Restrepo, 2019).*
- Continually assess for the presence of gag reflex after critical illness that required mechanical ventilation. EB: *In individuals with prolonged ventilation the presence of one or both gag reflexes could predict a reduction in extubation failure related to aspiration or excessive upper airway secretions (Howes et al, 2020).*
- Use central nervous system depressants cautiously; older clients may have an increased incidence of aspiration with altered levels of consciousness. EB: *Older clients have altered metabolism, distribution, and excretion of drugs. Many medications can interfere with the swallowing reflex, including antipsychotic drugs, proton pump inhibitors, and angiotensin-converting enzyme inhibitors (Yoon et al, 2019).*
- Keep an older, mostly bedridden client sitting upright for 45 minutes to 1 hour after meals.
- Recommend to families that enteral feedings may or may not be indicated for clients with advanced dementia. Instead, if possible, use hand-feeding assistance, modified food consistency as needed, and feeding favorite foods for comfort. EB: *The American Geriatrics Society (2014) recommends that when feeding difficulties arise in individuals with advanced dementia, feeding tubes should not be used as they can increase agitation and result in aspiration leading to pneumonia and death. Careful hand feeding is advised in this population.*

Home Care

- The above interventions may be adapted for home care use.
- For clients at high risk for aspiration, obtain complete information from the discharging institution regarding institutional management.
- Assess the client and family for willingness and cognitive ability to learn and cope with swallowing, feeding, and related disorders.
- Assess caregiver understanding and reinforce teaching regarding positioning and assessment of the client for possible aspiration.
- Provide the client with emotional support in dealing with fears of aspiration. *Fear of choking can provoke extreme anxiety, which can interfere with the client's ability or willingness to adhere to the treatment plan.* Refer to care plan for **Anxiety.**
- Establish emergency and contingency plans for care of the client. *Clinical safety of the client between visits is a primary goal of home care nursing.*
- Have a speech and occupational therapist assess the client's swallowing ability and other physiological factors and recommend strategies for working with the client in the home (e.g., pureeing foods served to the client; providing adequate adaptive equipment for independence in eating). *Successful strategies allow the client to remain part of the family.*

A

- Obtain suction equipment for the home as necessary.
- Teach caregivers safe, effective use of suctioning devices. Inform the client and family that only individuals instructed in suctioning should perform the procedure.
- Institute case management of frail elderly to support continued independent living.

Client/Family Teaching and Discharge Planning

- Teach the client and family signs of aspiration and precautions to prevent aspiration.
- Teach the client and family how to safely administer tube feeding.
- Teach the family about proper client positioning to facilitate feeding and reduce risk of aspiration.
- Verify client family/caregiver knowledge about feeding, aspiration precautions, and signs of aspiration.

REFERENCES

American Association of Critical Care Nurses. (2016a). AACN practice Alert-prevention of aspiration in adults. *American Association of Critical Care Nurses*. Retrieved from https://www.aacn.org/~/media/aacn-website/clinical-resources/practice-alerts/preventionaspirationpracticealert.pdf. [Accessed June 7, 2021].

American Association of Critical Care Nurses. (2016b). AACN practice Alert-Initial and Ongoing verification of feeding tube placement in adults. *American Association of Critical Care Nurses*. Retrieved from https://www.aacn.org/~/media/aacn-website/clinical-resources/practice-alerts/feedingtubepa.pdf. [Accessed June 7, 2021].

American Association of Critical Care Nurses. (2017a). AACN practice Alert-prevention of ventilator-associated pneumonia in adults. *American Association of Critical Care Nurses*. Retrieved from https://www.aacn.org/~/media/aacn-website/clinical-resources/practice-alerts/preventingvapinadults2017.pdf. [Accessed June 7, 2021].

American Association of Critical Care Nurses. (2017b). AACN practice Alert-oral care for acutely and critically ill patients. *American Association of Critical Care Nurses*. Retrieved from https://www.aacn.org/~/media/aacn-website/clinical-resources/practice-alerts/oralcarepractalert2017.pdf. [Accessed June 7, 2021].

American Geriatrics Society Ethics Committee and Clinical Practice and Models of Care Committee. (2014). American Geriatrics Society feeding tubes in advanced dementia position statement. *Journal of the American Geriatrics Society*, *62*(8), 1590–1593. https://doi.org/10.1111/jgs.12924.

Amirlak, B., Amirlak, I., Awad, Z., Zahmatkesh, M., Pipinos, I., & Forse, A. (2012). Pneumothorax following feeding tube placement: Precaution and treatment. *Acta Medica Iranica*, *50*(5), 355–358.

Boullata, J. I., Carrera, A. L., Harvey, L., et al. & ASPEN safe practices for enteral nutrition therapy Task Force, American Society for Parenteral and Enteral Nutrition. (2017). ASPEN Safe Practices for Enteral Nutrition Therapy [Formula: see text]. *JPEN Journal of Parenteral and Enteral Nutrition*, *41*(1), 15–103. https://doi.org/10.1177/0148607116673053.

Brodsky, M. B., Suiter, D. M., González-Fernández, et al. (2016). Screening accuracy for aspiration using bedside water swallow tests: A systematic review and meta-analysis. *Chest*, *150*(1), 148–163. https://doi.org/10.1016/j.chest.2016.03.059.

Carter, M., Roberts, S., & Carson, J. A. (2018). Small-bowel feeding tube placement at bedside: Electronic medical device placement and x-ray agreement. *Nutrition in Clinical Practice*, *33*(2), 274–280. doi:10.1002/ncp.10072.

Cipra, E. J. (2019). Implementation of a risk assessment tool to reduce aspiration pneumonia in nonstroke patients. *Clinical Nurse Specialist*, *33*(6), 279–283. doi:10.1097/NUR.0000000000000484.

Devlin, J. W., Skrobik, Y., Gélinas, C., et al. (2018). Clinical practice guidelines for the prevention and management of pain, agitation/sedation, delirium, immobility, and sleep disruption in adult patients in the ICU. *Critical Care Medicine*, *46*(9), e825–e873. doi:10.1097/CCM.0000000000003299.

DiLibero, J., Lavieri, M., O'Donoghue, S., & DeSanto-Madeya, S. (2015). Withholding or continuing enteral feedings during repositioning and the incidence of aspiration. *American Journal of Critical Care*, *24*(3), 258–262.

Elke, G., Felbinger, T. W., & Heyland, D. K. (2015). Gastric residual volume in critically ill patients: A dead marker or still alive? *Nutrition in Clinical Practice*, *30*(1), 59–71.

Ellett, M. L., Cohen, M. D., Perkins, S. M., et al. (2011). Predicting the insertion length for gastric tube placement in neonates. *Journal of Obstetric, Gynecologic, & Neonatal Nurses*, *40*(4), 412–421.

Gamache, J., & Kamangar, N. (2018). Aspiration pneumonitis and pneumonia. *Medscape*. https://emedicine.medscape.com/article/296198-overview.

Hasler, W., & Owyang, C. (2018). Approach to the patient with gastrointestinal disease. In J. Larry Jameson, A. S. Fauci, D. L. Kasper, et al. (Eds.), *Harrison's principles of internal medicine* (20th ed.). New York: McGraw-Hill.

Howes, S., Hartmann-Boyce, J., Livingstone-Banks, J., Hong, B., & Lindson, N. (2020). Antidepressants for smoking cessation. *Cochrane Database of Systematic Reviews*, *4*, CD000031.

Imam, S. S., Shinkar, D. M., Mohamed, N. A., & Mansour, H. E. (2019). Effect of right lateral position with head elevation on tracheal aspirate pepsin in ventilated preterm neonates: Randomized controlled trial. *Journal of Maternal-Fetal and Neonatal Medicine*, *32*(22), 3741–3746. doi:10.1080/14767058.2018.1471674.

Kemper, C., Haney, B., Oschman, A., Lee, B. R., et al. (2019). Acidity of enteral feeding tube aspirate in neonates: Do pH values meet the cutoff for predicting gastric placement? *Advances in Neonatal Care*, *19*(4), 333–341. doi:10.1097/ANC.0000000000000591.

Lee, K. C., & Huang, Y. H. (2019). To chew carefully and swallow slowly. *Journal of the Chinese Medical Association*, *82*(10), 745. https://doi.org/10.1097/JCMA.0000000000000167.

McGinnis, C. (2017). Nasogastric and orogastric tube insertion, care, and removal. In D. L. Wiegand (Ed.), *AACN procedure manual for high acuity, progressive, and critical care* (7th ed.). Philadelphia: Elsevier.

Metheny, N. A. (2011a). Turning tube feeding off while repositioning patients in bed: Ask the experts. *Critical Care Nurse*, *31*(2), 96–97.

Metheny, N. A. (2011b). Preventing aspiration in older adults with dysphagia. *Med-Surg Matters*, *20*(5), 6–7.

Metheny, N. A., Davis-Jackson, J., & Stewart, B. (2010). Effectiveness of an aspiration risk-reduction protocol. *Nursing Research*, *59*(1), 18–25.

Metheny, N. A., & Frantz, R. A. (2013). Head-of-bed elevation in critically ill patients: A review. *Critical Care Nurse*, *33*(3), 53–67.

Metheny, N. A., Mills, A. C., & Stewart, B. J. (2012). Monitoring for intolerance to gastric tube feedings: A national survey. *American Journal of Critical Care*, *21*(2), e33–e40.

Metheny, N. A., Pawluszka, A., Lulic, M., Hinyard, L. J., & Meert, K. L. (2017). Testing placement of gastric feeding tubes in infants. *American Journal of Critical Care*, *26*(6), 466–473.

Metheny, N. A., Stewart, B. J., & McClave, S. A. (2011). Relationship between feeding tube site and respiratory outcomes. *Journal of Parenteral and Enteral Nutrition*, *35*(3), 346–355.

Morata, L., & Walsh, M. (2021). Nutritional therapy. In M. Sole, D. Klein, M. Moseley, et al. (Eds.), *Introduction to critical care nursing* (pp. 94–104). St. Louis: Elsevier.

Munro, C. L. (2014). Oral health: Something to smile about. *American Journal of Critical Care, 23*(4), 282–289.
Powers, J., Luebbehusen, M., Aguirre, L., et al. (2018). Improved safety and efficacy of small-bore feeding tube confirmation using an electromagnetic placement device. *Nutrition in Clinical Practice, 33*(2), 268–273. doi:10.1002/ncp.10062.
Rodriguez, A. E., & Restrepo, M. I. (2019). New perspectives in aspiration community acquired pneumonia. *Expert Review of Clinical Pharmacology, 12*(10), 991–1002. https://doi.org/10.1080/17512433.2019.1663730.
Schallom, M., Dykeman, B., Metheny, N., Kirby, J., & Pierce, J. (2015). Head-of-bed elevation and early outcomes of gastric reflux, aspiration, and pressure ulcers: A feasibility study. *American Journal of Critical Care, 24*(1), 57–66.
Talbert, S., Detrick, C. W., Emery, K., et al. (2020). Intubation setting, aspiration, and ventilator-associated conditions. *American Journal of Critical Care, 29*(5), 371–378. doi:10.4037/ajcc2020129.
Taylor, S. J., Allan, K., Clemente, R., Marsh, A., & Toher, D. (2018). Feeding tube securement in critical illness: Implications for safety. *British Journal of Nursing, 27*(18), 1036–1041. https://doi.org/10.12968/bjon.2018.27.18.1036.
U.S. Food and Drug Administration. (2003). *FDA Public health advisory: Subject: Reports of blue discoloration and death in patients receiving enteral feedings tinted with the dye, FD&C blue No. 1.* Retrieved from https://www.fda.gov/industry/medical-devices/fda-public-health-advisory-subject-reports-blue-discoloration-and-death-patients-receiving-enteral. [Accessed June 7, 2021].
Veitz-Keenan, A., & Ferraiolo, D. M. (2017). Oral care with chlorhexidine seems effective for reducing the incidence of ventilator-associated pneumonia. *Evidence-Based Dentistry, 18*(4), 113–114. doi:10.1038/sj.ebd.6401272.
Velayutham, P., Irace, A. L., Kawai, K., et al. (2018). Silent aspiration: Who is at risk? *Laryngoscope, 128*(8), 1952–1957. https://doi.org/10.1002/lary.27070.
Wangen, T., Hatlevig, J., Pifer, G., & Vitale, K. (2019). Preventing aspiration complications, implementing a swallow screening tool. *Clinical Nurse Specialist, 33*(5), 237–243. doi:10.1097/NUR.0000000000000471.
Wen, Z., Xie, A., Peng, M., Bian, L., Wei, L., & Li, M. (2019). Is discard better than return gastric residual aspirates: A systematic review and meta-analysis. *BMC Gastroenterology, 19*(1), 113. https://doi.org/10.1186/s12876-019-1028-7.
Williams, T. A., Leslie, G., Mills, L., et al. (2014). Frequency of aspirating gastric tubes for patients receiving enteral nutrition in the ICU: A randomized controlled trial. *JPEN: Journal of Parenteral and Enteral Nutrition, 38*(7), 809–816.
Yasuda, H., Kondo, N., Yamamoto, R., et al. (2019). Monitoring of gastric residual volume during enteral nutrition. *Cochrane Database of Systematic Reviews, 5,* CD013335. https://doi.org/10.1002/14651858.CD013335.
Yoon, H. Y., Shim, S. S., Kim, S. J., et al. (2019). Long-term mortality and prognostic factors in aspiration pneumonia. *Journal of the American Medical Directors Association, 20*(9), 1098–1104.e4. https://doi.org/10.1016/j.jamda.2019.03.029.
Zhao, T., Wu, X., Zhang, Q., Li, C., Worthington, H. V., & Hua, F. (2020). Oral hygiene for critically ill patients to prevent ventilator-associated pneumonia. *Cochrane Database of Systematic Reviews, 12,* CD008367. doi:10.1002/14651858.CD008367.pub4.

Risk for Impaired Attachment

Domain 7 Role relationship Class 2 Family relationships

Margaret Quinn, DNP, CPNP, CNE

NANDA-I

Definition

Susceptible to disruption of the interactive process between parent or significant other and child that fosters the development of a protective and nurturing reciprocal relationship.

Risk Factors

Anxiety; child's illness prevents effective initiation of parental contact; disorganized infant behavior; inability of parent to meet personal needs; insufficient privacy; parent's illness prevents effective initiation of infant contact; parent-child separation; parental conflict resulting from disorganized infant behavior; physical barrier; substance misuse

At-Risk Population

Premature infants

NOC (Nursing Outcomes Classification)

Suggested NOC Outcomes

Parent-Infant Attachment; Parenting Performance: Psychosocial Adjustment: Life Change

Example NOC Outcomes with Indicators

Holds infant close, touches, strokes, pats infant, responds to infant cues, holds infant for feeding, vocalizes to infant. (Rate the outcome and indicators of appropriate parent and infant behaviors that demonstrate an enduring affectionate bond: 1 = never demonstrated, 2 = rarely demonstrated, 3 = sometimes demonstrated, 4 = often demonstrated, 5 = consistently demonstrated [see Section I].)

A

Client Outcomes

Parent(s)/Caregiver(s) Will (Specify Time Frame)

- Be willing to consider pumping breast milk (and storing appropriately) or breastfeeding, if feasible
- Demonstrate behaviors that indicate secure attachment to infant/child
- Provide a safe environment, free of physical hazards
- Provide nurturing environment sensitive to infant/child's need for nutrition/feeding, sleeping, comfort, and social play
- Read and respond contingently to infant/child's distress
- Support infant's self-regulation capabilities, intervening when needed
- Engage in mutually satisfying interactions that provide opportunities for attachment
- Give infant nurturing sensory experiences (e.g., holding, cuddling, stroking, rocking)
- Demonstrate an awareness of developmentally appropriate activities that are pleasurable, emotionally supportive, and growth fostering
- Avoid physical and emotional abuse and/or neglect as retribution for parent's perception of infant/child's misbehavior
- State appropriate community resources and support services

NIC (Nursing Interventions Classification)

Suggested NIC Interventions

Anticipatory Guidance; Attachment Promotion; Coping Enhancement; Counseling; Developmental Enhancement: Infant; Family Involvement Promotion; Parent Education: Infant; Parenting Promotion

Example NIC Activities—Anticipatory Guidance

Instruct about normal development and behavior, as appropriate; Provide a ready reference for the client (e.g., educational materials, pamphlets) as appropriate

Nursing Interventions and *Rationales*

Mother–Baby Dyad Interventions

- Establish a trusting relationship with parent/caregiver in the perinatal and postnatal period. EBN: *The early detection of deficiencies in the maternal-fetal relationship and the timely diagnosis of postpartum depression (PPD) can significantly improve the maternal-neonatal relationship in the future (Dubber et al, 2015).*
- Educate parents about the importance of the infant–caregiver relationship as a foundation for the development of the infant's self-regulation capacities. EB: *By showing the "calming and regulating effect" of moderate pressure massage, this study contributes to a greater understanding of the influence of self-regulation on the development of play and playfulness in preterm babies and on mothers' participation in such interventions with their infants (Hendel, 2017).*
- Educate parents in reading/responding sensitively to their infant's unique "body language" (behavior cues), which communicates approach ("I'm ready to play"), avoidance/stress ("I'm unhappy. I need a change."), and self-calming ("I'm helping myself"). EB: *Education about the principles of neurodevelopment and behavioral cues make individualized developmentally appropriate, neuroprotective care possible (Altimier & Phillips, 2016).*
- Encourage physical closeness using skin-to-skin experiences as appropriate. EBN: *Placing a newborn skin to skin on the mother is the essential first step to promote and establish successful breastfeeding (Jefferson & Bibb, 2019).*

Maternal/Parental Interventions

- Identify factors related to PPD/major depression and offer appropriate interventions/referrals. EBN: *A significant and inverse correlation was observed between PPD and all the domains of maternal-fetal attachment (Delvari et al, 2018).*
- Assess for additional comorbid factors related to depression and offer appropriate interventions/referrals. EB: *The combination of maternal depression and dual/disorganized attachment style may pose a special risk constellation for the developing mother–infant bond that should be addressed in prevention and early intervention programs (Nonnemacher et al, 2016).*

A

- Nurture parents so that they in turn can nurture their infant/child. EB: *Family-centered developmental care (FCDC) is designed to meet the needs of all babies, healthy newborns as well as hospitalized infants, and the needs of families coping with the crisis of the neonatal intensive care unit (NICU) experience (Craig et al, 2015).*
- Offer parents opportunities to verbalize their childhood fears associated with attachment. EBN: *Infants were more likely to form disorganized attachment relationships if their mothers had histories of attachment disorganization (Raby et al, 2015).*
- Identify mothers who may need assistance in enhancing maternal role attainment (MRA). EBN: *Peer support and role modeling may help mothers to develop maternal identity (Rossman et al, 2015).*
- Encourage positive involvement and relationship development between children and fathers. EBN: *Attachment between the father and child is significant (Frazier & Scharf, 2015).*

Premature Infants/Infants Requiring Specialty or Intensive Care

- Support mothers of preterm infants in providing pumped breast milk for their babies until they are ready for oral feedings and transitioning from gavage to breast. CEBN: *The Spatz Ten Steps model (Spatz, 2004) is associated with "significant improvements in parents' perception of nurses' support for mothers' efforts to breastfeed and [improvement] in the odds of the VLBW [very-low-birth-weight] infant receiving MOM [mother's own milk] at the time of hospital discharge" (Fugate et al, 2015).*
- Suggest journaling or scrapbooking as a way for parents of hospitalized infants to cope with stress and emotions. EB: *Narrative writing provides opportunities to remember and organize events in a meaningful and sensible manner. It helps create a feeling of problem-solving, stops unpleasant feelings, and gradually leads to the fading of negative experiences (Kadivar et al, 2015).*
- Offer parent-to-parent support to parents of infants in the NICU. EBN: *Quantitative studies showed parent-to-parent support increased perceptions of support, reduced maternal stress, and increased mothers' confidence in the ability to care for their baby (Hunt et al, 2019).*
- Plan ways for parents and their support system to interact/assist with infant/child caregiving. EB: *Full participation of parents is essential (Craig et al, 2015).*
- Educate and support parents' ability to relieve the infant/child's stress, distress, or pain. EBN: *Various studies demonstrate the efficacy of facilitated tucking as a nonpharmacological pain intervention in premature infants as young as 23 weeks' gestational age during such painful procedures as heel sticks, endotracheal suctioning, and venipuncture (Hartley et al, 2015).*
- Guide parents in adapting their behaviors/activities with infant/child cues and changing needs. EB: *Parents' emotional closeness to their preterm NICU infant "may be crucial to the well-being of the newborn, the development of mutual regulation, the establishment of a functioning parent–infant affective relationship and the parents' confidence in their ability to provide care for their baby" (Stefana & Lavelli, 2017).*
- Attend to both parents and infant/child to strengthen high-quality interactions. EBN: *NICU fathers of preterm infants have been found to exhibit coping strategies and needs different from NICU mothers. As a result, nursing support and intervention need to be tailored to parents individually to sustain caregiving engagement and the transition to post discharge parenting (Provenzi & Santoro, 2015).*
- Encourage opportunities for physical closeness. EB: *A study evaluating 11 NICUs in 6 European countries concluded that units providing facilities for parents to stay overnight had a higher level of parental presence, with younger mothers, in particular, staying close to their infants (Raisklia et al, 2017).*
- Recognize that fathers, compared with mothers, may have different starting points in the attachment process in the NICU because nurses encourage parents to have early skin-to-skin contact (SSC). EB: *Results of this Taiwanese study confirm the positive effects of father–infant SSC "in terms of exploring, talking, touching, and caring," as well as the enhancing of the relationship at 3 days postpartum (Chen et al, 2017).*

Pediatric

- Recognize and support infant/child's capacity for self-regulation and intervene when appropriate. *There is a significant yet weak association between attachment security and temperament, suggesting that attachment and temperament are relatively independent developmental constructs (Groh et al, 2017).*
- Provide lyrical, soothing music in the nursery and at home that is age appropriate (i.e., corrected, in the case of premature infants) and contingent with state or behavioral cues. EBN: *Implementing early intervention services, such as music therapy in the postpartum unit, can provide new mothers useful music applications that can enhance mother–infant interaction, especially mothers living in high-stress or negative environments (Robertson & Detmer, 2019).*
- Recognize and support infant/child's attention capabilities. EBN: *During social interactions, sensitive non-vocal behavior may serve to assist infants in coordinating their attention to objects differently than during*

A

social interactions where vocal behavior dominates, which draws infants' attention to the caregiver (Miller, Hurdish, & Gros-Louis, 2018).

- Encourage opportunities for mutually satisfying interactions between infant and parent. EB: *A secure attachment to a primary caregiver is necessary for the development of emotional security and the sense that one's needs are important (Berkowitz, 2020).*
- Encourage parents and caregivers to massage their infants and children. EB: *There is evidence that infant massage has beneficial effects on preterm infants in the NICU, including shorter length of stay; reduced pain; and improved weight gain, feeding tolerance, and neurodevelopment. Parents who performed massage with their infants in the NICU reported experiencing less stress, anxiety, and depression (Pados & McGlothen-Bell, 2019).*

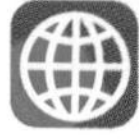

Multicultural

- Provide culturally sensitive parent support to new immigrant families and other non–native-English-speaking mothers and families. EB: *Culturally competent care must be considered and implemented as a separate standalone aspect when caring for new immigrant and non–native-English-speaking families (Hendson et al, 2015).*
- Discuss cultural norms with families to provide care that is appropriate for enhancing attachment with the infant/child. EB: *It is important to consider factors such as who makes decisions on the child's behalf, how the family prefers to communicate and interact with the medical and nursing team, and roles of family members in the home country (Langer et al, 2015).*

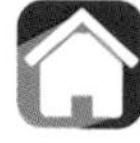

Home Care

- The previously mentioned interventions may be adapted for home care use.
- Observe the attachment style and pattern during all clinical encounters with infants and parents. EBN: *Health care professionals can teach parents the importance of quality of their interaction with their infant and the effect of attachment on the development of the child's sense of self-worth, comfort, and trust (Hagan et al, 2017).*
- Assess for social and environmental risk factors. EBN: *Global maternal insensitivity was associated with higher attachment disorganization for infants of mothers with higher sociodemographic risk, but not for those of mothers with lower sociodemographic risk (Gedaly & Leerkes, 2016).*
- Assess quality of interaction between parent and infant/child. *Within the parent–child relationship, parents' sensitive responsiveness to infant attachment signals is believed to be the principal organizing force shaping the quality of the early attachment relationship (Groh et al, 2017).*
- ▲ Assess for PPD at the pediatric primary care visit at 1-, 2-, 4-, and 6-month visits. EB: *Pediatric primary care providers are in a good position to recognize the signs of PPD because they are in frequent contact with parents of infants (Earls et al, 2019).*
- Empower family members to draw on personal strengths in which multiple worldviews/values are recognized, incorporated, and negotiated. EBN: *Infants develop different patterns of attachment to different caregivers depending on the quality of care received from a specific caregiver (Groh et al, 2017).*

Special Considerations

- Promote attachment process/development of maternal sensitivity in incarcerated women. EB: *Separation from and attachment to children correlate with higher levels of depression, the influence of the inmate's mother on the context of what is a good mother, and the dichotomous tension (i.e., good mother/bad mother) between expectations and reality for the incarcerated mother (Baker, 2019).*
- Promote the attachment process in women who have abused substances by providing a culturally based, family-centered, supportive treatment environment. EBN: *With support, mothers embraced opportunities to bond with their infants, and they frequently acknowledged fears that they may be separated from their infants due to their history of substance use (Kramlich et al, 2018).*
- ▲ Encourage custodial grandparents to use support groups available for caregivers of children. EBN: *In addition to providing useful parenting advice and direct support to custodial grandparents, pediatricians should refer these families as needed to local grandparenting groups, social service agencies, experienced legal counsel, and relevant national organizations for support and guidance (Ge & Adesman, 2017).*
- Provide options for communication for infants and children whose parents have been separated for military or work deployment EBN: *Video-mediated communication may be ideally suited when families are separated geographically during the perinatal period and early infancy (e.g., military/work deployment, hospitalization, educational opportunity and migrant/refugee families who send one parent ahead), as it provides communication context by adding visual cues and contextualizing auditory cues (Furukawa, Driessnack, & Kobori, 2020).*

REFERENCES

Altimier, L., & Phillips, R. (2016). The neonatal integrative developmental care model: Advanced clinical adaptations of the seven core measures for neuroprotective family-centered developmental care. *Newborn and Infant Nursing Reviews*, *16*(4), 230–244. https://doi.org/10.1053/j.nainr.2016.09.030.

Baker, B. (2019). Perinatal outcomes of incarcerated pregnant women: An integrative review. *Journal of Correctional Health Care*, *25*(2), 92–104. https://doi.org/10.1177/1078345819832366.

Berkowitz, C. D. (Ed.). (2020). *Berkowitz's pediatrics: A primary care approach* (6th ed.). Itasca, IL: American Academy of Pediatrics.

Chen, E. M., Gau, M. L., Liu, C. Y., & Lee, T. Y. (2017). Effects of father-neonatal skin-to-skin contact on attachment: A randomized controlled trial. *Nursing Research and Practice*, 8612024. https://doi.org/10.1155/2017/8612024.

Craig, J. W., Glick, C., Phillips, R., Hall, S. L., Smith, J., & Browne, J. (2015). Recommendations for involving the family in developmental care of the NICU baby. *Journal of Perinatology*, *35*, S5–S8. https://doi.org10.1038/jp.2015.142.

Delavari, M., Mohammad-Alizadeh-Charandabi, C., & Mirghafurvand, M. (2018). The relationship between maternal–fetal attachment and maternal self-efficacy in Iranian women: A prospective study. *Journal of Reproductive and Infant Psychology*, *36*(3), 302–311. https://doi.org/10.1080/02646838.2018.1436753.

Dubber, S., Reck, C., Müller, M., & Gawlik, S. (2015). Postpartum bonding: The role of perinatal depression, anxiety and maternal fetal bonding during pregnancy. *Archives of Women's Mental Health*, *18*(2), 187–195. https://doi.org/10.1007/s00737-014-0445-4.

Earls, M. F., Yogman, M. W., Mattson, G., & Rafferty, J. (2019). Incorporating recognition and management of perinatal depression into pediatric practice. *Pediatrics*, *143*(1), e20183259. https://doi.org/10.1542/peds.2018-3259.

Frazier, K. F., & Scharf, R. J. (2015). Parent-infant attachment. *Pediatrics in Review*, *36*(1), 41–42. https://doi.org/10.1542/pir.36-1-41.

Fugate, K., Hernandez, I., Ashmeade, T., Miladinovic, B., & Spatz, D. L. (2015). Improving human milk and breastfeeding practices in the NICU. *Journal of Obstetric, Gynecologic, and Neonatal Nursing*, *44*(3), 426–438. https://doi.org/10.1111/1552-6909.12563.

Furukawa, R., Driessnack, M., & Kobori, E. (2020). The effect of video-mediated communication on father-infant bonding and transition to fatherhood during and after Satogaeri Bunben. *International Journal of Nursing Practice*, *26*(4), e12828. https://doi.org/10.1111/ijn.12828.

Ge, W., & Adesman, A. (2017). Grandparents raising grandchildren: A primer for pediatricians. *Current Opinion in Pediatrics*, *29*, 379–384. https://doi.org/10.1097/MOP.0000000000000501.

Gedaly, L. R., & Leerkes, E. M. (2016). The role of sociodemographic risk and maternal behavior in the prediction of infant attachment disorganization. *Attachment & Human Development*, *18*(6), 554–569. https://doi.org/10.1080/14616734.2016.1213306.

Groh, A. M., Narayan, A. J., Bakermans-Kranenburg, M. J., et al. (2017). Attachment and temperament in the early life course: A meta-analytic review. *Child Development*, *88*(3), 770–795. https://doi.org/10.1111/cdev.12677.

Hagan, J., Shaw, J., Duncan, P., et al. (2017). *Bright futures: Guidelines for health supervision of infants, children, and adolescents. Bright futures* (4th ed.). Itasca, IL: American Academy of Pediatrics.

Hartley, K. A., Miller, C. S., & Gephart, S. M. (2015). Facilitated tucking to reduce pain in neonates: Evidence for best practice. *Advances in Neonatal Care*, *15*(3), 201–208. https://doi.org/10.1097/ANC.0000000000000193.

Hendel, C. (2017). *The effects of moderate pressure massage on self-regulation and play in preterm babies*. Nova Southeastern University, ProQuest Dissertations Publishing.

Hendson, L., Reis, M. D., & Nicholas, D. B. (2015). Health care providers' perspectives of providing cultural competent care in the NICU. *Journal of Obstetric, Gynecologic, and Neonatal Nursing*, *44*(1), 17–27. https://doi.org/10.1111/1552-6909.12524.

Hunt, H., Abbott, R., Boddy, K., et al. (2019). "They've walked the walk": A systematic review of quantitative and qualitative evidence for parent-to-parent support for parents of babies in neonatal care. *Journal of Neonatal Nursing*, *25*(4), 166–176. https://doi.org/10.1016/j.jnn.2019.03.011.

Jefferson, U. T., & Bibb, D. (2019). A breastfeeding algorithm to guide bedside health care practice for term newborns. *Nursing for Women's Health*, *23*(1), 49–58. https://doi.org/10.1016/j.nwh.2018.11.003.

Kadivar, M., Seyedfatemi, N., Akbari, N., & Haghani, H. (2015). The effect of narrative writing on maternal stress in neonatal intensive care settings. *Journal of Maternal-Fetal and Neonatal Medicine*, *28*(8), 938–943. https://doi.org/10.3109/1467058.2014.937699.

Kramlich, D., Kronk, R., Marcellus, L., Colbert, A., & Jakub, K. (2018). Rural postpartum women with substance use disorders. *Qualitative Health Research*, *28*(9), 1449–1461. https://doi.org/1049732318765720.

Langer, T., Cummings, C. L., & Meyer, E. C. (2015). When worlds intersect: Practical and ethical challenges when caring for international patients in the NICU. *Journal of Perinatology*, *35*, 982–984. https://doi.org/10.1038/jp.2015.106.

Miller, J. L., Hurdish, E., & Gros-Louis, J. (2018). Different patterns of sensitivity differentially affect infant attention span. *Infant Behavior and Development*, *53*, 1–4. https://doi.org/10.1016/j.infbeh.2018.10.001.

Nonnemacher, N., Doe, D., Ehrenthal, J. C., & Reck, C. (2016). Postpartum bonding: The impact of maternal depression and adult attachment style. *Archives of Women's Mental Health*, *19*(5), 927–935. https://doi.org/10.1007/s00737-016-0648-y.

Pados, B. F., & McGlothen-Bell, K. (2019). Benefits of infant massage for infants and parents in the NICU. *Nursing for Women's Health*, *23*(3), 265–271. https://doi.org/10.1016/j.nwh.2019.03.004.

Provenzi, L., & Santoro, E. (2015). The lived experience of fathers of preterm infants in the neonatal intensive care unit: A systematic review of qualitative studies. *Journal of Clinical Nursing*, *24*(13–14), 1784–1794. https://doi.org/10.1111/jocn.12828.

Raby, K. L., Steele, R. D., Carlson, E. A., & Sroufe, L. A. (2015). Continuities and changes in infant attachment patterns across two generations. *Attachment & Human Development*, *17*(4), 414–428. https://doi.org/10.1080/14616734.2015.1067824.

Raisklia, S., Axelin, A., Toome, L., et al. (2017). Parents' presence and parent-infant closeness in 11 neonatal intensive care units in six European countries vary between and within the countries. *Acta Paediatrica*, *106*(6), 878–888. https://doi.org/10.1111/apa.13798.

Robertson, A. M., & Detmer, M. R. (2019). The effects of contingent lullaby music on parent-infant interaction and amount of infant crying in the first six weeks of life. *Journal of Pediatric Nursing*, *46*, 33–38. https://doi.org/10.1016/j.pedn.2019.02.025.

Rossman, B., Greene, M. M., & Meier, P. P. (2015). The role of peer support in the development of maternal identity for "NICU moms." *Journal of Obstetric, Gynecologic, and Neonatal Nursing*, *44*(1), 3–16. https://doi.org/10.1111/1552-6909.1252.

Spatz, D. L. (2004). Ten steps for promoting and protecting breastfeeding for vulnerable infants. *Journal of Perinatal and Neonatal Nursing*, *18*(4), 385–396. https://doi.org/10.1097/00005237-200410000-00009.

Stefana, A., & Lavelli, M. (2017). Parental engagement and early interactions with preterm infants during the stay in the neonatal intensive care unit: Protocol of a mixed-method and longitudinal study. *BMJ Open*, *7*(2), e013824. https://doi.org/10.1136/bmjopen-2016-013824.

A

Autonomic Dysreflexia

Domain 9 Coping/stress tolerance Class 3 Neurobehavioral stress

Carla Aresco, MSL, CRNP

NANDA-I

Definition

Life-threatening, uninhibited sympathetic response of the nervous system to a noxious stimulus after a spinal cord injury at the 7th thoracic vertebra (T7) or above.

Defining Characteristics

Blurred vision; bradycardia; chest pain; chilling; conjunctival congestion; diaphoresis above the injury; diffuse pain in different areas of the head; Horner's syndrome; metallic taste in mouth; nasal congestion; pallor below injury; paresthesia; paroxysmal hypertension; pilomotor reflex; red blotches on skin above the injury; tachycardia

Related Factors

Gastrointestinal Stimuli

Bowel distention; constipation; difficult passage of feces; digital stimulation; enemas; fecal impaction; suppositories

Integumentary Stimuli

Cutaneous stimulation; skin irritation; sunburn; wound

Musculoskeletal-Neurological Stimuli

Irritating stimuli below level of injury; muscle spasm; painful stimuli below level of injury; pressure over bony prominence; pressure over genitalia; range of motion exercises

Regulatory-Situational Stimuli

Constrictive clothing; environmental temperature fluctuations; positioning

Reproductive-Urological Stimuli

Bladder distention; bladder spasm; instrumentation; sexual intercourse

Other Factors

Inadequate caregiver knowledge of disease process; inadequate knowledge of disease process

At-Risk Population

Individuals exposed to environmental temperature extremes; men with spinal cord injury or lesion who are experiencing ejaculation; women with spinal cord injury or lesion who are experiencing labor; women with spinal cord injury or lesion who are menstruating; women with spinal cord injury or lesion who are pregnant

Associated Conditions

Bowel fractures; detrusor sphincter dyssynergia; digestive system diseases; epididymitis; heterotopic bone; ovarian cyst; pharmaceutical preparations; renal calculi; substance withdrawal; surgical procedures; urinary catheterization; urinary tract infection; venous thromboembolism

NOC (Nursing Outcomes Classification)

Suggested NOC Outcomes

Neurological Status; Neurological Status: Autonomic; Vital Signs

Example NOC Outcome with Indicators

Neurological Status: Autonomic as evidenced by the following indicators: Systolic blood pressure/Diastolic blood pressure/Apical heart rate/Perspiration response pattern/Goose bumps response pattern/Pupil reactivity/Peripheral tissue perfusion. (Rate each indicator of **Neurological Status: Autonomic:** 1 = severely compromised, 2 = substantially compromised, 3 = moderately compromised, 4 = mildly compromised, 5 = not compromised [see Section I].)

Client Outcomes

Client Will (Specify Time Frame)

- Maintain baseline blood pressure
- Remain free of dysreflexia symptoms
- Explain symptoms, treatment, and prevention of dysreflexia

NIC (Nursing Interventions Classification)

Suggested NIC Intervention

Dysreflexia Management

Example NIC Activities—Dysreflexia Management

Identify and minimize stimuli that may precipitate dysreflexia; Monitor for signs and symptoms of autonomic dysreflexia

Nursing Interventions and *Rationales*

- ● Teach clients with a spinal cord injury (SCI) about potential causes, symptoms, treatment, and prevention of autonomic dysreflexia (AD). EB: *The nurse should inform the individual and his or her family about the signs and symptoms of AD. The nurse should also inform the client that the first occurrence of AD is often 3 to 6 months after injury (Perkins, 2020). Written material about AD treatment should be given to the client as well. The nurse should emphasize the importance of keeping a dysreflexia diary and encourage clients to carry an AD card at all times (Vatansever, 2015).*
- ● Monitor the client for symptoms of dysreflexia, particularly those with high-level and more complete SCIs. See Defining Characteristics. EB: *This condition most commonly occurs in individuals with lesions at or above the level of sympathetic splanchnic outflow (T6), with incidence increasing with more clinically complete SCI (Solinsky et al, 2016). The most common signs and symptoms of AD are a sudden increase in systolic blood pressure (SBP) of at least 20 mm Hg from baseline, bradycardia, pounding headache, diaphoresis, flushing, and piloerection above the level of injury (Vatansever, 2015; Liepvre et al, 2017). Although bradycardia is more common, it is not uncommon for clients to develop tachycardia and cardiac arrhythmias (ACOG Committee on Obstetric Practice, 2020).*
- ▲ Collaborate with providers and caregivers to identify the cause of dysreflexia. AD is triggered by a stimulus from below the level of injury, leading to systemic vasoconstriction. The most common triggers are bladder distention, kidney stones, kink in urinary catheter, urinary tract infection, fecal impaction, pressure ulcer, ingrown toenail, menstruation, hemorrhoids, tight clothing, invasive testing, and sexual intercourse (*ACOG Committee on Obstetric Practice, 2020; Perkins, 2020*). EB: *It is important to understand that untreated AD increases the risk of stroke, myocardial infarction, retinal detachment, hypertensive encephalopathy, cardiac arrest,' seizures, and death. Recurring AD can lead to chronic cardiovascular and immune problems (Perkins, 2020).*
- ● If dysreflexia symptoms are present, immediately place client in high Fowler's position, remove all support hoses or binders, loosen clothing, check the urinary catheter for kinks, and attempt to determine the noxious stimulus causing the response. Check the client's blood pressure every 3 to 5 minutes. If blood pressure cannot be decreased following these initial interventions, notify the provider emergently (i.e., STAT). EB: *Sitting allows some gravitational pooling of blood in the lower extremities. Survey the person for instigating causes beginning with the most common cause, the urinary system. To determine the stimulus for dysreflexia:*
    - ○ First, assess bladder function. Check for distention, and if present, catheterize the client using an anesthetic jelly as a lubricant. Do not use the Valsalva maneuver or Crede's method to empty the bladder because this form of reflex voiding could worsen AD. Ensure existing catheter patency and irrigate if

necessary. Also assess for signs of urinary tract infection. EB: *Bladder distention or irritation is responsible for up to 90% of AD cases (Vatansever, 2015; O'Stephenson & Berliner, 2017).*
  - Second, assess bowel function. Numb the bowel area with a topical anesthetic as ordered and gently check for impaction. EB: *Check the rectal vault. Instill lidocaine gel into the rectum, pause for 2 minutes, and gently remove any stool (Solinsky et al, 2016).*
  - Third, assess the skin. Look for any pressure points, wounds, and ingrown toenails. EB: *Any noxious stimuli can cause AD. Although bladder and intestinal problems are most common, approximately 2% of AD cases are attributed to skin issues (Vatansever, 2015).*

- ▲ Initiate antihypertensive therapy as soon as ordered and monitor for cardiac dysrhythmias. EB: *Because of the large amount of sympathetic discharge following AD, clients in hypertensive crisis are at risk for arrhythmias, myocardial infarction, cerebral hemorrhage, seizures, and death (Perkins, 2020). Antihypertensives should be administered when SBP remains at 150 mm Hg. Nitrates and nifedipine are most commonly used for acute episodes of AD, whereas clonidine is most effective for recurrent AD (Caruso et al, 2015; O'Stephenson & Berliner, 2017; Biering-Sørensen et al, 2018).*
- ● Monitor vital signs every 3 to 5 minutes during an acute event; continue to monitor vital signs after event is resolved (e.g., symptoms resolve and vital signs return to baseline, usually up to 2 hours after the event). EB: *Monitor pulse and blood pressure every 2 to 5 minutes during an episode of AD, keeping in mind that impaired autonomic function can lead to labile blood pressure. Monitor for rebound hypotension following antihypertensive administration (O'Stephenson & Berliner, 2017).*
- ● Watch for complications of dysreflexia, including signs of cerebral hemorrhage, seizures, cardiac dysfunction, or intraocular hemorrhage. EB: *Extremely high blood pressure can cause stroke, myocardial injury and dysfunction, and death (Perkins, 2020).*
- ● Accurately and completely record any incidences of dysreflexia; especially note the precipitating stimuli. *It is imperative to determine the noxious stimuli that precipitated AD and whether the condition is recurrent, requiring the client to take medications routinely or to implement different interventions to prevent repeat incidences (Perkins, 2020).*
- ● Use the following interventions to prevent dysreflexia:
  - Ensure catheter patency and empty urinary catheter bags frequently. Assess the client for signs and symptoms of urinary tract infection during every shift. EB: *Approximately 90% of AD episodes are caused by genitourinary issues (Vatansever, 2015).*
  - Ensure a regular pattern of defecation to prevent fecal impaction. EB: *Approximately 8% of AD episodes can be attributed to the gastrointestinal system (Vatansever, 2015). A regular bowel program is essential in preventing constipation, impaction, or ileus. Topical lidocaine is useful in preventing dysreflexia from occurring during a bowel program (O'Stephenson & Berliner, 2017).*
  - Frequently change position of client to relieve pressure and prevent formation of pressure injuries. EB: *Routine weight shifts while sitting and frequent skin checks are imperative in preventing pressure injury. Any skin breakdown should be addressed by a physician or wound care personnel (O'Stephenson & Berliner, 2017).*
- ▲ Notify all health care team members of recurrent AD episodes. EB: *Recurrent dysreflexia may be caused by an occult or insidious pathophysiological process, which requires a more comprehensive workup (Biering-Sørensen et al, 2018).*
- ▲ For female clients with SCI, assess the client for AD during menstrual cycle. If the client becomes pregnant, collaborate with obstetrical health care practitioners to monitor for signs and symptoms of dysreflexia. EB: *In a recent cohort study, 60% of pregnant women with a spinal cord lesion above T6 experienced AD, with two cases resulting in cerebral hemorrhage during labor (Liepvre et al, 2017). Pregnancy in the female SCI population must be preceded by preconceptional consultation with a multiprofessional team including both prenatal and neurological specialists (Hollenbach, et al, 2020).*

Home Care

- ● The previously mentioned interventions may be adapted for home care use.
- ● Provide the client and caregiver with written information on common causes of AD and initial treatment. EB: *Despite the availability of consensus-based resources, first responders and emergency department (ED) health care professionals (HCPs) have limited knowledge regarding AD (Krassioukov et al, 2016). An AD card is available from the Craig Hospital Autonomic Dysreflexia Resources page (see* https://craighospital.org/uploads/Educational-PDFs/624.CRADEnglishWalletID.pdf*), as well as from the Christopher and*

A

Dana Reeve Foundation (see https://www.christopherreeve.org/living-with-paralysis/free-resources-and-downloads/wallet-cards*) (Christopher and Dana Reeve Foundation, 2015; Craig, 2017).*

- ● Provide resources to clients with any known proclivity toward dysreflexia. Advise them to wear a medical alert bracelet and carry a medical alert wallet card when not accompanied by knowledgeable caregivers. **EB:** *Always keep an AD emergency kit on hand. Include the following items: blood pressure cuff, lubricating jelly (for rectal check), spare urinary catheter and insertion kit, bladder irrigation kit, and prescribed antihypertensives (Craig, 2020).*
- ▲ Establish an emergency plan: maintain a current prescription of antihypertensive medication, and administer antihypertensives when dysreflexia is refractory to nonmedicinal interventions. If SBP remains over 150 mm Hg following the previously mentioned interventions, go to the nearest ED and present the AD wallet card on arrival. **EB:** *A paucity of knowledge regarding AD diagnosis and treatment still exists among ED HCPs; therefore it is important to present the wallet card on arrival to ensure safe and effective care (Krassioukov et al, 2016).*
- ● When an episode of dysreflexia has resolved, continue to monitor blood pressure every 30 to 60 minutes for the next 2 hours or admit to an institution for observation. **EB:** *AD may resolve following administration of antihypertensive medication; however, if the underlying cause is not corrected, recurrence should be expected (O'Stephenson & Berliner, 2017).*

Client/Family Teaching and Discharge Planning

- ● Teach recognition of early dysreflexia symptoms, appropriate interventions, and the need to obtain help immediately. Give client a written card describing signs and symptoms of AD and initial actions. **EB:** *If AD occurs, sit at 90 degrees and lower legs if possible, as this will help decrease blood pressure; loosen or remove anything tight (abdominal binder, compression hose or tight socks, clothes, belts, shoes or leg bag strap, external catheter tape); find and correct the cause (check bladder; is your catheter tube kinked; do you need to be catheterized; if AD occurs during bowel program, stop digital stimulation, check skin); check blood pressure; if your blood pressure is elevated and does not come down within 20 to 30 minutes, go to the ED and bring your AD wallet card (Craig, 2017).*
- ● Teach steps to prevent dysreflexia episodes: routine bladder and bowel care, pressure injury prevention, and preventing other forms of noxious stimuli (e.g., not wearing clothing that is too tight, nail care). Discuss the potential impact of sexual intercourse and pregnancy on AD. **EB:** *Sperm retrieval methods used in men with SCI lesions at T6 and above can stimulate an episode of AD (Ibrahim et al, 2016).*

REFERENCES

ACOG Committee Opinion Committee on Obstetric Practice. (2020). Obstetric management of patients with spinal cord injuries. *Obstetrics & Gynecology, 135*(5), e230–e236. https://doi.org/10.1016/j.autneu.2017.02.004.

Biering-Sørensen, F., Biering-Sørensen, T., Liu, N., Malmqvist, L., Wecht, J. M., & Krassioukov, A. (2018). Alterations in cardiac autonomic control in spinal cord injury. *Autonomic Neuroscience, 209*, 4–18. https://doi.org/10.1016/j.autneu.2017.02.004.

Caruso, D., Gater, D., & Harnish, C. (2015). Prevention of recurrent autonomic dysreflexia: A survey of current practice. *Clinical Autonomic Research, 25*, 293. https://doi-org.aurarialibrary.idm.oclc.org/10.1007/s10286-015-0303-0.

Christopher and Dana Reeve Foundation. (2015). *Paralysis resource Center, AD card*. Retrieved from http://www.christopherreeve.org/site/c.mtKZKgMWKwG/b.7717499/k.D633/Autonomic_Dysreflexia_AD_Card__Send_to_a_Friend/apps/ka/ecard/choosecard.asp. [Accessed 7 June 2021].

Craig. (2017). *Craig Hospital spinal cord injury handbook*. Retrieved from www.craighospital.org. [Accessed 7 June 2021]. https://craighospital.org/spinal-cord-injury-resource-library.

Craig. (2020). *Autonomic dysreflexia*. Retrieved from www.craighospital.org. [Accessed 7 June 2021]. https://craighospital.org/resources/disreflexia-autónoma.

Hollenbach, P. M., Ruth-Sahd, L. A., & Hole, J. (2020). Management of the pregnant patient with a spinal cord injury. *American Association of Neuroscience Nurses, 52*(2), 53–57.

Ibrahim, E., Lynne, C. M., & Brackett, N. L. (2016). Male fertility following spinal cord injury: An update. *Andrology, 4*, 13–26. doi:10.1111/andr.12119.

Krassioukov, A., Tomasone, J. R., Pak, M., et al. (2016). "The ABCs of AD": A prospective evaluation of the efficacy of an educational intervention to increase knowledge of autonomic dysreflexia management among emergency health care professionals. *The Journal of Spinal Cord Medicine, 39*(2), 190–196.

Liepvre, H. L., Dinh, A., Idiard-Chamois, B., et al. (2017). Pregnancy in spinal cord-injured women: A cohort study of 37 pregnancies in 25 women. *Spinal Cord, 55*, 167–171. doi:10.1038/sc.2016.138.

O'Stephenson, R., & Berliner, J. (2017). Autonomic dysreflexia in spinal cord injury. *Medscape*. Retrieved from https://emedicine.medscape.com/article/322809-overview. [Accessed 7 June 2021].

Perkins, A. (2020). Spinal cord injury: A lifelong condition. *Nursing Made Incredibly Easy, 18*(5), 34–43. Retrieved from https://journals.lww.com/nursingmadeincrediblyeasy/Fulltext/2020/09000/Spinal_cord_injury__A_lifelong_condition.7.aspx. [Accessed 7 June 2021].

Solinsky, R., Svircev, J. N., James, J. J., Burns, S. P., & Bunnell, A. E. (2016). A retrospective review of safety using a nursing driven protocol for autonomic dysreflexia in patients with spinal cord injury. *The Journal of Spinal Cord Medicine, 39*(6), 713–719.

Vatansever, N. (2015). A nursing diagnosis: Autonomic dysreflexia. *International Journal of Caring Sciences, 8*(3), 837–842.

A

Risk for Autonomic Dysreflexia Domain 9 Coping/stress tolerance Class 3 Neurobehavioral stress

Mary Beth Flynn Makic, PhD, RN, CCNS, CCRN-K, FAAN, FNAP, FCNS

NANDA-I

Definition

Susceptible to life-threatening, uninhibited response of the sympathetic nervous system post–spinal shock, in an individual with spinal cord injury or lesion at the 6th thoracic vertebra (T6) or above (has been demonstrated in patients with injuries at the 7th thoracic vertebra [T7] and the 8th thoracic vertebra [T8]), which may compromise health.

Risk Factors

Gastrointestinal Stimuli

Bowel distention; constipation; difficult passage of feces; digital stimulation; enemas; fecal impaction; suppositories

Integumentary Stimuli

Cutaneous stimulations; skin irritation; sunburn; wound

Musculoskeletal-Neurological Stimuli

Irritating stimuli below level of injury; muscle spasm; painful stimuli below level of injury; pressure over bony prominence; pressure over genitalia; range of motion exercises

Regulatory-Situational Stimuli

Constrictive clothing; environmental temperature fluctuations; positioning

Reproductive-Urological Stimuli

Bladder distention; bladder spasm; instrumentation; sexual intercourse

Other Factors

Inadequate caregiver knowledge of disease process; inadequate knowledge of disease process

At-Risk Population

Individuals with spinal cord injury or lesion exposed to extremes of environmental temperature; men with spinal cord injury or lesion who are experiencing ejaculation; women with spinal cord injury or lesion who are experiencing labor; women with spinal cord injury or lesion who are menstruating; women with spinal cord injury or lesion who are pregnant

Associated Conditions

Bone fractures; detrusor sphincter dyssynergia; digestive system diseases; epididymitis; heterotopic bone; ovarian cyst; pharmaceutical preparations; renal calculi; substance withdrawal; surgical procedures; urinary catheterization; urinary tract infection; venous thromboembolism

NIC, NOC, Client Outcomes, Nursing Interventions and *Rationales,* Client/Family Teaching and Discharge Planning, and References

Refer to care plan for **Autonomic Dysreflexia.**

Risk for Bleeding Domain 11 Safety/projection Class 2 Physical injury

Kimberly Anne Rumsey, RN, MSN, CNE

NANDA-I

Definition

Susceptible to a decrease in blood volume, which may compromise health.

Risk Factors

Inadequate knowledge of bleeding precautions

At-Risk Population

Individuals with a history of falls

Associated Conditions

Aneurysm; circumcision; disseminated intravascular coagulopathy; gastrointestinal condition; impaired liver function; inherent coagulopathy; postpartum complication; pregnancy complication; trauma; treatment regimen

NOC (Nursing Outcomes Classification)

Suggested NOC Outcomes

Blood Coagulation; Blood Loss Severity; Circulation Status; Fall Prevention Behavior; Gastrointestinal Function; Knowledge: Personal Safety, Maternal Status, Physical Injury Severity, Risk Control, Safe Home Environment, Vital Signs

Example NOC Outcome with Indicators

Blood Coagulation as evidenced by the following indicators: Clot formation/International normalized ratio (INR)/Hemoglobin (Hgb)/Platelet Count/Bleeding/Bruising/Hematuria/Hematemesis. (Rate the outcome and indicators of **Blood Coagulation:** 1 = severe deviation from normal range, 2 = substantial deviation from normal range, 3 = moderate deviation from normal range, 4 = mild deviation from normal range, 5 = no deviation from normal range.)

Client Outcomes

Client Will (Specify Time Frame)

- Identify clients at risk for bleeding and implement precautions to prevent bleeding and subsequent complications
- Identify and implement interventions to alleviate bleeding episodes
- Discuss precautions to prevent bleeding complications
- Explain actions that should be taken if bleeding happens
- Maintain adherence to mutually agreed upon anticoagulant medication and follow-up laboratory regimen
- Monitor for signs and symptoms of bleeding

NIC (Nursing Interventions Classification)

Suggested NIC Interventions

Admission Care; Bleeding Precautions; Bleeding Reduction; Blood Product Administration; Circumcision Care; Fluid Management; Health Screening; Hemorrhage Control; Neurologic Monitoring; Postpartum Care; Risk Identification; Teaching: Disease Process; Prescribed Medication; Oxygen Therapy; Shock Prevention; Surveillance; Vital Signs Monitoring

Example NIC Activities—Bleeding Precautions

Monitor the client closely for hemorrhage; Monitor coagulation studies; Monitor orthostatic vital signs, including blood pressure; Instruct the client and/or family on signs of bleeding and appropriate actions in case bleeding occurs

Nursing Interventions and *Rationales*

B

- Identify clients at risk for bleeding episodes. Consider client-related and procedure-related risk factors. EBN: *Early identification of client at risk for bleeding episode decreases morbidity related to bleeding episodes (Lopes et al, 2015).*
- Perform admission fall risk assessment. Safety precautions should be implemented for all at-risk clients. EBN: *On client admission to any health care facility, nurses should assess for fall risk factors that could increase the risk of bleeding (Health Research & Educational Trust, 2016).*
- Monitor the client at increased risk for bleeding for signs or symptoms of bleeding, including bleeding of the gums; nosebleed; blood in sputum, emesis, urine, or stool; bleeding from a wound or site of invasive procedure; petechiae; ecchymosis; and purpura. EB: *Clients at increased risk for bleeding may include older individuals (>60 years of age) and individuals with active gastroduodenal ulcer, anemia, intrapartum and postpartum women, previous bleeding episode, hypertension, labile INRs or INR greater than 3.0, low platelet count, malignancy, renal or liver failure, intensive care unit stay, drug or alcohol use, coadministration of antiplatelets and nonsteroidal antiinflammatory drugs (NSAIDs), and antithrombotic and anticoagulant therapies (Chapman et al, 2019; Sheth et al, 2020).*
- ▲ Clients with a history of cancer, current cancer, or leukemias are at a higher risk of bleeding associated with the disease and/or interplay of treatment-related factors. Risk of bleeding may be higher because of associated thrombocytopenia, platelet dysfunction, infection, and liver disease. CEB/EB: *Ensure the client is aware of signs and symptoms of bleeding and informs health care provider of changes. Prophylactic platelet transfusions or administration of medications such as mesna or tranexamic acid may be prescribed (Damron et al, 2009; Corbitt et al, 2019).*
- If bleeding develops, apply pressure over the site or appropriate artery as needed. Apply pressure dressing; if unable to stop the bleeding, then consider a tourniquet if indicated. EB: *Nonpharmacological means, such as application of pressure, may reduce bleeding (Cassell, 2017; Raval et al, 2017).*
- ▲ Collaborate on an appropriate bleeding management plan, including nonpharmacological and pharmacological measures to stop bleeding based on the antithrombotic used. EB: *Recommendations for bleeding risk prevention and management carefully weigh the risks and benefits of nonpharmacological and pharmacological interventions (Gimbel, Minderhoud, & ten Berg, 2018).*
- ▲ Monitor coagulation studies, including prothrombin time, INR, activated partial thromboplastin time (aPTT), fibrinogen, fibrin degradation/split products, and platelet counts as appropriate. EB: *New direct oral anticoagulants (DOACs) often have no requirement for routine coagulation studies; however, vigilance is still warranted because the risk for bleeding without benefit of reversal agents exists, except for dabigatran (Pradaxa), which can be reversed with intravenous (IV) idarucizumab (Praxbind) (Barras, Hughes, & Ullner, 2016; Raval et al, 2017). INR is the preferred method to evaluate warfarin therapy, typically at least 16 hours after the last dose is administered. Dose adjustments will not result in a steady-state INR value for up to 3 weeks (Witt et al, 2016).*
- Assess vital signs at frequent intervals to assess for physiological evidence of bleeding, such as tachycardia, tachypnea, and hypotension. Symptoms may include dizziness, shortness of breath, altered mental status, and fatigue. EB: *Carefully assess for compensatory changes associated with bleeding, including increased heart rate and respiratory rate. Initially, blood pressure may be stable, before beginning to decrease. Assess for orthostatic blood pressure changes (drop in systolic by >20 mm Hg and/or a drop in diastolic by >10 mm Hg in 3 minutes) by taking blood pressure with the client in lying, sitting, and standing positions (Emergency Nurses Association, 2018).*
- ▲ Monitor all medications for potential to increase bleeding, including antiplatelets, NSAIDs, selective serotonin reuptake inhibitors (SSRIs), and complementary and alternative therapies such as coenzyme Q10 and ginger. EB: *Antiplatelet medications can increase the risk of bleeding in high-risk clients. Instruct clients that ginger, when taken with medicines that slow clotting, may increase the chances for bruising and bleeding. There is a multitude of medications including over-the-counter medications and herbs/natural supplements that can interact with anticoagulants. When any of these medications are stopped or started, closer monitoring of INR may be warranted (Witt et al, 2016; Melkonian et al, 2017; Sheth et al, 2020).*

Safety Guidelines for Anticoagulant Administration: The Joint Commission National Patient Safety Goals

- ✱ Follow approved protocol for anticoagulant administration:
- Use prepackaged medications and prefilled or premixed parenteral therapy as ordered.
- Check laboratory tests (i.e., INR) before administration.

- ● Use programmable pumps when using parenteral administration.
- ● Ensure appropriate education for client/family and all staff concerning anticoagulants used.
- ● Notify dietary services when warfarin is prescribed (to provide consistent vitamin K in diet).
- ● Monitor for any symptoms of bleeding before administration. **EB:** *Standard defined protocols can decrease errors in administration (Barras, Hughes, & Ullner, 2016; Witt et al, 2016; The Joint Commission, 2020).*
- ● Anticoagulation therapy is complex and requires consistent implementation of medication reconciliation in all settings. **EBN:** *Nurses have an integral role in medication management through the education of clients.* **EB:** *Medication reconciliation at clinical transition points reduces client safety concerns (Kern et al, 2017). Risk of bleeding is reduced in clients who receive appropriate education in anticoagulant therapy use (The Joint Commission, 2020).*
- ▲ Before administering anticoagulants, assess the clotting profile of the client. If the client is on warfarin, assess the INR. If the INR is outside of the recommended parameters, notify the provider. **EB:** *Target INR for warfarin is between 2 and 3 for nonvalvular atrial fibrillation and between 2.5 and 3.5 for valvular atrial fibrillation. Risk for bleeding increases when INR is >4 and risk for thromboembolism increases when INR is <1.7. A single slightly out of range INR <0.3 units above or below therapeutic range may just be monitored. It is not recommended to skip or boost doses for a slightly out of range INR in the absence of bleeding (Barras, Hughes, & Ullner, 2016; Witt et al, 2016).*
- ▲ Recognize that vitamin K for vitamin K antagonists (e.g., warfarin, phenprocoumon, Sinthrome, and phenindione) may be given orally or intravenously as ordered for INR levels greater than 4.5 without signs of bleeding. In the case of major bleeding, prohemostatic therapies may be warranted for the rapid reversal of vitamin K antagonists (tranexamic acid, fresh frozen plasma, cryoprecipitate, platelet transfusion, fibrinogen concentrate, factor IV prothrombin complex concentrate [Kcentra], and activated prothrombin complex concentrate) (Witt et al, 2016; Corbitt et al, 2019). **EB:** *With INR levels above 4.5, it is recommended to give vitamin K rather than withholding the warfarin; administration of vitamin K is by oral or IV route, because subcutaneous and intramuscular routes result in erratic absorption (Christos & Naples, 2016).*
- ▲ Manage fluid resuscitation and volume expansion as ordered. **EB:** *A Cochrane systematic review included 69 studies and more than 30,000 critically ill client comparing colloids (starches, dextrans, gelatins, albumin, or fresh frozen plasma) to crystalloids for fluid resuscitation found minimal evidence that either solution is safer or more effective than any other (Lewis et al, 2018). CEB: Blood products (including human albumin), nonblood products, or combinations can be used to restore circulating blood volume in individuals at risk for blood losses from trauma, burns, or surgery. Administration of albumin over normal sterile saline does not alter survival rates (Damron et al, 2009).*
- ▲ Consider use of permissive hypotension and restrictive transfusion strategies when treating bleeding episodes. **EB:** *The effectiveness of permissive hypotension/hypotensive resuscitation and restricted/controlled resuscitation is still inconclusive. Additional research is needed (Kudo, Yoshida, & Kushimoto, 2017).*
- ▲ Consider discussing the coadministration of a proton-pump inhibitor alongside traditional NSAIDs or with the use of a cyclooxygenase 2 inhibitor with the prescriber. **EB:** *Risk of NSAID-related bleeding may be reduced with the use of a proton-pump inhibitor or cyclooxygenase 2 inhibitor (Witt et al, 2016).*
- ✱ Ensure adequate nurse staffing to provide a high level of surveillance capability. **EB:** *A key component in surveillance is monitoring; additional research is warranted in this area to identify new technologies and processes to optimize surveillance. The number and skill of nurses staffed in hospitals have been demonstrated to have a direct effect on client outcomes. Lower levels of nurse staffing have been associated with higher rates of poor client outcomes (Cho et al, 2016).*

Pediatric

- ▲ Recognize that prophylactic vitamin K administration should be used in neonates for vitamin K deficiency bleeding (VKDB). **EB:** *A dose of 0.5 to 1 mg vitamin K remains a standard administration for neonates to avoid VKDB and associated problems (Marchili et al, 2018).*
- ▲ Recognize warning signs of VKDB, including minimal bleeds, evidence of cholestasis (icteric sclera, dark urine, and irritability), and failure to thrive. **EB:** *Signs of classic VKDB may be mild and include delayed or difficulty feeding or bruising in 24 hours to 1 week, whereas late VKDB associated with breastfeeding may occur at 2 to 12 weeks (Marchilli et al, 2018).*
- ▲ Use caution in administering NSAIDs in children. *Ensure adequate hydration before administration of NSAIDs.*
- ▲ Monitor children and adolescents for potential bleeding after blunt trauma. **EB:** *Blunt trauma in children has been associated with early coagulopathy and subsequent bleeding requiring close monitoring to reduce*

B

rate of blood loss and minimize need for transfusions (Hagedorn et al, 2019). **EB:** *Children and adolescents who take SSRIs need to be closely monitored because the potential for bleeding exists across age groups (Laporte et al, 2017).*

Client/Family Teaching and Discharge Planning

- Teach client and family or significant others about any anticoagulant medications prescribed, including when to take, how often to have laboratory tests done, signs of bleeding to report, dietary consistency, and need to wear medic alert bracelet and precautions to be followed. Instruct the client to report any adverse side effects to his or her health care provider. *Medication teaching includes the drug name, purpose, administration instructions (e.g., with or without food), necessary laboratory tests, and any side effects. Provision of such information using clear communication principles and an understanding of the client's health literacy level may facilitate appropriate adherence to the therapeutic regimen by enhancing knowledge base (National Institutes of Health [NIH], 2016; The Joint Commission, 2020).*
- Instruct the client and family on the disease process and rationale for care. When clients and their family members have sufficient understanding of their disease process, they can participate more fully in care and healthy behaviors. Knowledge empowers clients and family members, allowing them to be active participants in their care. **EB:** *Use of written, verbal, and/or video education enhances client retention of information needed when managing potent medications. Clients actively engaged in their health care report better experiences, improved outcomes, and lower health care costs (The Joint Commission, 2020).*
- Provide client and family or significant others with both oral and written educational materials that meet the standards of client education and health literacy. **EB:** *The use of clear communication, materials written at a fifth-grade level, and the teach-back method enhances the client's ability to understand important health-related information and improves self-care safety (NIH, 2016; Hull, Garcia, & Vazquez, 2021).*

REFERENCES

Barras, M. A., Hughes, D., & Ullner, M. (2016). Direct oral anticoagulants: New drugs with practical problems. How can nurses help prevent patient harm? *Nursing and Health Sciences*, *18*(3), 408–411. https://doi.org//10.1111/nhs.12263.

Cassell, P. (2017). Risk for bleeding: A nursing perspective. *Journal of Vascular Nursing*, *35*(2), 114–115. https://doi.org/10.1016/j.jvn.2017.04.003.

Chapman, W., Siau, K., Thomas, F., et al. (2019). Acute upper gastrointestinal bleeding: A guide for nurses. *British Journal of Nursing*, *28*(1), 53–59. https://doi.org:10.12968/bjon.2019.28.1.53.

Cho, E., Lee, N. J., Kim, E. Y., et al. (2016). Nurse staffing level and overtime associated with patient safety, quality of care and care left undone in hospitals: A cross-sectional study. *International Journal of Nursing Studies*, *60*, 263–271.

Christos, S., & Naples, R. (2016). Anticoagulation reversal and treatment strategies in major bleeding: Update 2016. *Western Journal of Emergency Medicine*, *17*(3), 264–270. doi.org/10.5811westjem.2016.3.29294.

Corbitt, N., Harrington, J., Kendall, T., et al. (2019). *Prevention of bleeding*. Oncology Nursing Society [website]. Retrieved from https://www.ons.org/pep/prevention-bleeding. [Accessed 8 June 2021].

Damron, B. H., Brent, J. M., Belansky, H. B., Friend, P. J., Samsonow, S., & Schaal, A. (2009). Putting evidence into practice: Prevention and management of bleeding in patients with cancer. *Clinical Journal of Oncology Nursing*, *13*(5), 573–583. https://doi.org:10.1188/09.CJON.573-583.

Emergency Nurses Association. (2018). *Emergency nursing core curriculum* (7th ed.). St. Louis: Elsevier.

Gimbel, M. E., Minderhoud, S. C. S., & ten Berg, J. M. (2018). A practical guide on how to handle patients with bleeding events while on oral antithrombotic treatment. *Netherlands Heart Journal*, *26*(6), 241–251. https://doi.org/10.1007/s12471-018-1117-1.

Hagedorn, J. C., Fox, N., Ellison, J. S., et al. (2019). Pediatric blunt renal trauma practice management guidelines: Collaboration between the Eastern association for the surgery of trauma and the Pediatric trauma Society. *The Journal of Trauma and Acute Care Surgery*, *86*(5), 916–925. https://doi.org/10.1097/TA.0000000000002209.

Health Research and Educational Trust. (2016). *Preventing patient falls: A systematic approach from The Joint Commission Center for Transforming Healthcare Project Health Research & Educational Trust*. Retrieved from http://www.hpoe.org/Reports-HPOE/2016/preventing-patient-falls.pdf.

Hull, R.D., Garcia, D.A., & Vazquez, S.R. (2021). Patient education: Warfarin (beyond the basics). In: UpToDate, Leung, L.L.K, eds., UpToDate, Waltham, MA. Retrieved from https://www.uptodate.com/contents/warfarin-beyond-the-basics. [Accessed 3 September 2021].

The Joint Commission. (2020). 2020 hospital national patient safety goals. Oakbrook Terrace, IL: The Joint Commission. Retrieved from https://www.jointcommission.org/-/media/tjc/documents/standards/national-patient-safety-goals/2020/simplified_2020-hap-npsgs-eff-july-final.pdf. [Accessed 8 June 2021].

Kern, E., Dingae, M. B., Langmack, E. L., Juarez, C., Cott, G., & Meadows, S. K. (2017). Measuring to improve medication reconciliation in a large subspecialty outpatient practice. *The Joint Commission on Quality and Patient Safety*, *43*, 212–223. https://doi.org/10.1016/j.jcjq.2017.02.00.

Kudo, D., Yoshida, Y., & Kushimoto, S. (2017). Permissive hypotension/hypotensive resuscitation and restricted/controlled resuscitation in patients with severe trauma. *Journal of Intensive Care*, *5*(11). https://doi/org/10.1186/s40560-016-0202-z.

Laporte, S., Chapelle, C., Caillet, P., et al. (2017). Bleeding risk under selective serotonin reuptake inhibitor (SSRI) antidepressants: A meta-analysis of observational studies. *Pharmacological Research*, *118*, 19–32. https://doi.org/10.1016/j.phrs.2016.08.017.

Lewis, S. R., Pritchard, M. W., Evans, D. J. W., et al. (2018). Colloids versus crystalloids for fluid resuscitation in critically ill people. *Cochrane Database of Systematic Reviews*, *8*, CD000567. https://doi.org/10.1002/14651858.CD000567.pub7.

Lopes, C. T., dos Santos, T. R., Brunori, E. H. F. R., Moorhead, S. A., Lopes, J. D. L., & de Barros, A. L. B. L. (2015). Excessive bleeding predictors after cardiac surgery in adults: Integrative review. *Journal of Clinical Nursing*, *24*(21), 3046–3062. https://doi.org/ 10.1111/jocn.12936.

Marchili, M. R., Santoro, E., Marchesi, A., Bianchi, S., Aufiero, L. R., & Villani, A. (2018). Vitamin K deficiency: A case report and review of current guidelines. *Italian Journal of Pediatrics, 44*(1), 36. https://www.doi.org/10.1186/s13052-018-0474-0.

Melkonian, M., Jarzebrowski, W., Pautas, E., Siguret, V., Belmin, J., & Lafuente-Lafuente, C. (2017). Bleeding risk of antiplatelet drugs compared with oral anticoagulants in older patients with atrial fibrillation: A systematic review and meta-analysis. *Journal of Thrombosis and Haemostatsis, 15*, 1500–1510. https://www.doi.org/10.1111/jth.13697.

National Institutes of Health (NIH). (2016). Clear communication: An NIH health literacy initiative. Retrieved from https://www.nih.gov/institutes-nih/nih-office-director/office-communications-public-liaison/clear-communication. [Accessed 8 June 2021].

Raval, A. N., Cigarroa, J. E., Chung, M. K., et al. (2017). Management of patients on non-vitamin K antagonist oral anticoagulants in the acute care and periprocedural setting: A scientific statement from the American heart association. *Circulation, 135*(10), e604–e633.

Sheth, K. R., Bernthal, N. M., Ho, H. S., et al. (2020). Perioperative bleeding and non-steroidal anti-inflammatory drugs: An evidence-based literature review, and current clinical appraisal. *Medicine (Baltimore), 99*(31), e20042. https://doi.org/10.1097/MD.0000000000020042.

Witt, D. M., Clark, N. P., Kaatz, S., Schnurr, T., & Ansell, J. E. (2016). Guidance for the practical management of warfarin therapy in the treatment of venous thromboembolism. *Journal of Thrombosis and Thrombolysis, 41*(1), 187–205.

B

Risk for Unstable Blood Pressure

Domain 4 Activity/rest Class 4 Cardiovascular/pulmonary responses

Mary Beth Flynn Makic, PhD, RN, CCNS, CCRN-K, FAAN, FNAP, FCNS

NANDA-I

Definition

Susceptible to fluctuating forces of blood flowing through arterial vessels, which may compromise health.

Risk Factors

Inconsistency with medication regimen; orthostasis

Associated Conditions

Adverse effects of pharmaceutical preparations; adverse effects of cocaine; cardiac dysrhythmia; Cushing's syndrome; fluid retention; fluid shifts; hormonal change; hyperparathyroidism; hyperthyroidism; hypothyroidism; increased intracranial pressure; pharmaceutical preparations; rapid absorption and distribution of pharmaceutical preparations; sympathetic responses

NOC (Nursing Outcomes Classification)

Suggested NOC Outcomes

Fatigue; Arrhythmia; Dizziness; Confusion; Blurred Vision; Circulation Status; Tissue Perfusion: Cardiac; Tissue Perfusion: Cellular; Vital Signs

Example NOC Outcome with Indicators

Tissue Perfusion: Cardiac as evidenced by the following indicators: Heart rate/Arrhythmia/Profuse diaphoresis/Nausea/Vomiting. (Rate the outcome and indicators of **Tissue Perfusion: Cardiac:** 1 = severe, 2 = substantial, 3 = moderate, 4 = mild, 5 = none [see Section I].)

Client Outcomes

Client Will (Specify Time Frame)

- Maintain vital signs within normal range
- Remain asymptomatic with cardiac rhythm (have absence of arrhythmias, tachycardia, or bradycardia)
- Be free from dizziness with changes in positions (lying to standing)
- Deny fatigue, nausea, vomiting
- Deny chest pain

NIC (Nursing Interventions Classification)

Suggested NIC Interventions

Cardiac Care; Cardiac Precautions; Hypertension Management; Hypotension Management; Dysrhythmia Management; Vital Signs Monitoring

Example NIC Activity—Vital Signs Monitoring

Note trends and wide fluctuations in blood pressure; Monitor blood pressure while client is lying, sitting, and standing before and after position change as appropriate; Monitor blood pressure after client has taken medications if possible; Monitor for central and peripheral cyanosis

Nursing Interventions and *Rationales*

- ▲ Hypertension (HTN) is a major risk factor for cardiovascular disease, placing the client at increased risk of myocardial infarction and stroke (Whelton et al, 2017). EB: *The 2017 clinical practice guidelines for the management of adults with HTN now defines HTN as a blood pressure above 130/80 mm Hg for anyone at risk of a myocardial infarction or stroke. Significant emphasis is placed on ensuring the client understands the importance of lifestyle modifications, including regular exercise and dietary changes (Whelton et al, 2017).*
- ● Provide client-specific education about the importance of a healthy lifestyle to reduce complications associated with HTN. EB: *A heart-healthy diet with low-sodium content, maintaining a normal weight, limiting alcohol consumption, and a regular exercise program can lower the client's blood pressure and associated risk of cardiovascular disease (Whelton et al, 2017).*
- ● Provide drug- and client-specific education if medications are prescribed to manage the client's HTN. *Blood pressure medications may cause hypotension or secondary complications such as electrolyte imbalances, dehydration, and orthostasis (Whelton et al, 2017).*
- ▲ Screen clients for secondary causes of HTN with abrupt onset or age <30 years. EB: *Secondary HTN should be explored so that the primary cause of the HTN is treated. The client should be evaluated for undetected renal disease, primary aldosteronism, obstructive sleep apnea (OSA), thyroid disease, and alcohol-induced HTN (Whelton et al, 2017; Wolf et al, 2018).*
- ▲ Review the client's medical history. EB: *Understanding the client's risk for secondary causes of HTN is important to establish a proper plan of care and follow-up treatments (Wolf et al, 2018).*
- ● Explore the client's subjective statements concerning poor sleep, report of snoring, and daytime fatigue. EB: *OSA compromises cardiovascular health. Assessment of OSA can be easily incorporated into practice using valid and reliable assessment tools such as STOP Bang (Nagappa et al, 2015; Miller & Berger, 2016). If OSA is assessed, the nurse should notify the provider for additional monitoring to address OSA and HTN management.*
- ● Review the client's history of arrhythmias, especially a history of atrial fibrillation. EB: *Atrial fibrillation alters cardiac output and can cause hypotension and HTN episodes that result in client falls and/or altered mentation, chest pain, and increased stroke risk (Gumprecht et al, 2019).*
- ● Review the client's current medications, both prescribed and over the counter. EB: *Many medications and over-the-counter agents can cause HTN and interfere with antihypertension treatments (Gumprecht et al, 2019).*
- ● Steroid agents, administered at higher doses (e.g., 80–200 mg/day), can trigger HTN. EB: *Teach the client to monitor blood pressure and report changes to the prescribing provider (Johns Hopkins Medicine, 2021).* EB: *Individuals who have abused anabolic steroids have been found to have HTN and aortic stiffness (Rasmussen et al, 2018).*
- ● Ask the client if they are prescribed antidepressant agents. EB: *Several antidepressant agents cause an elevation in blood pressure that may be progressively clinically significant if the diastolic blood pressure rises above 90 mm Hg (Whelton et al, 2017).*
- ● Nonsteroidal antiinflammatory drugs (NSAIDs) can induce HTN and/or interfere with antihypertensive therapy. EB: *Ask if the client uses NSAIDS, including dose and frequency of consuming these over-the-counter drugs (Whelton et al, 2017; MedlinePlus, 2021).*
- ● Overconsumption of caffeine stimulates sympathetic activity, which causes a rise in blood pressure that can be followed by a decrease in blood pressure once the effects of the caffeine have worn off. EB: *Ask the client to describe their caffeine consumption, including frequency, dose, and physical effects when consuming products containing caffeine (Turnbull et al, 2017).*
- ● Licorice consumption may trigger HTN in some clients. EB: *A systematic review and meta-analysis found that chronic licorice consumption can prolong cortisol metabolism associated with an 11β-hydroxysteroid dehydrogenase deficiency leading to HTN and a drop in plasma potassium levels. Ask the client about typical consumption of licorice and teach the client about risks associated with chronic licorice consumption (Penninkilampi et al, 2017).*

B

- Some herbal products may induce HTN and/or interfere with antihypertensive treatment. CEB/EB: *Over-the counter herbal agents are poorly regulated; however, some agents such as arnica, bitter orange, blue-cohosh, dong quai, ephedra, ginkgo, ginseng, guarana, licorice, pennyroyal oil, Scotch broom, senna, southern bayberry, St. John's wort, and yohimbine are known stimulants that may elevate blood pressure (Jalili et al, 2013; Jain et al, 2018). Ask the client about herbal agents, including dose, frequency, and reason for taking the herbal agent.*
- Alcohol is known to elevate blood pressure and increases the client's risk of HTN. EB: *Inquire about the client's typical alcohol consumption. Current recommendations suggest men should be limited to no more than two drinks per day and women to no more than one standard alcohol drink per day (Whelton et al, 2017).*
- Blood pressure may be unstable with substance abuse disorders (SUDs). Certain drugs have specific effects on the cardiovascular system. EB: *Clients may experience tachycardia along with severe hypotension or HTN with an overdose of opioid, cocaine, and synthetic cannabinoids (Akerele & Olupona, 2017).*
- Cocaine use causes increased alertness and feelings of euphoria, along with dilated pupils, increased body temperature, tachycardia, and increased blood pressure. EB: *Tachyarrhythmias and marked elevated blood pressure can be life-threatening. Cocaine overdose can present as a myocardial infarction or arterial dissection (Akerele & Olupona, 2017).*
- Cocaine overdose is a medical emergency because of the risk of cardiac toxicity. EB: *Treatment is focused on lowering body temperature with external cooling devices and antipyretic medications, administering sedation agents to treat hyperactivity, oxygen to address increased myocardial oxygen needs, and possible administration of antithrombotic agents if a myocardial infarction is suspected (Akerele & Olupona, 2017).*
- Opioid intoxication results in changes in heart rate, slowed breathing, and decrease in blood pressure leading to loss of alertness. EB: *Opioid intoxication and overdose lead to primarily respiratory arrest with subsequent cardiovascular arrest (Jones et al, 2015; Akerele & Olupona, 2017).*
- Synthetic cannabinoids are manmade, mind-altering chemicals that may be added to foods or inhaled. There is a growing availability of these designer drugs in which adverse effects are not well known. EB: *The primary effect of synthetic cannabinoid intoxication results in severe anxiety, paranoia, nausea, vomiting, and cardiovascular symptoms to include slurred speech, HTN, chest pain, skin pallor, muscle twitches, and hypokalemia that may lead to arrhythmias (Weaver, Hooper, & Gunderson, 2015; Akerele & Olupona, 2017).*
- Explore client use of wearable technology for self-monitoring heart rhythm irregularities. EB: *There is a growing body of evidence that smartwatch wearable devices are increasingly more accurate at detecting heart rate abnormalities, atrial fibrillation, and associated changes in blood pressure (Wasserlauf et al, 2019; Seshadri et al, 2020).*

Critical Care

- Monitor the client for symptoms associated with chest pain, myocardial infarction, acute HTN, and hypotension. EB: *Alterations in blood pressure, HTN, and hypotension adversely affect cardiac function and myocardial oxygen consumption that can result in myocardial muscle injury. Nursing interventions to monitor cardiac function and reduce oxygen needs should be implemented along with continuous cardiac function monitoring (Habib, 2018).*
- Clients with hypertensive crisis will require close monitoring for signs and symptoms consistent with acute renal failure, stroke, myocardial infarction, and acute heart failure. EB: *Many conditions may cause hypertensive crisis; however, uncontrolled HTN is the most common cause. Subjective symptoms include severe headache, shortness of breath, faintness, and severe anxiety (Habib, 2018).*
- Myxedema coma is an acute emergency associated with hypothyroidism that manifests with severe hypotension, bradycardia, hypothermia, seizures, and coma. EB: *Treatment focuses on supporting the client's blood pressure and restoring thyroid function by administering levothyroxine as prescribed and supporting other organ systems (Munir, 2018).*
- Thyroid storm (thyrotoxicosis) is an acute, life-threatening, hypermetabolic state induced by excessive release of thyroid-stimulating hormone (TSH). Symptoms are severe and include fever, tachycardia, HTN, congestive heart failure leading to hypotension and shock, profuse sweating, respiratory distress, nausea and vomiting, diarrhea, abdominal pain, jaundice, anxiety, seizures, and coma. EB: *Nursing care focuses on symptom management, including reducing fever and cardiovascular support (Munir, 2018).*

Pediatric

- HTN is an underrecognized disease in children. Current recommendations include annual blood pressure monitoring with more focused monitoring in high-risk children. EB: *Blood pressure monitoring should be initiated starting at age 3. Client risk factors that include obesity and inactivity should be addressed during well-child visits to reduce the cardiovascular risks associated with childhood HTN (Dionne, 2017).*
- ▲ Secondary causes of HTN should be explored in the absence of childhood obesity, known cardiovascular disease, and family history. EB: *Kidney disease should be explored as a possible etiology of unexplained HTN (Dionne, 2017).*
- Normal ranges for child and adolescent blood pressure measurements were recently updated to reflect age, gender, and weight considerations. *Revisions to the blood pressure table are intended to facilitate earlier detection of abnormal blood pressure allowing for earlier intervention to reduce the risk of end-organ injury (Flynn et al, 2017).*

Geriatric

- Risk of cardiac arrhythmias increases with advanced age, placing the client at increased risk of HTN and hypotension. EB: *Ask the client about a history of arrhythmias, feeling his or her heart "skip beats," history of falls, lightheadedness, and any associated pain or discomfort during these episodes (Gumprecht et al, 2019).*
- Comorbid cardiovascular disease risks increase with advanced age. EB: *Clients, regardless of age, should be encouraged to engage in daily physical activity, consume a heart-healthy diet, maintain ideal body weight, and monitor effects of prescribed cardiovascular medications (Whelton et al, 2017).*
- Polypharmacy is a risk for both hypotension and HTN in older clients. *Review the client's medications frequently, including prescribed and over-the-counter medications and herbal agents.*

Client/Family Teaching and Discharge Planning

- Nutritional education has been found to be an important variable in an individual maintaining cardiovascular health. EB: *Assumptions have been made that individuals understand what a healthy diet means. Current guidelines suggest that using props such as a plate and food types/portions along with practicing reading food labels are essential to client nutritional education/learning (Allison, 2017).*
- Teach the client to monitor blood pressure and to report changes in blood pressure to the provider and with each health care visit. EB: *A recent systematic review and meta-analysis found that teaching the client to properly self-monitor blood pressure, along with other cardiovascular treatments (i.e., diet, exercise, medications), has been found to clinically lower blood pressure for up to a year (Tucker et al, 2017).*

REFERENCES

Akerele, E., & Olupona, T. (2017). Drugs of abuse. *Psychiatric Clinics of North America*, *40*(3), 501–517.

Allison, R. L. (2017). Back to basics: The effect of healthy diet and exercise on chronic disease management. *South Dakota Medicine: The Journal of the South Dakota State Medical Association*, *5*, 10–18.

Dionne, J. M. (2017). Updated guideline may improve the recognition and diagnosis of hypertension in children and adolescents: Review of the 2017 AAP blood pressure clinical practice guideline. *Current Hypertension Reports*, *19*(10), 84.

Flynn, J. T., Kaelber, D. C., & Baker-Smith, C. M. (2017). Clinical practice guideline for screening and management of high blood pressure in children and adolescents. *Pediatrics*, *140*(3), e20171904.

Gumprecht, J., Domek, M., Lip, G. Y. H., & Shantsila, A. (2019). Invited review: Hypertension and atrial fibrillation: Epidemiology, pathophysiology, and implications for management. *Journal of Human Hypertension*, *33*(12), 824–836. https://doi.org/10.1038/s41371-019-0279-7.

Habib, G. B. (2018). Hypertension. In G. N. Levine (Ed.), *Cardiology secrets* (5th ed.; pp. 369–376). St. Louis: Elsevier.

Jain, S., Buttar, H. S., Chintameneni, M., & Kaur, G. (2018). Prevention of cardiovascular diseases with anti-inflammatory and anti-oxidant nutraceuticals and herbal products: An overview of pre-clinical and clinical studies. *Recent Patents on Inflammation & Allergy Drug Discovery*, *12*(2), 145–157. https://doi.org/10.2174/1872213X12666180815144803.

Jalili, J., Askeroglu, U., Alleyne, B., & Guyuron, B. (2013). Herbal products that may contribute to hypertension. *Plastic and Reconstructive Surgery*, *131*(1), 168–173.

Johns Hopkins Medicine. (2021). *Prednisone*. Johns Hopkins Vasculitis Center [website]. Retrieved from https://www.hopkinsvasculitis.org/vasculitis-treatments/prednisone/. [Accessed 8 June 2021].

Jones, C. M., Campopiano, M., Baldwin, G., & McCance-Katz, E. (2015). National and state treatment need and capacity for opioid agonist medication-assisted treatment. *American Journal of Public Health*, *105*(8), E55–E63.

MedlinePlus. (2021). *Over-the-counter pain relievers*. U.S. National Library of Medicine. Retrieved from https://medlineplus.gov/ency/article/002123.htm. [Accessed 8 June 2021].

Miller, J. N., & Berger, A. M. (2016). Screening and assessment for obstructive sleep apnea in primary care. *Sleep Medicine Reviews*, *29*, 41–51.

Munir, A. (2018). Myxedema coma. *Journal of Ayub Medical College, Abbottabad*, *30*(1), 119–120.

Nagappa, M., Liao, P., Wong, J., et al. (2015). Validation of the STOP bang questionnaire as a screening tool for obstructive sleep apnea among different populations: A systematic review and meta-analysis. *PLoS One*, *10*(12), e014367 doi:10.1371/journal.pone.0143697.

Penninkilampi, R., Eslick, E. M., & Eslick, G. D. (2017). The association between consistent licorice ingestion, hypertension and hypokalaemia: A systematic review and meta-analysis. *Journal of Human Hypertension*, *31*(11), 699–707. https://doi.org/10.1038/jhh.2017.45.

Rasmussen, J. J., Schou, M., Madsen, P. L., et al. (2018). Increased blood pressure and aortic stiffness among abusers of anabolic androgenic steroids: Potential effect of suppressed natriuretic peptides in plasma? *Journal of Hypertension, 36*(2), 277–285. https://doi.org/10.1097/HJH.0000000000001546.

Seshadri, D. R., Bittel, B., Browsky, D., Houghtaling, P., et al. (2020). Accuracy of Apple watch for detection of atrial fibrillation. *Circulation, 141*(8), 702–703. https://doi.org/10.1161/CIRCULATIONAHA.119.044126.

Tucker, K. L., Sheppard, J. P., Stevens, R., et al. (2017). Self-monitoring of blood pressure in hypertension: A systematic review and individual patient data meta-analysis. *PLoS Medicine, 14*(9), e1002389 doi:10.1371/journal.pmed.1002389.

Turnbull, D., Rodricks, J. V., Mariano, G. F., et al. (2017). Caffeine and cardiovascular health. *Regulatory Toxicology and Pharmacology, 89*, 165–185.

Wasserlauf, J., You, C., Patel, R., Valys, A., Albert, D., & Passman, R. (2019). Smartwatch performance for the detection and quantification of atrial fibrillation. *Circulation. Arrhythmia and Electrophysiology, 12*(6), e006834. https://doi.org/10.1161/CIRCEP.118.006834.

Weaver, M. F., Hooper, J. A., & Gunderson, E. W. (2015). Designer drugs 2015: Assessment and management. *Addiction Science & Clinical Practice, 10*(1), 1–9.

Whelton, P. K., Carey, R. M., Aronow, W. S., et al. (2017). ACC/AHA/AAPA/ABC/ACPM/AGS/APha/ASH/ASPC/NMA/PCNA guidelines for the prevention, detection, evaluation, and management of high blood pressure in adults: A report of the American College of Cardiology/American Heart Association Task forces on clinical practice guidelines. *Journal of the American College of Cardiology, 71*, e127–e248. Retrieved from http://www.onlinejacc.org/content/71/19/e127?_ga=2.66372653.2004839219.1542569578-506177100.1542569578. [Accessed 6 February 2022].

Wolf, M., Ewen, S., Mahfoud, F., & Böhm, M. (2018). Hypertension: History and development of established and novel treatments. *Clinical Research in Cardiology, 107*(Suppl. 2), S16–S29.

Disturbed Body Image Domain 6 Self-perception Class 3 Body image

Marina Martinez-Kratz, MS, RN, CNE

NANDA-I

Definition

Negative mental picture of one's physical self.

Defining Characteristics

Altered proprioception; altered social involvement; avoids looking at one's body; avoids touching one's body; consistently compares oneself with others; depressive symptoms; expresses concerns about sexuality; expresses fear of reaction by others; expresses preoccupation with change; expresses preoccupation with missing body part; focused on past appearance; focused on past function; focused on past strength; frequently weighs self; hides body part; monitors changes in one's body; names body part; names missing body part; neglects nonfunctioning body part; nonverbal response to body changes; nonverbal response to perceived body changes; overexposes body part; perceptions that reflect an altered view of appearance; refuses to acknowledge change; reports feeling one has failed in life; social anxiety; uses impersonal pronouns to describe body part; uses impersonal pronouns to describe missing body part

Related Factors

Body consciousness; conflict between spiritual beliefs and treatment regimen; conflict between values and cultural norms; distrust of body function; fear of disease recurrence; low self-efficacy; low self-esteem; obesity; residual limb pain; unrealistic perception of treatment outcome; unrealistic self-expectations

At-Risk Population

Cancer survivors; individuals experiencing altered body weight; individuals experiencing developmental transition; individuals experiencing puberty; individuals with altered body function; individuals with scars; individuals with stomas; women

Associated Conditions

Binge-eating disorder; chronic pain; fibromyalgia; human immunodeficiency virus infections; impaired psychosocial functioning; mental disorders; surgical procedures; treatment regimen; wounds and injuries

NOC (Nursing Outcomes Classification)

Suggested NOC Outcomes

Body Image; Self-Esteem; Acceptance Health Status: Coping, Personal Identity

B

Example NOC Outcome with Indicators

Body Image as evidenced by the following indicators: Congruence between body reality, body ideal, and body presentation/Satisfaction with body appearance/Adjustment to changes in physical appearance. (Rate the outcome and indicators of **Body Image:** 1 = never positive, 2 = rarely positive, 3 = sometimes positive, 4 = often positive, 5 = consistently positive [see Section I].)

Client Outcomes

Client Will (Specify Time Frame)

- Demonstrate adaptation to changes in physical appearance or body function as evidenced by adjustment to lifestyle change
- Identify and change irrational beliefs and expectations regarding body size or function
- Recognize health-destructive behaviors and demonstrate willingness to adhere to treatments or methods that will promote health
- Verbalize congruence between body reality and body perception
- Describe, touch, or observe affected body part
- Demonstrate social involvement rather than avoidance and use adaptive coping and/or social skills
- Use cognitive strategies or other coping skills to improve perception of body image and enhance functioning
- Use strategies to enhance appearance (e.g., wig, clothing)

NIC (Nursing Interventions Classification)

Suggested NIC Interventions

Body Image Enhancement; Counseling; Eating Disorders Management; Referral; Self-Awareness Enhancement; Self-Esteem Enhancement; Support Group; Therapy Group; Weight Gain Assistance

Example NIC Activities—Body Image Enhancement

Determine client's body image expectations based on developmental stage; Assist client to identify actions that will enhance appearance

Nursing Interventions and *Rationales*

- Incorporate psychosocial questions related to body image as part of nursing assessment to identify clients at risk for body image disturbance.
- Maintain awareness of conditions or changes that are likely to cause a disturbed body image: removal of a body part or change/loss of body function such as blindness or hearing loss, cancer survivors, clients with eating disorders, burns, skin disorders, or those with stomas or other disfiguring conditions, or a loss of perceived attractiveness such as hair loss.
- Incorporate an appropriate body image assessment tool or questions to identify clients at risk for body image disturbance. EB: *A systematic review of body image assessments supported the majority of measures in terms of reliability and validity, but suitability varied across populations and some measurement properties were insufficiently evaluated (Kling et al, 2019).*
- Assess the impact of body image on sexual function and sexuality. EB: *A study of clients with urticaria found that 57.8% of the clients reported that their sexual life was affected by chronic urticaria. These individuals had lower body image and sexual self-confidence scores (Simsek et al, 2020).*
- Be aware of the impact of treatments and surgeries that involve the face and neck and be prepared to address the client's psychosocial needs. EB: *A cross-sectional survey of 150 clients with head and neck cancer demonstrated that radical neck surgery has a significant impact on their body image (Hung et al, 2017).*
- Maintain understanding that age, gender, and other demographic identifiers may be associated with higher degrees of body image disturbance. EB: *A study of body image disturbance in clients with stomas was demonstrated to be higher in males, younger adults, and overweight clients (Jayarajah & Samarasekera, 2017).*
- Consideration should be given to providing counseling for women with breast cancer to assist with acceptance of the reality of the disease and to increase their resilience against breast surgery. EB: *Current*

B

research supports previous findings regarding the change in body image satisfaction following breast surgery (Mushtaq & Naz, 2017).

- Offer breast cancer clients with appearance-related treatment side effects a beauty care intervention. Beauty care interventions can consist of make-up, hair care, or a photo shoot. **EB:** *A study found that clients with breast cancer who received beauty care interventions reported fewer symptoms of depression, higher quality of life, and higher self-esteem (Richard et al, 2019).*
- Encourage individuals to express self-compassion related to their body image through writing. **EB:** *A study found that a self-compassion writing intervention improved body dissatisfaction (Moffitt, Neumann, & Williamson, 2018).*
- Nurses and other health professionals should support clients with stomas in problem-focused coping strategies. **EBN:** *It is also important for nurses to encourage clients to have contact with their friends and family, as well as stoma support groups (Burch, 2017).*

Pediatric

- Many of the previously mentioned interventions are appropriate for the pediatric client.
- Educate parents on the role their own attitudes play in a child's body perception and acceptance. **EB:** *A recent study confirms previous research demonstrating that body dissatisfaction is related to internalization of a socially acceptable body size and the pressure to change body shape among parents. There is an elevated risk that parents can model negative body attitudes to their children (Kościcka et al, 2016).*
- Avoid or redirect fat talk or negative comments about one's body. **EB:** *A meta-analysis found that fat talk is related to a broader range of body image constructs and suggests that fat talk is a risk factor for body image issues (Mills & Fuller-Tyszkiewicz, 2017).*
- For adolescent clients, incorporate media literacy interventions to promote a healthy body image. Media literacy interventions are designed to influence media-related beliefs and attitudes to prevent risky behaviors. **EB:** *A study using media literacy-based healthy body image interventions found change in positive embodiment and health-related quality of life among participants (Sundgot-Borgen et al, 2019).*
- When caring for adolescents, be aware of the impact of acne vulgaris on body image and mental health. Assess for symptoms of social withdrawal, limited eye contact, and expressions of low self-esteem. Provide education on skin care and hygiene, and assist with referrals to a dermatologist as needed. **EB:** *A review of studies indicated that acne vulgaris has a substantial negative impact on clients' self-esteem and body image (Gallitano & Berson, 2017).*

Geriatric

- Assess older adults with chronic illness for body image issues. **EB:** *Research suggests that chronic illness may elevate risk for body dissatisfaction in older adults (Rakhkovskaya & Holland, 2017).*

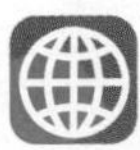

Multicultural

- Acknowledge that body image disturbances can affect all individuals regardless of culture, race, or ethnicity. Assess for the influence of cultural beliefs, regional norms, and values on the client's body image. **EB:** *A study of Indian college students found that males were slightly more at risk for eating disorders than female students (Chaudhari et al, 2017), and another study found some discrepancies in body image perception correlated to ethnicity (Goldzak-Kunik & Leshem, 2017). A study of Brazilian women found that a significant number of those studied reported having a worse quality of life associated with being overweight or underweight (Medeiros de Morais et al, 2017).*

Home Care

- The previously mentioned interventions may be adapted for home care use.
- Assess client's level of social support. Social support is one of the determinants of the client's recovery and emotional health.
- Assess family/caregiver level of acceptance of the client's body changes.
- Encourage clients to discuss concerns related to sexuality and provide support or information as indicated. Many conditions that affect body image also affect sexuality.
- Teach all aspects of care. Involve clients and caregivers in self-care as soon as possible. Do this in stages if clients still have difficulty looking at or touching a changed body part.

Client/Family Teaching and Discharge Planning

B

- Advise clients with a stoma about the support available to them. EBN: *Proper discharge preparation for clients with a stoma involves the anticipation of psychological issues and depression and support to manage these issues (Burch, 2017).*

REFERENCES

Burch, J. (2017). Post-discharge care for patients following stoma formation: What the nurse needs to know. *Nursing Standard, 31*(51), 41–45. https://doi.org/10.7748/ns.2017.e10198.

Chaudhari, B., Tewari, A., Vanka, J., Kumar, S., & Saldanha, D. (2017). The relationship of eating disorders risk with body mass index, body image and self-esteem among medical students. *Annals of Medical and Health Sciences Research, 7*(3), 144–149.

Gallitano, S. M., & Berson, D. S. (2017). How acne bumps cause the blues: The influence of acne vulgaris on self-esteem. *International Journal of Women's Dermatology, 4*(1), 12–17. https://doi.org/10.1016/j.ijwd.2017.10.004.

Goldzak-Kunik, G., & Leshem, M. (2017). Body image drawings dissociate ethnic differences and anorexia in adolescent girls. *Child and Adolescent Psychiatry and Mental Health, 11*, 13. https://doi.org/10.1186/s13034-017-0150-y.

Hung, T. M., Lin, C. R., Chi, Y. C., et al. (2017). Body image in head and neck cancer patients treated with radiotherapy: The impact of surgical procedures. *Health and Quality of Life Outcomes, 15*(1), 165.

Jayarajah, U., & Samarasekera, D. N. (2017). Psychological adaptation to alteration of body image among stoma patients: A descriptive study. *Indian Journal of Psychological Medicine, 39*(1), 63–68. https://doi.org/10.4103/0253-7176.198944.

Kling, J., Kwakkenbos, L., Diedrichs, P. C., et al. (2019). Systematic review of body image measures. *Body Image, 30*, 170–211. https://doi.org/10.1016/j.bodyim.2019.06.006.

Kościcka, K., Czepczor, K., & Brytek-Matera, A. (2016). Body size attitudes and body image perception among preschool children and their parents: A preliminary study. *Archives of Psychiatry and Psychotherapy, 18*(4), 28–34. https://doi.org/10.1371/journal.pone.0184031.

Medeiros de Morais, M. S., Andrade do Nascimento, R., Vieira, M. C. A., et al. (2017). Does body image perception relate to quality of life in middle-aged women? *PLoS One, 12*(9), 1–12.

Mills, J., & Fuller-Tyszkiewicz, M. (2017). Fat talk and body image disturbance. *Psychology of Women Quarterly, 41*(1), 114–129. https://doi.org/10.1177/0361684316675317.

Moffitt, R. L., Neumann, D. L., & Williamson, S. P. (2018). Comparing the efficacy of a brief self-esteem and self-compassion intervention for state body dissatisfaction and self-improvement motivation. *Body Image, 27*, 67–76. https://doi.org/10.1016/j.bodyim.2018.08.008.

Mushtaq, M., & Naz, F. (2017). Body image satisfaction, distress and resilience in women with breast cancer surgery: A within group study. *Journal of Postgraduate Medical Institute, 31*(1), 39–43.

Rakhkovskaya, L. M., & Holland, J. M. (2017). Body dissatisfaction in older adults with a disabling health condition. *Journal of Health Psychology, 22*(2), 248–254. https://doi.org/10.1177/1359105315600237.

Richard, A., Harbeck, N., Wuerstlein, R., & Wilhelm, F. H. (2019). Recover your smile: Effects of a beauty care intervention on depressive symptoms, quality of life, and self-esteem in patients with early breast cancer. *Psycho-Oncology, 28*(2), 401–407. https://doi.org/10.1002/pon.4957.

Simsek, N., Evli, M., Uzdil, N., Albayrak, E., & Kartal, D. (2020). Body image and sexual self-confidence in patients with chronic urticaria. *Sexuality and Disability, 38*(1), 147–159. https://doi.org/10.1007/s11195-019-09610-6.

Sundgot-Borgen, C., Friborg, O., Kolle, E., et al. (2019). The healthy body image (HBI) intervention: Effects of a school-based cluster-randomized controlled trial with 12-months follow-up. *Body Image, 29*, 122–131. https://doi.org/10.1016/j.bodyim.2019.03.007.

Insufficient Breast Milk Production **Domain 2 Nutrition Class 1 Ingestion**

Barbara A. Reyna, PhD, RN, NNP-BC

NANDA-I

Definition

Inadequate supply of maternal breast milk to support nutritional state of an infant or child.

Defining Characteristics

Absence of milk production with nipple stimulation; breast milk expressed is less than prescribed volume for infant; delayed milk production; infant constipation; infant frequently crying; infant frequently seeks to suckle at breast; infant refuses to suckle at breast; infant voids small amounts of concentrated urine; infant weight gain <500 g in a month; prolonged breastfeeding time; unsustained suckling at breast

Related Factors

Ineffective latching on to breast; ineffective sucking reflex; infant's refusal to breastfeed; insufficient maternal fluid volume; insufficient opportunity for suckling at the breast; insufficient suckling time at breast; maternal alcohol consumption; maternal malnutrition; maternal smoking; maternal treatment regimen

At-Risk Population

Women who become pregnant while breastfeeding

B

NOC (Nursing Outcomes Classification)

Suggested NOC Outcomes

Breastfeeding Establishment: Infant, Maternal; Breastfeeding Maintenance; Anxiety Self-Control; Parent-Infant Attachment

Example NOC Outcome with Indicators

Breastfeeding Establishment: as evidenced by the following indicators: Proper alignment/Latch on/Areolar compression/Suck reflex/Nursing minimum of 15 minutes per breast/Urinations and stools appropriate for age/Weight gain appropriated for age. (Rate the outcome and indicators of **Breastfeeding Establishment:** 1 = not adequate, 2 = slightly adequate, 3 = moderately adequate, 4 = substantially adequate, 5 = totally adequate [see Section I].)

Client Outcomes

Client Will (Specify Time Frame)

- State knowledge of indicators of adequate milk supply
- State and demonstrate measures to ensure adequate milk supply

NIC (Nursing Interventions Classification)

Suggested NIC Interventions

Lactation Counseling; Lactation Suppression; Kangaroo Care; Parent Education: Infant

Example NIC Activities—Lactation Counseling

Correct misconceptions, misinformation, and inaccuracies about breastfeeding; Provide educational material, as needed; Encourage attendance at breastfeeding classes and support groups

Nursing Interventions and *Rationales*

- Provide lactation support at all phases of lactation. EB: *Lactation support for early breastfeeding challenges can improve breastfeeding initiation, duration, and exclusivity rates (Patel & Patel, 2016; Anstey et al, 2018).*
- Assess maternal intention regarding breastfeeding and communicate routine advice to mothers without making them feel pressured or guilty. CEB: *Interactions with providers about milk supply concern evoked strong emotions among mothers (Flaherman et al, 2012).*
- Verify mothers' understanding and reinforce critical information. EB: *Ensuring mothers receive and understand the fundamental breastfeeding information is a modifiable factor to increase breastfeeding duration (Leurer & Misskey, 2015).*
- Initiate skin-to-skin holding at birth and undisturbed contact for the first hour following birth. EBN: *Immediate or early skin-to-skin holding should be common practice for healthy newborns, including those delivered by cesarean and those born at 35 weeks or more (Moore et al, 2016; Yilmaz et al, 2019).*
- Encourage postpartum women to start breastfeeding based on infant need as early as possible and reduce formula use to increase breastfeeding frequency. Use nonnarcotic analgesics as early as possible. EBN: *Mothers with intention to fully breastfeed whose infants receive formula supplementation may need additional support to attain exclusive breastfeeding by hospital discharge (Bentley et al, 2017; Huang & Chih, 2020).*
- Provide suggestions for mothers on how to increase milk production and how to determine the infant is receiving sufficient milk. EBN: *Increase in breastfeeding frequency is associated with elevated prolactin levels, increased milk production, and improved infant weight gain (Huang & Chih, 2020).*
- Instruct mothers that breastfeeding frequency, sucking times, and volume produced are variable and normal. EBN: *Implementing more effective informational, emotional, and practical support can reduce common problems experienced by multiparous mothers (Demirtas, 2015). Breastfeeding rates may be affected by a maternal perception of insufficient milk production and improved with interventions that develop maternal confidence in their breastfeeding capacity (Galipeau et al, 2018).*

B

▲ Consider the use of medication for mothers of preterm infants with insufficient expressed breast milk. **EB:** *There is inconclusive evidence supporting the efficacy and safety of natural and pharmacological galactogogues for mothers breastfeeding their healthy term infants and the effect on continued breastfeeding (Foong et al, 2020). Use of domperidone in mothers of preterm infants lacks evidence for optimal timing and dose, and safety has not been established (Asztalos et al, 2017).*

▲ *Not in the scope of practice for International Board of Lactation Consultants (IBLC) to recommend galactagogues (Brodribb & The Academy of Breastfeeding Medicine, 2018).*

Pediatric

- Provide individualized follow-up with extra home visits or outpatient visits for teen mothers within the first few days after hospital discharge and encourage schools to be more compatible with breastfeeding. **EBN:** *In a study of Hispanic and non-Hispanic White teen mothers, few breastfed to 6 months. Most common reasons for stopping included latch or suck difficulties, insufficient milk volume, painful, and competing demands of work (Cota-Robles et al, 2017).*

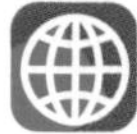

Multicultural

✱ Provide information and support to mothers on benefits of breastfeeding at antenatal visits. **EBN:** *Rates of breastfeeding initiation and duration vary based on ethnicity and race. In a study of Mexican American mothers, breastfeeding decisions were influenced by their cultural beliefs and practices, and continued breastfeeding was challenged by competing demands outside of the home, limited breastmilk supply, and personal concerns (Wambach et al, 2016).*

- Refer to care plans Interrupted **Breastfeeding** and Readiness for Enhanced **Breastfeeding** for additional interventions.

REFERENCES

Anstey, E. H., Coulter, M., Jevitt, C. M., et al. (2018). Lactation consultants' perceived barriers to providing professional breastfeeding support. *Journal of Human Lactation*, *34*(1), 51–67. https://doi.org/10.1177/0890334417726305.

Asztalos, E. V., Campbell-Yeo, M., da Silva, O. P., et al. (2017). Enhancing human milk production with domperidone in mothers of preterm infants: Results from the EMPOWER trial. *Journal of Human Lactation*, *33*(1), 181–187. https://doi.org/10.1177/0890334416680176.

Bentley, J. P., Nassar, N., Porter, M., de Vroome, M., Yip, E., & Ampt, A. J. (2017). Formula supplementation in hospital and subsequent feeding at discharge among women who intended to exclusively breastfeed: An administrative data retrospective cohort study. *Birth*, *44*(4), 352–362. https://doi.org/10.1111/birt.12300.

Brodribb, W., & The Academy of Breastfeeding Medicine (2018). ABM Clinical Protocol #9: Use of galactagogues in initiating or augmenting the rate of maternal milk production, second revision 2018. *Breastfeeding Medicine*, *13*(5), 307–314. https://doi.org/10.1089/bfm.2018.29092.wjb.

Cota-Robles, S., Pedersen, L., & LeCroy, C. W. (2017). Breastfeeding initiation and duration for teen mothers. *MCN. The American Journal of Maternal Child Nursing*, *42*(3), 173–178. https://doi.org/10.1097/NMC.0000000000000327.

Demirtas, B. (2015). Multiparous mothers: Breastfeeding support provided by nurses. *International Journal of Nursing Practice*, *21*(5), 493–504. http://doi.org/10.1111/ijn.12353.

Flaherman, V. J., Hicks, K. G., Cabana, M. D., & Lee, K. A. (2012). Maternal experience of interactions with providers among mothers with milk supply concern. *Clinical Pediatrics*, *51*(8), 778–784. https://doi.org/10.1177/0009922812448954.

Foong, S. C., Tan, M. L., Foong, W. C., Marasco, L. A., Ho, J. J., & Ong, J. H. (2020). Oral galactagogues (natural therapies or drugs) for increasing breast milk production in mothers of non-hospitalised term infants. *Cochrane Database of Systematic Reviews*, *5*, CD011505. https://doi.org/10.1002/14651858.CD011505.pub2.

Galipeau, R., Baillot, A., Trottier, A., & Lemire, L. (2018). Effectiveness of interventions on breastfeeding self-efficacy and perceived insufficient milk supply: A systematic review and meta-analysis. *Maternal and Child Nutrition*, *14*(3), e12607. https://doi.org/10.1111/mcn.12607.

Huang, S.-K., & Chih, M.-H. (2020). Increased breastfeeding frequency enhances milk production and infant weight gain: Correlation with the basal maternal prolactin level. *Breastfeeding Medicine*, *15*(10), 639–645. http://doi.org/10.1089/bfm.2020.0024.

Leurer, M. D., & Misskey, E. (2015). "Be positive as well as realistic": A qualitative description analysis of information gaps experienced by breastfeeding mothers. *International Breastfeeding Journal*, *10*, 10. https://doi.org/10.1186/s13006-015-0036-7.

Moore, E. R., Bergman, N., Anderson, G. C., & Medley, N. (2016). Early skin-to-skin contact for mothers and their healthy newborn infants. *Cochrane Database of Systematic Reviews*, *11*, CD003519. https://doi.org/10.1002/14651858.CD003519.pub4.

Patel, S., & Patel, S. (2016). The effectiveness of lactation consultants and lactation counselors on breastfeeding outcomes. *Journal of Human Lactation*, *32*(3), 530–541. https://doi.org/10.1177/0890334415618668.

Wambach, K., Domian, E. W., Page-Goertz, S., Wurtz, H., & Hoffman, K. (2016). Exclusive breastfeeding experiences among Mexican American women. *Journal of Human Lactation*, *32*(1), 103–111. https://doi.org/10.1177/0890334415599400.

Yilmaz, F., Küçükoglu, S., Özdemir, A. A., Oğul, T., & Aşki, N. (2019). The effect of kangaroo mother care, provided in the early postpartum period, on the breastfeeding self-efficacy level of mothers and the perceived insufficient milk supply. *Journal of Perinatal & Neonatal Nursing*, *34*(1), 80–87. https://doi.org/10.1097/JPN.0000000000000434.

Ineffective Breastfeeding Domain 2 Nutrition Class 1 Ingestion

Barbara A. Reyna, PhD, RN, NNP-BC

NANDA-I

Definition

Difficulty providing milk from the breast, which may compromise nutritional status of the infant/child.

Defining Characteristics

Infant or Child

Arching at breast; crying at breast; crying within 1 hour after breastfeeding; fussing within 1 hour after breastfeeding; infant inability to latch on to maternal breast correctly; inadequate stooling; inadequate weight gain; resisting latching on to breast; sustained weight loss; unresponsive to other comfort measures; unsustained suckling at breast

Mother

Insufficient emptying of each breast during feeding; insufficient signs of oxytocin release; perceived inadequate milk supply; sore nipples persisting beyond first week

Related Factors

Delayed stage II lactogenesis; inadequate family support; inadequate parental knowledge regarding breastfeeding techniques; inadequate parental knowledge regarding importance of breastfeeding; ineffective infant suck-swallow response; insufficient breast milk production; insufficient opportunity for suckling at breast; interrupted breastfeeding; maternal ambivalence; maternal anxiety; maternal breast anomaly; maternal fatigue; maternal obesity; maternal pain; pacifier use; supplemental feedings with artificial nipple

At-Risk Population

Individuals with history of breast surgery; individuals with history of breastfeeding failure; premature infants; women with short maternity leave

Associated Conditions

Oropharyngeal defect

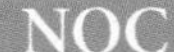

NOC (Nursing Outcomes Classification)

Suggested NOC Outcomes and Example

Breastfeeding Establishment: Infant/Maternal; Breastfeeding Maintenance; Knowledge: Breastfeeding; Refer to care plan for Readiness for Enhanced **Breastfeeding**

Client Outcomes

Client Will (Specify Time Frame)

- Achieve effective milk transfer (dyad)
- Verbalize/demonstrate techniques to manage breastfeeding problems (mother)
- Manifest signs of adequate intake at the breast (infant)
- Manifest positive self-esteem in relation to the infant feeding process (mother)
- Explain alternative method of infant feeding if unable to continue exclusive breastfeeding (mother)

NIC (Nursing Interventions Classification)

Suggested NIC Interventions

Referral; Lactation Counseling; Teaching Infant Nutrition 0-3 Months

B

Nursing Interventions and *Rationales*

- Identify women with risk factors for lower breastfeeding initiation and continuation rates, as well as factors contributing to ineffective breastfeeding (see conditions listed in the section Related Factors) as early as possible in the perinatal experience. EBN: *Health care professionals are well positioned to identify mothers at risk for breastfeeding challenges and to provide accurate information and support the development of breastfeeding skills, which facilitates breastfeeding confidence and success (Balogun et al, 2016; Ogbo et al, 2017).* CEB: *The Breastfeeding Self-Efficacy Scale Short Form (BSES-SF) is a reliable measure of breastfeeding self-efficacy and can be used to identify mothers who are likely to be successful and mothers needing additional support to ensure success (Dennis, 2003).*
- Provide time for clients to express expectations and concerns, and provide emotional support as needed. EBN: *Lactation consultants, nurses, and peers play a key role in the establishment and continuation of breastfeeding (Balogun et al, 2016; McFadden et al, 2017).*
- Encourage skin-to-skin holding, beginning immediately after delivery. EBN: *Skin-to-skin holding is associated with improved milk supply, early initiation of breastfeeding, and improved breastfeeding duration (Moore et al, 2016; Yilmaz et al, 2020).*
- Use valid and reliable tools to assess breastfeeding performance and identify dyads at risk for breastfeeding failure. CEB: *A study to evaluate the validity and reliability of the Infant Breastfeeding Assessment Tool (IBFAT), the Mother Baby Assessment (MBA) Tool, and the LATCH scoring system found them to be reliable and compatible to assess the efficiency of breastfeeding (Altuntas et al, 2014).* EBN: *Casal et al (2017) examined 16 instruments measuring breastfeeding attitudes, knowledge, and social support and found that not all scales demonstrated content, construct, and predictive validity.*
- Promote comfort and relaxation to reduce pain and anxiety. EB: *Women experiencing postpartum anxiety and negative postpartum mood are less likely to breastfeed exclusively and more likely to terminate breastfeeding earlier (Fallon et al, 2016).*
- Avoid supplemental feedings. EBN: *A correlation exists between formula and/or water supplements and failure to succeed with exclusive breastfeeding (Tarrant et al, 2015).*
- Teach mother to observe for infant behavioral cues and responses to breastfeeding. EBN: *Providing support and education to mother will build her confidence and knowledge base, and it is associated with improved breastfeeding duration and exclusivity (McFadden et al, 2017).*
- ▲ Provide necessary equipment/instruction/assistance for milk expression as needed. EB: *Expressing breast milk by hand may be more effective in the removal of milk, particularly in the immediate postpartum period, than the use of electric pumps (Becker et al, 2016).*
- ▲ Provide referrals and resources: lactation consultants, nurse and peer support programs, community organizations, and written and electronic sources of information. EBN: *Systematic reviews support the use of professionals with special skills in breastfeeding, peer support programs, and written and electronic information to promote continued breastfeeding (McFadden et al, 2017). Novel approaches to education, such as text messages to mothers and interactive online education programs for fathers/partners, have demonstrated improved breastfeeding knowledge base and self-efficacy and improved breastfeeding exclusivity rates (Abbass-Dick et al, 2017; Harari et al, 2018).*
- See care plan for Readiness for Enhanced **Breastfeeding.**

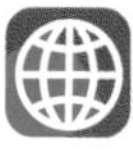

Multicultural

- Assess whether the client's cultural beliefs about breastfeeding are contributing to ineffective breastfeeding. EB: *Women from different cultures may add formula as a result of concerns that the infant is not getting enough to eat and the perception that "big is healthy" (Kuswara et al, 2016; Wandel et al, 2016).* EB: *Some traditional cultures consider colostrum unsuitable for feeding the newborn, and liquids other than breast milk may be substituted. These feedings may significantly increase the risk of infection, particularly in developing countries in which sanitation may be poor. In addition, failure to empty the breasts regularly in the early hours and days after delivery may result in suboptimal milk supply (Agho et al, 2016).*
- Assess the influence of family support on the decision to continue or discontinue breastfeeding. EBN: *Family members' impressions and ideas about breastfeeding influence breastfeeding initiation, duration, and exclusivity in Chinese mothers (Lok et al, 2017).*
- See care plan for Readiness for Enhanced **Breastfeeding.**

Home Care

- The previously mentioned interventions may be adapted for home care use.

B

- Provide anticipatory guidance in relation to home management of breastfeeding. EB: *The two most common problems experienced by breastfeeding women are nipple and/or breast pain and low (or perceived low) milk supply; these problems may be preventable with anticipatory guidance (Cleugh & Langseth, 2017; Wood & Sanders, 2018).* EBN: *For mothers returning to the workforce, longer maternity leaves and regularly pumping milk during the workday are associated with enhanced work–life balance and longer breastfeeding duration (Jantzer et al, 2018).*
- ▲ Investigate availability of support services and refer to public health department, hospital home follow-up breastfeeding program, or other postdischarge support. EBN: *Postdischarge follow-up has been associated with improved breastfeeding duration (Wood & Sanders, 2018).*
- See care plan for Risk for Impaired **Attachment.**

Client/Family Teaching and Discharge Planning

- Instruct the client on maternal breastfeeding behaviors/techniques (preparation for, positioning, initiation of/promoting latch-on, burping, completion of session, and frequency of feeding) using a variety of strategies such as written materials, videos, and online resources. EB: *Assessing breastfeeding mothers to determine knowledge deficits and providing individualized teaching facilitates breastfeeding success (Cleugh & Langseth, 2017; Nilsson et al, 2017).*
- Teach the mother self-care measures (e.g., breast care, management of breast/nipple discomfort, nutrition/fluid, rest/activity). EBN: *Painful nipples, mastitis, inadequate hydration, and fatigue are some potentially modifiable problems a breastfeeding woman may experience (McFadden et al, 2017).*
- Provide information regarding infant feeding cues and behaviors and appropriate maternal responses, as well as measures of infant feeding adequacy. EBN: *Improved knowledge base and ongoing support to learn psychomotor skills facilitate effective breastfeeding (McFadden et al, 2017).*
- Provide education to partner/family/significant others as needed. EBN: *Family members' impressions and ideas about breastfeeding influence breastfeeding initiation and duration (Lok et al, 2017).*

REFERENCES

See Readiness for Enhanced **Breastfeeding** for additional references.

Abbass-Dick, J., Xie, F., Koroluk, J., et al. (2017). The development and piloting of an eHealth breastfeeding resource targeting fathers and partners as co-parents. *Midwifery, 50*, 139–147. https://doi.org/10.1016/j.midw.2017.04.004.

Agho, K. E., Ogeleka, P., Ogbo, F. A., Ezeh, O. K., Eastwood, J., & Page, A. (2016). Trends and predictors of prelacteal feeding practices in Nigeria (2003–2013). *Nutrients, 8*(8), E462. https://doi.org/ 10.3390/nu8080462.

Altuntas, N., Turkyilmaz, C., Yildiz, H., et al. (2014). Validity and reliability of the Infant Breastfeeding Assessment Tool, the Mother Baby Assessment tool, and the LATCH scoring system. *Breastfeeding Medicine, 9*(4), 191–195. https://doi.org/ 10.1089/bfm.2014.0018.

Balogun, O. O., O'Sullivan, E. J., McFadden, A., et al. (2016). Interventions for promoting the initiation of breastfeeding. *Cochrane Database of Systematic Reviews, 11*, CD001688. https://doi.org/10.1002/14651858.CD001688.pub3.

Becker, G. E., Smith, H. A., & Cooney, F. (2016). Methods of milk expression for lactating women. *Cochrane Database of Systematic Reviews, 9*, CD006170. https://doi.org/ 10.1002/14651858.CD006170.pub5.

Casal, C. S., Lei, A., Young, S. L., & Tuthill, E. L. (2017). A critical review of instruments measuring breastfeeding attitudes, knowledge, and social support. *Journal of Human Lactation, 33*(1), 21–47. https://doi.org/10.1177%2F0890334416677029.

Cleugh, F., & Langseth, A. (2017). Fifteen-minute consultation on the healthy child: Breast feeding. Archives of Disease in Childhood. *Education and Practice Edition, 102*(1), 8–13. https://doi.org/10.1136/archdischild-2016-311456.

Dennis, C. L. (2003). The breastfeeding self-efficacy scale: Psychometric assessment of the short form. *Journal of Obstetric, Gynecologic, and Neonatal Nursing, 32*(6), 734–744. https://doi.org/ 10.1177/0884217503258459.

Fallon, V., Groves, R., Halford, J. C. G., Bennett, K. M., & Harrold, J. A. (2016). Postpartum anxiety and infant-feeding outcomes. *Journal of Human Lactation, 32*(4), 740–758. https://doi.org/10.1177/0890334416662241.

Harari, N., Rosenthal, M. S., Bozzi, V., et al. (2018). Feasibility and acceptability of a text message intervention used as an adjunct tool by WIC breastfeeding peer counsellors: The LATCH pilot. *Maternal and Child Nutrition, 14*(1), e12488. https://doi.org/10.1111/mcn.12488.

Jantzer, A. M., Anderson, J., & Kuehl, R. A. (2018). Breastfeeding support in the workplace: The relationships among breastfeeding support, work-life balance, and job satisfaction. *Journal of Human Lactation, 34*(2), 379–385. https://doi.org/10.1177/0890334417707956.

Kuswara, K., Laws, R., Kremer, P., Hesketh, K. D., & Campbell, K. J. (2016). The infant feeding practices of Chinese immigrant mothers in Australia: A qualitative exploration. *Appetite, 105*(1), 375–384. https://doi.org/10.1016/j.appet.2016.06.008.

Lok, K. Y. W., Bai, D. L., & Tarrant, M. (2017). Family members' infant feeding preferences, maternal breastfeeding exposures and exclusive breastfeeding intentions. *Midwifery, 53*, 49–54. https://doi.org/10.1016/j.midw.2017.07.003.

McFadden, A., Gavine, A., Renfrew, M. J., et al. (2017). Support for healthy breastfeeding mothers with healthy term babies. *Cochrane Database of Systematic Reviews, 2*, CD001141. https://doi.org/10.1002/14651858.CD001141.pub5.

Moore, E. R., Bergman, N., Anderson, G. C., & Medley, N. (2016). Early skin-to-skin contact for mothers and their healthy newborn infants. *Cochrane Database of Systematic Reviews, 11*, CD003519. https://doi.org/10.1002/14651858.CD003519.pub4.

Nilsson, I. M. S., Strandberg-Larsen, K., Knight, C. H., Hansen, A. V., & Kronborg, H. (2017). Focused breastfeeding counselling improves short- and long-term success in an early-discharge setting: A cluster-randomized study. *Maternal and Child Nutrition, 13*(4), e12432. https://doi.org/ 10.1111/mcn.12432.

Ogbo, F. A., Eastwood, J., Page, A., et al. (2017). Prevalence and determinants of cessation of exclusive breastfeeding in the early postnatal period in Sydney, Australia. *International Breastfeeding Journal, 12*, 16. https://doi.org/10.1186/s13006-017-0110-4.

Tarrant, M., Lok, K. Y. W., Fong, D. Y. T., et al. (2015). Effect of a hospital policy of not accepting free infant formula on in-hospital formula supplementation rates and breastfeeding duration. *Public Health Nutrition*, *18*(14), 2689–2699. https://doi.org/10.1017/S1368980015000117.

Wandel, M., Terragni, L., Nguyen, C., Lyngstad, J., Amundsen, M., & de Paoli, M. (2016). Breastfeeding among Somali mothers living in Norway: Attitudes, practices and challenges. *Women and Birth*, *29*(6), 487–493. https://doi.org/10.1016/j.wombi.2016.04.006.

Wood, N. K., & Sanders, K. A. (2018). Mothers with perceived insufficient milk: Preliminary evidence of home interventions to boost mother-infant interactions. *Western Journal of Nursing Research*, *40*(8), 1184–1202. https://doi.org/10.1177/0193945916687552.

Yilmaz, F., Küçükoglu, S., Özdemir, A. A., Oğul, T., & Aşki, N. (2020). The effect of kangaroo mother care, provided in the early postpartum period, on the breastfeeding self-efficacy level of mothers and the perceived insufficient milk supply. *Journal of Perinatal & Neonatal Nursing*, *34*(1), 80–87. https://doi.org/10.1097/JPN.0000000000000434.

Interrupted Breastfeeding Domain 2 Nutrition Class 1 Ingestion

Barbara A. Reyna, PhD, RN, NNP-BC

NANDA-I

Definition

Break in the continuity of feeding milk from the breasts, which may compromise breastfeeding success and/or nutritional status of the infant/child.

Defining Characteristics

Nonexclusive breastfeeding

Related Factors

Abrupt weaning of infant; maternal-infant separation

At-Risk Population

Employed mothers; hospitalized children; hospitalized infants; premature infants

Associated Conditions

Contraindications to breastfeeding; infant illness; maternal illness

NOC (Nursing Outcomes Classification)

Suggested NOC Outcomes

Breastfeeding Maintenance; Knowledge: Breastfeeding; Parent-Infant Attachment

Example NOC Outcome with Indicators

Breastfeeding Maintenance as evidenced by the following indicators: Infant's growth and development in normal range/Ability to safely collect and store breast milk/Awareness that breastfeeding can continue beyond infancy/Knowledge of benefits from continued breastfeeding. (Rate the outcome and indicators of **Breastfeeding Maintenance: Infant:** 1 = not adequate, 2 = slightly adequate, 3 = moderately adequate, 4 = substantially adequate, 5 = totally adequate [see Section I].)

Client Outcomes

Client Will (Specify Time Frame)

Infant

- Receive mother's breast milk if not contraindicated by maternal conditions (e.g., certain drugs, infections) or infant conditions (e.g., galactosemia)

Maternal

- Maintain lactation
- Achieve effective breastfeeding or satisfaction with the breastfeeding experience
- Demonstrate effective methods of breast milk collection and storage

B

NIC (Nursing Interventions Classification)

Suggested NIC Interventions

Bottle Feeding; Cup Feeding: Newborn; Emotional Support; Lactation Counseling

Example NIC Activities—Lactation Counseling

Instruct client to contact health care provider (lactation consultant, nurse, midwife, or physician) to assist in determining status of milk supply (i.e., whether insufficiency is perceived or actual); Encourage employers to provide opportunities and private facilities for lactating mothers to pump and store breast milk during the workday

Nursing Interventions and *Rationales*

- Provide information and support to mother and partner/family regarding mother's desire/intention to begin or resume breastfeeding. EBN: *Mothers who perceived that care providers, partners, and other family members favored exclusive breastfeeding achieved significantly higher rates of breastfeeding compared with those who perceived that care providers and family were neutral about the method of infant feeding (Radzyminski & Callister, 2015; Lok et al, 2017).*
- Clarify the indication for interrupting breastfeeding is warranted. EB: *Use of gadolinium or iodinated contrast with magnetic resonance imaging (MRI) is not an indication to interrupt breastfeeding (ACOG, 2017). LactMed is a resource to obtain the most current data on a prescribed medication during lactation. Rare exceptions exist in regard to maternal immunization and lactation (Sachs & AAP, 2013).*
- Provide anticipatory guidance to the mother/family regarding potential duration of the interruption when possible/feasible, ensuring that measures to sustain or restart lactation and promote parent–infant attachment can make it possible to resume breastfeeding when the condition/situation requiring interruption is resolved. EB: *Factors contributing to the establishment of relactation are motivation of the mother to reinitiate breastfeeding, nipple stimulation, and strong support and encouragement (Mehta et al, 2018).*
- Reassure the mother/family that the infant will benefit from any amount of breast milk provided. EBN: *One of the most common reasons mothers supplement or stop breastfeeding is their perception of the baby not getting milk and/or enough milk (Wood & Sanders, 2018).*
- Assess mother's concerns, and observe mother performing psychomotor skills (expression, storage, alternative feeding, skin-to-skin care, and/or breastfeeding) and assist as needed. EBN: *Individualized support and instruction improves likelihood of breastfeeding success (Becker et al, 2016; McFadden et al, 2017).*
- Collaborate with mother/family/health care providers (as needed) to develop a plan for skin-to-skin contact. EBN: *Skin-to-skin contact between mothers and newborns results in improved rates of exclusive breastfeeding (McFadden et al, 2017).*
- Collaborate with the mother/family/health care provider/employer (as needed) to develop a plan for expression/pumping of breast milk and/or infant feeding. EB: *Individualized education focused on evidence-based strategies to optimize milk production and extraction enhances milk quality and quantity (Becker et al, 2016).* EBN: *A supportive employee lactation program can ease the transition of returning to work (Froh & Spatz, 2016; Snyder et al, 2018).*
- Monitor for signs indicating infant's ability to breastfeed and interest in breastfeeding. EBN: *Teach the mother to recognize and respond to her baby's feeding cues and signs that her breasts are filling (McFadden et al, 2017).*
- ▲ Use formula supplementation only as medically indicated. EB: *Reducing the number of formula supplements given to infants in the hospital is associated with increased rates of exclusive breastfeeding and breastfeeding duration (Tarrant et al, 2015; Bentley et al, 2017).*
- Provide anticipatory guidance for common problems associated with interrupted breastfeeding (e.g., incomplete emptying of milk glands, diminishing milk supply, infant difficulty with resuming breastfeeding, or infant refusal of alternative feeding method). EBN: *Emotional support, as well as information regarding how to prevent and respond to breastfeeding problems, contributes to promotion of exclusive breastfeeding (Wood & Sanders, 2018; Gianni et al, 2019).*
- ▲ Initiate follow-up and make appropriate referrals.
- Provide emotional support for the mother if effective breastfeeding is not achieved and assist with learning an alternative method of infant feeding. EB: *The inability to breastfeed can be devastating for a mother and can be best supported with unconditional respect (McGuire, 2016).*
- See care plans for Readiness for Enhanced **Breastfeeding** and Ineffective **Breastfeeding.**

B

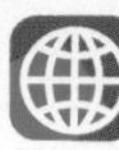

Multicultural

- Assess the client's cultural beliefs about breastfeeding and the ability to exclusively breastfeed. EBN: *A study examining breastfeeding exclusivity among immigrant and Canadian-born Chinese women found that immigrant women are at increased risk for discontinuation of exclusive breastfeeding (Dennis et al, 2019).* EB: *Some traditional cultures consider colostrum unsuitable to feed the newborn and substitute other liquids. Breast expression/pumping is needed to ensure breasts are regularly emptied and to facilitate an optimal milk supply (Agho et al, 2016).*
- See care plans for Readiness for Enhanced **Breastfeeding** and Ineffective **Breastfeeding.**

Home Care

- The previously mentioned interventions may be adapted for home care use.

Client/Family Teaching and Discharge Planning

- Teach mother effective methods to express breast milk. EB: *Expressing breast milk by hand may be more effective in the removal of milk, particularly in the immediate postpartum period, than the use of electric pumps (Becker et al, 2016).*
- Teach mother/parents about skin-to-skin care. EBN: *Skin-to-skin care promotes attachment, facilitates improved milk production, and contributes to improved rate and duration of breastfeeding (Moore et al, 2016; Crenshaw, 2019).*
- Instruct mother on safe breast milk handling and storage. EB: *Breastfeeding mothers can retain the high quality of breast milk and the health of their infant by using safe preparation guidelines and storage methods (Eglash et al, 2017).*
- See care plans for Readiness for Enhanced **Breastfeeding** and Ineffective **Breastfeeding.**

REFERENCES

See Readiness for **Enhanced Breastfeeding** for additional references.

Agho, K. E., Ogeleka, P., Ogbo, F. A., Ezeh, O. K., Eastwood, J., & Page, A. (2016). Trends and predictors of prelacteal feeding practices in Nigeria (2003–2013). *Nutrients*, *8*(8), E462. https://doi.org/ 10.3390/nu8080462.

American College of Obstetricians and Gynecologists (ACOG). (2017). Guidelines for diagnostic imaging during pregnancy and lactation. Committee opinion No. 723. *Obstetrics & Gynecology*, *130*(4), e210–e216. https://doi.org/10.1097/AOG.0000000000002355.

Becker, G. E., Smith, H. A., & Cooney, F. (2016). Methods of milk expression for lactating women. *Cochrane Database of Systematic Reviews*, *9*, CD006170. https://doi.org/ 10.1002/14651858.CD006170.pub5.

Bentley, J. P., Nassar, N., Porter, M., de Vroome, M., Yip, E., & Ampt, A. J. (2017). Formula supplementation in hospital and subsequent feeding at discharge among women who intended to exclusively breastfeed: An administrative data retrospective cohort study. *Birth*, *44*(4), 352–362. https://doi.org/10:1111/birt.12300.

Crenshaw, J. T. (2019). Healthy birth practice #6: Keep mother and newborn together—It's best for mother, newborn, and breastfeeding. *Journal of Perinatal Education*, *28*(2), 108–115. https://doi.org/ 10.1891/1058-1243.28.2.108.

Dennis, C.-L., Brown, H. K., Chung-Lee, L., et al. (2019). Prevalence and predictors of exclusive breastfeeding among immigrant and Canadian-born Chinese women. *Maternal and Child Nutrition*, *15*(2), e12687. https://doi.org/ 10.1111/mcn.12687.

Eglash, A., Simon, L., & The Academy of Breastfeeding Medicine. (2017). ABM Clinical Protocol #8: Human milk storage information for home use for full-term infants, revised 2017. *Breastfeeding Medicine*, *12*(7), 390–395. https://doi.org/10.1089/bfm.2017.29047.aje.

Froh, E. B., & Spatz, D. L. (2016). Navigating return to work and breastfeeding in a hospital with a comprehensive employee lactation program: The voices of mothers. *Journal of Human Lactation*, *32*(4), 689–694. https://doi.org/ 10.1177/0890334416663475.

Gianni, M. L., Bettinelli, M. E., Manfra, P., et al. (2019). Breastfeeding difficulties and risk for early breastfeeding cessation. *Nutrients*, *11*(10), 2266. https://doi.org/ 10.3390/nu11102266.

Lok, K. Y. W., Bai, D. L., & Tarrant, M. (2017). Family members' infant feeding preferences, maternal breastfeeding exposures and exclusive breastfeeding intentions. *Midwifery*, *53*, 49–54. https://doi.org/10.1016/j.midw.2017.07.003.

McFadden, A., Gavine, A., Renfrew, M. J., et al. (2017). Support for healthy breastfeeding mothers with healthy term babies. *Cochrane Database of Systematic Reviews*, *2*, CD001141. http://doi.org/10.1002/14651858.CD001141.pub5.

McGuire, E. (2016). Feelings of failure: Early weaning. *Breastfeeding Review*, *24*(2), 21–26. https://doi.org/10.24911/SJP.2018.1.6.

Mehta, A., Rathi, A. K., Kushwaha, K. P., & Singh, A. (2018). Relactation in lactation failure and low milk supply. *Sudanese Journal of Paediatrics*, *18*(1), 39–47. https://doi.org/10.24911/SJP.2018.1.6.

Moore, E. R., Bergman, N., Anderson, G. C., & Medley, N. (2016). Early skin-to-skin contact for mothers and their healthy newborn infants. *Cochrane Database of Systematic Reviews*, *11*, CD003519. https://doi.org/10.1002/14651858.CD003519.pub4.

Radzyminski, S., & Callister, L. C. (2015). Health professionals' attitudes and beliefs about breastfeeding. *Journal of Perinatal Education*, *24*(2), 102–109. https://doi.org/ 10.1891/1058-1243.24.2.102.

Sachs, H. C., & American Academy of Pediatrics (AAP) Committee on Drugs. (2013). The transfer of drugs and therapeutics into human breast milk: An update on selected topics. *Pediatrics*, *132*(3), e796–e809. https://doi.org/10.1542/peds.2013-1985.

Snyder, K., Hansen, K., Brown, S., Portratz, A., White, K., & Dinkel, D. (2018). Workplace breastfeeding support varies by employment type: The service workplace disadvantage. *Breastfeeding Medicine*, *13*(1), 23–27. https://doi.org/ 10.1089/bfm.2017.0074.

Tarrant, M., Lok, K. Y. W., Fong, D. Y. T., et al. (2015). Effect of a hospital policy of not accepting free infant formula on in-hospital formula supplementation rates and breastfeeding duration. *Public Health Nutrition*, *18*(14), 2689–2699. https://doi.org/10.1017/S1368980015000117.

Wood, N. K., & Sanders, K. A. (2018). Mothers with perceived insufficient milk: Preliminary evidence of home interventions to boost mother-infant interactions. *Western Journal of Nursing Research*, *40*(8), 1184–1202. https://doi.org/10.1177/0193945916687552.

Readiness for Enhanced Breastfeeding Domain 2 Nutrition Class 1 Ingestion

Barbara A. Reyna, PhD, RN, NNP-BC

B

NANDA-I

Definition

A pattern of providing milk from the breasts to an infant or child, which can be strengthened.

Defining Characteristics

Expresses desire to enhance ability to exclusively breastfeed; expresses desire to enhance ability to provide breast milk for child's nutritional needs

NOC (Nursing Outcomes Classification)

Suggested NOC Outcomes

Breastfeeding Establishment: Infant, Maternal; Breastfeeding Maintenance

Example NOC Outcome with Indicators

Breastfeeding Establishment: Infant as evidenced by the following indicators: Proper alignment and latch-on/Proper areolar grasp/Effective areolar compression/Correct suck and tongue placement/Audible swallow/Breastfeeding a minimum of 5 to 10 minutes per breast/Minimum eight feedings per day/Urinations per day appropriate for age/Weight gain appropriate for age. (Rate the outcome and indicators of **Breastfeeding Establishment: Infant:** 1 = not adequate, 2 = slightly adequate, 3 = moderately adequate, 4 = substantially adequate, 5 = totally adequate [see Section I].)

Client Outcomes

Client Will (Specify Time Frame)

- Maintain effective breastfeeding
- Maintain normal growth patterns (infant)
- Verbalize satisfaction with breastfeeding process (mother)

NIC (Nursing Interventions Classification)

Suggested NIC Intervention

Lactation Counseling

Example NIC Activities—Lactation Counseling

Provide information about psychological and physiological benefits of breastfeeding; Provide mother the opportunity to breastfeed after birth, when possible

Nursing Interventions and *Rationales*

- Encourage expectant mothers to learn about breastfeeding during pregnancy. EBN: *Individualized, needs-based health education by a health care professional, provided in the antenatal and perinatal period, is most likely to increase breastfeeding initiation rates (Jacobsen, 2018; Huang et al, 2019).*
- Encourage and facilitate early skin-to-skin contact. EBN: *Skin-to-skin holding is associated with improved milk supply, early initiation of breastfeeding, and improved breastfeeding duration (Moore et al, 2016; Yilmaz et al, 2020).*
- Encourage breastfeeding on demand and rooming-in. EB: *Breastfeeding on demand supports continued breastfeeding (Colombo et al, 2018).* EB: *Effects of rooming-in on breastfeeding duration is uncertain but there is some evidence that mothers who room-in with their infants are more likely to be exclusively breastfeeding in the short term (Jaafar et al, 2016; Ng et al, 2019).*

- Monitor the breastfeeding process, identify opportunities to enhance knowledge and experience, and provide direction as needed. **EBN:** *Individualized education focused on evidence-based strategies improves breastfeeding duration and exclusivity (McFadden et al, 2017).*
- Provide encouragement and positive feedback to mothers as they learn to breastfeed. **EBN:** *A mother's belief that she can breastfeed successfully will be more likely to lead her to exclusively breastfeed and for longer duration (Brockway et al, 2017).* **EBN:** *Lactation consultants, nurses, and peers play a key role in the establishment and continuation of breastfeeding (Balogun et al, 2016; McFadden et al, 2017).*
- Discuss prevention and treatment of common breastfeeding problems, such as nipple pain and/or trauma. **EBN:** *Emotional support, as well as information regarding how to prevent and respond to breastfeeding problems, contributes to promotion of exclusive breastfeeding (Wood & Sanders, 2018; Gianni et al, 2019).*
- Teach mother to observe for infant behavioral cues and responses to breastfeeding. **EBN:** *Providing support and education to mother will build her confidence and knowledge base, and it is associated with improved breastfeeding duration and exclusivity (McFadden et al, 2017).*
- Identify current support-person network and opportunities for continued breastfeeding support. **EB:** *Family members' impressions and ideas about breastfeeding influence breastfeeding initiation and duration (Lok et al, 2017).*
- Use formula supplementation only as medically indicated, and do not provide samples of formula on discharge from hospital. **EB:** *Reducing the number of formula supplements given to infants in hospital, and refraining from sending formula samples home, is associated with increased rates of exclusive breastfeeding and increased breastfeeding duration (Tarrant et al, 2015; Bentley et al, 2017).*

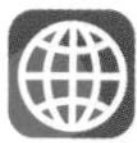

Multicultural

- Assess for the influence of cultural beliefs, norms, and values on current breastfeeding practices. **EBN:** *Women from different cultures, such as Chinese, Somali, and Hispanic women, may add formula as a result of concerns that the infant is not getting enough to eat and the perception that "big is healthy" (Kuswara et al, 2016; Wandel et al, 2016).* **EB:** *Some traditional cultures consider colostrum unsuitable for feeding the newborn and liquids other than breast milk may be substituted; thus, formula may be required to prevent hypoglycemia and dehydration, and breast expression/pumping is needed to ensure breasts are regularly emptied to facilitate an optimal milk supply (Agho et al, 2016).*

Home Care

- The previously mentioned interventions may be adapted for home care use.

Client/Family Teaching and Discharge Planning

- Include the partner and other family members in education about breastfeeding. **EB:** *Family members' impressions and ideas about breastfeeding influence breastfeeding initiation and duration (Lok et al, 2017).*
- Teach the client the importance of maternal nutrition and self-care. **CEB:** *Breastfeeding mothers should consume about 500 calories more per day than nonpregnant, nonnursing women, with a focus on nutrient-dense foods, including 200 to 300 mg docosahexaenoic acid (DHA) (the amount ingested with consumption of one to two portions of fish per week) (AAP & Section on Breastfeeding, 2012).* **EB:** *Consuming a balanced diet with adequate nutrient intakes during the breastfeeding period can affect healthy body weight and some nutrients with breastmilk (Koletzko et al, 2019).*
- Teach mother to observe for the infant's hunger cues (e.g., rooting, sucking, mouthing, hand-to-mouth and hand-to-hand activity) and encourage her to breastfeed on demand. **EBN:** *Evidence-based practice guidelines support the teaching/reinforcement of these skills as important to effective breastfeeding (McFadden et al, 2017).*
- Review guidelines for frequency of feeds (at least every 2–3 hours, or 8–12 feedings per 24 hours) and feeding duration (until suckling and swallowing slow down and satiety is reached). **EBN:** *In the first few days, frequent and regular stimulation of the breasts is important to establish an adequate milk supply; after breastfeeding is established, feeding lasts until the breasts are drained (McFadden et al, 2017).*

▲ Provide referrals and resources: lactation consultants, nurse and peer support programs, community organizations, and written and electronic sources of information. **EBN:** *Systematic reviews support the use of professionals with special skills in breastfeeding and peer support programs to promote continued breastfeeding (McFadden et al, 2017; Wood & Sanders, 2018).*

B

REFERENCES

Agho, K. E., Ogeleka, P., Ogbo, F. A., Ezeh, O. K., Eastwood, J., & Page, A. (2016). Trends and predictors of prelacteal feeding practices in Nigeria (2003–2013). *Nutrients*, *8*(8), E462. https://doi.org/10.3390/nu8080462.

American Academy of Pediatrics (AAP), & Section on Breastfeeding. (2012). Breastfeeding and the use of human milk. *Pediatrics*, *129*(3), e827–e841. https://doi.org/10.1542/peds.2011-3552.

Balogun, O. O., O'Sullivan, E. J., McFadden, A., et al. (2016). Interventions for promoting the initiation of breastfeeding. *Cochrane Database of Systematic Reviews*, *11*, CD001688. https://doi.org/10.1002/14651858.CD001688.pub3.

Bentley, J. P., Nassar, N., Porter, M., de Vroome, M., Yip, E., & Ampt, A. J. (2017). Formula supplementation in hospital and subsequent feeding at discharge among women who intended to exclusively breastfeed: An administrative data retrospective cohort study. *Birth*, *44*(4), 352–362. https://doi.org/10:1111/birt.12300.

Brockway, M., Benzies, K., & Hayden, K. A. (2017). Interventions to improve breastfeeding self-efficacy and resultant breastfeeding rates: A systematic review and meta-analysis. *Journal of Human Lactation*, *33*(3), 486–499. https://doi.org/ 10.1177/0890334417707957.

Colombo, L., Crippa, B. L., Consonni, D., et al. (2018). Breastfeeding determinants in healthy term newborns. *Nutrients*, *10*(1), 48. https://doi.org/ 10.3390/nu10010048.

Gianni, M. L., Bettinelli, M. E., & Manfra, P. (2019). Breastfeeding difficulties and risk for early breastfeeding cessation. *Nutrients*, *11*(10), 1–10. https://doi.org/10.3390/nu11102266.

Huang, P., Yao, J., Liu, X., & Luo, B. (2019). Individualized intervention to improve rates of exclusive breastfeeding. *Medicine*, *98*(47), e17822. http://doi.org/ 10.1097/MD.0000000000017822.

Jaafar, S. H., Ho, J. J., & Lee, K. S. (2016). Rooming-in for new mother and infant versus separate care for increasing duration of breastfeeding. *Cochrane Database of Systematic Reviews*, 8, CD006641. https://doi.org/10.1002/14651858.CD006641.pub3.

Jacobsen, N. (2018). Antenatal breastfeeding education and support: Summary and analysis of 2 Cochrane publications. *Journal of Perinatal and Neonatal Nursing*, *32*(2), 144–152. https://doi.org/10.1097/JPN.0000000000000323.

Koletzko, B., Godfrey, K. M., Poston, L., et al. (2019). Nutrition during pregnancy, lactation, and early childhood and its implications for maternal and long-term child health: The Early Nutrition Project recommendations. *Annals of Nutrition and Metabolism*, *74*(2), 93–106. https://doi.org/ 10.1159/000496471.

Kuswara, K., Laws, R., Kremer, P., Hesketh, K. D., & Campbell, K. J. (2016). The infant feeding practices of Chinese immigrant mothers in Australia: A qualitative exploration. *Appetite*, *105*(1), 375–384. https://doi.org/10.1016/j.appet.2016.06.008.

Lok, K. Y. W., Bai, D. L., & Tarrant, M. (2017). Family members' infant feeding preferences, maternal breastfeeding exposures and exclusive breastfeeding intentions. *Midwifery*, *53*, 49–54. https://doi.org/10.1016/j.midw.2017.07.003.

McFadden, A., Gavine, A., Renfrew, M. J., et al. (2017). Support for healthy breastfeeding mothers with healthy term babies. *Cochrane Database of Systematic Reviews*, *2*, CD001141. https://doi.org/10.1002/14651858.CD001141.pub5.

Moore, E. R., Bergman, N., Anderson, G. C., & Medley, N. (2016). Early skin-to-skin contact for mothers and their healthy newborn infants. *Cochrane Database of Systematic Reviews*, *11*, CD003519. https://doi.org/10.1002/14651858.CD003519.pub4.

Ng, C. A., Ho, J. J., & Lee, Z. H. (2019). The effect of rooming-in on duration of breastfeeding: A systematic review of randomized and non-randomised prospective controlled studies. *PLoS One*, *14*(4), e0215869. https://doi.org/10.1371/journal.pone.0215869.

Tarrant, M., Lok, K. Y. W., Fong, D. Y. T., et al. (2015). Effect of a hospital policy of not accepting free infant formula on in-hospital formula supplementation rates and breastfeeding duration. *Public Health Nutrition*, *18*(14), 2689–2699. https://doi.org/10.1017/S1368980015000117.

Wandel, M., Terragni, L., Nguyen, C., Lyngstad, J., Amundsen, M., & de Paoli, M. (2016). Breastfeeding among Somali mothers living in Norway: Attitudes, practices and challenges. *Women and Birth*, *29*(6), 487–493. https://doi.org/10.1016/j.wombi.2016.04.006.

Wood, N. K., & Sanders, K. A. (2018). Mothers with perceived insufficient milk: Preliminary evidence of home interventions to boost mother-infant interactions. *Western Journal of Nursing Research*, *40*(8), 1184–1202. doi:10.1177/0193945916687552.

Yilmaz, F., Küçükoglu, S., Özdemir, A. A., Oğul, T., & Aşki, N. (2020). The effect of kangaroo mother care, provided in the early postpartum period, on the breastfeeding self-efficacy level of mothers and the perceived insufficient milk supply. *The Journal of Perinatal & Neonatal Nursing*, *34*(1), 80–87. https://doi.org/10.1097/JPN.0000000000000434.

Ineffective Breathing Pattern **Domain 4 Activity/rest Class 4 Cardiovascular/pulmonary responses**

Debra Siela, PhD, RN, ACNS-BC, CCRN-K, CNE, RRT

NANDA-I

Definition

Inspiration and/or expiration that does not provide adequate ventilation.

Defining Characteristics

Abdominal paradoxical respiratory pattern; altered chest excursion; altered tidal volume; bradypnea; cyanosis; decreased expiratory pressure; decreased inspiratory pressure; decreased minute ventilation; decreased vital capacity; hypercapnia; hyperventilation; hypoventilation; hypoxemia; hypoxia; increased anterior-posterior chest diameter; nasal flaring; orthopnea; prolonged expiration phase; pursed-lip breathing; subcostal retraction; tachypnea; use of accessory muscles to breathe; use of three-point position

Related Factors

Anxiety; body position that inhibits lung expansion; fatigue; increased physical exertion; obesity; pain

At-Risk Population

Young women

B

Associated Conditions

Bony deformity; chest wall deformity; chronic obstructive pulmonary disease; critical illness; heart diseases; hyperventilation syndrome; hypoventilation syndrome; increased airway resistance; increased serum hydrogen concentration; musculoskeletal impairment; neurological immaturity; neurological impairment; neuromuscular diseases; reduced pulmonary complacency; sleep-apnea syndromes; spinal cord injuries

NOC (Nursing Outcomes Classification)

Suggested NOC Outcomes

Respiratory Status: Airway Patency, Ventilation; Vital Signs

Example NOC Outcome with Indicators

Respiratory Status: Ventilation as evidenced by the following indicators: Respiratory rate/Moves sputum out of airway/Adventitious breath sounds not present/Shortness of breath not present/Auscultated breath sounds/Auscultated vocalization/Chest x-ray findings (Rate each indicator of **Respiratory Status: Ventilation:** 1 = severe deviation from normal range, 2 = substantial deviation from normal range, 3 = moderate deviation from normal range, 4 = mild deviation from normal range, 5 = no deviation from normal range [see Section I].)

Client Outcomes

Client Will (Specify Time Frame)

- Demonstrate a breathing pattern that supports blood gas results within the client's normal parameters
- Report ability to breathe comfortably
- Demonstrate ability to perform pursed-lip breathing and controlled breathing
- Identify and avoid specific factors that exacerbate episodes of ineffective breathing patterns

NIC (Nursing Interventions Classification)

Suggested NIC Interventions

Airway Management; Respiratory Monitoring

Example NIC Activities—Airway Management

Encourage slow, deep breathing, turning, and coughing; Monitor respiratory and oxygenation status as appropriate

Nursing Interventions and *Rationales*

- Monitor respiratory rate, depth, and ease of respiration. *Normal respiratory rate is 10 to 20 breaths per minute in the adult (Jarvis, 2019).*
- Note pattern of respiration. If client is dyspneic, note what seems to cause the dyspnea, the way in which the client deals with the condition, and how the dyspnea resolves or gets worse. **EB:** *Ask the client if they are short of breath (Mahler & O'Donnell, 2015).* **EBN:** *When possible, use a valid and reliable objective tool, such as the Respiratory Distress Observation Scale, a numerical scale, or a visual analog scale that allows assessment of intensity of dyspnea when the client cannot self-report (Campbell, 2017).*
- Note amount of anxiety associated with the dyspnea. **EB:** *A normal respiratory pattern is regular in a healthy adult. To assess dyspnea, it is important to consider all of its dimensions, including antecedents, mediators, reactions, and outcomes (Sauls, 2021).*
- Attempt to determine if client's dyspnea is physiological or psychological in cause. **EB:** *The evaluation of a client with dyspnea continues to be dependent on a thorough history and physical examination. In the client with acute worsening of chronic breathlessness, the health care provider must be attuned to the possibility of a new pathophysiological derangement superimposed on a known disorder. Instruments or sections of instruments pertaining to dyspnea should be classified as addressing domains of sensory-perceptual experience, affective distress, or symptom/disease impact or burden (Mahler & O'Donnell, 2015; Budhwar, & Syed, 2020).*

- The rapidity of which the onset of dyspnea is noted is also an indicator of the severity of the pathological condition. EB: *Evaluate the rate and depth along with changes in mentation when assessing a client with dyspnea (Sauls, 2021).*

Psychological Dyspnea—Hyperventilation

- Monitor for symptoms of hyperventilation, including rapid respiratory rate, sighing breaths, lightheadedness, numbness and tingling of hands and feet, palpitations, and sometimes chest pain (Bickley et al, 2020).
- Assess cause of hyperventilation by asking client about current emotions and psychological state.
- Pulmonary rehabilitation programs that contain components of behavioral, cognitive, or psychosocial components have been shown to improve dyspnea and reduce anxiety and depression, particularly in clients with COPD (GOLD, 2020).
- Pharmacological treatment to reduce anxiety and panic disorders that likely increase dyspnea may not be recommended for clients with asthma and COPD (GOLD, 2020).
- Ask the client to breathe with you to slow down respiratory rate. EB: *Maintain eye contact and give reassurance. By making the client aware of respirations and giving support, the client may gain control of the breathing rate (Sauls, 2021).*
- ▲ Consider having the client breathe in and out of a paper bag as tolerated. *This simple treatment helps associated symptoms of hyperventilation, including helping to retain carbon dioxide, which will decrease associated symptoms of hyperventilation (Bickley et al, 2020).*
- ▲ If client has chronic problems with hyperventilation, numbness and tingling in extremities, dizziness, and other signs of panic attacks, refer for counseling or pulmonary rehabilitation. EB: *A systematic review and meta-analysis found that continued supervised pulmonary rehabilitation programs compared with usual care resulted in significant reduction in symptoms, improved self-report of dyspnea, and reduced risk of respiratory-cause hospital admission (Jenkins et al, 2018).*

Physiological Dyspnea

- ▲ Ensure that clients in acute dyspneic state have received any ordered medications, oxygen, and any other treatment needed. EB: *Providing oxygen and opioids is often immediately helpful in relieving acute dyspnea, and cooling the room or use of a fan has been reported by clients to ease symptoms (Baldwin & Cox, 2016).* EB: *It is important for the nurse to know different modes of oxygen delivery and percent of oxygen to avoid risks associated with oxygen toxicity (Siela & Kidd, 2017).*
- Use valid and reliable tools to evaluate perceived dyspnea. CEB/EB: *Determine intensity, unpleasantness, or distress of dyspnea using a rating scale such as an intensity-focused modified Borg scale or Respiratory Distress Observation Scale visual analog scale (Parshall et al, 2012; Campbell, 2017).*
- Ask the client to describe the quality of breathing effort. EB: *Dyspnea and breathlessness are subjective symptoms; thus asking questions as to triggers for dyspneic events, chest tightness, air hunger, inability to breathe deeply, urge to breathe, starved for air, or feeling of suffocation is important to understand and more fully address the client's dyspnea (Baldwin & Cox, 2016; Campbell, 2017).*
- Acute onset of dyspnea is often accompanied by signs of respiratory distress, which include tachypnea, cough, stridor, wheezing, cyanosis, impaired speech, tachycardia, hypotension, peripheral edema, frothy sputum, pursed-lip breathing, accessory respiratory muscle use, crackles, tripod positioning, and other signs.
- Observe color of tongue, oral mucosa, and skin for signs of cyanosis. *In central cyanosis, both the skin and mucous membranes are affected due to seriously impaired pulmonary function from unventilated or underventilated alveoli. Peripheral cyanosis (skin only) usually indicates vasoconstriction or obstruction to blood flow (Loscalzo, 2018).*
- Auscultate breath sounds, noting decreased or absent sounds, crackles, or wheezes. *These abnormal lung sounds can indicate a respiratory pathology associated with an altered breathing pattern (Bickley et al, 2020).*
- Assess for hemodynamic stability for the client with acute dyspnea. EB: *Rapid evaluation for impending respiratory failure is essential and includes fragmented speech, tripod positioning, diaphoresis, cyanosis, Pao_2 less than 50 mm Hg, $Paco_2$ greater than 70, and use of accessory muscles. Hypotension along with dyspnea indicates threat of cardiopulmonary collapse (Baldwin & Cox, 2016).*
- Monitor oxygen saturation continuously using pulse oximetry. Note blood gas results as available. *An oxygen saturation of less than 90% (normal: 95%–100%) or a partial pressure of oxygen of less than 80 mm Hg (normal: 80–100 mm Hg) indicates significant oxygenation problems (Loscalzo, 2018).*

- Using touch on the shoulder, coach the client to slow respiratory rate, demonstrating slower respirations, making eye contact with the client, and communicating in a calm, supportive fashion. The nurse's presence, reassurance, and help in controlling the client's breathing can be beneficial in decreasing anxiety. EB: *Anxiety is an important indicator of severity of client's disease with chronic obstructive pulmonary disease (COPD) (Baldwin & Cox, 2016; Campbell, 2017).*
- Support the client in using pursed-lip and controlled breathing techniques. EB: *Pursed-lip breathing may relieve dyspnea in advanced COPD. Pursed-lip breathing results in increased use of intercostal muscles, decreased respiratory rate, increased tidal volume, and improved oxygen saturation levels (Nguyen & Duong, 2020).*
- If the client is acutely dyspneic, consider having the client lean forward over a bedside table, resting elbows on the table if tolerated. EB: *Leaning forward can help decrease dyspnea, possibly because gastric pressure allows better contraction of the diaphragm. This is called the tripod position and is used during times of distress, including when walking (Baldwin & Cox, 2016; Nguyen & Duong, 2020).*
- Position the client in a semi-Fowler's position to address dyspnea symptoms. EB: *Most clients will have optimal vital capacity, when upright with arms elevated on pillows or a bedside table; however, semi-Fowler's position can facilitate better oxygen diffusion and reduce air hunger (Baldwin & Cox, 2016; Campbell, 2017; Loscalzo, 2018).*

▲ Administer oxygen as ordered. EB: *Supplemental oxygen may not relieve all dyspnea. Other interventions such as exercise, behavioral therapy, mindfulness exercises, treating anxiety, opioids, and a fan have been found to provide relief to clients with dyspnea who are not hypoxemic (Baldwin & Cox, 2016; Campbell, 2017).*

- Opioids may be used for both acute and terminal dyspnea, considering careful safe dosing for relief and side effect of constipation (Baldwin & Cox, 2016; Campbell, 2017).
- Use of music as a distraction may reduce the perception of dyspnea. EB: *A randomized control trial found that using music reduced the perceived severity of dyspnea and anxiety but did not positively affect vital signs. Using music was found to be an easy and effective intervention in addressing acute dyspnea (Ergin et al, 2018).*
- Increase client's activity to walking three times per day as tolerated. Assist the client in using oxygen during activity as needed. EB: *Walking 20 minutes per day is recommended for those unable to be in a structured program. Supervised exercise has been shown to decrease dyspnea and increase tolerance to activity (GOLD, 2020).*
- Schedule rest periods before and after activity. EB: *Respiratory clients with dyspnea are easily exhausted and need additional rest. Nurses coordinate all client care and are integral to ensuring spacing of activity to minimize or prevent dyspnea (Campbell, 2017).*

▲ Evaluate the client's nutritional status. Refer to a dietitian if needed. Use nutritional supplements to increase nutritional level if needed. EB: *The Academy of Nutrition and Dietetics strongly recommends that people with COPD have their body weight and medical nutrition therapy assessed and monitored by a registered dietitian nutritionist (Hanson et al, 2021).*

- Provide small, frequent feedings. EB: *Small feedings are given to avoid compromising ventilatory effort and to conserve energy. Clients with dyspnea often do not eat sufficient amounts of food because their priority is breathing (Hanson et al, 2021).*
- Encourage the client to take deep breaths at prescribed intervals and do controlled coughing. EB: *Pulmonary exercises, including practice with pursed-lip breathing, have been found to facilitate the client's self-care management of dyspnea symptoms (Nguyen & Duong, 2020).*
- Help the client with chronic respiratory disease to evaluate dyspnea experience to determine whether previous incidences of dyspnea were similar and to recognize that the client survived those incidences. Encourage the client to be self-reliant if possible, use problem-solving skills, and maximize use of social support. EB: *The focus of attention on sensations of breathlessness has an impact on judgment used to determine the intensity of the sensation (Campbell, 2017).*
- See care plan for Ineffective **Airway** Clearance if client has a problem with increased respiratory secretions.

▲ Refer the client with COPD for pulmonary rehabilitation. EB: *Clients receiving pulmonary rehabilitation have a significant and clinically meaningful improvement in dyspnea discomfort and also an improvement in the effect of dyspnea on activities of daily living and overall quality of life. Among the beneficial effects of pulmonary rehabilitation are a reduction in exertional dyspnea during exercise and improved exercise tolerance, as well as decreases in self-reported dyspnea with activity. Pulmonary rehabilitation benefits for COPD clients include reduction of the perceived intensity of breathlessness (GOLD, 2020).*

B

Geriatric

- Assess respiratory systems in older adults with the understanding that inspiratory muscles weaken, resulting in a slight barrel chest. EB: *Expiratory muscles work harder with use of accessory muscles (Mahler, 2017).*
- Encourage ambulation as tolerated. EB: *Immobility is harmful to older adults because it decreases ventilation, increases stasis of secretions, and worsens dyspnea symptoms* (Brummel et al, 2015).
- Encourage older clients to sit upright or stand and to avoid lying down for prolonged periods during the day. EB: *Encouraging the older adult to engage in activities of daily living fosters independence and movement, which is important to increase pulmonary capacity and reduce breathlessness* (Brummel et al, 2015; Mahler, 2017).

Home Care

- Work with the client to determine what strategies are most helpful during times of dyspnea. Educate and empower the client to self-manage the disease associated with impaired gas exchange.
- Assist the client and family with identifying other factors that precipitate or exacerbate episodes of ineffective breathing patterns (e.g., stress, allergens, stairs, activities that have high energy requirements). EB: *Awareness of precipitating factors helps clients avoid them and decreases risk of ineffective breathing episodes (Baldwin & Cox, 2016; Campbell, 2017).*
- Assess client knowledge of and compliance with medication regimen. *Client/family may need repetition of instructions received at hospital discharge and may require reiteration as fear of a recent crisis decreases. Fear interferes with the ability to assimilate new information.*
- ▲ Refer the client for telemonitoring with a pulmonologist as appropriate, with use of an electronic spirometer or an electronic peak flowmeter.
- Teach the client and family the importance of maintaining the therapeutic regimen and having as-needed drugs easily accessible at all times. EB: *Appropriate and timely use of medications can decrease the risk of exacerbating ineffective breathing. The 2020 GOLD Report states that bronchodilator medications are central to management of dyspnea (GOLD, 2020).*
- Provide the client with emotional support in dealing with symptoms of respiratory difficulty. Provide family with support for care of a client with chronic or terminal illness. *Witnessing breathing difficulties and facing concerns of dealing with chronic or terminal illness can create fear in caregiver. Fear inhibits effective coping (Campbell, 2017).* Refer to care plan for **Anxiety.**
- When electrically based equipment for respiratory support is being implemented, evaluate home environment for electrical safety, such as proper grounding. Ensure that notification is sent to the local utility company, the emergency medical team, and police and fire departments. *Notification is important to provide priority service. Identify an emergency plan including when to call the health care provider or 911. Having a ready emergency plan reassures the client and promotes client safety.*
- Support clients' efforts at self-care. Ensure they have all the information they need to participate in care.
- ▲ Referral for in-home occupational therapy evaluation and teaching of energy conservation techniques and appropriate home safety (GOLD, 2020).
- ▲ Institute case management of frail elderly to support continued independent living (Mahler, 2017).

Client/Family Teaching and Discharge Planning

- Teach pursed-lip and controlled breathing techniques. EB: *Studies have demonstrated that pursed-lip breathing was effective in decreasing breathlessness and improving respiratory function* (Nguyen & Duong, 2020).
- Teach about dosage, actions, and side effects of medications. *Inhaled steroids and bronchodilators can have undesirable side effects, especially when taken in inappropriate doses.*
- Teach client progressive muscle relaxation techniques. EB: *Relaxation therapy may help reduce dyspnea and anxiety Benefits of pulmonary rehabilitation include reduction of anxiety and depression associated with COPD* (*GOLD, 2020*).
- Teach the client to identify and avoid specific factors that exacerbate ineffective breathing patterns, such as exposure to other sources of air pollution, especially smoking. If client smokes, refer to a smoking cessation program. EB: *A systematic review and meta-analysis found that multimodal smoking cessation plans (group work and medications) are often required to support a client change in smoking behavior and successful efforts to quit (Chen & Wu, 2015).*

C

REFERENCES

Baldwin, J., & Cox, J. (2016). Treating dyspnea: Is oxygen therapy the best option for all patients? *Medical Clinics of North America, 100*(5), 1123–1130. https://doi.org/10.1016/j.mcna.2016.04.018.

Bickley, L. S., Szilagyi, P., Hoffman, R. M., & Soriano, R. P. (2020). Foundations of health assessment. In *Bate's guide to physical examination* (13th ed.). Philadelphia: Lippincott, Williams and Wilkins.

Brummel, N. E., Balas, M. C., Morandi, A., Ferrante, L. E., Gill, T. M., & Ely, E. W. (2015). Understanding and reducing disability in older adults following critical illness. *Critical Care Medicine, 43*(6), 1265–1275. https://doi.org/10.1097/CCM.0000000000000924.

Budhwar, N., & Syed, Z. (2020). Chronic dyspnea: Diagnosis and evaluation. *American Family Physician, 101*(9), 542–548.

Campbell, M. L. (2017). Dyspnea. *Critical Care Nursing Clinics of North America, 29*(4), 461–470. https://doi.org/10.1016/j.cnc.2017.08.006.

Chen, D., & Wu, L. T. (2015). Smoking cessation interventions for adults aged 50 or older: A systematic review and meta-analysis. *Drug and Alcohol Dependence, 154*, 14–24. https://doi.org/10.1016/j.drugalcdep.2015.06.004.

Ergin, E., Sagkal Midilli, T., & Baysal, E. (2018). The effect of music on dyspnea severity, anxiety, and hemodynamic parameters in patients with dyspnea. *Journal of Hospice and Palliative Nursing, 20*(1), 81–87. https://doi.org/10.1097/NJH.0000000000000403.

Global Initiative for Chronic Obstructive Lung Disease (GOLD). (2020). Global strategy for the diagnosis, management, and prevention of COPD (revised 2020). *Global Initiative for Chronic Obstructive Lung Disease*. Retrieved from https://goldcopd.org/wp-content/uploads/2019/12/GOLD-2020-FINAL-ver1.2-03Dec19_WMV.pdf. [Accessed 8 June 2021].

Hanson, C., Bowser, E. K., Frankenfield, D. C., & Piemonte, T. A. (2021). Chronic obstructive pulmonary disease: A 2019 evidence analysis center evidence-based practice guideline. *Journal of the Academy of Nutrition and Dietetics, 121*(1), 139–165.e15. doi:10.1016/j.jand.2019.12.001.

Jarvis, C. (2019). General survey, measurement, vital signs. In C. Jarvis (Ed.), *Physical examination & health assessment* (8th ed.). St. Louis: Elsevier.

Jenkins, A. R., Gowler, H., Curtis, F., Holden, N. S., Bridle, C., & Jones, A. W. (2018). Efficacy of supervised maintenance exercise following pulmonary rehabilitation on health care use: A systematic review and meta-analysis. *International Journal of Chronic Obstructive Pulmonary Disease, 13*, 257–273. https://doi.org/10.2147/COPD.S150650.

Loscalzo, J. (2018). Hypoxia and cyanosis. In J. Larry Jameson, A. S. Fauci, D. L. Kasper, et al. (Eds.), *Harrison's principles of internal medicine* (20th ed.). New York: McGraw-Hill.

Mahler, D. A. (2017). Evaluation of dyspnea in the elderly. *Clinics in Geriatric Medicine, 33*(4), 503–521. https://doi.org/10.1016/j.cger.2017.06.004.

Mahler, D. A., & O'Donnell, D. E. (2015). Recent advances in dyspnea. *Chest, 147*(1), 232–241.

Nguyen, J., & Duong, H. (2020). Pursed-lip breathing. *StatPearls. Treasure Island*, FL: StatPearls Publishing. Retrieved from https://www.ncbi.nlm.nih.gov/books/NBK545289/. [Accessed 8 June 2021].

Parshall, M. B., Schwartzstein, R. M., Adams, L., et al. (2012). An official American thoracic society statement: Update on the mechanisms, assessment, and management of dyspnea. *American Journal of Respiratory and Critical Care Medicine, 185*(4), 435–452.

Sauls, J. L. (2021). Acute respiratory failure. In M. Sole, D. Klein, M. Moseley, et al. (Eds.), *Introduction to critical care nursing* (pp. 375–403). St. Louis: Elsevier.

Siela, D., & Kidd, M. (2017). Oxygen requirements for acutely and critically ill patients. *Critical Care Nurse, 37*(4), 58–70.

Decreased Cardiac Output Domain 4 Activity/rest Class 4 Cardiovascular/pulmonary responses

Ann Will Poteet, MS, RN, CNS, AGNP-C

NANDA-I

Definition

Inadequate volume of blood pumped by the heart to meet the metabolic demands of the body.

Defining Characteristics

Altered Heart Rate/Rhythm

Bradycardia, electrocardiogram change; heart palpitations; tachycardia

Altered Preload

Decrease in central venous pressure; decrease in pulmonary artery wedge pressure; edema; fatigue; heart murmur; increased central venous pressure; increased pulmonary artery wedge pressure; jugular vein distention; weight gain

Altered Afterload

Abnormal skin color; altered blood pressure; clammy skin; decreased peripheral pulses; decreased pulmonary vascular resistance; decreased systemic vascular resistance; dyspnea; increased pulmonary vascular resistance; increased systemic vascular resistance; oliguria; prolonged capillary refill

Altered Contractility

Adventitious breath sounds; coughing; decreased cardiac index; decreased ejection fraction; decreased left ventricular stroke work index; decreased stroke volume index; orthopnea; paroxysmal nocturnal dyspnea; presence of S3 heart sound; presence of S4 heart sound

Behavioral/Emotional

Anxiety; psychomotor agitation

Related Factors

To be developed

Associated Conditions

Altered afterload, altered contractility; altered heart rate; altered heart rhythm; altered preload; altered stroke volume

NOC (Nursing Outcomes Classification)

Suggested NOC Outcomes

Cardiac Pump Effectiveness; Circulation Status; Tissue Perfusion: Abdominal Organs, Peripheral; Vital Signs

Example NOC Outcome with Indicators

Cardiac Pump Effectiveness as evidenced by the following indicators: Blood pressure/Heart rate/Cardiac index/Ejection fraction/Activity tolerance/Peripheral pulses/Neck vein distention not present/Heart rhythm/Heart sounds/Angina not present/Peripheral edema not present/Pulmonary edema not present. (Rate the outcome and indicators of **Cardiac Pump Effectiveness:** 1 = severe deviation from normal range, 2 = substantial deviation from normal range, 3 = moderate deviation from normal range, 4 = mild deviation from normal range, 5 = no deviation from normal range [see Section I].)

Client Outcomes

Client Will (Specify Time Frame)

- Demonstrate adequate cardiac output as evidenced by blood pressure, pulse rate, and rhythm within normal parameters for client; strong peripheral pulses; maintained level of mentation; lack of chest discomfort, dyspnea, or edema; maintain adequate urinary output; maintain an ability to tolerate activity without symptoms of dyspnea, syncope, or chest pain
- Remain free of side effects from the medications used to achieve adequate cardiac output
- Explain actions and precautions to prevent primary or secondary cardiac disease

NIC (Nursing Interventions Classification)

Suggested NIC Interventions

Cardiac Care; Cardiac Care: Acute

Example NIC Activities—Cardiac Care

Evaluate chest pain (e.g., intensity, location, radiation, duration, precipitating and alleviating factors); Document cardiac dysrhythmias

Nursing Interventions and *Rationales*

- Recognize characteristics of decreased cardiac output including, but not limited to, fatigue, dyspnea, edema, orthopnea, paroxysmal nocturnal dyspnea, chest pain, decreased exercise capacity, weight gain, hepatomegaly, jugular venous distention, palpitations, lung rhonchi, cough, clammy skin, skin color changes, dysuria, altered mental status, anemia, and hemodynamic changes.
- Monitor and report presence and degree of symptoms including dyspnea at rest, reduced exercise capacity, difficulty with activities of daily living, orthopnea, paroxysmal nocturnal dyspnea, cough, palpitations, chest pain, distended abdomen, early satiety, fatigue, presyncope/syncope, or weakness. Monitor

and report signs including jugular vein distention, peripheral edema, firm or distended abdomen, prominent S2, S3 gallop, rales, positive hepatojugular reflux, ascites, laterally displaced or pronounced point of maximal impact, holosystolic murmur, narrow pulse pressure, cool extremities, tachycardia with pulsus alternans, pulsus paradoxus, and irregular heartbeat. CEB/EB: *These are symptoms and signs consistent with heart failure (HF) and decreased cardiac output (Yancy et al, 2013; Konstam et al, 2018).*

- ● Monitor orthostatic blood pressures, oxygenation, hemodynamic values, urine output, and daily weights. CEB/EB: *These interventions assess for fluid volume status. Peripheral edema or the lack of peripheral edema is not always indicative of hypervolemia or decreased cardiac output (Yancy et al, 2013; Konstam et al, 2018).*
- ● Recognize that decreased cardiac output can occur in a number of noncardiac disorders such as septic shock, electrolyte imbalances, and hypovolemia. Expect variation in orders for differential diagnoses related to decreased cardiac output, because orders will be distinct to address the primary cause of the altered cardiac output.
- ● Obtain a thorough client-specific and familial history. CEB/EB: *It is important to assess for cardiac and noncardiac disorders and/or behaviors that might accelerate the progression of HF symptoms, such as high-sodium diet, excess fluid intake, substance abuse, missed medication doses, hypertension, diabetes mellitus, metabolic syndrome, obesity, hyperlipidemia, hormonal abnormalities, genetic disorders, coronary artery disease, sleep disordered breathing, congenital heart disease, cancer, immune disorders, and pregnancy (Yancy et al, 2013, 2017; Bozkurt et al, 2016).*
- ▲ Monitor pulse oximetry and administer oxygen as needed per health care provider's order. Supplemental oxygen increases oxygen availability to the myocardium and can relieve symptoms of hypoxemia. Resting hypoxia or oxygen desaturation may indicate fluid overload or concurrent pulmonary disease.
- ● Place client in semi-Fowler's or high Fowler's position with legs down or in a position of comfort. Elevating the head of the bed and legs in the down position may decrease the work of breathing and may decrease venous return and preload.
- ● During acute events, ensure client remains on short-term bed rest or maintains activity level that does not compromise cardiac output.
- ● Provide a restful environment by minimizing controllable stressors and unnecessary disturbances. Reducing stressors decreases cardiac workload and oxygen demand.
- ▲ Apply graduated compression stockings or intermittent pneumatic compression (IPC) leg sleeves as ordered. Ensure proper fit by measuring accurately. Remove stockings at least twice a day, and then reapply. Assess the condition of the extremities frequently. Graduated compression stockings may be contraindicated in clients with peripheral arterial disease. CEB: *A Cochrane review that assessed use of knee-length graduated compression stockings versus thigh-length graduated compression stockings found no difference in effectiveness. Type of stocking should be determined by client preference, cost, and ease of use (Sajid et al, 2012).* EB: *Graduated compression stockings, alone or used in conjunction with other prevention modalities, help promote venous return and reduce the risk of deep vein thrombosis in hospitalized clients who have undergone general or orthopedic surgery. Further research is needed in regard to* graduated compression stockings *in medical clients not undergoing surgical procedures (Sachdeva et al, 2018).*
- ▲ Check blood pressure, pulse, and condition before administering cardiac medications (e.g., angiotensin-converting enzyme inhibitors, angiotensin receptor blockers, angiotensin receptor-neprilysin inhibitors, calcium channel blockers, diuretics, digoxin, and beta-blockers). Notify health care provider if heart rate or blood pressure is low before holding medications. It is important that the nurse evaluate how well the client is tolerating current medications before administering cardiac medications; do not hold medications without health care provider input. The health care provider may decide to have medications administered even though the blood pressure or pulse rate has lowered. EB: *Clients with preserved ejection heart failure (HFpEF) or reduced ejection fraction heart failure (HFrEF) and persistent hypertension, and those with HF and increased cardiovascular risk (age >75 years old, established vascular disease, chronic renal disease, or Framingham risk score >15%), should receive guideline-directed medical therapy (GDMT) to maintain a systolic blood pressure less than 130 mm Hg (Yancy et al, 2017).*
- ● Observe for and report chest pain or discomfort; note location, radiation, severity, quality, duration, and associated manifestations such as nausea, indigestion, or diaphoresis; also note precipitating and relieving factors. Chest pain/discomfort may indicate an inadequate blood supply to the heart, which can further compromise cardiac output. CEB: *Clients with decreased cardiac output may present with myocardial ischemia. Those with myocardial ischemia may present with decreased cardiac output and HF (Yancy et al, 2013; Amsterdam et al, 2014).*

▲ If chest pain is present, refer to the interventions in Risk for Decreased **Cardiac** Tissue Perfusion care plan.

• Recognize the effect of sleep disordered breathing in HF and that sleep disorders are common in clients with HF (Yancy et al, 2013, 2017). EB: *Central sleep apnea is recognized as an independent risk factor for worsening HF and reduced survival in clients with HF. The pathological effects of sleep apnea that contribute to worsening cardiac function include sympathetic nervous system stimulation, systemic inflammation, oxidative stress, and endothelial dysfunction (Costanzo et al, 2015).* EB: *For obstructive sleep apnea, continuous positive airway pressure (CPAP) can reduce apneic events, improve nocturnal oxygenation, and improve sleep quality (Yancy et al, 2017).*

• Administer CPAP or supplemental oxygen at night as ordered for management of suspected or diagnosed sleep disordered breathing. EB: *Both CPAP and nocturnal oxygen supplementation have been shown to reduce episodes of sleep apnea, reduce sympathetic nervous system stimulation, reduce occurrence of atrial arrhythmias, and improve cardiac function (Costanzo et al, 2015; Yancy et al, 2017).*

▲ Closely monitor fluid intake, including intravenous lines. Maintain fluid restriction if ordered. Clients with decreased cardiac output, poorly functioning ventricles, and ventricular dysfunction may not tolerate increased fluid volumes. CEB: *Fluid restriction along with sodium restriction can enhance volume management with diuretics, and in some clients can improve outcomes (Yancy et al, 2013).*

• Monitor intake and output (I&O). If client is acutely ill, measure hourly urine output and note decreases in output. Decreased cardiac output results in decreased perfusion of the kidneys, with a resulting decrease in urine output. CEB: *Clinical practice guidelines cite that monitoring I&O is useful for monitoring effects of HF treatment, including diuretic therapy (Yancy et al, 2013).*

▲ Note results of initial diagnostic studies, including electrocardiography, echocardiography, and chest radiography. CEB: *Clinical practice guidelines suggest that chest radiography, echocardiography, and electrocardiogram are recommended in the initial assessment of HF (Yancy et al, 2013).*

▲ Note results of further diagnostic imaging studies such as radionuclide imaging, stress echocardiography, cardiac catheterization, computed tomography (CT), or magnetic resonance imaging (MRI). CEB: *Clinical practice guidelines state that radionuclide and MRI are useful studies when assessing left ventricular ejection fraction and volume if echocardiography is not sufficient (Yancy et al, 2013).*

▲ Review laboratory data as needed, including arterial blood gases, complete blood count, serum electrolytes (sodium, potassium, magnesium, and calcium), blood urea nitrogen, creatinine, iron studies, urinalysis, glucose, fasting lipid profile, liver function tests, thyroid-stimulating hormone, B-type natriuretic peptide assay (BNP), or N-terminal pro-B-type natriuretic peptide (NTpro-BNP). Routine blood work can provide insight into the etiology of HF and extent of decompensation. EB: *Clinical practice guidelines recommend that BNP or NTpro-BNP assay should be measured in clients to determine prognosis or disease severity in chronic or acute decompensated HF, guide treatment during hospitalization, and establish a baseline at time of hospital discharge. BNP can also be evaluated in at-risk clients for prevention in the outpatient setting (Chow et al, 2017; Yancy et al, 2017).* EB: *Iron-deficiency anemia is related to decreased exercise capacity, and anemia is a strong indication of HF severity (Yancy et al, 2017).*

• Gradually increase activity when the client's condition is stabilized by encouraging slower-paced activities, or shorter periods of activity, with frequent rest periods after exercise prescription; observe for symptoms of intolerance. Take blood pressure and pulse before and after activity and note changes. Activity of the cardiac client should be closely monitored. See care plan Decreased **Activity** Tolerance.

▲ Encourage a diet that promotes cardiovascular health and reduces risk of hypertension, atherosclerotic disease, renal impairment, insulin resistance, and hypervolemia, within the context of an individual's cultural preferences (Van Horn et al, 2016; Whelton et al, 2018; Arnett et al, 2019). EB: *Reduced sodium intake, weight loss, healthy diet (low sugar, legumes, whole grains, fruits and vegetables, low total fat, fish), and avoidance of excess caloric intake is recommended for individuals with elevated blood pressure and prevention of cardiovascular disease (Van Horn et al, 2016; Whelton et al, 2018).* EB: *Replacing saturated fats with polyunsaturated or monounsaturated fats, and reducing intake of processed meats, refined carbohydrates, and sweetened beverages, will help to decrease atherosclerotic cardiovascular disease (ASCVD) risk (Sacks et al, 2017; Arnett et al, 2019).*

▲ Monitor bowel function. Provide stool softeners as ordered. Caution client not to strain when defecating, as this may cause vasovagal syncope. Decreased activity, pain medication, and diuretics can cause constipation.

- Weigh the client at the same time daily (after voiding). Daily weight is a good indicator of fluid balance. Use the same scale if possible when weighing clients for consistency. Increased weight and severity of symptoms can signal decreased cardiac function with retention of fluids. CEB: *Clinical practice guidelines state that weighing at the same time daily is useful to assess effects of diuretic therapy (Yancy et al, 2013).*
- ▲ Provide influenza and pneumococcal vaccines as needed before client discharge for those who have yet to receive those inoculations (Centers for Disease Control and Prevention, 2020).
- Evaluate a client's social determinants of health (SDOH), including race, gender identity, socioeconomic position, insurance coverage, living condition, food security, access to transportation, social support, and health literacy, among other factors. EB: *The "downstream" effects of SDOH can negatively affect clients by reducing access to care and contributing to poor HF outcomes. By assessing a client's SDOH you can reduce health care disparities (White-Williams et al, 2020).*
- Assess for presence of depression and/or anxiety and refer for treatment if present. See Nursing Interventions and Rationales for Anxiety to facilitate reduction of anxiety in clients and family. CEB: *Depression is common in clients with HF, and it has been found that individuals with depressive symptoms have poorer quality of life, use health care services more frequently, have poorer self-care, and have worse clinical outcomes (Yancy et al, 2013).*
- ▲ Refer to a cardiac rehabilitation program for education and monitored exercise. EB/CEB: Exercise training or regular physical activity is recommended for HF clients. Cardiac rehabilitation can improve quality of life and functional capacity (*Yancy et al, 2013*; *Anderson et al, 2016*). EB: A systematic review of outcomes of exercise-based interventions in clients with HF found that cardiac rehabilitation likely reduces hospital admissions and can improve quality of life, but does not appear to have an effect on mortality (*Long et al, 2019*).
- ▲ Refer to an HF program for education, evaluation, and guided support to increase activity and rebuild quality of life. Support for the HF client should be client centered, culturally sensitive, and include family and social support. CEB: Multiprofessional systems of care that are designed to support clients with HF can improve outcomes (*Yancy et al, 2013*).

Critically Ill

- ▲ Observe for symptoms of cardiogenic shock, including impaired mentation, hypotension, decreased peripheral pulses, cold clammy skin, signs of pulmonary congestion, and decreased organ function. If present, notify the health care provider immediately. Cardiogenic shock is a state of circulatory failure from loss of cardiac function associated with inadequate organ perfusion and a high mortality rate. CEB: *Critical cardiogenic shock presents with severe hypotension, increasing inotropic and vasopressor support, organ hypoperfusion, and worsening acidosis and lactate levels (Yancy et al, 2013).*
- ▲ If shock is present, monitor hemodynamic parameters for an increase in pulmonary wedge pressure, an increase in systemic vascular resistance, or a decrease in stroke volume, cardiac output, and cardiac index. CEB: *Hemodynamic monitoring with a pulmonary artery catheter can be beneficial in clients with respiratory distress, impaired systemic perfusion, and dependence on intravenous inotropic support, and when clinical assessment is inadequate or severe symptoms persist despite recommended therapies (Yancy et al, 2013).*
- ▲ Titrate inotropic and vasoactive medications within defined parameters to maintain contractility, preload, and afterload per health care provider's order. By following parameters, the nurse ensures maintenance of a delicate balance of medications that stimulate the heart to increase contractility while maintaining adequate perfusion of the body. CEB: *Clinical practice guidelines recommend that intravenous inotropic drugs might be reasonable for HF clients presenting with low blood pressure and low cardiac output to maintain systemic perfusion and preserve end-organ performance (Yancy et al, 2013).*
- ▲ Identify significant fluid overload and initiate intravenous diuretics as ordered. Monitor I&O, daily weight, and vital signs, as well as signs and symptoms of congestion. Watch laboratory data, including cardiac biomarkers, serum electrolytes, creatinine, and urea nitrogen. CEB: *Intravenous loop diuretics should be initiated in the HF client who presents with significant fluid overload as either intermittent boluses or continuous infusion to reduce morbidity (Yancy et al, 2013).* EB: *Monitor for acute kidney injury and cardiorenal syndrome, as well as diuretic resistance (Rangaswami et al, 2019).*
- ▲ When using pulmonary arterial catheter technology, be sure to appropriately level and zero the equipment, use minimal tubing, maintain system patency, perform square wave testing, position the client appropriately, and consider correlation to respiratory and cardiac cycles when assessing waveforms and integrating data into client assessment. CEB: *Clinical practice guidelines recommend that invasive hemodynamic monitoring can be useful in acute HF with persistent symptoms when therapy is refractory, fluid status*

is unclear, systolic pressures are low, renal function is worsening, vasoactive agents are required, or when considering advanced device therapy or transplantation (Yancy et al, 2013).

- ▲ Observe for worsening signs and symptoms of respiratory compromise. Recognize that invasive or noninvasive ventilation may be required for clients with acute cardiogenic pulmonary edema. EB/CEB: *Clinical practice guidelines for HF state that CPAP improves daily functional capacity and quality of life for those with HF and obstructive sleep apnea and is reasonable for clients with refractory HF not responding to other medical therapies (Yancy et al, 2013; Costanzo et al, 2015).* EB: *Noninvasive positive pressure ventilation (NPPV), including CPAP and bilevel NPPV, can reduce hospital mortality, intensive care unit (ICU) length of stay, and intubation rate, and result in faster client improvement (Berbenetz et al, 2019).*
- ▲ Monitor client for signs and symptoms of fluid and electrolyte imbalance when clients are receiving ultrafiltration or continuous renal replacement therapy (CRRT). Clients with refractory HF may have ultrafiltration or CRRT ordered as a mechanical method to remove excess fluid volume. CEB: *Clinical practice guidelines cite that ultrafiltration is reasonable for clients with obvious volume overload and congestion, and refractory congestion not responsive to medical therapy (Yancy et al, 2013).*
- ● Recognize that hypoperfusion from low cardiac output can lead to altered mental status and decreased cognition. CEB: *A study that assessed an association among cardiac index and neuropsychological ischemia found that decreased cardiac function, even with normal cardiac index, was associated with accelerated brain aging (Jefferson et al, 2010).*
- ● Recognize that clients with severe HF may undergo additional therapies, such as internal pacemaker or defibrillator placement, and/or placement of a ventricular assist device (VAD). CEB: *The use of VADs is a reasonable treatment as a bridge to recovery, transplant, or decision-making in selected HF clients with reduced ejection fraction and profound hemodynamic compromise (Yancy et al, 2013).*

Geriatric

- ● Recognize that older clients may demonstrate fatigue and depression as signs of HF and decreased cardiac output.
- ● Recognize that older adults in the critical care setting often have geriatric syndromes such as polypharmacy, multimorbidity, cognitive decline, and frailty that can be exacerbated in the critical care setting and contribute to prolonged hospitalization, increased mortality, increased HF, increased disability, and decreased quality of life (Damluji et al, 2019).
- ▲ If the client has heart disease–causing activity intolerance, refer for cardiac rehabilitation. EB: *Cardiac rehabilitation can positively affect an individual's quality of life and reduce hospitalizations regardless of age (Anderson et al, 2016; Long et al, 2019).*
- ▲ Recognize that edema can present differently in the older population. CEB: *In the older population, lower extremity edema is often related to peripheral causes, such as dependency, rather than cardiac causes (Yancy et al, 2013).*
- ▲ Recognize that blood pressure control is beneficial for older clients to reduce the risk of worsening HF. CEB: *Hypertension treatment is particularly beneficial in the older population, and control of both systolic and diastolic hypertension has been shown to reduce the risk of HF (Yancy et al, 2013).* CEB: *Clients with stage A HF and hypertension, with increased cardiovascular risk (age >75 years old, established vascular disease, chronic renal disease, or Framingham risk score >15%), should have a target systolic blood pressure less than 130 mm Hg (Yancy et al, 2017).* EB: *Older clients are at higher risk for resistant hypertension and may require multiple antihypertensive medications for blood pressure control (Carey et al, 2018).*
- ▲ Recognize that renal function is not always accurately represented by serum creatinine in the older population because of less muscle mass (Yancy et al, 2013).
- ▲ Observe for side effects from cardiac medications. Older adults can have difficulty with metabolism and excretion of medications because of decreased function of the liver and kidneys; therefore, toxic side effects are more common. EB: *Older adults are at increased risk for digoxin toxicity, especially at larger doses, because of lower body mass and impaired renal function (Yancy et al, 2013).*
- ▲ Older adults may require more frequent visits, closer monitoring of medication dose changes, and more gradual increases in medications *because of changes in the metabolism of medications and impaired renal function (Yancy et al, 2013).*
- ▲ Recognize that older adults still benefit from smoking cessation *to reduce risk of worsening cardiovascular disease (Arnett et al, 2019).*
- ▲ As older adults approach end of life, clinicians should help to facilitate a comprehensive plan of care that incorporates the client and family's values, goals, and preferences (Allen et al, 2012; National Consensus

Project for Quality Palliative Care, 2018). EB: *For older adults (>65 years old) with multiple comorbidities and limited life expectancy, it is reasonable to use a team-based approach to weigh the risks and benefits of tight blood pressure control and choice of antihypertensive medication (Whelton et al, 2018).*

Home Care

- Some of the previously mentioned interventions may be adapted for home care use. Home care agencies may use specialized staff and methods to care for chronic HF clients. CEB: *A study assessing HF outcomes over a 10-year period between a multiprofessional home care intervention and usual care found significantly improved survival and prolonged event-free survival and was both cost and time effective (Ingles et al, 2006).*
- Assess for fatigue and weakness frequently. Assess home environment for safety, as well as resources/obstacles to energy conservation.
- Help family adapt daily living patterns to establish life changes that will maintain improved cardiac functioning in the client. Take the client's perspective into consideration and use a holistic approach in assessing and responding to client planning for the future.
- Assist client to recognize and exercise power in using self-care management to adjust to health change. Refer to care plan for **Powerlessness.**
- ▲ Refer to medical social services, cardiac rehabilitation, telemonitoring, and case management as necessary for assistance with home care, access to resources, and counseling about the impact of severe or chronic cardiac diseases. EB/CEB: *Access to systems that promote care coordination is essential for successful care of the HF client. Good communication and documentation between services, health care providers, and transitions of care is essential to ensure improved outcomes in HF clients (Yancy et al, 2013; Albert et al, 2015).*
- ▲ As the client chooses, refer to palliative care, which can begin earlier in the care of the HF client. Palliative care can be used to increase comfort and quality of life in the HF client before end-of-life care. EB/CEB: *Palliative care should address quality of life, ongoing symptom control, preferences about end of life, psychosocial distress, and caregiver support (Yancy et al, 2013; National Consensus Project for Quality Palliative Care, 2018).*
- ▲ If the client's condition warrants, refer to hospice. CEB: *The palliative care and HF teams are best suited to determine when end-of-life care is appropriate for the client and family (Yancy et al, 2013).*

Client/Family Teaching and Discharge Planning

- Begin discharge planning as soon as possible on admission to the emergency department (ED) if appropriate with a case manager or social worker to assess home support systems and the need for community or home health services. EB: *Discharge planning should include adherence to the treatment plan, medication management, follow-up with health care providers and care coordination, dietary and physical activities, cardiac rehabilitation, and secondary prevention recommendations (Yancy et al, 2013; Albert et al, 2015).*
- Discharge education should be comprehensive, evidence based, culturally sensitive, and include both the client and family (Yancy et al, 2013).
- Teach the client about any medications prescribed. Medication teaching includes the drug name; its purpose; administration instructions, such as taking it with or without food; and any side effects. Instruct the client to report any adverse side effects to his or her health care provider.
- Teach the importance of performing and recording daily weights on arising for the day, and to report weight gain. Ask if client has a scale at home; if not, assist in getting one. EB: *Clinical practice guidelines suggest that daily weight monitoring leads to early recognition of excess fluid retention, which, when reported, can be offset with additional medication to avoid hospitalization from HF decompensation (Yancy et al, 2013).*
- Teach the types and progression patterns of worsening HF symptoms, when to call a health care provider for help, and when to go to the hospital for urgent care (Yancy et al, 2013).
- Stress the importance of ceasing tobacco use (Whelton et al, 2018). CEB/EB: *Effects of nicotine include increasing pulse and blood pressure and constricting blood vessels. Tobacco use is a primary factor in heart disease (Amsterdam et al, 2014; Whelton et al, 2018).* EB: *To facilitate cessation, a combination of behavioral and pharmacotherapy is recommended to improve cessation rates (Arnett et al, 2019).*
- ▲ Individuals should be screened for electronic cigarette use (e-cigarette). CEB: *Although more studies are needed regarding the health effects of e-cigarette use, the American Heart Association recommends that all health care providers educate their clients regarding the long-term use of e-cigarettes given the known toxicities present in e-cigarettes, as well as the presence of nicotine in most types of e-cigarettes (Bhatnagar et al, 2014).*

C

- On hospital discharge, educate clients about low-sodium, low–saturated fat diet, with consideration of client education, literacy, and health literacy level.
- Educate clients that comorbidities, including obesity, hypertension, metabolic syndrome, diabetes mellitus, and hyperlipidemia, are common in individuals with HF and can affect clinical outcomes related to HF if not controlled (Bozkurt et al, 2016). EB: *One of the most important factors in preventing HF is to promote a healthy lifestyle (Arnett et al, 2019).*
- For clients with diabetes mellitus, educate about the importance of glycemic control. EB: *Individuals with diabetes mellitus are at increased risk for HF and should be managed according to recommended guidelines. Thiazolidinediones should be avoided in individuals with class III or IV HF because of increased fluid retention (Bozkurt et al, 2016).* EB: *To reduce the risk of worsening HF outcomes, educate clients with type 2 diabetes mellitus about the importance of improving dietary habits and regular exercise. Clients should also be initiated on metformin, a sodium-glucose cotransporter 2 inhibitor (SGLT2i), or a glucagon-like peptide-1 receptor agonist (GLP-1) to improve glycemic control and reduce risk for worsening cardiovascular disease or cardiorenal syndrome (Arnett et al, 2019; Rangaswami et al, 2019).*
- Instruct client and family on the importance of regular follow-up care with health care providers. EB: *Post-discharge support can significantly reduce hospital readmissions and improve health care outcomes, quality of life, and costs (Yancy et al, 2013).*
- ▲ Teach stress reduction (e.g., meditation, imagery, controlled breathing, muscle relaxation techniques). EB: *Meditation is a reasonable adjunct to GDMT for reduction of cardiovascular risk and lifestyle modification (Levine et al, 2017).*
- Discuss advance directives with the HF client, including resuscitation preferences. EB/CEB: *Evidence suggests that advance directives can help to reduce overall health care costs, reduce in-hospital deaths, and increase hospice use (Yancy et al, 2013; National Consensus Project for Quality Palliative Care, 2018).*
- Clients should be provided with education regarding the influenza vaccine and pneumococcal vaccine before discharge. EB: *The influenza vaccine is recommended for all adults, and the pneumococcal vaccine is recommended for individuals more than 65 years old and for individuals who are at high risk for cardiovascular disease (Centers for Disease Control and Prevention, 2020).*
- Teach the importance of physical activity as tolerated. EB: *Exercise helps control blood pressure and weight, which are the most important controlled risk factors for cardiovascular disease. Individuals should engage in aerobic physical activity of varying intensity as tolerated and incorporate variable anaerobic activities such as resistance training (Bozkurt et al, 2016; Arnett et al, 2019).* EB: *Exercise is beneficial in the prevention of cardiovascular disease and HF. Ideally, clients should engage in 150 minutes per week of moderate-intensity aerobic exercise if able. At minimum, any aerobic moderate-intensity exercise is ideal (Bozkurt et al, 2016; Arnett et al, 2019).* EB: *Clients with arrhythmias or advanced HF may require supervision or monitoring during exercise (Bozkurt et al, 2016).*

REFERENCES

Albert, N. M., Barnason, S., Deswal, A., et al. (2015). Transitions of care in heart failure: A scientific statement from the American Heart Association. *Circulation Heart Failure*, *8*(2), 384–409.

Allen, L. A., Stevenson, L. W., Grady, K. L., et al. (2012). Decision making in advanced heart failure: A scientific statement from the American Heart Association. *Circulation*, *125*(15), 1928–1952.

Amsterdam, E. A., Wenger, N. K., Brindis, R. G., et al. (2014). 2014 AHA/ACC guideline for the management of patients with non-ST elevation acute coronary syndromes: A report of the American College of Cardiology/American Heart Association Task Force on Practice Guidelines. *Circulation*, *130*(25), e344–e426.

Anderson, L., Oldridge, N., Thompson, D. R., et al. (2016). Exercise-based cardiac rehabilitation for coronary heart disease: Cochrane systematic review and meta-analysis. *Journal of the American College of Cardiology*, *67*(1), 1–12.

Arnett, D. K., Blumenthal, R. S., Albert, M. A., et al. (2019). 2019 ACC/AHA guideline on the primary prevention of cardiovascular disease: A report of the American College of Cardiology/American Heart Association Task Force on Clinical Practice Guidelines. *Circulation*, *140*(11), e596–e646.

Berbenetz, N., Wang, Y., Brown, J., et al. (2019). Non-invasive positive pressure ventilation (CPAP or bilevel NPPV) for cardiogenic pulmonary oedema. *Cochrane Database of Systematic Reviews*, *4*, CD005351 https://www.cochranelibrary.com/cdsr/doi/10.1002/14651858.CD005351.pub4/full.

Bhatnagar, A., Whitsel, L. P., Ribisl, K. M., et al. (2014). Electronic cigarettes: A policy statement from the American Heart Association. *Circulation*, *130*(16), 1418–1436.

Bozkurt, B., Aguilar, D., Deswal, A., et al. (2016). Contributory risk and management of comorbidities of hypertension, obesity, diabetes mellitus, hyperlipidemia, and metabolic syndrome in chronic heart failure: A scientific statement from the American Heart Association. *Circulation*, *134*(23), e535–e578.

Carey, R. M., Calhoun, D. A., Bakris, G. L., et al. (2018). Resistant hypertension: Detection, evaluation, and management: A scientific statement from the American Heart Association. *Hypertension*, *72*(5), e53–e90.

Centers for Disease Control and Prevention. (2020). *Adult immunization schedules for ages 19 years or older, United States, 2020*. Retrieved from http://www.cdc.gov/vaccines/schedules/hcp/imz/adult.html. Accessed June 9, 2021.

Chow, S. L., Maisel, A. S., Anand, I., et al. (2017). Role of biomarkers for the prevention, assessment, and management of heart failure: A scientific statement from the American Heart Association. *Circulation*, *135*(22), e1054–e1091.

Costanzo, M. R., Khayat, R., Ponikowski, P., et al. (2015). Mechanisms and clinical consequences of untreated central sleep apnea in heart failure. *Journal of American Colleges of Cardiology*, *65*(1), 72–84.

Damluji, A. A., Forman, D. E., van Diepen, S., et al. (2019). Older adults in the cardiac intensive care unit: Factoring geriatric syndromes in the management, prognosis, and process of care: A scientific statement from the American Heart Association. *Circulation*, *141*(2), e6–e32.

Ingles, S. C., Pearson, S., Treen, S., Gallasch, T., Horowitz, J. D., & Stewart, S. (2006). Extending the horizon in chronic heart failure: Effects of multidisciplinary, home-based intervention relative to usual care. *Circulation*, *114*(23), 2466–2473.

Jefferson, A. L., Himali, J. J., Beiser, A. S., et al. (2010). Cardiac index is associated with brain aging: The Framingham Heart Study. *Circulation*, *122*(7), 690–697.

Konstam, M. A., Kiernan, M. S., Bernstein, D., et al. (2018). Evaluation and management of right-sided heart failure: A scientific statement from the American Heart Association. *Circulation*, *137*(20), e578–e622.

Levine, G. N., Lange, R. A., Bairey-Merz, C. N., et al. (2017). Meditation and cardiovascular risk reduction: A scientific statement from the American Heart Association. *Journal of the American Heart Association*, *6*(10), e002218.

Long, L., Mordi, I. R., Bridges, C., et al. (2019). Exercise-based cardiac rehabilitation for adults with heart failure. *Cochrane Database of Systematic Reviews*, *1*, CD003331 https://www.cochranelibrary.com/cdsr/doi/10.1002/14651858.CD003331.pub5/full.

National Consensus Project for Quality Palliative Care. (2018). *Clinical practice guidelines for quality palliative care* (4th ed.). Retrieved from. https://www.nationalcoalitionhpc.org/ncp/. Accessed June 9, 2021.

Rangaswami, J., Bhalla, V., Blair, J. E. A., et al. (2019). Cardiorenal syndrome: Classification, pathophysiology, diagnosis, and treatment strategies. *Circulation*, *139*(16), e840–e878.

Sachdeva, A., Dalton, M., & Lees, T. (2018). Graduated compression stockings for prevention of deep vein thrombosis. *Cochrane Database of Systematic Reviews*, *11*, CD001484 https://www.cochranelibrary.com/cdsr/doi/10.1002/14651858.CD001484.pub4/full.

Sacks, R. M., Lichtenstein, A. H., Wu, J. H. Y., et al. (2017). Dietary fats and cardiovascular disease: A presidential advisory from the American Heart Association. *Circulation*, *136*(3), e1–e23.

Sajid, M. S., Desai, M., Morris, R. W., & Hamilton, G. (2012). Knee length versus thigh length graduated compression stockings for prevention of deep vein thrombosis in postoperative surgical patients. *Cochrane Database of Systematic Reviews*, 5, CD007162 https://www.cochranelibrary.com/cdsr/doi/10.1002/14651858.CD007162.pub2/full.

Van Horn, L., Carson, J. S., Appel, L. J., et al. (2016). Recommended dietary pattern to achieve adherence to the American Heart Association/American College of Cardiology (AHA/ACC) guidelines: A scientific statement from the American Heart Association. *Circulation*, *134*(22), e505–e529.

Whelton, P. K., Carey, R. M., Aronow, W. S., et al. (2018). 2017 ACC/AHA/AAPA/ABC/ACPM/AGS/APhA/ASH/ASPC/NMA/PCNA guideline for the prevention, detection, evaluation, and management of high blood pressure in adults; executive summary: A report of the American College of Cardiology/American Heart Association Task Force on Clinical Practice Guidelines. *Hypertension*, *71*(6), 1269–1324.

White-Williams, C., Rossi, L. P., Bittner, V. A., et al. (2020). Addressing social determinants of health in the care of patients with heart failure: A scientific statement from the American Heart Association. *Circulation*, *141*(22), e841–e863.

Yancy, C. W., Jessup, M., Bozkurt, B., et al. (2013). 2013 ACCF/AHA guideline for the management of heart failure: A report of the American College of Cardiology Foundation/American Heart Association Task Force on Practice Guidelines. *Circulation*, *128*(16), e240–e327.

Yancy, C. W., Jessup, M., Bozkurt, B., et al. (2017). 2017 ACCF/AHA/HFSA focused update of the 2013 ACCF/AHA guideline for the management of heart failure: A report of the American College of Cardiology Foundation/American Heart Association Task Force on Clinical Practice Guidelines and the Heart Failure Society of America. *Circulation*, *136*(6), e137–e161.

Risk for Decreased Cardiac Output **Domain 4 Activity/rest Class 4 Cardiovascular/pulmonary responses**

Mary Beth Flynn Makic, PhD, RN, CCNS, CCRN-K, FAAN, FNAP, FCNS

NANDA-I

Definition

Susceptible to inadequate blood pumped by the heart to meet metabolic demands of the body, which may compromise health.

Risk Factors

To be developed

Associated Conditions

Altered afterload; altered contractility; altered heart rate; altered heart rhythm; altered preload; altered stroke volume

NIC, NOC, Client Outcomes, Nursing Interventions and *Rationales,* Client/Family Teaching and Discharge Planning, and References

Refer to care plan for Decreased **Cardiac** Output.

Risk for Decreased Cardiac Tissue Perfusion Domain 4 Activity/rest Class 4 Cardiovascular/pulmonary responses

Ann Will Poteet, MS, RN, CNS, AGNP-C

NANDA-I

Definition

Susceptible to a decrease in cardiac (coronary) circulation, which may compromise health.

Risk Factors

Inadequate knowledge of modifiable factors; substance misuse

At-Risk Population

Individuals with a family history of cardiovascular disease

Associated Conditions

Cardiac tamponade; cardiovascular surgery; coronary artery spasm; diabetes mellitus; elevated C-reactive protein; hyperlipidemia; hypertension; hypovolemia; hypoxemia; hypoxia; pharmaceutical preparations

NOC (Nursing Outcomes Classification)

Suggested NOC Outcomes

Cardiac Pump Effectiveness; Circulation Status; Tissue Perfusion: Cardiac; Tissue Perfusion: Cellular; Vital Signs

Example NOC Outcome with Indicators

Tissue Perfusion: Cardiac as evidenced by the following indicators: Angina/Arrhythmia/Tachycardia/Bradycardia/Nausea/Vomiting/Profuse diaphoresis. (Rate the outcome and indicators of **Tissue Perfusion: Cardiac:** 1 = severe, 2 = substantial, 3 = moderate, 4 = mild, 5 = none [see Section I].)

Client Outcomes

Client Will (Specify Time Frame)

- Maintain vital signs within normal range
- Retain an asymptomatic cardiac rhythm (have absence of arrhythmias, tachycardia, or bradycardia)
- Be free from chest and radiated discomfort as well as associated symptoms related to acute coronary syndromes (ACSs)
- Deny nausea and be free of vomiting or gastrointestinal distress
- Have skin that is dry and of normal temperature
- Maintain normal cognition
- Maintain healthy lifestyle behaviors that promote primary prevention of cardiovascular disease

NIC (Nursing Interventions Classification)

Suggested NIC Interventions

Cardiac Care; Cardiac Precautions; Embolus Precautions; Dysrhythmia Management; Vital Signs Monitoring; Shock Management: Cardiac

Example NIC Activity—Cardiac Precautions

Avoid causing intense emotional situations; Avoid overheating or chilling the client; Provide small frequent meals; Substitute artificial salt and limit sodium intake if appropriate; Promote effective techniques for reducing stress; Restrict smoking

Nursing Interventions and *Rationales*

- Be aware that the primary cause of ACS which include unstable angina (UA), non–ST-elevation myocardial infarction (NSTEMI), and ST-elevation myocardial infarction (STEMI), is an imbalance between myocardial oxygen consumption and demand that is associated with partially or fully occlusive thrombus development in coronary arteries (Amsterdam et al, 2014).
- Assess for symptoms of coronary hypoperfusion and possible ACS, including chest discomfort (pressure, tightness, crushing, squeezing, dullness, or achiness), with or without radiation (or originating) in the retrosternal area, back, neck, jaw, shoulder, or arm discomfort or numbness; shortness of breath (SOB); associated diaphoresis; abdominal pain; dizziness, lightheadedness, loss of consciousness, or unexplained fatigue; nausea or vomiting with chest discomfort, heartburn, or indigestion; and associated anxiety. EB/CEB: *These symptoms are signs of decreased cardiac perfusion and ACSs, such as UA, NSTEMI, or STEMI, as well as other cardiovascular disorders such as aortic aneurysm, valve disorders, myocarditis, spontaneous coronary artery dissection (SCAD), heart failure, and pericarditis. A physical assessment will aid in the assessment of the extent, location, and presence of, and complications resulting from, a myocardial infarction (MI). It will promote rapid triage and treatment. It is also important to assess whether the client had a prior stroke, heart failure, or other cardiovascular disorder. It is important to note that certain psychiatric disorders (somatoform disorders, panic attack, and anxiety disorders) can mimic ACS, but they are typically noncardiac causes of chest pain (Amsterdam et al, 2014; Mehta et al, 2016).*
- Evaluate client for noncardiac causes of chest pain, other than psychiatric disorders, including gastrointestinal disorders (reflux disease, esophagitis), pleuritic pain (secondary to pulmonary embolus, infection), costochondritis, and musculoskeletal disorders.
- Consider atypical presentations of ACS for women, older adults, and individuals with diabetes mellitus, impaired renal function, and dementia. EB/CEB: *Women, older adults, and individuals with diabetes mellitus, impaired renal function, and dementia may present with atypical findings (Amsterdam et al, 2014; Mieres et al, 2014; McSweeney et al, 2016; Mehta et al, 2016). Research continues to confirm that that women had significantly less chest discomfort and were more likely to present with fatigue, neck pain, syncope, nausea, right arm pain, abdominal and back pain, dizziness, and jaw pain (Lau et al, 2016). Delaying identification of atypical presentations can have negative effects on timely intervention and management of ACS, resulting in poorer outcomes and higher mortality (Mehta et al, 2016).*
- Evaluate the client for socioeconomic or race/ethnicity factors that put them at higher risk for atherosclerotic cardiovascular disease (ASCVD). EB: *Understanding a client's socioeconomic factors leads to shared decision-making between the client and clinician, thereby guiding treatment decisions that meet the client's needs. Socioeconomic factors are strong determinants of CVD risk, and failure to identify these factors may lead to poor treatment adherence or decrease the efficacy of known prevention recommendations (Arnett et al, 2019).*
- Review the client's medical, surgical, social, and familial history. CEB: *A medical history must be concise and detailed to determine the possibility of ACS and to help determine the possible cause of cardiac symptoms and pathology (Amsterdam et al, 2014).*
- Perform physical assessments for both coronary artery disease (CAD) and noncoronary findings related to decreased coronary perfusion, including vital signs, pulse oximetry, equal blood pressure in both arms, heart rate, respiratory rate, and pulse oximetry. Check bilateral pulses for quality and regularity. Report tachycardia, bradycardia, hypotension or hypertension, pulsus alternans or pulsus paradoxus, tachypnea, or abnormal pulse oximetry reading. Assess cardiac rhythm for arrhythmias; skin and mucous membrane color, temperature, and dryness; and capillary refill. Assess for peripheral vascular disease. Assess neck veins for elevated central venous pressure, cyanosis, and pericardial or pleural friction rub. Examine client for cardiac S4 gallop, new heart murmur, lung crackles, altered mentation, pain on abdominal palpation, abdominal distention, decreased bowel sounds, or decreased urinary output. CEB: *These indicators help assess for cardiac and noncardiac etiologies of symptoms and differential diagnoses (Amsterdam et al, 2014).*

▲ Administer supplemental oxygen as ordered and needed for clients presenting with ACS, respiratory distress, or other high-risk features of hypoxemia to maintain a Po_2 of at least 90%. EB: *American Heart Association guidelines for emergency cardiovascular care during ACS recommend administering oxygen for breathlessness, hypoxemia, signs of heart failure, or if signs of shock are present, and the need for oxygen should be guided by noninvasive monitoring of oxygen saturation. There is limited evidence to support or refute the use of high-flow or low-flow supplemental oxygen if a normal oxygen level (>90%) is present, but it is reasonable to withhold supplemental oxygen in normoxic individuals (O'Connor et al, 2015).* EB: *A Cochrane review found there was limited evidence to support or refute the use of routine supplemental oxygen with acute MI, and that harm from excess supplemental oxygen cannot be ruled out, recommending further studies (Cabello et al, 2016).*

- ▲ Use continuous pulse oximetry as ordered. CEB: *Prevention and treatment of hypoxemia include maintaining arterial oxygen saturation over 90% (Amsterdam et al, 2014).*
- ▲ Insert one or more large-bore intravenous catheters to keep the vein open. Routinely assess saline locks for patency. Clients who come to the hospital with possible decrease in coronary perfusion or ACS may have intravenous fluids and medications ordered routinely or emergently to maintain or restore adequate cardiac function and rhythm.
- ▲ Observe the cardiac monitor for hemodynamically significant arrhythmias, ST depressions or elevations, T-wave inversions, and/or Q-waves as signs of ischemia or injury. Be aware that clients with prior cardiothoracic surgery may have abnormal electrocardiogram (ECG) changes at baseline. Report abnormal findings. CEB: *Arrhythmias and ECG changes indicate myocardial ischemia, injury, and/or infarction. Note that left ventricular hypertrophy, ventricular pacing, and bundle branch blocks can mask signs of ischemia or injury (Amsterdam et al, 2014).*
- • Have emergency equipment and defibrillation capability nearby and be prepared to defibrillate immediately if ventricular tachycardia with clinical deterioration or ventricular fibrillation occurs.
- ▲ Perform a 12-lead ECG as ordered to be interpreted within 10 minutes of emergency department arrival and during episodes of chest discomfort or angina equivalent. CEB: *A 12-lead ECG should be performed within 10 minutes of emergency department arrival for all clients who are having chest discomfort. ECGs are used to identify the area of ischemia or injury, such as ST depressions or elevations, new left-bundle branch block, T-wave inversions, and/or Q-waves, and to guide treatment (O'Gara et al, 2013; Amsterdam et al, 2014).*
- ▲ Administer non–enteric-coated aspirin as ordered, as soon as possible after presentation and for maintenance. CEB: *Aspirin has been shown to prevent platelet clumping, aggregation, and activation that leads to thrombus formation, which in coronary arteries leads to ACSs. Contraindications include active peptic ulcer disease, bleeding disorders, and aspirin allergy (O'Gara et al, 2013; Amsterdam et al, 2014).*
- ▲ Administer nitroglycerin tablets sublingually as ordered, every 5 minutes until the chest pain is resolved while monitoring the blood pressure for hypotension, for a maximum of three doses as ordered. Administer nitroglycerin paste or intravenous preparations as ordered. CEB: *Nitroglycerin causes coronary arterial and venous dilation, and at higher doses peripheral arterial dilation, reducing preload and afterload and decreasing myocardial oxygen demand while increasing oxygen delivery (Amsterdam et al, 2014).*
- • Do not administer nitroglycerin preparations to individuals with hypotension, or individuals who have received phosphodiesterase type 5 inhibitors, such as sildenafil, tadalafil, or vardenafil, in the last 24 hours (48 hours for long-acting preparations). CEB: *Synergistic effect causes marked exaggerated and prolonged vasodilation/hypotension (Amsterdam et al, 2014).*
- ▲ Administer morphine intravenously as ordered, every 5 to 30 minutes until pain is relieved while monitoring blood pressure when nitroglycerin alone does not relieve chest discomfort. EB: *Morphine has potent analgesic and antianxiolytic effects and causes mild reductions in blood pressure and heart rate that reduce myocardial oxygen consumption. Hypotension and respiratory depression are the most serious complications of morphine use, and naloxone may be administered as ordered for morphine overdose (Amsterdam et al, 2014).*
- ▲ Assess and report abnormal laboratory work results of cardiac enzymes, specifically troponin I or high-sensitivity troponin T, B-type natriuretic peptide, chemistries, hematology, coagulation studies, arterial blood gases, finger stick blood sugar, elevated C-reactive protein, or drug screen. CEB: *Abnormalities can identify the cause of the decreased perfusion and identify complications related to the decreased perfusion such as anemia, hypovolemia, coagulopathy, drug abuse, hyperglycemia, kidney (renal) failure, and heart failure. Markedly elevated cardiac enzymes are usually indicative of an MI, and the cardiac enzymes can help determine short- and long-term prognosis (Amsterdam et al, 2014).*
- • Assess for individual risk factors for CAD, such as hypertension, dyslipidemia, cigarette smoking, diabetes mellitus, metabolic syndrome, obesity, or family history of heart disease. Other risk factors including socioeconomic factors, sedentary lifestyle, obesity, or cocaine or amphetamine use. Note age and gender as risk factors. EB/CEB: *Certain conditions place clients at higher risk for decreased cardiac tissue perfusion (Amsterdam et al, 2014; Mieres et al, 2014; Mehta et al, 2016; Arnett et al, 2019).* EB: *Screening with ASCVD risk estimator evidence-based tools can help to inform treatment decisions. Frequency of screening for ASCVD risk should be based on age categories (Arnett et al, 2019).*
- ▲ Administer additional heart medications as ordered, including beta-blockers, calcium channel blockers, angiotensin-converting enzyme inhibitors, angiotensin II receptor blockers, aldosterone antagonists, antiarrhythmics, diuretics, antiplatelet agents, and anticoagulants. Always check blood pressure and pulse rate before administering these medications. If the blood pressure or pulse rate is low, contact the health care provider to establish whether the medication should be withheld. Also check platelet counts, renal

function, and coagulation studies as ordered to assess proper effects of these agents. CEB: *These medications are useful to optimize cardiac and kidney function, including blood pressure, heart rate, myocardial oxygen demand, intravascular fluid volume, and cardiac rhythm (Amsterdam et al, 2014).*

- ▲ Administer lipid-lowering therapy as ordered. EB/CEB: *Use of statin drugs and/or combination therapy with other nonstatin lipid-lowering agents (ezetimibe, bile acid sequestrants, and PCSK9 inhibitors) has been shown to reduce an individual's risk of recurrent MI, stroke, and coronary heart disease mortality, especially with high-intensity statins that lower low-density lipoprotein cholesterol levels (Amsterdam et al, 2014; Grundy et al, 2019).* EB: *The decision to start drug therapy should be based on 10-year ASCVD risk and lifetime risk estimation as well as comorbidities, including diabetes mellitus, and other risk-enhancing factors (Arnett et al, 2019; Grundy et al, 2019).*
- ▲ Prepare client with education, withholding of meals and/or medications, and intravenous access for early invasive therapy with cardiac catheterization, reperfusion therapy, and possible percutaneous coronary intervention in individuals with refractory angina or hemodynamic or electrical instability, and first medical contact to device time of less than 90 minutes if STEMI is suspected. CEB: *First medical contact to device time of less than 90 minutes was associated with improved client outcomes (O'Gara et al, 2013; Amsterdam et al, 2014).*
- ▲ Prepare clients with education, withholding of meals and/or medications, and intravenous access for noninvasive cardiac diagnostic procedures such as echocardiogram, exercise, or pharmacological stress test, and cardiac computed tomography scan as ordered. CEB: *Clients suspected of decreased coronary perfusion should receive these diagnostic procedures as appropriate to evaluate for CAD (Fletcher et al, 2013; Amsterdam et al, 2014; Mieres et al, 2014).*
- ▲ Request a referral to a cardiac rehabilitation program. CEB: *Cardiac rehabilitation programs are designed to limit the physiological and psychological effects of cardiac disease, reduce the risk for sudden cardiac death and reinfarction, control symptoms and stabilize or reverse the process of plaque formation, and enhance psychosocial and vocational status of clients (Amsterdam et al, 2014).* EB: *Cardiac rehabilitation can improve quality of life and functional capacity, and decrease cardiovascular mortality, hospitalizations, and associated health care costs (Anderson et al, 2016).*

Geriatric

- • Consider atypical presentations of possible ACS in older adults. EB/CEB: *Older adults may present with atypical signs and symptoms such as weakness, stroke, syncope, or change in mental status (Amsterdam et al, 2014; McSweeney et al, 2016; Mehta et al, 2016).*
- ▲ Ask the prescriber about possible reduced dosage of medications for older clients, considering weight, creatinine clearance, and glomerular filtration rate. EB/CEB: *Older clients can have reduced pharmacokinetics and pharmacodynamics, including reduced muscle mass, reduced renal and hepatic function, and reduced volume of distribution, which can alter drug dosing, efficacy, and safety, as well as some drug–drug interactions (Amsterdam et al, 2014; Grundy et al, 2019).*
- • Consider issues such as quality of life, palliative care, end-of-life care, and differences in sociocultural aspects for clients and families when supporting them in decisions regarding aggressiveness of care. Ask about living wills, as well as medical and durable power of attorney. EB/CEB: *Management decisions, including decisions regarding invasive treatment, should be client-centered and take into account client preferences and goals, cultural considerations, comorbidities, cognitive and functional status, and life expectancy (Amsterdam et al, 2014; McSweeney et al, 2016; Mehta et al, 2016; National Consensus Project for Quality Palliative Care, 2018; Grundy et al, 2019).*

Client/Family Teaching and Discharge Planning

- ▲ Client and family education regarding a multiprofessional plan of care should start early. Special attention to client and family education should occur during transitions of care. CEB: *It is important to provide the client and family with a comprehensive plan of care and education materials that are evidence based to assist with client compliance and to potentially reduce hospital readmissions related to ACS. The plan of care should take into consideration the client's psychosocial and socioeconomic status, access to care, risk for depression and/or social isolation, and health care disparities (Amsterdam et al, 2014).*
- • Teach the client and family to call 911 for symptoms of new angina, existing angina unresponsive to rest and sublingual nitroglycerin tablets, or heart attack, or if an individual becomes unresponsive.
- • On discharge, instruct clients about symptoms of ischemia, when to cease activity, when to use sublingual nitroglycerin, and when to call 911.

- Teach client about any medications prescribed. Medication teaching includes the drug name, its purpose, administration instructions such as taking it with or without food, and any side effects. Instruct the client to report any adverse side effects to the health care provider.
- On hospital discharge, educate clients and significant others about discharge medications, including nitroglycerin sublingual tablets or spray, with written, easy to understand, culturally sensitive information. CEB: *Clients and significant others need to be prepared to act quickly and decisively to relieve ischemic discomfort (Amsterdam et al, 2014).*
- Provide client education related to risk factors for decreased cardiac tissue perfusion, such as hypertension, hyperlipidemia, metabolic syndrome, diabetes mellitus, tobacco use, obesity, advanced age, and female gender. EB/CEB: *Those with two or more risk factors should have a 10-year risk screening for development of symptomatic coronary heart disease. Client education is a vital part of nursing care for the client. Start with the client's base level of understanding and use that as a foundation for further education. It is important to factor in cultural and/or religious beliefs in the education provided (Amsterdam et al, 2014; Barnason et al, 2017; Arnett et al, 2019).*
- Instruct the client on antiplatelet and anticoagulation therapy, and about signs of bleeding, need for ongoing medication compliance, and international normalized ratio monitoring. CEB: *Special attention and education should be provided to older individuals because they are at greater risk for bleeding (Amsterdam et al, 2014).*
- After discharge, continue education and support for client blood pressure and diabetes control, weight management, and resumption of physical activity. EB/CEB: *Reducing risk factors acts as secondary prevention of CAD (Amsterdam et al, 2014; Arnett et al, 2019).* EB: *Participation in cardiac rehabilitation therapy reduces cardiovascular mortality (Anderson et al, 2016).*

▲ Clients should be provided with education regarding the influenza vaccine and pneumococcal vaccine before hospital discharge. EB/CEB: *The influenza vaccine is recommended for all adults, and the pneumococcal vaccine is recommended for individuals older than 65 years and for individuals who are at high risk for cardiovascular disease (Amsterdam et al, 2014; Centers for Disease Control and Prevention, 2020).*

▲ Stress the importance of ceasing tobacco use. EB/CEB: *Tobacco use can cause or worsen decreased blood flow in the coronaries, as well as cause vasoconstriction, which can lead to atherosclerotic disease. Effects of nicotine include increasing pulse and blood pressure and constricting blood vessels. Tobacco use is a primary factor in heart disease (Amsterdam et al, 2014; Whelton et al, 2018).* EB: *To facilitate cessation, a combination of behavioral and pharmacotherapy is recommended to improve cessation rates (Arnett et al, 2019).*

▲ Individuals should be screened for electronic cigarette (e-cigarette) use. CEB: *Although more studies are needed regarding the health effects of e-cigarette use, the American Heart Association recommends that all health care providers educate their clients regarding the long-term use of e-cigarettes given the known toxicities present in e-cigarettes, as well as the presence of nicotine in most types of e-cigarettes (Bhatnagar et al, 2014).*

▲ On hospital discharge, educate clients about a low-sodium, low–saturated fat diet, with consideration to client education, literacy, and health literacy level. CEB: *Reducing risk factors acts as secondary prevention of CAD (Amsterdam et al, 2014).*

- Teach the importance of exercise and physical activity as tolerated. EB/CEB: *Aerobic and resistance exercise help to control blood pressure, reduce weight, improve physical functioning, and improve glycemic control, all of which lower ASCVD risk. Individuals should engage in moderate or vigorous aerobic and/or anaerobic physical activity as tolerated to reduce ASCVD risk (Amsterdam et al, 2014; Bozkurt et al, 2016; Arnett et al, 2019).* EB: Clients with arrhythmias or advanced heart failure may require supervision or monitoring during exercise (*Bozkurt et al, 2016*).

REFERENCES

Amsterdam, E. A., Wenger, N. K., Brindis, R. G., et al. (2014). 2014 AHA/ACC guideline for the management of patients with non-ST elevation acute coronary syndromes: A report of the American College of Cardiology/American Heart Association Task Force on Practice Guidelines. *Circulation, 130*(25), e344–e426.

Anderson, L., Oldridge, N., Thompson, D. R., et al. (2016). Exercise-based cardiac rehabilitation for coronary heart disease: Cochrane systematic review and meta-analysis. *Journal of the American College of Cardiology, 67*(1), 1–12.

Arnett, D. K., Blumenthal, R. S., Albert, M. A., et al. (2019). 2019 ACC/AHA guideline on the primary prevention of cardiovascular disease: A report of the American College of Cardiology/American Heart Association Task Force on Clinical Practice Guidelines. *Circulation, 140*(11), e596–e646.

Barnason, S., White-Williams, C., Rossi, L. P., et al. (2017). Evidence for therapeutic patient interventions to promote cardiovascular patient self-management: A scientific statement for healthcare professionals from the American Heart Association. *Circulation Cardiovascular Quality and Outcomes, 10*(6), e000025.

Bhatnagar, A., Whitsel, L. P., Ribisl, K. M., et al. (2014). Electronic cigarettes: A policy statement from the American Heart Association. *Circulation, 130*(16), 1418–1436.

Bozkurt, B., Aguilar, D., Deswal, A., et al. (2016). Contributory risk and management of comorbidities of hypertension, obesity, diabetes mellitus, hyperlipidemia, and metabolic syndrome in chronic heart failure: A scientific statement from the American Heart Association. *Circulation, 134*(23), e535–e578.

Cabello, J. B., Burls, A., Emparanza, J. I., Bayliss, S. E., & Quinn, T. (2016). Oxygen therapy for acute myocardial infarction. *Cochrane Database of Systematic Reviews, 12*, CD007160.
Centers for Disease Control and Prevention. (2020). Adult immunization schedules for ages 19 years or older, United States, 2020. Retrieved from http://www.cdc.gov/vaccines/schedules/hcp/imz/adult.html. Accessed June 9, 2021.
Fletcher, G. F., Ades, P. A., Kligfield, P., et al. (2013). Exercise standards for testing and training: A scientific statement from the American Heart Association. *Circulation, 128*(8), 873–934.
Grundy, S. M., Stone, N. J., Bailey, A. L., et al. (2019). 2018 AHA/ACC/AACVPR/AAPA/ABC/ACPM/ADA/AGS/APhA/ASPC/NLA/PCNA guideline on the management of blood cholesterol: A report of the American College of Cardiology/American Heart Association Task Force on Clinical Practice Guidelines. *Circulation, 139*(25), e1082–e1143.
Lau, E. S., O'Donoghue, M. L., Hamilton, M. A., & Goldhaber, S. Z. (2016). Women and heart attacks. *Circulation, 133*(10), e428–e429 https://doi.org/10.1161/CIRCULATIONAHA.115.018973.
McSweeney, J. C., Rosenfeld, A. G., Abel, W. M., et al. (2016). Preventing and experiencing ischemic heart disease as a woman: State of the science: A scientific statement from the American Heart Association. *Circulation, 133*(13), 1302–1331.
Mehta, L. S., Beckie, T. M., DeVon, H. A., et al. (2016). Acute myocardial infarction in women: A scientific statement from the American Heart Association. *Circulation, 133*(9), 916–947.
Mieres, J. H., Gulati, M., Bairey Merz, N., et al. (2014). Role of noninvasive testing in the clinical evaluation of women with suspected ischemic heart disease: A consensus statement from the American heart association. *Circulation, 130*(4), 350–379.
National Consensus Project for Quality Palliative Care. (2018). In *Clinical Practice guidelines for quality palliative care* (4th ed.). Retrieved from https://www.nationalcoalitionhpc.org/ncp/. Accessed June 9, 2021.
O'Connor, R. E., Al Ali, A. S., Brady, W. J., et al. (2015). Part 9: Acute coronary syndromes: 2015 American Heart Association guidelines update for cardiopulmonary resuscitation and emergency cardiovascular care. *Circulation, 132*(18 Suppl. 2), S483–S500.
O'Gara, P. T., Kushner, F. G., Ascheim, D. D., et al. (2013). 2013 ACCF/AHA guideline for the management of ST-elevation myocardial infarction: Executive summary: A report of the American College of Cardiology Foundation/American Heart Association Task Force on Practice guidelines. *Circulation, 127*(4), 529–555.
Whelton, P. K., Carey, R. M., Aronow, W. S., et al. (2018). 2017 ACC/AHA/AAPA/ABC/ACPM/AGS/APhA/ASH/ASPC/NMA/PCNA guideline for the prevention, detection, evaluation, and management of high blood pressure in adults; executive summary: A report of the American College of Cardiology/American Heart Association Task Force on clinical Practice Guidelines. *Hypertension, 71*(6), 1269–1324.

Risk for Impaired Cardiovascular Function Domain 4 Activity/rest Class 4 Cardiovascular/pulmonary responses

Mary Beth Flynn Makic, PhD, RN, CNS, CCNS, CCRN-K, FAAN, FNAP, FCNS

NANDA-I

Definition

Susceptible to disturbance in substance transport, body homeostasis, tissue metabolic residue removal, and organ function, which may compromise health.

Risk Factors

Anxiety; average daily physical activity is less than recommended for age and gender; body mass index above normal range for age and gender; excessive accumulation of fat for age and gender; excessive alcohol intake; excessive stress; inadequate dietary habits; inadequate knowledge of modifiable factors; inattentive to second-hand smoke; ineffective blood glucose level management; ineffective blood pressure management; ineffective lipid balance management; smoking; substance misuse

At-Risk Population

Economically disadvantaged individuals; individuals with family history of diabetes mellitus; individuals with family history of dyslipidemia; individuals with family history of hypertension; individuals with family history of metabolic syndrome; individuals with family history of obesity; individuals with history of cardiovascular event; men; older adults; postmenopausal women

Associated Conditions

Depression; diabetes mellitus; dyslipidemia; hypertension; insulin resistance; pharmaceutical preparations

NIC, NOC, Client Outcomes, Nursing Interventions and *Rationales,* Client/Family Teaching and Discharge Planning and References

See the care plans for Decreased **Cardiac** Output; Risk for Decreased **Cardiac** Tissue Perfusion; Risk for **Metabolic Syndrome;** and Risk for **Thrombosis**

Caregiver Role Strain Domain 7 Role relationship Class 1 Caregiving roles

Olga F. Jarrín, PhD, RN and Mary Velahos, BSN

C

NANDA-I

Definition

Difficulty in fulfilling care responsibilities, expectations and/or behaviors for family or significant others.

Defining Characteristics

Caregiving Activities

Apprehensive about future ability to provide care; apprehensive about future health of care receiver; apprehensive about potential institutionalization of care receiver; apprehensive about well-being of care receiver if unable to provide care; difficulty completing required tasks; difficulty performing required tasks; dysfunctional change in caregiving activities; preoccupation with care routine

Caregiver Health Status

Physiological: Fatigue; gastrointestinal distress; headache; hypertension; rash; reports altered sleep-wake cycle; weight change
Emotional: Depressive symptoms; emotional lability; expresses anger; expresses frustration; impatience; insufficient time to meet personal needs; nervousness; somatization
Socioeconomic: Altered leisure activities; isolation; low work productivity; refuses career advancement

Caregiver-Care Receiver Relationship

Difficulty watching care receiver with illness; sadness about altered interpersonal relations with care receiver; uncertainty about alteration in interpersonal relations with care receiver

Family Processes

Family conflict; reports concern about family member(s)

Related Factors

Caregiver

Competing role commitments; depressive symptoms; inadequate fulfillment of others' expectations; inadequate fulfillment of self-expectations; inadequate knowledge about community resources; inadequate psychological resilience; inadequate recreation; ineffective coping strategies; inexperience with caregiving; insufficient physical endurance; insufficient privacy; not developmentally ready for caregiver role; physical conditions; social isolation; stressors; substance misuse; unrealistic self-expectations

Care Receiver Factors

Discharged home with significant needs; increased care needs; loss of independence; problematic behavior; substance misuse; unpredictability of illness trajectory; unstable health status

Caregiver-Care Receiver Relationship

Abusive interpersonal relations; codependency; inadequate interpersonal relations; unaddressed abuse; unrealistic care receiver expectations; violent interpersonal relations

Caregiving Activities

Altered nature of care activities; around-the-clock care responsibilities; complexity of care activities; excessive caregiving activities; extended duration of caregiving required; inadequate assistance; inadequate equipment for providing care; inadequate physical environment for providing care; inadequate respite for caregiver; insufficient time; unpredictability of care situation

Family Processes

Family isolation; ineffective family adaptation; pattern of family dysfunction; pattern of family dysfunction prior to the caregiving situation; pattern of ineffective family coping

Socioeconomic

C

Difficulty accessing assistance; difficulty accessing community resources; difficulty accessing support; inadequate community resources; inadequate social support; inadequate transportation; social alienation

At-Risk Population

Care receiver with developmental disabilities; caregiver delivering care to partner; caregiver with developmental disabilities; female caregiver; individuals delivering care to infants born prematurely; individuals experiencing financial crisis

Associated Conditions

Care Receiver

Impaired health status; psychological disorder

Caregiver

Chronic disease; congenital disorders; illness severity; mental disorders

NOC (Nursing Outcomes Classification)

Suggested NOC Outcomes

Caregiver Adaptation to Patient Institutionalization; Caregiver Emotional Health; Caregiver Home Care Readiness; Caregiver Lifestyle Disruption; Caregiver-Patient Relationship; Caregiver Performance: Direct Care; Caregiver Performance: Indirect Care; Caregiver Physical Health; Caregiver Role Endurance; Caregiver Stressors; Caregiver Well-Being; Family Resiliency; Family Coping

Example NOC Outcome with Indicators

Caregiver Emotional Health with plans for a positive future as evidenced by the following indicators: Satisfaction with life/Sense of control/Self-esteem/Certainty about future/Perceived social connectedness/Perceived spiritual well-being/Perceived adequacy of resources. (Rate the outcome and indicators of **Caregiver Emotional Health:** 1 = severely compromised, 2 = substantially compromised, 3 = moderately compromised, 4 = mildly compromised, 5 = not compromised [see Section I].)

Client Outcomes

Throughout the Care Situation, the Caregiver Will

- Be able to express feelings of strain
- Feel supported by health care professionals, family, and friends; feel they have adequate information to provide care
- Report reduced or acceptable feelings of burden or distress
- Take part in self-care activities to maintain own physical and psychological/emotional health; identify resources (family and community) available to help in giving care
- Verbalize mastery of the care activities; feel confident and competent to provide care; have the skills to provide care
- Ask for help when needed
- Not refuse help when offered

Throughout the Care Situation, the Care Recipient Will

- Obtain quality and safe physical care and emotional care
- Be treated with respect and dignity

NIC (Nursing Interventions Classification)

Suggested NIC Intervention

Caregiver Support

Example NIC Activities—Caregiver Support

Determine caregiver's acceptance of role; Accept expressions of negative emotion

Nursing Interventions and *Rationales*

- Assess for caregiver role strain at the onset of the care situation, at regular intervals throughout the care situation, at care transitions, and with changes in care recipient status. EBN: *Changes in the care recipient's health status necessitate new skills and monitoring from the caregiver and affect the caregiver's ability to continue to provide care and may affect caregiver health (Trevino et al, 2018).* EB: *Valid and reliable instruments to assess caregiver health include the Caregiver Strain Risk Index, Positive Aspects of Caregiving Questionnaire (Abdollahpour et al, 2017), Caregiver Burden Inventory, Caregiver Reaction Assessment (Given et al, 1992), Screen for Caregiver Burden, Subjective and Objective Scale, Family Caregiver Self Expectations, Caregiver Preparedness Scale (Petruzzo et al, 2017), the Family Caregiver Activation in Transitions (FCAT) Tool, and DECAFTM Family Caregiver Tool (Coleman et al, 2015).*
- Monitor overall health of the caregiver at regular intervals for signs and symptoms of depression, anxiety, role strain, hopelessness, posttraumatic stress, and deteriorating physical health, particularly their control over chronic diseases and comorbid conditions. EB: *Caregivers of stroke survivors had difficulty dealing with depressive feelings, feelings of guilt, anxious/panic episodes, feelings of uncertainty and hopelessness, posttraumatic stress symptoms, and feelings of role strain from commitments (McCurley et al, 2019).* EB: *Caregivers with high levels of depressive symptoms have demonstrated poor health and increased health care utilization and cost (Shaffer et al, 2017).*
- Identify caregiver personal resources such as resilience, proficiency in caregiving skills, social support, optimism, positive aspects of care and resilience, and utilization or availability of social services (e.g., state-funded senior services, veterans' services, Area Agency on Aging resources). EB: *Identification and appreciation of resources may help buffer the negative effects of providing care on caregivers' emotional health and increase the effectiveness of interventions to reduce strain (Joling et al, 2017).*
- Encourage the caregiver to share feelings, concerns, uncertainties, and fears; support groups, including Internet-based ones, can be helpful to gain support. EB: *Internet social support groups can be an effective form of support (Parker Oliver et al, 2017).*
- Regularly assess for any evidence of caregiver or care recipient violence or abuse, especially emotional and verbal abuse; risk factors include substance abuse, poor premorbid relationship, and psychiatric illness. EB: *Caregivers are often unaware of the effect of their behavior on care recipient, and the definition of abuse (Liu et al, 2019).*
- ♦ Ensure appropriate referrals for physical, occupational, and speech-language therapy, as well as social work, including referrals for outpatient therapy or skilled home health care if needed (including therapy needed to maintain functional abilities and prevent decline). EB: *Improvement in client physical function resulted in better physical and psychological quality of life for both client and caregiver (Pucciarelli et al, 2017).*
- Talk with caregivers early and often about palliative care as a means of symptom management for the care recipient. EB: *Many care recipients and their families do not know what palliative care means, which may lead to underutilization of comfort measures (Scott et al, 2017).*
- Help the caregiver learn mindfulness stress management techniques, which can reduce psychological distress. EB: *Mindfulness stress reduction interventions can result in improvement in quality of life, self-compassion, caregiver burden, and relationship satisfaction (Schellekens et al, 2017).*
- Assist the client to identify spiritual beliefs and engage in spiritual practices. EB: *Spiritual beliefs and practices may help caregivers cope because it protects them from depression (Penman, 2018).*
- Encourage regular and open communication with the care recipient and with the health care team. EB: *Care transitions are a critical point to ensure that caregivers have adequate information for client safety and efficient and effective care (Scott et al, 2017).*

C

Geriatric

- The interventions described previously may be adapted for use with geriatric clients.
- Monitor the caregiver for psychological distress and signs of depression, especially if there was an unsatisfactory family relationship before caregiving. EB: *Family caregivers report higher levels of resiliency in providing care when their relationship with care recipient was harmonious before the caregiving role (Joling et al, 2017).*
- To improve the ability to provide safe care: assess caregiver's support and learning needs and provide skills training related to direct care, perform complex monitoring tasks, supervise, and interpret client symptoms, assist with decision-making, assist with medication adherence. EB: *Caregivers need individualized resources and support to master skills needed for care management, care coordination, and medical/nursing tasks (Polenick et al, 2017).*

Pediatric

- Assess parents for perceived self-blame or worsened relationship with their child, especially if their child's condition is psychiatric in nature, and assist them to seek social support, instill hope, and identify how they might grow. EB: *Parents of children with severe mental illness including self-mutilation, suicidal ideation, obsessive compulsive disorders, eating disorders, and so on, often placed a high amount of responsibility on themselves and reported feeling the psychiatric disorder pushed them and their child apart (Whitlock et al, 2018).*
- Assess for partner support of the caregiver in dual-earning households, and provide resources related to couples' or family therapy if needed. EB: *Perceived lack of support from a partner is associated with greater caregiver role strain and psychological distress, and strain between partners leads to further stress (DePasqale et al, 2017).*

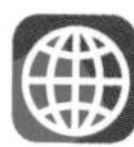

Multicultural

- Assess for cultural and spiritual needs of client and caregiver. EB: *Culturally competent care can improve client care quality and outcomes; cultural competence refers to the ability of health providers and organizations to deliver services that meet the cultural, social, and religious needs of clients and their families (Mahdavi et al, 2017; Swihart et al, 2021).*

Home Care

- Assess the client and caregiver at every visit for the quality of their relationship and for the quality and safety of the care provided. EB: *Education, social support, and behavioral management are the most effective support for caregivers of dementia clients (Clarkson et al, 2017).*
- Encourage use of respite care, which may include regular care and assistance at home, or a brief period of total care (24/7) at home or in an inpatient facility to allow the caregiver to recover from an illness, attend a wedding, or go on a short vacation. EB: *Respite care provides time away from the care situation and may help alleviate some caregiver distress (Vandepitte et al, 2016; Sakurai & Kohno, 2020).*

Client/Family Teaching and Discharge Planning

- Identify client and caregiver factors that necessitate the use of skilled home health care services or need to be addressed before the client can be safely discharged. EBN: *Interventions to be considered needed at discharge may include medication management, medication reconciliation, symptom monitoring, identification of community-based resources, skills training for clients and caregivers, and specific client or caregiver concerns about home health care (Mollica et al, 2017).*
- Collaborate with the caregiver and discuss the care needs of the client, disease processes, medications, and what to expect as part of discharge planning and transition care. EBN: *Components of comprehensive and effective transitional care may require adaptation and include client and caregiver well-being, caregiver engagement, caregiver education, client engagement, client education, complexity/medication management, care continuity, and accountability (Naylor et al, 2017, 2018).*
- Involve the family caregiver in care transitions and discharge from institutions; use a multiprofessional team to provide medical and social services for detailed instruction and planning specific to the care need. EB: *Family members need education specific to their situation at discharge, and this educational approach should be based on the cltient's needs. The postdischarge visit serves as an important vehicle to prevent readmissions and improve quality of care for clients (Rodakowski et al, 2017; Soufer et al, 2017).*

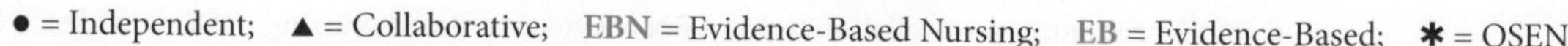

REFERENCES

Abdollahpour, I., Nedjat, S., Noroozian, M., Salimi, Y., & Majdzadeh, R. (2017). Positive aspects of caregiving questionnaire: A validation study in caregivers of patients with dementia. *Journal of Geriatric Psychiatry and Neurology*, *30*(2), 77–83. https://doi.org/10.1177/0891988716686831.

Clarkson, P., Davies, L., Jasper, R., Loynes, N., Challis, D., & Home Support in Dementia (HoSt-D) Programme Management Group. (2017). A systematic review of the economic evidence for home support interventions in dementia. *Value in Health*, *20*(8), 1198–1209 https://doi.org/10.1016/j.jval.2017.04.004.

Coleman, E. A., Ground, K. L., & Maul, A. (2015). The Family Caregiver Activation in Transitions (FCAT) tool: A new measure of family caregiver self-efficacy. *Joint Commission Journal on Quality and Patient Safety*, *41*(11), 502–507. https://doi.org/10.1016/S1553-7250(15)41066-9.

DePasquale, N., Polenick, C. A., Davis, K. D., Moen, P., Hammer, L. B., & Almeida, D. M. (2017). The psychosocial implications of managing work and family caregiving roles: Gender differences among information technology professionals. *Journal of Family Issues*, *38*(11), 1495–1519. https://doi.org/10.1177/0192513X15584680.

Given, C. W., Given, B., Stommel, M., Collins, C., King, S., & Franklin, S. (1992). The caregiver reaction assessment (CRA) for caregivers to persons with chronic physical and mental impairments. *Research in Nursing & Health*, *15*(4), 271–283.

Joling, K. J., Windle, G., Dröes, R. M., Huisman, M., Hertough, C. M. P. M., & Woods, R. T. (2017). What are the essential features of resilience for informal caregivers of people living with dementia? A Delphi consensus examination. *Aging & Mental Health*, *21*(5), 509–517. https://doi.org/10.1080/13607863.2015.1124836.

Liu, P. J., Conrad, K. J., Beach, S. R., Iris, M., & Schiamberg, L. B. (2019). The importance of investigating abuser characteristics in elder emotional/psychological abuse: Results from adult protective services data. *Journals of Gerontology Series B: Psychological Sciences and Social Sciences*, *74*(5), 897–907. https://doi.org/10.1093/geronb/gbx064.

Mahdavi, B., Fallahi-Khoshknab, M., Mohammadi, F., Hosseini, M. A., & Haghi, M. (2017). Effects of spiritual group therapy on caregiver strain in home caregivers of the elderly with Alzheimer's disease. *Archives of Psychiatric Nursing*, *31*(3), 269–273. https://doi.org/10.1016/j.apnu.2016.12.003.

McCurley, J. L., Funes, C. J., Zale, E. L., et al. (2019). Preventing chronic emotional distress in stroke survivors and their informal caregivers. *Neurocritical Care*, *30*(3), 581–589. https://doi.org/10.1007/s12028-018-0641-6.

Mollica, M. A., Litzelman, K., Rowland, J. H., & Kent, E. E. (2017). The role of medical/nursing skills training in caregiver confidence and burden: A CanCORS study. *Cancer*, *123*(22), 4481–4487. https://doi.org/10.1002/cncr.30875.

Naylor, M. D., Hirschman, K. B., Toles, M. P., Jarrín, O. F., Shaid, E., & Pauly, M. V. (2018). Adaptations of the evidence-based transitional care model in the U.S. *Social Science & Medicine*, *213*, 28–36. https://doi.org/10.1016/j.socscimed.2018.07.023.

Naylor, M. D., Shaid, E. C., Carpenter, D., et al. (2017). Components of comprehensive and effective transitional care. *Journal of the American Geriatrics Society*, *65*(6), 1119–1125. https://doi.org/10.1111/jgs.14782.

Oliver, D. P., Patil, S., Benson, J. J., et al. (2017). The effect of internet group support for caregivers on social support, self-efficacy, and caregiver burden: A meta-analysis. *Telemedicine Journal and e-Health*, *23*(8), 621–629. https://doi.org/10.1089/tmj.2016.0183.

Penman, J. (2018). Finding paradise within: How spirituality protects palliative care clients and caregivers from depression. *Journal of Holistic Nursing*, *36*(3), 243–246. https://doi.org/10.1177/0898010117714665.

Petruzzo, A., Paturzo, M., Buck, H. G., et al. (2017). Psychometric evaluation of the Caregiver Preparedness Scale in caregivers of adults with heart failure. *Research in Nursing & Health*, *40*(5), 470–478. https://doi.org/10.1002/nur.21811.

Polenick, C. A., Leggett, A. N., & Kales, H. C. (2017). Medical care activities among spouses of older adults with functional disability: Implications for caregiving difficulties and gains. *American Journal of Geriatric Psychiatry*, *25*(10), 1085–1093. https://doi.org/10.1016/j.jagp.2017.05.001.

Pucciarelli, G., Vellone, E., Savini, S., et al. (2017). Roles of changing physical function and caregiver burden on quality of life in stroke: A longitudinal dyadic analysis. *Stroke*, *48*(3), 733–739. https://doi.org/10.1161/STROKEAHA.116.014989.

Rodakowski, J., Rocco, P. B., Ortiz, M., et al. (2017). Caregiver integration during discharge planning for older adults to reduce resource use: A metaanalysis. *Journal of the American Geriatrics Society*, *65*(8), 1748–1755. https://doi.org/10.1111/jgs.14873.

Sakurai, S., & Kohno, Y. (2020). Effectiveness of respite care via short-stay services to support sleep in family caregivers. *International Journal of Environmental Research and Public Health*, *17*(7), 2428. https://doi.org/10.3390/ijerph17072428.

Schellekens, M. P. J., van den Hurk, D. G. M., Prins, J. B., et al. (2017). Mindfulness-based stress reduction added to care as usual for lung cancer patients and/or their partners: A multicentre randomized controlled trial. *Psycho-Oncology*, *26*(12), 2118–2126. https://doi.org/10.1002/pon.4430.

Scott, A. M., Li, J., Oyewole-Eletu, S., et al. (2017). Understanding facilitators and barriers to care transitions: Insights from Project ACHIEVE site visits. *Joint Commission Journal on Quality and Patient Safety*, *43*(9), 433–447. https://doi.org/10.1016/j.jcjq.2017.02.012.

Shaffer, K. M., Kim, Y., Carver, C. S., & Cannady, R. S. (2017). Depressive symptoms predict cancer caregivers' physical health decline. *Cancer*, *123*, 4277–4285. https://doi.org/10.1002/cncr.30835.

Soufer, A., Riello, R. J., Desai, N. R., Testani, J. M., & Ahmad, T. (2017). A blueprint for the post discharge clinic visit after an admission for heart failure. *Progress in Cardiovascular Diseases*, *60*(2), 237–248. https://doi.org/10.1016/j.pcad.2017.08.004.

Swihart, D. L., Yarrarapu, S. N. S., & Martin, R. L. (2021). Cultural religious competence in clinical practice. *StatPearls*. Treasure Island, FL: StatPearls Publishing. Last updated Feb 18, 2021. Retrieved from https://www.ncbi.nlm.nih.gov/books/NBK493216/. Accessed June 9, 2021.

Trevino, K. M., Prigerson, H. G., & Maciejewski, P. K. (2018). Advanced cancer caregiving as a risk for major depressive episodes and generalized anxiety disorder. *Psycho-Oncology*, *27*(1), 243–246. https://doi.org/10.1002/pon.4441.

Vandepitte, S., Van Den Noortgate, N., Putman, K., Verhaeghe, S., Verdonck, C., & Annemans, L. (2016). Effectiveness of respite care in supporting informal caregivers of persons with dementia: A systematic review. *International Journal of Geriatric Psychiatry*, *31*(12), 1277–1288. https://doi.org/10.1002/gps.4504.

Whitlock, J., Lloyd-Richardson, E., Fisseha, F., & Bates, T. (2018). Parental secondary stress: The often hidden consequences of nonsuicidal self-injury in youth. *Journal of Clinical Psychology*, *74*(1), 178–196. https://doi.org/10.1002/jclp.22488.

Risk for Caregiver Role Strain Domain 7 Role relationship Class 1 Caregiving roles

Marina Martinez-Kratz, MS, RN, CNE

C

NANDA-I

Definition

Susceptible to difficulty in fulfilling care responsibilities, expectations, and/or behaviors for family or significant others, which may compromise health.

Risk Factors

Caregiver Factors

Competing role commitments; depressive symptoms; inadequate fulfillment of others' expectations; inadequate fulfillment of self-expectations; inadequate knowledge about community resources; inadequate psychological resilience; inadequate recreation; ineffective coping strategies; inexperience with caregiving; insufficient physical endurance; insufficient privacy; not developmentally ready for caregiver role; physical conditions; stressors; substance misuse; unrealistic self-expectations; unstable health status

Care Receiver Factors

Discharged home with significant needs; increased care needs; loss of independence; problematic behavior; substance misuse; unpredictability of illness trajectory; unstable health condition

Caregiver-Care Receiver Relationship

Abusive interpersonal relations; codependency; inadequate interpersonal relations; unaddressed abuse; unrealistic care receiver expectations; violent interpersonal relations

Caregiving Activities

Altered nature of care activities; around-the-clock care responsibilities; complexity of care activities; excessive caregiving activities; extended duration of caregiving required; inadequate assistance; inadequate equipment for providing care; inadequate physical environment for providing care; inadequate respite for caregiver; insufficient time; unpredictability of care situation

Family Processes

Family isolation; ineffective family adaptation; pattern of family dysfunction; pattern of family dysfunction prior to the caregiving situation; pattern of ineffective family coping

Socioeconomic

Difficulty accessing assistance; difficulty accessing community resources; difficulty accessing support; inadequate community resources; inadequate social support; inadequate transportation; social alienation; social isolation

At-Risk Population

Care receiver with developmental disabilities; care receiver's condition inhibits conversation; caregiver delivering care to partner; caregiver with developmental disabilities; female caregiver; individuals delivering care to infants born prematurely; individuals experiencing financial crisis

Associated Conditions

Caregiver Factors

Impaired health status; psychological disorder

Care Receiver Factors

Chronic disease; congenital disorders; illness severity; mental disorders

NIC, NOC, Client Outcomes, Nursing Interventions and *Rationales,* Client/Family Teaching, and References

Refer to care plan for **Caregiver Role Strain.**

Risk for Ineffective Cerebral Tissue Perfusion

Domain 4 Activity/rest Class 4 Cardiovascular/pulmonary responses

Kimberly S. Meyer, PhD, ACNP-BC, CNRN

C

NANDA-I

Definition

Susceptible to a decrease in cerebral tissue circulation, which may compromise health.

Risk Factors

Substance misuse

At-Risk Population

Individuals with history of recent myocardial infarction

Associated Conditions

Abnormal serum partial thromboplastin time; abnormal serum prothrombin time; akinetic left ventricular wall segment; atherosclerosis; atrial fibrillation; atrial myxoma; brain injuries; brain neoplasm; carotid stenosis; cerebral aneurysm; coagulopathy; dilated cardiomyopathy; disseminated intravascular coagulopathy; embolism; hypercholesterolemia; hypertension; infective endocarditis; mechanical prosthetic valve; mitral stenosis; pharmaceutical preparations; sick sinus syndrome; treatment regimen

NOC (Nursing Outcomes Classification)

Suggested NOC Outcomes

Acute Confusion Level; Tissue Perfusion: Cerebral; Agitation Level; Neurological Status; Cognition; Seizure Control; Motor Strength

Example NOC Outcome with Indicators

Tissue Perfusion: Cerebral as evidenced by the following indicators: Headache/Restlessness/Listlessness/Agitation/Vomiting/Fever/Impaired cognition/Decreased level of consciousness/Motor weakness/Dysphagia/Slurred speech. (Rate the outcome and indicators of **Tissue Perfusion: Cerebral:** 1 = severe, 2 = substantial, 3 = moderate, 4 = mild, 5 = none [see Section I].)

Client Outcomes

Client Will (Specify Time Frame)

- State stable or improved headache
- Demonstrate appropriate orientation to person, place, time, and situation
- Demonstrate ability to follow simple commands
- Demonstrate equal bilateral motor strength
- Demonstrate adequate swallowing ability
- Maintain (or improve) neurological examination

NIC (Nursing Interventions Classification)

Suggested NIC Interventions

Medication Management; Neurologic Monitoring; Positioning: Neurologic; Cerebral Perfusion Promotion; Fall Prevention; Cognitive Stimulation; Environmental Management: Safety

Example NIC Activities—Neurologic Monitoring

Monitor pupillary size, shape, symmetry, and reactivity; Monitor level of consciousness; Monitor level of orientation; Monitor trend of Glasgow Coma Scale; Monitor facial symmetry; Note complaint of headache; Monitor blood pressure (BP) and heart rate; Monitor respiratory function

C

Nursing Interventions and *Rationales*

- To decrease risk of reduced cerebral perfusion related to stroke or transient ischemic attack (TIA):
  - Obtain a family history of hypertension, diabetes, and stroke to identify persons who may be at increased risk of stroke. EB: *A positive family history of stroke increases risk of stroke significantly (Pourasgari & Mohamadkhani, 2020).*
  - Monitor BP regularly because hypertension is a major risk factor for both ischemic and hemorrhagic stroke. EB: *Systolic BP should be treated to a goal of less than 140 mm Hg and diastolic BP to less than 90 mm Hg, whereas clients with diabetes or renal disease have a BP goal of less than 130/80 mm Hg (Flack & Adekola, 2020).*
  - Teach hypertensive clients the importance of taking their health care provider–ordered antihypertensive agent to prevent stroke. EB: *Treatment of hypertension in adults with diabetes with a calcium channel blocker or angiotensin-converting enzyme (ACE) inhibitor may be useful (Flack & Adekola, 2020).*
  - Stress smoking cessation at every encounter with clients, using multimodal techniques to aid in quitting, such as counseling, nicotine replacement, and oral smoking cessation medications. Provide client and family education to reduce lifestyle-associated risk factors for stroke. EB: *Studies show that a consistent and overwhelming relationship between lifestyle risk factors such as smoking, physical inactivity, and poor diet associated with obesity increases the client risk of both ischemic and hemorrhagic stroke (Ding et al, 2019; Parikh et al, 2020).*
  - Teach clients who experience a transient TIA that they are at increased risk for a stroke. Instruct clients that adherence to medication therapy decreases recurrent TIA/stroke risk. EB: *The 90-day risk for stroke after a TIA is as high as 17%, with the greatest risk occurring in the first week (Heron, 2016).* EB: *Dual antiplatelet therapy decreases the incidence of subsequent ischemic events (Johnston et al, 2020).*
  - Screen clients 65 years of age and older for atrial fibrillation with pulse assessment. EB: *Atrial fibrillation is associated with a fivefold increase in stroke. Systematic pulse assessment in a primary care setting resulted in a 60% increase in the detection of atrial fibrillation (Jones et al, 2020).*
  - Instruct the client regarding the appropriate use and side effects of anticoagulation in the prevention of cardioembolic stroke. EB: *With therapeutic dosing, vitamin K agonists and non–vitamin K agonists reduce the stroke risk in client with atrial fibrillation (Wutzler et al, 2019).*
  - Call 911 or activate the rapid response team of a hospital immediately when clients display symptoms of stroke as determined by the Cincinnati Stroke Scale (F: facial drooping; A: arm drift on one side; S: speech slurred), being careful to note the time of symptom appearance. Additional symptoms of stroke include sudden numbness/weakness of face, arm, or leg, especially on one side; sudden confusion; trouble speaking or understanding; sudden difficulty seeing with one or both eyes; sudden trouble walking, dizziness, loss of balance, or coordination; or sudden severe headache (Jauch et al, 2013). EB: *The Cincinnati Stroke Scale (derived from the National Institutes of Health [NIH] Stroke Scale) is used to identify clients having a stroke who may be candidates for thrombolytic therapy or mechanical thrombectomy (De Luca et al, 2019; Crowe et al, 2021). Emergency medical services (EMS) activation results in faster health care provider assessment, computed tomography, and neurological evaluation, which facilitates administering thrombolytics to eligible individuals who had a stroke within the required 3- to 4.5-hour time period (Jauch et al, 2013).*
  - Use clinical practice guidelines for glycemic control and BP targets to guide the care of clients with diabetes who have had a stroke or TIA. EB: *The American Stroke Association recommends that evidence-based guidelines be used in the care of clients with diabetes. Good glycemic control has been associated with decreased incidence of strokes (Zhu et al, 2019).* EB: *Hypoglycemia (blood sugar <60 mg/dL) should be corrected immediately to improve stroke outcomes (Powers et al, 2019).* EB: *Persistent hyperglycemia (blood sugar >180 mg/dL) should be avoided because hyperglycemia is associated with worse stroke outcomes (Powers et al, 2019; Zheng & Zhou, 2020).*
  - Maintain head of bed less than 30 degrees in the acute phase (<72 hours of symptom onset) of ischemic stroke. EB: *Cerebral blood flow is decreased when head of bed is elevated from 0 to 30 degrees in clients with acute ischemic stroke but the effects on recovery outcomes are unclear (Anderson & Olivarría, 2018).*
  - Head of bed may be elevated to sitting position without detrimental effect to cerebral blood flow in clients with ischemic stroke or hemorrhagic stroke at 72 hours after symptom onset. EB: *Head of bed elevation of 45 and 70 degrees in the subacute phase of ischemic stroke resulted in minor changes in cerebral blood flow velocities (Aries et al, 2013).* EB: *Cerebral blood flow had no significant changes in head of bed elevations from 0 to 90 degrees in clients with subarachnoid hemorrhage at days 3, 7, and 10 (Kung et al, 2013).*

- ○ Administer enteric/oral nimodipine as prescribed by the health care provider after aneurysmal subarachnoid hemorrhage for 21 days. EB: *Nimodipine, a calcium channel blocker, has been shown by multiple randomized clinical trials to improve outcome by limiting delayed cerebral ischemia after subarachnoid hemorrhage strokes (Pal'a et al, 2019).* EB: *If hypotension occurs following nimodipine administration, vasopressor support and modification of the dosing schedule to include smaller, more frequent dosages should be implemented as missed doses result in adverse outcomes (Ehrlich et al, 2019; Pal'a et al, 2019).*
- ○ Monitor neurological function frequently in the first 2 weeks after subarachnoid hemorrhage because subtle declines may be related to cerebral vasospasm. EB: *Cerebral vasospasm occurs in up to two-thirds of clients with subarachnoid hemorrhage and can lead to delayed cerebral ischemia (Reynolds et al, 2020; Thomas & Petrone, 2020).*
- ○ Maintain cerebral perfusion pressure (CPP) 60 to 70 mm Hg in clients with traumatic brain injury. EB: *When injury-related impaired autoregulation is present, CPP less than 60 is associated with worse outcomes (Carney et al, 2017; Güiza et al, 2017).*

▲ To decrease risk of reduced CPP: CPP = Mean arterial pressure – intracranial pressure (CPP = MAP – ICP)

- ○ Maintain euvolemia. EB: Infusing isotonic intravenous fluids to sustain normal circulating volume helps maintain normal cerebral blood flow and reduces the incidence of vasospasm (Hemphill et al, 2015; Rumalla et al, 2021).

▲ To treat decreased CPP:

- ○ Clients with subarachnoid hemorrhagic stroke experiencing delayed cerebral ischemia, as evidenced by declining neurological examination, should undergo a stepwise trial of induced hypertension up to 220 mm Hg. EB: *Medically managed hypertension increased cerebral blood flow and produced neurological improvement in the majority of clients (Suwatcharangkoon et al, 2019).*
- ○ Administer vasopressor infusions to raise MAP per collaborative protocol. EB: *Clients with delayed cerebral ischemia treated with norepinephrine or phenylephrine have better BP augmentation and better clinical outcomes than clients treated with other vasopressors (Roy et al, 2017; Rouanot & Silva, 2019).*
- ○ Mobilize clients with subarachnoid hemorrhage as early as 1 day after aneurysm is secured. EB: *Clients undergoing early mobilization are less likely to develop severe cerebral vasospasm, have a shorter hospital length of stay, and are more likely to discharge to home or acute rehabilitation (Karic et al, 2017; Young et al, 2019).*

REFERENCES

Anderson, C. S., & Olavarría, V. V. (2018). Head positioning in acute stroke. *Stroke, 50*(1), 224–228 https://doi.org/10.1161/STROKEAHA.118.020087.

Aries, M. J., Elting, J. W., Stewart, R., De Keyser, J., Kremer, B., & Vroomen, P. (2013). Cerebral blood flow velocity changes during upright positioning in bed after acute stroke: An observational study. *British Medical Journal Open, 3*, 1–4 http://dx.doi.org/10.1136/bmjopen-2013-002960.

Carney, N., Totten, A. M., O'Reilly, C., et al. (2017). Guidelines for the management of severe traumatic brain injury, fourth edition. *Neurosurgery, 80*(1), 6–15.

Crowe, R. P., Myers, J. B., Fernandez, A. R., Bourn, S., & McMullan, J. T. (2021). The Cincinnati Prehospital Stroke Scale compared to stroke severity tools for large vessel occlusion stroke prediction. *Prehospital Emergency Care, 25*(1), 67–75. https://doi.org/10.1080/10903127.2020.1725198

De Luca, A., Mariani, M., Riccardi, M. T., & Damiani, G. (2019). The role of the Cincinnati Prehospital Stroke Scale in the emergency department: Evidence from a systematic review and meta-analysis. *Open Access Emergency Medicine, 11*, 147–159 https://doi.org/10.2147/OAEM.S178544.

Ding, N., Sang, Y., Chen, J., et al. (2019). Cigarette smoking, smoking cessation, and long-term risk of 3 major atherosclerotic diseases. *Journal of the American College of Cardiology, 74*(4), 498–507 https://doi.org/10.1016/j.jacc.2019.05.049.

Erlich, G., Kirschning, T., Wenz, J., Hegewald, A. A., Neumaier-Probst, E., & Seiz-Rosenhagen, M. (2019). Outcome of oral and intra-arterial nimodipine administration after aneurysmal subarachnoid hemorrhage: A single centre study. *In Vivo, 33*(6), 1967–1975 doi:10.21873/invivo.11692.

Flack, J. M., & Adekola, B. (2020). Blood pressure and the new ACC/AHA hypertension guidelines. *Trends in Cardiovascular Medicine, 30*(3), 160–164 https://doi.org/10.1016/j.tcm.2019.05.003.

Güiza, F., Meyfroidt, G., Piper, I., et al. (2017). Cerebral perfusion pressure insults and associations with outcome in adult traumatic brain injury. *Journal of Neurotrauma, 34*(16), 2425–2431.

Hemphill, J. C., 3rd, Greenburg, S. M., Anderson, C. S., et al. (2015). Guidelines for the management of spontaneous intracerebral hemorrhage. *Stroke, 46*(7), 2032–2060.

Heron, N. (2016). Optimizing secondary prevention in the acute period following a TIA of ischaemic origin. *BMJ Open Sport & Exercise Medicine, 2*(1), e000161 doi:10.1136/bmjsem-2016-000161.

Jauch, E. C., Saver, J. L., Adams, H. P., Jr., et al. (2013). Guidelines for the early management of patients with acute ischemic stroke: A guideline for healthcare professionals from the American heart association/American stroke association. *Stroke, 44*(3), 870–947.

Johnston, S. C., Amarenco, P., Denison, H., et al. (2020). Ticagrelor and aspirin or aspirin alone in acute ischemic stroke or TIA. *New England Journal of Medicine, 383*, 207–217.

Jones, N. R., Taylor, C. J., Hobbs, F. D. R., Bowman, L., & Casadei, B. (2020). Screening for atrial fibrillation: A call for evidence. *European Heart Journal, 41*(10), 1075–1085 https://doi.org/10.1093/eurheartj/ehz834.

Karic, T., Røe, C., Nordenmark, T. H., Becker, F., Sorteberg, W., & Sorteberg, A. (2017). Effect of early mobilization and rehabilitation on complications in aneurysmal subarachnoid hemorrhage. *Journal of Neurosurgery*, *126*(2), 518–526.

Kung, D. K., Chalouhi, N., Jabbour, P. M., et al. (2013). Cerebral blood flow dynamics and head-of-bed changes in the setting of subarachnoid hemorrhage. *BioMed Research International*, *2013*, 640638 http://dx.doi.org/10.1155/2013/640638.

Pal'a, A., Schick, J., Klein, M., et al. (2019). The influence of nimodipine and vasopressors on outcome in patients with delayed cerebral ischemia after spontaneous subarachnoid hemorrhage. *Journal of Neurosurgery*, *132*(4), 1096–1104 Retrieved from https://thejns.org/view/journals/j-neurosurg/132/4/article-p1096.xml. [Accessed 29 November 2020].

Parikh, N. S., Omran, S. S., Kamel, H., Elkind, M. S. V., & Willey, J. Z. (2020). Smoking-cessation pharmacotherapy for patients with stroke and TIA: Systematic review. *Journal of Clinical Neuroscience*, *78*, 236–241 https://doi.org/10.1016/j.jocn.2020.04.026.

Pourasgari, M., & Mohamadkhani, A. (2020). Heritability for stroke: Essential for taking family history. *Caspian Journal of Internal Medicine*, *11*(3), 237–243 https://doi.org/10.22088/cjim.11.3.237.

Powers, W. J., Rabinstein, A. A., Ackerson, T., et al. (2019). Guidelines for the early management of patients with acute ischemic stroke: 2019 update to the 2018 guidelines for the early management of acute ischemic stroke: A guideline for healthcare professionals from the American heart association/American stroke association. *Stroke*, *50*(12), e344–e418 https://10.1161/STR.0000000000000211.

Reynolds, R. A., Amin, S. N., Jonathan, S. V., et al. (2020). Hyperoxemia and cerebral vasospasm in aneurysmal subarachnoid hemorrhage. *Neurocritical Care*, *35*(1), 30–38 https://doi.org/10.1007/s12028-020-01136-6.

Rouanet, C., & Silva, G. S. (2019). Aneurysmal subarachnoid hemorrhage: Current concepts and updates. *Arquivos de Neuro-Psiquiatria*, *77*(11), 806–814 https://doi.org/10.1590/0004-282x20190112.

Roy, B., McCullough, L. D., Dhar, R., Grady, J., Wang, Y. B., & Brown, R. J. (2017). Comparison of initial vasopressors used for delayed cerebral ischemia after subarachnoid hemorrhage. *Cerebrovascular Disease*, *43*(5–6), 266–271.

Rumalla, K., Lin, M., Ding, L., et al. (2021). Risk factors for cerebral vasospasm in aneurysmal subarachnoid hemorrhage: A population-based study of 8346 patients. *World Neurosurgery*, *145*, e233–e241 https://doi.org/10.1016/j.wneu.2020.10.008.

Suwatcharangkoon, S., De Marchis, G. M., Witsch, J., et al. (2019). Medical treatment failure for symptomatic vasospasm after subarachnoid hemorrhage threatens long-term outcome. *Stroke*, *50*(7), 1686–1702 doi:10.1161/STROKEAHA.118.022536.

Thomas, C., & Petrone, A. (2020). Incidence of cerebral vasospasm and delayed cerebral ischemia following non–traumatic aneurysmal subarachnoid hemorrhage. *FASEB Journal*, *34*(S1), 1-1 https://doi.org/10.1096/fasebj.2020.34.s1.04288.

Wutzler, A., Krogias, C., Grau, A., Veltkamp, R., Heuschmann, P. U., & Haeusler, K. G. (2019). Stroke prevention in patients with acute ischemic stroke and atrial fibrillation in Germany—a cross sectional survey. *BMC Neurology*, *19*(1), 25 https://doi.org/10.1186/s12883-019-1249-y.

Young, B., Moyer, M., Pino, W., Kung, D., Zager, E., & Kumar, M. A. (2019). Safety and feasibility of early mobilization in patients with subarachnoid hemorrhage and external ventricular drain. *Neurocritical Care*, *31*(1), 88–96 https://doi.org/10.1007/s12028-019-00670-2.

Zheng, D., & Zhao, X. (2020). Intensive versus standard glucose control in patients with ischemic stroke: A meta-analysis of randomized controlled trials. *World Neurosurgery*, *136*, e487–e495. https://doi.org/10.1016/j.wneu.2020.01.042.

Zhu, B., Pan, Y., Jing, J., et al. (2019). Stress hyperglycemia and outcome of non-diabetic patients after acute ischemic stroke. *Frontiers in Neurology*, *10*, 1003. https://doi.org/10.3389/fneur.2019.01003.

Ineffective Childbearing Process Domain 8 Sexuality Class 3 Reproduction

Dianne F. Hayward, RN, MSN, WHNP

NANDA-I

Definition

Inability to prepare for and/or maintain a healthy pregnancy, childbirth process, and care of the newborn for ensuring well-being.

Defining Characteristics

During Pregnancy

Failure to utilize social support; inadequate attachment behavior; inadequate prenatal care; inadequate prenatal lifestyle; inadequate preparation of newborn care items; inadequate preparation of the home environment; inadequate respect for unborn baby; ineffective management of unpleasant symptoms in pregnancy; unrealistic expectations about labor and delivery

During Labor and Delivery

Decreased proactivity during labor and delivery; failure to utilize social support; inadequate attachment behavior; inadequate lifestyle for stage of labor; inappropriate response to onset of labor

After Birth

Failure to utilize social support; inadequate attachment behavior; inadequate baby care techniques; inadequate infant clothing; inappropriate baby feeding techniques; inappropriate breast care; inappropriate lifestyle; unsafe environment for an infant

C

Related Factors

Domestic violence; inadequate knowledge of childbearing process; inadequate mental preparation for parenting; inadequate parental role model; inadequate prenatal care; inadequate social support; inconsistent prenatal health visits; low maternal confidence; maternal malnutrition; maternal powerlessness; maternal psychological distress; substance misuse; unrealistic birth plan; unsafe environment

At-Risk Population

Individuals experiencing unplanned pregnancy; individuals experiencing unwanted pregnancy

NOC (Nursing Outcomes Classification)

Suggested NOC Outcomes

Fetal Status: Antepartum, Intrapartum; Maternal Status: Antepartum, Intrapartum; Depression Level; Family Resiliency; Knowledge: Substance Use Control; Social Support; Spiritual Support; Risk for Infection

Example NOC Outcome with Indicators

Maternal Status: Antepartum as evidenced by the following indicators: Emotional attachment to fetus/Coping with discomforts of pregnancy/Mood lability/Has realistic birth plan/Has support system. (Rate each indicator of **Maternal Status: Antepartum:** 1 = severe deviation from normal range, 2 = substantial deviation from normal range, 3 = moderate deviation from normal range, 4 = mild deviation from normal range, 5 = no deviation from normal range [see Section I].)

Client Outcomes

Client Will (Specify Time Frame)

Antepartum

- Obtain early prenatal care in the first trimester and maintain regular visits
- Demonstrate appropriate care of oneself during pregnancy including good nutrition and psychological health
- Attend prenatal education either virtual or in person with significant other or involved family member
- Understand the risks of substance abuse and resources available
- Feel empowered to seek social and spiritual support for emotional well-being during pregnancy
- Prepare home for baby (e.g., crib, diapers, infant car seat, outfits, blankets) before due date
- Use support systems for emotional support
- Develop a realistic birth plan, taking into account any high-risk pregnancy issues before due date
- Understand the labor and delivery process and comfort measures to manage labor pain before due date

Intrapartum

- Use support system for emotional support during labor and delivery
- Demonstrate appropriate understanding of choices in labor and delivery
- Demonstrate effective coping strategies during labor and delivery

Postpartum

- Provide a safe environment for self and infant
- Demonstrate appropriate newborn care and postpartum care of self
- Demonstrate appropriate bonding and parenting skills

NIC (Nursing Interventions Classification)

Suggested NIC Interventions

High-Risk Pregnancy Care; Intrapartal Care; Infant Care: Newborn

C

Example NIC Activities—High-Risk Pregnancy Care

Instruct client in self-care techniques to increase the chance of a healthy outcome (e.g., hydration, diet, activity modifications, importance of regular prenatal checkups, normalization of blood sugars, and sexual precautions, including abstinence).

Monitor physical and psychosocial status closely throughout pregnancy. Refer as appropriate for specific programs (e.g., smoking cessation, substance abuse treatment, diabetes education, preterm birth prevention education, abuse shelter as needed).

Nursing Interventions and *Rationales*

- ● Encourage early prenatal care (PNC) and regular prenatal visits. EB: *PNC is essential for a good pregnancy outcome for mothers and infants. Many women in the United States receive late or no PNC, resulting in avoidable adverse health outcomes (Oghogho & Beck-Sagué, 2020). The World Health Organization (WHO) guidelines for antenatal care include a minimum of eight contacts to reduce perinatal mortality and improve women's experience of care, counseling about healthy eating, and keeping physically active during pregnancy (World Health Organization, 2016).*
- ● Identify any high-risk factors that may require additional surveillance, such as preterm labor, hypertensive disorders of pregnancy, diabetes, depression, other chronic medical conditions, presence of fetal anomalies, virus exposure, homelessness (resources can be accessed through the HUD exchange [https://www.hudexchange.info/resources] and Homeless Prenatal Program [www.homelessprenatal.org]), or other high-risk factors. EB: *Preeclampsia is a major cause of maternal morbidity and is associated with adverse fetal outcomes, including intrauterine growth restriction, preterm birth, placental abruption, fetal distress, and fetal death in utero (Fox et al, 2019).* EBN: *It is exceedingly difficult for homeless pregnant women to access prenatal care, often leading to poorer maternal and neonatal outcomes. Nurses need to be prepared to make timely referrals to support services as an important first step (Azarmehr et al, 2018).*
- ▲ Assess and screen for signs and symptoms of depression during pregnancy and in the postpartum period and refer for behavioral-cognitive counseling and/or medication. EB: *Susser et al (2016) reported that nearly 20% of women in pregnancy and in the postpartum period are affected with depression.*
- ▲ Observe for signs of alcohol misuse and counsel women to stop drinking during pregnancy. Give appropriate referral for treatment if needed. EBN: *There is no safe time to drink alcohol during pregnancy and can fetal alcohol spectrum disorder (FASD). FASD is a range of physical, mental, behavioral, and/or learning disabilities with potential lifelong implications that occur after exposure to alcohol in utero (Association of Women's Health, Obstetric and Neonatal Nurses [AWHONN] Position Statement, 2019).*
- ▲ Obtain a smoking history and counsel women to stop smoking for the safety of the baby. Give appropriate referral to a smoking cessation program if needed. EBN: *Many women who do stop smoking during their pregnancies relapse in the postpartum period. Smoking is a major cause of adverse pregnancy and birth outcomes (Fallin-Bennett et al, 2019). A free and helpful website for quitting smoking is available at* https://women.smokefree.gov/tools-tips-women/text-programs/smokefreemom *(U.S. Department of Health and Human Services, n.d.).*
- ▲ Monitor for substance misuse with recreational drugs. Refer to a treatment program as needed. Refer opiate-dependent women to methadone clinics to improve maternal and fetal pregnancy outcomes. EB: *Pregnancy is an opportune time to identify substance misuse dependence, facilitate conversion to maintenance treatment, and coordinate comprehensive prenatal care with specialists in addiction medicine, behavioral health, and social services (Krans et al, 2015).*
- ● Monitor for psychosocial issues, including lack of social support system, loneliness, depression, lack of confidence, maternal powerlessness, and socioeconomic problems. EBN: *Expanded screening of at-risk women should include significant risk factors other than depression and anxiety symptoms (Ruyak et al, 2017).*
- ▲ Monitor for signs of domestic violence. Refer to a community program for abused women that provides safe shelter as needed. EBN: *Abuse during pregnancy can result in poor maternal, neonatal, and early childhood outcomes; routine screening and assessment may interrupt further abuse and promote positive outcomes (Bianchi et al, 2016).*
- ● Provide antenatal education to increase the woman's knowledge needed to make informed choices during pregnancy, labor, and delivery and to promote a healthy lifestyle. Encourage pregnant women to use digital resources such as Text4Baby (see https://www.text4baby.org or https://www.whattoexpect.com)

to track pregnancy progress and provide education and motivation to make healthy lifestyle choices in nutrition (abstinence from poor nutrition, smoking, and alcohol, and illicit drugs). EBN: *Multiple digital sources of health-related information are available and women may need help to identify those that are most reputable and useful (Lowe & Hartley, 2018).*

- Encourage expectant parents to prepare a realistic birth plan or "birth preferences" to prepare for the physical and emotional aspects of the birth process and to plan ahead for how they want various situations handled. EBN: *The birth plan allows the woman to communicate her expectations and needs (Biescas et al, 2017). A flexible approach to the birth plan is necessary, including the consideration of using alternative approaches and allowing for unexpected circumstances (Divall et al, 2017).*
- Encourage good nutritional intake during pregnancy to facilitate proper growth and development of the fetus. Women should consume an additional 300 calories per day during pregnancy, take a multimicronutrient supplement containing at least 400 μg folic acid, and achieve a total weight gain of 25 to 30 pounds. EB: *Nutritional information during pregnancy can be found at* choosemyplate.gov, *which presents healthy choices from each food group (U.S. Department of Agriculture [USDA], 2020). The U.S. Preventive Services Task Force (USPSTF) has updated its recommendation that all women who are planning a pregnancy or capable of becoming pregnant take a daily supplement containing 0.4 to 0.8 mg (400–800 μg) of folic acid (USPSTF as cited in Bibbins-Domingo et al, 2017).*

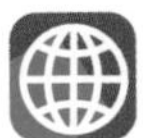

Multicultural

- ▲ Provide for a translator as needed. EBN: *In most Middle Eastern cultures female translators would be necessary because they are reluctant or sometimes forbidden to discuss female concerns with men (Meyer et al, 2016).* EBN: *The appropriate use of translation services and good communication skills are necessary to make women feel heard and have the opportunity to make choices (Rowland-Neve, 2017).*
- ▲ Provide depression screening. EB: *A 2015 study found that Mexican American women exhibit higher prenatal maternal depressive symptoms. Depressive symptoms increased when the women tried to mesh American and Mexican cultural values, and incorporation of the Anglo value of self-reliance and independence was a risk factor for depression (D'Anna-Hernandez et al, 2015).*
- Perform a cultural assessment and provide care that is culturally appropriate. EBN: *Nonjudgmental care that promotes equality can be accomplished through the appropriate use of translation services and good communication skills to make certain that women feel heard and have the opportunity to make choices (Rowland-Neve, 2017).*

Postpartal

- Assess client's beliefs and concerns about the postpartum period to provide culturally appropriate health and nutrition information and guidance on contemporary postpartum practices. EB: *Encourage women to adopt a healthy diet with protein-rich foods (Chakona & Shackleton, 2019).*

REFERENCES

Association of Women's Health, Obstetric and Neonatal Nurses (AWHONN) Position Statement. (2019). Optimizing outcomes for women with substance use disorders in pregnancy and the postpartum period. *Journal of Obstetric Gynecologic and Neonatal Nursing, 48*(5), 583–585 https://doi.org/10.1016/j.jogn.2019.06.001.

Azarmehr, H., Lowry, K., Sherman, A., Smith, C., & Zuñiga, J. A. (2018). Nursing practice strategies for prenatal care of homeless pregnant women. *Nursing for Womens Health, 22*(6), 489–498 https://doi.org/10.1016/j.nwh.2018.09.005.

Bianchi, A., Cesario, S. K., & McFarlane, J. (2016). Interrupting intimate partner violence during pregnancy with an effective screening and assessment program. *Journal of Obstetric Gynecologic and Neonatal Nursing, 45*(4), 579–591. https://doi.org/10.1016/j.jogn.2016.02.012.

Bibbins-Domingo, K., Grossman, D. C., Curry, S. J., et al. (2017). Folic acid supplementation for the prevention of neural tube defects. *JAMA, 317*(2), 183–189. https://doi.org/10.1001/jama.2016.19438.

Biescas, H., Benet, M., Pueyo, M. J., et al. (2017). A critical review of the birth plan use in Catalonia. *Sexual Reproductive Healthcare: Official Journal of the Swedish Association of Midwives, 13*, 41–50. https://doi.org/10.1016/j.srhc.2017.05.006.

Chakona, G., & Shackleton, C. (2019). Food taboos and cultural beliefs influence food choice and dietary preferences among pregnant women in the Eastern Cape, South Africa. *Nutrients, 11*(11), 2668. https://doi.org/10.3390/nu11112668.

D'Anna-Hernandez, K. L., Aleman, B., & Flores, A. M. (2015). Acculturative stress negatively impacts maternal depressive symptoms in Mexican-American women during pregnancy. *Journal of Affective Disorders, 176*, 35–42. https://doi.org/10.1016/j.jad.2015.01.036.

Divall, B., Spiby, H., Nolan, M., & Slade, P. (2017). Plans, preferences or going with the flow: An online exploration of women's views and experiences of birth plans. *Midwifery, 54*, 29–34. https://doi.org/10.1016/j.nwh.2016.08.001.

Fallin-Bennett, A., Scott, T., Fallin-Bennett, K., & Ashford, K. (2019). Call to action to reduce tobacco use during pregnancy. *Journal of Obstetric Gynecologic and Neonatal Nursing, 48*(5), 563–567. https://doi.org/10.1016/j.jogn.2019.02.009.

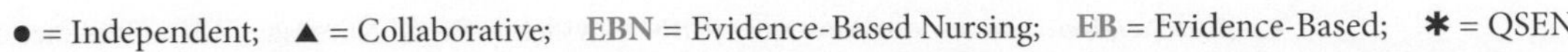

Fox, R., Kitt, J., Leeson, P., Aye, C. Y. L., & Lewandowski, A. J. (2019). Preeclampsia: Risk factors, diagnosis, management, and the cardiovascular impact on the offspring. *Journal of Clinical Medicine*, *8*(10), 1625. https://doi.org/10.3390/jcm8101625.

Krans, E. E., Cochran, G., & Bogen, D. L. (2015). Caring for opioid dependent pregnant women prenatal and postpartum care considerations. *Clinical Obstetrics and Gynecology*, *58*(2), 370–379. https://doi.org/10.1097/GRF.0000000000000098.

Lowe, N. K., & Hartley, A. K. (2018). Evolving landscape of mHealth apps. *Journal of Obstetric Gynecologic Neonatal Nursing*, *47*(6), 725–727. https://doi.org/10.1016/j.jogn.2018.10.001.

Meyer, J., Pomeroy, M., Reid, D., & Zuniga, J. (2016). Nursing care of pregnant Muslim women during Ramadan. *Nursing for Womens Health*, *20*(5), 456–462. https://doi.org/10.1016/j.nwh.2016.08.001.

Oghogho, E. S., & Beck-Sagué, C. (2020). Effect of Medicaid expansion status on risk of late or no prenatal care in black and white US mothers: Analysis of US natality data, 2010–17. *Lancet Global Health*, *8*(Suppl. 1), S27. https://doi.org/10.1016/s2214-109x(20)30168-6.

Rowland-Neve, K. (2017). Seeking asylum while pregnant. *British Journal of Midwifery*, *25*(9), 598–602. https://doi.org/10.12968/bjom.2017.25.9.598.

Ruyak, S. L., Flores-Montoya, A., & Boursaw, B. (2017). Antepartum services and symptoms of postpartum depression in at-risk women. *Journal of Obstetric Gynecologic, and Neonatal Nursing*, *46*(5), 696–708. https://doi.org/10.1016/j.jogn.2017.07.006.

Susser, L. C., Sansone, S. A., & Hermann, A. D. (2016). Selective serotonin reuptake inhibitors for depression in pregnancy. *American Journal of Obstetrics and Gynecology*, *215*(6), 722–730. https://doi.org/10.1016/j.ajog.2016.07.011.

U.S. Department of Agriculture (USDA). (2020). *MyPlate*. Choosemyplate.gov. Accessed June 10, 2021.

U.S. Department of Health and Human Services. (n.d.). *SmokefreeMOM*. https://women.smokefree.gov/tools-tips-women/text-programs/smokefreemom. Accessed June 10, 2021.

World Health Organization. (2016). *New guidelines on antenatal care for a positive pregnancy experience*. Geneva, Switzerland: WHO. Retrieved from http://www.who.int/reproductivehealth/news/antenatal-care/en/. Accessed June 10, 2021.

Readiness for Enhanced Childbearing Process Domain 8 Sexuality Class 3 Reproduction

Gail B. Ladwig, MSN, RN and Dianne F. Hayward, RN, MSN, WHNP

NANDA-I

Definition

A pattern of preparing for and maintaining a healthy pregnancy, childbirth process and care of the newborn for ensuring well-being which can be strengthened.

Defining Characteristics

During Pregnancy

Expresses desire to enhance knowledge of childbearing process; expresses desire to enhance management of unpleasant pregnancy symptoms; expresses desire to enhance prenatal lifestyle; expresses desire to enhance preparation for newborn

During Labor and Delivery

Expresses desire to enhance lifestyle appropriate for stage of labor; expresses desire to enhance proactivity during labor and delivery

After Birth

Expresses desire to enhance attachment behavior; expresses desire to enhance baby care techniques; expresses desire to enhance baby feeding techniques; expresses desire to enhance breast care; expresses desire to enhance environmental safety for the baby; expresses desire to enhance postpartum lifestyle; expresses desire to enhance use of support system

NOC (Nursing Outcomes Classification)

Suggested NOC Outcomes

Knowledge: Pregnancy; Knowledge: Infant Care; Knowledge: Postpartum Maternal Health; Knowledge: Breastfeeding, Parent-Infant Attachment

C

Example NOC Outcome with Indicators

Knowledge: Pregnancy as evidenced by client conveying understanding of the following indicators: Importance of frequent prenatal care/Importance of prenatal education/Benefits of regular exercise/Healthy nutritional practices/Anatomic and physiological changes of pregnancy/Psychological changes associated with pregnancy/Birthing options/Effective labor techniques/Signs and symptoms of labor. (Rate the outcome and indicators of **Knowledge: Pregnancy:** 1 = no knowledge, 2 = limited knowledge, 3 = moderate knowledge, 4 = substantial knowledge, 5 = extensive knowledge [see Section I].)

Client Outcomes

Client Will (Specify Time Frame)

Antepartum

- Attend all scheduled prenatal visits and attend prenatal education either with significant other or involved family member
- Use appropriate self-care for discomforts of pregnancy
- Prepare home for baby (e.g., crib, diapers, infant car seat, outfits, blankets) before due date
- Develop a realistic birth plan, taking into account any high-risk pregnancy issues before due date
- Feel empowered to seek social and spiritual support for emotional well-being during pregnancy
- Make healthy lifestyle choices prenatally: activity and exercise/healthy nutritional practices
- Use strategies to balance activity and rest

Intrapartum

- Demonstrate appropriate lifestyle choices during labor
- State knowledge of birthing options, signs and symptoms of labor before due date
- Demonstrate effective labor techniques
- Use support systems for labor and emotional support

Postpartum

- Demonstrate appropriate lifestyle choices postpartum
- Report normal physical sensations after delivery
- State understanding of recommended nutrient intake, strategies to balance activity and rest, appropriate exercise, time frame for resumption of sexual activity, strategies to manage stress
- Demonstrate bonding with infant
- Demonstrate proper handling and positioning of infant/infant safety
- Demonstrate feeding technique and bathing of infant

NIC (Nursing Interventions Classification)

Suggested NIC Interventions

Prenatal Care; Intrapartal Care; Postpartal Care; Attachment Promotion; Infant Care: Newborn; Lactation Counseling; Family Support

Example NIC Activities—Prenatal Care

Encourage prenatal class attendance either virtual or in person and encourage involvement of client's partner or involved family member; Discuss nutritional needs and concerns (e.g., balanced diet, folic acid, food safety, and supplements); Discuss activity level with client (e.g., appropriate exercise, activities to avoid, and importance of rest); Discuss importance of participating in prenatal care throughout entire pregnancy

Nursing Interventions and *Rationales*

▲ Refer to care plans Risk for Impaired **Attachment;** Readiness for Enhanced **Breastfeeding;** Readiness for Enhanced Family **Coping;** Readiness for Enhanced **Family** Processes; Readiness for Enhanced **Nutrition;** Readiness for Enhanced **Parenting;** and Ineffective **Role** Performance.

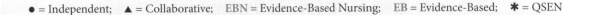

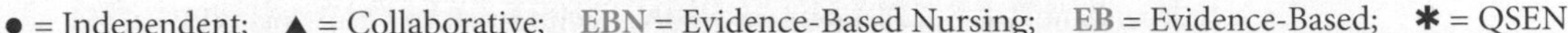

Prenatal Care

- Encourage early prenatal care (PNC) and regular prenatal visits. EB: *PNC is essential for a good pregnancy outcome for mothers and infants. In the United States, many women receive late or no PNC, resulting in avoidable adverse health outcomes (Oghogho & Beck-Sagué, 2020).* EB: *The World Health Organization (WHO) guidelines for antenatal care include a minimum of eight contacts to reduce perinatal mortality and improve women's experience of care, counseling about healthy eating, and keeping physically active during pregnancy (World Health Organization, 2016).*
- ▲ Ensure that pregnant clients have an adequate diet and take multimicronutrient supplements containing at least 400 µg of folic acid, especially during early pregnancy. EB: *Nutritional information can be found at* choosemyplate.gov. *which presents healthy choices from each food group needed for a healthy pregnancy (U.S. Department of Agriculture [USDA], 2020).* EB: *The U.S. Preventive Services Task Force (USPSTF) has updated its recommendation that all women who are planning or capable of pregnancy take a daily supplement containing 0.4 to 0.8 mg (400–800 µg) of folic acid to prevent neural tube deficits (Bibbins-Domingo et al, 2017).*
- Assess smoking status of pregnant clients and offer effective smoking-cessation interventions. EBN: *Many women who do stop smoking during their pregnancies relapse in the postpartum period. Smoking is a major cause of adverse pregnancy and birth outcomes (Fallin-Bennett et al, 2019). A free and helpful website for quitting smoking is available at* https://women.smokefree.gov/tools-tips-women/text-programs/smokefreemom *(U.S. Department of Health and Human Services, n.d.).*
- ▲ Assess all pregnant clients for signs of depression and make appropriate referral for inadequate weight gain, underutilization of PNC, substance misuse, and premature birth. EBN: *Maternal depression is associated with adverse perinatal outcomes, including an increased risk of poor adherence to treatment regimen, inadequate nutrition, loss of interpersonal and financial resources, smoking and substance misuse (Kendig et al, 2017).*
- Provide the pregnant client with breastfeeding education. EB: *Early initiation, exclusive, and continued breastfeeding are among the most effective interventions to reduce infant and child morbidity and mortality. Breastfeeding also improves early childhood development and reduces the risks of childhood obesity and noncommunicable disease (Rollins & Doherty, 2019).*

Intrapartal Care

Provide a calm, relaxing, and supportive birth environment. EBN: *The client's outcome and safety are affected by the birth environment and culture. The care providers, whether midwives, doulas, and/or the nursing staff, must be knowledgeable and committed to providing labor support (Stark et al, 2016).*

Offer the client in labor a clear liquid diet and water if allowed. EB: *The American College of Obstetricians and Gynecologists now endorses clear liquids during labor; however, current recommendations suggest that solid food intake should be avoided. According to Sperling et al, recent evidence from a systematic review involving 3130 women in active labor suggests that oral intake should not be restricted in women at low risk of complications (Sperling et al, 2016).*

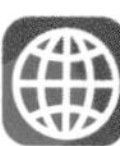

Multicultural

Prenatal

- ▲ Provide for an appropriate translator if needed. EBN: *In the Arab and most Middle Eastern cultures female translators would be necessary because they are reluctant or sometimes forbidden to discuss female concerns with men (Meyer et al, 2016).* EBN: *The appropriate use of translation services and good communication skills are necessary to make women feel heard and have the opportunity to make choices (Rowland-Neve, 2017).*
- Assess the client's beliefs and concerns to inform culturally appropriate PNC. EBN: *When caring for a woman of a different culture recognize the danger of making assumptions about the health care needs of the group to which she belongs. Identify the specific needs of the individual (Rowland-Neve, 2017).*

Intrapartal

- Assess client's beliefs and concerns about labor. EBN: *Instead of reducing the choices available to women during the birth experience, providers should understand, respect, and integrate cultural interpretations of childbirth and the needs of women and their families (Withers et al, 2018).*

Postpartal

- Assess client's beliefs and concerns about the postpartum period to provide culturally appropriate health and nutrition information and guidance on contemporary postpartum practices. EB: *Encourage women to adopt a healthy diet with protein-rich foods (Chakona & Shackleton, 2019).*

Home Care

Prenatal

▲ As needed refer pregnant clients to drug treatment programs that include coordinated interventions in several areas, such as drug misuse, infectious diseases, mental health, personal and social welfare, and gynecological/obstetric care. EB: *Pregnancy is an opportune time to identify substance misuse, facilitate conversion to maintenance treatment, and coordinate comprehensive PNC with specialists in addiction medicine, behavioral health, and social services (Krans et al, 2015).*

Postpartal

Provide information about parenting websites approved by the health care provider to support new parents with postpartum advice, newborn care, and breastfeeding. EB: *Online family support websites afford parents an alternative, cost-effective service that can be accessed from anywhere, increasing opportunities for parents to become active in their own support (Lamberton, Devaney, & Bunting, 2016).*

Client/Family Teaching and Discharge Planning

Prenatal

- Provide dietary and lifestyle counseling as part of PNC to pregnant women. EBN: *Pregnancy is an opportunity to address health behavior change. Recognizing both barriers and motivators during this time frame can allow for more focused interventions to be created and applied to the population (McCloud, 2018).*

Postpartal

- Encourage physical activity in postpartum women, after being cleared by the health care provider. EBN: *By becoming more physically active, a woman can see benefits of this self-care in her sense of well-being and perceived fitness (Shelton & Lee, 2018).*

▲ Provide breastfeeding mothers contact information for a lactation consultant, phone numbers, and website information for the La Leche League (http://www.lalecheleague.org), and local breastfeeding support groups. EBN: *In 2015 the Association of Women's Health, Obstetric and Neonatal Nurses (AWHONN) published its position statement on breastfeeding: it "supports, protects, and promotes breastfeeding as the ideal and most normal method for feeding infants" (Henry et al, 2017).*

- Teach mothers of young children principles to substitute foods high in saturated fat with foods moderate in PUFAs such as avocados, tuna, walnuts, and olive oil. Include lean protein, fruits and vegetables, and complex carbohydrates. EB: *Parental feeding behavior has a significant influence on the development of children's food preferences (Russell, Worsley, & Campbell, 2015).*

REFERENCES

Bibbins-Domingo, K., Grossman, D. C., Curry, S. J., et al. (2017). Folic acid supplementation for the prevention of neural tube defects. *JAMA*, *317*(2), 183–189 https://doi.org/10.1001/jama.2016.19438.

Chakona, G., & Shackleton, C. (2019). Food taboos and cultural beliefs influence food choice and dietary preferences among pregnant women in the Eastern Cape, South Africa. *Nutrients*, *11*(11), 2668 https://doi.org/10.3390/nu11112668.

Fallin-Bennett, A., Scott, T., Fallin-Bennett, K., & Ashford, K. (2019). Call to action to reduce tobacco use during pregnancy. *Journal of Obstetric, Gynecologic, and Neonatal Nursing*, *48*(5), 563–567 https://doi.org/10.1016/j.jogn.2019.02.009.

Henry, L. S., Hansson, M. C., Haughton, V. C., et al. (2017). Application of Kotter's theory of change to achieve baby-friendly designation. *Nursing for Women's Health*, *21*(5), 372–382.

Kendig, S., Keats, J. P., Hoffman, M. C., et al. (2017). Consensus bundle on maternal mental health: Perinatal depression and anxiety. *Obstetrics & Gynecology*, *129*(3), 422–430 https://doi.org/10.1097/aog.0000000000001902.

Krans, E. E., Cochran, G., & Bogen, D. L. (2015). Caring for opioid dependent pregnant women prenatal and postpartum care considerations. *Clinical Obstetrics and Gynecology*, *58*(2), 370–379 https://doi,org10.1097/GRF.0000000000000098.

Lamberton, L., Devaney, J., & Bunting, L. (2016). New challenges in family support: The use of digital technology in supporting parents. *Child Abuse Review*, *25*(5), 359–372 https://doi.org/wayne.edu/10.1002/car.2451A.

McCloud, M. B. (2018). Health behavior change in pregnant women with obesity. *Nursing for Women's Health*, *22*(6), 471–480 https://doi.org/10.1016/j.nwh.2018.09.002.

Meyer, J., Pomeroy, M., Reid, D., & Zuniga, J. (2016). Nursing care of pregnant Muslim women during Ramadan. *Nursing for Womens Health*, *20*(5), 456–462 https://doi.org/10.1016/j.nwh.2016.08.001.

Oghogho, E. S., & Beck-Sagué, C. (2020). Effect of Medicaid expansion status on risk of late or no prenatal care in black and white US mothers:

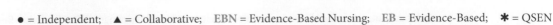

Analysis of US natality data, 2010–17. *The Lancet Global Health, 8*(Suppl. 1), S27 https://doi.org/10.1016/s2214-109x(20)30168-6.
Rollins, N., & Doherty, T. (2019). Improving breastfeeding practices at scale. *The Lancet Global Health, 7*(3), e292–e293 https://doi.org/10.1016/s2214-109x(18)30557-6.
Rowland-Neve, K. (2017). Seeking asylum while pregnant. *British Journal of Midwifery, 25*(9), 598–602 https://doi.org/10.12968/bjom.2017.25.9.598.
Russell, C. G., Worsley, A., & Campbell, K. J. (2015). Strategies used by parents to influence their children's food preferences. *Appetite, 90*, 123–130 https://doi.org/10.1016/j.appet.2015.02.038.
Shelton, S. L., & Lee, S. (2018). Women's self-reported factors that influence their postpartum exercise levels. *Nursing for Womens Health, 22*(2), 148–157 https://doi.org10.1016/j.nwh.2018.02.003.
Sperling, J. D., Dahlke, J. D., & Sibai, B. M. (2016). Restriction of oral intake during labor: Whither are we bound? *American Journal of Obstetrics and Gynecology, 214*(5), 592–596 https://doi.org/10.1016/j.ajog.2016.01.166.
Stark, M. A., Remynse, M., & Zwelling, E. (2016). Importance of the birth environment to support physiologic birth. *Journal of Obstetric, Gynecologic, and Neonatal Nursing, 45*(2), 285–294 https://doi.org/10.1016/j.jogn.2015.12.008.
U.S. Department of Agriculture (USDA). (2020). *MyPlate.* Choosemyplate.gov. Accessed June 10, 2021.
U.S. Department of Health and Human Services. (n.d.). SmokefreeMOM. https://women.smokefree.gov/tools-tips-women/text-programs/smokefreemom. Accessed June 10, 2021.
Withers, M., Kharazmi, N., & Lim, E. (2018). Traditional beliefs and practices in pregnancy, childbirth and postpartum: A review of the evidence from Asian countries. *Midwifery, 56*, 158–170 https://doi.org/10.1016/j.midw.2017.10.019.
World Health Organization. (2016). *New guidelines on antenatal care for a positive pregnancy experience*. Geneva: WHO. Retrieved from https://www.who.int/reproductivehealth/news/antenatal-care/en/. Accessed June 10, 2021.

C

Risk for Ineffective Childbearing Process Domain 8 Sexuality Class 3 Reproduction

Dianne F. Hayward, RN, MSN, WHNP

NANDA-I

Definition

Susceptible to an inability to prepare for and/or maintain a healthy pregnancy, childbirth process and care of the newborn for ensuring well-being.

Risk Factors

Inadequate knowledge of childbearing process; inadequate mental preparation for parenting; inadequate parental role model; inadequate prenatal care; inadequate social support; inconsistent prenatal health visits; low maternal confidence; maternal malnutrition; maternal powerlessness; maternal psychological distress; substance misuse; unaddressed domestic violence; unrealistic birth plan; unsafe environment

At-Risk Population

Individuals experiencing unplanned pregnancy; individuals experiencing unwanted pregnancy

NOC, NIC, Client Outcomes, Nursing Interventions and *Rationales,* Client/Family Teaching, and References

Refer to care plan for Ineffective **Childbearing** Process.

Impaired Comfort Domain 12 Comfort Class 1 Physical comfort

Gail B. Ladwig, MSN, RN and Julianne E. Doubet, BSN, RN, EMT-B

NANDA-I

Definition

Perceived lack of ease, relief, and transcendence in physical, psychospiritual, environmental, cultural, and/or social dimensions.

Defining Characteristics

Anxiety; crying; difficulty relaxing; expresses discomfort; expresses discontentment with situation; expresses fear; expresses feeling cold; expresses feeling warm; expresses itching; expresses psychological distress;

irritable mood; moaning; psychomotor agitation; reports altered sleep-wake cycle; reports hunger; sighing; uneasy in situation

Related Factors

Inadequate control over environment; inadequate health resources; inadequate situational control; insufficient privacy; unpleasant environmental stimuli

C

Associated Conditions

Illness-related symptoms; treatment regimen

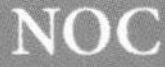

NOC (Nursing Outcomes Classification)

Suggested NOC Outcomes

Client Satisfaction; Symptom Control; Comfort Status; Coping; Hope; Pain Control; Anxiety Level Personal Well-Being; Spiritual Health

Example NOC Outcomes with Indicators

Comfort Status as evidenced by the following indicators: Physical and psychological well-being/Symptom control/Enhanced comfort. (Rate the outcome and indicators of **Comfort Status:** 1 = severely compromised, 2 = substantially compromised, 3 = moderately compromised, 4 = mildly compromised, 5 = not compromised [see Section I].)

Client Outcomes

Client Will (Specify Time Frame)

- Provide evidence for improved comfort compared to baseline
- Identify strategies, with or without significant others, to improve and/or maintain acceptable comfort level
- Perform appropriate interventions, with or without significant others, as needed to improve and/or maintain acceptable comfort level
- Evaluate the effectiveness of strategies to maintain/and or reach an acceptable comfort level
- Maintain an acceptable level of comfort when possible

NIC (Nursing Interventions Classification)

Suggested NIC Interventions

Calming Techniques; Massage; Healing Touch; Heat/Cold Application; Hope Inspiration; Humor; Meditation Facilitation; Music Therapy; Pain Management; Acute/Chronic; Presence; Progressive Muscle Relaxation; Spiritual Growth Facilitation; Distraction

Example NIC Activities—Hope Inspiration

Assist the client/significant others to identify areas of hope in life; Help expand spiritual self; Involve the client actively in own care

Nursing Interventions and *Rationales*

- Assess client's understanding of ranking his or her comfort level. EB: *Teachings that are easily understood (as well as client participation in discussions before discharge), which target client comprehension of instructions, have the potential to increase client knowledge and strengthen the ability to self-manage (Flink & Ekstedt, 2016).* EBN: *Routine pain assessments should be encouraged, and the significance of the results explained to the client (Dequeker et al, 2018).*
- Ask about client's current level of comfort. This is the first step in helping clients achieve improved comfort. EBN: *Vuille et al (2018) found in their study that the assessment of pain intensity using a validated pain scale/tool should be the initial step in evaluating a client's level of discomfort: client's self-reporting of pain quality is widely accepted as the key to effective pain management.*

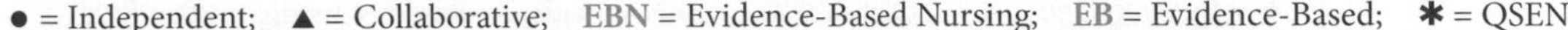

C

- Comfort is a holistic state under which pain management is included. EBN: *Nurses have a responsibility to promote optimal comfort for clients and to intercede in certain situations to protect the client's level of comfort (Karabulut et al, 2015).*
- Manipulate the environment as necessary to improve comfort. EBN: *The theoretical foundation of holistic comfort, which consists of relief, ease, and transcendence, in the settings of physical, psychological, social, and environmental experiences, enables the nurse to meet the individual comfort needs of the client (Ng, 2017).*
- Encourage early mobilization and provide routine position changes. Range of motion and weight-bearing decrease physical discomforts and disability associated with bed rest. EBN: *It has been shown that immobility is linked to many unacceptable client outcomes in critical care units. Mobility takes many forms (e.g., passive and active range of motion exercises, sitting up, dangling legs on side of bed), along with walking, and these should be included in client care (Crowe et al, 2017).*
- Provide simple massage. Massage has many therapeutic effects, including improved relaxation, circulation, and well-being. EBN: *Lind (2017), in his theses on the use of massage as a complementary therapy in client relaxation techniques, found that massage has shown the most potential in helping to alleviate the client's pain and comfort issues.*
- Provide a healing touch, which is well suited for clients who cannot tolerate more stimulating interventions. EBN: *According to Anderson et al (2017), providing nurses with the knowledge of healing touch and demonstrating its use in acute client care gives the nurse another means of ensuring positive client outcomes.*
- Encourage clients to use relaxation techniques to reduce pain, anxiety, depression, and fatigue. EBN: *Ju et al (2019) state that administration of analgesics for client comfort is a fundamental part of nursing practice, but the use of nonpharmacological interventions such as massage, music, guided imagery, and relaxation as adjuncts to support pain control is becoming increasingly more common.*

Geriatric

- Use hand massage for older adults. Most older adults respond well to touch and the health care provider's presence. Lines of communication open naturally during hand massage. EBN: *Hand massage has been found to ease apprehension, generate a positive effect on vital signs, and enhance the client's comfort (Çavdar et al, 2020).*
- Discomfort from cold can be treated with warmed blankets. There are physiological dangers associated with hypothermia. EBN: *The nurse plays an effective role in advocating for clients' well-being by monitoring the individual client's environment and adjusting it, as necessary, to fit the client's specific comfort needs (Hussein & Karim, 2020).*
- Use complementary therapies such as doll therapy in clients with dementia to increase comfort and reduce stress. EBN: *Both staff and families of clients with advanced dementia confined to a nursing care facility found that complementary therapies were supportive in reducing loneliness and in offering interventions that afforded companionship for residents in distress (Mitchell et al, 2020).*
- Address any unmet physical, psychological, emotional, spiritual, and environmental needs when attempting to mediate the behavior of an older client with dementia. EBN: *As nursing and health care adjust to serve an aging population, there is a renewed interest in providing holistic nursing care appropriate to the client's mental and physical conditions (Pryor & Clarke, 2017).*

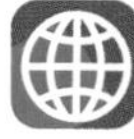

Multicultural

- Identify and clarify cultural language used to describe pain and other discomforts. Expressions of pain and discomfort vary across cultures. EBN: *Nurses today are challenged to find means to facilitate culturally harmonious care for all clients; according to Jeffreys and Zoucha (2017), this can be accomplished "through ongoing assessment, education, research, and practice initiatives."*
- Encourage and allow clients to practice their own cultural beliefs and recognize the impact that diverse cultures have on a client's belief about health care, comforting measures, and decision-making. EBN: *Cultural competence is a necessary element of complete nursing care and is achieved by establishing good communication, having skill in making the correct diagnosis, and recognition of clients' language and beliefs as they relate to health and illness (Debiasi & Selleck, 2017).*
- Assess for cultural and religious beliefs when providing care. EB: *According to Schweda et al (2017), in their study of cultural stereotyping, it was found that there is not just one perspective on culture and/or religion, but each individual's stance is formed by political, social, and situation beliefs.*

Client/Family Teaching and Discharge Planning

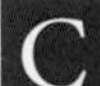

- Teach techniques to use when the client is uncomfortable, including relaxation techniques, guided imagery, hand massage, and music therapy. EBN: *Many complementary therapies can be conducted by the nurse and then taught to the client and family for use at home (Blackburn et al, 2019).*
- At end of life, the dying client is comforted by having a companion. EBN: *Most clients questioned by Thompson et al (2019), in their study regarding dying alone, acknowledged that they would welcome social connections as they neared the end of their life.*
- Teach the client to follow up with the health care provider if problems persist. EBN: *Dahlberg et al (2018), in their study of follow-up for postoperative clients discharged home, found that it is essential for clients to feel secure, assured, and responded to during their recovery.*
- Use nonpharmacological strategies to enhance comfort. EBN: *Supplementing pain management by nonpharmacological means can enhance pain control and reduce unpleasant side effects, thus leading to improved client and nurse satisfaction (Blackburn et al, 2019).*
- Encourage clients to use the Internet as a means of providing education to complement medical care for those who may be homebound or unable to attend face-to-face education. EB: *According to a study by Sánchez-Valle et al (2017), use of the Internet by older adults can offer a means of dynamic aging and could affect their lifestyle and could have a positive effect on the community as well.*
- Encourage clients to use guided imagery techniques. Guided imagery helps distract clients from stressful situations and facilitates relaxation. EBN: *The use of guided imagery by nurses is economical, uncomplicated, and easily accessible and has shown effectiveness in the delivery of comfort care (Coelho et al, 2018).*
- Provide psychospiritual support and a comforting environment to enhance comfort during emotional crises. EBN: *As health care professionals, nurses should intervene and provide care that recognizes and reduces strain for the client, caregiver, and family during a mental health crisis (Naseimento et al, 2016).*
- When nurses attend to the comfort of perioperative clients, the clients' sense of hope for a full recovery increases. EBN: *Fowler (2020) states that nurses can "assess, inspire, and evaluate hope" and that nurses, no matter what their area of expertise, use comparable approaches to foster hope in their clients.*
- Providing music and verbal relaxation therapy enhances holistic comfort by reducing anxiety. EBN: *Music is one of the complementary and alternative medicine therapies that has shown positive results in easing anxiety, pain, and the use of opioids (Poulsen & Coto, 2018).*
- Caregivers should not hesitate to use humor when caring for their clients. EBN: *Zhao et al (2019), in their analysis of laughter and humor use as a complementary medicine intervention, observed that humor is valuable in easing depression and anxiety, and has shown value in augmenting sleep quality in adults.*

REFERENCES

Anderson, J. G., Friesen, M. A., Swengros, D., Herbst, A., & Mangione, L. (2017). Examination of the use of healing touch by registered nurses in the acute care setting. *Journal of Holistic Nursing, 35*(1), 97–107. https://doi.org/10.1177/0898010116644834.

Blackburn, L. M., Abel, S., Green, L., Johnson, K., & Panda, S. (2019). The use of comfort kits to optimize adult cancer pain management. *Pain Management Nursing, 20*(1), 25–31. https://doi.org/10.1016/j.mn.2018.01.004 on 10/13/2020.

Çavdar, A. U., Yilmaz, E., & Baydur, H. (2020). The effect of hand massage before cataract surgery on patient anxiety and comfort: A randomized controlled study. *Journal of Perinesthesia Nursing, 35*(1), 54–59. https://doi.org/10.1016/j.jopan.2019.06.012.

Coelho, A., Parola, V., Sandgren, A., Fernandes, O., Kolcaba, K., & Apóstolo, J. (2018). The effects of guided imagery on comfort in palliative care. *Journal of Hospice and Palliative Nursing, 20*(4), 392–399. https://doi.org/10.1097/NJH.0000000000000460.

Crowe, S., Brook, A., & Reynolds, J. (2017). You want me to do what? Mobility and continuous renal replacement therapy (CRRT) patients (Abstract). *Canadian Journal of Critical Care Nursing, 28*(2), 29.

Dahlberg, K., Jaensson, M., Nilsson, U., Eriksson, M., & Odencrants, S. (2018). Holding it together—Patients' perspectives on postoperative recovery when using an e-assesed follow-up: Qualitative study. *JMIR mHealth and uHealth, 6*(5), e10387. https://doi.org/10.2196/10387.

Debiasi, L., & Selleck, C. (2017). Cultural competence training for primary care nurse practioners: An intervention to increase culturally competent care. *Journal of Cultural Diversity, 24*(2), 39–45.

Dequeker, S., Van Lancker, A., & Van Hecke, A. (2018). Hospitalized patients' vs nurses' assessments of pain intensity and barriers to pain management. *Journal of Advanced Nursing, 74*(1), 160–171. https://doi.org/10.1111/jan.13395.

Flink, M., & Ekstedt, M. (2016). Prerequisites for patient self-management learning at hospital discharge: An observational multiple case study (Abstract). *International Journal of Integrated Care, 16*(6), A220. https://doi.org/10.5334/ijic.2768.

Fowler, S. B. (2020). Critical care nurses' perceptions of hope: Original qualitative research. *Dimensions of Critical Care Nursing, 39*(2), 110–115. https://doi.org/10.1097/DCC.0000000000000405.

Hussein, A., & Karim, K. (2020). Enhancing patient's surrounding: Application of nightingale's environmental theory into nursing practice. *i-Manager's Journal on Nursing, 10*(1), 45–49. https://doi.org/10.16843/jnurs.10.1.1668.

Jeffreys, M. R., & Zoucha, R. (2017). Revisiting "the invisible culture of the multiracial, multiethnic individual: A transcultural imperative. *Journal of Cultural Diversity, 24*(1), 3–5. PMID:11855217.

Ju, W., Ren, L., Chen, J., & Du, Y. (2019). Efficacy of relaxation therapy as an effective nursing intervention for post-operative pain relief in patients undergoing abdominal surgery: A systematic review and meta-analysis. *Experimental and Therapeutic Medicine*, *18*(4), 2909–2916. https://doi.org/10.3892/etm.2019.7915.

Karabulut, N., Aktaş, Y., Gürçayir, D., Yilmaz, D., & Gökmen, V. (2015). Patient satisfaction with their pain management and comfort level after open heart surgery. *Australian Journal of Advanced Nursing*, *32*(3), 16–24.

Lind, B. R. (2017). *The use of massage as an adjuvant nursing intervention. Nursing Capstones* (Vol. 223). University of North Dakota. Retrieved from https://commons.und.edu/nurs-capstones/223. Accessed June 10, 2021.

Mitchell, B., Jackson, G. A., Sharp, B., & Tolson, D. (2020). Complimentary therapy for advanced dementia palliation in nursing homes. *Journal of Integrated Care*, *28*(4), 419–432. https://doi.org/10.1108/JICA-02-2020-0009.

Naseimento, K., Kolhs, M., Mells, S., et al. (2016). The family challenge in for people suffering from mental disorder. *Journal of Nursing UFPE Online*, *10*(3), 940–948. https://doi.org/10.5205/reuol.8702-76273-4-SM.1003201601.

Ng, S. H. (2017). Application of Kolkaba's Comfort Theory to the management of a patient with heptacellular carcinoma. *Singapore Nursing Journal*, *44*(1), 16–23.

Poulsen, M. J., & Coto, J. (2018). Nursing music protocol and postoperative pain. *Pain Management Nursing*, *19*(2), 172–176. https://doi.org/1016/j.pm.2017.09.003.

Pryor, C., & Clarke, A. (2017). Nursing care for people with delirium superimposed on dementia. *Nursing Older People*, *29*(3), 18–21. https://doi.org/10.7748/nop.2017.e887.

Sánchez-Valle, M., Vinarás Abad, M., & Llorente-Barroso, C. (2017). Empowering the elderly and promoting active ageing through the internet: The benefit of e-inclusion programmes. In I. Kollak (Ed.), *Safe at home with assistive technology* (pp. 95–108). New York: Springer. https://doi.org/10.1007/978-3-319-42890-1_7.

Schweda, M., Schicktanz, S., Raz, A., & Silvers, A. (2017). Beyond cultural stereotyping: Views on end-of-life decision making among religious and secular persons in the USA, Germany, and Israel. *BMC Medical Ethics*, *18*(1), 13. https://doi.org/10.1186/s12910-017-0170-4.

Thompson, G., Shindruck, C., Wickson-Griffiths, et al. (2019). "Who would want to die like that?" Perspectives on dying alone in a long-term care facility. *Death Studies*, *43*(8), 509–520. https://doi.org/10.1080/07481187.2018.1491484.

Vuille, M., Foerster, M., Foucault, E., & Hugli, O. (2018). Pain assessment by emergency nurses at triage in the emergency department: A qualitative study. *Journal of Clinical Nursing*, *27*(3–4), 669–676. https://doi.org/10.1111/jocn:13992.

Zhao, J., Yin, H., Zhang, G., et al. (2019). A meta-analysis of randomized controlled trials of laughter and humour interventions on depression, anxiety and sleep quality in adults. *Journal of Advanced Nursing*, *75*(11), 2435–2448. https://doi.org/10.1111/jan.14000.

Readiness for Enhanced Comfort Domain 12 Comfort Class 2 Environmental comfort

Gail B. Ladwig, MSN, RN and Julianne E. Doubet, BSN, RN, EMT-B

NANDA-I

Definition

A pattern of ease, relief, and transcendence in physical, psychospiritual, environmental, and/or social dimensions, which can be strengthened.

Defining Characteristics

Expresses desire to enhance comfort; expresses desire to enhance feelings of contentment; expresses desire to enhance relaxation; expresses desire to enhance resolution of complaints

NOC (Nursing Outcomes Classification)

Suggested NOC Outcomes

Client Satisfaction: Caring; Symptom Control; Comfort Status; Coping; Hope; Motivation; Pain Control; Participation in Health Care Decisions; Spiritual Health

Example NOC Outcomes with Indicators

Comfort Status as evidenced by the following indicators: Physical well-being/Symptom control/ Psychological well-being. (Rate the outcome and indicators of **Comfort Level:** 1 = not at all satisfied, 2 = somewhat satisfied, 3 = moderately satisfied, 4 = very satisfied, 5 = completely satisfied [see Section I].)

Client Outcomes

Client Will (Specify Time Frame)

- Assess current level of comfort as acceptable
- Express the need to achieve an enhanced level of comfort

- Identify strategies to enhance comfort
- Perform appropriate interventions as needed for increased comfort
- Evaluate the effectiveness of interventions at regular intervals
- Maintain an enhanced level of comfort when possible

NIC (Nursing Interventions Classification)

Suggested NIC Interventions

Calming Technique; Cutaneous Stimulation; Environmental Management: Comfort; Heat/Cold Application; Hope Inspiration; Humor; Meditation Facilitation; Music Therapy; Pain Management: Acute and Chronic; Presence; Guided Imagery; Massage; Relaxation Therapy; Spiritual Growth Facilitation; Therapeutic Play; Therapeutic Touch; Touch; Distraction

Example NIC Activities—Spiritual Growth Facilitation

Assist the client with identifying barriers and attitudes that hinder growth or self-discovery; Assist the client to explore beliefs as related to healing of the body, mind, and spirit; Model healthy relating and reasoning skills

Nursing Interventions and *Rationales*

- Assess clients' comfort needs and current level of comfort in various contexts, as outlined in Kolcaba's comfort theory and practice: physical, psychospiritual, sociocultural, and environmental. EBN: *By using the comfort theory's framework, the nurse can recognize the client's physical, psychosocial, sociocultural, and environmental needs; bringing these aspects into play will aid in identifying nursing problems and the necessary interventions that can be implemented to enrich the client's environment (Ng, 2017).*
- Educate clients about the various contexts of comfort and help them understand that enhanced comfort is a desirable, positive, and achievable goal. EBN: *According to Silveira Mendes et al (2016), nursing care should incorporate all aspects of the client's comfort needs and not just the physical, which are both expressed and unexpressed.*
- Enhance feelings of trust between the client and the health care provider to maintain an effective and therapeutic relationship. EBN: *Kornhaber et al (2016) found that the ability to deliver person-centered care is essential for nurses; connecting with clients therapeutically will augment positive health-related results.*
- Maintain an open and effective communication with clients and keep them informed about their health, their plan of care, and their environment. EBN: *By asking relevant questions, the nurse can first build trust with the client, but Price (2017) also maintains that as care evolves, it will be necessary for the nurse to continue to support the client's sense of psychological well-being.*
- Implement comfort rounds that regularly assess for clients' comfort needs. EBN: *Regular nurse–client contact advances client–nurse interactions and augments the early recognition of client comfort and safety needs (Sims et al, 2018).*
- Collaborate with other health care professionals, such as health care providers, pharmacists, social workers, chaplains, occupational and physical therapists, and dietitians, among others, in planning interventions that address comfort needs in various contexts: physical, psychospiritual, sociocultural, and environmental. EBN: *Kolcaba's comfort theory can be used as a guide for client care in offering uncomplicated and holistic standards that assist the nurse in recognizing clients' needs, developing interventions to satisfy those needs, assessing the outcomes of these interventions, and meeting goals of quality client and family care. These goals may also encompass discharge planning and follow-up with various health and spiritual providers (Boudiab & Kolcaba, 2015).*
- Educate clients about and encourage the use of various integrative therapies and modalities to provide options that enhance comfort, beyond the traditional plan of care.
    - Massage. EBN: *Zhao et al (2020)* noted that the use of massage therapy, alone or in combination with other nonpharmaceutical interventions (e.g., aromatherapy, calming music), can noticeably reduce symptoms of anxiety and agitation for clients with dementia.
    - Guided imagery. EBN: *Guided imagery is effective in relieving postoperative pain in adults (Álvarez-García & Yaban, 2020).*

C

- ❍ Mindfulness and mindfulness-based interventions. EBN: *Mindfulness-based stress reduction (MBSR) is a beneficial approach offering clients a plan for self-management that can be employed when challenged by the potential for stress and disease (El Aoufy et al, 2018).*
- ❍ Energy therapy or biofield therapy such as healing touch, therapeutic touch, and Reiki. EBN: *According to Mangione et al (2017), biofield practices that include healing touch and Reiki encourage relaxation, ease anxiety and stress, and positively complement mood.*
- ❍ Acupuncture and auricular acupuncture. EBN: *Faircloth (2015) stated that acupuncture and acupressure have been found to decrease apprehension preoperatively, reduce intraoperative anesthetic requirements, diminish postoperative discomfort, lower the occurrence of postoperative nausea and vomiting, and fortify the treatment of chronic pain management.*
- ❍ Aromatherapy. EB: *In their study of individuals exposed to the lemon grass scent, Costa Goes et al (2015) found that there was a reduction in anxiety and subjective stress within minutes of the aroma's administration.*
- ❍ Music. EBN: *Music, as a nursing intervention, has been shown to be beneficial in relieving clients' discomfort, apprehension, and distress (Waterworth & Rickson, 2017).*
- ❍ Other mind–body therapies such as meditation or yoga. EB: *Meditation is a strategy of self-care that offers potential usefulness in mental health situations, behavioral self-regulation, and integrative medical care (Burke et al, 2017).*

- ● Foster and instill hope in clients whenever possible. See the care plan for **Hopelessness**. EBN: *Fowler (2020) found, in her study of critical-care nurses and hope, that nurses can "assess, inspire, and evaluate hope."*
- ● Provide opportunities for and enhance spiritual care activities. EBN: *As spirituality has been acknowledged by numerous health care professionals as a vital component in health and healing, Hawthorne and Gordon (2020) state that holistic nursing care should then incorporate the assessment and response of clients' essential spiritual needs.*
- ▲ Enhance social support and family involvement. EBN: In their survey (based on Kolcaba's enhanced comfort theory) addressing family experiences, when a loved one is hospitalized in an intensive care unit, *Twohig et al (2015)* found that there was an elevated level of satisfaction among family members in all aspects of client care, including communication and the opportunity to be involved in decision-making.
- ▲ Promote participation in creative arts and activity programs. EB: *Adult education classes in creative arts were found to improve well-being by boosting mood and providing a feeling of belonging. It also supported members in developing self-confidence, in the development of new relationships, and in general, it encouraged more active lives (Pearce, 2017).*
- ▲ Encourage clients to use health information technology (HIT) as needed. EB: *In a European Union study, Internet users in the United Kingdom validated the concept that the Internet was a good option in gaining knowledge of self-care and care of others and was valuable in positive health care outcomes (Marton, 2015).*
- ● Evaluate the effectiveness of all comfort interventions at regular intervals and adjust therapies as necessary. EBN: *In a study by Coelho et al (2016), clients were asked how they sensed a feeling of comfort, and their responses included individualized care, symptom containment, need for a comfortable environment, and hope and relationships. Recognition of these needs gives the nurse the opportunity to construct personalized interventions that meet these needs as well as to evaluate and revise them as needed.*

Geriatric

- ● Refer to previously mentioned interventions for geriatric interventions.

Pediatric

- ● Assess and evaluate the child's level of comfort at frequent intervals. With assessment of pain in children, it is best to use input from the parents or a primary caregiver. EBN: *According to Shaw et al (2017), skillful communication with clients and families is necessary for proficient, personalized comfort care in the pediatric environment.*
- ● Skin-to-skin contact (SSC) in the comfort of newborns, especially those at risk. EBN: Newborn SSC practice is natural and instinctive and has been found to have positive effects on health outcomes and comfort, especially for at-risk newborns in low-support environments (Hubbard & Gattman, 2017).
- ● Encourage parental presence whenever possible. EBN: There is an increasing awareness by health care professionals that parents play a vital function in promoting the positive health outcomes of low-birth-weight and preterm infants (*Franck & O'Brien, 2019*).

- Promote use of alternative comforting strategies such as positioning, presence, massage, spiritual care, music therapy, art therapy, and storytelling to enhance comfort when needed. EB: *In their study of comfort measures and sedation/analgesics used in pediatric intensive care units (PICUs), Guerra et al (2016) found that enhanced comfort care is offered through music, swaddling, pacifiers, television, and sucrose solutions.*
- Support the child's spirituality. EBN: It is becoming generally acknowledged that spiritual care for children with chronic illness is necessary to support them in dealing with their illness and/or disabilities (Bakker et al, 2018).

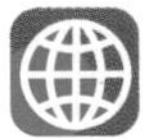

Multicultural

- Identify cultural beliefs, values, lifestyles, practices, and problem-solving strategies when assessing a client's comfort. EBN: *According to Moore (2017), it is a necessity for nurses to recognize that culture and language are the basis for the realization of health awareness and should make it a goal to work within the cultural perspective of the client.*
- Enhance cultural knowledge by actively seeking out information regarding different cultural and ethnic groups EBN: *As the multicultural population of the United States continues to expand, there is a growing need for outreach and culturally sensitive education that will better serve these communities (Sanchez Elminowski, 2015).*
- ▲ Recognize the impact of culture on communication styles and techniques EBN: *Livesay et al (2017) surmised that growing diversification of societies places increasing emphasis on the demand for culturally suitable communication, which both addresses the needs of the health care consumer and the provider.*

Home Care

- The nursing interventions described for Readiness for Enhanced **Comfort** may be used with clients in the home care setting. When needed, adaptations can be made to meet the needs of specific clients, families, and communities.
- ▲ Make appropriate referrals to other organizations or health care providers as needed to enhance comfort. EBN: *Nurses performing holistic assessments as the center of client care and then making appropriate referrals and providing beneficial health promotions, have made a noticeable improvement in the physical health outcomes for people with mental illness (Tranter & Robertson, 2019).*
- ▲ Promote an interdisciplinary (e.g., home care nurses, physicians, pharmacy) approach to home care. EBN: *Imhof et al (2016), in their study of nurse-led interdisciplinary team approach to palliative care, found that the nurse specialist was an important player in establishing and sustaining an interdisciplinary complex system of care.*
- Evaluate regularly if enhanced comfort is attainable in the home care setting. EB: *A study by Seow et al (2016) found that home care nurses provided comfort and support to cancer clients who wished to die at home and not in the hospital.*

Client/Family Teaching and Discharge Planning

- Teach client how to regularly assess levels of comfort.
- Instruct client that a variety of interventions may be needed at any given time to enhance comfort. EBN: *Health care professionals involved in home care should be proficient in medical technology to preserve a feeling of safety and allay fears in both clients and their caregivers (Munck & Sandgren, 2017).*

REFERENCES

Álvarez-García, C., & Yaban, Z. Ş. (2020). The effects of preoperative guided imagery interventions on preoperative anxiety and postoperative pain: A meta-analysis. *Complementary Therapies in Clinical Practice*, *38*, 101077. https://doi.org/10.1016/j.ctcp.2019.101077.

Bakker, A. A. D., van Leeuwen, R. R. R., & Roodbol, P. F. P. (2018). The spirituality of children with chronic conditions: A qualitative meta-synthesis. *Journal of Pediatric Nursing*, *43*, e106–e113. https://doi.org/10.1016/j.pedn.2018.08.003.

Boudiab, L. D., & Kolcaba, K. (2015). Comfort theory: Unraveling the complexities of veterans' health care needs. *Advances in Nursing Practice*, *38*(4), 270–278. https://doi.org/10.1097/ANS.0000000000000089.

Burke, A., Lam, C., Stussman, B., et al. (2017). Mind-body therapies. *Journal of the Australian Traditional-Medicine Society, Spring*, *23*(3) 169–170.

Coelho, A., Parola, V., Escobar-Bravo, M., & Apóstolo, J. (2016). Comfort experience in palliative care: A phenomenological study. *BMC Palliative Care*, *15*, 71. https://doi.org/10.1186/s12904-016-0145-0.

Costa Goes, T., Reis Carvalho Ursulino, F., Almeida-Souza, T. H., Alves, P. B., & Teixeira-Silva, F. (2015). Effect of lemongrass aroma on experimental anxiety in humans. *Journal of*

Alternative & Complementary Medicine, *21*(12), 766–773. https://doi.org/10.1089/acm.2015.0099.

El Aoufy, K., Pollina, A., Pezzutto, A., Matucci Cerinic, M., & Maddali Bongi, S. (2018). AB1432-HPR mindfulness-based stress reduction (MBSR) protocol applied to systemic sclerosis (SSC) patients: A pilot interventional study focused on nursing assessment and perceived stress. *Annals of the Rheumatic Diseases*, *77*, 1849–1850. https://doi.org/10.1016/j.ctcp.2019.101077.

Faircloth, A. (2015). Acupuncture: History from the Yellow Emperor to modern anesthesia practice. *AANA Journal*, *83*(4), 289–295.

Fowler, S. B. (2020). Critical care nurses' perceptions of hope: Original qualitative research. *Dimensions of Critical Care Nursing*, *39*(2), 110–115. https://doi.org/10.1097/DCC.0000000000000405.

Franck, L. S., & O'Brien, K. (2019). The evolution of family-centered care: From supporting patient-delivered care interventions to a model of family integrated care. *Birth Defects Research*, *111*(15), 1044–1059. https://doi.org/10.1002/bdr2.1521.

Guerra, G. G., Joffe, A. R., Cave, D., et al. (2016). Survey of sedation and analgesia practice among Canadian pediatric critical care physicians. *Pediatric Critical Care Medicine*, *17*(9), 823–830. https://doi.org/10.1097/PCC.0000000000000864.

Hawthorne, D. M., & Gordon, S. C. (2020). The invisibility of spiritual nursing care in clinical practice. *Journal of Holistic Nursing*, *38*(1), 147–155. https://doi.org/10.1177/0898010119889704.

Hubbard, J. M., & Gattman, K. R. (2017). Parent-infant skin-to-skin contact following birth: History, benefits, and challenges. *Neonatal Network*, *36*(2), 89–97. https://doi.org/10.1891/0730-0832.36.2.89.

Imhof, L., Kipfer, S., & Waldboth, V. (2016). Nurse-led palliative care services facilitate an interdisciplinary network of care. *International Journal of Palliative Nursing*, *22*(8), 404–410. https://doi.org/10.12968/ijpn.2016.22.8.404.

Kornhaber, R., Walsh, K., Duff, J., & Walker, K. (2016). Enhancing adult therapeutic interpersonal relationships in the acute healthcare setting: An integrative review. *Journal of Multidisciplinary Healthcare*, *9*, 537–546. https://doi.org/10.2147/JMDH.S116957.

Livesay, K., Lau, P., McNair, R., & Chiminello, C. (2017). The culturally and linguistically diverse SPs' evaluation of simulation experience. *Clinical Simulation in Nursing*, *13*(5), 228–237. https://doi.org/10.1016/j.ecns.2017.01.004.

Mangione, L., Swengros, D., & Anderson, J. G. (2017). Mental health wellness and biofield therapies: An integrative review. *Issues in Mental Health Nursing*, *38*(11), 930–944. https://doi.org/10.1080/01612840.2017.1364808.

Marton, C. (2015). Understanding the health information needs of British internet users seeking health information online and their perceptions of the quality of the internet as a source of health information. *Journal of Hospital Librarianship*, *15*(2), 175–188. https://doi.org/10.1080/15323269.2015.1015092.

Moore, P. (2017). *Cultural and health literacy assessment of the Hispanic/Latino patient population: Presentation of a cultural competence toolkit for acute care nurses. Doctor of nursing practice (DNP) Projects.* Scholarworks@UMassAmherst [Internet]. Retrieved from https://scholarworks.umass.edu/nursing_dnp_capstone/114/. Accessed June 10, 2021.

Munck, B., & Sandgren, A. (2017). The impact of medical technology on sense of security in the palliative home care setting. *British Journal of Community Nursing*, *22*(3), 130–135. https://doi.org/10.12968/bjcn.2017.22.3.130.

Ng, S. H. (2017). Application of Kolcaba's Comfort Theory to the management of a patient with hepatocellular carcinoma. *Singapore Nursing Journal*, *44*(1), 16–23.

Pearce, E. (2017). Participants' perspectives on the social bonding and well-being effects of creative arts adult education classes. *Arts & Health: An International Journal of Research, Policy & Practice*, *9*(1), 42–59. https://doi.org/10.1080/17533015.2016.1193550.

Price, B. (2017). Developing patient rapport, trust and therapeutic relationships. *Nursing Standard*, *31*(50), 52–63. https://doi.org/10.7748/ns.2017.e10909.

Sanchez Elminowski, N. (2015). Developing and implementing a cultural awareness workshop for nurse practitioners. *Journal of Cultural Diversity*, *22*(3), 105–113 PMID:26647489.

Seow, H., Sutradhar, R., McGrail, K., et al. (2016). End-of-life cancer care: Temporal association between homecare nursing and hospitalizations. *Journal of Palliative Medicine*, *19*(3), 263–270. https://doi.org/10.1089/jpm.2015.0229.

Shaw, A., Lind, C., & Ewashen, C. (2017). Harlequin-inspired story-based learning: An educational innovation for pediatric nursing communication. *Journal of Nursing Education*, *56*(5), 300–303. https://doi.org/10.3928/01484834-20170421-09.

Silveira Mendes, R., Cruz, M., Palva, R., et al. (2016). Comfort theory as support for a safe clinical nursing care. *Ciência, Cuidado e Saúde*, *15*(2), 390–395.

Sims, S., Leamy, M., Davies, N., et al. (2018). Realist synthesis of intentional rounding in hospital wards: Exploring the evidence of what works, for whom, in what circumstances and why. *BMJ Quality and Safety*, *27*(9), 743–757. https://doi.org/10.1136/bmjqs-2017-006757.

Tranter, S., & Robertson, M. (2019). Improving the physical health of people with a mental illness: Holistic nursing assessments. *Mental Health Practice*, *23*(4), 34–41. https://doi.org/10.7748/mhp.2019.e1334.

Twohig, B., Manasia, A., Bassily-Marcus, A., et al. (2015). Family experience survey in the surgical intensive care unit. *Applied Nursing Research*, *28*(4), 281–284. https://doi.org/10.1016/j.apnr.2015.02.009.

Waterworth, C., & Rickson, D. (2017). Music in nursing. *Kai Tiaki: Nursing New Zealand*, *23*(7), 28–41.

Zhao, H., Gu, W., & Zhang, M. (2020). Massage therapy in nursing as nonpharmacological intervention to control agitation and stress in patients with dementia. *Alternative Therapies in Health & Medicine*, *26*(6), 29–33. https://pubmed.ncbi.nlm.nih.gov/32088672.

Readiness for Enhanced Communication **Domain 5 Perception/cognition Class 5 Communication**

Stacey M. Carroll, PhD, APRN-BC and Suzanne White, DNP, RN, PHCNS-BC

NANDA-I

Definition

A pattern of exchanging information and ideas with others, which can be strengthened.

● = Independent; ▲ = Collaborative; EBN = Evidence-Based Nursing; EB = Evidence-Based; ✱ = QSEN

Defining Characteristics

Expresses desire to enhance communication

NOC (Nursing Outcomes Classification)

Suggested NOC Outcomes

Communication; Communication: Expressive, Receptive

Example NOC Outcome with Indicators

Communication as evidenced by the following indicators: Use of spoken language/Use of written language/Acknowledgment of messages received/Exchanges messages accurately with others. (Rate the outcome and indicators of **Communication:** 1 = severely compromised, 2 = substantially compromised, 3 = moderately compromised, mildly compromised, 5 = not compromised [see Section I].)

Client Outcomes

Client Will (Specify Time Frame)

- Express willingness to enhance communication
- Demonstrate ability to speak or write a language
- Form words, phrases, and language
- Express thoughts and feelings
- Use and interpret nonverbal cues appropriately
- Express satisfaction with ability to share information and ideas with others

NIC (Nursing Interventions Classification)

Suggested NIC Interventions

Active Listening; Communication Enhancement: Hearing Deficit; Communication Enhancement: Speech Deficit

Example NIC Activities—Communication Enhancement

Hearing Deficit

Listen attentively; Allow patient adequate time to process communication and respond; Verify what was said or written using patient's response before continuing

Nursing Interventions and *Rationales*

- Assess the client's health literacy level so information can be tailored accordingly. EBN: *The Rapid Estimate of Adult Literacy in Medicine–Short Form (REALM-SF) provides a quick, valid assessment (Nowak, 2019).*
- ▲ Provide resources for communication for those who are deaf or hard of hearing, ensuring applications are HIPAA compliant. For a comprehensive list of available resources, see http://connect-hear.com/.
- ▲ Refer clients with autism spectrum disorder (ASD) to augmentative and alternative communication (AAC) specialists for employment, as appropriate. EB: *Clients with ASD who used mobile AAC devices in their place of employment had increased communicative support and participation (Richardson et al, 2019).*
- ▲ Refer couples in maladjusted relationships for psychosocial intervention and social support to strengthen communication; consider nurse specialists. EB: *The Couple Communication Satisfaction Scale showed high levels of reliability across genders (Jones et al, 2018).*
- ▲ Encourage communication partner training. EB: *Unresponsive partner communication led to negative emotional responses in people with aphasia (Harmon et al, 2020).* **EB:** *Communication skills training of clients with traumatic brain injuries and their partners resulted in improved communication in both parties (Rietdijk et al, 2020).*
- Use social media as a means to facilitate communication. EB: *Individuals who use AAC methods may benefit from integration of social media to further enhance communication (Caron, 2016).*
- Teach clients mindfulness meditation. EB: *Mindfulness meditation enhanced language production in clients with aphasia (Dickinson et al, 2017).*

C

- Use photographs as a communication aid. EB: *Use of photographs during conversation resulted in people with aphasia talking more about the topic and staying on that topic (Ulmer et al, 2017).*
- Encourage clients with aphasia to join communication groups. EB: *Gavel Clubs, emphasizing public speaking and leadership skills, increased quality of communication life and communication confidence in clients with aphasia, regardless of aphasia severity (Plourde et al, 2019).*
- ▲ Use telephonic (with or without video) health care to promote communication, especially in areas with lower access or when infection control precautions are in place. EBN: *Registered nurses effectively practiced person-centered care, including communication and presence, in telehealth (Boström et al, 2020).* EB: *Telehealth was equivalent to in-person delivery of social communication training for people with traumatic brain injury and their communication partners (Rietdijk et al, 2020).*
- ▲ Refer transgender clients for voice therapy if the client desires voice modification. EB: *Voice therapy assisted transgender clients in adjusting their voice to match their identified gender (Smith, 2020).*
- See care plan for Impaired Verbal **Communication.**

Pediatric

- Use social media as appropriate. EB: *Russell et al (2016) identified social media as a method for pediatric communication having numerous benefits, including increasing accessibility, interactions with others, and access to information.*
- Implement a collaborative approach to communication. EBN: *McKean et al (2017) found that when practitioners embraced services and systems that enabled more fluid forms of collaboration, trust and reciprocity developed.*
- See care plan for Impaired Verbal **Communication.**

Geriatric

- Facilitate communication through reminiscence. EB: *Reminiscence improved cognitive abilities and social engagement in older adults (Shropshire, 2020).* EB: *Clients with dementia used life story work to communicate memories with others (O'Philbin et al, 2020).*
- ▲ Encourage group singing activities and music therapy interventions in clients with dementia. EB: *"Singing for the Brain" is a group singing activity developed by the Alzheimer's Society and the program resulted in increased social inclusiveness and improvements in relationships (Osman et al, 2016).*
- Encourage drawing by caregivers of clients with dementia. EBN: *Drawing by caregivers of clients with dementia enhanced the communication experience (McEvoy & Bellass, 2017).*
- See care plan for Impaired Verbal **Communication.**

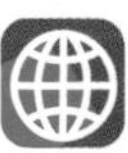

Multicultural

- See care plan for Impaired Verbal **Communication.**

Home Care and Client/Family Teaching and Discharge Planning

- The interventions described previously may be used in home care, discharge planning, and client and family teaching.
- See care plan for Impaired Verbal **Communication.**

REFERENCES

Boström, E., Ali, L., Fors, A., Ekman, I., & Andersson, A. E. (2020). Registered nurses' experiences of communication with patients when practicing person-centered care over the phone: A qualitative interview study. *BMC Nursing, 19*, 54 https://doi.org/10.1186/s12912-020-00448-4.

Caron, J. (2016). Engagement in social media environments for individuals who use augmentative and alternative communication. *NeuroRehabilitation, 39*(4), 499–506 https://doi.org/10.3233/NRE-161381.

Dickinson, J., Friary, P., & McCann, C. M. (2017). The influence of mindfulness meditation on communication and anxiety. *Aphasiology, 31*(9), 1044–1058 https://doi.org/10.1080/02687038.2016.1234582.

Harmon, T. G., Jacks, A., Haley, K. L., & Bailliard, A. (2020). How responsiveness from a communication partner affects story retell in aphasia: Quantitative and qualitative findings. *American Journal of Speech-Language Pathology, 29*(1), 142–156 https://doi.org/10.1044/2019_AJSLP-19-0091.

Jones, A. C., Jones, R. L., & Morris, N. (2018). Development and validation of the Couple Communication Satisfaction Scale. *American Journal of Family Therapy, 46*(5), 505–524 https://doi.org/10.1080/01926187.2019.1566874.

McEvoy, P., & Bellass, S. (2017). Using drawings as a reflective tool to enhance communication in dementia care. *Nursing Standard, 31*(19), 46–52.

McKean, C., Law, J., Laing, K., et al. (2017). A qualitative case study in the social capital of co-professional collaborative co-practice for children with speech, language and communication needs. *International Journal of Language & Communication Disorders, 52*(4), 514–527 https://doi.org/10.1111/1460-6984.12296.

Nowak, T. J. (2019). Implementation of a health literacy universal toolkit to improve postdischarge care at an urban trauma center. *Journal of Trauma Nursing, 26*(4), 180–185 https://doi.org/10.1097/JTN.0000000000000446.

O'Philbin, L., Woods, B., & Holmes, E. (2020). People with dementia and caregiver preferences for digital life story work service interventions: A discrete choice experiment and digital survey. *Aging & Mental Health, 24*(2), 353–361 https://doi.org/10.1080/13607863.2018.1525606.

Osman, S. E., Tischler, V., & Schneider, J. (2016). "Singing for the brain": A qualitative study exploring the health and well-being benefits of singing for people with dementia and their carers. *Dementia, 15*(6), 1326–1339 https://doi.org/10.1177/1471301214556291.

Plourde, J. M. H., Purdy, S. C., Moore, C., Friary, P., Brown, R., & McCann, C. M. (2019). Gavel Club for people with aphasia: Communication confidence and quality of communication life. *Aphasiology, 33*(1), 73–93 https://doi.org/10.1080/02687038.2018.1453043.

Richardson, L., McCoy, A., & McNaughton, D. (2019). "He's worth the work": The employment experiences of adults with ASD who use augmentative and alternative communication. *Work, 62*(2), 205–219 https://doi.org/10.3233/WOR-192856.

Rietdijk, R., Power, E., Attard, M., Heard, R., & Togher, L. (2020). Improved conversation outcomes after social communication skills training for people with traumatic brain injury and their communication partners: A clinical trial investigating in-person and telehealth delivery. *Journal of Speech, Language, and Hearing Research, 63*(2), 615–632 https://doi.org/10.1044/2019_JSLHR-19-00076.

Russell, D. J., Sprung, J., McCauley, D., et al. (2016). Knowledge exchange and discovery in the age of social media: The journey from inception to establishment of a parent-led web-based research advisory community for childhood disability. *Journal of Medical Internet Research, 18*(11), e293 https://doi.org/10.2196/jmir.5994.

Shropshire, M. (2020). Reminiscence intervention for community-dwelling older adults without dementia: A literature review. *British Journal of Community Nursing, 25*(1), 40–44 https://doi.org/10.12968/bjcn.2020.25.1.40.

Smith, C. J. (2020). Culturally competent care for transgender voice and communication intervention. *Perspectives of the ASHA Special Interest Groups, 5*(2), 457–462 https://doi.org/10.1044/2020_PERSP-19-00117.

Ulmer, E., Hux, K., Brown, J., Nelms, T., & Reeder, C. (2017). Using self-captured photographs to support the expressive communication of people with aphasia. *Aphasiology, 31*(10), 1183–1204 https://doi.org/10.1080/02687038.2016.1274872.

Impaired Verbal Communication **Domain 5 Perception/cognition Class 5 Communication**

Stacey M. Carroll, PhD, APRN-BC and Suzanne White, DNP, RN, PHCNS-BC

NANDA-I

Definition

Decreased, delayed, or absent ability to receive, process, transmit, and/or use a system of symbols.

Defining Characteristics

Absence of eye contact; agraphia; alternative communication; anarthria; aphasia; augmentative communication; decline of speech productivity; decline of speech rate; decreased willingness to participate in social interaction; difficulty comprehending communication; difficulty establishing social interaction; difficulty maintaining communication; difficulty using body expressions; difficulty using facial expressions; difficulty with selective attention; displays negative emotions; dysarthria; dysgraphia; dyslalia; dysphonia; fatigued by conversation; impaired ability to speak; impaired ability to use body expressions; impaired ability to use facial expressions; inability to speak language of caregiver; inappropriate verbalization; obstinate refusal to speak; slurred speech

Related Factors

Altered self-concept; dyspnea; emotional lability; environmental constraints; inadequate stimulation; low self-esteem; perceived vulnerability; psychological barriers; values incongruent with cultural norms

At-Risk Population

Individuals facing physical barriers; individuals in the early postoperative period; individuals unable to verbalize; individuals with communication barriers; individuals without a significant other

Associated Conditions

Altered perception, developmental disabilities; flaccid facial paralysis; hemifacial spasm; motor neuron disease; neoplasms; neurocognitive disorders; oropharyngeal defect; peripheral nervous system diseases; psychotic disorders; respiratory muscle weakness; sialorrhea; speech disorders; tongue diseases; tracheostomy; treatment regimen; velopharyngeal insufficiency; vocal cord dysfunction

NOC (Nursing Outcomes Classification)

Suggested NOC Outcomes

Communication; Communication: Expressive, Receptive

C

Example NOC Outcome with Indicators

Communication as evidenced by the following indicators: Use of spoken and written language/Acknowledgment of messages received/Exchanges messages accurately with others. (Rate the outcome and indicators of **Communication:** 1 = severely compromised, 2 = substantially compromised, 3 = moderately compromised, 4 = mildly compromised, 5 = not compromised [see Section I].)

Client Outcomes

Client Will (Specify Time Frame)

- Use effective communication techniques
- Use alternative methods of communication effectively
- Demonstrate congruency of verbal and nonverbal behavior
- Demonstrate understanding even if not able to speak
- Express desire for social interactions

NIC (Nursing Interventions Classification)

Suggested NIC Interventions

Active Listening; Communication Enhancement: Hearing Deficit; Communication Enhancement: Speech Deficit; Presence; Touch

Example NIC Activities—Communication Enhancement

Hearing Deficit
Listen attentively; Allow client adequate time to process communication and respond; Verify what was said or written using client's response before continuing

Nursing Interventions and *Rationales*

- Use a comprehensive nursing assessment to determine the language spoken, cultural considerations, satisfaction with communication, literacy level, cognitive level, and use of glasses and/or hearing aids; avoid making assumptions about clients' communication preferences. EB: *Asking specific assessment questions, including assessing client understanding, can garner more variable and useful responses from clients (Street & Mazor, 2017).* EB: *Clients want to be involved in decisions about their health through communication with providers (Ninnoni, 2019).*
- Determine client's own perception of communication difficulties and potential solutions, in accordance with the Healthy People 2030 goal to decrease the number of clients who report poor client–provider communication. EB: *The Communication Confidence Rating Scale for Aphasia (CCRSA) was used to measure self-reported communication confidence in clients with aphasia (Plourde et al, 2019).* EB: *The Healthcare Communication Distress Scale showed preliminary reliability and validity in assessing client distress with communication in healthcare (Lum et al, 2020).*
- Involve a familiar person when attempting to communicate with a client who has difficulty with communication, if accepted by the client. EB: *Training communication partners of clients with traumatic brain injury improved the communication experience of the client and family member (Togher et al, 2016).* EB: *Retaining valued relationships facilitated communication in people with dementia (Alsawy et al, 2017).*
- Listen carefully and validate verbal and nonverbal expressions particularly when dealing with pain and use appropriate scales for pain when appropriate. EBN: *The Pain Assessment Tool in Cognitively Impaired Elders showed preliminary reliability and validity for assessing nonverbal pain behaviors in African American and Caucasian nursing home residents with dementia (Richey et al, 2020).* EB: *The Revised Nonverbal Pain Scale and the Original Nonverbal Pain Scale both demonstrated reliability and validity for assessing pain in clients who are nonverbal and ventilated (Chookalayi et al, 2017).*

- Use communication programs to improve communication in clients who are nonvocal and mechanically ventilated. EB: *Implementing a program to facilitate communication with clients who are nonvocal significantly increased ease of communication scores (Trotta et al, 2020).*
- Be mindful of word choice when communicating with clients. EBN: *Using neutral and nonjudgmental terms facilitates respect and empowerment in vulnerable populations (Carroll, 2019).*
- Avoid ignoring the client with verbal impairment and place call light within reach of client who cannot verbally call for help, in order to promote safety and concern. EB: *Clients perceived being ignored when health professionals' nonverbal communication did not convey active presence (Timmerman et al, 2017).*
- Validate clients' feelings, focus on their strengths, and assist them in gaining confidence in identifying needs. EBN: *Viewing clients with communicative difficulties in a holistic manner cultivates empowering communication (Parsloe & Carroll, 2020).*
- Explain all health care procedures, be persistent in deciphering what the client is saying, and do not pretend to understand when the message is unclear. CEBN: *Persons who were nonvocal and ventilated appreciated persistence on the nurses' part with respect to being understood, found it bothersome when others pretended to understand them, and appreciated explanations from the nurse (Carroll, 2007).*
- ▲ Use an individualized and creative multiprofessional approach to augmentative and alternative communication (AAC) assistance and other communication interventions. EB: *Speech-language pathologists (SLPs) often introduce AAC measures, and the multiprofessional team needs to be aware of the client's attitude, socioeconomic status, and culture when choosing AAC (Moorcroft et al, 2019).* EB: *High-technology AAC use by those with intellectual and development disabilities and complex communication needs resulted in some positive effects on communication outcomes (Ganz et al, 2017).*
- Use consistent nursing staff for those with communication impairments. EB: *Among linguistically and culturally diverse clients with dementia, other communication methods (e.g., body language) along with spoken language can develop over time, indicating the importance of the continuity of providers (Strandroos & Antelius, 2017).*
- ▲ Consult communication specialists from various disciplines as appropriate. SLPs, audiologists, and translators provide comprehensive communication assistance for those with impaired communication. EBN: *Use of interpreter services increased clients' perception that their communication needs were met (Lopez-Bushnell et al, 2020).*
- ▲ When the client is having difficulty communicating, assess and refer for audiology consultation for hearing loss (American Academy of Audiology, 2021). Suspect hearing loss when:
  - Client frequently complains that people mumble and that others' speech is not clear.
  - Client often asks people to repeat what they said and hears only parts of conversations.
  - Client's friends or relatives state that the client does not seem to hear very well or plays the television or radio too loudly.
  - Client does not laugh at jokes because of missing too much of the story.
  - Client needs to ask others about the details of a meeting that the client attended.
  - Client cannot hear the doorbell or the telephone.
  - Client finds it easier to understand others when facing them, especially in a noisy environment.
- When communicating with a client with a hearing loss:
  - Obtain client's attention before speaking and face toward his or her unaffected side or better ear while allowing client to see the speaker's face at a reasonably close distance, provide sufficient light, do not stand in front of a window, use gestures as appropriate to aid in communication, do not raise voice or over enunciate, and minimize extraneous noise. *Correct positioning and an optimal listening environment increase the client's awareness of the interaction and enhance the client's ability to communicate. Light facing the speaker makes expressions and lip movements clearer whereas light behind the speaker causes glare, impeding visibility of the speaker's face (UCSF Health, 2020).*
  - Encourage the client to wear hearing aids, if appropriate. EB: *Hearing aids reduced communicative efforts of those with hearing loss and their communicative partners (Beechey et al, 2020).*
  - Remove masks if safe, or use see-through anti-fog masks to allow for visibility of the mouth and less muffling of sound which enhances communication. *For information on see-through masks, see www.amphl.org.*

Pediatric

- Observe behavioral communication cues in infants. EB: *Kupán et al (2017) found that infants' choice behavior is affected by the adult's presence or absence.*

C

- Identify and define at least two forms of augmentative and alternative communication modalities that may be used by children with significant disabilities. EB: *Drager et al (2019) found that augmentative and alternative communication with visual scene displays and Just In Time programming may be effective in increasing symbolic communication for students with severe developmental disability.* EB: *Pitt and Brumberg (2018) determined that brain–computer interfaces (BCIs) have the potential to provide an alternate modality for accessing augmentative and alternative communication for individuals with profound speech and motor impairments, including paralysis and akinetic mutism.*
- Teach children with severe disabilities functional communication skills. EB: *Quinn and Kidd (2019) found that symbolic play provides a rich context for the exchange and negotiation of meaning, and thus may contribute to the development of important skills underlying communicative development.*
- ▲ Refer children with primary speech and language delay/disorder for speech and language therapy interventions. EB: *McManus et al (2020) determined that early intervention is needed to improve integrated systems of care affecting primary care processes and coordination.*

Geriatric

- Be aware of nonverbal communication. EBN: *Older adults had both positive and negative responses to nurses' nonverbal communication (Wanko Keutchafo et al, 2020).*
- Perform hearing screenings and refer for hearing evaluations in accordance with Healthy People 2030 goal to encourage increasing both the proportion of older adults having hearing examination and the number of referrals for hearing evaluation and treatment. EBN: *Hearing loss was often missed during admission and nursing assessments of older adults, necessitating the increased use of screening measures (Mormer et al, 2020).* EB: *Simple screening procedures such as questioning about hearing loss, the finger-rub test, and the whisper test can be used for identification of hearing loss in older adults and referrals for evaluation (Strawbridge & Wallhagen, 2017).*
- Avoid use of "elderspeak," which is a speech style similar to baby talk. EB: *Avoiding elderspeak reduces resistiveness to care in clients with dementia (Zhang et al, 2020).* EB: *A brief communication training intervention resulted in lower use of elderspeak by staff and less resistiveness to care among clients with dementia (Williams et al, 2018).*
- Initiate communication with the client with dementia and give client time to respond, use eye contact, speak in shorter sentences, and use music. EBN: *The Verbal and Nonverbal Interaction Scale is valid and reliable and can assess sociable and unsociable communication in clients with dementia (Williams et al, 2017).* EB: *Using music in people with late stage dementia resulted in an increase in their nonverbal communication and quality of life (Clare et al, 2020).*

Use touch, a therapeutic communication strategy, as appropriate. EBN: *Touch resulted in positive responses from older adults (Wanko Keutchafo et al, 2020).*

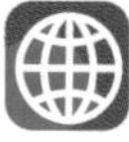

Multicultural

- ▲ Attend to the meaning of a culture's nonverbal communication modes, such as eye contact, facial expression, touch, and body language. EB: *Attending to nonverbal interactions facilitated communication among culturally and linguistically diverse clients with dementia (Strandroos & Antelius, 2017).*
- ▲ Use instruments to determine culturally appropriate therapeutic communication. EBN: *The Global Interprofessional Therapeutic Communication Scale measures culturally appropriate client–provider communication and has demonstrated preliminary reliability and validity (Campbell & Aredes, 2019).*
- ▲ Assess for the influence of cultural beliefs, norms, and values on the client's communication process. EBN: *Misunderstandings and conflicts can arise when there is a difference in language and/or culture of the provider and client (Crawford et al., 2017).*
- ▲ Assess personal space needs, acceptable communication styles, acceptable body language, interpretation of eye contact, perception of touch, and use of paraverbal modes when communicating with the client. EB: *When caring for clients of varied ethnicities and languages, nurses used nonverbal means such as pointing, smiling, modeling, and touch to convey information and calm clients in long-term care (Small et al, 2015).*
- ▲ Assess how language barriers contribute to health disparities among ethnic and racial minorities. EBN: *Client safety was compromised when language barriers were present (van Rosse et al, 2016).*
- ▲ The Office of Minority Health of the U.S. Department of Health and Human Services' national standards on culturally and linguistically appropriate services (CLAS) in health care should be used. EB: *CLAS standards aim to improve health care quality and advance health equity by establishing a framework for*

organizations to serve the nation's increasingly diverse communities (Office of Minority Health, U.S. Dept. of Health & Human Services, n.d.).

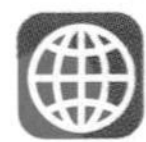

Home Care

- The interventions described previously may be adapted for home care use.

Client/Family Teaching and Discharge Planning

▲ Refer the client to a SLP or audiologist. Audiological assessment quantifies and qualifies hearing in terms of the degree of hearing loss, the type of hearing loss, and the configuration of the hearing loss. Once a particular hearing loss has been identified, a treatment and management plan can be put into place by an SLP. EB: *Audiological services can improve communication in clients with dementia and hearing loss (Mamo et al, 2017).* EB: *SLPs often introduce AAC to those with communication needs but this needs to be done in collaboration with a multiprofessional team (Moorcroft et al, 2019).*

REFERENCES

Alsawy, S., Mansell, W., McEvoy, P., & Tai, S. (2017). What is good communication for people living with dementia? A mixed methods systematic review. *International Psychogeriatrics, 29*(11), 1785–1800 https://doi.org/10.1017/S1041610217001429.

American Academy of Audiology. (2021). *How's your hearing?* Retrieved from https://www.audiology.org/consumers-0. [Accessed 10 June 2021].

Beechey, T., Buchholz, J. M., & Keidser, G. (2020). Hearing aid amplification reduces communication effort of people with hearing impairment and their conversation partners. *Journal of Speech, Language, and Hearing Research, 63*(4), 1299–1311 https://doi.org/10.1044/2020_JSLHR-19-00350.

Campbell, S. H., & Aredes, N. D. A. (2019). Global Interprofessional Therapeutic Communication Scale© (GITCS©): Development and validation. *Clinical Simulation in Nursing, 34*, 30–42 https://doi.org/10.1016/j.ecns.2019.05.006.

Carroll, S. M. (2007). Silent, slow lifeworld: The communication experiences of nonvocal ventilated patients. *Qualitative Health Research, 17*(9), 1165–1177 https://doi.org/10.1177/1049732307307334.

Carroll, S. M. (2019). Respecting and empowering vulnerable populations: Contemporary terminology. *Journal for Nurse Practitioners, 15*(3), 228–231 https://doi.org/10.1016/j.nurpra.2018.12.031.

Chookalayi, H., Heidarzadeh, M., Hasenpour, M., Jabrailzadeh, S., & Sadeghpour, F. (2017). A study on the psychometric properties of Revised-nonverbal pain scale and original-nonverbal pain scale in Iranian nonverbal-ventilated patients. *Indian Journal of Critical Care Medicine, 21*(7), 429–435 https://doi.org/10.4103/ijccm.IJCCM_114_17.

Clare, A., Camic, P. M., Crutch, S. J., West, J., Harding, E., & Brotherhood, E. (2020). Using music to develop a multisensory communicative environment for people with late-stage dementia. *The Gerontologist, 60*(6), 1115–1125 https://doi.org/10.1093/geront/gnz169.

Crawford, T., Candlin, S., & Roger, P. (2017). New perspectives on understanding cultural diversity in nurse-patient communication. *Collegian, 24*(1), 63–69 https://doi.org/10.1016/j.colegn.2015.09.001.

Drager, K. D. R., Light, J., Currall, J., et al. (2019). AAC technologies with visual scene displays and "just in time" programming and symbolic communication turns expressed by students with severe disability. *Journal of Intellectual & Developmental Disability, 44*(3), 321–336 https://doi.org/10.3109/13668250.2017.1326585.

Ganz, J. B., Morin, K. L., Foster, M. J., et al. (2017). High-technology augmentative and alternative communication for individuals with intellectual disabilities and complex communication needs: A meta-analysis. *Augmentative and Alternative Communication, 33*(4), 224–238 https://doi.org/10.1080/07434618.2017.1373855.

Kupán, K., Király, I., Kupán, K., Krekó, K., Miklósi, Á., & Topál, J. (2017). Interacting effect of two social factors on 18-month-old infants' imitative behavior: Communicative cues and demonstrator presence. *Journal of Experimental Child Psychology, 161*, 186–194 https://doi.org/10.1016/j.jecp.2017.03.019.

Lopez-Bushnell, F. K., Guerra-Sandoval, G., Schutzman, E. Z., Langsjoen, J., & Villalobos, N. E. (2020). Increasing communication with healthcare providers for patients with limited English proficiency through interpreter language services education. *Medsurg Nursing, 29*(2), 89–95.

Lum, M., Garnett, M., Sheridan, J., O'Connor, E., & Meuter, R. (2020). Healthcare communication distress scale: Pilot factor analysis and validity. *Patient Education and Counseling, 103*(7), 1302–1310 https://doi.org/10.1016/j.pec.2020.02.010.

Mamo, S. K., Oh, E., & Lin, F. R. (2017). Enhancing communication in adults with dementia and age-related hearing loss. *Seminars in Hearing, 38*(2), 177–183 https://doi.org/10.1055/s-0037-1601573.

McManus, B. M., Richardson, Z., Schenkman, M., et al. (2020). Child characteristics and early intervention referral and receipt of services: A retrospective cohort study. *BMC Pediatrics, 20*(1), 84 https://doi.org/10.1186/s12887-020-1965-x.

Moorcroft, A., Scarinci, N., & Meyer, C. (2019). A systematic review of the barriers and facilitators to the provision and use of low-tech and unaided AAC systems for people with complex communication needs and their families. *Disability and Rehabilitation Assistive Technology, 14*(7), 710–731 https://doi.org/10.1080/17483107.2018.1499135.

Mormer, E., Bubb, K. J., Alrawashdeh, M., & Cipkala-Gaffin, J. A. (2020). Hearing loss and communication among hospitalized older adults: Prevalence and recognition. *Journal of Gerontological Nursing, 46*(6), 34–42 https://doi.org/10.3928/00989134-20200316-03.

Ninnoni, J. P. K. (2019). A qualitative study of the communication and information needs of people with learning disabilities and epilepsy with physicians, nurses and carers. *BMC Neurology, 19*(1), 12 https://doi.org/10.1186/s12883-018-1235-9.

Office of Minority Health, U.S. Department of Health & Human Services. (n.d.). *CLAS (Culturally and Linguistically Appropriate Services)*. Retrieved from https://thinkculturalhealth.hhs.gov/clas/what-is-clas. [Accessed June 10, 2021].

Parsloe, S., & Carroll, S. M. (2020). Accessibility, acceptance, and equity: Examining disability-linked health disparities as nursing and communication scholars. *Communication in Nursing, 1*(1), 1–14.

Pitt, K. M., & Brumberg, J. S. (2018). Guidelines for feature matching assessment of brain-computer interfaces for augmentative and alternative communication. *American Journal of Speech-Language Pathology, 27*(3), 950–964 https://doi.org/10.1044/2018_AJSLP-17-0135.

Plourde, J. M. H., Purdy, S. C., Moore, C., Friary, P., Brown, R., & McCann, C. M. (2019). Gavel Club for people with aphasia: Communication confidence and quality of communication life. *Aphasiology, 33*(1), 73–93 https://doi.org/10.1080/02687038.2018.1453043.

Quinn, S., & Kidd, E. (2019). Symbolic play promotes non-verbal communicative exchange in infant-caregiver dyads. *British Journal of Developmental Psychology*, *37*(1), 33–50 https://doi.org/10.1111/bjdp.12251.

Richey, S. A., Capezuti, E., Cron, S. G., Reed, D., Torres-Vigil, I., & de Oliveira Otto, M. C. (2020). Development and testing of the Pain Assessment Tool in Cognitively Impaired Elders (PATCIE): Nonverbal pain behaviors in African American and Caucasian nursing home residents with dementia. *Pain Management Nursing*, *21*(2020), 187–193 https://doi.org/10.1016/j.pmn.2019.08.004.

Small, J., Chan, S. M., Drance, E., et al. (2015). Verbal and nonverbal indicators of quality of communication between care staff and residents in ethnoculturally and linguistically diverse long-term care settings. *Journal of Cross Cultural Gerontology*, *30*(3), 285–304 https://doi.org/10.1007/s10823-015-9269-6.

Strandroos, L., & Antelius, E. (2017). Interaction and common ground in dementia: Communication across linguistic and cultural diversity in a residential dementia care setting. *Health*, *21*(5), 538–554 https://doi.org/10.1177/1363459316677626.

Strawbridge, W. J., & Wallhagen, M. I. (2017). Simple tests compare well with a hand-held audiometer for hearing loss screening in primary care. *Journal of the American Geriatrics Society*, *65*(10), 2282–2284 https://doi.org/10.1111/jgs.15044.

Street, R. L., Jr., & Mazor, K. M. (2017). Clinician-patient communication measures: Drilling down into assumptions, approaches, and analyses. *Patient Education and Counseling*, *100*(8), 1612–1618 https://doi.org/10.1016/j.pec.2017.03.021.

Timmermann, C., Uhrenfeldt, L., & Birkelund, R. (2017). Ethics in the communicative encounter: Seriously ill patients' experiences of health professionals' nonverbal communication. *Scandinavian Journal of Caring Sciences*, *31*(1), 63–71 https://doi.org/10.1111/scs.12316.

Togher, L., McDonald, S., Tate, R., Rietdijk, R., & Power, E. (2016). The effectiveness of social communication partner training for adults with severe chronic TBI and their families using a measure of perceived communication ability. *NeuroRehabilitation*, *38*(2016), 243–255 https://doi.org/10.3233/NRE-151316.

Trotta, R. L., Hermann, R. M., Polomano, R. C., & Happ, M. B. (2020). Improving nonvocal critical care patients' ease of communication using a modified SPEACS-2 program. *Journal for Healthcare Quality*, *42*(1), e1–e9 https://doi.org10.1097/JHQ.0000000000000163.

UCSF Health. (2020). *Communicating with people with hearing loss. [Internet]*. Retrieved from https://www.ucsfhealth.org/education/communicating_with_people_with_hearing_loss/. Accessed June 10, 2021.

van Rosse, F., de Bruijne, Suurmond, J., Essink-Bot, M. L., & Wagner, C. (2016). language barriers and patient safety risks in hospital care: A mixed methods study. *International Journal of Nursing Studies*, *54*, 45–53 https://doi.org/10.1016/j.ijnurstu.2015.03.012.

Wanko Keutchafo, E. L., Kerr, J., & Jarvis, M. A. (2020). Evidence of nonverbal communication between nurses and older adults: A scoping review. *BMC Nursing*, *19*, 53 https://doi.org/10.1186/s12912-020-00443-9.

Williams, C. L., Newman, D., & Hammar, L. M. (2017). Preliminary psychometric properties of the Verbal and Nonverbal Interaction Scale: An observational measure for communication in persons with dementia. *Issues in Mental Health Nursing*, *38*(5), 381–390 https://doi.org/10.1080/01612840.2017.1279248.

Williams, K. N., Perkhounkova, Y., Jao, Y. L., et al. (2018). Person-centered communication for nursing home residents with dementia: Four communication analysis methods. *Western Journal of Nursing Research*, *40*(7), 1012–1031 https://doi.org/10.1177/0193945917697226.

Zhang, M., Zhao, H., & Fan-Ping, M. (2020). Elderspeak to resident dementia patients increases resistiveness to care in health care profession. *Inquiry: A Journal of Medical Care Organization, Provision, and Financing*, *57*, 46958020948668 https://doi.org/10.1177/0046958020948668.

Acute Confusion Domain 5 Perception/cognition Class 4 Cognition

Kimberly S. Meyer, PhD, ACNP-BC, CNRN

NANDA-I

Definition

Reversible disturbances of consciousness, attention, cognition, and perception that develop over a short period of time, and which last less than 3 months.

Defining Characteristics

Altered psychomotor functioning; difficulty initiating goal-directed behavior; difficulty initiating purposeful behavior; hallucinations; inadequate follow-through with goal-directed behavior; inadequate follow-through with purposeful behavior; misperception; neurobehavioral manifestations; psychomotor agitation

Related Factors

Altered in sleep-wake cycle; dehydration; impaired physical mobility, inappropriate use of physical restraint; malnutrition, pain, sensory deprivation; substance misuse; urinary retention

At-Risk Population

Individuals aged ≥60 years; individuals with history of cerebral vascular accident; men

Associated Conditions

Decreased level of consciousness; impaired metabolism; infections; neurocognitive disorders; pharmaceutical preparations

C

NOC (Nursing Outcomes Classification)

Suggested NOC Outcomes

Improved Cognitive Function; Improved Sensory Perception; Improved Thought Processes

Example NOC Outcome with Indicators

Cognition as evidenced by the following indicators: Communication clear for age/Comprehension of the meaning of situations/Attentiveness/Concentration/Cognitive orientation. (Rate the outcome and indicators of **Cognition:** 1 = severely compromised, 2 = substantially compromised, 3 = moderately compromised, 4 = mildly compromised, 5 = not compromised [see Section I].)

Client Outcomes

Client Will (Specify Time Frame)

- Demonstrate restoration of cognitive status to baseline
- Be oriented to time, place, and person
- Demonstrate appropriate motor behavior
- Maintain functional capacity
- Remain free from injury

NIC (Nursing Interventions Classification)

Suggested NIC Interventions

Delirium Management; Delusion Management

Example NIC Activities—Delirium Management

Inform client of time, place, and person as needed; Provide information slowly and in small doses with frequent rest periods; Ensure client has appropriate assistive sensory devices (e.g., glasses, hearing aids)

Nursing Interventions and *Rationales*

- Recognize that delirium is characterized by an acute onset, a fluctuating course, inattention, and disordered thinking. EBN: *Delirium is often underrecognized and can have significant adverse consequences for clients, including increase in length of hospitalization, cognitive deficits, and increased mortality. Common conditions that place clients at risk for delirium include advanced age, pain, dehydration, infections, metabolic disturbances, medication use/withdrawal, mechanical ventilation, invasive lines, and surgery (Xing et al, 2019; Wilson et al, 2020).*
- Use a validated screening tool to assess for delirium. EBN: *The Confusion Assessment Method (CAM) and the Delirium Observation Screening (DOS) Scale are brief evaluations that can be used for the assessment of delirium in most clients. The CAM-ICU can be used to screen for delirium in critically ill clients (Ho et al, 2020).*
- Identify the three distinct types of delirium: hyperactive (easy to recognize), hypoactive (commonly missed), and mixed (the most commonly occurring) (Wilson et al, 2020).
  - Hyperactive: delirium characterized by restlessness, agitation, irritability, hypervigilance, hallucinations, and delusions; client may be combative or may attempt to remove tubes, lines.
  - Hypoactive: delirium characterized by decreased motor activity, decreased vocalization, detachment, apathy, lethargy, somnolence, reduced awareness of surroundings, and confusion.
  - Mixed: delirium characterized by the client fluctuating between periods of hyperactivity and agitation and hypoactivity and sedation. EB: *Delirium is underrecognized by both medical and nursing staff, particularly the hypoactive form (Morandi et al, 2020).*
- Perform a comprehensive nursing assessment and mental status examination that includes the following assessment (Solà-Miravete et al, 2018):
  - History from a reliable source that documents an acute and fluctuating change in cognitive function, attention, and behavior from baseline.

C

- ❍ Cognition as evidenced by level of consciousness; orientation to time, person, and place; thought process (thinking may be disorganized, distorted, fragmented, slow, or accelerated with delirium; conversation may be irrelevant or rambling); and content (perceptual disturbances such as visual, auditory, or tactile delusions or hallucinations).
- ❍ Level of attention (may be decreased or may fluctuate with delirium; may be unable to focus, shift, or sustain attention; may be easily distracted or may be hypervigilant).
- ❍ Behavior characteristics and level of psychomotor behavior (activity may be increased or decreased and may include restlessness, finger tapping, picking at bedclothes, changing position frequently, spastic movements or tremors, or decreased psychomotor activity such as sluggishness, staring into space, remaining in the same position for prolonged periods).
- ❍ Level of consciousness (may be easily aroused, lethargic, drowsy, difficult to arouse, unarousable, hyperalert, easily startled, and overly sensitive to stimuli).
- ❍ Mood and affect (may be paranoid or fearful with delirium; may have rapid mood swings).
- ❍ Insight and judgment (may be impaired).
- ❍ Memory (recent and immediate memory is impaired with delirium; unable to register new information).
- ❍ Language (may have rapid, rambling, slurred, incoherent speech).
- ❍ Altered sleep-wake cycle (insomnia, excessive daytime sleepiness).
- ❍ Nutrition status.
- ❍ Bowel and bladder elimination habits.
- ❍ Mobility status.

EBN: *Establishing the client's baseline mental status by obtaining an accurate history and performing a brief cognitive assessment observing for key diagnostic criteria are important in the diagnosis of delirium (Solà-Miravete et al, 2018). Encourage family presence to facilitate assessment of subtle changes in cognition (Devlin et al, 2018).*

- ● Identify predisposing factors that may precede the development of delirium: dementia, cognitive impairment, functional impairment, visual impairment, alcohol misuse, multiple comorbidities, severe illness, history of transient ischemic attack or stroke, depression, history of delirium, and advanced age (older than 65). EB: *Delirium is a multifactorial syndrome most commonly seen in the intensive care unit (ICU), palliative care, and postoperative settings; identification of risk factors is important for prevention (Devlin et al, 2018).*
- ● Surgical procedures increase the risk of delirium postoperatively. EB: *Assess the client for risk factors and implement interventions to reorient client postoperatively. Effectively treat pain and anxiety with the lowest effective dose. Avoid benzodiazepine agents if possible (Devlin et al, 2018).*
- ● Identify iatrogenic factors that may precede the development of delirium, especially for individuals with predisposing factors: use of restraints, indwelling bladder catheter, metabolic disturbances, polypharmacy, pain, infection, dehydration, blood loss, constipation, electrolyte imbalances, immobility, general anesthesia, mechanical ventilation, hospital admission for fractures or hip surgery, anticholinergic medications, anxiety, sleep deprivation, lack of use of vision and/or hearing aids, and environmental factors. EB: *Prevention of delirium needs to remain a high priority in light of frequency of occurrence, high treatment costs, longer hospital length of stay, higher rates of functional decline and resultant institutional care, and greater mortality; delirium may persist and lead to long-term cognitive decline (Davidson et al, 2015).*
- ● Facilitate appropriate extended visitation for clients at risk of delirium. EBN: *Extended visitation is associated with decreased incidence of delirium and shorter length of stay (Liang et al, 2021). In the absence of family availability, simulated presence using prerecorded video or audio messages may decrease agitation (Waszynski et al, 2018).*
- ▲ Assess for and report possible physiological alterations (e.g., sepsis, hypoglycemia, hypoxia, hypotension, infection, changes in temperature, fluid and electrolyte imbalance, use of medications with known cognitive and psychotropic side effects). CEB: *Systemic disturbances, including immunological, metabolic, neuroinflammatory, endocrinological, and neurological factors, lead to alterations in neurotransmitter synthesis and availability, which leads to delirium (Maldonado, 2013).*
  - ❍ Treat the underlying risk factors or the causes of delirium in collaboration with the health care team: establish/maintain normal fluid and electrolyte balance, normal body temperature, normal oxygenation (if the client experiences low oxygen saturation, deliver supplemental oxygen), normal blood glucose levels, and normal blood pressure, and address malnutrition and anemia. EB: *Early recognition of risk factors may help to prevent the negative sequelae of delirium (Burry et al., 2019).*

- ❍ Monitor for any trends occurring in these manifestations, including laboratory tests. EB: *Careful monitoring of laboratory tests assessing for metabolic abnormities is important to identify the potential etiological factors for delirium (Davidson et al, 2015).*

▲ Conduct a medication review and eliminate unnecessary medications; potentially inappropriate medications for older adults at risk for delirium include anticholinergics, benzodiazepines, corticosteroids, H_2 receptor antagonists, sedative hypnotics, and tricyclic antidepressants (American Geriatrics Society, 2015). EB: *Polypharmacy is associated with delirium, and a elimination of high-risk medications improves agitation and cognitive function (Aloisi et al, 2019).*

▲ Recognize that delirium is frequently treated with antipsychotic medications or sedatives; if there is no other way to keep the client safe, administer these medications cautiously, as ordered, while monitoring for medication side effects. EB: *Studies show that routine use of antipsychotic medications does not decrease the duration and severity of delirium and increases the risk of cardiac side effects (Nikooie et al, 2019).*

- Locate at risk-clients in private (single-bed) rooms when possible. EB: *Studies in the long-term care population suggest that the incidence of delirium is decreased when there is no roommate (Blandfort et al, 2020).*
- Identify, evaluate, and treat pain quickly and adequately (see care plans for Acute **Pain** or Chronic **Pain**). EB: *Untreated pain is a potential cause of delirium (Blair et al, 2019; Daoust et al, 2020). The use of nonopioid analgesia (acetaminophen, antiinflammatory medications) reduces the need for opiates, continuous observation, and the development of delirium (Connolly et al, 2020).*
- Facilitate sleep hygiene. Establish day/night routines and plan care to allow for appropriate sleep-wake cycles (Lu et al, 2019). EBN: *The use of ear plugs and eye masks may improve sleep and decrease the risk of delirium (Hu et al, 2015; Reznik & Slooter, 2019).* EB: *Administration of melatonin is associated with reduced risk of delirium in at-risk ICU and surgical clients (Baumgartner et al, 2019; Campbell et al, 2019).*
- Promote regulation of bowel and bladder function; use bladder scanning to identify retention, avoid prolonged insertion of urinary catheters, and remove catheters as soon as possible (Bounds et al, 2016).
- Ensure adequate nutritional and fluid intake. EB: *Malnutrition is significantly associated with delirium. Attending to correct levels of B vitamins, antioxidants, glucose, water, and lipids may lead to resolution of delirium (Rosted et al, 2018).*
- Promote early mobilization and rehabilitation in a progressive manner. EB: *Early, aggressive mobilization is associated with decreased incidence of delirium (Liang et al, 2021).*
- Promote continuity of care; avoid frequent changes in staff and surroundings. EB: *Changes may contribute to feelings of disorientation and confusion (Mazur et al, 2016).*
- Facilitate appropriate sensory input by having clients use aids (e.g., glasses, hearing aids, dentures) as needed; check for impacted ear wax. EB: *Delirium can be addressed with nonpharmacological interventions, such as decreasing sensory impairment (Javedan & Tulebaev, 2014; Burry et al, 2019) or avoiding sensory overload for clients with agitation.* EB: *A systematic review of interventions to help reduce delirium risk included multicomponent interventions, such as encouraging use of vision and hearing aids, and may assist in the prevention of delirium in individuals who are not cognitively impaired (Trogrlić et al, 2015).*
- Modulate sensory exposure; eliminate excessive noise, use appropriate lighting based on the time of day, and establish a calm environment.
- Provide cognitive stimulation through conversation about current events, viewpoints, and relationships and encourage reminiscence or word games. EBN: *Daily cognitive stimulation can prevent cognitive decline and promote cognitive recovery (Trogrlić et al, 2015).*
- Provide reality orientation, including identifying self by name at each encounter with the client, calling the client by their preferred name, and the gentle use of orientation techniques; when reorientation is not effective, use distraction. Gently correct misperceptions. EB: *Efforts to reorient may agitate some clients; changing the subject may help calm the client (Davidson et al, 2015; Trogrlić et al, 2015).*
- Provide clocks and calendars, update dry erase white boards each shift, encourage family to visit regularly and to bring familiar objects from home, such as family photos or an afghan. EB: *Persons at risk for delirium should be provided clocks and calendars that are easily visible; family and friends may help with reorientation (Bannon et al, 2016).*
- Use gentle, caring communication; provide reassurance of safety; and give simple explanations of procedures.
- Provide supportive nursing care, including meeting basic needs, such as feeding, regular toileting, and ensuring adequate hydration; closely observe behaviors that provide clues as to what might be distressing the client. Delirious clients are unable to care for themselves because of their confusion. EB: *Understanding and anticipating behaviors promotes client comfort and safety (Faught, 2014).*

- If clients know that they are not thinking clearly, acknowledge the concern. Fear is frequently experienced by people with delirium. EB: *Confusion is frightening; the memory of the delirium can be distressing to clients and families (Bannon et al, 2016).*

Critical Care

- Recognize admission risk factors for delirium. EB: *ICU clients are at increased risk for delirium because of greater use of sedatives, analgesics, severity of illness, age, infection, multiorgan failure, sleep deprivation, surgery, fracture, restraint use, immobility, tubes, catheters, hypovolemia, polypharmacy, malnutrition, electrolyte imbalance, and stroke (Devlin et al, 2018).*
- Assess level of arousal using the Richmond Agitation Sedation Scale (RASS); clients receiving a score of −5 to −4 are comatose and unable to be assessed for delirium. CEB: *Establishing level of arousal before using the CAM for the ICU (CAM-ICU) decreases the incidence of inappropriate "unable to assess" (UTA) ratings on the CAM-ICU; it was found that noncomatose clients were inappropriately determined to be UTA (Swan, 2014).*
- Assess for pain every 2 to 3 hours or more frequently as needed with a standardized assessment tool, which includes either a numerical rating scale or one with behavioral indicators, such as the Behavioral Pain Scale (BPS) or Critical Care Pain Observation Tool (CPOT). EB: *Behavioral pain scales provide reliable assessments in critically ill clients (Bouajram et al, 2020).* EBN: *Uncontrolled pain is associated with a threefold increase in the development of delirium (Daoust et al, 2020).*
- ▲ Incorporate the Awakening and Breathing Coordination, Delirium Monitoring and Management, and Early Mobility (ABCDE) ICU delirium and weakness prevention bundle in conjunction with the interdisciplinary team. EB: *Implementation of the ABCDE bundle leads to fewer incidence of ICU delirium and short durations of delirium (Bounds et al, 2016).*
  - Assess safety and implementation of a spontaneous awakening trial (SAT) using an established protocol. EB: Daily interruption of sedation may be beneficial when it results in a reduced total dose of sedative administered; minimizing the depth and duration of sedation is beneficial for reducing delirium (*Bounds et al, 2016*).
  - Assess sedation and agitation level using a valid and reliable tool; titrate sedation to target sedation level. EB: Sedatives and analgesics prescribed to improve client–ventilator dyssynchrony and treat anxiety and pain may precipitate delirium (*Davidson et al, 2015*).

Geriatric

- The interventions described previously are relevant to the geriatric client.
- Recognize that delirium may be superimposed on dementia; the nurse must be aware of the client's baseline cognitive function. EB: *Dementia increases the risk and severity of delirium, and current research suggests delirium is an independent risk for subsequent dementia (Parrish, 2019).*
- Understand that delirium is common in frail, older adults and leads to increased lengths of stay and mortality. EBN: *Delirium is underrecognized in older adults but routine screening improves identification and treatment (Geriatric Medicine Research Collaborative, 2019).*
- Provide feeding assistance as needed. See care plan for Imbalanced **Nutrition:** Less than Body Requirements. EB: *Modified food consistencies and nutritional supplements can improve nutritional status and decrease development of delirium in older adults (Volkert et al, 2019).*
- Promote adequate hydration; keep a glass of water within easy reach of the client and offer fluids frequently. EBN: *Older adults are at high risk for dehydration (Volkert et al, 2019).*
- Avoid use of restraints; remove all nonessential equipment such as telemetry, blood pressure cuffs, catheters, and intravenous lines as soon as possible. EBN: *The use of restraints contributes to the development of delirium and posttraumatic stress disorder in critically ill clients (Franks et al, 2021).*
- Consider use of music to decrease the development of delirium, especially in surgical clients. EB: *Listening to music has been found to decrease delirium during acute hospitalization of older clients (Cheong et al, 2016).*
- ▲ Assess risk for falls and implement fall prevention strategies. EB: *Falls are an independent predictor of delirium-inducing hospitalizations and a consequence of delirium in the hospitalized client (Mazur et al, 2016).*
- ▲ Determine whether the client is nourished; watch for protein-calorie malnutrition. Consult with health care provider or dietitian as needed. EB: *Malnutrition is significantly associated with delirium. Attending to*

correct levels of B vitamins, antioxidants, glucose, water, and lipids may lead to resolution of delirium (Rosted et al, 2018).

- Explain hospital routines and procedures slowly and in simple terms; repeat information as necessary.
- Educate family members about delirium assessment and strategies to use to prevent and lessen delirium. EBN: *Delirium increases caregiver burden (Fong et al, 2019).*

C

Home Care

- The interventions described previously are relevant to home care use.
- Assess and monitor for acute changes in cognition and behavior.
- Recognize that delirium is reversible but can contribute to early cognitive decline in many clients (Goldberg et al, 2020).
- Avoid preconceptions about the source of acute confusion; assess each occurrence on the basis of available evidence.
- ▲ Institute case management of frail elderly clients to support continued independent living if possible once delirium has resolved.

Client/Family Teaching and Discharge Planning

- Teach the family to recognize signs of early confusion and seek medical help.
- Counsel the client and family regarding the management of delirium and its sequelae. Increased care requirements at discharge may be needed for clients who have experienced delirium. EB: *Frailty and delirium can lead to functional decline and institutionalization (Geriatric Medicine Research Collaborative, 2019; Goldberg et al, 2020).*

REFERENCES

Aloisi, G., Marengoni, A., Morandi, A., et al. (2019). Drug prescriptions and delirium in older inpatients: Results from the Nationwide Multicenter Italian Delirium Day 2015–2016. *Journal of Clinical Psychiatry*, *80*(2), 18m12430. https://doi.org/10.4088/JCP.18m12436.

American Geriatrics Society. (2015). American Geriatrics Society 2015 Updated Beers criteria for potentially inappropriate medication use in older adults. *Journal of the American Geriatrics Society*, *63*(11), 2227–2246. https://doi.org/10.1111/jgs.13702.

Bannon, L., McGaughey, J., Clarke, M., McAuley, D. F., & Blackwood, B. (2016). Impact of non-pharmacological interventions on prevention and treatment of delirium in critically ill patients: Protocol for a systematic review of quantitative and qualitative research. *Systematic Reviews*, *5*, 75. https://doi.org/10.1186/s13643-016-0254-0.

Baumgartner, L., Lam, K., Lai, J., et al. (2019). Effectiveness of melatonin for the prevention of intensive care unit delirium. *Pharmacotherapy: The Journal of Human Pharmacology and Drug Therapy*, *39*(3), 280–287. https://doi.org/10.1002/phar.2222, 10.1002/phar.2222.

Blair, G. J., Mehmood, T., Rudnick, M., Kuschner, W. G., & Barr, J. (2019). Nonpharmacologic and medication minimization strategies for the prevention and treatment of ICU delirium: A narrative review. *Journal of Intensive Care Medicine*, *34*(3), 183–190. https://doi.org/10.1177/0885066618771528.

Blandfort, S., Gregersen, M., Rahbek, K., Juul, S., & Damsgaard, E. M. (2020). Single-bed rooms in a geriatric ward prevent delirium in older patients. *Aging-Clinical & Experimental Research*, *32*(1), 141–147.

Bouajram, R. H., Sebat, C. M., Love, D., Louie, E. L., Wilson, M. D., & Duby, J. J. (2020). Comparison of self-reported and behavioral pain assessment tools in critically ill patients. *Journal of Intensive Care Medicine*, *35*(5), 453–460. https://doi.org/10.1177/0885066618757450.

Bounds, M., Kram, S., Speroni, K. G., et al. (2016). Effect of ABCDE bundle implementation on prevalence of delirium in intensive care unit patients. *American Journal of Critical Care*, *25*(6), 535–544. https://doi.org/10.4037/ajcc2016209.

Burry, L., Hutton, B., Williamson, D. R., et al. (2019). Pharmacological interventions for the treatment of delirium in critically ill adults. *Cochrane Database of Systematic Reviews*, *9*, CD011749. https://doi.org/10.1002/14651858.CD011749.pub2.

Campbell, A. M., Axon, D. R., Martin, J. R., Slack, M. K., Mollon, L., & Lee, J. K. (2019). Melatonin for the prevention of postoperative delirium in older adults: A systematic review and meta-analysis. *BMC Geriatrics*, *19*(1), 272. https://doi.org/10.1186/s12877-019-1297-6.

Cheong, C. Y., Tan, J. A., Foong, Y. L., et al. (2016). Creative music therapy in an acute care setting for older patients with delirium and dementia. *Dementia and Geriatric Cognitive Disorders Extra*, *6*(2), 268–275. https://doi.org/10.1159/000445883.

Connolly, K. P., Kleinman, R. S., Stevenson, K. L., Neuman, M. D., & Mehta, S. N. (2020). Delirium reduced with intravenous acetaminophen in geriatric hip fracture patients. *Journal of the American Academy of Orthopaedic Surgeons*, *28*(8), 325–331. https://doi.org/10.5435/JAAOS-D-17-00925.

Daoust, R., Paquet, J., Boucher, V., Pelletier, M., Gouin, E., & Emond, M. (2020). Relationship between pain, opioid treatment, and delirium in older emergency department patients. *Academic Emergency Medicine*, *27*(8), 708–716.

Davidson, J. E., Winkelman, C., Gélinas, C., & Dermenchyan, A. (2015). Pain, agitation, and delirium guidelines: Nurses' involvement in development and implementation. *Critical Care Nurse*, *35*(3), 17–31.

Devlin, J. W., Skrobik, Y., Gelinas, C., et al. (2018). Clinical practice guidelines for the prevention and management of pain, agitation/sedation, delirium, immobility, and sleep disruption in adult patients in the ICU. *Critical Care Medicine*, *46*(9), e825–e873.

Faught, D. D. (2014). Delirium: The nurse's role in prevention, diagnosis, and treatment. *Medsurg Nursing*, *23*(5), 301–305.

Fong, T. G., Racine, A. M., Fick, D. M., et al. (2019). The caregiver burden of delirium in older patients with Alzheimer's disease and related disorders. *Journal of the American Geriatric Society*, *67*(12), 2587–2592. https://doi.org/10.1111/jgs.16199.

Franks, Z. M., Alcock, J. A., Lam, T., Haines, K. J., Arora, N., & Ramanan, M. (2021). Physical restraints and post-traumatic stress disorder in survivors of critical illness. A systematic review and meta-analysis. *Annals of the American Thoracic Society*, *18*(4), 689–697. https://doi.org/10.1513/AnnalsATS.202006-738OC.

Geriatric Medicine Research Collaborative. (2019). Delirium is prevalent in older hospital inpatients and associated with adverse outcomes: Results of a prospective multi-centre study on World Delirium Awareness Day. *BMC Medicine, 17*(1), 229. https://doi.org/10.1186/s12916-019-1458-7.

Goldberg, T. E., Chen, C., Wang, Y., et al. (2020). Association of delirium with long-term cognitive decline: A meta-analysis. *JAMA Neurology, 77*(11), 1373–1381. https://doi.org/10.1001/jamaneurol.2020.2273.

Ho, M. H., Montgomery, A., Traynor, V., et al. (2020). Diagnostic performance of delirium assessment tools in critically ill patients: A systematic review and meta–analysis. *Worldviews on Evidence-Based Nursing, 17*(4), 301–310. https://doi.org/10.1111/wvn.12462.

Hu, R. F., Jiang, X. Y., Chen, J., et al. (2015). Non–pharmacological interventions for sleep promotion in the intensive care unit. *Cochrane Database of Systematic Reviews, 10*, CD008808. https://doi.org/10.1002/14651858.CD008808.pub2.

Javedan, H., & Tulebaev, S. (2014). Management of common postoperative complications: Delirium. *Clinics in Geriatric Medicine, 30*(2), 271–278.

Liang, S., Chau, J. P. C., Lo, S. H. S., Zhao, J., & Choi, K. C. (2021). Effects of nonpharmacological delirium-prevention interventions on critically ill patients' clinical, psychological, and family outcomes: A systematic review and meta-analysis. *Australian Critical Care, 34*(4), 378–387. https://doi.org/10.1016/j.aucc.2020.10.004.

Lu, Y., Li, Y.-W., Wang, L., et al. (2019). Promoting sleep and circadian health may prevent postoperative delirium: A systematic review and meta-analysis of randomized clinical trials. *Sleep Medicine Reviews, 48*, 101207. https://doi.org/10.1016/j.smrv.2019.08.001.

Maldonado, J. R. (2013). Neuropathogenesis of delirium: Review of current etiologic theories and common pathways. *American Journal of Geriatric Psychiatry, 21*(12), 1190–1222.

Mazur, K., Wilczyński, K., & Szewieczek, J. (2016). Geriatric falls in the context of a hospital fall prevention program: Delirium, low body mass index, and other risk factors. *Clinical Interventions in Aging, 11*, 1253–1261. https://doi.org/10.2147/CIA.S115755.

Morandi, A., Zambon, A., Di Santo, S. G., et al. (2020). Understanding factors associated with psychomotor subtypes of delirium in older inpatients with dementia. *Journal of the American Medical Directors Association, 21*(4), 486–492.e7.

Nikooie, R., Neufeld, K. J., Oh, E. S., et al. (2019). Antipsychotics for treating delirium in hospitalized adults: A systematic review. *Annals of Internal Medicine, 171*(7), 485–495. https://doi.org/10.7326/M19-1860.

Parrish, E. (2019). Delirium superimposed on dementia: Challenges and opportunities. *Nursing Clinics of North America, 54*(4), 541–550. https://doi.org/10.1016/j.cnur.2019.07.004.

Reznik, M. E., & Slooter, A. J. C. (2019). Delirium management in the ICU. *Current Treatment Options in Neurology, 21*(11), 59. https://doi.org/10.1007/s11940-019-0599-5.

Rosted, E., Prokofieva, T., Sanders, S., & Schultz, M. (2018). Serious consequences of malnutrition and delirium in frail older patients. *Journal of Nutrition in Gerontology & Geriatrics, 37*(2), 105–116. https://doi.org/10.1080/21551197.2018.147055.

Solà-Miravete, E., López, C., Martínez-Segura, E., Adell-Lleixà, M., Juvé-Udina, M. E., & Lleixà-Fortuño, M. (2018). Nursing assessment as an effective tool for the identification of delirium risk in older in-patients: A case-control study. *Journal of Clinical Nursing, 27*(1–2), 345–354.

Swan, J. T. (2014). Decreasing inappropriate unable-to-assess ratings for the confusion assessment method for the intensive care unit. *American Journal of Critical Care, 23*(1), 60–69.

Trogrlić, Z., van der Jagt, M., Bakker, J., et al. (2015). A systematic review of implementation strategies for assessment, prevention, and management of ICU delirium and their effect on clinical outcomes. *Critical Care, 19*(1), 157. https://doi.org/10.1186/s13054-015-0886-9.

Volkert, D., Beck, A. M., Cederholm, T., et al. (2019). ESPEN guideline on clinical nutrition and hydration in geriatrics. *Clinical Nutrition, 38*(1), 10–47. https://doi.org/10.1016/j.clnu.2018.05.024.

Waszynski, C. M., Milner, K. A., Staff, I., & Molony, S. L. (2018). Using simulated family presence to decrease agitation in older hospitalized delirious patients: A randomized controlled trial. *International Journal of Nursing Studies, 77*, 154–161. https://doi.org/10.1016/j.ijnurstu.2017.09.018.

Wilson, J. E., Mart, M. F., Cunningham, C., et al. (2020). Delirium. *Nature Reviews Disease Primers, 6*(1), 90. https://doi.org/10.1038/s41572-020-00223-4.

Xing, J., Yuan, Z., Jie, Y., Liu, Y., Wang, M., & Sun, Y. (2019). Risk factors for delirium: Are therapeutic interventions part of it? *Neuropsychiatric Disease and Treatment, 15*, 1321–1327. https://doi.org/10.2147/NDT.S192836.

Chronic Confusion **Domain 5 Perception/cognition Class 4 Cognition**

Linda J. Hassler, DNP, RN, GCNS-BC, FGNLA, Philemon Tedros, BSN, RN, and Olga F. Jarrín, PhD, RN

NANDA-I

Definition

Irreversible, progressive, insidious disturbances of consciousness, attention, cognition, and perception, which last more than 3 months.

Defining Characteristics

Altered personality; difficulty retrieving information when speaking; difficulty with decision-making; impaired executive functioning skills; impaired psychosocial functioning; inability to perform at least one daily activity; incoherent speech; long-term memory loss; marked change in behavior; short-term memory loss

Related Factors

Chronic sorrow; sedentary lifestyle; substance misuse

At-Risk Population

Individuals aged ≥60 years

Associated Conditions

Human immunodeficiency virus infections; mental disorders; neurocognitive disorders; stroke

NOC (Nursing Outcomes Classification)

Suggested NOC Outcomes

Cognition; Cognitive Orientation; Agitation Level; Comfort Status; Dementia Level; Dementia Management; Social Support

Example NOC Outcome with Indicators

Cognition as evidenced by the following indicators: Cognitive orientation/Communicates clearly for age/ Comprehends the meaning of situations/Attentiveness/Concentration. (Rate the outcome and indicators of **Cognition:** 1 = severely compromised, 2 = substantially compromised, 3 = moderately compromised, 4 = mildly compromised, 5 = not compromised [see Section I].)

Client Outcomes

Client Will (Specify Time Frame)

- Remain content and free from harm
- Function at maximal cognitive level
- Participate in activities of daily living at the maximum of functional ability
- Have minimal episodes of agitation (agitation occurs in up to 70% of clients with dementia)

NIC (Nursing Interventions Classification)

Suggested NIC Interventions

Dementia Management; Environmental Management; Surveillance: Safety; Validation Therapy

Example NIC Activities—Dementia Management

Use distraction rather than confrontation to manage behavior; Give one simple direction at a time

Nursing Interventions and *Rationales*

Note: Nursing science has a rich history of conceptualizing behavioral and psychological symptoms of dementia (BPSD), which include delusions, hallucinations, misidentification of depression, sleeplessness, anxiety, physical aggression, wandering, restlessness, agitation, pacing, screaming, culturally inappropriate behavior, sexual disinhibition, crying, cursing, apathy, repetitive questioning, and shadowing (stalking), as expressions of unmet pathophysiological and psychological needs related to environmental and caregiver factors (Kolanowski et al, 2017).

- Assess for BPSD using the BEHAVE-AD or Neuropsychiatry Inventory (NPI-Q), and determine cause(s) of symptoms, which may include changes in the environment, caregiver, or routine; demands to perform beyond capacity; multiple competing stimuli, including discomfort. EBN: *Agitated behaviors can be an expression of a need that is not being met; needs assessment is facilitated through methods to enhance communication so that needs may be expressed (Kolanowski et al, 2017).*
- Assess the client for delirium (physiological causes of delirium include acute hypoxia, pain, medication effects, malnutrition, and infections such as urinary tract infection, fatigue, electrolyte disturbances, constipation, and urinary retention). EB: *Delirium is a medical emergency that can often be confused for chronic confusion and lead to increased mortality/morbidity rates, thus screening for delirium superimposed on dementia is fundamental to client safety (Steensma et al, 2019).*
- If the client is suspected of delirium (presenting as inattention, and impaired arousal or vigilance), initiate three-part delirium screener, which includes questions: "What are the days of the week backward?" and

"What type of place is this?" If either question is incorrect or the client appears sleepy proceed to diagnostic delirium testing such as the Confusion Assessment Method (CAM). EB: *Delirium superimposed on dementia is a common clinical syndrome in hospital and institutional settings that often results in poor outcomes (Morandi et al, 2017).*

C

- Assess the client for signs of depression and anxiety (including sadness, irritability, agitation, somatic complaints, tension, loss of concentration, insomnia, poor appetite, apathy, flat affect, and withdrawn behavior) with an instrument appropriate for the cognitive level. EB: *The Cornell Scale for Depression in Dementia (CSDD) and Hamilton Depression Rating Scale (HDRS) have the highest sensitivity for screening clients with dementia (Goodarzi et al, 2017). The Geriatric Anxiety Inventory (GAI), Hospital Anxiety and Depression Scale (HADS-A), and Rating Anxiety in Dementia (RAID) scale are reliable and valid instruments for identifying and measuring anxiety in dementia (Creighton et al, 2019).*
- Assess for pain, including pain with movement, using a method appropriate to the client's level of cognition. EBN: *Pain assessment tools appropriate for client's living with cognitive impairments include the Pain Assessment in Advanced Dementia Scale (PAINAD) (Masman et al, 2018) and the Rotterdam Elderly Pain Observation Scale (REPOS) for noncommunicative clients (Boerlage et al, 2019).*
- Begin each interaction with the client calmly and empathetically, maintain eye contact, identify yourself, and call the client by their name; talk slowly, keep communication simple, give clear choices, and one-step instructions; if indicated, use gestures, prompts, cues, or visual aids. CEB: *These communication techniques assist in focusing attention, incorporate nonverbal means of communication, simplify memory demands, compensate for cognitive slowing, and assist with retrieval and comprehension (Feil & de Klerk-Rubin, 2012).*
- To promote completion of activity of daily living tasks, focus on what the client can still do (e.g., comb their hair, brush their teeth), as opposed to what they cannot do. Using a hand-under-hand technique, a caregiver can guide the client to complete tasks with less challenging behaviors exhibited, giving the client a sense of independence and completion of a task. EB: *By focusing on the retained skills, the caregiver is better able to accomplish other tasks and establish positive relationships between the client and caregiver (Batchelor-Murphy et al, 2015; Snow, 2019).*
- Promote person-centered care, which includes getting to know the unique and complete person, recognizing/accepting the person's reality, supporting their ongoing opportunities for meaningful engagement, and evaluating care practices regularly. EBN: *Understanding the individual's past and sharing memories enhances communication and client and staff satisfaction (Scales et al, 2018).*
- Obtain information about the client's life history, interests, routines, needs, and preferences from the family or significant others to plan care and facilitate reminiscence and validation therapy; collaborate with family members to engage in reminiscence using personal photographs and belongings to stimulate memories and improve sense of self. CEB: *When more recent memory fails, earlier memories are retrieved to restore balance; when eyesight fails, the mind's eye is used to see; when hearing goes, sounds from the past are heard (Feil & de Klerk-Rubin, 2012).*
- Utilize validation therapy techniques to meet clients where they are in their mind; instead of correcting their thoughts, guide them through the reminiscence of that thought. CEB: *Painful feelings that are expressed, acknowledged, and validated by a trusted listener will diminish, and those that are ignored or suppressed will gain strength; decreasing stress of both the care recipient and the family/caregiver (Feil & de Klerk-Rubin, 2012).*
- Facilitate the use of music therapy via activities staff, or electronic sources (e.g., Amazon Echo/Alexa and Google Home); identify the client's music preferences and interview family members if necessary. EB: *Music therapy is beneficial and improves behavior disorders, anxiety, depression, and agitation in people living with dementia (Moreno-Morales et al, 2020).*
- Use multisensory stimulation (e.g., exercise, nature, arts, group activities, music, aromas) to improve mood, behavior, and quality of life; engage assistance of volunteers and family caregivers in one-on-one activities. EB: *Multisensory interventions can improve mood, behaviors, and quality of life, particularly when a personalized approach is taken. Do not correct their thoughts, but guide, when cognitive stimulation is combined with recreational activities, occupational therapy, and physical exercise (Zucchella et al, 2018; Cheng et al, 2019).*
- Promote regular, supervised physical activity and exercise. EB: *Regular physical exercise is recommended for all adults and may improve physical and mental health, reduce frailty, and improve cognitive function (Groot, 2016; Zucchella et al, 2018).*
- Provide opportunities for contact with nature gardens or nature-based stimuli, such as facilitating time spent outdoors with a safe walking path or indoor gardening. EBN: *Improvements in mood among clients*

with dementia were associated with exposures to nature of relatively short duration (Scales et al, 2018; White et al, 2018).

- Facilitate the use of doll therapy for clients with advanced dementia and challenging dementia related behaviors. EB: *Doll therapy is associated with reducing cognitive, behavioral, and emotional symptoms of dementia; improving overall well-being; and the ability to relate with an external environment (Ng et al, 2017).*
- Provide pet therapy and other animal-assisted activities when possible. EBN: *Animal-assisted activities and interventions (including use of centrally located aquariums) showed a strong positive effect on social behaviors, physical activity, and dietary intake in dementia clients and a positive effect on agitation/aggression and quality of life (Scales et al, 2018; Yakimicki et al, 2019).*
- Use individual or group reminiscence therapy. EBN: *Reminiscence therapy can positively affect quality of life, attitudes toward old age, and symptoms of depression in elderly adults with cognitive impairment (Scales et al, 2018).*
- Use an environmental audit tool to evaluate and optimize the living environment in group home and assisted living facilities (e.g., provide unobtrusive safety features, reduce unnecessary stimulation, enhance useful stimulation, provide wayfinding cues, and encourage safe wandering). EB: *Moderate evidence supports environmental design, noise/sound and light regulation, and the use of cognitively stimulating activity stations (such as folding towels or socks and setting the table) and memory boxes (with personal photos and mementos) to support well-being, daytime activity, nighttime sleep, and wayfinding (Jensen & Padilla, 2017). The Built Environment Assessment Tool (BEAT-D) is a free app for iOS and Google/Android that includes original versions of the Environmental Assessment Tool (EAT and EAT-HC).*
- Use appropriate lighting to support regulation of sleep-wake patterns and associated behavioral issues. EB: *Ambient lighting and bright light therapy interventions encourage proper sleep-wake cycles and improve sleep efficiency in persons with dementia and their caregivers, and may help prevent sundowning (confusion in late afternoon and evening) (Figueiro et al, 2019).*
- Provide the client and family information regarding advance directives, palliative and hospice care options, and discuss/document goals of care in the early stages of illness when further cognitive decline is anticipated. EB: *Discussion of delicate and important end-of-life issues should be discussed with clients early in the course of their illness, when decision-making capacity is less likely to be impaired, so that goals of care may more accurately reflect their true personal preferences (Abu Snineh et al, 2017).* EBN: *Advantages of advanced care planning with dementia include increased communication and documentation about end-of-life care preferences; increased concordance between care preferences documented and provided; and lower rates of unwanted, burdensome treatments at end of life (Kim et al, 2015).*
- Refer to the care plans for Impaired **Memory, Wandering,** Feeding **Self-Care** Deficit, Dressing **Self-Care** Deficit, Toileting **Self-Care** Deficit, and Bathing **Self-Care** Deficit as needed.

Geriatric

Note: All interventions are appropriate for geriatric clients.

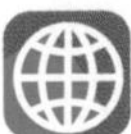

Multicultural

- Provide culturally and linguistically appropriate care. EB: *Linguistic and cultural isolation may cause or worsen agitation in people living with dementia (Cooper et al, 2018).*
- Facilitate cultural congruity, defined as the match of the client's cultural values, preferences (language, food, music, customs), and traditions within the care environment, which may include companion care, adult day care, board and care homes, or nursing homes, including state veterans' homes. EB: *Culturally congruent care is associated with greater satisfaction, well-being, social stimulation, and happiness (Martin et al, 2019; Richardson et al, 2019).*
- Assess for the influence of cultural beliefs, norms, and values on the client and the family's understanding of chronic confusion or dementia; assist the family or caregiver in identifying and accessing available social services or other supportive services. EB: *In some cultures, traditional family caregiving (which may be the responsibility of an adult child) is both an obligation and provided from one's heart, which may complicate discussions regarding topics of caregiver role strain, caregiver burnout, or decisions related to use of nursing home level care (Richardson et al, 2019; Yaghmour et al, 2019).*

Home Care

- The interventions described previously may be adapted for home care use.

C

- Provide education and support to the family regarding effective communication, home safety, fall prevention, engagement in meaningful activities, ways to manage cognitive and behavioral changes, and comprehensive health care for both client and caregiver(s), including screening for depression and caregiver role strain. EB: *Among clients with mild-to-moderate dementia living in the community, a multimodal occupational therapy approach (including cognitive and behavioral interventions for clients and their caregivers) was effective in improving clients' ability to participate in activities of daily living and reducing caregiver burden (Zucchella et al, 2018).*
- Provide information about respite care to family caregivers. EB: *Although many caregivers report that they derive significant emotional and spiritual rewards from their caregiving role, many also experience physical and emotional problems directly related to the stress and demands of daily care. Caregiver resilience can be enhanced through the use of respite programs, including day care, overnight respite, support groups, and counseling services (Roberts & Struckmeyer, 2018).*
- Refer to the care plans for Feeding **Self-Care Deficit;** Dressing **Self-Care** Deficit; Toileting **Self-Care** Deficit; Bathing **Self-Care** Deficit; and **Caregiver Role Strain** as needed.

Client/Family Teaching and Discharge Planning

- In the client's early stages of dementia, provide the caregiver with information on illness processes, needed care, available services, role changes, and importance of advance directives discussion; facilitate family cohesion. EBN: *Education provided to caregivers early in the disease trajectory may assist them to anticipate care needs and role changes and to facilitate involving the individual with dementia in care decisions (Kim et al, 2015; Abu Snineh et al, 2017).*
- Provide education and support to the family regarding effective communication, home safety, fall prevention, engagement in meaningful activities, ways to manage cognitive and behavioral changes, and comprehensive health care, including screening for depression. Be prepared to offer support and information to family members who also live at a distance. EB: *The need for care, services, and support for individuals in the community with dementia and their caregivers is often unmet; evaluation and diagnosis of dementia, personal and home safety, physical and mental health care, advanced care planning, and legal issues are needs that should be addressed (Roberts & Struckmeyer, 2018).*
- Refer for home care services before discharge as needed.

REFERENCES

Abu Snineh, M., Camicioli, R., & Miyasaki, J. M. (2017). Decisional capacity for advanced care directives in Parkinson's disease with cognitive concerns. *Parkinsonism & Related Disorders, 39*, 77–79. https://doi.org/10.1016/j.parkreldis.2017.03.006.

Batchelor-Murphy, M., Amella, E. J., Zapka, J., Mueller, M., & Beck, C. (2015). Feasibility of a web-based dementia feeding skills training program for nursing home staff. *Geriatric Nursing, 36*(3), 212–218. https://doi.org/10.1016/j.gerinurse.2015.02.003.

Boerlage, A. A., van Rosmalen, J., Cheuk-Alam-Balrak, J., Goudzwaard, J. A., & van Dijk, M. (2019). Validation of the Rotterdam Elderly Pain Observation Scale in the hospital setting. *Pain Practice, 19*(4), 407–417. https://doi.org/10.1111/papr.12756.

Cheng, C., Baker, G. B., & Dursun, S. M. (2019). Use of multisensory stimulation interventions in the treatment of major neurocognitive disorders. *Psychiatry and Clinical Psychopharmacology, 29*(4), 916–921. https://doi.org/10.1080/24750573.2019.1699738.

Cooper, C., Rapaport, P., Robertson, S., et al. (2018). Relationship between speaking English as a second language and agitation in people with dementia living in care homes: Results from the MARQUE (Managing Agitation and Raising Quality of life) English national care home survey. *International Journal of Geriatric Psychiatry, 33*(3), 504–509. https://doi.org/10.1002/gps.4786.

Creighton, A. S., Davison, T. E., & Kissane, D. W. (2019). The psychometric properties, sensitivity and specificity of the Geriatric Anxiety Inventory, Hospital Anxiety and Depression Scale, and Rating Anxiety in Dementia scale in aged care residents. *Aging & Mental Health, 23*(5), 633–642. https://doi.org/10.1080/13607863.2018.1439882.

Feil, N., & de Klerk-Rubin, V. (2012). *The validation Breakthrough: Simple techniques for communicating with people with Alzheimer's and other dementias* (3rd ed.). Baltimore, MD: Health Professions Press.

Figueiro, M. G., Plitnick, B., Roohan, C., Sahin, L., Kalsher, M., & Rea, M. S. (2019). Effects of a tailored lighting intervention on sleep quality, rest-activity, mood, and behavior in older adults with Alzheimer disease and related dementias: A randomized clinical trial. *Journal of Clinical Sleep Medicine, 15*(12), 1757–1767. https://doi.org/10.5664/jcsm.8078.

Goodarzi, Z. S., Mele, B. S., Roberts, D. J., & Holroyd-Leduc, J. (2017). Depression case finding in individuals with dementia: A systematic review and meta-analysis. *Journal of the American Geriatrics Society, 65*(5), 937–948. https://doi.org/10.1111/jgs.14713.

Groot, C., Hooghiemstra, A. M., Raijmakers, P. G., et al. (2016). The effect of physical activity on cognitive function in patients with dementia: A meta-analysis of randomized control trials. *Ageing Research Reviews, 25*, 13–23. https://doi.org/10.1016/j.arr.2015.11.005.

Jensen, L., & Padilla, R. (2017). Effectiveness of environment-based interventions that address behavior, perception, and falls in people with Alzheimer's disease and related major neurocognitive disorders: A systematic review. *American Journal of Occupational Therapy, 71*(5), 7105180030. https://doi.org/10.5014/ajot.2017.027409.

Kim, H., Ersek, M., Bradway, C., & Hickman, S. E. (2015). Physician orders for life-sustaining treatment for nursing home residents with dementia. *Journal of the American Association of Nurse Practitioners, 27*(11), 606–614. https://doi.org/10.1002/2327-6924.12258.

Kolanowski, A., Boltz, M., Galik, E., et al. (2017). Determinants of behavioral and psychological symptoms of dementia: A scoping review of the evidence. *Nursing Outlook*, *65*(5), 515–529. https://doi.org/10.1016/j.outlook.2017.06.006.

Martin, C., Woods, B., & Williams, S. (2019). Language and culture in the caregiving of people with dementia in care homes—What are the implications for well-being? A scoping review with a Welsh perspective. *Journal of Cross-Cultural Gerontology*, *34*(1), 67–114. https://doi.org/10.1007/s10823-018-9361-9.

Masman, A. D., van Dijk, M., van Rosmalen, J., Baar, F. P. M., Tibboel, D., & Boerlage, A. A. (2018). The Rotterdam Elderly Pain Observation Scale (REPOS) is reliable and valid for non-communicative end-of-life patients. *BMC Palliative Care*, *17*(1), 34. https://doi.org/10.1186/s12904-018-0280-x.

Morandi, A., Davis, D., Bellelli, G., et al. (2017). The diagnosis of delirium superimposed on dementia: An emerging challenge. *Journal of the American Medical Directors Association*, *18*(1), 12–18. https://doi.org/10.1016/j.jamda.2016.07.014.

Moreno-Morales, C., Calero, R., Moreno-Morales, P., & Pintado, C. (2020). Music therapy in the treatment of dementia: A systematic review and meta-analysis. *Frontiers of Medicine*, *7*, 160. https://doi.org/10.3389/fmed.2020.00160.

Ng, Q. X., Ho, C. Y. X., Koh, S. S., Tan, W. C., & Chan, H. W. (2017). Doll therapy for dementia sufferers: A systematic review. *Complementary Therapies in Clinical Practice*, *26*, 42–46. https://doi.org/10.1016/j.ctcp.2016.11.007.

Richardson, V. E., Fields, N., Won, S., Bradley, E., Gibson, A., Rivera, G., et al. (2019). At the intersection of culture: Ethnically diverse dementia caregivers' service use. *Dementia*, *18*(5), 1790–1809. https://doi.org/10.1177/1471301217721304.

Roberts, E., & Struckmeyer, K. M. (2018). The impact of respite programming on caregiver resilience in dementia care: A qualitative examination of family caregiver perspectives. *Inquiry: A Journal of Medical Care Organization, Provision and Financing*, *55*, 46958017751507. https://doi.org10.1177/0046958017751507.

Scales, K., Zimmerman, S., & Miller, S. J. (2018). Evidence-based nonpharmacological practices to address behavioral and psychological symptoms of dementia. *Gerontologist*, *58*(Suppl. 1), S88–S102. https://doi.org/10.1093/geront/gnx167.

Snow, T. (2019). *Bathing and dementia—With Teepa Snow of positive approach to care (PAC) [video]*. YouTube.com. Available at https://youtu.be/iKT9YIVPREE. [Accessed 11 June 2021].

Steensma, E., Zhou, W., Ngo, L., et al. (2019). Ultra-brief screeners for detecting delirium superimposed on dementia. *Journal of the American Medical Directors Association*, *20*(11), 1391–1396. https://doi.org/10.1016/j.jamda.2019.05.011.

White, P. C., Wyatt, J., Chalfont, G., et al. (2018). Exposure to nature gardens has time-dependent associations with mood improvements for people with mid- and late-stage dementia: Innovative practice. *Dementia*, *17*(5), 627–634. https://doi.org/10.1177/1471301217723772.

Yaghmour, S. M., Bartlett, R., & Brannelly, T. (2019). Dementia in Eastern Mediterranean countries: A systematic review. *Dementia*, *18*(7), 2635–2661. https://doi.org/10.1177/1471301217753776.

Yakimicki, M. L., Edwards, N. E., Richards, E., & Beck, A. M. (2019). Animal-assisted intervention and dementia: A systematic review. *Clinical Nursing Research*, *28*(1), 9–29. https://doi.org/10.1177/1054773818756987.

Zucchella, C., Sinforiani, E., Tamburin, S., et al. (2018). The multidisciplinary approach to Alzheimer's disease and dementia: A narrative review of non-pharmacological treatment. *Frontiers in Neurology*, *9*, 1058. https://doi.org/10.3389/fneur.2018.01058.

Risk for Acute Confusion Domain 5 Perception/cognition Class 4 Cognition

Marina Martinez-Kratz, MS, RN, CNE

NANDA-I

Definition

Susceptible to reversible disturbances of consciousness, attention, cognition, and perception that develop over a short period of time, which may compromise health.

Risk Factors

Alteration in sleep-wake cycle; dehydration; impaired physical mobility; inappropriate use of physical restraint; malnutrition; pain; sensory deprivation; substance misuse; urinary retention

At-Risk Population

Individuals aged ≥60 years; individuals with history of cerebral vascular accident; men

Associated Conditions

Decreased level of consciousness; impaired metabolism; infections; neurocognitive disorders; pharmaceutical preparations

NIC, NOC, Client Outcomes, Nursing Interventions and *Rationales,* Client/Family Teaching, and References

Refer to care plan for Acute **Confusion.**

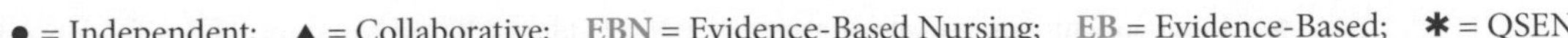

Constipation Domain 3 Elimination and exchange Class 2 Gastrointestinal function

Amanda Andrews, BSc (Hons), MA and Bernie St Aubyn, BSc (Hons), MSc

NANDA-I

Definition

Infrequent or difficult evacuation of feces.

Defining Characteristics

Evidence of symptoms in standardized diagnostic criteria; hard stools; lumpy stools; need for manual maneuvers to facilitate defecation; passing fewer than three stools a week; sensation of anorectal obstruction; sensation of incomplete evacuation; straining with defecation

Related Factors

Altered regular routine; average daily physical activity is less than recommended for age and gender; communication barriers; habitually suppresses urge to defecate; impaired physical mobility; impaired postural balance; inadequate knowledge of modifiable factors; inadequate toileting habits; insufficient fiber intake; insufficient fluid intake; insufficient privacy; stressors; substance misuse

At-Risk Population

Individuals admitted to hospital; individuals experiencing prolonged hospitalization; individuals in aged care settings; individuals in the early postoperative period; older adults; pregnant women; women

Associated Conditions

Blockage in the colon; blockage in the rectum; depression; developmental disabilities; digestive system diseases; endocrine diseases; heart diseases; mental disorders; muscular diseases; nervous system diseases; neurocognitive disorders; pelvic floor disorders; pharmaceutical preparations; radiotherapy; urogynecological disorders

NOC (Nursing Outcomes Classification)

Suggested NOC Outcomes

Bowel Elimination; Hydration

Example NOC Outcome with Indicators

Bowel Elimination as evidenced by the following indicators: Elimination pattern/Stool soft and formed/ Passage of stool without aids/Ease of stool passage. (Rate each indicator of **Bowel Elimination:** 1 = severely compromised, 2 = substantially compromised, 3 = moderately compromised, 4 = mildly compromised, 5 = not compromised [see Section I].)

Client Outcomes

Client Will (Specify Time Frame)

- Maintain passage of soft, formed stool (i.e., Bristol Stool Scale Type 4) every 1 to 3 days without straining
- State relief from discomfort of constipation
- Identify measures that prevent or treat constipation

NIC (Nursing Interventions Classification)

Suggested NIC Intervention

Constipation/Impaction Management

Example NIC Activities—Constipation/Impaction Management

Identify factors (e.g., medications, bed rest, diet) that may cause or contribute to constipation/impaction; Institute a toileting schedule, as appropriate

Nursing Interventions and *Rationales*

C

- Introduce yourself to the client and any companions and inform them of your role. *Introducing yourself to a client helps establish and develop a therapeutic relationship that recognizes the person within the client and forms the basis for building trust on which to base the provision of care (Ellis et al, 2020).*
- Gain consent to perform care before proceeding further with the assessment. *Clients have the right of autonomy both legally and morally and therefore should be fully involved in the decision-making process (Griffith & Tengnah, 2020).*
- Wash hands using a recognized technique. EB: *Performing strict hand-hygiene regimens significantly reduces the incidence of infection with methicillin-resistant Staphylococcus aureus and Clostridium difficile infection (Goldberg, 2017).*
- Assess usual pattern of defecation and establish the extent of the constipation problem. EB: *A thorough and holistic assessment of the client enables effective treatment of constipation to be delivered. A thorough assessment allows the nurse to identify the cause, plan interventions, monitor outcomes, and evaluate care (Mitchell, 2019).*
- Assess the client's bowel habits:
  - Time of day of bowel evacuation
  - Amount and frequency of stool
  - Consistency of stool (using the Bristol Stool Scale)
  - Bleeding/passing mucus on defecation
  - History of bowel habits and/or laxative use

  EB: *Assess usual pattern of defecation, including time of day; amount and frequency of stool; consistency of stool; history of bowel habits or laxative use; and diet, including fiber and fluid intake. A nursing assessment that identifies the client's usual bowel habits will assist in the identification and management of their constipation (Lee, 2015).*
- Assess the client's lifestyle factors that may influence constipation:
  - Fiber content in diet
  - Daily fluid intake
  - Exercise patterns
  - Personal remedies for constipation
  - Recently stopped smoking
  - Alcohol consumption/recreational drug use

  EB: *When undertaking an assessment of a client with suspected constipation, it is important to discuss their lifestyle factors, which can be useful in establishing a clinical diagnosis. The main lifestyle factors to consider and record include the client's food and fluid intake, the fiber content of their diet, smoking, physical activity level, and mood (Andrews & St Aubyn, 2020).*
- Review the client's medical history:
  - Obstetrical/gynecological/urological history and surgeries
  - Diseases that affect bowel motility
  - Bleeding/passing mucus on defecation
  - Current medications

  EB: *Review the client's medical history for conditions that may contribute to constipation, obstetrical/gynecological history, surgeries, diseases that affect bowel motility, alterations in perianal sensation, and the present bowel regimen. It is imperative to establish a nursing history that identifies the client's bowel habits because this will assist in the identification and management of their constipation (Lee, 2015).*
- Assess the client for emotional influences that may be contributing to constipation:
  - Anxiety and depression
  - Long-term defecation issues
  - Stress

  EB: *Consider emotional influences (e.g., depression and anxiety) on defecation. Anxiety and depression are related to the occurrence of constipation; however, this is often a neglected aspect of client assessment and care in clinical practice (Jing & Jia, 2019).*
- Complete a physical examination (palpation for abdominal distention, percussion for dullness, and auscultation for bowel sounds). EB: *Research recommends the use of a standardized constipation assessment and management pathway. The key elements of such a pathway include a physical examination for the detection of any palpable fecal mass or abnormalities (Sandweiss et al, 2018).*

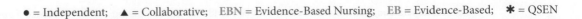

C

- Complete a digital rectal examination (DRE) if competent and suitably trained to do so, to identify hemorrhoids, rectal prolapse, anal fissure, rectocele, the anal tone, and fecal impaction. EBN: *A DRE should be performed by nurses who have received suitable training and demonstrated a level of competence determined by their professional governing body (Mitchell, 2019). A DRE is essential aid to identify any abnormalities and/or constipation (Bardsley, 2017).*
- Check for impaction; if present, use a combination of oral laxatives and enemas initially to remove fecal loading and impaction (National Institute for Health and Care Excellence, 2020). Clients with neurogenic bowel dysfunction (e.g., spinal cord injury) commonly require manual evacuation of stool (McClurg & Norton, 2016).
- Encourage the client or family to keep a 7-day diary of bowel habits, including time of day, length of time spent on the toilet, consistency, amount and frequency of stool, and any straining (using the Bristol Stool Scale). EBN: *Keeping a diary helps establish a client's bowel pattern and helps with recall and accuracy (Andrews & St Aubyn, 2020).*
- Encourage the client or family to keep a 7-day diary of lifestyle issues in relation to bowel habits, including fluid consumption, fiber content in diet, usual bowel stimulus, and exercise regimen. EB: *The use of bowel diaries for efficiently and reliably characterizing bowel habits cannot be over emphasized (Bharucha & Wald, 2019).*
- Use the Bristol Stool Scale to assess stool consistency. EB: The Bristol Stool Scale is widely used as a more objective measure to describe stool consistency (DerSarkissian, 2020).
- ▲ Review the client's current medications. EB: *A review of current medication should be requested, including recently started medications and any over-the-counter or herbal medications the client is taking. Medications associated with chronic constipation include opioid analgesics, anticholinergics, antipsychotics, antispasmodics, and calcium channel blockers (Joint Formulary Committee, 2016). This baseline information is key to gaining a comprehensive client assessment (Bardsley, 2017).*
- Discuss with clients already taking opioids (temporarily or long term) that constipation is a common side effect. If the client is receiving temporary opioids (e.g., for acute postoperative pain), request an order for routine stool softeners from the primary care provider, monitor bowel movements, and request a laxative for the client if constipation develops. If the client is receiving around-the-clock opiates (e.g., for palliative care), laxatives, then softeners, stimulants, or osmotic laxatives should be requested. EB: *Constipation is the most common opioid-related adverse effect. Opioids cause a lack of peristalsis in the large intestine and decrease fluid in the stool and increase anal muscle tone. Clients should be prescribed a stool softener and a bowel stimulant prophylactically to prevent constipation (Brant, 2018).*
- ▲ If the client is terminally ill and is receiving around-the-clock opioids for palliative care, speak with the prescribing health care provider about ordering low-dose naloxone, which is a drug that blocks opioid effects on the gastrointestinal tract without interfering with analgesia *(Sanders et al, 2015).*
- If new onset of constipation, determine whether the client has recently stopped smoking. EB: *Constipation is common, but usually transient, when people stop smoking. A 2016 study surveyed 16,840 individuals between 45 and 75 years of age and found that smoking was associated with abdominal pain, bloating, and constipation (Lundström et al, 2016).*
- ▲ Advise a fiber intake of 18 to 25 g daily and suggest foodstuffs high in fiber (e.g., prune juice, leafy green vegetables, whole meal bread and pasta). EB: *Fiber creates bulky feces and stretches the bowel wall to stimulate peristalsis, thus shortening bowel transit time (Bardsley, 2017).*
- Add fiber gradually to the diet to decrease bloating and flatus. EB: *The National Institute for Care and Excellence recommends that fiber intake must be increased slowly to minimize bloating and flatulence, enhancing Client comfort (NICE Guidelines, 2020).*
- Recommend prunes or prune juice daily. Each 100 g of prunes contains about 6 g of fiber, 15 g of sorbitol, and 184 mg of polyphenol, which all have laxative effects. EB: *Prunes are generally perceived to have a laxative effect. They are high in fiber, including hemicellulose, pectin, and cellulose. These fibers resist colonic fermentation and increase stool water and volume (Lever et al, 2019).*
- Advise a fluid intake of 1.5 to 2 L of fluid per day (ideally, 6–8 glasses of water), unless contraindicated by comorbidities, such as kidney or heart disease. *The recommended intake of fluid is 1.5 to 2 L daily, if the client presents with clinical signs of dehydration (Shen et al, 2019).*
- ▲ If the client is uncomfortable or in pain because of constipation or has acute or chronic constipation that does not respond to increased fiber, fluid, activity, and appropriate toileting, refer the client to the primary care provider for an evaluation of bowel function and health status. EB: *The main aim of referral is to rule out any serious causes of changes in bowel habits (e.g., the presence of tumors, old scarring, and megacolon).*

Red flags (anemia, rectal bleeding, and a family history of bowel cancer or inflammatory bowel disease) are commonly used in general practice to identify the need for further referral (Lee, 2015).

- Encourage physical activity within the client's current ability to mobilize. Encourage turning and changing position in bed if immobile. For clients with reduced mobility, encourage knee to chest raises, waist twists, and stretching the arms away from the body. For fully mobile clients, encourage walking and swimming. EB: *Physical activity can help stimulate peristaltic waves in the colon and encourage the transit of feces to the rectum (Mihara et al, 2020).*
- Demonstrate the use of gentle external abdominal massage, following the direction of colon activity. EB: *Abdominal massage accelerates peristalsis by changing the intraabdominal pressure, thereby mechanically and reflexively acting on the intestines to evacuate the intestine (Okuyan & Bilgili, 2019).*
- Recommend that clients establish a regular elimination routine that includes activity, diet and fluids, and scheduled toilet visits. If required, assist clients to the bathroom at the same time every day; always be mindful of the need for privacy (closing of bathroom doors). EBN: *A daily routine should begin with mild physical activity, consumption of a hot and preferably caffeinated beverage, and a breakfast that includes a form of soluble fiber to induce peristaltic contractions to take advantage of colonic motility and the gastrocolic reflex (Baffy et al, 2017).*
- Educate the client about how to adopt the best posture for defecation. Keep knees slightly higher than hips, keep feet flat on the floor, and lean forward, putting elbows onto knees, thus adopting a squatting position. EB: *Adopting the squatting position helps with the angle of the anorectal section of the colon by lifting the sigmoid colon. The puborectalis muscles work most effectively when they are able to relax in the squatting position (Mercola, 2018).*
- Teach clients about the importance of responding promptly to the urge to defecate. EB: *The body's natural "call to stool" should be heeded in that it is a response to the stimulation of nerve endings in the rectum when a stool is present. Failure to respond to the urge of defecation or waiting until a more suitable time leads to stool retropulsion and worsening of the constipation (George & Borello-France, 2017).*
- Consider the use of laxatives, suppositories, enemas, and bowel irrigation as required if other more natural interventions are not effective. EBN/EB: *The overall aim of laxative therapy is to enable the client to defecate in a manner that promotes comfort and enhances symptom management. A fast active stimulant laxative should be considered to provide short-term relief and longer term management, including the use of an osmotic laxative (Andrews & St Aubyn, 2020). A systematic review identified that bowel irrigation is effective for chronic constipation in around 50% of clients (Emmett et al, 2015).*
- Discourage the use of long-term laxatives and enemas and advise clients to gradually reduce their use if taken regularly. EB: *Long-term use or overuse of laxatives can cause health problems (e.g., electrolyte imbalance) or hide symptoms that may be from a serious medical condition. The evidence base does not support use of stimulant laxatives for more than 4 weeks as associated with long-term colonic effects and possible carcinogenic risks (Noergaard et al, 2019).*

Geriatric

- Assess older adults for the presence of factors that contribute to constipation, including dietary fiber and fluid intake (<1.5 L/day), physical activity, use of constipating medications, and diseases that are associated with constipation. EB: *Constipation is a private problem and the need for health care professionals to be attentive to this issue and initiate assessment with clients in order to advise on the management of constipation is paramount to person-centered care (Munch et al, 2016).*
- Explain the importance of adequate fiber intake, fluid intake, activity, and established toileting routines to ensure soft, formed stool. EB: *In the prevention of constipation in older adults, evidence suggests that the majority of clients would respond to lifestyle modifications reinforced by bowel training measures (De Giorgio et al, 2015).*
- Determine the client's perception of normal bowel elimination and laxative use; promote adherence to a regular schedule. EB: *A systematic review on older people's experiences of living with constipation showed that older people had individual and personal strategies relative to their own beliefs. Clients reported bodily experiences of everyday life shadowed by constipation and adverse psychological effects, which need to be explored to prevent and treat constipation (Tvistholm et al, 2017).*
- Explain why straining (Valsalva maneuver) should be avoided. EB: *Excessive straining can cause syncope or cardiac dysrhythmias in susceptible people (Pstras et al, 2016).*
- Respond quickly to the client's call for assistance with toileting.

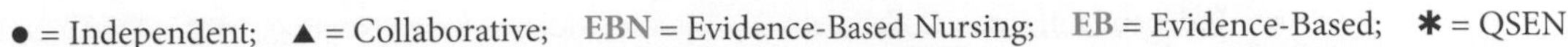

● = Independent; ▲ = Collaborative; EBN = Evidence-Based Nursing; EB = Evidence-Based; ✱ = QSEN

C

- Offer food, fluids, activity, and toileting opportunities to older clients who are cognitively impaired. EB: *Even cognitively impaired individuals who are unable to initiate a request for food, fluids, and so forth may respond when opportunities are offered. A recent research study concluded that 25% of the studied population had functional constipation with the most important risk factors being cited as nutritional impairment and cognitive impairment with advanced age (Farahat et al, 2019).*
- Avoid regular use of enemas in older adults. EB: *Enemas can cause fluid and electrolyte imbalances and damage to the colonic mucosa. However, judicious enema use may help prevent impactions (De Giorgio et al, 2015).*
- Advise the client against attempting to remove impacted feces on his or her own. *Older or confused clients in particular may attempt to remove feces and cause rectal damage.*
- ▲ Use opioids cautiously. EB: *Intestinal constipation is the main secondary effect to the use of opioids (Bezerra de Lima & Pereira, 2017).*
- Position the client on the toilet or commode and place a small footstool under the feet. *Placing a small footstool helps the client assume a squatting posture to facilitate defecation.*

Home Care

- The interventions described previously may be adapted for home care use.
- Take complaints seriously and evaluate claims of constipation in a matter-of-fact manner. EB: *Continued constipation can lead to bowel obstruction, which is a medical emergency. Use of a matter-of-fact manner will limit positive reinforcement of the behavior if actual constipation does not exist. (Tvistholm et al, 2017).*
- Assess the self-care management activities the client is already using. EB: *Many older adults seek solutions to constipation, with laxative use a frequent remedy that creates its own problems (Tvistholm et al, 2017).*
- Offer the following treatment recommendations:
  - Acknowledge the client's lifelong experience of bowel function; respect beliefs, attitudes, and preferences, and avoid patronizing responses.
  - Make available comprehensive, useful written information about constipation and possible solutions.
  - Make available empathetic and accessible professional care to provide treatment and advice; a multiprofessional approach (including health care provider, nurse, and pharmacist) should be used.
  - Institute a bowel management program.
  - Consider affordability when suggesting solutions to constipation; discuss cost-effective strategies.
  - Discuss a range of solutions to constipation and allow the client to choose the preferred options.
  - Have orders in place for a suppository and enema as needed. As part of a bowel management program, suppositories or enemas may become necessary.
- Although the use of a bedside commode may be necessitated by the client's condition, allow the client to use the toilet in the bathroom when possible and provide assistance. *Bowel elimination is a private act, and a lack of privacy can contribute to constipation.*
- In older clients, routinely advise consumption of fluids, fruits, and vegetables as part of the diet, and ambulation if the client is able. EB: *Introduce a bowel management program at the first sign of constipation. Constipation is a major problem for terminally ill or hospice clients who may need very high doses of opioids for pain management (De Giorgio et al, 2015).*
- ▲ Refer for consideration of the use of polyethylene glycol 3350 (PEG-3350) for constipation. EB: *There is good evidence to support the use of PEG-3350 for both chronic constipation and constipation associated with irritable bowel syndrome. PEG 3350 resolved constipation in the short term, was well tolerated, and led to sustained improvement in bowel function in the long-term treatment of clients with chronic constipation (Nakajima et al, 2019).*
- Use a bowel program to establish a pattern that is regular, thereby allowing the client to be part of the family unit. EB: *Regularity of the program promotes psychological and/or physiological readiness to evacuate stool. Families of home care clients often cannot proceed with normal daily activities until bowel programs are complete (Tvistholm et al, 2017).*

Client/Family Teaching and Discharge Planning

- Instruct the client on normal bowel function and the need for adequate fluid and fiber intake, activity, and a defined toileting pattern in a bowel program.

- Encourage the client to heed defecation warning signs and develop a regular schedule of defecation by using a stimulus such as a warm drink or prune juice. *Most cases of constipation are mechanical and result from habitual neglect of impulses that signal the appropriate time for defecation.*
- Encourage the client to avoid long-term use of laxatives and enemas and to gradually withdraw from their use if they are used regularly. EB: *Long-term use or overuse of laxatives can cause health problems (e.g., electrolyte imbalance) or hide symptoms that may be from a serious medical condition. The evidence base does not support use of stimulant laxatives for more than 4 weeks as associated with long-term colonic effects and possible carcinogenic risks (Noergaard et al, 2019).*
- If not contraindicated, teach the client how to do bent-leg sit-ups to increase abdominal tone; also encourage the client to contract the abdominal muscles frequently throughout the day. Help the client develop a daily exercise program to increase peristalsis.
- Provide client with comprehensive written information about constipation and its management. EB: *Providing clients with well-written, evidence-based information about their condition and treatment can have a beneficial effect on the outcomes of treatment. A research study suggests that the use of family-friendly colorful and informative leaflets can have a direct effect on health-related issues (Shabde & Harrison, 2016).*
- ▲ Collaborate with members of the multiprofessional team to provide treatment and advice to clients and caregivers. EB: *Teamwork is a central process in health care organizations. Effective organization and delivery of health care services depends on a wide range of professionals, families, clients, and carers working together to achieve the best health outcomes and quality of life (Flynn & Mercer, 2018).*
- ▲ Consider referral to other specialist practitioners if constipation persists. EB: *A diagnosis of primary chronic constipation is made after the exclusion of secondary causes of constipation and managed effectively. If unsuccessful, subspecialist referrals should be considered (Rao et al, 2016).*
- Document all care and advice given in a factual and comprehensive manner. EB: *Good record keeping is an integral part of nursing practice and is essential to the provision of safe and effective care (St Aubyn & Andrews, 2015).*

C

REFERENCES

Andrews, A., & St Aubyn, B. (2020). Assessment, diagnosis and management of constipation. *Nursing Standard*, *35*(9), 59–65. doi:10.7748/ns.2020.e11512.

Baffy, N., Foxx-Orenstein, A., Harris, L., & Sterler, S. (2017). Intractable constipation in the elderly. *Current Treatment Options in Gastroenterology*, *15*(3), 363–381.

Bardsley, A. (2017). Assessment and treatment options for patients with constipation. *British Journal of Nursing*, *26*(6), 312–318.

Bezerra de Lima, M., & Pereira, M. (2017). Constipation in patients treated with opioids: An integrative review. *Brazilian Journal in Health Promotion*, *30*(2), 275–282.

Bharucha, A. E., & Wald, A. (2019). Chronic constipation. *Mayo Clinic Proceedings*, *94*(11), 2340–2357.

Brant, J. M. (2018). Assessment and management of cancer pain in older adults: Strategies for success. *Asia-Pacific Journal of Oncology Nursing*, *5*(3), 248–253.

De Giorgio, R., Ruggeri, E., Stanghellini, V., Eusebi, L. H., Bazzoli, F., & Chiarioni, G. (2015). Chronic constipation in the elderly: A primer for the gastroenterologist. *BMC Gastroenterology*, *15*, 130.

DerSarkissian, C. (2020). *What kind of poop do I have?* WebMD [Internet]. Retrieved from https://www.webmd.com/digestive-disorders/poop-chart-bristol-stool-scale. Accessed June 11, 2021.

Ellis, P., Standing, M., & Roberts, S. (2020). *Patient assessment and care planning in nursing (Transforming nursing practice series)*. London: Sage Publications.

Emmett, C. D., Close, H. J., Yiannakou, Y., & Mason, J. M. (2015). Trans-anal irrigation therapy to treat adult chronic functional constipation: Systematic review and meta-analysis. *BMC Gastroenterology*, *15*, 139.

Farahat, T. M., El-Esrigy, F. A., & Salama, W. E. I. (2019). Risk factors for constipation among elderly attending family health center in Damietta District, Damietta Governorate, Egypt. *Menoufia Medical Journal*, *32*(1), 145–150.

Flynn, M., & Mercer, D. (Eds.). (2018). *Oxford handbook of adult nursing*. Oxford: Oxford University Press.

George, S. E., & Borello-France, D. F. (2017). Perspective on physical therapist management of functional constipation. *Physical Therapy*, *97*(4), 478–493.

Goldberg, J. L. (2017). Guideline implementation; hand hygiene. *AORN Journal*, *105*(2), 203–212.

Griffith, R., & Tengnah, C. (2020). *Law and professional issues in nursing (Transforming nursing practice series)*. London: Sage Publications.

Jing, D., & Jia, L. (2019). Assessment of patients' psychological state and self-efficacy associated with post-operative constipation of the thoracolumbar fracture surgery. *Journal of International Medical Research*, *47*(9), 4215–4224 https://doi.org/10.1177%2F0300060519859732.

Joint Formulary Committee. (2016). *British National Formulary (BNF) No. 72*. London: Pharmaceutical Press.

Lee, A. (2015). Combatting the causes of constipation. *Nursing and Residential Care*, *117*(6), 327–331.

Lever, E., Scott, S. M., Louis, P., Emery, P. W., & Whelan, K. (2019). The effect of prunes on stool output, gut transit time and gastrointestinal microbiota: A randomized control trial. *Clinical Nutrition*, *38*(1), 165–173.

Lundström, O., Manjer, J., & Ohlsson, B. (2016). Smoking is associated with several functional gastrointestinal symptoms. *Scandinavian Journal of Gastroenterology*, *51*(8), 914–922.

McClurg, D., & Norton, C. (2016). What is the best way to manage neurogenic bowel dysfunction? *BMJ*, *354*, i3931. https://doi.org/10.1136/bmj.i3931. (Clinical research ed.).

Mercola, J. (2018). *Perfect position to poop*. Mercola.com [Internet]. Retrieved from https://articles.mercola.com/sites/articles/archive/2018/09/22/proper-pooping-position.aspx. Accessed June 11, 2021.

Mihara, H., Murayama, A., Nanjo, S., et al. (2020). Factors correlated with drug use for constipation: Perspectives from the 2016 open Japanese National Database. *BMC Gastroenterology*, *20*(1), 284.

Mitchell, A. (2019). Carrying out a holistic assessment of a patient with constipation. *British Journal of Nursing, 28*(4), 230–232.

Munch, L., Tvistholm, N., Trosborg, I., & Konradsen, H. (2016). Living with constipation—older people's experiences and strategies with constipation before and during hospitalization. *International Journal of Qualitative Studies on Health and Well-Being, 11*, 30732.

Nakajima, A., Shinbo, K., Oota, A., & Kinoshita, Y. (2019). Polyethylene glycol 3350 plus electrolytes for chronic constipation: A 2-week, randomized, double-blind, placebo-controlled study with a 52-week open-label extension. *Journal of Gastroenterology, 54*(9), 792–803.

National Institute for Health and Care Excellence. (2020). *Constipation. Clinical knowledge summaries*. Retrieved from https://www.nice.org.uk/guidance/conditions-and-diseases/digestive-tract-conditions/constipation. Accessed November 2, 2020.

Noergaard, M., Andersen, J. T., Jimenez-Solem, E., & Christensen, M. B. (2019). Long term treatment with stimulant laxatives- clinical evidence for effectiveness and safety? *Scandinavian Journal of Gastroenterology, 54*(1), 27–34.

Okuyan, C. B., & Bilgili, N. (2019). Effect of abdominal massage on constipation and quality of life in older adults: A randomized controlled trial. *Complimentary Therapies in Medicine, 47*, 102219.

Pstras, L., Thomaseth, K., Waniewski, J., Balzani, I., & Bellavere, F. (2016). The Valsalva manoeuvre: Physiology and clinical examples. *Acta Physiologica, 217*(2), 103–119.

Rao, S. S. C., Rattanakovit, K., & Patcharatrakul, T. (2016). Diagnoses and management of chronic constipation on adults. *Nature Reviews Gastroenterology & Hepatology, 13*(5), 295–305.

Sanders, M., Jones, S., Löwenstein, O., Jansen, J.-P., Miles, H., & Simpson, K. (2015). New formulation of sustained released naloxone can reverse opioid induced constipation without compromising the desired opioid effects. *Pain Medicine, 16*(8), 1540–1550.

Sandweiss, D. R., Allen, L., Deneau, M., et al. (2018). Implementing a standardized constipation—Management pathway to reduce resource utilization. *Academic Pediatrics, 18*(8), 957–964.

Shabde, N., & Harrison, H. (2016). G331(P) developing parental pathways: The most effective way to care for children with constipation- a cumbrian experience. *Archives of Disease in Childhood, 101*, A192–A193.

Shen, L., Huang, C., Lu, X., Xu, X., Juang, Z., & Zhu, C. (2019). Lower dietary fibre intake, but not total water consumption, is associated with constipation: A population-based analysis. *Journal of Human Nutrition and Dietetics, 32*(4), 422–431.

St Aubyn, B., & Andrews, A. (2015). If it's not written down it didn't happen. *British Journal of Community Nursing, 29*(5), 20–22.

Tvistholm, N., Munch, L., & Danielsen, A. K. (2017). Constipation is casting a shadow over everyday life—a systematic review of older people's experience living with constipation. *Journal of Clinical Nursing, 26*(7–8), 902–914.

Risk for Constipation Domain 3 Elimination and exchange Class 2 Gastrointestinal function

Mary Beth Flynn Makic, PhD, RN, CCNS, CCRN-K, FAAN, FNAP, FCNS

NANDA-I

Definition

Susceptible to infrequent or difficult evacuation of feces, which may compromise health.

Risk Factors

Altered regular routine; average daily physical activity is less than recommended for age and gender; communication barriers; habitually suppresses urge to defecate; impaired physical mobility; impaired postural balance; inadequate knowledge of modifiable factors; inadequate toileting habits; insufficient fiber intake; insufficient fluid intake; insufficient privacy; stressors; substance misuse

At-Risk Population

Individuals admitted to hospital; individuals experiencing prolonged hospitalization; individuals in aged care settings; individuals in the early postoperative period; older adults; pregnant women; women

Associated Conditions

Blockage in the colon; blockage in the rectum; depression; developmental disabilities; digestive system diseases; endocrine system diseases; heart diseases; mental disorders; muscular diseases; nervous system diseases; neurocognitive disorders; pelvic floor disorders; pharmaceutical preparations; radiotherapy; urogynecological disorders

NIC, NOC, Client Outcomes, Nursing Interventions and *Rationales,* Client/Family Teaching, and References

Refer to care plan for **Constipation.**

Perceived Constipation Domain 3 Elimination and exchange Class 2 Gastrointestinal function

Amanda Andrews, BSc (Hons), MA and Bernie St Aubyn, BSc (Hons), MSc

C

NANDA-I

Definition

Self-diagnosis of infrequent or difficult evacuation of feces combined with abuse of methods to ensure a daily bowel movement.

Defining Characteristics

Enema misuse; expects bowel movement at same time daily; laxative misuse; suppository misuse

Related Factors

Cultural health beliefs; deficient knowledge about normal evacuation patterns; disturbed thought processes; family health beliefs

NOC (Nursing Outcomes Classification)

Suggested NOC Outcomes

Bowel Elimination; Health Beliefs; Health Beliefs: Perceived Threat

Example NOC Outcome with Indicators

Bowel Elimination as evidenced by the following indicators: Elimination pattern/Stool soft and formed/ Passage of stool without aids/Ease of stool passage. (Rate each indicator of **Bowel Elimination:** 1 = severely compromised, 2 = substantially compromised, 3 = moderately compromised, 4 = mildly compromised, 5 = not compromised [see Section I].)

Client Outcomes

Client Will (Specify Time Frame)

- Regularly defecate soft, formed stool without use of aids (i.e., Bristol Stool Scale Type 4) every 1 to 3 days without straining
- Understand the need to decrease or eliminate the use of stimulant laxatives, suppositories, and enemas
- Identify alternatives to stimulant laxatives, enemas, and suppositories for ensuring defecation
- Understand that defecation does not have to occur every day

NIC (Nursing Interventions Classification)

Suggested NIC Interventions

Bowel Management; Medication Management

Example NIC Activities—Bowel Management

Note preexistent bowel problems, bowel routine, and use of laxatives; Initiate a bowel training program, as appropriate

Nursing Interventions and *Rationales*

- Introduce yourself to the client and any companions and inform them of your role. EB: *Introducing yourself to a client helps establish and develop a therapeutic relationship that recognizes the person within the client and forms the basis for building trust on which to base the provision of care (Ellis et al, 2020).*
- Gain consent to perform care before proceeding further with the assessment. EB: *Clients have the right of autonomy both legally and morally and therefore should be fully involved in the decision-making process (Griffith & Tengnah, 2020).*

- Wash hands using a recognized technique. EB: *Performing strict hand-hygiene regimens significantly reduces the incidence of infection with methicillin-resistant* Staphylococcus aureus *and* Clostridium difficile (i.e., *Clostridioides difficile) infections (Goldberg, 2017).*
- Assess usual pattern of defecation and establish the extent of the perceived constipation problem. Assess the client's bowel habits:
  - Time of day
  - Amount and frequency of stool
  - Consistency of stool (using the Bristol Stool Scale)
  - Bleeding/passing mucus on defecation
  - Client history of bowel habits and/or laxative use
  - Family history of bowel habits and/or laxative use

  EB: *A nursing assessment that identifies the client's usual bowel habits will assist in the identification and management of their constipation (Lee, 2015).*
- ▲ Assess the client's lifestyle factors that may affect bowel function:
  - Fiber content in diet
  - Daily fluid intake
  - Exercise patterns
  - Personal remedies for constipation
  - Cultural remedies for constipation
  - Recently stopped smoking
  - Alcohol consumption/recreational drug use

  EB: *One of the key causes of constipation is dehydration of stools. A lack of water in the bowel leads to hard fecal matter, which is difficult to pass (Bardsley, 2017). Alcohol has a dehydrating effect on the body.*
- ▲ Review the client's medical history:
  - Obstetrical/gynecological/urological history and surgeries
  - Diseases that affect bowel motility
  - Bleeding/passing mucus on defecation
  - Current medications

  EB: *Review the client's medical history for conditions that may contribute to constipation, obstetrical/gynecological history, surgeries, diseases that affect bowel motility, alterations in perianal sensation, and the present bowel regimen (Lee, 2015).*
- ▲ Emotional influences:
  - Anxiety and depression/psychological disorders
  - History of eating disorders
  - History of physical/or sexual abuse
  - Long-term defecation issues
  - Stress

  EB: *Consider emotional influences (e.g., depression and anxiety) on defecation. Anxiety and depression are related to the occurrence of constipation; however, this is often a neglected aspect of client assessment and care in clinical practice (Jing & Jia, 2019).*
- Encourage the client or family to keep a 7-day diary of bowel habits, including time of day, length of time spent on the toilet, consistency, amount and frequency of stool, and any straining (using the Bristol Stool Scale). EBN: *Keeping a diary helps establish a client's bowel pattern and helps with recall and accuracy (Andrews & St Aubyn, 2020).*
- Encourage the client or family to keep a 7-day diary of lifestyle issues in relation to bowel habits, including fluid consumption, fiber content in diet, usual bowel stimulus, and exercise regimen. EB: *Enabling clients to present their condition in their own words ensures that they feel the health care professionals understand their concerns (Bharucha & Wald, 2019).*
- Educate the client that it is not necessary to have a daily bowel movement. EB: *A healthy bowel function can vary from three stools each day to three stools each week. The criteria of choice used for establishing a diagnosis of constipation are often the Rome IV criteria. The criteria-based definition calls for the presence of two or more of the symptoms for at least 3 months for a definition of constipation (Drossman, 2016).*
- Encourage the client to record use of laxatives, suppositories, or enemas, and suggest replacing them with an increase in fluid and fiber intake. EB: *Laxatives available for the treatment of constipation are generally safe when used at established doses under medical supervision. Their long-term use should be monitored by*

health care professionals and clients to optimize treatment on an individualized basis, enhancing efficacy and minimizing adverse effects (Serrano-Falcón & Rey, 2017).

- Advise a fiber intake of 18 to 30 g daily in adults and suggest foodstuffs high in fiber (e.g., prune juice, leafy green vegetables, whole meal bread and pasta). EB: *Fiber creates bulky feces and stretches the bowel wall to stimulate peristalsis, thus shortening bowel transit time (Bardsley, 2017). For further information on use of fiber, see the care plan for* **Constipation.**
- Advise a fluid intake of 1.5 to 2 L of fluid per day (ideally, 6–8 glasses of water), unless contraindicated by comorbidities, such as kidney or heart disease. EB: *Water passes into the gut to promote the formation of a softer fecal mass and provides lubrication to prevent a blockage of the gut. The recommended intake of fluid is 1.5 to 2 L daily, if the client presents with clinical signs of dehydration (Shen et al, 2019).*
- Obtain a referral to a dietitian for analysis of the client's diet and fluid intake *to provide strategies to improve diet and nutrition.*
- Encourage physical activity within the client's current ability to mobilize. Encourage turning and changing position in bed if immobile. For clients with reduced mobility, encourage knee to chest raises, waist twists, and stretching the arms away from the body. For fully mobile clients, encourage walking and swimming. EB: *Physical activity can help stimulate peristaltic waves in the colon and encourage the transit of feces to the rectum (Mihara et al, 2020).*
- Demonstrate the use of gentle external abdominal massage, using aroma therapy oils, following the direction of colon activity. EB: *Abdominal massage accelerates peristalsis by changing the intraabdominal pressure, thereby mechanically and reflexively acting on the intestines to evacuate the intestine (Okuyan & Bilgili, 2019).*
- Recommend that clients establish a regular elimination routine that includes activity, diet and fluids, and scheduled toilet visits. If required, assist clients to the bathroom at the same time every day; always be mindful of the need for privacy (closing of bathroom doors). EB: *A daily routine should begin with mild physical activity, consumption of a hot and preferably caffeinated beverage, and a breakfast that includes a form of soluble fiber to induce peristaltic contractions to take advantage of colonic motility and the gastrocolic reflex (Baffy et al, 2017).*
- Observe for the presence of an eating disorder by using laxatives to control or decrease weight; refer for counseling if needed. *People with eating disorders suffer from constipation and other gastrointestinal symptoms, or use laxatives as part of inducing weight loss (Sato & Fukudo, 2015).*
- Observe family cultural patterns related to eating and bowel habits. Cultural patterns may control bowel habits.

Client/Family Teaching and Discharge Planning

- Educate the client about how to adopt the best posture for defecation. Keep knees slightly higher than hips, keep feet flat on the floor, and lean forward putting elbows onto knees, thus adopting a squatting position. EB: *Adopting the squatting position helps with the angle of the anorectal section of the colon by lifting the sigmoid colon. The puborectalis muscles work most effectively when they are able to relax in the squatting position (Mercola, 2018).*
- Teach clients about the importance of responding promptly to the urge to defecate. EB: *The body's natural "call to stool" should be heeded in that it is a response to the stimulation of nerve endings in the rectum when a stool is present. Failure to respond to the urge of defecation or waiting until a more suitable time leads to stool retropulsion and worsening of the constipation (George & Borello-France, 2017).*
- Discourage the use of long-term laxatives and enemas and explain the potential harmful effects of the continual use of defecation aids such as laxatives and enemas. EB: *"Lazy bowel syndrome" may occur if laxatives are used too frequently, causing the bowel to become dependent on laxatives to stimulate a bowel movement. Overuse of laxatives can also lead to poor absorption of vitamins and other nutrients, and to damage of the gastrointestinal tract (Elran-Barak et al, 2017).*
- Discourage the long-term use of laxatives and enemas and advise clients to gradually reduce their use if taken regularly. EB: *Long-term use or overuse of laxatives can cause health problems (e.g., electrolyte imbalance) or hide symptoms that may be from a serious medical condition. The evidence base does not support use of stimulant laxatives for more than 4 weeks as associated with long-term colonic effects and possible carcinogenic risks (Noergaard et al, 2019).*
- Provide client with comprehensive written information about constipation and its management. EB: *Providing clients with well-written, evidence-based information about their condition and treatment can have a beneficial effect on the outcomes of treatment. A research study suggests that the use of family-friendly colorful and informative leaflets can have a direct effect on health-related issues (Shabde & Harrison, 2016).*

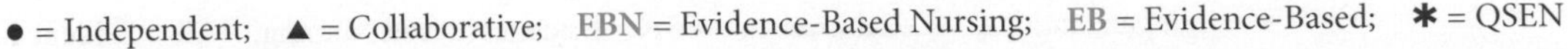

C

- Collaborate with members of the multiprofessional team to provide treatment and advice to clients and caregivers. *Teamwork is a central process in health care organizations. Effective organization and delivery of health care services depends on a wide range of professionals, families, clients, and carers working together to achieve the best health outcomes and quality of life (Flynn & Mercer, 2018).*
- Document all care and advice given in a factual and comprehensive manner. *Good record keeping is an integral part of nursing practice and is essential to the provision of safe and effective care (St Aubyn & Andrews, 2015).*

REFERENCES

Andrews, A., & St Aubyn, B. (2020). Assessment, diagnosis and management of constipation. *Nursing Standard, 35*(9), 59–65. https://doi.org/10.7748/ns.2020.e11512.

Baffy, N., Foxx-Orenstein, A., Harris, L., & Sterler, S. (2017). Intractable constipation in the elderly. *Current Treatment Options in Gastroenterology, 15*(3), 363–381.

Bardsley, A. (2017). Assessment and treatment options for patients with constipation. *British Journal of Nursing, 26*(6), 312–318.

Bharucha, A. E., & Wald, A. (2019). Chronic constipation. *Mayo Clinic Proceedings, 94*(11), 2340–2357.

Drossman, D. A. (2016). Functional gastrointestinal disorders: History, pathophysiology, clinical features and Rome IV. *Gastroenterology, 150*(6), 1262–1279.e2.

Ellis, P., Standing, M., & Roberts, S. (2020). *Patient assessment and care planning in nursing (Transforming nursing practice series)*. London: Sage Publications.

Elran-Barak, R., Goldschmidt, A., Scott, J., et al. (2017). Is laxative misuse associated with binge eating? Examination of laxative misuse among individuals seeking treatment for eating disorders. *International Journal of Eating Disorders, 50*(9), 1114–1118.

Flynn, M., & Mercer, D. (Eds.). (2018). *Oxford handbook of adult nursing*. Oxford: Oxford University Press.

George, S. E., & Borello-France, D. F. (2017). Perspective on physical therapist management of functional constipation. *Physical Therapy, 97*(4), 478–493.

Goldberg, J. L. (2017). Guideline implementation; hand hygiene. *AORN Journal, 105*(2), 203–212.

Griffith, R., & Tengnah, C. (2020). *Law and professional issues in nursing (Transforming nursing practice series)*. London: Sage Publications.

Jing, D., & Jia, L. (2019). Assessment of patients' psychological state and self-efficacy associated with post-operative constipation of the thoracolumbar fracture surgery. *Journal of International Medical Research, 47*(9), 4215–4224. https://doi.org/10.1177%2F0300060519859732.

Lee, A. (2015). Combatting the causes of constipation. *Nursing and Residential Care, 117*(6), 327–331.

Mercola, J. (2018). *Perfect position to poop*. Mercola.com [Internet]. Retrieved from: https://articles.mercola.com/sites/articles/archive/2018/09/22/proper-pooping-position.aspx. Accessed June 11, 2021.

Mihara, H., Murayama, A., Nanjo, S., et al. (2020). Factors correlated with drug use for constipation: Perspectives from the 2016 open Japanese National Database. *BMC Gastroenterology, 20*(1), 284.

Noergaard, M., Andersen, J. T., Jimenez-Solem, E., & Christensen, M. B. (2019). Long term treatment with stimulant laxatives—Clinical evidence for effectiveness and safety? *Scandinavian Journal of Gastroenterology, 54*(1), 27–34.

Okuyan, C. B., & Bilgili, N. (2019). Effect of abdominal massage on constipation and quality of life in older adults: A randomized controlled trial. *Complementary Therapies in Medicine, 47*, 102219.

Sato, Y., & Fukudo, S. (2015). Gastrointestinal symptoms and disorders in patients with eating disorders. *Clinical Journal of Gastroenterology, 8*(5), 255–263.

Serrano-Falcón, B., & Rey, E. (2017). The safety of available treatments for chronic constipation. *Expert Opinion on Drug Safety, 16*(11), 1243–1253.

Shabde, N., & Harrison, H. (2016). G331(P) Developing parental pathways: The most effective way to care for children with constipation—A cumbrian experience. *Archives of Disease in Childhood, 101*, A192–A193.

Shen, L., Huang, C., Lu, X., Xu, X., Juang, Z., & Zhu, C. (2019). Lower dietary fibre intake, but not total water consumption, is associated with constipation: A population-based analysis. *Journal of Human Nutrition and Dietetics, 32*(4), 422–431.

St Aubyn, B., & Andrews, A. (2015). If it's not written down it didn't happen. *British Journal of Community Nursing, 29*(5), 20–22.

Chronic Functional Constipation **Domain 3 Elimination and exchange Class 2 Gastrointestinal function**

Amanda Andrews, BSc (Hons), MA and Bernie St Aubyn, BSc (Hons), MSc

NANDA-I

Definition

Infrequent or difficult evacuation of feces, which has been present for at least 3 of the prior 12 months.

Defining Characteristics

General

Distended abdomen; fecal impaction; leakage of stool with digital stimulation; pain with defecation; palpable abdominal mass; positive fecal occult blood test; prolonged straining; Type 1 or 2 on Bristol Stool Chart

Adult: *Presence of ≥2 of the following symptoms on Rome III classification system:*

Lumpy or hard stools in ≥25% defecations; manual maneuvers to facilitate ≥25% of defecations (digital manipulation, pelvic floor support); sensation of anorectal obstruction/blockage for ≥25% of defecations; sensation of incomplete evacuation for ≥25% of defecations; ≤3 evacuations per week

Child >4 years: *Presence of ≥2 criteria on the Rome III Pediatric classification system for ≥2 months:*

Large diameter stools that may obstruct the toilet; painful or hard bowel movements; presence of large fecal mass in the rectum; stool retentive posturing; ≤2 defecations per week; ≥1 episode of fecal incontinence per week

Child ≤4 years: *Presence of ≥2 criteria on the Rome III Pediatric classification system for ≥1 month:*

Large diameter stools that may obstruct the toilet; painful or hard bowel movements; presence of large fecal mass in the rectum; stool retentive posturing; ≤2 defecations per week; ≥1 episode of fecal incontinence per week

Related Factors

Decreased food intake; dehydration; diet disproportionally high in fat; diet disproportionally high in protein; frail elderly syndrome; habitually suppresses urge to defecate; impaired physical mobility; inadequate dietary intake; inadequate knowledge of modifiable factors; insufficient fiber intake; insufficient fluid intake; low caloric intake; sedentary lifestyle

At-Risk Population

Older adults; pregnant women

Associated Conditions

Amyloidosis; anal fissure; anal stricture; autonomic neuropathy; chronic intestinal pseudo-obstruction; chronic renal insufficiency; colorectal cancer; depression; dermatomyositis; diabetes mellitus; extra intestinal mass; hemorrhoids; Hirschsprung's disease; hypercalcemia; hypothyroidism; inflammatory bowel disease; ischemic stenosis; multiple sclerosis; myotonic dystrophy; neurocognitive disorders; panhypopituitarism; paraplegia; Parkinson's disease; pelvic floor disorders; perineal damage; pharmaceutical preparations; polypharmacy; porphyria; postinflammatory stenosis; proctitis; scleroderma; slow colon transit time; spinal cord injuries; stroke; surgical stenosis

NOC (Nursing Outcomes Classification)

Suggested NOC Outcomes

Bowel Elimination; Symptom Severity

Example NOC Outcome with Indicators

Bowel Elimination as evidenced by the following indicators: Elimination pattern/Stool soft and formed/ Passage of stool without aids/Ease of stool passage. (Rate each indicator of **Bowel Elimination:** 1 = severely compromised, 2 = substantially compromised, 3 = moderately compromised, 4 = mildly compromised, 5 = not compromised [see Section I].)

Client Outcomes

Client Will (Specify Time Frame)

- Maintain passage of soft, formed stool (i.e., Bristol Stool Scale Type 4) every 1 to 3 days without straining.
- Identify measures that prevent or treat constipation

NIC (Nursing Interventions Classification)

Suggested NIC Intervention

Constipation/Impaction Management

Example NIC Activities—Constipation/Impaction Management

Identify factors (e.g., medications, bed rest, diet) that may cause or contribute to constipation/impaction; Institute a toileting schedule, as appropriate

C

Nursing Interventions and *Rationales*

All Client Ages

- Introduce yourself to the client and any companions and inform them of your role. EB: *Introducing yourself to a client helps establish and develop a therapeutic relationship that recognizes the person within the client and forms the basis for building trust on which to base the provision of care (Ellis et al, 2020).*
- Gain consent to perform care before proceeding further with the assessment. EB: *Clients have the right of autonomy both legally and morally and therefore should be fully involved in the decision-making process (Griffith & Tengnah, 2020).*
- Wash hands using a recognized technique. EB: *Performing strict hand-hygiene regimens significantly reduces the incidence of infection with methicillin-resistant* Staphylococcus aureus *and* Clostridium difficile *infection (Goldberg, 2017).*
- Assess usual pattern of defecation and establish the extent of the constipation problem. EB: *A thorough and holistic assessment of the client enables effective treatment of constipation to be delivered. A thorough assessment allows the nurse to identify the cause, plan interventions, monitor outcomes, and evaluate care (Mitchell, 2019).*
- Assess bowel habits:
  - Time of day
  - Amount and frequency of stool
  - Consistency of stool (using the Bristol Stool Scale)
  - Bleeding/passing mucus on defecation
  - History of bowel habits and/or laxative use
  - Assess children younger than 4 years using the Rome III pediatric classification (for at least 1 month)
  - Assess children older than age 4 years using the Rome III pediatric classification (for at least 2 months)

  EB: *Assess adults using the Rome IV classification. The Rome Foundation updated the criteria with the release of Rome IV criteria, devised in 2016, which specify that clients must be symptomatic with at least two or more of the criteria that are relevant to their specific age range (Drossman, 2016).*
- ▲ Assess the client's lifestyle factors that may affect bowel function:
  - Fiber content in diet
  - Daily fluid intake
  - Exercise patterns
  - Personal remedies for constipation
  - Recently stopped smoking
  - Alcohol consumption/recreational drug use
  - Personal habits related to defecation

  EB: *Alcohol has a dehydrating effect on the body. One of the key causes of constipation is dehydration of stools. A lack of water in the bowel leads to hard fecal matter, which is difficult to pass (Bardsley, 2017). When undertaking an assessment of a client with suspected constipation, it is important to discuss their lifestyle factors, which can be useful in establishing a clinical diagnosis. The main lifestyle factors to consider and record include the client's food and fluid intake, the fiber content of their diet, smoking, physical activity level, and mood (Andrews & St Aubyn, 2020).*
- ▲ Review the client's medical history:
  - Obstetrical/gynecological/urological history and surgeries
  - Existing anatomical anomalies (e.g., anal fissures, anal strictures and hemorrhoids)
  - Diseases that affect bowel motility (e.g., colorectal cancer, chronic intestinal pseudo-obstruction, and Hirschsprung's disease)
  - Bleeding/passing mucus on defecation
  - Current medications

  EB: *A full review of a client's medical history is essential. Within this assessment the inclusion of family history of inflammatory bowel disease or colorectal cancer will identify red flag symptoms leading to the need for further investigations and referral (Mitchell, 2019).*
- ▲ Review emotional influences with the client:
  - Anxiety and depression
  - Long-term defecation issues
  - Stress

EB: *A detailed and accurate assessment of the client enables the nurse to plan interventions, monitor outcomes, and evaluate care, ensuring no unnecessary treatment is performed. Consider emotional influences (e.g., depression and anxiety) on defecation. Anxiety and depression are related to the occurrence of constipation; however, this is often a neglected aspect of client assessment and care in clinical practice (Jing & Jia, 2019).*

- Complete a physical examination (palpation for abdominal distention, percussion for dullness, and auscultation for bowel sounds). EB: *Research recommends the use of a standardized constipation assessment and management pathway. The key elements of such a pathway include a physical examination for the detection of any palpable fecal mass or abnormalities (Sandweiss et al, 2018).*
- Encourage the client or family to keep a 7-day diary of bowel habits, including time of day, length of time spent on the toilet, consistency, amount and frequency of stool, and any straining (using the Bristol Stool Scale). EBN: *Keeping a diary helps establish a client's bowel pattern and helps with recall and accuracy (Andrews & St Aubyn, 2020).*
- Encourage the client or family to keep a 7-day diary of lifestyle issues in relation to bowel habits, including fluid consumption, fiber content in diet, usual bowel stimulus, and exercise regimen. EB: *The importance of using bowel diaries for efficiently and reliably characterizing bowel habits cannot be overemphasized (Bharucha & Wald, 2019).*
- Actively encourage children and families to attend bowel management programs to aid the establishment of regular bowel routines. EB: *Research shows that children who followed a structured program can experience successful treatment of severe constipation (Kilpatrick et al, 2020).*
- Discuss with clients already taking opioids (temporarily or long term) that constipation is a common side effect. If the client is receiving temporary opioids (e.g., for acute postoperative pain), request an order for routine stool softeners from the primary care provider, monitor bowel movements, and request a laxative for the client if constipation develops. If the client is receiving around-the-clock opiates (e.g., for palliative care), laxatives, then softeners, stimulants, or osmotics, should be requested. EB: *Constipation is the most common opioid-related adverse effect. Opioids cause a lack of peristalsis in the large intestine and decrease fluid in the stool and increase anal muscle tone. Clients should be prescribed a stool softener and a bowel stimulant prophylactically to prevent constipation (Brant, 2018).*
- Advise a fiber intake of 18 to 30 g of fiber daily in adults and suggest foodstuffs to facilitate this diet (e.g., prune juice, leafy green vegetables, whole meal bread and pasta). EB: *Fiber creates bulky feces and stretches the bowel wall to stimulate peristalsis, thus shortening bowel transit time (Bardsley, 2017).*
- Advise clients to drink at least 6–8 glasses of water a day, unless contraindicated by comorbidities, such as kidney or heart disease. EB: *The recommended intake of fluid is 1.5 to 2 L daily (e.g., 6-8 glasses), if the client presents with clinical signs of dehydration (Shen et al, 2019).*
- Encourage physical activity within the client's current ability to mobilize. Encourage turning and changing position in bed if immobile. For clients with reduced mobility, encourage knee to chest raises, waist twists, and stretching the arms away from the body. For fully mobile clients, encourage walking and swimming. EB: *Physical activity can help stimulate peristaltic waves in the colon and encourage the transit of feces to the rectum (Mihara et al, 2020).*
- Demonstrate the use of gentle external abdominal massage, following the direction of colon activity. EB: *Abdominal massage accelerates peristalsis by changing the intraabdominal pressure, thereby mechanically and reflexively acting on the intestines to evacuate the intestine (Okuyan & Bilgili, 2019).*
- Recommend that clients establish a regular elimination routine that includes activity, diet and fluids, and scheduled toilet visits. If required, assist clients to the bathroom at the same time every day; always be mindful of the need for privacy (closing of bathroom doors). EB: *A daily routine should begin with mild physical activity, consumption of a hot and preferably caffeinated beverage, and a breakfast that includes a form of soluble fiber to induce peristaltic contractions to take advantage of colonic motility and the gastrocolic reflex (Baffy et al, 2017).*
- Educate the client about how to adopt the best posture for defecation. Keep knees slightly higher than hips, keep feet flat on the floor, and lean forward putting elbows onto knees, thus adopting a squatting position. EB: *Adopting the squatting position helps with the angle of the anorectal section of the colon by lifting the sigmoid colon. The puborectalis muscles work most effectively when they are able to relax in the squatting position (Mercola, 2018).*
- Consider the teaching of biofeedback therapy to encourage a "new normal" bowel routine for clients to adopt. EB: *A literature review concluded that the use of biofeedback therapy in chronic constipation was successful and remains the safest option to successfully manage chronic constipation (Chiarioni, 2016).*

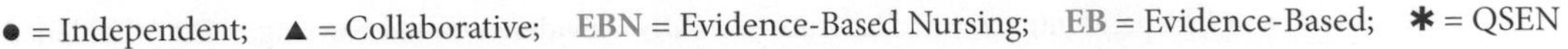

C

- Teach clients about the importance of responding promptly to the urge to defecate. EB: *The body's natural "call to stool" should be heeded in that it is a response to the stimulation of nerve endings in the rectum when a stool is present. Failure to respond to the urge of defecation or waiting until a more suitable time leads to stool retropulsion and worsening of the constipation (George & Borello-France, 2017).*
- Consider the use of laxatives, suppositories, enemas, and bowel irrigation as required if other more natural interventions are not effective. EB: *The overall aim of laxative therapy is to enable the client to defecate in a manner that promotes comfort and enhances symptom management. A fast active stimulant laxative should be considered to provide short-term relief and longer-term management including the use of an osmotic laxative (Andrews & St Aubyn, 2020). A systematic review identified that bowel irrigation is effective for chronic constipation in around 50% of clients (Emmett et al, 2015).*
- Discourage the long-term use of laxatives and enemas and advise clients to gradually reduce their use if taken regularly. EB: *Long-term use or overuse of laxatives can cause health problems (e.g., electrolyte imbalance) or hide symptoms that may be from a serious medical condition. The evidence base does not support use of stimulant laxatives for more than 4 weeks as associated with long-term colonic effects and possible carcinogenic risks (Noergaard et al, 2019).*
- Provide client with comprehensive written information about constipation and its management. EB: *Providing clients with well-written, evidence-based information about their condition and treatment can have a beneficial effect on the outcomes of treatment. A research study suggests that the use of family-friendly colorful and informative leaflets can have a direct effect on health-related issues (Shabde & Harrison, 2016).*
- Provide written instructions for children about taking their medication and about how the bowel works. *Written clear information provided to children with chronic functional constipation will help them understand and therefore recognize when they are at risk for constipation recurrence (National Institute for Health and Care Excellence, 2017).*
- Collaborate with members of the multiprofessional team to provide treatment and advice to clients and caregivers. EB: *Teamwork is a central process in health care organizations. Effective organization and delivery of health care services depends on a wide range of professionals, families, clients, and carers working together to achieve the best health outcomes and quality of life (Flynn & Mercer, 2018).*
- Consider referral to other specialist practitioners if constipation persists. *A diagnosis of primary chronic constipation is made after the exclusion of secondary causes of constipation and managed effectively. If unsuccessful, subspecialist referrals should be considered (Rao et al, 2016).*
- Document all care and advice given in a factual and comprehensive manner. EBN: *Good record keeping is an integral part of nursing practice and is essential to the provision of safe and effective care (St Aubyn & Andrews, 2015).*

REFERENCES

Andrews, A., & St Aubyn, B. (2020). Assessment, diagnosis and management of constipation. *Nursing Standard, 35*(9), 59–65. https://doi:10.7748/ns.2020.e11512.

Baffy, N., Foxx-Orenstein, A., Harris, L., & Sterler, S. (2017). Intractable constipation in the elderly. *Current Treatment Options in Gastroenterology, 15*(3), 363–381.

Bardsley, A. (2017). Assessment and treatment options for patients with constipation. *British Journal of Nursing, 26*(6), 312–318.

Bharucha, A. E., & Wald, A. (2019). Chronic constipation. *Mayo Clinic Proceedings, 94*(11), 2340–2357.

Brant, J. M. (2018). Assessment and management of cancer pain in older adults: Strategies for success. *Asia-Pacific Journal of Oncology Nursing, 5*(3), 248–253.

Chiarioni, G. (2016). Biofeedback treatment of chronic constipation: Myths and misconceptions. *Techniques in Coloproctology, 20*(9), 611–618.

Drossman, D. A. (2016). Functional gastrointestinal disorders: History, pathophysiology, clinical features and Rome IV. *Gastroenterology, 150*(6), 1262–1279.e2.

Ellis, P., Standing, M., & Roberts, S. (2020). *Patient assessment and care planning in nursing (Transforming nursing practice series).* London: Sage Publications.

Emmett, C. D., Close, H. J., Yiannakou, Y., & Mason, J. M. (2015). Trans-anal irrigation therapy to treat adult chronic functional constipation: Systematic review and meta-analysis. *BMC Gastroenterology, 15*, 139.

Flynn, M., & Mercer, D. (Eds.). (2018). *Oxford handbook of adult nursing.* Oxford: Oxford University Press.

George, S. E., & Borello-France, D. F. (2017). Perspective on physical therapist management of functional constipation. *Physical Therapy, 97*(4), 478–493.

Goldberg, J. L. (2017). Guideline implementation; hand hygiene. *AORN Journal, 105*(2), 203–212.

Griffith, R., & Tengnah, C. (2020). *Law and professional issues in nursing (Transforming nursing practice series).* London: Sage Publications.

Jing, D., & Jia, L. (2019). Assessment of patients' psychological state and self-efficacy associated with post-operative constipation of the thoracolumbar fracture surgery. *Journal of International Medical Research, 47*(9), 4215–4224.

Kilpatrick, J. A., Zobell, S., Leeflang, E. J., Cao, D., Mammen, L., & Rollins, M. D. (2020). Intermediate and long-term outcomes of a bowel management program for children with severe constipation or fecal incontinence. *Journal of Pediatric Surgery, 55*(3), 545–548.

Mercola, J. (2018). *Perfect position to poop*. Mercola.com [Internet]. Retrieved from: https://articles.mercola.com/sites/articles/archive/2018/09/22/proper-pooping-position.aspx. Accessed June 11, 2021.

Mihara, H., Murayama, A., Nanjo, S., et al. (2020). Factors correlated with drug use for constipation: Perspectives from the 2016 open Japanese National Database. *BMC Gastroenterology*, *20*(1), 284.

Mitchell, A. (2019). Carrying out a holistic assessment of a patient with constipation. *British Journal of Nursing*, *28*(4), 230–232.

National Institute for Health and Care Excellence. (2017). *Constipation in children and young people: Diagnosis and management*. Retrieved from https://www.nice.org.uk/guidance/cg99. Accessed December 26, 2020.

Noergaard, M., Andersen, J. T., Jimenez-Solem, E., & Christensen, M. B. (2019). Long term treatment with stimulant laxatives—clinical evidence for effectiveness and safety? *Scandinavian Journal of Gastroenterology*, *54*(1), 27–34.

Okuyan, C. B., & Bilgili, N. (2019). Effect of abdominal massage on constipation and quality of life in older adults: A randomized controlled trial. *Complimentary Therapies in Medicine*, *47*, 102219.

Rao, S. S. C., Rattanakovit, K., & Patcharatrakul, T. (2016). Diagnoses and management of chronic constipation on adults. *Nature Reviews Gastroenterology & Hepatology*, *13*(5), 295–305.

Sandweiss, D. R., Allen, L., Deneau, M., et al. (2018). Implementing a standardized constipation—management pathway to reduce resource utilization. *Academic Pediatrics*, *18*(8), 957–964.

Shabde, N., & Harrison, H. (2016). G331(P) Developing parental pathways: The most effective way to care for children with constipation—a cumbrian experience. *Archives of Disease in Childhood*, *101*, A192–A193.

Shen, L., Huang, C., Lu, X., Xu, X., Juang, Z., & Zhu, C. (2019). Lower dietary fibre intake, but not total water consumption, is associated with constipation: A population-based analysis. *Journal of Human Nutrition and Dietetics*, *32*(4), 422–431.

St Aubyn, B., & Andrews, A. (2015). If it's not written down it didn't happen. *British Journal of Community Nursing*, *29*(5), 20–22.

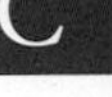

Risk for Chronic Functional Constipation

Domain 3 Elimination and exchange Class 2 Gastrointestinal function

Mary Beth Flynn Makic, PhD, RN, CCNS, CCRN-K, FAAN, FNAP, FCNS

NANDA-I

Definition

Susceptible to infrequent or difficult evacuation of feces, which has been present nearly 3 of the prior 12 months, which may compromise health.

Risk Factors

Decreased food intake; dehydration; diet disproportionally high in fat; diet disproportionally high in protein; frail elderly syndrome; habitually suppresses urge to defecate; impaired physical mobility; inadequate dietary intake; inadequate knowledge of modifiable factors; insufficient fiber intake; insufficient fluid intake; low caloric intake; sedentary lifestyle

At-Risk Population

Older adults; pregnant women

Associated Conditions

Amyloidosis; anal fissure; anal stricture; autonomic neuropathy; chronic intestinal pseudo-obstruction; chronic renal insufficiency; colorectal cancer; depression; dermatomyositis; diabetes mellitus; extra intestinal mass; hemorrhoids; Hirschsprung's disease; hypercalcemia; hypothyroidism; inflammatory bowel disease; ischemic stenosis; multiple sclerosis; myotonic dystrophy; neurocognitive disorders; panhypopituitarism; paraplegia; Parkinson's disease; pelvic floor disorders; perineal damage; pharmaceutical preparations; polypharmacy; porphyria; postinflammatory stenosis; proctitis; scleroderma; slow colon transit time; spinal cord injuries; stroke; surgical stenosis

NIC, NOC, Client Outcomes, Nursing Interventions and *Rationales,* Client/Family Teaching and Discharge Planning, and References

Refer to care plan for Chronic Functional **Constipation.**

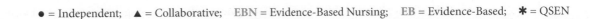

Contamination Domain 11 Safety/protection Class 4 Environmental hazards

Pauline McKinney Green, PhD, RN, CNE

C

NANDA-I

Definition

Exposure to environmental contaminants in doses sufficient to cause adverse health effects.

Defining Characteristics

Pesticides

Dermatological effects of pesticide exposure; gastrointestinal effects of pesticide exposure; neurological effects of pesticide exposure; pulmonary effects of pesticide exposure; renal effects of pesticide exposure

Chemicals

Dermatological effects of chemical exposure; gastrointestinal effects of chemical exposure; immunological effects of chemical exposure; neurological effects of chemical exposure; pulmonary effects of chemical exposure; renal effects of chemical exposure

Biologics

Dermatological effects of biologic exposure; gastrointestinal effects of biologic exposure; neurological effects of biologic exposure; pulmonary effects of biologic exposure; renal effects of biologic exposure

Pollution

Neurological effects of pollution exposure; pulmonary effects of pollution exposure

Waste

Dermatological effects of waste exposure; gastrointestinal effects of waste exposure; hepatic effects of waste exposure; pulmonary effects of waste exposure

Radiation

Genetic effects of radiotherapy exposure; immunological effects of radiotherapy exposure; neurological effects of radiotherapy exposure; oncological effects of radiotherapy exposure

Related Factors

External Factors

Carpeted flooring; chemical contamination of food; chemical contamination of water; flaking, peeling surface in presence of young children; inadequate breakdown of contaminant; inadequate household hygiene practices; inadequate municipal services; inadequate personal hygiene practices; inadequate protective clothing; inappropriate use of protective clothing; individuals who ingested contaminated material; playing where environmental contaminants are used; unprotected exposure to chemical; unprotected exposure to heavy metal; unprotected exposure to radioactive material; use of environmental contaminant in the home; use of noxious material in inadequately ventilated area; use of noxious material without effective protection

Internal Factors

Concomitant exposure; malnutrition; smoking

At-Risk Population

Children aged <5 years; economically disadvantaged individuals; individuals exposed perinatally; individuals exposed to areas with high concomitant level; individuals exposed to atmospheric pollutants; individuals exposed to bioterrorism; individuals exposed to disaster; individuals with history of exposure to contaminant; older adults; pregnant women; women

Associated Conditions

Pre-existing disease; radiotherapy

NOC (Nursing Outcomes Classification)

Suggested NOC Outcomes

Community Health Status; Family Physical Environment; Anxiety Level; Fear Level

Example NOC Outcome with Indicators

Community Health Status as evidenced by the following indicators: Evidence of health protection measures/Compliance with environmental health standards/Health status of population. (Rate the outcome and indicators of **Community Health Status:** 1 = poor, 2 = fair, 3 = good, 4 = very good, 5 = excellent [see Section I].)

Client Outcomes

Client Will (Specify Time Frame)

- Have minimal health effects associated with contamination
- Cooperate with appropriate decontamination protocol
- Participate in appropriate isolation precautions
- Use health surveillance data system to monitor for contamination incidents
- Use disaster plan to evacuate and triage affected members
- Have minimal health effects associated with contamination
- Use measures to reduce household environmental risks

NIC (Nursing Interventions Classification)

Suggested NIC Interventions

Triage: Disaster; Infection Control; Anxiety Reduction; Crisis Intervention; Health Education

Example NIC Activities—Triage: Disaster

Initiate appropriate emergency measures, as indicated; Monitor for and treat life-threatening injuries or acute needs

Nursing Interventions and Rationales

▲ Help individuals cope with contamination incident by doing the following:
  - ❍ Use organizations and groups that have survived terrorist attacks as a useful resource for victims
  - ❍ Provide accurate information on risks involved, preventive measures, and use of antibiotics and vaccines
  - ❍ Assist to deal with feelings of fear, vulnerability, and grief
  - ❍ Encourage individuals to talk to others about their fears
  - ❍ Assist victims to think positively and to move toward the future

▲ In a crisis situation, interventions aimed at supporting an individual's coping help the person deal with feelings of fear, helplessness, and loss of control that are normal reactions in a crisis situation.

- Triage, stabilize, transport, and treat affected community members. EB: *Accurate triage and early treatment provide the best chance of survival to affected persons (Goodwin Veenema, 2019).*
- Prioritize mental health care for highly vulnerable risk groups or those with special needs (women, older persons, children and adolescents, displaced persons, especially those living in shelters; persons with pre-existing mental health disorders, including those living in institutions, those significantly exposed to contaminants). CEB: *Persons with special needs are vulnerable to marginalization during emergencies and are exposed to greater stress (Pan American Health Organization, 2012).*

✱ Collaborate with members of the health care delivery system and outside agencies (local health department, emergency medical services [EMS], state and federal agencies). EB: *Communication among agencies increases the ability to handle a crisis efficiently by disseminating evidence-based information (Centers for Disease Control and Prevention [CDC], 2018; Goodwin Veenema, 2019).*

C

- Use approved procedures for decontamination of persons, clothing, and equipment. *Victims may first require decontamination before entering health facility to receive care to prevent the spread of contamination (U.S. Army Medical Research Institute of Infectious Diseases, 2014).*
- Use appropriate isolation precautions: universal, airborne, droplet, and contact isolation to prevent cross-contamination by contaminating agents (U.S. Army Medical Research Institute of Infectious Diseases, 2014). EB: *Client contact is a major risk factor for provider contamination and transmission (Jackson et al, 2018).*
- Monitor individuals for therapeutic effects, side effects, and compliance with postexposure drug therapy that may extend over a long period of time and require monitoring for compliance and for therapeutic and side effects (Adalja, Toner, & Inglesby, 2015; Goodwin Veenema, 2019).
- Perform effective handwashing using 60% to 90% alcohol-based hand rub before and after touching a client, after touching client's immediate environment, aseptic tasks, contact with body fluids or contaminated surfaces, and immediately after glove removal (CDC, 2020a).
- Prevent cross-contamination by systematically disinfecting stethoscopes (diaphragm and tubing) after each use. EB: *A descriptive study using cultures and bioluminescence to visualize contamination demonstrated improve stethoscope hygiene among providers (Holleck et al, 2020).*
- Minimize occupational exposure to antineoplastic agents by following National Institute for Occupational Safety and Health (NIOSH) guidelines regarding personal protective equipment (PPE) and correct handling of hazardous drugs. CEB: *Nurse safety is directly related to knowledge of hazard assessment, decontamination, and proper use of PPE (NIOSH, 2013; Crickman, 2017).*
- Adhere to standards and transmission-based precautions when caring for clients with SARS-CoV-2 and use correct donning and doffing procedure with PPE (CDC, 2020b).
- Follow institutional policy and procedure for optimizing supply of PPE during surges or instances of low or inadequate PPE (CDC, 2020b).

Geriatric

- Help the client identify age-related factors that may affect response to contamination incidents.
- Advise older adults to follow public notices related to drinking water. *Contaminated water can harm the health of older persons and those with chronic conditions (CDC, 2014).*
- Encourage older adults to receive influenza vaccination when it is available, beginning as early as late August and continuing through the end of February. *Flu vaccination protects persons against influenza, protects those in proximity who are more vulnerable to serious flu illness, and reduces flu-associated hospitalizations among older adults (CDC, 2019a).*
- Instruct older adults with special needs or chronic conditions to create and share a plan with family and friends for emergencies and keep medications, prescriptions, and special devices on hand. *Sharing a plan for emergencies helps older adults create a social network that will be available for support and assistance (Federal Emergency Management Agency, 2020).*

Pediatric

- Provide environmental health hazard information. *Developing children are more vulnerable to environmental toxicants because of greater and longer exposure and particular susceptibility windows (Children's Environmental Health Network, 2017).*
- Reduce risks from exposure to environmental contaminants by identifying the ages and life stages of children. CEB: *Coordinate hazard and exposure assessment using children's ages and life stages to accommodate for children's physiology and developmental stage, which contribute to opportunities for environmental exposure and contamination (Hubal et al, 2014).*
- Screen newly arrived immigrant and refugee children, adolescents, pregnant and lactating women, and children for elevated blood lead levels secondary to lead hazards in country of origin and residence in older housing. EB: *Lead exposure is common in newly arrived refugees and those residing in older housing (CDC, 2020c).*
- Be aware that the risk for lead exposure is much higher in many countries from which children are adopted than in the United States; screening should then be conducted for those identified from 6 months and up to 16 years of age (CDC, 2019b).
- The current reference level of 5 μg/dL is used to identify children and environments associated with lead-exposure hazards. EB: *The CDC currently recommends using 5 μg/dL as the reference value in place of the previously recommended level of 10 μg/dL; reference values are updated every 4 years based on the most recent population-based blood lead surveys among children (CDC, 2020d).*

- Encourage flu vaccination among children. CEB: *Children vaccinated against flu were 74% less likely to be admitted to a pediatric intensive care for influenza compared with controls (Ferdinands et al, 2014).*

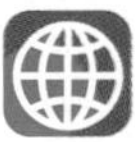

Multicultural

- Ask about use of imported or culture-specific products that contain lead, such as greta and azarcon (Hispanic folk medicine for upset stomach and diarrhea), ghasard (Indian folk medicine tonic), ba-baw-san (Chinese herbal remedy), and daw-tway (Thai and Myanmar [Burmese] remedy). *Immigrant children are at increased risk for contamination, particularly from lead related to exposure to imported culture-specific products (CDC, 2019c).*
- ✱ Nurses need to consider the cultural and social factors that affect access to and understanding of the health care system, particularly for groups such as migrant workers who do not have consistent health care providers. CEB: *Subtle cultural biases in how nurses approach care can affect outcomes (Holmes, 2012; Hubal et al, 2014).*

Home Care

- Assess current environmental stressors and identify community resources. *Accessing resources decreases stress and increases ability to cope.*
- Recognize that relocated and unemployed individuals/families are at risk for psychological distress. EB: *People who lose their social network are at a very high risk for postevent psychological distress and require appropriate care and resources to respond and recover from disasters (Substance Abuse and Mental Health Services Administration [SAMHSA], 2020).*
- Support policy and program initiatives that integrate case identification, triage, and mental health interventions into emergency care response following large scale disaster events. EB: *A skills-based mental health program using front-line workers was found feasible and beneficial in reducing psychological symptoms among disaster survivors (O'Donnell et al, 2020).*
- Instruct community members concerned about lead in drinking water from plumbing pipes and fixtures to have the water tested by calling the US Environmental Protection Agency (EPA) drinking water hotline at 1-800-424-8802.
- Educate community members to reduce exposure to lead by inquiring about lead-based paint before buying a home or renting an apartment built before 1978; *federal law requires disclosure of known information about lead-based paint (U. S. EPA, 2020).*
- Instruct individuals and families that food contamination occurs through a variety of mechanisms and that food safety is associated with proper washing of hands, surfaces, and utensils; prompt refrigeration of food; and cooking foods at the correct temperature. EB: *Pathogens can be introduced into food from infected humans who handle food without thoroughly washing their hands, from food that touches surfaces or utensils contaminated by pathogens in raw food, and improper refrigeration or heating of food (CDC, 2020e).*

Client/Family Teaching and Discharge Planning

- Provide truthful information to the person or family affected.
- Discuss signs and symptoms of contamination.
- Explain decontamination protocols.
- Explain need for isolation procedures.
- *Well-managed efforts at communication of contamination information ensure messages are correctly formulated, transmitted, and received and result in meaningful actions.*
- Emphasize the importance of prehospital exposure and postexposure treatment of contamination. CEB: *Early treatment decreases associated complications related to contamination (Agency for Toxic Substances and Disease Registry [ATSDR], 2014).*
- Provide parents with actionable information to reduce environmental contamination in the home. CEBN: *A randomized educational intervention to reduce contamination in the home demonstrated significant reduction in biomarker levels and improved environmental health self-efficacy and precaution adoption (Butterfield et al, 2011).*

REFERENCES

Adalja, A., Toner, E., & Inglesby, T. V. (2015). Clinical management of bioterrorism-related conditions. *New England Journal of Medicine, 372*(10), 954–962. https://doi:10.1056/NEJMra409755.

Agency for Toxic Substances and Disease Registry (ATSDR). (2014). *Medical management guidelines for parathion*. Retrieved from https://wwwn.cdc.gov/TSP/MMG/MMGDetails.aspx?mmgid=1140&toxid=246. Accessed 14 June 2021.

Butterfield, P. G., Hill, W., Postma, J., Butterfield, P. W., & Odom-Maryon, T. (2011). Effectiveness of a household environmental health intervention delivered by rural public health nurses. *American Journal of Public Health, 101*(Suppl. 1), S262–S270. https://doi:10.2105/AJPH.2011.3001.

Centers for Disease Control and Prevention. (2014). *Water-related diseases and contaminants in public water systems*. Retrieved from

https://www.cdc.gov/healthywater/drinking/public/water_diseases.html. Accessed 14 June 2021.
Centers for Disease Control and Prevention. (2018). *Emergency Preparedness and Response. Clinical outreach and communication activity (COCA)*. Retrieved from ht tps://emergency.cdc.gov/coca/index.asp. Accessed 14 June 2021.
Centers for Disease Control and Prevention. (2019a). Key facts about seasonable flu vaccine. What are the benefits of flu vaccination? Retrieved from https://www.cdc.gov/flu/prevent/keyfacts.htm. Accessed 14 June 2021.
Centers for Disease Control and Prevention. (2019b). *International adoption*. Retrieved from https://www.cdc.gov/nceh/lead/prevention/adoption.htm. Accessed 14 June 2021.
Centers for Disease Control and Prevention. (2019c). *Lead in food, cosmetics, and medicines*. Retrieved from https://www.cdc.gov/nceh/lead/prevention/sources/foods-cosmetics-medicines.htm. Accessed 14 June 2021.
Centers for Disease Control and Prevention. (2020a). *Hand hygiene guidance*. Retrieved from ht tps://www.cdc.gov/handhygiene/providers/guideline.html. Accessed 14 June 2021.
Centers for Disease Control and Prevention. (2020b). *Optimizing personal protective equipment (PPE) supplies*. Retrieved from https://www.cdc.gov/coronavirus/2019-ncov/hcp/ppe-strategy/index.html. Accessed 14 June 2021.
Centers for Disease Control and Prevention. (2020c). *Screening for lead during the domestic medical examination for newly arrived refugees*. Retrieved from https://www.cdc.gov/immigrantrefugeehealth/guidelines/lead-guidelines.html. Accessed 14 June 2021.
Centers for Disease Control and Prevention. (2020d). *Blood lead levels in children*. Retrieved from https://www.cdc.gov/nceh/lead/prevention/blood-lead-levels.htm. Accessed 14 June 2021.
Centers for Disease Control and Prevention. (2020e). *Foodborne outbreaks. Prevention and education*. Retrieved from https://www.cdc.gov/foodsafety/outbreaks/prevention-education/index.html. Accessed 14 June 2021.
Children's Environmental Health Network. (2017). *Children's environmental health 101*. Retrieved from https://cehn.org/resources/for-parents-families-and-other-child-health-advocates/childrens-environmental-health-101/. Accessed 14 June 2021.
Crickman, R. (2017). Chemotherapy safe handling. Limiting nursing exposure with a hazardous drug control program. *Clinical Journal of Oncology Nursing*, *21*(1), 73–78. https://doi:10.1188/17.CJON.73-78.
Federal Emergency Management Agency (FEMA). (2020). *Preparing makes sense for people with disabilities, others with access and functional needs and the whole community.* Retrieved from https://oes.ucsc.edu/emergency-preparedness/procedures/femaada.pdf.
Ferdinands, J. M., Olsho, L. E., Agan, A. A., et al. (2014). Effectiveness of influenza vaccine against life-threatening RT-PCR-confirmed influenza in U. S. children, 2010-2012. *Journal of Infectious Diseases, 210*(5), 674–683. https://doi:10/1093/infdis/j.iu185.
Goodwin Veenema, T. (2019). *Disaster nursing and emergency preparedness for chemical, biological, radiological terrorism and other hazards* (4th ed.). New York: Springer.
Holleck, J. L., Campbell, S., Alrawili, H., et al. (2020). Stethoscope hygiene: Using cultures and real-time feedback with bioluminescence-based adenosine triphosphate technology to change behavior. *American Journal of Infection Control*, *48*(4), 380–385. https://doi.org/10.1016/j.ajic.2019.10.005.
Holmes, S. M. (2012). The clinical gaze in the practice of migrant health: Mexican migrants in the United States. *Social Science & Medicine*, *74*(6), 873–881. https://doi:10.1016/j.socscimed.2011.06.067.
Hubal, E., de Wet, T., Du Toit, L., et al. (2014). Identifying important life stages for monitoring and assessing risks from exposures to environmental contaminants: Results of a World Health Organization review. *Regulatory Toxicology and Pharmacology*, *69*(1), 113–124. https://doi:10.1016/j.yrtph.2013.09.008.
Jackson, S. S., Thom, K. A., Madger, L. S., et al. (2018). Patient contact is main risk factor for vancomycin-resistant enterococcus contamination of healthcare workers' gloves and gowns in the intensive care unit. *Infection Control and Hospital Epidemiology*, *39*, 1063–1067. https://doi:10.1017.ice/2018.160.
National Institute for Occupational Safety and Health. (NIOSH). (2013). *Medical surveillance for healthcare workers exposed to hazardous drugs*. Retrieved from ht tps://www.cdc.gov/niosh/docs/wp-solutions/2013-103/pdfs/2013-103.pdf?id=10.26616/NIOSHPUB2013103. Accessed 14 June 2021.
O'Donnell, M. L., Lau, W., Fredrickson, J., et al. (2020). An open label pilot study of a brief psychological intervention for disaster and trauma survivors. *Frontiers in Psychiatry*, *11*, 483. doi:10.3389/fpsyt.2020.00483.
Pan American Health Organization. (2012). *Mental health and psychosocial support in disaster situations in the Caribbean: Core knowledge for emergency preparedness and response*. Washington, DC: PAHO.
Substance Abuse and Mental Health Services Administration (SAMHSA). (2020). *Disaster preparedness, response, and recovery*. Retrieved from https://www.samhsa.gov/disaster-preparedness. Accessed 14 June 2021.
U.S. Army Medical Research Institute of Infectious Diseases. (2014). *USAMRIID's medical management of biological casualties handbook* (8th ed.). Frederick, MD: USAMRIID. Retrieved from https://www.usamriid.army.mil/education/bluebookpdf/USAMRIID%20BlueBook%208th%20Edition%20-%20Sep%202014.pdf. Accessed 14 June 2021.
U.S. Environmental Protection Agency (EPA). (2020). *Protect your family from lead in your home*. Retrieved from ht tps://www.epa.gov/lead/protect-your-family-lead-your-home-english. Accessed 14 June 2021.

Risk for Contamination **Domain 11 Safety/protection Class 4 Environmental hazards**

Mary Beth Flynn Makic, PhD, RN, CCNS, CCRN-K, FAAN, FNAP, FCNS

NANDA-I

Definition

Susceptible to exposure to environmental contaminants, which may compromise health.

Risk Factors

External Factors

Carpeted flooring; chemical contamination of food; chemical contamination of water; flaking, peeling surface in presence of young children; inadequate breakdown of contaminant; inadequate household hygiene practices; inadequate municipal services; inadequate personal hygiene practices; inadequate protective clothing; inappropriate use of protective clothing; individuals who ingested contaminated material; playing where environmental contaminants are used; unprotected exposure to chemical; unprotected exposure to heavy metal; unprotected exposure to radioactive material; use of environmental contaminant in the home; use of noxious material in inadequately ventilated area; use of noxious material without effective protection

Internal Factors

Concomitant exposure; malnutrition; smoking

At-Risk Population

Children aged <5 years; economically disadvantaged individuals; individuals exposed perinatally; individuals exposed to areas with high contaminant level; individuals exposed to atmospheric pollutants; individuals exposed to bioterrorism; individuals exposed to disaster; individuals with history of exposure to contaminant; older adults; pregnant women; women

Associated Conditions

Pre-existing disease; radiotherapy

NIC, NOC, Client Outcomes, Nursing Interventions and *Rationales,* Client/Family Teaching, and References

Refer to care plan for **Contamination.**

Impaired Bowel Continence

Domain 3 Elimination and exchange Class 2 Gastrointestinal function

Kim L. Paxton, DNP, APRN, ANP-BC, LHIT-C

NANDA-I

Definition

Inability to hold stool, to sense the presence of stool in the rectum, to relax and store stool when having a bowel movement is not convenient.

Defining Characteristics

Abdominal discomfort; bowel urgency; fecal staining; impaired ability to expel formed stool despite recognition of rectal fullness; inability to delay defecation; inability to hold flatus; inability to reach toilet in time; inattentive to urge to defecate; silent leakage of stool during activities

Related Factors

Avoidance of non-hygienic toilet use; constipation; dependency for toileting; diarrhea; difficulty finding the bathroom; difficulty obtaining timely assistance to bathroom; embarrassment regarding toilet use in social situations; environmental constraints that interfere with continence; generalized decline in muscle tone; impaired physical mobility; impaired postural balance; inadequate dietary habits; inadequate motivation to maintain continence; incomplete emptying of bowel; laxative misuse; stressors

At-Risk Population

Older adults; women giving birth vaginally; women giving birth with obstetrical extraction

Associated Conditions

Anal trauma; congenital abnormalities of the digestive system; diabetes mellitus; neurocognitive disorders; neurological diseases; physical inactivity; prostatic diseases; rectum trauma; spinal cord injuries; stroke

C

NOC (Nursing Outcomes Classification)

Suggested NOC Outcomes

Bowel Continence; Bowel Elimination

Example NOC Outcome with Indicators

Bowel Continence as evidenced by the following indicators: Maintains predictable pattern of stool evacuation/Maintains control of stool passage/Evacuates stool at least every 3 days. (Rate the outcome and indicators of **Bowel Continence:** 1 = never demonstrated, 2 = rarely demonstrated, 3 = sometimes demonstrated, 4 = often demonstrated, 5 = consistently demonstrated [see Section I].)

Client Outcomes

Client Will (Specify Time Frame)

- Have regular, complete evacuation of fecal contents from the rectal vault (pattern may vary from every day to every 3 days)
- Have regulation of stool consistency (soft, formed stools)
- Reduce or eliminate frequency of incontinent episodes
- Exhibit intact skin in the perianal/perineal area
- Demonstrate the ability to isolate, contract, and relax pelvic muscles (when incontinence related to sphincter incompetence or high-tone pelvic floor dysfunction)
- Increase pelvic muscle strength (when incontinence related to sphincter incompetence)
- Identify triggers that precipitate change in bowel continence

NIC (Nursing Interventions Classification)

Suggested NIC Interventions

Bowel Incontinence Care; Bowel Incontinence Care: Encopresis; Bowel Training

Example NIC Interventions—Bowel Incontinence Care

Determine physical or psychological cause of fecal incontinence; Instruct client/family to record fecal output, as appropriate

Nursing Interventions and *Rationales*

- In a private setting, directly question client about the presence of fecal incontinence. If the client reports altered bowel elimination patterns, problems with bowel control, or "uncontrollable diarrhea," complete a focused nursing history including previous and present bowel elimination routines, dietary history, frequency and volume of uncontrolled stool loss, and aggravating and alleviating factors. EB: *Unless questioned directly or the client is experiencing bothersome fecal incontinence, clients are often hesitant or withhold reporting the presence of fecal incontinence (Menees et al, 2018). The nursing history determines the patterns of stool elimination, to characterize involuntary stool loss and the possible causation of the incontinence (Yates, 2018).*
- Recognize that risk factors for fecal incontinence include older individuals, female sex, impaired mobility, cognitive impairment, obesity, individuals who have undergone pelvic surgery, diabetes, and structural or functional impairment of bowel function and medications (Young et al, 2017; Menees et al, 2018). *Although fecal incontinence is more common in women, it is also a problem for men and should not be overlooked when obtaining a health history. Men are more likely to report increased frequency of stool leakage episodes compared with women (Young et al, 2017; Menees et al, 2018).*
- Physiological changes of the female pelvis that occur with aging, along with those that occur with childbirth and anoreceptive intercourse increase the risk of elimination problems, both constipation and

incontinence (Young et al, 2017; Brown et al, 2020). EBN: *While most people associate incontinence automatically with urinary incontinence, it is often forgotten that at least 1 out of 10 women suffers from fecal incontinence as well who are over the age of 20 (Gass et al, 2019).*

- Recognize that additional risk factors for bowel incontinence in hospitalized clients include antibiotic therapy, medications, enteral feeding, indwelling urinary catheter placement, immobility, inability to communicate elimination needs, acute disease processes and procedures (e.g., cancer, abdominal surgery), sedation, and mechanical ventilation (Eman & Lohrmann, 2015; Pitta et al, 2019).
- ▲ Conduct a health history assessment that includes a review of current bowel patterns/habits, including constipation and use of laxatives; diarrhea; pelvic floor injury with childbirth; acute trauma to organs, muscles, or nerves involved in defecation; gastrointestinal inflammatory disorders; functional disability; and medications (Whitehead et al, 2016; Musa et al, 2019).
- Closely inspect the perineal skin and skinfolds for evidence of skin breakdown in clients with incontinence. EBN: *An expert consensus statement defined moisture-associated skin damage as inflammation and erosion of the skin caused by prolonged exposure to various sources of moisture (Coyer et al, 2017; McNichol et al, 2018). Incontinence-associated dermatitis (IAD) is a form of skin irritation that develops from chronic exposure to urine or liquid stool (Bliss et al, 2015; Coyer et al, 2017; McNichol et al, 2018). A recent meta-analysis found a strong association between IAD and a client developing a pressure ulcer (Manderlier et al, 2019).*
- Use a validated tool that focuses on bowel elimination patterns. EB: *Valid and reliable assessment tools help provide a clearer understanding of the client's individual challenges and perceptions of symptoms associated with fecal incontinence (Brown et al, 2020; McNichol et al, 2018).*
- Complete a focused physical assessment, including inspection of perineal skin, pelvic muscle strength assessment, digital examination of the rectum for the presence of impaction and anal sphincter strength, and evaluation of functional status (mobility, dexterity, and visual acuity).
- Complete an assessment of cognitive function; explore for a history of dementia, delirium, or acute confusion (Bliss et al, 2015; Blekken et al, 2018). EBN: *A study found that critically ill clients who were less cognitively aware were 50% more likely to develop IAD than clients who were more cognitively aware (Bliss et al, 2015; McNichol et al, 2018).*
- Document patterns of stool elimination and incontinent episodes through a bowel record, including frequency of bowel movements, stool consistency, frequency and severity of incontinent episodes, precipitating factors, and dietary and fluid intake. EB: *Documented patterns of elimination are used to narrow the likely etiology of stool incontinence and serve as a baseline to evaluate treatment efficacy (Rao et al, 2016; Yates, 2018).*
- Assess stool consistency and its influence on risk for stool loss. Several classification systems for stool exist and may assist the nurse and client to differentiate among normal soft, formed stool, hardened stools associated with constipation, and liquid stools associated with diarrhea. EB/EBN: *A study of stool consistency found good reliability when evaluated by nurses and clients. Word-only descriptors yielded equivocal consistency when assessed by subjects, as did tools that combined words with illustrations of various stool consistencies (Bliss et al, 2015). Less well-formed (loose or liquid) stool is associated with an increased severity and frequency of fecal incontinence episodes and potential for compromised skin integrity (Bliss et al, 2015; Beeckman, 2017; Coyer et al, 2017; Yates, 2018).*
- Identify conditions contributing to or causing fecal incontinence. *Fecal incontinence is frequently multifactorial. Accurate assessment of the probable etiology of fecal incontinence is necessary to select a treatment plan likely to control or eliminate the condition (Yates, 2018; Pitta et al, 2019).*
- Improve access to toileting:
  - Identify usual toileting patterns and plan opportunities for toileting accordingly.
  - Provide assistance with toileting for clients with limited access or impaired functional status (mobility, dexterity, and access).
  - Institute a prompted toileting program for persons with impaired cognitive status.
  - Provide adequate privacy for toileting.
  - Respond promptly to requests for assistance with toileting.

  EB: *Acute or transient fecal incontinence frequently occurs in the acute care or long-term care facility secondary to cognition changes, mentation changes associated with environment change, inadequate access to toileting facilities, insufficient assistance with toileting, inability to perform activities of daily living, or inadequate privacy when attempting to toilet (Blekken et al, 2016; Musa et al, 2019).*
- Review the client's nutritional history and evaluate methods to normalize stool consistency with dietary adjustments (e.g., avoiding high-fat foods) and use of fiber along with assessing for use of caffeine, lactose,

and sugar replacements (Paquette et al, 2017; Da Silva & Sirany, 2019; International Foundation for Functional Gastrointestinal Disorders [IFFGD], 2019; O'Donnell, 2020). EB: *Diet modifications have been found to be helpful in the management of fecal incontinence, including restrictions of some foods, adding fiber to the diet, and establishing consistent eating patterns (National Institute for Diabetes and Digestive and Kidney Diseases, 2017; Da Silva & Sirany, 2019; O'Donnell, 2020).*

- Encourage the client to keep a nutrition log to track foods that irritate the bowel (Paquette et al, 2017).
- For hospitalized clients with tube feeding–associated fecal incontinence, involve the nutrition specialist to evaluate the formula composition, osmolality, and fiber content.
- For the client with intermittent episodes of fecal incontinence related to acute changes in stool consistency, begin a bowel reeducation program consisting of the following:
  - Cleansing the bowel of impacted stool if indicated
  - Normalizing stool consistency by adequate intake of fluids (30 mL/kg of body weight per day) and dietary or supplemental fiber
  - Establishing a regular routine of fecal elimination based on established patterns of bowel elimination (patterns established before onset of incontinence)

  EB: *Education on bowel patterns and strategies to establish normal defecation patterns and stool consistency to reduce or eliminate the risk of recurring fecal incontinence have been found to be beneficial in controlling fecal incontinence associated with changes in stool consistency (NHS Choices Information, 2018; IFFGD, 2019).*
- Implement a scheduled stimulation defecation program for persons with neurological conditions causing fecal incontinence:
  - Cleanse the bowel of impacted fecal material before beginning the program.
  - Implement strategies to normalize stool consistency, including adequate intake of fluid and fiber and avoidance of foods associated with diarrhea.
  - Determine a regular schedule for bowel elimination (typically every day or every other day) based on prior patterns of bowel elimination.
  - Provide a stimulus before assisting the client to a position on the toilet; digital stimulation, a stimulating suppository, "mini-enema," or pulsed evacuation enema may be used for stimulation.

  EB: *The scheduled, stimulated program relies on consistency of stool and a mechanical or chemical stimulus to produce a bolus contraction of the rectum with evacuation of fecal material (Duelund-Jakobsen et al, 2016; Paquette et al, 2017).*
- Begin a reeducation or pelvic floor muscle exercise program for the person with sphincter incompetence or high-tone pelvic floor muscle dysfunction of the pelvic muscles, or refer persons with fecal incontinence related to sphincter dysfunction to a nurse specialist or other therapist with clinical expertise in these techniques of care. EB: *Although evidence of overall effectiveness of pelvic floor muscle exercise programs is inconclusive as a treatment strategy for fecal incontinence, the programs are not harmful (Brown et al, 2020).*
- ▲ Consider a sacral nerve stimulation program in clients with urgency to defecate and fecal incontinence related to weakened sphincter muscles or sphincter defect. EB: *Sacral nerve stimulation has been found to significantly reduce incontinence for some clients (Da Silva & Sirany, 2019; Brown et al, 2020).*
- Institute a structured skin care regimen that incorporates three essential steps: cleanse, moisturize, and protect:
  - Select a cleanser with a pH range comparable to that of normal skin (usually labeled "pH balanced").
  - Moisturize with an emollient to replace lipids removed with cleansing and protect with a skin. Products containing petrolatum, dimethicone, or zinc oxide base or a no-sting skin barrier should be used.
  - Routine incontinence care should include daily perineal skin cleansing and after each episode of incontinence.
  - When feasible, select a product that combines two or all three of these processes into a single step. Ensure that products are available at the bedside when caring for a client with total incontinence in an inpatient facility.
- Use of absorptive pads or adult containment briefs that are applied next to the client's skin increases the risk of IAD. Absorbent underpads that wick moisture away from skin may be used with immobile clients. EB/EBN: *A structured skin care regimen based on a three-step process (cleanse, moisturize, and protect) is effective for the prevention of IAD (Gray et al, 2016; Beeckman, 2017; Coyer et al, 2017; Manderlier et al, 2019).*

C

- ▲ Consult the provider if a fungal infection is suspected. An antifungal cream or powder beneath a protective ointment may be indicated (Gray et al, 2016; Coyer et al, 2017).
- • Assist the client to select and apply a containment device for occasional episodes of fecal incontinence. A fecal containment device will prevent soiling of clothing and reduce odors in the client with uncontrolled stool loss. EBN: *A study of community persons with fecal incontinence who used an absorptive dressing to contain mucus and stool leakage after surgery revealed that the device was preferred over traditional pads by 92% (Bliss et al, 2015).*
- • In the client with frequent episodes of fecal incontinence and limited mobility, monitor the sacrum and perineal area for pressure ulcerations. EBN: *Limited mobility, particularly when combined with fecal incontinence and increased moisture, increases the risk of pressure ulceration. Routine cleansing, pressure reduction techniques, and management of fecal and urinary incontinence reduce this risk (Beeckman, 2017; Manderlier et al, 2019).*
- • With acutely ill clients, anticipate and evaluate the cause of acute diarrhea. Anticipate diarrhea associated with treatment or specific interventions (e.g., medications, initiation of tube feedings). *Interventions to manage acute diarrhea include use of absorbent pads and skin protectant moisturizers or fecal collector/pouch (Beeckman, 2017; Pather et al, 2017).*
- ▲ Consult a provider or the standing orders before inserting a bowel management system (BMS) in the critically ill client when conservative measures have failed and fecal incontinence is excessive and/or produces perianal skin injury or IAD. *Indwelling BMSs, also called fecal management systems (FMSs), are commercially available and designed to direct, collect, and contain liquid stool in immobile clients. BMS devices are approved by the Food and Drug Administration for up to 29 days for management of liquid stool (Da Silva & Sirany, 2019).* EBN: *Devices other than BMSs should not be used for indwelling bowel/feces diversion (Da Silva & Sirany, 2019).*

Geriatric

- • Evaluate all older clients for established or acute fecal incontinence when the older client enters the acute or long-term care facility and intervene as indicated. EB: *Fecal incontinence often coexists with urinary incontinence, necessitating evidence-based interventions to prevent skin breakdown and/or pressure ulcer development in the older client (Shahin & Lohrmann, 2015; Blekken et al, 2018; McNichol et al, 2018).*
- • Determine the client's cognitive level using a screening tool such as the Mini-Mental State Exam (MMSE), Montreal Cognitive Assessment (MoCA), the Confusion Assessment Method (CAM), or Mini-Cog. EB: *Use of a standard evaluation tool such as the MMSE or MoCA can help determine the client's abilities and assist in planning appropriate nursing interventions. Acute or established dementias increase the risk of fecal incontinence among older adults (Jerez-Roig et al, 2015; Trzepacz et al, 2015).*
- • Teach nursing colleagues, nonprofessional care providers, family, and clients the importance of providing toileting opportunities and adequate privacy for the client in an acute or long-term care facility.

Home Care

- • The preceding interventions may be adapted for home care use.
- • Assess and teach a bowel management program to support continence. Address timing, diet, fluids, and actions taken independently to deal with bowel incontinence. *Identifying factors that change level of incontinence may guide interventions. If the client has been taking over-the-counter medications or home remedies, it is important to consider their influence.*
- • Instruct the caregiver to provide clothing that is nonrestrictive, can be manipulated easily for toileting, and can be changed with ease. *Avoidance of complicated maneuvers increases the chance of success in toileting programs and decreases the client's risk for embarrassing incontinent episodes.*
- • Evaluate self-care strategies of community-dwelling older adults, strengthen adaptive behaviors, and counsel older adults about altering strategies that compromise general health.
- • Assist the family in arranging care in a way that allows the client to participate in family or favorite activities without embarrassment. *Careful planning can both help the client retain dignity and maintain integrity of family patterns.*
- ▲ If the client is limited to bed (or bed and chair), provide a commode or bedpan that can be easily accessed. Involve occupational and physical therapy services as indicated to promote safe transfers.
- ▲ If the client is frequently incontinent, refer for home health aide services to assist with hygiene and skin care.
- ▲ Refer the family to support services to assist with in-home management of fecal incontinence as indicated.
- • Refer to care plans for **Diarrhea** and **Constipation** for detailed management of these related conditions.

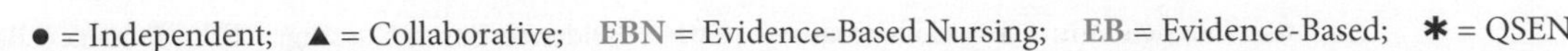

C

REFERENCES

Beeckman, D. (2017). A decade of research on incontinence-associated dermatitis (IAD): Evidence, knowledge gaps and next steps. *Journal of Tissue Viability*, *26*(1), 47–56. https://doi.org/10.1016/j.jtv.2016.02.004.

Blekken, L. E., Vinsnes, A. G., Gjeilo, K. H., & Bliss, D. Z. (2018). Management of fecal incontinence in older adults in long-term care. In D. Z. Bliss (Ed.), *Management of fecal incontinence for the advanced practice nurse* (pp. 149–169). New York: Springer. https://doi.org/10.1007/978-3-319-90704-8_8.

Blekken, L. E., Vinsnes, A. G., Gjeilo, K. H., et al. (2016). Exploring faecal incontinence in nursing home patients: A cross-sectional study of prevalence and associations derived from the Residents assessment Instrument for long term care facilities. *Journal of Advanced Nursing*, *72*(7), 1579–1591. https://doi.org/10.1111/jan.1293.

Bliss, D. Z., Funk, T., Jacobson, M., & Savik, K. (2015). Incidence and characteristics of incontinence-associated dermatitis in community-dwelling persons with fecal incontinence. *Journal of Wound, Ostomy and Continence Nursing*, *42*(5), 525–530. https://doi.org/10.1097/WON.0000000000000159.

Brown, H. W., Dyer, K. Y., & Rogers, R. G. (2020). Management of fecal incontinence. *Obstetrics & Gynecology*, *136*(4), 811–822. https://doi.org/10.1097/AOG.0000000000004054.

Coyer, F., Gardner, A., & Doubrovsky, A. (2017). An interventional skin care protocol (InSPiRE) to reduce incontinence-associated dermatitis in critically ill patients in the intensive care unit: A before and after study. *Intensive and Critical Care Nursing*, *40*, 1–10. https://doi.org/10.1016/j.iccn.2016.12.001.

Da Silva, G., & Sirany, A. (2019). *Recent advances in managing fecal incontinence*. F1000Research [online], 8, F1000 Faculty Rev-1291. https://doi.org/10.12688/f1000research.15270.2.

Duelund-Jakobsen, J., Worsoe, J., Lundby, L., Christensen, P., & Krogh, K. (2016). Management of patients with faecal incontinence. *Therapeutic Advances in Gastroenterology*, *9*(1), 86–97. https://doi.org/10.1177/1756283X15614516.

Eman, S. M., & Lohrmann, C. (2015). Prevalence of fecal and double fecal and urinary incontinence in hospitalized patients. *Journal of Wound, Ostomy and Continence Nursing*, *42*(1), 89–93. https://doi.org/10.1097/WON.0000000000000082.

Gass, F., Kuhn, M., Koening, I., Radlinger, L., & Koehler, B. (2019). Development of an ICF-based questionnaire for urinary and/or fecal incontinence (ICF-IAF): The female patients' perspective using focus groups (subproject). *Neurourology and Urodynamics*, *38*(6), 1657–1662. https://doi.org/10.1002/nau.24031.

Gray, M., McNickol, L., & Nix, D. (2016). Incontinence-associated dermatitis progress, promises, and ongoing challenges. *Journal of Wound, Ostomy and Continence Nursing*, *43*(2), 188–192. https://doi.org/10.1097/WON.0000000000000217.

International Foundation for Functional Gastrointestinal Disorders. (2019). *Diet strategies for managing chronic diarrhea*. Retrieved from https://www.iffgd.org/lower-gi-disorders/diarrhea/nutrition-strategies.html. Accessed 14 June 2021.

Jerez-Roig, J., Souza, D., Amaral, F., & Lima, K. C. (2015). Prevalence of fecal incontinence (FI) and associated factors in institutionalized older adults. *Archives of Gerontology and Geriatrics*, *60*(3), 425–430. https://doi.org/10.1016/j.archger.2015.02.003.

Manderlier, B., Van Damme, N., Verhaeghe, S., et al. (2019). Modifiable patient-related factors associated with pressure ulcers on the sacrum and heels: Secondary data analyses. *Journal of Advanced Nursing*, *75*(11), 2773–2785. https://doi.org/10.1111/jan.14149.

McNichol, L. L., Ayello, E. A., Phearman, L. A., Pezzella, P. A., & Culver, E. A. (2018). Incontinence-associated dermatitis: State of the science and knowledge translation. *Advances in Skin & Wound Care*, *31*(11), 502–513. https://doi.org/10.1097/01.ASW.0000546234.12260.61.

Menees, S. B., Almario, C. V., Spiegel, B. M., & Chey, W. D. (2018). Prevalence of and factors associated with fecal incontinence: Results from a population-based survey. *Gastroenterology*, *154*(6), 1672–1681.e3. https://doi.org/10.1053/j.gastro.2018.01.062.

Musa, M. K., Saga, S., Blekken, L. E., Harris, R., Goodman, C., & Norton, C. (2019). The prevalence, incidence, and correlates of fecal incontinence among older people residing in care homes: A systematic review. *Journal of the American Medical Directors Association*, *20*(8), 956–962. https://doi.org/10.1016/j.jamda.2019.03.033.

National Institute for Diabetes and Digestive and Kidney Diseases. (2017). *Treatment of fecal incontinence*. Retrieved from https://www.niddk.nih.gov/health-information/digestive-diseases/bowel-control-problems-fecal-incontinence/treatment. Accessed 14 June 2021.

NHS Choices Information. (2018). *Bowel incontinence: Treatment*. Retrieved from http://www.nhs.uk/Conditions/Incontinence-bowel/Pages/Treatment.aspx. Accessed 14 June 2021.

O'Donnell, K. F. (2020). Fecal incontinence: A stepwise approach to primary care management. *The Journal for Nurse Practitioners*, *16*(8), 586–589. https://doi.org/10.1016/j.nurpra.2020.05.006.

Paquette, I. M., Varma, M. G., Kaiser, A. M., Steele, S. R., & Rafferty, J. F. (2017). The American Society of Colon and Rectal Surgeons' clinical practice guideline for the treatment of fecal incontinence. *Diseases of the Colon & Rectum*, *58*(7), 623–636. https://doi.org/10.1097/DCR.0000000000000397.

Pather, P., Hines, S., Kynoch, K., & Coyer, F. (2017). Effectiveness of topical skin products in the treatment and prevention of incontinence-associated dermatitis: A systematic review. *JBI Database of Systematic Reviews and Implementation Reports*, *15*(5), 1473–1496. https://doi.org/10.11124/JBISRIR-2016-003015.

Pitta, M. R., Campos, F. M., Monteiro, A. G., Cunha, A. F., Porto, J. D., & Gomes, R. R. (2019). Tutorial on diarrhea and enteral nutrition: A comprehensive step-by-step approach. *Journal of Parenteral and Enteral Nutrition*, *43*(8), 1008–1019. https://doi.org/10.1002/jpen.1674.

Rao, S. C., Bharucha, A. E., Chiarioni, G., et al. (2016). Anorectal disorders. *Gastroenterology*, *150*(6), 1430–1442. https://doi.org/10.1053/j.gastro.2016.02.009.

Shahin, E. S. M., & Lohrmann, C. (2015). Prevalence of fecal and double fecal and urinary incontinence in hospitalized patients. *Journal of Wound, Ostomy and Continence Nursing*, *42*(1), 89–93.

Trzepacz, P. T., Hochstetler, H., Wong, S., Walker, B., Saykin, A. J., & Alzheimer's Disease Neuroimaging Initiative. (2015). Relationship between the Montreal Cognitive Assessment and Mini-Mental State Examination for assessment of mild cognitive impairment in older adults. *BMC Geriatrics*, *15*, 107. https://doi.org/10.1186/s12877-015-0103-3.

Whitehead, W. E., Palsson, O. S., & Simren, M. (2016). Treating fecal incontinence: An unmet need in primary care medicine. *North Carolina Medical Journal*, *77*(3), 211–215.

Yates, A. (2018). How to perform a comprehensive baseline continence assessment. *Nursing Times*, *114*(5), 26–29. Retrieved from https://www.nursingtimes.net/clinical-archive/continence/how-to-perform-a-comprehensive-baseline-continence-assessment-16-04-2018/. Accessed 14 June 2021.

Young, C. J., Zahid, A., Koh, C. E., & Young, J. M. (2017). Hypothesized summative anal physiology score correlates but poorly predicts incontinence severity. *World Journal of Gastroenterology*, *23*(31), 5732–5738.

Risk for Adverse Reaction to Iodinated Contrast Media Domain 11 Safety/protection Class 5 Defensive processes

Pauline McKinney Green, PhD, RN, CNE

NANDA-I

Definition

Susceptible to noxious or unintended reaction that can occur within seven days after contrast agent injection, which may compromise health.

Risk Factors

Dehydration; generalized weakness

At-Risk Population

Individuals at extremes of age; individuals with history of adverse effect from iodinated contrast media; individuals with a history of allergy

Associated Conditions

Chronic disease; concurrent use of pharmaceutical preparations; decreased level of consciousness; individuals with fragile veins

NOC (Nursing Outcomes Classification)

Suggested NOC Outcomes

Tissue Perfusion: Renal; Kidney Function

Example NOC Outcome with Indicators

Kidney Function as evidenced by 24-hour intake and output balance/Blood urea nitrogen/Serum creatinine/Urine color/Serum electrolytes. (Rate the outcome and indicators of **Kidney Function:** 1 = severely compromised, 2 = substantially compromised, 3 = moderately compromised, 4 = mildly compromised, 5 = not compromised [see Section I].)

Client Outcomes

Client Will (Specify Time Frame)

- Maintain normal blood urea nitrogen and serum creatinine levels
- Maintain urine output of 0.5 mL/kg/hr
- Maintain serum electrolytes (K^+, PO_4, Na^+) within normal limits

NIC (Nursing Interventions Classification)

Suggested NIC Interventions

Fluid/Electrolyte Management; Laboratory Data Interpretation

Example NIC Activities—Fluid/Electrolyte Management

Monitor for serum electrolytes levels, as available; Weigh daily and monitor trends; Monitor vital signs, as appropriate

Nursing Interventions and *Rationales*

Recognize that iodinated contrast media can be harmful to clients in a number of ways, including onset of contrast-induced nephropathy (CIN), allergic reactions to the dye, and damage to veins and vascular access devices.

Contrast-Induced Nephropathy

Protect clients from contrast media-induced nephropathy by taking the following actions:

- ● Advocate for high-risk clients who are prone to develop contrast-induced acute kidney injury.
- ● Assess client's baseline kidney function, including serum creatinine, creatinine clearance, estimated glomerular filtration rate, and blood urea nitrogen (Nahar, 2017). EB: *Baseline renal values are critical for comparison purposes following contrast media; estimated glomerular filtration rate is a biomarker for CIN risk (American College of Radiology, 2021).*
- ▲ Assess clients for risk factors for adverse reactions to contrast media: preexisting renal insufficiency, diabetes mellitus, dehydration, cardiovascular disease, diuretic use, advanced age, multiple myeloma, hypertension, hyperuricemia, multiple doses of iodinated contrast media in less than 24 hours (American College of Radiology, 2021).
- ● Communicate information about at-risk clients to provider and procedure team in the hand-off report and electronic medical record. EBN: *A study of clients undergoing percutaneous coronary interventions with contrast media demonstrated significant reduction in acute kidney injury rates when evidence-based practices in nursing were introduced/standardized (Lambert et al, 2017).*
- ▲ Ensure that clients having diagnostic testing with contrast are well hydrated with isotonic intravenous (IV) fluids for volume expansion as ordered before and after the examination. EB: *Incidence of CIN is reduced by IV hydration with isotonic fluids (lactated Ringer's solution or 0.9% normal saline) before and after IV contrast administration (American College of Radiology, 2021).*
- ▲ Assess clients with symptoms of heart failure on an individual basis to determine tolerance for IV fluids used for hydration in the periprocedure period (Lambert et al, 2017).
- ▲ Monitor for and report signs of acute kidney injury for 48 hours after iodinated contrast administration in clients at risk: absolute serum creatinine increase ≥0.3 mg/dL, percentage increase in serum creatinine ≥50%, or urine output reduced to ≤0.5 mL/kg/hr for at least 6 hours. (Refer to your institution policy for specific clinical parameters.) *These clinical parameters are suggestive of acute kidney injury (Mehta et al, 2007; American College of Radiology, 2021).*
- ▲ Clients known to have acute kidney injury who are taking metformin should temporarily discontinue its use at the time of or before the procedure using contrast media, withhold metformin for 48 hours following, and reinstitute use only when renal function is found to be normal (Rose & Choi, 2015; American College of Radiology, 2021).

Allergic Reaction to Contrast Media

- ▲ Previous allergic reactions to contrast material, history of asthma, and other allergies are factors that may increase the client's risk of developing an adverse reaction. Discuss premedication with prednisone, methylprednisolone, or hydrocortisone with the provider for clients who have had previous reactions to contrast media or known asthma or allergies. EB: *Premedication may reduce the incidence of allergic reaction in some clients (Wang & Soloff, 2020; American College of Radiology, 2021).*
- ● Monitor carefully for symptoms of a hypersensitivity reaction, which can be mild, moderate, or severe. Report all symptoms to the provider because symptoms can advance rapidly from mild to severe.
    - ❍ *Mild reactions:* Nausea, vomiting, headache, itchy throat or eyes, flushing, mild skin rash, or hives.
    - ❍ *Moderate reactions:* Diffuse skin rash or hives, itchiness, erythema, wheezing but no hypoxia, facial edema but no dyspnea, throat tightness but no dyspnea.
    - ❍ *Severe reactions:* Diffuse hives with hypotension, diffuse itchiness or erythema with hypotension, diffuse edema including facial edema, wheezing with hypoxia, laryngeal edema with stridor and or hypoxia, anaphylactic shock (hypotension and tachycardia).
    - ❍ *Both allergic and allergic-like (anaphylactoid) reactions can occur. Life-threatening events usually occur within 20 minutes after injection. Delayed reactions may occur with rash that appears hours or days afterward (American College of Radiology, 2021).*

Vein Damage and Damage to Vascular Access Devices

- ● Recognize that *only* vascular access devices labeled "power injectable" can be used to administer power-injected contrast media. These include a power port, a power peripherally inserted central catheter (PICC) line, and a power central venous catheter (UCSF Department of Radiology and Biomedical Imaging, 2020a). *A regular vascular access device used for administration of contrast media can rupture from the high pressures used to administer the contrast media.*

- Reduce the risk of vein and vascular access device damage with the following:
  - Maintain constant communication with the client during the injection and monitor client for report of pain or swelling at the injection site, paresthesia, or tenderness. *These are signs of complications that require the injection to be discontinued (American College of Radiology, 2021).*
  - Monitor access site for extravasation during and after the procedure; be vigilant for clients at increased risk of extravasation. *Clients at increased risk include those who cannot communicate, such as infants, older adults, or those with altered consciousness; severely ill or debilitated clients; clients with abnormal circulation in the affected limb; clients receiving the injection via a peripheral IV line that has been in place for more than 24 hours or into a vein that has been punctured multiple times; and clients with arterial insufficiency or compromised venous or lymphatic drainage in the affected extremity (American College of Radiology, 2021).*
  - Assess for venous backflow before injecting contrast. *If backflow is not obtained, the catheter may need adjustment (American College of Radiology, 2021).*
  - Directly monitor and palpate the venipuncture site during the first 15 seconds of injection. *A critical step in preventing significant extravasation is direct monitoring of the venipuncture site (American College of Radiology, 2021).*

C

Geriatric

- Screen the older client thoroughly before diagnostic testing using contrast media. *Adults over 60 years of age are considered at risk for acute adverse reactions to contrast media (Beckett, Moriority, & Langer, 2015).*

Pediatric

- Contrast medium can be safely administered intravenously by power injector at high flow rates of up to 2 mL/second (depending on size of client). A short peripheral IV catheter in the antecubital or forearm is the preferred route for intravenous contrast administration (UCSF Department of Radiology and Biomedical Imaging, 2020b). *Neonates and small children are especially susceptible to fluid shifts and have lower tolerance for intravascular osmotic loads compared with adults (American College of Radiology, 2021).* EB: *A retrospective study of pediatric clients who underwent computed tomography scan with iodinated contrast media injection found CIN incidents of 10.3% and 30-day unfavorable outcomes in 45.8% of clients (Cantais et al, 2016).*

Client/Family Teaching and Discharge Teaching

✱ Discharge instructions should include the importance of self-hydration after the procedure; reporting of symptoms of fluid retention or decrease in urine output; identifying which medications to take, withhold, or discontinue; scheduling laboratory evaluation 48 to 72 hours after the procedure; and scheduling follow-up with the provider (Lambert et al, 2017). *Client education contributes to client safety and greater compliance with self-care measures.*

REFERENCES

American College of Radiology. (2021). *ACR manual on contrast media.* Retrieved from https://www.acr.org/-/media/ACR/files/clinical-resources/contrast_media.pdf. Accessed 14 June 2021.

Beckett, K. R., Moriority, A. K., & Langer, J. M. (2015). Safe use of contrast media: What the radiologist needs to know. *RadioGraphics, 35*(6), 1738–1750. https://doi.org/10.1148/rg.2015150033.

Cantais, A., Hammouda, Z., Mory, O., et al. (2016). Incidence of contrast-induced acute kidney injury in a pediatric setting: A cohort study. *Pediatric Nephrology, 31*(8), 1355–1362. https://doi.org/10.1007/s0047-016-3313-9.

Lambert, P., Chaisson, K., Horton, S., et al. (2017). Reducing acute kidney injury due to contrast material: How nurses can improve patient safety. *Critical Care Nurse, 37*(1), 13–26. https://doi.org/10.4037/ccn2017178.

Mehta, R. L., Kellum, J. A., Shah, S. V., et al. (2007). Acute Kidney Injury Network: Report of an initiative to improve outcomes in acute kidney injury. *Critical Care, 11*(2), R31. https://doi.org/10.1186/cc5713.

Nahar, D. (2017). Prophylactic management of contrast-induced kidney injury in high-risk patients. *Nephrology Nursing Journal, 43*(3), 244–249.

Rose, T. A., Jr., & Choi, J. W. (2015). Intravenous imaging contrast media complications: The basics that every clinician needs to know. *American Journal of Medicine, 128*(9), 943–949. https://doi.org/10.1016/j.amjmed.2015.02.018.

UCSF Department of Radiology and Biomedical Imaging. (2020a). *Vascular access and use of central lines and ports in adults.* University of California San Francisco. Retrieved from ht tps://radiology.ucsf.edu/patient-care/patient-safety/contrast/iodinated/vascular-access-adults. Accessed 14 June 2021.

UCSF Department of Radiology and Biomedical Imaging. (2020b). *Vascular access and use of central lines and ports in pediatrics.* University of California San Francisco. Retrieved from https://radiology.ucsf.edu/patient-care/patient-safety/contrast/iodinated/vacular-access-pediatrics. Accessed 14 June 2021.

Wang, C. L., & Soloff, E. V. (2020). Contrast reaction readiness for your department or facility. *Radiology Clinics of North America, 58*(5), 841–850. https://doi.org/10.1016/jrcl.2020.04.002.

Readiness for Enhanced Community Coping

Domain 9 Coping/stress tolerance Class 2 Coping responses

Marina Martinez-Kratz, MS, RN, CNE

C

NANDA-I

Definition

A pattern of community activities for adaptation and problem-solving for meeting the demands or needs of the community, which can be strengthened.

Defining Characteristics

Expresses desire to enhance availability of community recreation programs; expresses desire to enhance availability of community relaxation programs; expresses desire to enhance communication among community members; expresses desire to enhance communication between groups and larger community; expresses desire to enhance community planning for predictable stressors; expresses desire to enhance community resources for managing stressors; expresses desire to enhance community responsibility for stress management; expresses desire to enhance problem-solving for identified issue

NOC (Nursing Outcomes Classification)

Suggested NOC Outcomes

Community Competence; Community Health Status

Example NOC Outcome with Indicators

Community Health Status as evidenced by the following indicators: Prevalence of health promotion programs, health status of infants, children, adolescents, adults, elders, participation rates in community health programs. (Rate the outcome and indicators of **Community Health Status:** 1 = poor, 2 = fair, 3 = good, 4 = very good, 5 = excellent [see Section I].)

Community Outcomes

Community Will (Specify Time Frame)

- Develop enhanced coping strategies
- Maintain effective coping strategies for management of stress

NIC (Nursing Interventions Classification)

Suggested NIC Interventions

Environmental Management: Community; Health Policy Monitoring: Program Development

Example NIC Activities—Program Development

Assist the group or community in identifying significant health needs or problems; Identify alternative approaches to address the need(s) or problem(s)

Nursing Interventions and *Rationales*

Note: Interventions depend on the specific aspects of community coping that can be enhanced (e.g., planning for stress management, communication, development of community power, community perceptions of stress, community coping strategies).

▲ Establish a collaborative partnership with the community. EB: *A recent study found that counties whose Area Agencies for the Aging (AAAs) maintained informal partnerships with a broad range of organizations in health care and other sectors had significantly lower hospital readmission rates compared with counties whose AAAs had informal partnerships with fewer types of organizations (Brewster et al, 2018).*

- Assess community needs with the use of concept mapping methodology. EB: *The findings of a recent study showed that an integration of several concept mapping methods into a community engagement process was able to increase the input from a wide range of populations (Velonis et al, 2018).*
- Assess for the impact of social determinants of health on community health. EB: *A validated multivariate social determinants of health index score was used to accurately classify counties with high cardiovascular burden (Hong & Mainous, 2020).*

C

- Encourage participation in faith-based organizations that want to improve community stress management. EBN: *A recent study showed that coaching by faith community nurses created an environment of sustained support that promoted improved lifestyles and blood pressure changes over time (Cooper & Zimmerman, 2017).*
- ▲ Identify the health services and information resources that are currently available in the community through network analysis. EB: *A study found that network analysis served as a useful tool to evaluate community partnerships and facilitate coalition building (An et al, 2017).*
- Work with community members to increase problem-solving abilities. EBN: *Problem-solving is essential for effective coping. Findings from a recent study showed positive outcomes from a direct and tailored problem-solving training program (Easom et al, 2018).*
- Provide support to the community and help community members identify and mobilize additional supports. EB: *A community mobilization project demonstrated how cross-sector, coordinated efforts focused on vulnerable populations can leverage local strengths to establish and enhance breastfeeding support services customized to local needs (Colchamiro et al, 2015).*
- Advocate for the community in multiple arenas (e.g., multimedia, social media, and governmental agencies). EB: *A recent study explored how social media can help community organizations engage in advocacy work (Guo et al, 2018).*
- Work with communities to ensure that vulnerable individuals with access and functional needs are included in preparations for, response to, and recovery from disasters. EB: *Analysis of recent disasters has identified that a combination of strategic and operational methods, appropriate planning tools, and planning for the entire community will prevent individuals with access and functional needs from being disproportionately and negatively affected by disasters (Franks & Seaton, 2017).*
- Partner with community pharmacies to provide community education and health prevention services. EB: *A review of reviews found support for the development of community pharmacy health services focused on primary disease prevention (Thomson et al, 2019).*

Pediatric

- Protect children and adolescents from exposure to community violence. EB: *A systematic review found evidence for a positive association between community violence exposure and cardiovascular and sleep problems in children and adolescents (Wright et al, 2017).*
- Assess children and adolescents for the effects of direct and indirect crime exposure rather than only focusing solely on violent victimization. EB: *A study found poor behavioral health outcomes for adolescents with self-reported crime exposure (Grinshteyn et al, 2018).*

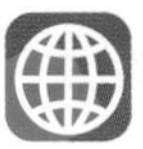

Multicultural

- Acknowledge the stressors unique to racial/ethnic communities. EB: *A recent study of Hispanic and African American women found that neighborhood context was an important factor in examining the determinants of health, survivorship, and quality of life outcomes among cancer clients (Wu et al, 2018).*
- Identify community strengths with community members. EBN: *A community-based participatory research approach was used to obtain Native American community input and identify strengths to address youth suicide and substance abuse. The results led to the development of a strengths-based intervention incorporating the Gathering of Native Americans curriculum (Holliday et al, 2018).*
- Use an empowerment approach to address health behaviors in diverse communities. An empowerment approach includes increasing clients' self-efficacy and capacity to make informed decisions about their health care. EB: *A recent study found use of an empowerment approach was effective in changing nonadherent Latinas' breast screening behaviors and promoting them to become agents of change in their communities (Molina et al, 2018). The empowerment intervention has three sessions focused on early detection, sharing information with family/friends, and health volunteerism.*

C

- • Work with members of the community to prioritize and target health goals specific to the community. EB: *Recent research found that members of underserved communities, in informed deliberations, prioritized research on quality of life, client-doctor, special needs, access, and compare approaches (Goold et al, 2017).*
- • Establish and sustain partnerships with key individuals within communities when developing and implementing programs. EB: *A study of community engagement strategies found the following techniques to be effective: proactively engaging stakeholders in informational meetings, webinars, social media, the promising practice process, and community advisory council meetings (D'Angelo et al, 2017).*
- • Use mentoring strategies for community members. EB: *A recent study showed parent mentors are highly effective in insuring uninsured Latino children and eliminating disparities (Flores et al, 2018).*
- • Use community church settings as a forum for advocacy, teaching, and program implementation. EBN: *A recent study found that trust, respect, open dialog with participants, and commitment to address community health needs contributed to successful engagement and recruitment of African American churches to serve as participants in cancer research projects (Slade et al, 2018).*

REFERENCES

An, R., Khan, N., Loehmer, E., & McCaffrey, J. (2017). Assessing the network of agencies in local communities that promote healthy eating and lifestyles among populations with limited resources. *American Journal of Health Behavior, 41*(2), 127–138.

Brewster, A. L., Kunkel, S., Straker, J., & Curry, L. A. (2018). Curry cross-sectoral partnerships by area agencies on aging: Associations with health care use and spending. *Health Affairs, 37*(1), 15–21 https://doi.org/10.1377/hlthaff.2017.1346.

Colchamiro, R., Edwards, R. A., Nordstrom, C., et al. (2015). Mobilizing community resources to enhance post discharge support for breastfeeding in Massachusetts (USA): Results of a catalyst grant approach. *Journal of Human Lactation, 31*(4), 631–640 https://doi.org/10.1177/089033441559768.

Cooper, J., & Zimmerman, W. (2017). The effect of a faith community nurse network and public health collaboration on hypertension prevention and control. *Public Health Nursing, 34*(5), 444–453 https://doi.org/10.1111/phn.12325.

D'Angelo, G., Pullmann, M. D., & Lyon, A. R. (2017). Community engagement strategies for implementation of a policy supporting evidence-based practices: A case study of Washington state. *Administration and Policy in Mental Health and Mental Health Services Research, 44*(1), 6–15 https://doi.org/10.1007/s10488-015-0664-7.

Easom, L. R., Wang, K., Moore, R. H., Wang, H., & Bauer, L. (2018). Operation family caregiver: Problem-solving training for military caregivers in a community setting. *Journal of Clinical Psychology, 74*(4), 536–553 https://doi.org/10.1002/jclp.22536.

Flores, G., Lin, H., Walker, C., et al. (2018). Parent mentoring program increases coverage rates for uninsured Latino children. *Health Affairs, 37*(3), 403–412 https://doi.org/10.1377/hlthaff.2017.1272.

Franks, S., & Seaton, E. (2017). Utilizing strategic and operational methods for whole-community disaster planning. *Disaster Medicine and Public Health Preparedness, 11*(6), 741–746 https://doi.org/10.1017/dmp.2017.6.

Goold, S. D., Myers, C. D., Szymecko, L., et al. (2017). Priorities for patient-centered outcomes research: The views of minority and underserved communities. *Health Services Research, 52*(2), 599–615 https://doi.org/10.1111/1475-6773.12505.

Grinshteyn, E. G., Xu, H., Manteuffel, B., & Ettner, S. L. (2018). The associations of area-level violent crime rates and self-reported violent crime exposure with adolescent behavioral health. *Community Mental Health Journal, 54*(3), 252–258 https://doi.org/10.1007/s10597-017-0159-y.

Guo, C., & Saxton, G. D. (2018). Speaking and being heard: How nonprofit advocacy organizations gain attention on social media. *Nonprofit and Voluntary Sector Quarterly, 47*(1), 5–26 https://doi.org/10.1177/0899764017713724.

Holliday, C. E., Wynne, M., Katz, J., Ford, C., & Barbosa-Leiker, C. (2018). A CBPR approach to finding community strengths and challenges to prevent youth suicide and substance abuse. *Journal of Transcultural Nursing, 29*(1), 64–73 https://doi.org/10.1177/1043659616679234.

Hong, Y. R., & Mainous, A. G., 3rd. (2020). Development and validation of a county-level social determinants of health risk assessment tool for cardiovascular disease. *The Annals of Family Medicine, 18*(4), 318–325 https://doi.org/10.1370/afm.2534.

Molina, Y., San Miguel, L. G., Tamayo, L., et al. (2018). Empowering Latinas to obtain breast cancer screenings: Comparing intervention effects, part 2. Cancer epidemiology, biomarkers & prevention. *A Publication of the American Association for Cancer Research, 27*(3), 353–354 https://doi.org/10.1158/1055-9965.EPI-18-0048.

Slade, J., Holt, C. L., Bowie, J., et al. (2018). Recruitment of African American churches to participate in cancer early detection interventions: A community perspective. *Journal of Religion and Health, 57*(2), 751–761 https://doi.org/10.1007/s10943-018-0586-2.

Thomson, K., Hillier-Brown, F., Walton, N., Bilaj, M., Bambra, C., & Todd, A. (2019). The effects of community pharmacy-delivered public health interventions on population health and health inequalities: A review of reviews. *Preventive Medicine, 124*, 98–109 https://doi.org/10.1016/j.ypmed.2019.04.003.

Velonis, A. J., Molnar, A., Lee-Foon, N., Rahim, A., Boushel, M., & O'Campo, P. (2018). "One program that could improve health in this neighbourhood is _?" Using concept mapping to engage communities as part of a health and human services needs assessment. *BMC Health Services Research, 18*(1), 150 https://doi.org/10.1186/s12913-018-2936-x.

Wright, A. W., Austin, M., Booth, C., & Kliewer, W. (2017). Systematic review: Exposure to community violence and physical health outcomes in youth. *Journal of Pediatric Psychology, 42*(4), 364–378 https://doi.org/10.1093/jpepsy/jsw088.

Wu, C., Ashing, K. T., Jones, V. C., & Barcelo, L. (2018). The association of neighborhood context with health outcomes among ethnic minority breast cancer survivors. *Journal of Behavioral Medicine, 41*(1), 52–61 https://doi/10.1007/s10865-017-9875-6.

Defensive Coping Domain 9 Coping/stress tolerance Class 2 Coping responses

Arlene T. Farren, PhD, RN, AOCN, CTN-A

C

NANDA-I

Definition

Repeated projection of falsely positive self-evaluation based on a self-protective pattern that defends against underlying perceived threats to positive self-regard.

Defining Characteristics

Altered reality testing; denies problems; denies weaknesses; difficulty establishing interpersonal relations; difficulty maintaining interpersonal relations; grandiosity; hostile laughter; hypersensitivity to a discourtesy; hypersensitivity to criticism; inadequate follow through with treatment regimen; inadequate participation in treatment regimen; projection of blame; projection of responsibility; rationalization of failures; reality distortion; ridicules others; superior attitude toward others

Related Factors

Conflict between self-perception and value system; fear of failure; fear of humiliation; fear of repercussions; inadequate confidence in others; inadequate psychological resilience; inadequate self-confidence; inadequate social support; uncertainty; unrealistic self-expectations

NOC (Nursing Outcomes Classification)

Suggested NOC Outcomes

Coping; Decision-Making; Impulse Self-Control; Information Processing

Example NOC Outcome with Indicators

Coping as evidenced by the following indicators: Identifies effective and ineffective coping patterns/Modifies lifestyle to reduce stress. (Rate the outcome and indicators of **Coping:** 1 = never demonstrated, 2 = rarely demonstrated, 3 = sometimes demonstrated, 4 = often demonstrated, 5 = consistently demonstrated [see Section I].)

Client Outcomes

Client Will (Specify Time Frame)

- Acknowledge need for change in coping style
- Accept responsibility for own behavior
- Establish realistic goals with validation from caregivers
- Solicit caregiver validation in decision-making

NIC (Nursing Interventions Classification)

Suggested Nursing Interventions

Body Image Enhancement; Complex Relationship Building; Coping Enhancement; Patient Contracting; Resiliency Promotion; Self-Awareness Enhancement; Self-Esteem Enhancement; Socialization Enhancement; Surveillance

Example NIC Activities—Self-Awareness Enhancement

Encourage client to recognize and discuss thoughts and feelings; Assist client in identifying behaviors that are self-destructive

Nursing Interventions and *Rationales*

- Assess for possible symptoms associated with defensive coping: depressive symptoms, excessive self-focused attention, negativism and anxiety, hypertension, posttraumatic stress disorder (e.g., exposure

C

to terrorism), substance use symptoms, unjust world beliefs. EBN: *In one study, 45% of nurse educators (212/470) experienced workplace bullying and coped with avoidance behaviors such as disengagement; the researcher recommended development of more effective ways to assess workplace bullying and further research exploring coping strategies in this population (Wunnenberg, 2020).* EBN: *Toxic stress may be associated with physiological disruptions that play roles of stressor, promotor of effects of stressful environments, and inhibitor of positive coping responses in mothers with personal history of trauma (Condon & Sadler, 2019).*

▲ Use cognitive behavioral interventions. EBN: *Cajanding (2016) conducted a randomized control trial of a nurse-led cognitive behavioral intervention in Filipino heart failure* (n =100) *clients (48-control group and 52-intervention group participants) and found a positive effect on quality of life, self-esteem, and improved mood.*

- Ask appropriate questions to assess whether denial (defensive coping) is being used in association with health problems including alcoholism, myocardial infarction (MI), or other diagnoses EBN: *Rogers et al (2017) conducted a study of 244 newly diagnosed colorectal cancer clients to determine coping with symptoms before diagnosis and found that denial was used by those with lower education and income levels and that denial was a factor in delaying care and time to diagnosis.*
- Promote interventions with multisensory stimulation approaches (MSA). EB: *MSA has been studied in a variety of health situations including anorexia (Provenzano et al, 2019) and in a review of randomized controlled trials in older adults (Silva et al, 2018) both suggesting MSA provides promise as interventions to reduce negative coping strategies such as denial, distortions, agitation, and anxiety; researchers recommend future research.*
- Empower the client/caregiver's self-knowledge. EB: In a qualitative study of adults receiving medications for rheumatoid arthritis, researchers found that self-efficacy in managing the medication regimen was associated with self-knowledge and medication knowledge and was influenced by initial denial and future acceptance (*Oshotse et al, 2018*).

Geriatric

▲ Identify problems with alcohol in older adults with the appropriate tools and make suitable referrals. EB: *Using valid and reliable tools including the Daily Drinking Questionnaire (DDQ) revised version subscale of drinking to cope motives, researchers found that older adults* (n = 98) *with higher drinking to cope motives and low expectancies drank more; the researchers recommended examining drinking to cope motives so more targeted interventions could be formulated (Wilson et al, 2019).* CEB: *Tools such as the Alcohol Use Disorders Identification Test (AUDIT), Michigan Alcohol Screening Test—Geriatric Version (MAST-G), and the Alcohol-Related Problems Survey (ARPS) may have additional use in this population. Brief interventions have been shown to be effective in producing sustained abstinence or reducing levels of consumption, decreasing hazardous and harmful drinking (Culberson, 2006).*

- Encourage exercise for positive coping. EB: *In a pilot randomized clinical trial of a physical activity intervention in sedentary obese older adults* (n = 66), *researchers found the intervention improved activity levels and coping while reducing stress; researchers recommended future research of the intervention (Matson et al, 2019).*
- Use individual and/or group reminiscence therapy (RT). EBN: *In a literature review of studies examining both individual and group RT in older adults without dementia, findings indicated that both approaches to RT showed promise for enhancing coping and social engagement and reducing depressive symptoms (Shropshire, 2020).*

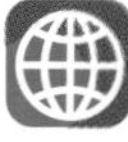

Multicultural

- Acknowledge racial/ethnic differences at the onset of care. EB: *In a quantitative study of women who experienced intimate partner violence (IPV), researchers found racial/ethnic differences in the use of coping strategies such that African American women used more problem solving and avoidance coping than their Latina and White participants; researchers reported that their findings were consistent with earlier studies in the literature (Weiss et al, 2017).*
- Assess an individual's sociocultural backgrounds in teaching self-management and self-regulation. EB: *A study of problem gambling in South Pacific and Asian cultures found a relationship between problem gambling between parents and participants, such that expectancies and motives about gambling may help targeted interventions for offspring of problem gamblers (Dowling et al, 2018).*

C

- Encourage the client to use spiritual coping mechanisms such as faith and prayer. EBN: *In a qualitative study of Hispanic older adults (n = 17) and coping with mental health issues most participants described spiritual beliefs and religious practices, including a reliance on God, deep faith, and prayer, as their primary coping strategies (Curtin et al, 2019).* EB: *In a study of renal cell carcinoma clients' (n = 117) expressive writing, positive religious coping was found to be a common coping strategy; however, negative religious coping was associated with psychological distress (Narayanan et al, 2020).*
- Encourage spirituality as a source of support for coping. EBN: *Experts in hospice and palliative care recommend spiritual assessment and encourage client preferred interventions that may include prayer, meditation, and meaning-focused therapy (Ferrell, 2017).* EB: *In a study of religion and coping with racial discrimination among African Americans (n = 2032) and Caribbean Blacks (n = 857), researchers found that both groups were similar in their likelihood of using prayer for coping with discrimination (Hayward & Krause, 2015).*

Home Care

▲ Refer the client for programs that teach coping skills. EB: *Researchers explored binge drinking in American Indian adolescents and found that in addition to findings supporting previous research about the role of peer influence, cultural identity was associated with the level of binge drinking behavior; recommendations included culturally appropriate coping skills training for youth and their families and identified an effective program, the American Indian Life Skills Development Curriculum for this population (Cwik et al, 2017).*

Client/Family Teaching and Discharge Planning

- Teach coping skills to clients and caregivers. EBN: *In a longitudinal study of a psychoeducation program versus standard education in Spanish clients with Parkinson's disease (n = 140) and their caregivers (n = 127), researchers found that in the short-term the psychoeducation program improved quality of life of clients and coping in caregivers (Navarta-Sánchez et al, 2020).*
- Teach reflexive and expressive writing to address emotions. EBN: *A collaborative diary writing intervention was studied to examine its effectiveness for clients with critical illness at risk of critical care posttraumatic stress (PTS) (n = 66) compared with standard care (n = 68); researchers found the clients in the intervention group had lower incidence of PTS (Torres et al, 2020).* EBN: *Kim-Godwin et al (2020) conducted a mixed method pretest, post-test design study of mothers (n = 37) of children with behavioral or emotional problems and a 6-week journaling intervention; researchers found increases in measures of optimism and gratitude and themes included positive thinking and emotional well-being, leading the researchers to conclude that positive writing intervention can contribute to well-being and self-care.*

REFERENCES

Refer to Ineffective **Coping** for additional references.

Cajanding, R. J. M. (2016). The effectiveness of a nurse-led cognitive-behavioral therapy on the quality of life, self-esteem, and mood among Filipino patients living with heart failure: A randomized controlled trial. *Applied Nursing Research*, *31*, 86–93.

Condon, E. M., & Sadler, L. S. (2019). Toxic stress and vulnerable mothers: A multilevel framework of stressors and strengths. *Western Journal of Nursing Research*, *41*(6), 872–900. https://doi.org/10.1177/0193945918788676.

Culberson, J. W. (2006). Alcohol use in the elderly: Beyond the CAGE. Part 2: Screening instruments and treatment strategies. *Geriatrics*, *61*(11), 20–26.

Curtin, A., Martins, D. C., & Schwartz-Barcott, D. (2019). Coping with mental health issues among Hispanic older adults. *Geriatric Nursing*, *40*(2), 123–128. https://doi.org/10.1016/j.gerinurse.2018.07.003.

Cwik, M. F., Rosenstock, S., Tingey, L., et al. (2017). Exploration of pathways to binge drinking among American Indian adolescents. *Prevention Science*, *18*, 545–554. https://doi.org/10.1007/s11121-017-0752-x.

Dowling, N. A., Oldenhof, E., Shandley, K., et al. (2018). The intergenerational transmission of problem gambling: The mediating role of offspring gambling expectancies and motives. *Addictive Behaviors*, *77*, 16–20. https://doi.org/10.1016/j.addbeh.2017.09.003.

Ferrell, B. R. (2017). Spiritual care in hospice and palliative care. *Korean Journal of Hospice and Palliative Care*, *20*(4), 215–220. https://doi.org/10.14475/Kjhpc.2017.20.4.215.

Hayward, R. D., & Krause, N. (2015). Religion and strategies for coping with racial discrimination among African Americans and Caribbean blacks. *International Journal of Stress Management*, *22*(1), 70–91.

Kim-Godwin, Y. S., Kim, S.-S., & Gil, M. (2020). Journaling for self care and coping in mothers of troubled children in the community. *Archives of Psychiatric Nursing*, *34*(2), 50–57. https://doi.org/10.1016/j.apnu.2020.02.005.

Matson, T. E., Anderson, M. L., Renz, A. D., Greenwood-Hickman, M. A., McClure, J. B., & Rosenberg, D. E. (2019). Changes in self-reported health and psychosocial outcomes in older adults enrolled in sedentary behavioral intervention study. *American Journal of Health Promotion*, *33*(7), 1053–1057. https://doi.org/10.1177/0890117119841405.

Narayanan, S., Milbury, K., Wagner, R., & Cohen, L. (2020). Religious coping in cancer: A quantitative analysis of expressive writing samples from patients with renal cell carcinoma. *Journal of Pain and Symptom Management*, *60*(4), 737–745. e3. https://doi.org/10.1016/j.jpainsymman.2020.04.029.

Navarta-Sánchez, M. V., Ambrosio, L., Portillo, M. C., Ursúa, M. E., Senosiain, J. M., & Riverol, M. (2020). Evaluation of a psychoeducational intervention compared with education in people with Parkinson's disease and their informal caregivers: A quasi-experimental study. *Journal of Advanced Nursing*, *76*(10), 2719–2732. https://doi.org/10.1111/jan.14476.

Oshotse, C., Zullig, L. L., Bosworth, H. B., Tu, P., & Lin, C. (2018). Self-efficacy and adherence behaviors in rheumatoid arthritis patients. *Preventing Chronic Disease*, *15*, E127.
Provenzano, L., Pociello, G., Ciccarone, S., et al. (2019). Characterizing body image distortion and bodily self-plasticity in anorexia nervosa via visuo-tactile stimulation in virtual reality. *Journal of Clinical Medicine*, *9*(1), 98. https://doi.org10.3390/jcm9010098.
Rogers, H. L., Siminoff, L. A., Longo, D. R., & Thomson, M. D. (2017). Coping with pre-diagnosis symptoms of colorectal cancer: A study of 244 individuals with recent diagnosis. *Cancer Nursing*, *40*(2), 145–151. https://doi.org/10.1097/ncc.0000000000000361.
Shropshire, M. (2020). Reminiscence intervention for community dwelling older adults without dementia: A literature review. *British Journal of Community Nursing*, *25*(1), 40–44. https://doi.org/10.12968/bjcn.2020.25.1.40.
Silva, R., Abrunheiro, S., Cardoso, D., et al. (2018). Effectiveness of multisensory stimulation in managing neuropsychiatric symptoms in older adults with major neurocognitive disorder: A systematic review. *JBI Database of Systematic Reviews & Implementation Reports*, *16*(8), 1663–1708. https://doi.org/10.11124/JBISRIR-2017-003483.
Torres, L., Nelson, F., & West, G. (2020). Original research: Exploring the effects of a nurse-initiated diary intervention on post-critical care posttraumatic stress disorder. *American Journal of Nursing*, *120*(5), 24–33. https://doi.org/10.1097/01.naj.0000662804.81454.66.
Weiss, N. H., Johnson, C. D., Contractor, A., Peasant, C., Swan, S. C., & Sullivan, T. P. (2017). Racial/ethnic differences moderate associations of coping strategies and posttraumatic distress disorder symptom clusters among women experiencing partner violence: A multigroup path analysis. *Anxiety, Stress & Coping*, *30*(3), 347–363. https://doi.org/10.1080/10615806.2016.1228900.
Wilson, T. D., Wray, L. A., & Turrisi, R. J. (2019). Positive alcohol expectancies and injunctive drinking norms in drinking to cope motives and alcohol use among older adults. *Addictive Behavior Reports*, *10*, 100207. https://doi.org/10.1016/j.abrep.2019.100207.
Wunnenberg, M. (2020). Psychosocial bullying among nurse educators: Exploring coping strategies and intent to leave. *Journal of Nursing Scholarship*, *52*(5), 574–582. https://doi.org/10.1111/jnu.12581.

Ineffective Coping **Domain 9 Coping/stress tolerance Class 2 Coping responses**

Arlene T. Farren, PhD, RN, AOCN, CTN-A

NANDA-I

Definition

A pattern of invalid appraisal of stressors, with cognitive and/or behavioral efforts, that fails to manage demands related to well-being.

Defining Characteristics

Altered affective responsiveness; altered attention; altered communication pattern; destructive behavior toward others; destructive behavior toward self; difficulty organizing information; fatigue; frequent illness; impaired ability to ask for help; impaired ability to attend to information; impaired ability to deal with a situation; impaired ability to meet basic needs; impaired ability to meet role expectation; inadequate follow-through with goal-directed behavior; inadequate problem resolution; inadequate problem-solving skills; reports altered sleep-wake cycle; reports inadequate sense of control; risk-taking behavior; substance misuse

Related Factors

High degree of threat; inability to conserve adaptive energies; inaccurate threat appraisal; inadequate confidence in ability to deal with a situation; inadequate health resources; inadequate preparation for stressor; inadequate sense of control; inadequate social support; ineffective tension release strategies

At-Risk Population

Individuals experiencing maturational crisis; individuals experiencing situational crisis

NOC (Nursing Outcomes Classification)

Suggested NOC Outcomes

Coping; Decision-Making; Impulse Self-Control; Information Processing

Example NOC Outcome with Indicators

Coping as evidenced by the following indicators: Identifies effective and ineffective coping patterns/Modifies lifestyle to reduce stress. (Rate the outcome and indicators of **Coping:** 1 = never demonstrated, 2 = rarely demonstrated, 3 = sometimes demonstrated, 4 = often demonstrated, 5 = consistently demonstrated [see Section I].)

Client Outcomes

Client Will (Specify Time Frame)

- Use effective coping strategies
- Use behaviors to decrease stress
- Remain free of destructive behavior toward self or others
- Report decrease in physical symptoms of stress
- Report increase in psychological comfort
- Seek help from a health care professional as appropriate

NIC (Nursing Interventions Classification)

Suggested NIC Interventions

Coping Enhancement; Decision-Making Support

Example NIC Activities—Coping Enhancement

Assist the client in developing an objective appraisal of the event; Explore with the client previous methods of dealing with life problems

Nursing Interventions and *Rationales*

- Appraise the presence of contributing factors for ineffective coping such as poor self-concept, grief, lack of problem-solving skills, lack of support, recent change in life situation, and maturational or situational crises. EBN: *Contributing factors may include experiences such as intimate partner violence in sexual minority men (Goldberg-Looney et al, 2016) and lifestyle behaviors such as high TV viewing in women experiencing trauma with or without symptoms (Jung et al, 2019).*
- Use presence and other verbal and nonverbal therapeutic communication approaches including empathy, active listening, calm approach, and acceptance. EBN: *Clients feel cared for and listened to with nurse presence as measured by the Presence of Nursing Scale (PONS) (Hansbrough & Georges, 2019).*
- Collaborate with the client to identify strengths such as the ability to relate the facts and to recognize the source of stressors. EBN: *Strength-based nursing (SBN) is a philosophical approach that includes eight values, including a collaborative partnership with clients and families (Gottlieb & Gottlieb, 2017).* EB: *Self-compassion in parents (n = 139) of children with autism spectrum disorders was associated with decreased stress and improved quality of life (Bohadana et al, 2019).*
- Explore the client's previous stressors and coping methods. EBN: *Caregivers of young adults with early psychosis experience stress due to client's behaviors and fear of harm to the client or themselves (Cheng et al, 2020b).* EB: *A review examining endometriosis and behavioral, cognitive, and emotional coping strategies demonstrated that despite mixed results, clinicians should engage in an evaluation of women's coping strategies to promote well-being and minimize poor mental health outcomes (Zarbo et al, 2018).*
- Provide opportunities to discuss the meaning the situation might have for the client. EBN: *A qualitative study of the coping experiences of spouses of people with dementia found that spouses search each day for meaning while experiencing stress and using coping strategies (Myhre et al, 2018).*
- Assist the client to set realistic goals and identify personal skills and knowledge. EBN: *Setting realistic goals is recommended as part of the support needed during weight loss programs (Fruh, 2017).* EB: *In a qualitative study of nurses and other health care providers (n = 10), researchers found that assisting clients to set realistic goals was essential to successful coaching interventions (Brandt et al, 2018).*
- Provide information regarding care, including diagnoses, treatments, and anticipated expectations. EBN: *Clients and caregivers of persons hospitalized for a cancer diagnosis reported that meeting their information needs assisted them to cope with (Abuatiq et al, 2020).*
- Discuss changes with the client before making them. EBN: *In a review of evidence about minimally invasive, robotic-assisted cancer surgery, researchers recommended that nursing care should focus on providing information and preparation to clients and families for shorter hospital stays (Sun & Fong, 2017).* EB: *In a study (n = 451) about transfer of clients from an intensive care unit to inpatient unit, clients/family were more satisfied and less stressed if they were informed in advance about impending transfers and nurses met with the client shortly after transfer (Stelfox et al, 2017).*
- Provide mental and physical activities within the client's ability (e.g., reading, television, radio, crafts, outings, movies, dinners out, social gatherings, exercise, sports, games). EB: *In a study of health care workers*

(n = 657) dealing with the stress of the COVID-19 pandemic, physical exercise was the preferred coping strategy for the majority of participants (Shechter et al, 2020).

- Discuss the power of the client and family to change a situation or the need to accept a situation. EBN: *Power as knowing participation in change was statistically significantly associated with client's (n = 98) engagement in health decision-making and resulted in satisfaction with the decisions (Sheikh, 2019).*
- Offer instruction regarding alternative coping strategies. EBN: *Motivational interviewing is a supportive strategy that helps elicit client perspectives and can promote coping (Carr, 2016).* EBN: *Mills, Wong-Anuchit, and Poogpan (2017) conducted a concept analysis of Thum-jai, a Thai coping strategy, and discussed the consequences or outcomes, which include emotional stability, positive thought, and productive change. It is recommended as an alternate coping strategy.*
- Encourage use of spiritual resources as desired. EBN: *Clark and Hunter (2019) conducted a literature review regarding spiritual coping in clients with advanced heart failure and recommended Reed's Theory of Self-Transcendence as a foundation for examining individuals' perspectives of their vulnerability and understanding one's sense of meaning.* EB: *Finding meaning after breast cancer treatment and experiencing post-traumatic growth was a significant source of coping and continued for as long as 2 years after treatment (Hamama-Raz et al, 2019).*
- Encourage use of social support resources. EBN: Based on a study of informal caregivers (n = 108) of persons with dementia, researchers recommended health care providers assist caregivers of persons with dementia build a broad-based support system because availability of social support predicted resilient coping (*Jones et al, 2019*).
- ▲ Refer for additional or more intensive therapies as needed. EB: *More complex interventions are available to assist with coping; for example, a randomized controlled trial of older adults in the community found that mindfulness and a self-compassion program consisting of 10, 2-hour sessions were successful in improving coping strategies (Perez-Blasco et al, 2016).*

Pediatric

- ✱ Monitor the client's risk of harming self or others and intervene appropriately. See care plan for Risk for **Suicidal Behavior**. EBN: *In a study of 140 Taiwanese secondary school students, resourcefulness as a coping strategy was inversely associated with depressive symptoms (Yang et al, 2017).*
- Monitor pediatric clients for exposure to community violence. EBN: *Researchers found that stressors such as violence and other traumatic disruptions in early childhood may interfere with the child's stress-response patterns and mental health in later life (Condon & Sadler, 2019).*
- Engage adolescents during stressful periods with comforting activities. EB: *In an experimental study that compared watching a video on cellphone, sitting quietly, or texting a friend after a stressful event, researchers found improved mood and decreased stress in adolescents (average age 12.4 years) only with the texting activity (Yau et al, 2021).*

Geriatric

- ▲ Assess and report possible physiological alterations (e.g., sepsis, hypoglycemia, hypotension, infection, changes in temperature, fluid and electrolyte imbalances, use of medications with known cognitive and psychotropic side effects). EBN: *Physical and mental comorbidities were found to be stressors for well older adults (ages 55–99) (Rubio et al, 2016) and for caregivers of older adults after stroke (Eeseung et al, 2016).*
- Screen for elder neglect or other forms of elder mistreatment. EBN/EB: *There is no gold standard for assessment of elder neglect, abuse, or mistreatment. There are several literature reviews exploring best practices for assessment and intervention (Hirst et al, 2016; Fearing et al, 2017; Moore & Browne, 2017).*
- Encourage the client to make choices (as appropriate) and participate in planning care and scheduled activities. EB: *Researchers found older adults preferred active engagement in making health care decisions, but the preference may be different for those with four or more comorbidities (Chi et al, 2017).*
- Target selected coping mechanisms for older persons based on client features, use, and preferences. EB: *Qualitative researchers, Birtwell and Dubrow-Marshall (2018), found older adults with mild dementia used coping mechanisms such as engaging in new activities and using humor.* EB: *In a quantitative study, older adult Internet users experiencing lockdown during a pandemic reported improved well-being associated with coping by hobby and interest-based Internet use (Nimrod, 2020).*
- Increase and mobilize support available to older persons by encouraging a variety of mechanisms involving family, friends, peers, and health care providers. EB: *Families give older adults important psychological support for coping with functional disabilities, pain, and other health issues (Honn Qualls, 2016).*

- Actively listen to complaints and concerns. EBN: *During the working phase of Peplau's theory, holistic communication includes the use of active listening to promote the older adult patient's development of a deeper connection with the nurse; active listening and focusing are essential holistic communication skills (Deane & Fain, 2016).*
- Engage the client in reminiscence. EBN: *A study of older adults with dementia living in a nursing home examined an intervention of music reminiscence therapy with reality orientation techniques, resulting in positive improvements in depression in the intervention group (Onieva-Zafra et al, 2018).*

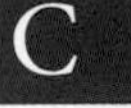

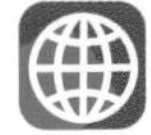

Multicultural

- Assess for the influence of cultural beliefs, norms, and values on the client's perceptions of effective coping. EBN: *One integrative review found evidence to support culture as a factor in coping with multiple chronic conditions; for example, the cultural belief of Arabic people includes multiple chronic conditions as sent by God and a sign of their relation with God (Cheng et al, 2020a).*
- Assess for intergenerational family problems that can overwhelm coping abilities. EBN: *A study of Chinese family caregivers revealed family expectations to provide care, but family resources contributed to coping, and a sense of self-sacrifice by the caregivers (Qiu et al, 2018).*
- ✱ Negotiate with the client regarding aspects of coping behavior that will need to be modified. EBN: *Adolescents are less likely to engage in help-seeking behaviors, which places them at greater risk for self-harm and suicide; resourcefulness has been found to be negatively and significantly related to self-harm in Taiwanese adolescents (Yang et al, 2017).* EB: *Researchers conducted two studies of Australian adolescents' online coping and found that those who engaged in frequent use of online technology for coping had poorer recovery from worry and jealousy (Duvenage et al, 2020).*
- Refer families experiencing race-based stress and trauma to evidence-based programs. EB: *The EMBRace program is based on racial socialization theory and is used to assist Black youth and their families to develop coping strategies to deal with the stress and trauma of discrimination (Anderson et al, 2019).*
- Identify which family members the client can count on for support. EBN: *In Madurai women who underwent hysterectomy (n = 60), researchers found that family support was associated with coping and quality of life and concluded that support from the partner is especially important to both coping and quality of life (Shanthi & Jeyapal, 2016).*
- Support the inner resources that clients use for coping. EBN: *Researchers in the United States and Asia have found evidence that supports that self-transcendence is an inner resource for coping and well-being in a variety of populations and situations; the effects of inner resources, such as resilience, self-adjustments, and getting out of oneself for the interest of others, are ways to enhance self-transcendence and meaning in life (Ho et al, 2016; Haase et al, 2017).*
- Use an empowerment framework to redefine coping strategies. EBN: *Canadian researchers tested an intervention based on a Caregiver Grief Model that enhanced empowerment and coping in caregivers of people with dementia (MacCourt et al, 2017).*

Home Care

- The interventions described previously may be adapted for home care use.
- ✱ Assess for suicidal tendencies. Refer for mental health care immediately if indicated.
- ✱ Identify an emergency plan should the client become suicidal. Ineffective coping can occur in a crisis situation and can lead to suicidal ideation if the client sees no hope for a solution. A suicidal client is not safe in the home environment unless supported by professional help. Refer to the care plan for Risk for **Suicidal Behavior.**
- Discuss preferred coping strategies of family caregivers. EBN: *Researchers found that family caregivers of dying persons used a variety of problem- and emotion-based coping strategies to achieve a sense of death preparedness (Durepos et al, 2019).*
- Encourage clients to participate knowingly in their care. Refer to the care plan for **Powerlessness.** EBN: *Power enhances coping when patients and caregivers participate knowingly to care for others and for those engaged in health care decision-making (Leveille-Tulce, 2017; Sheikh, 2019).*
- ▲ Refer the client and family to support groups. EB: *In a study of adolescents and adults with neurofibromatosis type 1 (NF1), a genetic, progressive disorder, researchers found that participation in support groups had an influence on self-esteem and recommended that health care professionals inform clients about support groups (Rosnau et al, 2017).*

C

▲ If monitoring medication use, discuss the barriers and facilitators to adapting and coping with the regimen. EBN: *Researchers found that patients with heart failure have stressors, often associated with social determinants of health that affect their ability to adhere to their medication and treatment regimens (Dickens et al, 2019).*

▲ Institute case management for frail elderly clients to support continued independent living. EBN: *Nurse-led community care for the oldest-old that includes care coordination and follow-up could preserve functioning in the oldest-old in the community (Bleijenberg et al, 2017).* EB: *A study examining tablet and Skype use in a case management program for frail older adults found that the participants had positive experiences with the technology as a means of communicating with case managers (Berner et al, 2016).*

Client/Family Teaching and Discharge Planning

• Teach the client to problem solve. Have the client define the problem and cause, and list the advantages and disadvantages of the options. EB: *A problem-solving intervention that included defining the problem and goals, listing multiple solutions, and selecting a solution found improved task-oriented coping, avoidant coping, and generic health-related quality of life (Visser et al, 2016).*

• Teach relaxation techniques. EBN: *A combination intervention of relaxation techniques and sleep hygiene training statistically significantly reduced insomnia, a source of stress, in postmenopausal women (Duman & Taşhan, 2018).*

• Work closely with the client to develop appropriate educational tools that address individualized needs. EB: *A participatory project to develop client education materials for older adults about lung stereotactic body radiotherapy (SBRT) involved clients at each step of the process. Participants had high health literacy and home Internet access, but researchers found that the participants had a preference for written and verbal teaching about the SBRT procedure (Jewitt et al, 2016).*

▲ Teach the client about available community resources (e.g., therapists, ministers, counselors, self-help groups). EBN: *Easom, Cotter, and Ramos (2018) conducted a post-participation examination of the Resources for Enhancing Alzheimer's Caregiver Health (REACH II) program provided to African American and Caucasian caregivers of people with Alzheimer's disease and found it to be a culturally appropriate and effective program.*

REFERENCES

Abuatiq, A., Brown, R., Wolles, B., & Randall, R. (2020). Perceptions of stress: Patient and caregiver experiences with stressors during hospitalization. *Clinical Journal of Oncology Nursing, 24*(1), 51–57. https://doi.org/10.1188/20.CJON.

Anderson, R. E., McKenny, M. C., & Stevenson, H. C. (2019). EMBRace: Developing a racial socialization intervention to reduce racial stress and enhance racial coping among Black parents and adolescents. *Family Process, 58*(1), 53–67. https://doi.org/10.1111/famp.12412.

Berner, J., Anderberg, P., Rennemark, M., & Berglund, J. (2016). Case management for frail older adults through tablet computers and Skype. *Informatics for Health and Social Care, 41*(4), 405–416. https://doi.org/10.3109/17538157.2015.1033528.

Birtwell, K., & Dubrow-Marshall, L. (2018). Psychological support for people with dementia: A preliminary study. *Counseling & Psychotherapy Research, 18*(1), 79–88. https://doi.org/10.1002/capr.12154.

Bleijenberg, N., Imhof, L., Mahrer-Imhof, R., Wallhagen, M. I., de Wit, N. J., & Schuurmans, M. J. (2017). Patient characteristics associated with a successful response to nurse-led care programs targeting the oldest-old: A comparison of two RCTs. *Worldviews on Evidence-Based Nursing, 14*(3), 210–222.

Bohadana, G., Morrissey, S., & Paynter, J. (2019). Self-compassion: A novel predictor of stress and quality of life in parents of children with autism spectrum disorder. *Journal of Autism and Developmental Disorders, 49*(10), 4039–4052. https://doi.org/10.1007/s10803-019-04121-x.

Brandt, C. J., Søgaard, G. I., Clemensen, J., Søndergaard, J., & Nielsen, J. B. (2018). Determinants of successful ehealth coaching for consumer lifestyle changes: Qualitative interview study among health care professionals. *Journal of Medical Internet Research, 20*(7), 76–85. http://dx.doi.org/10.2196/jmir.9791.

Carr, D. D. (2016). Motivational interviewing supports patient centered-care and communication. *Journal of the New York State Nurses Association, 25*(1), 39–43.

Cheng, C., Inder, K., & Chan, S. W. (2020a). Coping with multiple chronic conditions: An integrative review. *Nursing and Health Sciences, 22*(3), 486–497. https://doi.org/10.1111/nhs.12695.

Cheng, S. C., Backonja, U., Buck, B., Monroe-DeVita, M., & Walsh, E. (2020b). Facilitating pathways to care: A qualitative study of self-reported needs and coping skills of caregivers of young adults diagnosed with early psychosis. *Journal of Psychiatric and Mental Health Nursing, 27*(4), 368–379. https://doi.org/10.1111.jpm.12591.

Chi, W. C., Wolff, J., Greer, R., & Dy, S. (2017). Multimorbidity and decision-making preferences among older adults. *The Annals of Family Medicine, 15*(6), 546–551. https://doi.org/10.1370/afm.2106.

Clark, C. C., & Hunter, J. (2019). Spirituality, spiritual well-being, and spiritual coping in advanced heart failure: Review of the literature. *Journal of Holistic Nursing, 37*(1), 56–73. https://doi.org./10.1177/0898010118761401.

Condon, E. M., & Sadler, L. S. (2019). Toxic stress and vulnerable mothers: A multilevel framework of stressors and strengths. *Western Journal of Nursing Research, 41*(6), 872–900. https://doi.org/10.1177/0193945918788676.

Deane, W. H., & Fain, J. A. (2016). Incorporating Peplau's theory of interpersonal relations to promote holistic communication between older adults and nursing students. *Journal of Holistic Nursing, 34*(1), 35–41. https://doi.org/10.1177/0898010115577975.

Dickens, C., Dickson, V. V., & Piano, M. R. (2019). Perceived stress among patients with heart failure who have low socioeconomic status: A mixed methods study. *The Journal of*

Cardiovascular Nursing, *34*(3), E1–E8. https://doi.org/10.1097/JCN.0000000000000562.

Duman, M., & Taşhan, S. T. (2018). The effect of sleep hygiene education and relaxation exercises on insomnia among postmenopausal women: A randomized clinical trial. *International Journal of Nursing Practice*, *24*(4), e12650. https://doi.org/10.1111/ijn.12650.

Durepos, P., Sussman, T., Ploeg, J., Akhtar-Danesh, N., Punia, H., & Kaasalainen, S. (2019). What does death preparedness mean for family caregivers of persons with dementia? *American Journal of Hospice and Palliative Medicine*, *36*(5), 436–446. https://doi.org/10.1177/1049909118814240.

Duvenage, M., Correia, H., Uink, B., Barber, B. L., Donovan, C. L., & Modecki, K. L. (2020). Technology can sting when reality bites: Adolescents' frequent online coping is ineffective with momentary stress. *Computers in Human Behavior*, *102*, 248–259. https://doi.org/10.1016/j.chb.2019.08.024.

Easom, L., Cotter, E., & Ramos, A. (2018). Comparison of African American and Caucasian caregiver self-efficacy. *Journal of Gerontological Nursing*, *44*(3), 16–21. https://doi.org/10.3928/00989134-20171023-01.

Eeseung, B., Riegel, B., Sommers, M., Tkacs, N., & Evans, L. (2016). Caregiving immediately after stroke: A student of uncertainty in caregivers of older adults. *Journal of Neuroscience Nursing*, *48*(6), 343–351. https://doi.org/10.1097/JNN.0000000000000238.

Fearing, G., Sheppard, C. L., McDonald, L., Beaulieu, M., & Hitzig, S. L. (2017). A systematic review on community-based interventions for elder abuse and neglect. *Journal of Elder Abuse & Neglect*, *29*(2–3), 102–133. https://doi.org/10.1080/08946566.2017.1308286.

Fruh, S. M. (2017). Obesity: Risk factors, complications, and strategies for sustainable long-term weight management. *Journal of the American Association of Nurse Practitioners*, *29*(S1) S3–S14. https://doi.org/10.1002/2327-6924.12510.

Goldberg-Looney, L. D., Perrin, P. B., Snipes, D. J., & Calton, J. M. (2016). Coping styles used by sexual minority men who experience intimate partner violence. *Journal of Clinical Nursing*, *25*(23–24), 3687–3696. https://doi.org/10.1111/jocn.13388.

Gottlieb, L. N., & Gottlieb, B. (2017). Strengths-based nursing: A process for implementing a philosophy into practice. *Journal of Family Nursing*, *23*(3), 319–340. https://doi.org/10.1177/1074840717717731.

Haase, J. E., Kintner, E. K., Robb, S. L., et al. (2017). The resilience in illness model part 2: Confirmatory evaluation in adolescents and young adults with cancer. *Cancer Nursing*, *40*(6), 454–463. https://doi.org/10.1097/NCC.0000000000000450.

Hamama-Raz, Y., Pat-Horenczyk, R., Roziner, I., Perry, S., & Stemmer, S. M. (2019). Can posttraumatic growth after breast cancer promote positive coping? A cross-lagged study. *Psycho-Oncology*, *28*(4), 767–774. https://doi,org/10.1002/pon.5017.

Hansbrough, W. B., & Georges, J. M. (2019). Validation of presence of nursing Scale using data triangulation. *Nursing Research*, *68*(6), 439–444. https://doi.org/10.1097/NNR/0000000000000381.

Hirst, S. P., Penney, T., McNeil, S., Boscart, V. M., Podnieks, E., & Sinha, S. K. (2016). Best practice guidelines for prevention of abuse/neglect of older adults. *Canadian Journal on Aging*, *35*(2), 242–260. https://doi.org/10.1017/S0714980816000209.

Ho, H., Tseng, Y., Hsin, Y., Chou, F. H., & Lin, W. T. (2016). Living with illness and self-transcendence: The lived experience of patients with spinal muscular atrophy. *Journal of Advanced Nursing*, *72*(11), 2695–2705. https://doi.org/10.1111/jan.13042.

Honn Qualls, S. (2016). Caregiving families within the long-term services and support systems for older adults. *American Psychologist*, *71*(4), 283–293. https://doi.org/10.1037/a0040252.

Jewitt, N., Hope, A. J., Milne, R., et al. (2016). Development and evaluation of patient education materials for elderly lung cancer patients. *Journal of Cancer Education*, *31*(1), 70–74. https://doi.org/10.1007/s12187-014-0780-1.

Jones, S. M., Woodward, M., & Mioshi, E. (2019). Social support and high resilient coping in carers of people with dementia. *Geriatric Nursing*, *40*(6), 584–589. https://doi.org/10.1016/j.gerinurse.2019.05.011.

Jung, S. J., Winning, A., Roberts, A. L., et al. (2019). Posttraumatic stress disorder symptoms and television viewing patterns in the nurses' health study II: A longitudinal analysis. *PLoS One*, *14*(3), e0213441. https://doi.org/10.1371/journal.pone.0213441.

Leveille-Tulce, A. M. B. (2017). *A quasi-experimental study of a health patterning modality about childhood vaginitis and power in Haitian primary caregivers*. Unpublished doctoral dissertation.

MacCourt, P., McLennan, M., Somers, S., & Krawczyk, M. (2017). Effectiveness of a grief intervention for caregivers of people with dementia. *Omega*, *75*(3), 230–247. https://doi.org/10.1177/0030222816652802.

Mills, A. C., Wong-Anuchit, C., & Poogpan, J. (2017). A concept analysis of Thum-jai: A Thai coping strategy. *Pacific Rim International Journal of Nursing Research*, *21*(3), 234–243. https://he02.tci-thaijo.org/index.php/PRIJNR/article/view/78114.

Moore, C., & Browne, C. (2017). Emerging innovations, best practices, and evidence-based practices in elder abuse and neglect: A review of recent developments in the field. *Journal of Family Violence*, *32*(4), 383–397. https://doi.org/10.1007/s10896-016-9812-4.

Myhre, J., Tonga, J. B., Ulstein, I. D., Høye, S., & Kvaal, K. (2018). The coping experiences of spouses of persons with dementia. *Journal of Clinical Nursing*, *27*(3–4), e495–e502. https://doi.org/10.1111/jocn.14047.

Nimrod, G. (2020). Changes in internet use when coping with stress: Older adults during the COVID-19 pandemic. *American Journal of Geriatric Psychiatry*, *28*(10), 1020–1024. https://doi.org/10.1016/j.jagp.2020.07.010.

Onieva-Zafra, M. D., Hernández-Garcia, L., Gonzalez-del-Valle, M. T., Parra-Fernández, M. L., & Fernandez-Martinez, E. (2018). Music intervention with reminiscence therapy, and reality orientation for elderly people with Alzheimer's dementia living in a nursing home: A pilot study. *Holistic Nursing Practice*, *32*(1), 43–50. https://doi.org/10.1097/HNP.0000000000000247.

Perez-Blasco, J., Sales, A., Meléndez, J. C., & Mayordomo, T. (2016). The effects of mindfulness and self-compassion on improving the capacity to adapt to stress situations in elderly people living in the community. *Clinical Gerontologist*, *39*(2), 90–103. https://doi.org/10.1080/07317115.2015.1120253.

Qiu, X., Sit, J. W. H., & Koo, F. K. (2018). The influence of Chinese culture on family caregivers of stroke survivors: A qualitative study. *Journal of Clinical Nursing*, *27*(1–2), e309–e319. https://doi.org/10.1111/jocn.13947.

Rosnau, K., Hashmi, S. S., Northrup, H., Slopis, J., Noblin, S., & Ashfaq, M. (2017). Knowledge and self-esteem of individuals with neurofibromatosis type 1 (NF1). *Journal of Genetic Counseling*, *26*(3), 620–627. https://doi.org/10.1007/s10897-016-0036-9.

Rubio, L., Dumitrache, C., Cordon-Pozo, E., & Rubio-Herrera, R. (2016). Coping: Impact of gender and stressful life events in middle and in old age. *Clinical Gerontologist*, *39*(5), 468–488. https://doi.org/10.1080/07317115.2015.1132290.

Shanthi, P., & Jeyapal, M. (2016). Assess the level of coping, family support, and quality of life of women who had undergone hysterectomy in selected hospitals at Madurai. *Asian Journal of Nursing Education and Research*, *6*(3), 347–350.

Shechter, A., Diaz, F., Moise, N., et al. (2020). Psychological distress, coping behaviors, and preferences for support among New York healthcare workers during the COVID-19 pandemic. *General Hospital Psychiatry*, *66*, 1–8. https://doi.org/10.1016/j.genhosppsych.2020.06.007.

Sheikh, K. R. (2019). Knowing participation in change, engagement, and satisfaction with healthcare decision-making. *Visions: The Journal of Rogerian Science*, *25*(1), 1–14.

Stelfox, H., Leigh, J., Dodek, P., et al. (2017). A multi-center prospective cohort study of patient transfers from the intensive care unit to the hospital ward. *Intensive Care Medicine*, *43*(10), 1485–1494. http://doi.org/10.1007/s00134-017-4910-1.

Sun, V., & Fong, Y. (2017). Minimally invasive cancer surgery: Indications and outcomes. *Seminars in Oncology Nursing*, *33*(1), 23–36. https://doi.org/10.1016/j.soncn.2016.11.003.

Visser, M. M., Heijenbrok-Kal, M. H., van't Spijker, A., Lannoo, E., Busschbach, J. J. V., & Ribbers, G. M. (2016). Problem-solving therapy during outpatient stroke rehabilitation improves coping and health-related quality of life: Randomized controlled trial. *Stroke*, *47*(1), 135–142. https://doi.org/10.1161/STROKEAHA.115.010961.

Yang, F., Lai, C. Y., Yen, C., Hsu, Y. Y., & Zauszniewski, J. A. (2017). The depressive symptoms, resourcefulness, and self-harm behaviors of adolescents. *Journal of Nursing Research*, *25*(1), 41–49. https://doi.org/10.1097/jnr.0000000000000127.

Yau, J. C., Reich, S. M., & Lee, T. Y. (2021). Coping with stress through texting: An experimental study. *Journal of Adolescent Health*, *68*(3), 565–571. https;//doi.org/10.1016/j.jadohealth.2020.07.004.

Zarbo, C., Brugnera, A., Friegerio, L., et al. (2018). Behavioral, cognitive, and emotional coping strategies of women with endometriosis: A critical narrative review. *Archives of Women's Mental Health*, *21*(1), 1–13. https://doi.org/10.1007/s00737-017-0779-9.

Readiness for Enhanced Coping

Domain 9 Coping/stress tolerance Class 2 Coping responses

Arlene T. Farren, PhD, RN, AOCN, CTN-A

NANDA-I

Definition

A pattern of valid appraisal of stressors with cognitive and/or behavioral efforts to manage demands related to well-being, which can be strengthened.

Defining Characteristics

Expresses desire to enhance knowledge of stress management strategies; expresses desire to enhance management of stressors; expresses desire to enhance social support; expresses desire to enhance use of emotion-oriented strategies; expresses desire to enhance use of problem-oriented strategies; expresses desire to enhance use of spiritual resource

NOC (Nursing Outcomes Classification)

Suggested NOC Outcomes

Coping; Personal Well-Being; Social Interaction Skills; Quality of life

Example NOC Outcome with Indicators

Coping as evidenced by the following indicators: Identifies effective coping patterns/Uses effective coping strategies. (Rate the outcome and indicators of **Coping:** 1 = never demonstrated, 2 = rarely demonstrated, 3 = sometimes demonstrated, 4 = often demonstrated, 5 = consistently demonstrated [see Section I].)

Client Outcomes

Client Will (Specify Time Frame)

- Acknowledge personal power
- State awareness of possible environmental changes that may contribute to decreased coping
- State that stressors are manageable
- Seek new effective coping strategies
- Seek social support for problems associated with coping
- Demonstrate ability to cope, using a broad range of coping strategies
- Use spiritual support of personal choice

NIC (Nursing Interventions Classification)

Suggested NIC Interventions

Coping Enhancement; Health Education; Decision-Making Support

Example NIC Activities—Coping Enhancement

Assist client in developing an objective appraisal of the event; Explore with client previous methods of dealing with life problems

C

Nursing Interventions and *Rationales*

- Assess and support positive psychological strengths, that is, hope, optimism, self-efficacy, resiliency, and social support. EB: *Researchers found that young adults demonstrating resilience use coping strategies such as strategic planning, positive refocusing, and restructuring and view situations with an optimistic perspective (Kim & Lee, 2018).*
- Be physically and emotionally present for the client while using a variety of therapeutic communication techniques. EBN: *A qualitative study using focus groups to understand nurses' (*N = 27*) experiences of presence found empathy, active listening, and use of silence were among the therapeutic communication approaches that were required to implement presence and improve client outcomes (Stockmann et al, 2018).* EBN: *Clients feel cared for and listened to with nurse presence as measured by the Presence of Nursing Scale (PONS) (Hansbrough & Georges, 2019).*
- Empower the client to set realistic goals and to engage in problem-solving. EBN: *Power as knowing participation in change was reported by a sample of adults (*n = 98*) with at least one chronic condition; the researcher found that freedom to act with intention was associated with engagement and satisfaction with health decisions and recommended that nurses increase their awareness of power as it can enhance person-centered care (Sheikh, 2019).* EB: *In a quantitative study of African American women (*n = 290*) who successfully increased their physical activity, coping behaviors such as setting goals, self-monitoring, and self-regulation were associated with their success; researchers recommended that the findings can be helpful to create interventions for other African-American women who may need to improve their level of physical activity (Kinsey et al, 2019).*
- Encourage expression of positive thoughts and emotions. EBN: *In a study of nurses working in the Philippines (*n = 227*), researchers found high levels of optimism and proactive coping; recommendations included creating policies and interventions to ensure continued levels of well-being of nurses to promote quality nursing care (Cruz et al, 2018).* EB: *Positive thinking was found to be associated with health, optimism, and problem-focused coping in a sample of cancer survivors (*n = 603*); researchers concluded that positive thinking and optimism promote resilience and healthy coping in cancer survivors (Gallagher et al, 2019).*
- Encourage the client to use spiritual coping mechanisms such as faith and prayer. EBN: *In a cross-sectional study of women living with human immunodeficiency virus (HIV)/acquired immunodeficiency syndrome (AIDS), researchers found that prayer and spirituality were associated with coping and health outcomes (Dalmida et al, 2018).*
- Help the client with serious and chronic conditions such as depression, cancer diagnosis, and chemotherapy treatment to maintain social support networks or assist in building new ones. EBN: *In a secondary analysis of longitudinal data, researchers examined illness uncertainty for clients with prostate cancer and their partners; researchers found social support reduced uncertainty and recommended providers promote social support networks for clients and their partners (Guan et al, 2020).*
- ▲ Refer for cognitive-behavioral therapy (CBT) to enhance coping skills. EBN: *In a randomized control trial of a nurse-led cognitive behavioral intervention in a sample of heart failure clients (*n = 48*, control, and* n = 52*, intervention group), researchers found a positive effect on quality of life, self-esteem, and mood (Cajanding, 2016). Refer to the care plans for Readiness for Enhanced* **Communication** *and Readiness for Enhanced* **Spiritual** *Well-Being.*

Pediatric

- Encourage children and adolescents to engage in diversional activities and exercise to promote self-esteem, enhance coping, and prevent behavioral and other physical and psychosocial problems. EBN: *Researchers examining physical activity in children attending school (*n = 133*) found that enjoyment and self-efficacy were important influences in promoting physical activity in children (Ling et al, 2015).* EBN: *In a qualitative study of hospitalized children (*n = 10*) receiving chemotherapy for cancer, researchers found that engaging children in entertaining activities and having fun were among positive coping strategies (Sposito et al, 2015).*
- Provide families of children with chronic illness with education, transitional assistance, and psychosocial support to enhance coping. EBN: *An integrative literature review found that interventions should be*

directed toward education and psychosocial support for clients and families dealing with a new diagnosis of chronic illnesses (Gunter & Duke, 2018).

Geriatric

C

- Encourage active, meaning-based coping strategies for older adults with chronic illness. EBN: *In a qualitative study of older adults living with HIV (*n = 40*) residing in an urban environment, researchers uncovered four themes: accessing support, helping oneself and others, and tapping into their own spirituality. These address successful coping for the participants (DeGrezia & Scrandis, 2015).* EB: *Using a case study and evidence-based approach, experts identified meaning-based interventions to engage older adults, such as life-review, reminiscence, honoring wisdom, and engaging in mindfulness; experts recommended providers encourage these activities with older adults (Yang et al, 2018).*
- Consider the use of Web-based and technological resources for older adults in the community. EBN: *In a pilot study to explore the feasibility of an Internet health education program for older adults, researchers found improved attitudes toward Internet sources of health information and improved e-health literacy; researchers concluded that this educational intervention showed promise for enhancing e-health literacy in older adults (Chang et al, 2021).*
- Refer the older client to self-help support groups that address health, psychosocial, and/or social support. EB: *In a qualitative study of a reading and writing group for the well-being of older adults (*n = 12*), researchers categorized themes in relational terms including relation to self with subthemes of acknowledgment and achievement, as well as time for self; the reading and writing allowed for eliciting insight and working on emotions; researchers concluded the group enhanced well-being in older adults and recommended bibliotherapy and writing in a variety of community groups (Malyn et al, 2020).*

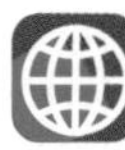

Multicultural

- Assess an individual's sociocultural backgrounds to identify factors that support coping. EBN: *Using qualitative, narrative methods to explore positive identity in First Nation men, participants described themselves as living a balanced life that engaged coping approaches such as having positive mentors and connections with positive aboriginal communities; researchers concluded that supporting positive identity and supporting culturally safe care can promote strength-based coping and well-being (Carter et al, 2017).* EB: *Researchers found that in a sample of African American college students (*n = 191*), a variety of past messages regarding racial socialization may predict race-specific coping in African-American college students (Blackmon et al, 2016).*
- Encourage spirituality as a source of support for coping. EBN: *Living with the unity of God and nature was one of the essential themes found in a hermeneutic study of Afro-Caribbean adults (*n = 14*) using folklore practices for healing and well-being (Joseph, 2020).*
- Facilitate positive ethnocultural identity to enhance coping. EBN: *The importance of a positive ethnocultural identity emerged in the qualitative study of Carter et al (2017) of First Nation men with themes regarding balance in life and engaging with positive aboriginal communities.*
- Foster family support. EBN: *In Madurai women who underwent hysterectomy (*N = 60*), researchers found that family support was associated with coping and quality of life and concluded that support from the partner is especially important to both coping and quality of life (Shanthi & Jeyapal, 2016). Refer to the care plan for Ineffective* ***Coping.***

Home Care

- The interventions described previously may be adapted for home care use.
- Engage both clients and their caregivers as a dyad. CEBN: *In a review of a program of research about helping clients and family caregivers cope with cancer, Northouse (2012) related lessons learned about caring for client and family caregiver dyad. Recommendations included identifying strengths; three-way, open communication and alliances; and promoting active coping (versus avoidant coping).*
- ▲ Institute case management for frail elderly clients to support continued independent living. EBN: *Nurse-led community care for the oldest-old that includes care coordination and follow-up could preserve functioning in the oldest-old in the community (Bleijenberg et al, 2017).* EB: *A study examining tablet and Skype use in a case management program for frail older adults found that the participants had positive experiences with the technology as a means of communicating with case managers (Berner et al, 2016).*
- Refer the client and family to support groups. EB: *A study of adolescents and adults with neurofibromatosis type 1 (NF1), a genetic, progressive disorder, explored knowledge of the disease, self-esteem, and the effect of support groups. Researchers found that participation in support groups had an influence on*

self-esteem and recommended that health care professionals inform clients about support groups (Rosnau et al, 2017).

- Refer prostate cancer clients and their spouses to family programs that include family-based interventions of communication, hope, coping, uncertainty, and symptom management. EBN: *In their longitudinal secondary data analysis of uncertainty in prostate cancer clients and their partners, Guan et al (2020) found that those with lower social support had greater uncertainty; researchers recommended nurses tailor interventions that include opportunities for social support of clients and their partners.*
- ▲ Refer military members, veterans, and family members for appropriate health services. EB: *Research found veterans with and without posttraumatic stress disorder (PTSD) enrolled in the Veterans Administration Program of Comprehensive Assistance for Family Caregivers (PCAFC) accessed more mental health, primary, and specialty care services than weighted comparisons (Shepherd-Banigan et al, 2018).*

Client/Family Teaching and Discharge Planning

- Teach the client about available community resources (e.g., therapists, ministers, counselors, self-help groups, family education groups). EBN: *Easom, Cotter, and Ramos (2018) conducted a postparticipation examination of the Resources for Enhancing Alzheimer's Caregiver Health (REACH II) program provided to African American and Caucasian caregivers of people with Alzheimer's disease and found it to be a culturally appropriate and effective program.*
- Teach caregivers using a variety of interventions that contribute to coping. EBN: *In one quasi-experimental study to examine the effectiveness of an education program for informal caregivers of persons with stroke, researchers found the intervention group gained practical skills, reported lower burden levels, and had better general mental health (Araujo et al, 2018).*
- Teach expressive writing, journaling, and education about emotions. EBN: *In a mixed-method study of a 6-week journaling intervention of mothers (n =37), researchers found increases in reports of optimism and gratitude; qualitative themes included positive thinking and emotional well-being (Kim-Godwin et al, 2020).*

REFERENCES

Araujo, O., Lage, I., Cabrita, J., & Teixeira, L. (2018). Training informal caregivers to care for older people after stroke: A quasi-experimental study. *Journal of Advanced Nursing, 74*, 2196–2206. https://doi.org/10.1111/jan.13714.

Berner, J., Anderberg, P., Rennemark, M., & Berglund, J. (2016). Case management for frail older adults through tablet computers and Skype. *Informatics for Health and Social Care, 41*(4), 405–416. https://doi.org/10.3109/17538157.2015.1033528.

Blackmon, S. M., Coyle, L. D., Davenport, S., Owens, A. C., & Sparrow, C. (2016). Linking racial-ethnic socialization to culture and race-specific coping among African-American college students. *Journal of Black Psychology, 42*(6), 549–576. https://doi.org/10.1177/0095798415617865.

Bleijenberg, N., Imhof, L., Mahrer-Imhof, R., Wallhagen, M. I., de Wit, N. J., & Schuurmans, M. J. (2017). Patient characteristics associated with a successful response to nurse-led care programs targeting the oldest-old: A comparison of two RCTs. *Worldviews on Evidence-Based Nursing, 14*(3), 210–222.

Cajanding, R. J. M. (2016). The effect of nurse-led cognitive behavioral therapy on quality of life, self-esteem, and mood among Filipino patients living with heart failure: A randomized control trial. *Applied Nursing Research, 31*, 86–93.

Carter, C., Lapum, J., Lavallée, L., Martin, L. S., & Restoule, J. P. (2017). Urban First Nations men: Narratives of positive identity and implications for culturally safe care. *Journal of Transcultural Nursing, 28*(5), 445–454. https://doi.org/10.1177/1043659616659348.

Chang, S. J., Yang, E., Lee, K. E., & Ryu, H. (2021). Internet health information education for older adults: A pilot study. *Geriatric Nursing, 42*(2), 533–539. https://doi.org/10.1016/j.gerinurse.2020.10.002.

Cruz, J. P., Cabrera, D. N. C., Hufana, O. D., Alquwez, N., & Almazan, J. (2018). Optimism, proactive coping, and quality of life of nurses: A cross-sectional study. *Journal of Clinical Nursing, 27*(9–10), 2098–2108. https://doi.org/10.1111/jocn.14363.

Dalmida, S. G., Kraemer, K. R., Unguary, S., Di Valerio, E., Koenig, H. G., & Holstad, M. M. (2018). The psychosocial and clinical wellbeing of women living with human immunodeficiency virus/AIDS. *Nursing Clinics of North America, 53*(2), 203–225. https://doi.org/10.1016/j.cnur.2018.01.008.

DeGrezia, M. G., & Scrandis, D. (2015). Successful coping in urban, community-dwelling older adults with HIV. *Journal of the Association of Nurses in AIDS Care, 26*(12), 151–163. https://doi.org/10.1016/j.jana.2014.11.008.

Easom, L., Cotter, E., & Ramos, A. (2018). Comparison of African American and Caucasian caregiver self-efficacy. *Journal of Gerontological Nursing, 44*(3), 16–21. https://doi.org/10.3928/00989134-20171023-01.

Gallagher, M. W., Long, L. J., Richardson, A., & D'Souza, J. M. (2019). Resilience and coping in cancer survivors: The unique effects of optimism and mastery. *Cognitive Therapy and Research, 43*(1), 32–44. https://doi.org/10.1007/s10608-018-9975-9.

Guan, T., Guo, P., Santacroce, S. J., Chen, D. G., & Song, L. (2020). Illness uncertainty and its antecedents for patients with prostate cancer and their partners. *Oncology Nursing Forum, 47*(6), 721–731. https://doi.org/10.1188/20.ONF.721-731.

Gunter, M. D., & Duke, G. (2018). Reducing uncertainty in families dealing with childhood cancers: An integrative literature review. *Pediatric Nursing, 44*(1), 21. https://link.gale.com/apps/doc/A529906622/AONE?u=cuny_statenisle&sid=AONE&xid=20649a06.

Hansbrough, W. B., & Georges, J. M. (2019). Validation of the Presence of Nursing Scale using data triangulation. *Nursing Research, 68*(6), 439–444. https://doi.org/10.1097/NNR/0000000000000381.

Joseph, M. A. (2020). The lived experiences of folklore healing practices as a health patterning modality. *Journal of Holistic Nursing, 38*(3), 262–277. https://doi.org/10.1177/0898010119880116.

Kim, S. R., & Lee, S. M. (2018). Resilient college students in school-to-work transition. *International Journal of Stress Management*, *25*(2), 195–207. https://doi.org/10.1037/str0000060.
Kim-Godwin, Y. S., Kim, S.-S., & Gil, M. (2020). Journaling for self-care and coping in mothers of troubled children in the community. *Archives of Psychiatric Nursing*, *34*(2), 50–57. https://doi.org/10.1016/j.apnu. 2020.02.005.
Kinsey, A. W., Segar, M. L., Barr-Anderson, D. J., Whitt-Glover, M. C., & Affuso, O. (2019). Positive outliers among African American women and the factors associated with long-term physical activity maintenance. *Journal of Racial and Ethnic Health Dispartities*, *6*(3), 603–617. https://doi.org/10.1007/s40615-018-00559-4.
Ling, J., Robbins, L. B., McCarthy, V. L., & Speck, B. J. (2015). Psychosocial determinants of physical activity in children attending afterschool programs: A path analysis. *Nursing Research*, *64*(3), 190–199. https://doi.org/10.1097/NNR.0000000000000084.
Malyn, B. O., Thomas, E., & Ramsey-Wade, C. E. (2020). Reading and writing for well-being: A qualitative exploration of the experience of older adult participants in a bibliotherapy and creative writing group. *Counseling & Psychotherapy Research*, *20*(4), 715–724. https://doi.org/10.1002/capr.12304.
Northouse, L. L. (2012). Helping patients and their family caregivers cope with cancer. *Oncology Nursing Forum*, *39*(5), 500–506. https://doi.org/10.1188/12.ONF.500-506.
Rosnau, K., Hashmi, S. S., Northrup, H., Slopis, J., Noblin, S., & Ashfaq, M. (2017). Knowledge and self-esteem of individuals with neurofibromatosis type 1 (NF1). *Journal of Genetic Counseling*, *26*(3), 620–627. https://doi.org/10.1007/s10897-016-0036-9.
Shanthi, P., & Jeyapal, M. (2016). Assess the level of coping, family support, and quality of life of women who had undergone hysterectomy in selected hospitals at Madurai. *Asian Journal of Nursing Education and Research*, *6*(3), 347–350. https://doi.org/10.5958/2349-2996.2016.00065.3.
Sheikh, K. R. (2019). Knowing participation in change, engagement, and satisfaction with health care decision-making. *Visions: The Journal of Rogerian Science*, *25*(1), 1–14.
Shepherd-Banigan, M., Smith, V. A., Maciejewski, M. L., et al. (2018). The effect of support and training for family members on access to outpatient services for veterans with posttraumatic stress disorder (PTSD). *Administration and Policy in Mental Health*, *45*(4), 550–564. https://doi.org/10.1007/s10488-017-0844-8.
Sposito, A., Silva-Rodriques, F., Sparapani, V., Pfeifer, L. L., de Lima, R. A. G., & Nascimento, L. C. (2015). Coping strategies used by hospitalized children with cancer undergoing chemotherapy. *Journal of Nursing Scholarship*, *47*(2), 143–151. https://doi.org/10.1111/jnu.12126.
Stockmann, C., Gabor, O., Divito-Thomas, P., & Ehlers, C. (2018). The use and intended outcomes of presence: A focus group study. *International Journal of Nursing Knowledge*, *29*(1), 59–65. https://doi.org/10.1111/2047-3095.12153.
Yang, J. A., Wilhelm, B. L., & McGlynn, K. (2018). Enhancing meaning when facing later life losses. *Clinical Gerontologist*, *41*(5), 498–507. https://doi.org/10.1080/07317115.2018.1432735.

Ineffective Community Coping

Domain 9 Coping/stress tolerance Class 2 Coping responses

Marina Martinez-Kratz, MS, RN, CNE

NANDA-I

Definition

A pattern of community activities for adaptation and problem-solving that is unsatisfactory for meeting the demands or needs of the community.

Defining Characteristics

Community does not meet expectations of its members; deficient community participation; elevated community illness rate; excessive community conflict; excessive community stress; high incidence of community problems; perceived community powerlessness; perceived community vulnerability

Related Factors

Inadequate community problem-solving resources; inadequate community resources; nonexistent community systems

At-Risk Population

Community that has experienced a disaster

NOC (Nursing Outcomes Classification)

Suggested NOC Outcomes

Community Competence; Community Health Status; Community Violence Level

Example NOC Outcome with Indicators

Community Competence as evidenced by the following indicators: Participation rates in community activities/Consideration of common and competing interests among groups when solving community problems/Representation of all segments of the community in problem-solving/Effective use of conflict management strategies. (Rate the outcome and indicators of **Community Competence:** 1 = poor, 2 = fair, 3 = good, 4 = very good, 5 = excellent [see Section I].)

Community Outcomes

A Broad Range of Community Members Will (Specify Time Frame)

- Participate in community actions to improve power resources
- Develop improved communication among community members
- Participate in problem-solving
- Demonstrate cohesiveness in problem-solving
- Develop new strategies for problem-solving
- Express power to deal with change and manage problems

NIC (Nursing Interventions Classification)

Suggested NIC Interventions

Community Health Development; Program Development

Example NIC Activities—Community Health Development

Enhance community support networks; Identify and develop potential community leaders; Unify community members behind a common mission; Ensure that community members maintain control over decision-making

Nursing Interventions and *Rationales*

Note: The diagnosis of Ineffective **Coping** does not apply and should not be used when stress is being imposed by external sources or circumstance. If the community is a victim of circumstances, using the nursing diagnosis Ineffective **Coping** is equivalent to blaming the victim. See the care plan for Readiness for Enhanced Community **Coping.**

- ▲ Establish a collaborative partnership with the community (see the care plan for Readiness for Enhanced Community **Coping** for additional references). EB: *A recent study found that counties whose Area Agencies for the Aging (AAAs) maintained informal partnerships with a broad range of organizations in health care and other sectors had significantly lower hospital readmission rates compared with counties whose AAAs had informal partnerships with fewer types of organizations (Brewster et al, 2018).*
- ● Assess community needs with the use of concept mapping methodology. EB: *The findings of a recent study showed that an integration of several concept mapping methods into a community engagement process was able to increase the input from a wide range of populations (Velonis et al, 2018).*
- ● Assess for the impact of social determinants of health on community health. EB: *A validated multivariate social determinants of health index score was used to accurately classify counties with high cardiovascular burden (Hong & Mainous, 2020).*
- ● Encourage participation in faith-based organizations that want to improve community stress management. EBN: *A recent study showed that coaching by faith community nurses created an environment of sustained support that promoted improved lifestyles and blood pressure changes over time (Cooper & Zimmerman, 2017).*
- ▲ Identify the health services and information resources that are currently available in the community through network analysis. EB: *A study found that network analysis served as a useful tool to evaluate community partnerships and facilitate coalition building (An et al, 2017).*
- ● Work with community members to increase problem-solving abilities. EBN: *Problem-solving is essential for effective coping. Findings from a recent study showed positive outcomes from a direct and tailored problem-solving training program (Easom et al, 2018).*

C

- Provide support to the community and help community members identify and mobilize additional supports. EB: *A community mobilization project demonstrated how cross-sector, coordinated efforts focused on vulnerable populations can leverage local strengths to establish and enhance breastfeeding support services customized to local needs (Colchamiro et al, 2015).*
- Advocate for the community in multiple arenas (e.g., multimedia, social media, governmental agencies). EB: *A recent study explored how social media can help community organizations engage in advocacy work (Guo & Saxton, 2018).*
- Work with communities to ensure that vulnerable individuals with access and functional needs are included in preparations for, response to, and recovery from disasters. EB: *Analysis of recent disasters has identified that a combination of strategic and operational methods, appropriate planning tools, and planning for the entire community will prevent individuals with access and functional needs from being disproportionately and negatively affected by disasters (Franks & Seaton, 2017).*
- Partner with community pharmacies to provide community education and health prevention services. EB: *A review of reviews found support for the development of community pharmacy health services focused on primary disease prevention (Thomson et al, 2019).*

Pediatric

- Protect children and adolescents from exposure to community violence. EB: *A systematic review found evidence for a positive association between community violence exposure and cardiovascular and sleep problems in children and adolescents (Wright et al, 2017).*
- Assess children and adolescents for the effects of direct and indirect crime exposure rather than only focusing solely on violent victimization. EB: *A study found poor behavioral health outcomes for adolescents with self-reported crime exposure (Grinshteyn et al, 2018).*

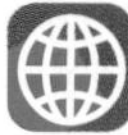

Multicultural

- Acknowledge the stressors unique to racial/ethnic communities. EB: *A recent study of Hispanic and African American women found that neighborhood context was an important factor in examining the determinants of health, survivorship, and quality of life outcomes among cancer clients (Wu et al, 2018).*
- Identify community strengths with community members. EBN: *A community-based participatory research approach was used to obtain Native American community input and identify strengths to address youth suicide and substance abuse. The results led to the development of a strengths-based intervention incorporating the Gathering of Native Americans curriculum (Holliday et al, 2018).*
- Use an empowerment approach to address health behaviors in diverse communities. An empowerment approach includes increasing clients' self-efficacy and capacity to make informed decisions about their health care. EB: *A recent study found use of an empowerment approach was effective in changing nonadherent Latinas' breast screening behaviors and promoting them to become agents of change in their communities (Molina et al, 2018). The empowerment intervention has three sessions focused on early detection, sharing information with family/friends, and health volunteerism.*
- Work with members of the community to prioritize and target health goals specific to the community. EB: *Recent research found that members of underserved communities, in informed deliberations, prioritized research categories on quality of life, client-doctor relationships, special needs, access, and compare approaches (Goold et al, 2017).*
- Establish and sustain partnerships with key individuals within communities when developing and implementing programs. EB: *A study of community engagement strategies found the following techniques to be effective: proactively engaging stakeholders in informational meetings, webinars, social media, the promising practice process, and community advisory council meetings (D'Angelo et al, 2017).*
- Use mentoring strategies for community members. EB: *A recent study showed parent mentors are highly effective in insuring uninsured Latino children and eliminating disparities (Flores et al, 2018).*
- Use community church settings as a forum for advocacy, teaching, and program implementation. EBN: *A recent study found that trust, respect, open dialog with participants, and commitment to address community health needs contributed to successful engagement and recruitment of African American churches to serve as participants in cancer research projects (Slade et al, 2018).*

REFERENCES

An, R., Khan, N., Loehmer, E., & McCaffrey, J. (2017). Assessing the network of agencies in local communities that promote healthy eating and lifestyles among populations with limited resources. *American Journal of Health Behavior, 41*(2), 127–138.

Brewster, A. L., Kunkel, S., Straker, J., & Curry, L. A. (2018). Cross-sectoral partnerships by area agencies on aging: Associations with health care use and spending. *Health Affairs, 37*(1), 15–21. https://doi.org/10.1377/hlthaff.2017.1346.

Colchamiro, R., Edwards, R. A., Nordstrom, C., et al. (2015). Mobilizing community resources to enhance postdischarge support for breastfeeding in Massachusetts (USA): Results of a catalyst grant approach. *Journal of Human Lactation, 31*(4), 631–640. https://doi.org/10.1177/089033441559768.

Cooper, J., & Zimmerman, W. (2017). The effect of a faith community nurse network and public health collaboration on hypertension prevention and control. *Public Health Nursing, 34*(5), 444–453. https://doi.org/10.1111/phn.12325.

D'Angelo, G., Pullmann, M. D., & Lyon, A. R. (2017). Community engagement strategies for implementation of a policy supporting evidence-based practices: A case study of Washington state. *Administration and Policy in Mental Health, 44*(1), 6–15. https://doi.org/10.1007/s10488-015-0664-7.

Easom, L. R., Wang, K., Moore, R. H., Wang, H., & Bauer, L. (2018). Operation family caregiver: Problem-solving training for military caregivers in a community setting. *Journal of Clinical Psychology, 74*(4), 536–553. https://doi.org/10.1002/jclp.22536.

Flores, G., Lin, H., Walker, C., et al. (2018). Parent mentoring program increases coverage rates for uninsured Latino children. *Health Affairs, 37*(3), 403–412. https://doi.org/10.1377/hlthaff.2017.1272.

Franks, S., & Seaton, E. (2017). Utilizing strategic and operational methods for whole-community disaster planning. *Disaster Medicine and Public Health Preparedness, 11*(6), 741–746. https://doi.org/10.1017/dmp.2017.6.

Goold, S. D., Myers, C. D., Szymecko, L., et al. (2017). Priorities for patient-centered outcomes research: The views of minority and underserved communities. *Health Services Research, 52*(2), 599–615. https://doi.org/10.1111/1475-6773.12505.

Grinshteyn, E. G., Xu, H., Manteuffel, B., & Ettner, S. L. (2018). The associations of area-level violent crime rates and self-reported violent crime exposure with adolescent behavioral health. *Community Mental Health Journal, 54*(3), 252–258. https://doi.org/10.1007/s10597-017-0159-y.

Guo, C., & Saxton, G. D. (2018). Speaking and being heard: How nonprofit advocacy organizations gain attention on social media. *Nonprofit and Voluntary Sector Quarterly, 47*(1), 5–26. http://doi.org/10.1177/0899764017713724.

Holliday, C. E., Wynne, M., Katz, J., Ford, C., & Barbosa-Leiker, C. (2018). A CBPR approach to finding community strengths and challenges to prevent youth suicide and substance abuse. *Journal of Transcultural Nursing, 29*(1), 64–73. http://doi.org/10.1177/1043659616679234.

Hong, Y. R., & Mainous, A. G., 3rd. (2020). Development and validation of a county-level social determinants of health risk assessment tool for cardiovascular disease. *Annals of Family Medicine, 18*(4), 318–325. https://doi.org/10.1370/afm.2534.

Molina, Y., San Miguel, L. G., Tamayo, L., et al. (2018). Empowering Latinas to obtain breast cancer screenings: Comparing intervention effects, part 2. *Cancer Epidemiology, Biomarkers & Prevention, 27*(3), 353–354. https://doi.org /10.1158/1055-9965.EPI-18-0048.

Slade, J. L., Holt, C. L., Bowie, J., et al. (2018). Recruitment of African American churches to participate in cancer early detection interventions: A community perspective. *Journal of Religion and Health, 57*(2), 751–761. http://doi.org/10.1007/s10943-018-0586-2.

Thomson, K., Hillier-Brown, F., Walton, N., Bilaj, M., Bambra, C., & Todd, A. (2019). The effects of community pharmacy-delivered public health interventions on population health and health inequalities: A review of reviews. *Preventive Medicine, 124*, 98–109. https://doi.org/10.1016/j.ypmed.2019.04.003.

Velonis, A. J., Molnar, A., Lee-Foon, N., Rahim, A., Boushel, M., & O'Campo, P. (2018). "One program that could improve health in this neighbourhood is _?" Using concept mapping to engage communities as part of a health and human services needs assessment. *BMC Health Services Research, 18*(1), 150. http://doi.org/10.1186/s12913-018-2936-x.

Wright, A. W., Austin, M., Booth, C., & Kliewer, W. (2017). Systematic review: Exposure to community violence and physical health outcomes in youth. *Journal of Pediatric Psychology, 42*(4), 364–378. http://doi.org.proxy.lib.umich.edu/10.1093/jpepsy/jsw088.

Wu, C., Ashing, K. T., Jones, V. C., & Barcelo, L. (2018). The association of neighborhood context with health outcomes among ethnic minority breast cancer survivors. *Journal of Behavioral Medicine, 41*(1), 52–61. http://doi.org/10.1007/s10865-017-9875-6.

C

Compromised Family Coping

Domain 9 Coping/stress tolerance Class 2 Coping responses

Katherina Nikzad-Terhune, PhD, MSW

NANDA-I

Definition

An usually supportive primary person (family member, significant other, or close friend) provides insufficient, ineffective, or compromised support, comfort, assistance, or encouragement that may be needed by the client to manage or master adaptive tasks related to his or her health challenge.

Defining Characteristics

Client complaint about support person's response to health problem; client reports concern about support person's response to health problem; limitation in communication between support person and client; protective behavior by support person incongruent with client's abilities; protective behavior by support person incongruent with client's need for autonomy; support person reports inadequate knowledge; support person reports inadequate understanding; support person reports preoccupation with own reaction to client's need; support person withdraws from client; unsatisfactory assistive behaviors of support person

Related Factors

C

Coexisting situations affecting support person; depleted capacity of support person; family disorganization; inaccurate information presented by others; inadequate information available to support person; inadequate reciprocal support; inadequate support given by client to support person; inadequate understanding of information by support person; misunderstanding of information by support person; preoccupation by support person with concern outside of family

At-Risk Population

Families with member with altered family role; families with support person experiencing depleted capacity due to prolonged disease; families with support persons experiencing developmental crisis; families with support persons experiencing situational crisis

NOC (Nursing Outcomes Classification)

Suggested NOC Outcomes

Caregiver Emotional Health; Caregiver-Client Relationship; Family Coping; Family Participation in Professional Care; Family Support During Treatment

Example NOC Outcome with Indicators

Family Coping as evidenced by the following indicators: Confronts family problems/Manages family problems/Reports needs for family assistance. (Rate each indicator of **Family Coping:** 1 = never demonstrated, 2 = rarely demonstrated, 3 = sometimes demonstrated, 4 = often demonstrated, 5 = consistently demonstrated [see Section I].)

Client Outcomes

Family/Significant Person Will (Specify Time Frame)

- Verbalize internal resources to help deal with the situation
- Verbalize knowledge and understanding of illness, disability, or disease
- Provide support and assistance as needed
- Identify need for and seek outside support

NIC (Nursing Interventions Classification)

Suggested NIC Interventions

Caregiver Support; Coping Enhancement; Family Involvement Promotion; Family Mobilization; Family Support; Mutual Goal Setting; Normalization Promotion; Sibling Support

Example NIC Activities—Family Support

Appraise family's emotional reaction to client's condition; Promote trusting relationship with family

Nursing Interventions and *Rationales*

- Assess the strengths and deficiencies of the family system. Consider using Family Systems Nursing, which emphasizes collaboration and a strength-focused relationship between health care professionals and the entire family as a unit of care. EBN: *A Family Systems Approach in nursing, as well as multiprofessional collaboration, is effective in facilitating illness management and improving communication and support between family members (Duhamel, 2017).*
- Establish rapport with families by providing accurate communication.
- Assist family members to recognize the need for help and teach them how to ask for it.
- Encourage family members to verbalize feelings. Spend time with them, sit down and make eye contact, and offer coffee and other nourishment.

- Provide family support interventions in situations in which caregiving is involved in the family. EB: *A comprehensive review of caregiving literature in both the fields of aging and developmental disabilities revealed that family-support interventions improved participant well-being, improved service access and satisfaction, reduced caregiver burden, and delayed institutional placement (Heller, Gibbons, & Fisher, 2015).*
- Provide privacy during family visits. If possible, maintain flexible visiting hours to accommodate more frequent family visits. If possible, arrange staff assignments so the same staff members have contact with the family. Familiarize other staff members with the situation in the absence of the usual staff member. *Providing privacy, maintaining flexible hours, and arranging consistent staff assignments reduce stress, enhance communication, and facilitate the building of trust.*
- Provide education to clients regarding active coping strategies to use in situations involving chronic illnesses. EB: *Mindfulness-based activities and cognitive behavioral therapy strategies can improve emotional, behavioral, and cognitive functioning in individuals experiencing various stressors (Gu et al, 2015).*
- Provide psychoeducation interventions and support for families providing palliative care to help reduce caregiver stress and burden. EB: *Brief psychoeducation interventions helped reduce stress in caregivers caring for a dying relative (Hudson et al, 2015).*
- Refer the family with ill family members to appropriate resources for assistance as indicated (e.g., counseling, psychotherapy, financial assistance, spiritual support).

Pediatric

- Provide screening for postpartum depression (PPD) during the prenatal period and during the 6-week postpartum checkup to identify symptoms of depression in mothers. EB: *The Edinburgh Postnatal Depression Scale (EPDS) is the most widely used screening tool for detecting PPD and has been shown to be effective both prenatally and postnatally for detecting symptoms of depression in women. The EPDS is also considered an adequate tool for identifying depressive symptoms in Spanish pregnant women (Vázquez & Míguez, 2019).*
- Consider medication management and psychosocial interventions, including individual therapy, group therapy, support groups, and brief psychotherapy. EB: *These are effective treatment strategies for managing PPD (Stewart & Vigod, 2019).*
- ▲ Use preventive strategies, such as screening, psychoeducation, postpartum debriefing, and companionship in the delivery room (e.g., community volunteer). Continuing education is also recommended for health care professionals to improve knowledge regarding PPD. EBN: *New mothers viewed depression screening and receiving community resource information as a positive part of their care (Logsdon et al, 2018).*
- Use technology-based education to help increase knowledge and support for parents performing care procedures for their children. EBN: *Research suggests that smartphone-based education should be considered as an effective educational intervention in providing nursing support for parents of children with respiratory disease (Lee, Kim, & Min, 2017).*
- Use best practices and participate in training to help make communication and environmental adaptations when interacting with children with autism spectrum disorder (ASD) to enhance communication, improve quality of care, and reduce behavioral problems and frustration. EBN: *Nursing students who participated in a simulation using a standardized client role-playing an adolescent with ASD reported increased knowledge and improved clinical skills for responding to behavior and communication challenges in children with ASD (McIntosh et al, 2018b).* EBN: *School nurses can help reduce and manage problematic behaviors in children with ASD by using extrinsic motivation and reinforcement techniques, as well as communicating clear expectations, providing the child with choices, and using visual activity schedules (McIntosh et al, 2018a).*
- Effectively engaging and collaborating with parents is essential for supporting parents of children with long-term health conditions, and it may enhance the parent–professional relationship and communication. EBN: *Smith, Swallow, and Coyne (2015) provided a framework for involving parents in the care of a child with long-term health conditions, which includes valuing the parent's knowledge and expertise of their child, supporting parents in their role, establishing rapport, mutually exchanging information with parents, sharing decisions, collaborating during care planning, and designing services around both the needs of the child and the family.*
- Provide evidence-based psychological therapies for parents with children with chronic conditions. EB: *Psychological therapies, such as cognitive behavioral therapy, can lead to improvements in mood and behavior in parents of children diagnosed with attention-deficit hyperactivity disorder (ADHD) (Wong et al, 2018).*
- When performing pediatric diabetes care, be attentive to the mother's experience, including burnout experienced as a result of caregiving for the child. EBN: *The well-being of the mother has the potential to*

affect the well-being of the child and the well-being of the family unit. Focusing on the well-being of mothers of children with pediatric diabetes may lead to improvements in overall family functioning, and referrals for appropriate interventions (Lindström et al, 2017).

- Provide options for home-based interventions when severe childhood illnesses make it difficult for children and families to participate in interventions. In-home visits, assessments, and interventions may help improve self-management among the client and family and reduce emergency department visits and inpatient hospitalizations. EBN: *The delivery of a home visit program for pediatric asthma clients enhanced early communication, reduced response time between problem identification and resolution, and reduced inpatient care over the course of 1 year (McClure et al, 2017).*

Geriatric

- ▲ Perform a holistic assessment of all needs of informal family caregivers. EBN: *Nurse-led caregiver-centered intervention may help prevent decompensation in caregiver well-being. Results from a recent study reveal that caregivers view a trusting relationship with mental health nurses as being crucial, and that collaboration with nurses can lead to increased well-being in both care recipients and caregivers (Zegwaard et al, 2017).*
- ▲ Assist informal caregivers with reducing unmet needs by helping them obtain the information, education, and support necessary for caring for an older adult with a chronic health condition. EB: *Internet interventions can help meet the educational and support needs of informal dementia caregivers. Results from a systematic review demonstrate that Internet-based interventions can help improve mental health outcomes for informal caregivers of individuals with dementia (Egan et al, 2018).*
- In situations in which familial caregiving is being provided, assess current coping strategies utilized within the family. Provide interventions for family caregivers that are designed specifically to enhance coping skills, including problem-solving strategies and emotional support. EB: *Psychosocial interventions that incorporated problem-solving skills, emotional support, knowledge of dementia, and social resources helped caregivers develop more effective coping strategies, which have the potential to reduce caregiver burden (Chen et al, 2015).*

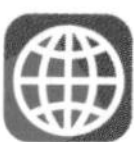

Multicultural

- Acknowledge sociocultural differences and health care disparities at the onset of care. EBN: *Consider using Almutairi's critical cultural competence (CCC) model as a comprehensive approach for addressing challenges that may arise from sociocultural and linguistic issues during cross-cultural interactions. Research support use of the Critical Cultural Competence Scale (CCCS) to measure health care providers' perceptions of their CCC (Almutairi & Dahinten, 2017).*
- Use valid and culturally competent assessment tools and procedures when working with families with different racial/ethnic backgrounds. EBN: *The cultural information in nursing models and assessments should encompass health beliefs and practices, communication styles, religious orientation, and the degree of acculturation among others (Shen, 2015).*
- Assess for the influence of cultural beliefs, norms, and values on the individual/family/community's perceptions of coping. EB: *The Cross-Cultural Depression Coping Inventory (CCD-CI) is recommended to assess how individuals from different cultures prefer to cope with depression. Empirical results designate the CCD-CI as a reliable and valid measure of coping strategies for depression that are appropriate for adults from different ethnic groups (Markova, Sandal, & Guribye, 2020).*
- Provide opportunities for clients and families to discuss spirituality. EBN: *Spiritual interventions and coping strategies that focus on meaning, purpose, and connectedness are recommended in the nursing literature, and have been found to be effective in particular with clients experiencing heart failure (Clark & Hunter, 2019).*
- Ensure culturally responsive approaches to end-of-life care. EBN: *Providing culturally informed nursing care allows elderly immigrants the opportunity to make choices during their end-of-life care that are congruent with their cultural beliefs and expectations (Johnstone et al, 2016).*

Home Care

- The interventions described previously may be adapted for home care use.
- Assess the reason behind the breakdown of family coping. *Knowledge of the reasons behind compromised coping will assist in identification of appropriate interventions. Refer to the care plan for* ***Caregiver Role Strain.***
- ▲ During the time of compromised coping, increase visits to ensure the safety of the client, support of the family, and reassurance regarding expectations for prognosis as appropriate.

- ▲ Assess the needs of the caregiver in the home, and intervene to meet needs as appropriate; explore all available resources that may be used to provide adequate home care (e.g., parish nursing as an effective adjunct, home health aide services to relieve the caregiver's fatigue).
- ▲ Encourage caregivers to attend to their own physical, mental, and spiritual health, and give more specific information about the client's needs and ways to meet them.
- ▲ Refer the family to medical social services for evaluation and supportive counseling. Serve as an advocate, mentor, and role model for caregiving; provide written information for the care needed by the client.
- ▲ A positive approach and caring by the nurse and concrete task definition and assignment reinforce positive coping strategies and allow caregivers to feel less guilty when tasks are delegated to multiple caregivers.
- ▲ When a terminal illness is the precipitating factor for ineffective coping, offer hospice services and support groups as possible resources. EB: *Research suggests that clients and their families value home hospice care services and report experiencing beneficial outcomes as a result of using hospice services (Ong et al, 2016).*
- ● Encourage the client and family to discuss changes in daily functioning and routines created by the client's illness, and validate discomfort resulting from changes. *Individuals who live together for a long period tend to become familiar with each other's patterns; for example, meals are expected at certain times or a spouse becomes accustomed to the client's sleep habits.*
- ● Support positive individual and family coping efforts. *Positive feedback reinforces desired behaviors and supports the family unit.*
- ● Screen for mental health disorders (MHDs) in the elderly home care population. EBN: *Approximately one-third of elderly clients with MHDs received mental health services during a 60-day home care episode. Regular screening and intervention protocols can improve psychiatric care for the homebound elderly (Wang et al, 2016).*
- ● During home care visits and assessments, provide individuals and families with information for Internet-based interventions, including information on using social media as a health communications tool. EB: *A systematic review supports the effectiveness of online interventions (Web and app based) for clients with severe psychiatric disorders as well as their families as evidenced by improvements in knowledge, allowing for experiences to be shared, reported symptom relief for the client, fewer hospitalizations, and an increase in perceived social support (Barbeito et al, 2020).*

Client/Family Teaching and Discharge Planning

- ● Assess grief in parents who have lost a child to help determine parental needs, especially in the first year after the death of a child. EB: *The presentation of grief may differ in mothers and fathers, resulting in different needs during the first year after a child's death (Youngblut et al, 2017).*
- ▲ Refer women with breast cancer and their family caregivers to support groups (including social network sites and online communities), and to other services that provide assistance with daily coping. EB: *Online support groups and communities are feasible and useful tools that may enhance the overall well-being of breast cancer survivors by providing information and opportunities to engage and connect with other cancer survivors (Falisi et al, 2017).*
- ▲ For families dealing with childhood illnesses, developmental disorders, or other psychosocial stressors, refer parents to training, support, and education groups to provide opportunities for parents to access support, learn new parenting skills, and obtain additional coping resources. EB: *Empirical evidence reveals that support groups for parents of children with ASD are effective in reducing stress and enhancing professional knowledge and peer support (Tzur Bitan, 2018). Consider referring parents of children with ASD to parent training programs, which systematic reviews and a randomized clinical trials have revealed are effective for improving parent-child interaction, disruptive behaviors in children, and the mental health of the mother (Iida et al, 2018).* EBN: *Since youth present to health care professionals with symptoms related to cyberbullying, a systematic review supports educating both parents and youth on cyberbullying as an evidence-based practice for enhancing coping skills, communication, and digital citizenship (Hutson, Kelly, & Militello, 2018).*
- ● Provide comprehensive discharge planning for individuals and families to help improve quality of life at home. EBN: *Ensuring high-quality discharge planning and assessing parental readiness for discharge can result in identifying at-risk families and mobilizing anticipatory services to support the family's transition home. Assessing discharge readiness is also linked to enhanced parental coping and reduced child hospital readmission (Weiss et al, 2017).* EB: *A meta-analysis reveals that when older adults are discharged to a community setting, integrating caregivers into the discharge planning process reduces the risk of hospital readmission (Rodakowski et al, 2017).*

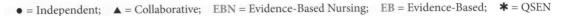

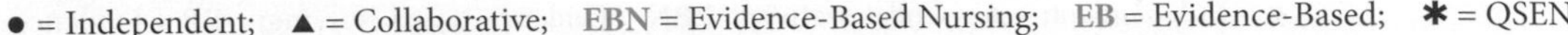

C

- Individuals diagnosed with a developmental disability and a mental illness and their families frequently experience multiple challenges and insufficient resources and support. EBN: *Best practices include providing person- and family-centered care; navigation support; prevention strategies; emergency and crisis care services; and housing and vocation assistance to help address gaps in services and enhance familial coping (Nicholas et al, 2017).*
- Nurses can help clients with type 2 diabetes with self-management education and support (DSME/S), which includes the facilitation of knowledge, skills, and abilities necessary to manage diabetes, as well as obtaining the support necessary for executing and maintaining the coping and behavioral skills needed for self-management. EB: *Self-management education and support has been shown to improve health outcomes in clients with type 2 diabetes (Powers et al, 2017).*

REFERENCES

Almutairi, A. F., & Dahinten, V. S. (2017). Construct validity of Almutairi's critical cultural competence scale. *Western Journal of Nursing Research*, *39*(6), 784–802. https://doi.org/10.1177/0193945916656616.

Barbeito, S., Sánchez-Gutiérrez, T., Becerra-García, J. A., Pinto, A. G., Caletti, E., & Calvo, A. (2020). A systematic review of online interventions for families of patients with severe mental disorders. *Journal of Affective Disorders*, *263*, 147–154. https://doi.org/10.1016/j.jad.2019.11.106.

Chen, H. M., Huang, M. F., Yeh, Y. C., Huang, W. H., & Chen, C. S. (2015). Effectiveness of coping strategies intervention on caregiver burden among caregivers of elderly patients with dementia. *Psychogeriatrics*, *15*(1), 20–25. https://doi.org/10.1111/psyg.12071.

Clark, C. C., & Hunter, J. (2019). Spirituality, spiritual well-being, and spiritual coping in advanced heart failure: Review of the literature. *Journal of Holistic Nursing*, *37*(1), 56–73. https://doi.org/10.1177/0898010118761401.

Duhamel, F. (2017). Translating knowledge from a family systems approach to clinical practice: Insights from knowledge translation research experiences. *Journal of Family Nursing*, *23*(4), 461–487. https://doi.org/10.1177/1074840717739030.

Egan, K. J., Pinto-Bruno, Á. C., Bighelli, I., et al. (2018). Online training and support programs designed to improve mental health and reduce burden among caregivers of people with dementia: A systematic review. *Journal of the American Medical Directors Association*, *19*(3), 200–206. https://doi.org/10.1016/j.jamda.2017.10.023.

Falisi, A. L., Wiseman, K. P., Gaysynsky, A., Scheideler, J. K., Ramin, D. A., & Chou, W. Y. S. (2017). Social media for breast cancer survivors: A literature review. *Journal of Cancer Survivorship*, *11*(6), 808–821. https://doi.org/10.1007/s11764-017-0620-5.

Gu, J., Strauss, C., Bond, R., & Cavanagh, K. (2015). How do mindfulness-based cognitive therapy and mindfulness-based stress reduction improve mental health and wellbeing? A systematic review and meta-analysis of mediation studies. *Clinical Psychology Review*, *37*, 1–12. https://doi.org/10.1016/j.cpr.2015.01.006.

Heller, T., Gibbons, H. M., & Fisher, D. (2015). Caregiving and family support interventions: Crossing networks of aging and developmental disabilities. *Intellectual and Developmental Disabilities*, *53*(5), 329. https://doi.org/10.1352/1934-9556-53.5.329.

Hudson, P., Trauer, T., Kelly, B., et al. (2015). Reducing the psychological distress of family caregivers of home based palliative care patients: Longer term effects from a randomised controlled trial. *Psycho-Oncology*, *24*(1), 19–24. https://doi.org/10.1002/pon.3610.

Hutson, E., Kelly, S., & Militello, L. K. (2018). Systematic review of cyberbullying interventions for youth and parents with implications for evidence–based practice. *Worldviews on Evidence-Based Nursing*, *15*(1), 72–79. https://doi.org/10.1111/wvn.12257.

Iida, N., Wada, Y., Yamashita, T., Aoyama, M., Hirai, K., & Narumoto, J. (2018). Effectiveness of parent training in improving stress-coping capability, anxiety, and depression in mothers raising children with autism spectrum disorder. *Neuropsychiatric Disease and Treatment*, *14*, 3355–3362. https://doi.org/10.2147/NDT.S188387.

Johnstone, M. J., Hutchinson, A. M., Redley, B., & Rawson, H. (2016). Nursing roles and strategies in end-of-life decision making concerning elderly immigrants admitted to acute care hospitals: An Australian study. *Journal of Transcultural Nursing*, *27*(5), 471–479. https://doi.org/10.1177/1043659615582088.

Lee, J. M., Kim, S. J., & Min, H. Y. (2017). The effects of smartphone-based nebulizer therapy education on parents' knowledge and confidence of performance in caring for children with respiratory disease. *Journal of Pediatric Nursing*, *36*, 13–19. https://doi.org/10.1016/j.pedn.2017.04.012.

Lindström, C., Åman, J., Norberg, A. L., Forssberg, M., & Anderzén-Carlsson, A. (2017). "Mission impossible"; the mothering of a child with type 1 diabetes—From the perspective of mothers experiencing burnout. *Journal of Pediatric Nursing*, *36*, 149–156. https://doi.org/10.1016/j.pedn.2017.06.002.

Logsdon, M. C., Vogt, K., Davis, D. W., Myers, J., Hogan, F., Eckert, D., et al. (2018). Screening for postpartum depression by hospital-based perinatal nurses. *MCN: American Journal of Maternal/Child Nursing*, *43*(6), 324–329. https://doi.org/10.1097/NMC.0000000000000470.

Markova, V., Sandal, G. M., & Guribye, E. (2020). What do immigrants from various cultures think is the best way to cope with depression? Introducing the cross-cultural coping inventory. *Frontiers in Psychology*, *11*, 1599. https://doi.org/10.3389/fpsyg.2020.01599.

McClure, N., Lutenbacher, M., O'Kelley, E., & Dietrich, M. S. (2017). Enhancing pediatric asthma care and nursing education through an academic practice partnership. *Journal of Pediatric Nursing*, *36*, 64–69. https://doi.org/10.1016/j.pedn.2017.04.008.

McIntosh, C. E., Gundlach, J., Brelage, P., & Snyder, S. (2018a). School nurses increasing the compliance of hygiene routines for students with autism spectrum disorder. *NASN School Nurse*, *33*(5), 319–323. https://doi.org/10.1177/1942602x18779412.

McIntosh, C. E., Thomas, C. M., Wilczynski, S., & McIntosh, D. E. (2018b). Increasing nursing students' knowledge of autism spectrum disorder by using a standardized patient. *Nursing Education Perspectives*, *39*(1), 32–34. https://doi.org/10.1097/01.nep.0000000000000179.

Nicholas, D. B., Calhoun, A., McLaughlin, A. M., Shankar, J., Kreitzer, L., & Uzande, M. (2017). Care experiences of adults with a dual diagnosis and their family caregivers. *Global Qualitative Nursing Research*, *4*, 2333393617721646. https://doi.org/10.1177/2333393617721646.

Ong, J., Brennsteiner, A., Chow, E., & Hebert, R. S. (2016). Correlates of family satisfaction with hospice care: General inpatient hospice care versus routine home hospice care. *Journal of Palliative Medicine*, *19*(1), 97–100. https://doi.org/10.1089/jpm.2015.0055.

Powers, M. A., Bardsley, J., Cypress, M., et al. (2017). Diabetes self-management education and support in type 2 diabetes: A joint position statement of the American Diabetes Association, the American Association of Diabetes Educators, and the Academy of Nutrition and Dietetics. *Diabetes Educator*, *43*(1), 40–53. https://doi.org/10.2337/diaclin.34.2.70.

Rodakowski, J., Rocco, P. B., Ortiz, M., et al. (2017). Caregiver integration during discharge planning for older adults to reduce resource use: A metaanalysis. *Journal of the American Geriatrics Society*, *65*(8), 1748–1755. https://doi.org/10.1111/jgs.14873.

Shen, Z. (2015). Cultural competence models and cultural competence assessment instruments in nursing: A literature review. *Journal of Transcultural Nursing*, *26*(3), 308–321. https://doi.org/10.1177/1043659614524790.

Smith, J., Swallow, V., & Coyne, I. (2015). Involving parents in managing their child's long-term condition—a concept synthesis of family-centered care and partnership-in-care. *Journal of Pediatric Nursing*, *30*(1), 143–159. https://doi.org/10.1016/j.pedn.2014.10.014.

Stewart, D. E., & Vigod, S. N. (2019). Postpartum depression: Pathophysiology, treatment, and emerging therapeutics. *Annual Review of Medicine*, *70*, 183–196. https://doi.org/10.1146/annurev-med-041217-011106.

Tzur Bitan, D., Zilcha-Mano, S., Ganor, O., Biran, L., & Bloch, Y. (2018). Routine measurement and feedback in support groups for parents of children with autistic spectrum disorder. *Psychotherapy*, *55*(2), 191–195. https://doi.org/10.1037/pst0000140.

Vázquez, M. B., & Míguez, M. C. (2019). Validation of the Edinburgh postnatal depression scale as a screening tool for depression in Spanish pregnant women. *Journal of Affective Disorders*, *246*, 515–521. https://doi.org/10.1016/j.jad.2018.12.075.

Wang, J., Kearney, J. A., Jia, H., & Shang, J. (2016). Mental health disorders in elderly people receiving home care: Prevalence and correlates in the national U.S. population. *Nursing Research*, *65*(2), 107–116. https://doi.org/10.1097/NNR.0000000000000147.

Weiss, M. E., Sawin, K. J., Gralton, K., et al. (2017). Discharge teaching, readiness for discharge, and post-discharge outcomes in parents of hospitalized children. *Journal of Pediatric Nursing*, *34*, 58–64. https://doi.org/10.1016/j.pedn.2016.12.021.

Wong, D. F., Ng, T. K., Ip, P. S. Y., Chung, M. L., & Choi, J. (2018). Evaluating the effectiveness of a group CBT for parents of ADHD children. *Journal of Child and Family Studies*, *27*, 227–239. https://doi.org/10.1007/s10826-017-0868-4.

Youngblut, J. M., Brooten, D., Glaze, J., Promise, T., & Yoo, C. (2017). Parent grief 1–13 months after death in neonatal and pediatric intensive care units. *Journal of Loss & Trauma*, *22*(1), 77–96. https://doi.org/10.1080/15325024.2016.1187049.

Zegwaard, M. I., Aartsen, M. J., Grypdonck, M. H., & Cuijpers, P. (2017). Trust: An essential condition in the application of a caregiver support intervention in nursing practice. *BMC Psychiatry*, *17*(1), 47. https://doi.org/10.1186/s12888-017-1209-2.

C

Disabled Family Coping Domain 9 Coping/stress tolerance Class 2 Coping responses

Marina Martinez-Kratz, MS, RN, CNE

NANDA-I

Definition

Behavior of primary person (family member, significant other, or close friend) that disables his or her capacities and the client's capacities to effectively address tasks essential to either person's adaptation to the health challenge.

Defining Characteristics

Abandons client; adopts illness symptoms of client; aggressive behaviors; depressive symptoms; difficulty structuring a meaningful life; disregards basic needs of client; disregards family relations; distorted reality about client's health problem; expresses feeling abandoned; family behaviors detrimental to well-being; hostility; impaired individualism; inadequate ability to tolerate client; loss of client independence; neglects treatment regimen; performing routines without regard for client's needs; prolonged hyperfocus on client; psychomotor agitation; psychosomatic symptoms

Related Factors

Ambivalent family relationships; chronically unexpressed feelings by support person; differing coping styles between support person and client; differing coping styles between support persons

NOC (Nursing Outcomes Classification)

Suggested NOC Outcomes

Caregiver Well-Being; Family Coping; Family Normalization; Neglect Recovery

C

Example NOC Outcome with Indicators

Family Normalization as evidenced by the following indicators: Adapts family routines to accommodate needs of affected member/Meets physical and psychosocial needs of family members/Provides activities appropriate to age and ability for affected family member/Uses community support groups. (Rate the outcome and indicators of **Family Normalization:** 1 = never demonstrated, 2 = rarely demonstrated, 3 = sometimes demonstrated, 4 = often demonstrated, 5 = consistently demonstrated [see Section I].)

Client Outcomes

Family/Significant Person Will (Specify Time Frame)

- Identify normal family routines that will need to be adapted
- Participate positively in the client's care within the limits of his or her abilities
- Identify responses that may be harmful
- Acknowledge and accept the need for assistance with circumstances
- Identify appropriate activities for affected family member

NIC (Nursing Interventions Classification)

Suggested NIC Interventions

Family Process Maintenance; Caregiver Support; Family Support; Family Therapy; Respite Care

Example NIC Activities—Family Process Maintenance

Determine typical family processes; Minimize family routine disruption by facilitating family routines and rituals such as private meals together or family discussions for communication and decision-making; Design schedules of home care activities that minimize disruption of family routine

Nursing Interventions and *Rationales*

- Families dealing with acute trauma are susceptible to mild to very severe levels of anxiety. Support should be offered through necessary channels, which are appropriate to the situation, such as providing frequent information, offering social services, or counseling. EB: *Findings from one study suggest that a large percentage of caregivers of clients with trauma suffered from mild to very severe levels of anxiety (Rahnama et al, 2017).*
- Assess coping strategies of family members. EBN: *A study found that assessment of family coping during a hospitalization of their child with cancer can help nurses develop and implement supportive interventions (Lyu et al, 2017).*
- Cancer caregiving interventions should include communication skill building, including strategies for self-care. EB: *Findings from this study confirmed that caregiver quality of life is affected by stress about communication across all domains (Wittenberg et al, 2017).*
- Provide ideas for positive child coping and consider collaboration with mental health providers for children with chronic illnesses who are facing emotional problems. EBN: *One study suggested that negative child coping may have deleterious effects on the family (Woodson et al, 2015).*
- Assess social support of family members caring for survivors of traumatic brain injuries (TBIs). Facilitate realistic expectations about caregiving. EB: *TBI survivors and caregivers had multiple self-reported unaddressed needs after their discharge from facility-based treatment. They expressed the need for further education regarding potential post-TBI challenges and strategies for addressing them, including a need for community and mental health resources (Adams & Dahdah, 2016).*
- Respect and promote the spiritual needs of the client and family. EB: *Spiritual well-being is associated with better mental health and positive coping skills of family caregivers (Kelley & Morrison, 2015).*

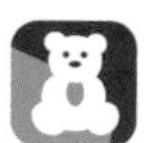

Pediatric

- Assist parents and children suffering from chronic illness to develop accommodative coping skills (adapting to stressors rather than attempting to change the stressors). EB: *A study of child and family coping with pediatric inflammatory bowel disease found participants coped through social support, cognitive strategies (positive attitude), behavioral strategies for managing emotions, and confidence in medical care (Easterlin et al, 2020).*

- Assess discharge readiness of parents of ill children and construct high-quality parent teaching to address educational attainment. EBN: *A study found a sequential effect of the quality of discharge teaching delivery on parent discharge readiness, which is associated with parent coping difficulty and child readmission (Weiss et al, 2017).*

C

Geriatric

- Assess the emotional well-being of family members who are caring for clients with long-term illnesses, such as stroke. EB: *Ali and Kausar (2016) studied levels of psychological distress experienced by the caregivers of clients who had a stroke, concluding that distress can be reduced by providing greater social support.*
- Be aware of age-related deterioration in coping skills. EB: *A study that compared executive functioning, short-term memory, and coping in a sample of young and older adults found young participants scored higher than older adults on executive functioning and short-term memory (Nieto et al, 2020).*

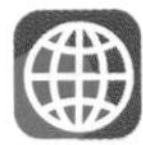

Multicultural

- Acknowledge racial/ethnic differences at the onset of care. EBN: *Acknowledgment of race/ethnicity issues will enhance communication, establish rapport, and promote treatment outcomes (Giger & Davidhizar, 2021).*
- Be sensitive to the stigma attached to particular illness in various cultures. EB: *Iseselo, Kajula, and Yahya-Malima (2016) studied families coping with mental illness in Tanzania and concluded that the psychosocial challenges of families and caregivers require a collaborative approach.*

Home Care

The interventions described previously may be adapted for home care use:

- Assess for strain in family caregivers.
- Assess for "caregiver fatigue" and provide information related to available respite care.
- Consult social services for available home resources related to the client's age and illness.

Client/Family Teaching and Discharge Planning

- Provide psychoeducational family teaching for families impacted by mental illness. EB: *A study found that psychoeducational family intervention was effective in improving the adaptive coping strategies of relatives of clients with a diagnosis of bipolar I disorder (Sampogna et al, 2018).*
- Involve the client and family in the planning of care as often as possible.
- Recognize that family decision makers may need additional psychosocial support services.

REFERENCES

Adams, D., & Dahdah, M. (2016). Coping and adaptive strategies of traumatic brain injury survivors and primary caregivers. *NeuroRehabilitation, 39*(2), 223–237. https://doi.org/10.3233/NRE-161353.

Ali, N., & Kausar, R. (2016). Social support and coping as predictors of psychological distress in family caregivers of stroke patients. *Pakistan Journal of Psychological Research, 31*(2), 587–608.

Easterlin, M. C., Berdahl, C. T., Rabizadeh, S., et al. (2020). Child and family perspectives on adjustment to and coping with pediatric inflammatory bowel disease. *Journal of Pediatric Gastroenterology and Nutrition, 71*(1), e16–e27. https://doi.org/10.1097/MPG.0000000000002693.

Giger, J., & Davidhizar, R. (2021). *Transcultural nursing: Assessment and intervention* (8th ed.). St. Louis: Elsevier.

Iseselo, M. K., Kajula, L., & Yahya-Malima, K. I. (2016). The psychosocial problems of families caring for relatives with mental illnesses and their coping strategies: A qualitative urban based study in dar es salaam, Tanzania. *BMC Psychiatry, 16*, 146. https://doi.org/10.1186/s12888-016-0857-y.

Kelley, A. S., & Morrison, R. S. (2015). Palliative care for the seriously ill. *New England Journal of Medicine, 373*(8), 747–755. https://doi.org/10.1056/nejmra140468.

Lyu, Q., Kong, S. K. F., Wong, F. K. Y., et al. (2017). Psychometric validation of an instrument to measure family coping during a child's hospitalization for cancer. *Cancer Nursing, 40*(3), 194–200. https://doi.org/10.1097/NCC.0000000000000382.

Nieto, M., Romero, D., Ros, L., et al. (2020). Differences in coping strategies between young and older adults: The role of executive functions. *International Journal of Aging and Human Development, 90*(1), 28–49. https://doi.org/10.1177/0091415018822040.

Rahnama, M., Shahdadi, H., Bagheri, S., Moghadam, M. P., & Absalan, A. (2017). The relationship between anxiety and coping strategies in family caregivers of patients with trauma. *Journal of Clinical and Diagnostic Research, 11*(4), 6–9. https://doi.org/10.7860/JCDR/2017/25951.9673.

Sampogna, G., Luciano, M., Del Vecchio, V., et al. (2018). The effects of psychoeducational family intervention on coping strategies of relatives of patients with bipolar I disorder: Results from a controlled, real-world, multicentric study. *Neuropsychiatric Disease and Treatment, 14*, 977–989. https://doi.org/10.2147/NDT.S159277.

Weiss, M. E., Sawin, K. J., Gralton, K., et al. (2017). Discharge teaching, readiness for discharge, and post-discharge outcomes in parents of hospitalized children. *Journal of Pediatric Nursing, 34*, 58–64. https://doi.org/10.1016/j.pedn.2016.12.021.

Wittenberg, E., Borneman, T., Koczywas, M., Del Ferraro, C., & Ferrell, B. (2017). Cancer communication and family caregiver quality of life. *Behavioral Sciences, 7*(1), 12. https://doi.org/10.3390/bs7010012.

Woodson, K. D., Thakkar, S., Burbage, M., Kichler, J., & Nabors, L. (2015). Children with chronic illnesses: Factors influencing family hardiness. *Issues in Comprehensive Pediatric Nursing, 38*(1), 57–69. https://doi.org/10.3109/01460862.2014.988896.

Readiness for Enhanced Family Coping

Domain 9 Coping/stress tolerance Class 2 Coping responses

Keith A. Anderson, PhD, MSW and Marina Martinez-Kratz, MS, RN, CNE

C

NANDA-I

Definition

A pattern of management of adaptive tasks by primary person (family member, significant other, or close friend) involved with the client's health challenge, which can be strengthened.

Defining Characteristics

Expresses desire to acknowledge growth impact of crisis; expresses desire to choose experiences that optimize wellness; expresses desire to enhance connection with others who have experienced a similar situation; expresses desire to enhance enrichment of lifestyle; expresses desire to enhance health promotion

NOC (Nursing Outcomes Classification)

Suggested NOC Outcomes

Family Coping; Health-Seeking Behavior; Participation in Health Care Decisions

Example NOC Outcome with Indicators

Family Coping as evidenced by the following indicators: Confronts and manages family problems/Cares for needs of all family members. (Rate the outcome and indicators of **Family Coping:** 1 = never demonstrated, 2 = rarely demonstrated, 3 = sometimes demonstrated, 4 = often demonstrated, 5 = consistently demonstrated [see Section I].)

Client Outcomes

Client Will (Specify Time Frame)

- State a plan indicating coping strengths, abilities, and resources, as well as areas for growth and change
- Perform tasks and engage resources needed for growth and change
- Evaluate changes and continually reevaluate plan for continued growth

NIC Interventions (Nursing Interventions Classification)

Suggested NIC Interventions

Family Integration Promotion; Family Involvement Promotion; Family Support; Mutual Goal Setting

Example NIC Activities—Family Coping

Facilitate communication of concerns and feelings between clients and family or among family members; Provide resources that support and encourage adaptive family coping; Respect and support adaptive coping mechanisms used by family

Nursing Interventions and *Rationales*

▲ Assess the structure, resources, and coping abilities of families and use these assessments in selecting interventions and formulating care plans. EBN: *It is critical to understand the resiliency and coping capabilities of families; the use of established assessment instruments (e.g., Family Assessment Device, Family Assessment Measure) can provide insight into family dynamics, coping styles, and resources of family systems (Sawin, 2016).*

▲ Acknowledge, assess, and support the spiritual needs and resources of families and clients. EB/EBN: *Spirituality has been found to be an important, yet often overlooked, coping resource for families and clients during illness and recovery (Hodge, 2015; Prouty et al, 2016).*

- ▲ Establish rapport with families and empower their decision-making through effective communication and person/family-centered care. EBN: *Effective communication and person/family-centered care approaches can help to establish rapport, personalize treatment plans, and empower families in their caregiving activities and decision-making capacities (Mitchell et al, 2016; Coombs et al, 2017).*
- ▲ Provide family members with educational and skill-building interventions to alleviate caregiving stress and to facilitate adherence to prescribed plans of care. EBN: *The provision of psychoeducational and supportive interventions may enable family members to gain a sense of control in the caregiving role and become more comfortable in providing care and making informed decisions (Dockham et al, 2016).*
- ▲ Develop, provide, and encourage family members to use counseling services and interventions. EBN: *Family-centered counseling interventions have been shown to be effective, particularly in situations regarding serious illness and difficult family decisions (Creasy et al, 2015).*
- ▲ Identify and refer to support programs that discuss experiences and challenges similar to those faced by the family (e.g., cancer support groups). EB: *Although there is wide diversity in the format of support programs, couples and family support approaches can be beneficial and enhance coping (Inhestern et al, 2016).*
- ▲ Incorporate the use of emerging technologies to increase the reach of interventions to support family coping. EBN: *Emerging computer and Internet-based supportive and educational interventions may hold promise in enhancing family members' well-being and informational needs (Risling, Risling, & Holtslander, 2017; Salem et al, 2017).*
- ▲ Refer to **Compromised Family Coping** for additional interventions.

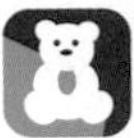

Pediatric

- ▲ Identify and assess the management styles of families and facilitate the use of more effective ways of coping with childhood illness. EB: *Understanding the dominant characteristics of each family's coping styles and resources and helping them to use more effective management styles can result in better family functioning and treatment outcomes (McCarthy et al, 2016; Ketelaar et al, 2017).*
- ▲ Provide educational and supportive interventions for families caring for children with illness and disability. EBN: *Providing information, training parents in care management, and offering supportive programs can reduce stress levels in parents and lead to better outcomes for children (Golfenshtein, Srulovici, & Deatrick, 2016).*

Geriatric

- ▲ Encourage family caregivers to participate in counseling and support groups. EB/EBN: *Although a wide variety of programs exist, certain counseling and support group programs have been found to be effective in increasing family resourcefulness and lowering caregiver burden, anxiety, depression, and family conflict (Dam et al, 2016; Muller et al, 2017).*
- ▲ Provide educational and therapeutic interventions to family caregivers that focus on knowledge and skill building. EBN: *Psychoeducational interventions that are accessible and tailored to individual needs can be highly valued and useful to family caregivers (Bakas, McCarthy, & Miller, 2017).*

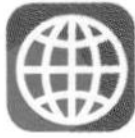

Multicultural

- ● Acknowledge the importance of cultural influences in families and ensure that assessments and assessment tools account for such cultural differences. EB: *Family coping tends to vary across cultures and may affect the fit, reliability, and validity of existing family functioning and coping assessment tools (Desai, Rivera, & Backes, 2016).*
- ● Understand and incorporate cultural differences into interventions to enhance the impact of family interventions. EB: *Tailoring interventions to the customs, beliefs, preferences, and strengths of specific groups may increase effectiveness (McCalman et al, 2017).*

REFERENCES

Bakas, T., McCarthy, M., & Miller, E. T. (2017). Update on the state of evidence for stroke family caregiver and dyad interventions. *Stroke, 48*(5), e122–e125. https://doi.org/10.1161/STROKEAHA.117.016052.

Coombs, M., Puntillo, K. A., Franck, L. S., et al. (2017). Implementing the SCCM Family-Centered Care Guidelines in critical care nursing practice. *AACN Advanced Critical Care, 28*(2), 138–147. https://doi.org/10.4037/aacnacc2017766.

Creasy, K. R., Lutz, B. J., Young, M. E., & Stacciarini, J. M. R. (2015). Clinical implications of family-centered care in stroke rehabilitation. *Rehabilitation Nursing, 40*(6), 349–359. https://doi.org/10.1002/rnj.188.

Dam, A. E. H., de Vugt, M. E., Klinkenberg, I. P. M., Verhey, F. R. J., & van Boxtel, M. P. J. (2016). A systematic review of social support interventions for caregivers of people with dementia: Are they doing what they promise? *Maturitas, 85*, 117–130. https://doi.org/10.1016/j.maturitas.2015.12.008.

Desai, P. P., Rivera, A. T., & Backes, E. M. (2016). Latino caregiver coping with children's chronic health conditions: An integrative

C

literature review. *Journal of Pediatric Health Care, 30*(2), 108–120. https://doi.org/10.1016/j.pedhc.2015.06.001.

Dockham, B., Schafenacker, A., Yoon, H., et al. (2016). Implementation of a psychosocial program for cancer survivors and family caregivers at a cancer support community affiliate: A pilot effectiveness study. *Cancer Nursing, 39*(3), 169–180. https://doi.org/10.1097/NCC.0000000000000311.

Golfenshtein, N., Srulovici, E., & Deatrick, J. A. (2016). Interventions for reducing parenting stress in families with pediatric conditions: An integrative review. *Journal of Family Nursing, 22*(4), 460–492. https://doi.org/10.1177/1074840716676083.

Hodge, D. R. (2015). Administering a two-stage spiritual assessment in healthcare settings: A necessary component of ethical and effective care. *Journal of Nursing Management, 23*(1), 27–38. https://doi.org/10.1111/jonm.12078.

Inhestern, L., Haller, A. C., Wlodararczyk, O., & Bergelt, C. (2016). Psychosocial interventions for families with parental cancer and barriers and facilitators to implementation and use: A systematic review. *PLoS One, 11*(6), e0156967. https://doi.org/10.1371/journal.pone.0156967.

Ketelaar, M., Bogossian, A., Saini, M., Visser-Meily, A., & Lach, L. (2017). Assessment of the family environment in pediatric neurodisability: A state-of-the-art review. *Developmental Medicine and Child Neurology, 59*(3), 259–269. https://doi.org/10.1111/dmcn.13287.

McCalman, J., Heyeres, M., Campbell, S., et al. (2017). Family-centred interventions by primary healthcare services for Indigenous early childhood well-being in Australia, Canada, New Zealand, and the United States: A systematic scoping review. *BMC Pregnancy and Childbirth, 17*(1), 71. https://doi.org/10.1186/s12884-017-1247-2.

McCarthy, M. C., Wakefield, C. E., DeGraves, S., Bowden, M., Eyles, D., & Williams, L. K. (2016). Feasibility of clinical psychosocial screening in pediatric oncology: Implementing the PAT2.0. *Journal of Psychosocial Oncology, 34*(5), 363–375. https://doi.org/10.1080/07347332.2016.1210273.

Mitchell, M. L., Coyer, F., Kean, S., Stone, R., Murfield, J., & Dwan, T. (2016). Patient, family-centred care interventions within the adult ICU setting: An integrative review. *Australian Critical Care, 29*(4), 179–193. https://doi.org/10.1016/j.aucc.2016.08.002.

Muller, C., Lautenschlager, S., Meyer, G., & Stephan, A. (2017). Interventions to support people with dementia and their caregivers during the transition from home care to nursing home care: A systematic review. *International Journal of Nursing Studies, 71*, 139–152.

Prouty, A. M., Fischer, J., Purdom, A., Cobos, E., & Helmeke, K. B. (2016). Spiritual coping: A gateway to enhancing family communication during cancer treatment. *Journal of Religion and Health, 55*(1), 269–287. https://doi.org/10.1007/s10943-015-0108-4.

Risling, T., Risling, D., & Holtslander, L. (2017). Creating a social media assessment tool for family nursing. *Journal of Family Nursing, 23*(1), 13–33. https://doi.org/10.1177/1074840716681071.

Salem, H., Johansen, C., Schmiegelow, K., et al. (2017). FAMily-Oriented Support (FAMOS): Development and feasibility of a psychosocial intervention for families of childhood cancer survivors. *Acta Oncologica, 56*(2), 367–374. https://doi.org/10.1080/0284186X.2016.1269194.

Sawin, K. J. (2016). Measurement in family nursing: Established instruments and new directions. *Journal of Family Nursing, 22*(3), 287–297. https://doi.org/10.1177/1074840716656038.

Readiness for Enhanced Decision-Making

Domain 10 Life principles
Class 3 Value/belief/action congruence

Dawn Fairlie, PhD, NP and Marina Martinez-Kratz, MS, RN, CNE

NANDA-I

Definition

A pattern of choosing a course of action for meeting short- and long-term health-related goals, which can be strengthened.

Defining Characteristics

Expresses desire to enhance congruency of decisions with sociocultural goal; expresses desire to enhance congruency of decisions with sociocultural value; expresses desire to enhance congruency of decisions with goal; expresses desire to enhance congruency of decisions with values; expresses desire to enhance decision-making; expresses desire to enhance risk-benefit analysis of decisions; expresses desire to enhance understanding of choices; expresses desire to enhance understanding of meaning of choices; expresses desire to enhance use of reliable evidence for decisions

NOC (Nursing Outcomes Classification)

Suggested NOC Outcomes

Decision-Making; Participation in Health Care Decisions; Personal Autonomy

Example NOC Outcome with Indicators

Participation in Health Care Decisions as evidenced by the following indicators: Claims decision-making responsibility/Exhibits self-direction in decision-making/Seeks reputable information/Specifies health outcome preferences. (Rate the outcome and indicators of **Participation in Health Care Decisions:** 1 = never demonstrated, 2 = rarely demonstrated, 3 = sometimes demonstrated, 4 = often demonstrated, 5 = consistently demonstrated [see Section I].)

Client Outcomes

Client Will (Specify Time Frame)

- Review treatment options with providers
- Ask questions about the benefits and risks of treatment options
- Communicate decisions about treatment options to providers in relation to personal preferences, values, and goals

NIC (Nursing Interventions Classification)

Suggested NIC Interventions

Decision-Making Support; Mutual Goal Setting; Support System Enhancement; Values Clarification

Example NIC Activities—Decision-Making Support

Help client identify the advantages and disadvantages of each alternative; Facilitate collaborative decision-making; Help client explain decisions to others, as needed

Nursing Interventions and *Rationales*

- Support and encourage clients and their representatives to engage in health care decisions. EB: *Decisional conflict was assessed using the Decisional Conflict Scale (DCS) among 186 Dutch mental health clients. They concluded that client participation in decision-making and measuring decisional conflict and knowledge about influencing factors could improve adherence to treatment and clinical outcomes (Metz et al, 2018).* EBN: *Decision aids are intended to help people participate in decisions that involve weighing the benefits and harms of treatment options, often with scientific uncertainty. Hart, Tofthagen, and Hsiao-Lan (2016) developed a decision aid that could be adapted and used in a variety of settings with a focus on initiating a conversation between the client and provider on lung cancer screening. Respect personal preferences, values, needs, and rights.* EBN: *"Clarifying values can be a rewarding exercise, as it not only ensures the best possible decision but demonstrates to patients that we are genuinely interested in incorporating their views and how they value the outcomes from screening options" (Lang et al, 2018, p 29).*
- Provide information that is appropriate, relevant, and timely. EBN: *Decisional conflict was assessed using the DCS among surrogate decision-makers to compare end-of-life terminologies "Do Not Resuscitate" (DNR) and "Allow Natural Death" (AND). Findings included that the framing of the decision influenced decision satisfaction and decision-making. Additionally, prior experience with end-of-life decision-making demonstrated lower mean total DCS scores and lower mean subscores, indicating that prior experience is an important aspect of end-of-life decision-making (Fairlie, 2017).*
- Determine the health literacy of clients and their representatives before helping with decision-making. EB: *An online decision aid for a low health literacy population will be pilot tested with 30 women diagnosed with early breast cancer with the anticipation that the low health literacy decision aid will be useful and acceptable to young women with low health literacy who have been diagnosed with breast cancer and it will be preferred over the high literacy decision aid (Peate et al, 2017).*
- Tailor information to the specific needs of individual clients, according to principles of health literacy. EB: *Altin and Stock (2016) sampled 1125 German adults to examine the contributions of health literacy, shared decision-making, person-centered communication, and satisfaction with care received by the general practitioner. Respondents with sufficient health literacy skills were 2.06 times as likely to be satisfied with their care.*
- Motivate clients to be as independent as possible in decision-making. EB: *A study of shared decision-making and autonomy among clients with multiple sclerosis revealed that person-centered decision-making was most commonly preferred by study participants, followed by shared decision-making (Cofield et al, 2017).*

- Facilitate communication between the client and family members regarding the final decision; offer support to the person actually making the decision. EBN: *A study of surrogate decision-makers' decisional conflict with end-of-life decision-making found that surrogates who had discussed end-of-life preferences with their loved one experienced less decisional conflict than those who had not discussed preferences (Fairlie, 2017).*
- Design educational interventions for decision support. EBN: *The goal of client decision aids is to engage clients in health care decisions by providing evidence-based information in plain language. The goal is to assist clients in understanding the risks and benefits of all available treatment/diagnosis options and engage clients in health care decisions to improve alignment of treatment choices with clients' preferences (Madden & Kleinlugtenbelt, 2017).*

Geriatric

- The previously mentioned interventions may be adapted for geriatric use.
- Facilitate collaborative decision-making. EB: *A systematic review of randomized controlled trials evaluating the efficacy of decision aids compared with the usual care for older adults facing treatment, screening, or care decisions found that decision aids improve older adults' knowledge, increase their risk perception, decrease decisional conflict, and seem to enhance participation in shared decision-making (van Weert et al, 2016).*

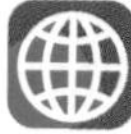

Multicultural

- Use existing decision aids for particular types of decisions or develop decision aids as indicated. EB: *Hoffman et al (2017) measured decisional conflict as a primary measure of decision quality and an intermediate measure in the process of screening uptake in a sample of 88 African American males. The purpose of client decision was to prepare clients for a consultation with their doctor. The entertainment–education decision aid significantly improved African American clients' knowledge, reduced their decisional conflict, and increased their sense of self-advocacy regarding colorectal cancer screening.*

Home Care

- The previously mentioned interventions may be adapted for home care use.
- Develop clinical practice guidelines that include shared decision-making. EBN: *Thoma-Lürken et al (2018) reported that people with dementia who wish to age in place are susceptible to nursing home admission. Nurses can intervene by detecting practical problems people with dementia and caregivers face. They identified three domains, decreased self-reliance, safety-related problems, and informal caregiver/social network-related problems, and proposed addressing these domains to facilitate aging in place.*

Client/Family Teaching and Discharge Planning

- Instruct the client and family members to provide advance directives in the following areas:
  - Person to contact in an emergency
  - Preference (if any) to die at home or in the hospital
  - Desire to initiate advance directives, such as a living will or medical power of attorney
  - Desire to donate an organ
  - Funeral arrangements (i.e., burial, cremation)

  EBN: *Shared decision-makers experienced less decisional conflict when they had discussed end-of-life preferences with the client (Fairlie, 2017).*

REFERENCES

Altin, S., & Stock, S. (2016). The impact of health literacy, patient-centered communication and shared decision-making on patients' satisfaction with care received in German primary care practices. *BMC Health Services Research, 16*(1), 450. https://doi.org/10.1186/s12913-016-1693-y.

Cofield, S., Thomas, N., Tyry, T., Fox, R. J., & Salter, A. (2017). Shared decision making and autonomy among US participants with multiple sclerosis in the NARCOMS Registry. *International Journal of MS Care, 19*(6), 303–312. https://doi.org/10.7224/1537-2073.2016-091.

Fairlie, D. E. (2017). Specific words and experience matter to surrogates when making end of life decisions. *Health Communication, 33*(5), 537–543. https://doi.org/10.1080/10410236.2017.1283560.

Hart, K., Tofthagen, C., & Hsiao-Lan, W. (2016). Development and evaluation of a lung cancer screening decision aid. *Clinical Journal of Oncology Nursing, 20*(5), 557–559. https://doi.org/10.1188/16.CJON.557-559.

Hoffman, A., Lowenstein, L., Kamath, G., et al. (2017). An entertainment-education colorectal cancer screening decision aid for African American patients: A randomized controlled trial. *Cancer, 123*(8), 1401–1408. https://doi.org/10.1002/cncr.30489.

Lang, E., Bell, N., Dickinson, J., et al. (2018). Eliciting patient values and preferences to inform shared decision making in preventive screening. *Canadian Family Physician, 64*(1), 28–31. PMID:29358246.

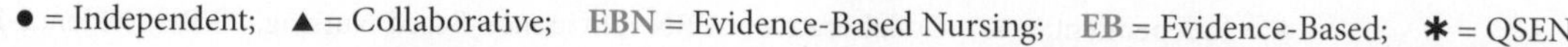

Madden, K., & Kleinlugtenbelt, Y. V. (2017). Cochrane in CORR: Decision aids for people facing health treatment or screening decisions. *Clinical Orthopaedics and Related Research, 475*(5), 1298–1304. https://doi.org/10.1007/s11999-017-5254-4.

Metz, M. J., Veerbeek, M. A., van der Feltz-Cornelis, C. M., de Beurs, E., & Beekman, A. T. F. (2018). Decisional conflict in mental health care: A cross-sectional study. *Social Psychiatry and Psychiatric Epidemiology, 53*(2), 161–169. https://doi.org/10.1007/s00127-017-1467-9.

Peate, M., Smith, S. K., Pye, V., et al. (2017). Assessing the usefulness and acceptability of a low health literacy online decision aid about reproductive choices for younger women with breast cancer: The aLLIAnCE pilot study protocol. *Pilot and Feasibility Studies, 3*, 31. https://doi.org/10.1186/s40814-017-0144-9.

Thoma-Lürken, T., Bleijlevens, M. H. C., Lexis, M. A. S., de Witte, L. P., & Hamers, J. P. H. (2018). Facilitating aging in place: A qualitative study of practical problems preventing people with dementia from living at home. *Geriatric Nursing, 39*(1), 29–38. https://doi.org/10.1016/j.gerinurse.2017.05.003.

van Weert, J. C. M., van Munster, B. C., Sanders, R., Spijker, R., Hooft, L., & Jansen, J. (2016). Decision aids to help older people make health decisions: A systematic review and meta-analysis. *BMC Medical Informatics and Decision Making, 16*(1), 45. https://doi.org/10.1186/s12911-016-0281-8.

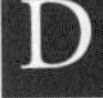

Decisional Conflict Domain 10 Life principles Class 3 Value/belief/action congruence

Dawn Fairlie, PhD, NP and Marina Martinez-Kratz, MS, RN, CNE

NANDA-I

Definition

Uncertainty about course of action to be taken when choice among competing actions involves risk, loss, or challenge to values and beliefs.

Defining Characteristics

Delayed decision-making; expresses distress during decision making; physical sign of distress; physical sign of tension; questions moral principle while attempting a decision; questions moral rule while attempting a decision; questions moral values while attempting a decision; questions personal beliefs while attempting a decision; questions personal values while attempting a decision; recognizes undesired consequences of potential actions; reports uncertainty about choices; self-focused; vacillating among choices

Related Factors

Conflict with moral obligation; conflicting information sources; inadequate information; inadequate social support; inexperience with decision-making; interference in decision-making; moral principle supports mutually inconsistent actions; moral rule supports mutually inconsistent actions; moral value supports mutually inconsistent actions; unclear personal beliefs; unclear personal values

NOC (Nursing Outcomes Classification)

Suggested NOC Outcomes

Decision-Making; Information Processing; Participation in Health Care Decisions; Personal Autonomy

Example NOC Outcome with Indicators

Decision-Making as evidenced by the following indicators: Identifies relevant information/Identifies alternatives/Identifies potential consequences of each alternative/Identifies needed resources to support each alternative. (Rate the outcome and indicators of **Decision-Making:** 1 = severely compromised, 2 = substantially compromised, 3 = moderately compromised, 4 = mildly compromised, 5 = not compromised [see Section I].)

Client Outcomes

Client Will (Specify Time Frame)

- State the advantages and disadvantages of choices
- Share fears and concerns regarding choices and responses of others

- Seek resources and information necessary for making an informed choice
- Make an informed choice

NIC (Nursing Interventions Classification)

Suggested NIC Intervention

D

Decision-Making Support

Example NIC Activities—Decision-Making Support

Inform client of alternative views or solutions in a clear and supportive manner; Provide information requested by client

Nursing Interventions and *Rationales*

- Observe for factors causing or contributing to conflict (e.g., value conflicts, fear of outcome, poor problem-solving skills). EB: *When studying clients with prostate cancer, Hoffman et al (2018) assessed differences across four treatment groups and asked about decision-making.*
- Provide emotional support. EB: *O'Neill et al (2018) assessed the information needs and levels of distress and correlates of this distress of young women with breast cancer. They reported lower distress and significantly lower decisional conflict and greater endorsement of an array of healthy coping strategies and suggested that young adult women have unmet cancer genetic information and support needs.*
- Use decision aids or computer-based decision aids to assist clients in making decisions. EB: *Baptista et al (2018) found that Web-based decision aids performed similarly to alternative formats for decision-quality outcomes. Additionally, because of anonymity, Web-based decision aids increased access to decision aids that support prostate cancer screening decisions among men. Initiate health teaching and referrals when needed.* EB: *Lopez-Olivo et al (2018) developed and tested multimedia education tools (video tools) for clients with knee osteoarthritis, osteoporosis, and rheumatoid arthritis. They found that multimedia educational tools that incorporate videos increase client understanding and management of their disease.*
- Facilitate communication between the client and family members regarding the final decision; offer support to the person actually making the decision. EBN: *A study of surrogate decision makers' decisional conflict with end-of-life decision-making found that surrogates who had discussed end-of-life preferences with their loved ones experienced less decisional conflict than those who had not discussed their preferences (Fairlie, 2018).*

Geriatric

- Carefully assess clients with dementia regarding ability to make decisions. EBN: *A study of the shared decision-making process of persons with dementia identified a broad spectrum of the shared decision-making process. Results indicated that not all persons with dementia are excluded from participating in the decision-making process. Loizeau et al (2018) tested the effect of fact box decision support tools on decisional conflict and preferences in advanced dementia. They found that fact boxes reduced decisional conflict, increased knowledge, and promoted preferences to forego antibiotics in advanced dementia in decision makers.*
- Discuss the purpose of advance directives such as a living will or medical power of attorney. EB: *Basile et al (2018) studied a Web-based decision aid in clients with severe chronic obstructive pulmonary disease to assist in preparation for decision-making about invasive mechanical ventilation for respiratory failure. Increased knowledge and opportunity to deliberate and discuss treatment choices after using the decision aid improved decision-making at the time of critical illness.*

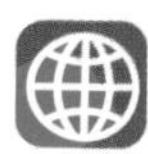

Multicultural

- Assess for the influence of cultural beliefs, norms, and values on the client's decision-making conflict. EB: *A study of couples undergoing genetic counseling found that factors associated with conflict during decision-making included cultural customs, age, emotional state, religious beliefs, and being forced to attend counseling. Provide support for client's decision-making (Schoeffel et al, 2018).*

Home Care

- The interventions described previously may be adapted for home care use.
- Encourage discussion of life-sustaining treatments and advance directives. EB: *Torke et al (2019) conducted a feasibility study of the Physician Orders for Life-Sustaining Treatment (POLST) with community-dwelling adults age 65 and older enrolled in a complex care management program. They found that 87.5% of decision makers agreed or strongly agreed that "talking about the (POLST) form helped me think about what I really want."*

D

Client/Family Teaching and Discharge Planning

- Instruct the client and family members to provide advance directives in the following areas:
  - ❍ Person to contact in an emergency
  - ❍ Preference (if any) to die at home or in the hospital
  - ❍ Desire to initiate advance directives, such as a living will or medical power of attorney
  - ❍ Desire to donate an organ
  - ❍ Funeral arrangements (i.e., burial, cremation)

  EBN: *Shared decision makers experienced less decisional conflict when they had discussed the client's preferences with the client (Fairlie, 2018).*
- Inform the family of treatment options; encourage and defend self-determination. EB: *Hwang et al (2018) surveyed clients seeking treatment for a lumbar herniated disc and measured decisional conflict using the SURE questionnaire. They found that participants with decisional conflict were less satisfied with their treatment decision and found a high level of decisional conflict when choosing a treatment option. They concluded that there is a need to implement tools and strategies to improve decisional quality, such as decision aids before consultation.*
- Recognize and allow the client to discuss the selection of complementary therapies available, such as spiritual support, relaxation, imagery, exercise, lifestyle changes, diet (e.g., macrobiotic, vegetarian), and nutritional supplementation. EB: *Hippman and Balneaves (2018) studied women's decision-making for treatment of depression during pregnancy and found that women require a nonjudgmental environment when choosing among medications, psychotherapy, electroconvulsive therapy, deep brain stimulation, and complementary and alternative medicine options.*

▲ Provide the POLST form for clients and families faced with end-of-life choices across the health care continuum. EB: *Torke et al (2019) found that a large majority of decision makers agreed or strongly agreed that talking about the (POLST) form helped with decision-making.*

REFERENCES

Baptista, S., Sampaio, E. T., Heleno, B., Azevedo, L. F., & Martins, C. (2018). Web-based versus usual care and other formats of decision aids to support prostate cancer screening decisions: Systematic review and meta-analysis. *Journal of Medical Internet Research, 20*(6), e228. https://doi.org/10.2196/jmir.9070.

Basile, M., Andrews, J., Jacome, S., Zhang, M., Kozikowski, A., & Hajizadeh, N. (2018). A decision aid to support shared decision making about mechanical ventilation in severe chronic obstructive pulmonary disease patients (InformedTogether): Feasibility study. *Journal of Participatory Medicine, 10*(2), e7. https://jopm.jmir.org/2018/2/e7/.

Fairlie, D. E. (2018). Specific words and experience matter to surrogates when making end of life decisions. *Health Communication, 33*(5), 537–543. https://doi.org/10.1080/10410236.2017.1283560.

Hippman, C., & Balneaves, L. G. (2018). Women's decision making about antidepressant use during pregnancy: A narrative review. *Depression and Anxiety, 35*(12), 1158–1167. https://doi.org/10.1002/da.22821.

Hoffman, R. M., Van Den Eeden, S. K., Davis, K. M., et al. (2018). Decision-making processes among men with low-risk prostate cancer: A survey study. *Psycho-Oncology, 27*(1), 325–332. https://doi.org/10.1002/pon.4469.

Hwang, R., Lambrechts, S., Liu, H., et al. (2018). Decisional conflict among patients considering treatment options for lumbar herniated disc. *World Neurosurgery, 116*, e680–e690. https://doi.org/10.1016/j.wneu.2018.05.068.

Loizeau, A. J., Theill, N., Cohen, S. M., et al. (2018). Fact box decision support tools reduce decisional conflict about antibiotics for pneumonia and artificial hydration in advanced dementia: A randomized controlled trial. *Age and Ageing, 48*(1), 67–74. https://doi.org/10.1093/ageing/afy149.

Lopez-Olivo, M. A., Ingleshwar, A., Volk, R. J., et al. (2018). Development and pilot testing of multimedia patient education tools for patients with knee osteoarthritis, osteoporosis, and rheumatoid arthritis. *Arthritis Care & Research, 70*(2), 213–220. https://doi.org/10.1002/acr.23271.

O'Neill, S. C., Evans, C., Hamilton, R. J., et al. (2018). Information and support needs of young women regarding breast cancer risk and genetic testing: Adapting effective interventions for a novel population. *Familial Cancer, 17*(3), 351–360. https://doi.org/10.1007/s10689-017-0059-x.

Schoeffel, K., Veach, P. M., Rubin, K., & LeRoy, B. (2018). Managing couple conflict during prenatal counseling sessions: An investigation of genetic counselor experiences and perceptions. *Journal of Genetic Counseling, 27*(5), 1275–1290. https://doi.org/10.1007/s10897-018-0252-6.

Torke, A. M., Hickman, S. E., Hammes, B., et al. (2019). POLST facilitation in complex care management: A feasibility study. *American Journal of Hospice and Palliative Care, 36*(1), 5–12. https://doi.org/10.1177/1049909118797077.

Risk for Elopement Attempt Domain 1 Health promotion Class 2 Health management

Marina Martinez-Kratz, MS, RN, CNE

D

NANDA-I

Definition

Susceptible to leaving a health care facility or a designated area against recommendation or without communicating to health care professionals or caregivers, which may compromise safety and/or health.

Risk Factors

Anger behaviors; exit-seeking behavior; frustration about delay in treatment regimen; inadequate caregiver vigilance; inadequate interest in improving health; inadequate social support; perceived complexity of treatment regimen; perceived excessive family responsibilities; perceived excessive responsibilities in interpersonal relations; perceived lack of safety in surrounding environment; persistent wandering; psychomotor agitation; self-harm intent; substance misuse

At-Risk Population

Economically disadvantaged individuals; homeless individuals; individuals brought to designated area against own wishes; individuals frequently requesting discharge; individuals hospitalized <three weeks; individuals with history of elopement; individuals with history of non-adherence to treatment regimen; individuals with history of self-harm; individuals with impaired judgment; men; older adults with cognitive disorders; unemployed individuals; young adults

Associated Conditions

Autism spectrum disorder; developmental disabilities; mental disorders

NOC (Nursing Outcomes Classification)

Suggested NOC Outcomes

Elopement Propensity Risk; Elopement Occurrence

Example NOC Outcome with Indicators

Elopement Propensity Risk as evidenced by the following indicators: Wanders/Attempts to leave secure area/Attempts to leave with visitors/States wants to go home/Threatens to leave. (Rate the outcome and indicators of **Elopement Propensity Risk:** 1 = consistently demonstrated, 2 = often demonstrated, 3 = sometimes demonstrated, 4 = rarely demonstrated, 5 = never demonstrated [see Section I.)

Client Outcomes

Client Will (Specify Time Frame)

- Remain safely and securely in treatment area
- Remain at scheduled activities
- Identify the consequences of leaving treatment
- Make a commitment to continuing treatment
- Accept discharge date and process

NIC (Nursing Interventions Classification)

Suggested NIC Intervention

Elopement Precautions

Example NIC Activities—Elopement Precautions

Monitor client for indicators of elopement potential (e.g., verbal indicators, loitering near exits, multiple layers of clothing, disorientation, separation anxiety, and homesickness); Limit patient to a physically-secure environment (e.g., locked or alarmed doors at exits and locked windows); Discuss with patient why he/she desires to leave the treatment setting; Encourage the patient, when appropriate, to make a commitment to continue treatment (e.g., contracting)

Nursing Interventions and *Rationales*

- Identify client factors associated with elopement risk and implement appropriate precautions. EB: *A systematic review regarding elopement in forensic clients found that previous elopements, aggression, substance use, high Historical Clinical Risk Management–20 score, antisocial tendencies, psychiatric symptoms, sexual offending, and poor treatment adherence were factors with predictive value for elopement (Olagunju et al, 2020).*
- Assess the client's stress level and coping. EB: *A retrospective chart review was completed on reported elopement events for over a 2-year period by clients on forensic units in a public psychiatric hospital. Results indicated that the best indicator of a client's risk for elopement was having experienced a stressful, significant event in the 2 weeks before the elopement (Martin et al, 2018).*
- Assess for and ask about the client's responsibilities and commitments outside of the hospital setting. EBN: *A systematic review found that clients who abscond from the hospital view their elopement as a means to meet their needs to address outside responsibilities and commitments (Voss & Bartlett, 2019).*
- Offer the client time and information so they can be involved in decision-making related to their care. EBN: *A systematic review found that clients who abscond from the hospital view their elopement as a positive means to exert power and control over their situation (Voss & Bartlett, 2019).*
- For clients admitted involuntarily to a psychiatric setting, implement elopement precautions to maintain client safety. EB: *Involuntary admission has been identified as a risk factor for elopement (Gowda et al, 2019).*

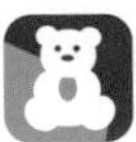

Pediatric

- Assess for factors associated with risk for elopement. EB: *A study examined predictors of initial elopement from residential care settings (RCSs) in a large sample of youth receiving residential treatment (n = 1261) and found 3 categories of elopement motivation. Youth with a diagnosis of disruptive behavior disorders were most likely to elope as were youth who were motivated by peer influence, escape from negative stimuli inside the RCS, and reinforcing stimuli outside the RCS (Milette-Winfree, Ku, & Mueller, 2017).*
- Counsel families of children diagnosed with autism spectrum disorder (ASD) about the danger related to elopement. EB: *Elopement behavior is exhibited by many children with a diagnosis of ASD. A study of elopement prevention for children diagnosed with ASD identified child and family characteristics that were related to elopement, the use of modifications, and stressed the importance of counseling families about elopement (Pereira-Smith et al, 2019).*
- ▲ If interested, refer families of children diagnosed with ASD for a consultation regarding electronic tracking device (ETD) technology. EB: *A recent study of families and caregivers of children with ASD found that in current (n = 361) and past (n = 96) ETD users, ETD use was associated with decreased frequency and duration of elopement and decreased risk for serious injury because of elopement (all p < 0.001) (McLaughlin et al, 2020).*

Geriatric

- Many of the previous interventions can be adapted for use with geriatric clients.
- Assess for behaviors that may indicate the client with dementia may elope or wander away. EB: *A study found six antecedent behaviors to wandering/elopement: stating intent to leave, door lingering/tampering, preparing to go outside, packing up belongings, calling to be picked up, and draw to outside stimuli (Neubauer & Liu, 2020).*
- Implement elopement precautions for clients who exhibit critical wandering behaviors. EB: *A systematic review calculated a rate of 82 deaths and 61 injuries per 1000 incidents of unexplained absence in nursing home clients (Woolford, Weller, & Ibrahim, 2017).*

- Use a unique room door design for individuals living with dementia in a residential care. EBN: *Internal doors were transformed using a giant adhesive poster created by a commercial graphic designer to replicate the look of traditional front doors. The Revised Algase Wandering Scale (RAWS) was used to identify the effects of introducing the doors on persistent walking, eloping behaviors, and spatial disorientation and found a reduction in all (Varshawsky & Traynor, 2021).*
- Implement a structured physical activity program for with dementia. EBN: *A study found that clients with dementia who participated in a structured physical activity program showed a statistically significant reductions in agitation ($p < 0.001$) and eloping ($p = 0.001$) (Traynor et al, 2018).*

D

- ▲ Refer to occupational therapy for assistive technology to address elopement safety for clients diagnosed with dementia. EB: *Study findings suggest that assistive technology devices are often used by occupational therapists to address safety concerns related to elopement with this population (Collins, 2018).*
- See the care plan for **Wandering.**

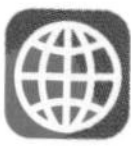

Multicultural

- The previous interventions can be adapted for use with multicultural clients.

Home Care

- The previous interventions can be adapted for use with home care clients.
- ▲ Refer families of clients with dementia to smart home technologies to manage nighttime wandering. EB: *The Night-time Wandering Detection and Diversion system detects when the person with dementia gets out of bed and automatically provides cue lighting to guide them safely to the bathroom, uses prerecorded audio prompts if individuals leave their bedroom, and wakes the caregiver when the person with dementia opens an exit door. A study found that the system is successful in supporting the safety of persons with dementia, as well as their caregivers (Ault et al, 2020).*

Client/Family Teaching and Discharge Planning

- Assess family reactions to the client's elopement attempts or wandering behavior. EBN: *A study found caregivers' health outcomes were negatively affected by the client's elopement behaviors. Specifically, clients getting lost outside of the house influenced caregivers' mental fatigue ($\beta = 0–0.215$, $p < .05$) and eloping behavior influenced caregivers' sleep disturbance ($\beta = 0.231$, $p < .05$) (Peng et al, 2018).*
- Provide family and caregivers information about elopement precautions. EB: *A home-based missing incident prevention program (HMIPP) was effective in reducing the number of missing incidents, searching time, and caregivers' stress at 3 months and 1 year. Interventions included dementia education, prescription of assistive devices, on-site skills training, environmental modifications, community service referrals, and redesigning of daily life routine tasks (Lau, Chan, & Szeto, 2019).*

REFERENCES

Ault, L., Goubran, R., Wallace, B., Lowden, H., & Knoefel, F. (2020). Smart home technology solution for night-time wandering in persons with dementia. *Journal of Rehabilitation and Assistive Technologies Engineering, 7*. https://doi.org/10.1177/2055668320938591.

Collins, M. E. (2018). Occupational therapists' experience with assistive technology in provision of service to clients with Alzheimer's disease and related dementias. *Physical & Occupational Therapy in Geriatrics, 36*(2–3), 179–188. https://doi.org/10.1080/02703181.2018.1458770.

Gowda, G. S., Thamby, A., Basavaraju, V., Nataraja, R., Kumar, C. N., & Math, S. B. (2019). Prevalence and clinical and coercion characteristics of patients who abscond during inpatient care from psychiatric hospital. *Indian Journal of Psychological Medicine, 41*(2), 144–149.

Lau, W. M., Chan, T. Y., & Szeto, S. L. (2019). Effectiveness of a home-based missing incident prevention program for community-dwelling elderly patients with dementia. *International Psychogeriatrics, 31*(1), 91–99. https://doi.org/10.1017/S1041610218000546.

Martin, K., McGeown, M., Whitehouse, M., & Stanyon, W. (2018). Who's going to leave? An examination of absconding events by forensic inpatients in a psychiatric hospital. *Journal of Forensic Psychiatry and Psychology, 29*(5), 810–823. https://doi.org/10.1080/14789949.2018.1467948.

McLaughlin, L., Rapoport, E., Keim, S., & Adesman, A. (2020). Wandering by children with autism spectrum disorders: Impact of electronic tracking devices on elopement behavior and quality of life. *Journal of Developmental and Behavioral Pediatrics, 41*(7), 513–521. https://doi.org/10.1097/DBP.0000000000000817.

Milette-Winfree, M., Ku, J., & Mueller, C. W. (2017). Predictors and motivational taxonomy of youth elopement from residential mental health placement. *Residential Treatment for Children & Youth, 34*(2), 135–154. https://doi.org/10.1080/0886571X.2017.1329643.

Neubauer, N. A., & Liu, L. (2020). Evaluation of antecedent behaviors of dementia-related wandering in community and facility settings. *Neurodegenerative Disease Management, 10*(3), 125–135. https://doi.org/10.2217/nmt-2019-0030.

Olagunju, A., Bouskill, S., Olagunju, T., Prat, S. S., Mamak, M., & Chaimowitz, G. A. (2020). Absconsion in forensic psychiatric services: A systematic review of literature. *CNS Spectrums, 27*(1), 1–12. https://doi.org/10.1017/S1092852920001881.

Peng, L., Chiu, Y., Liang, J., & Chang, T. H. (2018). Risky wandering behaviors of persons with dementia predict family caregivers' health outcomes. *Aging & Mental Health, 22*(12), 1650–1657. https://doi.org/10.1080/13607863.2017.1387764.

Pereira-Smith, S., Boan, A., Carpenter, L. A., Macias, M., & LaRosa, A. (2019). Preventing elopement in children with autism spectrum disorder. *Autism Research, 12*(7), 1139–1146. https://doi.org/10.1002/aur.2114.

Traynor, V., Veerhuis, N., Johnson, K., Hazelton, J., & Gopalan, S. (2018). Evaluating the effects of a physical activity on agitation and wandering (PAAW) experienced by individuals living with a dementia in care homes. *Journal of Research in Nursing, 23*(2–3), 125–138. https://doi.org/10.1177/1744987118756479.

Varshawsky, A. L., & Traynor, V. (2021). Graphic designed bedroom doors to support dementia wandering in residential care homes: Innovative practice. *Dementia, 20*(1), 348–354. https://doi.org/10.1177/1471301219868619.

Voss, I., & Bartlett, R. (2019). Seeking freedom: A systematic review and thematic synthesis of the literature on patients' experience of absconding from hospital. *Journal of Psychiatric and Mental Health Nursing, 26*, 289–300. https://doi.org/10.1111/jpm.12551.

Woolford, M. H., Weller, C., & Ibrahim, J. E. (2017). Unexplained absences and risk of death and injury among nursing home residents: A systematic review. *Journal of the American Medical Directors Association, 18*(4), 366.e1–366.e15. https://doi.org/10.1016/j.jamda.2017.01.007.

Impaired Emancipated Decision-Making Domain 10 Life principles Class 3 Value/belief/action congruence

Ruth A. Wittmann-Price, PhD, RN, CNS, CNE, CNEcl, CHSE, ANEF, FAAN

NANDA-I

Definition

A process of choosing a health care decision that does not include personal knowledge and/or consideration of social norms, or does not occur in a flexible environment, resulting in decisional dissatisfaction.

Defining Characteristics

Delayed enactment of health care option; difficulty choosing a health care option that best fits current lifestyle; expresses constraint in describing own opinion; expresses distress about others' opinion; expresses excessive concern about others' opinions; expresses excessive fear of what others think about a decision; impaired ability to describe how option will fit into current lifestyle; limited verbalization about health care option in others' presence

Related Factors

Decreased understanding of available health care options; difficulty adequately verbalizing perceptions about health care options; inadequate confidence to openly discuss health care options; inadequate information regarding health care options; inadequate privacy to openly discuss health care options; inadequate self-confidence in decision-making; insufficient time to discuss health care options

At-Risk Population

Individuals with limited decision making experience; women accessing health care from systems with patriarchal hierarchy; women living in families with patriarchal hierarch

NOC (Nursing Outcomes Classification)

Suggested NOC Outcomes

Decision-Making; Self-Esteem; Coping; Health Promoting Behavior; Stress Level; Communication; Self-Care Status; Participation in Health Care Decisions; Health-Seeking Processing; Personal Autonomy; Psychosocial Adjustment: Life Change

Example NOC Outcome with Indicators

Participation in Health Care Decisions as evidenced by the following indicator: Claims decision making responsibility. (Rate the outcome and indicators of **Participation in Health Care Decisions:** 1 = never demonstrated, 2 = rarely demonstrated, 3 = sometimes demonstrated, 4 = often demonstrated, 5 = consistently demonstrated [see Section I].)

Client Outcomes

Client Will (Specify Time Frame)

- Verbalize option outcomes freely before making a health care decision
- Freely verbalize own opinion with health care providers before making a health care decision
- Choose the health care option that fits his or her lifestyle within an appropriate amount of time that allows enactment of the choice
- Describe how the chosen option fits into his or her current lifestyle before or after the decision has been made
- Verbalizes appropriate concern about others' opinions before making the health care choice
- Remains stress-free when listening to others' opinions before making the health care choice
- Arrives at a decision in a timely manner

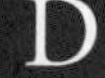

NIC (Nursing Interventions Classification)

Suggested NIC Interventions

Decision-Making Support; Health Coaching; Cognitive Restructuring; Self-Awareness Enhancement

Example NIC Activities—Emancipated Decision-Making

Assist client in making an emancipated decision about health care options by discussing social norms with the client; Provide a flexible environment; Encourage the client to use personal knowledge

Nursing Interventions and *Rationales*

- Assess client's readiness to openly discussing the decision-making process. EBN: *Using a qualitative approach, Huang et al (2020) studied shared decision-making in clients (n =12) with mental illness. The researchers found that clients preferred to use a shared decision-making approach to issues and actively sought health care information to make decisions.* EB: *Chen (2017) conducted a study with 15 clients with cancer about the decision-making process within three stages of cancer treatment and found that different decision-making approaches to provided information were taken by clients and ranged from informed to paternalistic to shared.*
- Use active listening in a nonjudgmental manner to provide the client with a flexible decision-making environment. EBN: *Through a literature review, van der Heijden et al (2020) found that adults rooming-in with hospitalized family members had a positive emotional effect on clients' well-being.* EB: *Park and colleagues (2020) studied (1) whether clients were invited into clinical decision-making processes and (2) whether administrators fostered person-centered health care and shared decision-making practices. The survey results disclosed that only 23% of substance abuse treatment clinics invited clients into treatment meetings.*
- Use anticipatory guidance by proactively providing the client with information. EB: *Williams et al (2020) completed an integrated review of the literature regarding decisions made by chronically ill clients and found four themes. The themes all suggested that effective communication and having clients involved in care decisions improved affect and promoted positive care outcomes.* CEB: *Wittmann-Price, Fliszar, and Bhattacharya (2011) found in a mixed method study that the majority of pregnant clients (N = 50) reported they had been provided with information prenatally, but not all clients felt they were given enough information at the time of delivery to make an informed choice.*
- Establish a purposeful provider–client relationship. EB: *A mixed methods study with clients who have Parkinson's disease (N = 65) demonstrated that the provider–client relationship was important for the client in the decision-making process (Zizzo et al, 2017).* EBN: *Sun et al (2020) completed a study to examine the relationship of client–provider communication (N = 320) in relation to treatment outcomes and clients' risk perception. The study demonstrated that client–provider communication has a significant influence on client treatment outcomes and their risk perception of the chosen treatments.*
- ▲ Refer to counseling as needed. EB: *Klausen et al (2017) studied clients in the outpatient setting (N = 25) who were referred for mental health issues and found four key components to shared decision-making: (1) during admission, (2) in individualized treatment, (3) in different treatment contexts, and (4) in user–professional relationships.* CEB: *Wittmann-Price (2006) demonstrated in a quantitative correlational study that women's (N = 97) decision-making was empowered when they were provided resources and information to arrive at an emancipated choice.*
- Provide decision-making support. EBN: *Quinn et al (2020) studied veteran women's (N = 2,302) decisions about contraception and found significant differences in unintended pregnancies and use of specific contraception in different ethnic and racial women. The study highlights the need for improved teaching,*

decision-making, and access to assist women in reaching their reproductive goals. EBN: *Lazenby et al (2017) studied 15 physicians and 5 nurses about their involvement in end-of-life conversations and decisions with hemodialysis clients and found that advanced decision-making planning was deficit and needed attention to accommodate clients' wishes.*

- Provide a flexible environment by encouraging others to accept the client's choice. EB: *Gerbasi et al (2020) studied women with postpartum depression in a randomized trial and how they reported symptoms in relation to the tool their provider was using. The researchers found that some tools actually promoted shared decision-making for women better than other postpartum assessment tools.* CEB: *Wittmann-Price and Bhattacharya (2008) quantitatively studied pain management decisions for clients in labor (N = 92) and found that a flexible environment was needed for the client to make a supported and emancipated decision.*
- Encourage the client to use personal knowledge as part of the decision-making process to increase decisional satisfaction. CEB: *Women can make health care decisions that are right for them if they can use personal knowledge to overcome oppressive social forces (Stepanuk et al, 2013).* CEB: *Using personal knowledge is the best indicator to making an emancipated decision and correlates strongly and positively with satisfaction with the decision (Wittmann-Price, 2006).*

Pediatric

- When able, involve the client in health care decision-making when possible. EBN: *Sedig et al (2020) studied decision-making in families with terminally ill children (N = 28) and found that the majority (61%) wanted shared decision-making. Being able to participate in end-of-life decision-making for their child significantly affected the parents' perception of the child's death.* EBN: *Craske et al (2017) studied how 12 nurses decide on withdrawal of pediatric sedation and found in complex pediatric cases that there is a variation in assessing client behavior and response to treatment.*
- Provide parental information in the decision-making process. EBN: *Richards et al (2017) performed an integrative review of family-centered behaviors that were experienced in the intensive care unit and found that there were five salient themes needed to engage parents in decision-making: (1) sharing information, (2) hearing parental voices, (3) making decisions for or with parents, (4) negotiating roles, and (5) individualizing communication.* EB: *Lin et al (2020) completed a qualitative study to understand parents' (N = 27) perspectives of shared decision-making for children with complex health care needs. The three themes that emerged from the parental interviews were participation, knowledge, and context.*
- Enhance client decision-making in the critical care setting. EBN: *Petrinec (2017) studied the family decision makers (N = 30) for long-term critical care clients and found they had post–intensive care syndrome, which warrants nursing awareness and interventions to support family decision makers.* EB: *A study completed by Kim et al (2020) compared clients' (N = 58) end-of-life decisions with the recommendations made by the rapid response team. Clients who used a rapid response team intervention were more successful in carrying out their end-of-life preferences for allowing a natural death.*

Geriatric

- Include geriatric clients in the decisional process. EB: *Lippe et al (2020) conducted a pilot study to assess a communication guide on clients' understanding of prognosis. The findings demonstrated that a communication guide can bridge the gap of understanding between provider and client allowing the client a more informed decision-making process.* EB: *Using a case study method, Strohschein et al (2020) found that implementing a program of comprehensive care can promote decision-making, facilitate communication, and contribute to personalization of care.*

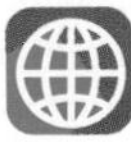

Multicultural

- Consider cultural influences on decision-making. EB: *Nogami et al (2020) studied the factors that influenced the decision-making processes of Japanese women (N = 44) facing end-of-life care due to metastatic breast cancer. The study demonstrated that younger clients and those with shorter recurrence-free time had more difficulty with decision-making.* EBN: *Adefris et al (2017) studied women (N = 384) who delayed treatment for uterine prolapse in sub-Saharan Africa and found that it was related to the "social stigma" within the culture.*

Home Care

- Use open communication to assist clients to develop health care plans to which they can adhere. EBN: *An integrative review of the literature by Bayless et al (2017) found that men who choose active surveillance rather than surgical intervention for prostate cancer take a more active, communicative role in the decision-making process.* EB: *Lussier et al (2020) investigated the effects of using ambient assisted living*

(AAL) technologies as part of home care monitoring. The researchers found that AAL monitoring helped health care professionals to have information that they may not have had otherwise and the information gained assisted the health care providers in caring for the clients.

REFERENCES

Adefris, M., Abebe, S. M., Terefe, K., et al. (2017). Reasons for delay in decision making and reaching health facility among obstetric fistula and pelvic organ prolapse patients in Gondar University Hospital, Northwest Ethiopia. *BMC Women's Health, 17*(1), 64. https://doi.org/10.1186/s12905-017-0416-9.

Bayless, D. R., Duff, J., Stricker, P., & Walker, K. (2017). Decision-making in prostate cancer—Choosing active surveillance over other treatment options: A literature review. *Urologic Nursing, 37*(1), 15–22. https://doi.org/10.7257/1053-816X.2017.37.1.15.

Chen, S. (2017). Information behaviour and decision-making in patients during their cancer journey. *The Electronic Library, 35*(3), 494–506. https://doi.org/10.1108/EL-03-2016-0062.

Craske, J., Carter, B., Jarman, I. H., & Tume, L. N. (2017). Nursing judgement and decision-making using the Sedation Withdrawal Score (SWS) in children. *Journal of Advanced Nursing, 73*(10), 2327–2338. https://doi.org/10.1111/jan.13305.

Gerbasi, M. E., Elder-Lissai, A., Acaster, S., et al. (2020). Associations between commonly used patient-reported outcome tools in postpartum depression clinical practice and the Hamilton Rating Scale for Depression. *Archives of Women's Mental Health, 23*(5), 727–735. https://doi.org/10.1007/s00737-020-01042-y.

Huang, C., Plummer, V., Wang, Y., Lam, L., & Cross, W. (2020). I am the person who knows myself best: Perception on shared decision-making among hospitalized people diagnosed with schizophrenia in China. *International Journal of Mental Health Nursing, 29*(5), 846–855. https://doi.org/10.1111/inm.12718.

Kim, J. S., Lee, M. J., Park, M. H., Park, J. Y., & Kim, A. J. (2020). Role of the rapid response System in end-of-life care decisions. *American Journal of Hospice & Palliative Care, 37*(11), 943–949. https://doi.org/10.1177/1049909120927372.

Klausen, R. K., Blix, B. H., Karlsson, M., Haugsgjerd, S., & Lorem, G. F. (2017). Shared decision making from the service users' perspective: A narrative study from community mental health centers in northern Norway. *Social Work in Mental Health, 15*(3), 354–371. https://doi.org/10.1080/15332985.2016.1222981.

Lazenby, S., Edwards, A., Samuriwo, R., Riley, S., Murray, M. A., & Carson-Stevens, A. (2017). End-of-life care decisions for haemodialysis patients—We only tend to have that discussion with them when they start deteriorating. *Health Expectations, 20*(2), 260–273. https://doi.org/10.1111/hex.12454.

Lin, J., Clark, C. L., Halpern-Felsher, B., et al. (2020). Parent perspectives in shared decision-making for children with medical complexity. *Academic Pediatrics, 20*(8), 1101–1108. https://doi.org/10.1016/j.acap.2020.06.008.

Lippe, M., Phillips, F., McCulloch, J., Alexandra, S., Jones, B., & Goodgame, B. (2020). Communicating oncologic prognosis with empathy: A pilot study of a novel communication guide. *American Journal of Hospice and Palliative Medicine, 37*(12), 1029–1036. https://doi.org/10.1177/1049909120921834.

Lussier, M., Couture, M., Moreau, M., et al. (2020). Integrating an ambient assisted living monitoring system into clinical decision-making in home care: An embedded case study. *Gerontechnology, 19*(1), 77–92. https://doi.org/10.4017/gt.2020.19.1.008.00.

Nogami, N., Nakai, K., Horimoto, Y., Mizushima, A., & Saito, M. (2020). Factors affecting decisions regarding terminal care locations of patients with metastatic breast cancer. *American Journal of Hospice and Palliative Medicine, 37*(10), 853–858. https://doi.org/10.1177/1049909119901154.

Park, S., Mosley, J. E., Grogan, C. M., et al. (2020). Patient-centered care's relationship with substance use disorder treatment utilization. *Journal of Substance Abuse Treatment, 118*, 108125. https://doi.org/10.1016/j.jsat.2020.108125.

Petrinec, A. (2017). Post-intensive care syndrome in family decision makers of long-term acute care hospital patients. *American Journal of Critical Care, 26*(5), 416–422. https://doi.org/10.4037/ajcc2017414.

Quinn, D. A., Sileanu, F. E., Zhoa, X., et al. (2020). History of unintended pregnancy and patterns of contraceptive use among racial and ethnic minority women veterans. *American Journal of Obstetrics and Gynecology, 223*(4), 564.e1–564.e13. https://doi.org/10.1016/j.ajog.2020.02.042.

Richards, C. A., Starks, H., O'Connor, M. R., & Doorenbos, A. Z. (2017). Elements of family-centered care in the pediatric intensive care unit: An integrative review. *Journal of Hospice and Palliative Nursing, 19*(3), 238–246. https://doi.org/10.1097/NJH.0000000000000335.

Sedig, L. K., Spruit, J. L., Paul, Y. K., et al. (2020). Supporting pediatric patients and their families at the end of life: Perspectives from bereaved parents. *American Journal of Hospice and Palliative Medicine, 37*(12), 1009–1015. https://doi.org/10.1177/1049909120922973.

Stepanuk, K. M., Fisher, K. M., Wittmann-Price, R., Posmontier, B., & Bhattacharya, A. (2013). Women's decision-making regarding medication use in pregnancy for anxiety and/or depression. *Journal of Advanced Nursing, 69*(11), 2470–2480.

Strohschein, F. J., Loucks, A., Jin, R., & Vanderbyl, B. (2020). Comprehensive geriatric assessment: A case report on personalizing cancer care of an older adult patient with head and neck cancer. *Clinical Journal of Oncology Nursing, 24*(5), 514–525. https://doi.org/10.1188/20.CJON.514-525.

Sun, C., Wei, D., Gong, H., Ding, X., & Wu, X. (2020). How does patient provider communication affect patients' risk perception? A scenario experiment and an exploratory investigation. *International Journal of Nursing Practice, 26*(5), e12872. 10.1111/ijn.12872.

van der Heijden, M. J. E., van Mol, M. M. C., Witkamp, E. F. E., Osse, R. J., Ista, E., & van Dijk, M. (2020). Perspectives of patients, relatives and nurses on rooming-in for adult patients: A scoping review of the literature. *Applied Nursing Research, 55*, 151320. https://doi.org/10.1016/j.apnr.2020.151320.

Williams, M. T., Kozachik, S. L., Karlekar, M., & Wright, R. (2020). Advance care planning in chronically ill persons diagnosed with heart failure or chronic obstructive pulmonary disease: An integrative review. *American Journal of Hospice and Palliative Medicine, 37*(11), 950–956. https://doi.org/10.1177/1049909120909518.

Wittmann-Price, R. A. (2006). Exploring the subconcepts of the Wittmann-Price Theory of Emancipated Decision-Making in women's health care. *Journal of Nursing Scholarship, 38*(4), 377–382. https://doi.org/10.1111/j.1547-5069.2006.00130.x.

Wittmann-Price, R. A., & Bhattacharya, A. (2008). Reexploring the subconcepts of the Wittmann-Price Theory of Emancipated Decision-Making in women's healthcare. *Advances in Nursing Science, 31*(3), 225–236. https://doi.org/10.1097/01.ANS.0000334286.81354.16.

Wittmann-Price, R. A., Fliszar, R., & Bhattacharya, A. (2011). Elective cesarean births: Are women making emancipated decisions? *Applied Nursing Research, 24*, 147–152. https://doi.org/10.1016/j.apnr.2009.08.002.

Zizzo, N., Bell, E., LaFontaine, A. L., & Racine, E. (2017). Examining chronic care patient preferences for involvement in health-care decision making: The case of Parkinson's disease patients in a patient-centered clinic. *Health Expectations, 20*(4), 655–664. https://doi.org/10.1111/hex.12497.

Readiness for Enhanced Emancipated Decision-Making

Domain 10 Life principles Class 3 Value/belief/action congruence

Ruth A. Wittmann-Price, PhD, RN, CNS, CNE, CNEcl, CHSE, ANEF, FAAN

D

NANDA-I

Definition

A process of choosing a health care decision that includes personal knowledge and/or consideration of social norms, which can be strengthened.

Defining Characteristics

Expresses desire to enhance ability to choose health care options that enhance current lifestyle; expresses desire to enhance ability to enact chosen health care option; expresses desire to enhance ability to understand all available health care options; expresses desire to enhance ability to verbalize own opinion without constraint; expresses desire to enhance comfort to verbalize health care options in the presence of others; expresses desire to enhance confidence in decision-making; expresses desire to enhance confidence to discuss health care options openly; expresses desire to enhance decision-making; expresses desire to enhance privacy to discuss health care options

NOC (Nursing Outcomes Classification)

Suggested NOC Outcomes

Decision-Making; Self-Esteem; Coping; Health Promotion Behavior; Stress Level; Communication; Self-Care; Participation in Health Care Decisions; Health-Seeking Behavior; Knowledge: Treatment Options; Psychosocial Adjustment

Example NOC Outcome with Indicators

Participation in Health Care Decisions as evidenced by the following indicator: Claims decision-making responsibility. (Rate the outcome and indicators of **Participation in Health Care Decisions:** 1 = never demonstrated, 2 = rarely demonstrated, 3 = sometimes demonstrated, 4 = often demonstrated, 5 = consistently demonstrated [see Section I].)

Client Outcomes

Client Will (Specify Time Frame)

- Verbalize option of outcomes freely before making a health care decision
- Freely verbalize own opinion with health care providers before making a health care decision
- Choose the health care option that best fits his or her lifestyle within an appropriate amount of time that allows enactment of the choice
- Describe how the chosen option fits into his or her current lifestyle before or after the decision has been made
- Verbalizes appropriate concern about others' opinions before making the health care choice
- Remains stress-free when listening to others' opinions before making the health care choice
- Arrives at a decision in a timely manner

NIC (Nursing Interventions Classification)

Suggested NIC Intervention

Decision-Making Support

Example NIC Activities—Emancipated Decision-Making

Assist client in making an emancipated decision about health care options by discussing social norms with the client; Provide a flexible environment; Encourage the client to use personal knowledge

Nursing Interventions and *Rationales*

- Assess client's readiness to choose through active listening. EBN: *Chen et al (2017) applied a home-based, individually tailored intervention, which included nursing education, skills training, listening/counseling, and resources for family caregivers of cognitively impaired individuals. Listening skills and interventions improved caregiving skills and increased the family's quality of life.* EB: *Barnett, Sivam, and Easthall (2020) studied the confidence of pharmacy students in using a person-centered care approach that included shared decision-making. The researchers successfully provided professional development about shared decision-making and it increased scores on participants self-confidence post-test. Information included in the professional development to enhance pharmacists use of shared decision-making were active listening, using open questions, method to empower clients, developing a shared agenda, and encouraging clients to be accountable.*
- Use anticipatory guidance by proactively providing the client with information. (Refer to Impaired Emancipated **Decision-Making.**)
- Establish a purposeful provider–client relationship. EB: *Researchers examined the quality of the client–provider relationship and its effect on attachment and self-management of clients with multiple chronic diseases (N = 209). The study results demonstrated that client–provider relationships with attachment and communication provide that client with information and improve decisions about self-management (Brenk-Franz et al, 2017).* EB: *Stanley et al (2020) studied the effects of client–provider relationship on health care decisions of African American women. The researchers found that communication is key to improving client–provider trust. The focus groups discussed that the lack of commitment by the provider was a barrier to the client–provider relationship.*
- ▲ Include multiprofessional health care team members as needed to increase knowledge of chosen option. EB: *Wong et al (2017) studied the lived experience of emergency department (ED) staff (N = 31) members caring for agitated clients and found three themes from the focus groups: (1) ED staff provide high-quality care to marginalized clients, (2) teamwork is critical to safely managing clients and hierarchy and professional silos hinder care, and (3) environmental challenges increase threats to staff safety.* EB: *Labuschagne et al (2020) studied the spiritual needs of clients and their families (N = 254) admitted to the intensive care unit (ICU). Of all the clients and families seen for spiritual care by hospital Chaplains only 15% requested assistance in decision-making. The researchers suggest that Chaplains should be a more prominent part of the client's decision-making process, especially during times that include end-of-life care.*
- Provide decision-making support. (Refer to Impaired Emancipated **Decision-Making.**)
- Continue to provide a flexible environment for client to enact choice. EB: *Investigators studied shared decision-making about health care options with spinal cord injury (SCI) clients (N = 22) during the clients' first rehabilitation experience and found that decision-making capabilities were reduced in the first few days of hospitalizations because of physical, psychological, and environmental factors. Additionally, they stated that understandable, personalized information was necessary to participate in decision-making (Scheek-Sailer et al, 2017).* EB: *Li et al (2021) studied the Internet environment in relation to client decision-making. The researchers found that clients using the Internet had better follow-up outcomes and factors that assisted follow-up decisions included technical quality and interpersonal connectivity.*
- Encourage the client to use personal knowledge as part of the decision-making process to increase decisional satisfaction. EB: *Hultberg and Rudebeck (2017) explored client agency and resistance in decision-making about cardiovascular treatments in primary care settings. The study described client resistance as part of the decision-making process and it can be passive or aggressive. Health care providers need to allow client agency and open communication to establish a working relationship in shared decision-making.* EB: *Melzer et al (2020) qualitatively studied practitioners' (N = 24) views about shared decision-making for clients who are eligible for lung cancer screening. Interviews verified that practitioners agreed that screening should be congruent with clients' values and preferences.*

Pediatric

- Understand interventions that parents prefer when in the decision-making process. EBN: *Craske et al (2017) studied withdrawal syndrome in children and how nurses (N = 12) make decisions about treatment and qualitatively found each stage of decision-making described as noticing, interpreting, and responding.* EB: *Yamaji et al (2020) completed a meta-synthesis about children's decision-making related to palliative care, treatment, and family involvement. The four themes were (1) facing changes, (2) preparing for action, (3) asserting one's choice, and (4) internal and external influences. The results demonstrated that children's preferences, values, and emotions are part of building a relationship with health care providers and this enhances their decision-making ability.*

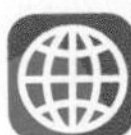

Multiculturai

- Use open communication to assist clients to develop health care plans to which they can adhere. EBN: *Rodrigo, Caïs, and Monforte-Rovo (2017) used grounded theory to examine nurses' participation in decision-making in Spain and found that the health care system still functions mainly from a disease-focused view making it difficult for nurses to take responsibility for decision-making.*

D

Home Care/Nursing Home Care

- Optimize self-care personal knowledge for home care. EB: *Mariani et al (2017) studied shared decision-making in clients with dementia and found that team collaboration and communication skills assisted shared decision-making. Lack of funding and lack of family involvement hindered shared decision-making in nursing home care, but findings can be applicable to home care.* EBN: *Coburn (2018) used a grounded theory study to understand the reasons why women (N = 11) choose a home birth rather than a traditional hospital delivery. The study was based on the Emancipated Decision-Making Theory, and the women revealed the reasons for choosing a home birth fell into the following themes: (1) realizing an alternative, (2) deciding to call the shots, and (3) building a shelter.*
- Refer to care plan Impaired Emancipated **Decision-Making** for additional interventions for pediatric, critical care, geriatric, and multicultural care.

REFERENCES

Barnett, N. L., Sivam, R., & Easthall, C. (2020). Pilot study to evaluate knowledge of person-centred care, before and after a skill development programme, in a cohort of preregistration pharmacists within a large London hospital. *European Journal of Hospital Pharmacy: Science and Practice*, *27*(4), 222–225. https://doi.org/10.1136/ejhpharm-2018-001704.

Brenk-Franz, K., Strauß, B., Tiesler, F., Fleischhauer, C., Schneider, N., & Gensichen, J. (2017). Patient-provider relationship as mediator between adult attachment and self-management in primary care patients with multiple chronic conditions. *Journal of Psychosomatic Research*, *97*, 131–135. https://doi.org/10.1016/j.jpsychores.2017.04.007.

Chen, M. C., Chiu, Y. C., Wei, P. M., & Hsu, W. C. (2017). Reducing the care-related burdens of a family caregiver of a person with mild cognitive impairment: A home-based case management program. *Hu Li Za Zhi: The Journal of Nursing*, *64*(3), 105–111. https://doi.org/10.6224/JN.000046.

Coburn, J. (2018). Deciding to call the shots: Awareness, agency, and shelter-building during home birth planning. *Theses and Dissertations, 1776*. Retrieved from https://dc.uwm.edu/etd/1776. [Accessed June 21, 2021].

Craske, J., Carter, B., Jarman, I. H., & Tume, L. N. (2017). Nursing judgement and decision-making using the Sedation Withdrawal Score (SWS) in children. *Journal of Advanced Nursing*, *73*(10), 2327–2338. https://doi.org/10.1111/jan.13305.

Hultberg, J., & Rudebeck, C. E. (2017). Patient participation in decision-making about cardiovascular preventive drugs—resistance as agency. *Scandinavian Journal of Primary Health Care*, *35*(3), 231–239. https://doi.org/10.1080/02813432.2017.1288814.

Labuschagne, D., Torke, A., Grossoehme, D., et al. (2020). Chaplaincy care in the MICU: Describing the spiritual care provided to MICU patients and families at the end of life. *American Journal of Hospice and Palliative Medicine*, *37*(12), 1037–1044. https://doi.org/10.1177/1049909120912933.

Li, C., Zhang, E., & Han, J. (2021). Adoption of online follow-up service by patients: An empirical study based on the elaboration likelihood model. *Computers in Human Behavior*, *114*, 106581. https://doi.org/10.1016/j.chb.2020.106581.

Mariani, E., Vernooij-Dassen, M., Koopmans, R., Engels, Y., & Chattat, R. (2017). Shared decision-making in dementia care planning: Barriers and facilitators in two European countries. *Aging & Mental Health*, *21*(1), 31–39. https://doi.org/10.1080/13607863.2016.1255715.

Melzer, A. C., Golden, S. E., Ono, S. S., Datta, S., Crothers, K., & Slatore, C. G. (2020). What exactly is shared decision-making? A qualitative study of shared decision-making in lung cancer screening. *Journal of General Internal Medicine*, *35*(2), 546–553. https://doi.org/10.1007/s11606-019-05516-3.

Rodrigo, O., Caïs, J., & Monforte-Rovo, C. (2017). Professional responsibility and decision-making in the context of a disease-focused model of nursing care: The difficulties experienced by Spanish nurses. *Nursing Inquiry*, *24*(4). https://doi.org/10.1111/nin.12202.

Scheek-Sailer, A., Post, M. W., Michel, F., Weidmann-Hügle, T., & Hölzle, R. B. (2017). Patients' views on their decision making during inpatient rehabilitation after newly acquired spinal cord injury—A qualitative interview-based study. *Health Expectations*, *20*(5), 1133–1142. https://doi.org/10.1111/hex.12559.

Stanley, S. J., Chatham, A. P., Trivedi, N., & Aldoory, L. (2020). Communication and control: Hearing the voices of low-income African American adults to improve relationships with healthcare providers. *Health Communication*, *35*(13), 1633–1642. https://doi.org/10.1080/10410236.2019.1654177.

Wong, A. H., Combellick, J., Wispelwey, B. A., Squires, A., & Gang, M. (2017). The patient care paradox: An interprofessional qualitative study of agitated patient care in the emergency department. *Academic Emergency Medicine*, *24*(2), 226–235. https://doi.org/10.1111/acem.13117.

Yamaji, N., Suto, M., Takemoto, Y., Suzuki, D., da Silva Lopes, K., & Ota, E. (2020). Supporting the decision making of children with cancer: A meta-synthesis. *Journal of Pediatric Oncology Nursing*, *37*(6), 431–443. https://doi.org/10.1177/1043454220919711.

Risk for Impaired Emancipated Decision-Making

Domain 10 Life principles Class 3 Value/belief/action congruence

Ruth A. Wittmann-Price, PhD, RN, CNS, CNE, CNEcl, CHSE, ANEF, FAAN

D

NANDA-I

Definition

Susceptible to a process of choosing a health care decision that does not include personal knowledge and/or consideration of social norms, or does not occur in a flexible environment, resulting in decisional dissatisfaction.

Risk Factors

Decreased understanding of available health care options; difficulty adequately verbalizing perceptions about health care options; inadequate confidence to openly discuss health care options; inadequate information regarding health care options; inadequate privacy to openly discuss health care options; inadequate self-confidence in decision-making; insufficient time to discuss health care options

At-Risk Population

Individuals with limited decision making experience; women accessing health care from systems with patriarchal hierarchy; women living in families with patriarchal hierarchy

NOC (Nursing Outcomes Classification)

Suggested NOC Outcomes

Decision-Making; Self-Confidence; Coping; Health Promotion Behavior; Stress Level; Communication; Self-Care; Participation in Health Care Decisions; Health-Seeking Behavior; Knowledge; Treatment Options; Psychosocial Adjustment

Example NOC Outcome with Indicators

Participation in Health Care Decisions as evidenced by the following indicator: Claims decision-making responsibility. (Rate the outcome and indicators of **Participation in Health Care Decisions:** 1 = never demonstrated, 2 = rarely demonstrated, 3 = sometimes demonstrated, 4 = often demonstrated, 5 = consistently demonstrated [see Section I].)

Client Outcomes

Client Will (Specify Time Frame)

- Verbalize option outcomes freely before making a health care decision in a private setting with in which he or she feels comfortable
- Freely verbalize own opinion with health care providers before making a health care decision
- Discuss how options fit or hinder his or her lifestyle within an appropriate amount of time that allows enactment of the choice
- Discuss concerns about others' opinions before making the health care choice
- Decrease stress about others' opinions by placing options in perspective through informational resources
- Discuss the time frame in which the decision needs to be made

NIC (Nursing Interventions Classification)

Suggested NIC Interventions

Establish Rapport; Decision-Making Support

Example NIC Activities—Emancipated Decision-Making

Assist client to verbalize and discuss barriers that she or he perceives in making an emancipated decision about health care options; Acknowledge social norms about decision options; Provide a flexible environment that is safe and private for the discussions; Use empathy to understand the client's personal point of view about the options

Nursing Interventions and *Rationales*

- Assess client's vulnerability for an impaired decision-making process. EBN: *Scheepmans et al (2017) studied the decision-making process of placing older adults (N = 5) in restraints at home and found through a cross-sectional survey that the main decision-making variables were safety, keeping the client home longer, and to provide respite for the caregiver.* EB: *Hell and Nielsen (2020) did a literature review (N = 6) about informed decisions related to alcohol-addicted clients and their choice of rehabilitation. The researchers examined four variables: (1) drinking outcome, (2) quality of life (QOL), (3) enrollment, and (4) adherence. The researchers found that involving clients in the choice of treatment improved QOL, increased enrollment, and promoted adherence.*
- Assess the client's experience with decision-making. EBN: *Smith et al (2017) studied cancer clients (N = 21) perceptions of their involvement in treatment decisions and found that most clients just consented to radiation because of oncologist recommendations. The study recommends that clients be provided with more opportunities to ask questions to be empowered in decisions about their uncertainties and concerns.* EBN: *Lippe et al (2020) completed a study to pilot a communication guide for clients with terminal cancer because they often needed to engage in prompt decision-making. The communication guide was developed by a multiprofessional team that included nurses. The research team found that clients wanted detailed information and welcomed different perspectives when making prompt decisions about their care.*
- Recognize the traditional hierarchical family and health care system. EBN: *Petrinec (2017) studied the effect of clients' long-term care experiences on the family decision maker (N = 30) and found, using a qualitative descriptive study method, that family decision makers need support and often have post–intensive care syndrome caused by the stress.* EBN: *Virdun et al (2020) used an exploratory qualitative method with semi-structured interviews (N = 21) to ascertain if palliative care clients perceived their needs were met and their decisions were respected by health care professionals. The important themes that emerged about decision-making were the need for effective communication and shared decision-making; the need for expert care; and family involvement, financial assistance, maintaining self-identity, decreasing burden, respect, compassion, and trust.*
- Provide privacy to discuss health care options. EBN: *Chang et al (2017) studied the decision-making of nurses who triage clients in an emergency department and what factors were considered in their decision-making. The study results indicated that the clients' privacy was an important consideration in choosing care options and prioritizing during a triage situation.* EBN: *Frey et al (2020) investigated palliative care services and found, through a cross-sectional survey (N = 4778), that factors that increased client satisfaction with care included being treated with dignity and respect, adequate privacy, pain relief, and decisions in line with clients' wishes.*
- Allow the client time to choose. EB: *Simmons et al (2017) studied an online decision aid for youth (N = 66) with depression and their ability to make decisions and found that it assisted clients to feel involved in their decision and providing them with time to make the decision and accessibility.* EBN: *Chan et al (2020) studied a hope intervention and its effect of decisional conflict with clients with stage 5 chronic kidney disease. The study is a randomized control trial in which a 4-week Brief Hope Intervention will be completed in the control group. Hope has been associated with decreasing depression and increasing positive expectations and this study will examine its effect on optimizing decision-making and attain better health.*
- ▲ Understand the primary health care providers' role in the decision-making process. EB: *Hyde et al (2017) did a systematic review about shared decision-making and prescribing analgesia by primary care practitioners for musculoskeletal pain and identified important factors in shared decision-making that mainly focus on client emotions and conditions that required analgesics.* EBN: *Asif et al (2020) completed a literature review (N = 11) about the experiences of clients with hip fractures and their caregivers during the transitions in care. The results found that barriers to decision-making were lack of information, role confusion, and disorganized discharge planning. The study results encourage health care providers to collaborate with clients with hip fracture and caregivers on decision-making about plans after the acute care hospital stay.*
- Provide informational resources. EBN: *Asiodu et al (2017) completed a critical ethnographic research study to describe breastfeeding perceptions of African American mothers (N = 21) and key themes that were identified about the high percentage of early weaning, which were expressed as guilt and shame for not breastfeeding, stressors, lack of breastfeeding role models, limited experiences, and changes to the family dynamics.* EBN: *Parker et al (2020) used the theory of planned behavior (attitudes, perceived control, and social norms) to qualitatively study mothers (N = 23) of preterm infants experiences related to breastfeeding. The study found that mothers felt that breastfeeding was a way to bond, that breast milk was healthy and protective, and that breast milk alone was insufficient for a growing preterm infant. For perceived control, mothers felt*

D

empowered to breastfeed due to encouragement from hospital staff, friends, and family. Social norms were aligned with support for and against breastfeeding among providers, family, friends, and the media.

- Provide encouragement so clients increase their confidence in the decision-making process. EB: *Knox, Douglas, and Bigby (2017) studied how clients with traumatic brain injury (TBI) participated in decision-making and discovered that self-conceptualization was a theme and that TBI clients wanted a sense of autonomy.* EBN: *Şengün İnan et al (2020) investigated women's (n = 12) perceptions about returning to work after being treated for breast cancer. The interviews revealed four themes: the decision-making process, difficulties in work life, sources of motivation, and benefits of working. The women's perspectives showed that support from family, colleagues, and employers was important in making the decision to successfully return to work.*

Pediatric

- Understand the parent/guardian's vulnerability when making health care decisions for their children. EB: *O'Hare et al (2016) studied a tool to evaluate children and young client's (n = 151) participation in decision-making. The pilot demonstrated that the reliability and validity of the Child and Adolescent Participation in Decision-Making Questionnaire (CAP-DMQ) showed promise as a useful tool to evaluate decision-making participation, which can assist the family when decisions need to be made.* EBN: *Sedig et al (2020) surveyed parents (n = 28) of children with cancer diagnoses about their decision-making, services, and communications. Parents reported a desire for shared decision-making, and shared decision-making was correlated positively with the parents' perception of how well the child's death was handled.*
- Understand the adolescent decision-making processes. EBN: *Lu et al (2020) retrospectively studied dialectical behavior therapy for adolescents (DBT-A) and if it was offered in a child and youth psychiatric outpatient clinic, and examined the variables of those who were and were not offered DBT-A. Forty-four healthcare records were reviewed for (1) initial mental health intake assessment, (2) age 13 to 16 years, and (3) active suicidal ideation. The decision to offer DBT-A increased with multiple suicide risks and youth who experienced significant childhood trauma. The study recommends that decision-making to use DBT-A be based on multiple factors, not just risk and adverse childhood experiences, since the treatment has been demonstrated to be effective.* EB: *Mosner et al (2017) investigated vicarious effort-based decision-making in adolescents (N = 50) with autism spectrum disorders (ASDs) in a comparison study. Group comparisons demonstrated that adolescents with ASDs were better choosing for themselves than making choices that involved other people, indicating the participants had decreased sensitivity toward others.*
- Refer to care plan Impaired Emancipated **Decision-Making** for additional interventions for critical care, geriatric, multicultural care, and home care.

REFERENCES

Asif, M., Cadel, L., Kuluski, K., Everall, A. C., & Guilcher, S. J. T. (2020). Patient and caregiver experiences on care transitions for adults with a hip fracture: A scoping review. *Disability & Rehabilitation, 42*(24), 3549–3558. https://doi.org/10.1080/09638288.2019.1595181.

Asiodu, I. V., Waters, C. M., Dailey, D. E., & Lyndon, A. (2017). Infant feeding decision-making and the influences of social support persons among first-time African American mothers. *Maternal and Child Health Journal, 21*(4), 863–872. https://doi.org/10.1007/s10995-016-2167-x.

Chan, K., Wong, F., Tam, S. L., Kwok, C. P., Fung, Y. P., & Wong, P. N. (2020). The effects of a brief hope intervention on decision–making in chronic kidney disease patients: A study protocol for a randomized controlled trial. *Journal of Advanced Nursing, 76*(12), 3631–3640. https://doi.org/10.1111/jan.14520.

Chang, W., Liu, H. E., Goopy, S., Chen, L. C., Chen, H. J., & Han, C. Y. (2017). Using the five-level Taiwan triage and acuity scale computerized system: Factors in decision making by emergency department triage nurses. *Clinical Nursing Research, 26*(5), 651–666. https://doi.org/10.1177/1054773816636360.

Frey, R., Robinson, J., Old, A., Raphael, D., & Gott, M. (2020). Factors associated with overall satisfaction with care at the end-of-life: Caregiver voices in New Zealand. *Health and Social Care in the Community, 28*(6), 2320–2330. https://doi.org/10.1111/hsc.13053.

Hell, M. E., & Nielsen, A. S. (2020). Does patient involvement in treatment planning improve adherence, enrollment and other treatment outcome in alcohol addiction treatment? A systematic review. *Addiction Research and Theory, 28*(6), 537–545. https://doi.org/10.1080/16066359.2020.1723083.

Hyde, C., Dunn, K. M., Higginbottom, A., & Chew-Graham, C. A. (2017). Process and impact of patient involvement in a systematic review of shared decision making in primary care consultations. *Health Expectations, 20*(2), 298–308. https://doi.org/10.1111/hex.12458.

Knox, L., Douglas, J. M., & Bigby, C. (2017). "I've never been a yes person": Decision-making participation and self-conceptualization after severe traumatic brain injury. *Disability & Rehabilitation, 39*(22), 2250–2260. https://doi.org/10.1080/09638288.2016.1219925.

Lippe, M., Phillips, F., McCulloch, J., Alexandra, S., Jones, B., & Goodgame, B. (2020). Communicating oncologic prognosis with empathy: A pilot study of a novel communication guide. *American Journal of Hospice and Palliative Medicine, 37*(12), 1029–1036. https://doi.org/10.1177/1049909120921834.

Lu, J., Dyce, L., Hughes, D., DeBono, T., Cometto, J., & Boylan, K. (2020). Outpatient psychiatric care for youth with suicide risk: Who is offered dialectical behavioural therapy? *Child and Youth Care Forum, 49*(6), 839–852. https://doi.org/10.1007/s10566-020-09560-7.

Mosner, M. G., Kinard, J. L., McWeeny, S., et al. (2017). Vicarious effort-based decision-making in autism spectrum disorders. *Journal of Autism and Developmental Disorders, 47*(10), 2992–3006. https://doi.org/10.1007/s10803-017-3220-3.

O'Hare, L., Santin, O., Winter, K., & McGuinness, C. (2016). The reliability and validity of a Child and Adolescent Participation in Decision-Making Questionnaire. *Child: Care, Health and Development*, *42*(5), 692–698. https://doi.org/10.1111/cch.12369.

Parker, M. G., Hwang, S. S., Forbes, E. S., Colvin, B. N., Brown, K. R., & Colson, E. R. (2020). Use of the theory of planned behavior framework to understand breastfeeding decision-making among mothers of preterm infants. *Breastfeeding Medicine*, *15*(10), 608–615. https://doi.org/10.1089/bfm.2020.0127.

Petrinec, A. (2017). Post-intensive care syndrome in family decision makers of long-term acute care hospital patients. *American Journal of Critical Care*, *26*(5), 416–422. https://doi.org/10.4037/ajcc2017414.

Scheepmans, K., Dierckx de Casterlé, B., Paquay, L., Van Gansbeke, H., & Milisen, K. (2017). Restraint use in older adults receiving home care. *Journal of the American Geriatrics Society*, *65*(8), 1769–1776. https://doi.org/10.1111/jgs.14880.

Sedig, L. K., Spruit, J. L., Paul, Y. K., et al. (2020). Supporting pediatric patients and their families at the end of life: Perspectives from bereaved parents. *American Journal of Hospice and Palliative Medicine*, *37*(12), 1009–1015. https://doi.org/10.1177/1049909120922973.

Şengün İnan, F., Günüşen, N., Özkul, B., & Aktürk, N. (2020). A dimension in recovery: Return to working life after breast cancer. *Cancer Nursing*, *43*(6), E328–E334. https://doi.org/10.1097/NCC.0000000000000757.

Simmons, M. B., Elmes, A., McKenzie, J. E., Trevena, L., & Hetrick, S. E. (2017). Right choice, right time: Evaluation of an online decision aid for youth depression. *Health Expectations*, *20*(4), 714–723. https://doi.org/10.1111/hex.12510.

Smith, S. K., Nathan, D., Taylor, J., et al. (2017). Patients' experience of decision-making and receiving information during radiation therapy: A qualitative study. *European Journal of Oncology Nursing*, *30*, 97–106. https://doi.org/10.1016/j.ejon.2017.08.007.

Virdun, C., Luckett, T., Lorenz, K., Davidson, P. M., & Phillips, J. (2020). Hospital patients' perspectives on what is essential to enable optimal palliative care: A qualitative study. *Palliative Medicine*, *34*(10), 1402–1415. https://doi.org/10.1177/0269216320947570.

Readiness for Enhanced Exercise Engagement

Domain 1 Health promotion

Class 2 Health management

Stacey M. Carroll, PhD, APRN-BC

NANDA-I

Definition

A pattern of attention to physical activity characterized by planned, structured, repetitive body movements, which can be strengthened.

Defining Characteristics

Expresses desire to enhance autonomy for activities of daily living; expresses desire to enhance competence to interact with physical and social environments; expresses desire to enhance knowledge about environmental conditions for participation in physical activity; expresses desire to enhance knowledge about group opportunities for participation in physical activity; expresses desire to enhance knowledge about physical settings for participation in physical activity; expresses desire to enhance knowledge about the need for physical activity; expresses desire to enhance physical abilities; expresses desire to enhance physical appearance; expresses desire to enhance physical conditioning; expresses desire to maintain motivation to participate in a physical activity plan; expresses desire to maintain physical abilities; expresses desire to maintain physical well-being through physical activity; expresses desire to meet others' expectations about physical activity plans

NOC (Nursing Outcomes Classification)

Suggested NOC Outcomes

Exercise Participation; Physical Fitness; Exercise Promotion; Endurance

Example NOC Outcome with Indicators

Exercise Participation as evidenced by the following indicators: Plans appropriate exercise with health provider before starting exercise/Identifies barriers to exercise program/Balances life routine to include exercise/Participates in regular exercise. (Rate the outcome and indicators of: 1 = never demonstrated, 2 = rarely demonstrated, 3 = sometimes demonstrated, 4 = often demonstrated, 5 = consistently demonstrated.)

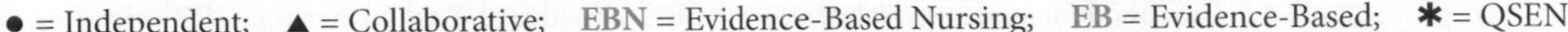

Client Outcomes

Client Will (Specify Time Frame)

- Engage in purposeful moderate-intensity cardiorespiratory (aerobic) exercise for 30 to 60 minutes/day on 5 or more days per week for a total of 2 hours and 30 minutes (150 minutes) per week
- Increase pedometer step counts by 1000 steps per day every 2 weeks to reach a daily step count of at least 7000 steps per day, with a daily goal for most healthy adults of 10,000 steps per day
- Perform resistance exercises that involve all major muscle groups (legs, hips, back, chest, abdomen, shoulders, and arms) performed 2 to 3 days/week
- Perform flexibility exercise (stretching) for each of the major muscle-tendon groups 2 days/week for 10 to 60 seconds to improve joint range of motion; greatest gains occur with daily exercise

NIC (Nursing Interventions Classification)

Suggested NIC Interventions

Exercise Promotion; Exercise Promotion: Strength Training; Exercise Promotion: Stretching

Example NIC Activities—Exercise Promotion

Assist individuals to develop an appropriate exercise program to meet needs; Assist individual to set short-term and long-term goals for the exercise program; Assist individual to schedule regular periods for the exercise program into weekly routine

Nursing Interventions and *Rationales*

- ✱ Determine whether the client needs a physical examination, with a focus on cardiac health, before engaging in additional exercise. EB: *Per the American College of Sports Medicine, a physical examination is warranted if the client is sedentary; has a heart condition, diabetes, kidney disease, or lung disease; and/or plans to begin high-intensity exercise (Chokshi, 2017).*
- ▲ Highlight benefits of exercise on health outcomes to increase motivation. EB: *Benefits of physical activity were fou nd, via an overview of systematic reviews, to be decreased mortality and increased quality of life, with very few safety concerns (Posadzki et al, 2020).* EB: *Varying levels of intensity of exercise were all positively related to cognitive ability and health-related quality of life (Alsubaie et al, 2020).*
- ▲ Use theories to guide increasing motivation and engagement in physical activity. EB: *Self-determination theory was used to study dance and walking programs in older women; the programs were highly attended and participants expressed satisfaction and a desire to continue (Gray et al, 2018).* EB: *A health belief model–guided educational program on exercise and motivation resulted in a significantly higher physical activity level in middle-aged Iranian women (Shariati et al, 2021).*
- ● Support the client's autonomous (internal) motivation with regard to physical activity by discussing the value of positive health behaviors. EB: *Autonomous motivation was associated with physical activity engagements in clients with type 2 diabetes (Koponen et al, 2017).*
- ● Provide motivational support and encourage positive thinking to facilitate exercise engagement. EB: *Clients with heart failure who received motivational support felt more encouraged to be physically active (Klompstra et al, 2021).* EB: *Positive thinking regarding self-image as well as physical activity being a way to achieve goals resulted in increased motivation to continue with physical activity (Hall-McMaster et al, 2016).*
- ● Encourage activities the client finds enjoyable, to promote continued engagement. EB: *A qualitative analysis resulted in a proposal by the authors that joyful activities can result in a more positive body image (Alleva et al, 2019).*
- ● Develop exercise plans that allow for flexibility for the client. EB: *When clients with chronic illness had an activity plan with flexibility in its execution, they were more likely to enact the plan (Fleig et al, 2017).* EB: *Giving clients flexibility in choosing physical activity routines with regular follow-up resulted in increased motivation (Joelsson et al, 2020).*
- ▲ Provide resources for technology options, such as phone applications (which continue to be developed and tested), to increase exercise engagement. EB: *Use of a phone application while walking resulted in more steps walked by community adults (Samendinger et al, 2018).* EB: *Use of an electronic tracking device during physical activity resulted in increased health motivation (Bice et al, 2016).*

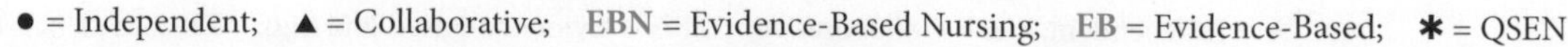

- Administer the Physical Self-Description Questionnaire short form (PSDQ-s) to assess physical self-concept. EB: *Sports competence scores on the PSDQ-s were associated with more frequent participation in a music exercise program (Aasa et al, 2017).*
- ▲ Consider sports programs to increase motivation regarding exercise. EB: *Teachers who participated in a team sport intervention reported increased motivation toward physical activity (Kim & Gurvitch, 2020).*
- Write a "prescription" for exercise for the client. EB: *Having a written prescription for physical activity served as a reminder and increased motivation (Joelsson et al, 2020).*
- ▲ Educate clients about modified or adaptive activities available. EB: *In clients who were status post–major trauma, facilitating access to modified activities such as clinical Pilates and hydrotherapy was appreciated (Ekegren et al, 2020).* EB: *Research supports aquatic therapy as helpful in neurorehabilitation (Becker, 2020). See https://www.moveunitedsport.org/ for resources on adaptive sports.*
- ▲ Incorporate genetically tailored physical activity interventions to individualize plan. EB: *Subjects in the group with genetically tailored physical activity interventions had greater physical activity energy expenditure than the standard program intervention group (Horne et al, 2020).*

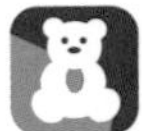

Pediatric

- Assess the child's current activity status using the Pediatric Inactivity Triad (Faigenbaum et al, 2018). EB: *Components of the Pediatric Inactivity Triad include (1) exercise deficit disorder (less than 60 minutes of recommended physical activity daily), (2) pediatric dynapenia (decreased muscle strength and power), and (3) physical illiteracy (low competence and confidence). Addressing these components collectively will enhance effective change (Faigenbaum et al, 2018).*
- Assess parent's perceptions of children's screen time and active play. EB: *A study identified that parental perceptions of the benefits and risks of screen time and active play were not always consistent with current research (Hinkley & McCann, 2018).*
- Children and adolescents should participate in 60 minutes (1 hour) or more of physical activity daily.
  - Aerobic: Sixty or more minutes a day should be either moderate-intensity or vigorous-intensity aerobic physical activity, and should include vigorous-intensity physical activity at least 3 days a week.
  - Muscle-strengthening: As part of daily physical activity, children and adolescents should include muscle-strengthening physical activity at least 3 days of the week.
  - Bone-strengthening: As part of daily physical activity, children and adolescents should include bone-strengthening physical activity at least 3 days of the week.
  - Providing activities that are age appropriate, enjoyable, and varied will encourage young people to participate in physical activities (US Department of Health and Human Services, 2018).
- Assist families to develop family-based interventions to increase child physical activity. EB: *A meta-analysis of family-based interventions found a small effect on physical activity when interventions were tailored to the ethnicity, motivation, and time constraints of the family; combined goal-setting and reinforcement techniques were used; educational strategies were used to increase knowledge as needed; and consideration of the family psychosocial environment (Brown et al, 2016).*
- Encourage participation in youth sports. EB: *A systematic review found that participation in youth sport was positively associated with children's physical activity levels, and that youth participating in sports were more likely to persist in their physical activity (Lee, Pope, & Gao, 2018).*
- Encourage parents and caregivers to adhere to the following American Academy of Pediatrics guidelines for children's media use (Chassiakos et al, 2016):
  - For children younger than 18 months, avoid use of screen media other than video-chatting.
  - Parents of children 18 to 24 months of age who want to introduce digital media should choose high-quality programming and watch it with their children to help them understand what they are seeing.
  - For children ages 2 to 5 years, limit screen use to 1 hour/day of high-quality programs. Parents should co-view media with children to help them understand what they are seeing and apply it to the world around them.
  - For children ages 6 and older, place consistent limits on the time spent using media, and the types of media, and make sure media does not take the place of adequate sleep, physical activity, and other behaviors essential to health.
  - Designate media-free times together, such as dinner or driving, and media-free locations at home, such as bedrooms.
  - Have ongoing communication about online citizenship and safety, including treating others with respect online and off-line.

- ❍ Encourage parents and caregivers to create their personalized family media plan from the American Academy of Pediatrics (see https://www.healthychildren.org/English/media/Pages/default.aspx).

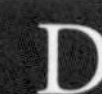

Geriatric

- ● Engage older adults in determining creative ways to exercise. EB: *Older adults co-developed strategies for staying active, including intergenerational purposeful activities (botanical walks) and activity companions (dog walking program) (Guell et al, 2018).*
- ● Explain that shorter periods of activity can still be beneficial, to increase engagement in exercise. EB: *Older adults who engaged in just 6 minutes of self-paced walking had an increase in motivation for more physical activity (Boolani et al, 2021).*
- ▲ Encourage participation in physical activity programs to increase motivation and engagement, even when living in a facility. EBN: *A physical activity program for older adults in a long-term care hospital resulted in improved physical outcomes and happiness (Ryu & Kim, 2020).*
- ▲ Educate older men about testosterone to increase physical activity. EB: *Testosterone treatment in men over 65 years of age resulted in a slight improvement in physical activity (Snyder et al, 2016).*

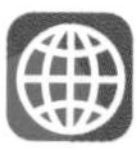

Multicultural

- ▲ Incorporate spirituality into physical activity plans to individualize them to the client's culture, to facilitate continued engagement. EB: *A pilot study combining Christian meditation with physical activity showed preliminary support for the intervention's effect on reducing stress (Knabb et al, 2020).*

Home Care

- ● The interventions described previously may be used in home care.

Client/Family Teaching and Discharge Planning

- ▲ Refer clients returning to sports after an injury for on-field physical therapy rehabilitation after gym rehabilitation is completed. EB: *On-field rehabilitation assists with transition back to a competitive team environment and includes restoring movement, physical conditioning, restoring specific skills, and increasing training load (Buckthorpe et al, 2019).*
- ▲ Encourage activity programs after the cardiac rehabilitation phase to increase physical activity. EB: *Interventions related to exercise shortly after cardiac rehabilitation ended overall showed that clients with cardiac issues maintained physical activity and had better physical activity outcomes than those receiving no specific interventions (Graham et al, 2020).*

REFERENCES

Aasa, U., Paulin, J., & Maidson, G. (2017). Correspondence between physical self-concept and participation in, and fitness change after, biweekly body conditioning classes in sedentary women. *Journal of Strength & Conditioning Research*, *31*(2), 451–461. https://doi.org/10.1519/JSC.0000000000001721.

Alleva, J. M., Gattario, K. H., Martijn, C., & Lunde, C. (2019). What can my body do vs. how does it look? A qualitative analysis of young women and men's descriptions of their body functionality or physical appearance. *Body Image*, *31*, 71–80. https://doi.org/10.1016/j.bodyim.2019.08.008.

Alsubaie, S. F., Alkathiry, A. A., Abdelbasset, W. K., & Nambi, G. (2020). The physical activity type most related to cognitive function and quality of life. *BioMed Research International*, *2020*, 8856284. https://doi.org/10.1155/2020/8856284.

American Academy of Pediatrics. (2021). *Family media plan*. Healthychildren.org [website]. Retrieved from https://www.healthychildren.org/English/media/Pages/default.aspx. [Accessed 21 June 2021].

Becker, B. E. (2020). Aquatic therapy in contemporary neurorehabilitation: An update. *PM & R: Journal of Injury, Function, and Rehabilitation*, *12*(12), 1251–1259. https://doi.org/10.1002/pmrj.12435.

Bice, M. R., Ball, J. W., & McClaran, S. (2016). Technology and physical activity motivation. *International Journal of Sport and Exercise Physiology*, *14*(4), 295–304. https://doi.org/10.1080/1612197X.2015.1025811.

Boolani, A., Sur, S., Yang, D., et al. (2021). Six minutes of physical activity improves mood in older adults: A pilot study. *Journal of Geriatric Physical Therapy*, *44*(1), 18–24. https://doi.org/10.1519/JPT.0000000000000233.

Brown, H. E., Atkin, A. J., Panter, J., Wong, G., Chinapaw, M. J. M., & van Sluijs, E. M. F. (2016). Family-based interventions to increase physical activity in children: A systematic review, meta-analysis and realist synthesis. *Obesity Reviews*, *17*(4), 345–360. https://doi.org/10.1111/obr.12362.

Buckthorpe, M., Della Villa, F., Della Villa, S., & Roi, G. S. (2019). On-field rehabilitation part 1: Four pillars of high-quality on-field rehabilitation are restoring movement quality, physical conditioning, restoring sport-specific skills, and progressively developing chronic training load. *Journal of Orthopaedic & Sports Physical Therapy*, *49*(8), 565–569. https://doi.org/10.2519/jospt.2019.8954.

Chassiakos, Y. L. R., Radesky, J., Christakis, D., Moreno, M. A., Cross, C., & Council on Communications and Media.. (2016). Children and adolescents and digital media. *Pediatrics*, *138*(5), e20162593. https://doi.org/10.1542/peds.2016-2593.

Chokshi, N. (2017). *Do you need a heart check-up before starting an exercise program?* Penn Medicine [website]. Retrieved from https://www.pennmedicine.org/updates/blogs/heart-and-vascular-blog/2017/february/do-you-need-a-heart-check-up-before-starting-an-exercise-program. [Accessed 21 June 2021].

Ekegren, C. L., Braaf, S., Ameratunga, S., et al. (2020). Adaptation, self-motivation and support services are key to physical activity participation three to five years after major trauma: A qualitative study. *Journal of Physiotherapy*, *66*(3), 188–195. https://doi.org/10.1016/j.jphys.2020.06.008.

Faigenbaum, A. D., Rebullido, T. R., & MacDonald, J. P. (2018). Pediatric inactivity triad: A risky PIT. *Current Sports Medicine Reports*, *17*(2), 45–47. https://doi.org/10.1249/JSR.0000000000000450.

Fleig, L., Gardner, B., Keller, J., Lippke, S., Pomp, S., & Wiedemann, A. U. (2017). What contributes to action plan enactment? Examining characteristics of physical activity plans. *British Journal of Health Psychology*, *22*(4), 940–957. https://doi.org/10.1111/bjhp.12263.

Graham, H., Prue-Owens, K., Kirby, J., & Ramesh, M. (2020). Systematic review of interventions designed to maintain or increase physical activity post-cardiac rehabilitation phase II. *Rehabilitation Process and Outcome*, *9*, 1–14. https://doi.org/10.1177/1179572720941833.

Gray, S. M., Higgins, J. W., & Rhodes, R. E. (2018). Understanding physical activity motivation and behavior through self-determination and servant leadership theories in a feasibility study. *Journal of Aging and Physical Activity*, *26*(3), 419–429. https://doi.org/10.1123/japa.2017-0066.

Guell, C., Panter, J., Griffin, S., & Ogilvie, D. (2018). Towards co-designing active ageing strategies: A qualitative study to develop a meaningful physical activity typology for later life. *Health Expectations*, *21*(5), 919–926. https://doi.org/10.1111/hex.12686.

Hall-McMaster, S. M., Treharne, G. J., & Smith, C. M. (2016). Positive thinking and physical activity motivation for one individual with multiple sclerosis: A qualitative case-study. *New Zealand Journal of Physiotherapy*, *44*, 26–32. Retrieved from https://12218-console.memberconnex.com/Folder?Action=View%20File&Folder_id=385&File=44.1.04.pdf. [Accessed 21 June 2021].

Hinkley, T., & McCann, J. R. (2018). Mothers' and father's perceptions of the risks and benefits of screen time and physical activity during early childhood: A qualitative study. *BMC Public Health*, *18*(1), 1271. https://doi.org/10.1186/s12889-018-6199-6.

Horne, J. R., Gilland, J., Leckie, T., O'Connor, C., Seabrook, J. A., & Madill, J. (2020). Can a lifestyle genomics intervention motivate patients to engage in greater physical activity than a population-based intervention? Results from the NOW randomized control trial. *Lifestyle Genomics*, *13*(6), 180–186. https://doi.org/10.1159/000510216.

Joelsson, M., Lundqvist, S., & Larsson, M. E. H. (2020). Tailored physical activity on prescription with follow-ups improved motivation and physical activity levels: A qualitative study of a 5-year Swedish primary care intervention. *Scandinavian Journal of Primary Care*, *38*(4), 399–410. https://doi.org/10.1080/02813432.2020.1842965.

Kim, G., & Gurvitch, R. (2020). The effect of sports-based physical activity programme on teachers' relatedness, stress and exercise motivation. *Health Education Journal*, *79*(6), 658–670. https://doi.org/10.1177/0017896920906185.

Klompstra, L., Liljeroov, M., Jaarsma, T., & Strömberg, A. (2021). Experience of physical activity described by patients with heart failure who have received individualized exercise advice: A qualitative study. *Journal of Rehabilitative Medicine*, *53*(1), jrm00139. https://doi.org/10.2340/16501977-2771.

Knabb, J., Pate, J., Sullivan, S., Salley, E., Miller, A., & Boyer, W. (2020). "Walking with God": Developing and pilot testing a manualized four-week program combining Christian meditation and light-to-moderate physical activity for daily stress. *Mental Health, Religion & Culture*, *23*(9), 756–776. https://doi.org/10.1080/13674676.2020.1819221.

Koponen, A. M., Simonsen, N., & Suominen, S. (2017). Determinants of physical activity among patients with type 2 diabetes: The role of perceived autonomy support, autonomous motivation and self-care competence. *Psychology Health & Medicine*, *22*(3), 332–344. https://doi.org/10.1080/13548506.2016.1154179.

Lee, J. E., Pope, Z., & Gao, Z. (2018). The role of youth sports in promoting children's physical activity and preventing pediatric obesity: A systematic review. *Behavioral Medicine*, *44*(1), 62–76. https://doi.org/10.1080/08964289.2016.1193462.

Posadzki, P., Pieper, D., Bajpai, R., et al. (2020). Exercise/physical activity and health outcomes: An overview of Cochrane systematic reviews. *BMC Public Health*, *20*(1), 1724. https://doi.org/10.1186/s12889-020-09855-3.

Ryu, S. I., & Kim, A. (2020). Development and effects of a physical activity promotion program for elderly patients hospitalized in a long-term care hospital. *Journal of Korean Academy of Fundamental Nursing*, *27*(4), 400–412. https://doi.org/10.7739/jkafn.2020.27.4.400.

Samendinger, S., Pfeiffer, K. A., & Felz, D. L. (2018). Testing group dynamics with a virtual partner to increase physical activity motivation. *Computers in Human Behavior*, *88*, 168–175. https://doi.org/10.1016/j.chb.2018.07.004.

Shariati, M., Astenah, H. P., Khedmat, L., & Khatami, F. (2021). Promoting sustainable physical activity among middle-aged Iranian women: A conceptual model-based interventional study. *BMC Women's Health*, *21*(1), 1. https://doi.org/10.1186/s12905-020-01152-w.

Snyder, P. J., Bhasin, S., Cunningham, G. R., et al. (2016). Effects of testosterone treatment in older men. *New England Journal of Medicine*, *374*(7), 611–624. https://doi.org/10.1056/NEJMoa1506119.

US Department of Health and Human Services. (2018). *Physical activity guidelines for Americans: Youth physical activity recommendations*. Washington, DC: US Department of Health and Human Services.

Ineffective Denial **Domain 9 Coping/stress tolerance Class 2 Coping responses**

Lorraine Chiappetta, MSN, RN, CNE and Julianne E. Doubet, BSN, RN, EMT-B

NANDA-I

Definition

Conscious or unconscious attempt to disavow the knowledge or meaning of an event to reduce anxiety and/or fear, leading to the detriment of health.

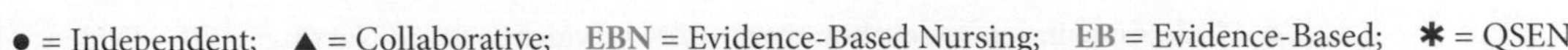

Defining Characteristics

Delayed search for health care; denies fear of death; denies fear of disability; displaced source of symptoms; does not admit impact of disease on life; does not perceive relevance of danger; does not perceive relevance of symptoms; fear displacement regarding impact of condition; inappropriate affect; minimizes symptoms; refuses health care; uses dismissive comments when speaking of distressing event; uses dismissive gestures when speaking of distressing event; uses treatment not advised

D

Related Factors

Anxiety; excessive stress; fear of death; fear of losing personal autonomy; fear of separation; inadequate emotional support; inadequate sense of control; ineffective coping strategies; perceived inadequacy in dealing with strong emotions; threat of unpleasant reality

NOC (Nursing Outcomes Classification)

Suggested NOC Outcomes

Acceptance: Health Status; Anxiety Self-Control; Health Beliefs: Perceived Threat; Symptom Control

Example NOC Outcome with Indicators

Anxiety Self-Control as evidenced by the following indicators: Eliminates precursors of anxiety/Monitors physical manifestations of anxiety/Controls anxiety response. (Rate the outcome and indicators of **Anxiety Self-Control:** 1 = never demonstrated, 2 = rarely demonstrated, 3 = sometimes demonstrated, 4 = often demonstrated, 5 = consistently demonstrated [see Section I].)

Outcomes

Client Will (Specify Time Frame)

- Demonstrate understanding of a crisis event or change in health status
- Seek out appropriate health care attention when needed
- Demonstrate adherence to treatment regimen
- Display appropriate affect and verbalize fears
- Actively engage in treatment program related to substance misuse as needed
- Remain substance free
- Demonstrate alternate adaptive coping mechanism

NIC (Nursing Interventions Classification)

Suggested NIC Intervention

Anxiety Reduction

Example NIC—Activities Anxiety Reduction

Use a calm, reassuring approach; Stay with the patient to promote safety and reduce fear

Nursing Interventions and *Rationales*

- Establish a trusting nurse–client relationship. EBN: *Establishing a trusting relationship between nurses and clients improves outcomes and has been shown to increase clients' adaptation to the state of illness or disability (Polansky, 2019).*
- Assess the client's and family's understanding of the illness the person is experiencing and the feeling states evoked. EBN: *Clients may have complex feelings about their health, especially when living with chronic illnesses. Nursing assessments help nurses provide more individualized care (Polansky, 2019).*
- Express empathetic concern for the anxiety that can be evoked as a person considers the forced adjustments and potential limitations imposed due to the development of a chronic illness or stressful event that leads to a change in lifestyle. EB: *Health providers who offer empathy tend to be more effective in guiding clients and fostering behavior change and medication adherence. Clients are more likely to reveal nonadherence when they believe their provider cares about them (Kourakos et al, 2018).*

- Function as a knowledgeable resource for clients who rely on home remedies or complementary and alternative medicine. EB: *Alternative therapies are not free from risks and contraindications. Without guidance from a care provider, clients are left to self-educate, leading to a potential risk to the client's health (Wojciechowski, 2020).*
- ▲ Support referral to a medical or mental health professional when the use of denial or extreme levels of anxiety significantly interfere with health care needs; the use of motivational interviewing is one counseling method to facilitate change. EB: *Implementing motivational interviewing has been shown to facilitate the establishment of rapport and potentially improve long-term health outcomes for individuals with chronic illness (Schaefer & Kavookjian, 2017).*
- Aid the client in making choices regarding treatment and actively involve him or her in the decision-making process. EBN: *Nurses must encourage a client's participation in shared decision-making by providing the client with balanced, evidence-based treatment alternatives and endeavor to identify what is most important to the client and then support their choices (Dawn & Légaré, 2015).*
- Allow the client to express and use denial as a coping mechanism if appropriate to treatment. EB: *According to Werner and Steihaug (2017), it is important for the health care provider to respect the client's autonomy and realize that the client has the right to refuse information regarding his or her condition.*
- Assist the client in using existing and additional sources of support. EBN: *In their study of men with brain tumors who did not access social services, Longbecker, Eckberg, and Yates (2017) opined that there is a divide between clients' needs and utilization of services; this may be a result of the client's expectancy of what the medical system would offer, alternations in standards for well-being, changes in cognition, and difficulties accessing services.*
- Refer to care plans for Defensive **Coping** and Dysfunctional **Family** Processes.

Geriatric

- Engage the person in any decision making about health care issues. EB: *A pilot study found that a communication guide can bridge the gap of understanding between provider and client, allowing the client a more informed decision-making process (Lippe et al, 2020).*
- Enlist the family and significant others to help support the individual. EB: *Family and friends have significant potential to influence clients' chronic illness self-management (Lee et al, 2017).*
- Allow the client to explain his or her concepts of health care needs, and then use reality-focused techniques whenever possible to provide feedback. EB: *Clients should be made aware that primary medical treatment, even when associated with a positive prognosis, does not predict how well clients will fare during their lifetime (Linden et al, 2015).*
- Encourage communication among family members. EB: *According to Hays, Maliski, and Warner (2017), family can be the most important means of support for those diagnosed with health problems, if they are made aware of the client's medical issues.*

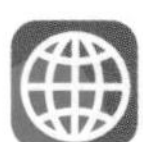

Multicultural

- Discuss with the client those aspects of his or her health behavior/lifestyle that will remain unchanged by health status and those aspects of health behavior that need to be modified to improve health status. EBN: *"Culturally sensitive interventions are required to ensure people of culturally and linguistically diverse backgrounds have the appropriate skills to self-manage their complex medical conditions" (Williams et al, 2015).*
- Establish a trusting relationship. Recognize the role that *medical mistrust* plays in the client's and family's ability to acknowledge health status. Groups who have faced exploitation and discrimination at the hands of the medical/health care community are at greater risk of struggling with this potential barrier. EB: *Trust in one's health care providers is vital to optimal client outcomes. In establishing trust the responsibility lies with providers, and the answer requires recognizing and attending to the mistrust (Sullivan, 2020).*
- Support the client's spiritual coping. EB: *The aim of spiritual care is to facilitate meaning making, providing clients guidance to adequately deal with difficult situations (Kruizinga et al, 2018).*

Home Care

- Previously mentioned interventions may be adapted for home care utilization.
- Provide family with education about the individual's disease process, the grief process, and how to support a loved one through a difficult situation to encourage meaningful family support. EB: *People with chronic conditions who have more support from family and friends are more successful in managing their health (Lee et al, 2017).*

D

- Observe family interaction and roles. Encourage effective communication between family members. EB: *Family can be a key site of support for individuals who are diagnosed with a health issue, as long as the health condition is known within the family unit (Hays et al, 2017).*
- ✱ Support the use of peer support networks, including formal support groups, community group-based programs, and online social media platforms. EB: *Peer support is especially effective at engaging people into needed services and empowering them to play an active role in their own recovery (Davidson et al, 2018).*
- ▲ Observe family interaction and roles. Refer the client/family for follow-up if prolonged denial is a risk. EBN: *Nurses are mentors and guides who can support caregivers of dying family members with coordination of care, symptom management education, and making referrals to other agencies as needed (Hartnett, Thom, & Kline, 2016).*

Client/Family Teaching and Discharge Planning

- Instruct client and family to recognize the signs and symptoms of recurring illness and the appropriate responses to alterations in client's health status. EB: *Giving necessary client education can boost chronic disease management, gives clients knowledge and skills regarding their chronic disease, and improves client-provider communication (Stoner et al, 2018).*
- ▲ Inform family of available community support resources. EBN: *According to study findings by Mendes and Palmer (2016), nurses, especially those involved with the community, can play a pivotal part in aiding caregivers by furnishing useful information, connecting caregivers to community resources, and contributing essential emotional support.*

REFERENCES

See Defensive **Coping** for additional references.

Davidson, L., Bellamy, C., Chinman, M., et al. (2018). Revisiting the rationale and evidence for peer support. *Psychiatric Times, 35*(6), 11–12. Retrieved from https://www.mentalhealthexcellence.org/revisiting-rationale-evidence-peer-support/. [Accessed June 21, 2021].

Dawn, S., & Légaré, F. (2015). Engaging patients using an interprofessional approach to decision making. *Canadian Oncology Nursing Journal, 25*(4), 455–461.

Hartnett, J., Thom, B., & Kline, N. (2016). Caregiver burden in end stage ovarian. *Clinical Journal of Oncology Nursing, 20*(2), 169–173. https://doi.org/10.1188/16.CJON.169-173.

Hays, A., Maliski, R., & Warner, B. (2017). Analyzing the effects of family communication patterns to disclose a health issue to a parent: The benefits of conversation and danger of conformity. *Health Communication, 32*(7), 837–844. https://doi.org/10.1080/10410236.2016.1177898.

Kourakos, M. I., Vlachou, E. D., & Kelesi, M. N. (2018). Empathy in the health professions: An ally in the care of patients with chronic diseases. *International Journal of Health Sciences & Research, 8*(2), 233–240.

Kruizinga, R., Scherer-Rath, M., Schilderman, H. J. B. A.M., Puchalski, C. M., & van Laarhoven, H. H. W. M. (2018). Toward a fully fledged integration of spiritual care and medical care. *Journal of Pain and Symptom Management, 55*(3), 1035–1040. https://doi.org/10.1016/j.jpainsymman.2017.11.015.

Lee, A. A., Piette, J. D., Heisler, M., Janevic, M. R., Langa, K. M., & Rosland, A. M. (2017). Family members' experiences supporting adults with chronic illness: A national survey. Families, systems & health. *Families Systems and Health, 35*(4), 463–473. https://doi.org/10.1037/fsh0000293.

Linden, W., MacKenzie, R., Rnic, K., Marshall, C., & Vodermaier, A. (2015). Emotional adjustment over 1 year post-diagnosis on patients with cancer: Understanding and predicting adjustment trajectories. *Supportive Care in Cancer, 123*(5), 1391–1399. https://doi.org/10.1007/s00520-014-2492-9.

Lippe, M., Phillips, F., McCulloch, J., Alexandra, S., Jones, B., & Goodgame, B. (2020). Communicating oncologic prognosis with empathy: A pilot study of a novel communication guide. *American Journal of Hospice and Palliative Medicine, 37*(12), 1029–1036. https://doi.org/10.1177/1049909120921834.

Longbecker, D., Eckberg, S., & Yates, P. (2017). Don't need help, don't want help, can't get help: How patients with brain tumors account for not using rehabilitation, psychosocial and community services. *Patient Education and Counseling, 100*(7), 1744–1750. https://doi.org/10.1016/j.pec.2017.04.004.

Mendes, A., & Palmer, S. (2016). Supporting unpaid carers in the community. *British Journal of Community Nursing, 21*(7), 364. https://doi.org/10.12968/bjcn.2016.21.7.364.

Polansky, M. (2019). Building trust in home healthcare. *Nursing2020, 49*(10), 16–17.

Schaefer, M. R., & Kavookjian, J. (2017). The impact of motivational interviewing on adherence and symptom severity in adolescents and young adults with chronic illness: A systematic review. *Patient Education and Counseling, 100*(12), 2190–2199. https://doi.org/10.1016/j.pec.2017.05.037.

Stoner, A. M., Cannon, M., Shan, L., Plewa, D., Caudell, C., & Johnson, L. (2018). The other 45: Improving patients' chronic disease self-management and medical students' communication skills. *Journal of the American Osteopathic Association, 118*(11), 703–712. https://doi.org/10.7556/jaoa.2018.155.

Sullivan, L. S. (2020). Trust, risk, and race in American medicine. *Hastings Center Report, 50*(1), 18–26. https://doi.org/10.1002/hast.1080.

Werner, A., & Steihaug, S. (2017). Conveying hope in consultation with life-threatening diseases: The balance supporting and challenging the patient. *Scandinavian Journal of Primary Health Care, 35*(2), 143–152. https://doi.org/10.1080/02813432.2017.1333322.

Williams, A., Manias, E., Cross, W., & Crawford, K. (2015). Motivational interviewing to explore culturally and linguistically diverse people's comorbidity medication self-efficacy. *Journal of Clinical Nursing, 24*(9–10), 1269–1279. https://doi.org/10.1111/jocn.12700.

Wojciechowski, M. (2020). Complementary and alternative medicine: What nurses need to know. *Minority Nurse*. January 28, 2020. Retrieved from https://minoritynurse.com/complementary-and-alternative-medicine-what-nurses-need-to-know/. [Accessed June 21, 2021].

Impaired Dentition Domain 11 Safety/protection Class 2 Physical injury

Morgan Nestingen, MSN, APRN, AGCNS-BC, OCN, ONN-CG

NANDA-I

Definition

Disruption in tooth development/eruption pattern or structural integrity of individual teeth.

Defining Characteristics

Abraded teeth; absence of teeth; dental caries; enamel discoloration; eroded enamel; excessive oral calculus; excessive oral plaque; facial asymmetry; halitosis; incomplete tooth eruption for age; loose tooth; malocclusion; premature loss of primary teeth; root caries; tooth fracture; tooth misalignment; toothache

Related Factors

Difficulty accessing dental care; difficulty performing oral self-care; excessive intake of fluoride; excessive use of abrasive oral cleaning agents; habitual use of staining substance; inadequate dietary habits; inadequate knowledge of dental health; inadequate oral hygiene habits; malnutrition

At-Risk Population

Economically disadvantaged individuals; individuals with genetic predisposition to dental disorders

Associated Conditions

Bruxism; chronic vomiting; oral temperature sensitivity; pharmaceutical preparations

NOC (Nursing Outcomes Classification)

Suggested NOC Outcomes

Oral Health

Example NOC Outcome with Indicators

Oral Health as evidenced by the following indicators: Cleanliness of teeth/Cleanliness of gums/Cleanliness of dentures/Tongue integrity/Gum integrity. (Rate the outcome and indicators of **Oral Health:** 1 = severely compromised, 2 = substantially compromised, 3 = moderately compromised, 4 = mildly compromised, 5 = not compromised [see Section I].)

Client Outcomes

Client Will (Specify Time Frame)

- Have clean teeth, healthy pink gums
- Be free of halitosis
- Explain and demonstrate how to perform oral care
- Demonstrate ability to masticate foods without difficulty
- State absence of pain in mouth

NIC (Nursing Interventions Classification)

Suggested NIC Interventions

Oral Health Maintenance; Oral Health Promotion; Oral Health Restoration

Example NIC Activities—Oral Health Maintenance

Establish a mouth care routine; Arrange for dental care and check-ups as needed

Nursing Interventions and *Rationales*

D

- ▲ Inspect oral cavity/teeth/gingiva at least once daily and note any discoloration, presence of debris, amount of plaque buildup, presence of lesions such as white lesions or patches, edema, or bleeding, and intactness of teeth. Refer to a dentist or periodontist as appropriate. EB: *Inspection is a critical diagnostic tool; observations can identify impending problems. Leukoplakia is the presence of uncharacterized white lesions, which can be a precursor to squamous cell carcinoma. If leukoplakia is observed, prompt referral for diagnosis and potential biopsy is indicated (Lingen et al, 2017; Abadeh et al, 2019).*
- • If the client is free of bleeding disorders and able to swallow, encourage toothbrushing with a soft toothbrush using fluoride-containing toothpaste at least two times per day. Do not use foam swabs or lemon glycerin swabs to clean the teeth. EB: *Oral bacteria cause caries and periodontal disease. Plaque is a biofilm of bacteria, which often becomes contaminated with antibiotic-resistant bacteria in the hospitalized client (Featherstone & Chaffee, 2018; Kearney et al, 2020). Lemon glycerin swabs are no longer recommended for use in tooth cleaning, prevention of ventilator-associated pneumonia, or treating xerostomia as they may cause disturbances in the pH and microbial balance within the oral cavity, may cause decalcification, and may worsen xerostomia (Lavigne & Lavigne, 2019).*
- • The toothbrush is the most important tool for oral care. Twice daily mechanical toothbrushing is the most effective method of reducing plaque and controlling periodontal disease (Pitchika et al, 2019). EB: *A recent systematic review found no difference in oral health outcomes including cleanliness, gingival health, and ventilator-assisted pneumonia when toothbrushes were used versus oral swabs; limited evidence suggests a soft toothbrush may be preferred in mechanically ventilated children and should be used unless toothbrushing causes pain (Narain & Felipe, 2017; Gadepalli & Hirschl, 2020).*
- • Normal gums should be pink and firm. *Gingivitis is characterized by changes in gingival tissue, including redness, sponginess, bleeding, and changes in contour, and weakening of dental attachment (Trombelli et al, 2018).*
- • Encourage the client to perform interdental hygiene by flossing or cleaning between teeth with interdental brushes, woodsticks, or oral irrigation at least once per day if free of a bleeding disorder. If the client is unable to floss, assist with flossing or encourage the use of an oral irrigator (i.e., "water flossing"). EB: *A Cochrane review determined that all forms of interdental cleaning performed in addition to toothbrushing are associated with decreased gingivitis; no specific method of interdental cleaning was found to be superior (Worthington et al, 2019). Some interdental cleaning techniques may also assist with interdental plaque removal, but current findings are inconsistent (Ng & Lim, 2019; Slot, Valkenburg, & Van der Weijden, 2020).*
- • Use a rotation-oscillation power toothbrush for removal of dental plaque. If the client has a fixed orthodontic appliance, particularly any appliance that limits access or toothbrushing motion, a manual toothbrush may be used. EB: *Use of a rotation-oscillation power toothbrush more effectively removes plaque and reduces gingivitis versus manual toothbrushing (Elkerbout et al, 2020; Grender, Adam, & Erb, 2020). A systematic review and meta-analysis found strong, consistent evidence that rotation-oscillation power toothbrushes are more effective at reducing plaque and gingivitis than ultrasonic and other power toothbrushes (Clark-Perry & Levin, 2020). Recent systematic reviews and meta-analyses fail to show a significant difference between manual toothbrushing use of a powered toothbrush when the client has a fixed orthodontic appliance (Tilliss & Carey, 2018; ElShehaby et al, 2020).*
- • Determine the client's mental status and manual dexterity; if the client is unable to care for self, nursing personnel must provide dental hygiene. The nursing diagnosis **Bathing Self-Care Deficit** is then applicable.
- • If the client is unable to brush his or her own teeth, follow this procedure:
  - ○ Position the client sitting upright or on side.
  - ○ Use a soft bristle toothbrush.
  - ○ Use fluoride toothpaste and tap water or saline as a solution.
  - ○ Brush teeth with a manual toothbrush by positioning the brush at a 45-degree angle and directing the bristle tips just below the gingival margin.
  - ○ Brush teeth with an oscillating toothbrush by positioning the brush over the teeth and directing the edge of the oscillating bristle head just below the gingival margin.
  - ○ Suction as needed.

  EB: *Each client must receive oral care including toothbrushing twice daily to maintain healthy teeth and oral tissues and to prevent complications associated with periodontitis (the advanced form of gum disease that can cause tooth loss), which is associated with health problems such as cardiovascular disease, stroke, and bacterial pneumonia (Zimmermann et al, 2015; Kumar, Tadakamadla, & Johnson, 2016).*

- Monitor the client's nutritional and fluid status to determine if adequate. Recommend the client eat a balanced diet and limit between-meal snacks. EB: *Poor nutrition and frequent snacking predispose clients to dental disease (Hujoel & Lingström, 2017; Blostein et al, 2020).*
- Recommend that the client maintain a healthy diet with limited sugar intake; in particular, the client should limit sugary beverages and snacks. EB: *Diets high in sugar are strongly associated with formation of caries in adults and children (Laniado et al, 2020).*
- Instruct the client with halitosis to clean the tongue when performing oral hygiene. Brush tongue with a tongue scraper or toothbrush and follow with a mouth rinse. EB: *A Cochrane review found limited evidence that tongue cleaning, chewing gum, systemic deodorizing agents, topical agents, or specialized toothpastes/mouth rinses were effective in controlling halitosis; toothbrushing combined with tongue cleaning and mouthwash has been identified as the most effective method of control (Van der Sluijs et al, 2018; Nagraj et al, 2019).*
- Determine the client's usual method of oral care. Whenever possible, build on the client's existing knowledge base and current practices to develop an individualized plan of care, including strategies to support oral hygiene as a routine habit. EB: *Teaching oral hygiene during childhood is associated with long-term benefits in plaque score, periodontal health, and caries formation (Lai et al, 2016). Habits play a key role in sustaining twice daily oral hygiene (Raison et al, 2020).*
- Instruct the client on effective toothbrushing technique. A manual toothbrush should be held at a 45-degree angle to the gums; clients should brush using short lateral strokes, gently directing the bristle tips just below the gingival margin, brushing all surfaces of each tooth. An oscillating toothbrush should be placed directly over each tooth with the bristled head just below the gingival margin; the client should brush all surfaces of each tooth. EB: *Several toothbrushing methods have been evaluated for impact on oral health outcomes; there is little evidence to suggest one method is clearly superior, but angled brushing and gentle agitation at the gingival margin have been associated with disruption of biofilm and prevention of gingival pockets. Oscillating toothbrushes provide sufficient action without specialized toothbrushing techniques (American Dental Association, 2019a; Perry, Takei, & Do, 2019).*
- Instruct the client to use a soft-bristled toothbrush, which should be replaced every 3 to 4 months or sooner if bristles begin to appear splayed or worn. EB: *Worn toothbrushes are less effective at removing plaque (American Dental Association, 2019a; Van Leeuwen et al, 2019).*
- Recommend appropriate therapeutic mouthwashes to prevent or reduce symptoms of periodontal disease, including plaque, gingivitis, caries, and halitosis. Over-the-counter mouthwashes containing mint or essential oils may be used in combination with toothbrushing and interdental cleaning to maintain oral health. Avoid routine use of hydrogen peroxide, chlorhexidine, or alcohol-based mouthwashes. EB: *Mint and essential oil mouthwashes have been shown to exert an antimicrobial effect on biofilm, reduce loss of mineralization, and improve halitosis when used with toothbrushing and interdental cleaning with minimal discomfort and other adverse effects (Alaee et al, 2017; Albuquerque et al, 2018; Kulaksiz et al, 2018). Although hydrogen peroxide in mouthwash has been linked with chemical gastritis and colitis, it has been shown to be an effective preprocedural virucidal during the SARS-CoV-2 pandemic (Sabau et al, 2017; Zanelli, Ragazzi, & De Marco, 2017; Kulaksiz et al, 2018; Bidra et al, 2020). Chlorhexidine may be beneficial in reducing plaque, gingivitis, and bacterial aerosolization; however, its use is associated with tooth staining, microbial resistance, and anaphylaxis (Rashed, 2016; Brookes et al, 2020). Routine use of alcohol-based mouthwashes may be associated with oral cancers (Argemí et al, 2020; Ustrell-Borràs, Traboulsi-Garet, & Gay-Escoda, 2020).*
- Recommend client see a dentist at prescribed intervals, generally two times per year (recommended frequency depends on overall oral health and potential comorbidities). EB: *Twice yearly dental visits for assessment of dental health and preventive and restorative treatment are associated with a lower incidence of tooth loss (Hahn, Kraus, & Hooper-Lane, 2017).*
- If there are any signs of bleeding when the teeth are brushed, refer the client to a dentist. If bleeding accompanies apparently inflamed gums, refer client to a periodontist. EB: *Early gingivitis can often be reversed with good oral hygiene; advanced cases may require treatment by a periodontist (Trombelli et al, 2018).*
- If platelets are low, use a soft-bristled toothbrush with a fluoride-containing toothpaste to maintain oral hygiene. Flossing should be avoided if it stimulates gingival bleeding. Moistened toothettes and mild cleaning fluids (e.g., saline rinse) may be used if thrombocytopenia is severe. EB: *Use of toothettes is not an adequate substitute for toothbrushing but may be used to improve oral cleanliness and appearance (Onubogu et al, 2019). Adequate cleaning with toothbrush and fluoride toothpaste helps to reduce biofilm and prevent*

secondary infection of mucosal ulcers; if thrombocytopenia is severe, toothettes with saline may reduce mucosal trauma to damaged tissues (Madeswaran et al, 2019).

- Provide meticulous dental care/oral care to prevent hospital-acquired (or extended care–acquired) pneumonia. EB: *Numerous references have found oral care effective in preventing new-onset pneumonia, although heterogeneity in interventions weakens the level and consistency of evidence (Mitchell et al, 2019; Quinn, Giuliano, & Baker, 2020; Satheeshkumar, Papatheodorou, & Sonis, 2020).*
- Provide scrupulous dental care to critically ill clients, including ventilated clients to prevent ventilator-associated pneumonia. EB/EBN: *Numerous studies have demonstrated decreased incidence of ventilator-associated pneumonia with good oral care. Germicides (i.e., chlorhexidine gluconate) may further reduce risk of ventilator-associated pneumonia in addition to toothbrushing (de Camargo, da Silva, & Chambrone, 2019; Kocaçal Güler & Türk, 2019; Kusumasari & Achadi, 2019; Pechilis, 2019).*
- If teeth are nonfunctional for chewing, modification of oral intake (e.g., edentulous diet, soft diet) may be necessary. The nursing diagnosis Imbalanced **Nutrition:** Less Than Body Requirements may apply.
- If the client is unable to swallow, keep suction nearby when providing oral care.
- See care plan for Impaired **Oral Mucous Membrane** Integrity.

Pregnant Client

- Encourage the expectant mother to eat a healthy, balanced diet that is rich in calcium and abstain from alcohol during pregnancy. The teeth usually start to form in the gums during the second trimester of pregnancy. EB: *Maternal dietary imbalance leading to malnutrition or obesity may be associated with changes in the health of infants' deciduous teeth and subsequent caries in children (Badruddin et al, 2017; Behie & Miszkiewicz, 2019; Wu et al, 2019; Yenen & Ataçağ, 2019).*
- Instruct the pregnant mother to perform twice-daily meticulous oral care. EB: *Pregnancy is associated with hormonal changes, emesis, changes in dietary patterns, and altered metabolism of nutrients, which may lead to poor periodontal maternal outcomes during pregnancy, including gingivitis, caries, erosion, and granulomas. Meticulous, twice-daily oral care is critical to maternal health and pregnancy outcomes (Yenen & Ataçağ, 2019).*
- Advise the pregnant mother not to smoke. EB: *Maternal smoking during pregnancy has been associated with caries formation and tooth loss in the child (Kellesarian et al, 2017; Nakagawa Kang et al, 2019).*

Infant Oral Hygiene

- Gently wipe the infant's gums with a clean washcloth or sterile gauze at least once a day. EB: *Wiping infant gums is recommended by the American Dental Association as part of routine infant oral care (American Dental Association, 2020a).*
- Never allow the infant to fall asleep with a bottle containing milk, formula, fruit juice, or sweetened liquids. Instead, parents may give the infant a bottle filled with cool water or provide a clean pacifier recommended by the dentist or health care provider. Do not dip pacifiers in sweet liquids. Avoid filling the infant's bottle with liquids such as sugar water and soft drinks. EB: *Decay occurs when sweetened liquids such as milk, formula, and fruit juice are left to pool in the infant's mouth during sleep. Cariogenic bacteria in the mouth feed on these sugars and promote early childhood caries (Brecher & Lewis, 2018).*
- Maintain meticulous parental and infant oral hygiene and avoid use of shared utensils or prechewing food when feeding the infant. EB: *Certain feeding habits including use of shared utensils are associated with transfer of Streptococcus mutans from mother to infant (Esra et al, 2020).*
- Instruct parents to begin toothbrushing at first tooth eruption, twice daily using a small, soft toothbrush with a rice grain–sized amount of fluoride-containing toothpaste (a pea-sized amount should be used in children older than 3 years of age). EB: *Parental toothbrushing and use of fluoride have been shown to be effective in reducing the formation of early childhood caries (Brecher & Lewis, 2018).*
- Advise parents to begin regular dental visits at 12 months; parents should establish a "dental home" for routine care, including early application of dental fluoride. EB: *Dental care should be established early to support routine preventive care, evaluate infant anatomic concerns (e.g., frenum attachments), and effective approaches to feeding, sucking, and weaning (American Academy of Pediatric Dentistry, 2017; Brecher & Lewis, 2018).*

Older Children

▲ Encourage the family to talk with the dentist about dental sealants or fluoride varnishes, which can help reduce biofilm and prevent cavities in permanent teeth. EB: *A Cochrane review found that dental sealants and fluoride varnishes are both effective in preventing caries (Kashbour et al, 2020).*

- Teach children to brush teeth twice a day and begin flossing when directed by their dentist; instruct parents to provide support and guidance as needed until children are independent in the task. EB: *The American Dental Association recommends brushing twice daily beginning in early childhood and flossing between ages 7 and 12 (American Dental Association, 2020a).*
- Recommend that parents should not allow the child to smoke or chew tobacco, and stress the importance of setting a good example by not using tobacco products themselves. EB: *Smoking is associated with dental caries (Jiang et al, 2019). Secondary exposure to tobacco is associated with increased risk for dental caries in children (Drummond et al, 2017).*
- Recommend the child drink fluoridated water when possible and use fluoride-containing toothpaste. EB: *The American Dental Association strongly endorses use of fluoridated water as an effective, low-risk public health strategy to reduce tooth decay. Other sources of fluoride including fluoride-containing toothpastes and topical fluoride applications are safe methods of preventing tooth decay (American Dental Association, 2019c).*

D

Geriatric

- Provide dentists with accurate medication history to avoid drug interactions and client harm. If the client is taking anticoagulants, laboratory values should be reviewed before providing dental care. EB: *Older adults are at higher risk for medication errors, drug interactions, and sensitivity to medications used in dentistry (e.g., anesthetics) (American Dental Association, 2019b).*
- Help clients brush their own teeth twice daily; if clients lack dexterity, provide assistance or modified equipment to support self-care.
- If the client has dementia or delirium and exhibits care-resistant behavior such as fighting, biting, or refusing care, use the following method:
  - Ensure client is in a quiet environment, such as his or her own bathroom, and sitting or standing at the sink to prime memory for appropriate actions.
  - Approach the client at eye level within his or her range of vision.
  - Approach with a smile, and begin conversation with a touch of the hand and gradually move up.
  - Use mirror–mirror technique, standing behind the client, and brush and floss teeth.
  - Use respectful adult speech. Avoid "elderspeak," a style of speech characterized by short phrases and questions uttered in a sing-song voice and use of collective pronouns and intimate terms (e.g., first name, nicknames, "deary" or "honey"). *Elderspeak is perceived as demeaning and is a documented trigger for care-resistant behavior (Schnabel et al, 2020; Zhang, Zhao, & Meng, 2020).*
  - Promote self-care when client brushes own teeth if possible.
  - Use distractors when needed: talking, reminiscing, singing.

  EB: Use of specific techniques can decrease resistance to nursing care and increase the effectiveness of nurses providing oral care to older clients. (National Institute for Health and Care Excellence [NICE], 2016).
- ▲ Ensure that dentures are removed and cleaned regularly, after each meal and before bedtime. Brush and rinse dentures to remove debris and soak overnight in a peroxide-based cleaning solution. Dentures left in the mouth at night impede circulation to the palate and predispose the client to oral lesions. EB: *Brushing combined with immersion in a peroxide-based cleaning solution reduces the number of microorganisms surviving on the surface of dentures (Shastri et al, 2018).*
- ▲ Support other caregivers by providing oral hygiene. Physical and cognitive impairment in older adults can interfere with the client's ability to perform oral hygiene, and oral hygiene should be provided by a caregiver. If no caregiver is available, the client is prone to dental problems such as dental caries, tooth abscess, tooth fracture, and gingival and periodontal disease.

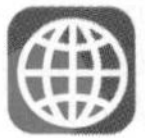

Multicultural

- Assess for the influence of cultural beliefs, norms, and values on the client's understanding of dental care. EBN: *What the client considers normal and abnormal dental health and appropriate care may be based on cultural perceptions (Attanasi, 2017; Updegraff et al, 2017).*
- Assess for barriers to access to dental care, such as lack of insurance. EB: *Social determinants of health including ethnic minority, low socioeconomic status, impaired family structure, and low health literacy are associated with limited access to care and poor oral health outcomes, including caries and tooth loss (Zhou, Elyasi, & Amin, 2017).*

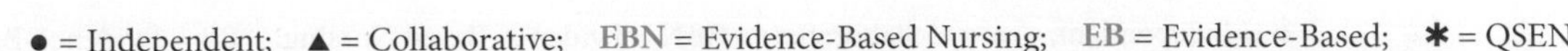

Home Care

- Assess client patterns for daily and professional dental care and related patterns (e.g., smoking, nail biting). Assess for environmental influences on dental status (e.g., fluoride).
- Assess client facilities and financial resources for providing dental care. *Lack of appropriate facilities or financial resources is a barrier to positive dental care patterns. Provision for dental care may be missing from health care plans or unavailable to the uninsured.*
- Request dietary log from the client, adding column for type of food (i.e., soft, pureed, regular).
- Observe a typical meal to assess first-hand the effect of impaired dentition on nutrition. *Clients, especially older adults, are often hesitant to admit nutritional changes that may be embarrassing because of poor dentition.*
- Assist the client with accessing financial or other resources *to support optimum dental and nutritional status.*

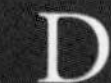

D

Client/Family Teaching and Discharge Planning

- Teach how to inspect the oral cavity and monitor for problems with the teeth and gums. EB: *Education is key to supporting clients' understanding of their oral health and thus their self-care behaviors (Albano et al, 2019).*
- Teach clients to implement a personal plan of dental hygiene, including appropriate toothbrushing and interdental cleaning. Consider motivational interviewing sessions to promote self-care. EB: *Recent systematic reviews have demonstrated an association between motivational interviewing with improved adherence to oral hygiene self-care and may decrease gingival bleeding times and plaque scores; results are more significant among high-risk groups (Carra et al, 2020; Colvara et al, 2020). See Appendix C, Motivational Interviewing, on Evolve.*
- Educate clients to change their toothbrush every 3 to 4 months to ensure effective plaque removal. EB: *Worn toothbrushes are less effective at removing plaque (American Dental Association, 2019a; Van Leeuwen et al, 2019).*
- Teach the client the value of having an optimal fluoride concentration in drinking water and to brush teeth twice daily with toothpaste containing fluoride.
- Teach clients of all ages about the need to decrease intake of sugary foods and to brush teeth regularly. EB: *The World Health Organization recommends limiting sugar to no more than 5% of energy intake to preserve oral health; client education plays a key role in client adherence (Moynihan et al, 2018).*
- Inform individuals who are considering oral piercing or body modification of the potential complications such as infection, development of oral "tic" behaviors, tooth chipping, or gingival recession. If client undergoes oral body modification, teach the client how to care for the wound and prevent complications. EB: *Oral piercings and modifications are associated with infection and oral trauma, including increased risk of gingival recession and tooth injuries (American Dental Association, 2020b; Magno et al, 2020).*
- Advise clients to avoid smoking. EB: *A PRISMA systematic review and meta-analysis found a positive and consistent association between smoking and dental caries (Jiang et al, 2019).*

REFERENCES

Abadeh, A., Ali, A. A., Bradley, G., & Magalhaes, M. A. (2019). Increase in detection of oral cancer and precursor lesions by dentists: Evidence from an oral and maxillofacial pathology service. *Journal of the American Dental Association*, *150*(6), 531–539.

Alaee, A., Aghayan, S., Kamalinejad, M., & Arezoomand, M. (2017). The comparison of mint mouthwash effect on microbial plaque with chlorhexidine, and acceptance of persons. *Journal of Research in Dental Sciences*, *14*(2), 97–102.

Albano, M. G., d'Ivernois, J. F., de Andrade, V., & Levy, G. (2019). Patient education in dental medicine: A review of the literature. *European Journal of Dental Education*, *23*(2), 110–118.

Albuquerque, Y. E., Danelon, M., Salvador, M. J., et al. (2018). Mouthwash containing Croton doctoris essential oil: In vitro study using a validated model of caries induction. *Future Microbiology*, *13*(06), 631–643.

American Academy of Pediatric Dentistry. (2017). Perinatal and infant oral health care. *Pediatric Dentistry*, *39*(6), 208–212.

American Dental Association (ADA). (2019a). *Oral health topics: Toothbrushes*. Retrieved from https://www.ada.org/en/member-center/oral-health-topics/toothbrushes. [Accessed June 24, 2021].

American Dental Association (ADA). (2019b). *Oral health topics: Aging and dental health*. Retrieved from ht tps://www.ada.org/en/member-center/oral-health-topics/aging-and-dental-health. [Accessed June 24, 2021].

American Dental Association (ADA). (2019c). *Oral health topics: Fluoride: Topical and systemic Supplements*. Retrieved from https://www.ada.org/en/member-center/oral-health-topics/fluoride-topical-and-systemic-supplements. [Accessed June 24, 2021].

American Dental Association (ADA). (2020a). *Babies and kids: Healthy habits. Mouth healthy*. Retrieved from https://www.mouthhealthy.org/en/babies-and-kids/healthy-habits.

American Dental Association (ADA). (2020b). *Oral health topics: Oral piercing/jewelry*. Retrieved from https://www.ada.org/en/member-center/oral-health-topics/oral-piercing-jewelry. [Accessed June 24, 2021].

Argemí, R. A., Navarro, B. G., García-Seisdedos, P. O., Devesa, A. E., & López-López, J. (2020). Mouthwash with alcohol and oral carcinogenesis: Systematic review and meta-analysis. *Journal of Evidence-Based Dental Practice, 20*(2), 101407.

Attanasi, K. (2017). *Perceived parental barriers to preventive dental care programs for children. [Doctoral Dissertation]*. Minneapolis, MN: Walden University College of Health Sciences.

Badruddin, I. A., Khansa, M., Rina, R., & Rahardjo, A. (2017). The relation of mothers' nutritional status to primary teeth dental caries. *International Journal of Applied Pharmaceutics, 9*(Special Issue 2), 141–143.

Behie, A. M., & Miszkiewicz, J. J. (2019). Enamel neonatal line thickness in deciduous teeth of Australian children from known maternal health and pregnancy conditions. *Early Human Development, 137*, 104821.

Bidra, A. S., Pelletier, J. S., Westover, J. B., Frank, S., Brown, S. M., & Tessema, B. (2020). Comparison of in vitro inactivation of SARS CoV-2 with hydrogen peroxide and povidone-iodine oral antiseptic rinses. *Journal of Prosthodontics, 29*(7), 599–603.

Blostein, F. A., Jansen, E. C., Jones, A. D., Marshall, T. A., & Foxman, B. (2020). Dietary patterns associated with dental caries in adults in the United States. *Community Dentistry and Oral Epidemiology, 48*(2), 119–129.

Brecher, E. A., & Lewis, C. W. (2018). Infant oral health. *Pediatric Clinics of North America, 65*(5), 909–921.

Brookes, Z. L., Bescos, R., Belfield, L. A., Ali, K., & Roberts, A. (2020). Current uses of chlorhexidine for management of oral disease: A narrative review. *Journal of Dentistry, 103*, 103497.

de Camargo, L., da Silva, S. N., & Chambrone, L. (2019). Efficacy of toothbrushing procedures performed in intensive care units in reducing the risk of ventilator-associated pneumonia: A systematic review. *Journal of Periodontal Research, 54*(6), 601–611.

Carra, M. C., Detzen, L., Kitzmann, J., Woelber, J. P., Ramseier, C. A., & Bouchard, P. (2020). Promoting behavioural changes to improve oral hygiene in patients with periodontal diseases: A systematic review. *Journal of Clinical Periodontology, 47*(Suppl. 22), 72–89.

Clark-Perry, D., & Levin, L. (2020). Systematic review and meta-analysis of randomized controlled studies comparing oscillating-rotating and other powered toothbrushes. *Journal of the American Dental Association, 151*(4), 265–275.e6.

Colvara, B. C., Faustino-Silva, D. D., Meyer, E., Hugo, F. N., Celeste, R. K., & Hilgert, J. B. (2020). Motivational interviewing for preventing early childhood caries: A systematic review and meta-analysis. *Community Dentistry and Oral Epidemiology, 49*(1), 10–16.

Drummond, B., Milne, T., Cullinan, M., Meldrum, A., & Coates, D. (2017). Effects of environmental tobacco smoke on the oral health of preschool children. *European Archives of Paediatric Dentistry, 18*(6), 393–398.

Elkerbout, T. A., Slot, D. E., Rosema, N. M., & Van der Weijden, G. (2020). How effective is a powered toothbrush as compared to a manual toothbrush? A systematic review and meta-analysis of single brushing exercises. *International Journal of Dental Hygiene, 18*(1), 17–26.

ElShehaby, M., Mofti, B., Montasser, M. A., & Bearn, D. (2020). Powered vs manual tooth brushing in patients with fixed orthodontic appliances: A systematic review and meta-analysis. *American Journal of Orthodontics and Dentofacial Orthopedics, 158*(5), 639–649.

Esra, K., Nurhan, O., Yilmaz, A. D., & Berrin, O. (2020). Vertical and horizontal transmission of *Streptococcus mutans* and effective factors: An in vivo study. *Journal of Advanced Oral Research, 11*(2), 172–179.

Featherstone, J. D. B., & Chaffee, B. W. (2018). The evidence for caries management by risk assessment (CAMBRA®). *Advances in Dental Research, 29*(1), 9–14. https://doi.org/10.1177/0022034517736500.

Gadepalli, S. K., & Hirschl, R. B. (2020). Mechanical ventilation in pediatric surgical disease. In G. W. Holcomb, 3rd, J. P. Murphy, & S. D. S. Peter (Eds.), *Holcomb and Ashcraft's pediatric surgery* (7th ed.). Philadelphia: Elsevier.

Grender, J., Adam, R., & Erb, J. (2020). Randomized controlled trial assessing plaque removal of an oscillating-rotating electric toothbrush with micro-vibrations. *International Dental Journal, 70*(Suppl. 1), S22–S27.

Hahn, T. W., Kraus, C., & Hooper-Lane, C. (2017). Clinical inquries: What is the optimal frequency for dental checkups for children and adults? *Journal of Family Practice, 66*(11), 699–700.

Hujoel, P. P., & Lingström, P. (2017). Nutrition, dental caries and periodontal disease: A narrative review. *Journal of Clinical Periodontology, 44*(Suppl. 18), S79–S84.

Jiang, X., Jiang, X., Wang, Y., & Huang, R. (2019). Correlation between tobacco smoking and dental caries: A systematic review and meta-analysis. *Tobacco Induced Diseases, 17*, 34.

Kashbour, W., Gupta, P., Worthington, H. V., & Boyers, D. (2020). Pit and fissure sealants versus fluoride varnishes for preventing dental decay in the permanent teeth of children and adolescents. *Cochrane Database of Systematic Reviews, 11*, CD003067.

Kearney, A., Kinnevey, P., Shore, A., et al. (2020). The oral cavity revealed as a significant reservoir of *Staphylococcus aureus* in an acute hospital by extensive patient, healthcare worker and environmental sampling. *Journal of Hospital Infection, S0195-6701*(20), 30103–30111.

Kellesarian, S.-V., Malignaggi, V.-R., de Freitas, P., Ahmed, H.-B., & Javed, F. (2017). Association between prenatal maternal cigarette smoking and early childhood caries. A systematic review. *Journal of Clinical and Experimental Dentistry, 9*(9), e1141.

Kocaçal Güler, E., & Türk, G. (2019). Oral chlorhexidine against ventilator-associated pneumonia and microbial colonization in intensive care patients. *Western Journal of Nursing Research, 41*(6), 901–919.

Kulaksiz, B., Sevda, E., Üstündağ-Okur, N., & Saltan-İşcan, G. (2018). Investigation of antimicrobial activities of some herbs containing essential oils and their mouthwash formulations. *Turkish Journal of Pharmaceutical Sciences, 15*(3), 370.

Kumar, S., Tadakamadla, J., & Johnson, N. (2016). Effect of toothbrushing frequency on incidence and increment of dental caries: A systematic review and meta-analysis. *Journal of Dental Research, 95*(11), 1230–1236.

Kusumasari, F., & Achadi, A. (2019). *Dental and oral care to reduce the incidence of ventilator associated pneumonia among patients with ventilator in intensive care unit: A systematic review*. Solo, Indonesia: Paper presented at the 6th International Conference on Public Health. October 23, 2019.

Lai, H., Fann, J. C. Y., Yen, A. M. F., Chen, L. S., Lai, M. H., & Chiu, S. Y. H. (2016). Long–term effectiveness of school–based children oral hygiene program on oral health after 10–year follow–up. *Community Dentistry and Oral Epidemiology, 44*(3), 209–215.

Laniado, N., Sanders, A. E., Godfrey, E. M., Salazar, C. R., & Badner, V. M. (2020). Sugar-sweetened beverage consumption and caries experience: An examination of children and adults in the United States, National Health and Nutrition Examination Survey 2011-2014. *Journal of the American Dental Association, 151*(10), 782–789.

Lavigne, P. S., & Lavigne, M. C. (2019). A performance summary of agents used in oral care for non-ventilated and mechanically-ventilated patients. *Annals of Pulmonary and Critical Care Medicine, 2*(2), 1–34.

Lingen, M. W., Abt, E., Agrawal, N., et al. (2017). Evidence-based clinical practice guideline for the evaluation of potentially malignant disorders in the oral cavity: A report of the American dental association. *Journal of the American Dental Association, 148*(10), 712–727.e710.

D

D

Madeswaran, S., Saravanan, D., Rethinam, S., & Muthu, K. (2019). Oral mucositis: Role of the dentist. *Journal of Oral Health and Community Dentistry*, *13*(3), 107.

Magno, M. B., Nadelman, P., de França Leite, K. L., Ferreira, D. M., Pithon, M. M., & Maia, L. C. (2020). Associations and risk factors for dental trauma: A systematic review of systematic reviews. *Community Dentistry and Oral Epidemiology*, *48*(6), 447–463.

Mitchell, B. G., Russo, P. L., Cheng, A. C., et al. (2019). Strategies to reduce non-ventilator-associated hospital-acquired pneumonia: A systematic review. *Infection Disease & Health*, *24*(4), 229–239.

Moynihan, P., Makino, Y., Petersen, P. E., & Ogawa, H. (2018). Implications of WHO guideline on sugars for dental health professionals. *Community Dentistry and Oral Epidemiology*, *46*(1), 1–7.

Nagraj, S. K., Eachempati, P., Uma, E., Singh, V. P., Ismail, N. M., & Varghese, E. (2019). Interventions for managing halitosis. *Cochrane Database of Systematic Reviews*, *12*, CD012213.

Nakagawa Kang, J., Unnai Yasuda, Y., Ogawa, T., et al. (2019). Association between maternal smoking during pregnancy and missing teeth in adolescents. *International Journal of Environmental Research and Public Health*, *16*(22), 4536.

Narain, T., & Felipe, E. (2017). *Soft toothbrushes versus foam swabs for oral care: A review of the comparative clinical effectiveness, cost-effectiveness, and guidelines.* [Internet]. Ottawa, Ontario: Canadian Agency for Drugs and Technologies in Health.

National Institute for Health and Care Excellence (NICE). (2016). *Oral health for adults in care homes. NICE guideline [NG48]*. Retrieved from https://www.nice.org.uk/guidance/ng48. [Accessed June 24, 2021].

Ng, E., & Lim, L. P. (2019). An overview of different interdental cleaning aids and their effectiveness. *Dentistry Journal*, *7*(2), 56.

Onubogu, U., Mansfield, W., & Ozbek, I. (2019). Oral healthcare measures to improve overall health in older adults. *Journal of Comprehensive Nursing Research and Care*, *4*, 156.

Pechilis, K. (2019). *Implementation of oral care guidelines to reduce incidences of ventilator-associated pneumonia: A systematic review of the literature. [Honors Thesis]*. Salem, MA: Salem State University School of Nursing.

Perry, D. A., Takei, H. H., & Do, J. H. (2019). Plaque biofilm control for the periodontal patient. In M. G. Newman, H. H. Takei, P. R. Klokkevold, & F. A. Carranza (Eds.), *Newman and Carranza's clinical periodontology* (13th ed.). Philadelphia: Elsevier.

Pitchika, V., Pink, C., Völzke, H., Welk, A., Kocher, T., & Holtfreter, B. (2019). Long-term impact of powered toothbrush on oral health: 11-year cohort study. *Journal of Clinical Periodontology*, *46*(7), 713–722.

Quinn, B., Giuliano, K. K., & Baker, D. (2020). Non-ventilator health care-associated pneumonia (NV-HAP): Best practices for prevention of NV-HAP. *American Journal of Infection Control*, *48*(5), A23–A27.

Raison, M., Corcoran, R., Burnside, G., & Harris, R. (2020). Oral hygiene behaviour automaticity: Are tooth-brushing and inter-dental cleaning habitual behaviours? *Journal of Dentistry*, *102*, 103470.

Rashed, H. T. (2016). Evaluation of the effect of hydrogen peroxide as a mouthwash in comparison with chlorhexidine in chronic periodontitis patients: A clinical study. *Journal of International Society of Preventive and Community Dentistry*, *6*(3), 206.

Sabau, R., Ormenisan, A., Monea, A., et al. (2017). Effect of essential oil mouthwash on halitosis. *Revista de Chimie*, *68*(3), 518–521.

Satheeshkumar, P. S., Papatheodorou, S., & Sonis, S. (2020). Enhanced oral hygiene interventions as a risk mitigation strategy for the prevention of non-ventilator-associated pneumonia: A systematic review and meta-analysis. *British Dental Journal*, *228*(8), 615–622.

Schnabel, E.-L., Wahl, H.-W., Streib, C., & Schmidt, T. (2020). Elderspeak in acute hospitals? The role of context, cognitive and functional impairment. *Research on Aging*, 0164027520949090.

Shastri, M., Joshi, S., Sajjan, C., & Konin, P. (2018). Denture disinfection by brushing and 6% hydrogen peroxide immersion on denture base resin after biofilm formation: An in vitro study. *Indian Journal of Dental Sciences*, *10*(2), 83.

Slot, D. E., Valkenburg, C., & Van der Weijden, G. (2020). Mechanical plaque removal of periodontal maintenance patients: A systematic review and network meta-analysis. *Journal of Clinical Periodontology*, *47*, 107–124.

Tilliss, T., & Carey, C. M. (2018). Insufficient evidence within a systematic review and meta-analysis of powered toothbrushes over manual toothbrushes for soft tissue health during orthodontic treatment. *Journal of Evidence-Based Dental Practice*, *18*(2), 176–177.

Trombelli, L., Farina, R., Silva, C. O., & Tatakis, D. N. (2018). Plaque-induced gingivitis: Case definition and diagnostic considerations. *Journal of Clinical Periodontology*, *45*(Suppl. 20), S44–S67.

Updegraff, K. A., Kuo, S. I., McHale, S. M., Umaña-Taylor, A. J., & Wheeler, L. A. (2017). Parents' traditional cultural values and Mexican-Origin Young adults' routine health and dental care. *Journal of Adolescent Health: Official Publication of the Society for Adolescent Medicine*, *60*(5), 513–519. https://doi.org/10.1016/j.jadohealth.2016.10.012.

Ustrell-Borràs, M., Traboulsi-Garet, B., & Gay-Escoda, C. (2020). Alcohol-based mouthwash as a risk factor of oral cancer: A systematic review. *Medicina Oral, Patología Oral Y Cirugía Bucal*, *25*(1), e1.

Van der Sluijs, E., Van der Weijden, G., Hennequin-Hoenderdos, N., & Slot, D. (2018). The effect of a tooth/tongue gel and mouthwash regimen on morning oral malodour: A 3-week single-blind randomized clinical trial. *International Journal of Dental Hygiene*, *16*(1), 92–102.

Van Leeuwen, M. P., Van der Weijden, F. A., Slot, D. E., & Rosema, M. A. (2019). Toothbrush wear in relation to toothbrushing effectiveness. *International Journal of Dental Hygiene*, *17*(1), 77–84.

Worthington, H. V., MacDonald, L., Pericic, T. P., et al. (2019). Home use of interdental cleaning devices, in addition to toothbrushing, for preventing and controlling periodontal diseases and dental caries. *Cochrane Database of Systematic Reviews*, *4*, CD012018.

Wu, H., Chen, T., Ma, Q., Xu, X., Xie, K., & Chen, Y. (2019). Associations of maternal, perinatal and postnatal factors with the eruption timing of the first primary tooth. *Scientific Reports*, *9*(1), 1–8.

Yenen, Z., & Ataçağ, T. (2019). Oral care in pregnancy. *Journal of the Turkish-German Gynecological Association*, *20*(4), 264.

Zanelli, M., Ragazzi, M., & De Marco, L. (2017). Chemical gastritis and colitis related to hydrogen peroxide mouthwash. *British Journal of Clinical Pharmacology*, *83*(2), 427.

Zhang, M., Zhao, H., & Meng, F.-P. (2020). Elderspeak to resident dementia patients increases resistiveness to care in health care profession. *Inquiry*, *57*, 0046958020948668.

Zhou, J. Y., Elyasi, M., & Amin, M. (2017). Associations among dental insurance, dental visits, and unmet needs of US children. *Journal of the American Dental Association*, *148*(2), 92–99.

Zimmermann, H., Zimmermann, N., Hagenfeld, D., Veile, A., Kim, T. S., & Becher, H. (2015). Is frequency of tooth brushing a risk factor for periodontitis? A systematic review and meta-analysis. *Community Dentistry and Oral Epidemiology*, *43*(2), 116–127.

Delayed Child Development Domain 13 Growth/development Class 2 Development

Daniela Moscarella, DNP, APN, CPNP-PC, CCRN-K

D

NANDA-I

Definition

Child who continually fails to achieve developmental milestones within the expected timeframe.

Defining Characteristics

Consistent difficulty performing cognitive skills typical of age group; consistent difficulty performing language skills typical of age group; consistent difficulty performing motor skills typical of age group; consistent difficulty performing psychosocial skills typical of age group

Related Factors

Infant or Child Factors

Inadequate access to health care provider; inadequate attachment behavior; inadequate stimulation; unaddressed abuse; unaddressed psychological neglect

Caregiver Factors

Anxiety; decreased emotional support availability; depressive symptoms; excessive stress; unaddressed domestic violence

At-Risk Population

Children aged 0-9 years; children born to economically disadvantaged families; children exposed to community violence; children exposed to environmental pollutants; children whose caregivers have developmental disabilities; children whose mothers had inadequate prenatal care; children with below normal growth standards for age and gender; institutionalized children; low birth weight infants; premature infants

Associated Conditions

Antenatal pharmaceutical preparations; congenital disorders; depression; inborn genetic diseases; maternal mental disorders; maternal physical illnesses; prenatal substance misuse; sensation disorders

NOC (Nursing Outcomes Classification)

Suggested NOC Outcomes

Abuse Recovery; Child Development: 1 Month, 2 Months, 4 Months, 6 Months, 12 Months, 2 Years, 3 Years, 4 Years, 5 Years, Middle Childhood, Adolescence; Development: Late Adulthood, Middle Adulthood, Young Adulthood; Knowledge: Parenting, Neglect Recovery

Example NOC Outcome with Indicators

Child Development as evidenced by the following indicators: Appropriate milestones of physical, cognitive, and psychosocial age-appropriate progression. (Rate the outcome and indicators of **Child Development:** 1 = never demonstrated, 2 = rarely demonstrated, 3 = sometimes demonstrated, 4 = often demonstrated, 5 = consistently demonstrated [see Section I].)

Client Outcomes

Client/Parents/Primary Caregiver Will (Specify Time Frame)

- Child will achieve expected milestones in all areas of development (physical, cognitive, academic, and psychosocial)
- Parent/caregiver will verbalize understanding of potential impediments to normal development and demonstrate actions or environmental/lifestyle changes necessary to provide appropriate care in a safe, nurturing environment

NIC (Nursing Interventions Classification)

Suggested NIC Interventions

Abuse Protection Support: Child; Caregiver Support; Developmental Enhancement: Child/Adolescent; Home Maintenance Assistance; Immunization/Vaccination Management; Infant Care; Kangaroo Care; Lactation Counseling; Learning Facilitation; Newborn Care; Newborn Monitoring; Nonnutritive Sucking; Normalization Promotion; Nutrition Management; Parent Education: Infant/Adolescent/Childbearing Family; Parenting Promotion; Referral; Risk Identification: Childbearing Family; Teaching: (Infant) Nutrition/Safety/Stimulation; (Toddler) Nutrition/Safety; Temperature Regulation (Infant); Therapeutic Play

Example NIC Activities—Parent Education

Instruct parent on normal physiological, emotional, and behavioral characteristics of child

Nursing Interventions and *Rationales*

Preconception/Pregnancy

- Assess for nutritional status during pregnancy. Review the importance of iron, folate, iodine, choline, and essential fatty acids. EB: *Maternal nutrition during pregnancy is essential for the health of an infant. Deficiencies in iron, folate, iodine, choline, and essential fatty acids can lead to neural tube defects, abnormal brain development, and preventable developmental delays (Black et al, 2020).*
- Assess for alcohol/drug use during pregnancy. Expectant mothers should be instructed that no amount of alcohol consumption is safe during pregnancy. EBN: *Alcohol is a well-established teratogen that can cause variable physical and behavioral effects on the fetus. Increased fetal exposure to alcohol and sustained alcohol intake during any trimester of pregnancy are associated with an increased risk of fetal alcohol syndrome (FAS) (Gupta, Gupta, & Shirasaka, 2016).*
- Assess and educate about consumption of marijuana use in pregnancy. EB: *Marijuana crosses the placenta and has been found to affect fetal neurodevelopment, which may cause problems with neurological development resulting in hyperactivity and poor cognitive function (Metz & Stickrath, 2015).*
- Educate expectant mothers to stop smoking and assist with methods of smoking cessation. Smoking is an avoidable risk factor for low birth weight and other significant prenatal issues. EB: *Reese et al (2017) noted that pregnant women disproportionately underreport smoking and smokers tend to have lower follow-up rates to repeat questionnaires.*
- Educate that it is recommended that women of childbearing age take 400 mcg of folic acid daily, along with a healthy, well-balanced diet, to reduce the risk of neural tube and other birth defects. EB: *The recommended supplementation of folic acid is 0.4 mg/400 mcg taken once per day, before attempting conception and continuing throughout pregnancy (Atrash & Jack, 2020).* EB: *The benefits of using folic acid supplements during the periconception period are to prevent neural tube defects and to ensure normal brain development (Valera-Gran et al, 2017).* EB: *Additionally, a comprehensive meta-analysis suggested that maternal use of folic acid supplements during pregnancy could significantly reduce the risk of autism spectrum disorders in children regardless of ethnicity compared with those women who did not supplement with folic acid (Wang et al, 2017).*

Neonate/Infant

- Educate new mothers about the importance of breastfeeding. EB: *Breast milk and the act of breastfeeding may benefit children's cognitive development (Black et al, 2020).*
- Assess the neonate/infant for age-appropriate milestones. EB: *Early identification of developmental delays expedites a referral for therapeutic services such as early intervention, which encourages gains in developmental milestones (Scharf et al, 2016).*
- Assess for maternal depression when caring for a newborn infant. EB: *It is essential to address maternal mental health and promote parenting strategies that encourage play-based interactions, which would reduce the risk of behavior and social-emotional problems in childhood (McDonald et al, 2018).*
- Provide information to parents about the importance of health supervision visits at the following intervals: first week of life, 1 month, 2 months, 4 months, 6 months, 9 months, and 12 months, with standardized developmental screen at 9 months old. EB: *Early identification of and intervention for developmental disorders are critical to the well-being of childhood development (Lipkin & Macias, 2020).*

- Teach parents about the necessity of daily tummy time for infants less than 6 months old. EB: *Tummy time has a positive effect related to infant development with an emphasis on motor development (Hewitt et al, 2017).*
- Explain the use of developmentally appropriate toys for play. EB: *Toys that match a child's developmental skills and abilities will further encourage the development of new skills. That is important in early childhood to facilitate cognitive development, language interactions, symbolic and pretend play, problem-solving, social interactions, and physical activity (Healey & Mendelsohn, 2019).*
- Monitor mother–baby interactions when caring for premature infants. EBN: *Posttraumatic stress disorder (PTSD) induced by preterm delivery has a significant impact on the infant–mother attachment dyad. Mothers often have attachment issues, and the infant may be affected, resulting in delayed development (Anderson & Cacola, 2017).*

D

Toddler/Preschooler/School-Age

- Assess for the effects of social disruption on cognitive abilities. EB: *A study found delayed negative effects on the academic achievement of children living in postdisaster communities (Gibbs et al, 2019).*
- Educate about the importance of eating a well-balanced diet in early childhood. EB: *Brain development is rapid in the early years of childhood and therefore adequate nutrition has a significant impact on neurodevelopment (Black et al, 2020).*
- Assess for age-appropriate milestones and developmental history at every visit.
- Autism spectrum disorder (ASD) screening should be conducted at the 18-month and 24-month visits. EB: *A developmental screen is recommended at the 18-month visit because delays in fine motor, communication, and language development are often evident by 18 months of age and may be indicative of ASD (Lipkin & Macias, 2020).*
- Educate parents about the importance of health supervision visits yearly with standardized developmental screening at 30 months' old and then again at the 4- to 5-year-old visit. EB: *Close attention to developmental skills necessary for school readiness should be performed at the 4- or 5-year visit. This is the opportunity to capture mild delays that may have been previously missed (Lipkin & Macias, 2020).*
- Monitor preterm infants more closely for developmental delays. EBN: *Children born prematurely have a higher risk of chronic health conditions, including attention deficit disorder and attention deficit hyperactivity disorder, speech problems, learning disability, anxiety, asthma, and developmental delays (Kelly, 2018).*
- Provide support and education to parents of toddlers with developmental disabilities (e.g., Down's syndrome [DS], cerebral palsy). EB: *A recent study of infants with DS affirmed previous findings showing that the rate of attainment of motor skills is delayed in children with DS compared with children with typical development; however, the developmental sequence is the same. The delayed development is more prominent in more complex skills (Beqaj, Jusaj, & Živković, 2017).*
- Provide parents and caregivers with information about speech-language development, play development, and speech-language stimulation strategies for children with language delay. Refer to speech and language specialists as needed. EB: *A study that implemented a low-intensity training program for parents, supported by a manual focusing on developmentally appropriate play and speech-language stimulation, found increased verbal interaction and changes in language input to children with language delay (Rajesh & Vankatesh, 2019).*
- Monitor for maternal eating disorders because they have a direct effect on childhood development. EB: *Sadeh-Sharvit, Levy-Shiff, and Lock (2016) found that children of mothers with eating disorders showed delayed mental and psychomotor development. Severity of maternal eating disorder symptoms emerged as a significant predictor of child development, but other maternal psychopathology did not. Findings suggest that maternal eating disorder history may play a unique role in the development of neurodevelopmental functions in their children.*
- Educate parents about the importance of avoiding lead-based paints in the home and other sources of lead in the environment. EB: *Low-level lead exposure has been shown to significantly increase the risk for learning disabilities, behavioral problems, and developmental delay (Hamp et al, 2018).*

▲ Refer parents and caregivers of children with language delays to Enhanced Milieu Teaching (EMT). EB: *EMT is an evidence-based, conversation-based intervention that uses child interests and initiations as opportunities to model and prompt language in everyday contexts. A study of EMT with language-delayed young children found gains in expressive language (Hatcher & Page, 2020).* EB: *Another study found that 12 months after the EMT intervention ended, children in the EMT intervention group displayed lower rates of parent-reported problem behaviors (Curtis et al, 2019).*

REFERENCES

Anderson, C., & Cacola, P. (2017). Implications of preterm birth for maternal mental health and infant development. *MCN American Journal of Maternal Child Nursing*, *42*(2), 108–114. https://doi.org/10.1097/nmc.0000000000000311.

Atrash, H., & Jack, B. (2020). Preconception care to improve pregnancy outcomes: Clinical practice guidelines. *Journal of Human Growth and Development*, *30*(3), 4017–4416.

Beqaj, S., Jusaj, N., & Živković, V. (2017). Attainment of gross motor milestones in children with Down syndrome in Kosovo—Developmental perspective. *Medicinski Glasnik: Official Publication of the Medical Association of Zenica-Doboj Canton, Bosnia and Herzegovina*, *14*(2), 189–198. https://doi.org/10.17392/917-17.

Black, M. M., Trude, A. C., & Lutter, C. K. (2020). All children thrive: Integration of nutrition and early childhood development. *Annual Review of Nutrition*, *40*(1), 375–406. https://doi.org/10.1146/annurev-nutr-120219-023757.

Curtis, P. R., Kaiser, A. P., Estabrook, R., & Roberts, M. Y. (2019). The longitudinal effects of early language intervention on children's problem behaviors. *Child Development*, *90*(2), 576–592. https://doi.org/10.1111/cdev.12942.

Gibbs, L., Nursey, J., Cook, J., et al. (2019). Delayed disaster impacts on academic performance of primary school children. *Child Development*, *90*(4), 1402–1412. https://doi.org/10.1111/cdev.13200.

Gupta, K. K., Gupta, V. K., & Shirasaka, T. (2016). An update on fetal alcohol syndrome—Pathogenesis, risks, and treatment. *Alcoholism: Clinical and Experimental Research*, *40*(8), 1594–1602. https://doi.org/10.1111/acer.13135.

Hamp, N., Zimmerman, A., & Hoffen, J. (2018). Advocating for automatic eligibility for early intervention services for children exposed to lead. *Pediatric Annals*, *47*(10), e413–e418. https://doi.org/10.3928/19382359-20180924-01.

Hatcher, A., & Page, J. (2020). Parent-implemented language intervention for teaching enhanced milieu teaching strategies to parents of low-socioeconomic status. *Journal of Early Intervention*, *42*(2), 122–142. https://doi.org/10.1177/1053815119873085.

Healey, A., & Mendelsohn, A. (2019). Selecting appropriate toys for young children in the digital era. *Pediatrics*, *143*(1), e20183348. https://doi.org/10.1542/peds.2018-3348.

Hewitt, L., Stanley, R. M., & Okely, A. D. (2017). Correlates of tummy time in infants aged 0–12 months old: A systematic review. *Infant Behavior and Development*, *49*, 310–321. https://doi.org/10.1016/j.infbeh.2017.10.001.

Kelly, M. M. (2018). Health and educational implications of prematurity in the United States: National Survey of Children's Health 2011/2012 data. *Journal of the American Association of Nurse Practitioners*, *30*(3), 131–139. https://doi.org/10.1097/jxx.0000000000000021.

Lipkin, P. H., & Macias, M. M. (2020). Promoting optimal development: Identifying infants and young children with developmental disorders through developmental surveillance and screening. *Pediatrics*, *145*(1), e20193449. https://doi.org/10.1542/peds.2019-3449.

McDonald, S. W., Kehler, H. L., & Tough, S. C. (2018). Risk factors for delayed social-emotional development and behavior problems at age two: Results from the All Our Babies/Families (AOB/F) cohort. *Health Science Reports*, *1*(10), e82. https://doi.org/10.1002/hsr2.82.

Metz, T. D., & Stickrath, E. H. (2015). Marijuana use in pregnancy and lactation: A review of the evidence. *American Journal of Obstetrics and Gynecology*, *213*(6), 761–778. https://doi.org/10.1016/j.ajog.2015.05.025.

Rajesh, V., & Venkatesh, L. (2019). Preliminary evaluation of a low-intensity parent training program on speech-language stimulation for children with language delay. *International Journal of Pediatric Otorhinolaryngology*, *122*, 99–104.

Reese, S. E., Zhao, S., Wu, M. C., et al. (2017). DNA methylation score as a biomarker in newborns for sustained maternal smoking during pregnancy. *Environmental Health Perspectives*, *125*(4), 760–766. https://doi.org/10.1289/ehp333.

Sadeh-Sharvit, S., Levy-Shiff, R., & Lock, J. D. (2016). Maternal eating disorder history and toddlers' neurodevelopmental outcomes: A brief report. *Eating Disorders*, *24*(2), 198–205. https://doi.org/10.1080/10640266.2015.1064280.

Scharf, R. J., Scharf, G. J., & Stroustrup, A. (2016). Developmental milestones. *Pediatrics in Review*, *37*(1), 25–38. https://doi.org/10.1542/pir.2014-0103.

Valera-Gran, D., Navarrete-Muñoz, E. M., Garcia de la Hera, M., et al. (2017). Effect of maternal high dosages of folic acid supplements on neurocognitive development in children at 4–5 years of age: The prospective birth cohort Infancia y Medio Ambiente (INMA) study. *American Journal of Clinical Nutrition*, *106*(3), 878–887. https://doi.org/10.3945/ajcn.117.152769.

Wang, M., Li, K., Zhao, D., & Li, L. (2017). The association between maternal use of folic acid supplements during pregnancy and risk of autism spectrum disorders in children: A meta-analysis. *Molecular Autism*, *8*, 51. https://doi.org/10.1186/s13229-017-0170-8.

Risk for Delayed Child Development Domain 13 Growth/development Class 2 Development

Marina Martinez-Kratz, MS, RN, CNE

NANDA-I

Definition

Child who is susceptible to failure to achieve developmental milestones within the expected timeframe.

Risk Factors

Infant or Child Factors

Inadequate access to health care provider; inadequate attachment behavior; inadequate stimulation; unaddressed abuse; unaddressed psychological neglect

Caregiver Factors

Anxiety; decreased emotional support availability; depressive symptoms; excessive stress; unaddressed domestic violence

At-Risk Population

Children aged 0-9 years; children born to economically disadvantaged families; children exposed to community violence; children exposed to environmental pollutants; children whose caregivers have developmental disabilities; children whose mothers had inadequate prenatal care; children with below normal growth standards for age and gender; institutionalized children; low birth weight infants; premature infants

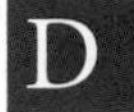

Associated Conditions

Antenatal pharmaceutical preparations; congenital disorders; depression; inborn genetic diseases; maternal mental disorders; maternal physical illnesses; prenatal substance misuse; sensation disorders

NIC, NOC, Client Outcomes, Nursing Interventions and *Rationales,* Client/Family Teaching, and References

Refer to care plan for Delayed Child **Development**.

Delayed Infant Motor Development Domain 13 Growth/development Class 2 Development

Daniela Moscarella, DNP, APN, CPNP-PC, CCRN-K

NANDA-I

Definition

Individual who consistently fails to achieve developmental milestones related to the normal strengthening of bones, muscles and ability to move and touch one's surroundings.

Defining Characteristics

Difficulty lifting head; difficulty maintaining head position; difficulty picking up blocks; difficulty pulling self to stand; difficulty rolling over; difficulty sitting with support; difficulty sitting without support; difficulty standing with assistance; difficulty transferring objects; difficulty with hand-and-knee crawling; does not engage in activities; does not initiate activities

Related Factors

Infant Factors

Difficulty with sensory processing; insufficient curiosity; insufficient initiative; insufficient persistence

Caregiver Factors

Anxiety about infant care; carries infant in arms for excessive time; does not allow infant to choose physical activities; does not allow infant to choose toys; does not encourage infant to grasp; does not encourage infant to reach; does not encourage sufficient infant play with other children; does not engage infant in games about body parts; does not teach movement words; insufficient fine motor toys for infant; insufficient gross motor toys for infant; insufficient time between periods of infant stimulation; limits infant experiences in the prone position; maternal postpartum depressive symptoms; negative perception of infant temperament; overstimulation of infant; perceived infant care incompetence

At-Risk Population

Boys; infants aged 0-12 months; infants born to economically disadvantaged families; infants born to large families; infants born to parents with low educational levels; infants in intensive care units; infants living in home with inadequate physical space; infants whose mothers had inadequate antenatal diet; infants with below normal growth standards for age and gender; low birth weight infants; premature infants; premature infants who do not receive physiotherapy during hospitalization

Associated Conditions

5 Minute Appearance, Pulse, Grimace, Activity, & Respiration (APGAR) score < 7; antenatal pharmaceutical preparations; complex medical conditions; failure to thrive; maternal anemia in late pregnancy; maternal mental health disorders in early pregnancy; maternal prepregnancy obesity; neonatal abstinence syndrome; neurodevelopmental disorders; postnatal infection of preterm infant; sensation disorders

NOC (Nursing Outcomes Classification)

D

Suggested NOC Outcomes

Abuse Recovery; Child Development: 1 Month, 2 Months, 4 Months, 6 Months, 12 Months; Knowledge: Infant Care, Pre-term Infant Care, Parenting; Neglect Cessation; Neglect Recovery

Example NOC Outcome with Indicators

Child Development as evidenced by the following indicators: Appropriate milestones of physical, cognitive, and psychosocial age-appropriate progression. (Rate the outcome and indicators of **Child Development:** 1 = never demonstrated, 2 = rarely demonstrated, 3 = sometimes demonstrated, 4 = often demonstrated, 5 = consistently demonstrated [see Section I].)

Client Outcomes

Client/Parents/Primary Caregiver Will (Specify Time Frame)

- Infant will achieve expected milestones in all areas of physical and motor development
- Parent/caregiver will verbalize understanding of potential impediments to normal development and demonstrate actions or environmental/lifestyle changes necessary to provide appropriate care in a safe, nurturing environment

NIC (Nursing Interventions Classification)

Suggested NIC Interventions

Abuse Protection Support; Caregiver Support; Developmental Enhancement: Infant; Immunization/Vaccination Management; Infant Care: Newborn/Pre-term; Kangaroo Care; Lactation Counseling; Learning Facilitation; Nonnutritive Sucking; Normalization Promotion; Nutrition Management; Parent Education: Infant/Childbearing Family; Parenting Promotion; Referral; Risk Identification: Childbearing Family; Teaching: (Infant) Nutrition/Safety/Stimulation; Temperature Regulation (Infant); Therapeutic Play

Example NIC Activities—Parent Education

Instruct parent on normal physiological, emotional, and behavioral characteristics of infant

Nursing Interventions and *Rationales*

Preconception/Pregnancy

- Assess for nutritional status during pregnancy. Review the importance of iron, folate, iodine, choline, and essential fatty acids. EB: *Maternal nutrition during pregnancy is essential for the health of an infant. Deficiencies in iron, folate, iodine, choline, and essential fatty acids can lead to neural tube defects, abnormal brain development, and preventable developmental delays (Black et al, 2020).*
- Assess for alcohol/drug use during pregnancy. Expectant mothers should be instructed that no amount of alcohol consumption is safe during pregnancy. EBN: *Alcohol is a well-established teratogen that can cause variable physical and behavioral effects on the fetus. Increased fetal exposure to alcohol and sustained alcohol intake during any trimester of pregnancy are associated with an increased risk of fetal alcohol syndrome (FAS) (Gupta, Gupta, & Shirasaka, 2016).*
- Assess and educate about consumption of marijuana use in pregnancy. EB: *Marijuana crosses the placenta and has been found to affect fetal neurodevelopment, which may cause problems with neurological development resulting in hyperactivity and poor cognitive function (Metz & Stickrath, 2015).*

- Educate expectant mothers to stop smoking and assist with methods of smoking cessation. Smoking is an avoidable risk factor for low birth weight and other significant prenatal issues. EB: *Reese et al (2017) noted that pregnant women disproportionately underreport smoking and smokers tend to have lower follow-up rates to repeat questionnaires.*
- Educate that it is recommended that women of childbearing age take 400 mcg of folic acid daily, along with a healthy, well-balanced diet, to reduce the risk of neural tube and other birth defects. EB: *The recommended supplementation of folic acid is 0.4 mg/400 mcg taken once per day, beginning at least 1 month before attempting conception and continuing throughout pregnancy (Kerr et al, 2017).* EB: *The benefits of using folic acid supplements during the periconception period are to prevent neural tube defects and to ensure normal brain development (Valera-Gran et al, 2017).*

Neonate/Infant

- Educate new mothers about the importance of breastfeeding. EB: *Breast milk and the act of breastfeeding may benefit children's cognitive development (Black et al, 2020).*
- Assess the neonate/infant for age-appropriate milestones. EB: *Early identification of developmental delays expedites a referral for therapeutic services such as early intervention, which encourages gains in developmental milestones (Scharf et al, 2016).*
- Assess for maternal depression. EB: *It is essential to address maternal mental health and promote parenting strategies that encourage play-based interactions, which would reduce the risk of behavior and social-emotional problems in childhood (McDonald et al, 2018).*
- Provide information to parents about the importance of health supervision visits at the following intervals: first week of life, 1 month, 2 months, 4 months, 6 months, 9 months, and 12 months, with standardized developmental screen at 9 months old. EB: *Early identification of and intervention for developmental disorders are critical to the well-being of childhood development (Lipkin & Macias, 2020).*
- Teach parents about the necessity of daily tummy time for infants less than 6 months old. EB: *Tummy time has a positive effect related to infant development with an emphasis on motor development (Hewitt et al, 2017).*
- Explain the use of developmentally appropriate toys for play. EB: *Toys that match a child's developmental skills and abilities will further encourage the development of new skills. That is important in early childhood to facilitate cognitive development, language interactions, symbolic and pretend play, problem-solving, social interactions, and physical activity (Healey & Mendelsohn, 2019).*
- Monitor mother–baby interactions when caring for premature infants. EBN: *Posttraumatic stress disorder (PTSD) induced by preterm delivery has a significant impact on the infant–mother attachment dyad. Mothers often have attachment issues, and the infant may be affected, resulting in delayed development (Anderson & Cacola, 2017).*
- Educate about the importance of eating a well-balanced diet in early childhood. EB: *Brain development is rapid in the early years of childhood and therefore adequate nutrition has a significant impact on neurodevelopment (Black et al, 2020).*
- Monitor preterm infants more closely for developmental delays. EBN: *Children born prematurely have a higher risk of chronic health conditions, including attention deficit disorder and attention deficit hyperactivity disorder, speech problems, learning disability, anxiety, asthma, and developmental delays (Kelly, 2018).*
- Provide parents or caregiver with teaching to provide postural support and opportunities for movement with support during parent–infant interactions with the goal of increasing infant movement quality and quantity. EB: *A study found that parent-delivered motor interventions (PDMI) were more effective in improving motor and cognitive outcomes than other interventions (Kharuna et al, 2020).*
- Provide support and education to parents of infants with developmental disabilities (e.g., Down syndrome [DS], cerebral palsy). EB: *A recent study of infants with DS affirmed previous findings showing that the rate of attainment of motor skills is delayed in children with DS compared with children with typical development; however, the developmental sequence is the same. The delayed development is more prominent in more complex skills (Beqaj, Jusaj, & Živković, 2017).*
- Provide education and support for parents of infants with tracheostomy to promote early motor development. EB: *A study found that infants with tracheostomy showed delayed gross motor milestones in head control in a supine position and rolling from a prone to a supine position compared with nontracheostomized infants. Parents should be instructed on the importance of time spent in the prone position (using a wedge or other support as needed) and exercises that strengthen the neck flexor muscle (Shin & Shin, 2020).*
- Monitor for maternal eating disorders because they have a direct effect on childhood development. EB: *Sadeh-Sharvit, Levy-Shiff, and Lock (2016) found that children of mothers with eating disorders showed*

delayed mental and psychomotor development. Severity of maternal eating disorder symptoms emerged as a significant predictor of child development, but other maternal psychopathology did not. Findings suggest that maternal eating disorder history may play a unique role in the development of neurodevelopmental functions in their children.

- Educate parents about the importance of avoiding lead-based paints in the home and other sources of lead in the environment. EB: *Low-level lead exposure has been shown to significantly increase the risk for learning disabilities, behavioral problems, and developmental delay (Hamp et al, 2018).*

D

REFERENCES

Anderson, C., & Cacola, P. (2017). Implications of preterm birth for maternal mental health and infant development. *MCN American Journal of Maternal Child Nursing*, *42*(2), 108–114. https://doi.org/10.1097/nmc.0000000000000311.

Beqaj, S., Jusaj, N., & Živković, V. (2017). Attainment of gross motor milestones in children with Down syndrome in Kosovo—Developmental perspective. *Medicinski Glasnik: Official Publication of the Medical Association of Zenica-Doboj Canton, Bosnia and Herzegovina*, *14*(2), 189–198. https://doi.org/10.17392/917-17.

Black, M. M., Trude, A. C., & Lutter, C. K. (2020). All children thrive: Integration of nutrition and early childhood development. *Annual Review of Nutrition*, *40*(1), 375–406. https://doi.org/10.1146/annurev-nutr-120219-023757.

Gupta, K. K., Gupta, V. K., & Shirasaka, T. (2016). An update on fetal alcohol syndrome—Pathogenesis, risks, and treatment. *Alcoholism: Clinical and Experimental Research*, *40*(8), 1594–1602. https://doi.org/10.1111/acer.13135.

Hamp, N., Zimmerman, A., & Hoffen, J. (2018). Advocating for automatic eligibility for early intervention services for children exposed to lead. *Pediatric Annals*, *47*(10), e413–e418. https://doi.org/10.3928/19382359-20180924-01.

Healey, A., & Mendelsohn, A. (2019). Selecting appropriate toys for young children in the digital era. *Pediatrics*, *143*(1), e20183348. https://doi.org/10.1542/peds.2018-3348.

Hewitt, L., Stanley, R. M., & Okely, A. D. (2017). Correlates of tummy time in infants aged 0–12 months old: A systematic review. *Infant Behavior and Development*, *49*, 310–321. https://doi.org/10.1016/j.infbeh.2017.10.001.

Kelly, M. M. (2018). Health and educational implications of prematurity in the United States: National Survey of Children's Health 2011/2012 data. *Journal of the American Association of Nurse Practitioners*, *30*(3), 131–139. https://doi.org/10.1097/jxx.0000000000000021.

Kerr, S. M., Parker, S. E., Mitchell, A. A., Tinker, S. C., & Werler, M. M. (2017). Periconceptional maternal fever, folic acid intake, and the risk for neural tube defects. *Annals of Epidemiology*, *27*(12), 777–782.e1. https://doi.org/10.1016/j.annepidem.2017.10.010.

Khurana, S., Kane, A. E., Brown, S. E., Tarver, T., & Dusing, S. C. (2020). Effect of neonatal therapy on the motor, cognitive, and behavioral development of infants born preterm: A systematic review. *Developmental Medicine and Child Neurology*, *62*(6), 684–692. https://doi.org/10.1111/dmcn.14485.

Lipkin, P. H., & Macias, M. M. (2020). Promoting optimal development: Identifying infants and young children with developmental disorders through developmental surveillance and screening. *Pediatrics*, *145*(1), e20193449. https://doi.org/10.1542/peds.2019-3449.

McDonald, S. W., Kehler, H. L., & Tough, S. C. (2018). Risk factors for delayed social-emotional development and behavior problems at age two: Results from the All Our Babies/Families (AOB/F) cohort. *Health Science Reports*, *1*(10), e82. https://doi.org/10.1002/hsr2.82.

Metz, T. D., & Stickrath, E. H. (2015). Marijuana use in pregnancy and lactation: A review of the evidence. *American Journal of Obstetrics and Gynecology*, *213*(6), 761–778. https://doi.org/10.1016/j.ajog.2015.05.025.

Reese, S. E., Zhao, S., Wu, M. C., et al. (2017). DNA methylation score as a biomarker in newborns for sustained maternal smoking during pregnancy. *Environmental Health Perspectives*, *125*(4), 760–766. https://doi.org/10.1289/ehp333.

Sadeh-Sharvit, S., Levy-Shiff, R., & Lock, J. D. (2016). Maternal eating disorder history and toddlers' neurodevelopmental outcomes: A brief report. *Eating Disorders*, *24*(2), 198–205. https://doi.org/10.1080/10640266.2015.1064280.

Scharf, R. J., Scharf, G. J., & Stroustrup, A. (2016). Developmental milestones. *Pediatrics in Review*, *37*(1), 25–38. https://doi.org/10.1542/pir.2014-0103.

Shin, H. I., & Shin, H. I. (2020). Delayed development of head control and rolling in infants with tracheostomies. *Frontiers in Pediatrics*, *8*, 571573. https://doi.org/10.3389/fped.2020.571573.

Valera-Gran, D., Navarrete-Muñoz, E. M., Garcia de la Hera, M., et al. (2017). Effect of maternal high dosages of folic acid supplements on neurocognitive development in children at 4–5 years of age: The prospective birth cohort Infancia y Medio Ambiente (INMA) study. *American Journal of Clinical Nutrition*, *106*(3), 878–887. https://doi.org/10.3945/ajcn.117.152769.

Risk for Delayed Infant Motor Development **Domain 13 Growth/development**

Class 2 Development

Marina Martinez-Kratz, MS, RN, CNE

NANDA-I

Definition

Individual susceptible to fails to achieve developmental milestones related to the normal strengthening of bones, muscles and ability to move and touch one's surroundings.

Risk Factors

Infant Factors

Difficulty with sensory processing; insufficient curiosity; insufficient initiative; insufficient persistence

Caregiver Factors

Anxiety about infant care; carries infant in arms for excessive time; does not allow infant to choose physical activities; does not allow infant to choose toys; does not encourage infant to grasp; does not encourage infant to reach; does not encourage sufficient infant play with other children; does not engage infant in games about body parts; does not teach movement words; insufficient fine motor toys for infant; insufficient gross motor toys for infant; insufficient time between periods of infant stimulation; limits infant experiences in the prone position; maternal postpartum depressive symptoms; negative perception of infant temperament; overstimulation of infant; perceived infant care incompetence

At-Risk Population

Boys; infants aged 0-12 months; infants born to economically disadvantaged families; infants born to large families; infants born to parents with low educational levels; infants in intensive care units; infants living in home with inadequate physical space; infants whose mothers had inadequate antenatal diet; infants with below normal growth standards for age and gender; low birth weight infants; premature infants; premature infants who do not receive physiotherapy during hospitalization

Associated Conditions

5 Minute Appearance, Pulse, Grimace, Activity, & Respiration (APGAR) score < 7; antenatal pharmaceutical preparations; complex medical conditions; failure to thrive; maternal anemia in late pregnancy; maternal mental health disorders in early pregnancy; maternal prepregnancy obesity; neonatal abstinence syndrome; neurodevelopmental disorders; postnatal infection of preterm infant; sensation disorders

NIC, NOC, Client Outcomes, Nursing Interventions and *Rationales,* Client/Family Teaching, and References

Refer to care plan for Delayed Infant Motor **Development.**

Diarrhea Domain 3 Elimination and exchange Class 2 Gastrointestinal function

Rosemary Timmerman, DNP, APRN, CCNS, CCRN-CSC-CMC

NANDA-I

Definition

Passage of three or more loose or liquid stools per day.

Defining Characteristics

Abdominal cramping; abdominal pain; bowel urgency; dehydration; hyperactive bowel sounds

Related Factors

Anxiety; early formula feeding; inadequate access to safe drinking water; inadequate access to safe food; inadequate knowledge about rotavirus vaccine; inadequate knowledge about sanitary food preparation; inadequate knowledge about sanitary food storage; inadequate personal hygiene practices; increased stress level; laxative misuse; malnutrition; substance misuse

At-Risk Population

Frequent travelers; individuals at extremes of age; individuals exposed to toxins

Associated Conditions

Critical illness; endocrine system diseases; enteral nutrition; gastrointestinal diseases; immunosuppression; infections; pharmaceutical preparations; treatment regimen

NOC (Nursing Outcomes Classification)

Suggested NOC Outcomes

D

Bowel Elimination; Electrolyte and Acid-Base Balance; Fluid Balance; Hydration; Risk Control: Environmental Hazards; Community Risk Control: Communicable Disease

Example NOC Outcome with Indicators

Bowel Elimination as evidenced by the following indicators: Elimination pattern/Stool soft and formed/Bowel sounds/Liquid stool. (Rate each indicator of **Bowel Elimination:** 1 = severely compromised, 2 = substantially compromised, 3 = moderately compromised, 4 = mildly compromised, 5 = not compromised [see Section I].)

Client Outcomes

Client Will (Specify Time Frame)

- Defecate formed, soft stool every 1 to 3 days
- Maintain the perirectal area free of irritation
- State relief from cramping and less or no diarrhea
- Explain cause of diarrhea and rationale for treatment
- Maintain good skin turgor and weight at usual level
- Have negative stool cultures

NIC (Nursing Interventions Classification)

Suggested NIC Intervention

Diarrhea Management

Example NIC Activities—Diarrhea Management

Evaluate medication profile for gastrointestinal side effects; Suggest trial elimination of foods containing lactose

Nursing Interventions and *Rationales*

- Recognize that diarrhea is defined as the passage of three or more loose or liquid stools in a 24-hour period (Shane et al, 2017).
- Assess pattern of defecation or have the client keep a diary that includes the following: time of day defecation occurs; usual stimulus for defecation; consistency, amount, and frequency of stool; type of, amount of, and time food consumed; fluid intake; history of bowel habits and laxative use; diet; exercise patterns; obstetrical/gynecological, medical, and surgical histories; medications; alterations in perianal sensations; and present bowel regimen. EB: *Assessment of defecation pattern and factors surrounding diarrhea episode, including changes in diet, medications, exercise, and health history, will help direct interventions and treatment (Gale & Wilson, 2016; Shane et al, 2017).*
- Recommend use of standardized tool to consistently assess, quantify, and then treat diarrhea. EB: *Stool classification systems include the Hart and Dobb Diarrhea Scale, the Guenther and Sweed Stool Output Assessment Tool, the Bristol Stool Scale, and the Diarrhea Grading Scale (Dag et al, 2015; Ford & Talley, 2016).*
- Although the abdominal examination has been historically performed in the order of inspection, auscultation, palpation, and percussion, recent scientific investigations have found that palpation and percussion do not affect the number of bowel sounds (Calis et al, 2019; Vizioli et al, 2020). EB: *Expect increased frequency of bowel sounds with diarrhea (Lattimer, Chandler, & Borum, 2017).*

- ▲ Use an evidence-based bowel management protocol that includes identifying and treating the cause of the diarrhea, obtaining a stool specimen if infectious etiology is suspected, evaluating current medications and osmolality of enteral feedings, assessing and treating hydration status of client, reviewing and stopping ordered and/or over-the-counter (OTC) laxatives, assessing food preparation practices, assessing home environment, providing good skin care and applying barrier creams to prevent skin irritation from diarrhea, and evaluating the need for antidiarrheal agents and possible fecal containment device with provider. EB: *The possible cause of the diarrhea needs to be assessed and client hydration and skin protective interventions put into place rapidly to prevent secondary complications associated with the client's diarrhea episodes (Gale & Wilson, 2016; Shane et al, 2017).*
- • Identify the cause of diarrhea if possible based on history (e.g., infection, gastrointestinal inflammation, medication effect, malnutrition or malabsorption, laxative abuse, osmotic enteral feedings, anxiety, stress).
- • Identification of the underlying cause is important because the treatment is determined based on the cause of diarrhea.
- ▲ Testing for diarrhea may consist of laboratory work such as a complete blood count with differential and blood cultures if the client is febrile. Also obtain stool specimens as ordered to either rule out or diagnose an infectious process (e.g., ova and parasites, *Clostridioides [Clostridium] difficile* infection [CDI], bacterial cultures for food poisoning). EB: *Assessing for signs of systemic infection and inflammatory response and evaluation of the stool for infection are important first steps in identifying the cause of diarrhea (Shane et al, 2017).*
- • Consider the possibility of CDI if the client over the age of 2 years has any of the following: watery diarrhea, low-grade fever, abdominal cramps, history of antibiotic therapy, history of gastrointestinal tract surgery, and if the client is taking medications that reduce gastric acid, including proton-pump inhibitors (PPIs), or if diarrhea occurs in the hospital setting. Any antibiotic can cause CDI, but clindamycin, cephalosporins, β-lactam/β-lactamase inhibitors, and fluoroquinolones pose the greatest risk, as do multiple antibiotics and longer duration of antibiotics (Shane et al, 2017; McDonald et al, 2018). EB: *CDIs have become increasingly common because of the frequent use of broad-spectrum antibiotics. Antibiotics and gastric acid–reducing medications can change normal gut flora, increasing the risk for development of CDI, diarrhea, and colitis (Shane et al, 2017; McDonald et al, 2018).*
- • Use standard precautions when caring for clients with diarrhea to prevent spread of infectious diarrhea; for individuals with a CDI, employ contact precautions until 48 hours after diarrhea has resolved; use gloves, gowns, and, when able, disposable equipment; perform handwashing with soap and water; perform routine room and equipment decontamination with a *C. difficile* sporicidal agent; provide a private room or cohort with other clients with a CDI; and provide a dedicated toilet to reduce transmission. *C. difficile* and viruses causing diarrhea have been shown to be highly contagious. *C. difficile* is difficult to eradicate because of spore formation (Shane et al, 2017; McDonald et al, 2018). EB: *Alcohol rubs are not effective in killing* C. difficile *spores (Shane et al, 2017; Centers for Disease Control and Prevention [CDC], 2018).* C. difficile *can survive for at least 24 hours on inanimate surfaces, and spores can survive for months on objects such as toilets, sinks, and bed rails (CDC, 2018).*
- ▲ Antibiotic stewardship is an important aspect in the prevention of *C. difficile* infections. *Antibiotics should be used judiciously (CDC, 2018; McDonald et al, 2018).* If the client has diarrhea associated with antibiotic therapy, consult with the health care provider regarding the use of probiotics, such as yogurt with active cultures, to treat diarrhea, or probiotic dietary supplements, or preferably use probiotics to prevent diarrhea when first beginning antibiotic therapy. EB: *Although conclusive evidence on the effectiveness of probiotic in treating and preventing CDI and diarrhea is lacking, evidence suggests that probiotics may be helpful for reducing the severity and duration of infectious diarrhea in immunocompetent adults and children; probiotics may be used in an attempt to balance intestinal flora and restrict the colonization of* C. difficile, *but the efficacy is influenced by the strain composition of the probiotic as well as the type and duration of antibiotic therapy (Agamennone et al, 2018; McDonald et al, 2018).*
- ▲ Probiotics may also be ordered for immunocompetent clients to prevent a CDI when high-risk antibiotics are prescribed; if a probiotic is ordered, administer it with food. Recommend that it should be taken through the antibiotic course and 10 to 14 days afterward. EB: *Food tends to buffer the stomach acids, allowing more of the probiotic ingredients to pass through the stomach for absorption in the intestines. Beginning this therapy early helps prevent antibiotic-associated diarrhea (McDonald et al, 2018).*
- ▲ Recognize that a CDI can commonly recur and that reculturing of stool is often required before initiating retreatment. EB: *High reinfection rates have been reported within the first 2 months of initial diagnosis. Repeat courses of antibiotics, usually metronidazole or vancomycin, are necessary to treat repeat CDIs. Fecal*

D

microbiota transplantation may be used for clients with severe recurrent or refractory CDIs who have failed antibiotic treatments (Eliakim-Raz & Bishara, 2019; Hui et al, 2019).

- Have the client complete a diet diary for 7 days and monitor the intake of high-fructose corn syrup and fructose sweeteners in relation to onset of diarrhea symptoms. If diarrhea is associated with fructose ingestion, intake should be limited or eliminated. EB: *High-fructose corn syrup or fructose sweeteners from fruit juices can cause gastrointestinal symptoms of bloating, rumbling, flatulence, and diarrhea (Pitta et al, 2019).*

D

- ▲ If the client has infectious diarrhea, consider avoiding use of medications that slow peristalsis. EB: *If an infectious process is occurring, such as a CDI or food poisoning, medication to slow peristalsis should generally not be given. The increase in gut motility helps eliminate the causative factor, and use of antidiarrheal medication could result in a toxic megacolon (Shane et al, 2017; McDonald et al, 2018).*
- Assess for dehydration by observing skin turgor over sternum or delayed capillary refill and inspecting for longitudinal furrows of the tongue. Watch for excessive thirst, fever, dizziness, lightheadedness, palpitations, excessive cramping, bloody stools, hypotension, and symptoms of shock. EB: *Severe diarrhea can cause deficient fluid volume, electrolyte imbalance, extreme weakness, and a possible shock state (Gale & Wilson, 2016; Shane et al, 2017).*
- ▲ Administer oral rehydration solution, consisting of a balanced sodium, potassium, and glucose solution, for individuals with mild to moderate dehydration or in individuals with mild dehydration associated with vomiting or severe diarrhea; provide isotonic intravenous solutions for severe dehydration, shock, or altered mental states (Shane et al, 2017; Ofei & Fuchs, 2019).
- Refer to care plans for Deficient **Fluid** Volume and Risk for Imbalanced **Fluid** Volume if appropriate.
- ▲ If the client has frequent or chronic diarrhea, consider suggesting use of dietary fiber after consultation with a nutritionist and/or provider. EB: *Use of a fiber supplement decreases the number of incontinent stools and improves stool consistency (Pitta et al, 2019).*
- ▲ If diarrhea is chronic and there is evidence of malnutrition, consult with the provider for a dietary consultation and possible nutrition supplementation to maintain nutrition while the gastrointestinal system heals (Pitta et al, 2019).
- Encourage the client to eat small, frequent meals, eating foods that are easy to digest at first (e.g., bananas, crackers, pretzels, rice, potatoes, clear soups, applesauce), but switch to a regular diet as soon as tolerated. Also recommend avoiding milk products, foods high in fiber, and caffeine (dark sodas, tea, coffee, chocolate). EB: *The bananas, rice, applesauce, and toast (BRAT) diet has been traditionally recommended but may be nutritionally incomplete (Schiller, Pardi, & Sellin, 2017; Bonci, & Almario, 2020).*
- Provide a readily available bathroom, commode, or bedpan; provide individuals with a CDI with a dedicated toilet to reduce transmission to other clients (McDonald et al, 2018).
- Thoroughly cleanse and dry the perianal and perineal skin daily as needed using a cleanser capable of stool removal. Apply skin moisture barrier cream as needed. Refer to perirectal skin care in the care plan for Bowel **Incontinence.**
- ▲ If the client has enteral tube feedings and diarrhea, consider infusion rate; position of feeding tube; tonicity of formula; fiber content in the formula; possible formula contamination; and excessive intake of hyperosmolar medications, such as sorbitol commonly found in the liquid version of medications; administer antidiarrheal medications such as loperamide as prescribed (Tatsumi, 2019; Pitta et al, 2019). Consider changing the formula to a lower osmolarity, lactose-free, or high-fiber feeding. *Determination of the cause of diarrhea should include an abdominal examination, fecal leukocytes, quantification of stool, stool culture for* C. difficile *(and/or toxin assay), serum electrolyte panel, and review of medications (Pitta et al, 2019; Tatsumi, 2019).*
- Avoid administering bolus enteral feedings or hyperosmolar formulas directly into the small bowel. EB: *The stomach has a larger capacity for large fluid volumes, whereas the small bowel can usually only tolerate up to 150 mL/h (Tatsumi, 2019; Pitta et al, 2019).*
- ▲ Dilute liquid medications before administration through the enteral tube and flush the enteral feeding tube with sufficient water before and after medication administration. *Because many liquid medications contain sorbitol or are hyperosmotic, diluting the medication may help decrease occurrence of diarrhea (Pitta et al, 2019).*
- Teach clients with cancer the types of diarrhea they may encounter, emphasizing not only chemotherapy- and radiation-induced diarrhea but also *C. difficile,* along with associated signs and symptoms and treatments. EB: *Diarrhea in cancer clients is a common complication that causes dehydration, electrolyte imbalances, nutritional deficits, and hospitalization for treatment. Providing the client education focusing on early*

recognition of diarrhea necessitating early interventions is important in preventing adverse client outcomes (Escalante et al, 2017; Schiller, Pardi, & Sellin, 2017).

- ▲ For chemotherapy-induced diarrhea (CID) and radiation-induced diarrhea (RID), review rationale for pharmacological interventions, along with soluble fiber and probiotic supplements. Consult a registered dietitian to assist with recommendations to alleviate diarrhea, decrease dehydration, and maintain nutritional status. EBN: *Both CID and RID can occur as often as or more than 50% of the time, depending on the chemotherapy regimen or combination with radiation (Escalante et al, 2017; Schiller, Pardi, & Sellin, 2017).*
- ▲ Acute traveler's diarrhea is the most common illness affecting individuals traveling to, usually, low-income regions of the world. EB: *Improved hygiene, avoidance of foods for which preparation methods are unknown (e.g., street food) as well as raw fruits or vegetables, water, drinks with ice, and use of bismuth salicylates can mitigate the severity of gastric distress. Clients should be counseled about precautions they can take while traveling to reduce the severity of the diarrhea, and a self-treatment antibiotic series may be prescribed by the health care provider for at-risk clients (Porter et al, 2017; Shane et al, 2017).*

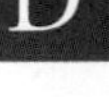

Pediatric

- ▲ Assess for mild or moderate signs of dehydration with both acute and persistent diarrhea: mild (increased thirst and dry mouth or tongue) and moderate (decreased urination; no wet diapers for 3+ hours; feeling of weakness/lightheadedness, irritability, or listlessness; few or no tears when crying) (Gupta, 2016). Refer to primary care provider for treatment.
- ▲ Recommend that parents give the child oral rehydration fluids to drink in the amounts specified by the health care provider, especially during the first 4 to 6 hours to replace lost fluid; avoid sodas, fruit juices, and clear liquids such as water and chicken broth. Once the child is rehydrated, an orally administered maintenance solution should be used along with food. Continue even if child vomits. EB: *Treatment with oral rehydration fluids for children is generally as effective as intravenous fluids (Shane et al, 2017; Ofei & Fuchs, 2019). Oral rehydration therapy (ORT) is an iso-osmolar, glucose-electrolyte solution that has been recognized for more than 40 years to be effective in treating children with dehydration caused by acute infectious diarrhea. Vomiting is not a contraindication to ORT but antinausea and antiemetic agents may be given to children older than 4 years to facilitate tolerance of oral rehydration. Adequate ORT is absorbed by most clients during vomiting (Shane et al, 2017; Rehydration Project, 2019).*
- ● Recommend that the mother resume breastfeeding as soon as possible.
- ● Recommend that parents avoid giving the child flat soda, fruit juices, sports drinks, gelatin dessert, broth, or instant fruit drink. EB: *These fluids have a high osmolality from carbohydrate contents and can exacerbate diarrhea. In addition, they have low sodium concentrations that can aggravate existing hyponatremia (Ofei & Fuchs, 2019; Rehydration Project, 2019).*
- ● Recommend that parents give children foods with complex carbohydrates, such as potatoes, rice, bread, cereal, yogurt, fruits, and vegetables. Avoid fatty foods, foods high in simple sugars, and milk products.
- ● Advise parents to return for assistance if fever, bloody diarrhea, or signs of severe dehydration such as decreased urine output, lightheadedness, or lethargy occur.
- ● Recommend CDC principles of safe food preparation, which include clean, separate, cook, chill, and report, particularly for children under the age of 5 years (US Department of Health and Human Services, 2019).
- ▲ Recommend rotavirus vaccine within the child's vaccination schedule. EB: *Two vaccines, Rotarix and RotaTeq, have undergone comprehensive studies with findings that they can significantly prevent severe rotavirus diarrhea and death caused by dehydration in children (Mwenda et al, 2017; Shane et al, 2017).*

Geriatric

- ▲ Evaluate medications the client is taking. Recognize that many medications can result in diarrhea, including digitalis, propranolol, angiotensin-converting enzyme inhibitors, histamine-receptor antagonists, nonsteroidal antiinflammatory drugs, anticholinergic agents, oral hypoglycemia agents, antibiotics, and so forth. EB: *Numerous medications can cause diarrhea. Evaluate changes in the client's medications as a possible cause of the diarrhea (DuPont, 2016; Schiller, Pardi, & Sellin, 2017).*
- ▲ Monitor the client closely to detect whether an impaction is causing diarrhea; remove impaction as ordered. Clients with fecal impaction commonly experience leakage of mucus or liquid stool from the rectum, rectal irritation, distention, and impaired anal sensation (Schiller, Pardi, & Sellin, 2017; Pitta et al, 2019).
- ▲ Seek medical attention if diarrhea is severe or persists for more than 24 hours, or if the client has a history of dehydration or electrolyte disturbances, such as lassitude, weakness, or prostration. EB: *Older adult*

clients can dehydrate rapidly; especially serious is the development of hypokalemia with dysrhythmias. C. difficile *is a common cause of diarrhea in older clients when they have been subjected to long-term antibiotic therapy (Gale & Wilson, 2016; Shane et al, 2017).*

- Provide emotional support for clients who are having trouble controlling unpredictable episodes of diarrhea. *Diarrhea can be a great source of embarrassment to older clients and can lead to social isolation and a feeling of powerlessness.*

Home Care

- Previously mentioned interventions may be adapted for home care use to keep the client well hydrated.
- Assess the home for general sanitation and methods of food preparation. Reinforce principles of sanitation for food handling. *Poor sanitation or mishandling of food may cause bacterial infection or transmission of dangerous organisms from utensils to food.*
- Assess for methods of handling soiled laundry if the client is bed bound or has been incontinent. Instruct or reinforce universal precautions with family and bloodborne pathogen precautions with agency caregivers. *The Bloodborne Pathogen Regulations of the Occupational Safety and Health Administration (OSHA) identify legal guidelines for caregivers.*
- When assessing medication history, include OTC drugs, both general and those currently being used to treat the diarrhea. Instruct clients not to mix OTC medications when self-treating. *Mixing OTC medications can further irritate the gastrointestinal system, intensifying the diarrhea or causing nausea and vomiting.*
- Evaluate current medications for indications that specific interventions are warranted. Blood levels of medications may increase during prolonged episodes of diarrhea, indicating the need for close monitoring of the client or direct intervention.
- Teach client importance of food safety practices and hand hygiene after using the toilet, changing a diaper, handling garbage or soiled laundry, and touching animals or their feces or their environment (Shane et al, 2017).
- Teach the client experiencing diarrhea to avoid swimming, water-related activities, and sex with other people while symptomatic (Shane et al, 2017).
- ▲ Evaluate the need for a home health aide or homemaker service referral. Caregiver may need support for maintaining client cleanliness to prevent skin breakdown.
- Evaluate the need for durable medical equipment in the home. The client may need a bedside commode, call bell, or raised toilet seat to facilitate prompt toileting.

Client/Family Teaching and Discharge Planning

- Encourage avoidance of coffee, spices, milk products, and foods that irritate or stimulate the gastrointestinal tract.
- Teach the appropriate method of taking ordered antidiarrheal medications; explain side effects.
- Explain how to prevent the spread of infectious diarrhea (e.g., careful handwashing, appropriate handling and storage of food, and thoroughly cleaning the bathroom and kitchen). EB: *Good hand hygiene has repeatedly been found to be the first step in preventing the spread of infectious diarrhea (CDC, 2018).*
- Help the client to determine stressors and set up an appropriate stress reduction plan, if stress is the cause of diarrhea.
- Teach signs and symptoms of dehydration and electrolyte imbalance.
- Teach perirectal skin care.
- ▲ Consider teaching clients about complementary therapies, such as probiotics, after consultation with primary care provider.

REFERENCES

Agamennone, V., Krul, C., Rijkers, G., & Kort, R. (2018). A practical guide for probiotics applied to the case of antibiotic-associated diarrhea in The Netherlands. *BMC Gastroenterology*, *18*(1), 103. https://doi.org/10.1186/s12876-018-0831-x.

Bonci, L., & Almario, C. (2020). *Diet strategies for managing chronic diarrhea*. International Foundation for Functional Gastrointestinal Disorders. Retrieved from https://mk0iffgd43a85spvyq6.kinstacdn.com/wp-content/uploads/208-Diarrhea-11.29.20.pdf.

Çalış, A. S., Kaya, E., Mehmetaj, L., et al. (2019). Abdominal palpation and percussion maneuvers do not affect bowel sounds. *Turkish Journal of Surgery*, *35*(4), 309–313. https://doi.org/10.5578/turkjsurg.4291.

Centers for Disease Control and Prevention (CDC). (2018). *C. diff (Clostridioides difficile)*. Retrieved from https://www.cdc.gov/hai/organisms/cdiff/cdiff_clinicians.html. [Accessed 24 June 2021].

Dag, G. S., Dicle, A., Saka, O., & Whelan, K. (2015). Assessment of the Turkish version of the King's stool chart for evaluating stool output and diarrhea among patients receiving enteral nutrition. *Gastroenterology Nursing*, *38*(3), 218–225. doi:10.1097/SGA.0000000000000114.

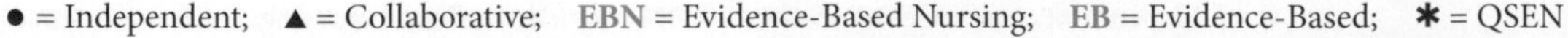

DuPont, H. L. (2016). Persistent diarrhea: A clinical review. *The Journal of the American Medical Association*, *315*(24), 2712–2723. doi:10.1001/jama.2016.7833.
Eliakim-Raz, N., & Bishara, J. (2019). Prevention and treatment of *Clostridium difficile* associated diarrhea by reconstitution of the microbiota. *Human Vaccines & Immunotherapeutics*, *15*(6), 1453–1456. doi:10.1080/21645515.2018.1472184.
Escalante, J., McQuade, R. M., Stojanovska, V., & Nurgali, K. (2017). Impact of chemotherapy on gastrointestinal functions and the enteric nervous system. *Maturitas*, *105*, 23–29. https://doi.org/10.1016/j.maturitas.2017.04.021.
Ford, A. C., & Talley, N. J. (2016). Irritable bowel syndrome. In M. Feldman, L. Friedman, & L. J. Brandt (Eds.), *Sleisenger and Fordtran's gastrointestinal and liver disease* (10th ed.) (pp. 2139–2153). Philadelphia: Elsevier.
Gale, A. R., & Wilson, M. (2016). Diarrhea: Initial evaluation and treatment in the emergency department. *Emergency Clinics of North America*, *34*(2), 293–308. http://dx.doi.org/10.1016/j.emc.2015.12.006.
Gupta, R. (2016). Diarrhea. In R. Wyllie, J. S. Hyams, & M. Kay (Eds.), *Pediatric gastrointestinal and liver disease* (5th ed.) (pp. 104–114). Philadelphia: Elsevier.
Hui, W., Li, T., Liu, W., Zhou, C., & Gao, F. (2019). Fecal microbiota transplantation for treatment of recurrent C. difficile infection: An updated randomized controlled trial meta-analysis. *PLoS One*, *14*(1), e0210016. https://doi.org/10.1371/journal.pone.0210016.
Lattimer, L. D. N., Chandler, M., & Borum, M. L. (2017). Chronic diarrhea. In F. J. Domino (Ed.), *The 5-minute clinical consult premium 2018*. Philadelphia: Lippincott Williams & Wilkins.
McDonald, L. C., Gerding, D. N., Johnson, S., et al. (2018). Clinical practice guidelines for *Clostridium difficile* infection in adults and children: 2017 update by the Infectious Diseases Society of America (IDSA) and Society for Healthcare Epidemiology of America (SHEA). *Clinical Infectious Disease*, *66*(7), e1–e48. https://doi.org/10.1093/cid/cix1085.
Mwenda, J. M., Burke, R. M., Shaba, K., et al. (2017). Implementation of rotavirus surveillance and vaccine introduction—World Health Organization, 2007–2016. *Morbidity and Mortality Weekly Report*, *66*(43), 1192–1196.
Ofei, S. Y., & Fuchs, G. J., 3rd. (2019). Principles and practice of oral rehydration. *Current Gastroenterology Reports*, *21*(12), 67. https://doi.org/10.1007/s11894-019-0734-1.
Pitta, M. R., Campos, F. M., Monteiro, A. G., Cunha, A., Porto, J. D., & Gomes, R. R. (2019). Tutorial on diarrhea and enteral nutrition: A comprehensive step-by-step approach. *JPEN: Journal of Parenteral and Enteral Nutrition*, *43*(8), 1008–1019. https://doi.org/10.1002/jpen.1674.
Porter, C. K., Olson, S., Hall, A., & Riddle, M. S. (2017). Travelers' diarrhea: An update on the incidence, etiology, and risk in military deployments and similar travel populations. *Military Medicine*, *182*(S2), 4–10.
Rehydration Project. (2019). Retrieved from http://rehydrate.org/ors/ort.htm. [Accessed 24 June 2021].
Schiller, L. R., Pardi, D. S., & Sellin, J. H. (2017). Chronic diarrhea: Diagnosis and management. *Clinical Gastroenterology and Hepatology*, *15*(2), 182–193. http://dx.doi.org/10.1016/j.cgh.2016.07.028.
Shane, A. L., Mody, R. K., Crump, J. A., et al. (2017). 2017 Infectious Diseases Society of America clinical practice guidelines for the diagnosis and management of infectious diarrhea. *Clinical Infectious Diseases*, *65*(12), e45–e80. https://doi.org/10.1093/cid/cix669.
Tatsumi, H. (2019). Enteral tolerance in critically ill patients. *Journal of Intensive Care*, *7*, 30. https://doi.org/10.1186/s40560-019-0378-0.
US Department of Health and Human Services. (2019). *People at risk: Children under five*. FoodSafety.gov [website]. Retrieved from ht tps://www.foodsafety.gov/people-at-risk/children-under-five. [Accessed 24 June 2021].
Vizioli, L. H., Winckler, F. D., da Luz, L. C., Marques, G. K., Callegari-Jacques, S. M., & Fornari, F. (2020). Abdominal palpation does not modify the number of bowel sounds in healthy volunteers and gastrointestinal outpatients. *The American Journal of the Medical Sciences*, *360*(4), 378–382. https://doi.org/10.1016/j.amjms.2020.05.041.

Risk for Disuse Syndrome **Domain 4 Activity/rest Class 2 Activity/exercise**

Darcy O'Banion, RN, MS, ACCNS-AG

NANDA-I

Definition

Susceptible to deterioration of body systems as the result of prescribed or unavoidable musculoskeletal inactivity, which may compromise health.

Risk Factors

Pain

Associated Conditions

Decreased level of consciousness; immobilization; paralysis; prescribed movement restrictions

NOC (Nursing Outcomes Classification)

Suggested NOC Outcomes

Pain Level; Endurance; Immobility Consequences: Physiological; Mobility; Neurological Status: Consciousness; Progressive Mobility

Example NOC Outcome with Indicators

Immobility Consequences: Physiological as evidenced by the following indicators: Pressure injury/ Constipation/Compromised nutrition status/Urinary calculi/Compromised muscle strength. (Rate the outcome and indicators of **Immobility Consequences: Physiological:** 1 = severe, 2 = substantial, 3 = moderate, 4 = mild, 5 = none [see Section I].)

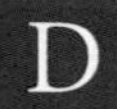

Client Outcomes

Client Will (Specify Time Frame)

- Express pain level that is tolerable to allow for desired mobility
- Maintain full range of motion in joints
- Maintain intact skin, good peripheral blood flow, and normal pulmonary function
- Maintain normal bowel and bladder function
- Express feelings about imposed immobility
- Explain methods to prevent complications of immobility

NIC (Nursing Interventions Classification)

Suggested NIC Interventions

Energy Management; Exercise Therapy: Joint Mobility; Muscle Control; Positioning; Pain Management

Example NIC Activities—Energy Management

Determine the client's significant other's perception of causes of fatigue; Use valid instruments to measure fatigue, as indicated

Nursing Interventions and *Rationales*

- Screen for mobility skills in the following order: (1) bed mobility; (2) supported and unsupported sitting; (3) transitional movements such as sit to stand, stand to sit, and transfers to chair from bed, from chair to bed, and so forth; and (4) standing and walking activities. Use a mobility assessment tool such as the Banner Mobility Assessment Tool (Boynton et al, 2014) or the ICU Mobility Scale (Hodgson et al, 2014). EB: *A systematic review showed that early mobilization led to a greater probability of walking without assistance at time of discharge and more days alive and out of hospital (Tipping et al, 2017).* EB: *Early mobilization is associated with decrease in intensive care unit (ICU) length of stay and hospital length of stay (Laurent et al, 2016).*
- Assess the level of assistance needed by the client and express in terms of amount of effort expended by the person assisting the client. The range is as follows: total assist, meaning client performs 0% to 25% of task and, if client requires the help of more than one caregiver, it is referred to as a dependent transfer; maximum assist, meaning client gives 25% of effort while the caregiver performs the majority of the work; moderate assist, meaning client gives 50% of effort; minimal assist, meaning client gives 75% of effort; contact guard assist, meaning no physical assist is given but caregiver is physically touching client for steadying, guiding, or in case of loss of balance; standby assist, meaning caregiver's hands are up and ready in case needed; supervision, meaning supervision of task is needed even if at a distance; modified independent, meaning client needs assistive device or extra time to accomplish task; and independent, meaning client is able to complete task safely without instruction or assistance. EB: *Functional status is often based on rating from the Functional Independence Measure. It is an 18-item instrument that measures care burden associated with physical and cognitive functioning on a scale from 1 (total assistance) to 7 (complete independence) based on assessments of memory, comprehension, self-care, transfers, and locomotion (Pretz et al, 2016).*
- ▲ Request a referral to a physical therapist (PT) as needed so that client's range of motion, muscle strength, balance, coordination, endurance, and early mobilization can be part of the initial evaluation. The PT may provide the client with bed exercises, including stretching, flexing/extending muscle groups, or using bands to maintain muscle strength and tone. Collaboration with nursing staff, therapy, and respiratory therapy as needed to mobilize clients as early and as safely possible. EB: *Muscle atrophy from disuse is associated with disability, functional decline, metabolic derangements, and early mortality (Atherton et al, 2016).*
- Passive range of motion can be done as the client tolerates. EBN: *Although there is evidence to support early mobility in reducing complications, recent literature shows that passive range of motion and stretching does not improve joint mobility (Harvey et al, 2017).*

- Use specialized boots to prevent pressure injury on the heels and foot drop; remove boots twice daily to assess the skin and to provide foot care as needed. Elevate heels off the bed as the client tolerates when boots are not in place. EB: *Boots help keep the foot in normal anatomical alignment to prevent foot drop and off-loading prevents pressure injury formation on the heel. Although no single support surface has been shown to be more effective than another, off-loading the heel will prevent heel pressure injuries (EPUAP/NPUAP, 2019; McNichol et al, 2020; Rivolo et al, 2020).*
- When positioning a client on the side, tilt client 30 degrees or less while lying on the side. EB: *There is insufficient evidence to support which particular positions or repositioning frequencies are most effective in reducing pressure injuries (Gillespie et al, 2020).*

D

- Assess skin condition every shift and more frequently if needed. Use a risk assessment tool such as the Braden Scale or Waterlow scale to predict the risk of developing pressure ulcers (now referred to as pressure injury). EBN: *There is insufficient evidence to support the effect of risk assessment on pressure ulcer incidence (such as the Braden Scale or Waterlow tool) when compared with training and risk assessment using clinical judgment (Moore & Patton, 2019). Refer to care plan for Risk for Impaired **Skin** Integrity.*
- Discuss with staff and management a "safe patient handling" policy that may include a "no lift" policy to prevent staff injury. EB: *Safe patient handling and mobilization programs are effective in reducing injuries; however, evidence is insufficient to identify the most effective interventions for the various levels of client care (Teeple et al, 2017).*
- Turn clients at high risk for pressure/shear/friction frequently and apply pressure-relieving devices when able. EB: *Although there are varying results around the most appropriate turning frequency and positions, the combination of frequent repositioning with the use of pressure-relieving devices is most effective in reducing pressure ulcers/injury in hospitalized clients (Chew et al, 2018; Gillespie et al, 2020).*
- Provide the client with appropriate pressure-relieving devices. For further interventions on skin care, refer to the care plan for Impaired **Skin** Integrity.
- Help the client out of bed as soon as able. EB: *Prolonged immobilization leads to harmful consequences in musculoskeletal, cardiovascular, respiratory, and integumentary systems, as well as cognition (Parry & Puthucheary, 2015; Atherton et al, 2016). However, there is insufficient evidence on the effect of early mobilization on functional outcome, adverse events, muscle strength, and quality of life (Doiron et al, 2018).*
- When getting the client up after bed rest, do so slowly and watch for signs and symptoms of postural (orthostatic) hypotension, including dizziness, tachycardia, nausea, diaphoresis, or syncope. EB: *To assess orthostatic vital signs, take the first blood pressure and heart rate measurements once the client has been lying supine for 5 minutes. Then have the client stand and check blood pressure and heart rate 1 and 3 minutes after standing. A decrease in systolic blood pressure by 20 mm Hg, a decrease in diastolic pressure of 10 mm Hg or more, or an increase in heart rate by 20 beats per minute or more is indicative of intravascular volume loss (Whelton et al, 2017). Compression wraps to abdomen and/or lower limbs can facilitate venous return if hypotension is an issue (Logan et al, 2017).*
- Obtain assistive devices such as braces, crutches, or canes to help the client reach and maintain as much mobility as possible. *Assistive devices can help increase mobility (Boynton et al, 2014).*
- ▲ Apply graduated compression stockings as ordered, if indicated for orthostatic hypotension. Ensure proper fit by measuring accurately. Remove the stockings at least twice a day, in the morning with the bath and in the evening to assess the condition of the extremity and skin, then reapply. Knee length is preferred rather than thigh length. EB: *The American College of Chest Physicians (Stevens et al, 2021) does not recommend graduated compression stockings to prevent deep vein thrombosis (DVT). Intermittent pneumatic compression devices alone are insufficient in preventing venous thromboembolism (VTE) compared with chemoprophylaxis or a combination of the two in high-risk surgical clients or medical inpatients who are not high bleeding risk (O'Connell et al, 2016; Schünemann et al, 2018). Refer to the CHEST guidelines for use of mechanical prophylaxis for specific client situations (Stevens et al, 2021).*
- Observe for signs of DVT, including pain, tenderness, redness, and swelling in the calf and thigh. Also observe for signs and symptoms of pulmonary embolism, including sudden onset of dyspnea, chest pain, syncope, dizziness, tachycardia, or tachypnea. EB: *Because of poor specificity of signs and symptoms of VTE, the diagnosis based on clinical manifestation alone is unreliable (Di Nisio, van Es, & Büller, 2016).*
- Have the client cough and deep breathe or use incentive spirometry every 2 hours while awake. EB: *Bed rest compromises breathing and can lead to atelectasis and pneumonia because of decreased chest expansion, decreased cilia activity, pooling of mucus, and the effects of organ shift (such as the diaphragm and heart and pressure on the esophagus when in the supine position) and leads to partial or complete atelectasis usually of the left lower lobe (Parry & Puthucheary, 2015).*

- Monitor respiratory functions, noting breath sounds, work of breathing, and respiratory rate. Percuss for new onset of dullness in lungs.
- Note bowel function daily. Provide fluids, fiber, and natural laxatives such as prune juice as needed. *Constipation is common in immobilized clients because of decreased activity and reduced fluid and food intake. Refer to care plan for* ***Constipation.***
- Increase fluid intake to 2000 mL/day within the client's cardiac and renal reserve. *Adequate fluids help prevent kidney stones and constipation, both of which are associated with bed rest.*
- Encourage intake of a balanced diet with adequate amounts of fiber and protein. Consider recommending Practical Interventions to Achieve Therapeutic Lifestyle Changes (TLC), which includes monounsaturated and polyunsaturated fats, oils, margarines, beans, peas, lentils, soy, skinless poultry, lean fish, trimmed cuts of meat, fat-free and low-fat dairy foods, omega-3 polyunsaturated fat sources, and whole grains, including soluble fiber sources such as oats, oat bran, and barley (Osborne et al, 2013).

Critical Care

▲ Recognize that the client who has been in an intensive care environment may develop a neuromuscular dysfunction acquired in the absence of causative factors other than the underlying critical illness and its treatment, resulting in ICU-acquired weakness, with an approximate incidence of 40% requiring more than 1 week of mechanical ventilation (Appleton, Kinsella, & Quasim, 2015). The client may need a workup to determine the cause before satisfactory ambulation can begin. EB: *Critical care clients can develop neuromuscular weakness, polyneuropathy, and delirium (Appleton, Kinsella, & Quasim, 2015; Wintermann et al, 2015).*

▲ Consider the use of a continuous lateral rotation therapy bed. EB: *A systematic review demonstrated limited evidence of the effects of routine lateral repositioning for critically ill clients, although mostly because of poor-quality studies (Hewitt, Bucknall, & Faraone, 2016).*

▲ For the stable client in the ICU, consider mobilizing the client in a four-phase method from dangling at the side of the bed to walking if there is sufficient knowledgeable staff available to protect the client from harm. Even ICU clients receiving mechanical ventilation can be mobilized safely if a multiprofessional team is present to support, protect, and monitor the client for intolerance to activity (Green et al, 2016; Agency for Healthcare Research and Quality, 2017). EBN: *Critical care clients are at high risk for complications related to immobility such as ventilator-associated pneumonia (VAP), atelectasis, and long-lasting functional limitations. Early mobility may reduce length of stay and improve functional outcomes but there is low quality of evidence in the current studies and many barriers to early mobility (Doiron, Hoffmann & Beller, 2018; Hodgson, Capell & Tipping, 2018).*

Geriatric

- Get the client out of bed as early as possible and ambulate frequently after consultation with the health care provider. EB: *Immobility is a risk factor for VTE; immobilization is a major risk factor for VTE, especially in people over 70 years old (Stevens et al, 2021; Talec, Gaujoux, & Samama, 2016). Functional decline from hospital-associated deconditioning is common in older adults, particularly because they are already more deconditioned with less muscle mass, and early rehabilitation can be effective in preventing this condition in addition to other comorbidities (Heldmann et al, 2019; Wald et al, 2019).*
- Consider physical and occupational therapy referrals to guide with environmental safety assessment and home exercise programs.
- Monitor nutrition status in the elderly to prevent malnutrition. EB: *Malnutrition is common in the elderly and can interfere with functional recovery (Agarwalla, Saikia, & Baruah, 2015; Engelheart & Brummer, 2018).*
- Monitor for signs of depression: flat affect, poor appetite, insomnia, and many somatic complaints. EB: *Depression can commonly accompany decreased mobility and function in older adults, and mobilization has a positive effect on depressive mood and enhances quality of life (López-Torres Hidalgo & DEP-EXERCISE Group, 2019).*
- Keep careful track of bowel function in older adults; do not allow the client to become constipated. EB: *Older adults can easily develop impactions as a result of immobility. Refer to* ***Constipation*** *care plan.*

Home Care

- Some of the previous interventions may be adapted for home care use.

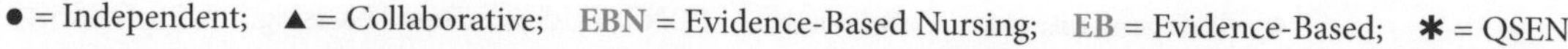

- ▲ Begin discharge planning at time of admission with case manager or social worker and input from physical and occupational therapy as appropriate to assess need for home support systems and community or home health services.
- ▲ Become oriented to all programs of care for the client before discharge from institutional care.
- ▲ Confirm the immediate availability of all necessary assistive devices for home.
- ● Perform complete physical assessment and recent history at initial home visit.
- ▲ Refer to physical and occupational therapies for immediate evaluations of the client's potential for independence and functioning in the home setting and for follow-up care.
- ● Allow the client to have as much input and control of the plan of care as possible. *Client perception of control increases self-esteem and motivation to follow medical plan of care.*
- ● Assess knowledge of all care with caregivers. Review as necessary. *Having the necessary knowledge and skills to perform care decreases caregiver role strain and supports safety of the client.*
- ▲ Support the family of the client in the assumption of caregiver activities. Refer for home health aide services for assistance and respite as appropriate. Refer to medical social services as appropriate.
- ▲ Institute case management of frail elderly to support continued independent living, if possible in the home environment.

Client/Family Teaching and Discharge Planning

- ● Teach client/family how to perform range-of-motion exercises in bed if not contraindicated; this is referred to as a home exercise program.
- ● Teach the family how to turn and position the client and provide all care necessary.

Note: Nursing diagnoses that are commonly relevant when the client is on bed rest include **Constipation,** Risk for Impaired **Skin** Integrity, Disturbed **Sleep** Pattern**, Frail Elderly** Syndrome, and **Powerlessness.**

REFERENCES

Agarwalla, R., Saikia, A. M., & Baruah, R. (2015). Assessment of the nutritional status of the elderly and its correlates. *Journal of Family and Community Medicine, 22*(1), 39–43.

Agency for Healthcare Research and Quality. (2017). *Early mobility guide for reducing ventilator-associated events in mechanically ventilated patients.* Retrieved from https://www.ahrq.gov/sites/default/files/wysiwyg/professionals/quality-patient-safety/hais/tools/mvp/modules/technical/early-mobility-mvpguide.pdf. [Accessed June 25, 2021].

Appleton, R. T., Kinsella, J., & Quasim, T. (2015). The incidence of intensive care unit-acquired weakness syndromes: A systematic review. *Journal of the Intensive Care Society, 16*(2), 126–136.

Atherton, P. J., Greenhaff, P. L., Phillips, S. M., Bodine, S. C., Adams, C. M., & Lang, C. H. (2016). Control of skeletal muscle atrophy in response to disuse: Clinical/preclinical contentions and fallacies of evidence. *American Journal of Physiology Endocrinology and Metabolism, 311*(3), e594–e604. doi:10.1152/ajpendo.00257.2016.

Boynton, T., Kelly, L., Perez, A., Miller, M., An, Y., & Trudgen, C. (2014). Banner mobility assessment tool for nurses: Instrument validation. *American Journal of Safe Patient Handling & Movement, 4*(3), 86–92.

Chew, H. S. J., Thiara, E., Lopez, V., & Shorey, S. (2018). Turning frequency in bedridden patients to prevent hospital-acquired pressure ulcer: A scoping review. *International Wound Journal, 15*(2), 225–236. https://doi.org/10.1111/iwj.12855.

Di Nisio, M., van Es, N., & Büller, H. R. (2016). Deep vein thrombosis and pulmonary embolism. *Lancet, 388*(10063), 3060–3073.

Doiron, K. D., Hoffmann, T. C., & Beller, E. M. (2018). Early intervention (mobilization or active exercise) for critically ill adults in the intensive care unit. *Cochrane Database of Systematic Reviews, 3*, CD010754. https://doi.org/10.1002/14651858.CD010754.pub2.

Engelheart, S., & Brummer, R. (2018). Assessment of nutritional status in the elderly: A proposed function-driven model. *Food & Nutrition Research, 62*.

European Pressure Ulcer Advisory Panel, National Pressure Injury Advisory Panel, and Pan Pacific Pressure Injury Alliance. (2019). *Prevention and treatment of pressure ulcers/injuries: Quick reference guide.* Emily Haesler (Ed.). EPUAP/NPIAP/PPPIA.

Gillespie, B. M., Walker, R. M., Latimer, S. L., et al. (2020). Repositioning for pressure injury prevention in adults. *Cochrane Database of Systematic Reviews, 6*, CD009958. doi:10.1002/14651858.CD009958.pub3.

Green, M., Marzano, V., Leditschke, I. A., Mitchell, I., & Bissett, B. (2016). Mobilization of intensive care patients: A multidisciplinary practical guide for clinicians. *Journal of Multidisciplinary Healthcare, 9*, 247–256. https://doi.org/10.2147/JMDH.S99811.

Harvey, L. A., Katalinic, O. M., Herbert, R. D., Moseley, A. M., Lannin, N. A., & Schurr, K. (2017). Stretch for the treatment and prevention of contracture: An abridged republication of a Cochrane Systematic Review. *Journal of Physiotherapy, 63*(2), 67–75.

Heldmann, P., Werner, C., Belala, N., Bauer, J. M., & Hauer, K. (2019). Early inpatient rehabilitation for acutely hospitalized older patients: A systematic review of outcome measures. *BMC Geriatrics, 19*(1), 189. https://doi.org/10.1186/s12877-019-1201-4.

Hewitt, N., Bucknall, T., & Faraone, N. M. (2016). Lateral positioning for critically ill adult patients. *Cochrane Database of Systematic Reviews, 5*, CD007205. doi:10.1002/14651858.CD007205.pub2.

Hodgson, C. L., Capell, E., & Tipping, C. J. (2018). Early mobilization of patients in intensive care: Organization, communication and safety factors that influence translation into clinical practice. *Critical Care, 22*(1), 77. https://doi.org/10.1186/s13054-018-1998-9.

Hodgson, C. L., Needham, D., Haines, K., et al. (2014). Feasibility and inter-rater reliability of the ICU mobility scale. *Heart & Lung, 43*(1), 19–24.

Laurent, H., Aubreton, S., Richard, R., et al. (2016). Systematic review of early exercise in intensive care: A qualitative approach. *Anaesthesia Critical Care & Pain Medicine, 35*(2), 133–149.

Logan, A., Marsden, J., Freeman, J., & Kent, B. (2017). Effectiveness of non-pharmacological interventions in treating orthostatic hypotension in the elderly and people with a neurological condition: A systematic review. *JBI Database of Systematic Reviews and Implementation Reports*, *15*(4), 948–960.

López-Torres Hidalgo, J., & DEP-EXERCISE Group. (2019). Effectiveness of physical exercise in the treatment of depression in older adults as an alternative to antidepressant drugs in primary care. *BMC Psychiatry*, *19*(1), 21. https://doi.org/10.1186/s12888-018-1982-6.

McNichol, L., Mackey, D., Watts, C., & Zuecca, N. (2020). Choosing a support surface for pressure injury prevention and treatment. *Nursing*, *50*(2), 41–44. doi:10.1097/01.NURSE.0000651620.87023.d5.

Moore, Z. E., & Patton, D. (2019). Risk assessment tools for the prevention of pressure ulcers. *Cochrane Database System Reviews*, *1*, CD006471.

O'Connell, S., Bashar, K., Broderick, B. J., et al. (2016). The use of intermittent pneumatic compression in orthopedic and neurosurgical postoperative patients: A systematic review and meta-analysis. *Annals of Surgery*, *263*(5), 888–889. doi:10.1097/SLA.0000000000001530.

Osborne, K. S., Wraa, C. E., Watson, A. S., et al. (2013). In *Nutrition. Medical-surgical nursing, preparation for practice* (2nd ed.). Upper Saddle River, NJ: Pearson.

Parry, S. M., & Puthucheary, Z. A. (2015). The impact of extended bed rest on the musculoskeletal system in the critical care environment. *Extreme Physiology & Medicine*, *4*, 16. doi:10.1186/s13728-015-0036-7.

Pretz, C. R., Kean, J., Heinemann, A. J., Kozlowski, A. J., Bode, R. K., & Gebhardt, E. (2016). A multidimensional Rasch analysis of the functional independence measure based on the National Institute on Disability, Independent Living, and Rehabilitation Research Traumatic Brain Injury Model Systems National Database. *Journal of Neurotrauma*, *33*(14), 1358–1362. https://doi.org/10.1089/neu.2015.4138.

Rivolo, M., Dionisi, S., Olivari, D., et al. (2020). Heel pressure injuries: Consensus-based recommendations for assessment and management. *Advances in Wound Care*, *9*(6), 332–347.

Schünemann, H. J., Cushman, M., Burnett, A. E., et al. (2018). American Society of Hematology 2018 guidelines for management of venous thromboembolism: Prophylaxis for hospitalized and nonhospitalized medical patients. *Blood Advances*, *2*(22), 3198–3225.

Stevens, S. M., Woller, S. C., Baumann Kreuziger, L., et al. (2021). Antithrombotic therapy for VTE disease: Second update of the CHEST guideline and Expert Panel report—Executive summary. [Advance online publication.] *Chest*, *S0012-3692*(21), 01507–1515. https://doi.org/10.1016/j.chest.2021.07.056.

Talec, P., Gaujoux, S., & Samama, C. M. (2016). Early ambulation and prevention of post-operative thrombo-embolic risk. *Journal of Visceral Surgery*, *153*(6S), S11–S14.

Teeple, E., Collins, J. E., Shrestha, S., Dennerlein, J. T., Losina, E., & Katz, J. N. (2017). Outcomes of safe patient handling and mobilization programs: A meta-analysis. *Work*, *58*(2), 173–184.

Tipping, C. J., Harrold, M., Holland, A., Romero, L., Nisbet, T., & Hodgson, C. L. (2017). The effects of active mobilization and rehabilitation in ICU on mortality and function: A systematic review. *Intensive Care Medicine*, *43*(2), 171–183.

Wald, H. L., Ramaswamy, R., Perskin, M. H., et al. (2019). The case for mobility assessment in hospitalized older adults: American Geriatrics Society white paper executive summary. *Journal of American Geriatric Society*, *67*(1), 11–16. https://doi.org/10.1111/jgs.15595.

Whelton, P. K., Carey, R. M., Aronow, W. S., et al. (2017). 2017 ACC/AHA/AAPA/ABC/ACPM/AGS/APhA/ASH/ASPC/NMA/PCNA guideline for the prevention, Detection, evaluation, and management of high blood pressure in adults: A report of the American College of Cardiology/American Heart Association task Force on clinical practice guidelines. *Journal of the American College of Cardiology*, *71*(19), e127–e248.

Wintermann, G. B., Brunkhorst, F. M., Petrowski, K., et al. (2015). Stress disorders following prolonged critical illness survivors of severe sepsis. *Critical Care Medicine*, *43*(6), 1213–1222.

Decreased Diversional Activity Engagement

Domain 1 Health promotion Class 1 Health awareness

Nadia Ali Muhammad Ali Charania, PhD, RN

NANDA-I

Definition

Reduced stimulation, interest, or participation in recreational or leisure activities.

Defining Characteristics

Alteration in mood; boredom; expresses discontentment with situation; flat affect; frequent naps; physical deconditioning

Related Factors

Current setting does not allow engagement in activities; environmental constraints; impaired physical mobility; inadequate available activities; inadequate motivation; insufficient physical endurance; physical discomfort; psychological distress

At-Risk Population

Individuals at extremes of age; individuals experiencing prolonged hospitalization; individuals experiencing prolonged institutionalization

Associated Conditions

Prescribed movement restrictions; therapeutic isolation

NOC (Nursing Outcomes Classification)

Suggested NOC Outcomes

Leisure Participation; Play Participation; Social Involvement

Example NOC Outcome with Indicators

Leisure Participation as evidenced by the following indicators: Expresses satisfaction with leisure activities/Feels relaxed from leisure activities/Enjoys leisure activities. (Rate the outcome and indicators of **Leisure Participation:** 1 = never demonstrated, 2 = rarely demonstrated, 3 = sometimes demonstrated, 4 = often demonstrated, 5 = consistently demonstrated [see Section I].)

Client Outcomes

Client Will (Specify Time Frame)

- Engage in personally satisfying diversional activities

NIC (Nursing Interventions Classification)

Suggested NIC Interventions

Recreation Therapy; Self-Responsibility Facilitation

Example NIC Activities—Recreation Therapy

Assist the client to identify meaningful recreational activities; Provide safe recreational equipment

Nursing Interventions and *Rationales*

- Assess the client's needs through mapping to assess existing networks, current activities, and the impact on well-being. EB: *Mapping allows nurse and client to examine the quality of existing relationships and activities to identify where intervention is needed (Mann et al, 2017).*
- ▲ Encourage the client to share feelings of boredom. EB: *A better understanding of boredom will allow the development and implementation of interventions to address the client's needs (Kenah et al, 2018).*
- Encourage the client to participate in any available social or recreational opportunities in the health care environment. EB: *Client interviews revealed that participation in occupational therapy activity-based groups was associated with the themes of therapeutic relationship, connection with others, and the opportunity to engage (Ngooi et al, 2021).*
- Promote relaxation through guided imagery, visual imagery, and music interventions. EB: *Qualitative interviews on the effects of hospitalized bed rest on well-being found that relaxation interventions improved physical well-being and sleep (Yeager, 2019).*
- Use art making and music listening. EBN: *A randomized trial did not show a significant difference among the control, art making, and diversional music groups in reducing symptoms related to blood and marrow transplantation. It was asserted that art making and music listening are safe and desirable diversional activities for clients undergoing blood and marrow transplant in an outpatient clinic (Lawson et al, 2016).*
- Be creative, for example, use of the activity pillowcases with soft fabric pieces, plastic zipper, and a pouch to hold a picture as a diversional intervention that could be used in inpatient and hospice care settings. EBN: *Considered to be a helpful aid for adult clients who have intellectual and developmental disabilities and need a distraction and sensory input or modulation (Bahle et al, 2016).*
- Engage clients in physical activity or exercise programs as an adjunct treatment modality for a variety of mental illnesses; for example, depression, schizophrenia, anxiety, disorders, posttraumatic stress disorders, and substance abuse. EB: *The narrative synthesis of systematic reviews and clinical trials endorsed the integration of physical activity programs as part of the mental health treatment plan (Rosenbaum et al, 2016).*
- Engage clients in leisure activities such as art and coloring; puzzles, games, and reading; meditation, deep breathing, and relaxation techniques; and music as ways to reduce screen time during hospitalization.

EBN: *Decreasing screen time and engaging in leisure activities could contribute to short-term benefits during hospitalization and long-term health benefits after hospitalization if they continue to be used (Nelson, 2018).*

- • Engage antepartum women and families in diversional fun promoting activities including scrapbooking, game night, book clubs, movie night, and prayer services during hospitalization. EB: *Integration of diversional activities programs to promote socialization and family support can contribute to improving clients' satisfaction and promote nurses' engagement and empowerment (Lankford, 2017).*
- ▲ Hospitalized clients, particularly quarantined clients, are at risk for isolation and boredom and must be engaged in meaningful activities including technology-based (iPad with games or reactional-based applications) and non–technology-based (e.g., books, magazines, crafts, puzzles, games, adult coloring books, mind-stimulating activity books) activities. EB: *Availability of resources to engage clients in meaningful activities contributes to a decrease in clients' complaints of isolation and boredom (Knowles et al, 2020).*
- ▲ Refer to recreational, occupational, or art therapist to assist with activities. EB: *An evaluation of an art therapy program found overwhelming support for art therapy as one element within multiprofessional services available to clients in the acute psychiatry setting. The qualitative feedback associated art therapy with improvements in quality of life, individual support, and a nonverbal intervention for those who find talking therapy difficult (Brady, Moss, & Kelly, 2017).*

Pediatric

- • Assess for the child's interests, preferences, and hobbies. EBN: *A phenomenological study of nurses who care for children with cancer found that understanding the client helps the nurse identify ways to meet the child's needs (Nukpezah et al, 2020).*
- • Engage preschool children in play therapy. EBN: *The result of a prospective randomized controlled study supported the role of play therapy among preschoolers in promoting their social, emotional, and behavioral skills. Moreover, play therapy might be beneficial in reducing fear and anxiety and promoting communication, coping skills, and self-esteem (Sezici, Ocakci, & Kadioglu, 2017).*
- • Engage school-age children in origami during hospitalization. EB: *Origami as a play therapy was reported to be effective in reducing the level of hospitalization-associated anxiety among school-age children (Mathew & Daly, 2018) and assist them in better adapting to unpleasant situations during hospitalization (Varghese et al, 2018).*
- ▲ Refer to a music therapist. EBN: *A review of evidence found a beneficial effect of music medicine, music therapy, and other music-based interventions (Stegemann et al, 2019).*
- • Provide technology access for children to connect with family and friends, play computer games, and engage in virtual reality experiences for children. EBN: *A qualitative study of computer use in hospitalized children found benefits that included distraction from unpleasant treatments, social support, and normalization of experience (Nicholas & Chahauver, 2017).*
- • Provide animal-assisted therapy for hospitalized children. EB: *A study of an animal-assisted therapy program on physiological and psychosocial variables of pediatric oncology clients found a decrease in pain, irritation, and stress and an improvement in depression scores (Silva & Osório, 2018).*
- ▲ Refer to a child life specialist, play therapist, recreational therapist, or occupational therapist. EBN: *Child life therapists provide opportunities for self-expression and play for hospitalized children and may help to normalize the environment. Qualitative study of pediatric nurses found that nurses often do not have enough time to develop any playful activity and stressed the importance of having an adequate number of professionals to address the needs of the child (Ribeiro et al, 2020).*

Geriatric

- • Many of the previously listed interventions may be used with geriatric clients.
- • If the client is able, arrange for participation in group community activities. EB: *Research found that geriatric participation in group activities was important in offering social support as a platform to develop friendships, as well as create a sense of belonging and connectedness (Dare et al, 2018).*
- • Promote activity for older adults through the use of emerging information and communication technologies. EB: *Emerging information and communication technologies can be combined with high-intensity interval exercise regimens to make rehabilitation for impaired older adults more effective and enjoyable (McCaskey et al, 2018).*
- • Engage nursing home residents with dementia in music therapy. EB: *Evidence suggests that music therapy significantly contributes to decreasing depressive symptoms among nursing home residents with dementia and particularly improves the well-being of residents with moderate to severe dementia (Ray & Götell, 2018).*

- Engage hospitalized clients with dementia/delirium in a person-centered activity program including (1) the use of "Pleasant Events Schedule," (2) implementation of "Identity Cards," and (3) engaging in "Occupational Workstations and Programs." EB: *A person-centered activity program has been reported to reduce the behavioral and psychological symptoms of dementia. Moreover, the use of "Identify Cards" promoted client/family connections in the subacute inpatient unit setting (Goonan et al, 2019).*

Home Care

- Many of the previously listed interventions may be administered in the home setting.

D

Client/Family Teaching and Discharge Planning

- Offer group-based educational workshops such as the "Creative Ways to Care" for family and friends to learn strategies to engage their family or friends with dementia in diversional activities. "Creative Ways to Care" is a series of a total of seven workshops: (1) Introduction Session, (2)Dementia Behavior and Activities, (3) Reminiscence, (4) Stimulating and Soothing the Senses, (5) Music, (6) Creative Activities, and (7) Review Session. EB: *The program "Creative Ways to Care" contributes to carers' confidence in responding to changed behavior, decreases the occurrence of changed behaviors, improves the relationship between carers and the person with dementia, and improves carers' quality of life (Allen, 2017).*
- If the client is in isolation, give the client complete information on why isolation is needed and how it should be accomplished, especially guidelines for visitors; provide diversional activities and encourage visitation. EBN: *Most reviewed studies reported negative psychological effects of isolation, including posttraumatic stress symptoms, confusion, and anger. Stressors included longer quarantine duration, infection fears, frustration, boredom, inadequate supplies, inadequate information, financial loss, and stigma (Brooks et al, 2020).*

REFERENCES

Allen, J. (2017). Creative ways to care: Strategies for carers of people living with dementia—An evidence-based education program for family and friends carers to use activities and diversional strategies at home [Poster presentation]. July 18, 2017, Alzheimer's Association International Conference. *Alzheimer's & Dementia, 13*(7S Part 24), P1162-P1162. https://doi.org/10.1016/j.jalz.2017.06.1706.

Bahle, J., Ludwick, R., Govazzi, G., & Faler, C. (2016). Beyond folding washcloths: An innovation for diversional activity. *American Nurse, 48*(6), 10. PMID:29790706.

Brady, C., Moss, H., & Kelly, B. D. (2017). A fuller picture: Evaluating an art therapy programme in a multidisciplinary mental health service. *Medical Humanities, 43*(1), 30–34. http://dx.doi.org/10.1136/medhum-2016-011040.

Brooks, S. K., Webster, R. K., Louise E Smith, L. E., et al. (2020). The psychological impact of quarantine and how to reduce it: Rapid review of the evidence. *Lancet, 395*(10227), 912–920. https://doi.org/10.1016/S0140-6736(20)30460-8.

Dare, J., Wilkinson, C., Marquis, R., & Donovan, R. J. (2018). "The people make it fun, the activities we do just make sure we turn up on time." Factors influencing older adults' participation in community-based group programmes in Perth, Western Australia. *Health and Social Care in the Community, 26*(6), 871–881. https://doi.org/10.1111/hsc.12600.

Goonan, R., Nicks, R., Jolliffe, L., & Pritchard, E. (2019). Implementation of a person-centred activity program on a sub-acute inpatient dementia ward. *Physical & Occupational Therapy in Geriatrics, 37*(1), 171–182.

Kenah, K., Bernhardt, J., Cumming, T., Spratt, N., Luker, J., & Janssen, H. (2018). Boredom in patients with acquired brain injuries during inpatient rehabilitation: A scoping review. *Disability & Rehabilitation, 40*(22), 2713–2722. https://doi.org/10.1080/09638288.2017.1354232.

Knowles, E., O'Donnell, C., Lynch, A., & Snethen, G. (2020). Providing opportunities for meaningful activities for isolated, hospitalized COVID-19 patients at Temple University Hospital. *Case Report, 1*(3), 132–137. doi:10.15367/ch.v1i3.418.

Lankford, D. N. (2017). *Improving antepartum care by implementing schedule of fun activities* [Poster presentation]. Atlanta: Association of Women's Health, Obstetric and Neonatal Nurses Convention, April 3-5, 2017. Retrieved from https://issuu.com/awhonn/docs/con-003-17_final_program-forweb/12.

Lawson, L. M., Glennon, C., Fiscus, V., et al. (2016). Effects of making art and listening to music on symptoms related to blood and marrow transplantation. *Oncology Nursing Forum, 43*(2), E56–E63. https://doi.org/10.1188/16.ONF.E56-E63.

Mann, F., Bone, J. K., Lloyd-Evans, B., et al. (2017). A life less lonely: The state of the art in interventions to reduce loneliness in people with mental health problems. *Social Psychiatry and Psychiatric Epidemiology, 52*(6), 627–638. https://doi.org /10.1007/s00127-017-1392-y.

Mathew, C. S., Daly, C. H., Mookambika, S., et al. (2018). Effectiveness of origami on hospitalized anxiety among children. *International Journal of Advance Research and Development, 3*(8), 169–173.

McCaskey, M. A., Shättin, A., Martin-Niedeken, A. L., & de Bruin, E. D. (2018). Making more of IT: Enabling intensive motor cognitive rehabilitation exercises in geriatrics using information technology solutions. *BioMed Research International, 2018*, 4856146. https://doi.org/10.1155/2018/4856146.

Nelson, L. M. (2018). Turn off the TV: Benefits of offering alternative activities on medical-surgical units. *Medsurg Nursing, 27*(1), 9–13.

Ngooi, B. X., Wong, S. R., Chen, J. D., et al. (2021). Benefits of occupational therapy activity-based groups in a Singapore acute psychiatric ward: Participants' perspectives. *Occupational Therapy in Mental Health, 37*(1), 38–55. https://doi.org/10.1080/0164212X.2021.1874591.

Nicholas, D. B., & Chahauver, A. (2017). Examining computer use by hospitalized children and youth. *Journal of Technology in Human Services, 35*(4), 277–291. https://doi.org/10.1080/15228835.2017.1366886.

Nukpezah, R. N., Khoshnavay, F. F., Hasanpour, M., & Nasrabadi, A. N. (2020). Striving to reduce suffering: A phenomenological study of nurses experience in caring for children with cancer in Ghana. *Nursing Open, 8*(1), 473–481. https://doi.org/10.1002/nop2.650.

Ray, K. D., & Götell, E. (2018). The use of music and music therapy in ameliorating depression symptoms and improving well-being in nursing home residents with dementia. *Frontiers of Medicine*, *5*, 287. doi:10.3389/fmed.2018.00287.

Ribeiro, N., Maria, A., Ribeiro, C., et al. (2020). The nurse's perception of playing and the impact of these practices in pediatric assistance. *Revista de Pesquisa Cuidado e Fundamental*, *12*(1), 1017–1021.

Rosenbaum, S., Tiedemann, A., Stanton, R., et al. (2016). Implementing evidence-based physical activity interventions for people with mental illness: An Australian perspective. *Australasian Psychiatry*, *24*(1), 49–54. https://doi.org/10.1177/1039856215590252.

Sezici, E., Ocakci, A. F., & Kadioglu, K. (2017). Use of play therapy in nursing process: A prospective randomized controlled study. *Journal of Nursing Scholarship*, *49*(2), 162–169. https://doi.org/10.1111/jnu.12277.

Silva, N. B., & Osório, F. L. (2018). Impact of an animal-assisted therapy programme on physiological and psychosocial variables of paediatric oncology patients. *PLoS One*, *13*(4), e0194731. https://doi.org/10.1371/journal.pone.0194731.

Stegemann, T., Geretsegger, M., Phan Quoc, E., Riedl, H., & Smetana, M. (2019). Music therapy and other music-based interventions in pediatric health care: An overview. *Medicines*, *6*(1), 25. https://doi.org/10.3390/medicines6010025.

Varghese, J. S., Ravichandran, Samson, R., & Sujatha, S. (2018). Origami and manifested behaviour in hospitalized children. *International Journal of Advances in Nursing Management*, *6*(2), 115–119. https://doi.org/10.5958/2454-2652.2018.00027.6.

Yeager, J. (2019). Relaxation interventions for antepartum mothers on hospitalized bedrest. *American Journal of Occupational Therapy*, *73*(1), 7301205110. https://doi.org/10.5014/ajot.2019.025692.

E

Ineffective Adolescent Eating Dynamics Domain 2 Nutrition Class 1 Ingestion

Marina Martinez-Kratz, MS, RN, CNE

NANDA-I

Definition

Altered eating attitudes and behaviors resulting in over or under eating patterns that compromise nutritional health.

Defining Characteristics

Avoids participation in regular mealtimes; complains of hunger between meals; depressive symptoms; food refusal; frequent snacking; frequently consumes fast food; frequently eating processed food; frequently eats low quality food; inadequate appetite; overeating; undereating

Related Factors

Altered family relations; anxiety; changes to self-esteem upon entering puberty; eating disorder; eating in isolation; excessive family mealtime control; excessive stress; inadequate dietary habits; irregular mealtime; media influence on eating behaviors of high caloric unhealthy foods; media influence on knowledge of high caloric unhealthy foods; negative parental influences on eating behaviors; psychological neglect; stressful mealtimes; unaddressed abuse

Associated Conditions

Depression; parental psychiatric disorder; physical challenge with eating; physical challenge with feeding; physical health issue of parent; psychological health issue of parent

NOC (Nursing Outcomes Classification)

Suggested NOC Outcomes

Nutritional Status; Nutritional Status: Food and Fluid Intake; Nutrient Intake; Weight Control; Knowledge: Healthy Diet; Knowledge: Weight Management; Eating Disorder Self-Control; Body Image

Example NOC Outcome with Indicators

Knowledge: Healthy Diet as evidenced by the following indicators: Caloric intake appropriate for metabolic needs/Nutrient intake appropriate for individual needs/Guidelines for food portions/Importance of eating breakfast/Strategies to avoid foods with high caloric value. (Rate the outcome and indicators of **Nutritional Status:** 1 = no knowledge, 2 = limited knowledge, 3 = moderate knowledge, 4 = substantial knowledge, 5 = extensive knowledge [see Section I].)

Client Outcomes

Client Will (Specify Time Frame)

- Maintain weight within normal range for height and age
- Eat breakfast daily
- Participate in meal planning and preparation
- Consume healthy and nutritious foods

NIC (Nursing Interventions Classification)

Suggested NIC Interventions

Nutrition Counseling; Nutrition Monitoring; Family Involvement Promotion; Parenting Promotion

Example NIC Activities—Nutritional Counseling

Establish a therapeutic relationship based on trust and respect; Facilitate identification of eating behaviors to be changed; Discuss the meaning of food to client

Nursing Interventions and *Rationales*

- ● Assess for goals and motives related to eating behaviors. EB: *A study found that appearance-focused goals and controlled eating regulation were positively related to disordered eating symptoms (Verstuyf et al, 2016)*
- ▲ Assess the adolescent client for comorbid psychological disorders and make appropriate referrals for treatment. EB: *A long-term evolution study's findings suggested a reciprocal relationship between depressive symptoms and unhealthy eating behaviors (Wu et al, 2016). A cross-sectional study found that binge eating was associated with trait anxiety in Korean adolescent girls (Jung et al, 2017).*
- ● Assess the adolescent for experiences of cyberbullying and the strength of friendship dynamics. EB: *A study found that adolescents who were cyberbullied were almost twice as likely to consider themselves too fat. Stronger friendship dynamics were associated with decreased levels of body dissatisfaction, with friendship dynamics partially mediating the relationship between cyberbullying and body dissatisfaction (Kenny et al, 2018).*
- ● Offer obese or overweight adolescents healthy methods for weight loss. EB: *A study showed statistically significant health behavior improvements after implementing a developmentally informed intervention to increase positive health diet and exercise behaviors (Issner et al, 2017).*
- ● Offer families of obese or overweight adolescents bias-free, individually accepting, and supportive interventions to address weight loss. EBN: *Optimal weight loss practices that encourage healthy eating and exercise must be mindful of the possible negative implications of inducing overweight or obesity perceptions (Lucibello et al, 2020).*
- ● Recommend that families eat together for at least one meal per day. EB: *Research findings show a significant relationship between frequent family meals and better nutritional health in younger and older children (Dallacker, Hertwig, & Mata, 2018).*
- ● Recommend involving the adolescents in planning family meals and food preparation. EB: *Results suggested that involving adolescents in food preparation for the family is related to better adolescent dietary quality and eating patterns (Berge et al, 2016).*
- ● Assist parents at being good role models of healthy eating. EB: *The Healthy Home Offerings via the Mealtime Environment Plus program showed significantly improved parental self-efficacy for identifying appropriate portion sizes (Fulkerson et al, 2014).*
- ● Recommend that the family try new foods, such as either a new food or recipe every week. EB: *The Healthy Home Offerings via the Mealtime Environment Plus program showed decreasing child neophobia scores over time that were developmentally appropriate (Fulkerson et al, 2014).*
- ● Frame healthy eating as consistent with the adolescent values of autonomy from adult control and the pursuit of social justice. EB: *A study with eighth-graders framed healthy eating as a way to take a stand against manipulative practices of the food industry, such as engineering addictive junk food and marketing to young children. These youth would forgo unhealthy foods for healthier options after associating healthy eating with autonomy-assertive and social justice–oriented behavior (Bryan et al, 2016).*

- Explore the adolescent's friendship dynamics. EB: *Findings from a recent study indicated that adolescent friendships play an integral role in the development of unhealthy weight control and are a useful method to identify adolescents at risk (Simone, Long, & Lockhart, 2018).*

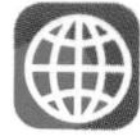

Multicultural

- Assess racial-ethnic minority overweight adolescents for disordered eating behaviors. EB: *A study found that across diverse cultural groups, overweight adolescents are at risk for disordered eating (Rodgers et al, 2017).*
- Encourage racial-ethnic minority families to refrain from weight-based teasing. EB: *A study found that family weight-based teasing was common and was associated with negative well-being among youth from all ethnic groups studied (Eisenberg et al, 2019).*

E

Home Care

- The interventions previously described may be adapted for home care use.

Client/Family Teaching and Discharge Planning

▲ Refer the adolescent and family to family treatment-behavior (FT-B) for treatment of eating disorders. EB: *A review found that FT-B is the only well-established treatment for adolescent eating disorders (Lock, 2015).*

▲ Teach the family that hospitalization of the adolescent may be indicated for medical stabilization of serious physical complications and refer as needed. EB: *A study found that inpatient medical stabilization for adolescent eating disorders addresses acute medical complications and also appears to activate the client and family regarding the need for ongoing treatment (Bravender, Elkus, & Lange, 2017).*

REFERENCES

Berge, J. M., MacLehose, R. F., Larson, N., Laska, M., & Neumark-Sztainer, D. (2016). Family food preparation and its effects on adolescent dietary quality and eating patterns. *Journal of Adolescent Health*, *59*(5), 530–536. https://doi.org/10.1016/j.jadohealth.2016.06.007.

Bravender, T., Elkus, H., & Lange, H. (2017). Inpatient medical stabilization for adolescents with eating disorders: Patient and parent perspectives. *Eating and Weight Disorders*, *22*(3), 483–489. https://doi.org/10.1007/s40519-016-0270-z.

Bryan, C. J., Yeager, D. S., Hinojosa, C. P., et al. (2016). Harnessing adolescent values to motivate healthier eating. *Proceedings of the National Academy of Sciences of the United States of America*, *113*(39), 10830–10835. https://doi.org/10.1073/pnas.1604586113.

Dallacker, M., Hertwig, R., & Mata, J. (2018). The frequency of family meals and nutritional health in children: A meta-analysis. *Obesity Reviews*, *19*(5), 638–653. https://doi.org/10.1111/obr.12659.

Eisenberg, M. E., Puhl, R., Areba, E. M., & Neumark-Sztainer, D. (2019). Family weight teasing, ethnicity and acculturation: Associations with well-being among Latinx, Hmong, and Somali adolescents. *Journal of Psychosomatic Research*, *122*, 88–93. https://doi.org/10.1016/j.jpsychores.2019.04.007.

Fulkerson, J. A., Larson, N., Horning, M., & Neumark-Sztainer, D. (2014). A review of associations between family or shared meal frequency and dietary and weight status outcomes across the lifespan. *Journal of Nutrition Education and Behavior*, *46*(1), 2–19. https://doi.org/10.1016/j.jneb.2013.07.012.

Issner, J. H., Mucka, L. E., & Barnett, D. (2017). Increasing positive health behaviors in adolescents with nutritional goals and exercise. *Journal of Child and Family Studies*, *26*(2), 548–558. https://doi.org/10.1007/s10826-016-0585-4.

Jung, J. Y., Kim, K. H., Woo, H. Y., et al. (2017). Binge eating is associated with trait anxiety in Korean adolescent girls: A cross sectional study. *BMC Women's Health*, *17*(8), 8. https://doi.org/10.1186/s12905-017-0364-4.

Kenny, U., Sullivan, L., Callaghan, M., Molcho, M., & Kelly, C. (2018). The relationship between cyberbullying and friendship dynamics on adolescent body dissatisfaction: A cross-sectional study. *Journal of Health Psychology*, *23*(4), 629–639. https://doi.org/10.1177/1359105316684939.

Lock, J. (2015). An update on evidence-based psychosocial treatments for eating disorders in children and adolescents. *Journal of Clinical Child and Adolescent Psychology*, *44*(5), 707–721. https://doi.org/10.1080/15374416.2014.971458.

Lucibello, K. M., Sabiston, C. M., O'Loughlin, E. K., & O'Loughlin, J. L. (2020). Mediating role of body-related shame and guilt in the relationship between weight perceptions and lifestyle behaviours. *Obesity Science and Practice*, *6*(4), 365–372. https://doi.org/10.1002/osp4.415.

Rodgers, R. F., Watts, A. W., Austin, S. B., Haines, J., & Neumark-Sztainer, D. (2017). Disordered eating in ethnic minority adolescents with overweight. *International Journal of Eating Disorders*, *50*(6), 665–671. https://doi.org/10.1002/eat.22652.

Simone, M., Long, E., & Lockhart, G. (2018). The dynamic relationship between unhealthy weight control and adolescent friendships: A social network approach. *Journal of Youth and Adolescence*, *47*(7), 1373–1384. https://doi.org/10.1007/s10964-017-0796-z.

Verstuyf, J., Vansteenkiste, M., Soetens, B., & Soenens, B. (2016). Motivational dynamics underlying eating regulation in young and adult female dieters: Relationships with healthy eating behaviours and disordered eating symptoms. *Psychology and Health*, *31*(6), 711–729. https://doi.org/10.1080/08870446.2016.1143942.

Wu, W. C., Luh, D. L., Lin, C. I., et al. (2016). Reciprocal relationship between unhealthy eating behaviours and depressive symptoms from childhood to adolescence: 10-year follow-up of the child and adolescent behaviors in long-term evolution study. *Public Health Nutrition*, *19*(9), 1654–1665. https://doi.org/10.1017/S1368980015003675.

Ineffective Child Eating Dynamics Domain 2 Nutrition Class 1 Ingestion

Marina Martinez-Kratz, MS, RN, CNE

E

NANDA-I

Definition

Altered attitudes, behaviors, and influences on child eating patterns resulting in compromised nutritional health.

Defining Characteristics

Avoids participation in regular mealtimes; complains of hunger between meals, food refusal, frequent snacking; frequently consumes fast food; frequently eating processed food; frequently eats low quality food; inadequate appetite; overeating; undereating

Related Factors

Eating Habit

Abnormal eating habit patterns; bribing child to eat; consumption of large volumes of food in a short period of time; eating in isolation; excessive parental control over child's eating experience; excessive parental control over family mealtime; forcing child to eat; inadequate dietary habits; lack of regular mealtimes; limiting child's eating; rewarding child to eat; stressful mealtimes; unpredictable eating patterns; unstructured eating of snacks between meals

Family Process

Abusive interpersonal relations; anxious parent-child relations; disengaged parenting; hostile parent-child relations; insecure parent-child relations; intrusive parenting; tense parent-child relations; uninvolved parenting

Parental

Anorexia; inability to divide eating responsibility between parent and child; inability to divide feeding responsibility between parent and child; inability to support healthy eating patterns; ineffective coping strategies; lack of confidence in child to develop healthy eating habits; lack of confidence in child to grow appropriately; substance misuse

Unmodified Environmental Factors

Media influence on eating behaviors of high caloric unhealthy foods; media influence on knowledge of high caloric unhealthy foods

At-Risk Population

Children born to economically disadvantaged families; children experiencing homelessness; children experiencing life transition; children living in foster care; children whose parents are obese

Associated Conditions

Depression; parental psychiatric disorder; physical challenge with eating; physical challenge with feeding; physical health issue of parent; psychological health issue of parent

NOC (Nursing Outcomes Classification)

Suggested NOC Outcomes

Appetite; Parenting Performance; Knowledge: Healthy Diet; Health Beliefs; Nutritional Status

Example NOC Outcome with Indicators

Appetite as evidenced by the following indicators: Desire to eat/Food intake/Nutrient intake/Fluid intake/Stimulus to eat. (Rate the outcome and indicators of **Appetite:** 1 = severely compromised, 2 = substantially compromised, 3 = moderately compromised, 4 = mildly compromised, 5 = not compromised [see Section I].)

Client Outcomes

Client Will (Specify Time Frame)

- Identify hunger and satiety cues
- Consume healthy and nutritious foods
- Consume adequate calories to support growth and development
- Engage in positive interactions with caregiver during meals

NIC (Nursing Interventions Classification)

Suggested NIC Interventions

Nutrition management; Nutrition Counseling; Nutritional Monitoring

Example NIC Activities—Nutritional Counseling

Establish a therapeutic relationship based on trust and respect; Determine attitudes and beliefs of significant others about food, eating, and the client's needed nutritional change

Nursing Interventions and *Rationales*

- ▲ Use a nutritional screening tool designed for nurses, such as Subjective Global Nutrition Assessment (SGNA), and refer to a dietitian for scores of moderate or severe. EB: *A study found that SGNA can be a reliable tool for assessing nutritional status in children (Minocha et al, 2018).*
- Assess parents for food or eating concerns, aberrant feeding behavior, or inappropriate feeding practices. EB: *Caregiver concerns about food or child eating warrant additional assessment (Kerzner et al, 2015).*
- Assess child for type of eating difficulty. Children can present with limited appetite, food selectivity, and fear of feeding. EB: *Identifying the eating issue will enable appropriate intervention (Kerzner et al, 2015).*
- Assess the caregiver's feeding style by asking three questions: How anxious are you about your child's eating? How would you describe what happens during mealtime? What do you do when your child will not eat? EB: *Kerzner et al (2015) identify three feeding styles that have negative consequences: neglectful, controlling, and indulgent. Responses from neglectful parents will be vague, and controlling parents will describe pressuring/forcing their child to eat. Indulgent parents will describe pleading, begging, and preparing special foods.*
- Assess the child for persistent picky eating with three questions/answers: Is your child a picky eater? (yes). Does she or he have strong likes with regard to food? (yes). Does your child accept new foods readily? (no). EB: *A study found that 3 of 18 feeding behavior questions were significantly associated with persistent picky eaters (Toyama & Agras, 2016). Early identification of picky eating will allow early intervention.*
- Assess child for symptoms of malnutrition, including short stature, thin arms and legs, poor condition of skin and hair, visible vertebrae and rib cage, wasted buttocks, wasted facial appearance, lethargy, and, in extreme cases, edema.
- Assess weight and height of the child and use a growth chart to help determine growth pattern, which reflects nutrition. Age-related growth charts are available from www.cdc.gov/growthcharts/ (Centers for Disease Control and Prevention, 2016).
- Recommend that families turn off the television during meal times. EB: *A study found that the presence of television during meals was negatively associated with the dietary healthfulness and emotional atmosphere of the meal and the child's overall dietary quality. Television was also positively associated with serving fast food for family meals (Trofholz et al, 2017).*
- Recommend that families eat together for at least one meal per day. EB: *A family meals intervention led to improvements in children's weight status, food preparation skills, and TV viewing during meals (Gunther et al, 2019).*
- Encourage parent–child interactions that promote attachment. EB: *A study found that insecure attachment was significantly associated with higher body mass index (Maras et al, 2016).*
- Recommend that the child eats breakfast daily. EB: *A systemic review of children and adolescents found that breakfast eaters had higher energy intake, higher fiber intake, and higher consumption of fruits and vegetables and lower consumption of soft drinks than breakfast skippers (Giménez-Legare et al, 2020).*
- Recommend involving the family in planning meals and food preparation. Children can learn about nutrition as they help plan and make meals. EB: *The Healthy Home Offerings via the Mealtime Environment Plus program showed increased cooking skills among the children participating (Fulkerson et al, 2018).*

- Assist parents at being good role models of healthy eating. EB: *The Healthy Home Offerings via the Mealtime Environment Plus program showed significantly improved parental self-efficacy for identifying appropriate portion sizes (Fulkerson et al, 2018).*
- Recommend that the family try new foods, either a new food or recipe every week. EB: *The Healthy Home Offerings via the Mealtime Environment Plus program showed decreasing child neophobia scores over time that were developmentally appropriate (Fulkerson et al, 2018).*
- ▲ Refer children with highly selective food behaviors and sensory food aversion to a nutritional specialist. EB: *Refusal to eat entire categories of foods related to their taste, texture, smell, temperature, and/or appearance can interrupt normal development and have negative health consequences (Kerzner et al, 2015).*
- ▲ Refer children with feeding difficulties caused by a medical condition to the appropriate specialist. EB: *Organic conditions may contribute to feeding difficulties and express as food aversions, fear of feeding, and selective eating (Kerzner et al, 2015).*

E

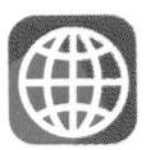

Multicultural

- Assess for the meanings, attitudes, and behaviors related to feeding practices in culturally diverse families. EB: *A qualitative study of Hispanic mothers found that feeding attitudes were central to the maternal responsibility of having well-fed children, and feeding practices included the use of coercive/negative reinforcement strategies (Martinez et al, 2015).*
- Assess the feeding styles of Hispanic and African American mothers for congruence with current child feeding recommendations. EB: *A study showed that Hispanic and African American mothers seldom spoke to their children about food characteristics, rarely referred to feelings of hunger and fullness, encouraged more eating, and made more attempts to enforce table manners than to teach eating skills (Power et al, 2015).*

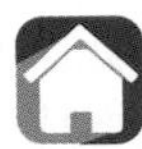

Home Care

- The interventions previously described may be adapted for home care use.

Client/Family Teaching and Discharge Planning

- Provide parents with the following guidelines: avoid distractions during mealtimes (e.g., television, cell phones), maintain a pleasant neutral attitude throughout meal, feed to encourage appetite, limit meal duration (20–30 minutes), limit to 4 to 6 meals/snacks a day with only water in between, serve age-appropriate foods, systematically introduce new foods (up to 8–15 times), encourage self-feeding, and tolerate age-appropriate mess. EB: *Guidelines will prevent and/or resolve feeding difficulties, whether mild or severe (Kerzner et al, 2015).*
- Teach families to provide a feeding environment that sets boundaries around food, through meal timing and the types of foods offered. EB: *Evidence suggests that children's eating self-regulation is best supported when caregivers provide a structured feeding environment (Wood et al, 2020).*
- Teach parents to recognize the difference between hunger and satiety in their children. EB: *Parents may misperceive the child's appetite despite normal growth and need encouragement to accept the child's interpretation of their hunger and satiety (Kerzner et al, 2015).*
- Teach parents of children with limited appetites to establish a feeding schedule with a maximum of five meals per day and nothing but water in between. Parents must be taught to model healthy eating, adhere to the established feeding schedule, and set limits/consequences for mealtime behavior. EB: *A feeding schedule will provide adequate nutrition and assist the child with recognizing and responding appropriately to hunger and satiety (Kerzner et al, 2015).*
- Teach parents of children with food selectivity to refrain from coercive and indulgent feeding practices. EB: *Coercive and indulgent feeding practices may create family discord and subsequent child behavioral problems (Kerzner et al, 2015).*
- Teach parents to use nondirective feeding strategies such as repeatedly offering foods, offering a familiar and accepted food (e.g., ketchup) alongside novel or refused foods, and having family and/or peers model eating the food with enjoyment. EB: *Nondirective feeding strategies have been demonstrated to increase the consumption of a given food and maintain responsivity in the feeding environment (Wood et al, 2020).*
- Teach parents to avoid restrictive feeding practices such as limiting intakes of certain foods. EB: *Restrictive feeding practices have been associated with eating when not hungry (Bauer et al, 2017).*
- Teach parents the concept of being a responsive feeder, in which the parent determines where, when, and what the child is fed and the child determines how much to eat. Responsive feeders guide the child's eating, set limits, model appropriate eating, talk positively about food, and respond appropriately to the

child's feeding cues. EB: *Research has reported that a responsive feeding style has resulted in children developing a lower risk of being overweight through consumption of more fruits, vegetables, and dairy products and less unhealthy foods (Kerzner et al, 2015).*

REFERENCES

Bauer, K. W., Haines, J., Miller, A. L., et al. (2017). Maternal restrictive feeding and eating in the absence of hunger among toddlers: A cohort study. *International Journal of Behavioral Nutrition and Physical Activity*, *14*(1), 172. https://doi.org/10.1186/s12966-017-0630-8.

Centers for Disease Control and Prevention (CDC). (2016). *National Center for Health Statistics [website]*. Resources for the General Public. Atlanta: CDC. Retrieved from ht tps://www.cdc.gov/nchs/nchs_for_you/general_public.htm. [Accessed 28 June 2021].

Fulkerson, J. A., Friend, S., Horning, M., et al. (2018). Family home food environment and nutrition-related parent and child personal and behavioral outcomes of the Healthy Home Offerings via the Mealtime Environment (HOME) Plus program: A randomized controlled trial. *Journal of the Academy of Nutrition and Dietetics*, *118*(2), 240–251. https://doi.org/10.1016/j.jand.2017.04.006.

Giménez-Legarre, N., Flores-Barrantes, P., Miguel-Berges, M. L., Moreno, L. A., & Santaliestra-Pasías, A. M. (2020). Breakfast characteristics and their association with energy, macronutrients, and food intake in children and adolescents: A systematic review and meta-analysis. *Nutrients*, *12*(8), 2460. https://doi.org/10.3390/nu12082460.

Gunther, C., Rogers, C., Holloman, C., et al. (2019). Child diet and health outcomes of the simple suppers program: A 10-week, 2-group quasi-experimental family meals trial. *BMC Public Health*, *19*(1), 1657. https://doi.org/10.1186/s12889-019-7930-7.

Kerzner, B., Milano, K., Maclean, W. C., Jr., Berall, G., Stuart, S., & Chatoor, I. (2015). A practical approach to classifying and managing feeding difficulties. *Pediatrics*, *135*(2), 344–353. https://doi.org/10.1542/peds.2014-1630.

Maras, D., Obeid, N., Flament, M., et al. (2016). Attachment style and obesity: Disordered eating behaviors as a mediator in a community sample of Canadian youth. *Journal of Developmental and Behavioral Pediatrics*, *37*(9), 762–770. https://doi.org/10.1097/DBP.0000000000000361.

Martinez, S. M., Rhee, K., Blanco, E., & Boutelle, K. (2015). Maternal attitudes and behaviors regarding feeding practices in elementary school-aged Latino children: A pilot qualitative study on the impact of the cultural role of mothers in the US-Mexican border region of San Diego, California. *Journal of the Academy of Nutrition and Dietetics*, *115*(Suppl. 5), S34–S41. https://doi.org/10.1016/j.jand.2015.02.028.

Minocha, P., Sitaraman, S., Choudhary, A., & Yadav, R. (2018). Subjective Global nutritional assessment: A reliable screening tool for nutritional assessment in cerebral palsy children. *Indian Journal of Pediatrics*, *85*(1), 15–19. https://doi.org/10.1007/s12098-017-2501-3.

Power, T. G., Hughes, S. O., Goodell, L. S., et al. (2015). Feeding practices of low-income mothers: How do they compare to current recommendations? *International Journal of Behavioral Nutrition and Physical Activity*, *12*, 34. https://doi.org/10.1186/s12966-015-0179-3.

Toyama, H., & Agras, W. S. (2016). A test to identify persistent picky eaters. *Eating Behaviors*, *23*, 66–69. https://doi.org/10.1016/j.eatbeh.2016.07.003.

Trofholz, A. C., Tate, A. D., Miner, M. H., & Berge, J. M. (2017). Associations between TV viewing at family meals and the emotional atmosphere of the meal, meal healthfulness, child dietary intake, and child weight status. *Appetite*, *108*, 361–366. https://doi.org/10.1016/j.appet.2016.10.018.

Wood, A. C., Blisset, J. M., Brunstrom, J. M., et al. (2020). Caregiver influences on eating behaviors in young children: A scientific statement from the American Heart association. *Journal of the American Heart Association*, *9*(10), e014520. https://doi.org/10.1161/JAHA.119.014520.

Risk for Electrolyte Imbalance Domain 2 Nutrition Class 5 Hydration

Dina M. Hewett, PhD, RN, NEA-BC

NANDA-I

Definition

Susceptible to changes in serum electrolyte levels, which may compromise health.

Risk Factors

Diarrhea; excessive fluid volume; inadequate knowledge of modifiable factors; insufficient fluid volume; vomiting

Associated Conditions

Compromised regulatory mechanism; endocrine regulatory dysfunction; renal dysfunction; treatment regimen

NOC (Nursing Outcomes Classification)

Suggested NOC Outcomes

Electrolyte and Acid-Base Balance; Fluid Balance; Hydration; Nutritional Status: Biochemical Measures; Nutritional Status: Food and Fluid Intake; Nutritional Status: Nutrient Intake; Kidney Function

Example NOC Outcome with Indicators

Electrolyte and Acid-Base Balance as evidenced by the following indicators: Apical heart rate/Apical heart rhythm/Serum potassium/Serum sodium/Serum calcium, serum magnesium, serum phosphorus. (Rate the outcome and indicators of **Electrolyte and Acid-Base Balance:** 1 = severe deviation from normal range, 2 = substantial deviation from normal range, 3 = moderate deviation from normal range, 4 = mild deviation from normal range, 5 = no deviation from normal range [see Section I].)

Client Outcomes

Client Will (Specify Time Frame)

- Maintain a normal sinus heart rhythm with a regular rate
- Have a decrease in edema
- Maintain an absence of muscle cramping
- Maintain normal serum potassium, sodium, calcium, magnesium and phosphorus
- Maintain normal serum pH

NIC (Nursing Interventions Classification)

Suggested NIC Interventions

Electrolyte Monitoring; Electrolyte Management: Hypokalemia, Hyperkalemia, Hypocalcemia, Hypercalcemia, Hyponatremia, Hypernatremia, Hypomagnesemia, Hypermagnesemia, Hypophosphatemia, and Hyperphosphatemia; Electrolyte Management: Hyponatremia; Fluid/Electrolyte Management; Laboratory Data Interpretation

Example NIC Activities—Electrolyte Monitoring

Identify possible causes of electrolyte imbalances; Monitor the serum level of electrolytes

Nursing Interventions and *Rationales*

- ▲ Monitor vital signs at least three times a day, or more frequently as needed. Notify health care provider of significant deviation from baseline. EB: *Electrolyte imbalance can lead to clinical manifestations such as respiratory failure, arrhythmias, edema, muscle weakness, and altered mental status (Shrimanker & Bhattarai, 2020)*
- ▲ Monitor cardiac rate and rhythm. Report changes to provider. Hypokalemia and hyperkalemia can result in electrocardiogram (ECG) changes that can lead to cardiac arrest and ventricular dysrhythmias. EB: *Hypophosphatemia can cause ventricular arrhythmias, derangements of cardiac and respiratory function, and death. It can also cause cardiomyopathy (Ariyoshi et al, 2016; Christopoulou et al, 2017). Magnesium and calcium imbalances also can cause cardiac arrhythmias. Low serum magnesium (≤2 mEq/L) is associated with hypokalemia and ECG changes, and high phosphate may indicate kidney injury (Shrimanker & Bhattarai, 2020). Low magnesium also may impair respiratory function. It has been associated with higher mortality, the need for mechanical ventilation, and increased length of stay (Upala et al, 2016). Low magnesium also is common in clients with heart failure (Shrimanker & Bhattarai, 2020).*
- ● Monitor intake and output and daily weights using a consistent scale. EB: *Weight gain is a sensitive and consistent sign of fluid volume excess (Shrimanker & Bhattarai, 2020).*
- ● Monitor for abdominal distention and discomfort. A focused assessment should be done on any client presenting with hepatic, gastrointestinal, or pancreatic dysfunction (Shrimanker & Bhattarai, 2020). EB: *Abdominal distention and intraabdominal swelling can lead to compression of the abdominal contents and acute kidney injury, especially in the postoperative period (Raghavendra Prasad et al, 2017).*
- ● Monitor the client's respiratory status and muscle strength. Phosphorus is an essential element in cell structure, metabolism, and maintenance of acid-base processes. EB: *Consequences of hypophosphatemia include cardiac failure, respiratory failure, and alterations in sensorium (Diringer, 2017).*
- ● Assess cardiac status and neurological alterations. EB: *Hypophosphatemia can cause myocardial dysfunction, hematological dysfunction, respiratory depression, and neurological changes (Diringer, 2017).*
- ● Imbalances of sodium, potassium, calcium, and magnesium all can cause neurological disturbances (Kear, 2017). EB: *Hyperphosphatemia is associated with hypocalcemia (because it is inversely related to calcium), causing tetany, muscle spasms, and cardiac arrhythmias, as well as vascular mineralization (Marcuccilini, Chonchol, & Jovanovich, 2017).*

- ▲ Review laboratory data as ordered and report deviations to provider. Laboratory studies may include serum electrolytes potassium, chloride, sodium, bicarbonate, magnesium, phosphate, and calcium; serum pH; comprehensive metabolic panel; and arterial blood gases.
- • Review the client's medical and surgical history for possible causes of altered electrolytes. EB: *Periods of excess fluid loss can lead to dehydration and resulting loss of electrolytes; fluid can be lost through gastrointestinal illness, renal failure, hyperthermia, blood loss, and perspiration caused by strenuous exercise (Hew-Butler et al, 2017; Kear, 2017). Additional causes of electrolyte imbalances include excessive use of antacids, burns, trauma, sepsis, diabetic ketoacidosis, extensive surgeries, and changes in acid-base balance (Shrimanker & Bhattarai, 2020).*
- ▲ Complete pain assessment. Assess and document the onset, intensity, character, location, duration, aggravating factors, and relieving factors. Notify the provider of any increase in pain or discomfort or if comfort measures are not effective. EB: *Symptoms of electrolyte imbalance and dehydration can include muscle cramps, paresthesias, abdominal cramps, skin manifestations, cardiac arrhythmias, and tetany (Shrimanker & Bhattarai, 2020).*
- ▲ Monitor the effects of ordered medications such as diuretics and heart medications. EB: *Medications can have adverse effects on kidney function and electrolyte balance, particularly contrast agents, chemotherapeutic agents, amphotericin B, aminoglycosides, phosphate ingestion, loop diuretics, and vitamin D (Kear, 2017; Alfarouk et al, 2020).*
- ▲ Administer parenteral fluids as ordered and monitor their effects. EB: *Rapid resuscitation with fluids can cause adverse effects such as electrolyte imbalance, increased bleeding, and coagulopathies (Shrimanker & Bhattarai, 2020). Administration of fluids should be done to improve the plasma electrolytes and pH and hemodynamic improvement (Bedreag et al, 2016).*

Geriatric

- • Monitor electrolyte levels carefully, including sodium levels and potassium levels, with both increased and decreased levels possible. EB: *Older adults are prone to electrolyte abnormalities because of failure of regulatory mechanisms associated with heart and kidney disease, a decrease in the ability to reabsorb sodium, and a loss of diluting capacity in the kidneys (Kear, 2017). Dehydration in the elderly is attributable to inadequate water intake caused by dysfunction of the central nervous system controlling thirst. Data also suggest that sodium appetite is reduced in aged rats and therefore also in the elderly (Begg, 2017). Many older clients receive selective serotonin reuptake inhibitors for treatment of depression, which can result in hyponatremia (Varela-Piñón & Adán-Manes, 2017).*

Client/Family Teaching and Discharge Planning

- • Teach client/family the signs of low potassium and the risk factors. EB: *Signs and symptoms of low potassium include muscle weakness, nausea, vomiting, constipation, and irregular pulse (Shrimanker & Bhattarai, 2020).*
- • Teach client/family the signs of high potassium and the risk factors. EB: *Signs and symptoms of high potassium include restlessness, muscle weakness, slow heart rate, diarrhea, and cramping (Shrimanker & Bhattarai, 2020).*
- • Teach client/family the signs of low sodium and the risk factors. EB: *Early signs of low sodium include nausea, muscle cramps, disorientation, and mental status changes (Shrimanker & Bhattarai, 2020).*
- • Teach client/family the signs of high sodium and the risk factors. EB: *Signs of high sodium include thirst, dry mucous membranes, rapid heartbeat, low blood pressure, and mental status changes; symptoms can progress to confusion, delirium, and seizures (Shrimanker & Bhattarai, 2020).*
- • Teach client/family the importance of hydration during exercise. Dehydration occurs when the amount of water leaving the body is greater than the amount consumed. EB: *The body can lose large amounts of fluid when it tries to cool itself by sweating (Begg, 2017).*
- • Teach client/family the warning signs of dehydration. Early signs of dehydration include thirst and decreased urine output. As dehydration increases, symptoms may include dry mouth, muscle cramps, nausea and vomiting, lightheadedness, and orthostatic hypotension. EB: *Severe dehydration can cause confusion, weakness, coma, and organ failure (Shrimanker & Bhattarai, 2020).*
- • Teach client about any medications prescribed. Medication teaching includes the drug name, its purpose, administration instructions such as taking it with or without food, and any side effects. EB: *Studies have shown that insufficient and ineffective client education, leading to poor treatment adherence, and suboptimal*

use of guideline-recommended drug regimens have been identified as contributing factors to client nonadherence to antiplatelet therapy and high hospital acute coronary syndrome (ACS) readmission rates (Larkin et al, 2017). Clients on a diuretic should understand side effects such as those for low potassium. Diuretic use remains a primary cause of low serum potassium levels (Kear, 2017). Clients on warfarin should also be educated on dietary interactions to improve medication efficacy (Jenner et al, 2015).

▲ Instruct the client to report any adverse medication side effects to his or her health care provider. Assessing and instructing clients about medications and focusing on important details can help prevent client medication errors. EB: *Pharmacist involvement with client education can improve medication efficacy and decrease hospital readmissions (Phatak et al, 2016).*

E

REFERENCES

Alfarouk, K. O., Ahmed, S. B. M., Ahmed, A., et al. (2020). The interplay of dysregulated pH and electrolyte imbalance in cancer. *Cancers, 12*(4), 898. https://doi.org/10.3390/cancers12040898.

Ariyoshi, N., Nogi, M., Ando, A., Watanabe, H., & Umekawa, S. (2016). Hypophosphatemia-induced cardiomyopathy. *The American Journal of the Medical Sciences, 352*(3), 317–323.

Bedreag, O. H., Papurica, M., Rogobete, A. F., et al. (2016). New perspectives of volemic resuscitation in polytrauma patients: A review. *Burns & Trauma, 4*, 5. https://doi.org/10.1186/s41038-016-0029-9.

Begg, D. P. (2017). Disturbances of thirst and fluid balance associated with aging. *Physiology & Behavior, 178*, 28–34. https://doi.org/10.1016/j.physbeh.2017.03.003.

Christopoulou, E. C., Fillapatos, T. D., Megapanou, E., Elisaf, M. S., & Liamis, G. (2017). Phosphate imbalance in patients with heart failure. *Heart Failure Reviews, 22*(3), 349–356.

Diringer, M. (2017). Neurologic manifestations of major electrolyte abnormalities. *Handbook of Clinical Neurology, 141*, 705–713.

Hew-Butler, T., Loi, V., Pani, A., & Rosner, M. H. (2017). Exercise-associated hyponatremia: 2017 update. *Frontiers of Medicine, 4*, 21.

Jenner, K. M., Simmons, B. J., Delate, T., Clark, N. P., Kurz, D., & Witt, D. M. (2015). An education program for patient self-management of warfarin. *The Permanente Journal, 19*(4), 33–38.

Kear, T. M. (2017). Fluid and electrolyte management across the age continuum. *Nephrology Nursing Journal, 44*(6), 491–496.

Larkin, A., LaCouture, M., Geissel, K., et al. (2017). Quality improvement in management of acute coronary syndrome: Continuing medical education and peer coaching improve antiplatelet medication adherence and reduce hospital readmissions. *Critical Pathways in Cardiology, 16*(3), 96–101.

Marcuccilini, M., Chonchol, M., & Jovanovich, A. (2017). Phosphate binders and targets over decades: Do we have it right now? *Seminars in Dialysis, 30*(2), 134–141.

Phatak, A., Prusi, R., Ward, B., et al. (2016). Impact of pharmacist involvement in the transitional care of high-risk patients through medication reconciliation, medication education, and post-discharge call-backs (IPITCH Study). *Journal of Hospital Medicine, 11*(1), 39–44.

Raghavendra Prasad, G., Subba Rao, J. V., Aziz, A., & Rashmi, T. M. (2017). The role of routine measurement of intra-abdominal pressure in preventing abdominal compartment syndrome. *Journal of Indian Association of Pediatric Surgeons, 22*(3), 134–138.

Shrimanker, I., & Bhattarai, S. (2020). *Electrolytes*. StatPearls [Internet]. Treasure Island, FL: StatPearls Publishing.

Upala, S., Jaruvongvanic, V., Wijarnpreecha, K., & Sanguankeo, A. (2016). Hypomagnesemia and mortality in patients admitted to intensive care unit: A systematic review and meta-analysis. *QJM: Monthly Journal of the Association of Physicians, 109*(7), 453–459.

Varela Piñón, M., & Adán-Manes, J. (2017). Selective serotonin reuptake inhibitor-induced hyponatremia: Clinical implications and therapeutic alternatives. *Clinical Neuropharmacology, 40*(4), 177–179.

Labile Emotional Control Domain 5 Perception/cognition Class 4 Cognition

Marina Martinez-Kratz, MS, RN, CNE

NANDA-I

Definition

Uncontrollable outbursts of exaggerated and involuntary emotional expression.

Defining Characteristics

Absence of eye contact; crying; excessive crying without feeling sadness; excessive laughing without feeling happiness; expresses embarrassment regarding emotional expression; expression of emotion incongruent with triggering factor; impaired nonverbal communication; involuntary crying; involuntary laughing; social alienation; uncontrollable crying; uncontrollable laughing; withdrawal from occupational situation

Related Factors

Altered self-esteem; excessive emotional disturbance; fatigue; inadequate knowledge about symptom control; inadequate knowledge of disease; insufficient muscle strength; social distress; stressors; substance misuse

Associated Conditions

Brain injuries; functional impairment; mental disorders; mood disorders; musculoskeletal impairment; pharmaceutical preparations; physical disability

E

NOC (Nursing Outcomes Classification)

Suggested NOC Outcomes

Coping; Knowledge: Disease Process; Impulse; Self-Control; Self-Esteem; Quality of Life; Personal Well-Being; Stress Level

Example NOC Outcome with Indicators

Knowledge: Disease Process as evidenced by the following indicator: Specific disease process. (Rate the outcome and indicators of **Knowledge: Disease Process:** 1 = no knowledge, 2 = limited knowledge, 3 = moderate knowledge, 4 = substantial knowledge, 5 = extensive knowledge [see Section I].)

Client Outcomes

Client Will (Specify Time Frame)

- Improve coping strategies
- Improve knowledge about disease process, signs and symptoms, triggers, symptom control
- Use mechanisms to control impulses and ask for help when feeling impulses
- Improve feelings of dignity
- Enhance and improve response to social and environmental stimuli

NIC (Nursing Interventions Classification)

Suggested NIC Interventions

Coping Enhancement; Teaching: Disease Process; Enhance Self-Esteem; Improved Quality of Life; Improved Well-Being

Example NIC Activities—Labile Emotional Control

Coping Enhancement: Assist the patient to solve problems in a constructive manner; Instruct the patient on the use of relaxation techniques, as needed; Assist the patient to identify positive strategies to deal with limitations and manage needed lifestyle or role changes

Nursing Interventions and *Rationales*

- Identify clients at risk of having labile emotional control. EB: *Clients with traumatic brain injury (TBI), Parkinson's disease (PD), multiple sclerosis (MS), amyotrophic lateral sclerosis (ALS), stroke, and schizophrenia (including schizoaffective and schizophreniform disorders) were most closely associated with pseudobulbar affect (PBA) diagnosis, which is associated with emotional lability (Allen et al, 2018).*
- Assess clients with an appropriate screening tool such as the Pathological Laughter and Crying Scale (PLACS), Center for Neurologic Study-Lability Scale (CNS-LS), or the Emotional Lability Questionnaire (ELQ). EB: *A review found that these tools have been used with success in both academic research and clinical trials (Finegan et al, 2019).*
- Offer client the choice of email and/or videoconferencing for delivery of therapy. EBN: *A cross-sectional study found that virtually delivered therapy can be a beneficial alternative to face-to-face meetings for people with PBA (Bentley, O'Connor, & Breen, 2017).*
- Assess clients for use of experiential avoidance, which is the process of negatively evaluating, escaping, or avoiding unwanted thoughts, emotions, or sensations. EB: *A recent study found experiential avoidance was*

associated with both higher levels of negative affect (P < .001) and increased emotional lability (P = .021) (Gerhart et al, 2018).

- Offer the client choices when possible in emotional situations. EB: *A study found that choice appears to be a powerful tool that permits regulation of negative emotions in an adaptive fashion (Thuillard & Dan-Glauser, 2017).*
- Encourage clients to verbalize their emotional reactions and lability. EB: *Encouraging clients to talk about their emotional reactions could help normalize their experiences and may prevent the development of responses that could delay or negatively affect their recovery (Gillespie et al, 2020).*
- Encourage clients to talk about their emotional reactions and acknowledge that the unpredictable and uncontrollable nature of emotional lability can be embarrassing and cause distress. EB: *A qualitative study found that embarrassment and social withdrawal were commonly reported and had a detrimental effect on participant's mood and quality of life (McAleese et al, 2021).*
- Encourage the client to use distraction, humor, optimism, and social support as a way to manage the episodes. EB: *A qualitative study found that positive experiences were shaped by a better understanding of the condition, an increased sense of control, social support, and optimism (McAleese et al, 2021).*
- Consider using motive-oriented therapeutic relationship (MOTR). EB: *A randomized controlled study using MOTR found that early expressions of distress were shown to significantly decrease with adaptive emotions emerging in clients diagnosed with borderline personality disorder (Berthoud et al, 2017).*
- Provide progressive muscle relaxation (PMR) exercise and guided imagery (GI) techniques. EB: *A nursing study found that PMR and GI were effective in reducing anxiety and improving mood states in parents of children with malignancy (Tsitsi et al, 2017).*
- Consider using cognitive-behavioral therapy (CBT). EB: *A current study of youth with anxiety disorders found that CBT resulted in decreased sadness and anger dysregulation and increases in adaptive coping with anger (Suveg et al, 2018).*

Pediatric

- Assess adolescents with high emotional dysregulation for substance use disorders. EB: *Study results indicated that adolescents scoring high on emotional dysregulation are at risk for substance dependence because of more externalizing and internalizing symptomatology (Wills et al, 2016).*
- Teach parents that their reactions to their children's emotions play a critical role in teaching children effective emotion regulation. EB: *A recent study suggested that supportive parent emotion socialization practices are associated with parent-rated emotion regulation skills (Breaux et al, 2018).*
- Provide parents with emotion coaching strategies to manage their children's emotional outbursts. Emotion coaching includes fostering parental awareness and acceptance of their children's emotions with behaviors that acknowledge their children's emotions and teaches understanding, coping with, and appropriately expressing emotion. EB: *Study results suggested that when children with oppositional defiant disorder (ODD) experience more frequent, intense, and unstable emotions, families are better able to benefit from treatment and reduce children's behavior problems when mothers begin treatment or are already engaging in emotion coaching (Dunsmore et al, 2016).*
- ▲ Refer adolescent clients to a dialectical behavior therapy (DBT) group. EB: *Research shows that DBT is an effective means of assisting adolescents in learning to enhance their emotion-regulation skills (Gill et al, 2018).*

Geriatric

- Many of the previous interventions may be adapted for geriatric use.
- Evaluate geriatric clients suspected of PBA with the following three-step model: (1) crying inconsistent with environment/stimuli; (2) diagnosis of any of the following neurological disorders: TBI, PD, MS, ALS; or (3) at least two of the following disorders: stroke, schizophrenia (including schizoaffective and schizophreniform disorders), or documentation of spinal cord injury (SCI) as most closely associated with the PBA diagnosis. EB: *Based on analysis, this three-item checklist to facilitate PBA risk assessment in the nursing home setting was developed (Allen et al, 2018).*

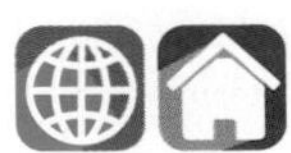

Multicultural and Home Care

- The previous interventions may be adapted for multicultural and home care.

E

Client/Family Teaching and Discharge Planning

- Instruct client and family to monitor for cutaneous adverse effects of the neurological medications used to treat PBA and report occurrence to their health care provider. EB: *A review of the literature found that cutaneous reactions were associated with medications approved by the US Food and Drug Administration (FDA) to treat PBA (Bahrani et al, 2016).*
- Inform client and family about the emotional lability and talk with them about how to cope with the situation. EBN: *Clients and families need more information about this syndrome so they can recognize the signs and symptoms, get a diagnosis, and obtain treatment (Schneider & Schneider, 2017).*
- For clients with neurological disorders, provide teaching that emotionalism is a neurological condition and not a clinical mood disorder to promote better understanding for clients, their families, and significant others. EB: *For poststroke clients, positive experiences were shaped by a better understanding of the condition (McAleese et al, 2021).*
- Use verbal and nonverbal therapeutic communication approaches including empathy, active listening, and confrontation to encourage the client and family to express emotions such as sadness, guilt, and anger (within appropriate limits); verbalize fears and concerns; and set goals. *Solution-focused communication with clients helps focus on goals and helps find solutions.*
- Offer instruction to the client and family to wait for emotional episodes to pass. EB: *A qualitative study found that positive experiences were shaped by an increased sense of control (McAleese et al, 2021).*

REFERENCES

Allen, C., Zarowitz, B., O'Shea, T., Peterson, E., Yonan, C., & Waterman, F. (2018). Identification of pseudobulbar affect symptoms in the nursing home setting: Development and assessment of a screening tool. *Geriatric Nursing, 39*(1), 54–59. https://doi.org/10.1016/j.gerinurse.2017.06.002.

Bahrani, E., Nunneley, C. E., Hsu, S., & Kass, J. S. (2016). Cutaneous adverse effects of neurologic medications. *CNS Drugs, 30*(3), 245–267. https://doi.org/10.1007/s40263-016-0318-7.

Bentley, B., O'Connor, M., & Breen, L. (2017). *Counselling people with amyotrophic lateral sclerosis. Presented at 5th Annual Worldwide nursing Conference (WNC2017), July 24th–25*th, 2017. Singapore: Annual Worldwide Nursing Conference, 279–285. https://doi.org/10.5176/2315-4330_WNC17.131.

Berthoud, L., Pascual-Leone, A., Caspar, F., et al. (2017). Leaving distress behind: A randomized controlled study on change in emotional processing in borderline personality disorder. *Psychiatry, 80*(2), 139–154. https://doi.org/10.1080/00332747.2016.1220230.

Breaux, R. P., McQuade, J. D., Harvey, E. A., & Zakarian, R. J. (2018). Longitudinal associations of parental emotion socialization and children's emotion regulation: The moderating role of ADHD symptomatology. *Journal of Abnormal Child Psychology, 46*(4), 671–683. https://doi.org/10.1007/s10802-017-0327-0.

Dunsmore, J. C., Booker, J. A., Ollendick, T. H., & Greene, R. W. (2016). Emotion socialization in the context of risk and psychopathology: Maternal emotion coaching predicts better treatment outcomes for emotionally labile children with oppositional defiant disorder: Emotion coaching and treatment outcomes for ODD. *Social Development, 25*(1), 8–26. https://doi.org/10.1111/sode.12109.

Finegan, E., Chipika, R. H., Shing, S. L. H., Hardiman, O., & Bede, P. (2019). Pathological crying and laughing in motor neuron disease: Pathobiology, screening, intervention. *Frontiers in Neurology, 10*, 260. https://doi.org/10.3389/fneur.2019.00260.

Gerhart, J., Vaclavik, E., Lillis, T. A., Miner, J., McFadden, R., & O'Mahony, S. (2018). A daily diary study of posttraumatic stress, experiential avoidance, and emotional lability among inpatient nurses. *Psycho-Oncology, 27*(3), 1068–1071. https://doi.org/10.1002/pon.4531.

Gill, D., Warburton, W., Simes, D., & Sweller, N. (2018). Group therapy for emotional dysregulation: Treatment for adolescents and their parents. *Child and Adolescent Social Work Journal, 35*(2), 169–180. https://doi.org/10.1007/s10560-017-0510-8.

Gillespie, D. C., Cadden, A. P., West, R. M., & Broomfield, N. M. (2020). Non-pharmacological interventions for post-stroke emotionalism (PSE) within inpatient stroke settings: A theory of planned behavior survey. *Topics in Stroke Rehabilitation, 27*(1), 15–24. https://doi.org/1080/10749357.2019.1654241.

McAleese, N., Guzman, A., O'Rourke, S. J., & Gillespie, D. C. (2021). Post-stroke emotionalism: A qualitative investigation. *Disability & Rehabilitation, 43*(2), 192–200. https://doi.org/10.1080/09638288.2019.1620876.

Schneider, M. A., & Schneider, D. A. (2017). Pseudobulbar affect: What nurses, stroke survivors, and caregivers need to know. *Journal of Neuroscience Nursing, 49*(2), 114–117.

Suveg, C., Jones, A., Davis, M., et al. (2018). Emotion-focused cognitive-behavioral therapy for youth with anxiety disorders: A randomized trial. *Journal of Abnormal Child Psychology, 46*(3), 569–580. https://doi.org/10.1007/s10802-017-0319-0.

Thuillard, S., & Dan-Glauser, E. S. (2017). The regulatory effect of choice in situation selection reduces experiential, exocrine and respiratory arousal for negative emotional stimulations. *Scientific Reports, 7*(1), 12626. https://doi.org/10.1038/s41598-017-12626-7.

Tsitsi, T., Charalambous, A., Papastavrou, E., & Raftopoulos, V. (2017). Effectiveness of a relaxation intervention (progressive muscle relaxation and guided imagery techniques) to reduce anxiety and improve mood of parents of hospitalized children with malignancies: A randomized controlled trial in Republic of Cyprus and Greece. *European Journal of Oncology Nursing, 26*, 9–18. https://doi.org/10.1016/j.ejon.2016.10.007.

Wills, T. A., Simons, J. S., Sussman, S., & Knight, R. (2016). Emotional self-control and dysregulation: A dual-process analysis of pathways to externalizing/internalizing symptomatology and positive well-being in younger adolescents. *Drug and Alcohol Dependence, 163*(Suppl.1), S37–S45. https://doi.org/10.1016/j.drugalcdep.2015.08.039.

Imbalanced Energy Field Domain 4 Activity/rest Class 3 Energy balance

Gail B. Ladwig, MSN, RN and Julianne E. Doubet, BSN, RN, EMT-B

NANDA-I

Definition

A disruption in the vital flow of human energy that is normally a continuous whole and is unique, dynamic, creative and nonlinear.

E

Defining Characteristics

Arrhythmic energy field patterns; blockage of the energy flow; congested energy field patterns; congestion of the energy flow; dissonant rhythms of the energy field patterns; energy deficit of the energy flow; expression of the need to regain the experience of the whole; hyperactivity of the energy flow; irregular energy field patterns; magnetic pull to an area of the energy field; pulsating to pounding frequency of the energy field patterns; pulsations sensed in the energy flow; random energy field patterns; rapid energy field patterns; slow energy field patterns; strong energy field patterns; temperature differentials of cold in the energy flow; temperature differentials of heat in the energy flow; tingling sensed in the energy flow; tumultuous energy field patterns; unsynchronized rhythms sensed in the energy flow; weak energy field patterns

Related Factors

Anxiety; discomfort; excessive stress; interventions that disrupt the energetic pattern or flow; pain

At-Risk Population

Individuals experiencing life transition; individuals experiencing personal crisis

Associated Conditions

Impaired health status; injury

NOC (Nursing Outcomes Classification)

Suggested NOC Outcomes

Personal Well-Being, Personal Health Status; Psychomotor Energy; Quality of Life

Example NOC Outcome with Indicators

Personal Well-Being as evidenced by the following indicators: Psychological health/Spiritual life/Ability to relax/Level of happiness. (Rate the outcome and indicators of **Personal Well-Being:** 1 = not all satisfied, 2 = somewhat satisfied, 3 = moderately satisfied, 4 = very satisfied, 5 = completely satisfied [see Section I].)

NIC (Nursing Interventions Classification)

Suggested NIC Interventions

Therapeutic Touch (TT); Hope Inspiration; Reiki

Nursing Interventions and *Rationales*

- Consider using complementary health approaches (CHAs), such as energy medicine (TT/healing touch, hope inspiration, and reiki), for clients with anxiety, tension, pain, or other conditions that indicate a disruption in the flow of energy. EBN: *Developing evidence suggests that there is biological support for the lessening of pain and anxiety for clients who receive CHAs in acute care settings (Kramlich, 2017).*
- Refer to care plans for **Anxiety,** Acute **Pain,** and Chronic **Pain.**

Guidelines for Complementary Health Approaches

- CHAs may be practiced by anyone with the requisite preparation, desire, and commitment. EBN: *Acute and critical care nurses who are certified to practice CHAs in the acute care setting must adhere to their scope of practice, be conscious of their role, and recognize their professional boundaries (Kramlich, 2017).*

- Volunteers who are not licensed health care professionals may practice in the home, but not in the health care setting unless they undertake a rigorous training program. EBN: *Because client safety is of utmost concern in the acute and critical care settings, volunteer complementary health professionals (CHPs) must support infection control, client privacy, and client security (Kramlich, 2017).*

Pediatric

- Consider using CHAs for pediatric clients with adjunct therapies to decrease stress, anxiety, and pain. EB: *McClafferty et al (2017) encouraged health care providers who care for children to foster the utilization of "relevant, safe, effective, and age-appropriate health services and therapies," whether conventional or complementary (McClafferty et al, 2017).*

E

Geriatric

- Consider CHAs for elderly with pain. EBN: *Bruckenthal et al (2016) found that comorbidities in older adults cause difficulties with relief of chronic pain due to polypharmacy, the number of painful conditions, and age-related disparities and especially in the use of opioids. The addition of complementary and alternative medicine (CAM) alternatives was recognized as effective in support of chronic pain respite for older adults (Bruckenthal et al, 2016).*

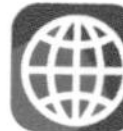

Multicultural

- Assess for the influence of cultural beliefs, norms, and values on the client's use of CAM. EBN: *The popularity of CAM fluctuates from country to country depending on economic, cultural, and social influences (Walker & Tangkiakumjat, 2018).*

Home Care

- Help the client and family accept CAM therapies as natural healing interventions. EBN: *Kramlich (2016) found, in her study of nurses employing CAM therapies in the treatment of acute illness, that these interventions adhere to the nursing standards of person- and family-centered care and in shared decision-making.*
- ▲ In the presence of a psychiatric disorder, refer for psychiatric home health care services for client reassurance and implementation of therapeutic regimens. EB: *It has been shown that a home visit intervention (HoVI) of psychiatric clients generates positive outcomes shown by the documented decrease in rehospitalization rates and number of days hospitalized, leading to health care cost savings (Chang & Chou, 2015).*

Client/Family Teaching and Discharge Planning

- Teach the client how to use guided imagery. EBN: *Assisting the client in the use of guided imagery may lead to progression in their comfort (Coelho et al, 2018).*
- Consider the use of progressive muscle relaxation, autogenic training, relaxation response, biofeedback, emotional freedom technique, guided imagery, diaphragmatic breathing, transcendental meditation, cognitive behavioral therapy, mindfulness-based stress reduction, and emotional freedom technique. EBN: *Family caregivers of the elderly who have received training in the practice of reflexology found that this technique had a substantial and affirmative effect on the health management of their elderly family member (Ali et al, 2017).*
- The practice of CAM therapies, both giving and receiving, can improve well-being. EBN: *In her honors thesis concerning the use of healing touch by nurses, Nunez (2017) found that nurses felt a genuine connection with their clients as they provided a holistic component in client care and helped to improve the clients' feeling of well-being.*

Nurses/Staff

- See the Evolve website for weblinks for client education resources.

REFERENCES

Ali, S. M., Boughdady, A. M., Elkhodary, T. R., & Hassnaen, A. A. (2017). Effect of reflexology training for family caregivers on health status of elderly patients with colorectal cancer. *International Journal of Nursing Didactics*, *7*(9), 13–27. https://doi.org/10.15520/ijnd.2017.vol7.iss9.248.13-27.

Bruckenthal, P., Marino, M. A., & Snelling, L. (2016). Complimentary and integrative therapies for persistent pain management on older adults: A review. *Journal of Gerontological Nursing*, *42*(12), 40–48. https://doi.org/10.3928/00989134-20161110-08.

Chang, Y. C., & Chou, F. H. C. (2015). Effects of home visit intervention on re-hospitalization rates of psychiatric patients. *Community Mental Health*, *51*(5), 598–605. https://doi.org/10.1007/s10597-014-9807-7.

Coelho, A., Parola, V., Sandgren, A., Fernandes, O., Kolcaba, K., & Apóstolo, J. (2018). The effects of guided imagery on comfort in palliative care. *Journal of Hospice and Palliative Nursing*, *20*(4), 392–399. https://doi.org/10.1097/NJH.0000000000000460.

Kramlich, D. (2016). Strategies for acute and critical care nurses implementing complimentary therapies requested

by patients and families. *Critical Care Nurse, 36*(6), 52–58. https://doi.org/10.4037/ccn2017181.
Kramlich, D. (2017). Complementary health practitioners in the acute and critical care setting: Nursing considerations. *Critical Care Nurse, 37*(3), 60–65. https://doi.org/10.4037/ccn2016974.
McClafferty, H., Vohra, S., Baily, M., et al. (2017). Pediatric integrative medicine. *Pediatrics, 140*(3), e20171961. https://doi.org/10.1542/peds.2017-1961.
Nunez, A. (2017). *Integrating complimentary medicine: Attitudes, education, and challenges regarding healing touch.* [Thesis]. Long Beach, CA: California State University. Retrieved from https://hdl.handle.net/20.500.12680/ft848s90s. [Accessed October 20, 2020].
Walker, D. M., & Tangkiakumjat, M. (2018). CAM use from Western and Asian perspectives: Overview of different cultural beliefs of CAM medicine and prevalence of use. *Complementary and Alternative Medicine and Kidney Health*, 24–42. https://doi.org/10.4018/978-1-5225-2882-1.ch002.

Ineffective Dry Eye Self-Management Domain 11 Safety/protection Class 2 Physical injury

Mary Beth Flynn Makic, PhD, RN, CCNS, CCRN-K, FAAN, FNAP, FCNS

NANDA-I

Definition

Unsatisfactory management of symptoms, treatment regimen, physical, psychosocial, and spiritual consequences and lifestyle changes inherent in living with inadequate tear film.

Defining Characteristics

Dry Eye Signs

Chemosis; conjunctival hyperemia; epiphora; filamentary keratitis; keratoconjunctival staining with fluorescein; low aqueous tear production according to Schirmer I Test; mucous plaques

Dry Eye Symptoms

Expresses dissatisfaction with quality of life; reports blurred vision; reports eye fatigue; reports feeling of burning eyes; reports feeling of ocular dryness; reports feeling of ocular foreign body; reports feeling of ocular itching; reports feeling of sand in eye

Behaviors

Difficulty performing eyelid care; difficulty reducing caffeine consumption; inadequate maintenance of air humidity; inadequate use of eyelid closure device; inadequate use of prescribed medication; inappropriate use of contact lenses; inappropriate use of fans; inappropriate use of hairdryer; inappropriate use of moisture chamber goggles; inattentive to dry eye signs; inattentive to dry eye symptoms; inattentive to second-hand smoke; insufficient dietary intake of omega-3 fatty acids; insufficient dietary intake of vitamin A; insufficient fluid intake; nonadherence to recommended blinking exercises; nonadherence to recommended eye breaks; use of products with benzalkonium chloride preservatives

Risk Factors

Competing demands; competing lifestyle preferences; conflict between health behaviors and social norms; decreased perceived quality of life; difficulty accessing community resources; difficulty managing complex treatment regimen; difficulty navigating complex health care systems; difficulty with decision-making; inadequate commitment to a plan of action; inadequate health literacy; inadequate knowledge of treatment regimen; inadequate number of cues to action; inadequate role models; inadequate social support; limited ability to perform aspects of treatment regimen; low self efficacy; negative feelings toward treatment regimen; nonacceptance of condition; perceived barrier to treatment regimen; perceived social stigma associated with condition; unrealistic perception of seriousness of condition; unrealistic perception of susceptibility to sequelae; unrealistic perception of treatment benefit

At-Risk Population

Children; economically disadvantaged individuals; individuals experiencing prolonged hospitalization; individuals with history of ineffective health self-management; individuals with limited decision-making experience; individuals with low educational level; older adults; women experiencing menopause

Associated Conditions

Allergies; autoimmune diseases; chemotherapy; developmental disabilities; graft versus host disease; incomplete eyelid closure; leukocytosis; metabolic diseases; neurological injury with motor reflex loss; neurological injury with sensory reflex loss; oxygen therapy; pharmaceutical preparations; proptosis; radiotherapy; reduced tear volume; surgical procedures

NOC (Nursing Outcomes Classification)

Suggested NOC Outcomes (Visual)

E

Dry Eye Severity; Sensory Function: Vision; Vision Compensation Behavior

Example NOC Outcome with Indicators

Dry Eye Severity as evidenced by the following indicators: Decreased tear production/Redness of conjunctiva/Burning eye sensation/Itchy eye sensation/Eye pain/Excessive watering/Blurred vision. (Rate each indicator of **Dry Eye Severity:** 1 = severe, 2 = substantial, 3 = moderate, 4 = mild, 5 = none [see Section I].)

Client Outcomes

Client Will (Specify Time Frame)

- State eyes are comfortable with no itching, burning, or dryness
- Have corneal surface that is intact and without injury
- Demonstrate self-administration of eye drops if ordered
- State vision is clear

NIC (Nursing Interventions Classification)

Suggested NIC Interventions

Communication Enhancement: Visual Deficit; Environmental Management

Example NIC Activities—Communication Enhancement: Visual Deficit

Identify yourself when you enter the client's space; Provide adequate room lighting

Nursing Interventions and *Rationales*

- ▲ Assess for symptoms of dry eyes, such as "irritation, tearing, burning, stinging, dry or foreign body sensation, mild itching, photophobia, blurry vision, contact lens intolerance, redness, mucus discharge, increased frequency of blinking, eye fatigue, diurnal fluctuation, symptoms that worsen later in the day" (Boyd, 2018; Mukamal, 2020).
- ▲ If symptoms are present, refer client to an ophthalmologist for diagnosis and treatment. EB: *Clients with dry eye who are evaluated by nonophthalmologist health care providers should be referred promptly to the ophthalmologist if moderate or severe pain, lack of response to therapy, corneal infiltration or ulceration, or vision loss occurs (Churchill & Gudgel, 2021).*
- ▲ Administer ordered eye drops. EB: *As the severity of the dry eye increases, aqueous enhancement of the eye using topical agents is appropriate. Emulsions, gels, and ointments can be used (Boyd, 2018).*
- ● Consider use of eyeglass side shields or moisture chambers. EB: *Eyeglass side shields can protect the eyes from drafts. Moisture chambers are a type of eyeglasses that are frequently worn by motorcyclists and mountain climbers and can be purchased at stores or online (Boyd, 2018; Mukamal, 2020).*
- ▲ Watch for symptoms of blepharitis including crusting and irritation at the base of the lashes and adjacent redness of the eyelid, which may accompany dry eye; refer for treatment as needed. EB: *Contributing ocular factors such as blepharitis should be treated. Particularly effective treatments for evaporative tear deficiency include eyelid therapy for conditions such as blepharitis (Boyd, 2018; O'Neil et al, 2019).*
- ▲ Discuss use of caffeine with client's health care provider. EB: *Seltman (2020) and Wang et al (2021) found that caffeine consumption may be a protective factor with dry eye disease, increasing tear volume or eye moisture.*
- ● Provide education to the client about how limiting screen time, computers, smart devices, and television can assist with reducing eyestrain and dry eyes. EB: *Eye discomfort is associated with screen time and "digital eyestrain" because most people blink less when looking at screens, causing eyestrain and dryness (Vimont, 2021;*

Wang et al, 2021). For clients who engage in a lot of screen time, glasses that filter blue light may reduce eyestrain (Palavets & Rosenfield, 2019). Encourage the client to use natural tears if prolonged or frequent digital eyestrain is anticipated.

Critical Care

- ▲ Provide regular cleaning of the eyes, lubricating eye drops and ointments, and consultation with an ophthalmologist if infection is suspected in clients in the intensive care unit (ICU). ICU staff may miss ocular complications while caring for life-threatening conditions. Ocular complications can seriously impair vision and quality of life. EBN: *A nursing study that randomized clients (n = 70 in each group) to either liquid artificial tears or gel artificial tears found that gel tears resulted in less symptoms of dry eye (Dias de Araujo et al, 2019).*
- ● Avoid using adhesive tape to keep eyes closed in sedated clients. EBN: *In an audit of eye dryness and corneal abrasions of clients in four ICUs in Iran, clients receiving adhesive tape as an eye care method were twice as likely to develop corneal abrasion (Masoudi et al, 2014).* EB: *Apply lubricant and ophthalmology-approved eye covers to protect the eyes of high-risk critically ill clients who lack natural mechanism to blink or keep eye lids fully closed (Alansari et al, 2015; Marsden & Davies, 2016).*

Geriatric

- ● Recognize that symptoms of dry eye are more common in menopausal women and geriatric clients. EB: *Hormonal changes after menopause can disrupt tear production. It is estimated that one in three individuals older than 65 years experiences dry eyes (National Health Service [NHS], 2018).*
- ● Many clients as they age develop comorbidities in which the treatments can cause dry eyes. EB: *Medications used to manage cardiovascular diseases, type 2 diabetes, or depression can have secondary effects, causing dry eyes (de Paiva, 2017).*

Client/Family Teaching and Discharge Planning

- ● Teach client conditions that can exacerbate dry eye symptoms. EB: *Exacerbating conditions include wind, air travel, decreased humidity, air conditioning or heating, and prolonged activities that reduce blink rate such as reading and computer use (Marshall & Roach, 2016; Boyd, 2018).*
- ● Teach client good eye hygiene:
  - ❍ Apply warm compresses for 10-minute intervals using a clean cloth and water that has been boiled and cooled (or sterile water).
  - ❍ Gently massage around eyelids.
  - ❍ Gently clean eyelids to remove excess oil, crusts, and bacteria. Use a few drops of baby shampoo in water that has been boiled and cooled, or in sterile water.
  - ❍ Good hygiene can help improve dry eyes, especially dry eye associated with blepharitis (NHS, 2018).
- ● Teach clients methods to decrease problems with dry eye, including the following:
  - ❍ Avoid drafty (e.g., ceiling fans) and low-humidity environments.
  - ❍ Avoid smoking and exposure to secondhand smoke.
- ▲ Discuss avoidance of offending medications with health care provider.
- ● Drink plenty of water to keep well hydrated. EB: *For clients with a clinical diagnosis of mild dry eye, potentially exacerbating exogenous factors such as antihistamine or diuretic use, cigarette smoking or exposure to secondhand smoke, and environmental factors such as air drafts and low-humidity environments should be addressed (Boyd, 2018; Mukamal, 2020). Symptoms of dry eye may be exacerbated by the use of medications such as diuretics, antihistamines, anticholinergics, antidepressants, and systemic retinoids (Boyd, 2018; Mukamal, 2020). Self-care includes drinking plenty of water to stay hydrated (Boyd, 2018; Mukamal, 2020).*
- ● Teach client to lower the computer screen to below eye level and to blink more frequently. EB: *Measures such as lowering the computer screen to below eye level to decrease lid aperture, scheduling regular breaks, and increasing blink frequency may decrease the discomfort associated with computer and reading activities (Boyd, 2018; Mukamal, 2020).*
- ▲ Teach client to consult with the health care provider regarding use of omega-3 supplements to decrease dry eye. EB: *Omega-3 fatty acid products without ethyl esters may be beneficial in the treatment of dry eye, although they may increase the risk of prostate cancer (Boyd, 2018; Mukamal, 2020; Wang et al, 2020).*
- ● Teach client how to self-administer eye drops.
- ● Warn clients with dry eyes that driving at night can be dangerous. Clients with dry eyes have light sensitivity and decreased refraction.

REFERENCES

Alansari, M. A., Hijazi, M. H., & Maghrabi, K. A. (2015). Making a difference in eye care of the critically ill patients. *Journal of Intensive Care Medicine, 30*(6), 311–317. https://doi.org/10.1177/0885066613510674.

Boyd, K. (2018). *Remedies to reduce dry eye symptoms.* American Academy of Ophthalmology [website]. Retrieved from https://www.aao.org/eye-health/tips-prevention/dry-eye-tips. [Accessed June 25, 2021].

Churchill, J., & Gudgel, D. T. (2021). *What is an ophthalmologist?* American Academy of Ophthalmology [website]. Retrieved from https://www.aao.org/eye-health/tips-prevention/what-is-ophthalmologist. [Accessed June 25, 2021].

de Paiva, C. S. (2017). Effects of aging in dry eye. *International Ophthalmology Clinics, 57*(2), 47–64. https://doi.org/10.1097/IIO.0000000000000170.

Dias de Araujo, D., Silva, D., Rodrigues, C., Silva, P. O., Macieira, T., & Chianca, T. (2019). Effectiveness of nursing interventions to prevent dry eye in critically ill patients. *American Journal of Critical Care, 28*(4), 299–306. https://doi.org/10.4037/ajcc2019360.

Marsden, J., & Davies, R. (2016). How to care for a patient's eyes in critical care settings. *Nursing Standard, 31*(16–18), 42–45. https://doi.org/10.7748/ns.2016.e10571.

Marshall, L. L., & Roach, J. M. (2016). Treatment of dry eye disease. *The Consultant Pharmacist, 31*(2), 96–106. https://doi.org/10.4140/TCP.n.2016.96.

Masoudi Alavi, N., Sharifitabar, Z., Shaeri, M., & Adib Hajbaghery, M. (2014). An audit of eye dryness and corneal abrasion in ICU patients in Iran. *Nursing in Critical Care, 19*(2), 73–77. https://doi.org/10.1111/nicc.12052.

Mukamal, R. (2020). *12 treatments for dry eyes: What patients should know.* American Academy of Ophthalmology [website]. Retrieved from https://www.aao.org/eye-health/tips-prevention/how-to-treat-dry-eye-devices. [Accessed June 25, 2021].

National Health Service (NHS). (2018). *Dry eyes.* Retrieved from http://www.nhs.uk/Conditions/Dry-eye-syndrome/Pages/Prevention.aspx. [Accessed June 25, 2021].

O'Neil, E. C., Henderson, M., Massaro-Giordano, M., & Bunya, V. Y. (2019). Advances in dry eye disease treatment. *Current Opinion in Ophthalmology, 30*(3), 166–178. https://doi.org/10.1097/ICU.0000000000000569.

Palavets, T., & Rosenfield, M. (2019). Blue-blocking filters and digital eyestrain. *Optometry and Vision Science, 96*(1), 48–54. https://doi.org/10.1097/OPX.0000000000001318.

Seltman, W. (2020). *Caffeine and dry eye.* WebMD [website]. Retrieved from https://www.webmd.com/eye-health/caffeine-dry-eye#1. [Accessed June 25, 2021].

Vimont, C. (2021). *Should you be worried about blue light?* American Academy of Ophthalmology [website]. Retrieved from https://www.aao.org/eye-health/tips-prevention/should-you-be-worried-about-blue-light. [Accessed June 25, 2021].

Wang, M., Muntz, A., Lim, J., et al. (2020). Ageing and the natural history of dry eye disease: A prospective registry-based cross-sectional study. *Ocular Surface, 18*(4), 736–741. https://doi.org/10.1016/j.jtos.2020.07.003.

Wang, M. T. M., Muntz, A., Mamidi, B., Wolffsohn, J. S., & Craig, J. P. (2021). Modifiable lifestyle risk factors for dry eye disease. *Contact Lens & Anterior Eye*, 101409. https://doi.org/10.1016/j.clae.2021.01.004.

Risk for Dry Eye Domain 11 Safety/protection Class 2 Physical injury

Mary Beth Flynn Makic, PhD, RN, CCNS, CCRN-K, FAAN, FNAP, FCNS

NANDA-I

Definition

Susceptible to inadequate tear film, which may cause eye discomfort and/or damage ocular surface, which may compromise health.

Risk Factors

Air conditioning; air pollution; caffeine consumption; decreased blinking frequency; excessive wind; inadequate knowledge of modifiable factors; inappropriate use of contact lenses; inappropriate use of fans; inappropriate use of hairdryer; inattentive to second-hand smoke; insufficient fluid intake; low air humidity; omega-3 fatty acids deficiency; smoking; sunlight exposure; use of products with benzalkonium chloride preservatives; vitamin A deficiency

At-Risk Population

Contact lens wearer; individuals experiencing prolonged intensive care unit stay; individuals with history of allergy; older adults; women

Associated Conditions

Artificial respiration; autoimmune disease; chemotherapy; decreased blinking; decreased level of consciousness; hormonal change; incomplete eyelid closure; leukocytosis; metabolic diseases; neurological injury with sensory or motor reflex loss; neuromuscular blockade; oxygen therapy; pharmaceutical preparations; proptosis; radiotherapy; reduced tear volume; surgical procedures

NOC, NIC, Client Outcomes, Nursing Interventions and *Rationales,* Client/Family Teaching and Discharge Planning, and References

Refer to care plan for Ineffective Dry **Eye** Self-Management.

Risk for Adult Falls
Domain 11 Safety/protection Class 2 Physical injury

Sherry A. Greenberg, PhD, RN, GNP-BC, FGSA, FAANP, FAAN

NANDA-I

Definition

Adult susceptible to experiencing an event resulting in coming to rest inadvertently on the ground, floor, or other lower level, which may compromise health.

Risk Factors

Physiological Factors

Chronic musculoskeletal pain; decreased lower extremity strength; dehydration; diarrhea; faintness when extending neck; faintness when turning neck; hypoglycemia; impaired physical mobility; impaired postural balance; incontinence; obesity; sleep disturbances; vitamin D deficiency

Psychoneurological Factors

Agitated confusion; anxiety; depressive symptoms; fear of falling; persistent wandering; substance misuse

Unmodified Environmental Factors

Cluttered environment; elevated bed surface; exposure to unsafe weather-related condition; inadequate anti-slip material in bathroom; inadequate anti-slip material on floors; inadequate lighting; inappropriate toilet seat height; inattentive to pets; lack of safety rails; objects out of reach; seats without arms; seats without backs; uneven floor; unfamiliar setting; use of throw rugs

Other Factors

Factors identified by standardized, validated screening tool; getting up at night without help; inadequate knowledge of modifiable factors; inappropriate clothing for walking; inappropriate footwear

At-Risk Population

Economically disadvantaged individuals; individuals aged ≥60 years; individuals dependent for activities of daily living; individuals dependent for instrumental activities of daily living; individuals experiencing prolonged hospitalization; individuals in aged care settings; individuals in palliative care settings; individuals in rehabilitation settings; individuals in the early postoperative period; individuals living alone; individuals receiving home-based care; individuals with history of falls; individuals with low educational level; individuals with restraints

Associated Conditions

Anemia; assistive devices for walking; depression; endocrine system diseases; lower limb prosthesis; major injury; mental disorders; musculoskeletal diseases; neurocognitive disorders; orthostatic hypotension; pharmaceutical preparations; sensation disorders; vascular disease

NOC (Nursing Outcomes Classification)

Suggested NOC Outcomes

Fall Prevention Behavior; Knowledge: Fall Prevention; Risk Control: Falls

Example NOC Outcome with Indicators

Fall Prevention Behavior as evidenced by the following indicators: Uses assistive devices correctly/Eliminates clutter, spills, glare from floors/Uses safe transfer procedures. (Rate each indicator of **Fall Prevention Behavior:** 1 = never demonstrated, 2 = rarely demonstrated, 3 = sometimes demonstrated, 4 = often demonstrated, 5 = consistently demonstrated [see Section I].)

Client Outcomes

Client Will (Specify Time Frame)

- Remain free of falls
- Have a decreased risk of injury if sustains a fall
- Adapt environment to minimize the incidence of falls
- Explain methods to prevent injury

NIC (Nursing Interventions Classification)

Suggested NIC Interventions

Dementia Management; Fall Prevention; Post-Fall Assessment; Surveillance: Safety

F

Example NIC Activities—Fall Prevention

Assist unsteady individual with ambulation; Monitor gait, balance, and fatigue level with ambulation

Nursing Interventions and *Rationales*

- Safety guidelines suggest a fall-risk assessment be completed for older adults in any health care setting with national guidelines and action plans such as the Falls Free Initiative (National Council on Aging, 2021).
- Use a valid and reliable fall risk assessment tool to assess the client's risk for falling; for example, in the acute care setting use the Hendrich II Model (Hendrich, 2013). Recognize that risk factors for falling include recent history of falls, fear of falling, confusion, depression, altered elimination patterns, cardiovascular/respiratory disease impairing perfusion or oxygenation, postural hypotension, dizziness or vertigo, primary cancer diagnosis, and altered mobility (National Council on Aging, 2021; Gray-Miceli & Quigley, 2021). CEB: *The Hendrich II Fall Risk Model is quick to administer and provides a determination of risk for falling based on gender, mental and emotional status, symptoms of dizziness, and known categories of medications increasing risk (Hendrich, 2013). This tool screens for primary prevention of falls and is integral in a postfall assessment for the secondary prevention of falls (Hendrich, 2013).*
- Screen all clients for balance and mobility skills (i.e., supine to sit, sitting supported and unsupported, sit to stand, standing, walking and turning around, transferring, stooping to floor and recovering, and sitting down). Use tools such as the Balance Scale by Tinetti, the Performance-Oriented Mobility Assessment (POMA), or the Timed Up & Go Test. CEB/EB: *It is helpful to determine the client's functional abilities and then plan for ways to improve problem areas or determine methods to ensure safety (Podsiadlo & Richardson, 1991; Resnick, 2019; National Council on Aging, 2021; Gray-Miceli & Quigley, 2021).*
- Identify client mobility function deficits and consider appropriate equipment needed to safely mobilize clients while promoting self-care. The Bedside Mobility Assessment Tool 2.0 (BMAT 2.0) helps nurses assess client mobility status and standardize safe client handling and mobility equipment use. EB: *The BMAT 2.0 is used mainly in the inpatient setting; takes only a few minutes to complete; and is conducted on admission, once per shift, and at a change in client status. Four levels of mobility are assessed: strength, coordination, balance, and tolerance. These are assessed at different levels depending on the client's function and overall safety depending on the health condition(s) and client ability. Nurses may work with multiprofessional team members to help clients progress in terms of mobility, strength, and type and safe use of mobility aids (Boynton, Kumpar, & VanGilder, 2020).*
- Older adults and others who may have been immobile due to acute illnesses and changing medications may be at risk for orthostatic hypotension. This is a drop in systolic blood pressure of 20 mm Hg or more or a drop in diastolic blood pressure of 10 mm Hg or more when changing from lying to sitting or sitting to standing. A concurrent rise in heart rate may occur as well. The client may or may not experience lightheadedness or dizziness. EB: *Encourage clients to change positions slowly. Take a client's blood pressure and pulse after standing 1 and 3 minutes to assess for orthostatic hypotension (Centers for Disease Control and Prevention, 2017).*
- Carefully assist a mostly immobile client up. Be sure to lock the bed and wheelchair and have sufficient personnel to protect the client from falls. When rising from a lying position, have the client change positions slowly, dangle legs, and stand next to the bed before walking to prevent orthostatic hypotension. EB: *Encourage client engagement in a monitored exercise program that will strengthen core and lower extremities to reduce fall risk (Grabiner, 2014; Hirase et al, 2014; National Institute of Neurological Disorders and Stroke [NINDS], 2019).*

- Use a "high-risk fall" armband/bracelet and fall risk room sign to alert staff for increased vigilance and mobility assistance. EB: *These steps alert the nursing staff of the increased risk of falls (Goodwin et al, 2014).*

▲ Evaluate the client's medications to determine whether medications increase the risk of falling. Consult with health care provider regarding the client's need for medication if appropriate. EB: *Polypharmacy, or taking more than four medications, has been associated with increased falls. Medications such as benzodiazepines, as well as psychotropic, antipsychotic, and antidepressant medications given to promote sleep, actually increase the rate of falls (Goodwin et al, 2014; The 2019 American Geriatrics Society Beers Criteria Update Expert Panel, 2019; Greenberg 2019b; National Council on Aging, 2020).* EB: *Short- to intermediate-acting benzodiazepine and tricyclic antidepressants may produce ataxia, impaired psychomotor function, syncope, and additional falls (Greenberg et al, 2016; Resnick, 2019; The 2019 American Geriatrics Society Beers Criteria Update Expert Panel, 2019).*

- Orient the client to the environment. Place the call light within reach and show how to call for assistance; answer call light promptly.
- Use one-fourth to one-half length side rails only, and maintain bed in a low position. Ensure that wheels are locked on the bed and commode. Keep dim light in the room at night. CEB/EB: *Use of full side rails can result in the client climbing over the rails, leading with the head, and sustaining a head injury. Side rails with widely spaced vertical bars and side rails not situated flush with the mattress have been associated with asphyxiation deaths because of rail and in-bed entrapment and should not be used (Capezuti, 2004; Goodwin et al, 2014).*
- Routinely assist the client with toileting on his or her own schedule. Take the client to the bathroom on awakening and before bedtime (Goodwin et al, 2014).
- Keep the path to the bathroom clear, label the bathroom, and leave the door open.

▲ Avoid use of restraints if possible. Obtain health care provider's order if restraints are deemed necessary, and use the least restrictive device. EB: *The use of restraints has been associated with serious injuries, including rhabdomyolysis, brachial plexus injury, neuropathy, and dysrhythmias, as well as strangulation, asphyxiation, traumatic brain injuries, and all the consequences of immobility (Cotter & Evans, 2018).* CEB: *A study demonstrated that there was no increase in falls or injuries in a group of clients who were not restrained versus a similar group that was restrained in a nursing home (Capezuti, 2004). A study in two acute care hospitals demonstrated that when restraints were not used, there was no increase in client falls, injuries, or therapy disruptions (Mion et al, 2001).*

- In place of restraints, use the following:
  - Well-staffed and educated nursing personnel with frequent client contact with careful consideration during shift changes
  - Nursing units designed to care for clients with cognitive and/or functional impairments
  - Nonskid footwear, sneakers preferable
  - Glasses and/or hearing aids, as needed
  - Adequate lighting, night-light in bathroom
  - Frequent toileting
  - Frequently assess need for invasive devices, tubes, intravenous (IV) access
  - Hide tubes with bandages to prevent pulling of tubes
  - Consider alternative IV placement site to prevent pulling out IV line
  - Alarm systems with ankle, above-the-knee, or wrist sensors
  - Bed or wheelchair alarms
  - Wedge cushions on chairs to prevent slipping
  - Increased observation of the client
  - Locked doors to unit
  - Low Low- or very-low-height beds
  - Border-defining pillow/mattress to cue the client to stay in bed

  EB: *These alternatives to restraints can be helpful to prevent falls (Grabiner, 2014; Cotter & Evans, 2018).*
- If the client has an acute change in mental status (delirium), recognize that the cause is usually physiological and is a medical emergency. Consider possible causes for delirium. Consult with the health care provider immediately. See interventions for Acute **Confusion.**
- If the client has chronic confusion caused by dementia, implement individualized strategies to enhance communication. Assessment of specific receptive and expressive language abilities is needed to understand the client's communication difficulties and facilitate communication. See interventions for Chronic **Confusion.**

F

- Ask family to stay with the client to assist with activities of daily living and prevent the client from accidentally falling or pulling out tubes.
- ▲ If the client is unsteady on his or her feet, have two nursing staff members alongside when walking the client. Use facility-approved mobility devices to assist with client ambulation (e.g., gait belts, walkers). Consider referral to physical therapy for gait training and strengthening. EB: *The client can walk independently, but the nurse can rapidly ensure safety if the client becomes weak or unsteady. Multiprofessional care is most comprehensive and beneficial to the client (Grabiner, 2014).*
- Place a fall-prone client in a room that is near the nurses' station. Such placement allows more frequent observation of the client.
- Help clients sit in a stable chair with armrests. Avoid use of wheelchairs except for transportation as needed. Clients are likely to fall when left in a wheelchair because they may stand up without locking the wheels or removing the footrests.
- ▲ Refer to physical therapy or other programs for exercise programs that target strength, balance, flexibility, or endurance. EB: *Programs with at least two of these components have been shown to decrease the rate of falling and number of people falling (National Council on Aging, 2021).*

F

Geriatric

- Assess mobility and gait speed using the Timed Up & Go Test. Ask the client to stand up from a standard arm chair, walk 10 feet (or 3 meters), turn around, walk back to the chair, and sit down (Podsiadlo & Richardson, 1991). This should be done with the client wearing usual footwear. EB: *Performance on this screening examination demonstrates the client's mobility. If the client completes the test in less than 10 seconds, he or she is considered freely mobile. If completing the test takes 10 to 19 seconds, the client is considered to be mostly independent in mobility. If the client takes 20 to 29 seconds, the client is considered to have variable mobility. If the client takes 30 or more seconds, he or she is considered to have impaired mobility and is more likely to be dependent on others and more likely to sustain a fall (Podsiadlo & Richardson, 1991; Centers for Disease Control and Prevention, National Center for Injury Prevention and Control, 2020).*
- Mobility assessment and acting on findings are crucial in care of older adults. This is embedded in the Age-Friendly Health System's Model of Care, an initiative of the John A. Hartford Foundation and the Institute of Healthcare Improvement (IHI) in partnership with the American Hospital Association and the Catholic Health Association of the United States that began in 2017. The Age-Friendly Health System model promotes the evidence-based 4Ms framework: (1) **What Matters** to the older adult, considering what is most important to the older adult, family, and caregivers, in terms of goals and preferences; (2) **Medication**, making sure all medications have a clear indication, prescribed at the lowest effective dosage and frequency; (3) **Mentation**, assessing and managing dementia, delirium, and/or depression; and (4) **Mobility**, maintaining or improving mobility and function (Institute for Healthcare Improvement, 2019). EB: *The 4Ms framework is a guide to care of older adults in all care settings. The 4Ms are to be implemented together as a set of evidence-based elements of high-quality care for older adults. The Mobility component is included as an essential component to ensure that older adults move safely every day in order to maintain function and do What Matters to them (Institute for Healthcare Improvement, 2019).*
- Complete a fall risk assessment for older adults in acute care using a valid and reliable tool such as the Hendrich II Fall Risk Model. EB: *It is quick to administer and provides a determination of risk for falling based on gender, mental and emotional status, symptoms of dizziness, and known categories of medications increasing risk (Hendrich, 2013). This tool screens for primary prevention of falls and is integral in a postfall assessment for the secondary prevention of falls (Goodwin et al, 2014; Greenberg, 2020; Hendrich, 2013).*
- ▲ If there is new onset of falling, assess for laboratory abnormalities, signs and symptoms of infection and dehydration, and blood glucose level for diabetics, and check blood pressure and pulse rate with client in supine, sitting, and standing positions for hypotension and orthostatic hypotension. If the client has borderline high blood pressure, the risk of falling because of the administration of antihypertensives may outweigh the benefits of the antihypertensive medication. Discuss with the health care provider on a client-to-client basis. EB: *If orthostatic hypotension is present and there is minimal change in the heart rate, most likely the baroreceptors are not working to maintain blood pressure on arising. This is common in older adults and may be caused by hypovolemia resulting from the excessive use of diuretics, vasodilators, or other types of drugs; dehydration; or prolonged bed rest, as well as cardiovascular disease, neurological disease, or the adverse effects of another medication (NINDS, 2019).*
- Complete a fear of falling assessment for older adults. This includes measuring fear of falling, or the level of concern about falling, and falls self-efficacy, which is the degree of confidence a person has in

performing common activities of daily living without falling. Fear of falling may be measured by a single-item question asking about the presence of fear of falling or rating severity of fear of falling on a 1 to 4 Likert scale as is commonly done in studies. Falls self-efficacy may be measured using a valid and reliable tool such as the Falls Efficacy Scale—International (Yardley et al, 2005; Greenberg, 2012; Greenberg et al, 2016; Greenberg 2019a).

- ● Encourage the client to wear glasses and use walking aids when ambulating.
- ● If the client experiences dizziness because of orthostatic hypotension when getting up, teach methods to decrease dizziness, such as rising slowly, remaining seated several minutes before standing, flexing feet upward several times while sitting, sitting down immediately if feeling dizzy, and trying to have someone present when standing. EB: *Always have the client dangle at the bedside before standing to evaluate for postural hypotension. Watch the client closely for dizziness during increased activity. Postural hypotension can be detected in up to 30% of older clients. These methods can help prevent falls and maintain adequate fluid intake (Goodwin et al, 2014).*
- ▲ If the client is experiencing syncope, determine symptoms that occur before syncope and note medications that the client is taking. Refer for medical care. The circumstances surrounding syncope often suggest the cause. EB: *Use of many medications, including diuretics, antihypertensives, digoxin, beta-blockers, and calcium channel blockers, can cause syncope. Use of the tilt table can be diagnostic in incidences of syncope (Goodwin et al, 2014; Fick & Mion, 2018).*
- ▲ Observe client for signs of anemia, and refer to health care provider for testing if appropriate.
- ● Evaluate client for chronic alcohol intake and mental health and neurological function.
- ▲ Refer to physical therapy for strength training, using free weights or machines, and suggest participation in exercise programs. EB: *Exercise can prevent falls in older people. Greater relative effects are seen in programs that include exercises that challenge balance, use a higher dose of exercise, and do not include a walking program. Service providers can use these findings to design and implement exercise programs for falls prevention (Grabiner, 2014; Hirase et al, 2014; National Council on Aging, 2021).*
- ▲ Evidence-based guidelines for preventing falls in older adults were published by the American Geriatrics Society (AGS) and British Geriatrics Society (BGS) collaboratively and specify recommendations for all clinical settings. The Centers for Disease Control and Prevention's Stopping Elderly Accidents, Deaths, & Injuries (STEADI) initiative related to older adult fall prevention provides implementation strategies. These recommendations include screening and assessment and interventions. Examples of interventions include (1) exercise for balance and for gait and strength training, such as tai chi or physical therapy; (2) environmental adaptation to reduce fall risk factors in the home and in daily activities; (3) cataract surgery when indicated; (4) medication reduction with particular attention to medications that affect the brain such as sleeping medications and antidepressants; (5) assessment and treatment of postural hypotension; (6) identification and appropriate treatment of foot problems; and (7) vitamin D supplementation for those with vitamin D deficiency (American Geriatrics Society [AGS], 2011; Centers for Disease Control and Prevention & National Center for Injury Prevention and Control, 2020; Centers for Disease Control and Prevention, 2021)
- ▲ Refer community-dwelling older adults to evidence-based community-based programs (National Council on Aging, 2021). EB: *A Matter of Balance is a group intervention focusing on increasing activity levels and decreasing concerns about falling. The program helps community-based older adults gain confidence by setting goals to increase activity and mobility, decrease fall risk factors in the home, and promote exercise to increase strength and improve balance (Alexander et al, 2015). CAPABLE (Community Aging in Place—Advancing Better Living for Elders) is a 5-month structured program delivered at home to decrease fall risk, improve safe mobility, and improve the ability to safely conduct functional tasks and activities (Ruiz et al, 2017).*

Home Care

- ● Some of the previously mentioned interventions may be adapted for home care use.
- ● Implement evidence-based fall prevention practices in community settings and home health care programs for older adults (National Council on Aging, 2021).
- ▲ If delirium is present, assess for cause of delirium and/or falls with the use of an multiprofessional team. Consult with the health care provider immediately. Assess and monitor for acute changes in cognition and behavior. EB: *An acute and fluctuating change in cognition and behavior is the classic presentation of delirium. Delirium is reversible and should be considered a medical emergency. Delirium can become chronic if untreated, and clients may be discharged from hospitals to home care in states of undiagnosed delirium.* EB: *Falls may be a precipitating event or an indication of frailty consistent with delirium (Goodwin et al, 2014).*

- ● Assess home environment for threats to safety, including clutter, slippery floors, scatter rugs, and other potential hazards. Additionally, assess external environment (e.g., uneven pavement, unleveled stairs/steps). EB: *Clients suffering from impaired mobility, impaired visual acuity, and neurological dysfunction, including dementia and other cognitive functional deficits, are all at risk for injury from common hazards. These recommendations were shown to be effective to reduce falls (AGS, 2011; Goodwin et al, 2014; National Council on Aging, 2021).*
- ▲ Institute a home-based, nurse-delivered exercise program to reduce falls or refer to physical therapy services for client and family education of safe transfers and ambulation and for strengthening exercises for the client (Grabiner, 2014; National Council on Aging, 2021).
- ▲ Instruct the client and family or caregivers on how to correct identified hazards for those with visual impairment. Refer to physical and occupational therapy services for assistance if needed. EB: *Interventions to improve home safety were shown to be effective in people at high risk, such as those with severe visual impairment (National Council on Aging, 2021).*
- ▲ Use a multifactorial assessment along with interventions targeted to the identified risk factors. Key components of the interventions include evaluating need for all medications, balance, gait, and strength training, use of strategies to deal with postural hypotension if present, home safety evaluation with needed modifications, and any needed cardiovascular treatment. EB: *As people age, they may fall more often for multiple reasons including problems with balance, poor vision, and dementia. Fear of falling can result in self-restricted activity levels (National Council on Aging, 2021).*
- ● If the client lives alone or spends a great deal of time alone, teach the client what to do if he or she falls and cannot get up, and make sure he or she has a personal emergency response system or a mobile phone that is available from the floor (AGS, 2011; National Council on Aging, 2021).
- ● Ensure appropriate nonglare lighting in the home. Ask the client to install indoor strip or "runway" type of lighting to baseboards to help clients balance. Install motion-sensitive lighting that turns on automatically when the client gets out of bed to go to the bathroom.
- ● Have the client wear supportive, low-heeled shoes with good traction when ambulating. Avoid use of slip-on footwear. Wear appropriate footwear in inclement weather. EB: *Supportive shoes provide the client with better balance and protect the client from instability on uneven surfaces. Anti-slip shoe devices worn in icy conditions have been shown to reduce falls (AGS, 2011; National Council on Aging, 2021).*
- ● Provide a signaling device for clients who wander or are at risk for falls. Orienting a vulnerable client to a safety net relieves the anxiety of the client and caregiver and allows for rapid response to a crisis situation.
- ● Provide medical identification bracelet for clients at risk for injury from dementia, diabetes, seizures, or other medical disorders.
- ● Suggest a tai chi class designed for older adults and selected clients who have sufficient balance to participate. EB: *Participation in once-per-week tai chi classes for 16 weeks can prevent falls in relatively healthy community-dwelling older people (AGS, 2011; National Council on Aging, 2021).*

Client/Family Teaching and Discharge Planning

- ● Teach the client and the family about the fall reduction measures that are being used to prevent falls (The Joint Commission, 2020).
- ● Providing education on safety guidelines to prevent falls is an important nursing intervention that should be completed as part of discharge planning (*National Council on Aging, 2021*)
- ● Teach the client how to safely ambulate at home, including using safety measures such as handrails in bathroom, reaching for items on high shelves, and avoiding carrying things or performing other tasks while walking.
- ● Teach the client the importance of maintaining a regular exercise program. If the client is afraid of falling while walking outside, suggest that he or she walk the length of a local mall. EB: *Exercise can prevent falls in older people. Greater relative effects are seen in programs that include exercises that challenge balance and use a higher dose of exercise than just walking programs (AGS, 2011; Grabiner, 2014; Hirase et al, 2014).*

REFERENCES

Alexander, J. L., Sartor-Glittenberg, C., Bordenave, E., & Bordenave, L. (2015). Effect of the Matter of Balance program on balance confidence in older adults. *GeroPsych The Journal of Gerontopsychology and Geriatric Psychiatry, 28*(4), 183–189.

F

American Geriatrics Society (AGS). (2011). *2010 AGS/BGS clinical practice guideline. Prevention of falls in older persons. Summary of recommendations*. Retrieved from https://hsctc.org/wp-content/uploads/2017/07/2010-American-Geriatrics-Society-Guideline_-Prevention-of-Falls-in-Older-Persons.pdf. Accessed June 25, 2021.

Boynton, T., Kumpar, D., & VanGilder, C. (2020). The bedside mobility assessment tool 2.0: Advancing patient mobility. *American Journal of Nursing, 15*(7), 18–22.

Capezuti, E. (2004). Minimizing the use of restrictive devices in dementia patients at risk for falling. *Nursing Clinics of North America, 39*(3), 625–647.

Centers for Disease Control and Prevention (CDC). (2017). *Measuring orthostatic blood pressure*. Retrieved from https://www.cdc.gov/steadi/pdf/Measuring_Orthostatic_Blood_Pressure-print.pdf. Accessed June 25, 2021.

Centers for Disease Control and Prevention (CDC). (2021). *Older adult fall prevention*. Retrieved from https://www.cdc.gov/falls. Accessed June 25, 2021.

Centers for Disease Control and Prevention & National Center for Injury Prevention and Control. (2020). *STEADI program—Older adult fall prevention*. Retrieved from https://www.cdc.gov/steadi/materials.html. Accessed June 25, 2021.

Cotter, V. T., & Evans, L. K. (2018). *Try This:® Best practices in nursing care to older adults. Fall risk assessment for older adults: Avoiding restraints in older adults with dementia*. New York: Hartford Institute for Geriatric Nursing and Alzheimer's Association. Retrieved from https://hign.org/consultgeri/try-this-series/avoiding-restraints-patients-dementia. Accessed June 25, 2021.

Fick, D., & Mion, L. C. (2018). *Try This:® Best practices in nursing care to older adults. Fall risk assessment for older adults: Assessing and managing delirium in older adults with dementia*. New York: Hartford Institute for Geriatric Nursing. Retrieved from https://hign.org/consultgeri/try-this-series/assessing-and-managing-delirium-persons-dementia. Accessed June 25, 2021.

Goodwin, V. A., Abbott, R. A., Whear, R., et al. (2014). Multiple component interventions for preventing falls and fall related injuries among older people: Systematic review and meta-analysis. *BMC Geriatrics, 14*, 15–21.

Grabiner, M. D. (2014). Exercise-based fall prevention programmes decrease fall-related injuries. *Evidence-Based Nursing, 17*(4), 125.

Gray-Miceli, D., & Quigley, P. A. (2021). Assessing, managing, and preventing falls in acute care. In M. Boltz, E. Capezuti, D. Zwicker, & T. Fulmer (Eds.), *Evidence-based geriatric nursing protocols for best practice* (6th ed.). New York: Springer.

Greenberg, S. A. (2012). Analysis of measurement tools of fear of falling among high-risk, community-dwelling older adults. *Clinical Nursing Research, 21*(1), 113–130. https://doi.org/10.1177/1054773811433824.

Greenberg, S. A. (2019a). *Try This:® Best practices in nursing care to older adults. Assessment of fear of falling in older adults: The Falls Efficacy Scale-International (FES-I)*. New York: Hartford Institute for Geriatric Nursing. Retrieved from https://hign.org/consultgeri/try-this-series/assessment-fear-falling-older-adults-falls-efficacy-scale-international. Accessed June 25, 2021.

Greenberg, S. A. (2019b). The 2019 American Geriatrics Society Updated Beers Criteria® for potentially inappropriate medication use in older adults. *Try This®, issue 16*. New York: Hartford Institute for Geriatric Nursing and American Geriatrics Society. Retrieved from https://hign.org/consultgeri/try-this-series/2019-american-geriatrics-society-updated-beers-criteria-r-potentially. Accessed June 25, 2021.

Greenberg, S. A. (2020). Falls in older adults: Prevention and assessment of risk in primary care. *Advances in Family Practice Nursing, 2*, 1–9. https://doi.org/10.1016/j.yfpn.2019.12.001.

Greenberg, S. A., Sullivan-Marx, E., Sommers, M. L. S., Chittams, J., & Cacchione, P. Z. (2016). Measuring fear of falling among high-risk, urban, community-dwelling older adults. *Geriatric Nursing, 37*(6), 489–495. https://doi.org/10.1016/j.gerinurse.2016.08.018.

Hendrich, A. (2013). *Try This:® Best practices in nursing care to older adults. Fall risk assessment for older adults: The Hendrich II Fall Risk Model™*. New York: Hartford Institute for Geriatric Nursing. Retrieved from http://www.wsha.org/wp-content/uploads/Hendrich-II-Fall-Risk.pdf. Accessed September 18, 2021.

Hirase, T., Inokuchi, S., Matsusaka, N., Nakahara, K., & Okita, M. (2014). A modified fall risk assessment tool that is specific to physical function predicts falls in community-dwelling elderly people. *Journal of Geriatric Physical Therapy, 37*(4), 159–165.

Institute for Healthcare Improvement. (2019). *Age-friendly health systems: Guide to using the 4Ms in the care of older adults*. Massachusetts: Institute for Healthcare Improvement. Retrieved from http://www.ihi.org/Engage/Initiatives/Age-Friendly-Health-Systems/Documents/IHIAgeFriendlyHealthSystems_GuidetoUsing4MsCare.pdf. Accessed September 18, 2021.

The Joint Commission. (2020). *Home care. 2020 National Patient Safety Goals. Goal 9. Reduce the risk of patient harm resulting from falls*. Retrieved from https://www.jointcommission.org/-/media/tjc/documents/standards/national-patient-safety-goals/2020/npsg_chapter_ome_jul2020.pdf. Accessed June 25, 2021.

Mion, L. C., Fogel, J., Sandhu, S., et al. (2001). Outcomes following physical restraint reduction programs in two acute care hospitals. *Joint Commission Journal on Quality Improvement, 27*(11), 605–618.

National Council on Aging. (June, 2021). *Falls Free® initiative*. Retrieved from https://www.ncoa.org/article/about-the-falls-free-initiative Accessed September 18, 2021.

National Institute of Neurological Disorders and Stroke (NINDS). (2019). *Orthostatic hypotension information page*. Retrieved from https://www.ninds.nih.gov/Disorders/All-Disorders/Orthostatic-Hypotension-Information-Page. Accessed June 25, 2021.

Podsiadlo, D., & Richardson, S. (1991). The timed "up & go": A test of basic functional mobility for frail elderly persons. *Journal of the American Geriatrics Society, 39*(2), 142–148.

Resnick, B. (2019). *Geriatric nursing review syllabus: A core curriculum in advanced practice geriatric nursing* (6th ed.). New York: American Geriatrics Society.

Ruiz, S., Snyder, L. P., Rotondo, C., Cross-Barnet, C., Colligan, E. M., & Giuriceo, K. (2017). Innovative home visit models associated with reductions in costs, hospitalizations, and emergency department use. *Health Affairs, 36*(3), 425–432.

The 2019 American Geriatrics Society Beers Criteria® Update Expert Panel. (2019). American Geriatrics Society 2019 Updated AGS Beers Criteria® for potentially inappropriate medication Use in older adults. *Journal of the American Geriatrics Society, 67*(4), 674–694.

Yardley, L., Beyer, N., Hauer, K., Kempen, G., Piot-Ziegler, C., & Todd, C. (2005). Development and initial validation of the Falls Efficacy Scale-International (FES-I). *Age and Ageing, 34*(6), 614–619.

F

Risk for Child Falls

Domain 11 Safety/protection Class 2 Physical injury

Sherry A. Greenberg, PhD, RN, GNP-BC, FGSA, FAANP, FAAN and Mary Beth Flynn Makic, PhD, RN, CCNS, CCRN-K, FAAN, FNAP, FCNS

NANDA-I

Definition

Child susceptible to experiencing an event resulting in coming to rest inadvertently on the ground, floor, or other lower level, which may compromise health.

F

Risk Factors

Caregiver Factors

Changes diapers on raised surfaces; exhaustion; fails to lock wheels of child equipment; inadequate knowledge of changes in developmental stages; inadequate supervision of child; inattentive to environmental safety; inattentive to safety devices during sports activities; places child in bouncer seat on raised surfaces; places child in infant walkers; places child in mobile seat on raised surfaces; places child in seats without a seat belt; places child in shopping cart basket; places child on play equipment unsuitable for age group; postpartum depressive symptoms; sleeps with child in arms without protective measures; sleeps with child on lap without protective measures

Physiological Factors

Decreased lower extremity strength; dehydration; hypoglycemia; hypotension; impaired physical mobility; impaired postural balance; incontinence; malnutrition; neurobehavioral manifestations; obesity; sleep disturbances

Unmodified Environmental Factors

Absence of stairway gate; absence of stairway handrail; absence of wheel locks on child equipment; absence of window guard; cluttered environment; furniture placement facilitates access to balconies; furniture placement facilitates access to windows; high chairs positioned near tables or counters; inadequate anti-slip material on floors; inadequate automobile restraints; inadequate lighting; inadequate maintenance of play equipment; inadequate restraints on elevated surfaces; inattentive to pets; objects out of reach; seats without arms; seats without backs; uneven floor; unfamiliar setting; use of furniture without anti-tipping devices; use of non–age appropriate furniture; use of throw rugs

Other Factors

Factors identified by standardized, validated screening tool; inappropriate clothing for walking; inappropriate footwear

At-Risk Population

Boys; children <12 years of age; children born to economically disadvantaged families; children experiencing prolonged prescribed fasting period; children exposed to overcrowded environment; children in the labor force; children whose caregivers have low educational level; children whose caregivers have mental health issues; children with history of falls; children with stressed caregivers; children with young caregivers; children within the first week of hospitalization

Associated Conditions

Assistive devices for walking; feeding and eating disorders; musculoskeletal diseases; neurocognitive disorders; pharmaceutical preparations; sensation disorders

NOC (Nursing Outcomes Classification)

Suggested NOC Outcomes

Fall Prevention Behavior; Knowledge: Child Physical Safety; Knowledge: Fall Prevention; Risk Control: Falls

Example NOC Outcome with Indicators

Fall Prevention Behavior as evidenced by the following indicators: Uses assistive devices correctly/ Eliminates clutter, spills, glare from floors, places barriers to prevent falls (Rate each indicator of **Fall Prevention Behavior:** 1 = never demonstrated, 2 = rarely demonstrated, 3 = sometimes demonstrated, 4 = often demonstrated, 5 = consistently demonstrated [see Section I].)

Client Outcomes

Client Will (Specify Time Frame)

- Remain free of falls
- Verbalize environmental conditions to prevent falls
- Have a decreased risk of injury if sustains a fall
- Adapt environment to minimize the incidence of falls
- Explain methods to prevent injury

F

NIC (Nursing Interventions Classification)

Suggested NIC Interventions

Fall Prevention; Surveillance: Safety

Example NIC Activities—Fall Prevention

Provides close supervision and/or restraining device (e.g., infant seat with seat belt) when placing infants/ young children on elevated surfaces (e.g., highchair and hand securely on child when on changing table)

Nursing Interventions and *Rationales*

- Provide and review home safety plans with parents. **CEB:** *A Cochrane review found that home safety plans were an inexpensive and effective way to reduce child harm. Education that encouraged the use of fitted stair gates reduced the risk of child falls by more than 50% (Kendrick et al, 2012).*
- Follow national guidelines to teach parents and guardians about fall safety for children.
  - Playground safety includes ensuring surfaces under equipment are soft and well maintained.
  - Home safety addresses guards on windows that are above ground level and use of stair gates and guard rails.
  - Use helmets and wrist, knee, and elbow pads/protective gear during recreation and sports activities.
  - Keep fire safety ladder available near window on floors above ground level.
  - Close supervision of young children is essential to reduce fall risks.

  EB: *The Centers for Disease Control and Prevention (CDC, 2019) provides information for parents, guardians, and teachers to protect children from falls and fall-related injuries, including head injuries.*
- Explore possible concerns of harm indirectly or directly resulting in a child fall. **EB:** *Multiple factors influence violence against a child, including individual, community, and social factors. Assess characteristics of the fall that may not be consistent with history and inform provider for additional evaluation (CDC, 2021).*
- Children younger than 4 years of age and those with special needs that increase caregiver burden are at greater risk of harm from unintentional falls (Chaudhary et al, 2018; CDC, 2021).
- Assess height from which the child fell and possible impact. **EB:** *Research exploring the mechanism and risk of children who fell with injuries found that children younger than 1 more likely fell from a caregiver's arms or from a higher surface due to improper safety device use (e.g., safety straps/seatbelts); younger children ages 2 to 6 are more prone to falls from furniture, down stairs, on playgrounds, or from balconies; and older children ages greater than 10 fall from higher surfaces, trampolines, and so on (Chaudhary et al, 2018). Providing age-specific fall prevention information to parents and caregivers may reduce the risk of injury with pediatric falls (CDC, 2019, 2021).*
- Safety guidelines suggest that a pediatric fall risk assessment tool should be completed to assess fall risk. **EBN:** *An integrative review of pediatric fall risk tools identified that factors most associated with pediatric falls in hospital settings include medication use (e.g., seizure medications, sedation), cognitive impairment, prolonged length of stay, orthopedic diagnosis, environmental circumstances, and history of falls. The hospital environment is different than home, thus assessing a child for risk of falls using a valid and reliable tool is essential to reduce risk and harm from falls (DiGerolamo & Davis, 2017).*

- Use a valid and reliable fall risk assessment tool to assess the client risk for falling (DiGerolamo & Davis, 2017). CEBN: *The Humpty Dumpty Fall Scale (HDFS) places pediatric clients at low or high risk of falling based on age, gender, diagnosis, cognitive impairment, environmental changes, response to surgery/sedation/anesthesia, and medication (Hill-Rodriquez et al, 2009). Another pediatric fall assessment tool, the I'M SAFE tool, has been found to assist with fall risk assessment in children and evaluates risk variables of impairment, medications, sedation/anesthesia, admitting diagnosis, fall history, and environment of care (Neiman et al, 2011).* CEBN: *Another tool, CHAMPS looks, has been found to predict risk of falls and includes four risk factors: change in mental status, history of falls, age less than 36 months, and mobility impairment (Razmus & Davis, 2012).*
- Screen children for balance and mobility skills (i.e., supine to sit, sitting supported and unsupported, sit to stand, standing, walking and turning around, transferring, stooping to floor and recovering, and sitting down). Use tools such as the Pediatric Balance Scale (Franjoine et al, 2003) or the Performance-Oriented Mobility Assessment–Gait (POMA-G) (Phillips et al, 2018). CEB/EB: *It is helpful to determine the client's functional abilities and then plan for ways to improve problem areas or determine methods to ensure safety (Franjoine et al, 2003; Phillips et al, 2018).*

F

- Keep the path to the bathroom clear, label the bathroom, and leave the door open.
- ▲ Refer to physical therapy or other programs for exercise programs that target strength, balance, flexibility, or endurance. EB: *Balance training programs with sessions at least two times a week were found to have the greatest impact on improving balance and reducing falls in adolescents (Gebel et al, 2018).*

Home Care

- Some of the previously mentioned interventions may be adapted for home care use.
- Encourage the child to engage in exercise and activities that are appropriate for development age to strengthen balance and muscles. EB: *Engaging children with Down syndrome in regular exercise was found to reduce incidence of falls, improve overall balance, and reduce severity of falls (Maïano et al, 2019).*
- Assess home environment for threats to safety, including clutter, slippery floors, scatter rugs, and other potential hazards. Additionally, assess external environment (e.g., uneven pavement, unleveled stairs/steps). *Clients suffering from impaired mobility, impaired visual acuity, neurological dysfunction, and immaturity in age are all at risk for injury from common hazards.*
- ▲ Institute a home-based, balance performance program to improve youth core strength and balance. EB: *A systematic review and meta-analysis found that frequency of balance training improved youths' overall strength, endurance, balance, and health (Gebel et al, 2018).*
- ▲ Use a multifactorial assessment along with interventions targeted to the identified risk factors. Key components of the interventions include evaluating all medications, balance, gait and strength training, home safety evaluation with needed modifications, and any needed safety equipment. EB: *Reviewing in home safety should be completed as risks will vary from hospital settings. Understanding changes in the child's physical needs, including changes in treatment plans and pharmaceutical preparations, is essential to reduce fall risks at home (DiGerolamo & Davis, 2017).*
- Ensure appropriate nonglare lighting in the home. Ask the client to install indoor strip or "runway" type of lighting to baseboards to help clients balance. Install motion-sensitive lighting that turns on automatically when the client gets out of bed to go to the bathroom.
- Provide medical identification bracelet for clients at risk for injury from diabetes, seizures, or other medical disorders.

Client/Family Teaching and Discharge Planning

- Teach the client and the family about the fall reduction measures that are being used to prevent falls (CDC, 2019).
- Providing education on safety guidelines to prevent falls is an important nursing intervention that should be completed as part of discharge planning (CDC, 2019)
- Teach the child and parent how to safely ambulate at home, including using safety measures such as handrails, avoid reaching for items or performing other tasks while walking.

REFERENCES

Centers for Disease Control and Prevention (CDC). (2021). *Violence prevention: Risks and protective factors*. Retrieved from https://www.cdc.gov/violenceprevention/childabuseandneglect/riskprotectivefactors.html. Accessed June 25, 2021.

Centers for Disease Control and Prevention (CDC). (2019). *Protect the ones you love: Child injuries are preventable*. Retrieved from https://www.cdc.gov/safechild/falls/. Accessed June 25, 2021.

Chaudhary, S., Figueroa, J., Shaikh, S., et al. (2018). Pediatric falls ages 0-4: Understanding demographics, mechanisms, and injury severities. *Injury Epidemiology, 5*(Suppl. 1), 7. https://doi.org/10.1186/s40621-018-0147-x.

DiGerolamo, K., & Davis, K. F. (2017). An integrative review of pediatric fall risk assessment tools. *Journal of Pediatric Nursing, 34*, 23–28.

Franjoine, M. R., Gunther, J. S., & Taylor, M. J. (2003). Pediatric balance scale: A modified version of the berg balance scale for the school-age child with mild to moderate motor impairment. *Pediatric Physical Therapy, 15*(2), 114–128. https://doi.org/10.1097/01.PEP.0000068117.48023.18.

Gebel, A., Lesinski, M., Behm, D. G., & Granacher, U. (2018). Effects and dose-response relationship of balance training on balance performance in youth: A systematic review and meta-analysis. *Sports Medicine, 48*(9), 2067–2089. https://doi.org/10.1007/s40279-018-0926-0.

Hill-Rodriquez, D., Messmer, P. R., Williams, P. D., Zeller, et al. (2009). The Humpty Dumpty falls scale: A case–control study. *Journal for Specialists in Pediatric Nursing, 14*(1), 22–32.

Kendrick, D., Young, B., Mason–Jones, A. J., et al. (2012). Home safety education and provision of safety equipment for injury prevention. *Cochrane Database of Systematic Reviews, 9*, CD005014. doi:10.1002/14651858.CD005014.pub3.

Maïano, C., Hue, O., Lepage, G., Morin, A., Tracey, D., & Moullec, G. (2019). Do exercise interventions improve balance for children and adolescents with down syndrome? A systematic review. *Physical Therapy, 99*(5), 507–518. https://doi.org/10.1093/ptj/pzz012.

Neiman, J., Rannie, M., Thrasher, J., Terry, K., & Kahn, M. G. (2011). Development, implementation, and evaluation of a comprehensive fall risk program. *Journal for Specialists in Pediatric Nursing, 16*(2), 130–139.

Phillips, D., Griffin, D., Przybylski, T., et al. (2018). Development and validation of a modified performance-oriented mobility assessment tool for assessing mobility in children with hypophosphatasia. *Journal of Pediatric Rehabilitation Medicine, 11*(3), 187–192.

Razmus, I., & Davis, D. (2012). The epidemiology of falls in hospitalized children. *Pediatric Nursing, 38*(1), 31–35.

F

Dysfunctional Family Processes Domain 7 Role relationship Class 2 Family relationships

Marina Martinez-Kratz, MS, RN, CNE

NANDA-I

Definition

Family functioning which fails to support the well-being of its members.

Defining Characteristics

Behavioral

Altered academic performance; altered attention; conflict avoidance; contradictory communication pattern; controlling communication pattern; criticizing others; decreased physical contact; denies problems; difficulty accepting a wide range of feelings; difficulty accepting help; difficulty adapting to change; difficulty dealing constructively with traumatic experiences; difficulty expressing a wide range of feelings; difficulty having fun; difficulty meeting the emotional needs of members; difficulty meeting the security needs of members difficulty meeting the spiritual needs of its members; difficulty receiving help appropriately; difficulty with intimate interpersonal relations; difficulty with life-cycle transition; enabling substance misuse pattern; escalating conflict; harsh self-judgment; immaturity; inadequate communication skills; inadequate knowledge about substance misuse; inappropriate anger expression; loss of independence; lying; maladaptive grieving; manipulation; nicotine addiction; orientation favors tension relief rather than goal attainment; paradoxical communication pattern; pattern of broken promises; power struggles; psychomotor agitation; rationalization; refuses to accept personal responsibility; refuses to get help; seeks affirmation; seeks approval; self-blame; social isolation; special occasions centered on substance misuse; stress-related physical illness; substance misuse; unreliable behavior; verbal abuse of children; verbal abuse of parent; verbal abuse of partner

Feelings

Anxiety; confuses love and pity; confusion; depressive symptoms; dissatisfaction; emotionally controlled by others; expresses anger; expresses distress; expresses embarrassment; expresses fear; expresses feeling abandoned; expresses feeling of failure; expresses feeling unloved; expresses frustration; expresses insecurity; expresses lingering resentment; expresses loneliness; expresses shame; expresses tension; hopelessness; hostility; loss; loss of identity; low self-esteem; mistrust of others; moodiness; powerlessness; rejection; reports feeling different from others; reports feeling emotionally isolated; reports feeling guilty; reports feeling misunderstood; repressed emotions; taking responsibility for substance misuser's behavior; unhappiness; worthlessness

Roles and Relationships

Altered family relations; altered role function; chronic family problems; closed communication system; conflict between partners; deterioration in family relations; diminished ability of family members to relate to each other for mutual growth and maturation; disrupted family rituals; disrupted family roles; family denial; family disorganization; inadequate family cohesiveness; inadequate family respect for autonomy of its members; inadequate family respect for individuality of its members; inadequate interpersonal relations skills; inconsistent parenting; ineffective communication with partner; neglects obligation to family member; pattern of rejection; perceived inadequate parental support; triangulating family relations

Related Factors

Addictive personality; inadequate problem-solving skills; ineffective coping strategies; perceived vulnerability

At-Risk Population

Economically disadvantaged families; families with history of resistance to treatment regimen; families with member with history of substance misuse; families with members with genetic predisposition to substance misuse

Associated Conditions

Depression; developmental disabilities; intimacy dysfunction; surgical procedures

NOC (Nursing Outcomes Classification)

Suggested NOC Outcomes

Family Coping; Family Functioning; Family Health Status; Substance Addiction Consequences

Example NOC Outcome with Indicators

Family Coping as evidenced by the following indicators: Confronts/manages family problems/Involves family members in decision-making. (Rate the outcome and indicators of **Family Coping:** 1 = never demonstrated, 2 = rarely demonstrated, 3 = sometimes demonstrated, 4 = often demonstrated, 5 = consistently demonstrated [see Section I].)

Client Outcomes

Family/Client Will (Specify Time Frame)

- State one way that alcoholism has affected the health of the family
- Identify three healthy coping behaviors that family members can use to facilitate a shift toward improved family functioning
- Express feelings
- Meet physical, psychosocial, and spiritual needs of members
- Seek appropriate assistance
- Participate in the development of the plan of care

NIC (Nursing Interventions Classification)

Suggested NIC Interventions

Family Process Maintenance; Substance Use Treatment

Example Activities—Family Process Maintenance

Identify effects of role changes on family process; Assist family members to use existing support mechanisms

Nursing Interventions and *Rationales*

- Refer to care plans for Interrupted **Family** Process, Ineffective **Denial,** and Defensive **Coping** for additional interventions.

- Assess family members for adverse childhood experiences (ACEs). EB: *A systematic review found a cumulative impact of ACEs with higher ACE counts being associated with higher health risks (Hughes, Hardcastle, & Bellis, 2016).*
- Acknowledge the range of emotions and feelings that may be experienced when the health status of a family member changes. EBN: *A study of family involvement during hospitalization found family health decreased with hospitalization (Misto, 2019).*
- Adopt a strength-oriented psychoeducational approach to assist family functioning. EBN: *A randomized controlled trial of a strength-oriented psychoeducational program on conventional stroke rehabilitation for family caregivers showed improvements in caregiving competence, problem-solving coping abilities, social support satisfaction, and family functioning (Cheng, Chair, & Chau, 2018).*
- Allow and encourage family members to assist in the client's treatment. EBN: *A convenience sample of 374 critical care nurses in the United States found that there are barriers to family caregiver involvement despite the positive outcomes for client and family (Hetland et al, 2018).*
- Support family members during emotional and conflict-type situations in the clinical setting. EBN: *A study found that bereaved parents identified nurses as "good" if the nurses looked out for the parents by providing emotional support, comfort, and using presence (Butler et al, 2018).*
- Screen clients for at-risk drinking during routine primary care visits and before surgery using the US Alcohol Use Disorders Identification Test (USAUDIT). EB: *The USAUDIT adapts the WHO AUDIT to 14-g standard drink and the US low-risk drinking guidelines. It provides greater accuracy in measuring alcohol consumption than the AUDIT-C (Higgins-Biddle & Babor, 2018).*
- ▲ Refer for family therapy and other family-oriented resources. EB: *Evidence-based interventions targeting affected family members have been shown to improve health outcomes for all family members, result in better addiction treatment outcomes, and prevent adolescent substance use (Ventura & Bagley, 2017).*
- ▲ Behavioral screening and intervention (BSI) should be integrated into all health care settings. Different terminology has evolved for screening, intervention, and referral for various behavioral issues. The five As—ask, advise, assess, assist, and arrange—apply to tobacco use. Screening, brief intervention, and referral to treatment (SBIRT) pertains to alcohol and drug use. EB: *The US Preventive Services Task Force recommends universal screening and intervention for tobacco use, excessive drinking, and depression. These services improve health outcomes, decrease health care costs, enhance public safety, and generate substantial return on investment (Babor, Del Boca, & Bray, 2017).*

Pediatric

- ▲ Encourage early intervention. When parental depression, childhood exposure to conflict and violence, and childhood experience with abuse and neglect coexist with parental substance abuse, their children are more likely to engage in increased teacher-rated unfavorable student behavioral problems. EB: *Early intervention with children of substance abusers (COSAs) is necessary to reach children while they are more receptive to treatment (Usher, McShane, & Dwyer, 2015).*
- Assess for the illness beliefs of the pediatric client as well as illness beliefs of the family. EB: *A systematic review of family-based interventions used for pediatric clients with functional somatic symptoms found that illness beliefs present important treatment targets (Hulgaard, Dehlholm-Lambertsen, & Rask, 2019).*
- Educate family members about available educational and support programs and encourage no/limited alcohol use in the home. EBN: *Both individual and multiperson interventions exert an influential role in family-based therapy for treatment of adolescent drug abuse (Gilligan et al, 2019).*
- Encourage adolescents to attend a 12-step program as needed. EB: *Wendt et al (2017) demonstrated that adolescents who attend 12-step groups after alcohol and other drug (AOD) treatment are more likely to remain abstinent and to avoid relapse.*
- Provide interactive school-based drug-prevention program to middle school students. EB: *A meta-analysis found support for the use of interactive school-based programs to prevent cannabis use among middle school students in North America (Lize et al, 2017).*

Geriatric

- Include the assessment of possible alcohol abuse when assessing older family members. EB: *Alcohol abuse and dependence in older people are important problems that frequently remain undetected by health services (Draper et al, 2015). The majority of older alcoholics are married, have low education levels, and do not belong to high social classes (Draper et al, 2015).*

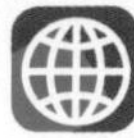

Multicultural

- Acknowledge racial/ethnic differences at the onset of care. **EBN:** *Acknowledgment of race/ethnicity issues will enhance communication, establish rapport, and promote treatment outcomes (Giger & Davidhizar, 2016).*
- Assess lesbian, gay, bisexual, or transgender (LGBTQ) youth for factors that contribute to family rejection. **EB:** *A recent study found that poverty and family instability are often precursors to family rejection and ultimately homelessness for LGBTQ youth (Robinson, 2018).*

Home Care

Note: In the community setting, alcoholism as a cause of dysfunctional family processes must be considered in two categories: (1) when the client suffers personally from the illness, and (2) when a significant other suffers from the illness, that is, the client is not the active alcoholic but may depend on the alcoholic for caregiving. The following considerations apply to both situations with appropriate adaptation for the circumstances.

- The previous interventions may be adapted for home care use.

F

Client/Family Teaching and Discharge Planning

- Provide education for the family. **EB:** *An intervention treatment focused on family education about bipolar disorder and the need for the caregiver health and mental health was found to reduce both caregiver and client depression scores (Perlick et al, 2018).*
- Facilitate participation in mutual help groups (MHGs). **EB:** *Client participation in 12-step groups is associated with lower substance use and problems over time (Humphreys et al, 2020).*

REFERENCES

Babor, T. F., Del Boca, F., & Bray, J. W. (2017). Screening, Brief Intervention and Referral to Treatment: Implications of SAMHSA's SBIRT initiative for substance abuse policy and practice. *Addiction*, *112*(Suppl. 2), 110–117. https://doi.org/10.1111/add.13675.

Butler, A. E., Copnell, B., & Hall, H. (2018). "Some were certainly better than others"—bereaved parents' judgements of healthcare providers in the paediatric intensive care unit: A grounded theory study. *Intensive and Critical Care Nursing*, *45*, 18–24. https://doi.org/10.1016/j.iccn.2017.12.003.

Cheng, H. Y., Chair, S. Y., & Chau, J. P. C. (2018). Effectiveness of a strength-oriented psychoeducation on caregiving competence, problem-solving abilities, psychosocial outcomes and physical health among family caregiver of stroke survivors: A randomised controlled trial. *International Journal of Nursing Studies*, *87*, 84–93. https://doi.org/10.1016/j.ijnurstu.2018.07.005.

Draper, B., Ridley, N., Johnco, C., et al. (2015). Screening for alcohol and substance use for older people in geriatric hospital and community health settings. *International Psychogeriatrics*, *27*(1), 157–166. https://doi.org/10.1017/S1041610214002014.

Giger, J., & Davidhizar, R. (2016). In *Transcultural nursing: Assessment and intervention* (7th ed.). St. Louis: Elsevier. https://doi.org/10.1111/add.13675.

Gilligan, C., Wolfenden, L., Foxcroft, D. R., et al. (2019). Family-based prevention programs for alcohol use in young people. *Cochrane Database of Systematic Reviews*, *3*(3), CD012287. https://doi.org/10.1002/14651858.CD012287.

Hetland, B., McAndrew, N., Perazzo, J., & Hickman, R. (2018). A qualitative study of factors that influence active family involvement with patient care in the ICU: Survey of critical care nurses. *Intensive and Critical Care Nursing*, *44*, 67–75. https://doi.org/10.1016/j.iccn.2017.08.008.

Higgins-Biddle, J. C., & Babor, T. F. (2018). A review of the Alcohol Use Disorders Identification Test (AUDIT), AUDIT-C, and USAUDIT for screening in the United States: Past issues and future directions. *American Journal of Drug and Alcohol Abuse*, *44*(6), 578–586. https://doi.org/10.1080/00952990.2018.1456545.

Hughes, K., Hardcastle, K., & Bellis, M. A. (2016). The impact of adverse childhood experiences on health: A systematic review and meta-analysis. *Injury Prevention*, *22*(Suppl. 2), A105. http://dx.doi.org/10.1136/injuryprev-2016-042156.286.

Hulgaard, D., Dehlholm-Lambertsen, G., & Rask, C. U. (2019). Family-based interventions for children and adolescents with functional somatic symptoms: A systematic review. *Journal of Family Therapy*, *41*(1), 4–28. https://doi.org/10.1111/1467-6427.12199.

Humphreys, K., Barreto, N. B., Alessi, S. M., et al. (2020). Impact of 12 step mutual help groups on drug use disorder patients across six clinical trials. *Drug and Alcohol Dependence*, *215*, 108213. https://doi.org/10.1016/j.drugalcdep.2020.108213.

Lize, S. E., Iachini, A. L., Tang, W., et al. (2017). A meta-analysis of the effectiveness of interactive middle school cannabis prevention programs. *Prevention Science*, *18*(1), 50–60. https://doi.org/10.1007/s11121-016-0723-7.

Misto, K. (2019). Family perceptions of family nursing in a magnet institution during acute hospitalizations of older adult patients. *Clinical Nursing Research*, *28*(5), 548–566. https://doi.org/10.1177/1054773817748400.

Perlick, D. A., Jackson, C., Grier, S., et al. (2018). Randomized trial comparing caregiver-only family-focused treatment to standard health education on the 6-month outcome of bipolar disorder. *Bipolar Disorders*, *20*(7), 622–633. https://doi.org/10.1111/bdi.12621.

Robinson, B. A. (2018). Conditional families and lesbian, gay, bisexual, transgender, and queer youth homelessness: Gender, sexuality, family instability, and rejection. *Journal of Marriage and Family*, *80*(2), 383–396. https://doi.org/10.1111/jomf.12466.

Usher, A. M., McShane, K. E., & Dwyer, C. (2015). A realist review of family-based interventions for children of substance abusing parents. *Systematic Reviews*, *4*, 177. https://doi.org/10.1186/s13643-015-0158-4.

Ventura, A. S., & Bagley, S. M. (2017). To improve substance use disorder prevention, treatment and recovery: Engage the family. *Journal of Addiction Medicine*, *11*(5), 339–341. https://doi.org/10.1097/ADM.0000000000000331.

Wendt, D. C., Hallgren, K. A., Daley, D. C., & Donovan, D. M. (2017). Predictors and outcomes of twelve-step sponsorship of stimulant users: Secondary analyses of a multisite randomized clinical trial. *Journal of Studies on Alcohol and Drugs*, *78*(2), 287–295. https://doi.org/10.15288/jsad.2017.78.287.

Interrupted Family Processes

Domain 7 Role relationship Class 2 Family relationships

Marina Martinez-Kratz, MS, RN, CNE

NANDA-I

Definition

Break in the continuity of family functioning which fails to support the well-being of its members.

Defining Characteristics

Altered affective responsiveness; altered communication pattern; altered family conflict resolution; altered family satisfaction; altered interpersonal relations; altered intimacy; altered participation in decision-making; altered participation in problem-solving; altered somatization; altered stress-reduction behavior; assigned tasks change; decreased emotional support availability; decreased mutual support; ineffective task completion; power alliance change; reports conflict with community resources; reports isolation from community resources; ritual change

Related Factors

Altered community interaction; altered family role; difficulty dealing with power shift among family members

At-Risk Population

Families with altered finances; families with altered social status; families with member experiencing developmental crisis; families with member experiencing developmental transition; families with member experiencing situational transition

Associated Conditions

Altered health status

NOC (Nursing Outcomes Classification)

Suggested NOC Outcomes

Family Coping; Family Functioning; Family Normalization; Psychosocial Adjustment: Life Change, Role Performance

Example NOC Outcome with Indicators

Family Coping as evidenced by the following indicators: Confronts/manages family problems/Involves family members in decision-making. (Rate the outcome and indicators of **Family Coping:** 1 = never demonstrated, 2 = rarely demonstrated, 3 = sometimes demonstrated, 4 = often demonstrated, 5 = consistently demonstrated [see Section I].)

Client Outcomes

Family/Client Will (Specify Time Frame)

- Express feelings (family)
- Identify ways to cope effectively and use appropriate support systems (family)
- Treat impaired family member as normally as possible to avoid overdependence (family)
- Meet physical, psychosocial, and spiritual needs of members or seek appropriate assistance (family)
- Demonstrate knowledge of illness or injury, treatment modalities, and prognosis (family)
- Participate in the development of the plan of care to the best of ability (significant person)

NIC (Nursing Interventions Classification)

Suggested NIC Interventions

Family Integrity Promotion; Family Process Maintenance; Normalization Promotion

F

Example NIC Activities—Family Integrity Promotion

Collaborate with family in problem-solving and decision-making; Counsel family members on additional effective coping skills for their own use

Nursing Interventions and *Rationales*

F

- Recognize informal roles in medical decision-making by family members. EBN: *Informal roles emerge in critical situations to help fill the gaps in how family members respond to the challenge of end-of-life decision-making (Connor & Chase, 2015).*
- Acknowledge the range of emotions and feelings that may be experienced when the health status of a family member changes. EBN: *A study of family involvement during hospitalization found that family health decreased with hospitalization (Misto, 2017).*
- Adopt a strength-oriented psychoeducational approach to assist family functioning. EBN: *A randomized controlled trial of a strength-oriented psychoeducational program on conventional stroke rehabilitation for family caregivers showed improvements in caregiving competence, problem-solving coping abilities, social support satisfaction, and family functioning (Cheng, Chair, & Chau, 2018).*
- Establish relationships among clients, their families, and health care professionals. EBN: *A progressively engaging approach to relationships with clients and their families emphasizes trust and reciprocity, which supports joint decision-making with nurses in acute care settings (Segaric & Hall, 2015).*
- Encourage family to visit the client; adjust visiting hours to accommodate the family's schedule. EBN: *A 10-month quality improvement collaborative was implemented to address person- and family-centered care engagement initiatives with open visitation, integration of families on rounds, establishing a client and family advisory committee, and using client and family diaries. After the implementation, family members reported statistically significant increases in overall family satisfaction, satisfaction with decision-making, and satisfaction with quality of care (Kleinpell et al, 2019).*
- Allow and encourage family members to assist in the client's treatment. EBN: *A convenience sample of 374 critical care nurses in the United States found that there are barriers to family caregiver involvement despite the positive outcomes for client and family (Hetland et al, 2018).*
- Support family members during emotional and conflict-type situations in the clinical setting. EBN: *A study found that bereaved parents identified nurses as "good" if the nurses looked out for the parents by providing emotional support, comfort, and using presence (Butler et al, 2018).*
- Anticipate and implement family reunification efforts after a disaster. EB: *Family reunification after disasters should be prioritized and included in plans at all emergency response levels. A family reunification tool can be accessed at https://www.aap.org/en-us/Documents/AAP-Reunification-Toolkit.pdf (American Academy of Pediatrics, 2018).*
- Refer to the care plan Readiness for Enhanced **Family** Processes for additional interventions.

Pediatric

- Carefully assess potential for reunifying children placed in foster care with their birth parents. EB: *Reunifying children placed in foster care with their birth parents is a primary goal of the child welfare system (Orsi et al, 2018).*
- Assess for the influence of family socioeconomic status on family processes. EB: *A study found that familial socioeconomic status was a significant factor in family processes and child behavior (Hosokawa & Katsura, 2017).*
- Provide prebirth risk assessments to identify prebirth and postbirth supports for high-risk pregnant women. EB: *Prebirth risk assessment is a process by which circumstances affecting an unborn child can be identified and support for mother and infant embedded into care (Harnett et al, 2018).*
- Provide parents with both general information and professional support by family-centered early childhood intervention services to their families. EB: *Providing families with general information in addition to specialized information about their children is most important to empower parents and increase family resiliency (Frantz et al, 2018).*
- Encourage and support parents/family to assist in client's care. EBN: *A study found that parental involvement in their child's care can improve the child's pain experience, reduce parental anxiety, and increase parents' satisfaction in care (Vasey et al, 2019).*

- Assess military families for the influence of deployment on family functioning. EB: *A study of families with a service member concurrently deployed at the time of a child neglect incident were at higher risk for failure to provide physical needs, lack of supervision, and educational neglect (Cozza et al, 2018).*
- ▲ Refer parents and other primary caregivers to a mindfulness-based stress reduction (MBSR) program. EB: *A systematic review found that caregivers, children, and adults who received MBSR all reported significant gains in subjective well-being immediately after the intervention (Hartley, Dorstyn, & Due, 2019).*

Geriatric

- Encourage family members to be involved in the care of relatives who are in residential care settings. EBN: *Family involvement and inclusion in residential long-term care represents person-centered care (Puurveen, Baumbusch, & Gandhi, 2018).*
- ▲ Refer for Family Life Review (FLR) therapy. EB: *A study of older adults who participated in FLR therapy found that it facilitated positive connections, enhanced existing relationships, and promoted self-acceptance (O'Hora & Roberto, 2018).*
- ▲ Refer family for counseling with a psychotherapist who is knowledgeable about gerontology.
- Refer to care plan for Readiness for Enhanced **Family** Processes for additional interventions.

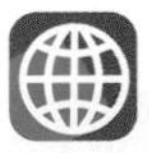

Multicultural

- Assess lesbian, gay, bisexual, transgender, and queer (LGBTQ) youth for factors that contribute to family rejection. EB: *A recent study found that poverty and family instability are often precursors to family rejection and ultimately homelessness for LGBTQ youth (Robinson, 2018a).*
- Refer to the care plan Readiness for Enhanced **Family** Processes for additional interventions.

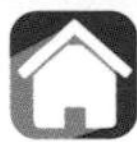

Home Care

- The nursing interventions described in the care plan for Compromised Family **Coping** should be used in the home environment with adaptations as necessary.
- Encourage family members to find meaning in life with a serious illness. EB: *A study found that families dealing with chronic illness move through the process of healing and eventually shift the focus away from illness and toward living (Robinson, 2018b).*

Client/Family Teaching and Discharge Planning

- Refer to Client/Family Teaching and Discharge Planning in Compromised Family **Coping** and Readiness for Enhanced Family **Coping** for suggestions that may be used with minor adaptations.

F

REFERENCES

American Academy of Pediatrics. (2018). *Family reunification following disasters: Planning tool for health care facilities.* American Academy of Pediatrics. https://www.aap.org/en-us/Documents/AAP-Reunification-Toolkit.pdf. Accessed June 11, 2021.

Butler, A. E., Copnell, B., & Hall, H. (2018). "Some were certainly better than others"—bereaved parents' judgements of healthcare providers in the paediatric intensive care unit: A grounded theory study. *Intensive and Critical Care Nursing, 45*, 18–24. https://doi.org/10.1016/j.iccn.2017.12.003.

Cheng, H. Y., Chair, S. Y., & Chau, J. P. C. (2018). Effectiveness of a strength-oriented psychoeducation on caregiving competence, problem-solving abilities, psychosocial outcomes and physical health among family caregiver of stroke survivors: A randomised controlled trial. *International Journal of Nursing Studies, 87*, 84–93. https://doi.org/10.1016/j.ijnurstu.2018.07.005.

Connor, N. E., & Chase, S. K. (2015). Decisions and caregiving: End of life among blacks from the perspective of informal caregivers and decision makers. *American Journal of Hospice and Palliative Care, 32*(4), 454–463. https://doi.org/10.1177/1049909114529013.

Cozza, S. J., Whaley, G. L., Fisher, J. E., et al. (2018). Deployment status and child neglect types in the U.S. Army. *Child Maltreatment, 23*(1), 25–33. https://doi.org/10.1177/1077559517717638.

Frantz, R., Hansen, S., Squires, J., & Machalicek, W. (2018). Families as partners: Supporting family resiliency through early intervention. *Infants & Young Children, 31*(1), 3–19.

Harnett, P. H., Barlow, J., Coe, C., Newbold, C., & Dawe, S. (2018). Assessing capacity to change in high-risk pregnant women: A pilot study. *Child Abuse Review, 27*(1), 72–84. https://doi.org/10.1002/car.2491.

Hartley, M., Dorstyn, D., & Due, C. (2019). Mindfulness for children and adults with autism spectrum disorder and their caregivers: A meta-analysis. *Journal of Autism and Developmental Disorders, 49*, 4306–4319. https://doi.org/10.1007/s10803-019-04145-3.

Hetland, B., McAndrew, N., Perazzo, J., & Hickman, R. (2018). A qualitative study of factors that influence active family involvement with patient care in the ICU: Survey of critical care nurses. *Intensive and Critical Care Nursing, 44*, 67–75. https://doi.org/10.1016/j.iccn.2017.08.008.

Hosokawa, R., & Katsura, T. (2017). A longitudinal study of socioeconomic status, family processes, and child adjustment from preschool until early elementary school: The role of social competence. *Child and Adolescent Psychiatry and Mental Health, 11*, 62. https://doi.org/10.1186/s13034-017-0206-z.

Kleinpell, R., Zimmerman, J., Vermoch, K., et al. (2019). Promoting family engagement in the ICU: Experience from a national collaborative of 63 ICUs. *Critical Care Medicine, 47*(12), 1692–1698. https://doi.org/10.1097/CCM.0000000000004009.

Misto, K. (2017). Family perceptions of family nursing in a magnet institution during acute hospitalizations of older adult patients. *Clinical Nursing Research, 28*(5), 548–566. https://doi.org/10.1177/1054773817748400.

O'Hora, K. A., & Roberto, K. A. (2018). Navigating emotions and relationship dynamics: Family life review as a clinical tool for older adults during a relocation transition into an assisted living facility. *Aging & Mental Health, 23*(4), 404–410. https://doi.org/10.1080/13607863.2017.1423028.

Orsi, R., Lee, C., Winokur, M., & Pearson, A. (2018). Who's been served and how? Permanency outcomes for children and youth involved in child welfare and youth corrections. *Youth Violence and Juvenile Justice, 16*(1), 3–17. https://doi.org/10.1177/1541204017721614.

Puurveen, G., Baumbusch, J., & Gandhi, P. (2018). From family involvement to family inclusion in nursing home settings: A critical interpretive synthesis. *Journal of Family Nursing, 24*(1), 60–85. https://doi.org/10.1177/1074840718754314.

Robinson, B. A. (2018a). Conditional families and lesbian, gay, bisexual, transgender, and queer youth homelessness: Gender, sexuality, family instability, and rejection. *Journal of Marriage and Family, 80*(2), 383–396. https://doi.org/10.1111/jomf.12466.

Robinson, C. A. (2018b). Families living well with chronic illness: The healing process of moving on. *Qualitative Health Research, 27*(4), 447–461.

Segaric, C. A., & Hall, W. A. (2015). Progressively engaging: Constructing nurse, patient, and family relationships in acute care settings. *Journal of Family Nursing, 21*(1), 35–56. https://doi.org/10.1177/1074840714564787.

Vasey, J., Smith, J., Kirshbaum, M. N., & Chirema, K. (2019). Tokenism or true partnership: Parental involvement in a child's acute pain care. *Journal of Clinical Nursing, 28*(9–10), 1491–1505. https://doi.org/10.1111/jocn.14747.

F

Readiness for Enhanced Family Processes

Domain 7 Role relationship Class 2 Family relationships

Marina Martinez-Kratz, MS, RN, CNE

NANDA-I

Definition

A pattern of family functioning to support the well-being of members, which can be strengthened.

Defining Characteristics

Expresses desire to enhance balance between personal autonomy and family cohesiveness; expresses desire to enhance communication pattern; expresses desire to enhance energy level of family to support activities of daily living; expresses desire to enhance family adaptation to change; expresses desire to enhance family dynamics; expresses desire to enhance family psychological resilience; expresses desire to enhance growth of family members; expresses desire to enhance interdependence with community; expresses desire to enhance maintenance of boundaries between family members; expresses desire to enhance respect for family members; expresses desire to enhance safety of family members

NOC (Nursing Outcomes Classification)

Suggested NOC Outcomes

Family Coping; Health-Promoting Behavior; Health-Seeking Behavior; Parent-Infant Attachment; Parenting Performance

Example NOC Outcome with Indicators

Family Coping as evidenced by the following indicators: Confronts/Manages family problems/Obtains family assistance. (Rate the outcome and indicators of **Family Coping:** 1 = never demonstrated, 2 = rarely demonstrated, 3 = sometimes demonstrated, 4 = often demonstrated, 5 = consistently demonstrated [see Section I].)

Client Outcomes

Family/Client Will (Specify Time Frame)

- Identify ways to cope effectively and use appropriate support systems (family)
- Meet physical, psychosocial, and spiritual needs of members or seek appropriate assistance (family)
- Demonstrate knowledge of potential environmental, lifestyle, and genetic risks to health and use appropriate measures to decrease possibility of risk (family)

- Focus on wellness, disease prevention, and maintenance (family and individual)
- Seek balance among exercise, work, leisure, rest, and nutrition (family and individual)

NIC (Nursing Interventions Classification)

Suggested NIC Interventions

Coping Enhancement; Decision-Making Support; Family Integrity Promotion; Family Involvement Promotion; Family Mobilization; Family Process Maintenance; Parent Education: Adolescent; Childrearing Family; Risk Identification; Role Enhancement

Example NIC Activities—Risk Identification

Determine availability and quality of resources (e.g., psychological, financial, education level, family and other social, and community)

F

Nursing Interventions and *Rationales*

- Assess the structure, resources, and coping abilities of families and use these assessments in selecting interventions and formulating care plans. EBN: *It is critical to understand the resiliency and coping capabilities of families; the use of established assessment instruments (e.g., Family Assessment Device, Family Assessment Measure) can provide insight into family dynamics, coping styles, and resources of family systems (Sawin, 2016).*
- Acknowledge, assess, and support the spiritual needs and resources of families and clients. EB/EBN: *Spirituality has been found to be an important, yet often overlooked, coping resource for families and clients during illness and recovery (Hodge, 2015; Prouty et al, 2016).*
- Develop, provide, and encourage family members to use counseling services and interventions. EBN: *Family-centered counseling interventions have been shown to be effective, particularly in situations regarding serious illness and difficult family decisions (Creasy et al, 2015).*
- Consider the use of family-centered theory as the conceptual foundation to help guide interventions. EBN: *Working closely with pediatric clients and their families helps the nurse to plan care with the family in mind (Cady et al, 2015).*
- Establish rapport with families and empower their decision-making through effective communication and person- and family-centered care. EBN: *Effective communication and person- and family-centered care approaches can help to establish rapport, personalize treatment plans, and empower families in their caregiving activities and decision-making capacities (Mitchell et al, 2016; Coombs et al, 2017).*
- Provide family members with educational and skill-building interventions to alleviate caregiving stress and to facilitate adherence to prescribed plans of care. EBN: *The provision of psychoeducational and supportive interventions may enable family members to gain a sense of control in the caregiving role and to become more comfortable in providing care and making informed decisions (Dockham et al, 2016).*

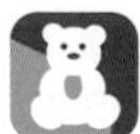

Pediatric

- Provide educational and supportive interventions for families caring for children with illness and disability. EBN: *Providing information, training parents in care management, and offering supportive programs can reduce stress levels in parents and lead to better outcomes for children (Golfenshtein, Srulovici, & Deatrick, 2016).*
- Encourage participation in virtual support groups. EB: *A study found that foster families viewed the virtual support group as usable and expressed satisfaction with group membership (Miller et al, 2019).*
- Encourage families with children and adolescents to have family meals. EB: *Research found that dinnertime rituals can potentially moderate the effects of parenting stress on child outcomes (Yoon et al, 2015).*

Geriatric

- Provide educational and therapeutic interventions to family caregivers that focus on knowledge and skill building. EBN: *Psychoeducational interventions that are accessible and tailored to individual needs can be highly valued and useful to family caregivers (Bakas, McCarthy, & Miller, 2017).*
- Encourage use of information and communications technologies (ICT) for social networking; social integration; and social engagement with friends, children, and relatives. EB: *Older adult use of ICT was*

associated with themes of connection, self-worth/esteem and personal development, productivity, occupation, self-sufficiency, being in control, and enjoyment in older adult ICT users (Hasan & Linger, 2016).

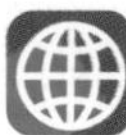

Multicultural

- Understand and incorporate cultural differences into interventions to enhance the impact of family interventions. EB: *Tailoring interventions to the customs, beliefs, preferences, and strengths of specific groups may increase effectiveness (McCalman et al, 2017).*
- With the client's consent, facilitate a group meeting for family members to discuss how the family is functioning. EBN: *Communication with the client and the family encourages discussion about the wants and needs of each individual and keeps each informed of what is occurring with the client (Kisvetrová et al, 2016).*
- Facilitate modeling and role playing for the client and family regarding healthy ways to start a discussion about the client's prognosis. EBN: *It is helpful to practice communication skills in a safe environment before trying them in a real-life situation (Waite & McKinney, 2016).*
- Encourage family mealtimes. EB: *Encouraging family mealtimes enhances the health and well-being of the family and can decrease parental stress (Yoon et al, 2015).*

Home Care

- The previous nursing interventions should be used in the home environment with adaptations as necessary.
- ▲ Encourage participation in virtual support groups to family caregivers. EB: *A systematic review of virtual support groups for informal caregivers of dementia found that participants identified many participation benefits (Armstrong & Alliance, 2019).*

Client/Family Teaching and Discharge Planning

- Refer to Client/Family Teaching and Discharge Planning for Readiness for Enhanced Family **Coping** for suggestions that may be used with minor adaptations.

F

REFERENCES

Armstrong, M. J., & Alliance, S. (2019). Virtual support groups for informal caregivers of individuals with dementia: A scoping review. *Alzheimer Disease and Associated Disorders*, *33*(4), 362–369. https://doi.org/10.1097/WAD.0000000000000349.

Bakas, T., McCarthy, M., & Miller, E. T. (2017). Update on the state of evidence for stroke family caregiver and dyad interventions. *Stroke*, *48*(5), e122–e125. https://doi.org/10.1161/STROKEAHA.117.016052.

Cady, R. G., Looman, W. S., Lindeke, L. L., et al. (2015). Pediatric care coordination: Lessons learned and future priorities. *Online Journal of Issues in Nursing*, *20*(3), 3. https://doi.org/10.3912/OJIN.Vol20No03Man03.

Coombs, M., Puntillo, K. A., Franck, L. S., et al. (2017). Implementing the SCCM Family-Centered Care Guidelines in critical care nursing practice. *AACN Advanced Critical Care*, *28*(2), 138–147. https://doi.org/10.4037/aacnacc2017766.

Creasy, K. R., Lutz, B. J., Young, M. E., & Stacciarini, J. M. R. (2015). Clinical implications of family-centered care in stroke rehabilitation. *Rehabilitation Nursing*, *40*(6), 349–359. https://doi.org/10.1002/rnj.188.

Dockham, B., Schafenacker, A., Yoon, H., et al. (2016). Implementation of a psychosocial program for cancer survivors and family caregivers at a cancer support community affiliate: A pilot effectiveness study. *Cancer Nursing*, *39*(3), 169–180. https://doi.org/10.1097/NCC.0000000000000311.

Golfenshtein, N., Srulovici, E., & Deatrick, J. A. (2016). Interventions for reducing parenting stress in families with pediatric conditions: An integrative review. *Journal of Family Nursing*, *22*(4), 460–492. https://doi.org/10.1177/1074840716676083.

Hasan, H., & Linger, H. (2016). Enhancing the wellbeing of the elderly: Social use of digital technologies in aged care. *Educational Gerontology*, *42*(11), 749–757. https://doi.org/10.1080/03601277.2016.1205425.

Hodge, D. R. (2015). Administering a two-stage spiritual assessment in healthcare settings: A necessary component of ethical and effective care. *Journal of Nursing Management*, *23*(1), 27–38. https://doi.org/10.1111/jonm.12078.

Kisvetrová, H., Školoudík, D., Joanovič, E., Konečná, J., & Mikšová, Z. (2016). Dying care interventions in the intensive care unit. *Journal of Nursing Scholarship*, *48*(2), 139–146. https://doi.org/10.1111/jnu.12191.

McCalman, J., Heyeres, M., Campbell, S., et al. (2017). Family-centred interventions by primary healthcare services for Indigenous early childhood well-being in Australia, Canada, New Zealand, and the United States: A systematic scoping review. *BMC Pregnancy and Childbirth*, *17*(1), 71. https://doi.org/10.1186/s12884-017-1247-2.

Miller, J. J., Cooley, M., Niu, C., et al. (2019). Virtual support groups among adoptive parents: Ideal for information seeking? *Journal of Technology in Human Services*, *37*(4), 347–361.

Mitchell, M. L., Coyer, F., Kean, S., Stone, R., Murfield, J., & Dwan, T. (2016). Patient, family-centred care interventions within the adult ICU setting: An integrative review. *Australian Critical Care*, *29*(4), 179–193. https://doi.org/10.1080/15228835.2019.1637320.

Prouty, A. M., Fischer, J., Purdom, A., Cobos, E., & Helmeke, K. B. (2016). Spiritual coping: A gateway to enhancing family communication during cancer treatment. *Journal of Religion and Health*, *55*(1), 269–287. https://doi.org/10.1007/s10943-015-0108-4.

Sawin, K. J. (2016). Measurement in family nursing: Established instruments and new directions. *Journal of Family Nursing*, *22*(3), 287–297. https://doi.org/10.1177/1074840716656038.

Waite, R., & McKinney, N. S. (2016). Capital we must develop: Emotional competence educating pre-licensure nursing students. *Nursing Education Perspectives*, *37*(2), 101–103. https://doi.org/10.5480/14-1343.

Yoon, Y., Newkirk, K., & Perry-Jenkins, M. (2015). Parenting stress, dinnertime rituals, and child and child well-being in working-class families. *Family Relations*, *64*(1), 93–107. https://doi.org/10.1111/fare.12107.

Fatigue Domain 4 Activity/rest Class 3 Energy balance

Barbara A. Given, PhD, RN, FAAN and David M. Wikstrom, BSN, RN, CMSRN

NANDA-I

Definition

An overwhelming sustained sense of exhaustion and decreased capacity for physical and mental work at the usual level.

Defining Characteristics

Altered attention; apathy; decreased aerobic capacity; decreased gait velocity; difficulty maintaining usual physical activity; difficulty maintaining usual routines; disinterested in surroundings; drowsiness; expresses altered libido; expresses demoralization; expresses frustration; expresses lack of energy; expresses nonrelief through usual energy-recovery strategies; expresses tiredness; expresses weakness; inadequate role performance; increased physical symptoms; increased rest requirement; insufficient physical endurance; introspection; lethargy; tiredness

Related Factors

Altered sleep-wake cycle; anxiety; depressive symptoms; environmental constraints; increased mental exertion; increased physical exertion; malnutrition; nonstimulating lifestyle; pain; physical deconditioning; stressors

At-Risk Population

Individuals exposed to negative life event; individuals with demanding occupation; pregnant women; women experiencing labor

Associated Conditions

Anemia; chemotherapy; chronic disease; chronic inflammation; dementia; fibromyalgia; hypothalamus-pituitary-adrenal axis dysregulation; myasthenia gravis; neoplasms; radiotherapy; stroke

NOC (Nursing Outcomes Classification)

Suggested NOC Outcomes

Concentration; Endurance; Energy Conservation/Restoration; Nutritional Status; Energy; Vitality

Example NOC Outcome with Indicators

Endurance as evidenced by the following indicators: Performance of daily activities/Energy restored after rest/Blood oxygen level with activity/Muscle endurance. (Rate the outcome and indicators of **Endurance:** 1 = severely compromised, 2 = substantially compromised, 3 = moderately compromised, 4 = mildly compromised, 5 = not compromised [see Section I].)

Client Outcomes

Client Will (Specify Time Frame)

- Identify potential etiology of fatigue
- Identify potential factors that precipitate, aggravate, and relieve fatigue
- Describe ways to assess and monitor patterns of fatigue over time (e.g., within a day, a few days, a week, a month)
- Describe ways in which fatigue affects the ability to accomplish activities of daily living (ADLs)
- Verbalize increased energy and improved vitality
- Explain energy conservation plan to offset fatigue
- Verbalize ability and capacity to concentrate and make decisions
- Verbalize strategies for energy restorative activities

NIC (Nursing Interventions Classification)

Suggested NIC Intervention

Energy management, including both conservation and restoration; conservation interventions are targeted at preserving an individual's energy, whereas restorative interventions are intended to reestablish vitality and energy

Example NIC Activities—Energy Management

Assess client's physiological and psychological status for deficits resulting in fatigue within the context of age, development, and stage of disease or illness. Determine client's/significant other's perception of causes of client's fatigue and factors that contribute to the relief. Assessing the pattern of reoccurrence and severity within a 24-hour period can be used to recommend usual daily activity.

F

Nursing Interventions and *Rationales*

- Assess severity of fatigue on a scale of 0 to 10 (average fatigue, worst and best levels); assess frequency of fatigue (number of days per week and time of day), activities and symptoms associated with increased fatigue (e.g., pain), activities that relieve, ability to perform ADLs and instrumental ADLs, interference with social and role function, times of the day for increased energy, ability to concentrate, mood, usual pattern of physical activity, and interference with sleep cycles. Consider use of an instrument such as the Profile of Mood State Short Form Fatigue Subscale (PROMIS), the Multidimensional Assessment of Fatigue, the Lee Fatigue Scale, the Fatigue Symptom Inventory, the Multidimensional Fatigue Inventory, the HIV-Related Fatigue Scale, the Brief Fatigue Inventory, Short Form Vitality Subscale, Fatigue Impact Scale, Fatigue Assessment Instrument, or Nottingham of Chronic Illness Therapy Fatigue Scale, Fatigue Severity Scale. EBN: *These assessments have all been shown to have good internal reliability. The Fatigue Severity Scale (9 items), Modified Fatigue Impact Scale (21 items), Brief Fatigue Inventory (9 items), and PROMIS Fatigue Scale (7 items) are short with good psychometric properties, making them clinically useful. These measures have shown the ability to detect changes in fatigue over time and the PROMIS measures appear to be the most commonly used and assess a range of symptoms from mild to overwhelming, debilitating, and sustained sense of exhaustion (Gibbons et al, 2017). PROMIS is a validated and effective survey for measuring fatigue in cancer clients (Jensen et al, 2017). Varying populations may respond differently to instruments and there are a number of scales for specific disease such as stroke, inflammatory bowel disease, rheumatoid arthritis, multiple sclerosis, Parkinson's disease, and sleep disorders (Matura et al, 2018). Poststroke clients may have severe fatigue without depression (Drummond et al, 2017).*
- Evaluate adequacy of nutrition and sleep hygiene (weight loss, anorexia, napping throughout the day, inability to fall asleep or stay asleep). Encourage the client to get adequate rest, limit naps (particularly in the late afternoon or evening), use a routine sleep/wake schedule, plan and prioritize for daily activities as tolerated, allow exposure to bright light during daytime hours, use relaxation techniques before bedtime such as meditation, music, or guided imagery (Dikmen & Terzioglu, 2019), avoid caffeine in the late afternoon or evening, and eat a well-balanced diet that includes fresh fruits, vegetables, and lean meats. Mindfulness interventions also result in improved sleep quality (Gok Metin et al, 2019). EBN: *Dysfunction in sleep (too much, too little, or too many interruptions) can aggravate fatigue (Silva et al, 2020).*
- Refer to **Imbalanced Nutrition: Less Than Body Requirements** or **Insomnia** if appropriate.
- Evaluate fluid status and assess for dehydration. Encourage at least eight glasses of water a day. Avoid caffeine, which can cause further dehydration. EB: *Dehydration may result in fatigue in acute stroke clients (Bahouth et al, 2018). Older adults and those with other medical conditions are more susceptible to dehydration, often due to symptoms such as diarrhea and vomiting or from treatments such as diuretics (Paulis et al, 2018).*

▲ Collaborate with the primary provider to identify physiological and/or psychological causes of fatigue that could be treated, such as nutritional deficit, pain, electrolyte imbalance (e.g., altered potassium levels, vitamin D deficiency), dehydration, thyroid disorders, anemia, arthritis, depression, anxiety, sleep disturbances (insomnia/sleep deprivation), acute or chronic infection, medication use or side effects, alcohol use/abuse, metabolic disorders (diabetes), or a preexisting comorbidity or disease (multiple sclerosis, cancer or cancer treatment, respiratory disease, fibromyalgia, cardiac disease, renal disease, Parkinson's disease). EB/EBN: *Vitamin D deficiency has been linked to fatigue in older clients (Pennisi et al, 2019). Fatigue is also related to psychological distress, medication side effects, and nutritional deficit (due to change in taste or cancer affecting swallowing or the digestive tract) (Baguley et al, 2019) and from chemotherapy and radiotherapy in cancer (Kolak et al, 2017). Fatigue also negatively affects a client's quality of life (Matura et al, 2018). Tumor necrosis and recently identified proinflammatory cytokines are associated with fatigue (Kolak et al, 2017; Matura et al, 2018).*

- ▲ Work with the primary care or specialty provider to determine if the client has chronic fatigue syndrome. Chronic fatigue syndrome is unexplained fatigue lasting 6 months or longer that is not associated with a diagnosed physical or psychological condition but may include muscle pain, memory problems, headaches, sleep problems, joint pain, and diarrhea (Milrad et al, 2018). EB: *Proinflammatory cytokines may contribute to these symptoms (Montoya et al, 2017). Studies also suggest there is a genetic component to chronic fatigue syndrome (Wang et al, 2017).*
- ● Encourage clients to express feelings, attribution of cause, and behaviors about fatigue, including potential causes of fatigue, and interventions that they use to alleviate or moderate the fatigue. Such interventions could include setting small, easily achieved short-term goals and developing energy management and energy conservation techniques; use active listening techniques to help identify sources of hope. In addition, help them determine the time of day when they have the most energy to do important things. Assess clients' level of motivation and willingness to adopt new behaviors or change behaviors that can improve symptoms of fatigue. EBN/EB: *Cognitive behavioral therapy (CBT) and self-efficacy interventions have been shown to be effective in reducing fatigue (Poort et al, 2020). Education and counseling have also been shown to be effective for identifying strategies to manage fatigue (Savina & Zaydiner, 2019).*
- ● Encourage the client to keep a journal of activities (or record using one of the many apps available) that contribute to symptoms of fatigue, patterns of symptoms across days/weeks/months, and feelings, including how fatigue affects the client's normal daily activities and roles. Have client identify the activities that contribute the most to fatigue. EB: *Clients may have physical activity enhanced by self-guided nutrition and physical activity (Henson et al, 2020) using technology that results in improvement of fatigue (Kiss et al, 2019).*
- ● Assist the client to identify sources of support and prioritize essential and nonessential tasks to determine which tasks need to be completed and which can be delegated and to whom. Give the client permission to limit or change or remove social and role demands if needed (e.g., switch to part-time employment, simplify meal preparation, give up activities for a short period, hire cleaning service). EBN: *Psychoeducational mindfulness, or behavioral therapy strategies, that include fatigue education, self-care, coping techniques, and activity management have been shown to be effective in reducing cancer-related fatigue (Corbett et al, 2019). Emotional support has been linked to decreased level of physical symptoms, including fatigue, for heart failure clients (Heo et al, 2018).*
- ▲ Collaborate with the primary provider regarding the appropriateness of referrals to physical therapy for carefully monitored and prescribed aerobic exercise program. EBN: *Physical activity and exercise, particularly aerobic exercise, can reduce cancer-related fatigue (Poort et al, 2020).*
- ● Encourage the client to use complementary and alternative therapies such as relaxation, meditation, and mindfulness to support other strategies. EB: *Mindfulness–CBT has exhibited improved outcomes for those experiencing cancer-related fatigue (Corbett et al, 2019).*
- ▲ Refer the client to diagnosis-appropriate support groups such as the American Parkinson Disease Association, National Chronic Fatigue Syndrome Association, National Parkinson Foundation, PatientsLikeMe, National Multiple Sclerosis Society, American Heart Association, American Cancer Society, National Comprehensive Cancer Network, Chronic Myalgic Encephalomyelitis, and Chronic Fatigue Society.
- ▲ For an individual with cardiac disease, recognize that fatigue is common with myocardial infarction, congestive heart failure, or chronic cardiac insufficiency (Matura et al, 2018). Refer to cardiac rehabilitation for a carefully prescribed and monitored exercise and rehabilitation program.
- ● If fatigue is associated with cancer or cancer-related treatment, assess for other symptoms that may increase fatigue (e.g., pain, insomnia, anemia, emotional distress, electrolyte imbalance [nausea, vomiting, diarrhea], or depression). EB: *There is evidence to support that depressive symptoms, anxiety, distress, sleep disturbances, lower physical activity levels, pain, difficulty coping, dysfunctional cognitions, and social support are related to fatigue and should be targets for intervention (Abrahams et al, 2018).*

- ▲ Refer the client for CBT to improve coping and self-management of fatigue. EB: *Fatigue associated with rheumatoid arthritis can affect a client's quality of life and coping. CBT has been shown to be effective in improving fatigue self-management, coping, and fatigue severity. CBT involves using self-management skills such as problem-solving to improve self-efficacy while achieving, priority planning, and pacing activities (Poort et al, 2020).*
- ▲ Collaborate with primary provider to identify attentional fatigue, which may manifest itself as the inability to direct attention necessary to perform usual activities. Attentional fatigue is associated with sleep disturbances, depressive symptoms, anxiety, and psychosocial stressors and can lead to inability to concentrate, plan goals, control emotions, or engage in social interactions. EBN: *A meta-analysis reported that persons with chronic fatigue syndrome had deficits in the areas of attention, memory, and reaction time (Geraghty et al, 2019).*
- ▲ Collaborate with primary providers to identify potential pharmacological treatment for fatigue. EBN: *Pharmacological treatment to reduce inflammation has been shown to reduce fatigue (Matura et al, 2018). Pharmacological therapy has not been shown to be effective in reducing fatigue in cancer clients (Mustian et al, 2017).*

Geriatric

- ● Evaluate fatigue in geriatric clients routinely, particularly in clients with limited physical function and lower levels of social support. EB: *Chronic conditions related to age can contribute to fatigue in the geriatric client, such as cancer, dyspnea, anemia, multiple medication usage and side effects from medication, depression, insomnia, nutritional deficiencies, electrolyte imbalance, and comorbidities and cardiac disease (Matura et al, 2018; Vardar-Yagli et al, 2019). Age-related changes in food consumption and body composition influence the perception of fatigue in the geriatric population (Azzolino et al, 2020).*
- ● Review medications to determine possible side effects or interaction effects that could cause fatigue. EB: *Polypharmacy may be related to frailty in older adults (Gutiérrez-Valencia et al, 2018).*
- ● Review comorbid conditions that may contribute to fatigue, such as congestive heart failure, pulmonary disease, cardiac disease, multiple sclerosis, arthritis, obesity, anemia, depression, Parkinson's disease, insomnia, cancer, and viral infections (e.g., COVID-19).
- ● Identify recent losses, even loss of physical function; monitor for depression or loneliness as a possible contributing factor to fatigue. EB: *Depression is associated with fatigue in geriatric clients and has a reciprocal relationship with frailty (Soysal et al, 2017).*
- ● Review other symptoms the client may be experiencing. Fatigue is often associated with other symptom clusters such as depression and sleep disturbances (National Comprehensive Cancer Network, 2021a). EB: *Clusters may be independent of age (Agasi-Idenburg et al, 2017). Depression, fatigue, and immune activation are interrelated (Lee & Giuliani, 2019).*
- ▲ Review medications for side effects. *Certain medications (e.g., diuretics with associated loss of potassium, antihypertensives, antihistamines, pain medications, anticonvulsants, chemotherapeutic agents, antipsychotics, antivirals, opioids, immune modulating agents, skeletal muscle relaxants, and corticosteroids) may result in fatigue in older adults (National Comprehensive Cancer Network, 2021b).*

Home Care

The previously mentioned interventions may be adapted for home care use as well.

- ● Assess the client's history and current patterns of fatigue as they relate to the home environment and environmental and behavioral triggers of increased fatigue. EB: *Fatigue may be more pronounced in specific settings for physical, environmental (e.g., stairs required to reach bathroom, patterns of movement around home, cleaning activities that require high energy), or psychological reasons (Gay et al, 2019). Frailty and or comorbidity may be related to the fatigue for the elderly (Soysal et al, 2017).*
- ▲ Encourage planned exercise regimens or physical activities such as walking or light aerobic exercises. This activity can be organized in the home, mall, on a treadmill, or in a setting such as senior centers or wellness facilities. EB: *Continued physical activity after cancer treatment has been associated with improved functioning in both physical and social realms (Hoffman et al, 2017). After a stroke, frail elderly also responded to an individualized exercise program with increased physical endurance and self-efficacy (Drummond et al, 2017; Liu et al, 2017).*
- ▲ Refer to occupational and/or physical therapy if substantial intervention is needed to assist the client in adapting to home and daily patterns. EB: *Interventions in older adults led by occupational and physical therapists have been associated with less difficulty in ADLs and instrumental ADLs, which may lead to lower*

levels of fatigue. Occupational and physical therapy rehabilitation has also been shown to decrease fatigue in cancer survivors (Dalzell et al, 2017). Home-based exercise in clients with stage IV lung and colorectal cancer has shown improvement in levels of fatigue (Hoffman et al, 2017).

- For clients receiving chemotherapy, intervene to:
  - Relieve symptom distress (anxiety, nausea and vomiting, diarrhea, lack of appetite, emotional distress, difficulty sleeping)
  - Encourage as much physical activity as possible with a specific recommendation (Hoffman et al, 2017)
- Teach the client and family the importance of and methods for setting priorities for activities, especially those with high energy demand (e.g., home or family events). Instruct in realistic expectations and behavioral pacing. EBN: *Prioritization of activities can be effective in restoring energy (Poort et al, 2020).*
  - Identify with clients ways in which they continue to be a valued part of their social environment.
  - Identify with clients ways in which they continue to maintain daily activity or social activities.
  - Encourage the client to maintain regular family routines (e.g., meals, daily activities, sleep patterns), as well as physical activity, as much as possible.

F

Client/Family Teaching and Discharge Planning

- Help the client to reframe cognitively; share information about fatigue, how to live with it, and how to moderate it, including need for positive self-talk. EBN: *Cognitive behavioral approaches to managing fatigue have been shown to have a positive effect with fatigue related to multiple sclerosis and cancer (Wendebourg et al, 2017; Poort et al, 2020).*
- Teach strategies for energy conservation that can result in improved fatigue level (e.g., sitting instead of standing during showering, limiting trips up and down stairs). EB: *Energy conservation strategies can decrease the amount of energy used (Blikman et al, 2017).*
- Teach the client to carry a pocket calendar, make lists of required activities, use electronic reminders, and post reminders around the house. *Apps that record steps will help clients understand their use of energy from moving around.*
- Teach the importance of following a healthy lifestyle with adequate nutrition, fluids, and rest; pain relief; insomnia correction; and appropriate exercise to decrease fatigue (i.e., energy restoration).
- Engage in outdoor relaxation and use of nature as an option to relieve fatigue.

REFERENCES

Abrahams, H. J. G., Gielissen, M. F. M., Verhagen, C. A. H. H. V. M., & Knoop, H. (2018). The relationship of fatigue in breast cancer survivors with quality of life and factors to address in psychological interventions: A systematic review. *Clinical Psychology Review, 63*, 1–11. https://doi.org/10.1016/j.cpr.2018.05.004.

Agasi-Idenburg, S. C., Thong, M. S. Y., Punt, C. J. A., Stuiver, M. M., & Aaronson, N. K. (2017). Comparison of symptom clusters associated with fatigue in older and younger survivors of colorectal cancer. *Supportive Care in Cancer, 25*(2), 625–632. https://doi.org/10.1007/s00520-016-3451-4.

Azzolino, D., Arosio, B., Marzetti, E., Calvani, R., & Cesari, M. (2020). Nutritional status as a mediator of fatigue and its underlying mechanisms in older people. *Nutrients, 12*(2), 444. https://doi.org/10.3390/nu12020444.

Baguley, B. J., Skinner, T. L., & Wright, O. R. L. (2019). Nutrition therapy for the management of cancer-related fatigue and quality of life: A systematic review and meta-analysis. *British Journal of Nutrition, 122*(5), 527–541. https://doi.org/10.1017/S000711451800363X.

Bahouth, M. N., Gottesman, R. F., & Szanton, S. L. (2018). Primary "dehydration" and acute stroke: A systematic research review. *Journal of Neurology, 265*(10), 2167–2181. https://doi.org/10.1007/s00415-018-8799-6.

Blikman, L. J., van Meeteren, J., Twisk, J. W., et al. (2017). Effectiveness of energy conservation management on fatigue and participation in multiple sclerosis: A randomized controlled trial. *Multiple Sclerosis, 23*(11), 1527–1541. https://doi.org/10.1177/1352458517702751.

Corbett, T. K., Groarke, A., Devane, D., Carr, E., Walsh, J. C., & McGuire, B. E. (2019). The effectiveness of psychological interventions for fatigue in cancer survivors: Systematic review of randomised controlled trials. *Systematic Reviews, 8*(1), 324. https://doi.org/10.1186/s13643-019-1230-2.

Dalzell, M. A., Smirnow, N., Sateren, W., et al. (2017). Rehabilitation and exercise oncology program: Translating research into a model of care. *Current Oncology, 24*(3), e191–e198. https://doi.org/10.3747/co.24.3498.

Dikmen, H. A., & Terzioglu, F. (2019). Effects of reflexology and progressive muscle relaxation on pain, fatigue, and quality of life during chemotherapy in gynecologic cancer patients. *Pain Management Nursing, 20*(1), 47–53. https://doi.org/10.1016/j.pmn.2018.03.001.

Drummond, A., Hawkins, L., Sprigg, N., et al. (2017). The Nottingham Fatigue after Stroke (NotFAST) study: Factors associated with severity of fatigue in stroke patients without depression. *Clinical Rehabilitation, 31*(10), 1406–1415. https://doi.org/10.1177/0269215517695857.

Gay, J. L., Cherof, S. A., LaFlamme, C. C., & O'Connor, P. J. (2019). Psychological aspects of stair use: A systematic review. *American Journal of Lifestyle Medicine*. https://doi.org/10.1177/1559827619870104.

Geraghty, K., Hann, M., & Kurtev, S. (2019). Myalgic encephalomyelitis/chronic fatigue syndrome patients' reports of symptom changes following cognitive behavioural therapy, graded exercise therapy and pacing treatments: Analysis of a primary survey compared with secondary surveys. *Journal of Health Psychology*, *24*(10), 1318–1333. https://doi.org/10.1177/1359105317726152.

Gibbons, L. E., Fredericksen, R., Batey, D. S., et al. (2017). Validity assessment of the PROMIS fatigue domain among people living with HIV. *AIDS Research and Therapy*, *14*(1), 21. https://doi.org/10.1186/s12981-017-0146-y.

Gok Metin, Z., Karadas, C., Izgu, N., Ozdemir, L., & Demirci, U. (2019). Effects of progressive muscle relaxation and mindfulness meditation on fatigue, coping styles, and quality of life in early breast cancer patients: An assessor blinded, three-arm, randomized controlled trial. *European Journal of Oncology Nursing*, *42*, 116–125. https://doi.org/10.1016/j.ejon.2019.09.003.

Gutiérrez-Valencia, M., Izquierdo, M., Cesari, M., Casas-Herrero, Á., & Martínez-Velilla, N. (2018). The relationship between frailty and polypharmacy in older people: A systematic review. *British Journal of Clinical Pharmacology*, *84*(7), 1432–1444. https://doi.org/10.1111/bcp.13590.

Henson, L. A., Maddocks, M., Evans, C., Davidson, M., Hicks, S., & Higginson, I. J. (2020). Palliative care and the management of common distressing symptoms in advanced cancer: Pain, breathlessness, nausea and vomiting, and fatigue. *Journal of Clinical Oncology*, *38*(9), 905–914. https://doi.org/10.1200/JCO.19.00470.

Heo, S., McSweeney, J., Ounpraseuth, S., Shaw-Devine, A., Fier, A., & Moser, D. K. (2018). Testing a holistic meditation intervention to address psychosocial distress in patients with heart failure: A pilot study. *Journal of Cardiovascular Nursing*, *33*(2), 126–134. https://doi.org/10.1097/JCN.0000000000000435.

Hoffman, A. J., Brintnall, R. A., Given, B. A., von Eye, A., Jones, L. W., & Brown, J. K. (2017). Using perceived self-efficacy to improve fatigue and fatigability in postsurgical lung cancer patients: A pilot randomized controlled trial. *Cancer Nursing*, *40*(1), 1–12. https://doi.org/10.1097/NCC.0000000000000378.

Jensen, R. E., Moinpour, C. M., Potosky, A. L., et al. (2017). Responsiveness of 8 Patient-Reported Outcomes Measurement Information System (PROMIS) measures in a large, community–based cancer study cohort. *Cancer*, *123*(2), 327–335. https://doi.org/10.1002/cncr.30354.

Kiss, N., Baguley, B. J., Ball, K., et al. (2019). Technology-supported self-guided nutrition and physical activity interventions for adults with cancer: Systematic review. *JMIR Mhealth Uhealth*, *7*(2), e12281. https://doi.org/10.2196/12281.

Kolak, A., Kamińska, M., Wysokińska, E., et al. (2017). The problem of fatigue in patients suffering from neoplastic disease. *Contemporary Oncology (Poznan Poland)*, *21*(2), 131–135. https://doi.org/10.5114/wo.2017.68621.

Lee, C.-H., & Giuliani, F. (2019). The role of inflammation in depression and fatigue. *Frontiers in Immunology*, *10*, 1696. https://doi.org/10.3389/fimmu.2019.01696.

Liu, J. Y., Lai, C. K., Siu, P. M., Kwong, E., & Tse, M. M. (2017). An individualized exercise programme with and without behavioural change enhancement strategies for managing fatigue among frail older people: A quasi-experimental pilot study. *Clinical Rehabilitation*, *31*(4), 521–531. https://doi.org/10.1177/0269215516649226.

Matura, L. A., Malone, S., Jaime-Lara, R., & Riegel, B. (2018). A systematic review of biological mechanisms of fatigue in chronic illness. *Biological Research For Nursing*, *20*(4), 410–421. https://doi.org/10.1177/1099800418764326.

Milrad, S. F., Hall, D. L., Jutagir, D. R., et al. (2018). Depression, evening salivary cortisol and inflammation in chronic fatigue syndrome: A psychoneuroendocrinological structural regression model. *International Journal of Psychophysiology*, *131*, 124–130. https://doi.org/10.1016/j.ijpsycho.2017.09.009.

Montoya, J. G., Holmes, T. H., Anderson, J. N., et al. (2017). Cytokine signature associated with disease severity in chronic fatigue syndrome patients. *Proceedings of the National Academy of Sciences of the USA*, *114*(34), E7150–E7158. https://doi.org/10.1073/pnas.1710519114.

Mustian, K. M., Alfano, C. M., Heckler, C., et al. (2017). Comparison of pharmaceutical, psychological, and exercise treatments for cancer-related fatigue: A meta-analysis. *JAMA Oncology*, *3*(7), 961–968. https://doi.org/10.1001/jamaoncol.2016.6914.

National Comprehensive Cancer Network. (2021a). *NCCN clinical practice guidelines in oncology: Cancer-related fatigue*. version 1. 2021. Retrieved from https://www.nccn.org/professionals/physician_gls/pdf/fatigue.pdf.

National Comprehensive Cancer Network. (2021b). *NCCN clinical practice guidelines in oncology: Older adult oncology*. version 1. 2021. Retrieved from https://www.nccn.org/professionals/physician_gls/pdf/senior.pdf.

Paulis, S. J. C., Everink, I. H. J., Halfens, R. J. G., Lohrmann, C., & Schols, J. M. G. A. (2018). Prevalence and risk factors of dehydration among nursing home residents: A systematic review. *Journal of the American Medical Directors Association*, *19*(8), 646–657. https://doi.org/10.1016/j.jamda.2018.05.009.

Pennisi, M., Malaguarnera, G., Di Bartolo, G., et al. (2019). Decrease in serum vitamin D level of older patients with fatigue. *Nutrients*, *11*(10), 2531. https://doi.org/10.3390/nu11102531.

Poort, H., Peters, M. E. W. J., van der Graaf, W. T. A., et al. (2020). Cognitive behavioral therapy or graded exercise therapy compared with usual care for severe fatigue in patients with advanced cancer during treatment: A randomized controlled trial. *Annals of Oncology*, *31*(1), 115–122. https://doi.org/10.1016/j.annonc.2019.09.002.

Savina, S., & Zaydiner, B. (2019). Cancer-related fatigue: Some clinical aspects. *Asia Pacific Journal of Oncology Nursing*, *6*(1), 7–9. https://doi.org/10.4103/apjon.apjon_45_18.

Silva, C. F. R., Duarte, C., Ferreira, R. J. O., Santos, E., & Pereira da Silva, J. A. (2020). Depression, disability and sleep disturbance are the main explanatory factors of fatigue in rheumatoid arthritis: A path analysis model. *Clinical & Experimental Rheumatology*, *38*(2), 314–321.

Soysal, P., Veronese, N., Thompson, T., et al. (2017). Relationship between depression and frailty in older adults: A systematic review and meta-analysis. *Ageing Research Reviews*, *36*, 78–87. https://doi.org/10.1016/j.arr.2017.03.005.

Vardar-Yagli, N., Calik-Kutukcu, E., Saglam, M., Inal-Ince, D., Arikan, H., & Coplu, L. (2019). The relationship between fear of movement, pain and fatigue severity, dyspnea level and comorbidities in patients with chronic obstructive pulmonary disease. *Disability & Rehabilitation*, *41*(18), 2159–2163. https://doi.org/10.1080/09638288.2018.1459886.

Wang, T., Yin, J., Miller, A. H., & Xiao, C. (2017). A systematic review of the association between fatigue and genetic polymorphisms. *Brain, Behavior, and Immunity*, *62*, 230–244. https://doi.org/10.1016/j.bbi.2017.01.007.

Wendebourg, M. J., Heesen, C., Finlayson, M., Meyer, B., Pöttgen, J., & Köpke, S. (2017). Patient education for people with multiple sclerosis-associated fatigue: A systematic review. *PLoS One*, *12*(3), e0173025. https://doi.org/10.1371/journal.pone.0173025.

Fear Domain 9 Coping/stress tolerance Class 2 Coping responses

Nadia Ali Muhammad Ali Charania, PhD, RN

NANDA-I

Definition

Basic, intense emotional response aroused by the detection of imminent threat, involving an immediate alarm reaction (American Psychological Association).

Defining Characteristics

Physiological Factors

Anorexia; diaphoresis; diarrhea; dyspnea; increased blood pressure; increased heart rate; increased respiratory rate; increased sweating; increased urinary frequency; muscle tension; nausea; pallor; pupil dilation; vomiting; xerostomia

Behavioral/Emotional

Apprehensiveness; concentration on the source of fear; decreased self-assurance; expresses alarm; expresses fear; expresses intense dread; expresses tension; impulsive behaviors; nervousness; psychomotor agitation

Related Factors

Communication barriers; learned response to threat; response to phobic stimulus; unfamiliar situation

At-Risk Population

Children; individuals exposed to traumatic situation; individuals living in areas with increased violence; individuals receiving terminal care; individuals separated from social support; individuals undergoing surgical procedure; individuals with family; individuals with history of falls; older adults; pregnant women; women; women experiencing childbirth

Associated Conditions

Sensation disorders

NOC (Nursing Outcomes Classification)

Suggested NOC Outcome

Fear Self-Control

Example NOC Outcome with Indicators

Fear Self-Control as evidenced by the following indicators: Eliminates precursors of fear/Seeks information to reduce fear/Plans coping strategies for fearful situations. (Rate the outcome and indicators of **Fear Self-Control:** 1 = never demonstrated, 2 = rarely demonstrated, 3 = sometimes demonstrated, 4 = often demonstrated, 5 = consistently demonstrated [see Section I].)

Client Outcomes

Client Will (Specify Time Frame)

- Verbalize known fears
- State accurate information about the situation
- Identify, verbalize, and demonstrate those coping behaviors that reduce own fear
- Report and demonstrate reduced fear

NIC (Nursing Interventions Classification)

Suggested NIC Interventions

Anxiety Reduction; Coping Enhancement; Security Enhancement

Example NIC Activities—Anxiety Reduction

Use a calm, reassuring approach; Stay with the client to promote safety and reduce fear

Nursing Interventions and *Rationales*

F

- Assess the source of fear in the client. EB: *A systematic review and meta-analysis found that fear of needles is common in clients requiring preventive care and in those undergoing treatment. Identifying sources of fear can promote interventions that alleviate fear in high-risk groups (McLenon & Rogers, 2019).*
- Assess for presence of fear avoidance beliefs. EB: *A study using the Fear Avoidance Beliefs Questionnaire (FABQ) found that a high level of fear avoidance is a risk factor for long-term sickness absence among workers with musculoskeletal pain regardless of the level of occupational physical activity (Jay et al, 2018).*
- Provide counseling to enhance client's self-efficacy. EBN: *A midwife-led study provided a series of counseling interventions for women with a fear of childbirth. Results indicated an increase in self-efficacy and a decrease in childbirth fears after the intervention (Firouzan et al, 2020).*
- Engage clients in skills that promote and contribute to their psychological flexibility, such as acceptance and openness to one's experience; cognitive defusion, or holding one's thoughts lightly; flexible attention to the here and now; having a stable and transcendental sense of self; clarification of and living based on deeply meaningful chosen values; and committed purposeful action. EB: *The use of psychological flexibility skills could address the rigid and repertoire narrowing effects of coronavirus-induced anxiety and fear (Presti et al, 2020).*
- Engage clients with a fear of cancer recurrence about cognitive-behavioral therapies that include teaching skills to identify patterns of thoughts, emotions, and behaviors; skills to identify triggers of fear of cancer recurrence; reframing skills to cope with cognitive appraisals of uncontrollability to make them as less threatening; skills for problem-solving; and behavioral exposure skills to confront avoidance of cancer-related stimuli. EB: *A systematic review and meta-analysis of randomized controlled trials (*n = 19*) pointed toward the effectiveness of mind-body interventions for reducing fear of cancer recurrence during the intervention, and after the intervention to some extent (small to medium effect sizes) (Hall et al, 2018).*
- Engage clients in a mindfulness-based training program. EBP: *A study found that mindfulness-based interventions enhance fear extinction and foster stress resilience (Sevinc et al, 2019).*
- Engage pregnant women with fear of childbirth in individual or group psychoeducation sessions or therapeutic conversations during pregnancy. EB: *A systematic review of research studies focused on interventions for relief of severe fear of childbirth in pregnancy and their underlying conceptual foundation pointed to the evidence that cognitive therapy sessions and theory-based group psychoeducation with relaxation are effective interventions (Striebich, Mattern, & Ayerle, 2018).*
- Provide antenatal education to women with fear of childbirth. EB: *A systematic review and meta-analysis of both quasi-randomized (*n = 2*) and randomized (*n = 8*) clinical trials supported that both educational-based interventions and self-hypnosis may reduce the fear of childbirth. Moreover, educational-based interventions appeared to be twice as effective as hypnosis-based interventions (Hosseinia, Nazarzadehb, & Jahanfar, 2018).*
- Provide brief psychoeducation to a client who has fear about surgery. EBN: *A systematic review and meta-analysis found that preoperative education can effectively decrease anxiety in clients undergoing cardiac surgery (Ramesh et al, 2017).*
- Offer psychological interventions for clients with a fear of public speaking. The psychological interventions can be delivered through traditional (face-to-face) or technology-assisted formats. EB: *The result of the meta-analysis of randomized control trials revealed that psychological interventions delivered using either traditional or technology-driven formats are effective in reducing fear of public speaking (Ebrahimi et al, 2019).*
- Assist clients with fear of lower back pain through a combination of strategies focused on reconceptualizing clients' knowledge about their lower back pain (e.g., "explain pain" and exposure in vivo). Strategies are targeted to assist clients to gain control over pain and responses to pain as a way to make sense of their lower back pain experience. EB: *The clinical commentary illustrated how Leventhal's common-sense model may assist physical therapists to understand the broader sense-making processes involved in the fear-avoidance cycle, and how they can be altered to facilitate a reduction in clients' fear by applying a combination of strategies (Bunzli et al, 2017).*

- Integrate psychologically informed practices for athletes who experience fear of reinjury through self-report questionnaires to quantify fear of reinjury at various key points of rehabilitation journey, education to reduce fear-avoidance beliefs, quota-based exercise, and graded exposure. EB: *Incorporating principles of psychologically informed practice into sports injury rehabilitation could improve rehabilitation outcomes for athletes with high fear of reinjury (Hsu et al, 2017).*
- ▲ Refer client for cognitive behavioral therapy (CBT). EB: *A systematic review and meta-analysis evaluating the effects of CBT on reducing fear of falling found that CBT appears to be effective in reducing fear of falling and improving balance among older people (Liu et al, 2018).*
- See care plan for **Anxiety.**

Pediatric

- Use distraction techniques to reduce fear of painful procedures. EBN: *The Buzzy device is a bee-shaped gadget producing vibrations and cooling through freezable wings. A study found a significant difference between the Buzzy intervention and control groups in terms of levels of pain and fear during intramuscular injections (Yilmaz & Alemdar, 2019).*
- Incorporate play therapy as an intervention to reduce fears during painful procedures. EBN: *The results of a systematic review found that the implementation of therapeutic play for hospitalized children decreases postoperative pain, improves behavior and attitude, and reduces anxiety during the hospital stay (Godino-Iáñez et al, 2020).*
- For adolescents with disordered eating behaviors, assess for a fear of food. EB: *Researchers found a specific, direct prospective relationship between fear of food and drive for thinness and conclude that intervening on fear of food may prevent drive for thinness (Levinson et al, 2017).*
- ▲ For children with cancer, refer children and families to screening for cancer-related posttraumatic stress symptoms (PTSS) and other stressors. EB: *Children with cancer may experience cancer-related PTSS and posttraumatic stress disorder (PTSD), which can lead to long-term impairment. Screening and referrals are necessary to enhance mental health throughout treatment and survivorship (Marusak et al, 2019).*

Geriatric

- Engage clients with a fear of falling in CBT-based multicomponent interventions, including cognitive restructuring, motivational interviewing, or goal-setting. EB: *A systematic review and meta-analysis of interventions used to reduce the fear of falling among community-dwelling older adults found that CBT-based multicomponent interventions appear to be effective in immediate, short-term (i.e., ≤6 months postintervention), and long-term (i.e., ≥6 months postintervention) periods. Moreover, CBT-based multicomponent interventions improve the confidence to perform activities requiring functional mobility, thus older adults with the fear of falling become more likely to engage in functional mobility–associated activities such as walking, getting up from a chair, bathing, and toileting (Chua et al, 2019).*
- Engage clients with a fear of falling in an intervention program that includes both CBT and exercise (focused primarily on balance and strength training or tai chi). EB: *The scoping review of the literature to identify effective evidence-based interventions for fear of falling among community-dwelling older adults found that the efficacious interventions typically were multicomponent programs including CBT and exercise (Whipple, Hamel, & Talley, 2018).*
- Provide mind-body interventions involving meditative movements (e.g., tai chi, qigong, yoga, and Pilates) for clients with fear of falling. EB: *Mind-body interventions encompassing meditative movements showed promising signs of improvements in psychological health including fear of falling among older adults without mental disorders (Weber et al, 2020).*
- Pair cognitive-behavioral strategies with exercises to improve physical skills and mobility to decrease fear of falling. EBN: *A study found that the combination of cognitive-behavioral strategies with exercises decreased fear of falling while increasing mobility and muscle strength (Huang et al, 2016).*
- Engage clients with the fear of death and dying in intervention strategies including psychotherapy, mindfulness exercises, and virtual reality. EB: *The review of literature on psychotherapy, mindfulness (traditional interventions), virtual reality, and use of psychedelics (innovative interventions) found that they might have a positive impact on addressing fear of death and dying, but was inconclusive in determining which out of the four is the most effective intervention strategy (Blomstroma et al, 2020).*
- See care plan for **Anxiety** or Death **Anxiety.**

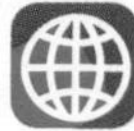

Multicultural

- Assess for fears of racism in culturally diverse clients. **EB:** *The differential experience of racism can contribute to posttraumatic stress and other fear-related responses (Williams, Peña, & Mier-Chairez, 2017).*
- Assess for fear of health care providers. **EB:** *A fear of physicians was associated with the client perceptions that physicians accommodated cultural differences related to issues of personal space and time and with perceptions of physicians' provision of person-centered care (Ahmed & Bates, 2017).*
- Provide education, support, and guidance to engage clients in their care. **EB:** *Research found that fears of serious medical diagnosis, stigma, medical distrust, and racism emerged as factors inhibiting health care utilization (Connell et al, 2019).*

Home Care

- The previous interventions may be adapted for home care use.
- Refer to care plan for **Anxiety.**

F

Client/Family Teaching and Discharge Planning

Assess for fears related to discharge from hospital. **EBN:** *A qualitative study of parents of premature infants found that the parents experience ambivalent feelings; joy is mixed with the fear of caring for a premature child at home (Osorio Galeano, Ochoa Marín, & Semenic, 2017).*

- See care plan for **Anxiety.**

REFERENCES

Ahmed, R., & Bates, B. R. (2017). Patients' fear of physicians and perceptions of physicians' cultural competence in healthcare. *Journal of Communication in Healthcare*, *10*(1), 55–60. https://doi.org/10.1080/17538068.2017.1287389.

Blomstroma, M., Burns, A., Larriviere, D., & Penberthy, J. K. (2020). Addressing fear of death and dying: Traditional and innovative interventions. *Mortality*. https://doi.org/10.1080/13576275.2020.1810649.

Bunzli, S., Smith, A., Schütze, R., Lin, I., & O'Sullivan, P. (2017). Making sense of low back pain and pain-related fear. *Journal of Orthopaedic & Sports Physical Therapy*, *47*(9), 628–636. https://www.jospt.org/doi/10.2519/jospt.2017.7434.

Chua, C. H. M., Jiang, Y., Lim, D. S., Wu, V. X., & Wang, W. (2019). Effectiveness of cognitive behaviour therapy–based multicomponent interventions on fear of falling among community–dwelling older adults: A systematic review and meta-analysis. *Journal of Advanced Nursing*, *75*(2), 3299–3315. https://doi.org/10.1111/jan.14150.

Connell, C. L., Wang, S. C., Crook, L., & Yadrick, K. (2019). Barriers to healthcare seeking and provision among african american adults in the rural mississippi delta region: Community and provider perspectives. *Journal of Community Health*, *44*(4), 636–645. https://doi.org/10.1007/s10900-019-00620-1.

Ebrahimi, O. V., Pallesen, S., Kenter, R. M. F., & Nordgreen, T. (2019). Psychological interventions for the fear of public speaking: A meta-analysis. *Frontiers in Psychology*, *10*, 488. https://doi.org/10.3389/fpsyg.2019.00488.

Firouzan, L., Kharaghani, R., Zenoozian, S., Moloodi, R., & Jafari, E. (2020). The effect of midwifery led counseling based on Gamble's approach on childbirth fear and self-efficacy in nulligravida women. *BMC Pregnancy and Childbirth*, *20*(1), 522. https://doi.org/10.1186/s12884-020-03230-1.

Godino-Iáñez, M. J., Martos-Cabrera, M. B., Suleiman-Martos, N., et al. (2020). Play therapy as an intervention in hospitalized children: A systematic review. *Healthcare*, *8*(3), 239. https://doi.org/10.3390/healthcare8030239.

Hall, D. L., Luberto, C. M., Philpotts, L. L., Song, R., Park, E. R., & Yeh, G. Y. (2018). Mind–body interventions for fear of cancer recurrence: A systematic review and meta–analysis. *Psycho-Oncology*, *27*(11), 2546–2558. https://doi.org/10.1002/pon.4757.

Hosseinia, V. M., Nazarzadehb, M., & Jahanfar, S. (2018). Interventions for reducing fear of childbirth: A systematic review and meta-analysis of clinical trials. *Women and Birth*, *31*(4), 254–262. https://doi.org/10.1016/j.wombi.2017.10.007.

Hsu, C.-J., Meierbachtol, A., George, S. Z., & Chmielewski, T. L. (2017). Fear of reinjury in athletes: Implications for rehabilitation. *Sports Health: A Multidisciplinary Approach*, *9*(2), 162–167.

Huang, T. T., Chung, M. L., Chen, F. R., Chin, Y. F., & Wang, B. H. (2016). Evaluation of a combined cognitive-behavioural and exercise intervention to manage fear of falling among elderly residents in nursing homes. *Aging & Mental Health*, *20*(1), 2–12. https://doi.org/10.1080/13607863.2015.1020411.

Jay, K., Thorsen, S. V., Sundstrup, E., et al. (2018). Fear avoidance beliefs and risk of long-term sickness absence: Prospective cohort study among workers with musculoskeletal pain. *Pain Research and Treatment*, 2018, 8347120. https://doi.org/10.1155/2018/8347120.

Levinson, C. A., Brosof, L. C., Ma, J., Fewell, L., & Lenze, E. J. (2017). Fear of food prospectively predicts drive for thinness in an eating disorder sample recently discharged from intensive treatment. *Eating Behaviors*, *27*, 45–51. https://doi.org/10.1016/j.eatbeh.2017.11.004.

Liu, T.-W., Ng, G. Y. F., Chung, R. C. K., & Ng, S. S. M. (2018). Cognitive behavioural therapy for fear of falling and balance among older people: A systematic review and meta-analysis. *Age and Ageing*, *47*(4), 520–527. https://doi.org/10.1093/ageing/afy010.

Marusak, H. A., Harper, F. W., Taub, J. W., & Rabinak, C. A. (2019). Pediatric cancer, posttraumatic stress and fear-related neural circuitry. *International Journal of Hematologic Oncology*, *8*(2), IJH17. https://doi.org/10.2217/ijh-2019-0002.

McLenon, J., & Rogers, M. A. M. (2019). The fear of needles: A systematic review and meta-analysis. *Journal of Advanced Nursing*, *75*(1), 30–42. https://doi.org/10.1111/jan.13818.

Osorio Galeano, S. P., Ochoa Marín, S. C., & Semenic, S. (2017). Preparing for post-discharge care of premature infants: Experiences of parents. *Investigación y Educación en Enfermería*, *35*(1), 100–106.

Presti, G., McHugh, L., Gloster, A., Karekla, M., & Hayes, S. C. (2020). The dynamics of fear at the time of COVID-19: A contextual behavioral science perspective. *Clinical Neuropsychiatry*, *17*(2), 65–71. https://doi.org/10.36131/CN20200206.

Ramesh, C., Nayak, B. S., Baburaya Pai, V., et al. (2017). Effect of preoperative education on postoperative outcomes among patients undergoing cardiac surgery: A systematic review and meta-analysis. *Journal of PeriAnesthesia Nursing, 32*(6), 518–529.e2. https://doi.org/10.1016/j.jopan.2016.11.011.

Sevinc, G., Hölzel, B. K., Greenberg, J., et al. (2019). Strengthened hippocampal circuits underlie enhanced retrieval of extinguished fear memories following mindfulness training. *Biological Psychiatry, 86*(9), 693–702. https://doi.org/10.1016/j.biopsych.2019.05.017.

Striebich, S., Mattern, E., & Ayerle, G. M. (2018). Support for pregnant women identified with fear of childbirth (FOC)/tokophobia—A systematic review of approaches and interventions. *Midwifery, 61*, 97–115. https://doi.org/10.1016/j.midw.2018.02.013.

Weber, M., Schnorr, T., Morat, M., Morat, T., & Donath, L. (2020). Effects of mind–body interventions involving meditative movements on quality of life, depressive symptoms, fear of falling and sleep quality in older adults: A systematic review with meta-analysis. *International Journal of Environmental Research and Public Health, 17*(18), 6556. https://doi.org/10.3390/ijerph17186556.

Whipple, M. O., Hamel, A. V., & Talley, K. M. C. (2018). Fear of falling among community-dwelling older adults: A scoping review to identify effective evidence-based interventions. *Geriatric Nursing, 39*(2), 170–177. https://doi.org/10.1016/j.gerinurse.2017.08.005.

Williams, M. T., Peña, A., & Mier-Chairez, J. (2017). Tools for assessing racism-related stress and trauma among Latinos. In L. T. Benuto (Ed.), *Toolkit for counseling Spanish-speaking clients* (pp. 71–95). New York: Springer. https://doi.org/10.1007/978-3-319-64880-4_4.

Yilmaz, G., & Alemdar, D. K. (2019). Using Buzzy, ShotBlocker, and bubble blowing in a pediatric emergency department to reduce the pain and fear caused by intramuscular injection: A randomized controlled trial. *Journal of Emergency Nursing, 45*(5), 502–511. https://doi.org/10.1016/j.jen.2019.04.003.

F

Ineffective Infant Feeding Dynamics

Domain 2 Nutrition Class 1 Ingestion

Marina Martinez-Kratz, MS, RN, CNE

NANDA-I

Definition

Altered parental feeding behaviors resulting in over or under eating patterns.

Defining Characteristics

Food refusal; inadequate appetite; inappropriate transition to solid foods; overeating; undereating

Related Factors

Abusive interpersonal relations; attachment issues; disengaged parenting; intrusive parenting; lack of confidence in child to develop healthy eating habits; lack of confidence in child to grow appropriately; lack of knowledge of appropriate methods of feeding infant for each stage of development; lack of knowledge of infant's developmental stages; lack of knowledge of parent's responsibility in infant feeding; media influence on feeding infant high caloric unhealthy foods; media influence on knowledge of high caloric unhealthy foods; multiple caregivers; uninvolved parenting

At-Risk Population

Abandoned infants; infants born to economically disadvantaged families; infants experiencing homelessness; infants experiencing life transition; infants experiencing prolonged hospitalization; infants living in foster care; infants who are small for gestational age; infants with history of hospitalization in neonatal intensive care; infants with history of unsafe eating and feeding experiences; premature infants

Associated Conditions

Chromosomal disorders; cleft lip; cleft palate; congenital heart disease; inborn genetic diseases; neural tube defects; parental psychiatric disorder; physical challenge with eating; physical challenge with feeding; physical health issue of parent; prolonged enteral nutrition; psychological health issue of parent; sensory integration dysfunction

NOC (Nursing Outcomes Classification)

Suggested NOC Outcomes

Bottle Feeding Establishment: Infant; Bottle Feeding Performance; Breastfeeding Establishment: Infant; Breastfeeding Maintenance; Breastfeeding Weaning; Parenting Performance: Infant; Knowledge: Parenting

Example NOC Outcome with Indicators

Parenting Performance Infant as evidenced by the following indicators: Exhibits a loving relationship/Interacts with infant to promote trust/Provides age-appropriate nutrition/Provides appropriate weaning. (Rate the outcome and indicators of **Nutritional Status:** 1 = never demonstrated, 2 = rarely demonstrated, 3 = sometimes demonstrated, 4 = often demonstrated, 5 = consistently demonstrated [see Section I].)

Client Outcomes

Client Will (Specify Time Frame)

- Infant will consume adequate calories to support growth and development
- Caregiver will follow healthy infant feeding practices
- Caregiver will identify infant behavioral cues related to hunger and satiety
- Caregiver and infant will engage in positive interactions during feeding

NIC (Nursing Interventions Classification)

Suggested NIC Interventions

Infant Care; Bottle Feeding; Teaching: Infant Nutrition

Example NIC Activities—Teaching: Infant Nutrition

Provide parents with written materials appropriate to identified knowledge needs; Instruct parent/caregiver to feed only breast milk or formula for first year (no solids before 4 months)

Nursing Interventions and *Rationales*

- Assess weight and height of the infant and use a growth chart to help determine growth pattern, which reflects nutrition. Age-related growth charts are available from www.cdc.gov/growthcharts/ (Centers for Disease Control and Prevention, 2016).
- Assess mothers for symptoms of postpartum depression. EB: *A study found an association between postpartum depression and poor infant nutritional status (Madeghe et al, 2016).*
- Encourage parent–child interactions that promote attachment. EB: *A study found that insecure attachment was significantly associated with higher body mass index (Maras et al, 2016).*
- Encourage overweight and obese mothers to follow current infant feeding guidelines. EB: *Research indicated that compared with normal weight mothers, overweight/obese mothers were less likely to breastfeed exclusively at infant age 2 months; they were more likely to breastfeed at low intensity during the first 2 months, and more likely to initiate early introduction of solid foods (Kitsantas et al, 2016).*
- Encourage individualized breastfeeding support as appropriate. EB: *A study highlights the need for individualized assistance to breastfeeding mothers, with special attention to personal experiences (Colombo et al, 2018).*
- Teach infant caregivers to recognize the following infant communication: infants signal appetite through interest or disinterest in food; infants use rapid and transient facial expressions to signal liking; and they use subtle or potent gestures, body movements, and vocalizations to express wanting. EB: *Research demonstrated the bidirectionality and interdependence of infant communication feeding, with more responsive feeding associated with more proficient communication by the infant (Hetherington, 2017).*
- Provide teaching and resources during pregnancy about recommended infant feeding practices. EB: *The results of a clinical trial testing a prenatal–postpartum individual nutrition/breastfeeding counseling program with follow-up nutrition and parenting support groups showed increased exclusive breastfeeding and reduced complementary foods and liquids in 3-month-old infants (Gross et al, 2016).*
- Provide caregivers of infants with teaching to encourage the early development of healthy eating patterns. EB: *Breastfed infants displayed more engagement and disengagement clues, which may make it easier to interpret the hunger/satiation cues (Wood et al, 2020).*
- Provide caregivers of infants with teaching on the importance of synchrony (offering the infant food and their willingness to eat) during the infant feeding time. EB: *A longitudinal study found that synchrony during feeding was related to the infant's willingness to eat (Costantini et al, 2018).*
- Encourage caregiver co-eating during infant feeding times. EB: *A longitudinal study found that co-eating during infant feeding was positively related to the infant's willingness to eat (Costantini et al, 2018).*

- Provide caregivers of infants with teaching about the strong association between sugar-sweetened beverages, obesity, and related chronic diseases. EB: *A systematic review suggests that consumption of sugar-sweetened beverages is positively associated with or has an effect on obesity indices in children (Luger et al, 2017).*
- Assist mothers to identify infant engagement and disengagement cues during breastfeeding or formula feeding. EB: *A study found that breastfeeding and formula-fed infants exhibited engagement and disengagement during feeding. Supporting a mother's ability to identify engagement and disengagement cues may promote more responsive feeding strategies (Shloim et al, 2017).*
- Provide mothers with unconditional positive regard in their choice of breast, formula, or mixed feeding of their infant. EB: *A study of breastfeeding women found that women experienced feelings of pressure and judgment around their infant feeding decisions (Hunt & Thomson, 2017).*

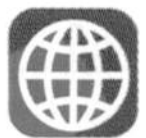

Multicultural

- Assess for cultural beliefs, values, and practices related to the feeding of infants. EB: *In a systematic review, familial and cultural influences provided the basis of many infant feeding decisions (Harrison, Brodribb, & Hepworth, 2017).*
- Identify the support persons of the infant caregiver and extend healthy infant feeding education and information to those support persons. EB: *A study of first-time African American mothers and breastfeeding indicated that over half of the mothers intended to exclusively breastfeed but were unable to because of life stressors and experiences. An informed support person could promote healthy infant feeding practices (Asiodu et al, 2017).*

Home Care

- The interventions previously described may be adapted for home care use.

Client/Family Teaching and Discharge Planning

- Many of the interventions previously described involve teaching.

REFERENCES

Asiodu, I. V., Waters, C. M., Dailey, D. E., & Lyndon, A. (2017). Infant feeding decision-making and the influences of social support persons among first-time African American mothers. *Maternal and Child Health Journal*, *21*(4), 863–872. https://doi.org/10.1007/s10995-016-2167-x.

Centers for Disease Control and Prevention (CDC). (2016). *National Center for health Statistics.* Growth charts. Retrieved from www.cdc.gov/growthcharts/. Accessed 16 September 2021.

Colombo, L., Crippa, B. L., Consonni, D., et al. (2018). Breastfeeding determinants in healthy term newborns. *Nutrients*, *10*(1), 48. https://doi.org/10.3390/nu10010048.

Costantini, C., Akehurst, L., Reddy, V., & Fasulo, A. (2018). Synchrony, co-eating and communication during complementary feeding in early infancy. *Infancy*, *23*(2), 288–304. doi.org/10.1111/infa.12220.

Gross, R. S., Mendelsohn, A. L., Gross, M. B., Scheinmann, R., & Messito, M. J. (2016). Randomized controlled trial of a primary care-based child obesity prevention intervention on infant feeding practices. *The Journal of Pediatrics*, *174*, 171–177.e2. https://doi.org/10.1016/j.jpeds.2016.03.060.

Harrison, M., Brodribb, W., & Hepworth, J. (2017). A qualitative systematic review of maternal infant feeding practices in transitioning from milk feeds to family foods. *Maternal and Child Nutrition*, *13*(2), e12360. https://doi.org/10.1111/mcn.12360.

Hetherington, M. M. (2017). Understanding infant eating behaviour—Lessons learned from observation. *Physiology & Behavior*, *176*, 117–124. doi:10.1016/j.physbeh.2017.01.022.

Hunt, L., & Thomson, G. (2017). Pressure and judgement within a dichotomous landscape of infant feeding: A grounded theory study to explore why breastfeeding women do not access peer support provision. *Maternal and Child Nutrition*, *13*(2), e12279. https://doi.org/10.1111/mcn.12279.

Kitsantas, P., Gallo, S., Palla, H., Nguyen, V., & Gaffney, K. (2016). Nature and nurture in the development of childhood obesity: Early infant feeding practices of overweight/obese mothers differ compared to mothers of normal body mass index. *Journal of Maternal-Fetal and Neonatal Medicine*, *29*(2), 290–293. https://doi.org/10.3109/14767058.2014.999035.

Luger, M., Lafontan, M., Bes-Rastrollo, M., Winzer, E., Yumuk, V., & Farpour-Lambert, N. (2017). Sugar-sweetened beverages and weight gain in children and adults: A systematic review from 2013 to 2015 and a comparison with previous studies. *Obesity Facts*, *10*(6), 674–693. doi.org/10.1159/000484566.

Madeghe, B. A., Kimani, V. N., Vander Stoep, A., Nicodimos, S., & Kumar, M. (2016). Postpartum depression and infant feeding practices in a low income urban settlement in Nairobi-Kenya. *BMC Research Notes*, *9*(1), 506. https://doi.org/10.1186/s13104-016-2307-9.

Maras, D., Obeid, N., Flament, M., et al. (2016). Attachment style and obesity: Disordered eating behaviors as a mediator in a community sample of Canadian youth. *Journal of Developmental and Behavioral Pediatrics*, *37*(9), 762–770. https://doi.org/10.1097/DBP.0000000000000361.

Shloim, N., Vereijken, C. M. J. L., Blundell, P., & Hetherington, M. M. (2017). Looking for cues—infant communication of hunger and satiation during milk feeding. *Appetite*, *108*, 74–82. https://doi.org/10.1016/j.appet.2016.09.020.

Wood, A. C., Blisset, J. M., Brunstrom, J. M., et al. (2020). Caregiver influences on eating behaviors in young children: A scientific statement from the American heart association. *Journal of the American Heart Association*, *9*(10), e014520. https://doi.org/10.1161/JAHA.119.014520.

Risk for Female Genital Mutilation

Domain 11 Safety/protection Class 3 Violence

Marina Martinez-Kratz, MS, RN, CNE

F

NANDA-I

Definition

Susceptible to full or partial ablation of the female external genitalia and other lesions of the genitalia, whether for cultural, religious or any other non-therapeutic reasons, which may compromise health.

Risk Factors

Lack of family knowledge about impact of practice on physical health; lack of family knowledge about impact of practice on psychosocial health; lack of family knowledge about impact of practice on reproductive health

At-Risk Population

Women belonging to ethnic group in which practice is accepted; women belonging to family in which any female member has been subjected to practice; women from families with favorable attitude towards practice; women planning to visit family's country of origin in which practice is accepted; women residing in country where practice is accepted; women whose family leaders belong to ethnic group in which practice is accepted

NOC (Nursing Outcomes Classification)

Suggested NOC Outcomes

Abuse Cessation; Abuse Protection; Abuse Recovery; Abuse Recovery: Emotional; Abuse Recovery: Physical

Example NOC Outcome with Indicators

Abuse Protection as evidenced by the following indicators: Plan for avoiding abuse/Implementation of plan to avoid abuse/Safety of self/Safety of child/Self-advocacy. (Rate the outcome and indicators of **Abuse Protection:** 1 = not adequate, 2 = slightly adequate, 3 = moderately adequate, 4 = substantially adequate, 5 = totally adequate [see Section I].)

Client/Family Outcomes

Client Will (Specify Time Frame)

- Express effects of family/culture on beliefs about female genital mutilation (FGM)
- Demonstrate evidence that FGM has not occurred
- Express/implement a plan for avoiding FGM
- Maintain safety of female children
- Demonstrate the ability to make decisions independent of cultural group
- Demonstrate self-advocacy skills

NIC (Nursing Interventions Classification)

Suggested NIC Interventions

Abuse Protection Support; Abuse Protection Support: Child; Abuse Protection Support: Religious

Example NIC Activities—Abuse Protection Support: Child

Identify parents who demonstrate an increased need for parent education; Determine whether a child demonstrates signs of physical abuse; Report suspected abuse or neglect to proper authorities; Refer families to human services and counseling professionals as needed

Nursing Interventions and *Rationales*

- Use therapeutic and culturally competent communication when asking women about FGM. EBN: *Asking about FGM with compassionate communication was a theme that emerged from the qualitative data of women living with FGM (Ormrod, 2019).*

- Identify the decision-making process related to the practice of FGM. EB: *The decision to undergo FGM is often a community decision and not an individual or family decision. Some survivors of FGM report that relatives or other community members performed FGM on them without their consent or the consent of their parents (Burrage, 2016).*
- Identify the type of FGM for which the female client is at risk. EB: *The World Health Organization (WHO) classifies types of FGM as follows.* ***Type 1:*** *Clitoridectomy, which is partial or total removal of the clitoris (a small sensitive and erectile part of the female genitals) and, in rare cases, removal of the prepuce only (the fold of skin surrounding the clitoris).* ***Type 2:*** *Excision, which is partial or total removal of the clitoris and labia minora with or without removal of the labia majora (the labia are "the lips" that surround the vagina).* ***Type 3:*** *Infibulation, which is narrowing of the vaginal opening through the creation of a covering seal. The seal is formed by cutting and repositioning the labia minora or majora with or without removal of the clitoris.* ***Type 4:*** *Other, which includes all other harmful procedures to the genitals for nonmedical reasons, for example, pricking, piercing, incision, scraping, and cauterizing the genital area (WHO, 2016). WHO's best practice standards indicated that nurses and health care providers are knowledgeable and aware of the types of FGM (WHO, 2016).*
- Assess and identify geographic, environmental, familial, religious, and/or other cultural factors that increase risk for FGM. EB: *Research indicated that the following are risk factors identified with FGM: older mothers, rural mothers, less educated mothers, maternal fears of social stigma, and mothers who have had FGM (Pashaei et al, 2016). FGM is most common in 30 countries of the western, eastern, and northeastern regions of Africa, in some countries in Asia and the Middle East, and among migrants from these areas. Countries with the highest rates of FGM are Egypt, Ethiopia, and Somalia (WHO, 2016).*
- Encourage the mothers of at-risk daughters to express their beliefs and attitudes toward FGM. EB: *Nurses and health care providers have to first understand the beliefs and attitudes toward FGM before implementing interventions to address the beliefs and attitudes. Among the beliefs for FGM are female cleanliness, beauty, safeguarding virginity, and as a rite of passage to adult womanhood (Pashaei et al, 2016).*
- Assess the mothers of at-risk daughters for positive affect (expression of feelings) and attitudes toward FGM. EB: *A recent Iranian study concluded that mothers' attitudes were the strongest predictor of their intention to allow their daughters to undergo FGM, suggesting that mothers with a more favorable attitude toward FGM are more likely to show the intention of mutilating their daughters (Pashaei et al, 2016).*
- In a respectful and nonjudgmental manner, provide men, fathers, and male partners with health education to address beliefs about FGM and provide information about the negative health outcomes associated with FGM. EB: *A study of anti-FGM advocates identified encouraging fathers' involvement in the upbringing of their daughters as an action to fight FGM (Mwenda et al, 2020).*
- In a respectful and nonjudgmental manner, convey accurate and clear information about FGM, using language and methods that can be readily understood by clients. EB: *Best practices indicated that individuals have the right to be fully informed by appropriately trained personnel with the assistance of an interpreter, if necessary (WHO, 2016).*
- In a respectful and nonjudgmental manner, provide the client, the client's parents, and the client's family with information that FGM is not a universal practice and that it is an illegal practice in many parts of the world. EB: *Women from countries that practice FGM may have inadequate knowledge of their bodies and biological facts and be shocked or angry to learn that FGM is not a universal practice and is illegal in the United States (Costello, 2015).*
- In a respectful and nonjudgmental manner, provide the client, the client's parents, and the client's family with health education to address false beliefs about female and clitoral anatomy and the physiology of women. EB: *Women from countries that practice FGM may have inadequate knowledge of their bodies and biological facts. Health education needs to convey that there are no known health benefits from FGM, and that women and children who experience FGM have lifelong health complications (WHO, 2016).*
- In a respectful and nonjudgmental manner, provide the client, the client's parents, and the client's family with health education to inform about the negative health outcomes associated with FMG. EB: *The negative health outcomes are both immediate and long-term. Immediate complications include bleeding, urinary retention, wound infection, sepsis, and death. Long-term complications include dysmenorrhea, dyspareunia, recurrent vaginal and urinary tract infections, infertility, difficult labor and delivery, and sexual dysfunction (Craven et al, 2016).*
- In a respectful and nonjudgmental manner, address false ideas or beliefs about FGM. EB: *A qualitative study found that FGM myths related to health, hygiene, religion, and the sexuality of women are used as justification by men and women in order to uphold the practice of FGM (Jiménez Ruiz, Almansa Martínez, & Alcón Belchí, 2017).*

F

F

- In a respectful and nonjudgmental manner, provide the client, the client's parents, and the client's family with health education to inform about the negative birth outcomes associated with mothers who have had FMG. EB: *A study found that mothers with FGM experienced the following obstetric complications: increased risk of neonatal resuscitation, low birth rate, stillbirth, and early neonatal death (Reisel & Creighton, 2015).*
- In a respectful and nonjudgmental manner, provide the client, the client's parents, and the client's family with health education to inform about the negative mental health outcomes associated with FGM. EB: *A cross-sectional study of female Somali refugees found that FGM was strongly associated with posttraumatic stress disorder, as well as depressive, anxiety, and somatic symptoms (Im et al, 2020).*
- Use therapeutic and culturally competent communication to focus on the current and future safety of the female child at risk for FGM. EB: *Therapeutic and culturally competent communication will acknowledge cultural practices without blame or judgment and will leverage parental love and concern to prevent harm to the child (Costello, 2015).*
- Use a cultural mediator to interpret cross-cultural norms about FGM. EB: *Cultural mediators are community leaders who are respected and known in their community for their opposition to FGM (Costello, 2015).*
- In a respectful and nonjudgmental manner, provide fathers with health education to address beliefs about FGM and provide information about the negative health outcomes associated with FGM. EB: *A systematic review found that the level of education of men was one of the most important indicators for men's support for the abandonment of FGM practices (Varol et al, 2015).*
- ▲ Refer families to counseling services. EB: *Family counseling will ensure that the family understands the reasons for the health care interventions and legislative/legal response and facilitate support of each other through the transition (Costello, 2015).*
- See care plans for **Post-Trauma** Syndrome, Impaired **Parenting,** and **Social** Isolation.

Pediatric

- Identify a system for assessment and referral of female infants at risk of FGM born to mothers who have undergone FGM. EB: *A British study assessed the effectiveness of a questionnaire to examine the level of risk of FGM if a girl is born to a mother who has undergone FGM. Study results indicated that the questionnaire formalized the referral process; identified infants at high risk; and helped to stratify risk into low, medium, and high. The questionnaire also indicated the demographics of those at highest risk (Flower et al, 2015).*
- For female children who may be survivors of FGM, or are at risk of FGM, notify Child Protective Services and other law enforcement authorities. EB: *FGM is child abuse. Nurses are mandated reporters and are legally obligated to report all instances of suspected child abuse and neglect. Notification of Child Protective Services and law enforcement allows appropriate health care intervention and may provide protection for siblings and other girls in the family against FGM (Creighton et al, 2016). All individuals have the right to the highest attainable standard of health and the right to life and physical integrity, including freedom from violence and the right to freedom from torture or cruel, inhumane, or degrading treatment (WHO, 2016).*
- Implement a school-based intervention to provide FGM health education to adolescent females. EB: *A study found that school-based health education had a positive impact on both the knowledge and attitude of female students toward FGM in Sudan (Mahgoub et al, 2019).*

REFERENCES

Burrage, H. (2016). *Female mutilation: The truth behind the horrifying global practice of female genital mutilation*. London: New Holland Publishers.

Costello, S. (2015). Female genital mutilation/cutting: Risk management and strategies for social workers and health care professionals. *Risk Management and Healthcare Policy*, *8*, 225–233. https://doi.org/10.2147/RMHP.S62091.

Craven, S., Kavanagh, A., & Khavari, R. (2016). Female genital mutilation management in the ambulatory clinic setting: A case study and review of the literature. *Journal of Surgical Case Reports*, *2016*(6), rjw104. https://doi.org/10.1093/jscr/rjw104.

Creighton, S. M., Dear, J., de Campos, C., Williams, L., & Hodes, D. (2016). Multidisciplinary approach to the management of children with female genital mutilation (FGM) or suspected FGM: Service description and case series. *BMJ Open*, *6*(2), e010311. https://doi.org/10.1136/bmjopen-2015-010311.

Flower, A., Palmer, C., & Hann, G. (2015). G48: A system for assessing the risk of female genital mutilation (FGM) for female infants born to mothers who have undergone FGM. *Archives of Disease in Childhood*, *100*(S3), A19–A20. https://doi.org/10.1136/archdischild-2015-308599.47.

Im, H., Swan, L. E. T., & Heaton, L. (2020). Polyvictimization and mental health consequences of female genital mutilation/circumcision (FGM/C) among Somali refugees in Kenya. *Women & Health*, *60*(6), 636–651. https://doi.org/10.1080/03630242.2019.1689543.

Jiménez Ruiz, I., Almansa Martínez, P., & Alcón Belchí, C. (2017). Dismantling the man-made myths upholding female genital mutilation. *Health Care for Women International*, *38*(5), 478–491. https://doi.org/10.1080/07399332.2017.1289211.

Mahgoub, E., Nimir, M., Abdalla, S., & Elhuda, D. A. (2019). Effects of school-based health education on attitudes of female students towards female genital mutilation in Sudan. *Eastern Mediterranean Health Journal, 25*(6), 406–412. https://doi.org/10.26719/emhj.18.053.

Mwendwa, P., Mutea, N., Kaimuri, M. J., et al. (2020). "Promote locally led initiatives to fight female genital mutilation/cutting (FGM/C)" lessons from anti-FGM/C advocates in rural Kenya. *Reproductive Health, 17*. Article 30.

Ormrod, J. (2019). The experience of NHS care for women living with female genital mutilation. *British Journal of Nursing, 28*(10), 628–633. https://doi.org/10.12968/bjon.2019.28.10.628.

Pashaei, T., Ponnet, K., Moeeni, M., Khazaee-pool, M., & Majlessi, F. (2016). Daughters at risk of female genital mutilation: Examining the determinants of mothers' intentions to allow their daughters to undergo female genital mutilation. *PLoS One, 11*(3), e0151630. https://doi.org/10.1371/journal.pone.0151630.

Reisel, D., & Creighton, S. M. (2015). Long term health consequences of female genital mutilation (FGM). *Maturitas, 80*(1), 48–51. https://doi.org/10.1016/j.maturitas.2014.10.009.

Varol, N., Turkmani, S., Black, K., Hall, J., & Dawson, A. (2015). The role of men in abandonment of female genital mutilation: A systematic review. *BMC Public Health, 15*, 1034. https://doi.org/10.1186/s12889-015-2373-2.

World Health Organization (WHO). (2016). *WHO guidelines on the management of health complications from female genital mutilation*. Geneva: WHO Press.

F

Risk for Imbalanced Fluid Volume

Domain 2 Nutrition Class 5 Hydration

Dina Hewett, PhD, RN, NEA-BC

NANDA-I

Definition

Susceptible to a decrease, increase, or rapid shift from one to the other of intravascular, interstitial, and/or intracellular fluid, which may compromise health.

Risk Factors

Altered fluid intake; difficulty accessing water; excessive sodium intake; inadequate knowledge about fluid needs; ineffective medication self-management; insufficient muscle mass; malnutrition

At-Risk Population

Individuals at extremes of weight; individuals with external conditions affecting fluid needs; individuals with internal conditions affecting fluid needs; women

Associated Conditions

Active fluid volume loss; deviations affecting fluid absorption; deviations affecting fluid elimination; deviations affecting fluid intake; deviations affecting vascular permeability; excessive fluid loss through normal route; fluid loss through abnormal route; pharmaceutical preparations; treatment regimen

NOC (Nursing Outcomes Classification)

Suggested NOC Outcomes

Fluid Balance; Electrolyte and Acid-Base Balance; Hydration

Example NOC Outcome with Indicators

Fluid Balance as evidenced by the following indicators: Blood pressure/Peripheral pulses palpable/Skin turgor/Moist mucous membranes/Serum electrolytes/Hematocrit/Body weight stable/24-hour intake and output balanced/Urine specific gravity. (Rate each indicator of **Fluid Balance:** 1 = severely compromised, 2 = substantially compromised, 3 = moderately compromised, 4 = mildly compromised, 5 = not compromised [see Section I].)

Client Outcomes

Client Will (Specify Time Frame)

- Lung sounds clear, respiratory rate 12 to 20 and free of dyspnea
- Urine output greater than 0.5 mL/kg/hr
- Blood pressure, pulse rate, temperature, and oxygen saturation within expected range

- Laboratory values within expected range, that is, normal serum sodium, hematocrit, and osmolarity
- Extremities and dependent areas free of edema
- Mental orientation appropriate based on previous condition

NIC (Nursing Interventions Classification)

Suggested NIC Interventions

Autotransfusion; Bleeding Precautions; Bleeding Reduction: Wound; Electrolyte Management; Fluid Management; Fluid Monitoring; Hemodynamic Regulation; Hypervolemia Management; Hypovolemia Management; Intravenous Therapy; Invasive Hemodynamic Monitoring; Shock Management: Volume; Vital Signs Monitoring

Example NIC Activities—Fluid Management

Maintain accurate intake and output record; Monitor vital signs

Nursing Interventions and *Rationales*

Surgical Clients

- Monitor the fluid balance. If there are symptoms of hypovolemia, refer to the interventions in the care plan for Deficient **Fluid** Volume. If there are symptoms of hypervolemia, refer to the interventions in the care plan for Excess **Fluid** Volume.

Preoperative

- Collect a thorough history and perform a preoperative assessment to identify clients with increased risk for hemorrhage or hypovolemia, that is, clients who take herbal supplements; those with recent traumatic injury, abnormal bleeding or altered clotting times, complicated kidney or liver disease, diabetes, cardiovascular disease, major organ transplant, history of aspirin and/or nonsteroidal antiinflammatory drug (NSAID) use, or anticoagulant therapy; or history of hemophilia, von Willebrand's disease, or disseminated intravascular coagulation. Assess the client's use of over-the-counter agents, including herbal products. EB: *Use of dietary herbal supplements (DHSs) causes the potential for DHS–drug interactions, which may lead to serious adverse events. Although drug-induced adverse events are thought to be responsible for up to 12% of hospitalizations, drug–drug interactions are estimated to be the direct cause of up to 2.8% of hospital admissions. Descriptions of adverse DHS–drug interactions in the surgical setting are found mostly in case reports and animal studies. These interactions mainly affected bleeding tendencies and level of sedation (Levy et al, 2017).*
- Recognize that nothing per mouth (NPO) at midnight may or may not be appropriate for each surgical client. Guidelines from the American Society of Anesthesiologists Committee (2011) recommended that healthy clients having elective surgery should be allowed to have clear liquids up to 2 hours before surgery. EB: *Current evidence has shown the value of allowing healthy clients to consume clear liquids up to 2 hours before surgery, but the practice is not consistent (Powers, 2017).* EB: *Many clients are unnecessarily dehydrated from lack of fluid for an extended period, which can complicate postoperative recovery. It is important to provide clear communication to the client that only clear liquids and/or carbohydrate-rich drinks can be safely consumed up to 2 hours before surgery (Myles et al, 2017).*
- Determine length of time the client has been without normal intake, been NPO, or experienced fluid loss (e.g., vomiting, diarrhea, bleeding). EB: *The length of time and severity of these factors, along with the presence of a fluid deficit, allow the health care provider to determine a general estimate of preoperative fluid loss, which can affect intraoperative fluid management. However, laboratory testing of hemoglobin, hematocrit, blood urea nitrogen (BUN), and creatinine should be used to corroborate the assessment (Kear, 2017).*
- Assess and document the client's mental status. A baseline assessment is important so that changes in mental status during the postoperative period can be easily identified.
- Recognize that there is conflicting evidence regarding liberal intraoperative fluid management versus restrictive fluid management. Fluid administration during surgery is more restrictive to prevent pulmonary complications associated with excessive fluid administration (Myles et al, 2017). CEB: *Hypovolemia and hypervolemia decrease tissue perfusion and may result in organ failure. Measurements to assess volume status include measuring mean arterial pressure (MAP), central venous pressure (CVP), and observing urine output. However, CVP shows a poor correlation to blood volume, is inadequate to detect hypovolemia*

reliably, and most notably cannot sense a decreased cardiac output (CO) and tissue oxygen debt in an early state. Furthermore, changes in CVP after volume administration do not allow any conclusions to changes in stroke volume (SV) or CO. Other signs such as hypotension and tachycardia may be more reliable indicators of volume assessment (Strunden et al, 2011). Urine output is a measure of glomerular filtration and can be an effective indicator of fluid status (Macedo et al, 2011; Strunden et al, 2011).

- To reduce fluid administration volume, colloids rather than crystalloid fluids may be administered during surgery (Myles et al, 2017).
- Recognize that an individualized fluid management plan would be developed incorporating client-specific assessment parameters (e.g., existing comorbid diseases, age) and type of surgical procedure (Myles et al, 2017; Lindahl, 2020). EB: *Perioperative hemodynamic and fluid management that is goal directed improved both short- and long-term outcomes and can be achieved easily (Lindahl, 2020).*
- Recognize the effects of general anesthetics, inhalational agents, and regional anesthesia on perfusion in the body and the potential for decreasing the blood pressure. EB: *In humans undergoing general anesthesia there is almost no relationship between mean arterial blood pressure and delivery of oxygen (DO_2), presumably because of widely varying systemic vascular resistance. Control of blood pressure requires measurement, an algorithm of action, and an intervention, such as medications or fluid administration (Bartels, Esper, & Thiele, 2016).*
- Monitor for signs of intraoperative hypovolemia such as dry skin, dry mucous membranes, tachycardia, decreased urinary output, decreased CVP, hypotension, increased pulse, and/or deep rapid respirations.
- Monitor for signs of intraoperative hypervolemia such as dyspnea, coarse crackles, increased pulse and respirations, decreased oxygenation, and decreased urinary output, all of which could progress to pulmonary edema.
- In the critically ill surgical client a pulmonary artery catheter or other minimally invasive CO monitoring device may be used to determine fluid balance and guide fluid and vasoactive intravenous (IV) drip administration. EB: *Devices that directly (pulmonary artery catheter or arterial line) or indirectly (minimally or noninvasive such as ongoing blood pressure monitoring) assess the client's cardiac status and fluid volume status may be used to "optimize" cardiac function by allowing better fluid regimens. Fluids must be individually titrated based on each client's changes in monitored variables (Bartels, Esper, & Thiele, 2016).*
- Monitor the client for hyponatremia with symptoms such as headache, anorexia, nausea and vomiting, diarrhea, tachycardia, general malaise, muscle cramps, weakness, lethargy, change in mental status, disorientation, seizures, and death. EB: *Many pathologies can predispose the client to hyponatremia, including adrenal insufficiency, brain tumor, cirrhosis, hypothyroidism, lung cancer, meningitis, renal disease, tuberculosis, use of complementary therapies, and head trauma (Icin et al, 2017).*
- Monitor clients undergoing laparoscopic or hysteroscopic procedures for the development of hyponatremia, hypervolemia, and pulmonary edema when an irrigation fluid is used. EB: *Use of local or spinal anesthesia for these operations can cause the client to develop symptoms of hyponatremia and hypervolemia sooner than with other anesthetics (Lindahl, 2020).*
- Monitor clients undergoing transurethral resection of the prostate (TURP) procedures for development of hyponatremia and hypervolemia with symptoms of TURP syndrome including headache, visual changes, agitation, lethargy, vomiting, muscle twitching, bradycardia, diminished pupillary reflexes, hypertension, and respiratory distress. EB: *Considerable fluid absorption occurs during TURP procedures and gynecological procedures, which can result in hyponatremia and/or hypervolemia (Pasha et al, 2015).*
- Measure the irrigation fluid used during urological and gynecological procedures accurately for volume deficit such as amount of irrigation used minus amount of irrigation recovered via suction. EB: *Absorption of large amounts of fluid can cause complications for the client (Lindahl, 2020).*
- Monitor intraoperative intake and output including blood loss, urine output, and third-space losses to provide an estimate of fluid volume. CEB: *Weighing used sponges can provide an estimate of blood loss (Blanchard & Burlingame, 2012).* EB: *Weighing fluid used and returned provides a more accurate measurement of fluid deficit than measuring the fluids (Silva et al, 2013). The use of balanced electrolyte IV solutions has been shown to be safer than the use of isotonic saline alone (Myles et al, 2017).*
- Observe the surgical client for hyperkalemia with symptoms including dysrhythmias, heart block, asystole, abdominal distention, and weakness. EB: *Hyperkalemia can occur intraoperatively because of massive blood transfusions, tissue breakdown from surgery, shifting of potassium from the cells into the extracellular fluid, decreased potassium excretion caused by renal failure or hypovolemia, crush injuries, or burns (Drury & Denker, 2020).*

F

- Maintain the client's core temperature at normal levels, using warming devices as needed. EB: *Hypothermia (body temperature <36°C) is present in the postoperative period in 26% to 90% of all clients who have undergone elective surgery. The risk of hypothermia is particularly high in clients over 60 years of age with poor nutritional status and preexisting disease that impairs thermoregulation (e.g., diabetes mellitus with polyneuropathy), and in those who have had major or lengthy surgery. Lower temperatures in the operating room also increase the risk of hypothermia: the lower the temperature, the higher the risk (Torossian et al, 2015).*
- Fluids administration during surgery can increase risk of hypothermia. EB: *Research has shown that perioperative hypothermia can adversely affect the cardiopulmonary system (Giuliano & Hendricks, 2017).*

Postoperative

- Continue to monitor fluids postoperatively. EB: *Restrictive fluid therapy and liberal conventional therapy were associated with similar rates of overall and cardiopulmonary complications; however, restrictive fluid therapy was associated with a more rapid recovery and a shorter length of hospital stay (Jia et al, 2017). Also, fluid overload is an independent risk factor for the development of acute kidney injury (Salahuddin et al, 2017).*
- Assess the client for development of tissue edema, especially after cataract surgery in clients with comorbidities such as diabetes. EB: *A history of diabetes mellitus has been found to be an independent risk factor for the development of postoperative cystoid macular edema in clients undergoing cataract surgery (Ovewole et al, 2017).*
- Recognize that IV fluid replacement decisions incorporate multiple assessment parameters such as hourly urine output, blood pressure, heart rate, respiratory rate, lung sounds, output from drains, and changes in laboratory results (e.g., hemoglobin/hematocrit, serum electrolytes).

Geriatric

- Check skin turgor of older clients on the forehead, subclavian area, or inner thigh; also look for the presence of longitudinal furrows on the tongue and dry mucous membranes. EB: *Older people commonly have decreased skin turgor from normal age-related loss of elasticity, and checking skin turgor on the arm is not reflective of fluid volume (Fingerhood, 2021).*
- Closely monitor urine output, concentration of urine, and serum BUN/creatinine results. EB: *Reduced renal perfusion and altered renal function as a normal or abnormal change in physiological aging can compromise the client's fluid volume status (Fingerhood, 2021).*
- Monitor older clients for excess fluid volume during the treatment of deficient fluid volume: auscultate lung sounds, assess for edema, and trend vital signs.
- Assess the older client's cognitive status. EB: *Cognitive impairment is a risk factor associated with dehydration, especially in the older adult (Fingerhood, 2021).*

Pediatric

- Assess the pediatric client's weight, length of NPO status, and underlying illness, and the surgical procedure to be performed.
- Recognize that newborns require very little fluid replacement when undergoing major surgical procedures during the first few days of life.
- Monitor pediatric surgical clients closely for signs of fluid loss.
- Administer fluids preoperatively until NPO status must be initiated so that fluid deficit is decreased.
- Perform an assessment for signs of fluid responsiveness in the pediatric client. EB: *A systematic review found that respiratory variation was the only assessment parameter to most reliably predict a pediatric client's responsiveness for fluid administration (Zeretzke-Bien, 2018).* EB: *Rehydration solutions such as low osmolality solutions have been shown to be safe and effective for correcting dehydration in children (Kumar et al, 2015).*

REFERENCES

American Society of Anesthesiologists Committee. (2011). Practice guidelines for preoperative fasting and the use of pharmacologic agents to reduce the risk of pulmonary aspiration: Application to healthy patients undergoing elective procedures: An updated report by the American Society of Anesthesiologists Committee on Standards and Practice Parameters. *Anesthesiology*, *114*(3), 495–511.

Bartels, K., Esper, S. A., & Thiele, R. H. (2016). Blood pressure monitoring for the anesthesiologist: A practical review. *Anesthesia & Analgesia*, *122*(6), 1866–1879.

Blanchard, J., & Burlingame, B. (2012). Perioperative standards and recommended practices. *AORN Journal*.

Drury, E. R., & Denker, B. M. (2020). Inpatient management of hyperkalemia. In R. K. Garg, J. V. Hennessey, A. O. Malabanan, & J.

R. Garber (Eds.), *Handbook of inpatient endocrinology* (pp. 189–198). Cham, Switzerland: Springer. https://doi-org.ezproxy.liberty.edu/10.1007/978-3-030-38976-5_16.

Fingerhood, M. L. (2021). Age-related changes in health. In M. Boltz, E. A. Capezuti, D. A. Zwicker, & T. Fulmer (Eds.), *Evidence-based geriatric nursing protocols for best practice* (6th ed.) (pp. 59–80). New York: Springer.

Giuliano, K. K., & Hendricks, J. (2017). Inadvertent perioperative hypothermia: Current nursing knowledge. *AORN Journal, 105*(5), 453–463.

Icin, T., Medic-Stojanoska, M., Ilic, T., et al. (2017). Multiple causes of hyponatremia: A case report. *Medical Principles and Practice, 26*(3), 292–295. doi:10.1159/000468938.

Jia, F. J., Yan, Q. Y., Sun, Q., Tuxun, T., Liu, H., & Shao, L. (2017). Liberal versus restrictive fluid management in abdominal surgery: A meta-analysis. *Surgery Today, 47*(3), 344–356.

Kear, T. M. (2017). Fluid and electrolyte management across the age continuum. *Nephrology Nursing Journal, 44*(6), 491–496.

Kumar, R., Kumar, P., Aneja, S., Kumar, V., & Rehan, H. S. (2015). Safety and efficacy of low-osmolarity ORS vs. modified rehydration solution for malnourished children for treatment of children with severe acute malnutrition and diarrhea: A randomized controlled trial. *Journal of Tropical Pediatrics, 61*(6), 435–441.

Levy, I., Attias, S., Ben-Arye, E., et al. (2017). Perioperative risks of dietary and herbal supplements. *World Journal of Surgery, 41*(4), 927–934.

Lindahl, S. B. (2020). Intraoperative irrigation: Fluid administration and management amidst conflicting evidence. *AORN Journal, 111*(5), 495–507. doi:10.1002/aorn.13010.

Macedo, E., Malhotra, R., Bouchard, J., Wynn, S. K., & Mehta, R. L. (2011). Oliguria is an early predictor of higher mortality in critically ill patients. *Kidney International, 80*(7), 760–767.

Myles, P. S., Andrews, S., Nicholson, J., Lobo, D. N., & Mythen, M. (2017). Contemporary approaches to perioperative IV fluid therapy. *World Journal of Surgery, 41*(10), 2457–2463. https://dx.doi.org.ezproxy.liberty.edu/10.1007/s00268-017-4055-y.

Oyewole, K., Tsogkas, F., Westcott, M., & Patra, S. (2017). Benchmarking cataract surgery outcomes in an ethnically diverse and diabetic population: Final post-operative visual acuity and rates of post-operative cystoid macular oedema. *Eye, 31*(12), 1672–1677.

Pasha, M. T., Khan, M. A., Jamal, Y., Wahab, F., & Naeem-Ullah, U. (2015). Postoperative complications with glycine and sterile distilled water after transurethral resection of prostate. *Journal of Ayub Medical College, Abbottabad, 27*(1), 135–139.

Powers, J. (2017). Changing guidelines for preoperative fasting. *Critical Care Nurse, 37*(1), 76–77.

Salahuddin, N., Sammani, M., Hamdan, A., et al. (2017). Fluid overload is an independent risk factor for acute kidney injury in critically ill patients: Results of a cohort study. *BMC Nephrology, 18*(1), 45.

Silva, J. M., Jr., Barros, M. A., Chahda, M. A. L., Santos, I. M., Marubayashi, L. Y., & Sá Malbouisson, L. M. (2013). Risk factors for perioperative complications in endoscopic surgery with irrigation. *Brazilian Journal of Anesthesiology, 63*(4), 327–333.

Strunden, M. S., Heckel, K., Goetz, A. E., & Reuter, D. A. (2011). Perioperative fluid and volume management: Physiological basis, tools and strategies. *Annals of Intensive Care, 1*(1), 2.

Torossian, A., Bräuer, A., Höcker, J., Bein, B., Wulf, H., & Horn, E. P. (2015). Preventing inadvertent perioperative hypothermia. *Deutsches Ärzteblatt International, 112*(10), 166–172.

Zeretzke-Bien, C. M. (2018). Resuscitation: Pediatric algorithms. In C. M. Zeretzke-Bien, T. B. Swan, & B. R. Allen (Eds.), *Quick hits for pediatric emergency medicine* (pp. 17–22). Cham, Switzerland: Springer. https://doi-org.ezproxy.liberty.edu/10.1007/978-3-319-93830-1_3.

F

Deficient Fluid Volume Domain 2 Nutrition Class 5 Hydration

Dina M. Hewett, PhD, RN, NEA-BC

NANDA-I

Definition

Decreased intravascular, interstitial, and/or intracellular fluid. This refers to dehydration, water loss alone without change in sodium.

Defining Characteristics

Altered mental status; altered skin turgor; decreased blood pressure; decreased pulse pressure; decreased pulse volume; decreased tongue turgor; decreased urine output; decreased venous filling; dry mucous membranes; dry skin; increased body temperature; increased heart rate; increased serum hematocrit levels; increased urine concentration; sudden weight loss; thirst; weakness

Related Factors

Difficulty meeting increased fluid volume requirement; inadequate access to fluid; inadequate knowledge about fluid needs; ineffective medication self-management; insufficient fluid intake; insufficient muscle mass; malnutrition

At-Risk Population

Individuals at extremes of weight; individuals with external conditions affecting fluid needs; individuals with internal conditions affecting fluid needs; women

Associated Conditions

Active fluid volume loss; deviations affecting fluid absorption; deviations affecting fluid elimination; deviations affecting fluid intake; excessive fluid loss through normal route; fluid loss through abnormal route; pharmaceutical preparations; treatment regimen

NOC (Nursing Outcomes Classification)

Suggested NOC Outcomes

Fluid Balance; Hydration; Nutritional Status: Food and Fluid Intake

Example NOC Outcome with Indicators

Fluid Balance as evidenced by the following indicators: Elastic skin turgor/Moist mucous membranes/ Orthostatic hypotension not present/24-hour intake and output balance/Urine specific gravity. (Rate each indicator of **Fluid Balance:** 1 = severely compromised, 2 = substantially compromised, 3 = moderately compromised, 4 = mildly compromised, 5 = not compromised [see Section I].)

F

Client Outcomes

Client Will (Specify Time Frame)

- Maintain urine output of 0.5 to 1.5 mL/kg/h or at least more than 1300 mL/day
- Maintain normal blood pressure, heart rate, and body temperature
- Maintain elastic skin turgor; moist tongue and mucous membranes; and orientation to person, place, and time
- Explain measures that can be taken to treat or prevent fluid volume loss
- Describe symptoms that indicate the need to consult with health care provider

NIC (Nursing Interventions Classification)

Suggested NIC Interventions

Fluid Management; Hypovolemia Management; Shock Management: Volume

Example NIC Activities—Fluid Management

Monitor hydration status (e.g., moist mucous membranes, adequacy of pulses, and orthostatic blood pressure) as appropriate; Administer intravenous (IV) therapy, as prescribed

Nursing Interventions and *Rationales*

- Watch for early signs of hypovolemia, including thirst, restlessness, headaches, and inability to concentrate. *Thirst is often the first sign of dehydration (Canfield, 2021).* CEB: *A study of healthy women showed heart rate was increased by fluid restriction along with increased urine specific gravity, darker urine color, and increased thirst. They also experienced decreased alertness and increased sleepiness, fatigue, and confusion (Pross et al, 2013).* EB: *A combination of biochemical markers that include serum osmolality (i.e., blood urea nitrogen and creatinine) and urine osmolality and specific gravity, blood pressure assessment and clinical symptoms such as thirst, dry mouth, lack of tears provide reliable assessment of dehydration (Armstrong et al, 2016).*
- Recognize symptoms of cyanosis, cold clammy skin, weak thready pulse, confusion, and oliguria as late signs of hypovolemia. EB: *These symptoms occur after the body has compensated for fluid loss by moving fluid from the interstitial space into the vascular compartment (Canfield, 2021).*
- Monitor pulse, respiration, and blood pressure of clients with deficient fluid volume every 15 minutes to 1 hour for the unstable client and every 4 hours for the stable client. *Vital sign changes seen with fluid volume deficit include tachycardia, tachypnea, decreased pulse pressure first, then hypotension, decreased pulse volume, and increased or decreased body temperature (Canfield, 2021).* CEB: *A systematic review demonstrated that hypotension and tachycardia, and occasionally fever, are clinical signs of dehydration (Jéquier & Constant, 2010).*
- Check orthostatic blood pressures with the client lying, sitting, and standing. EB: *A decrease in systolic blood pressure of 20 mm Hg or a decrease in diastolic blood pressure of 10 mm Hg within 3 minutes of*

standing when compared with blood pressure from the sitting position is considered orthostatic hypotension. This can occur with dehydration or cardiovascular disorders (Wedro & Stöppler, 2019).

- Note skin turgor over bony prominences such as the hand or shin.
- Monitor for the existence of factors causing deficient fluid volume (e.g., hypovolemia from vomiting, diarrhea, difficulty maintaining oral intake, fever, uncontrolled type 2 diabetes, diuretic therapy). EB: *Early identification of risk factors and early intervention can decrease the occurrence and severity of complications from deficient fluid volume and acute kidney injury (Dean, 2020; Canfield, 2021).*
- Observe for dry tongue and mucous membranes, and longitudinal tongue furrows. EB: *These are symptoms of decreased body fluids (Armstrong et al, 2016).*
- Recognize that checking capillary refill is an assessment of peripheral perfusion and may not be helpful in identifying fluid volume deficit. EB: *Capillary refill can appear to be normal in clients with sepsis or shock because increased body temperature dilates peripheral blood vessels and capillary return may be immediate (Canfield, 2021). A quick test is compression of the nail bed sufficient to cause blanching. If there is good blood flow to the nail bed, a pink color should return in less than 2 seconds after pressure is removed. Slow return to pink color can indicate dehydration (White, 2012; Bridges, 2017).* CEB: *Capillary refill has been shown to be a good clinical indicator to detect poor perfusion with good specificity but poor sensitivity (Shimizu et al, 2012).*
- Weigh client daily and watch for sudden decreases, especially in the presence of decreasing urine output or active fluid loss. EB: *Body weight changes of 1 kg (2.2 pounds) represent a fluid loss of 1 L (Canfield, 2021).*
- Monitor total fluid intake and output every 4 hours (or every hour for the unstable client or the client who has urine output equal to or less than 0.5 mL/kg/h). EB: *Recognize that urine output is an indicator of fluid balance. However, urine output alone does not differentiate between volume-sensitive reductions in glomerular filtration rate and structural kidney injury (Schrezenmeier et al, 2017).*
- A urine output of less than 0.5 mL/kg/h for more than 6 hours may be indicative of acute kidney injury (Dean, 2020; Molinari et al, 2020). Nevertheless, in any condition of hypovolemia, renal perfusion pressure falls. If it falls below the level of autoregulation (BP <80 mm Hg), renal blood flow and glomerular filtration will fall (Andreucchi et al, 2017). EB: *The RIFLE criteria define* oliguria *as urine output less than 0.5 mL/kg/hr for each of six or more consecutive hours, which is thought to confer "risk" of kidney injury; when urine output is less than 0.5 mL/kg/h and persists for 12 or more consecutive hours, the kidneys are considered to be "in injury" (James et al, 2016). The Kidney Disease: Improving Global Outcomes (KDIGO) guidelines indicate that acute kidney injury is an increase in creatinine 1.5 to 1.9 times baseline and urine output <0.5 mL/kg/h for 6 to 12 hours (Alseiari et al, 2016).*
- Note the color of urine, urine osmolality, and specific gravity. EB: *Normal urine is straw colored or amber. Dark-colored urine with a specific gravity greater than 1.030 and a high urine osmolality reflects fluid volume deficit (Kerber, 2021). Although these tools for dehydration screening have been advocated for use in the elderly, their diagnostic accuracy is low and may not be useful (Hooper et al, 2016b).*
- Provide fresh water and oral fluids preferred by the client (distribute over 24 hours [e.g., 1200 mL during days, 800 mL during evenings, and 200 mL during nights]), provide prescribed diet, offer snacks (e.g., frequent drinks, fresh fruits, fruit juice), and instruct significant other to assist the client with feedings as appropriate. EB: *Distributing the intake over the entire 24-hour period and providing snacks, specifically those with creatine and carnitine, and beverages including caffeine may improve muscular ability, endurance, and alertness (Somes, 2020).*

▲ Provide oral replacement therapy as ordered and tolerated with a hypotonic glucose-electrolyte solution when the client has acute diarrhea or nausea/vomiting. Provide small, frequent quantities of slightly chilled solutions. EB: *Maintenance of oral intake stabilizes the ability of the intestines to absorb nutrients and promote gastric emptying (Gaspar & Mentes, 2021); glucose-electrolyte solutions increase net fluid absorption while correcting deficient fluid volume. Use diluted carbohydrate-electrolyte solutions, such as sports replacement drinks, and ginger ale (Lešnik et al, 2017). The use of diluted oral replacement fluids has been found to reduce the need for IV hydration (Lešnik et al, 2017).*

▲ Administer antidiarrheals and antiemetics as ordered and appropriate. Consider what the client is eating to prevent further diarrhea (Bolen, 2020). The goal is to stop the loss that results from vomiting or diarrhea. Refer to care plan for **Diarrhea** or **Nausea.**

- If the client is on enteral feedings, evidence has shown either continuous or intermittent feedings had similar results regarding diarrhea and nausea (Houston & Fuldauer, 2017). EB: *Evaluate the rate of enteral feeding formula administration and other medications to address diarrhea and nausea (Houston & Fuldauer, 2017).*

- ▲ Hydrate the client with isotonic IV solutions as prescribed. EB: *For clients with mild to moderate fluid deficit, lactated Ringer's should be used for fluid volume replacement (Canfield, 2021).*
- • Assist with ambulation if the client has postural hypotension. EB: *Hypovolemia causes orthostatic hypotension, which can result in syncope when the client goes from a sitting to standing position (Canfield, 2021).*

Critically Ill

- ▲ Monitor stroke volume, passive leg lift, and ultrasound as trends for more accurate fluid volume status. EB: *Hemodynamic pressures such as central venous pressure (CVP) and pulmonary artery pressures have been demonstrated to be less predictive and specific of fluid volume responsiveness (Barlow et al, 2020), whereas changes in stroke volume measured by a number of noninvasive methods including passive leg lift may more accurately predict fluid volume responsiveness of a client (Bridges, 2017; Canfield, 2021).*
- ▲ Monitor serum and urine osmolality blood urea nitrogen (BUN)/creatinine ratio and hematocrit for elevations. EB: *These are all measures of concentration and will be elevated with decreased intravascular volume (Armstrong et al, 2016).*
- ▲ Insert an indwelling urinary catheter if ordered and measure urine output hourly. Notify health care provider if urine output is less than 0.5 mL/kg/h. EB: *A decrease in urine output is seen with poorly perfused kidneys and a drop in the glomerular filtration rate in the client with normal kidney function, and action, if taken early, can prevent further deterioration. Intensive monitoring of urine output is associated with increased detection of acute kidney injury and improved outcomes (Jin et al, 2017; Molinari et al, 2020; Kerber, 2021).*
- ▲ When ordered, initiate a fluid challenge of crystalloids (e.g., lactated Ringer's or 0.9% normal saline) for replacement of intravascular volume. EB: *Guidelines for early goal-directed therapy (EGDT) have been developed by the Surviving Sepsis campaign; however, EGDT in one study did not significantly decrease mortality (Zhang et al, 2017). A systematic review of the literature found that the passive leg raise intervention was valid and reliable in evaluating critically ill and mechanically ventilated clients' need for fluid resuscitation compared with IV fluid challenges that may result in fluid overload (Assadi, 2017).*
- ▲ Monitor the client's response to prescribed fluid therapy and fluid challenge, especially noting vital signs (mean arterial pressure [MAP] >65 mm Hg in the first 6 hours of treatment, systolic blood pressure >100 mm Hg) (Singer, 2016; Rhodes et al, 2017), urine output, blood lactate concentrations, and lung sounds. EB: *A fluid challenge can help the client with deficient fluid volume regain intravascular volume quickly, but the client must be carefully observed to ensure that he or she does not go into fluid volume overload because excess fluid volume can lead to organ edema and increased mortality (Assadi, 2017; Canfield, 2021).*
- • Position the client flat with legs elevated when hypotensive, if not contraindicated. EB: *This position enhances venous return and, coupled with stroke volume measurement, is a simple noninvasive technique to determine fluid responsiveness (Assadi, 2017).*
- ▲ Monitor trends in serum lactic acid levels and base deficit obtained from blood gases as ordered. EB: *A trend of increasing lactic acid levels >2.0 has been shown to increase mortality than levels less than 2.0 (Seymour et al, 2016; Rhodes et al, 2017).*
- ▲ Consult provider if signs and symptoms of deficient fluid volume persist or worsen. EB: *Prolonged deficient fluid volume increases the risk for development of complications, including decrease in cognitive function, weakness, tachycardia, hemodynamic instability, and kidney injury (Singer, 2016).*

Pediatric

- • Monitor the child for signs of deficient fluid volume, including sunken eyes, decreased tears, dry mucous membranes, poor skin turgor, and decreased urine output (Hockenberry et al, 2019). EB: *These assessment factors are more significant in identifying dehydration, but a combination of physical examination findings is a much better predictor than individual signs (Carson et al, 2017).*
- ▲ Reinforce the health care provider recommendation for the parents to give the child oral rehydration fluids to drink in the amounts specified, especially during the first 4 to 6 hours to replace fluid losses. Consider using diluted oral rehydration fluids. Once the child is rehydrated, an orally administered maintenance solution should be used along with food. EB: *A study demonstrated that treatment with oral rehydration fluids for children was generally as effective as IV fluids, and IV fluids did not shorten the duration of gastroenteritis and are more likely to cause adverse effects than oral rehydration therapy (Carson et al, 2016).* EB: *Current clinical practice guidelines have shown that diluted oral replacement fluids and some drugs resulted in reductions in stool output, decreased vomiting, and less need for IV hydration (Carson et al, 2017).*
- • Recommend that the mother resume breastfeeding as soon as possible.

- Recommend that parents not give the child carbonated soda, fruit juices, gelatin dessert, or instant fruit drink mix; instead, give the child oral rehydration fluids ordered and, when tolerated, food. EB: *Rehydration solutions such as low osmolality solutions have been shown to be safe and effective for correcting dehydration in children (Kumar et al, 2015). Antiemetic, antidiarrheal agents and probiotics have been shown to reduce the duration and severity of infectious diarrhea (Hockenberry et al, 2019).*
- Once the child has been rehydrated, begin feeding regular food, but avoid milk products (Guandalini et al, 2020).

Geriatric

- Monitor older clients for deficient fluid volume carefully, noting new onset of headache, weakness, dizziness, and postural hypotension. EB: *Older people are thought to be at greater risk of dehydration because thirst sensation and urinary concentrating ability frequently decline with age. Many older people use diuretics or laxatives, which encourage fluid loss, and reduced muscle volume leads to a smaller fluid reserve. Oral fluid intake may fall in older people for a variety of reasons, including reduced enjoyment of drinks, physical limitations, unmet activities of daily living needs, acute and chronic health problems, and decisions aimed at controlling continence (Oates & Price, 2017; Mantantzis et al, 2020). Additionally, those with dementia may forget to drink as daily routines are lost and social contact diminishes.*
- Implement fall precautions for clients experiencing weakness, dizziness, and/or postural hypotension. EB: *Falls are a serious risk in the elderly, especially those with hyponatremia (Kuo et al, 2017).*
- Dehydration in the older adult is associated with poor health outcomes, including fractures, heart disease, infections, and drug toxicity (Lešnik et al, 2017).
- Evaluate the risk for dehydration using the Dehydration Risk Appraisal Checklist. CEB: *A study demonstrated that the checklist has potential to predict the onset of dehydration in nursing home clients (Mentes & Wang, 2011).*
- Check skin turgor of older clients on the forehead and axilla; check for dry mucous membranes and dry tongue. EB: *A Cochrane review recommended in clinical practice to avoid the reliance on one clinical symptom as a sign of water-loss dehydration in older people (Hooper et al, 2016a). Older adults are susceptible to dehydration because of acute and chronic health problems, which impair thirst; reduce the ability to drink sufficiently; and/or increase urinary, skin, and respiratory fluid loss (Hooper et al, 2016b; Oates & Price, 2017). Older adults present with a constellation of signs and symptoms that need to be further evaluated for connection to dehydration. Signs and symptoms include fatigue, pallor, sunken periorbital area, chapped lips, hypotension, tachycardia, fever, orthostatic blood pressure, weight loss >4%, poor skin turgor over the sternum, and change in mental status (Miller, 2015).*
- Encourage fluid intake by offering fluids regularly to cognitively impaired clients. EB: *The single most common risk factor reported associated with dehydration in cognitively impaired clients was a worsening or change in mental state (Oates & Price, 2017).*
- Because older clients have low water reserves, they should be encouraged to drink regularly even when not thirsty. Frequent and varied beverage offerings should be made available by hydration assistants to routinely offer increased beverages to clients in extended care. EB: *Strategies to improve fluid intake include making healthy drinks and water easily available and accessible at all times and reminding and encouraging older adults to consume these fluids. Older people should not be encouraged to consume large amounts of fluids at once but rather small amounts throughout the day (Oates & Price, 2017).*
- Flag the food tray of clients with chronic dehydration to indicate if the client is identified as having chronic dehydration and indicate that they should finish 75% to 100% of their food and fluids. EB: *Offering beverages in brightly colored cups may improve fluid intake. Older clients often have a combination of both malnutrition and fluid deficit and may not have good taste sensation (Gaspar & Mentes, 2021).*
- Recognize that lower blood pressures and monitoring of an intake record over 24 hours are recommended to track oral intake and possible dehydration (Oates & Price, 2017).
- A higher BUN/creatinine ratio can be significant signs of dehydration in older adults. EB: *Structural changes of the kidney include alterations of renal blood flow of up to 50% from age 20 to 80. As people age, the kidney undergoes age-related changes, which translate to an inexorable and progressive decline in renal function.*
- In the United States more than 50% of seniors over the age of 75 are believed to have kidney disease (National Kidney Foundation, 2021).
- Monitor older clients for excess fluid volume during the treatment of deficient fluid volume: auscultate lung sounds, assess for edema, and note vital signs. EB: *The older client has a decreased ability to adapt to rapid increases in intravascular volume and can quickly develop fluid overload.*

Home Care

- Teach family members how to monitor output in the home (e.g., use of commode "hat" in the toilet, urinal, or bedpan, or use of catheter and closed drainage system). Instruct them to monitor both intake and output. Use common terms such as "cups" or "glasses of water a day" when providing education.
- When weighing the client, use same scale each day. Be sure scale is on a flat, not cushioned, surface. Do not weigh the client with a scale placed on any type of rug because scales provide more accurate readings when used on a hard surface.
- Teach family about complications of deficient fluid volume and when to call the health care provider.
- Teach the family the signs of hypovolemia, especially in older adults, and how to monitor for dizziness or unsteady gait.
- If the client is receiving IV fluids, there must be a responsible caregiver in the home. Teach caregiver about administration of fluids, complications of IV administration (e.g., fluid volume overload, development of phlebitis, speed of medication reactions), and when to call for assistance. Assist caregiver with administration for as long as necessary to maintain client safety. Administration of IV fluids in the home is a high-technology procedure and requires sufficient professional support to ensure safety of the client.
- Identify an emergency plan, including when to call 911. Some complications of deficient fluid volume cannot be reversed in the home and are life-threatening. Clients progressing toward hypovolemic shock will need emergency care.
- Deficient fluid volume may be a symptom of impending death in terminally ill clients. In palliative care situations, treatment of deficient fluid volume should be determined based on client/family goals. Information and support should be provided to assist the client/family in this decision. Support the family/client in a palliative care situation to decide if it is appropriate to intervene for deficient fluid volume or to allow the client to die without fluids. EB: *Deficient fluid volume may be a symptom of impending death in terminally ill clients. There is no defined gold standard for hydrating dying clients, and hydration and nutrition are considered basic acts for care of a dying client (Bear et al, 2017).*

Client/Family Teaching and Discharge Planning

- Instruct the client to avoid rapid position changes, especially from supine to sitting or standing.
- Teach the client and family about appropriate diet, fluid intake, and how to weight self weekly.
- Teach the client and family how to measure and record intake and output accurately.
- Teach the client and family about measures instituted to treat hypovolemia and to prevent or treat fluid volume loss.
- Instruct the client and family about signs of deficient fluid volume that indicate they should contact health care provider.

REFERENCES

Alseiari, M., Meyer, K. B., & Wong, J. B. (2016). Evidence underlying KDIGO (Kidney Disease: Improving Global Outcomes) guideline recommendations: A systematic review. *American Journal of Kidney Diseases*, *67*(3), 417–422.

Andreucci, M., Faga, T., Pisani, A., Perticone, M., & Michael, A. (2017). The ischemic/nephrotoxic acute kidney injury and the use of renal biomarkers in clinical practice. *European Journal of Internal Medicine*, *39*, 1–8.

Armstrong, L. E., Kavouras, S. A., Walsh, N. P., & Roberts, W. O. (2016). Diagnosing dehydration? Blend evidence with clinical observations. *Current Opinion in Clinical Nutrition and Metabolic Care*, *19*(6), 434–438. https://doi.org/10.1097/MCO.0000000000000320.

Assadi, F. (2017). Passive leg raising: Simple and reliable technique to prevent fluid overload in critically ill patients. *International Journal of Preventive Medicine*, *8*, 48.

Barlow, A., Barlow, B., Tang, N., Shah, B. M., & King, A. E. (2020). Intravenous fluid management in critically ill adults: A review. *Critical Care Nurse*, *40*(6), e17–e27. https://doi.org/10.4037/ccn2020337.

Bear, A. J., Bukowy, E. A., & Patel, J. J. (2017). Artificial hydration at the end of life. *Nutrition in Clinical Practice* (32), 628–632 5. https://doi-org.ezproxy.liberty.edu/10.1177/0884533617724741.

Bolen, B. B. (2020). *What to eat when you have diarrhea*. Verywell Health [website]. Retrieved from https://www.verywellhealth.com/what-to-eat-for-diarrhea-1944822. Accessed June 30, 2021.

Bridges, E. (2017). CE: Assessing patients during septic shock resuscitation. *American Journal of Nursing*, *117*(10), 34–40. https://doi.org/10.1097/01.NAJ.0000525851.44945.70.

Canfield, C. M. (2021). Shock, sepsis, and multiple organ dysfunction syndrome. In M. L. Sole, D. G. Klein, M. J. Moseley, M. B. F. Makic, & L. T. Morata (Eds.), *Introduction to critical care nursing* (8th ed.) (pp. 248–281). St. Louis: Elsevier.

Carson, R. A., Mudd, S. S., & Madati, P. J. (2016). Clinical practice guideline for the treatment of pediatric acute gastroenteritis in the outpatient setting. *Journal of Pediatric Health Care*, *6*(30), 610–616. https://doi.org/10.1016/j.

Carson, R. A., Mudd, S. S., & Madati, P. J. (2017). Evaluation of a nurse-initiated acute gastroenteritis pathway in the pediatric emergency department. *Journal of Emergency Nursing*, *43*(5), 406–412. https://doi.org/ezproxy.liberty.edu/10.1016/j.jen.2017.01.001.

Dean, E. (2020). Acute kidney injury: Who is at risk and how to care for patients. *Nursing Standard*, *35*(5), 67–68. https://doi.org/ezproxy.liberty.edu/10.7748/ns.35.5.67.s23.

Gaspar, P. M., & Mentes, J. C. (2021). Managing oral hydration in the older adult. In M. Boltz, E. A. Capezuti, D. A. Zwicker, & T. Fulmer (Eds.), *Evidence-based Geriatric nursing Protocols for best practice* (6th ed.) (pp. 157–178). New York: Springer.

Guandalini, S., Frye, R. E., & Tamer, M. A. (2020). *Diarrhea. Medscape [website]*. Retrieved from https://emedicine.medscape.com/article/928598-overview. Accessed June 30, 2021.

Hockenberry, M. J., Wilson, D., & Rodgers, C. C. (Eds.). (2019). *Wong's nursing care of infants and children* (11th ed.) St. Louis: Elsevier.

Hooper, L., Bunn, D. K., Abdelhamid, A., et al. (2016a). Water loss (intracellular) dehydration assessed using urinary tests: How well do they work? Diagnostic accuracy in older people. *American Journal of Clinical Nutrition, 104*(1), 121–131.

Hooper, L., Bunn, D. K., Downing, A., et al. (2016b). Which frail older people are dehydrated? The UK DRIE study. *Journals of Gerontology. Series A, Biological Sciences and Medical Sciences, 71*(10), 1341–1347.

Houston, A., & Fuldauer, P. (2017). Enteral feeding: Indications, complications, and nursing care. *American Nurse Today, 12*(1), 20–25. Retrieved from https://www.myamericannurse.com/wp-content/uploads/2016/12-ant1-CE-Enteral-Feeding-1219.pdf. Accessed February 16, 2022.

James, M. T., Hobson, C. E., Darmon, M., et al. (2016). Applications for detection of acute kidney injury using electronic medical records and clinical information systems: Workgroup statements from the 15th ADQI Consensus Conference. *Canadian Journal of Kidney Health and Disease, 3*, 9. https://doi.org/10.1186/s40697-016-0100-2.

Jéquier, E., & Constant, F. (2010). Water as an essential nutrient: The physiological basis of hydration. *European Journal of Clinical Nutrition, 64*(2), 115–123.

Jin, K., Murugan, R., Sileanu, F. E., et al. (2017). Intensive monitoring of urine output is associated with increased detection of acute kidney injury and improved outcomes. *Chest, 152*(5), 972–979.

Kerber, K. G. (2021). Acute kidney injury. In M. L. Sole, D. G. Klein, M. J. Moseley, M. B. F. Makic, & L. T. Morata (Eds.), *Introduction to critical care nursing* (8th ed.) (pp. 404–427). St. Louis: Elsevier.

Kumar, R., Kumar, P., Aneja, S., Kumar, V., & Rehan, H. S. (2015). Safety and efficacy of low-osmolarity ORS vs. modified rehydration solution for malnourished children for treatment of children with severe acute malnutrition and diarrhea: A randomized controlled trial. *Journal of Tropical Pediatrics, 61*(6), 435–441.

Kuo, S. C. H., Kuo, P. J., Rau, C. S., Wu, S. C., Hsu, S. Y., & Hsieh, C. H. (2017). Hyponatremia is associated with worse outcomes from fall injuries in the elderly. *International Journal of Environmental Research and Public Health, 14*(5), 460. PII:E460.

Lešnik, A., Piko, N., Železnik, D., & Bevc, S. (2017). Dehydration of older patients in institutional care and the home environment. *Research in Gerontological Nursing, 10*(6), 260–266. https://doi.org/ezproxy.liberty.edu/10.3928/19404921-20171013-03.

Mantantzis, K., Drewelies, J., Duezel, S., et al. (2020). Dehydration predicts longitudinal decline in cognitive functioning and well-being among older adults. *Psychology and Aging, 35*(4), 517–528.

Mentes, J. C., & Wang, J. (2011). Measuring risk for dehydration in nursing home residents: Evaluation of the dehydration risk appraisal checklist. *Research in Gerontological Nursing, 4*(2), 148–156.

Miller, H. J. (2015). Dehydration in the older adult. *Journal of Gerontological Nursing, 41*(9), 8–13.

Molinari, L., Sakhuja, A., & Kellum, J. A. (2020). Perioperative renoprotection: General mechanisms and treatment approaches. *Anesthesia & Analgesia, 131*(6), 1679–1692. https://doi.org/10.1213/ANE.0000000000005107.

National Kidney Foundation. (2021). *Aging and kidney disease*. Retrieved from https://www.kidney.org/news/monthly/wkd_aging. Accessed June 30, 2021.

Oates, L. L., & Price, C. I. (2017). Clinical assessments and care interventions to promote oral hydration amongst older patients: A narrative systematic review. *BMC Nursing, 16*, 4.

Pross, N., Demazières, A., Girard, N., et al. (2013). Influence of progressive fluid restriction on mood and physiological markers of dehydration in women. *British Journal of Nutrition, 109*(2), 313–321.

Rhodes, A., Evans, L. E., Alhazzani, W., et al. (2017). Surviving sepsis campaign: International guidelines for management of sepsis and septic shock: 2016. *Critical Care Medicine, 45*(3), 486–552.

Schrezenmeier, E. V., Barasch, J., Budde, K., Westhoff, T., & Schmidt-Ott, K. M. (2017). Biomarkers in acute kidney injury—Pathophysiological basis and clinical performance. *Acta Physiologica, 219*(3), 554–572.

Seymour, C. W., Liu, V. S., Iwashyna, T. J., et al. (2016). Assessment of clinical criteria for sepsis: For the Third International consensus definitions for sepsis and septic shock (Sepsis-3). *Journal of the American Medical Association, 315*(8), 762–774.

Shimizu, M., Kinoshita, K., Hattori, K., et al. (2012). Physical signs of dehydration in the elderly. *Internal Medicine (Tokyo, Japan), 51*(10), 1207–1210.

Singer, M. (2016). The new sepsis consensus definitions (Sepsis-3): The good, the not-so-bad, and the actually-quite-pretty. *Intensive Care Medicine, 42*(12), 2027–2029.

Somes, J. (2020). Weak and dizzy—another explanation to explore: Poor nutrition in the older adult. *Journal of Emergency Nursing, 46*(4), 541–545. https://doi.org/10.1016/j.jen.2020.02.016.

Wedro, B., & Stöppler, M. C. (2019). *Orthostatic hypotension (low blood pressure when standing)*. MedicineNet [website]. Retrieved from http://www.medicinenet.com/orthostatic_hypotension/article.htm. Accessed June 30, 2021.

White, C. J. (2012). Atherosclerotic peripheral arterial disease. In L. Goldman, & A. I. Schafer (Eds.), *Goldmans Cecil medicine* (25th ed.) (pp. 486–492). Philadelphia: Elsevier.

Zhang, Z., Hong, Y., Smischney, N. J., et al. (2017). Early management of sepsis with emphasis on early goal directed therapy: AME evidence series 002. *Journal of Thoracic Disease, 9*(2), 392–405.

F

Excess Fluid Volume Domain 2 Nutrition Class 5 Hydration

Dina Hewett, PhD, RN, NEA-BC

NANDA-I

Definition

Surplus retention of fluid.

Defining Characteristics

Adventitious breath sounds; altered blood pressure; altered mental status; altered pulmonary artery pressure; altered respiratory pattern; altered urine specific gravity; anxiety; azotemia; decreased serum hematocrit levels; decreased serum hemoglobin level; edema; hepatomegaly; increased central venous pressure; intake exceeds output; jugular vein distention; oliguria; pleural effusion; positive hepatojugular reflex; presence of S3 heart sound; psychomotor agitation; pulmonary congestion; weight gain over short period of time

Related Factors

Excessive fluid intake; excessive sodium intake; ineffective medication self-management

Associated Conditions

Deviations affecting fluid elimination; pharmaceutical preparations

NOC (Nursing Outcomes Classification)

F

Suggested NOC Outcomes

Electrolyte and Acid-Base Balance; Fluid Balance; Fluid Overload Severity; Hydration

Example NOC Outcome with Indicators

Fluid Balance as evidenced by the following indicators: Peripheral edema/Neck vein distention/Adventitious breath sounds/Body weight increase. (Rate each indicator of **Fluid Balance:** 1 = severe, 2 = substantial, 3 = moderate, 4 = mild, 5 = none [see Section I].)

Client Outcomes

Client Will (Specify Time Frame)

- Remain free of edema, effusion, and anasarca
- Maintain body weight appropriate for the client
- Maintain clear lung sounds; no evidence of dyspnea or orthopnea
- Remain free of jugular vein distention, positive hepatojugular reflex, and S3 heart sound
- Maintain normal central venous pressure, pulmonary artery pressure, cardiac output, and vital signs
- Maintain urine output of 0.5 mL/kg/h or more with normal urine osmolality and specific gravity
- Explain actions that are needed to treat or prevent excess fluid volume including fluid and dietary restrictions, and medications
- Describe symptoms that indicate the need to consult with health care provider

NIC (Nursing Interventions Classification)

Suggested NIC Interventions

Fluid Management; Fluid Monitoring

Example NIC Activities—Fluid Monitoring

Monitor weight; Monitor intake and output

Nursing Interventions and *Rationales*

- Monitor location and extent of edema using the 1+ to 4+ scale to quantify edema; also measure the legs using a millimeter tape in the same area at the same time each day. Note differences in measurement between extremities. EBN: *Numerous studies in clients and in experimental models of congestive heart failure (CHF) have established the important role of the renin-angiotensin-aldosterone system (RAAS) and the sympathetic nervous system (SNS) in the progression of cardiovascular and renal dysfunction in CHF. It is now accepted that excessive neurohormonal activation may adversely affect cardiac function and the hemodynamic condition by enhancement of systemic vasoconstriction and promoting salt and water retention by the kidneys (Azzam et al, 2017).*
- Monitor daily weight for sudden increases; use same scale and type of clothing at same time each day, preferably before breakfast. *Body weight changes reflect changes in body fluid volume.* EB: *Body weight is commonly used to monitor for fluid overload (Armstrong et al, 2016).*
- Monitor intake and output; note trends reflecting decreasing urine output in relation to fluid intake. EB: *Abnormally low urine output (oliguria) is a leading indicator of acute kidney injury (AKI), which increases*

mortality, cost of care, and length of stay (Robbins, 2018). The volume of all fluids should be measured. If the family is measuring, instruct them on common conversions between household measurements and metric. **EBN:** *Chronic heart failure (HF) is characterized by neurohumoral activation and sodium retention that leads to excessive fluid accumulation in the systemic and pulmonary circulations. Lung congestion increases dyspnea and impairs gas transfer (Melenovsky et al, 2015).*

- Chronic HF is characterized by neurohormonal activation and sodium retention that leads to excessive fluid accumulation in the systemic and pulmonary circulations. **EB:** *Monitor vital signs; note decreasing blood pressure, tachycardia, and tachypnea. Monitor for S3 heart sounds. If signs of HF are present, see the care plan for Decreased* **Cardiac** *Output.*
- Auscultate lung sounds for crackles, monitor respiration effort, and determine the presence and severity of orthopnea. **EB:** *The pulmonary system adapts to the increased post–central venous pressure, which is believed to be caused by reduced capillary filtration from pulmonary basal membrane thickening, enhanced alveolar fluid clearance, and increased lymphatic drainage (Melenovsky et al, 2015).*
- Monitor serum and urine osmolality, serum sodium, blood urea nitrogen (BUN)/creatinine ratio, and hematocrit for abnormalities. **EB:** *Fluid overload is a causative factor for the occurrence of AKI. Volume overload leads to organ congestion and a resultant decrease in renal blood flow (Salahuddin et al, 2017).*
- BUN and creatinine are monitored currently as biomarkers of kidney injury and failure. **EB:** *Serum creatinine is an imperfect marker because its levels reflect delayed functional consequences of the injury rather than direct cell injury and are not sensitive and specific in the early diagnosis of AKI (Salahuddin et al, 2017). BUN and creatinine are affected by fluid volume status and medications (Andreucci et al, 2017).*
- With head of bed elevated 30 to 45 degrees, monitor jugular veins for distention with the client in the upright position; assess for positive hepatojugular reflex. *Increased intravascular volume results in jugular vein distention as a result of backflow through the vena cava (Canfield, 2021).*
- Monitor the client's behavior for restlessness, anxiety, or confusion; use safety precautions if symptoms are present. *When excess fluid volume compromises cardiac output, the client may experience confusion, decreased consciousness, delirium, and HF (Canfield, 2021).*

▲ Monitor for the development of conditions that increase the client's risk for excess fluid volume, including HF, kidney failure, and liver failure, all of which result in decreased glomerular filtration rate and fluid retention. **EB:** *Other causes are increased intake of oral or intravenous (IV) fluids in excess of the client's cardiac and renal reserve levels, and increased levels of antidiuretic hormone (Tasler & Bruce, 2018). Many clients with fluid overload have AKI, and fluid balance is an important indicator of outcomes. One study of end-stage renal disease clients with chronic fluid overload showed a strong risk factor for death (Zoccali et al, 2017).*

▲ Provide a restricted-sodium diet as appropriate if ordered. **EB:** *Restricting the sodium in the diet will favor the renal excretion of excess fluid. Take care to avoid hyponatremia, which can cause serious complications, including nausea, seizures, coma, and death (Tasler & Bruce, 2018).*

▲ Monitor serum albumin level and provide protein intake as appropriate. **EB:** *When plasma proteins, especially albumin, no longer sustain sufficient colloid osmotic pressure to counterbalance hydrostatic pressure, edema develops (Canfield, 2021).*

▲ Administer prescribed diuretics as appropriate; ensure adequate blood pressure before administration. If diuretic is administered intravenously, note and record the blood pressure and urine output after the dose. Monitor serum sodium for hyponatremia. **EBN:** *Increased arginine vasopressin (AVP) levels in HF clients lead to fluid retention by its actions on vasopressin receptors. Hyponatremia is one of the commonly encountered clinical problems among HF clients with a prevalence of about 20% on hospitalization and has been associated with increased length of stay and in-hospital and postdischarge mortality rates. Hyponatremia in HF is mainly dilutional secondary to neurohormonal activation, especially AVP resulting in free water retention and volume overload (Vinod et al, 2017).* **EB:** *Clinical practice guidelines on HF state that daily weight along with monitoring input and output is useful for monitoring effects of diuretic therapy (Yancy et al, 2017).*

- Monitor for side effects of diuretic therapy, including orthostatic hypotension (especially if the client is also receiving angiotensin-converting enzyme [ACE] inhibitors), hypovolemia, and electrolyte imbalances (hypokalemia and hyponatremia). **EB:** *Observe for hyperkalemia in clients receiving a potassium-sparing diuretic and in those on beta-blockers and ACE inhibitors (Yancy et al, 2017).*

▲ Implement fluid restriction as ordered, especially when serum sodium is low; include all routes of intake. Schedule limited intake of fluids around the clock, and include the type of fluids preferred by the client. Fluid restriction may decrease intravascular volume and myocardial workload. Overzealous fluid restriction should not be used because hypovolemia can worsen HF. Client involvement in planning will enhance participation in the necessary fluid restriction.

- Maintain the rate of all IV infusions, using an IV pump. *This is done to prevent inadvertent exacerbation of excess fluid volume and to more accurately monitor fluid intake.*
- Turn clients with dependent edema at least every 2 hours and monitor for areas that may develop pressure ulcers. **EB:** *Decreased oncotic pressure caused by low levels of albumin affects distribution of total body fluids. The association between low levels of albumin and increased risk for pressure ulcers may be caused by a change in tissue tolerance, with redistribution of fluid and formation of edema (Saghaleini et al, 2018).*
- ▲ Provide ordered care for edematous extremities, including compression, elevation, and muscle exercises. **EB:** *Treatments for clients with peripheral edema include elevation of the extremities above heart level, use of a specialty bed, and offloading of the extremity by repositioning or the use of pressure-offloading devices (Bly et al, 2016).*
- Promote a positive body image and good self-esteem. Visible edema may alter the client's body image. Refer to the care plan for Disturbed **Body** Image.
- ▲ Consult with the health care provider if signs and symptoms of excess fluid volume persist or worsen. **EB:** *Pulmonary edema requires prompt treatment such as preload reducers, afterload reducers, and morphine to relieve anxiety (Yancy et al, 2017).*

F

Critically Ill

- Insert an indwelling urinary catheter if ordered and measure urine output hourly. Notify health care provider if output is less than 0.5 mL/kg/h. **EB:** *Urine output of less than 0.5 mL/kg/h for 6 or more hours is defined as oliguria (Schetz & Hoste, 2017).*
- ▲ Monitor blood pressure, heart rate, passive leg lift, mean arterial pressure, central venous pressure, pulmonary artery pressure, and cardiac output/index; note and report trends of increasing or decreasing pressures over time. **EB:** *Alterations in these parameters may indicate that the client is going into shock. Hemodynamic criteria for cardiogenic shock are sustained hypotension (systolic blood pressure less than 90 mm Hg for at least 30 minutes) and a reduced cardiac index (less than 2.2 L/min/m^2) in the presence of elevated pulmonary capillary occlusion pressure (greater than 15 mm Hg), pulmonary congestion, dyspnea, and hypoxemia (van Diepen et al, 2017; Walsh-Irwin, 2021).*
- ▲ Monitor the effects of infusion of diuretic drips. Perform continuous renal replacement therapy (CRRT) as ordered if the client is critically ill and hemodynamically unstable and excessive fluid must be removed. **EBN:** *CRRT is indicated for hypervolemia, metabolic acidosis, and hyperkalemia (Hewett, 2020).*

Geriatric

- Recognize that the presence of fluid volume excess is particularly serious in older adults. **EB:** *The kidney undergoes age-related changes that include structural and functional changes, which may increase the incidence of AKI (Fingerhood, 2021).*
- Monitor electrolyte levels carefully, including sodium levels and potassium levels, with both increased and decreased levels possible. **EB:** *Older adults are prone to electrolyte abnormalities caused by aging, decreased muscle mass, and decreased total body water (Fingerhood, 2021). Also, the large number of medications that are taken can affect electrolyte levels. Many older clients receive selective serotonin reuptake inhibitors (SSRIs) for treatment of depression, which can result in hyponatremia (Varela Piñón & Adán-Manes, 2017). SSRIs are also known to be responsible for many sexual side effects such as altered libido, erectile dysfunction, vaginal dryness, ejaculatory disorders, and orgasmic problems, which are frequently reported by clients (Reisman, 2017).*

Home Care

- Assess client and family knowledge of disease processes causing excess fluid volume.
- ▲ Teach about disease process and complications of excess fluid volume, including when to contact the health care provider.
- Assess client and family knowledge and compliance with medical regimen, including medications, diet, rest, and exercise. Assist family with integrating restrictions into daily living. Assistance with integration of cultural values, especially those related to foods, with medical regimen promotes compliance and decreased risk of complications.
- ▲ Teach and reinforce knowledge of medications. Instruct the client not to use over-the-counter medications (e.g., diet medications) without first consulting the provider.
- ▲ Instruct the client to make the primary health care provider aware of medications ordered by other health care providers.
- Identify emergency plan for rapidly developing or critical levels of excess fluid volume when diuresing is not safe at home. Excess fluid volume can be life-threatening.

▲ Teach about signs and symptoms of both excess and deficient fluid volume, such as darker urine, dry mouth, and peripheral edema, and when to call the health care provider. **EB:** *Urine color may be a simple indicator of hydration (Walsh-Irwin, 2021).*

Client/Family Teaching and Discharge Planning

- ● Describe signs and symptoms of excess fluid volume and actions to take if they occur.
- ▲ Teach client on diuretics to weigh self daily in the morning and to notify the health care provider if there is a 2.2 pound (1 kg) or more weight gain (Walsh-Irwin, 2021). **EB:** *Clinical practice guidelines on HF suggest that daily weight monitoring leads to early recognition of excess fluid retention, which, when reported, can be offset with additional medication to avoid hospitalization caused by HF decompensation (Yancy et al, 2017).*
- ▲ Teach the importance of fluid and sodium restrictions. Help the client and family devise a schedule for intake of fluids throughout the entire day. Refer to a dietitian concerning implementation of a low-sodium diet.
- ● Teach clients how to measure and document intake and output with common household measurements, such as cups.
- ▲ Teach how to take diuretics correctly: take one dose in the morning and second dose (if taken) no later than 4 p.m. **EB:** *Adjust potassium intake as appropriate for potassium-losing or potassium-sparing diuretics. Note the appearance of side effects such as weakness, muscle cramps, hypertension, or palpitations (Yancy et al, 2017).*
- ● For the client undergoing hemodialysis, teach client the required restrictions in dietary electrolytes, protein, and fluid. Spend time with the client to detect any factors that may interfere with the client's compliance with the fluid restriction or restrictive diet. **EBN:** *Nonadherence to fluid restrictions, especially in clients undergoing hemodialysis, has been linked to numerous deleterious outcomes, including client and provider frustration, treatment failure, illness complications and relapse, and mortality (Howren et al, 2016).*

REFERENCES

Andreucci, M., Faga, T., Pisani, A., Perticone, M., & Michael, A. (2017). The ischemic/nephrotoxic acute kidney injury and the use of renal biomarkers in clinical practice. *European Journal of Internal Medicine*, *39*, 1–8.

Armstrong, L. E., Kavouras, S. A., Walsh, N. P., & Roberts, W. O. (2016). Diagnosing dehydration? Blend evidence with clinical observations. *Current Opinion in Clinical Nutrition and Metabolic Care*, *19*(6), 434–438. https://doi.org/10.1097/MCO.0000000000000320.

Azzam, Z. S., Kinaneh, S., Bahouth, F., Ismael-Badarneh, R., Khoury, E., & Abassi, Z. (2017). Involvement of cytokines in the pathogenesis of salt and water imbalance in congestive heart failure. *Frontiers in Immunology*, *8*, 716.

Bly, D., Schallom, M., Sona, C., & Klinkenberg, D. (2016). A model of pressure, oxygenation, and perfusion risk factors for pressure ulcers in the intensive care unit. *American Journal of Critical Care*, *25*(2), 156–164.

Canfield, C. M. (2021). Shock, sepsis, and multiple organ dysfunction syndrome. In M. L. Sole, D. G. Klein, M. J. Moseley, M. B. F. Makic, & L. T. Morata (Eds.), *Introduction to critical care Nursing* (8th ed.) (pp. 248–281). St. Louis: Elsevier.

van Diepen, S., Katz, J. N., Albert, N. M., et al. (2017). Contemporary management of cardiogenic shock: A scientific statement from the American heart association. *Circulation*, *136*(16), e232–e268.

Fingerhood, M. L. (2021). Age-related changes in health. In M. Boltz, E. A. Capezuti, D. A. Zwicker, & T. Fulmer (Eds.), *Evidence-based geriatric nursing protocols for best practice* (6th ed.) (pp. 59–80). New York: Springer.

Hewett, D. (2020). *Fast facts for the critical care nurse* (2nd ed.). New York: Springer.

Howren, M. B., Kellerman, Q. D., Hillis, S. L., Cvengros, J., Lawton, W., & Christensen, A. J. (2016). Effect of a behavioral self-regulation intervention on patient adherence to fluid-intake restrictions in hemodialysis: A randomized controlled trial. *Annals of Behavioral Medicine*, *50*(2), 167–176.

Melenovsky, V., Andersen, M. J., Andress, K., Reddy, Y. N., & Borlaug, B. A. (2015). Lung congestion in chronic heart failure: Haemodynamic, clinical, and prognostic implications. *European Journal of Heart Failure*, *17*(11), 1161–1171.

Reisman, Y. (2017). Sexual consequences of post-SSRI syndrome. *Sexual Medicine Reviews*, *5*(4), 429–433.

Robbins, K. C. (2018). NNJ journal club: Read it, share it—Acute kidney injury. *Nephrology Nursing Journal*, *45*(4), 395–397.

Saghaleini, S. H., Dehghan, K., Shadvar, K., Sanaie, S., Mahmoodpoor, A., & Ostadi, Z. (2018). Pressure ulcer and nutrition. *Indian Journal of Critical Care Medicine*, *22*(4), 283–289. https://doi.org/10.4103/ijccm.IJCCM_277_17.

Salahuddin, N., Sammani, M., Hamdan, A., et al. (2017). Fluid overload is an independent risk factor for acute kidney injury in critically ill patients: Results of a cohort study. *BMC Nephrology*, *18*(1), 45.

Schetz, M., & Hoste, E. (2017). Understanding oliguria in the critically ill. *Intensive Care Medicine*, *43*(6), 914–916.

Tasler, T., & Bruce, S. D. (2018). Hyponatremia and SIADH: A case study for nursing consideration. *Clinical Journal of Oncology Nursing*, *22*(1), 17–19.

Varela Piñón, M., & Adán-Manes, J. (2017). Selective serotonin reuptake inhibitor-induced hyponatremia: Clinical implications and therapeutic alternatives. *Clinical Neuropharmacology*, *40*(4), 177–179.

Vinod, P., Krishnappa, V., Chauvin, A. M., Khare, A., & Raina, R. (2017). Cardiorenal syndrome: Role of arginine vasopressin and vaptans in heart failure. *Cardiology Research*, *8*(3), 87–95.

Walsh-Irwin, C. (2021). Cardiovascular alterations. In M. L. Sole, D. G. Klein, M. J. Moseley, M. B. F. Makic, & L. T. Morata (Eds.), *Introduction to critical care Nursing* (8th ed.) (pp. 282–330). St. Louis: Elsevier.

Yancy, C. W., Jessup, M., Bozkurt, B., et al. (2017). 2017 ACC/AHA/HFSA focused update of the 2013 ACCF/AHA guideline for the management of heart failure: A report of the American College of Cardiology/American Heart Association Task Force on Clinical Practice Guidelines and the Heart Failure Society of America. *Circulation*, *136*(6), e137–e161. https://doi.org/10.1161/CIR.0000000000000509.

Zoccali, C., Moissl, U., Chazot, C., et al. (2017). Chronic fluid overload and mortality in ESRD. *Journal of the American Society of Nephrology*, *28*(8), 2491–2497.

Risk for Deficient Fluid Volume Domain 2 Nutrition Class 5 Hydration

Mary Beth Flynn Makic, PhD, RN, CCNS, CCRN-K, FAAN, FNAP, FCNS

NANDA-I

Definition

Susceptible to experiencing decreased intravascular, interstitial, and/or intracellular fluid volumes, which may compromise health.

Risk Factors

F

Difficulty meeting increased fluid volume requirement; inadequate access to fluid; inadequate knowledge about fluid needs; ineffective medication self-management; insufficient fluid intake; insufficient muscle mass; malnutrition

At-Risk Population

Individuals at extremes of weight; individuals with external conditions affecting fluid needs; individuals with internal conditions affecting fluid needs; women

Associated Conditions

Active fluid volume loss; deviations affecting fluid absorption; deviations affecting fluid elimination; deviations affecting fluid intake; excessive fluid loss through normal route; fluid loss through abnormal route; pharmaceutical preparations; treatment regimen

NIC, NOC, Client Outcomes, Nursing Interventions and *Rationales,* Client/Family Teaching, and References

Refer to care plan for Deficient **Fluid** Volume.

Frail Elderly Syndrome Domain Health promotion Class 2 Health management

Marina Martinez-Kratz, MS, RN, CNE

NANDA-I

Definition

Dynamic state of unstable equilibrium that affects the older individual experiencing deterioration in one or more domains of health (physical, functional, psychological, or social) and leads to increased susceptibility to adverse health effects, in particular disability.

Defining Characteristics

Bathing self-care deficit (00108); decreased activity tolerance (00298); decreased cardiac output (00029); dressing self-care deficit (00109); fatigue (00093); feeding self-care deficit (00102); hopelessness (00124); imbalanced nutrition: less than body requirements (00002); impaired memory (00131); impaired physical mobility (00085); impaired walking (00088); social isolation (00053); toileting self-care deficit (00110)

Related Factors

Anxiety; decreased energy; decreased muscle strength; exhaustion; fear of falling; impaired postural balance; inadequate knowledge of modifiable factors; inadequate social support; malnutrition; neurobehavioral manifestations; obesity; sadness; sedentary lifestyle

At-Risk Population

Economically disadvantaged individuals; individuals aged >70 years; individuals experiencing prolonged hospitalization; individuals for whom walking 15 feet requires >6 seconds (4 meters > 5 seconds); individuals living alone; individuals living in constricted spaces; individuals with history of falls; individuals with low educational level; individuals with unintentional loss of 25% of body weight over one year; individuals with unintentional weight loss >10 pounds (>4.5 kg) in one year; socially vulnerable individuals; women

Associated Conditions

Anorexia; blood coagulation disorders; chronic disease; decreased serum 25-hydroxyvitamin D concentration; depression; endocrine regulatory dysfunction; mental disorders; sarcopenia; sarcopenic obesity; sensation disorders; suppressed inflammatory response

NOC (Nursing Outcomes Classification)

Suggested NOC Outcomes

Activity Tolerance; Balance; Exercise Participation; Hope; Physical Aging; Psychosocial Adjustment: Life Change; Client Satisfaction: Functional Assistance

F

Example NOC Outcome with Indicators

Client Satisfaction: Functional Assistance as evidenced by the following indicators: Included in planning for optimal mobility and self-care/Encouraged to be as active as possible/Assistance with physical activity/Allowed to choose food for meals. (Rate the outcome and indicators of **Client Satisfaction: Functional Assistance:** 1 = not at all satisfied, 2 = somewhat satisfied, 3 = moderately satisfied, 4 = very satisfied, 5 = completely satisfied [see Section I].)

Client Outcomes

Client Will (Specify Time Frame)

- Remain living as independently as possible in the home or care setting of his or her choice
- Maintain safety when engaging in activities of daily living and ambulation
- Increase exercise and/or daily physical activity to build muscle strength
- Maintain a healthy weight

NIC (Nursing Interventions Classification)

Suggested NIC Interventions

Exercise Promotion; Exercise Promotion: Balance; Exercise Promotion: Strength Training; Hope Inspiration; Nutrition Therapy

Example NIC Activities—Frail Elderly Syndrome

Promote physical activities that build strength and improve balance and endurance

Nursing Interventions and *Rationales*

- Establish a trusting relationship with the client. EBN: *A program for severely frail older people found that a person-centered approach with a focus on trust development and relationship building was a critical component of the care provided (Lhussier, Dalkin, & Hetherington, 2019).*
- Assess frailty with a tool such as the Frailty Index or the Edmonton Frail Scale. EB: *Apóstolo et al (2017) did a systematic review on diagnostic accuracy and predictive ability of frailty measures and found that the Frailty Index had good predictive reliability.* EB: *The Edmonton Frail Scale is a tool designed to identify frail older adults in clinical settings (Perna et al, 2017).*
- Perform a fall risk assessment on frail clients. EB: *The frailty group had the highest fall risk in a cohort of older adults living in a community-dwelling facility (Chittrakul et al, 2020).*
- Assess nutritional status using a validated nutritional screening assessment tool such as the Malnutrition Universal Screening Tool (MUST). EB: *Nutritional assessments can inform nursing care for frail clients (Murphy, Mayor, & Forde, 2018).*
- Assess for loneliness and implement measures to reduce feelings of loneliness. EB: *A prospective interventional study found that interventions to prevent loneliness have a positive effect on the frailty and independent living of the elderly (Ožić et al, 2020).*

- Encourage clients to engage in active lifestyles. EB: *The Longitudinal Aging Study Amsterdam (n = 1440) and the InCHIANTI Study (n = 998) found that physical inactivity was a component in the progression of frailty (Stenholm et al, 2019).*
- Recognize that balance and gait impairment are features of frailty and are risk factors for falls. EB: *By reversing frailty through exercise interventions that engender fitness, older adults will remain physically independent longer (Bray et al, 2016).*
- Address balance and gait impairments with a resistance based exercise program. EB: *A meta-analysis found that resistance-based exercise improved physical performance, improved gait speed, and increased leg strength in adults over the age of 60 (Macdonald et al, 2020).*
- Preserve physical functioning through individualized physical activity plans. EB: *Tomita et al (2018) found that frail older women who engaged in a high level of physical activity (>4000 kcal/week) can increase mobility and functional capacity.* EB: *de Labra et al (2015) did a systematic review of the literature and found that low physical activity has been shown to be one of the most common components of frailty.*

F

- Assess risk of fracture using tools such as the Cardiovascular Health Study (CHS) or Study of Osteoporotic Fracture (SOF) indicators. EBN: *Chen et al (2017) did a systematic review of the literature and in total five studies included 103,783 older people and recorded 2960 fractures.*
- Evaluate the client's medications to determine whether medications increase the risk of frailty and/or are potentially inappropriate medications (PIMs), and if appropriate, consult with the client's health care provider regarding the client's medications. EB: *Polypharmacy is associated with increased risk of mortality in elderly people (Gómez et al, 2015).* EB: *The number of medications prescribed can be useful to help physicians be aware of the high risk for PIMs (Tsao et al, 2016).*
- Use the Screening Tool of Older People's Prescriptions (STOPP) and the Screening Tool to Alert Right Treatment (START) to avoid omissions and inappropriateness in prescription. EB: *The STOPP criteria for frail older persons (>65 years) is largely associated with adverse drug events and recommends against taking medications to treat symptoms unassociated with selected illnesses (Nwadiugwu, 2020).*
- Assess and monitor vitamin D levels. EB: *Research participants with serum 25-hydroxyvitamin D levels less than 50 nmol/L were about two times more likely to be frail compared to participants with serum 25-hydroxyvitamin D levels greater than 50 nmol/L (Vaes et al, 2019).*
- ▲ Refer client to an exercise-training program. EB: *A randomized controlled trial found that participants in a frailty prevention program had a greater reduction in the combined frailty score and greater improvements in muscle endurance and balance than those in the control group (Yu et al, 2020).*
- Monitor weight loss. EB: *Weight loss is considered a main component of frailty syndrome (Yannakoulia et al, 2017).*
- Use an multiprofessional and person-centered approach for supporting frail older adults. EBN: *Engaging clients, their family members, or caregivers in care planning and goal setting during transitions is essential (Jeffs et al, 2017).*
- Refer to care plan for Readiness for Enhanced **Nutrition** for additional interventions.

Multicultural, Home Care, and Client/Family Teaching

- The previously mentioned interventions may be adapted for multicultural, home care, and client family teaching.
- Provide a home-based exercise-training program. EB: *The results of a randomized controlled trial indicate that a home-based physical training intervention conducted by nonprofessionals is feasible and can address frailty in older persons living at home (Luger et al, 2016).*

REFERENCES

Apóstolo, J., Cooke, R., Bobrowicz-Campos, E., et al. (2017). Predicting risk and outcomes for frail older adults: An umbrella review of frailty screening tools. *JBI Database of Systematic Reviews and Implementation Reports*, *15*(4), 1154–1208.

Bray, N. W., Smart, R. R., Jakobi, J. M., & Jones, G. R. (2016). Exercise prescription to reverse frailty. *Applied Physiology Nutrition and Metabolism*, *41*(10), 1112–1116.

Chen, K. W., Chang, S. F., & Lin, P. L. (2017). Frailty as a predictor of future fracture in older adults: A systematic review and meta-analysis. *Worldviews on Evidence-Based Nursing*, *14*(4), 282–293.

Chittrakul, J., Siviroj, P., Sungkarat, S., & Sapbamrer, R. (2020). Physical frailty and fall risk in community-dwelling older adults: A cross-sectional study. *Journal of Aging Research*, *2020*, 3964973. https://doi.org/10.1155/2020/3964973.

de Labra, C., Guimaraes-Pinheiro, C., Maseda, A., Lorenzo, T., & Millán-Calenti, J. C. (2015). Effects of physical exercise interventions in frail older adults: A systematic review of randomized controlled trials. *BMC Geriatrics*, *15*(1), 154.

Gómez, C., Vega-Quiroga, S., Bermejo-Pareja, F., Medrano, M. J., Louis, E. D., & Benito-León, J. (2015). Polypharmacy in the elderly: A marker of increased risk of mortality in a population-based prospective study (NEDICES). *Gerontology*, *61*(4), 301–309.

Jeffs, L., Kuluski, K., Law, M., et al. (2017). Identifying effective nurse-led care transition interventions for older adults with complex needs using a structured expert panel. *Worldviews on Evidence-Based Nursing, 14*(2), 136–144.

Lhussier, M., Dalkin, S., & Hetherington, R. (2019). Community care for severely frail older people: Developing explanations of how, why and for whom it works. *International Journal of Older People Nursing, 14*(1), e12217. https://doi.org/10.1111/opn.12217.

Luger, E., Dorner, T. E., Haider, S., Kapan, A., Lackinger, C., & Schindler, K. (2016). Effects of a home-based and volunteer-administered physical training, nutritional, and social support program on malnutrition and frailty in older persons: A randomized controlled trial. *Journal of the American Medical Directors Association, 17*(7), 671.e9–671.e16. https://doi.org/10.1016/j.jamda.2016.04.018.

Macdonald, S. H., Travers, J., Shé, É. N., et al. (2020). Primary care interventions to address physical frailty among community-dwelling adults aged 60 years or older: A meta-analysis. *PLoS One, 15*(2), e0228821. https://doi.org/10.1371/journal.pone.0228821.

Murphy, J., Mayor, A., & Forde, E. (2018). Identifying and treating older patients with malnutrition in primary care: The MUST screening tool. *British Journal of General Practice, 68*(672), 344–345. https://doi.org/10.3399/bjgp18X697853.

Nwadiugwu, M. C. (2020). Frailty and the risk of polypharmacy in the older person: Enabling and preventative approaches. *Journal of Aging Research, 2020*, 6759521. https://doi.org/10.1155/2020/6759521.

Ožić, S., Vasiljev, V., Ivković, V., Bilajac, L., & Rukavina, T. (2020). Interventions aimed at loneliness and fall prevention reduce frailty in elderly urban population. *Medicine, 99*(8), e19145. https://doi.org/10.1097/MD.0000000000019145.

Perna, S., Francis, M. D. A., Bologna, C., et al. (2017). Performance of Edmonton Frail Scale on frailty assessment: Its association with multi-dimensional geriatric conditions assessed with specific screening tools. *BMC Geriatrics, 17*(1), 2.

Stenholm, S., Ferrucci, L., Vahtera, J., et al. (2019). Natural course of frailty components in people who develop frailty syndrome: Evidence from two cohort studies. *Journals of Gerontology Series A: Biological Sciences & Medical Sciences, 74*(5), 667–674. https://doi.org?10.1093/gerona/gly132.

Tomita, M. R., Fisher, N. M., Nair, S., Ramsey, D., & Persons, K. (2018). Impact of physical activities on frailty in community-dwelling older women. *Physical & Occupational Therapy in Geriatrics, 36*(1), 107–119. https://doi.org/10.1080/02703181.2018.1443194.

Tsao, C. H., Tsai, C. F., Lee, Y. T., et al. (2016). Drug prescribing in the elderly receiving home care. *The American Journal of the Medical Sciences, 352*(2), 134–140.

Vaes, A. M. M., Brouwer-Brolsma, E. M., Toussaint, N., et al. (2019). The association between 25-hydroxyvitamin D concentration, physical performance and frailty status in older adults. *European Journal of Nutrition, 58*(3), 1173–1181.

Yannakoulia, M., Ntanasi, E., Anastasiou, C. A., & Scarmeas, N. (2017). Frailty and nutrition: From epidemiological and clinical evidence to potential mechanisms. *Metabolism: Clinical and Experimental, 68*, 64–76.

Yu, R., Tong, C., Ho, F., & Woo, J. (2020). Effects of a multicomponent frailty prevention program in prefrail community-dwelling older persons: A randomized controlled trial. *Journal of the American Medical Directors Association, 21*(2) 294.e1–294.e10. https://doi.org/10.1016/j.jamda.2019.08.024.

F

Risk for Frail Elderly Syndrome

Domain 1 Health promotion Class 2 Health management

Marina Martinez-Kratz, MS, RN, CNE

NANDA-I

Definition

Susceptible to a dynamic state of unstable equilibrium that affects the older individual experiencing deterioration in one or more domain of health (physical, functional, psychological, or social) and leads to increased susceptibility to adverse health effects, in particular disability.

Risk Factors

Anxiety; decreased energy; decreased muscle strength; exhaustion; fear of falling; impaired postural balance; inadequate knowledge of modifiable factors; inadequate social support; malnutrition; neurobehavioral manifestations; obesity; sadness; sedentary lifestyle

At-Risk Population

Economically disadvantaged individuals; individuals aged >70 years; individuals experiencing prolonged hospitalization; individuals for whom walking 15 feet requires >6 seconds (4 meters > 5 seconds); individuals living alone; individuals living in constricted spaces; individuals with history of falls; individuals with low educational level; individuals with unintentional loss of 25% of body weight over one year; individuals with unintentional weight loss >10 pounds (>4.5 kg) in one year; socially vulnerable individuals; women

Associated Conditions

Anorexia; blood coagulation disorders; chronic disease; decreased serum 25-hydroxyvitamin D concentration; depression; endocrine regulatory dysfunction; mental disorders; sarcopenia; sarcopenic obesity; sensation disorders; suppressed inflammatory response

NIC, NOC, Client Outcomes, Nursing Interventions and *Rationales*, and References

Refer to care plan for **Frail Elderly** Syndrome.

Impaired Gas Exchange

Domain 3 Elimination and exchange Class 4 Respiratory function

Debra Siela, PhD, RN, ACNS-BC, CCRN-K, CNE, RRT

G

NANDA-I

Definition

Excess or deficit in oxygenation and/or carbon dioxide elimination.

Defining Characteristics

Abnormal arterial pH; abnormal skin color; altered respiratory depth; altered respiratory rhythm; bradypnea; confusion; decreased carbon dioxide levels; diaphoresis; headache upon awakening; hypercapnia; hypoxemia; hypoxia; irritable mood; nasal flaring; psychomotor agitation; somnolence; tachycardia; tachypnea; visual disturbances

Related Factors

Ineffective airway clearance; ineffective breathing pattern; pain

At-Risk Population

Premature infants

Associated Conditions

Alveolar-capillary membrane changes; asthma; general anesthesia; heart diseases; ventilation-perfusion imbalance

NOC (Nursing Outcomes Classification)

Suggested NOC Outcomes

Respiratory Status: Gas Exchange, Ventilation

Example NOC Outcome with Indicators

Achieves appropriate **Respiratory Status: Gas Exchange** as evidenced by the following indicators: Cognitive status/Partial pressure of oxygen/Partial pressure of carbon dioxide/Arterial pH/Oxygen saturation. (Rate each indicator of **Respiratory Status: Gas Exchange:** 1 = severe deviation from normal range, 2 = substantial deviation from normal range, 3 = moderate deviation from normal range, 4 = mild deviation from normal range, 5 = no deviation from normal range [see Section I].)

Client Outcomes

Client Will (Specify Time Frame)

- Demonstrate improved ventilation and adequate oxygenation as evidenced by blood gas levels within normal parameters for that client
- Maintain clear lung fields and remain free of signs of respiratory distress
- Verbalize understanding of oxygen supplementation and other therapeutic interventions

NIC (Nursing Interventions Classification)

Suggested NIC Interventions

Acid-Base Management; Airway Management

Example NIC Activities—Acid-Base Management

Monitor for symptoms of respiratory failure (e.g., low Pa_{O_2} and elevated Pa_{CO_2} levels and respiratory muscle fatigue); Monitor determinants of tissue oxygen delivery (e.g., Pa_{O_2}, SaO_2, and hemoglobin levels, and cardiac output) if available

Nursing Interventions and *Rationales*

- Monitor respiratory rate, depth, and ease of respiration. Watch for use of accessory muscles and nasal flaring. EB: *Normal respiratory rate is 14 to 16 breaths per minute in the adult. When the respiratory rate exceeds 26 to 30 breaths per minute, along with other physiological measures, a significant cardiovascular or respiratory alteration exists (Bickley et al, 2020).*
- Auscultate breath sounds every 1 to 2 hours. The presence of crackles and wheezes may alert the nurse to airway obstruction, which may lead to or exacerbate existing hypoxia. EB: *In severe exacerbations of chronic obstructive pulmonary disease (COPD), lung sounds may be diminished or distant with air trapping (Bickley et al, 2020).*
- The nurse should consider respiratory rate, work of breathing, and lung sounds along with Pao_2 values, SaO_2, SpO_2, client tidal volume, and minute ventilation. EB: *Presence of dyspnea, asynchronous chest and abdominal movements, accessory muscles, and agitation indicate potential oxygenation problems (Barton, Vanderspank-Wright, & Shea, 2016).*
- Monitor the client's behavior and mental status for the onset of restlessness, agitation, confusion, and (in the late stages) extreme lethargy. EB: *Changes in behavior and mental status can be early signs of impaired gas exchange. In the late stages the client becomes lethargic and somnolent (Lee, 2017).*

▲ Monitor oxygen saturation continuously using pulse oximetry. Note blood gas results as available to determine correlation of pulse oximetry value with arterial blood gas oxygen saturation. EB: *An oxygen saturation of less than 88% (normal: 95%–100%) or a partial pressure of oxygen of less than 55 mm Hg (normal: 80–100 mm Hg) indicates significant oxygenation problems (Bein, Grasso, & Moerer, 2016; Siela & Kidd, 2017). Pulse oximetry is useful for tracking and/or adjusting supplemental oxygen therapy for clients with COPD (GOLD, 2020).*

- Monitor venous oxygen saturation to determine an index of oxygen balance to reflect between oxygen delivery and oxygen consumption (Dirks, 2017).
- Measurements of oxygenation supply in the macrocirculation include those made upstream from the tissue level. The parameters measured are arterial partial pressure of oxygen (Pao_2), arterial oxygen saturation (SaO_2) determined on the basis of arterial blood gas (ABG) analysis and pulse oximetry (SpO_2), and ratio of Pao_2 to fraction of inspired oxygen (FiO_2), or the P:F ratio. Measurements of oxygenation or oxygen extraction or consumption in the macrocirculation made downstream from tissues include tissue oxygen consumption, mixed venous oxygen saturation (SvO_2) or central venous oxygen saturation ($ScvO_2$), and blood levels of lactate (Siela & Kidd, 2017; Şanci, Coşkun, & Bayram, 2020).
- Observe for cyanosis of the skin; especially note color of the tongue and oral mucous membranes. EB: *In central cyanosis both the skin and mucous membranes are affected due to seriously impaired pulmonary function from unventilated or underventilated alveoli. Peripheral cyanosis (skin only) usually indicates vasoconstriction or obstruction to blood flow (Loscalzo, 2018). Central cyanosis of the tongue and oral mucosa is indicative of serious hypoxia and is a medical emergency. Peripheral cyanosis in the extremities may be due to activation of the central nervous system or exposure to cold and may or may not be serious (Bickley et al, 2020).*
- Position the client in a semirecumbent position with the head of the bed at a 30- to 45-degree angle to decrease the aspiration of gastric, oral, and nasal secretions. EB: *Evidence shows that mechanically ventilated clients have a decreased incidence of aspiration pneumonia if the client is placed in a 30- to 45-degree semirecumbent position as opposed to a supine position (American Association of Critical Care Nurses, 2016, 2017; Vollman, Sole, & Quinn, 2017b).*
- If the client has unilateral lung disease, position with head of bed at 30 to 45 degrees with "good lung down" in a side-lying position and affected lung up (Barton, Vanderspank-Wright, & Shea, 2016).

▲ If the client is acutely dyspneic, consider having the client lean forward over a bedside table, resting elbows on the table if tolerated. EB: *Leaning forward can help decrease dyspnea, possibly because gastric pressure allows better contraction of the diaphragm. This is called the tripod position and is used during times of distress, including when walking, leaning forward on the walker (Mahler, 2017).*

- Help the client deep breathe and perform controlled coughing. Have the client inhale deeply, hold the breath for several seconds, and cough two or three times with the mouth open while tightening the upper abdominal muscles as tolerated. Controlled coughing uses the diaphragmatic muscles, which makes the cough more forceful and effective.

▲ If the client has excessive fluid in the respiratory system based on auscultation, inform the prescribing provider to appropriate interventions.

▲ Monitor the effects of sedation and analgesics on the client's respiratory pattern; use judiciously. EB: *Both analgesics and medications that cause sedation can depress respiration at times. However, these medications*

G

can be very helpful for decreasing the sympathetic nervous system discharge that accompanies hypoxia (Barton, Vanderspank-Wright, & Shea, 2016).

- ● Schedule nursing care to provide rest and minimize fatigue. EB:*The hypoxic client has limited reserves; inappropriate activity can increase hypoxia (Barton, Vanderspank-Wright, & Shea, 2016; Mahler, 2017).*
- ▲ Administer humidified oxygen through an appropriate device (e.g., nasal cannula or venturi mask per the provider's order); aim for an oxygen (O_2) saturation level of 90% or above. Oxygen should be titrated to target an SpO_2 of >94%, except with carbon monoxide poisoning (100% oxygen), acute respiratory distress syndrome (ARDS) (88%–95%), those at risk for hypercapnia (88%–92%), and premature infants (88%–94%) (Bickley et al, 2020). Watch for onset of hypoventilation as evidenced by increased somnolence. EB: *There is a fine line between ideal and excessive oxygen therapy; increasing somnolence is caused by retention of CO_2 leading to CO_2 narcosis (Baldwin & Cox, 2016). Promote oxygen therapy during a COPD exacerbation. Supplemental oxygen should be titrated to improve the client's hypoxemia with a target of 88% to 92% (GOLD, 2020).*
- ● Once oxygen is started, arterial blood gases should be checked 30 to 60 minutes later to ensure satisfactory oxygenation without carbon dioxide retention or acidosis (GOLD, 2020). EB: *Use of high-flow nasal cannula oxygen therapy may improve gas exchange and oxygenation in acute hypoxemic respiratory failure (Siela & Kidd, 2017; Drake 2018) and hypercapnic hypoxemic respiratory failure (Şanci, Coşkun, & Bavram, 2020).*
- ● Supplemental oxygen can cause toxicity and should be administered at the lowest level that achieves an arterial saturation appropriate for a given client (Helmerhorst et al, 2015; Drake, 2018). EB: *Conservative oxygen strategies that target a goal of 88% to 92% SpO_2 levels in clients receiving invasive mechanical ventilation appear justified (Panwar et al, 2016). High-flow nasal cannula oxygen therapy decreases respiratory rate in acute respiratory failure (Marjanovic et al, 2020).*
- ● Assess nutritional status including serum albumin level and body mass index (BMI). EB: *Malnourishment in a client with COPD has a negative effect on the course of the disease; it can result in loss of muscle mass in the respiratory muscles, including the diaphragm, which can lead to respiratory failure (GOLD, 2020).* EB: *The Academy of Nutrition and Dietetics strongly recommend that people with COPD have their body weight and medical nutrition therapy be assessed and monitored by a registered dietitian nutritionist (Hanson et al, 2021).*
- ▲ Assist the client to eat small meals frequently and use dietary supplements as necessary. Engage dietary in evaluating and creating an optimal nutrition plan. For some clients, drinking 30 mL of a supplement every hour while awake can be helpful.
- ▲ If the client is severely debilitated from chronic respiratory disease, consider the use of a wheeled walker to help in ambulation. Request a physical therapy consultation to assist with mobility and strength training.
- ● Assess for signs of psychological distress, including anxiety, agitation, and insomnia.
- ▲ Refer the client with respiratory diseases, especially COPD, to a pulmonary rehabilitation program. Pulmonary rehabilitation is now considered a standard of care for the client with respiratory diseases (GOLD, 2020).

Critical Care

- ▲ Assess and monitor oxygen indices such as the P:F ratio (PaO_2 to FiO_2), venous oxygen saturation/oxygen consumption (SvO_2 or $ScvO_2$) (Dirks, 2017; Siela & Kidd, 2017; Lough et al, 2022).
- ▲ Turn the client every 2 hours. Monitor oxygen saturation closely after turning. If it drops by 10% or fails to return to baseline promptly, turn the client back into the supine position and evaluate oxygen status. If the client does not tolerate turning, consider use of a kinetic bed that rotates the client from side to side in a turn of at least 40 degrees (St. Clair & MacDermott, 2017).
- ▲ If the client has ARDS with difficulty maintaining oxygenation, consider positioning the client prone with the upper thorax and pelvis supported. Monitor oxygen saturation and turn the client back to supine position if desaturation occurs. EB: *Oxygenation levels have been shown to improve in the prone position, probably due to decreased shunting and better perfusion of the lungs (Drahnak & Custer, 2015; Barton, Vanderspank-Wright, & Shea, 2016; Bein, Grasso, & Moerer, 2016; Vollman, Dickinson, & Powers, 2017a).* EB: *A systematic review and meta-analysis found that prone position with mechanical ventilation significantly reduced mortality in clients with severe acute hypoxemic respiratory failure; however, clients should remain in the prone position for 12 hours daily (Munshi et al, 2017).*
- ▲ High levels of positive end-expiratory pressures may be prescribed to improve oxygenation and gas exchange (Barton, Vanderspank-Wright, & Shea, 2016). EB: *The delivery of positive end expiratory pressure can be provided through noninvasive or mechanical ventilation mechanisms (Siela & Kidd, 2017).*

Geriatric

- Use central nervous system depressants and other sedating agents carefully to avoid decreasing respiration rate.
- Teach the client how to cough and perform deep breathing exercises to enhance gas exchange.
- Maintain appropriate levels of supplemental oxygen therapy for clients with impaired gas exchange and hypoxemia (GOLD, 2020).

Home Care

- Work with the client to determine what strategies are most helpful during times of dyspnea. Educate and empower the client to self-manage the disease associated with impaired gas exchange. EB: *Use of oxygen, self-use of medication, handheld fan, behavioral modification, and music can assist clients dealing with dyspnea (Baldwin & Cox, 2016; Ergin et al, 2018). Evidence-based reviews have found that self-management offers COPD clients effective options for managing the illness, leading to more positive outcomes (GOLD, 2020).*
- Collaborate with health care providers regarding long-term oxygen administration for chronic respiratory failure clients with severe resting hypoxemia. Administer long-term oxygen therapy for Pa_{O2} less than 55 or SaO_2 at or below 88% (GOLD, 2020).
- Assess the home environment for irritants that impair gas exchange. Help the client adjust the home environment as necessary (e.g., install an air filter to decrease the level of dust).
- ▲ Refer the client to occupational therapy as necessary to assist the client in adapting to the home and environment and in energy conservation (GOLD, 2020).
- Assist the client with identifying and avoiding situations that exacerbate impairment of gas exchange (e.g., stress-related situations, exposure to pollution of any kind, proximity to noxious gas fumes such as chlorine bleach). Irritants in the environment decrease the client's effectiveness in accessing oxygen during breathing.
- Instruct the client to keep the home temperature above 68°F (20°C) and to avoid cold weather. EB: *Cold air temperatures cause constriction of the blood vessels, which impairs the client's ability to absorb oxygen (Bickley et al, 2020).*
- Instruct the client to limit exposure to persons with respiratory infections. EB: *Viruses, bacteria, and environmental pollutants are the main causes of exacerbations of COPD (GOLD, 2020).*
- Instruct the family on the complications of the disease and the importance of maintaining the medical regimen, including when to call a health care provider.
- ▲ Refer the client for home health aide services as necessary for assistance with activities of daily living. EB: *Clients with decreased oxygenation have decreased energy to carry out personal and role-related activities.*
- When respiratory procedures are being implemented, explain equipment and procedures to family members, and provide needed emotional support. Family members assuming responsibility for respiratory monitoring often find this stressful.
- When electrically based equipment for respiratory support is being implemented, evaluate home environment for electrical safety, proper grounding, and so on. Ensure that notification is sent to the local utility company, the emergency medical team, and police and fire departments. Notification is important to provide for priority service. Work with the family to have an emergency plan and ensure all individuals in the home are aware of the plan.
- ▲ Assess family role changes and coping ability. Refer the client to medical social services as appropriate for assistance in adjusting to chronic illness. EB: *Inability to maintain the level of social involvement experienced before illness leads to frustration and anger in the client and may create a threat to the family unit (Mahler, 2017).*
- Support the family of the client with chronic illness. EB: *Severely compromised respiratory functioning causes fear and anxiety in clients and their families. Reassurance from the nurse can be helpful (Baldwin & Cox, 2016; Mahler, 2017).*

Client/Family Teaching and Discharge Planning

- Teach the client how to perform pursed-lip breathing and inspiratory muscle training, and how to use the tripod position. Have the client watch the pulse oximeter to note improvement in oxygenation with these breathing techniques. EB: *Pursed-lip breathing results in increased use of intercostal muscles, decreased respiratory rate, and improved oxygen saturation levels. Pursed-lip breathing may relieve dyspnea in advanced respiratory diseases, such as COPD (Mahler, 2017; Nguyen & Duong, 2020).*
- Teach the client energy conservation techniques and the importance of alternating rest periods with activity. See nursing interventions for **Fatigue.**

- ▲ Teach the importance of not smoking. Refer to smoking cessation programs, and encourage clients who relapse to keep trying to quit. Ensure that clients receive appropriate medications to support smoking cessation from the primary health care provider. **EB:** *Clients should be referred to a comprehensive smoking cessation program, incorporating behavior change techniques that focus on enhancing client motivation and confidence, client education, and pharmacological and nonpharmacological interventions (GOLD, 2020).*
- ▲ Instruct the family regarding home oxygen therapy if ordered (e.g., delivery system, liter flow, safety precautions). **EB:** *Long-term oxygen therapy can improve survival, exercise ability, sleep, and ability to think in hypoxemic clients. Client education improves compliance with prescribed use of oxygen (GOLD, 2020).*
- ▲ Teach the client the need to receive a yearly influenza vaccine. Receiving a yearly influenza vaccine is helpful to prevent exacerbations of COPD (GOLD, 2020).
- ● Teach the client relaxation techniques to help reduce stress responses and panic attacks resulting from dyspnea. **EB:** *Relaxation therapy can help reduce dyspnea and anxiety (Baldwin & Cox, 2016; Mahler, 2017).*
- ● Teach the client to use music, along with a rest period, to decrease dyspnea and anxiety (Ergin et al, 2018; Loscalzo, 2018).

G

REFERENCES

American Association of Critical Care Nurses. (2016). AACN practice alert: Prevention of aspiration in adults. *Critical Care Nurse, 36*(1), e20–e24.

American Association of Critical Care Nurses. (2017). AACN Practice Alert: Prevention of ventilator-associated pneumonia in adults. *Critical Care Nurse, 37*(3), e22–e25.

Baldwin, J., & Cox, J. (2016). Treating dyspnea: Is oxygen therapy the best option for all patients? *Medical Clinics of North America, 100*(5), 1123–1130. https://doi.org/10.1016/j.mcna.2016.04.018.

Barton, G., Vanderspank-Wright, B., & Shea, J. (2016). Optimizing oxygenation in the mechanically ventilated patient: Nursing practice implications. *Critical Care Nursing Clinics of North America, 28*(4), 425–435.

Bein, T., Grasso, S., Moerer, O., et al. (2016). The standard of care of patients with ARDS: Ventilatory settings and rescue therapies for refractory hypoxemia. *Intensive Care Medicine, 42*(5), 699–711.

Bickley, L. S., Szilagyi, P., Hoffman, R. M., & Soriano, R. P. (2020). Thorax and lungs. In L. S. Bickley (Ed.), *Bates' guide to physical examination and history taking* (13th ed.) (pp. 441–487). Philadelphia: Wolters Kluwer.

Dirks, J. (2017). Continuous venous oxygen saturation monitoring. In D. L. Wiegand (Ed.), *AACN procedure Manual for high Acuity, Progressive, and Critical care* (7th ed.) (pp. 116–122). Philadelphia: Elsevier.

Drahnak, D. M., & Custer, N. (2015). Prone positioning of patients with acute respiratory distress syndrome. *Critical Care Nurse, 35*(6), 29–37.

Drake, M. G. (2018). High-flow nasal cannula oxygen in adults: An evidence-based assessment. *Annals of the American Thoracic Society, 15*(2), 145–155. https://doi.org/10.1513/AnnalsATS.201707-548FR.

Ergin, E., Sagkal Midilli, T., & Baysal, E. (2018). The effect of music on dyspnea severity, anxiety, and hemodynamic parameters in patients with dyspnea. *Journal of Hospice and Palliative Nursing, 20*(1), 81–87. https://doi.org/10.1097/NJH.0000000000000403.

Global Initiative for Chronic Obstructive Lung Disease (GOLD). (2020). *Global strategy for the diagnosis, management, and prevention of chronic obstructive pulmonary disease (2020 report).* Retrieved from https://goldcopd.org/wp-content/uploads/2019/12/GOLD-2020-FINAL-ver1.2-03Dec19_WMV.pdf. Accessed July 1, 2021.

Hanson, C., Bowser, E. K., Frankenfield, D. C., & Piemonte, T. A. (2021). Chronic obstructive pulmonary disease: A 2019 evidence analysis center evidence-based practice guideline. *Journal of the Academy of Nutrition and Dietetics, 121*(1), 139–165. e15. https://doi.org/10.1016/j.jand.2019.12.001.

Helmerhorst, H. J. F., Schultz, M. J., van der Voort, P. H. J., de Jong, E., & van Westerloo, D. J. (2015). Bench-to bedside review: The effects of hyperoxia during critical illness. *Critical Care, 19*(1), 284. https://doi.org/10.1186/s13054-015-0996-4.

Lee, D. B. (2017). Oxygen saturation monitoring with pulse oximetry. In D. L. Wiegand (Ed.), *AACN procedure Manual for high Acuity, Progressive, and Critical care* (7th ed.) (pp. 134–141). Philadelphia: Elsevier.

Loscalzo, J. (2018). Hypoxia and cyanosis. In J. L. Jameson, A. S. Fauci, D. L. Kasper, S. L. Hauser, D. L. Longo, & J. Loscalzo (Eds.), *Harrison's principles of internal medicine* (20th ed.). New York: McGraw-Hill.

Lough, M. E., Berger, S. J., Larsen, A., & Sandoval, C. P. (2022). Cardiovascular diagnostic procedures. In L. D. Urden, K. M. Stacy, & M. E. Lough (Eds.), *Critical care nursing Diagnosis and management* (8th ed.) (pp. 206–297). St. Louis: Elsevier.

Mahler, D. A. (2017). Evaluation of dyspnea in the elderly. *Clinics in Geriatric Medicine, 33*(4), 503–521. https://doi.org/10.1016/j.cger.2017.06.004.

Marjanovic, N., Guénézan, J., Frat, J. P., Mimoz, O., & Thille, A. W. (2020). High-flow nasal cannula oxygen therapy in acute respiratory failure at emergency departments: A systematic review. *American Journal of Emergency Medicine, 38*(7), 1508–1514. https://doi.org/10.1016/.akem.2020.04.091.

Munshi, L., Del Sorbo, L., Adhikari, N. K. J., et al. (2017). Prone position for acute respiratory distress syndrome. a systematic review and meta-analysis. *Annals of the American Thoracic Society, 14*(Suppl. 4), S280–S288. https://doi.org/10.1513/AnnalsATS.201704-343OT.

Nguyen, J. D., & Duong, H. (2020). Pursed-lip breathing. *StatPearls* [Internet]. Treasure Island, FL: StatPearls Publishing. https://www.ncbi.nlm.nih.gov/books/NBK545289/.

Panwar, R., Hardie, M., Bellomo, R., et al. (2016). Conservative versus liberal oxygenation targets for mechanically ventilated patients. A pilot multicenter randomized controlled trial. *American Journal of Respiratory and Critical Care Medicine, 193*(1), 43–51.

Şanci, E., Coşkun, F. E., & Bayram, B. (2020). Impact of high-flow nasal cannula on arterial blood gas parameters in the emergency department. *Cureus, 12*(9), e10516. https://doi.org/10.7759/cureus.10516.

Siela, D., & Kidd, M. (2017). Oxygen requirements for acutely and critically ill patients. *Critical Care Nurse, 37*(4), 58–70.

St. Clair, J., & MacDermott, J. (2017). Continuous lateral rotation therapy. In D. L. Wiegand (Ed.), *AACN procedure manual for high acuity, progressive, and critical care* (7th ed.) (pp. 111–115). Philadelphia: Elsevier.

Vollman, K., Dickinson, S., & Powers, J. (2017a). Pronation therapy. In D. L. Wiegand (Ed.), *AACN procedure Manual for high Acuity, Progressive, and Critical care* (7th ed.) (pp. 142–163). Philadelphia: Elsevier.

Vollman, K., Sole, M. L., & Quinn, B. (2017b). Endotracheal tube care and oral care practices for ventilated and non-ventilated patients. In D. L. Wiegánd (Ed.), *AACN procedure manual for high acuity, progressive, and critical care* (7th ed.) (pp. 32–39). Philadelphia: Elsevier.

Risk for Dysfunctional Gastrointestinal Motility

Domain 3 Elimination and exchange Class 2 Gastrointestinal function

Mary Beth Flynn Makic, PhD, RN, CCNS, CCRN-K, FAAN, FNAP, FCNS

NANDA-I

Definition

Susceptible to increased, decreased, ineffective, or lack of peristaltic activity within the gastrointestinal tract, which may compromise health.

Risk Factors

Altered water sources; anxiety; eating habit change; impaired physical mobility; malnutrition; sedentary lifestyle; stressors; unsanitary food preparation

At-Risk Population

Individuals who ingested contaminated material; older adults; premature infants

Associated Conditions

Decreased gastrointestinal circulation; diabetes mellitus; enteral nutrition; food intolerance; gastroesophageal reflux disease; infections; pharmaceutical preparations; treatment regimen

NIC, NOC, Client Outcomes, Nursing Interventions and *Rationales,* Client/Family Teaching and Discharge Planning, and References

Refer to care plan for Dysfunctional **Gastrointestinal** Motility.

Dysfunctional Gastrointestinal Motility

Domain 3 Elimination and exchange Class 2 Gastrointestinal function

Rosemary Timmerman, DNP, APRN, CCNS, CCRN-CSC-CMC

NANDA-I

Definition

Increased, decreased, ineffective, or lack of peristaltic activity within the gastrointestinal tract.

Defining Characteristics

Abdominal cramping; abdominal pain; absence of flatus; acceleration of gastric emptying; altered bowel sounds; bile-colored gastric residual; diarrhea; difficulty with defecation; distended abdomen; hard, formed stool; increased gastric residual; nausea; regurgitation; vomiting

Related Factors

Altered water source; anxiety; eating habit change; impaired physical mobility; malnutrition; sedentary lifestyle; stressors; unsanitary food preparation

At-Risk Population

Individuals who ingested contaminated material; older adults; premature infants

Associated Conditions

Decreased gastrointestinal circulation; diabetes mellitus; enteral nutrition; food intolerance; gastroesophageal reflux disease; infections; pharmaceutical preparations; treatment regimen

NOC (Nursing Outcomes Classification)

Suggested NOC Outcomes

Gastrointestinal Function; Electrolyte and Acid-Base Balance; Fluid Balance; Hydration; Nausea and Vomiting Control

Example NOC Outcome with Indicators

Gastrointestinal Function as evidenced by the following indicators: Bowel sounds/Stool soft and formed/Appetite present without evidence of reflux, nausea, or vomiting/Reported normal abdominal comfort/Abdomen soft to palpation without evidence of distention. (Rate the outcome and indicators of **Gastrointestinal Function:** 1 = severely compromised, 2 = substantially compromised, 3 = moderately compromised, 4 = mildly compromised, 5 = not compromised [see Section I].)

G

Client Outcomes

Client Will (Specify Time Frame)

- Be free of abdominal distention and pain
- Have normal bowel sounds
- Pass flatus rectally at intervals
- Defecate formed, soft stool every day to every third day
- State has an appetite
- Be able to eat food without nausea and vomiting

NIC (Nursing Interventions Classification)

Suggested NIC Intervention

Gastric Motility Management

Example NIC Activities—Gastric Motility Management

Evaluate use of prokinetics for delayed gastric motility; Suggest change in dietary habits to either increase or decrease gastric motility, depending on the presenting complaint

Nursing Interventions and *Rationales*

- Monitor for abdominal distention and presence of abdominal pain, weight loss, nausea, vomiting, obstipation, or diarrhea. EB: *The acute onset of abdominal distention in conjunction with symptoms of cramping pain, weight loss, nausea, vomiting, constipation, or diarrhea warrants further evaluation for disorders that cause intestinal obstruction (Nagarwala, Dev, & Markin, 2016).*
- Inspect, auscultate for bowel sounds noting characteristics and frequency; palpate and percuss the abdomen. Hypoactive bowel sounds are found with decreased motility as with peritonitis from paralytic ileus or from late bowel obstruction. EB: *Hyperactive bowel sounds are associated with increased motility (Nagarwala, Dev, & Markin, 2016).*
- Review history noting any anorexia or nausea and vomiting. Other symptoms may include relation of symptoms to meals, especially if aggravated by food, satiety, postprandial fullness/bloating, and weight loss or weight loss with severe gastroparesis. EB: *These are signs of abnormal gastric motility (Camilleri, 2016).*
- Monitor for fluid deficits by checking skin turgor and moisture of tongue, daily weights, input and output, and electrolyte values. Refer to care plan for Deficient **Fluid** Volume if relevant.
- ▲ Monitor for nutritional deficits by keeping close track of food intake. Review laboratory studies that affirm nutritional deficits, such as decreased albumin and serum protein levels, liver profile, glucose, fecal analysis, and an electrolyte panel. Refer to care plan for Imbalanced **Nutrition:** Less Than Body Requirements or Risk for **Electrolyte** Imbalance as appropriate.

Slowed Gastric Motility

- Monitor the client for signs and symptoms of decreased gastric motility, which may include nausea after meals, vomiting, early satiety, postprandial fullness, abdominal bloating, and abdominal pain (Grover et al, 2019; Vavricka & Greuter, 2019).

- ▲ Monitor daily laboratory studies and point of care testing blood glucose levels, ensuring ordered glucose levels are performed and evaluated. EB: *Elevated blood glucose levels can cause delayed gastric emptying; therefore it is important to normalize blood glucose levels (Shen et al, 2019; Sullivan et al, 2020).*
- • Obtain a thorough gastrointestinal history if the client has diabetes because he or she is at high risk for gastroparesis and gastric reflux. EB: *Gastroparesis with delayed emptying of the stomach is a well-known complication of diabetes but may also be idiopathic or caused by gastric surgery, medications, neurological disorders, connective tissue disorders, and mesenteric ischemia (Grover et al, 2019; Sullivan et al, 2020).*
- ▲ If client has nausea and vomiting, provide an antiemetic and intravenous fluids as ordered. Offer or perform oral hygiene after vomiting. Refer to the care plan for **Nausea.**
- ▲ Administer prokinetic, antisecretory, fundic relaxant, and neuromodulator medications as prescribed (Grover et al, 2019; Sullivan et al, 2020).
- ▲ Evaluate medications the client is taking. Recognize that opioids, calcium channel blockers, GLP-1 analogs, diphenhydramine, and anticholinergic medications can cause gastric slowing (Onyimba & Clarke, 2019; Shen et al, 2019).
- ▲ Review laboratory and other diagnostic tools, including complete blood count, amylase, and thyroid-stimulating hormone level, glucose with other metabolic studies, upper endoscopy, and gastric-emptying scintigraphy. EB: *The diagnosis of diabetic gastroparesis is made when other causes are excluded and postprandial gastric stasis is confirmed by gastric emptying scintigraphy, which is considered the gold standard for diagnosing gastroparesis (Grover et al, 2019; Sullivan et al, 2020).*
- ▲ Recognize that endoscopic and surgical therapies for severe gastroparesis include pyloric disruption, electrical stimulation, venting or bypass, and gastric resection (Onyimba & Clarke, 2019; Sullivan et al, 2020).
- ▲ Alternative and complementary therapies such as acupuncture, electroacupuncture, ginger, and massage may offer symptom relief for gastroparesis (Onyimba & Clarke, 2019).
- ▲ Obtain a nutritional consultation, considering a small particle size diet or diets lower or higher in liquids or solids, depending on gastric motility. CEB/EB: *A small (n = 45) randomized controlled trial found that diets with smaller particle size reduced the symptoms of gastroparesis in diabetic clients (Olausson et al, 2014; Grover et al, 2019).*
- ▲ If the client is unable to eat or retain food, consult with the registered dietitian and health care provider, considering further nutritional support in the form of enteral or parenteral feedings for the client with gastroparesis. EB: *Some clients require supplementation with either enteral or parenteral nutrition for survival (Vavricka & Greuter, 2019; Sullivan et al, 2020).*
- ▲ If the client is receiving gastric enteral nutrition, see the care plan Risk for **Aspiration.**
- ▲ Administer bulk-forming or osmotic laxative medications that increase gastrointestinal motility as ordered (Nagarwala, Dev, & Markin, 2016; Coutts, 2019).
- • Advise client to eat small meals low in fat and fiber four to five times each day to allow for adequate nutritional intake while limiting the sensation of fullness; avoid spicy food, carbonated beverages, alcohol, and acidic foods; avoid smoking (Grover et al, 2019; Sullivan et al, 2020).

Postoperative Ileus

- • Observe for complications of delayed intestinal motility. Symptoms include vague abdominal pain and distention, nausea, vomiting, anorexia, sometimes bloating, and tympany to percussion. Clients may or may not pass flatus and some stool (Eamudomkarn et al, 2018; Hedrick et al, 2018).
- ▲ Encourage the client to drink coffee three times per day postoperatively to decrease the time to first flatus and defecation after abdominal surgery (Eamudomkarn et al, 2018; Hedrick et al, 2018).
- ▲ Recommend chewing gum for the abdominal surgery client who is not at risk for aspiration and has normal dentition, particularly if oral intake is limited. EB: *Gum chewing may decrease postoperative ileus because it mimics dietary intake, potentially stimulating vagal tone and gastric and bowel motility (Eamudomkark et al, 2018; Hedrick et al, 2018).*
- ▲ Limit preoperative fasting to 6 hours for solid food and 2 hours for liquids; discontinue fasting and reintroduce oral nutrition postoperatively; if the client has difficulty with oral intake or experiences non-bilious emesis postoperatively, provide a clear liquid diet and advance as tolerated (Hedrick et al, 2018; Taurchini et al, 2018).
- • A preoperative walking program helps reduce time to first postoperative flatus and defecation for clients undergoing surgery for gynecological cancer (Özdemir et al, 2019).

Assist the client with early mobilization after surgery; encourage client to eat all meals in a chair. Exercise may increase gastrointestinal motility.

▲ Minimize the use of opioids and use a multimodal analgesic approach for pain as feasible (Hedrick et al, 2018; Özdemir et al, 2019).

▲ Administer alvimopan, a mu opioid receptor antagonist medication, as prescribed (Venara et al, 2016; Hedrick et al, 2018).

▲ Avoid routine use of prophylactic nasogastric tubes (Hedrick et al, 2018; Taurchini et al, 2018).

▲ Administer an antiemetic for nausea and nonbilious emesis; for clients experiencing bilious emesis with abdominal distention, tympany, and intolerance of oral intake, insert a nasogastric tube as prescribed and consider other etiologies for the symptoms (Hedrick et al, 2018).

▲ Maintain euvolemia and replace electrolytes as needed (Hedrick et al, 2018; Taurchini et al, 2018).

Increased Gastrointestinal Motility

▲ Observe for complications of gastric surgeries such as dumping syndrome. This syndrome is the effect of changes in size and function of the stomach, with rapid dumping of hyperosmolar food into the intestines (Vavricka & Greuter, 2019).

• Watch for signs and symptoms of early dumping syndrome that occur within 15 minutes to 1 hour after a meal, which might include nausea, vomiting, bloating, cramping, abdominal pain, epigastric fullness, borborygmi, diarrhea, dizziness, desire to lie down, palpitations, tachycardia, syncope, perspiration, headache, hypotension, flushing, pallor, and fatigue (Vavricka & Greuter, 2019).

• Monitor for low blood sugar, fatigue, weakness, confusion, hunger, syncope, perspiration, palpitations, tremor, irritability, and dizziness 1 to 3 hours after eating because this is when late rapid gastric emptying may occur; late rapid gastric emptying is associated with low blood sugar (Vavricka & Greuter, 2019).

▲ Order a nutritional consultation to discuss diet changes; the diet may vary depending on the kind of surgery causing dumping syndrome. **EB:** *Encourage small, frequent, high-fiber, high-protein meals; space fluids around meal times by at least 30 minutes (Vavricka & Greuter, 2019).*

• Encourage client to lie down for 30 minutes after a meal to delay gastric emptying (Vavricka & Greuter, 2019).

▲ Administer acarbose to decrease intraluminal digestion of carbohydrates and somatostatin to delay gastric emptying and decrease the release of insulin as prescribed (Vavricka & Greuter, 2019).

▲ Administer antiemetics and antidiarrhea medications as prescribed (Vavricka & Greuter, 2019).

▲ Give intravenous fluids as ordered for the client complaining of diarrhea with weakness and dizziness. Monitor electrolyte panel and acid-base balance. Severe diarrhea can cause deficient fluid volume with extreme weakness and metabolic acidosis.

- ❍ Offer bathroom, commode, or bedpan assistance, depending on frequency, amount of diarrhea, and condition of client.
- ❍ Monitor rectal area for altered skin integrity and apply barrier creams as needed to protect and treat skin.
- ❍ Consider a fecal management system for bedbound clients with frequent loose stools to protect the perineal skin and minimize spread of infection.

• Refer to the care plans for the nursing diagnoses of Deficient **Fluid** Volume, **Nausea,** Impaired **Skin** Integrity, and **Diarrhea** as relevant.

Pediatric

• Assess infants and children with suspected delayed gastric emptying for fullness and vomiting. **EB:** *Babies and children with delayed gastric emptying take longer to get hungry again and throw up undigested or partially digested food several hours after feeding (Westfal & Goldstein, 2017).*

▲ Observe for nutritional and fluid deficits with assessment of skin turgor, mucous membranes, fontanels, furrows of the tongue, electrolyte panel, fluid status, input and output, and daily weights (Islam, 2015).

▲ For pediatric clients age 6 months to 21 years with uncomplicated gastroenteritis, initiate oral rehydration therapy for mild (<5%) and moderate (5%–10%) dehydration with small, frequent volumes replacing ongoing losses with 2 ounces or 8 milliliters per kilogram for each episode of diarrhea or emesis; administer intravenous fluids as prescribed for severe (>10%) dehydration as prescribed; administer ondansetron for vomiting as prescribed (Carson et al, 2017).

- ▲ Recommend gentle massage for preterm infants as appropriate and to treat acute diarrhea in children. CEB/EB: *With massage, there was increased vagal activity. This was then associated with increased gastric motility and greater weight gain (Field, Diego, & Hernandez-Reif, 2011; Gao et al, 2018).*

Geriatric

- ● Closely monitor diet and medication use/side effects because they affect the gastrointestinal system; watch for constipation. EB: *Many gastrointestinal functions are slowed in older adults (Dumic et al, 2019).*
- ▲ Watch for symptoms of dysphagia, gastroesophageal reflux disease, dyspepsia, chronic atrophic gastritis, peptic ulcer disease, mesenteric ischemia, irritable bowel syndrome, inflammatory bowel disease, maldigestion, diverticular disease, and reduced absorption of nutrients. EB: *These are common gastrointestinal disorders in older adults (Dumic et al, 2019).*

Client/Family Teaching and Discharge Planning

- ● Teach the client and caregivers about medications, reinforcing side effects as they relate to gastrointestinal function.
- ● Teach client and caregivers to report signs and symptoms that may indicate further complications, including increased abdominal girth, projectile vomiting, and unrelieved acute cramping pain (bowel obstruction).
- ● Review signs and symptoms of dehydration with client and caregivers.

G

REFERENCES

Camilleri, M. (2016). Disorders of gastrointestinal motility. In L. Goldman, & A. I. Schafer (Eds.), *Goldman-Cecil medicine* (25th ed.) (pp. 884–890). Philadelphia: Elsevier.

Carson, R. A., Mudd, S. S., & Madati, P. J. (2017). Evaluation of a nurse-initiated acute gastroenteritis pathway in the pediatric emergency department. *Journal of Emergency Nursing, 43*(5), 406–412. https://doi.org/10.1016/j.jen.2017.01.001.

Coutts, A. (2019). Nursing management of irritable bowel syndrome. Nursing Standard. *Royal College of Nursing (Great Britain): 1987, 34*(5), 76–81. https://doi.org/10.7748/ns.2019.e11363.

Dumic, I., Nordin, T., Jecmenica, M., Stojkovic Lalosevic, M., Milosavljevic, T., & Milovanovic, T. (2019). Gastrointestinal tract disorders in older age. *Canadian Journal of Gastroenterology & Hepatology, 2019*, 6757524. https://doi.org/10.1155/2019/6757524.

Eamudomkarn, N., Kietpeerakool, C., Kaewrudee, S., Jampathong, N., Ngamjarus, C., & Lumbiganon, P. (2018). Effect of postoperative coffee consumption on gastrointestinal function after abdominal surgery: A systematic review and meta-analysis of randomized controlled trials. *Scientific Reports, 8*(1), 17349. https://doi.org/10.1038/s41598-018-35752-2.

Field, T., Diego, M., & Hernandez-Reif, M. (2011). Potential underlying mechanisms for greater weight gain in massaged preterm infants. *Infant Behavior and Development, 34*(3), 383–389.

Gao, L., Jia, C., & Huang, H. (2018). Paediatric massage for treatment of acute diarrhoea in children: A meta-analysis. *BMC Complementary and Alternative Medicine, 18*(1), 257. https://doi.org/10.1186/s12906-018-2324-4.

Grover, M., Farrugia, G., & Stanghellini, V. (2019). Gastroparesis: A turning point in understanding and treatment. *Gut, 68*(12), 2238–2250. https://doi.org/10.1136/gutjnl-2019-318712.

Hedrick, T. L., McEvoy, M. D., Mythen, M. M. G., et al. (2018). American Society for Enhanced Recovery and Perioperative Quality Initiative joint consensus statement on postoperative gastrointestinal dysfunction within an enhanced recovery pathway for elective colorectal surgery. *Anesthesia & Analgesia, 126*(6), 1896–1907. https://doi.org/10.1213/ANE.0000000000002742.

Islam, S. (2015). Gastroparesis in children. *Current Opinion in Pediatrics, 27*(3), 377–382. http://dx.doi.org/10.1016/j.emc.2015.12.005.

Nagarwala, J., Dev, S., & Markin, A. (2016). The vomiting patient: Small bowel obstruction, cyclic vomiting, and gastroparesis. *Emergency Medical Clinics of North America, 34*(2), 271–291.

Olausson, E. A., Störsrud, S., Grundin, H., Isaksson, M., Attvall, S., & Simrén, M. (2014). Small particle size diet reduces upper gastrointestinal symptoms in patients with diabetic gastroparesis: A randomized controlled trial. *American Journal of Gastroenterology, 109*(3), 375–385.

Onyimba, F. U., & Clarke, J. O. (2019). Helping patients with gastroparesis. *Medical Clinics of North America, 103*(1), 71–87. https://doi.org/10.1016/j.mcna.2018.08.013.

Özdemir, İ.A., Comba, C., Demirayak, G., et al. (2019). Impact of pre-operative walking on post-operative bowel function in patients with gynecologic cancer. *International Journal of Gynecological Cancer, 29*(8), 1311–1316. https://doi.org/10.1136/ijgc-2019-000633.

Shen, S., Xu, J., Lamm, V., Vachaparambil, C. T., Chen, H., & Cai, Q. (2019). Diabetic gastroparesis and nondiabetic gastroparesis. *Gastrointestinal Endoscopy Clinics of North America, 29*(1), 15–25. https://doi.org/10.1016/j.giec.2018.08.002.

Sullivan, A., Temperley, L., & Ruban, A. (2020). Pathophysiology, aetiology and treatment of gastroparesis. *Digestive Diseases and Sciences, 65*(6), 1615–1631. https://doi.org/10.1007/s10620-020-06287-2.

Taurchini, M., Del Naja, C., & Tancredi, A. (2018). Enhanced recovery after surgery: A patient centered process. *The Journal of Visualized Surgery, 4*, 40. https://doi.org/10.21037/jovs.2018.01.20.

Vavricka, S. R., & Greuter, T. (2019). Gastroparesis and dumping syndrome: Current concepts and management. *Journal of Clinical Medicine, 8*(8), 1127. https://doi.org/10.3390/jcm8081127.

Venara, A., Neunlist, M., Slim, K., et al. (2016). Postoperative ileus: Pathophysiology, incidence, and prevention. *Journal of Visceral Surgery, 153*(6), 439–446. https://doi.org/10.1016/j.jviscsurg.2016.08.010.

Westfal, M. L., & Goldstein, A. M. (2017). Pediatric enteric neuropathies: Diagnosis and current management. *Current Opinion in Pediatrics, 29*(3), 347–353.

Risk for Unstable Blood Glucose Level

Domain 2 Nutrition Class 4 Metabolism

Paula D. Hopper, MSN, RN, CNE

G

NANDA-I

Definition

Susceptible to variation in serum levels of glucose from the normal range, which may compromise health.

Risk Factors

Excessive stress; excessive weight gain; excessive weight loss; inadequate adherence to treatment regimen; inadequate blood glucose self-monitoring; inadequate diabetes self-management; inadequate dietary intake; inadequate knowledge of disease management; inadequate knowledge of modifiable factors; ineffective medication self-management; sedentary lifestyle

At-Risk Population

Individuals experiencing rapid growth period; individuals in intensive care units; individuals of African descent; individuals with altered mental status; individuals with compromised physical health status; individuals with delayed cognitive development; individuals with family history of diabetes mellitus; individuals with history of autoimmune disorders; individuals with history of gestational diabetes; individuals with history of hypoglycemia; individuals with history of pre-pregnancy overweight; low birth weight infants; Native American individuals; pregnant women >22 years of age; premature infants; women with hormonal shifts indicative of normal life stage changes

Associated Conditions

Cardiogenic shock; Diabetes mellitus; infections; pancreatic diseases; pharmaceutical preparations; polycystic ovary syndrome; pre-eclampsia; pregnancy-induced hypertension; surgical procedures

NOC (Nursing Outcomes Classification)

Suggested NOC Outcomes

Compliance Behavior: Prescribed Diet; Compliance Behavior: Prescribed Medication; Coping; Endurance; Knowledge: Diabetes Management; Knowledge: Treatment Regimen; Nutritional Status; Personal Health Status; Self-Management: Diabetes; Weight Maintenance Behavior

Example NOC Outcome with Indicators

Blood Glucose Level as evidenced by the following indicators: Blood glucose/Glycosylated hemoglobin/Fructosamine/Urine glucose/Urine ketones. (Rate the outcome and indicators of **Blood Glucose Level:** 1 = severe deviation from normal range, 2 = substantial deviation from normal range, 3 = moderate deviation from normal range, 4 = mild deviation from normal range, 5 = no deviation from normal range [see Section I].)

Client Outcomes

Client Will (Specify Time Frame)

- NOTE: All goals are general recommendations for most clients. Consult health care provider for client-specific goals.
- For most nonpregnant adults, maintain the following blood glucose targets (American Diabetes Association [ADA], 2021):
- A1C less than 7% (normal level <5.7%) or lower if it can be safely achieved
- A1C less than 8% in adults with limited life expectancy, or in those whom harms of treatment outweigh the benefits
- Preprandial glucose between 80 and 130 mg/dL
- Peak postprandial (1–2 hours after beginning of meal) glucose below 180 mg/dL
- For children and adolescents with diabetes, maintain the following blood glucose targets (ADA, 2021):
- A1C less than 6.5% if it can be achieved without excessive hypoglycemia (types 1 and 2)
- A1C less than 7% in most children (types 1 and 2)

- A1C less than 7.5% in children who are at higher risk of hypoglycemia (types 1 and 2)
- A1C less than 8% in children with history of severe life expectancy, short life expectancy, or in those whom harms of treatment outweigh the benefits (type 1)
- In pregnant mothers with gestational or preexisting type 1 or 2 diabetes, maintain blood glucose as follows (ADA, 2021):
- A1C less than 6% for most women, less than 7% if necessary to prevent hypoglycemia
- Fasting <95 mg/dL
- One-hour postprandial ≤140 mg/dL
- Two-hour postprandial ≤120 mg/dL
- In older adults, maintain blood glucose control as follows (ADA, 2021):
- Healthy older adults: A1C < 7 .0 to 7.5; preprandial blood glucose 80 to 130 mg/dL; bedtime 80 to 180 mg/dL
- Older adults with complex coexisting chronic illness, cognitive impairment, or functional dependence: A1C <8.0%, fasting or preprandial 90 to 150 mg/dL; bedtime 100 to 180 mg/dL
- Older adult end-stage chronic illness or moderate to severe cognitive impairment: A1C not pertinent; preprandial 100 to 180 mg/dL; bedtime 110 to 200 mg/dL
- Maintain blood glucose in the majority of hospitalized clients between 140 and 180 mg/dL; more stringent goals may be appropriate if hypoglycemia can be avoided (ADA, 2021)

G

NIC (Nursing Interventions Classification)

Suggested NIC Interventions

Hypoglycemia Management; Hyperglycemia Management

Example NIC Activities—Hypoglycemia Management

Monitor blood glucose levels, as indicated; Provide simple carbohydrate, as indicated

Nursing Interventions and *Rationales*

▲ Monitor blood glucose in hospitalized clients with diabetes who are eating, before meals; who are not eating, every 4 to 6 hours; and who are receiving intravenous (IV) insulin, every 30 minutes to 2 hours. EB: *Hypoglycemia and hyperglycemia in the hospitalized client are associated with adverse outcomes, including death (ADA, 2021).*

▲ In clients receiving multiple-dose insulin or insulin pump therapy, obtain blood glucose before meals and snacks, at bedtime, occasionally postprandially, before exercise or critical tasks such as driving, if low blood glucose is suspected, and after treatment for low blood glucose until normoglycemic. This may require checking up to 6 to 10 times daily. EB: *Self-monitoring of blood glucose (SMBG) helps clients evaluate their response to therapy and guide treatment and self-management decisions (ADA, 2021).*

▲ Consider SMBG in clients with type 2 diabetes not using insulin. EB: *SMBG for type 2 diabetes has showed limited improvement in outcomes. However, for some individuals, glucose monitoring can provide insight into the impact of diet, physical activity, and medication management on glucose levels (ADA, 2021).*

▲ Consider continuous glucose monitoring in clients with type 1 diabetes on intensive insulin regimens. EB: *When used properly, real-time continuous glucose monitors in conjunction with multiple daily injections and continuous subcutaneous insulin infusion and other forms of insulin therapy are a useful tool to lower and/or maintain A1C levels and/or reduce hypoglycemia in adults and youth with diabetes (ADA, 2021).*

▲ Evaluate A1C level for glucose control over previous 3 months. EB: *A1C reflects average glycemia over approximately 3 months and is used as a strong predictive value for diabetes complications (ADA, 2021).*

▲ Consider monitoring 2 hours after the start of meals in individuals who have premeal glucose values within target but have A1C values above target. EB: *Measuring postprandial plasma glucose 1–2 h after the start of a meal and using treatments aimed at reducing postprandial plasma glucose values to 180 mg/dL (10.0 mmol/L) may help to lower A1C (ADA, 2021).*

▲ Consult provider for insulin therapy orders for any client whose glucose is consistently above 180 mg/dL. EB: *Glucose control in critically and non–critically ill clients can reduce mortality, though very tight glucose control may increase risk of hypoglycemia and slightly increases risk of mortality (ADA, 2021).*

- Monitor for signs and symptoms of hypoglycemia, such as shakiness, irritability, confusion, tachycardia, hunger, headache, loss of consciousness, or seizures. EB: *Hypoglycemia may be inconvenient or frightening to clients with diabetes. Severe hypoglycemia can progress to loss of consciousness, seizure, coma, or death (ADA, 2021).*
- Identify level of hypoglycemia. Level 1 hypoglycemia is defined as a measurable glucose concentration <70 mg/dL (3.9 mmol/L) but ≥54 mg/dL (3.0 mmol/L) that can alert a person to take action" (Agiostratidou et al, 2017). Level 2 hypoglycemia is a blood glucose concentration <54 mg/dL (3.0 mmol/L), which is typically the threshold for neuroglycopenic symptoms. Level 3 hypoglycemia is a clinical event characterized by altered mental and/or physical functioning that requires assistance from another person for recovery. Levels 2 and 3 require immediate correction of low blood glucose (ADA, 2021). EB: *Hypoglycemia is a significant—and potentially fatal—complication of type 1 diabetes management and has been found to be a barrier to achieving glycemic goals. Repeated exposure to severe hypoglycemic events has been associated with an increased risk of cardiovascular events and all-cause mortality in people with type 1 or type 2 diabetes (Agiostratidou et al, 2017).*

G

- ▲ Raise glycemic targets in insulin-treated clients with hypoglycemia unawareness, one level 3 hypoglycemic event, or a pattern of unexplained level 2 hypoglycemia to strictly avoid hypoglycemia for at least several weeks. EB: *Several weeks of avoidance of hypoglycemia has been demonstrated to improve counterregulation and hypoglycemia awareness in many clients (ADA, 2021).*
- If the client is experiencing signs and symptoms of hypoglycemia, test glucose; if the result is below 70 mg/dL (level 1), administer 15 to 20 g glucose if the client is conscious. Pure glucose (e.g., three to four glucose tablets) is the preferred treatment, but any form of carbohydrate that contains glucose will suffice (a cup of fruit juice or regular [not diet] soda, one cup of milk, a small piece of fruit). Avoid treating with foods that contain fat, or in type 2 diabetes, avoid foods high in protein. Repeat test in 15 minutes and repeat treatment if indicated. Once blood glucose returns to normal, the individual should consume a meal or snack to prevent recurrence of hypoglycemia. EB: *Hypoglycemia treatment requires ingestion of glucose-containing or carbohydrate-containing foods. The acute glycemic response correlates better with the glucose content than with the carbohydrate content of the food. Pure glucose is the preferred treatment, but any form of carbohydrate that contains glucose will raise blood glucose. Added fat may slow and prolong the acute glycemic episode. In type 2 diabetes, ingested protein may increase insulin response without increasing plasma glucose concentrations. Carbohydrate sources high in protein should not be used to treat or prevent hypoglycemia (ADA, 2021).*
- ▲ Treat severe (level 3) hypoglycemia as follows, if client is unable to swallow glucose:
  - If the client has IV access, administer 25 g of 50% glucose IV (check agency protocol).
  - In the absence of IV access, administer 3 mg intranasal or 1 mg intramuscular or subcutaneous glucagon.
  - For the client at home with no IV glucose or glucagon access, contact emergency personnel and administer oral glucose or cake frosting into the buccal space. Tilt client's head to side to avoid aspiration.

  EB: *Severe hypoglycemia requires the assistance of another person to actively administer carbohydrate, glucagon, or other resuscitative actions. In a randomized, crossover trial comparing intranasal (3 mg) and intramuscular (1 mg) glucagon in 77 clients with type 1 diabetes and hypoglycemia … successful reversal of hypoglycemia occurred in 98.7 and 100 percent of intranasal glucagon and intramuscular glucagon visits, respectively. There is little evidence to support use of buccal glucose, but in the absence of other options it might be helpful while awaiting emergency personnel (Cryer, 2021).*
- ▲ Monitor for and report signs and symptoms of hyperglycemia, such as increased thirst or urination, high blood glucose levels, or elevated A1C. EB: *Achieving A1C targets of <7% has been shown to reduce microvascular (retinopathy, neuropathy, and diabetic kidney disease) complications of type 1 and type 2 diabetes when instituted early in the course of disease (ADA, 2021).*
- ▲ Monitor fluid balance and replace fluids in clients with diabetic ketoacidosis. EB: *Prompt rehydration is vital to restore circulating volume and tissue perfusion, clear ketones, and correct electrolyte imbalance. Restoring circulatory volume and tissue perfusion through aggressive rehydration improves glycemic control and acid base balance, and reduces counterregulatory hormones (Tran et al, 2017).*
- ▲ Avoid use of sliding scale insulin alone in hospitalized clients. EB: *A randomized controlled trial has shown that basal-bolus treatment improved glycemic control and reduced hospital complications compared with reactive, or sliding scale, insulin regimens (i.e., dosing given in response to elevated glucose rather than preemptively) in general surgery clients with type 2 diabetes (ADA, 2021).*

- Before administering IV insulin solution using polyethylene-lined tubing, precondition tubing with insulin solution and allow the solution to dwell for 30 minutes before completing a flush. Use an amount of solution equal to the volume of the tubing for the dwell and again for the flush. EB: *Adsorption of insulin into the IV bag and tubing can significantly reduce the concentration of delivered insulin. Less variability in insulin concentration is found in conditioned (with dwell time) tubing (Newby & Holmes, 2017).*
- ▲ Evaluate the client's medication regimen for medications that can alter blood glucose. EB: *Some asthma medications, some antipsychotic and antidepressant agents, thiazide diuretics, and glucocorticoids, among others, can cause hyperglycemia. Aspirin and beta-blockers are among agents that can cause hypoglycemia (National Prescribing Service Limited [NPS], 2019).*
- ▲ Refer client to a registered dietitian nutritionist (RDN) who is skilled in diabetes medical nutrition therapy (MNT) for individualized instruction. EB: *MNT delivered by an RD/RDN is associated with A1C absolute decreases of 1.0–1.9% for people with type 1 diabetes and 0.3%–2.0% for people with type 2 diabetes (ADA, 2021).*
- ▲ Refer people with type 1 diabetes and those with type 2 diabetes who are prescribed a flexible insulin therapy program for education on how to use carbohydrate counting (and in some cases fat and protein gram estimation) to determine mealtime insulin dosing. EB: *Education on how to use carbohydrate counting and on dosing for fat and protein content should be used to determine mealtime insulin dosing (ADA, 2021).*
- ▲ Refer overweight and obese clients with diabetes for diet and activity instruction. EB: *There is strong and consistent evidence that modest (5%–7%) persistent weight loss can delay the progression from prediabetes to type 2 diabetes (ADA, 2021).*
- Assist clients with periodontal disease to access dental care. EB: *Intensive periodontal treatment [is] associated with better glycemic control and reduction in inflammatory markers after 12 months of follow-up" (ADA, 2021).*
- ▲ Assist clients with depression or mental illness to gain access to mental health services, and ensure collaboration with the diabetes treatment team. EB: *Elevated depressive symptoms and depressive disorders affect one in four clients with type 1 or type 2 diabetes. Randomized controlled trials have shown improvements in diabetes and depression health outcomes when depression is simultaneously treated (ADA, 2021).*
- ▲ Advise all (clients) to avoid use of cigarettes and other tobacco products or e-cigarettes. EB: *Individuals with diabetes who smoke and/or are exposed to second-hand smoke have a heightened risk of cardiovascular disease, premature death, microvascular complications, and worse glycemic control when compared with those who do not smoke. Smoking may have a role in the development of type 2 diabetes (ADA, 2021).*
- For interventions regarding foot care, refer to the care plan Ineffective Peripheral **Tissue Perfusion.**

Geriatric

- Screen for geriatric syndromes (i.e., polypharmacy, cognitive impairment, depression, urinary incontinence, falls, and persistent pain) in older adults EB: *Geriatric syndromes may affect diabetes self-management and diminish quality of life (ADA 2021).*
- ▲ In clients with diabetes who require tube feedings, use a diabetes-specific formulation. EB: *For enteral nutritional therapy, diabetes-specific formulas appear to be superior to standard formulas in controlling postprandial glucose, A1C, and the insulin response (ADA 2020).*
- ▲ Refer older adults for diabetes self-management education and support. EB: *Management of frailty in diabetes includes optimal nutrition with adequate protein intake combined with an exercise program that includes aerobic and resistance training (ADA, 2021).*
- ▲ Collaborate with provider to ensure that diabetes treatment costs are affordable and cost-related nonadherence is avoided. EB: *Medication costs can be a major source of stress for clients with diabetes and contribute to worse adherence to medications; cost-reducing strategies may improve adherence in some cases (ADA, 2021).*

Pediatric

- ▲ Treat hypoglycemia in newborn infants with 0.5 mL/kg oral (buccal) dextrose gel. EB: *Neonatal hypoglycemia can be associated with brain injury. Treatment of infants with neonatal hypoglycemia with 40% dextrose gel reduces the incidence of mother-infant separation for treatment (Weston et al, 2016).*
- ▲ Teach parents of children with diabetes how to recognize and treat symptoms of hypoglycemia. EB: *Symptoms of hypoglycemia in the young result from adrenergic activation (e.g., shakiness, pounding heart, sweatiness) and neuroglycopenia (e.g., headache, drowsiness, difficulty in concentrating). In young children, behavioral changes such as irritability, agitation, quietness, and tantrums may be prominent (Abraham et al, 2018).*

- ▲ Begin screening youth with type 1 diabetes for eating disorders between 10 and 12 years of age. The Diabetes Eating Problems Survey—Revised (DEPS-R) is a reliable, valid, and brief screening tool for identifying disturbed eating behavior. EB: *Early detection of depression, anxiety, eating disorders, and learning disabilities can facilitate effective treatment options and help minimize adverse effects on diabetes management and disease outcomes (ADA, 2021).*
- ● Teach children and adolescents (and their parents) with type 1 diabetes to self-monitor glucose (with meter or continuous glucose monitoring) multiple times daily: before meals and snacks, at bedtime, before exercise, when they suspect low blood glucose, after treating low blood glucose until they are normoglycemic, and before critical tasks such as driving. EB: *A database study of almost 27,000 children and adolescents with type 1 diabetes showed that … increased daily frequency of SMBG was significantly associated with lower A1C (−0.2% per additional test per day) and with fewer acute complications (ADA, 2021).*
- ● Teach parents and children that children and adolescents with type 1 and 2 diabetes should spend 60 minutes or more per day in moderate to vigorous aerobic activity, and at least 3 days/week in muscle/bone-strengthening activity. EB: *The level of physical activity in children and adolescents with [type 1 diabetes] is lower than in their healthy peers (Czenczek-Lewandowska et al, 2019). Youth with type 1 diabetes who engage in more physical activity may have better health outcomes and health-related quality of life (ADA, 2021).*

G

Home Care

- ● Teach family and others having close contact with the person with diabetes how to use an emergency glucagon kit (intranasal, injection kit, or autoinjector, as prescribed). EB: *Glucagon should be prescribed for all individuals at increased risk of level 2 or 3 hypoglycemia so that it is available should it be needed. Caregivers, school personnel, or family members of these individuals should know where it is and how to administer it (ADA, 2021).* EB: *Nasal glucagon (NG) was non-inferior to intramuscular glucagon for successful treatment of insulin-induced hypoglycemia in Japanese clients with [type 1 and type 2 diabetes], supporting use of NG as a rescue treatment for severe hypoglycemia (Matsuhisa et al, 2020). In a validation study, 98.7% successfully administered the rescue injection using the glucagon autoinjector. Overall, there were no patterns of differences between trained versus untrained participants, between caregivers versus first responders or between adults versus adolescents (Valentine et al, 2019).*

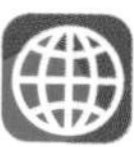

Multicultural

- ▲ Assess social context, including potential food insecurity, housing stability, and financial barriers, and collaborate with provider to apply the information to treatment decisions. EB: *Health inequities related to diabetes and its complications are well documented and are heavily influenced by social determinants of health. In those with diabetes and food insecurity, the priority is mitigating the increased risk for uncontrolled hyperglycemia and severe hypoglycemia (ADA, 2021).*
- ● Provide ethnically and culturally appropriate content that is person centered, considering such things as literacy levels, ethnic foods, and traditional remedies. EB: *Culturally tailored diabetes programs are an important strategy to overcome these health inequities, prevent diabetes complications, and improve care for ethnic minorities (Joo & Liu, 2021).*

Client/Family Teaching and Discharge Planning

- ● Provide "survival skills" education or review for hospitalized clients before discharge, including information about: (1) identification of the health care provider who will provide diabetes care after discharge; (2) level of understanding related to the diabetes diagnosis, self-monitoring of blood glucose, home blood glucose goals, and when to call the provider; (3) definition, recognition, treatment, and prevention of hyperglycemia and hypoglycemia; (4) information on making healthy food choices at home and referral to an outpatient RDN to guide individualization of meal plan, if needed. If relevant, when and how to take glucose-lowering medications, including insulin administration; (5) sick-day management; and (6) proper use and disposal of needles and syringes. Providing a structured discharge plan tailored to the individual client may reduce length of hospital stay and readmission rates and increase client satisfaction (ADA, 2021).
- ● Evaluate clients' monitoring technique and ability to use results to adjust therapy at regular intervals. EB: *Optimal use of SMBG requires proper review and interpretation of the data by both the client and provider, to ensure that data are used in an effective and timely manner (ADA, 2021).*

- Teach clients with type 2 diabetes the importance of reducing sedentary behavior, and to interrupt prolonged sitting at least every 30 minutes. EB: *Avoiding extended sedentary periods may help prevent type 2 diabetes for those at risk and may also aid in glycemic control for those with diabetes (ADA, 2021).*
- Teach adults with type 1 and type 2 diabetes to engage in 150 min or more of moderate to vigorous-intensity aerobic activity per week, spread over at least 3 days/week, with no more than 2 consecutive days without activity. Shorter durations (minimum 75 min/week) of vigorous intensity or interval training may be sufficient for younger and more physically fit individuals … Adults with type 1 and type 2 diabetes should engage in 2–3 sessions/week of resistance exercise on nonconsecutive days. EB: *Exercise has been shown to improve blood glucose control, reduce cardiovascular risk factors, contribute to weight loss, and improve well-being (ADA, 2021).*
- ▲ Discuss recommending resistance training with the client's provider. EB: *"Compared with no exercise, resistance training improves HbA1C by 0.34% and may modestly improve cardiorespiratory fitness" (Oyler et al, 2020).*
- Teach clients with type 1 diabetes to test for urine or blood ketones if they are ill, if their blood glucose is >240 mg/dL, and before exercise if blood glucose is >250 mg/dL. Advise to increase fluid intake and contact provider at first detection of ketones. EB: *Exercise should be postponed or suspended if blood ketone levels are elevated (≥1.5 mmol/L) as blood glucose levels and ketones may rise further with even mild activity (Colberg et al, 2016). Diabetic ketoacidosis onset and recurrence can largely be prevented through client education (Kreider, 2018).*
- ▲ Teach clients taking insulin or secretagogue medication to check blood glucose before and after exercise. Blood glucose levels before exercise should ideally be >90 mg/dL. Discuss carbohydrate use in relation to exercise with provider. EB: *Because of the variation in glycemic response to exercise bouts, clients need to be educated to check blood glucose levels before and after periods of exercise (ADA, 2021).*
- Teach clients to use alcohol with caution. EB: *Alcohol consumption may place people with diabetes at increased risk for delayed hypoglycemia, especially if taking insulin or insulin secretagogues (ADA, 2021).*
- Inform clients that use of smartphone applications may help them manage their diabetes care and glucose control. CEB/EB: *In adjunct to usual care, the use of a diabetes-related smartphone application combined with weekly text-message support from a health care professional can significantly improve glycemic control in adults with type 1 diabetes (Kirwan et al, 2013). Clients that used mobile platforms were found to test their blood glucose more often and demonstrated greater improvement in blood glucose compared to users who did not use the mobile platform (Offringa et al, 2018).*

REFERENCES

Abraham, M. B., Jones, T. W., Naranjo, D., et al. (2018). ISPAD Clinical Practice Consensus Guidelines 2018: Assessment and management of hypoglycemia in children and adolescents with diabetes. *Pediatric Diabetes, 19*(Suppl. 27), 178–192. https://doi.org/10.1111/pedi.12698.

Agiostratidou, G., Anhalt, H., Ball, D., et al. (2017). Standardizing clinically meaningful outcome measures beyond HbA1c for type 1 diabetes: A consensus report of the American Association of Clinical Endocrinologists, the American Association of Diabetes Educators, the American Diabetes Association, the Endocrine Society, JDRF International, The Leona M. and Harry B. Helmsley Charitable Trust, the Pediatric Endocrine Society, and the T1D Exchange. *Diabetes Care, 40*(12), 1622–1630. https://doi.org/10.2337/dc17-1624.

American Diabetes Association (ADA). (2020). Standards of medical care in diabetes—2020. *Diabetes Care, 43*(Suppl. 1).

American Diabetes Association (ADA). (2021). Standards of medical care in diabetes—2021. *Diabetes Care, 44*(Suppl. 1).

Colberg, S. R., Sigal, R. J., Yardley, J. E., et al. (2016). Physical activity/exercise and diabetes: A position statement of the American Diabetes Association. *Diabetes Care, 39*(11), 2065–2079.

Cryer, P.E. (2021). Hypoglycemia in adults with diabetes. *UpToDate.* I. B. Hirsch & J. E. Mulder (Eds.). Waltham: UpToDate. Retrieved from https://www.uptodate.com/contents/hypoglycemia-in-adults-with-diabetes-mellitus. Accessed July 1, 2021.

Czenczek-Lewandowska, E., Leszczak, J., Baran, J., et al. (2019). Levels of physical activity in children and adolescents with type 1 diabetes in relation to the healthy comparators and to the method of insulin therapy used. *International Journal of Environmental Research and Public Health, 16*(18), 3498. https://doi.org/10.3390/ijerph16183498.

Joo, J. Y., & Liu, M. F. (2021). Experience of culturally-tailored diabetes interventions for ethnic minorities: A qualitative systematic review. *Clinical Nursing Research, 30*(3), 253–262. https://doi.org/10.1177/1054773819885952.

Kirwan, M., Vandelanotte, C., Fenning, A., & Duncan, M. J. (2013). Diabetes self-management smartphone application for adults with type 1 diabetes: Randomized controlled trial. *Journal of Medical Internet Research, 15*(11), e235. https://doi.org/10.2196/jmir.2588.

Kreider, K. E. (2018). Updates in the management of diabetic ketoacidosis. *Journal for Nurse Practitioners, 14*(8), 591–597. https://doi.org/10.1016/j.nurpra.2018.06.013.

Matsuhisa, M., Takita, Y., Nasu, R., Nagai, Y., Ohwaki, K., & Nagashima, H. (2020). Nasal glucagon as a viable alternative for treating insulin-induced hypoglycaemia in Japanese patients with type 1 or type 2 diabetes: A phase 3 randomized crossover study. *Diabetes, Obesity and Metabolism, 22*(7), 1167–1175. https://doi.org/10.1111/dom.14019.

National Prescribing Service Limited (NPS). (2019). *Medicines that affect blood glucose levels.* Retrieved from https://www.nps.org.au/consumers/medicines-and-type-2-diabetes#medicines-that-affect-blood-glucose-levels. Accessed July 1, 2021.

Newby, B., & Holmes, D. T. (2017). Effect of tubing flush or preconditioning on available insulin concentration for IV infusion: A pilot project. *Canadian Journal of Hospital Pharmacy, 70*(4), 320–321. https://doi.org/10.4212/cjhp.v70i4.1685.

Offringa, R., Sheng, T., Parks, L., Clements, M., Kerr, D., & Greenfield, M. S. (2018). Digital diabetes management application improves glycemic outcomes in people with type 1 and type 2 diabetes. *Journal of Diabetes Science and Technology, 12*(3), 701–708. https://doi.org/10.1177/1932296817747291.

Oyler, V., Rahman, R., Barker, J., & Tran, M. H. (2020). In adults with type 2 diabetes, does a strength training program improve outcomes? *Evidence-Based Practice, 23*(9), 20–21. https://doi.org/10.1097/EBP.0000000000000721.

Tran, T. T. T., Pease, A., Wood, A. J., et al. (2017). Review of evidence for adult diabetic ketoacidosis management protocols. *Frontiers in Endocrinology, 8*, 106. http://doi.org/10.3389/fendo.2017.00106.

Valentine, V., Newswanger, B., Prestrelski, S., Andre, A. D., & Garibaldi, M. (2019). Human factors usability and validation studies of a glucagon autoinjector in a simulated severe hypoglycemia rescue situation. *Diabetes Technology & Therapeutics, 21*(9), 522–530. https://doi.org/10.1089/dia.2019.0148.

Weston, P. J., Harris, D. L., Battin, M., Brown, J., Hegarty, J. E., & Harding, J. E. (2016). Oral dextrose gel for the treatment of hypoglycaemia in newborn infants. *Cochrane Database of Systemic Reviews, 5*, CD011027. https://doi.org/10.1002/14651858.CD011027.pub2.

G

Maladaptive Grieving Domain 9 Coping/stress response Class 2 Coping responses

Ruth A. Wittmann-Price, PhD, RN, CNS, CNE, CNEcl, CHSE, ANEF, FAAN

NANDA-I

Definition

A disorder that occurs after the death of a significant other, in which the experience of distress accompanying bereavement fails to follow sociocultural expectations.

Defining Characteristics

Anxiety; decreased life role performance; depressive symptoms; diminished intimacy levels; disbelief; excessive stress; experiencing symptoms the deceased experienced; expresses anger; expresses being overwhelmed; expresses distress about the deceased person; expresses feeling detached from others; expresses feeling of emptiness; expresses feeling stunned; expresses shock; fatigue; gastrointestinal symptoms; grief avoidance; increased morbidity; longing for the deceased person; mistrust of others; nonacceptance of a death; persistent painful memories; preoccupation with thoughts about a deceased person; rumination about deceased person; searching for a deceased person; self-blame

Related Factors

Difficulty dealing with concurrent crises; excessive emotional disturbance; high attachment anxiety; inadequate social support; low attachment avoidance

At-Risk Population

Economically disadvantaged individuals; individuals experiencing socially unacceptable loss; individuals experiencing unexpected sudden death of significant other; individuals experiencing violent death of significant other; individuals unsatisfied with death notification; individuals who witnessed uncontrolled symptoms of the deceased

NOC (Nursing Outcomes Classification)

Suggested NOC Outcomes

Anxiety Level; Coping; Depression; Grief Resolution; Mood Equilibrium; Personal Well-Being; Psychosocial Adjustment: Life Change; Sleep

Example NOC Outcome with Indicators

Grief Resolution as evidenced by the following indicators: Resolves feelings/Verbalizes reality and acceptance of loss/Maintains living environment/Seeks Social support. (Rate the outcome and indicators of **Grief Resolution:** 1 = never demonstrated, 2 = rarely demonstrated, 3 = sometimes demonstrated, 4 = often demonstrated, 5 = consistently demonstrated [see Section I]).

Client Outcomes

Client Will (Specify Time Frame)

- Express appropriate feelings of guilt, fear, anger, or sadness
- Identify somatic distress associated with grief (e.g., anxiety, changes in appetite, insomnia, nightmares, loss of libido, decreased energy, altered activity levels)
- Seek support in dealing with grief-associated issues
- Identify personal strengths and effective coping strategies
- Function at a normal developmental level and begin to successfully and increasingly perform activities of daily living

NIC (Nursing Interventions Classification)

Suggested NIC Interventions

Grief Work Facilitation; Grief Work Facilitation: Perinatal Death; Guilt Work Facilitation; Hope Installation

G

Example NIC Activities—Grief Work Facilitation

Identify the loss; Encourage expression of feelings about the loss; Assist to identify personal coping strategies; Identify sources of community support

Nursing Interventions and *Rationales*

- Assess for signs of maladaptive grieving that include symptoms that persist at least 6 months after the death and are experienced at least daily or to a disabling degree. Symptoms include feeling emotionally numb, stunned, shocked, and that life is meaningless; dysfunctional thoughts and maladaptive behaviors; experiencing mistrust and estrangement from others; anger and bitterness over the loss; identity confusion; avoidance of the reality of the loss, or excessive proximity seeking to try to feel closer to the deceased, sometimes focused on wishes to die or suicidal statements and behavior; or difficulty moving on with life. Symptoms must be associated with psychosocial and physical impairments. EB: *Brown (2016) studied the recurrent grief in mothers caring for a child with intellectual disability and found that recurrent grief is correlated with coping and challenging behaviors of the child.* EB: *Buck et al (2020) studied complicated grieving and the effects of accelerated resolution therapy (ART) (a mind-body therapy). In a random control trial, one group of participants received four ART sessions, and the results demonstrated that the intervention group had decreased complicated grief and better grief resolution.*
- ▲ Determine the client's state of grieving. Use a tool such as the Prolonged Grief Disorder (PGD) scale (Jordan & Litz, 2014), the Grief Support in Health Care Scale (Anderson et al, 2010), the Hogan Grief Reaction Checklist (Hogan, Worden, & Schmidt, 2004), and the Beck Depression Inventory. EBN: *Researchers studied the grief of mothers (n = 130) and fathers (n = 52) after infant or child neonatal or pediatric intensive care unit death by completing the Hogan Grief Reaction Checklist at 1, 3, 6, and 13 months after the death, and found initial grief reactions decreased from 3 to 13 months for mothers and from 3 to 6 months for fathers (Youngblut et al, 2017).*
- ▲ Determine whether the client is experiencing depression, suicidal tendencies, or other emotional disorders. Refer the client for counseling or therapy as appropriate. EB: *The study also found that participants experiencing depression and maladaptive grief used grief services at a more frequent rate than participants who were not clinically depressed (Banyasz et al, 2017).* EB: *In a qualitative study (Titlestad et al, 2020) of Norwegian parents who experienced a drug-related death of a child, the researchers identified three salient themes. The first theme was processing grief emotions from the incident, the second theme was proactive coping, and the third theme was giving and receiving support and assistance from others and to others.*
- Educate the client and his or her support systems that grief resolution is not a sequential process and that the positive outcome of grief resolution is the integration of the deceased into the ongoing life of the griever. EB: *Mowll (2017) studied ways to support family members (n = 48) who needed to view the body of their relative after a traumatic death. Things that assisted the family members included support during interactions, giving permissions and possibilities, providing information and preparation, being caring, timing experiences appropriately, and tuning in to family needs.* EB: *Hanish, Margulies, and Cogan (2019) quantitatively studied the outcome of a residential retreat for women (n = 141) who experienced pregnancy or infant loss. The retreat included group discussions, yoga, meditation, crafts, and activities to facilitate grieving and healing. The study demonstrated statistically significant post-test improvements in participations' depression, self-compassion, and perceived social support.*

- ▲ Assess caregivers, particularly younger caregivers, for pessimistic thinking and additional stressful life events. Refer for appropriate support. EB: *Researchers studied African American caregivers (family members) (N = 108) of persons with dementia and found that negative thoughts increase depression and physical suffering (Schulz et al, 2017).* EB: *See et al (2020) qualitatively explored women's (N = 22) expectations when they entered an emergency department (ED) for early pregnancy bleeding and impending perinatal loss. Participant interviews revealed four themes: (1) need to inform clients of progress and explain treatments, (2) needing privacy to allow for grieving, (3) decreasing prolonged waiting time, and (4) recommending available services to support clients after they leave the ED.*
- ● See the interventions and rationales in the care plans for Readiness for Enhanced **Grieving** and Chronic **Sorrow.**

G

Pediatric/Parent

- ▲ Refer grieving children and parents to a program to help facilitate grieving if desired, especially if the death was traumatic. EB: *Schreiber, Sands, and Jordan (2017) studied children whose parents died of suicide and found that children felt isolated, abandoned, and responsible. Suggestions for nursing included developmentally appropriate education about suicide grief, depression, and normalizing.*
- ● Encourage grieving parents to take part in activities that are supportive, such as faith-based activities. EB: *Nuzum, Meaney, and O'Donoghue (2017) qualitatively studied parents who experienced the loss of a stillborn child, and study results indicated that stillbirth challenges parents' faith, usually one parent more than the other, indicating that all parents should be offered spiritual care after a stillbirth.*
- ● Encourage grieving parents to seek mental health services as needed. EBN: *Morris et al (2017) noted that bereaved parents are an "at-risk" group, and through anecdotal experiences they developed a hospital-wide, preventive model, bereavement program using education, guidance, and support. The model has been received by participants and staff with good results.*
- ● Help the adolescent determine sources of support and how to use them effectively. If the client is an adolescent exposed to a peer's suicide, watch for symptoms of traumatic grief and posttraumatic stress disorder, which include numbness, preoccupation with the deceased, functional impairment, and poor adjustment to the loss. EB: *Woollett et al (2017) qualitatively studied adolescents who were HIV-positive in Africa and their ability to disclose the disease and the bereavement process. The study found that most participants were orphaned and experiencing maladaptive grief that was related negatively to mental health and the ability to accept their HIV status and adhere to treatment.* EB: *Praetorius and Rivedal (2020) qualitatively studied stories about suicide survivors (N = 6) and found that stories could be equated to a theme such as sailing down the lazy river, which hit unexpected rapids, then getting to shore before going over a waterfall, waking in the ocean of why, and righting the ship and rescuing others. The story developed in this research project assisted others to understand the feelings of suicide survivors and help friends and family deal with the suicide.*

Geriatric

- ● Assess for deterioration in bereaved older adults' self-care. EBN: *Skritskaya et al (2017) investigated maladaptive cognitions and their relationship to complicated grief by developing a questionnaire called the Typical Beliefs Questionnaire (TBQ) and piloted the tool on bereaved adults (N = 394) with complicated grief. The new tool was effective in identifying specific maladaptive cognitions related to complicated grief.*
- ● Those who have lived with older adults with dementia and experienced significant feelings of loss before the loved one's death may be at risk for more intense feelings of grief after the death of the client with dementia. EB: *Berenbaum, Tziraki, and Cohen-Mansfield (2017) studied how people with dementia are told about the death of a peer. Adult daycare staff (N = 52) was qualitatively interviewed and felt that their clients have the emotional capacity to mourn despite their cognitive impairments.*
- ● Monitor the older client for complicated grieving manifesting in physical and mental health problems. EB: *Boer et al (2014) studied clients with chronic obstructive pulmonary disease (COPD) who have a grieving process because of loss of functioning and found that clients with COPD experience four stages of grief: denial, resistance, sorrow, and acceptance.*

Multicultural

- ● Assess for the influence of cultural beliefs, norms, and values on the client's grief and mourning practices. EBN: *Bravo (2017) studied undocumented Latino migrants (N = 12) living in the United States who have experienced coping with deaths of loved ones in their home countries. The participants experienced sadness and guilt, but communication with those in the home country was an important mechanism for coping.* EBN: *Kongsuwan et al (2019) completed a qualitative study of grieving Thai Buddhist husbands. Interviews revealed five themes: (1) loss of thoughtful focus and energy, (2) attachment to the children, (3) continuing social connections, (4) evaluating lived time, and (5) providing oneself healing time. The study results demonstrate that nurses can develop bereavement care processes by valuing the religious principles integrating social interaction for bereaved husbands.*

- Encourage discussion of the grief process. EBN: *Mun and Ow (2017) studied the grief process of mothers who lost a child in Singapore and found that qualitatively four themes were identified: (1) meaning to the child's life and death, (2) quality and assurance of an afterlife, (3) the function of crying, and (4) a continuing bond.*
- Identify whether the client had been notified of the health status of the deceased and was able to be present during illness and death. EB: *Young (2017) discussed cases related to people with profound intellectual and multiple disabilities (PIMD) that are bereaved and experience social, emotional, and physical constraints. Young found that people with PIMD are a high-risk group and at greater risk of maladaptive grieving.*

G

Home Care

- Previous interventions can be adapted for home care use.
- Consider providing support via the Internet. EB: *Researchers studied an Internet or telephone intervention with caregivers of veterans with dementia and found that in rural populations the Internet was effective if the caregiver was comfortable with technology (Hicken et al, 2017).* EB: *Pearce (2020) used the Internet to establish a "Tagboard" after a community crisis in which two people were killed. A content analysis of 493 images was completed and divulged a theme of authentic self in the grief of the community and was effective in promoting grief expression in a complicated situation that affected an entire community.*

REFERENCES

Anderson, K., Ewen, H., & Miles, E. (2010). The grief support in healthcare scale: Development and testing. *Nursing Research*, *59*(6), 372–379. https://doi.org/10.1097/NNR.0b013e3181fca9de.

Banyasz, A., Weikittle, R., Lorenz, A., Goodman, L., & Wells-Di Gregorio, S. (2017). Bereavement service preferences of surviving family members: Variation among next of kin with depression and complicated grief. *Journal of Palliative Medicine*, *20*(10), 1091–1097. https://doi.org/10.1089/jpm.2016.0235.

Berenbaum, R., Tziraki, C., & Cohen-Mansfield, J. (2017). The right to mourn in dementia: To tell or not to tell when someone dies in dementia day care. *Death Studies*, *41*(6), 353–359. https://doi.org/10.1080/07481187.2017.1284953.

Boer, L. M., Daudey, L., Peters, J. B., Molema, J., Prins, J. B., & Vercoulen, J. H. (2014). Assessing the stages of the grieving process in chronic obstructive pulmonary disease (COPD): Validation of the Acceptance of Disease and Impairments Questionnaire (ADIQ). *International Journal of Behavioral Medicine*, *21*(3), 561–570. https://doi.org/10.1007/s12529-013-9312-3.

Bravo, V. (2017). Coping with dying and deaths at home: How undocumented migrants in the United States experience the process of transnational grieving. *Mortality*, *22*(1), 33–44. https://doi.org/10.1080/13576275.2016.1192590.

Brown, J. M. (2016). Recurrent grief in mothering a child with an intellectual disability to adulthood: Grieving is the healing. *Child & Family Social Work*, *21*(1), 113–122. https://doi.org/10.1111/cfs.12116.

Buck, H. G., Cairns, P., Emechebe, N., et al. (2020). Accelerated resolution therapy: Randomized Controlled trial of a complicated grief intervention. *American Journal of Hospice and Palliative Medicine*, *37*(10), 791–799. https://doi.org/10.1177/1049909119900641.

Hanish, K. K., Margulies, I., & Cogan, A. M. (2019). Evaluation of an occupation-based retreat for women after pregnancy or infant loss. *American Journal of Occupational Therapy*, *73*(5), 7305345030p6. https://doi.org/10.5014/ajot.2019.034025.

Hicken, B. L., Daniel, C., Luptak, M., Grant, M., Kilian, S., & Rupper, R. W. (2017). Supporting caregivers of rural veterans electronically (SCORE). *The Journal of Rural Health*, *33*(3), 305–313. https://doi.org/10.1111/jrh.12195.

Hogan, N. S., Worden, J. W., & Schmidt, L. A. (2004). An empirical study of the proposed complicated grief disorder criteria. *Omega*, *48*(3), 263–277. https://doi.org/10.2190/GX7H-H05N-A4DN-RLU9.

Jordan, A. H., & Litz, B. T. (2014). Prolonged grief disorder: Diagnostic, assessment, and treatment considerations. *Professional Psychology: Research and Practice*, *45*(3), 180–187. https://doi.org/10.1037/a0036836.

Kongsuwan, W., Khaw, T., Chaiweeradet, M., & Locsin, R. (2019). Lived experience of grieving of Thai Buddhist husbands who had lost their wives from critical illness. *Journal of Nursing Scholarship*, *51*(4), 390–398. https://doi.org/10.1111/jnu.12477.

Morris, S. E., Dole, O. R., Joselow, M., Duncan, J., Renaud, K., & Branowicki, P. (2017). The development of a hospital-wide bereavement program: Ensuring bereavement care for all families of pediatric patients. *Journal of Pediatric Health Care*, *31*(1), 88–95. https://doi.org/10.1016/j.pedhc.2016.04.013.

Mowll, J. (2017). Supporting family members to view the body after a violent or sudden death: A role for social work. *Journal of Social Work in End-Of-Life and Palliative Care*, *13*(2–3), 94–112. https://doi.org/10.1080/15524256.2017.1331182.

Mun, S., & Ow, R. (2017). Death of a child: Perspective of Chinese mothers in Singapore. *Journal of Religion & Spirituality in Social Work*, *36*(3), 306–325. https://doi.org/10.1080/15426432.2017.1319781.

Nuzum, D., Meaney, S., & O'Donoghue, K. (2017). The spiritual and theological challenges of stillbirth for bereaved parents. *Journal of Religion and Health*, *56*(3), 1081–1095. https://doi.org/10.1007/s10943-017-0365-5.

Pearce, J. S. (2020). Lafayette strong: A content analysis of grief and support online following a theater shooting. *Illness, Crisis, and Loss, 28*(4), 299–320. https://doi.org/10.1177/1054137317742234.

Praetorius, R. T., & Rivedal, J. (2020). Navigating out of the ocean of "Why"—a qualitative study of the trajectory of suicide bereavement. *Illness, 28*(4), 347–362. https://doi.org/10.1177/1054137317741714.

Schreiber, J. K., Sands, D. C., & Jordan, J. R. (2017). The perceived experience of children bereaved by parental suicide. *Omega: The Journal of Death and Dying, 75*(2), 184–206. https://doi.org/10.1177/0030222815612297.

Schulz, R., Savla, J., Czaja, S. J., & Monin, J. (2017). The role of compassion, suffering, and intrusive thoughts in dementia caregiver depression. *Aging & Mental Health, 21*(9), 997–1004. https://doi.org/10.1080/13607863.2016.1191057.

See, S. Y. C., Blecher, G. E., Craig, S. S., & Egerton-Warburton, D. (2020). Expectations and experiences of women presenting to emergency departments with early pregnancy bleeding. *Emergency Medicine Australasia, 32*(2), 281–287. https://doi.org/10.1111/1742-6723.13403.

Skritskaya, N. A., Mauro, C., Olonoff, M., et al. (2017). Measuring maladaptive cognitions in complicated grief: Introducing the Typical Beliefs Questionnaire. *American Journal of Geriatric Psychiatry, 25*(5), 541–550. https://doi.org/10.1016/j.jagp.2016.09.003.

Titlestad, K. B., Stroebe, M., & Dyregrov, K. (2020). How do drug-death-bereaved parents adjust to life without the deceased? A qualitative study. *Omega: The Journal of Death and Dying, 82*(1), 141–164. https://doi.org/10.1177/0030222820923168.

Woollett, N., Black, V., Cluver, L., & Brahmbhatt, H. (2017). Reticence in disclosure of HIV infection and reasons for bereavement: Impact on perinatally infected adolescents' mental health and understanding of HIV treatment and prevention in Johannesburg, South Africa. *African Journal of AIDS Research: AJAR, 16*(2), 175–184. https://doi.org/10.2989/16085906.2017.1337646.

Young, H. (2017). Overcoming barriers to grief: Supporting bereaved people with profound intellectual and multiple disabilities. *International Journal of Developmental Disabilities, 63*(3), 131–137. https://doi.org/10.1080/20473869.2016.1158511.

Youngblut, J. M., Brooten, D., Glaze, J., Promise, T., & Yoo, C. (2017). Parent grief 1–13 months after death in neonatal and pediatric intensive care units. *Journal of Loss & Trauma, 22*(1), 77–96. https://doi.org/10.1080/15325024.2016.1187049.

G

Risk for Maladaptive Grieving

Domain 9 Coping/stress tolerance Class 2 Coping responses

Marina Martinez-Kratz, MS, RN, CNE

NANDA-I

Definition

Susceptible to a disorder that occurs after death of a significant other, in which the experience of distress accompanying bereavement fails to follow sociocultural expectations, which may compromise health.

Risk Factors

Difficulty dealing with concurrent crises; excessive emotional disturbance; high attachment anxiety; inadequate social support; low attachment avoidance

At-Risk Population

Economically disadvantaged individuals; individuals experiencing socially unacceptable loss; individuals experiencing unexpected sudden death of significant other; individuals experiencing violent death of significant other; individuals unsatisfied with death notification; individuals who witnessed uncontrolled symptoms of the deceased; individuals with history of childhood abuse; individuals with history of unresolved grieving; individuals with significant predeath dependency on the deceased; individuals with strong emotional proximity to the deceased; individuals with unresolved conflict with the deceased; individuals without paid employment; women

Associated Conditions

Anxiety disorders; depression

NIC, NOC, Client Outcomes, Nursing Interventions and *Rationales,* Client/Family Teaching and Discharge Planning, and References

Refer to care plan for Maladaptive **Grieving.**

Readiness for Enhanced Grieving

Domain 9 Coping/stress tolerance Class 2 Coping responses

Ruth A. Wittmann-Price, PhD, RN, CNS, CNE, CNEcl, CHSE, ANEF, FAAN

NANDA-I

Definition

A pattern of integration of a new functional reality that arises after an actual, anticipated or perceived significant loss, which can be strengthened.

Defining Characteristics

Expresses desire to carry on legacy of the deceased; expresses desire to engage in previous activities; expresses desire to enhance coping with pain; expresses desire to enhance forgiveness; expresses desire to enhance hope; expresses desire to enhance personal growth; expresses desire to enhance sleep-wake cycle; expresses desire to integrate feelings of anger; expresses desire to integrate feelings of despair; expresses desire to integrate feelings of guilt; expresses desire to integrate feelings of remorse; expresses desire to integrate positive feelings; expresses desire to integrate positive memories of deceased; expresses desire to integrate possibilities for a joyful life; expresses desire to integrate possibilities for a meaningful life; expresses desire to integrate possibilities for a purposeful life; expresses desire to integrate possibilities for a satisfactory life; expresses desire to integrate the loss; expresses desire to invest energy in new interpersonal relations

G

NOC (Nursing Outcomes Classification)

Suggested NOC Outcomes

Grief Resolution; Dignified Life Closure; Hope; Psychosocial Adjustment: Life Change

Example NOC Outcome with Indicators

Grief Resolution as evidenced by the following indicators: Resolves feelings about the loss/Verbalizes reality and acceptance of loss/Maintains living environment/Seeks social support. (Rate the outcome and indicators of **Grief Resolution:** 1 = never demonstrated, 2 = rarely demonstrated, 3 = sometimes demonstrated, 4 = often demonstrated, 5 = consistently demonstrated [see Section I].)

Client/Family Outcomes

Client/Family Will (Specify Time Frame)

- Express meaning of the loss to his or her life and the functioning of the family
- Identify ways to support family members and articulate methods of support he or she requires from family and friends
- Accept assistance in meeting the needs of the family from friends and/or extended family

NIC (Nursing Interventions Classification)

Suggested NIC Interventions

Grief Work Facilitation; Dying Care; Emotional Support: Perinatal Death; Hope Instillation; Support System Enhancement; Family Support; Family Integrity Promotion

Example NIC Activities—Grief Work Facilitation

Identify the loss; Encourage expression of feelings about the loss; Assist to identify personal coping strategies; Identify sources of community support

Nursing Interventions and *Rationales*

Anticipatory Grieving Interventions

- Acknowledge grieving of a critically ill or dying client and clients' family/relatives for the losses experienced during the deteriorating illness, and the future that will be filled with loss. EBN: *Johnson et al (2017)*

qualitatively studied anticipatory grieving associated with clients at the end of life and their families and found that less than 50% of the dying clients and their families were given an anticipatory grieving nursing diagnosis and met the nursing outcomes at the time of death (such as the spiritual health outcome), demonstrating that expected outcomes need additional nursing attention.

- Develop a trusting relationship both with the client and with the family by using presence and therapeutic communication techniques. **EBN:** *Al Mutair et al (2019) explored the impact of cultural diversity on how neonatal and pediatric intensive care nurses care for Muslim families before and after the death of infants. To overcome the challenges there was a commitment to respect everyone and an openness to differences.*
- Keep the family apprised of the client's ongoing condition as much as possible. Consult with the family for decision-making as appropriate. **EB:** *In a study of family caregiving of terminally ill clients, Ullrich et al (2020) found that difficult decision-making was related to moral distress in family members and having path options for choices assisted family caregivers to move toward acceptance.*
- Keep the family informed of client's needs for physical care and support in symptom control, and inform them about health care options at the end of life, including palliative care, hospice care, and home care. **EB:** *Brooks et al (2017) completed a study about communication and shared decision-making about end-of-life care in a 24-bed intensive care unit (ICU) using focus groups with 17 nurses and 11 physicians. Findings indicated that improvement was needed in initiating and communicating end-of-life care among health care professionals and with the families.*
- Ask family members about having adequate resources to care for themselves and the critically ill family member. **EBN:** *Eskola et al (2017) used a mixed-method study on parents' experiences and needs during a child's (N = 47) end-of-life care at home and found that parents created a sense of normality for the child, which caused parental exhaustion. Parents needed practical help with housekeeping and dealing with insurance.*
- Encourage family members to show their caring feelings and talk to the client. **EBN:** *The researchers completed a literature review about using transitional objects with parents for perinatal loss such as taking photographs for parents. The objects provide parents a brief sense of healing (LeDuff et al, 2017).*
- Recognize and respect different feelings and wishes from both the family members and the client. **EB:** *Immigrant families and their grieving related to COVID-19 family deaths were studied by Falicov et al (2020). The study found decreased family stress by providing families resources to Wi-Fi, smartphones, or computers, or sufficient living space.*
- If necessary, refer a family member for counseling or to a minister/priest to help him or her cope with the existential questions and current overwhelming reality. **EB:** *Parente and Ramos (2020) qualitatively studied Brazilian parents (N = 40) who experienced a death of a child and their spiritual-religious coping. The results demonstrated that spirituality was related to helping others after the death of a child and that 70% of parents reported volunteer work as a method to decrease the grief.* **EB:** *Thompson et al (2020) studied caregiver stress in family members caring for clients with Alzheimer's disease. The researchers examined stress, role strain, self-concept stress, and coping stress in relation to decision-making. The results demonstrated that strong family self-efficacy and high levels of coping skills assisted family members to make critical decisions.*
- Promote mutual goal setting in which decisions are made together that affect the family. **EBN:** *Kim et al (2017) descriptively studied end-of-life care decisions for cancer clients and found that 50% of caregivers did not agree on advance directives, and the overall recommendation is to better include caregivers in end-of-life decisions to decrease disagreement.*

Grieving Interventions When Death of a Loved One Occurs

Use the following activities when interacting with the bereaved person:

- Be present and attentive; use active empathetic listening. **EBN:** *Cheng and Fang (2018) completed a qualitative case study with a dialysis client who experienced the loss of her spouse. The investigators found three trends: dysfunctional grieving, hopelessness, and sleep pattern disturbance. The researchers used caring, active listening, and empathy to promote a positive grieving process by assisting participants to accept the reality of loss, work through the pain of grief, and adjust to an environment without her spouse.*
- Validate the client's feelings of grief and feeling hurt, stressful, anxious, out of control, and further symptoms of grieving with an appropriate tool. **EB:** *The Perinatal Bereavement Care Confidence Scale (PBCCS) has 43 items and is valid to elicit data about care knowledge, bereavement care skills, self-awareness, and*

organizational support (Kalu et al, 2020). The tool is recommended to be used by practitioners who care for bereaved perinatal parents.

- Provide time and space for the person to tell their story of loss. EB: *Lawrence (2017) completed a case study analysis with individuals who experienced catastrophic events as first responders of lost clients or victims. Telling their story assisted in the grieving process.*
- Offer condolences: "I am sorry that you lost your husband." EB: *Levi-Belz (2017) investigated the role of the ongoing relationship with the deceased family member comparing 58 suicide-loss survivors and 48 sudden-death and 53 natural-death bereaved individuals, and the suicide-loss family reported a lower positive ongoing relationship with the deceased.*
- Intentionally schedule meetings with family members to provide support during grieving. EB: *Parravicini (2017) completed a literature review about the protocols for newborns with life-limiting or life-threatening conditions and concluded that a multiprofessional team is needed to address the infant's needs, parental grieving process, and providers' distress.*
- Help the client use a method to give voice to his or her unique story of loss. Methods include keeping a personal journal to record feelings and insights; retelling of the loss narrative to a caring person; music therapy techniques with a trained therapist or listening to music that has significance to the relationship; and use of the "virtual dream," which is a dreamlike short story written by the grieving person to tell the narrative of the loss. EBN: *Beiermann et al (2017) studied families' (n = 50) bereavement reactions related to clients dying in the ICU and found that the majority of families responded positively to receiving an ECG Memento, which is a monitor strip of the clients' heart rhythm.*
- Discuss coping methods with the grieving person. Common coping techniques include exercise, telling the story of grief to a caring person, journaling, pets, and developing a legacy for the deceased. EB: *The researchers used kinetic sculpturing as a grief intervention in case studies to create visual examples of family equilibrium before, in the midst of, and after the deaths of family members. Family members found the creative expression beneficial (Brandon & Goldberg, 2017).*
- Encourage the family to create a quiet and comfortable healing environment, and follow comforting grief rituals such as prayer, interacting with nature, or lighting votive candles. EBN: *Barrett (2017) reviewed a case study related to how health care professionals provide empathy to grieving parents who lost a child and suggested nursing implications including being present and listening.*
- Help the family determine the best way and place to find social support. Encourage family members to continue to use support for as long as needed. EB: *Researchers studied spouses (n = 1224) whose partners died to examine (1) how life satisfaction changed; (2) whether sociodemographic factors and social and health resources moderate the effect on life satisfaction; and (3) whether anticipation, reaction, and adaptation are related to mortality. Life satisfaction decreases for about 2.5 years and older age was associated with more intense declines (Infurna et al, 2017).*
- Identify available community resources, including bereavement groups at local hospitals and hospice centers. Volunteers who provide bereavement support can also be effective. EB: *Gibson (2017) investigated the use of Second Life to symbolically bury and memorialize the real-life biological deaths of people. It was shown to not decrease the loss in real life; instead it provides a method to remember the person.*
- ▲ Refer the family members for spiritual counseling as desired. EB: *Ortega-Galán et al (2020) qualitatively studied the spiritual and religious beliefs of clients at the end of life by interviews (n = 87). Participants revealed that spirituality was important and that a variety of clergies in health units is needed so all clients and families get support that is comfortable.*
- ▲ Refer to mental health providers as needed. EB: *Lenger et al (2020) studied the health of grieving caregivers and its relation to prolonged grief. The researchers described the physical and mental health of people who were caring for clients at the end of life and found that caregivers scored lower on one physical subscale and all mental health measures when compared with the general population.*
- Refer to Maladaptive **Grieving** if the experience of distress accompanying bereavement fails to follow sociocultural expectations.

Pediatric/Parent

- Treat the child/parents with respect, and give them the opportunity to talk about concerns and answer questions honestly. EB: *Care providers can give anticipatory guidance to caregivers to support children who are grieving; to assist children to better understand what has happened; and to address any misinformation, misinterpretations, or misconceptions (Schonfeld & Demaria, 2016).*

- Listen to the child's expression of grief. **EBN:** *Schmidt et al (2020) studied 32 children who experienced a loss of a pet. The investigators found that children have continuing bonds with their pets after the loss. The continuing bonds vary depending on the attachment the child had with the pet and the age of the child.*
- Help parents recognize that the grieving child does not have to be "fixed"; instead they need support going through an experience of grieving just like adults. **EB:** *In a study of how bereaved students were perceived in a school setting by adults, the researchers found that 93% of adult participants interacted with bereaved students, provided emotional support, made classroom accommodations, interacted with the family/community, and referred the student for counseling (DeMuth et al, 2020).*
- Consider the use of art for children in hospice care who are dying or dealing with the death of a parent, sibling, or other family member. **EB:** *Hirschon et al (2018) used the "tree of life metaphor" and images to assist adolescents to express their grief. Participants were able to verbalize and share their grief reactions effectively using this technique.*

G

▲ Refer grieving children and parents to a program to help facilitate grieving if desired, especially if the death was traumatic. **EB:** *Testoni et al (2020) studied the grieving process of Italian mothers (n = 15) after a perinatal loss and identified three main themes during the interviews: continuing bonds between externalized and internalized presence, a difficult guilt to manage, and relationships are crucial support systems. The findings of this study demonstrate that there is a continuing bond after death between mother and the perinatal loss.*

- Help the adolescent determine sources of support and how to use them effectively. **EB:** *DeDiego, Wheat, and Fletcher (2017) explored Adventure Based Counseling (ABC) camps for grieving adolescents and children with positive results.* **EB:** *Dodd et al (2020) studied the Active Inhibition Scale (AIS), an 11-item, self-report measure of emotional suppression. The results revealed that emotional suppression scores were higher among girls compared to boys, Black and Hispanic youth compared to White youth, and older compared to younger age groups.*
- Encourage grieving parents to take good care of their own health. **EB:** *Albuquerque et al (2017) studied parental relationships (n = 17) after the death of a child by grounded theory method and identified three themes: search for meaning, communication with the partner, and care-in-relation that assisted couples to maintain a healthy relationship.*

▲ Refer grieving parents to seek mental health services as needed. The death of a child is regarded as among the most traumatic, incomprehensible, and devastating of losses, with the potential to precipitate a crisis of meaning for the bereaved parent. **EB:** *Researchers studied meaning reconstruction using a life-story interview with a Japanese woman who lost her son to suicide. The analysis revealed three themes: (1) making sense of her son's death and life, (2) relationships with other people, and (3) reconstruction of a bond with the deceased (Kawashima & Kawano, 2017).*

- Recognize that men and women often grieve differently, and explain this to parents as needed. **EB:** *Researchers used a mixed-method approach to investigate mothers' (n = 60) grief after losing a child, forgiveness, and posttraumatic growth. There was a negative correlation between forgiveness and grief and a positive correlation between forgiveness and posttraumatic growth (posttraumatic growth was viewed as changes in life) (Martinčeková & Klatt, 2017).*
- Recognize that mothers who have a miscarriage/stillbirth grieve and experience sorrow because of the loss of the child. **EBN:** *Rocha Catania et al (2017) performed a literature (n = 29) review about prenatal palliative care for parents carrying a fetus with malformations and found no long-term studies about the effects of prenatal palliative care.*

Geriatric

- Monitor an older adult who has been treated for bereavement-related depression for relapse or recurrence. **EB:** *Tanimukai et al (2015) studied the relationship between depression and insomnia in bereaved families and found that insomnia was highly correlated with depression.*
- Provide support for the family when the loss is associated with dementia of the family member. **EB:** *Researchers studied an intervention with caregivers of veterans with dementia. Caregivers were divided into groups of Internet or telephone intervention and found that in rural populations the Internet was effective if the caregiver was comfortable with technology (Hicken et al, 2017).*

- Determine the social supports of older adults. EBN: *Dunham, Allmark, and Collins (2017) investigated the experience of cancer pain in elderly clients (n = 9) and identified four themes for nursing consideration: better to be old than to be dying, maintaining independence, grieving for a former self, and denial of pain.*

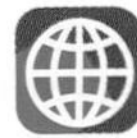

Multicultural

- See interventions and rationales in care plans for Maladaptive **Grieving** and Chronic **Sorrow.**

Home Care

- The interventions previously described may be adapted for home care use.
- Assessment of activities of daily living (ADLs) and instrumental ADLs is essential as part of comprehensive care after a home care client has suffered the loss of a loved one. EB: *Raitio, Kaunonen, and Aho (2015) explored parental grief intervention and its effects on maternal grief with health care provider intervention and found that support from the health care professionals was positively correlated with stronger personal growth at 6 months after the death.*
- Actively listen as the client grieves for his or her own death or for real or perceived loss. Normalize the client's expressions of grief for self. Demonstrate a caring and hopeful approach. EB: *Vergo et al (2017) measured the grief reactions of clients (n = 53) with advanced cancer using the Preparatory Grief in Advanced Cancer (PGAC) instrument and found that preparatory grief was common and 25% of participations had significant grief, and all clients demonstrated distress.*

G

- ▲ Refer the client to social services as necessary for losses not related to death. Support is helpful to grief work for all types of losses. Social workers can help the client plan for financial changes as a result of job losses and help with community referrals as appropriate. EB: *A study by social work researchers about women who experienced a miscarriage, stillbirth, or child's death compared self-esteem to maternal identity and found that stillbirth and death of a child negatively affected self-esteem, and that self-esteem levels were increased by stronger maternal identity (Hill et al, 2017).*
- ▲ Refer the bereaved to hospice bereavement programs or an Internet self-help group. Relief of the suffering of clients and families (physical, emotional, and spiritual) is the goal of hospice care. EB: *An ethnographic study was completed to understand the motivation for grieving mothers to start and maintain a blog. After reviewing 140 blogs the researchers identified themes such as sharing the loss and challenges, creating a network to support and comfort others, guaranteeing a space to express feelings, honoring and perpetuating the image of the child lost, and engaging in social activism (Figueiredo Frizzo et al, 2017).*

REFERENCES

Al Mutair, A., Al Ammary, M., Brooks, L. A., & Boomer, M. J. (2019). Supporting Muslim families before and after a death in neonatal and paediatric intensive care units. *Nursing in Critical Care, 24*(4), 192–200. https://doi.org/10.1111/nicc.12434.

Albuquerque, S., Cunha Ferreira, L., Narciso, I., & Pereira, M. (2017). Parents' positive interpersonal coping after a child's death. *Journal of Child and Family Studies, 26*(7), 1817–1830. https://doi.org/10.1007/s10826-017-0697-5.

Barrett, M. (2017). 'How would you feel ...?' A reflective case study. *British Journal of Cardiac Nursing, 12*(5), 219–222. https://doi.org/10.12968/bjca.2017.12.5.219.

Beiermann, M., Kalowes, P., Dyo, M., & Mondor, A. (2017). Family members' and intensive care unit nurses' response to the ECG Memento© during the bereavement period. *Dimensions of Critical Care Nursing: DCCN, 36*(6), 317–326. https://doi.org/10.1097/DCC.0000000000000269.

Brandon, K. E., & Goldberg, R. M. (2017). A kinetic sculpture intervention for individuals grieving the deaths of family members. *Journal of Creativity in Mental Health, 12*(1), 99 114. https://doi.org/10.1080/15401383.2016.1184114.

Brooks, L. A., Manias, E., & Nicholson, P. (2017). Communication and decision-making about end-of-life care in the intensive care unit. *American Journal of Critical Care, 26*(4), 336–341. https://doi.org/10.4037/ajcc2017774.

Cheng, P.-Y., & Fang, L. (2018). Applying the concept of grief counseling in caring for an elderly dialysis patient with bereavement due to the death of spouse: A nursing care experience. *Journal of Nursing, 65*(5), 98–104. https://doi.org/10.6224/JN.201810_65(5).12.

DeDiego, A. C., Wheat, L. S., & Fletcher, T. B. (2017). Overcoming obstacles: Exploring the use of adventure based counseling in youth grief camps. *Journal of Creativity in Mental Health, 12*(2), 230–241. https://doi.org/10.1080/15401383.2016.1191403.

DeMuth, M., Taggi-Pinto, A., Miller, E. G., & Alderfer, M. A. (2020). Bereavement accommodations in the classroom: Experiences and opinions of school staff. *Journal of School Health, 90*(3), 165–171. https://doi.org/10.1111/josh.12870.

Dodd, C. G., Hill, R. M., Alvis, L. M., et al. (2020). Initial validation and measurement invariance of the Active Inhibition Scale among traumatized and grieving youth. *Journal of Traumatic Stress, 33*(5), 843–849. https://doi.org/10.1002/jts.22529.

Dunham, M., Allmark, P., & Collins, K. (2017). Older people's experiences of cancer pain: A qualitative study. *Nursing Older People, 29*(6), 28–32. https://doi.org/10.7748/nop.2017.e943.

Eskola, K., Bergstraesser, E., Zimmermann, K., & Cignacco, E. (2017). Maintaining family life balance while facing a child's imminent death—a mixed methods study. *Journal of Advanced Nursing, 73*(10), 2462–2472. https://doi.org/10.1111/jan.13304.

Falicov, C., Niño, D., & D'Urso, S. (2020). Expanding possibilities: Flexibility and solidarity with under-resourced immigrant families during the COVID–19 pandemic. *Family Process*, *59*(3), 865–882. https://doi.org/10.1111/famp.12578.

Figueiredo Frizzo, H. C., Szylit Bousso, R., Rossi de Faria Ichikawa, C., & Nigro de Sá, N. (2017). Grieving mothers: Design of thematic blogs about loss of a child. *Acta Paulista de Enfermagem*, *30*(2), 116–121. https://doi.org/10.1590/1982-0194201700019.

Gibson, M. (2017). Grievable lives: Avatars, memorials, and family "plots" in Second Life. *Mortality*, *22*(3), 224–239. https://doi.org/10.1080/13576275.2016.1263941.

Hicken, B. L., Daniel, C., Luptak, M., Grant, M., Kilian, S., & Rupper, R. W. (2017). Supporting caregivers of rural veterans electronically (SCORE). *The Journal of Rural Health*, *33*(3), 305–313. https://doi.org/10.1111/jrh.12195.

Hill, P. W., Cacciatore, J., Shreffler, K. M., & Pritchard, K. M. (2017). The loss of self: The effect of miscarriage, stillbirth, and child death on maternal self-esteem. *Death Studies*, *41*(4), 226–235. https://doi.org/10.1080/07481187.2016.1261204.

Hirschson, S., Fritz, E., & Kilian, D. (2018). The tree of life as a metaphor for grief in AIDS-orphaned adolescents. *American Journal of Dance Therapy*, *40*(1), 87–109. https://doi.org/10.1007/s10465-017-9243-7.

Infurna, F. J., Wiest, M., Gerstorf, D., et al. (2017). Changes in life satisfaction when losing one's spouse: Individual differences in anticipation, reaction, adaptation and longevity in the German Socio-Economic Panel Study (SOEP). *Ageing and Society*, *37*(5), 899–934. https://doi.org/10.1017/S0144686X15001543.

Johnson, J., Lodhi, M. K., Cheema, U., et al. (2017). Outcomes for end-of-life patients with anticipatory grieving: Insights from practice with standardized nursing terminologies within an interoperable internet-based electronic health record. *Journal of Hospice and Palliative Nursing*, *19*(3), 223–231. https://doi.org/10.1097/NJH.0000000000000333.

Kalu, F. A., Larkin, P., & Coughlan, B. (2020). Development, validation and reliability testing of "Perinatal Bereavement Care Confidence scale (PBCCS)". *Women and Birth*, *33*(4), e311–e319. https://doi.org/10.1016/j.wombi.2019.07.001.

Kawashima, D., & Kawano, K. (2017). Meaning reconstruction process after suicide: Life-story of a Japanese woman who lost her son to suicide. *Omega: Journal of Death and Dying*, *75*(4), 360–375. https://doi.org/10.1177/0030222816652805.

Kim, S., Koh, S., Park, K., & Kim, J. (2017). End-of-life care decisions using a Korean advance directive among cancer patient-caregiver dyads. *Palliative & Supportive Care*, *15*(1), 77–87. http://dx.doi.org/10.1017/S1478951516000808.

Lawrence, M. (2017). Near-death and other transpersonal experiences occurring during catastrophic events. *American Journal of Hospice and Palliative Medicine*, *34*(5), 486–492. https://doi.org/10.1177/1049909116631298.

LeDuff, L. D., 3rd, Bradshaw, W. T., Blake, S. M., et al. (2017). Transitional objects to facilitate grieving following perinatal loss. *Advances in Neonatal Care*, *17*(5), 347–353. https://doi.org/10.1097/ANC.0000000000000429.

Lenger, M. K., Neergaard, M. A., Guldin, M. B., & Nielsen, M. K. (2020). Poor physical and mental health predicts prolonged grief disorder: A prospective, population-based cohort study on caregivers of patients at the end of life. *Palliative Medicine*, *34*(10), 1416–1424. https://doi.org/10.1177/0269216320948007.

Levi-Belz, Y. (2017). Relationship with the deceased as facilitator of posttraumatic growth among suicide-loss survivors. *Death Studies*, *41*(6), 376–384. https://doi.org/10.1080/07481187.2017.1285372.

Martinčeková, L., & Klatt, J. (2017). Mothers' grief, forgiveness, and posttraumatic growth after the loss of a child. *Omega: The Journal of Death and Dying*, *75*(3), 248–265. https://doi.org/10.1177/0030222816652803.

Ortega-Galán, A. M., Cabrera-Troya, J., Ibáñez-Masero, O., Carmona-Rega, M. I., & Ruiz-Fernández, M. D. (2020). Spiritual dimension at the end of life: A phenomenological study from the caregiver's perspective. *Journal of Religion and Health*, *59*(3), 1510–1523. https://doi.org/10.1007/s10943-019-00896-6.

Parente, N. T., & Ramos, D. G. (2020). The influence of spiritual-religious coping on the quality of life of Brazilian parents who have lost a child by homicide, suicide, or accident. *Journal of Spirituality in Mental Health*, *22*(3), 216–239. https://doi.org/10.1080/19349637.2018.1549525.

Parravicini, E. (2017). Neonatal palliative care. *Current Opinions Pediatrics*, *29*(2), 135–140. https://doi.org/10.1097/MOP.0000000000000464.

Raitio, K., Kaunonen, M., & Aho, A. L. (2015). Evaluating a bereavement follow-up intervention for grieving mothers after the death of a child. *Scandinavian Journal of Caring Sciences*, *29*(3), 510–520. https://doi.org/10.1111/scs.12183.

Rocha Catania, T., Bernardes, L., Guerra Benute, G. R., et al. (2017). When one knows a fetus is expected to die: Palliative care in the context of prenatal diagnosis of fetal malformations. *Journal of Palliative Medicine*, *20*(9), 1020–1031. https://doi.org/10.1089/jpm.2016.0430.

Schmidt, M., Naylor, P. E., Cohen, D., et al. (2020). Pet loss and continuing bonds in children and adolescents. *Death Studies*, *44*(5), 278–284. https://doi.org/10.1080/07481187.2018.1541942.

Schonfeld, D. J., & Demaria, T. (2016). Committee on Psychosocial Aspects of child and family health, Disaster Preparedness Advisory Council. Supporting the grieving child and family *Pediatrics*, *138*(3), e20162147. https://doi.org/10.1542/peds.2016-2147.

Tanimukai, H., Adachi, H., Hirai, K., et al. (2015). Association between depressive symptoms and changes in sleep condition in the grieving process. *Supportive Care in Cancer*, *23*(7), 1925–1931. https://doi.org/10.1007/s00520-014-2548-x.

Testoni, I., Bregoli, J., Pompele, S., & Maccarini, A. (2020). Social support in perinatal grief and mothers' continuing bonds: A qualitative study with Italian mourners. *Journal of Women & Social Work*, *35*(4), 485–502. https://doi.org/10.1177/0886109920906784.

Thompson, C. J., Bridier, N., Leonard, L., & Morse, S. (2020). Exploring stress, coping, and decision-making considerations of Alzheimer's family caregivers. *Dementia*, *19*(6), 1907–1926. https://doi.org/10.1177/1471301218809865.

Ullrich, A., Theochari, M., Bergelt, C., et al. (2020). Ethical challenges in family caregivers of patients with advanced cancer—A qualitative study. *BMC Palliative Care*, *19*(1), 70. https://doi.org/10.1186/s12904-020-00573-6.

Vergo, M. T., Whyman, J., Li, Z., et al. (2017). Assessing preparatory grief in advanced cancer patients as an independent predictor of distress in an American population. *Journal of Palliative Medicine*, *20*(1), 48–52. https://doi.org/10.1089/jpm.2016.0136.

Deficient Community Health

Domain 1 Health promotion Class 2 Health management

Marina Martinez-Kratz, MS, RN, CNE

NANDA-I

Definition

Presence of one or more health problems or factors that deter wellness or increase the risk of health problems experienced by a group or population.

Defining Characteristics

Health problem experienced by groups or populations; program unavailable to enhance wellness of a group or population; programs unavailable to eliminate health problems of a group or population; programs unavailable to prevent health problems of a group or population; programs unavailable to reduce health problems of a group or population; risk of hospitalization to a group or population; risk of physiological manifestations to a group or population; risk of psychological manifestations to a group or population

Related Factors

Inadequate access to health care provider; inadequate consumer satisfaction with programs; inadequate expertise within the community; inadequate health resources; inadequate program budget; inadequate program evaluation plan; inadequate program outcome data; inadequate social support for programs; programs incompletely address health problems

NOC (Nursing Outcomes Classification)

Suggested NOC Outcomes

Community Grief Response; Community Health Screening Effectiveness; Community Health Status Community Program Effectiveness; Community Resiliency; Community Risk Control: Obesity; Community Risk Control: Unhealthy Cultural Traditions

Example NOC Outcome with Indicators

Community Health Status as evidenced by the following indicators: Health status of infants/Children/Adolescents/Adults/Elders/Minority populations/Prevalence of health promotion programs. (Rate the outcome and indicators of **Community Health Status:** 1 = poor, 2 = fair, 3 = good, 4 = very good, 5 = excellent, NA [see Section I].)

Client Outcomes

Community/Adolescents/Minority Clients Will (Specify Time Frame)

- Provide programs for healthy behaviors
- Demonstrate goal setting
- Describe and comply with healthy behaviors

NIC (Nursing Interventions Classification)

Suggested NIC Interventions

Community health development: Identify health concerns, strengths, and priorities with community partners; Assist community members in raising awareness of health problems and concerns

Nursing Interventions and *Rationales*

- Refer to care plans for Readiness for Enhanced Community **Coping,** Ineffective Community **Coping,** Ineffective **Health** Maintenance Behaviors, Ineffective **Home** Maintenance Behaviors, and Risk for Other-Directed **Violence.**
- Assess for the presence of social determinants associated with community mortality. EB: *A study that evaluated associations between social determinants of health and life expectancy suggests that social determinants are associated with population health across the lifespan (Cohen, Broccoli, & Greaney, 2020).*

- Assess for needs related to the community's priority health concerns. EB: *In a community-based participatory research study with 3151 respondents, the five most identified health concerns were diabetes, cancer, hypertension, heart problems, and body weight (McElfish et al, 2018).*
- Assess clients accessing health services for a history of military service and provide the necessary referrals and information. EBN: *Many veterans eligible for Veterans Administration (VA) health benefits seek health care from community emergency departments and will benefit from information about VA resources (Merkl et al, 2016).*
- Implement community engagement techniques for collaboration with stakeholders to design, develop, and adapt relevant health interventions. EB: *In the Hearts of Sonoma County (HSC) initiative, clinical systems and communities worked to reduce cardiovascular disease risk (Cheadle et al, 2019).*
- Encourage attendance at community-based exercise programs. EBN: *In this study community-based exercise groups were perceived by pregnant women as a satisfactory and motivating form of exercise engagement (Ette, 2017).*
- Implement community engagement techniques in conjunction with tailored interventions to address health deficiencies. EB: *In this study, community engagement techniques were essential in coordinating interventions and engaging clients, the public, and local practitioners in delivery of mental health care (Lamb et al, 2015).*
- Collaborate with other community-based programs to use text messaging to broadcast targeted health messages to reach large numbers of community members. EB: *A cluster randomized controlled study showed that mobile text messaging had a positive effect on the gestational weights and hemoglobin levels of expectant mothers (Singh et al, 2020).*

H

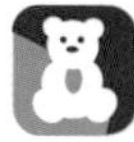

Pediatric

- ▲ Consider use of a clinical-community collaborative to address health deficiencies in underserved populations with children. EB: *Pediatric waiting rooms were redesigned to enhance families' engagement and connection to community resources. Caregivers were significantly more likely to perceive the redesigned waiting rooms as places to obtain help with connecting to community resources and clinical and educational information (Henize et al, 2018).*
- ▲ Screen at-risk pediatric populations for lead exposure. EB: *This study showed undertesting for lead exposure and no mandatory lead test screening in one-third of eligible children during the study period (Knighton, Payne, & Speedie, 2016).*

Geriatric

- ▲ Assess community-dwelling older individuals for cognitive impairment using the Brief Cognitive Assessment Tool-Short Form (BCAT-SF). EBN: *In this study, the BCAT-SF demonstrated sensitivity in differentiating between dementia and nondementia (Mace, Mansbach, & Clark, 2016).*
- ▲ Refer older clients with a diagnosis of dementia to a home-based missing incident prevention program (HMIPP). EB: *An HMIPP program was effective in reducing the number of missing incidents, searching time, and caregivers' stress at 3 months and 1 year (Lau, Chan, & Szeto, 2019).*
- ▲ Assess community-dwelling older individuals with the Identification of Seniors at Risk (ISAR) screening tool when they present for treatment in the emergency department. EB: *A systematic review and meta-analysis found the ISAR had modest predictive accuracy and may serve as a decision-making adjunct when determining which older adults can be safely discharged (Galvin et al, 2017).*
- ▲ Screen community-dwelling older individuals for fall risk with the Timed Up and Go Test (TUG) or the Functional Gait Assessment (FGA) and refer to a fall prevention program. EB: *A clinical review of research recommended the use of the TUG and FGA to identify fall risk in community-dwelling older individuals (Lee, Geller, & Strasser, 2013).* EBN: *A nurse practitioner–led fall prevention program was successful at reducing fall risk among older adults (Harrison, 2017).*

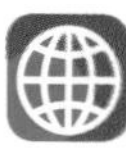

Multicultural

- Assess for the impact of race/ethnic-based segregation on health outcomes. EB: *Race-based residential segregation was associated with an increase in all-cause mortality that was mediated by education, income inequality, and exposure to air pollution (Schulz et al, 2020).*
- Provide culturally and linguistically appropriate community health programs. EB: *A systematic review found that culturally appropriate community-based physical activity programs appear to support and encourage engagement among culturally and linguistically diverse older adults (Montayre et al, 2020).*
- Use decision aids (DAs) (personal counseling, multimedia, and print materials) to facilitate communication between clients and health care providers to determine a plan for health care. EB: *A systematic review*

found 18 studies illustrating the effectiveness of DAs in improving client–provider communication and decision quality outcomes in minority populations (Nathan et al, 2016).

Home Care and Client/Family Teaching and Discharge Planning

- The previously mentioned interventions may be adapted for home care and client/family teaching.

REFERENCES

Cheadle, A., Rosaschi, M., Burden, D., et al. (2019). A community-wide collaboration to reduce cardiovascular disease risk: The Hearts of Sonoma County Initiative: Preventing chronic disease. *Preventing Chronic Disease*, *16*, E89. https://doi.org/10.5888/pcd16.180596.

Cohen, S. A., Broccoli, J. R., & Greaney, M. L. (2020). Community-based social determinants of three measures of mortality in Rhode Island cities and towns. *Archives of Public Health*, *78*, 56. https://doi.org/10.1186/s13690-020-00438-7.

Ette, L. (2017). Community-based exercise interventions during pregnancy are perceived as a satisfactory and motivating form of exercise engagement. *Evidence-Based Nursing*, *20*(3), 77–78.

Galvin, R., Gilleit, Y., Wallace, E., et al. (2017). Adverse outcomes in older adults attending emergency departments: A systematic review and meta-analysis of the Identification of Seniors at Risk (ISAR) screening tool. *Age and Ageing*, *46*(2), 179–186. https://doi.org/10.1093/ageing/afw233.

Harrison, B. E. (2017). Fall prevention program in the community: A nurse practitioner's contribution. *Journal for Nurse Practitioners*, *13*(8), e395–e397. https://doi.org/10.1016/j.nurpra.2017.06.017.

Henize, A. W., Beck, A. F., Klein, M. D., Morehous, J., & Kahn, R. S. (2018). Transformation of a pediatric primary care waiting room: Creating a bridge to community resources. *Maternal and Child Health Journal*, *22*(6), 779–785. https://doi.org/10.1007/s10995-018-2508-z.

Knighton, A. J., Payne, N. R., & Speedie, S. (2016). Lead testing in a pediatric population: Underscreening and problematic repeated tests. *Journal of Public Health Management and Practice*, *22*(4), 331–337. https://doi.org/10.1097/PHH.0000000000000344.

Lamb, J., Dowrick, C., Burroughs, H., et al. (2015). Community engagement in a complex intervention to improve access to primary mental health care for hard-to-reach groups. *Health Expectations: An International Journal of Public Participation in Health Care and Health Policy*, *18*(6), 2865–2879. https://doi.org/10.1111/hex.12272.

Lau, W. M., Chan, T. Y., & Szeto, S. L. (2019). Effectiveness of a home-based missing incident prevention program for community-dwelling elderly patients with dementia. *International Psychogeriatrics*, *31*(1), 91–99. https://doi.org/10.1017/S1041610218000546.

Lee, J., Geller, A. I., & Strasser, D. C. (2013). Analytical review: Focus on fall screening assessments. *P M & R: The Journal of Injury Function, and Rehabilitation*, *5*(7), 609–621. https://doi.org/10.1016/j.pmrj.2013.04.001.

Mace, R. A., Mansbach, W. E., & Clark, K. M. (2016). Rapid cognitive assessment of nursing home residents: A comparison of the Brief Interview for Mental Status (BIMS) and Brief Cognitive Assessment Tool-Short Form (BCAT-SF). *Research in Gerontological Nursing*, *9*(1), 35–44. https://doi.org/10.3928/19404921-20150522-05.

McElfish, P. A., Long, C. R., Stephens, R. M., et al. (2018). Assessing community health priorities and perceptions about health research: A foundation for a community-engaged research program. *Journal of Higher Education Outreach and Engagement*, *22*(1), 107–128.

Merkl, M. A., Tanabe, P., Sverha, J. P., 2nd, & Turner, B. (2016). A quality improvement initiative for designing and implementing a military service screening tool for a community emergency department. *Journal of Emergency Nursing*, *42*(5), 400–407. https://doi.org/10.1016/j.jen.2015.11.009.

Montayre, J., Neville, S., Dunn, I., Shrestha-Ranjit, J., & Wright-St Clair, V. (2020). What makes community-based physical activity programs for culturally and linguistically diverse older adults effective? A systematic review. *Australasian Journal on Ageing*, *39*(4), 331–340. https://doi.org/10.1111/ajag.12815.

Nathan, A. G., Marshall, I. M., Cooper, J. M., & Huang, E. S. (2016). Use of decision aids with minority patients: A systematic review. *Journal of General Internal Medicine*, *31*(6), 663–676. https://doi.org/10.1007/s11606-016-3609-2.

Schulz, A. J., Omari, A., Ward, M., et al. (2020). Independent and joint contributions of economic, social and physical environmental characteristics to mortality in the Detroit metropolitan area: A study of cumulative effects and pathways. *Health & Place*, *65*, 102391. https://doi.org/10.1016/j.healthplace.2020.102391.

Singh, J. K., Acharya, D., Paudel, R., et al. (2020). Effects of female community health volunteer capacity building and text messaging intervention on gestational weight gain and hemoglobin change among pregnant women in southern Nepal: A cluster randomized controlled trial. *Frontiers in Public Health*, *8*, 312. https://doi.org/10.3389/fpubh.2020.00312.

H

Risk-Prone Health Behavior

Domain 1 Health promotion Class 2 Health management

Marina Martinez-Kratz, MS, RN, CNE

NANDA-I

Definition

Impaired ability to modify lifestyle and/or actions in a manner that improves the level of wellness.

Defining Characteristics

Failure to achieve optimal sense of control; failure to take action that prevents health problem; minimizes health status change; nonacceptance of health status change; smoking; substance misuse

Related Factors

Inadequate social support; inadequate understanding of health information; low self efficacy; negative perception of health care provider; negative perception of recommended health care strategy; social anxiety; stressors

At-Risk Population

Economically disadvantaged individuals; individuals with family history of alcoholism

NOC (Nursing Outcomes Classification)

Suggested NOC Outcomes

Participation in Health Care Decisions; Psychosocial Adjustment: Life Change; Risk Detection

Example NOC Outcome with Indicators

Risk Detection as evidenced by the following indicators: Recognizes signs and symptoms that indicate risks/Identifies potential health risks/Participates in screening at recommended intervals/Obtains information about changes in health recommendations. (Rate the outcome and indicators of **Risk Detection:** 1 = never demonstrated, 2 = rarely demonstrated, 3 = sometimes demonstrated, 4 = often demonstrated, 5 = consistently demonstrated [see Section I].)

Client Outcomes

Client Will (Specify Time Frame)

- State acceptance of change in health status
- Request assistance in altering behaviors to adapt to change
- State personal goals for dealing with change in health status and means to prevent further health problems
- State experience of a period of grief that is proportional to the actual or perceived effect of the loss
- Report and/or demonstrate behavior changes mutually agreed upon with nurse as evidence of positive adaptation

NIC (Nursing Interventions Classification)

Suggested NIC Intervention

Self-Efficacy Enhancement

Example NIC Activities—Self-Efficacy Enhancement

Explore individual's perception of his or her capability to perform the desired behavior; Reinforce confidence in making behavior changes and taking action

Nursing Interventions and *Rationales*

- Assess the client's perceptions of health, wellness, disability, and major barriers to health and wellness. EB: *Understanding the differences in perceptions can direct how a provider talks to clients about their health, but it could also provide insight into how clients value and perceive their own disability and wellness (Morris et al, 2018).*
- Assess the client for adverse childhood experiences (ACEs) and refer for counseling and follow-up as appropriate. EB: *A study reported that an ACE score ≥4 was associated with increased odds for binge drinking, heavy drinking, smoking, behavior that increases the risk of HIV transmission, diabetes, myocardial infarction, coronary heart disease, stroke, and depression (Campbell, Walker, & Egede, 2016).*
- Assess the client for depression and refer for counseling and follow-up as appropriate. EB: *A study reported data indicating that depression may be a barrier to health-promoting behavior in middle-aged and older women with hypertension or heart disease (Cramer et al, 2020).*
- Use motivational interviewing to help the client identify and change unhealthy behaviors. EB: *Motivational interviewing predicted decreases in emerging adults' health-risk behaviors (DeVargas & Stormshak, 2020).*

- Encourage mindfulness and meditation to help the client cope with changes in health status. EB: *A study found mindfulness training improved levels of mindfulness, acceptance, and emotion regulation, and these increases were correlated with reductions in stress, depression, and overeating (Vieten et al, 2018).*
- Allow the client adequate time to express feelings about the change in health status. EB: *A longitudinal study of clients with newly diagnosed diabetes found that there was a perception of time pressure, and considerable time was spent with clients by health professionals repeating information that may not be relevant to client need (Dowell et al, 2018).*
- Encourage participation in work-based wellness programs. EB: *A 5-year retrospective study to measure health outcomes changes of wellness program participants found statistically significant improvement for cardiovascular disease risk (Pesis-Katz et al, 2020).*
- Provide the client with positive feedback for accomplishments. EB: *A study reported that providing feedback was one strategy that improved hand hygiene compliance in the emergency department (Seo et al, 2019).*
- Promote use of positive spiritual and religious experiences as appropriate. EB: *A study reported different dimensions of religiousness and spirituality are associated with positive health behaviors in breast cancer survivors (Park, Waddington, & Abraham, 2018).*
- Discuss the client's current goals and assist in modification as needed. Use a goal attainment scaling (GAS) approach, which is a therapeutic method that refers to the development of a written follow-up guide between the client and the nurse and is used for monitoring client progress. EB: *A study of clients enrolled in a geriatric day hospital (GDH) demonstrated short- and long-term effectiveness of GDHs in helping clients achieve individualized outcome measures using GAS (Moorhous et al, 2017).*

▲ Refer to community resources. Provide general and contact information for ease of use. EBN: *A study of oncology navigators identified that common barriers for clients obtaining assistance included lack of resources (50%), lack of knowledge about resources (46%), and complex/duplicative paperwork (20%) (Spencer et al, 2018).*

H

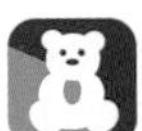

Pediatric

- Include social history in client assessment to help identify past abuse and traumatic experiences. EBN: *A systematic review found that only 28% of abuse or neglect cases identified by researchers are found in clients' files. This information is considered essential for developing comprehensive formulations and effective treatment plans (Read et al, 2018).*
- Encourage participation in school-based wellness programs. EB: *After a school-based health promotion intervention, participants demonstrated significant improvements in physiological measures and health behaviors (Jamerson et al, 2017).*
- Promote use of positive spiritual experiences and religious attendance, as appropriate. EB: *A study reported that high spirituality protects adolescents from health risk behaviors such as smoking and drinking alcohol when combined with religious attendance (Malinakova et al, 2019).*
- Encourage parents to process and express grief, uncertainty, and discouragement after learning about their child's diagnosis, prognosis, and treatments. Provide parents with resources and tools to help further their understanding of the illness. EB: *A study assessed the effectiveness of an intervention called the Nurturing Program for Parents and Their Children With Special Needs and Health Challenges (SNHC) and found that after the intervention families showed an increase in empathy toward their children's needs and an increase in empowerment as measured by the family empowerment scale (Burton et al, 2018).*
- Provide parents of critically ill children with individualized coping resources. EBN: *Research findings indicated that a range of diverse coping strategies are used by neonatal intensive care unit parents. The most common are acceptance, emotional support, active coping, positive reframing, religion, planning, and instrumental support. Despite this, 91% of participants indicated they would likely attend at least one type of parent support program, if offered according to their preferences (Huenink & Porterfield, 2017).*
- Use distraction with children undergoing procedures or treatment with unpleasant side effects. EB: *This review found that there was strong support for the use of distraction techniques with older children (Ali, McGrath, & Drendel, 2016).*

Geriatric

▲ Assess for signs of depression resulting from illness-associated changes and make appropriate referrals. EB: *A review of evidence related to depression in older individuals found that major depressive disorder (MDD) is less common in late life, but has a more chronic course compared with younger adults with MDD. A significant finding was that older adults with subclinical forms of depression report functional impairment similar to MDD (Haigh et al, 2018).*

- Support activities that promote a sense of purpose for older adults. EB: *Purpose in life (PIL) is strongly associated with improved mental and physical health outcomes among older adults. Thus interventions to improve and/or maintain higher levels of PIL over time may promote successful aging (Musich et al, 2018).*
- Encourage social support. EB: *In this study, social support was a prerequisite for success of the health-promoting intervention and perceived well-being in older adults (von Berens et al, 2018).*

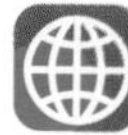

Multicultural

- Assess for the influence of cultural beliefs, norms, and values on the client's ability to modify health behavior. CEB: *What the client considers normal and abnormal health behavior may be based on cultural perceptions (Leininger & McFarland, 2002).*
- Assess the client's readiness for change. EBN: *A study reported readiness for change was highly correlated with health promotion behaviors in African American women (Hepburn, 2018).*
- Assess the role of fatalism on the client's ability to modify health behavior. Fatalistic perspectives, which involve the belief that you cannot control your own fate, may influence health behaviors in some cultures. EB: *A study found that clients with type 2 diabetes who exhibited more fatalistic attitudes were younger, were of lower education levels, had higher body mass index (BMI), and had fewer diabetes comorbidities. It is crucial for health care practitioners to identify fatalistic clients and to tailor culturally appropriate strategies in diabetes management (Sukkarieh-Haraty et al, 2018).*
- Encourage spirituality as a source of support for coping. EBN: *Findings from a study provided data to support an understanding of how African American women define spirituality, the role it plays, the purpose it serves, the function of spirituality in their lives, and the implications for breast health behaviors (Conway-Phillips & Janusek, 2016).*
- Acknowledge client's identified gender and sexual orientation and refer client and family members to support networks that have experience with lesbian, gay, bisexual, or transgender (LGBT) issues, as appropriate. EBN: *Disclosure and support systems are associated with better self-help perception; creating safe and accepting environments for LGBT clients has been shown to improve overall care in this underserved population (Kamen et al, 2015).*

Home Care

- The previously mentioned interventions may be adapted for home care use.
- Take the client's perspective into consideration and use a holistic approach in assessing and responding to client planning for the future. EB: *A recent qualitative study described the experience of the client with both type 1 diabetes and an eating disorder and that of their health care providers. Results demonstrated the need for multiprofessional, collaborative approaches to treatment (Macdonald et al, 2018).*
- Assist the client/family to adapt to his or her diagnosis and to live with their disease. EBN: *Research suggested that time-sensitive interventions directed toward education and psychosocial support for all clients and families dealing with a new diagnosis of chronic illnesses are needed (Gunter & Duke, 2018).*
- Ensure that evaluations of the client's ability to perform activities of daily living are age appropriate and consider existing, as well as new, diagnoses. EB: *This study used a geriatric-designed functional evaluation that took into account the age-related decrease in flexibility and strength by identifying additional areas for potential loss of function (Adamo, Talley, & Goldberg, 2015).*
- Refer to care plan for **Powerlessness.**

Client/Family Teaching and Discharge Planning

- Assess family/caregivers for coping and teaching/learning styles. EBN: *Recommendations for teaching family or caregivers include providing realistic expectations and nurturing psychological safety so caregivers feel comfortable asking questions, expressing their thoughts, and discussing mistakes (Lindauer, Sexson, & Harvath, 2017).*
- Foster communication between the client/family and medical staff. EBN: *A study of caregiver communication indicated that oncology nurses must be able to address questions posed by family caregivers and support family communication challenges (Wittenberg et al, 2017).*
- Educate and prepare families regarding the appearance and function of the client and the environment before initial exposure. EBN: *A study of mother-caregivers found that health care providers can help anchor family management by recognizing caregiver expectations and facilitating communication about realistic expectations (Lucas et al, 2016).*

- Teach clients and their family relaxation techniques (controlled breathing, guided imagery) and help them practice. EB: *A randomized controlled study reported a significant reduction in signs and symptoms of compulsive Internet use, anxiety, and depression (Quinones & Griffiths, 2019).*

REFERENCES

Adamo, D. E., Talley, S. A., & Goldberg, A. (2015). Age and task differences in functional fitness in older women: Comparisons with senior fitness test normative and criterion-referenced data. *Journal of Aging and Physical Activity*, *23*(1), 47–54.

Ali, S., McGrath, T., & Drendel, A. L. (2016). An evidence-based approach to minimizing acute procedural pain in the emergency department and beyond. *Pediatric Emergency Care*, *32*(1), 36–42. https://doi.org/10.1097/PEC.0000000000000669.

Burton, R. S., Zwahr-Castro, J., Magrane, C. L., Hernandez, H., Farley, L. G., & Amodei, N. (2018). The nurturing program: An intervention for parents of children with special needs. *Journal of Child and Family Studies*, *27*(4), 1137–1149. https://doi.org/10.1007/s10826-017-0966-3.

Campbell, J. A., Walker, R. J., & Egede, L. E. (2016). Associations between adverse childhood experiences, high-risk behaviors, and morbidity in adulthood. *American Journal of Preventive Medicine*, *50*(3), 344–352. https://doi.org/10.1016/j.amepre.2015.07.022.

Conway-Phillips, R., & Janusek, L. W. (2016). Exploring spirituality among African American women: Implications for promoting breast health behaviors. *Holistic Nursing Practice*, *30*(6), 322–329. https://doi.org/10.1097/HNP.0000000000000173.

Cramer, H., Lauche, R., Adams, J., Frawley, J., Broom, A., & Sibbritt, D. (2020). Is depression associated with unhealthy behaviors among middle-aged and older women with hypertension or heart disease? *Women's Health Issues*, *30*(1), 35–40. https://doi.org/10.1016/j.whi.2019.09.003.

DeVargas, E. C., & Stormshak, E. A. (2020). Motivational interviewing skills as predictors of change in emerging adult risk behavior. *Professional Psychology: Research and Practice*, *51*(1), 16–24. https://doi.org/10.1037/pro0000270.

Dowell, A., Stubbe, M., Macdonald, L., et al. (2018). A longitudinal study of interactions between health professionals and people with newly diagnosed diabetes. *Annals of Family Medicine*, *16*(1), 37–44. https://doi.org/10.1370/afm.2144.

Gunter, D. M., & Duke, G. (2018). Reducing uncertainty in families dealing with childhood cancers: An integrative literature review. *Pediatric Nursing*, *44*(1), 21–37.

Haigh, E. A. P., Bogucki, O. E., Sigmon, S. T., & Blazer, D. G. (2018). Depression among older adults: A 20-year update on five common myths and misconceptions. *American Journal of Geriatric Psychiatry*, *26*(1), 107–122.

Hepburn, M. (2018). The variables associated with health promotion behaviors among urban Black women. *Journal of Nursing Scholarship*, *50*(4), 353–366. https://doi.org/10.1111/jnu.12387.

Huenink, E., & Porterfield, S. (2017). Parent support programs and coping mechanisms in NICU parents. *Advances in Neonatal Care*, *17*(2), E10–E18. https://doi.org/10.1097/ANC.0000000000000359.

Jamerson, T., Sylvester, R., Jiang, Q., et al. (2017). Differences in cardiovascular disease risk factors and health behaviors between Black and non-Black students participating in a school-based health promotion program. *American Journal of Health Promotion*, *31*(4), 318–324. https://doi.org/10.1177/0890117116674666.

Kamen, C., Smith-Stoner, M., Heckler, C. E., Flannery, M., & Margolies, L. (2015). Social support, self-rated health, and lesbian, gay, bisexual, and transgender identity disclosure to cancer care providers. *Oncology Nursing Forum*, *42*(1), 44–51.

Leininger, M., & McFarland, M. (2002). *Transcultural nursing: Concepts, theories, research and practices* (3rd ed.). New York: McGraw-Hill.

Lindauer, A., Sexson, K., & Harvath, T. A. (2017). Teaching caregivers to administer eye drops, transdermal patches, and suppositories. *American Journal of Nursing*, *117*(5 Suppl. 1), S11–S16. https://doi.org/10.1097/01.NAJ.0000516388.97515.ca.

Lucas, M. S., Barakat, L. P., Ulrich, C. M., Jones, N. L., & Deatrick, J. A. (2016). Mother-caregiver expectations for function among survivors of childhood brain tumors. *Supportive Care in Cancer*, *24*(5), 2147–2154.

Macdonald, P., Kan, C., Stadler, M., et al. (2018). Eating disorders in people with type 1 diabetes: Experiential perspectives of both clients and healthcare professionals. *Diabetic Medicine*, *35*(2), 223–231. https://doi.org/10.1111/dme.13555.

Malinakova, K., Kopcakova, J., Madarasova Geckova, A., et al. (2019). "I am spiritual, but not religious": Does one without the other protect against adolescent health-risk behaviour? *International Journal of Public Health*, *64*(1), 115–124 https://doi.org/10.1007/s00038-018-1116-4.

Moorhous, P., Theou, O., Fay, S., McMillan, M., Moffatt, H., & Rockwoof, K. (2017). Treatment in a geriatric day hospital improve individualized outcome measures using goal attainment scaling. *BMC Geriatrics*, *17*(1), 9. https://doi.org/10.1186/s12877-016-0397-9.

Morris, M. A., Inselman, J., Rogers, J. M. G., Halverson, C., Branda, M., & Griffin, J. M. (2018). How do patients describe their disabilities? A coding system for categorizing patients' descriptions. *Disability and Health Journal*, *11*(2), 310–314. https://doi.org/10.1016/j.dhjo.2017.10.006.

Musich, S., Wang, S. S., Kraemer, S., Hawkins, K., & Wicker, E. (2018). Purpose in life and positive health outcomes among older adults. *Population Health Management*, *21*(2), 139–147. https://doi.org/10.1089/pop.2017.0063.

Park, C. L., Waddington, E., & Abraham, R. (2018). Different dimensions of religiousness/spirituality are associated with health behaviors in breast cancer survivors. *Psycho-Oncology*, *27*(10), 2466–2472. https://doi.org/10.1002/pon.4852.

Pesis-Katz, I., Smith, J. A., Norsen, L., DeVoe, J., & Singh, R. (2020). Reducing cardiovascular disease risk for employees through participation in a wellness program. *Population Health Management*, *23*(3), 212–219. https://doi.org/10.1089/pop.2019.0106.

Quinones, C., & Griffiths, M. D. (2019). Reducing compulsive Internet use and anxiety symptoms via two brief interventions: A comparison between mindfulness and gradual muscle relaxation. *Journal of Behavioral Addictions*, *8*(3), 530–536.

Read, J., Harper, D., Tucker, I., & Kennedy, A. (2018). Do adult mental health services identify child abuse and neglect? A systematic review. *International Journal of Mental Health Nursing*, *27*(1), 7–19. https://doi.org/:10.1111/inm.12369.

Seo, H.-J., Sohng, K.-Y., Chang, S. O., Chaung, S. K., Won, J. S., & Choi, M.-J. (2019). Interventions to improve hand hygiene compliance in emergency departments: A systematic review. *Journal of Hospital Infection*, *102*(4), 394–406 https://doi.org/10.1016/j.jhin.2019.03.013.

Spencer, J. C., Samuel, C. A., Rosenstein, D. L., et al. (2018). Oncology navigators' perceptions of cancer-related financial burden and financial assistance resources. *Supportive Care in Cancer*, *26*(4), 1315–1321. https://doi.org/10.1007/s00520-017-3958-3.

Sukkarieh-Haraty, O., Egede, L. E., Abi Kharma, J., & Bassil, M. (2018). Predictors of diabetes fatalism among Arabs: A cross-sectional study of Lebanese adults with type 2 diabetes. *Journal of Religion and Health, 57*(3), 858–868. https://doi.org/10.1007/s10943-017-0430-0.

Vieten, C., Laraia, B. A., Kristeller, J., et al. (2018). The mindful moms training: Development of a mindfulness-based intervention to reduce stress and overeating during pregnancy. *BMC Pregnancy and Childbirth, 18*(1). https://doi.org/10.1186/s12884-018-1757-6.

von Berens, Å., Koochek, A., Nydahl, M., et al. (2018). "Feeling more self-confident, cheerful and safe." Experiences from a health-promoting intervention in community dwelling older adults—A qualitative study. *Journal of Nutrition, Health & Aging, 22*(4), 541–548.

Wittenberg, E., Buller, H., Ferrell, B., Koczywas, M., & Borneman, T. (2017). Understanding family caregiver communication to provide family-centered cancer care. *Seminars in Oncology Nursing, 33*(5), 507–516. https://doi.org/10.1016/j.soncn.2017.09.001.

Ineffective Health Self-Management

Domain 1 Health promotion Class 2 Health management

Ruth A. Wittmann-Price, PhD, RN, CNS, CNE, CNEcl, CHSE, ANEF, FAAN

H

NANDA-I

Definition

Unsatisfactory management of symptoms, treatment regimen, physical, psychosocial, and spiritual consequences and lifestyle changes inherent in living with a chronic condition.

Defining Characteristics

Difficulty with prescribed regimen; failure to include treatment regimen in daily living; failure to take action to reduce risk factor; ineffective choices in daily living for meeting health goal

Related Factors

Competing demands; competing lifestyle preferences; conflict between cultural beliefs and health practices; conflict between health behaviors and social norms; conflict between spiritual beliefs and treatment regimen; decreased perceived quality of life; depressive symptoms; difficulty accessing community resources; difficulty managing complex treatment regimen; difficulty navigating complex health care systems; difficulty with decision-making; inadequate commitment to a plan of action; inadequate health literacy; inadequate knowledge of treatment regimen; inadequate number of cues to action; inadequate role models; inadequate social support; individuals with limited decision making experience; limited ability to perform aspects of treatment regimen; low self efficacy; negative feelings toward treatment regimen; neurobehavioral manifestations; nonacceptance of condition; perceived barrier to treatment regimen; perceived social stigma associated with condition; substance misuse; unrealistic perception of seriousness of condition; unrealistic perception of susceptibility to sequelae; unrealistic perception of treatment benefit

At-Risk Population

Children; economically disadvantaged individuals; individuals experiencing adverse reactions to medications; individuals with caregiving responsibilities; individuals with history of ineffective health self-management; individuals with low educational level; older adults

Associated Conditions

Asymptomatic disease; developmental disabilities; high acuity illness; neurocognitive disorders; polypharmacy; significant comorbidity

NOC (Nursing Outcomes Classification)

Suggested NOC Outcomes

Health Beliefs: Perceived Control, Perceived Threat; Knowledge: Disease Process; Knowledge: Treatment Regimen; Participation in Health Care Decisions

Example NOC Outcome with Indicators

Knowledge: Treatment Regimen as evidenced by the following indicators: Extent of understanding of prescribed medication, activity, exercise, and specific disease process. (Rate the outcome and indicators of **Knowledge: Treatment Regimen:** 1 = no knowledge, 2 = limited knowledge, 3 = moderate knowledge, 4 = substantial knowledge, 5 = extensive knowledge [see Section I].)

Client Outcomes

Client Will (Specify Time Frame)

- Describe daily food and fluid intake that meets therapeutic goals
- Describe activity/exercise patterns that meet therapeutic goals
- Describe scheduling of medications that meets therapeutic goals
- Verbalize ability to manage therapeutic regimens
- Collaborate with health professionals to decide on a therapeutic regimen that is congruent with health goals and lifestyle

NIC (Nursing Interventions Classification)

Suggested NIC Interventions

Adherence Behavior; Health Education; Health System Guidance; Learning Facilitation; Learning Readiness Enhancement; Teaching: Prescribed Diet, Prescribed Exercise, Prescribed Medication

Example NIC Activities—Learning Facilitation

Present the information in a stimulating manner; Encourage the client's active participation

H

Nursing Interventions and *Rationales*

- Establish a collaborative partnership with the client for purposes of meeting health-related goals. EBN: *Nurse researchers explored ways that nurses and clients can better understand postoperative pain management needs, and the results of a qualitative study revealed the following helpful interventions: (1) communication and knowledge and the clients' ability to communicate, (2) pain assessment using a numerical rating scale, and (3) client–nurse relationship consisting of frequent and direct contact (Kaptain, Bregnballe, & Dreyer, 2017).*
- Explore the client's perception of their illness experience and identify uncertainties and needs through open-ended questions. EBN: *A research team qualitatively explored perceptions and preferences of older adults (n = 13) and their family members about a fall risk assessment system when aging in place and to develop better technology to promote safety. Results demonstrated an acceptance of the technology after participants adapted, and acceptance was a process that grew in stages as the client became used to technology (Galambos et al, 2017).* EB: *Hertroijs et al (2020) investigated care preferences and their determinants in clients (n = 288) with type 2 diabetes. Participants were provided a choice of six diabetic care packages and the favorable choice was for the traditional care model because it included the most important issue for them, which was emotional support.*
- Assist the client to enhance self-efficacy or confidence in his or her own ability to manage the illness. EBN: *Banman and Sawatzky (2017) completed a literature review on cardiovascular disease prevention and uncovered several reasons women are not as active as men in preventive health management: (1) lower self-efficacy beliefs, (2) lack of social support and confidence in their ability to care for themselves, and (3) any findings of depression negatively correlated with women's self-efficacy beliefs related to health behavior.* EB: *Harel-Katz et al (2020) studied the Improving Participation After Stroke Self-Management (IPASS) program's effectiveness for stroke clients (n = 60). The results of the randomized intervention demonstrated that the IPASS was feasible for Israeli clients and had a positive effect on improving quality of life.*
- Review factors of the health belief model (HBM) (individual perceptions of seriousness and susceptibility, demographic and other modifying factors, and perceived benefits and barriers) with the client. EB: *Ahlers-Schmidt et al (2020) used the HBM to redesign community baby showers in order to promote infant safe sleep using the American Academy of Pediatrics Safe Sleep Guidelines. The study participants (n = 812) demonstrated positive changes about safe sleep after the community baby shower and better understood many of the safe sleep concepts such as sleeping with infant can cause death, loose blankets can cause death, infants should sleep alone, and infants should be placed on their back to sleep.*
- Help the client identify and modify barriers to effective self management. EB: *Researchers examined clients (n = 14) with type 2 diabetes and severe mental illness because this group of clients experiences significantly poorer health outcomes than type 2 diabetic clients without severe mental illness. Participants were aware of the risks and stated that family and health care provider support was important in their self-maintenance (Mulligan et al, 2017).*
- Help the client self-manage his or her own health through education about strategies for changing habits such as overeating, sedentary lifestyle, and smoking. EB: *Pappa et al (2017) investigated activity behavior*

and analyzed the message content participants (n = *107,886) in r/loseit, an online weight management community on the online social network Reddit, over 30 days and found that the most discussed topics were healthy food, clothing, calorie counting, workouts, looks, habits, support, and unhealthy food.* **EBN:** *Powell and Deroche (2020) studied variables that predicted clients'* (n = *500) use of an electronic portal to assist them in self-managing their health. The nurse researchers found that age, gender, or distance from provider did not make a difference in portal use.*

- Develop a contract with the client to maintain motivation for changes in behavior. **EBN:** *Leine et al (2017) studied clients* (n = *6) with chronic obstructive pulmonary disease (COPD) and their understanding and treatment adherence using a partnership-based nursing practice program. Interviews revealed two themes: feeling safe and comforted, and motivation to take better care of themselves.*
- Use focus groups to evaluate the implementation of self-management programs. **EB:** *Serwe et al (2017) used focus groups* (n = *4) to study caregivers' implementation of a telehealth self-maintenance program; the themes suggested that it promoted relationships, promoted positive interactions, and better explained the role.*
- Refer to the care plan Ineffective Family **Health** Self-Management.

Geriatric

H

- Identify the reasons for behaviors that are not therapeutic and discuss alternatives. **EBN:** *Lee et al (2017a) used the Theory of Planned Behavior with older adults to affect diabetes maintenance and found that older adults need adequate social support to sustain diabetes self-management practices.*

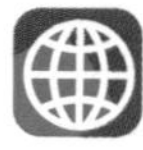

Multicultural

- Assess the influence of cultural beliefs, norms, and values on the individual's perceptions of the therapeutic regimen. **EBN:** *Mou (2017) explored traditional Chinese medicine (TCM) as a method for promoting health and found through an online survey in China with 800 responses that cultural orientation and spirituality predicted use of TCM to promote health.* **EB:** *Zuccarino et al (2020) studied older Italian clients'* (n = *2486) educational level and how it affected their rehabilitation outcome. The results demonstrated that older adults with less education had poorer rehabilitation and health management outcomes.*
- Provide health information that is consistent with the health literacy of clients. **EB:** *Sainato et al (2017) studied US adolescents with chronic conditions and found that this high-risk group was twice as likely not to receive routine vaccinations, indicating that additional education is needed in families with adolescents 16 to 18 years old with chronic illnesses.*
- Assess for barriers that may interfere with client follow-up of treatment recommendations. **EBN:** *Riley and Krüger (2017) examined the use of inhalers in clients with COPD and found that it is imperative to assess and teach clients about using a correct inhalation technique, assessing adequate dexterity to use the prescribed inhaler, if there is sufficient inspiratory flow rate to achieve adequate lung deposition, and if the inhaler is used by the client at all.*
- Validate the client's feelings regarding the ability to manage his or her own care and the impact on lifestyle. **EBN:** *Lee et al (2017b) qualitatively studied clients' perceptions of brisk walking as a method to reduce chronic disease symptomology in the community. Six focus groups were conducted* (n = *48), ages 48 to 81, and five themes were identified: (1) health promotion and maintenance, (2) relationship building and social interactions, (3) leaders' enthusiasm and peer pressure, (4) the nature of brisk walking, and (5) becoming part of one's daily life.*

Home Care

- Prepare and instruct clients and family members in the use of a medication box. Set up an appropriate schedule for filling the medication box, and post medication times and doses in an accessible area (e.g., attached by a magnet to the refrigerator). **EBN:** *Milner and Bonaventura (2017) used self-management for clients on anticoagulants at home and it increased client engagement in anticoagulant management, which resulted in better clinical outcomes.* **EB:** *Safren et al (2020) studied medication adherence in clients* (n = *27) with uncontrolled HIV and psychosocial problem using transdiagnostic adherence counseling and cognitive behavioral therapy. The interventions improved self-reported medication adherence and therefore health management.*
- Refer to health care professionals for questions and self-care management. **EB:** *Homsted, Magee, and Nesin (2017) studied the use of a comprehensive, medical-home approach to controlling clients'* (n = *1300) use of controlled substances. By using a program researchers decreased the use of controlled substances by 67.2% and 65.6%, with fewer clients receiving benzodiazepines.* **EB:** *Researchers studied the effects of a chronic disease self-management program on empowering hemodialysis clients* (n = *53) and their quality of life. Self-management increased the clients' quality of life in 3 months (Ahmadzadeh et al, 2017).*

Client/Family Teaching and Discharge Planning

- Identify the client's and/or family's current knowledge and adjust teaching accordingly. Teach the client and family about all aspects of the therapeutic regimen, providing as much knowledge as the client and family will accept, in a culturally congruent manner. EBN: *Sugiharto et al (2017) studied the client outcome of improving nurses' skills and confidence in delivering diabetes self-management education (DSME) among clients with type 2 diabetes and found that the diabetes training program for community health center nurses increased their skills and confidence in delivering DSME.* EB: *Chen, Flaherty, and Threats (2020) qualitatively studied complementary and integrative health (CIH) beliefs in 14 participants. The participants had chronic pain conditions and verbalized three thematic beliefs about CIH: (1) individual's beliefs; (2) approach to CIH, including how people view provider information and personalize their CIH use; and (3) factors that affect trust in the information encountered. The identified factors can be taken into account to improve health management.*
- Teach ways to adjust activities of daily living (ADLs) for inclusion in therapeutic regimens. EBN: *Jansons et al (2017) completed a randomized, controlled trial of clients with chronic conditions using a gym-based exercise program for health management and found improved health outcomes in the group that exercised when compared with the control group.* EBN: *Nestler et al (2017) performed a literature review* (n = *12) related to women's muscle strength and work health issues and found that weight training reduced pain and improved outcomes for women working in strenuous and nonstrenuous environments.*
- Teach safety in taking medications. EB: *Kim and Hubert (2017)* studied three groups with different levels of technology knowledge about accessing personal health information management (PHIM) by online survey and found that advanced PHIM users were significantly more likely to engage in emailing with providers, viewing test results online, and receiving summaries of hospital visits, indicating that technology knowledge is important for self-advocating.

H

REFERENCES

Ahlers-Schmidt, C. R., Schunn, C., Hervey, A. M., et al. (2020). Redesigned community baby showers to promote infant safe sleep. *Health Education Journal, 79*(8), 888–900. https://doi.org/10.1177/0017896920935918.

Ahmadzadeh, S., Matlabi, H., Allahverdipor, H., & Ashan, S. K. (2017). The effectiveness of self-management program on quality of life among haemodialysis patients. *Progress in Palliative Care, 25*(4), 177–184. https://doi.org/10.1080/09699260.2017.1345407.

Banman, L., & Sawatzky, J. V. (2017). The role of self-efficacy in cardiovascular disease prevention in women. *Canadian Journal of Cardiovascular Nursing, 27*(3), 11–19. https://doi.org/10.2147/PI.S12624.

Chen, A. T., Flaherty, M. G., & Threats, M. (2020). Attitudes, provider and treatment selection of complementary and integrative health among individuals with pain-related conditions. *Complementary Therapies in Medicine, 51*, 102410. https://doi.org/10.1016/j.ctim.2020.102410.

Galambos, C., Rantz, M., Back, J., Jun, J. S., Skubic, M., & Miller, S. J. (2017). Older adults' perceptions of and preferences for a fall risk assessment system: Exploring stages of acceptance model. *Computers, Informatics, Nursing, 35*(7), 331–337. https://doi.org/10.1097/CIN.0000000000000330.

Harel-Katz, H., Adar, T., Milman, U., & Carmeli, E. (2020). Examining the feasibility and effectiveness of a culturally adapted participation-focused stroke self-management program in a day-rehabilitation setting: A randomized pilot study. *Topics in Stroke Rehabilitation, 27*(8), 577–589. https://doi.org/10.1080/10749357.2020.1738676.

Hertroijs, D. F. L., Elissen, A. M. J., Brouwers, M. C. G. J., Hiligsmann, M., Schaper, N. C., & Ruwaard, D. (2020). Preferences of people with type 2 diabetes for diabetes care: A discrete choice experiment. *Diabetic Medicine, 37*(11), 1807–1815. https://doi.org/10.1111/dme.13969.

Homsted, F. A. E., Magee, C. E., & Nesin, N. (2017). Population health management in a small health system: Impact of controlled substance stewardship in a patient-centered medical home. *American Journal of Health-System Pharmacy, 74*(18), 1468–1475. https://doi.org/10.2146/ajhp161032.

Jansons, P., Robins, L., O'Brien, L., & Haines, T. (2017). Gym-based exercise and home-based exercise with telephone support have similar outcomes when used as maintenance programs in adults with chronic health conditions: A randomised trial. *Journal of Physiotherapy, 63*(3), 154–160. https://doi.org/10.1016/j.jphys.2017.05.018.

Kaptain, K., Bregnballe, V., & Dreyer, P. (2017). Patient participation in postoperative pain assessment after spine surgery in a recovery unit. *Journal of Clinical Nursing, 26*(19/20), 2986–2994. https://doi.org/10.1111/jocn.13640.

Kim, S., & Huber, J. T. (2017). Characteristics of personal health information management groups: Findings from an online survey using Amazon's mTurk. *Journal of the Medical Library Association, 105*(4), 361–375. https://doi.org/10.5195/jmla.2017.312.

Lee, L. T., Bowen, P. G., Mosley, M. K., & Turner, C. C. (2017a). Theory of Planned behavior: Social support and diabetes self-management. *The Journal for Nurse Practitioners, 13*(4), 265–270. https://doi.org/10.1016/j.nurpra.2016.07.013.

Lee, P. H., Chuang, Y. H., Chen, S. R., Fang, C. L., Lai, H. R., & Lee, P. I. (2017b). Perspectives of brisk walking among middle-aged and older persons in community: A qualitative study. *Collegian, 24*(2), 147–153. https://doi.org/10.1016/j.colegn.2015.11.001.

Leine, M., Wahl, A. K., Borge, C. R., Hustavenes, M., & Bondevik, H. (2017). Feeling safe and motivated to achieve better health: Experiences with a partnership-based nursing practice programme for in-home patients with chronic obstructive pulmonary disease. *Journal of Clinical Nursing, 26*(17/18), 2755–2764. https://doi.org/10.1111/jocn.13794.

Milner, K. A., & Bonaventura, K. R. (2017). Self-management of warfarin: An approach to increase patient engagement in care. *The Journal for Nurse Practitioners, 13*(8), e389–e393. https://doi.org/10.1016/j.nurpra.2017.06.016.

Mou, Y. (2017). Predicting the use of traditional Chinese medicine health maintenance approach from cultural and spiritual perspectives. *Journal of Religion and Health*, *56*(3), 971–985. https://doi.org/10.1007/s10943-016-0299-3.

Mulligan, K., McBain, H., Lamontagne-Godwin, F., et al. (2017). Barriers and enablers of type 2 diabetes self-management in people with severe mental illness. *Health Expectations*, *20*(5), 1020–1030. https://doi.org/10.1111/hex.12543.

Nestler, K., Witzki, A., Rohde, U., Rüther, T., Tofaute, K. A., & Leyk, D. (2017). Strength training for women as a vehicle for health promotion at work. *Deutsches Aerzteblatt International*, *114*(26), 439–446. https://doi.org/10.3238/arztebl.2017.0439.

Pappa, G. L., Cunha, T. O., Bicalho, P. V., et al. (2017). Factors associated with weight change in online weight management communities: A case study in the LoseIt Reddit community. *Journal of Medical Internet Research*, *19*(1), e17. https://doi.org/10.2196/jmir.5816.

Powell, K. R., & Deroche, C. (2020). Predictors and patterns of portal use in patients with multiple chronic conditions. *Chronic Illness*, *16*(4), 275–283. doi:10.1177/1742395318803663.

Riley, J., & Krüger, P. (2017). Optimising inhaler technique in chronic obstructive pulmonary disease: A complex issue. *British Journal of Nursing*, *26*(7), 391–397. https://doi.org/10.12968/bjon.2017.26.7.391.

Safren, S. A., Harkness, A., & Lee, J. S. (2020). Addressing syndemics and self-care in individuals with uncontrolled HIV: An open trial of a transdiagnostic treatment. *AIDS and Behavior*, *24*(11), 3264–3278. https://doi.org/10.1007/s10461-020-02900-7.

Sainato, R., Flores, M., Malloy, A., et al. (2017). Health maintenance deficits in a fully insured population of adolescents with chronic medical conditions. *Clinical Pediatrics*, *56*(6), 512–518. https://doi.org/10.1177/0009922816678183.

Serwe, K. M., Hersh, G. I., Pickens, N. D., & Pancheri, K. (2017). Caregiver perceptions of a telehealth wellness program. *American Journal of Occupational Therapy*, *71*(4), 1–5. https://doi.org/10.5014/ajot.2017.025619.

Sugiharto, S., Stephenson, M., Hsu, Y. Y., & Fajriyah, N. N. (2017). Diabetes self-management education training for community health center nurses in Indonesia: A best practice implementation project. *JBI Database of Systematic Reviews & Implementation Reports*, *15*(9), 2390–2397. https://doi.org/10.11124/JBISRIR-2016-003329.

Zuccarino, S., Fattore, G., Vitali, S., Antronaco, G., Frigerio, S., & Colombo, M. (2020). The association between education and rehabilitation outcomes: A population retrospective observational study. *Archives of Gerontology and Geriatrics*, *91*, 104218. https://doi.org/10.1016/j.archger.2020.104218.

Readiness for Enhanced Health Self-Management

Domain 1 Health promotion
Class 2 Health management

Ruth A. Wittmann-Price, PhD, RN, CNS, CNE, CNEcl, CHSE, ANEF, FAAN

NANDA-I

Definition

A pattern of satisfactory management of symptoms, treatment regimen, physical, psychosocial, and spiritual consequences and lifestyle changes inherent in living with a chronic condition, which can be strengthened.

Defining Characteristics

Expresses desire to enhance choices of daily living for meeting goals; expresses desire to enhance immunization/vaccination status; expresses desire to enhance management of illness; expresses desire to enhance management of prescribed regimens; expresses desire to enhance management of risk factors; expresses desire to enhance management of symptoms

NOC (Nursing Outcomes Classification)

Suggested NOC Outcomes

Health-Promoting Behavior; Health-Seeking Behavior; Knowledge: Health Behavior; Health Promotion; Health Resources; Illness Care; Medication; Prescribed Activity; Treatment Regimen

Example NOC Outcome with Indicators

Health-Promoting Behavior as evidenced by the following indicators: Monitors personal behavior for risks/Seeks balance activity and rest/Performs healthy behaviors routinely/Uses financial and social support resources to promote health. (Rate each indicator of **Health-Promoting Behavior:** 1 = never demonstrated, 2 = rarely demonstrated, 3 = sometimes demonstrated, 4 = often demonstrated, 5 = consistently demonstrated [see Section I].)

Client Outcomes

Client Will (Specify Time Frame)

- Describe integration of therapeutic regimen into daily living
- Demonstrate continued commitment to integration of therapeutic regimen into daily living routines

NIC (Nursing Interventions Classification)

Suggested NIC Interventions

Anticipatory Guidance; Mutual Goal Setting; Client Contracting; Self-Modification Assistance; Self-Responsibility Facilitation; Support System Enhancement

Example NIC Activities—Mutual Goal Setting

Assist client and significant others to develop realistic expectations of themselves in performance of their roles; Clarify with the client the roles of the health care provider and the client, respectively

H

Nursing Interventions and *Rationales*

- Acknowledge the expertise that the client and family bring to health management. EBN: *Nurse researchers compared hospitalized care need perceptions of clients (*n = 50*) with nurses (*n = 100*) and found that surveyed clients and nurses agreed on needed areas such as communication and basic care. Slightly lower agreement scores between nurses and clients were identified for care planning and organization (Fernanades Martins & Galan Perroca, 2017).* EB: *Kim et al (2019) studied factors related to health care readiness, including family support and self-management competencies in adults (*n = 87*) with type 1 diabetes mellitus. A cross-sectional survey found that family involvement in diabetes care enhanced self-management competencies.*
- Review factors that contribute to the likelihood of health promotion and health protection. Use Pender's Health Promotion Model and Becker's Health Belief Model to identify contributing factors (Pender et al, 2015). EBN: *Researchers used a quasi-experimental designed study with women (*n =108*) who were placed in two groups to examine nutritional behavior, and the nurse researchers found that Pender's Health Promotion Model–based nutritional training improved behavior better in the experimental group (Khodaveisi et al, 2017).* EBN: *Ali et al (2020) investigated the effect of sexual health education based on Pender and Health Belief on sexual function of females (*n = 80*) with type 2 diabetes. The researchers used a pre- and post-Rosen's sexual function questionnaire and provided an intervention group with 90-minute weekly educational sessions. The Pender group (interventional group) demonstrated an increase in the mean total score of sexual function and subscales.*
- Further develop and reinforce contributing factors that might change with ongoing self-management of the therapeutic regimen (e.g., knowledge, self-efficacy, self-esteem, and perceived benefits). EB: *Jiao et al (2017) studied the relationship between methadone maintenance treatment clients with mental health illnesses and resilience and found resilience to be negatively correlated with depression and anxiety, indicating that resilience in this population is important for mental health.* EB: *Ritzert et al (2020) studied the use of acceptance and commitment therapy (ACT) self-help bibliotherapy for anxiety and related problems. The researchers found that the ACT model for self-help supported positive change factors in the intervention group.*
- Review the client's strengths in the management of the therapeutic regimen. EB: *Liu et al (2020) researched disparities in access to online health-related technology among older adults (*n = 1497*). The research results identified social determinants that placed clients at risk for lower use of online health-management tools. The risk factors are (1) being a racial/ethnic minority, (2) being married, (3) being uninsured, (4) having low educational attainment, (5) having low income, and (6) being in poor health.*
- Collaborate with the client to identify strategies to maintain strengths and develop additional strengths as indicated. EB: *Researchers studied person-centered care by surveying and interviewing older clients (*n = 56*) in relation to being malnourished and found themes that affected dietary intake of older adults (>81 years): (1) dietetic follow-up, (2) interdisciplinary coordination, and (3) high-quality hospital food services. The nutritional recommendations from this study may facilitate evidence-based person-centered care for older malnourished clients (Hazzard et al, 2017).*
- Identify contributing factors that may need to be improved now or in the future. EB: *Kelsey et al (2020) studied clinical decision support systems (CDSSs) in the electronic medical record (EMR) in a primary care practice to identify and remind clients due for cancer screening tests. The CDSSs were*

piloted with clients (n = 37), and there was an increased cancer screening rate for the participants compared with nonparticipants in the CDSS system. EBN: *Schneider and Howard (2017) investigated the differences in discharge readiness and postdischarge coping in stroke clients (n = 128) using education provided via a technology package (including client online portal access, email/secure messaging) compared with current standard discharge teaching methods and found that there was no statistically significant difference between the groups in discharge readiness, but there was a significant increase in coping scores in the technology group.*

- Help the client maintain existing support and seek additional supports as needed. EBN: *Westcott and Welding (2017) documented case studies that support continuously reassessing home-bound clients' support surfaces in the house, educating clients, and providing appropriate resources to decrease pressure ulcers in community long-term care clients.* EB: *David et al (2019) investigated the relationship between family support, diabetes self-care, and health outcomes in older adults (n = 60). The findings indicated that family support or quality of family relations did not contribute significantly to client self-care.*

Geriatric

H

- Facilitate the client and family to obtain health insurance and drug payment plans whenever needed and possible. EBN: *Researchers used an multiprofessional approach to explore the needs of geriatric clients (n = 293) and found through surveys and interviews that the clients' needs included guidance around falls prevention, improved nutrition, medication management, and referrals to available community and social service supports (Hansen et al, 2017).* EB: *Kandagatla et al (2018) studied the effect of a postoperative ileostomy intervention (self-care checklist) on readmission and self-efficacy in older surgical clients (n = 288) compared with younger clients (n = 72). The researchers found that older and younger clients reported similar self-efficacy scores and similar rates of readmission.*

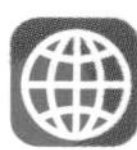

Multicultural

- Assess client's cultural perspectives on health management. EB: *Raffaele et al (2018) studied the Self-care Ability Scale for the Elderly (SASE) to assess the perceived self-care ability in older Italian adults (n = 402). The researchers used SASE to assess self-care ability to achieve well-being and to set personal goals and produced a 13-item version of the SASE with good psychometric properties.*
- Assess health literacy in clients of diverse backgrounds. EBN: *Lee, Lee, and Chung (2017) investigated the level of health literacy in different age groups of South Koreans (n = 1000) and found that for the 45 through 64 and the 65 and over age groups, education was positively associated with health literacy. Additionally, the oldest age group and gender also had a positive association with health literacy. Depression was negatively associated with health literacy.* EB: *Kes and Gökdoğan (2020) developed a Turkish version of the Hypertension Self-care Profile and tested the tool on 200 participants with known hypertension and found that the Turkish version of the Hypertension Self-care Profile had validity and reliability in that population and was successfully translated and cross-culturally adapted.*
- Validate the client's feelings regarding the ability to manage his or her own care and the impact on current lifestyle. EBN: *Araújo do Reis and de Oliva Menezes (2017) qualitatively studied religiosity and spirituality as a resilience strategy for improved lifestyles and health in aging clients (n = 14) and found that clients who revealed they participated in religious or spiritual habits achieved increased well-being and resiliency and were better able to cope with health and social problems.*

Client/Family Teaching and Discharge Planning

- Facilitate the client and family to obtain financial assistance in the form of health insurance and drug payment plans whenever needed and possible. EB: *Tumin et al (2017) studied the change in health insurance after heart transplants in adolescents (n = 366) and found through statistical analysis that changes in health insurance predicted a greater mortality risk compared with clients with continuous private insurance. Therefore assisting with insurance coverage maintenance may provide better health outcomes.*
- Use electronic monitoring to improve medication adherence. EB: *Madrasi et al (2017) studied medication adherence for preexposure prophylaxis for clients (n = 1147) using electronic adherence records recording the date and time of medication bottle cap opening and found that female clients and older clients had better adherence.* EBN: *Low et al (2017) studied medication adherence with post–kidney transplant clients (n = 25) in a descriptive exploratory study, and the themes identified were causes of distress and coping resources. Researchers concluded that regular reminders, such as alarms to take medications, will reduce the stress of managing a kidney transplant.*

- Review therapeutic regimens and their optimal integration with daily living routines. EBN: *Nurse researchers evaluated a family-based heart failure education program and performed a randomized controlled trial with clients (n = 50) and caretakers (n = 50) in a rural community and found that clients and family members who received the education program had higher knowledge scores at 3 and 6 months than those who received traditional outpatient education (Srisuk et al, 2017).*
- Teach disease processes and therapeutic regimens to clients and peer supporters for management of disease processes. EBN: *Kang et al (2018) investigated discharge information provided to surgical clients that addressed their self-management at home using a mixed method literature search (n = 7) design. The literature revealed that discharge education was delivered to clients in the studies at various times and most instructions were standardized. The researchers found that the quality of discharge education had a significant influence in the client's self-care management.*

REFERENCES

Ali, M., Iraj, S., Hajar, S., Naeleh, K., Faezeh, K., & Amin, H. M. (2020). Effect of sexual health education based on health belief and Pender health promotion models on the sexual function of females with type II diabetes. *Journal of Diabetic Nursing*, *8*(1), 992–1001. http://jdn.zbmu.ac.ir/article-1-383-en.html.

Araújo do Reis, L., & de Oliva Menezes, T. M. (2017). Religiosity and spirituality as resilience strategies among long-living older adults in their daily lives. *Revista Brasileira de Enfermagem*, *70*(4), 761–766. https://doi.org/10.1590/0034-7167-2016-0630.

David, D., Dalton, J., Magny-Normilus, C., Brain, M. M., Linster, T., & Lee, S. J. (2019). The quality of family relationships, diabetes self-care, and health outcomes in older adults. *Diabetes Spectrum*, *32*(2), 132–138. https://doi.org/10.2337/ds18-0039.

Fernanades Martins, P., & Galan Perroca, M. (2017). Care necessities: The view of the patient and nursing team. *Revista Brasileira de Enfermagem*, *70*(5), 1026–1032. https://doi.org/10.1590/0034-7167-2016-0197.

Hansen, K. T., McDonald, C., O'Hara, S., Post, L., Silcox, S., & Gutmanis, I. A. (2017). A formative evaluation of a nurse practitioner-led interprofessional geriatric outpatient clinic. *Journal of Interprofessional Care*, *31*(4), 546–549. https://doi.org/10.1080/13561820.2017.1303463.

Hazzard, E., Barone, L., Mason, M., Lambert, K., & McMahon, A. (2017). Patient-centred dietetic care from the perspectives of older malnourished patients. *Journal of Human Nutrition and Dietetics*, *30*(5), 574–587. https://doi.org/10.1111/jhn.12478.

Jiao, M., Gu, J., Xu, H., et al. (2017). Resilience associated with mental health problems among methadone maintenance treatment patients in Guangzhou, China. *AIDS Care*, *29*(5), 660–665. https://doi.org/10.1080/09540121.2016.1255705.

Kandagatla, P., Nikolian, V. C., Matusko, N., Mason, S., Regenbogen, S. E., & Hardiman, K. M. (2018). Patient-reported outcomes and readmission after ileostomy creation in older adults. *The American Surgeon*, *84*(11), 1814–1818. https://doi.org/10.1177/000313481808401141.

Kang, E., Gillespie, B. M., Tobiano, G., & Chaboyer, W. (2018). Discharge education delivered to general surgical patients in their management of recovery post discharge: A systematic mixed studies review. *International Journal of Nursing Studies*, *87*, 1–13. https://doi.org/10.1016/j.ijnurstu.2018.07.004.

Kelsey, E. A., Njeru, J. W., Chaudhry, R., Fischer, K. M., Schroeder, D. R., & Croghan, I. T. (2020). Understanding user acceptance of clinical decision support systems to promote increased cancer screening rates in a primary care practice. *Journal of Primary Care & Community Health*, *11*, 2150132720958832. https://doi.org/10.1177/2150132720958832.

Kes, D., & Gökdoğan, F. (2020). Reliability and validity of a Turkish version of the hypertension self-care profile. *Journal of Vascular Nursing*, *38*(3), 149–155. https://doi.org/10.1016/j.jvn.2020.05.001.

Khodaveisi, M., Omidi, A., Farokhi, S., & Soltanian, A. R. (2017). The effect of Pender's health promotion model in improving the nutritional behavior of overweight and obese women. *International Journal of Community Based Nursing & Midwifery*, *5*(2), 165–174. http://doi.org/10.1136/bmjopen-2016-015415.131.

Kim, G., Choi, E. K., Kim, H. S., Kim, H., & Kim, H. S. (2019). Healthcare transition readiness, family support, and self-management competency in Korean emerging adults with type 1 diabetes mellitus. *Journal of Pediatric Nursing*, *48*, e1–e7. https://doi.org/10.1016/j.pedn.2019.03.012.

Lee, E. J., Lee, H. Y., & Chung, S. (2017). Age differences in health literacy: Do younger Korean adults have a higher level of health literacy than older Korean adults? *Health & Social Work*, *42*(3), 133–141. https://doi.org/10.1093/hsw/hlx026.

Liu, D., Yamashita, T., Burston, B., & Keene, J. R. (2020). The use of online health-management tools and health care utilization among older Americans. *Gerontologist*, *60*(7), 1224–1232. https://doi.org/10.1093/geront/gnaa068.

Low, J. K., Crawford, K., Manias, E., & Williams, A. (2017). Stressors and coping resources of Australian kidney transplant recipients related to medication taking: A qualitative study. *Journal of Clinical Nursing*, *26*(11/12), 1495–1507. https://doi.org/10.1111/jocn.13435.

Madrasi, K., Chaturvedula, A., Haberer, J. E., et al. (2017). Markov mixed effects modeling using electronic adherence monitoring records identifies influential covariates to HIV preexposure prophylaxis. *Journal of Clinical Pharmacology*, *57*(5), 606–615. https://doi.org/10.1002/jcph.843.

Pender, N. J., Murdaugh, C. L., & Parsons, M. A. (2015). *Health promotion in nursing practice* (7th ed.). Upper Saddle River, NJ: Prentice Hall.

Raffaele, B., Biagiola, V., Cirillo, L., Grazia De Marinis, M., & Matarese, M. (2018). Cross-validation of the self-care ability Scale for Elderly (SASE) in a sample of Italian older adults. *Scandinavian Journal of Caring Sciences*, *32*(4), 1398–1408. https://doi.org/10.1111/scs.12585.

Ritzert, T. R., Berghoff, C. R., Tifft, E. D., & Forsyth, J. P. (2020). Evaluating ACT processes in relation to outcome in self-help treatment for anxiety-related problems. *Behavior Modification*, *44*(6), 865–890. https://doi.org/10.1177/0145445519855616.

Schneider, M., & Howard, K. A. (2017). Using technology to enhance discharge teaching and improve coping for patients after stroke. *Journal of Neuroscience Nursing*, *49*(3), 152–156. https://doi.org/10.1097/JNN.0000000000000275.

Srisuk, N., Caneron, J., Ski, C. F., & Thompson, D. R. (2017). Randomized controlled trial of family-based education for patients with heart failure and their carers. *Journal of Advanced Nursing*, *73*(4), 857–870. https://doi.org/10.1111/jan.13192.

Tumin, D., Li, S. S., Nandi, D., et al. (2017). Health insurance coverage among young adult survivors of pediatric heart transplantation. *The Journal of Pediatrics*, *188*, 82–86. https://doi.org/10.1016/j.jpeds.2017.06.014.

Westcott, S., & Welding, L. (2017). Support surface selection for long-term patients in the community. *Journal of Community Nursing*, *31*(4), 36–39. NLM UID:101090738.

Ineffective Family Health Self-Management

Domain 1 Health promotion Class 2 Health management

Gail B. Ladwig, MSN, RN and Julianne E. Doubet, BSN, RN, EMT-B

NANDA-I

Definition

Unsatisfactory management of symptoms, treatment regimen, physical, psychosocial and spiritual consequences and lifestyle changes inherent in living with one or more family members' chronic condition.

Defining Characteristics

Caregiver strain; decrease in attention to illness in one or more family members; depressive symptoms of caregiver; exacerbation of disease signs of one or more family members; exacerbation of disease symptoms of one or more family members; failure to take action to reduce risk factor in one or more family members; ineffective choices in daily living for meeting health goal of family unit; one or more family members report dissatisfaction with quality of life

H

Related Factors

Cognitive dysfunction of one or more caregivers; competing demands on family unit; competing lifestyle preferences within family unit; conflict between health behaviors and social norms; conflict between spiritual beliefs and treatment regimen; difficulty accessing community resources; difficulty dealing with role changes associated with condition; difficulty managing complex treatment regimen; difficulty navigating complex health care systems; difficulty with decision-making; family conflict; inadequate commitment to a plan of action; inadequate health literacy of caregiver; inadequate knowledge of treatment regimen; inadequate number of cues to action; inadequate social support; ineffective communication skills; ineffective coping skills; limited ability to perform aspects of treatment regimen; low self efficacy; negative feelings toward treatment regimen; nonacceptance of condition; perceived barrier to treatment regimen; perceived social stigma associated with condition; substance misuse; unrealistic perception of seriousness of condition; unrealistic perception of susceptibility to sequelae; unrealistic perception of treatment benefit; unsupportive family relations

At-Risk Population

Economically disadvantaged families; families with member experiencing delayed diagnosis; families with members experiencing low educational level; families with members who have limited decision-making experience; families with premature infant

Associated Conditions

Chronic disease; mental disorders; neurocognitive disorders; terminal illness

NOC (Nursing Outcomes Classification)

Suggested NOC Outcomes

Family Health-Status; Knowledge: Treatment Regimen; Family Participation in Professional Care

Example NOC Outcome with Indicators

Knowledge: Treatment Regimen as evidenced by the following indicator: Understanding conveyed about prescribed medication, activity, exercise, and specific disease process. (Rate the outcome and indicators of **Knowledge: Treatment Regimen:** 1 = no knowledge, 2 = limited knowledge, 3 = moderate knowledge, 4 = substantial knowledge, 5 = extensive knowledge [see Section I].)

Client Outcomes

Client Will (Specify Time Frame)

- Make adjustments in usual activities (e.g., diet, activity, stress management) to incorporate therapeutic regimens of its members

- Reduce illness symptoms of family members
- Express desire to manage therapeutic regimens of its members
- Describe a decrease in the difficulties of managing therapeutic regimens
- Describe actions to reduce risk factors

NIC (Nursing Interventions Classification)

Suggested NIC Interventions

Family Involvement Promotion; Family Mobilization; Teaching: Disease Process

Example NIC Activities—Family Involvement Promotion

Identify and respect coping mechanisms used by family members; Provide crucial information to family members about the client in accordance with client's preference

Nursing Interventions and *Rationales*

- Base family interventions on knowledge of the family, family context, family dynamics, family structure, and family function. EBN: *A family-centered advance care planning (ACP) information intervention for persons with mild dementia and their family caregivers (FCGs) found significant improvements among persons with dementia and FCGs for knowledge of end-stage dementia treatment, knowledge of ACP, and significant reductions in decisional conflicts (Huang et al, 2020).*
- Use a family approach when helping an individual with a health problem that requires therapeutic management. EBN: *According to Nunes de Paiva et al (2018), it is important for hemodialysis clients to contribute to the management of their own health care, but to be successful, they will need the support of family and friends.*
- Review with family members the congruence and incongruence of family behaviors and health-related goals. EBN: *Nurses are especially qualified to fill the roles of both mentor and coach, and to work with clients and families toward positive health outcomes (Orchard et al, 2017).*
- Acknowledge the challenge of integrating therapeutic regimens with family behaviors. EBN: *A study by McDonnell et al (2019) concerning African American cancer survivors details the stressors that affect family members and highlights their particular health care problems. These stressors compromise their ability to effectively alter health behaviors.*
- Review the symptoms of specific illnesses and work with the family toward development of greater self-efficacy in relation to these symptoms. EBN: *Nurses should prioritize family support: involve them in the care of the client by coaching them through the completion of multifaceted medical tasks, reducing the family's need for outside services (Funk et al, 2020).*
- Support family decisions to adjust therapeutic regimens as indicated. EB: *The National Institute of Neurological Disorders and Stroke (2018) published findings that concluded a woman suffering from epilepsy can have a healthy pregnancy and deliver a healthy child with planned adjustments in medication and the addition of certain supplements.*
- Help the family mobilize social supports. EBN: *Nurses in any capacity may detect a family/individual in crisis and are obliged to provide crisis intervention while connecting the family/individual to other needed support services (Parsons, 2016).*
- Help family members modify perceptions as indicated. EB: *Illness perception, family adaptability, and coping mechanisms are key factors for the quality of life of a client with a chronic disease (Postolica et al, 2017).*
- Use one or more theories of family dynamics to describe, explain, or predict family behaviors (e.g., theories of Bowen, Satir, and Minuchin). EBN: *Family plays a critical role in health and illness; it is crucial for nurses to evaluate and modify family dynamics by using theoretical framework (Yekatalab et al, 2017).*

▲ Collaborate with expert nurses or other consultants regarding strategies for working with families. EBN: *The findings underscore the need for researchers and health care professionals to engage in collaborative discussions and make cooperative efforts to help alleviate treatment burden and tailor treatment regimens to the realities of people's daily lives (Sav et al, 2015).*

- Coaching methods can be used to help families improve their health. EB: *Young et al (2020) determined in their controlled trial study that a system employing a health coaching program for those with type 2 diabetes had a positive impact on the "physiological, behavioral, psychological, and social outcomes for clients with chronic health conditions."*

Pediatric

- Support skin-to-skin care for infants at risk at birth. Keep infants in an upright position in skin-to-skin contact until they no longer tolerate it. EBN: *According to ten Ham-Baloyi, Ricks, and van Rooyen (2017), some of the benefits derived from kangaroo mother care (KMC) are improving mother–infant attachment; encouraging the continuance of breastfeeding; and helping to reduce mortality of preterm neonates.*

Geriatric

- Recommend that clients use the "Ask Me 3" program when communicating with their health providers (What is my main problem? What do I need to do? Why is it important for me to do this?). EBN: *Organized client education using the Ask Me 3 questions program, produced encouraging results confirmed by a reduction in hospital readmissions and an increase in client satisfaction (Smith, 2020).*

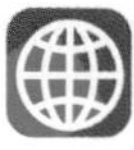

Multicultural

- Acknowledge racial and ethnic differences at the onset of care. EBN: *Markey et al (2018) surmised that a significant element in improving culturally sensitive, quality care was to first recognize, and then remedy, the nurse's insecurity and lack of confidence when delivering care for clients from a mixture of cultural and ethnic backgrounds.*
- Ensure that all strategies for working with the family are congruent with the culture of the family. EBN: *Cain et al (2018) emphasized that the nurse's obligation is to personalize care without stereotyping the client's—and the family's—principles and traditions; each person is unique, no matter the culture with which they identify.*
- Use the nursing intervention of cultural brokerage to help families deal with the health care system. EBN: *In their study of how culture shapes nursing practice, Crawford et al (2017) concluded that parents of pediatric clients count on nurses for cultural brokerage, to support them in bridging the daunting cultural restrictions found on a hospital unit.*

H

Client/Family Teaching and Discharge Planning

- Teach about all aspects of therapeutic regimens. Provide as much knowledge as family members will accept, adjust instruction to account for what the family already knows, and provide information in a culturally congruent manner. EBN: *Use "tailored to the client" instructions, which may include medical and disease education, skills training, and resource connection (Chin et al, 2017).*
- Teach ways to adjust family behaviors to include therapeutic regimens, such as safety in taking medications and teaching family members to act as self-advocates with health providers who prescribe therapeutic regimens. EBN: *By using continuous care interventions, a trusting relationship can be established with the FCG (Chin et al, 2017).*

REFERENCES

Cain, C. L., Surbone, A., Elk, R., & Kagawa-Singer, M. (2018). Cultural and palliative care preferences communication, meaning and mutual decision making. *Journal of Pain and Symptom Management, 55*(5), 1408–1419. https://doi.org/10.16/j.painsymman.2018.007.

Chin, M., Chiu, Y., Wei, A., & Hsu, W. C. (2017). Reducing the care-related burdens of a family caregiver of a person with mild cognitive impairment: A home-based care management program. *Hu Li Za Zhi The Journal of Nursing, 64*(3), 105–111. https://doi.org/10.6224/JN.000046.

Crawford, R., Stein-Parbury, J., & Dignam, D. (2017). Culture shapes nursing practice: From a New Zealand study. *Patient Education and Counseling, 100*(1), 2047–2053. https://doi.org/10.1016/j.pec.2017.06.017.

Funk, L. M., Stajduhar, K. I., Giesbrecht, M., Cloutier, D., Williams, A., & Wolse, F. (2020). Applying the concept of structural empowerment to interactions between families and home-care nurses. *Nursing Inquiry, 27*(1), e12313. https://doi.org/10.1111/nin.12313.

Huang, H. L., Lu, W. R., Liu, C. L., & Chang, H. J. (2020). Advance care planning information intervention for persons with mild dementia and their family caregivers: Impact on end-of-life care decision conflicts. *PLoS One, 15*(10), e0240684. https://doi.org/10.1371/journal.pone.0240684.

Markey, K., Tilki, M., & Taylor, G. (2018). Understanding nurses' concerns when caring for patients from different cultural and ethnic backgrounds. *Journal of Clinical Nursing, 27*(1–2), e259–e268. https://doi.org/10.1111/jocn.13926.

McDonnell, K. K., Owens, O. L., Hilfinger Messias, D. K., et al. (2019). Health behavior changes in African-American family members facing lung cancer: Tensions and compromises. *European Journal of Oncology Nursing, 38*, 57–64. https://doi.org/10.1016/j.ejon.2018.12.002.

National Institute of Neurological Disorders and Stroke. (2018). *The epilepsies and seizures: Hope through research.* Retrieved from https://www.ninds.nih.gov/disorders/patient-caregiver-education/hope-through-research/epilepsies-and-seizures-hope-through. Accessed 2 July 2021.

Nunes de Paiva, M. G. M., Dantas de Sá Tinôco, J., Lima e Silva, F. B. B., Rangel Dantas, J., Venícios de Oliveira Lopes, & Brandão de Carvalho Lira, A. L. (2018). Ineffective health management in hemodialysis patients: Content analysis. *Revista Brasileira de Enfermagem, 71*(4), 1825–1831. http://doi.org/10.1590/0034-7167-2016-0682.

Orchard, C. A., Sonibare, O., Morse, A., Collins, J., & Al-Hamad, A. (2017). Collaborative Leadership Part 2 the role of the nurse leader in interprofessional team-based practice-shifting from task to collaborative patient/family focused care. *Nursing Leadership*, *30*(2), 26–38. http://doi:10.12927/cjnl.2017.25257.

Parsons, C. (2016). Evidence-based care of adolescents and families in crisis. *Nursing Clinics of North America*, *51*(2), 249–260. https://doi.org/10.1016/j.cnurs.2016.01.008.

Postolica, R., Iorga, M., Petrariu, F., & Azoicai, D. (2017). Cognitive-behavioral coping, illness perception, and family adaptability in oncological patients with a family history of cancer. *BioMed Research International*, *2017*, 8104397.

Sav, A., King, M. A., Whitty, J. A., et al. (2015). Burden of treatment for chronic illness: A concept analysis and review of the literature. *Health Expectations*, *18*(3), 312–324. https://doi.org/10.1111/hex.12046.

Smith, C. R. (2020). *Improving healthcare transitions: Using Ask Me 3 to structure patient education [Doctor of nursing practice project]*. Sophia, St. Catherine University School of Nursing. Retrieved from https://sophia.stkate.edu/dnp_projects/120/. Accessed 2 July 2021.

ten Ham-Baloyi, W., Ricks, E., & van Rooyen, D. (2017). An educational strategy supporting kangaroo mother care: Interviews with health care practitioners. *Africa Journal of Nursing and Midwifery*, *19*(3). https://doi.org/10.25159/2520-5293/1859.

Yektatalab, S., Oskouee, F. S., & Sodani, M. (2017). Efficacy of the Bowen theory of marital conflict in the family nursing practice: A randomized controlled trial. *Issues in Mental Health Nursing*, *38*(3), 253–260. https://doi.org/10.1080/0612840.2016.1261210.

Young, H. M., Miyamoto, S., Dharmar, M., & Tang-Feldman, Y. (2020). Nurse coaching and mobile health compared with usual care to improve diabetes self-efficacy of persons with type 2 diabetes: A randomized controlled trial. *JMIR mHealth uHealth*, *8*(3), e16665. https://doi.org/10.2196/16665.

Ineffective Health Maintenance Behaviors **Domain 1 Health promotion Class 2 Health management**

Kathaleen C. Bloom, PhD, CNM and Lauren McAlister, MSN, FNP-BC, DNP

NANDA-I

Definition

Management of health knowledge, attitudes, and practices underlying health actions that is unsatisfactory for maintaining or improving well-being, or preventing illness and injury.

Defining Characteristics

Failure to take action that prevents health problem; failure to take action that reduces risk factor; inadequate commitment to a plan of action; inadequate health literacy; inadequate interest in improving health; inadequate knowledge about basic health practices; ineffective choices in daily living for meeting health goal; pattern of lack of health-seeking behavior

Related Factors

Competing demands; competing lifestyle preferences; conflict between cultural beliefs and health practices; conflict between health behaviors and social norms; conflicts between spiritual beliefs and health practices; depressive symptoms; difficulty accessing community resources; difficulty navigating complex health care systems; difficulty with decision-making; inadequate health resources; inadequate social support; inadequate trust in health care professional; individuals with limited decision making experience; ineffective communication skills; ineffective coping strategies; ineffective family coping; low self efficacy; maladaptive grieving; neurobehavioral manifestations; perceived prejudice; perceived victimization; spiritual distress

At-Risk Population

Economically disadvantaged individuals; individuals from families with ineffective family coping; individuals with history of violence; men; older adults; young adult

Associated Conditions

Chronic disease; developmental disabilities; mental disorders

NOC (Nursing Outcomes Classification)

Suggested NOC Outcomes

Health Orientation; Health Beliefs: Perceived Resources; Health-Promoting Behavior; Health-Seeking Behavior

Example NOC Outcome with Indicators

Health-Seeking Behavior as evidenced by the following indicators: Completes health-related tasks/Performs self-screening/Obtains assistance from health professional. (Rate the outcome and indicators of **Health-Seeking Behavior:** 1 = never demonstrated, 2 = rarely demonstrated, 3 = sometimes demonstrated, 4 = often demonstrated, 5 = consistently demonstrated [see Section I].)

Client Outcomes

Client Will (Specify Time Frame)

- Discuss fear of or blocks to implementing health regimen
- Follow mutually agreed on health care maintenance plan
- Meet goals for health care maintenance

NIC (Nursing Interventions Classification)

Suggested NIC Interventions

H

Health Education; Health System Guidance; Support System Enhancement

Example NIC Activities—Health Education

Prioritize identified learner needs based on client preference, skills of nurse, resources available, and likelihood of successful goal attainment; Emphasize immediate or short-term positive health benefits to be received by positive lifestyle behaviors, rather than long-term benefits or negative effects of noncompliance

Nursing Interventions and *Rationales*

- ● Provide support to clients in making their health care decisions and provide information about options and associated benefits/harms. EB: *A Cochrane review of 105 studies involving 31,043 clients found that people who used simple decision aids were more knowledgeable about options, less conflicted in making decisions, more accurate in their perception of risk, and more apt to be active in decision-making (Stacey et al, 2017).*
- ● Assess for family patterns, economic issues, and spiritual and cultural patterns that influence compliance with a given medical regimen. EBN: *A systematic review of 42 studies found knowledge, motivation, health and safety concerns, lack of social support, and monetary costs associated with exercise facilities to be among the barriers to physical activity among African American women (Joseph et al, 2015).*
- ● Involve the client in shared decision-making regarding health maintenance. CEB: *A meta-analysis of 32 clinical trials revealed that assessing client preferences and involving them in shared decision-making had higher adherence, higher satisfaction, and better clinical outcomes (Lindhiem et al, 2014).* EB: *A study of US veterans with mental illnesses found collaboration in decision-making positively influenced satisfaction with care and that such decision-making is best done by tailoring therapeutic approaches to consumer preferences for shared decision-making (Klingaman et al, 2015).*
- ● Show genuine interest in the client's individual needs. EB: *A systematic review of 10 qualitative studies concluded that clients' perceptions of the health care professional's responsiveness, interest in their individual needs, and shared information positively influence self-care (Fu et al, 2016).*
- ● Assist the client in finding methods to reduce stress. EB: *Analysis of the US National Health Interview data of 1997 to 2016 indicated that those who experience psychological distress were more likely to report high-risk behaviors such as alcohol consumption, physical inactivity, and tobacco use (Jokela et al, 2020).*
- ● Identify complementary healing modalities, such as herbal remedies, acupuncture, healing touch, yoga, or cultural shamans that the client uses in addition to or instead of the prescribed allopathic regimen along with the client's perception of the complementary healing modalities. EB: *Results of a mailed survey of health practices of 1825 US veterans indicated common use of acupuncture, chiropractic, massage, and manual physical therapy for pain as well as yoga, meditation, mindfulness, and exercise for well-being and/or general health (Donaldson et al, 2018).*
- ▲ Refer the client to appropriate and accessible medical and social services as needed, providing adequate information on details about the service. EBN: *A systematic review of 43 studies found that nonparticipation in cardiac rehabilitation (CR) was associated more with logistical and health system factors than with interpersonal or CR program factors (Resurrección et al, 2019).*

- Identify in-person and teleconferenced support groups related to the disease process. EB: *A systematic review of 17 studies concluded that outcomes of professional-led teleconferenced support groups are similar to in-person groups (Banbury et al, 2018).*
- Use social media such as text messaging to remind clients of scheduled appointments. EB: *Evaluation of compliance with treatment plans found 59% higher odds of attendance at a scheduled follow-up clinic visit with text message reminders and overall decreased cost as compared with telephone reminders (Anthony et al, 2019).* CEB: *A Cochrane review of eight randomized controlled trials concluded that text messaging reminders increase attendance at health care appointments similar to telephone reminders but better than no reminders or postal reminders (Gurol-Urganci et al, 2013).*
- Use telehealth interventions to facilitate self-care. EB: *In a study with 641 individuals with cardiovascular risk, telehealth services including telephone calls facilitating self-management through the use of targeted online resources were associated with reductions in blood pressure, weight, and body mass index, as well as improvements in diet, physical activity, drug adherence, and satisfaction (Salisbury et al, 2016).*

Geriatric

- Assess the client's perception of health and health maintenance. EB: *In a survey of 828 community-dwelling individuals at risk for cardiovascular disease, slightly more than half had an accurate perception of their risk, with one-third underestimating their risk (Lee et al, 2019).*
- Assist client to identify realistic health-related goals. EB: *A systematic review and meta-synthesis of 9 qualitative studies found that engagement in individually tailored goal-setting processes based on client preferences, and in conjunction with knowledgeable and skilled clinicians, facilitated setting of realistic goals and avoidance of disappointment in rehabilitative processes (Plant et al, 2016).*
- Encourage and facilitate informed decision-making. EB: *Although physicians generally inform clients and families of the risks and benefits of treatment options, incorporation of client/family preferences in the decision-making process, although essential to shared decision-making, is practiced much less frequently (Holmes-Rovner et al, 2015).*
- Educate the client about the symptoms of life-threatening illness, such as myocardial infarction (MI), and the need for timeliness in seeking care. EB: *An Australian mass media campaign focused on warning signs of MI was significantly associated with decreased prehospital delay time from onset of symptoms (Bray et al, 2015).*

H

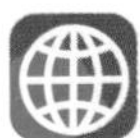

Multicultural

- Assess influence of cultural beliefs, norms, and values on the client's ability to modify health behavior. EB: *A survey of 1445 young Hispanic adults found the cultural concept of respeto (respect for and deferential treatment of family members based on age and status) to be associated with decreased binge drinking and marijuana and hard drug use and that fatalistic beliefs were associated with alternative tobacco product use (Escobedo et al, 2018).*
- Assess the effect of fatalism on the client's ability to modify health behavior. EB: *Analysis of data from a national survey (n = 2657) found a high prevalence of fatalistic beliefs related to cancer: everything causes cancer (66%), thinking about cancer makes you think about death (58%), and there's not much you can do to prevent cancer; such fatalism was associated with lack of information seeking, especially among those with low health literacy (Kobayashi & Smith, 2016).*
- Clarify culturally related health beliefs and practices. EB: *A qualitative study with 24 self-employed and uninsured Korean immigrant adults indicated that these individuals sought health information from social networks made up of primarily other Koreans or through organizations exclusively serving Korean immigrants. These individuals felt that non-Koreans would not understand the circumstances of Korean immigrants (Oh & Jeong, 2017).*
- Provide culturally appropriate education and health care services. EB: *Culturally tailored educational sessions with 159 culturally and linguistically diverse individuals in Australia were found to be associated with improved knowledge and attitudes about cancer screening as well as increased intention to participate in such screenings (Cullerton et al, 2016).*

Home Care

- The interventions described previously may be adapted for home care use.

▲ Provide nurse-led case management. EBN: *A retrospective chart review of 307 clients found that those who utilized a nurse-led community case management system had 55% fewer emergency department visits and 61% fewer hospital admissions than those who did not (Armold, 2017).*

• Provide a health promotion focus for the client with disabilities, with the goals of reducing secondary conditions (e.g., obesity, hypertension, pressure sores), maintaining functional independence, providing opportunities for leisure and enjoyment, and enhancing overall quality of life. EB: *A secondary analysis of data from the Medical Expenditure Panel Survey revealed that individuals with cognitive, physical, and multiple disabilities are more likely to have unmet health care needs, including being less likely to receive preventive services, dental care, and cancer screening (Mahmoudi & Meade, 2015).*

• Provide support and individual training for caregivers before the client is discharged from the hospital. EBN: *In a study of 138 caregiver–client dyads, caregiver training was found to enhance caregivers' preparedness for caregiving and decrease caregiver stress (Hendrix et al, 2016).*

Client/Family Teaching and Discharge Planning

H

• Provide the client and family with credible social media sources from which health information can be obtained. EB: *In a study with 457 clients, 99.1% reported searching online for health information; there was a significant relationship between the type of health information seeking (online versus non-online) and problem-solving (changing decisions, consulting others, promoting self-efficacy) with the highest correlation with online health information searches (Chen et al, 2018).*

▲ Develop collaborative multiprofessional partnerships. EBN: *Multiprofessional and multifactorial interventions are likely to be more effective in achieving desired outcomes. In a retrospective cohort study of readmission rates for 660 clients with pneumonia, clients receiving a postdischarge visit by a multiprofessional team consisting of health care providers, nurses, and social workers had significantly fewer 30-day readmissions (Otsuka et al, 2019).*

• Tailor both the information provided and the method of delivery of information to the specific client and/or family. EB: *A structured program for engaging parents of children with chronic conditions in preparation for hospital discharge using an iPad-based intervention found that parents had improved quality of discharge teaching and showed promise in helping parents prepare for transition to home (Lerret et al, 2020).*

REFERENCES

Anthony, N., Molokwu, J., Alozie, O., & Magallanes, D. (2019). Implementation of a text message to improve adherence to clinic and social service appointments. *Journal of the International Association of Providers of AIDS Care, 18* 2325958219870166. https://doi.org/10.1177/2325958219870166.

Armold, S. (2017). Utilization of the health care system of community case management patients. *Professional Case Management, 22*(4), 155–162. https://doi.org/10.1097/NCM.0000000000000197.

Banbury, A., Nancarrow, S., Dart, J., Gray, L., & Parkinson, L. (2018). Telehealth interventions delivering home-based support group videoconferencing: Systematic review. *Journal of Medical Internet Research, 20*(2), e25. https://doi.org/10.2196/jmir.8090.

Bray, J. E., Stub, D., Ngu, P., et al. (2015). Mass media campaigns' influence on prehospital behavior for acute coronary syndromes: An evaluation of the Australian Heart Foundation's Warning Signs Campaign. *Journal of the American Heart Association, 4*(7), e001927. https://doi.org/10.1161/JAHA.115.001927.

Chen, Y. Y., Li, C. M., Liang, J. C., & Tsai, C. C. (2018). Health information obtained from the internet and changes in medical decision making: Questionnaire development and cross-sectional survey. *Journal of Medical Internet Research, 20*(2), e47. https://doi.org/10.2196/jmir.9370.

Cullerton, K., Gallegos, D., Ashley, E., et al. (2016). Cancer screening education: Can it change knowledge and attitudes among culturally and linguistically diverse communities in Queensland, Australia? *Health Promotion Journal of Australia, 27*(2), 140–147. https://doi.org/10.1071/HE15116.

Donaldson, M. T., Polusny, M. A., MacLehose, R. F., et al. (2018). Patterns of conventional and complementary non-pharmacological health practice use by US military veterans: A cross-sectional latent class analysis. *BMC Complementary and Alternative Medicine, 18*(1), 246. https://doi.org/10.1186/s12906-018-2313-7.

Escobedo, P., Allem, J. P., Baezconde-Garbanati, L., & Unger, J. B. (2018). Cultural values associated with substance use among Hispanic emerging adults in Southern California. *Addictive Behaviors, 77*, 267–271. https://doi.org/10.1016/j.addbeh.2017.07.018.

Fu, Y., McNichol, E., Marczewski, K., & Closs, S. J. (2016). Patient-professional partnerships and chronic back pain self-management: A qualitative systematic review and synthesis. *Health and Social Care in the Community, 24*(3), 247–259. https://doi.org/10.1111/hsc.12223.

Gurol-Urganci, I., de Jongh, T., Vodopivec-Jamsek, V., Atun, R., & Car, J. (2013). Mobile phone messaging reminders for attendance at healthcare appointments. *Cochrane Database of Systematic Reviews, 12*, CD007458. https://doi.org/10.1002/14651858.CD007458.pub3.

Hendrix, C. C., Bailey, D. E., Jr., Steinhauser, K. E., et al. (2016). Effects of enhanced caregiver training program on cancer caregiver's self-efficacy, preparedness, and psychological well-being. *Supportive Care in Cancer, 24*(1), 327–336. https://doi.org/10.1007/s00520-015-2797-3.

Holmes-Rovner, M., Montgomery, J. S., Rovner, D. R., et al. (2015). Informed decision making: Assessment of the quality of physician communication about prostate cancer diagnosis and treatment. *Medical Decision Making, 35*(8), 999–1009. https://doi.org/10.1177/0272989X15597226.

Jokela, M., García-Velázquez, R., Gluschkoff, K., Airaksinen, J., & Rosenström, T. (2020). Health behaviors and psychological distress: Changing associations between 1997 and 2016 in the United States. *Social Psychiatry and Psychiatric Epidemiology, 55*(3), 385–391. https://doi.org/10.1007/s00127-019-01741-7.

Joseph, R. P., Ainsworth, B. E., Keller, C., & Dodgson, J. E. (2015). Barriers to physical activity among African American women: An integrative review of the literature. *Women & Health, 55*(6), 679–699. https://doi.org/10.1080/03630242.2015.1039184.

Klingaman, E. A., Medoff, D. R., Park, S. G., et al. (2015). Consumer satisfaction with psychiatric services: The role of shared decision making and the therapeutic relationship. *Psychiatric Rehabilitation Journal, 38*(3), 242–248. https://doi.org/10.1037/prj0000114.

Kobayashi, L. C., & Smith, S. G. (2016). Cancer fatalism, literacy, and cancer information seeking in the American public. *Health Education & Behavior, 43*(4), 461–470. https://doi.org/10.1177/1090198115604616.

Lee, K. S., Feltner, F. J., Bailey, A. L., et al. (2019). The relationship between psychological states and health perception in individuals at risk for cardiovascular disease. *Psychology Research and Behavior Management, 12*, 317–324. https://doi.org/10.2147/PRBM.S198280.

Lerret, S. M., Johnson, N. L., Polfuss, M., et al. (2020). Using the engaging parents in education for discharge (ePED) iPad application to improve parent discharge experience. *Journal of Pediatric Nursing, 52*, 41–48. https://doi.org/10.1016/j.pedn.2020.02.041.

Lindhiem, O., Bennett, C. B., Trentacosta, C. J., & McLear, C. (2014). Client preferences affect treatment satisfaction, completion, and clinical outcome: A meta-analysis. *Clinical Psychology Review, 34*(6), 506–517. https://doi.org/10.1016/j.cpr.2014.06.002.

Mahmoudi, E., & Meade, M. A. (2015). Disparities in access to health care among adults with physical disabilities: Analysis of a representative national sample for a ten-year period. *Disability and Health Journal, 8*(2), 182–190. https://doi.org/10.1016/j.dhjo.2014.08.007.

Oh, H., & Jeong, C. H. (2017). Korean immigrants don't buy health insurance: The influences of culture on self-employed Korean immigrants focusing on structure and functions of social networks. *Social Science & Medicine, 191*, 194–201. https://doi.org/10.1016/j.socscimed.2017.09.012.

Otsuka, S., Smith, J. N., Pontiggia, L., Patel, R. V., Day, S. C., & Grande, D. T. (2019). Impact of an interprofessional transition of care service on 30-day hospital reutilizations. *Journal of Interprofessional Care, 33*(1), 32–37. https://doi.org/10.1080/13561820.2018.1513466.

Plant, S. E., Tyson, S. F., Kirk, S., & Parsons, J. (2016). What are the barriers and facilitators to goal-setting during rehabilitation for stroke and other acquired brain injuries? A systematic review and meta-synthesis. *Clinical Rehabilitation, 30*(9), 921–930. https://doi.org/10.1177/0269215516655856.

Resurrección, D. M., Moreno-Peral, P., Gómez-Herranz, M., et al. (2019). Factors associated with non-participation in and dropout from cardiac rehabilitation programmes: A systematic review of prospective cohort studies. *European Journal of Cardiovascular Nursing, 18*(1), 38–47. https://doi.org/10.1177/1474515118783157.

Salisbury, C., O'Cathain, A., Thomas, C., et al. (2016). Telehealth for patients at high risk of cardiovascular disease: Pragmatic randomised controlled trial. *BMJ, 353*, i2647. https://doi.org/10.1136/bmj.i2647.

Stacey, D., Légaré, F., Lewis, K., et al. (2017). Decision aids for people facing health treatment or screening decisions. *Cochrane Database of Systematic Reviews, 4*, CD001431. https://doi.org/10.1002/14651858.CD001431.pub5.

H

Ineffective Home Maintenance Behaviors

Domain 1 Health promotion Class 2 Health management

Kathaleen C. Bloom, PhD, CNM and Lauren McAlister, MSN, FNP-BC, DNP

NANDA-I

Definition

An unsatisfactory pattern of knowledge and activities for the safe upkeep of one's residence.

Defining Characteristics

Cluttered environment; difficulty maintaining a comfortable environment; failure to request assistance with home maintenance; home task-related anxiety; home task-related stress; impaired ability to regulate finances; negative affect toward home maintenance; neglected laundry; pattern of hygiene-related diseases; trash accumulation; unsafe cooking equipment; unsanitary environment

Related Factors

Competing demands; depressive symptoms; difficulty with decision-making; environmental constraints; impaired physical mobility; impaired postural balance; inadequate knowledge of home maintenance; inadequate knowledge of social resources; inadequate organizing skills; inadequate role models; inadequate social support; insufficient physical endurance; neurobehavioral manifestations; powerlessness; psychological distress

At-Risk Population

Economically disadvantaged individuals; individuals living alone; older adult

Associated Conditions

Depression; mental disorders; neoplasms; neurocognitive disorders; sensation disorders; vascular diseases

NOC (Nursing Outcomes Classification)

Suggested NOC Outcomes

Safe Home Environment; Self-Care: Activities of Daily Living (ADLs)

Example NOC Outcome with Indicators

Safe Home Environment as evidenced by the following indicators: Elimination of pests/Smoke detector maintenance/Accessibility of assistive devices/Elimination of tobacco smoke. (Rate the outcome and indicators of **Safe Home Environment:** 1 = not adequate, 2 = slightly adequate, 3 = moderately adequate, 4 = substantially adequate, 5 = totally adequate [see Section I].)

H

Client Outcomes

Client Will (Specify Time Frame)

- Maintain a healthy home environment
- Use community resources to assist with home care needs
- Maintain a safe home environment

NIC (Nursing Interventions Classification)

Suggested NIC Intervention

Home Maintenance Assistance

Example NIC Activities—Home Maintenance Assistance

Involve client/family in deciding home maintenance requirements; Provide information on how to make home environment safe and clean; Help family use social support network

Nursing Interventions and *Rationales*

- Assess the knowledge and concerns of family members, especially the primary caregiver, about home care maintenance and management. EBN: *A qualitative descriptive study of 40 caregivers of clients with heart failure concluded that caregivers contributed to both the self-care maintenance and self-care management of the family member, but sometimes lacked necessary skill and/or confidence in decision-making (Durante et al, 2019).*
- Provide home safety education and safety equipment when possible. EB: *A program evaluation of a home safety program found that providing safety devices as well as education strategies, including videos and checklists, significantly decreased injuries in the home (Stewart et al, 2016).*
- Assess injury prevention knowledge and practices of the client and caregivers and provide information as appropriate. EB: *An evaluation of parental descriptions of the mechanism and perceived cause of 104 childhood home injuries revealed house features, furnishings, foods and/or beverages, and toys as primary causes of injury; 56% reported making changes in the home environment to prevent further injury, including eliminating or replacing hazardous items and increasing adult supervision (Jones et al, 2018).*

▲ Consider a predischarge home assessment referral to determine the need for accessibility and safety-related environmental changes. EB: *A randomized controlled trial (RCT) of 1848 individuals in 842 households found significantly fewer falls and fall-related injuries in those households that had specific low-cost home modifications such as alterations in steps inside and outside the house, grab rails and nonslip bath mats in bathrooms, outside lighting, and alterations in carpeting (Keall et al, 2015).*

- Use an assessment tool to identify environmental safety hazards in the home. EB: *A scoping review of 136 articles and 4 environmental hazard checklists highlighted the importance of inclusion of objective measurement of structural hazards in the home (Blanchet & Edwards, 2018).*
- Establish an individualized plan of care for improved home maintenance with the client and family based on the client's needs and the caregiver's capabilities. EB: *In a study of 86 low-income older adults with*

asthma, inclusion of education on asthma, its environmental triggers, and environmental remediation was found to be significantly improve health care visits, asthma control, and quality of life (Turcotte et al, 2019).

- Set up a system of relief for the main caregiver in the home and a plan for sharing household duties and/or outside assistance. EBN: *In a qualitative study, parents of children with special health care needs involved in a respite care program underlined the benefits of respite care to the family as a whole, emphasizing the value of tailoring respite care to the specific family (Whitmore & Snethan, 2018).*
- ▲ Provide a multiprofessional approach to target the home environment and the client's ability to function in the home. EBN: *The Community Aging in Place: Advancing Better Living for Elders, a program involving teams of nurses, occupational therapists, and handymen that targets the home environment and individual physical function, found that 75% of the participants significantly improved their performance of ADLs and had improved ability to do their own shopping and manage their medications (Szanton et al, 2016).*

Geriatric

- All of the previously mentioned interventions are applicable for the geriatric population.
- Assess functional ability to manage safely after hospital discharge. EB: *A qualitative metasummary of 13 studies exploring the perceptions of older persons as they adapt to life after hospital discharge highlighted the importance of involvement of the client and caregiver in assessment, planning, and preparation of the home environment (Hestevik et al, 2019).*
- Explore community resources to assist with home maintenance (e.g., senior centers, Department of Aging, hospital case managers, friends and relatives, the Internet, or church parish nurse). CEB: *In a qualitative study with 43 older adults living at home, participants perceived that they were both capable of and willing to manage many home maintenance tasks using compensatory means, such as tools and technologies, making home maintenance and repairs themselves, hiring someone, or having friends, neighbors, or family do the task (Kelly et al, 2014).*
- Provide education related to home modification. EB: *A systematic review of 36 articles examining home modifications of older adults found strong evidence in support of home modifications in reducing both the rate and risk of falls (Stark et al, 2017).*
- Focus on the interaction between the older client and the technology, assisting the client to be an active participant in choices of and uses for technology. EB: *A qualitative study with older adults, care professionals, home care or social work managers, and technology designers and suppliers found that all groups believed success was enhanced when the older adult's needs and wishes are prioritized and that the technology is accepted by the older adults and perceived as beneficial (Peek et al, 2016).*
- See the care plans for Risk for **Injury** and Risk for **Falls.**

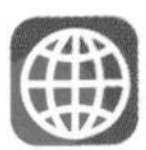

Multicultural

- Acknowledge the stresses unique to racial/ethnic communities. EB: *A systematic review of 36 qualitative and 88 quantitative studies focused on medical mistrust concluded that low trust or distrust in the health care system and/or health care providers is a contributing factor to health-related beliefs, utilization, and outcomes (Benkert et al, 2019).*

Home Care

- The previously mentioned interventions incorporate these resources.
- See care plans **Contamination** and Risk for **Contamination.**

Client/Family Teaching and Discharge Planning

- Identify support groups within the community to assist families in the caregiver role. EBN: *A qualitative study with 20 family caregivers of clients with Alzheimer's disease involved in a caregiver support group found positive associations with psychological support from professionals and others in similar situations leading to practical help, a feeling of companionship, and solution-focused optimism (Rosenberg & Tokovská, 2017).*
- Incorporate the perspectives of clients and their caregivers in the definition and description of safety. EBN: *In a triangulation study of clients in home care, their caregivers, and case management nurses, clients and caregivers recognized their role in ensuring safety, and tended to focus their definition of safety as it relates to meeting the clients' needs, underlining emphasis on empowerment as a model of case management (Jones, 2016).*

H

- Focus teaching on environmental hazards identified in the nursing assessment. Areas may include, but are not limited to, the following:
  - **Home Safety.** Identify the need for and use of common safety measures in the home. EB: *An RCT of an injury prevention briefing designed to improve fire safety found numerous risk factors for falls, poisonings, and scalds. Families in the intervention arm were less likely to report match play and more likely to report bedtime fire safety routines (Kendrick et al, 2017).*
  - **Food Safety.** Instruct client to avoid microbial foodborne illness by storing and cooking food at the proper temperature; regularly washing hands, food contact surfaces, and fruits and vegetables; and monitoring expiration dates. EB: *A cross-sectional study of 725 homebound older adults receiving home-delivered meals identified four potential areas of concern with food safety: lack of understanding of safe food storage times, inadequate freezer and/or refrigerator temperatures, overall poor kitchen conditions, and clients' visual difficulties (McWilliams et al, 2017).*
- Teach clients to assess their homes for potential environmental health hazards in the home, including risks related to structure, moisture/mold, fire, pets, electrical, ventilation, pests, and lifestyle. EB: *The results of visual in-home inspections of 106 homes using the Healthy Homes Rating System were compared to existing self-reports using the American Housing Survey. The in-home assessment was found to be more reflective of actual conditions, especially in very low income housing (Sokolowsky et al, 2017).*
- See care plans **Contamination,** Risk for **Contamination,** Risk for Adult **Falls,** Risk for Child **Falls**, Risk for **Infection,** and Risk for **Injury.**

H

REFERENCES

Benkert, R., Cuevas, A., Thompson, H. S., Dove-Meadows, E., & Knuckles, D. (2019). Ubiquitous yet unclear: A systematic review of medical mistrust. *Behavioral Medicine*, *45*(2), 86–101. https://doi.org/10.1080/08964289.2019.1588220.

Blanchet, R., & Edwards, N. (2018). A need to improve the assessment of environmental hazards for falls on stairs and in bathrooms: Results of a scoping review. *BMC Geriatrics*, *18*(1), 272. https://doi.org/10.1186/s12877-018-0958-1.

Durante, A., Paturzo, M., Mottola, A., Alvaro, R., Dickson, V. V., & Vellone, E. (2019). Caregiver contribution to self-care in patients with heart failure: A qualitative descriptive study. *Journal of Cardiovascular Nursing*, *34*(2), E28–E35. https://doi.org/10.1097/JCN.0000000000000560.

Hestevik, C. H., Molin, M., Debesay, J., Bergland, A., & Bye, A. (2019). Older persons' experiences of adapting to daily life at home after hospital discharge: A qualitative metasummary. *BMC Health Services Research*, *19*(1), 224. https://doi.org/10.1186/s12913-019-4035-z.

Jones, S. (2016). Alternative perspectives of safety in home delivered health care: A sequential exploratory mixed method study. *Journal of Advanced Nursing*, *72*(10), 2536–2546. https://doi.org/10.1111/jan.13006.

Jones, V. C., Shields, W., Ayyagari, R., Frattaroli, S., McDonald, E. M., & Gielen, A. C. (2018). Association between unintentional child injury in the home and parental implementation of modifications for safety. *JAMA Pediatrics*, *172*(12), 1189–1190. https://doi.org/10.1001/jamapediatrics.2018.2781.

Keall, M. D., Pierse, N., Howden-Chapman, P., et al. (2015). Home modifications to reduce injuries from falls in the home injury prevention intervention (HIPI) study: A cluster-randomised controlled trial. *Lancet*, *385*(9964), 231–238. https://doi.org/10.1016/S0140-6736(14)61006-0.

Kelly, A. J., Fausset, C. B., Rogers, W., & Fisk, A. D. (2014). Responding to home maintenance challenge scenarios: The role of selection, optimization, and compensation in aging-in-place. *Journal of Applied Gerontology*, *33*(8), 1018–1042. https://doi.org/10.1177/0733464812456631.

Kendrick, D., Ablewhite, J., Achana, F., et al. (2017). Keeping children safe: A multicentre programme of research to increase the evidence base for preventing unintentional injuries in the home in the under-fives. *NIHR Journals Library, 2017*(7). https://doi.org/10.3310/pgfar05140.

McWilliams, R. M., Hallman, W. K., Cuite, C. L., et al. (2017). Food safety practices of homebound seniors receiving home-delivered meals. *Topics in Clinical Nutrition*, *32*(4), 268–281. https://doi.org/10.1097/TIN.0000000000000117.

Peek, S. T. M., Wouters, E. J. M., Luijkx, K. G., & Vrijhoef, H. J. M. (2016). What it takes to successfully implement technology for aging in place: Focus groups with stakeholders. *Journal of Medical Internet Research*, *18*(5), e98. https://doi.org/10.2196/jmir.5253.

Rosenberg, A., & Tokovská, M. (2017). Participation in a support group from the perspective of family caregivers of Alzheimer's disease patients. *Nursing: Theory, Research, Education/Osetrovateľstvo: Teória, Výskum, Vzdelávanie*, *7*(2), 53–57.

Sokolowsky, A., Marquez, E., Sheehy, E., Barber, C., & Gerstenberger, S. (2017). Health hazards in the home: An assessment of a southern Nevada community. *Journal of Community Health*, *42*(4), 730–738. https://doi.org/10.1007/s10900-016-0311-6.

Stark, S., Keglovits, M., Arbesman, M., & Lieberman, D. (2017). Effect of home modification interventions on the participation of community-dwelling adults with health conditions: A systematic review. *American Journal of Occupational Therapy*, *71*(2), 1–11. https://doi.org/10.5014/ajot.2017.018887.

Stewart, T. C., Clark, A., Gilliland, J., et al. (2016). Home safe home: Evaluation of a childhood home safety program. *Journal of Trauma and Acute Care Surgery*, *81*(3), 533–540. https://doi.org/10.1097/TA.0000000000001148.

Szanton, S. L., Leff, B., Wolff, J. L., Roberts, L., & Gitlin, L. N. (2016). Home-based care program reduces disability and promotes aging in place. *Health Affairs*, *35*(9), 1558–1563. https://doi/10.1377/hlthaff.2016.0140.

Turcotte, D. A., Woskie, S., Gore, R., Chaves, E., & Adejumo, K. (2019). Asthma, COPD, and home environments: Interventions with older adults. *Annals of Allergy, Asthma, & Immunology*, *122*(5), 486–491. https://doi.org/10.1016/j.anai.2019.02.026.

Whitmore, K. E., & Snethen, J. (2018). Respite care services for children with special healthcare needs: Parental perceptions. *Journal for Specialists in Pediatric Nursing*, *23*(3), e12217. https://doi.org/10.1111/jspn.12217.

Readiness for Enhanced Home Maintenance Behaviors

Domain 1 Health promotion Class 2 Health management

Kathaleen C. Bloom, PhD, CNM

NANDA-I

Definition

A pattern of knowledge and activities for the safe upkeep of one's residence, which can be strengthened.

Defining Characteristics

Expresses desire to enhance affect toward home tasks; expresses desire to enhance attitude toward home maintenance; expresses desire to enhance comfort of the environment; expresses desire to enhance home safety; expresses desire to enhance household hygiene; expresses desire to enhance laundry management skills; expresses desire to enhance organizational skills; expresses desire to enhance regulation of finances; expresses desire to enhance trash management

H

NOC (Nursing Outcomes Classification)

Suggested NOC Outcomes

Safe Home Environment; Self-Care: Activities of Daily Living (ADLs)

Example NOC Outcome with Indicators

Safe Home Environment as evidenced by the following indicators: Elimination of pests/Smoke detector maintenance/Accessibility of assistive devices/Elimination of tobacco smoke. (Rate the outcome and indicators of **Safe Home Environment:** 1 = not adequate, 2 = slightly adequate, 3 = moderately adequate, 4 = substantially adequate, 5 = totally adequate [see Section I].)

Client Outcomes

Client Will (Specify Time Frame)

- Maintain a healthy home environment
- Use community resources to assist with home care needs
- Maintain a safe home environment

NIC (Nursing Interventions Classification)

Suggested NIC Intervention

Home Maintenance Assistance

Example NIC Activities—Home Maintenance Assistance

Involve client/family in deciding home maintenance requirements; Provide information on how to make home environment safe and clean; Help family use social support network

Nursing Interventions and *Rationales*

- Assess the client's level of readiness for change in home maintenance. EB: *A qualitative study using interview data from 30 participants concluded that assessing readiness to change was key to improving occupational safety and health (Cunningham & Jacobson, 2018).*
- Take the client's age and level of disability into account when determining need for housing adaptations. EB: *A qualitative analysis of interview data outlined five client profile clusters based on age and level of disability that can be useful in determining home-based interventions and follow-up processes (Luther et al, 2020). These clusters are (1) older adults with low level of disability, (2) older adults with medium/high level of disability, (3) adults with low level of disability, (4) adults with high level of disability, and (5) older adults with medium level of disability including at least moderate cognitive impairment.*

- Engage the client in decisions related to home modifications. EB: *In a qualitative study that included 10 older adults, the client often felt frustrated by the lack of attention to their voice in decisions and the aesthetics of the home environment (Lo Bianco et al, 2020).*
- Consider the expectations of individuals living with/caring for the client in determining home adaptations. EB: *Granbom et al (2017) used grounded theory to examine the expectations and experiences of nine partners of older persons and individuals with disabilities and found that the expectations of home adaptation centered around concern for mobility, safety, and independence in activities for their partner, as well as benefits to their own everyday life.*
- Reduce injury hazards for children in the home and implement use of safety devices. EB: *A systematic review and meta-analysis of four clinical trials concluded that there is evidence that home inspection, safety education, and safety devices reduce home hazards for children (Bhatta et al, 2020).*
- Encourage home rules regarding a smoke free environment. EB: *Data from smokers in the Global Adult Tobacco Survey indicate that there are 29.3% fewer cigarettes per day smoked by individuals who live in homes where smoking is not allowed in the home (Owusu et al, 2020).*

Geriatric

All of the previously mentioned interventions are applicable for the geriatric population.

- Provide information to older adults and their families to promote independent living. EB: *A review of 5-year longitudinal data indicates that structured advice and home modifications helped prevent transfer of care from home to long-term care facilities in moderately to severely frail older adults (Hollinghurst et al, 2020).*
- Focus on fall prevention in the home. EBN: *A quality improvement project designed to enhance awareness of fall risks in the home focused on promoting exercise, home safety, and regular check-up with the primary care provider. This approach was found to increase safety awareness and knowledge of fall prevention (Minnier et al, 2019).*
- Monitor the ways in which home adaptations and equipment are used in the home to ensure continuing safety. EB: *In a qualitative study, six older adults who had received a major home adaptation in the past 24 months wore body cameras for 1 day and participated in an interview. Results indicated that these individuals modified the home adaptations and equipment to fit their individual needs (Wilson et al, 2019).*

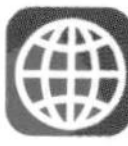

Multicultural

- Encourage maintenance of personal and cultural possessions in the home even as adaptations are made to the structure and function of the home. EB: *In a phenomenological study, participants described how their interaction with cherished possessions helped them connect with their past selves and cope with present changes and challenges. This has the potential to improve quality of life (Coleman & Wiles, 2020).*

Home Care

- Use principles of client-centeredness in home care. EBN: *A thematic analysis from an integrative review of 24 articles on home care approaches found four themes defining client-centered care and service in home care: (1) client involvement, (2) family and caregiver participation, (3) communication and collaboration, and (4) evidence-based service competence (Sanerma et al, 2020).*

Client/Family Teaching and Discharge Planning

- Provide the client and family with sufficient, quality information and resources before discharge to ensure a feeling of confidence in home care. EBN: *In a qualitative analysis of 14 clients' perception of the discharge process, clients revealed a desire to be involved in a discharge process that focused on communication, information, and participation (Krook et al, 2020).*
- Promote good communication between older persons, hospital providers, and home care providers to improve coordination of care and a seamless transition to home. EB: *A metasummary of qualitative data from 13 studies found that clients' concerns include the transition process, settling in at home, their caretaker, and lack of involvement in the process (Hestevik et al, 2019). This is especially true of communications relative to medication management (Tobiano et al, 2019).*

REFERENCES

Bhatta, S., Mytton, J., & Deave, T. (2020). Environmental change interventions to prevent unintentional home injuries among children in low- and middle-income countries: A systematic review and meta-analysis. *Child: Care, Health and Development*, *46*(5), 537–551. https://doi.org/10.1111/cch.12772.

Coleman, T., & Wiles, J. (2020). Being with objects of meaning: Cherished possessions and opportunities to maintain aging in place. *The Gerontologist*, *60*(1), 41–49. https://doi.org/10.1093/geront/gny142.

Cunningham, T. R., & Jacobson, C. J. (2018). Safety talk and safety culture: Discursive repertoires as indicators of workplace safety and health practice and readiness to change. *Annals of Work Exposures and Health*, *62*(1), S55–S64. https://doi.org/10.1093/annweh/wxy035.

Granbom, M., Taei, A., & Ekstam, L. (2017). Cohabitants' perspective on housing adaptations: A piece of the puzzle. *Scandinavian Journal of Caring Sciences*, *31*(4), 805–813. https://doi.org/10.1111/scs.12400.

Hestevik, C. H., Molin, M., Debesay, J., Bergland, A., & Bye, A. (2019). Older persons' experiences of adapting to daily life at home after hospital discharge: A qualitative metasummary. *BMC Health Services Research*, *19*(1), 224. https://doi.org/10.1186/s12913-019-4035-z.

Hollinghurst, J., Fry, R., Akbari, A., et al. (2020). Do home modifications reduce care home admissions for older people? A matched control evaluation of the care & repair cymru service in wales. *Age and Ageing*, *49*(6), 1056–1061. https://doi.org/10.1093/ageing/afaa158.

Krook, M., Iwarzon, M., & Siouta, E. (2020). The discharge process—From a patient's perspective. *SAGE Open Nursing*, *6*, 2377960819900707. https://doi.org/10.1177/2377960819900707.

Lo Bianco, M., Layton, N., Renda, G., & McDonald, R. (2020). "I think I could have designed it better, but I didn't think that it was my place": A critical review of home modification practices from the perspectives of health and of design. *Disability and Rehabilitation: Assistive Technology*, *15*(7), 781–788. https://doi.org/10.1080/17483107.2020.1749896.

Luther, A., Chiatti, C., Ekstam, L., Thordardottir, B., & Fänge, A. M. (2020). Identifying and validating housing adaptation client profiles—A mixed methods study. *Disability & Rehabilitation*, *42*(14), 2027–2034. https://doi.org/10.1080/09638288.2018.1550530.

Minnier, W., Leggett, M., Persaud, I., & Breda, K. (2019). Four Smart Steps: Fall prevention for community-dwelling older adults. *Creative Nursing*, *25*(2), 169–175. https://doi.org/10.1891/1078-4535.25.2.169.

Owusu, D., Quinn, M., Wang, K., Williams, F., & Mamudu, H. (2020). Smokefree home rules and cigarette smoking intensity among smokers in different stages of smoking cessation from 20 low-and-middle income countries. *Preventive Medicine*, *132*, 106000. https://doi.org/10.1016/j.ypmed.2020.106000.

Sanerma, P., Miettinen, S., Paavilainen, E., & Åstedt-Kurki, P. (2020). A client-centered approach in home care for older persons—An integrative review. *Scandinavian Journal of Primary Health Care*, *38*(4), 369–380. https://doi.org/10.1080/02813432.2020.1841517.

Tobiano, G., Chaboyer, W., Teasdale, T., Raleigh, R., & Manias, E. (2019). Patient engagement in admission and discharge medication communication: A systematic mixed studies review. *International Journal of Nursing Studies*, *95*, 87–102. https://doi.org/10.1016/j.ijnurstu.2019.04.009.

Wilson, G., Aitken, D., Hodgson, P., & Bailey, C. (2019). The hidden impact of home adaptations: Using a wearable camera to explore lived experiences and taken-for-granted behaviours. *Health and Social Care in the Community*, *27*(6), 1469–1480. https://doi.org/10.1111/hsc.12818.

H

Risk for Ineffective Home Maintenance Behaviors

Domain 1 Health promotion Class 2 Health management

Marina Martinez-Kratz, MS, RN, CNE

NANDA-I

Definition

Susceptible to an unsatisfactory pattern of knowledge and activities for the safe upkeep of one's residence, which may compromise health.

Defining Characteristics

Competing demands; depressive symptoms; difficulty with decision-making; environmental constraints; impaired physical mobility; impaired postural balance; inadequate knowledge of home maintenance; inadequate knowledge of social resources; inadequate organizing skills; inadequate role models; inadequate social support; insufficient physical endurance; neurobehavioral manifestations; powerlessness; psychological distress

At-Risk Population

Economically disadvantaged individuals; individuals living alone; older adults

Associated Conditions

Depression; mental disorders; neoplasms; neurocognitive disorders; sensation disorders; vascular disease

NOC, NIC, Client Outcomes, Nursing Interventions and *Rationales,* Client/Family Teaching and Discharge Planning, and References

Refer to care plans for Ineffective **Home** Maintenance Behaviors and Readiness for Enhanced **Home** Maintenance Behaviors.

Readiness for Enhanced Hope

Domain 6 Self-perception Class 1 Self-concept

Marina Martinez-Kratz, MS, RN, CNE

H

NANDA-I

Definition

A pattern of expectations and desires for mobilizing energy to achieve positive outcomes, or avoid a potentially threatening or negative situation, which can be strengthened.

Defining Characteristics

Expresses desire to enhance ability to set achievable goals; expresses desire to enhance belief in possibilities; expresses desire to enhance congruency of expectation with goal; expresses desire to enhance deep inner strength; expresses desire to enhance giving and receiving of care/love; expresses desire to enhance initiative; expresses desire to enhance involvement with self-care; expresses desire to enhance positive outlook on life; expresses desire to enhance problem-solving to meet goal; expresses desire to enhance sense of meaning in life; expresses desire to enhance spirituality

NOC (Nursing Outcomes Classification)

Suggested NOC Outcomes

Hope; Quality of Life

Example NOC Outcome with Indicators

Hope as evidenced by the following indicators: Expresses expectation of a positive future/Expresses faith/Expresses meaning in life/Exhibits a zest for life/Sets goals. (Rate the outcome and indicators of **Hope:** 1 = never demonstrated, 2 = rarely demonstrated, 3 = sometimes demonstrated, 4 = often demonstrated, 5 = consistently demonstrated [see Section I].)

Client Outcomes

Client Will (Specify Time Frame)

- Describe values, expectations, and meanings
- Set achievable goals that are consistent with values
- Design strategies to achieve goals
- Express belief in possibilities

NIC (Nursing Interventions Classification)

Suggested NIC Interventions

Emotional Support; Hope Inspiration; Presence; Support System Enhancement

Example NIC Activities—Hope Inspiration

Assist client and family to identify areas of hope in life; Demonstrate hope by recognizing the client's intrinsic worth; Encourage therapeutic relationships; Help the person expand spiritual self

Nursing Interventions and *Rationales*

- Spend one-on-one time with the client. Use empathy; try to understand what the client is saying and communicate this understanding to the client to create a nonjudgmental trusting environment to develop therapeutic relationships with the client. EB: *Client ratings of the therapeutic relationship predicted social inclusion through hopefulness (Berry & Greenwood, 2015).*
- Assist clients to identify sources of gratitude in their lives. EB: *A study found that gratitude predicted hope and happiness (vanOyen-Witvliet et al, 2019).*

- Screen the client for hope using a valid and reliable instrument as indicated. CEB: *The Herth Hope Index (HHI) is a brief instrument with good psychometric properties that has been developed for clinical use. It has been designed to facilitate the examination of hope at various intervals so that changes in levels of hope can be identified (Hunsaker et al, 2016).*
- Focus on the positive aspects of hope. EBN: *An integrative study found that when an institution provides a positive context, it promotes hope (e.g., sets goals, generates pathways, sustains motivation) in attaining educational objectives for college students (Griggs, 2017).*
- Assist the client to develop positive expectations outcomes and recognize the pathways to achieve the positive outcomes. EB: *Research findings suggest that lack of positive expectations account for the relationship between hopelessness and future depression and suicidal behavior among adolescents (Horwitz et al, 2017).*
- Explore the meanings, functions, objects, sources, and nature of hope with clients as they relate to their current situation. EBN: *A better understanding of clients' meanings of hope can assist nurses to foster hope and provide better support (Marco, Pérez, & García-Alandete, 2016).*
- Teach individuals how to become aware of attention that is focused on unwanted aspects of life and how to redirect attention toward things that feel more wanted or desired by using a future-directed approach. EB: *A study determined that the development of a future orientation led to a decline in hopelessness (Mac Giollabhui et al, 2018).*
- Review the client's strengths and resources in conjunction with the client. EBN: *A strengths-based perspective support group intervention reduced the participants' level of depressive symptoms and improved the pathway component of hope (Hou, Ko, & Shu, 2016).*
- Assist the client to consider alternatives and set long- and short-term goals that are important to him or her. EBN: *A mixed-method thematic review found that setting and achieving goals was a theme that increased hope (Broadhurst & Harrington, 2016).*
- Encourage engagement in positive and pleasant events. EB: *This study found that targeting both hopelessness and engagement in pleasant events may be helpful in improving the quality of life of vulnerable, rural, older adults (Scogin et al, 2016).*
- Facilitate sources of the client's resilience. EB: *Resilience has a mediating role in the relationship between risk factors involved in interpersonal functioning and hopelessness (Collazzoni et al, 2020).*
- Implement social supports and reintegration programs for postdeployment soldiers and veterans in a timely fashion. EB: *Research determined that hopelessness was moderated by timely implementation of postdeployment support and reintegration programs (Martin et al, 2016).*
- Encourage the client to adopt active coping strategies. EB: *In the current study, proactive coping predicted hope regardless of severity of spinal cord injury (Phillips et al, 2016).*
- Identify spiritual beliefs and practices. CEB: *Spirituality was identified as a factor in increasing hope in clients with mental illness (Schrank et al, 2012).*

Home Care

- The previously mentioned interventions may be adapted for home care use.

Client/Family Teaching and Discharge Planning

- Assist families to identify sources of gratitude in their lives. EB: *A study found that gratitude predicted hope and happiness (vanOyen-Witvliet et al, 2019).*
- Use a family-centered approach to provide information regarding the client's condition, treatment plan, and progress. EBN: *Clients reported increased hope after a planned family-centered discharge process (Ingram et al, 2017).*
- Teach alternative coping strategies such as physical activity. EB: *In a study of adults with congenital heart disease, regular physical activity was a protective factor against hopelessness (Eslami et al, 2017).*
- ▲ Refer the client to self-help groups. EB: *Support groups provided an experience of community in which hope was encouraged (Behler et al, 2017).*

REFERENCES

Behler, J., Daniels, A., Scott, J., & Mehl-Madrona, L. (2017). Depression/bipolar peer support groups: Perceptions of group members about effectiveness and differences from other mental health services. *Qualitative Report*, *22*(1), 213–236.

Berry, C., & Greenwood, K. (2015). Hope-inspiring therapeutic relationships, professional expectations and social inclusion for young people with psychosis. *Schizophrenia Research*, *168*(1–2), 153–160. https://doi.org/10.1016/j.schres.2015.07.032.

Broadhurst, K., & Harrington, A. (2016). A mixed method thematic review: The importance of hope to the dying patient. *Journal of Advanced Nursing, 72*(1), 18–32. https://doi.org/10.1111/jan.12765.

Collazzoni, A., Stratta, P., Pacitti, F., et al. (2020). Resilience as a mediator between interpersonal risk factors and hopelessness in depression. *Frontiers in Psychiatry, 11*, 10. https://doi.org/10.3389/fpsyt.2020.00010.

Eslami, B., Kovacs, A. H., Moons, P., Abbasi, K., & Jackson, J. L. (2017). Hopelessness among adults with congenital heart disease: Cause for despair or hope? *International Journal of Cardiology, 230*, 64–69. https://doi.org/10.1016/j.ijcard.2016.12.090.

Griggs, S. (2017). Hope and mental health in young adult college students: An integrative review. *Journal of Psychosocial Nursing and Mental Health Services, 55*(2), 28–35. https://doi.org/10.3928/02793695-20170210-04.

Horwitz, A. G., Berona, J., Czyz, E. K., Yeguez, C. E., & King, C. A. (2017). Positive and negative expectations of hopelessness as longitudinal predictors of depression, suicidal ideation, and suicidal behavior in high-risk adolescents. *Suicide and Life-Threatening Behavior, 47*, 168–176. https://doi.org/10.1111/sltb.12273.

Hou, W. L., Ko, N. Y., & Shu, B. C. (2016). Effects of a strengths-based perspective support group among Taiwanese women who left a violent intimate partner relationship. *Journal of Clinical Nursing, 25*, 543–554. https://doi.org/10.1111/jocn.13091.

Hunsaker, A. E., Terhorst, L., Gentry, A., & Lingler, J. H. (2016). Measuring hope among families impacted by cognitive impairment. *Dementia, 15*(4), 596–608. https://doi.org/10.1177/1471301214531590.

Ingram, J., Redshaw, M., Manns, S., et al. (2017). "Giving us hope": Parent and neonatal staff views and expectations of a planned family-centred discharge process (Train-to-Home). *Health Expectations, 20*, 751–759. https://doi.org/10.1111/hex.12514.

Mac Giollabhui, N., Nielsen, J., Seidman, S., Olino, T. M., Abramson, L. Y., & Alloy, L. B. (2018). The development of future orientation is associated with faster decline in hopelessness during adolescence. *Journal of Youth and Adolescence, 47*(10), 2129–2142. https://doi.org/10.1007/s10964-017-0803-4.

Marco, J. H., Pérez, S., & García-Alandete, J. (2016). Meaning in life buffers the association between risk factors for suicide and hopelessness in participants with mental disorders. *Journal of Clinical Psychology, 72*, 689–700. https://doi.org/10.1002/jclp.22285.

Martin, R. L., Houtsma, C., Green, B. A., & Anestis, M. D. (2016). Support systems: How post-deployment support impacts suicide risk factors in the United States Army National Guard. *Cognitive Therapy and Research, 40*, 14–21. https://doi.org/10.1007/s10608-015-9719-z.

Phillips, B. N., Smedema, S. M., Fleming, A. R., Sung, C., & Allen, M. G. (2016). Mediators of disability and hope for people with spinal cord injury. *Disability & Rehabilitation, 38*(17), 1672–1683. https://doi.org/10.3109/09638288.2015.1107639.

Schrank, B., Bird, V., Rudnick, A., & Slade, M. (2012). Determinants, self-management strategies and interventions for hope in people with mental disorders: Systematic search and narrative review. *Social Science & Medicine, 74*(4), 554–564.

Scogin, F., Morthland, M., DiNapoli, E. A., LaRocca, M. L., & Chaplin, W. (2016). Pleasant events, hopelessness, and quality of life in rural older adults. *The Journal of Rural Health, 32*, 102–109. https://doi.org/10.1111/jrh.12130.

vanOyen-Witvliet, C., Richie, F. J., Root Luna, L. M., & Van Tongeren, D. R. (2019). Gratitude predicts hope and happiness: A two-study assessment of traits and states. *The Journal of Positive Psychology, 14*(3), 271–282. https://doi.org/10.1080/17439760.2018.1424924.

H

Hopelessness **Domain 6 Self-perception Class 1 Self-concept**

Marina Martinez-Kratz, MS, RN, CNE

NANDA-I

Definition

The feeling that one will not experience positive emotions, or an improvement in one's condition.

Defining Characteristics

Anorexia; avoidance behaviors; decreased affective display; decreased initiative; decreased response to stimuli; decreased verbalization; depressive symptoms; expresses despondency; expresses diminished hope; expresses feeling of uncertain future; expresses inadequate motivation for the future; expresses negative expectations about self; expresses negative expectations about the future; expresses sense of incompetency in meeting goals; inadequate involvement with self care; overestimates the likelihood of unfortunate events; passivity; reports altered sleep-wake cycle; suicidal behaviors; unable to imagine life in the future; underestimates the occurrence of positive events

Related Factors

Chronic stress; fear; inadequate social support; loss of belief in spiritual power; loss of belief in transcendent values; low self efficacy; prolonged immobility; social isolation; unaddressed violence; uncontrolled severe disease symptoms

At-Risk Population

Adolescents; displaced individuals; economically disadvantaged individuals; individuals experiencing infertility; individuals experiencing significant loss; individuals with history of attempted suicide; individuals with history of being abandoned; older adults; unemployed individuals

Associated Conditions

Critical illness; depression; deterioration in physiological condition; feeding and eating disorders; mental disorders; neoplasms; terminal illness

NOC (Nursing Outcomes Classification)

Suggested NOC Outcomes

Decision-Making; Hope; Mood Equilibrium; Nutritional Status: Food and Fluid Intake; Quality of Life; Sleep

Example NOC Outcome with Indicators

Has a presence of **Hope** as evidenced by the following indicators: Expresses expectation of a positive future/Expresses faith/Expresses will to live. (Rate the outcome and indicators of **Hope:** 1 = never demonstrated, 2 = rarely demonstrated, 3 = sometimes demonstrated, 4 = often demonstrated, 5 = consistently demonstrated [see Section I].)

H

Client Outcomes

Client Will (Specify Time Frame)

- Verbalize feelings
- Participate in care
- Make positive statements (e.g., "I can" or "I will try")
- Set goals
- Make eye contact, focus on speaker
- Maintain appropriate appetite for age and physical health
- Sleep appropriate length of time for age and physical health
- Express concern for another
- Initiate activity

NIC (Nursing Interventions Classification)

Suggested NIC Intervention

Hope Inspiration

Example NIC Activities—Hope Inspiration

Assist client/family to identify areas of hope in life; Demonstrate hope by recognizing client's intrinsic worth and viewing client's illness as only one facet of the individual; Expand the client's repertoire of coping mechanisms

Nursing Interventions and *Rationales*

- Assess for, monitor, and document the potential for suicide. (Refer the client for appropriate treatment if a potential for suicide is identified.) Refer to the care plan Risk for **Suicidal** Behavior for specific interventions. EB: *A 10-year longitudinal study found that hopelessness predicts suicidal ideation (Qiu, Klonsky, & Klein, 2017).*
- Assess and monitor potential for depression. (Refer the client for appropriate treatment if depression is identified.) EB: *Hopelessness is associated with depressive and suicidal symptoms (Hallensleben et al, 2019).*
- Assess for hopelessness with the modified Beck Hopelessness Scale. CEB: *The modified Beck Hopelessness Scale is a valid and reliable tool to measure hopelessness (Fisher & Overholser, 2013).*
- Assess and monitor family caregivers for symptoms of hopelessness. EBN: *Significant correlations were found between hopelessness and coping strategies with a positive correlation between hopelessness and the helpless approaches (Tokem, Ozcelik, & Cicik, 2015).*
- Assess for pain and respond with appropriate measures for pain relief. EB: *In the present study, hopelessness played a central role in the relationship between pain and depression with pain intensity positively related to hopelessness (Hülsebusch, Hasenbring, & Rusu, 2016).*
- Facilitate sources of the client's resilience. EB: *Resilience has a mediating role in the relationship between risk factors involved in interpersonal functioning and hopelessness (Collazzoni et al, 2020).*

- Assist the adolescent client to develop positive expectations. EB: *Research findings suggest that lack of positive expectations account for the relationship between hopelessness and future depression and suicidal behavior among adolescents (Horwitz et al, 2017).*
- Assist the client to explore the meaning of his or her life, satisfaction with his or her life, and life goals. EB: *Research shows that a higher meaning of life buffers the association between suicide risk factors and hopelessness (Marco, Pérez, & García-Alandete, 2016).*
- Encourage adolescent clients to get 9 to 10 hours of sleep nightly. EB: *Research shows that among adolescents, as little as 1 hour less of weekday sleep was associated with significantly greater odds of feeling hopeless (Winsler et al, 2015).*
- Assist the client in looking at alternatives and setting long- and short-term goals that are important to him or her. EBN: *A mixed-method thematic review found that setting and achieving goals was a theme that increased hope (Broadhurst & Harrington, 2016).*
- Explore the meanings, functions, objects, sources, and nature of hope with clients as they relate to their current situation. EBN: *A better understanding of clients' meanings of hope can assist nurses to foster hope and provide better support (Marco, Pérez, & García-Alandete, 2016).*
- Spend one-on-one time with the client. Use empathy; try to understand what the client is saying and communicate this understanding to the client to create a nonjudgmental trusting environment to develop therapeutic relationships with the client. EB: *Client ratings of the therapeutic relationship predicted social inclusion through hopefulness (Berry & Greenwood, 2015).*
- Teach alternative coping strategies such as physical activity. EB: *In a study of adults with congenital heart disease, regular physical activity was a protective factor against hopelessness (Eslami et al, 2017).*
- Use a future-directed approach that teaches individuals how to become aware of attention that is focused on unwanted aspects of life and how to redirect attention toward things that feel more wanted or desired. EB: *A study determined that the development of a future orientation led to a decline in hopelessness (Mac Giollabhui et al, 2018).*
- Review the client's strengths and resources in conjunction with the client. EBN: *A strengths-based perspective support group intervention reduced the participants' level of depressive symptoms and improved the pathway component of hope (Hou, Ko, & Shu, 2016).*
- Encourage the client to adopt active coping strategies. EB: *In a current study, proactive coping predicted hope regardless of severity of spinal cord injury (Phillips et al, 2016).*
- Implement social supports and reintegration programs for postdeployment soldiers and veterans in a timely fashion. EB: *Research determined that hopelessness was moderated by timely implementation of postdeployment support and reintegration programs (Martin et al, 2016).*
- For additional interventions, see the care plans for Readiness for Enhanced **Hope, Spiritual** Distress, Readiness for Enhanced **Spiritual** Well-Being, and Disturbed **Sleep** Pattern.

Geriatric

- Previous interventions may be adapted for geriatric clients.
- ▲ If depression is suspected, confer with the primary health care provider regarding referral for mental health services. EB: *This study of older adults found that hopelessness was a significant predictor of death ideation (Guidry & Cukrowicz, 2016).*
- Take threats of self-harm or suicide seriously and intervene as needed. EB: *This study of older adults identified hopelessness as a significant predictor of death ideation (Guidry & Cukrowicz, 2016). Older adults have the highest risk of death by suicide in the United States (Fond et al, 2016).*
- Encourage engagement in positive and pleasant events. EB: *This study found that targeting both hopelessness and engagement in pleasant events may be helpful in improving the quality of life of vulnerable, rural older adults (Scogin et al, 2016).*

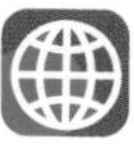

Multicultural

- Assess for the influence of cultural beliefs, norms, and values on the client's feelings of hopelessness. EB: *Research found that familial acculturative stress may exacerbate the effect of hopelessness on suicidal ideation (Lane & Miranda, 2018).*
- Assess for the effect of fatalism on the client's expression of hopelessness. EBN: *A systemic review of qualitative studies found that fatalistic perspectives were common among the cancer beliefs held by ethnic minority populations (Licqurish et al, 2017).*

- Use caution when highlighting health disparities of multicultural populations through public health campaigns and media broadcasts. EB: *This study found that media campaigns that broadcasted health disparities resulted in the targeted population feeling less hopeful about the future (Lee et al, 2017).*
- Encourage spirituality as a source of support for hopelessness. EB: *Structural equation modeling indicated that Malaysian adolescent students were high in hopelessness and depression, but were also high in spirituality and had less suicidal behavior than others (Talib & Abdollahi, 2017).*

Home Care

- Previously mentioned interventions may be adapted for home care use.
- Use in-person problem-solving therapy (PST) to address depressive symptoms and hopelessness. EB: *In-person PST reduced depressive symptoms and alleviated hopelessness in older homebound adults. PST focused on the participants' appraisal of specific problems, identification of the best possible solutions, and the practical implementation of those solutions (Choi, Marti, & Conwell, 2016).*

Client/Family Teaching and Discharge Planning

- Provide information regarding the client's condition, treatment plan, and progress. EBN: *Clients reported increased hope after a planned family-centered discharge process (Ingram et al, 2017).*
- ▲ Refer the client to self-help groups. EB: *Support groups provided an experience of community in which hope was encouraged (Behler et al, 2017).*

H

REFERENCES

Behler, J., Daniels, A., Scott, J., & Mehl-Madrona, L. (2017). Depression/bipolar peer support groups: Perceptions of group members about effectiveness and differences from other mental health services. *Qualitative Report, 22*(1), 213–236.

Berry, C., & Greenwood, K. (2015). Hope-inspiring therapeutic relationships, professional expectations and social inclusion for young people with psychosis. *Schizophrenia Research, 168*(1–2), 153–160. https://doi.org/10.1016/j.schres.2015.07.032.

Broadhurst, K., & Harrington, A. (2016). A mixed method thematic review: The importance of hope to the dying patient. *Journal of Advanced Nursing, 72*(1), 18–32. https://doi.org/10.1111/jan.12765.

Choi, N. G., Marti, C. N., & Conwell, Y. (2016). Effect of problem-solving therapy on depressed low-income homebound older adults' death/suicidal ideation and hopelessness. *Suicide Life Threat Behavior, 46*, 323–336. https://doi.org/10.1111/sltb.12195.

Collazzoni, A., Stratta, P., Pacitti, F., et al. (2020). Resilience as a mediator between interpersonal risk factors and hopelessness in depression. *Frontiers in Psychiatry, 11*, 10. https://doi.org/10.3389/fpsyt.2020.00010.

Eslami, B., Kovacs, A. H., Moons, P., Abbasi, K., & Jackson, J. L. (2017). Hopelessness among adults with congenital heart disease: Cause for despair or hope? *International Journal of Cardiology, 230*, 64–69. https://doi.org/10.1016/j.ijcard.2016.12.090.

Fisher, L. B., & Overholser, J. C. (2013). Refining the assessment of hopelessness: An improved way to look to the future. *Death Studies, 37*(3), 212–227.

Fond, G., Llorca, P. M., Boucekine, M., et al. (2016). Disparities in suicide mortality trends between United States of America and 25 European countries: Retrospective analysis of WHO Mortality Database. *Scientific Reports, 6*, 20256. https://doi.org/10.1038/srep20256.

Guidry, E. T., & Cukrowicz, K. C. (2016). Death ideation in older adults: Psychological symptoms of depression, thwarted belongingness, and perceived burdensomeness. *Aging & Mental Health, 20*(8), 823–830. https://doi.org/10.1080/13607863.2015.1040721.

Hallensleben, N., Glaesmer, H., Forkmann, T., et al. (2019). Predicting suicidal ideation by interpersonal variables, hopelessness and depression in real-time. An ecological momentary assessment study in psychiatric inpatients with depression. *European Psychiatry, 56*(1), 43–50. https://doi.org/10.1016/j.eurpsy.2018.11.003.

Horwitz, A. G., Berona, J., Czyz, E. K., Yeguez, C. E., & King, C. A. (2017). Positive and negative expectations of hopelessness as longitudinal predictors of depression, suicidal ideation, and suicidal behavior in high-risk adolescents. *Suicide and Life-Threatening Behavior, 47*, 168–176. https://doi.org/10.1111/sltb.12273.

Hou, W. L., Ko, N. Y., & Shu, B. C. (2016). Effects of a strengths-based perspective support group among Taiwanese women who left a violent intimate partner relationship. *Journal of Clinical Nursing, 25*, 543–554. https://doi.org/10.1111/jocn.13091.

Hülsebusch, J., Hasenbring, M. I., & Rusu, A. C. (2016). Understanding pain and depression in back pain: The role of catastrophizing, help-/hopelessness, and thought suppression as potential mediators. *International Journal of Behavavioral Medicine, 23*, 251. https://doi.org/10.1007/s12529-015-9522-y.

Ingram, J., Redshaw, M., Manns, S., et al. (2017). "Giving us hope": Parent and neonatal staff views and expectations of a planned family-centred discharge process (Train-to-Home). *Health Expectations, 20*, 751–759. https://doi.org/10.1111/hex.12514.

Lane, R., & Miranda, R. (2018). The effects of familial acculturative stress and hopelessness on suicidal ideation by immigration status among college students. *Journal of American College Health, 66*(2), 76–86. https://doi.org/10.1080/07448481.2017.1376673.

Lee, J. G. L., Landrine, H., Martin, R. J., Matthews, D. D., Averett, P. E., & Niederdeppe, J. (2017). Reasons for caution when emphasizing health disparities for sexual and gender minority adults in public health campaigns. *American Journal of Public Health, 107*(8), 1223–1225.

Licqurish, S., Phillipson, L., Chiang, P., Walker, J., Walter, F., & Emery, J. (2017). Cancer beliefs in ethnic minority populations: A review and meta-synthesis of qualitative studies. *European Journal of Cancer Care, 26*(1), e12556. https://doi.org/10.1111/ecc.12556.

Mac Giollabhui, N., Nielsen, J., Seidman, S., Olino, T. M., Abramson, L. Y., & Alloy, L. B. (2018). The development of future orientation is associated with faster decline in hopelessness during adolescence. *Journal of Youth and Adolescence, 47*(10), 2129–2142. https://doi.org/10.1007/s10964-017-0803-4.

Marco, J. H., Pérez, S., & García-Alandete, J. (2016). Meaning in life buffers the association between risk factors for suicide and hopelessness in participants with mental disorders. *Journal of Clinical Psychology, 72*, 689–700. https://doi.org/10.1002/jclp.22285.

Martin, R. L., Houtsma, C., Green, B. A., & Anestis, M. D. (2016). Support systems: How post-deployment support impacts suicide risk factors in the United States Army National Guard. *Cognitive Therapy and Research, 40*, 14–21. https://doi.org/10.1007/s10608-015-9719-z.

Phillips, B. N., Smedema, S. M., Fleming, A. R., Sung, C., & Allen, M. G. (2016). Mediators of disability and hope for people with spinal cord injury. *Disability & Rehabilitation, 38*(17), 1672–1683. https://doi.org/10.3109/09638288.2015.1107639.

Qiu, T., Klonsky, E. D., & Klein, D. N. (2017). Hopelessness predicts suicide ideation but not attempts: A 10-year longitudinal study. *Suicide and Life-Threatening Behavior, 47*(6), 718–722. https://doi.org/10.1111/sltb.12328.

Scogin, F., Morthland, M., DiNapoli, E. A., LaRocca, M. L., & Chaplin, W. (2016). Pleasant events, hopelessness, and quality of life in rural older adults. *Journal of Rural Health, 32*, 102–109. https://doi.org/10.1111/jrh.12130.

Talib, M. A., & Abdollahi, A. (2017). Spirituality moderates hopelessness, depression, and suicidal behavior among Malaysian adolescents. *Journal of Religion and Health, 56*, 784–795. https://doi.org/10.1007/s10943-015-0133-3.

Tokem, Y., Ozcelik, H., & Cicik, A. (2015). Examination of the relationship between hopelessness levels and coping strategies among the family caregivers of patients with cancer. *Cancer Nursing, 38*(4), E28–E34. https://doi.org/10.1097/NCC.0000000000000189.

Winsler, A., Deutsch, A., Vorona, R. D., Payne, P. A., & Szklo-Coxe, M. (2015). Sleepless in Fairfax: The difference one more hour of sleep can make for teen hopelessness, suicidal ideation, and substance use. *Journal of Youth and Adolescence, 44*(2), 362–378. https://doi.org/10.1007/s10964-014-0170-3.

Risk for Compromised Human Dignity

Domain 6 Self-perception Class 1 Self-concept

Mamilda Robinson, DNP, APN, PMHNP-BC and Kathleen L. Patusky, PhD, MA, RN, CNS

NANDA-I

Definition

Susceptible for perceived loss of respect and honor, which may compromise health.

Risk Factors

Dehumanization; disclosure of confidential information; exposure of the body; humiliation; inadequate understanding of health information; insufficient privacy; intrusion by clinician; loss of control over body function; perceived social stigma; values incongruent with cultural norms

At-Risk Population

Individuals with limited decision making experience

NOC (Nursing Outcomes Classification)

Suggested NOC Outcomes

Health Beliefs: Perceived Control; Decision-Making; Spiritual Control; Mental Control; Perceived Social Support

Example NOC Outcome with Indicators

Health Beliefs: Perceived Control as evidenced by the following indicators: Perceived responsibility for health decisions/Requested involvement in health decisions/Efforts at gathering information/Belief that own decisions control health outcomes/Willingness to designate surrogate decision maker. (Rate the outcome and indicators of **Health Beliefs: Perceived Control:** 1 = very weak, 2 = weak, 3 = moderate, 4 = strong, 5 = very strong [see Section I].)

Client Outcomes

Client/Caregiver Will (Specify Time Frame)

- Perceive that dignity is maintained throughout hospitalization/encounter
- Consistently call client by name and pronoun of choice
- Maintain client's privacy

NIC (Nursing Interventions Classification)

Suggested NIC Interventions

Presence; Decision-Making Support; Spiritual Support; Hope Instillation

Example NIC Activities—Presence

Demonstrate accepting attitude; Listen to client's concerns

Nursing Interventions and *Rationales*

- Use the person-centered approach for each client, while listening actively and addressing their individual needs. EBN: *It is important that the nurse remain cognizant of each person's health problem and recognizes their unique values. The nurse should determine why the person has developed the problem, what the individual wishes to achieve, and how the goal can best be achieved in a dignified manner (Nazarko, 2015).*
- Encourage client to enter into and stay in communication with others. Encourage connections with the inner life world of meaning and spirit of the other. Join in a mutual search for meaning and wholeness of being and becoming to potentiate comfort measures, pain control, a sense of well-being, wholeness, or even spiritual transcendence of suffering. EBN: *Human dignity is a central concept within nursing and the caring professions because it promotes client inclusivity. In a shared humanity, clients are included in professional responsibility and part of their care. Because nurses are eager to actualize the caring relationship with clients, they preserve dignity and respect integrity (Blomberg et al, 2015).*
- Determine the client's perspective about his or her health. Example questions include "Tell me about your health." "What is it like to be in your situation?" "Tell me how you perceive yourself in this situation." "What meaning are you giving to this situation?" "Tell me about your health priorities." "Tell me about the harmony you wish to reach." EBN: *Such questions usually contribute to promoting clients' dignity, as dignity has been established as one of the essential needs of those with life-threatening illnesses, as well as a measure to mediate the effect of physical symptoms on demoralization (Dose et al, 2017).*
- Determine the client's preferences for when and how nursing care is needed and follow the client's guidelines if possible. EBN: *The client's autonomy must be recognized as part of dignified nursing care. A Canadian study of decision-making during the pregnancy experience found that women reported lower autonomy when there were difficulties in communication with provider, feelings of pressure for certain interventions, and not feeling comfortable to ask the provider questions (Vedum et al, 2019).*
- Maintain the client's privacy at all times. EBN: *The results of a qualitative study found that preservation and promotion of the dignity of the client was an outcome of maintaining the privacy of hospitalized clients (Tehrani et al, 2020).*
- Encourage the client to share thoughts about spirituality and mortality as desired. EB: *The acceptance of mortality, using spirituality and mindfulness, allows clients to view themselves as mortal human beings who are supported by caring loved ones and health care professionals. When clients are dignified through this process, they gain a sense of spiritual healing despite the physicality of death (Nyatanga, 2018).*
- Use interventions to instill increased hope; see the care plan for Readiness for Enhanced **Hope.** EB: *When hope for a cure is no longer possible, clients should be reminded that despite the circumstance, they attain dignity in death that is centered to themselves and their loved ones. While dying cannot be stopped, efforts with support and instillation of hope provide comfort through the process of dying while minimizing distress in order to ensure dignity in death (Nyatanga, 2019).*
- ▲ Refer client for dignity therapy. EBN: *A systematic review and meta-analysis found that dignity therapy significantly improved dignity-related distress in existential distress domain and social support domain. The narrative summaries also indicated that dignity therapy exerted positive effects on clients' dignity, psychological well-being, and quality of life (Xiao et al, 2019).*
- See the care plan for Readiness for Enhanced **Spiritual** Well-Being.

Geriatric

- Always ask the client how he or she would like to be addressed. Avoid calling older clients "sweetie," "honey," "Gramps," "mama," or other terms that could be considered as demeaning unless this is acceptable in the client's culture or requested by the client. Appropriate forms of address and person-centered approaches must be used with older adults to maintain dignity. EB: *Addressing the client in a respectful manner promotes healthy relationships, which are important for mental well-being; this provides a sense of self-worth and belonging. The Care Act (2015) promotes person-centered outcomes as well as supporting families and older adults in order to maintain dignity along the care continuum (Stuart, 2020).*
- Treat the older client with the utmost respect, even if delirium or dementia is present with confusion. EB: *A narrative review found that providing respect to clients with dementia was a dignifying aspect of dementia care (van der Geugten & Goossensen, 2020).*

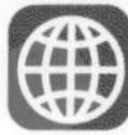

Multicultural

- Assess for the influence of cultural beliefs, norms, and values on the client's way of communicating, and follow the client's lead in communicating in matters of eye contact, amount of personal space, voice tones, and amount of touching. If in doubt, ask the client. EB: *Client dignity is promoted when staff provide privacy and use interactions that help clients feel comfortable, in control, and valued. When this is achieved, a personalized care plan can be developed with client's input to ensure dignity and support while addressing client's cultural beliefs, norms, and values (Hurtley, 2015).*
- Provide diverse clients with person-centered care that is responsive, respectful, and individualized. EB: *An Indonesian study found four major categories that described qualities of nursing care essential for maintaining a client's dignity in clinical care settings: (1) responsiveness; (2) respectful nurse–client relationships; (3) caring characteristics; and (4) personalized service. The researchers concluded that the ability to provide culturally competent care is important for nurses as a strategy to maintain client dignity during hospitalization (Asmaningrum & Tsai, 2018).*

Home Care

- Many of the previous intervention may be adapted for home care use.
- Encourage client participation in self-care and the management of one's own care process. EB: *An integrative review of client-centeredness in home care found that clients' involvement is the epicenter of successful home care. The researchers conclude that client-centeredness is supported by respect for individual persons' values, right to self-determination, mutual respect, and understanding (Sanerma et al, 2020).*

Client/Family Teaching and Discharge Planning

- Teach and support family and caregiver actions that maintain the dignity of the client. How an individual cognitively perceives and emotionally deals with the illness can depend on the person's family and social relationships, and ultimately can affect the ability to heal. EBN: *A qualitative study found that family members could identify when clients were deprived of dignity. The authors concluded that education, communication, and connections with family could prevent factors that may threaten dignified care (Sagbakken et al, 2017).*

REFERENCES

Asmaningrum, N., & Tsai, Y. –F. (2018). Patient perspectives of maintaining dignity in Indonesian clinical care settings: A qualitative descriptive study. *Journal of Advanced Nursing*, *74*(3), 591–602. https://doi.org/10.1111/jan.13469.

Blomberg, A., Bisholt, B., Nilsson, J., & Lindwall, L. (2015). Making the invisible visible—Operating theatre nurses' perceptions of caring in perioperative practice. *Scandinavian Journal of Caring Sciences*, *29*(2), 361–368. https://doi.org/10.1111/scs.12172.

Dose, A. M., Hubbard, J. M., Mansfield, A. S., McCabe, P. J., Krecke, C. A., & Sloan, J. A. (2017). Feasibility and acceptability of a dignity therapy/life plan intervention for patients with advanced cancer. *Oncology Nursing Forum*, *44*(5), E194–E202. https://doi.org/10.1188/17.ONF.E194-E202.

Hurtley, R. (2015). Ensuring dignity at the end of life: A personal perspective. *Nursing and Residential Care*, *17*(7), 380–384. https://doi.org/10.12968/nrec.2015.17.7.380.

Nazarko, L. (2015). Person-centered care of women with urinary incontinence. *Nurse Prescribing*, *13*(6), 288–293. https://doi.org/10.12968/npre.2015.13.6.288.

Nyatanga, B. (2018). Beginning with the end: The experience of dying in 2018. *British Journal of Community Nursing*, *23*(1), 48. https://doi.org/10.12968/bjcn.2018.23.1.48.

Nyatanga, B. (2019). Dignity in death: Implementing the NHS long term plan. *British Journal of Community Nursing*, *24*(3), 139. https://doi.org/10.12968/bjcn.2019.24.3.139.

Sagbakken, M., Nåden, D., Ulstein, I., Kvaal, K., Langhammer, B., & Rognstad, M. K. (2017). Dignity in people with frontotemporal dementia and similar disorders—A qualitative study of the perspective of family caregivers. *BMC Health Services Research*, *17*(1), 432. https://doi.org/10.1186/s12913-017-2378-x.

Sanerma, P., Miettinen, S., Paavilainen, E., & Åstedt-Kurki, P. (2020). A client-centered approach in home care for older persons—An integrative review. *Scandinavian Journal of Primary Health Care*, *38*(4), 369–380. https://doi.org/10.1080/02813432.2020.1841517.

Stuart, E. (2020). The importance of dining with dignity. *Journal of Community Nursing*, *34*(3), 22–23.

Tehrani, T. H., Maddah, S. S. B., Fallahi-Khoshknab, M., Shahboulaghi, F. M., & Ebadi, A. (2020). Outcomes of observance privacy in hospitalized patients: A qualitative content analysis. *Avicenna Journal of Nursing and Midwifery Care*, *27*(6), 441–450.

van der Geugten, W., & Goossensen, A. (2020). Dignifying and undignifying aspects of care for people with dementia: A narrative review. *Scandinavian Journal of Caring Sciences*, *34*(4), 818–838. https://doi.org/10.1111/scs.12791.

Vedum, S., Stoll, K., McRae, D. N., et al. (2019). Patient-led decision making: Measuring autonomy and respect in Canadian maternity care. *Patient Education and Counseling*, *102*(3), 586–594. https://doi.org/10.1016/j.pec.2018.10.023.

Xiao, J., Chow, K. M., Liu, Y., & Chan, C. W. H. (2019). Effects of dignity therapy on dignity, psychological well-being, and quality of life among palliative care cancer patients: A systematic review and meta-analysis. *Psycho-Oncology*, *28*(9), 1791–1802. https://doi.org/10.1002/pon.5162.

Neonatal Hyperbilirubinemia Domain 2 Nutrition Class 4 Metabolism

Maria Galletto, MSN, RN, CNL, CPHQ

NANDA-I

Definition

The accumulation of unconjugated bilirubin in the circulation (less than 15 mL/dL) that occurs after 24 hours of life.

Defining Characteristics

Abnormal liver function test results; bruised skin; yellow mucous membranes; yellow sclera; yellow-orange skin color

Related Factors

Delay in meconium passage; inadequate paternal feeding behavior; malnourished infants

H

At-Risk Population

East Asian neonates; low birth weight neonates; Native American neonates; Neonates aged ≤ 7 days; neonates who are breastfed; neonates whose blood groups are incompatible with mothers'; neonates whose mothers had gestational diabetes; neonates whose sibling had history of jaundice; neonates with significant bruising during birth; populations living at high altitudes; premature neonates

Associated Conditions

Bacterial infections; enzyme deficiency; impaired metabolism; internal bleeding; liver malfunction; prenatal infection; sepsis; viral infection

NOC (Nursing Outcomes Classification)

Suggested NOC Outcomes

Breastfeeding Establishment: Infant; Breastfeeding Maintenance; Bowel Elimination; Parent: Knowledge: Parenting/Infant Care; Risk Detection/Control

Example NOC Outcome with Indicators

Breastfeeding Establishment: Infant as evidenced by the following indicators: Proper alignment and latch-on/Proper areolar grasp/Proper areolar compression/Correct suck and tongue placement/Audible swallow/Minimum eight feedings per day/Urinations per day appropriate for age/Weight gain appropriate for age. (Rate the outcome and indicators of **Breastfeeding Establishment: Infant:** 1 = not adequate, 2 = slightly adequate, 3 = moderately adequate, 4 = substantially adequate, 5 = totally adequate [see Section I].)

Client Outcomes

Client (Infant) Will (Specify Time Frame)

- Establish effective feeding pattern (breast or bottle)
- Receive nursing assessments to determine risk for severity of jaundice
- Receive bilirubin assessment and screening within the first few days of life to identify potentially harmful levels of serum bilirubin
- Receive appropriate therapy to enhance indirect bilirubin excretion
- Maintain hydration: moist buccal membranes, four to six wet diapers in a 24-hour period, weight loss no greater than 10% of birth weight within the first week of life
- Evacuate stool within 48 hours of birth, and pass three or four stools per 24 hours by day 4 of life

Client (Parent[s]) Will (Specify Time Frame)

- Receive information on neonatal jaundice before discharge from birth hospital
- Verbalize understanding of physical signs of jaundice prior to discharge

- Verbalize signs requiring immediate health practitioner notification: sleepy infant who does not awaken easily for feedings, fewer than four to six wet diapers in 24-hour period by day 4, fewer than three to four stools in 24 hours by day 4, breastfeeds fewer than eight times per day
- Demonstrate ability to operate home phototherapy unit if prescribed

NIC (Nursing Interventions Classification)

Suggested NIC Interventions

Parent Education: Infant; Phototherapy: Neonate

Example NIC Activities—Phototherapy: Neonate

Review maternal and infant history for risk factors for hyperbilirubinemia (e.g., Rh or ABO incompatibility, polycythemia, sepsis, prematurity, malpresentation); Observe for signs of jaundice

H

Nursing Interventions and *Rationales*

- Evaluate maternal and delivery history for risk factors for neonatal jaundice (RhD, ABO, G6PD deficiency, direct Coombs). EB: *Assessment of maternal and neonatal risk factors that may cause jaundice is important in the detection of neonatal jaundice (Barrington & Sankaran, 2018).*
- Perform neonatal gestational age assessment once the newborn has had an initial period of interaction with mother and father. Gestational age is calculated using completed weeks of age. There are two major categories, preterm and term newborns, with further subdivisions in each category. Infants born before 34 weeks' completed gestation will be admitted to the neonatal intensive care unit (NICU). EB: *Infants who are born late preterm (34 to 36{6/7} weeks at birth) and early term (37 and 38{6/7} weeks at birth) are at significantly increased risk for problems related to hyperbilirubinemia, feeding problems, and hospital readmission (Reichman et al, 2015).*

PRETERM CATEGORY	TERM CATEGORY
Extremely preterm <28 weeks' completion	Early term 37 to 38 weeks' completion
Very preterm 28 to <32 weeks' completion	Term >38 to 42 weeks' completion
Late preterm 32 to <37 weeks' completion	Postterm >42 weeks' completion

- Encourage breastfeeding within the first hour (otherwise known as the Golden Hour) of the neonate's life. EB: *Early feedings increase neonatal intestinal activity, and infant begins establishing intestinal flora; in addition, early breastfeeding promotes enhanced maternal confidence in breastfeeding (Flaherman & Maisels, 2017).*
- Encourage skin-to-skin mother–newborn contact shortly after delivery to support the Golden Hour after birth. EB: *Early skin-to-skin mother–baby contact helps promote maternal confidence in nurturing abilities, and it is correlated with improved milk supply and milk transfer (Flaherman & Maisels, 2017).* EB: *The Golden Hour contributes to neonatal thermoregulation, decreased stress levels in a woman and her newborn, and improved mother–newborn bonding. Implementation of these actions is further associated with increased rates and duration of breastfeeding (Neczypor & Holley, 2017).*
- Encourage and assist mother with frequent breastfeeding. EB: *Increased frequency of breastfeeding accelerates weight gain and increases defecation frequency, reducing the severity of neonatal hyperbilirubinemia (Hassan & Zakerihamidi, 2018). Exclusive breastfeeding is recommended for neonatal feedings yet is associated with the development of hyperbilirubinemia and not directly as a result of the feeding substrate; perhaps it is caused by decreased caloric intake in the first week of life and a substance in breast milk that may interfere with bilirubin excretion (Flaherman & Maisels, 2017).*
- Assist parents who choose to bottle feed their neonate. EB: *Adequate caloric intake is essential for the promotion of stooling and the subsequent elimination of bilirubin from the intestine; bottle-feeding parents must be helped to optimize feedings (Hockenberry & Wilson, 2015).*
- Avoid feeding supplements such as water, dextrose water, or any other milk substitutes in breastfeeding neonate. EB: *Supplements may act to decrease the effective establishment of breastfeeding (Flaherman & Maisels, 2017).*

- Assess neonate's stooling pattern in first 48 hours of life. *Delayed stooling may indicate inadequate breast milk intake and may further increase reabsorption of bilirubin from neonate's intestine (Hockenberry, Wilson, & Rodgers, 2017).*
- Monitor infant's neurological status for any signs of emerging bilirubin encephalopathy. EB: *Initially, the infant may have lethargy, decreased activity, irritability, or poor feeding. As encephalopathy continues, the infant will develop rigid extension of extremities, fever, irritable cry, opisthotonos, and seizures (Green, 2016).*

▲ Monitor transcutaneous bilirubin level in jaundiced neonate per unit protocol. CEB/EB: *Noninvasive bilirubin monitoring is a safe and effective means for monitoring bilirubin levels and determining risk for increasing serum bilirubin levels in infants who are not treated with phototherapy (Bhutani et al, 2014; van den Esker-Jonker et al, 2016; Jain et al, 2017).*

▲ Collect and evaluate laboratory blood specimens as prescribed or per unit protocol. EB: *Because visual assessments of skin color alone are inadequate to determine rising levels of bilirubin, serum bilirubin measurement may be gathered to evaluate risk for pathology (Hockenberry, Wilson, & Rodgers, 2017). The purpose of monitoring, evaluating, and implementing treatment in moderate to severe cases of neonatal hyperbilirubinemia is to prevent acute bilirubin encephalopathy, which is an early acute central nervous system bilirubin toxicity that is related to the amount of unbound (indirect) bilirubin (Hockenberry, Wilson, & Rodgers, 2017).*

H

- Perform hour-specific total serum bilirubin (TSB) risk assessment before discharge from hospital or birth center and document the results. CEB: *The use of an hour-specific nomogram for designation of risk in healthy, late preterm, early term, and term infants, as well as clinical risk factors, may be used to determine the relative risk of rapidly increasing bilirubin levels requiring medical intervention such as phototherapy (American Academy of Pediatrics, 2004; Maisels et al, 2009). The hour-specific nomogram estimates the TSB in one of four risk zones: low risk, low intermediate risk, high intermediate risk (75th to 94th percentile), and high risk (95th percentile or greater). Infants with TSB values at or above the 75th percentile in addition to risk factors, such as preterm birth, may require medical intervention such as phototherapy (Maisels et al, 2009).*
- Monitor newborn for signs of inadequate breast milk or formula intake: dry oral mucous membranes, fewer than 4 to 6 wet diapers per 24 hours, no stool in 24 hours, and body weight loss greater than 10%. EB: *Inadequate intake of breast milk or formula in the neonatal period has been identified as a risk factor for the development of hyperbilirubinemia (Flaherman & Maisels, 2017).*
- Assess late preterm infant (born between 34 and 37 weeks' gestation) for ability to breastfeed successfully and adequate intake of breast milk. EB: *Late preterm infants are at higher risk for difficulty breastfeeding and suboptimal milk intake caused by physiological immaturity; thus such infants are also at a much higher risk for severe jaundice than term counterparts (Reichman et al, 2015; Barrington & Sankaran, 2018).*
- Assist mother with breastfeeding and assess latch-on. EB: *Successful breastfeeding in the first few weeks of life is associated with decreased levels of serum bilirubin (Flaherman & Maisels, 2017).* See Readiness for Enhanced **Breastfeeding.**
- Encourage alternate methods for providing expressed breast milk if maternal health status is compromised, such as assisting the mother with collection of breast milk via use of breast pump or hand expression. EB: *Alternate feeding methods for the ingestion of breast milk may be used to enhance milk intake necessary to promote stooling and enhance bilirubin excretion (Flaherman & Maisels, 2017).*
- Encourage partner's participation in newborn care by changing diapers, helping position newborn for breastfeeding, and holding newborn while mother rests. EB: *Paternal involvement in the care of the newborn helps solidify the father's role as a parent and strengthens the paternal–infant attachment process; paternal participation also helps the mother rest during the recovery from labor and delivery (Hockenberry & Wilson, 2015).*
- Weigh newborn daily. EB: *Daily weights assist in the detection of excess weight loss, which is often indicative of inadequate caloric intake (Flaherman & Maisels, 2017).*

▲ When phototherapy is ordered, place seminude infant (diaper only) under prescribed amount of phototherapy lights. CEB: *Phototherapy is the primary therapy used to treat mild to moderate neonatal indirect (unconjugated) hyperbilirubinemia; the infant must have a large skin surface area exposed to the light source for optimal effectiveness (Hockenberry, Wilson, & Rodgers, 2017).*

- Protect infant's eyes from phototherapy light source with eye shields; remove eye shields periodically when infant is removed from light source for feeding and parent–infant interaction. EB: *There is no evidence that removing the infant for parent–infant interaction during feedings and for brief caregiving activities prevents the effectiveness of phototherapy when the infant has mild to moderate hyperbilirubinemia (Hockenberry, Wilson, & Rodgers, 2017).*

- Monitor infant's hydration status, fluid intake, skin status, and body temperature while undergoing phototherapy. EB: *Transient side effects of phototherapy include increased body temperature, increased insensible water loss, increased gastrointestinal water loss (loose stools), lethargy, irritability, and poor feeding (Hockenberry, Wilson, & Rodgers, 2017).*
- ▲ Collect and evaluate laboratory blood specimens (TSB) while infant is undergoing phototherapy. CEB/EB: *Transcutaneous bilirubin measurements do not provide an adequate estimate of serum bilirubin level and are not effective once phototherapy has been initiated (American Academy of Pediatrics, 2004; Hockenberry, Wilson, & Rodgers, 2017). All bilirubin levels should be interpreted based on the newborn's age in hours (Hartman et al, 2018).*
- Encourage continuation of breastfeeding and brief infant care activities such as changing diapers while the infant is being treated with phototherapy; phototherapy may be interrupted for breastfeeding. EB: *Phototherapy can be used while continuing full breastfeeding, or it can be combined with supplementation of expressed breast milk or infant formula if maternal supply is insufficient. Only in extenuating circumstances is temporary interruption of breastfeeding with replacement feeding necessary (Flaherman & Maisels, 2017).*
- Provide emotional support for parents of infants undergoing phototherapy. EB: *Separation of the infant from the mother for phototherapy disrupts parent–infant interaction and may promote parental stress and decrease the effective establishment of breastfeeding (Hockenberry, Wilson, & Rodgers, 2017).* EBN: *The nursing staff must be prepared to hear and guide mothers throughout phototherapy, taking into consideration that it is a negative experience during the newborn hospitalization (de Souza Fernandes et al, 2016).*
- Provide for novel therapies that can be used in tandem with phototherapy to support parent–infant interaction during treatment. EB: *Massage therapy had significant effects on TSB levels, feeding, breastfeeding, defecation, and urination in newborns who received phototherapy for indirect hyperbilirubinemia (Korkmaz & Esenay, 2020).* EB: *Kangaroo Mother Care: Out of five trials, two trials reported a significant reduction in bilirubin and three trials reported a significant reduction in duration of phototherapy (Garg, Bansal, & Kabra, 2020).*

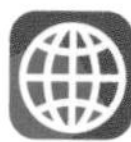

Multicultural

- Assess infants of Southeast Asian or Far East Asian and American Indian ethnicity for early rising bilirubin levels, especially when breastfeeding. EB: *Studies have shown Asian and American Indian newborns to have higher peak serum bilirubin levels than Caucasian and African American newborns (Hockenberry, Wilson, & Rodgers, 2017).* EB: *Mutations of the* UGT1A1 *gene have been shown to be linked to an increased risk of neonatal hyperbilirubinemia in Asian populations compared with white populations (Bentz et al, 2018).*

Client/Family Teaching and Discharge Planning

- Teach parents the signs of inadequate milk intake: fewer than three to four stools per day by day 4, fewer than four to six wet diapers in 24 hours, and dry oral mucous membranes; additional danger signs include a sleepy baby that does not awaken for breastfeeding or appears lethargic (decreased activity level from usual newborn pattern). EB: *Providing information about jaundice and effective breastfeeding may serve to decrease risk factors associated with increasing bilirubin levels (Flaherman & Maisels, 2017).*
- Teach parents about the transition in stool color and consistency starting with meconium, followed by green, seedy stool, to mustard-colored, seedy stool by the fourth day of life. EB: *Signs of adequate intake in breastfed infants include a transition to seedy, mustard-colored stools by the third or fourth day of life (Muchowski, 2014).*
- ▲ Teach parents and support persons about the appearance of jaundice (yellow or orange color of skin) after hospital or birth center discharge. Teach parents about the importance of medical follow-up in the first several days of life for the evaluation of jaundice. EB: *Most newborns who are discharged before 72 hours of age should have a follow-up visit in 2 days; a newborn who has a recognized risk factor for a health problem should be seen sooner (Hartman et al, 2018).*
- Teach parent about the use of phototherapy (hospital or home, as prescribed); the proper use of the phototherapy equipment; feedings; and assessment of hydration, body temperature, skin status, and urine and stool output. EB: *Provide information to the parents of the infant undergoing phototherapy to prevent misinformation about the infant's condition and treatment and to decrease parental anxiety and stress (Hockenberry & Wilson, 2015).* EBN: *Home-based phototherapy was more effective than hospital-based phototherapy in treatment of neonatal hyperbilirubinemia (Chu, Qiao, & Xu, 2020).*

REFERENCES

American Academy of Pediatrics. (2004). Management of hyperbilirubinemia in the newborn infant 35 or more weeks of gestation. *Pediatrics, 114*(1), 297–316.

Barrington, K. J., & Sankaran, K. (2018). The Canadian Paediatric Society Position Statement: Guidelines for detection, management and prevention of hyperbilirubinemia in term and late preterm newborn infants. Retrieved from https://www.cps.ca/en/documents/position/hyperbilirubinemia-newborn. Accessed 6 July 2021.

Bentz, M. G., Carmona, N., Bhagwat, M. M., et al. (2018). Beyond "Asian": Specific East and Southeast Asian races or ethnicities associated with jaundice readmission. *Hospital Pediatrics, 8*(5), 269–273. https://doi.org/10.1542/hpeds.2017-0234.

Bhutani, V. K., & Committee on Fetus and Newborn, & American Academy of Pediatrics. (2014). Phototherapy to prevent severe neonatal hyperbilirubinemia in the newborn infant 35 or more weeks of gestation. *Pediatrics,* 128(4), e1046–e1052. *Reaffirmed, 134*(3), e920.

Chu, L., Qiao, J., & Xu, C. (2020). Home-based phototherapy versus hospital-based phototherapy for treatment of neonatal hyperbilirubinemia: A systematic review and meta-analysis. *Clinical Pediatrics, 59*(6), 588–595. https://doi.org/10.1177/0009922820916894.

de Souza Fernandes, J. I., Teixeira Reis, A., da Silva, C. V., & Peixoto da Silva, A. (2016). Motherly challenges when facing neonatal phototherapy treatment: A descriptive study. *Online Brazilian Journal of Nursing, 15*(2), 188–195.

Flaherman, V. J., & Maisels, M. J. (2017). Academy of Breastfeeding Medicine clinical protocol #22: Guidelines for management of jaundice in the breastfeeding infant 35 weeks or more of gestation. *Breastfeeding Medicine, 12*(5), 250–257. doi:10.1089/bfm.2017.29042.vjf.

Garg, B. D., Bansal, A., & Kabra, N. S. (2020). Role of Kangaroo mother care in the management of neonatal hyperbilirubinemia in both term and preterm neonates: A systematic review. *The Journal of Perinatal Education, 29*(3), 123–133. http://dx.doi.org/10.1891/J-PE-D-18-00043.

Green, C. (2016). *Maternal newborn nursing care plans* (3rd ed.). Jones & Bartlett Learning.

Hartman, S., Loomis, E., Russell, H., & Brown, E. (2018). A guide to providing wide-ranging care to newborns. *Journal of Family Practice, 67*(4), E4–E15.

Hassan, B., & Zakerihamidi, M. (2018). The correlation between frequency and duration of breastfeeding and the severity of neonatal hyperbilirubinemia. *Journal of Maternal-Fetal and Neonatal Medicine, 31*(4), 457–463.

Hockenberry, M. J., & Wilson, D. (2015). *Wong's nursing care of infants and children* (10th ed.). St. Louis: Elsevier.

Hockenberry, M. J., Wilson, D., & Rodgers, C. C. (2017). *Wong's essentials of pediatric nursing* (10th ed.). St. Louis: Elsevier.

Jain, M., Bang, A., Tiwari, A., & Jain, S. (2017). Prediction of significant hyperbilirubinemia in term neonates by early non-invasive bilirubin measurement. *World J Pediatrics, 13*(3), 222–227.

Korkmaz, G., & Esenay, F. I. (2020). Effects of massage therapy on indirect hyperbilirubinemia in newborns who receive phototherapy. *Journal of Obstetric, Gynecologic, and Neonatal Nursing, 49*(1), 91–100. https://doi.org/10.1016/j.jogn.2019.11.004.

Maisels, M. J., Bhutani, V. K., Bogen, D., Newman, T. B., Stark, A. R., & Watchko, J. F. (2009). Hyperbilirubinemia in the newborn infant ≥35 weeks' gestation: An update with clarifications. *Pediatrics, 124*(4), 1193–1198.

Muchowski, K. E. (2014). Evaluation and treatment of neonatal hyperbilirubinemia. *American Family Physician, 89*(11), 873–878.

Neczypor, J. L., & Holley, S. L. (2017). Providing evidence-based care during the golden hour. *Nursing for Women's Health, 21*(6), 462–472. https://doi.org/10.1016/j.nwh.2017.10.011.

Reichman, N. E., Teitler, J. O., Moullin, S., Ostfeld, B. M., & Hegyi, T. (2015). Late-preterm birth and neonatal morbidities: Population-level and within-family estimates. *Annals of Epidemiology, 25*(2), 126–132.

van den Esker-Jonker, B., den Boer, L., Pepping, R. M. C., & Bekhof, J. (2016). Transcutaneous bilirubinometry in jaundiced neonates: A randomized controlled trial. *Pediatrics, 138*(6), e20162414. pii:e20162414.

H

Risk for Neonatal Hyperbilirubinemia

Domain 2 Nutrition Class 4 Metabolism

Maria Galletto, MSN, RN, CNL, CPHQ

NANDA-I

Definition

Susceptible to the accumulation of unconjugated bilirubin in the circulation (less than 15 ml/dl) that occurs after 24 hours of life, which may compromise health.

Risk Factors

Delay in meconium passage; inadequate paternal feeding behavior; malnourished infants

At-Risk Population

East Asian neonates; low birth weight neonates; Native American neonates; neonates aged ≤7 days; neonates who are breastfed; neonates whose blood groups are incompatible with mothers'; neonates whose mothers had gestational diabetes; neonates whose sibling had history of jaundice; neonates with significant bruising during birth; populations living at high altitudes; premature neonates

Associated Conditions

Bacterial infections; enzyme deficiency; impaired metabolism; internal bleeding; liver malfunction; prenatal infection; sepsis; viral infection

NOC (Nursing Outcomes Classification)

See care plan for Neonatal **Hyperbilirubinemia** for suggested NOC outcomes.

Client Outcomes

Client Will (Specify Time Frame)

- Neonatal total serum bilirubin (TSB) will be monitored and there will be no undetected TSB values in the high-risk (95th percentile or greater) or high-intermediate risk (75th to 94th percentile) zones (as determined by the hour-specific nomogram)
- Newborn will receive appropriate therapies to enhance bilirubin excretion
- Receive bilirubin assessment and screening within the first 24 hours of life with higher risk infants being reevaluated every 24 hours to detect increasing levels of serum bilirubin
- Receive nursing assessments to determine risk for severity of jaundice prior to discharge from birth hospital and schedule return clinic visit within 2 days of discharge for higher risk neonates
- Establish effective on-demand feeding pattern at least every 2 to 3 hours (breast or bottle)
- Maintain hydration: moist buccal membranes, four to six wet diapers in a 24-hour period, weight loss no greater than 10% of birth weight
- Evacuate stool within 48 hours of birth, and pass three to four stools per 24 hours by day 4 of life

NIC (Nursing Interventions Classification)

- See the care plan for Neonatal **Hyperbilirubinemia** for suggested NIC interventions.

Nursing Interventions and *Rationales*

- Identify clinical risk factors that place the infant at greater risk for development of neonatal jaundice: exclusive breastfeeding, isoimmune or hemolytic disease, preterm birth (37{6/7} weeks' gestation or less), weight loss of 10% or more from birth weight within the first week, neonatal sepsis, maternal diabetes, maternal obesity, previous sibling with jaundice, East Asian ethnicity, and significant bruising or cephalohematoma. EB: *Breastfeeding is often associated with a higher bilirubin level than is seen in infants fed formula exclusively; increasing the frequency of feeding usually reduces the bilirubin level (Flaherman & Maisels, 2017;. Hartman et al, 2018).* EB: *Preterm is defined as babies born before 37 weeks of pregnancy are completed. The subcategories of preterm birth are extremely preterm (less than 28 weeks), very preterm (28–32 weeks), and moderate to late preterm (32–37 weeks) (World Health Organization, 2018).*
- Measure transcutaneous bilirubin (TcB) of all newborns in the first 24 to 48 hours of life, using a noninvasive transcutaneous bilirubinometer. Plot TcB on a nomogram standardized for the appropriate client population; determine newborn's risk of subsequent significant hyperbilirubinemia. EB: *Transcutaneous measurement of bilirubin, in conjunction with use of a nomogram standardized for the appropriate client population, has been demonstrated to be an accurate predictor of subsequent hyperbilirubinemia (Jain et al, 2017). The use of TcB in jaundiced neonates is safe and results in a significant reduction of phlebotomy for serum bilirubin measurement (van den Esker-Jonker et al, 2016).*
- Refer to care plan for Neonatal **Hyperbilirubinemia** for additional interventions for multicultural and discharge planning.

Client/Family Teaching and Discharge Planning

- ▲ Teach parents about the importance of medical follow-up in the first several days of life for the evaluation of jaundice, especially in the late preterm infant. EB: *Late preterm infants (34–36 weeks' gestation) are at much greater risk for hyperbilirubinemia than infants born at term (37–41 weeks' gestation) and should be followed closely in the first few weeks of life (Reichman et al, 2015).*
- Refer to care plan for Neonatal **Hyperbilirubinemia** for additional interventions.

REFERENCES

Flaherman, V. J., & Maisels, M. J. (2017). Academy of Breastfeeding Medicine clinical protocol #22: Guidelines for management of jaundice in the breastfeeding infant 35 weeks or more of gestation. *Breastfeeding Medicine*, *12*(5), 250–257. http://dx.doi.org/10.1089/bfm.2017.29042.vjf.

Hartman, S., Loomis, E., Russell, H., & Brown, E. (2018). A guide to providing wide-ranging care to newborns. *Journal of Family Practice*, *67*(4), E4–E15.
Jain, M., Bang, A., Tiwari, A., & Jain, S. (2017). Prediction of significant hyperbilirubinemia in term neonates by early non-invasive bilirubin measurement. *World Journal of Pediatrics*, *13*(3), 222–227.
Reichman, N. E., Teitler, J. O., Moullin, S., Ostfeld, B. M., & Hegyi, T. (2015). Late-preterm birth and neonatal morbidities: Population-level and within-family estimates. *Annals of Epidemiology*, *25*(2), 126–132.
van den Esker-Jonker, B., den Boer, L., Pepping, R. M. C., & Bekhof, J. (2016). Transcutaneous bilirubinometry in jaundiced neonates: A randomized controlled trial. *Pediatrics*, *138*(6), e20162414. http://dx.doi.org/10.1542/peds.2016-2414.
World Health Organization (WHO). (2018). *Preterm birth, key facts*. Retrieved from https://www.who.int/news-room/fact-sheets/detail/preterm-birth. Accessed July 6, 2021.

Hyperthermia Domain 11 Safety/protection Class 6 Thermoregulation

Rosemary Timmerman, DNP, APRN, CCNS, CCRN-CSC-CMC

H

NANDA-I

Definition

Core body temperature above the normal diurnal range due to failure of thermoregulation.

Defining Characteristics

Abnormal posturing; apnea; coma; flushed skin; hypotension; infant does not maintain suck; irritable mood; lethargy; seizure; skin warm to touch; stupor; tachycardia; tachypnea; vasodilation

Related Factors

Dehydration; inappropriate clothing; vigorous activity

At-Risk Population

Individuals exposed to high environmental temperature

Associated Conditions

Decreased sweat response; impaired health status; increased metabolic rate; ischemia; pharmaceutical preparations; sepsis; trauma

NOC (Nursing Outcomes Classification)

Suggested NOC Outcomes

Thermoregulation; Thermoregulation: Newborn

Example NOC Outcome with Indicators

Thermoregulation as evidenced by the following indicators: Increased skin temperature/Decreased skin temperature/Skin color changes/Dehydration/Hyperthermia. (Rate the outcome and indicators of **Thermoregulation:** 1 = severe, 2 = substantial, 3 = moderate, 4 = mild, 5 = none [see Section I].)

Client Outcomes

Client Will (Specify Time Frame)

- Maintain core body temperature within adaptive levels (<40°C [104°F])
- Remain free of complications of malignant hyperthermia
- Remain free of complication of neuroleptic malignant syndrome
- Remain free of dehydration
- Remain free from infection
- Verbalize signs and symptoms of heat stroke and actions to prevent heat stroke
- Verbalize personal risks for malignant hyperthermia and neuroleptic malignant syndrome to be reported during health history reviews to all health care professionals, including pharmacists

NIC (Nursing Interventions Classification)

Suggested NIC Interventions

Fever Treatment; Malignant Hyperthermia Precautions; Temperature Regulation

Example NIC Activities—Hyperthermia Treatment

Monitor core body temperature using appropriate device; Monitor for abnormalities in mental status

Nursing Interventions and *Rationales*

Temperature Measurement

- ● Recognize that hyperthermia is a rise in body temperature above 40°C (104°F) that is not regulated by the hypothalamus, resulting in an uncontrolled increase in body temperature exceeding the body's ability to lose heat. EB: *It is a medical emergency (Gaudio & Grissom, 2016; Nakajima, 2016).*
- ● Continually measure a client's core temperature with a distal esophageal probe or obtain near core body temperature measurements with a rectal or bladder temperature probe and verify with a second method. EBN: *Obtaining an accurate core body temperature is essential for detecting heat stroke and monitoring the client's response to treatment; if a core temperature reading is not available or practical, a rectal or bladder temperature measurement provides a closer approximation of the core body temperature than temporal, axillary, oral, aural, or skin measurements (Lipman et al, 2019).* CEB: *Research is limited on the accuracy of temporal artery measurements outside normal ranges; axillary temperature is accurate in neonates but is not well supported in adults, and tympanic membrane measurements and chemical dot thermometers are least accurate and should be avoided in caring for the acutely ill adult client (Niven et al, 2015; Syrkin-Nikolau et al, 2017).*
- ● Use the same site and method (device) for temperature measurement for a given client so that temperature trends are assessed accurately; record site of temperature measurement. EBN/CEB: *There are differences in temperature depending on the site from which temperature measurement is obtained; however, differences between sites should not be greater than 0.3°C to 0.5°C (approximately 0.5°F–0.9°F) (Bridges & Thomas, 2009; Makic et al, 2011).*
- ▲ Work with the health care provider to help determine the cause of the temperature increase (hyperthermia), which will often help direct appropriate treatment. EB: *It is important to treat the underlying cause of the temperature to preserve neurological function of the client as well as implement interventions to rapidly lower the core temperature (Niven et al, 2015; Gaudio & Grissom, 2016).*
- ● Refer to care plan for Ineffective **Thermoregulation** for interventions managing fever (pyrexia).

Heat Stroke

- ● Recognize that heat stroke may be separated into two categories: classic and exertional. EB: *Classic heat stroke usually involves the very young or older client during environmental heat waves. Exertional heat stroke occurs in young adults performing strenuous physical activity in hot climates (Gaudio & Grissom, 2016; Knapik & Epstein, 2019).*
- ● Watch for risk factors for classic heat stroke, which include the following (Gaudio & Grissom, 2016; Knapik & Epstein, 2019):
    - ❍ Medications, especially diuretics, anticholinergic agents, beta-blockers, calcium channel blockers, anti-Parkinson's medications, antidepressants, thyroid agonists, and antihistamines
    - ❍ City dwellers who reside on top floors of buildings
    - ❍ Alcoholism
    - ❍ Diabetes mellitus
    - ❍ Mental illness
    - ❍ Obesity
    - ❍ Heart disease
    - ❍ Renal disease

  EB: *Physiologic effects of aging include lower onset of sweating and rate of sweating needed to help with dissipation of body heat; medications can dehydrate the client and blunt the physiologic responses necessary to assist with heat dissipation, increasing the risk of heat stroke in older clients (Gaudio & Grissom, 2016; Lipman et al, 2019).*

- Risk factors of exertional heat stroke include the following (Gaudio & Grissom, 2016; Lipman et al, 2019):
  - Preexisting illness
  - Drug use (e.g., alcohol, amphetamines, ecstasy)
  - Wearing protective clothing (uniforms and athletic gear) that limits heat dissipation
  - Obesity
  - Low physical fitness
  - Lack of sleep

  EB: *Recognize signs and symptoms of hyperthermia: core body temperature greater than 40°C (104°F), exercise-associated muscle cramps, tachycardia, tachypnea, orthostatic dizziness, weakness, fatigue, ataxia, vomiting, headache, confusion, delirium, seizures, coma, acute kidney injury (rhabdomyolysis), and hot dry skin (classic heat stroke) (Knapik & Epstein, 2019; Lipman et al, 2019).*
- Recognize that antipyretic agents are of little use in treatment of hyperthermia. EB: *Because the cause of the hyperthermia does not involve the hypothalamus, antipyretic agents are ineffective and not indicated in treatment of clients with hyperthermia (Leyk et al, 2019; Lipman et al, 2019).*

▲ Assess fluid loss and facilitate oral intake or administer intravenous fluids as prescribed to accomplish fluid replacement and support the cardiovascular system. EB: *Increased metabolic rate, diuresis, and diaphoresis-associated exertional hyperthermia cause loss of body fluids (Leyk et al, 2019; Lipman et al, 2019).* Refer to the care plan for Deficient **Fluid** Volume.

▲ Recognize use of alpha-adrenergic agents should be avoided if possible. EB: *Alpha-adrenergic agonist agents cause cutaneous vasoconstriction, which impairs cooling (Gaudio & Grissom, 2016).*

- Remove clothing and immerse young and healthy clients who have suffered exertional heat stroke in a cold water bath ensuring the head does not go underwater, or continuously douse the client with cold water. EB: *Cold water immersion rapidly cools the core temperature because of the high thermal conductivity of water but may not be practical because of client agitation and limited access for cardiovascular monitoring (Knapick & Epstein, 2019; Lipman et al, 2019).*
- For clients with classic heat stroke, remove clothes and spray or douse the skin with water and provide continual airflow over the body with a fan. EB: *Wetting the skin and directing airflow over the body promotes evaporative and convective cooling; this method is less effective for clients with exertional heat stroke (Cheshire, 2016; Lipman et al, 2019).*

▲ Recognize adjunctive cooling measures include administering cold (4°C [39.2°F]) intravenous fluids, ice sheeting (covering client with bed linens that have been soaked in ice water), water circulating hydrogel coated pads placed over the chest and legs, ice packs over the entire body, intravascular cooling catheter, and cooling blankets. EB: *There is insufficient evidence to recommend using adjunctive measures as a primary cooling method (Bursey et al, 2019; Lipman et al, 2019).*

▲ Continuously monitor the effects of cooling measures, stop cooling interventions once the body temperature is less than 39°C [102.2°F] , and benzodiazepines may be administered to control shivering. EB/EBN: *Hyperthermia must be treated aggressively to lower the body temperature to below 40°C [104°F] within 30 minutes; however, overshooting of the cooling process with resultant hypothermia must be prevented and avoidance of shivering is essential because of the associated increase in heat production, oxygen consumption, and cardiorespiratory effort (Leyk et al, 2019; Lipman et al, 2019).*

▲ Continually assess the client's neurologic and other organ function, especially kidney function (i.e., signs of rhabdomyolysis), for signs of injury from hyperthermia. EB/EBN: *Hyperthermia can cause permanent neurological injury, acute kidney injury, electrolyte imbalances, and coagulation disorders so continuous assessment of neurological and other organ function is essential (Knapik & Epstein, 2019; Lipman et al, 2019).*

Malignant Hyperthermia

▲ If the client has just received general anesthesia, especially halothane, sevoflurane, desflurane, enflurane, isoflurane, or succinylcholine, recognize that the hyperthermia may be caused by malignant hyperthermia and requires immediate treatment to prevent death. EB: *Malignant hyperthermia is often a fatal disease and must be treated promptly with rapid administration of the medication dantrolene, increasing oxygenation, assisting ventilation, initiating external cooling measures, and treating acid-base (e.g., metabolic acidosis) and electrolyte disorders (Riazi et al, 2018; Cieniewicz et al, 2019; Malignant Hyperthermia Association of the United States [MHAUS], 2020).*

- Monitor core temperature for all clients receiving general anesthetic agents for longer than 30 minutes. EB/EBN: *Hyperthermia typically occurs 30 minutes after induction of anesthesia and is associated with a higher mortality rate (Cieniewicz et al, 2019; MHAUS, 2020).*
- Recognize that signs and symptoms of malignant hyperthermia typically occur suddenly after exposure to the anesthetic agent and include rapid rise in core body temperature (as much as 1°C–2°C every 5 minutes [approximately 1.8°F–3.6°F]), hypercarbia (increase in end tidal carbon dioxide), muscle rigidity, masseter muscle spasm, dysrhythmias, tachycardia, tachypnea, rhabdomyolysis, acute kidney injury, and elevated serum calcium and potassium, progressing to disseminated intravascular coagulation and cardiac arrest (Riazi et al, 2018; Cieniewicz et al, 2019).
- ▲ If the client has malignant hyperthermia, begin treatment as prescribed, including cessation of the anesthetic agent and intravenous administration of dantrolene sodium, STAT, along with cooling measures, core body temperature monitoring, hyperventilation with 100% oxygen, antidysrhythmics, and continued support of the cardiovascular system. EB: *Dantrolene helps decrease the increased muscle activity associated with malignant hyperthermia and can be lifesaving (Cieniewicz et al, 2019; Riazi et al, 2018).*
- ▲ Recognize that dysrhythmias must not be treated with calcium channel blockers (e.g., verapamil) when the client has malignant hyperthermia. EB: *Calcium channel blockers in combination with dantrolene can lead to cardiac arrest (Riazi et al, 2018; Cieniewicz et al, 2019).*
- ▲ Recognize that antipyretics are not recommended. EB: *Antipyretics will not be effective for malignant hyperthermia because the hypothalamic set point is normal (Riazi et al, 2018; Cieniewicz et al, 2019).*
- Monitor for reoccurrence of malignant hyperthermia symptoms that correlates with the half-life of dantrolene, typically within 16 hours (Cieniewicz et al, 2019; MHAUS, 2020).
- Provide client and family education when malignant hyperthermia occurs because it is an inherited muscle disorder. EB: *Obtaining a thorough health history, including family history of adverse experiences with anesthesia or muscle disorders, is important in identifying clients at risk for malignant hyperthermia. Genetic counseling may also be indicated (Riazi et al, 2018; MHAUS, 2020).*

H

Neuroleptic Malignant Syndrome

- ▲ Recognize that neuroleptic malignant syndrome is a rare condition associated with clients who are taking typical and atypical antipsychotic agents or after abrupt discontinuation of dopaminergic agonist agents used for Parkinson's disorder (Pileggi & Cook, 2016; Ware et al, 2018). EB/EBN: *The most common agents associated with the condition are dopamine-2 inhibiting antipsychotic agents (e.g., haloperidol, fluphenazine, chlorpromazine, quetiapine, risperidone, olanzapine, aripiprazole, asenapine, clozapine, iloperidone, paliperidone, ziprasidone) and dopamine antagonists (e.g., metoclopramide, promethazine, prochlorperazine, droperidol); sudden cessation of dopamine agonists (amantadine, levodopa, lithium, and bromocriptine) has also been associated with neuroleptic malignant syndrome (Pileggi & Cook, 2016; Ware et al, 2018).*
- Watch for signs and symptoms that can range from mild to severe and include a sudden change in mental status, rapid rise in body temperature, muscle rigidity (lead pipe), tachycardia, tachypnea, elevated or labile blood pressure, diaphoresis, urinary incontinence rhabdomyolysis, and acute kidney injury (Kollmann-Camaiora et al, 2017; van Rensburg & Decloedt, 2019).
- ▲ Begin treatment when diagnosed, including cessation of the neuroleptic or dopamine antagonist agent or resumption of dopamine agonist agent that may have been abruptly discontinued; order administration of dantrolene, bromocriptine, amantadine, or benzodiazepine; initiate cooling measures; continue support of the cardiovascular, pulmonary, and renal systems; and electroconvulsive therapy if drug therapy fails or for severe symptoms (Kollmann-Camaiora et al, 2017; van Rensburg & Decloedt; 2019).
- A client health history that reports extrapyramidal reaction to any medication should be further explored for risk of neuroleptic malignant syndrome because this syndrome can occur at any time during a client's treatment with typical and atypical antipsychotic agents (Kollmann-Camaiora et al, 2017; Ware et al, 2018).
- Recognize that clients receiving rapid dose escalation of antipsychotic agents (e.g., haloperidol) intramuscularly for acute treatment of delirium may be at increased risk for neuroleptic malignant syndrome (Kollmann-Camaiora et al, 2017; Ware et al, 2018).

Drug Fever

- Recognize an elevated body temperature in response to a medication ranges from 37.2°C to 42.2°C [98.7°F–108°F) with a typical onset from 7 to 10 days after initiating the medication (Maddock & Connor, 2020).

- Recognize individuals suffering from a drug fever will appear clinically well with a lower heart rate relative to the body temperature (relative bradycardia) but may have a maculopapular rash, headache, myalgias, and an elevated eosinophil count (Maddock & Connor, 2020).
- ▲ Medications most commonly responsible for a drug fever include antimicrobials, antineoplastic agents, anticonvulsants, antiarrhythmics, and dexmedetomidine. **EB:** *Stopping the responsible medication should result in resolution of the fever within 72 hours; if the offending medication is not readily apparent all nonessential medications should be discontinued (Maddock & Connor, 2020).*

Pediatric

- Assess risk factors of malignant hyperthermia including a personal or family history of anesthesia-related complications or death or a history of muscle disorders. **EB:** *There is an increased prevalence of malignant hyperthermia in the pediatric population, and the administration of inhalation anesthesia and succinylcholine is common in this age group (Riazi et al, 2018; MHAUS, 2020).*
- ▲ Administer dantrolene, provide oxygen and assist with ventilation, monitor heart rate and rhythm, and treat electrolyte and acid-base disorders (i.e., metabolic acidosis) as ordered if malignant hyperthermia is present. **EB:** *Dantrolene and airway management/support are necessary during emergent treatment of malignant hyperthermia (MHAUS, 2020).*

H

Geriatric

- Help the client seek medical attention immediately if elevated core temperature is present. To diagnose the hyperthermia, assess for possible precipitating factors, including changes in medication, environmental changes, and recent medical interventions or infectious exposures. **EB:** *Older adults are more susceptible to environmentally and medication-induced hyperthermia because of the greater incidence of underlying chronic medical conditions that impair thermal regulation or prevent removal from a hot environment (Jain et al, 2018; Leyk et al, 2019).*
- In hot weather, encourage the client to wear lightweight cotton clothing (Jain et al, 2018; Leyk et al, 2019).
- Provide education on the importance of drinking eight glasses of fluid per day (within their cardiac and renal reserves) regardless of whether they are thirsty, wearing appropriate clothing for the environmental temperature, keeping the head covered, staying home in the afternoon, and avoiding direct sunlight and sitting in a parked vehicle in the sun; assess for the need for and presence of fans or air conditioning. **EB:** *Older adults are more susceptible to a hot environment than younger adults because of a decreased sensitivity to heat, decreased sweat gland function, decreased thirst, and decreased mobility (Jain et al, 2018; Leyk et al, 2019).*
- In hot weather, monitor the older client for signs of heat stroke such as rising temperature, orthostatic blood pressure drop, weakness, restlessness, mental status changes, faintness, thirst, nausea, and vomiting. If signs are present, move the client to a cool place, have the client lie down, give sips of water, check orthostatic blood pressure, spray with lukewarm water, cool with a fan, and seek medical assistance immediately. **EB:** *Older adults are predisposed to heat exhaustion and should be watched carefully for occurrence; if present, it should be treated promptly (Jain et al, 2018; Lipman et al, 2019).*
- During warm weather, help the client obtain a fan or an air conditioner to increase evaporation, as needed. Help the older client locate a cool environment to which they can go for safety in hot weather.
- Take the temperature of the older client in hot weather. **EB:** *Older clients may not be able to tell that they are hot because of decreased sensation.*

Home Care

- Some of the interventions described previously may be adapted for home care use.
- Determine whether the client or family has a functioning thermometer, and know how to use it. Refer to the previous interventions on taking a temperature.
- Help the client and caregivers prevent and monitor for heat stroke/hyperthermia during times of high outdoor temperatures. **EB:** *Preventive measures include minimizing time spent outdoors, use of air conditioning or fans, increasing fluid intake, and taking frequent rest periods (Centers for Disease Control and Prevention [CDC], 2020).*
- To prevent heat-related injury in athletes, laborers, and military personnel, instruct them to acclimate gradually to the higher temperatures, increase fluid intake, wear vapor-permeable clothing, and take frequent rests (Knapick & Epstein, 2019; CDC, 2020).

- In the event of temperature elevation above the adaptive range, institute measures to decrease temperature (e.g., get the client out of the sun and into a cool place, remove excess clothing, have the client drink fluids, spray the client with lukewarm water, fan with cool air, initiate emergency transport). EB: *Hyperthermia is an acute and possibly life-threatening situation (Lipman et al, 2019; CDC, 2020).*

Client/Family Teaching and Discharge Planning

▲ Instruct to increase fluids to prevent heat-induced hyperthermia and dehydration in the presence of fever. EB: *Liberal fluid intake replaces fluid lost through perspiration and respiration (Knapick & Epstein, 2019; Lipman et al, 2019).*

- Teach the client to stay in a cooler environment during periods of excessive outdoor heat or humidity. If the client does go out, instruct them to avoid vigorous physical activity; wear lightweight, loose-fitting clothing; and wear a hat to minimize sun exposure. EB: *Such methods reduce exposure to high environmental temperatures, which can cause heat stroke and hyperthermia (Jain et al, 2018; CDC, 2020).*

REFERENCES

H

Bridges, E., & Thomas, K. (2009). Noninvasive measurement of body temperature in critically ill patients. *Critical Care Nurse*, *29*(3), 94–97. doi:10.4037/ccn2009132.

Bursey, M. M., Galer, M., Oh, R. C., & Weathers, B. K. (2019). Successful management of severe exertional heat stroke with endovascular cooling after failure of standard cooling measures. *Journal of Emergency Medicine*, *57*(2), e53–e56. https://doi.org/10.1016/j.jemermed.2019.03.025.

Centers for Disease Control and Prevention (CDC). (2020). *Heat stress. NIOSH workplace safety and health tips*. Retrieved from https://www.cdc.gov/niosh/topics/heatstress/. Accessed 6 July 2021.

Cheshire, W. P., Jr. (2016). Thermoregulatory disorders and illness related to heat and cold stress. *Autonomic Neuroscience: Basic & Clinical*, *196*, 91–104. https://doi.org/10.1016/j.autneu.2016.01.001.

Cieniewicz, A., Trzebicki, J., Mayzner-Zawadzka, E., Kostera-Pruszczyk, A., & Owczuk, R. (2019). Malignant hyperthermia—What do we know in 2019? *Anaesthesiology Intensive Therapy*, *51*(3), 169–177. https://doi.org/10.5114/ait.2019.87646.

Gaudio, F. G., & Grissom, C. K. (2016). Cooling methods in heat stroke. *Journal of Emergency Medicine*, *50*(4), 607–616. doi:10.1016/j.jemermed.2015.09.014.

Jain, Y., Srivatsan, R., Kollannur, A., & Zachariah, A. (2018). Heatstroke: Causes, consequences and clinical guidelines. *The National Medical Journal of India*, *31*(4), 224–227. https://doi.org/10.4103/0970-258X.258224.

Knapik, J. J., & Epstein, Y. (2019). Exertional heat stroke: Pathophysiology, epidemiology, diagnosis, treatment, and prevention. *Journal of Special Operations Medicine*, *19*(2), 108–116.

Kollmann-Camaiora, A., Alsina, E., Domínguez, A., et al. (2017). Clinical protocol for the management of malignant hyperthermia. *Revista Espanola de Anestesiologia y Reanimacion*, *64*(1), 32–40. https://doi.org/10.1016/j.redar.2016.06.004.

Leyk, D., Hoitz, J., Becker, C., Glitz, K. J., Nestler, K., & Piekarski, C. (2019). Health risks and interventions in exertional heat stress. *Deutsches Arzteblatt International*, *116*(31–32), 537–544. https://doi.org/10.3238/arztebl.2019.0537.

Lipman, G. S., Gaudio, F. G., Eifling, K. P., Ellis, M. A., Otten, E. M., & Grissom, C. K. (2019). Wilderness medical Society clinical practice guidelines for the prevention and treatment of heat illness: 2019 update. *Wilderness and Environmental Medicine*, *30*(4S), S33–S46. https://doi.org/10.1016/j.wem.2018.10.004.

Maddock, K., & Connor, K. (2020). Drug fever: A patient case scenario and review of the evidence. *AACN Advanced Critical Care*, *31*(3), 233–238. https://doi.org/10.4037/aacnacc2020311.

Makic, M. B. F., VonRueden, K. T., Rauen, C. A., & Chadwick, J. (2011). Evidence-based practice habits: Putting more sacred cows out to pasture. *Critical Care Nurse*, *31*(2), 38–62. doi:10.4037/ccn2011908.

Malignant Hyperthermia Association of the United States (MHAUS). (2020). Website. Retrieved from http://www.mhaus.org/. Accessed 6 July 2021.

Nakajima, Y. (2016). Controversies in the temperature management of critically ill patients. *Journal of Anesthesia*, *30*(5), 873–883. https://doi.org/10.1007/s00540-016-2200-7.

Niven, D. J., Gaudet, J. E., Laupland, K. B., Mrklas, K. J., Roberts, D. J., & Stelfox, H. T. (2015). Accuracy of peripheral thermometers for estimating temperature: A systematic review and meta-analysis. *Annals of Internal Medicine*, *163*(10), 768–777. https://doi.org/10.7326/M15-1150.

Pileggi, D. J., & Cook, A. M. (2016). Neuroleptic malignant syndrome: Focus on treatment and rechallenge. *Annals of Pharmacotherapy*, *50*(11), 973–981. doi:10.1177/1060028016657553.

Riazi, S., Kraeva, N., & Hopkins, P. M. (2018). Updated guide for the management of malignant hyperthermia. *Canadian Journal of Anaesthesia*, *65*(6), 709–721. https://doi.org/10.1007/s12630-018-1108-0.

Syrkin-Nikolau, M. E., Johnson, K. J., Colaizy, T. T., Schrock, R., & Bell, E. F. (2017). Temporal artery temperature measurement in the neonate. *American Journal of Perinatology*, *34*(10), 1026–1031. https://doi.org/10.1055/s-0037-1601440.

van Rensburg, R., & Decloedt, E. H. (2019). An approach to the pharmacotherapy of neuroleptic malignant syndrome. *Psychopharmacology Bulletin*, *49*(1), 84–91.

Ware, M. R., Feller, D. B., & Hall, K. L. (2018). Neuroleptic malignant syndrome: Diagnosis and management. *Primary Care Companion for CNS Disorders*, *20*(1), 17r02185. https://doi.org/10.4088/PCC.17r02185.

Hypothermia Domain 11 Safety/protection Class 6 Thermoregulation

Rosemary Timmerman, DNP, APRN, CCNS, CCRN-CSC-CMC

NANDA-I

Definition

Core body temperature below normal diurnal range in individuals > 28 days of life.

Defining Characteristics

Acrocyanosis; bradycardia; cyanotic nail beds; decreased blood glucose level; decreased ventilation; hypertension; hypoglycemia; hypoxia; increased metabolic rate; increased oxygen consumption; peripheral vasoconstriction; piloerection; shivering; skin cool to touch; slow capillary refill; tachycardia

Related Factors

Alcohol consumption; excessive conductive heat transfer; excessive convective heat transfer; excessive evaporative heat transfer; excessive radiative heat transfer; inactivity; inadequate caregiver knowledge of hypothermia prevention; inadequate clothing; low environmental temperature; malnutrition

At-Risk Population

Economically disadvantaged individuals; individuals at extremes of age; individuals at extremes of weight

Associated Conditions

Damage to hypothalamus; decreased metabolic rate; pharmaceutical preparations; radiotherapy; trauma

NOC (Nursing Outcomes Classification)

Suggested NOC Outcomes

Thermoregulation; Thermoregulation: Newborn

Example NOC Outcome with Indicators

Thermoregulation as evidenced by the following indicators: Increased skin temperature/Decreased skin temperature/Skin color changes/Dehydration/Hypothermia. (Rate the outcome and indicators of **Thermoregulation:** 1 = severe, 2 = substantial, 3 = moderate, 4 = mild, 5 = none [see Section I].)

Client Outcomes

Client Will (Specify Time Frame)

- Maintain body temperature within normal range
- Identify risk factors of hypothermia
- State measures to prevent hypothermia
- Identify symptoms of hypothermia and actions to take when hypothermia is present
- If hypothermia is medically induced client/family will state goals for hypothermia treatment

NIC (Nursing Interventions Classification)

Suggested NIC Interventions

Hypothermia Treatment; Temperature Regulation; Temperature Regulation: Intraoperative; Vital Signs Monitoring

Example NIC Activities—Temperature Regulation

Institute use of a continuous core temperature-monitoring device, as appropriate; Promote adequate fluid and nutritional intake

Nursing Interventions and *Rationales*

Temperature Measurement

- Recognize hypothermia as a drop in core body temperature to 35°C (95°F) or lower (Zafren, 2017; Dow et al, 2019).
- Measure and record the client's temperature hourly or, if the client's temperature is less than 35°C (95°F), continuously. EB: *Ongoing temperature measurements are needed for timely treatment decisions (Paal et al, 2016; Zafren, 2017).*
- Select a core or a near core measurement site based on the clinical situation and ability to obtain an accurate measurement; verify the temperature reading with a second monitoring device as needed. EB: *Hypothermia can be a life-threatening crisis, and obtaining an accurate temperature measurement is essential for detecting hypothermia and monitoring the client's response to treatment. A core temperature measurement from a pulmonary artery catheter is considered the gold standard, but it is often not practical and may precipitate dysrhythmias in hypothermic clients. A probe placed in the distal esophagus correlates with the pulmonary artery temperature and can be used when the client has a decreased level of consciousness and the upper airway is secured. An indwelling urinary catheter with a temperature probe allows for simultaneous measurement of bladder temperatures and urine output but may not be accurate with a low urine output. Rectal and bladder probes provide near core temperature readings but may lag behind core temperatures during rapid cooling and rewarming. Tympanic measurements may give falsely low readings in clients with unstable or absent circulation; oral, skin, and temporal artery temperatures are inaccurate in hypothermic states (Paal et al, 2016; Zafren, 2017).*
- Use the same site and method (device) for a given client so that temperature trends are accurately assessed. CEB: *There are differences in temperature measurements depending on the site from which the temperature measurement is obtained; however, differences between sites should not be more than 0.3°C to 0.5°C (32.5°F–32.9°F) (Makic et al, 2011).*
- See the care plan for Ineffective **Thermoregulation** as appropriate.

Accidental Hypothermia

- Recognize that there are three categories of hypothermia based on the core temperature (Dow et al, 2019): mild—35°C to 32°C *(95°F–89.6°F),* where the individual is conscious and shivering; moderate—32°C to 28°C *(89.6°F–82.4°F),* where the individual exhibits altered mental status, paradoxical undressing, and loss of shivering and where thermoregulatory mechanisms are less effective, necessitating the application of exogenous heat; and severe—less than 28°C *(82.4°F),* resulting in unconsciousness, loss of shivering, and increased risk of cardiac arrest.
- Remove the client from the cause of the hypothermic episode (e.g., cold environment, cold or wet clothing), bring into a warm environment, cover the client with warm blankets, and apply a covering to the head and neck to conserve body heat. EB: *Layering of dry clothing, including wearing a hat, can be effective in warming a client with mild hypothermia; the goal is also to prevent any further heat loss (Zafren, 2017; Dow et al, 2019).*
- Keep the moderately and severely hypothermic client horizontal, limit limb movement, and handle gently during movements. EB: *Because cold myocardial tissue is irritable, rough or sudden movements or movement of the limbs of hypothermic clients can precipitate lethal ventricular dysrhythmias; a vertical position may cause severe cardiovascular stress* (*Zafren, 2017; Dow et al, 2019*).
- Monitor the client for signs of hypothermia: shivering, slurred speech, confusion, clumsy movements, fatigue progressing to a further decrease in level of consciousness, bradycardia, hypoventilation, hypotension, ventricular fibrillation, and asystole (Rischall & Rowland-Fisher, 2016; Zafren, 2017).
- Monitor the client's vital signs every hour and as appropriate, noting changes associated with hypothermia such as increased pulse rate, respiratory rate, and blood pressure, as well as diuresis with mild hypothermia, progressing to a decreased pulse rate, respiratory rate, and blood pressure, and oliguria with moderate to severe hypothermia. EB: *With mild hypothermia, the sympathetic nervous system is activated, which increases the heart rate and respiratory rate; as hypothermia progresses, decreased circulating volume develops, which results in decreased cardiac output and decreased oxygen delivery. Hypoxia, metabolic acidosis, and intrinsic irritability of a cold myocardium result in dysrhythmias (Zafren, 2017; Dow et al, 2019).*

- ▲ Attach electrodes and a cardiac monitor, increase the gain (QRS amplitude), and monitor for dysrhythmias. **EB:** *With hypothermia, the client is prone to dysrhythmias because of the cold myocardium; dysrhythmias may include atrial fibrillation, ventricular fibrillation, or asystole (Paal et al, 2016; Zafren, 2017).*
- ▲ Recognize that clients with a core temperature less than 30°C (86°F) are at a higher risk for cardiac arrest; if the client arrests:
  - ❍ Check the pulse for up to 1 minute because the pulse may be slow and weak.
  - ❍ Provide chest compressions unless the client has a frozen noncompressible chest.
  - ❍ Deliver ventilations at the same rate as recommended for a normothermic client if an advanced airway is not in place. If an advanced airway is in place, use an end-tidal CO_2 monitor to guide ventilations or provide ventilations at half the rate recommended for a normothermic client to avoid hyperventilation.
  - ❍ Limit defibrillations to one attempt at maximal power for clients with ventricular fibrillation or pulseless ventricular tachycardia until the client's core temperature is at least 30°C (86°F).
  - ❍ Medications may be withheld until the client has a core temperature greater than 30°C (86°F); double the interval between doses once the temperature is above 30°C (86°F); resume normal doses of medications once the temperature reaches 35°C (95°F).
  - ❍ Recognize prolonged cardiopulmonary resuscitation may be necessary as the client is rewarmed.

  EB: *Defibrillation and medications are less effective in the moderately or severely hypothermic client (Dow et al, 2019). Resuscitative efforts may be withheld if the client's serum potassium is greater than 12 mmol/L (12 mEq/L) from blood drawn from a central vein because a higher serum potassium level indicates that hypoxia and cell lysis preceded hypothermia (Pasquier et al, 2019; Rathjen et al, 2019).*
- ▲ Monitor for signs of coagulopathy (e.g., oozing of blood from any open areas or from intravascular catheter sites or mucous membranes) and note the results of clotting studies as available. **EB:** *Coagulopathy is a common occurrence during hypothermia because of reduced platelet function and coagulation enzymatic activity (Paal et al, 2016; Rischall & Rowland-Fisher, 2016).*
- ● Assess for localized cold injuries such as frostbite.
- ● For mild hypothermia (core temperature of 32.2°C–35°C [90°F–95°F]), rewarm client passively:
  - ❍ Set room temperature to 21°C to 24°C (70°F–75°F).
  - ❍ Keep the client dry; remove any damp or wet clothing.
  - ❍ Layer clothing and blankets and cover the client's head.
  - ❍ Offer warm fluids, particularly beverages high in carbohydrates for clients who are shivering and able to safely swallow; avoid alcohol or caffeine; avoid fluids that are so warm they might burn the esophagus (Zafren, 2017; Dow et al, 2019).
- ● For mild hypothermia, allow the client to rewarm at his or her own pace as heat is generated through the normal metabolism; *warm fluids help reduce further heat loss and carbohydrates help fuel metabolic processes (Rischall & Rowland-Fisher, 2016; Zafren, 2017).*
- ▲ For moderate hypothermia (core temperature 28°C–32.1°C [82.4°F–90°F]) or any client with a decreased level of consciousness, use active external rewarming methods, not exceeding an increase of more than 1°C to 2°C (approximately 1.8°F–3°F) per hour. **EB:** *Passive rewarming is not recommended for clients with temperatures lower than 32.2°C (90°F) because it is a slow process, requires sufficient glycogen stores to be used by the client's body, and may increase oxygen consumption, increasing the risk of adverse cardiac events (Zafren, 2017; Dow et al, 2019).*
- ● Methods to rewarm the client include the following (Dow et al, 2019; Rathjen et al, 2019):
  - ❍ Forced-air warming blankets
  - ❍ Circulation of warm water through external pads
  - ❍ Heated and humidified oxygen (42°C–46°C [107.6°F–114.8°F]) through the ventilator circuit as ordered
  - ❍ Warmed (40°C–42°C [104°F–107.6°F]) intravenous (IV) normal saline and blood products using a commercial IV fluid warmer (hypothermic clients cannot metabolize lactate so IV lactated Ringer's should not be administered)
  - ❍ Radiant heat sources; concentrate heat to axillae and upper torso
- ▲ For severe hypothermia (core temperature below 28°C [82.4°F]), use active core rewarming techniques as ordered (Dow et al, 2019; Rathjen et al, 2019):
  - ❍ Hemodialysis
  - ❍ Intravascular temperature management catheter
  - ❍ Body cavity (thorax, peritoneal, stomach, and bladder) lavage with warmed fluid

- ❍ Recognize that warming by extracorporeal life support (ECLS) using venoarterial extracorporeal membrane oxygenation (ECMO) or cardiopulmonary bypass is essential for clients experiencing hemodynamic instability or hypothermic cardiac arrest
- ● Rewarm clients slowly, generally at a rate of 1°C to 2°C every hour (approximately 1.8°F–3.6°F). EB: *Slow rewarming helps prevent a phenomenon called "afterdrop," in which cold, hyperkalemic blood from the periphery returns to the heart, resulting in a biochemical injury, leading to dysrhythmias and severe hypotension (Zafren, 2017; Dow et al, 2019).*
- ● Measure the blood pressure frequently when rewarming and monitor for hypotension. EB: *As the body warms, formerly vasoconstricted vessels dilate, resulting in hypotension; dehydration from cold diuresis worsens hypotension (Zafren, 2017).*
- ● After rewarming, monitor the client for afterdrop, or a decrease in body temperature due to return of colder blood from the periphery to the core.
- ▲ Administer isotonic IV normal saline warmed to 40°C to 42°C [104°F–107.6°F] as prescribed. EB: *Significant amounts of IV fluids are often needed to maintain adequate perfusion to vital tissues and organs because of hypovolemia from cold diuresis and vasodilation from rewarming; warmed IV fluid does not significantly raise the body temperature but does help prevent further heat loss (Rischall & Rowland-Fisher, 2016; Zafren, 2017).*
- ● Place a barrier between the client and the heating blanket and monitor the client's skin every 30 minutes. EB: *Cold skin is susceptible to pressure and thermal injury (Zafren, 2017; Dow et al, 2019).*
- ● Determine the factors leading to the hypothermic episode, particularly if the client fails to rewarm, and treat the underlying condition; see Related Factors. EB: *It is important to assess risk factors and precipitating events to prevent another incident of hypothermia and detect and treat underlying disease processes that impede thermoregulation (Rischall & Rowland-Fisher, 2016).*
- ▲ Request a social service referral to help the client obtain the heat, shelter, and food needed to maintain body temperature. EB: *A preventive approach that includes adequate food and fluid intake, shelter, heat, and clothing decreases the risk of hypothermia.*
- ▲ Encourage proper nutrition and hydration. EB: *Request a referral to a dietitian to identify appropriate dietary needs; insufficient calorie and fluid intake predisposes the client to hypothermia, especially in older adults (Rischall & Rowland-Fisher, 2016).*

Targeted Temperature Hypothermia

- ● Recognize that targeted temperature management, previously called therapeutic hypothermia, is the active lowering of the client's body temperature, in a controlled manner, to preserve neurological function after a cardiac arrest; targeted temperature management may also be considered for clients who have refractory intracranial hypertension. EB: *In the event the client is successfully resuscitated after a cardiac arrest, recognize that medically induced targeted temperature management has been shown to provide neurological protection against ischemic neuronal injury after cardiac arrest (Donnino et al, 2016; Cook, 2017).*
- ● Recognize that controlled cooling of clients should be considered for all unconscious survivors of in-hospital or out-of-hospital cardiac arrest with an initial shockable (ventricular fibrillation or pulseless ventricular tachycardia) or nonshockable (asystole or pulseless electrical activity) rhythm; achieve and maintain a constant target temperature between 32°C and 36°C (89.6°F–96.8°F) for at least 24 hours. EB: *The American Heart Association and the International Liaison Committee on Resuscitation have included therapeutic hypothermia as an intervention to be considered in the management of cardiac arrest clients to optimize neurological outcomes after return of spontaneous circulation (Donnino et al, 2016; Geocadin et al, 2017).*
- ● Monitor core or near core temperatures continuously using two methods of temperature monitoring. To ensure that the targeted temperature is achieved and maintained closely within the prescribed temperature range, two methods of core or near core temperature monitoring are recommended (*Cook, 2017; Taccone et al, 2020*).
- ● Recognize that cooling may be achieved noninvasively, using fluid-filled cooling pads or with an esophageal cooling catheter, or invasively, with an intravascular cooling catheter. EB/EBN: *Invasive cooling and surface cooling devices with temperature feedback mechanisms provide a more predictable and rapid cooling, minimizing adverse electrolyte shifts and shivering. Less optimal methods of cooling include the use of fans, ice packs, or blankets, which do not provide temperature regulation feedback between the machine and client (Calabró et al, 2019; Taccone et al, 2020).*
- ● Monitor for signs of infection and implement measures to prevent hospital-acquired infections. EB: *Hypothermia places the client at higher risk for infection because of immunosuppression (Cook, 2017; Wright et al, 2020).*

- Obtain vital signs hourly (or via continuous monitoring) and include continuous electrocardiogram monitoring, and observe for signs of hypotension, bradycardia, and dysrhythmias. Mechanical ventilation is required to protect the client's airway and breathing during treatment. EB: *Diuresis is more pronounced during the induction of hypothermia; hypotension may be more prominent as the client is rewarmed because of vasodilation, requiring close monitoring and interventions to support blood pressure. Bradycardia associated with hypothermia is often not responsive to atropine but does not need to be treated unless the client is hemodynamically unstable. If the client is overcooled (temperature drops below 32°C [89.6°F]), the risk of dysrhythmias will increase and ventricular fibrillation refractory to defibrillation may occur at temperatures below 30°C [86°F] (Cook, 2017; Wright et al, 2020).*
- ▲ Observe for shivering using a tool such as the Bedside Shivering Assessment Scale (BSAS) and implement skin counter-warming with blankets or a forced warm-air device; administer sedatives, opioids, neuromuscular blocking agents, α-agonists, buspirone, acetaminophen, nonsteroidal antiinflammatory agents, or magnesium sulfate as prescribed. EB: *Shivering typically occurs as the client transitions between 37°C and 35°C [98.6°F–95°F] and significantly increases the body's metabolic rate and oxygen consumption (Armahizer et al, 2020; Taccone et al, 2020).*
- ▲ Closely inspect the skin before and throughout the cooling intervention and implement frequent turning and other pressure reduction interventions as indicated. EB: *Lowering the body temperature causes vasoconstriction and can compromise perfusion to the skin, increasing the client's risk of skin breakdown and impaired wound healing (Cook, 2017; Ahtiala et al, 2018).*
- ▲ Monitor and treat serum electrolytes (e.g., potassium, magnesium, calcium, phosphorus) and serum glucose closely during targeted hypothermia and during rewarming of the client; electrolytes will fluctuate as the client is rewarmed. EB/EBN: *Hypokalemia can occur during the induction phase of targeted temperature management as potassium moves intracellularly and is also lost through diuresis; as the client is rewarmed, electrolyte replacements, especially potassium replacements, should be closely monitored to prevent rebound hyperkalemia that may occur as the body temperature rises (Cook, 2017; Wright et al, 2020).*
- ▲ Monitor blood cell counts and observe for signs and symptoms of coagulopathy during targeted hypothermia treatment. EB: *For every 1°C (approximately 1.8°F) decline in temperature, the hematocrit may increase by approximately 2%, requiring monitoring but not treatment. Platelet counts decrease during hypothermic states, but research has not found a significant risk of bleeding during targeted hypothermia treatment (Walker & Johnson, 2019; Wright et al, 2020).*
- Rewarming should occur in a controlled manner, with a rise in body temperature no faster than 0.5°C (approximately 0.9°F) per hour and a targeted goal of normothermia, 37°C [98.6°F] for 48 hours. EB: *Aggressive rewarming may cause rebound hyperthermia, cerebral edema, seizures, hypotension, and ventricular fibrillation; hyperthermia during the 36 hours after a cardiac arrest is associated with worse neurological outcomes and a higher mortality rate (Taccone et al, 2020; Wright et al, 2020).*
- ▲ Neurological and cognitive function should be assessed during targeted temperature treatment and after rewarming. EB: *The goal of targeted temperature treatment is neurological protection; close monitoring of neurological function after intervention and serial assessments are indicated (Donnino et al, 2016; Geocadin et al, 2017).*

Pediatric

- Recognize that pediatric clients have a decreased ability to adapt to temperature extremes; take the following actions to maintain body temperature in the infant/child:
  - Keep the head covered.
  - Use blankets to keep the client warm.
  - Keep the client covered during procedures, transport, and diagnostic testing.
  - Keep the room temperature at 22.2°C (72°F) for children and between 23°C and 25°C[73.4°F–77°F] for infants less than 32 weeks' gestation.
- The combination of a relatively smaller body surface area, smaller body fluid volume, less well-developed temperature control mechanisms, and smaller amount of protective body fat limits the infant's and child's ability to maintain normal temperatures (Sgro et al, 2016; Shah & Madhok, 2019).
- For the preterm or low-birth-weight newborn, set the room temperature to 25°C (77°F) before the delivery; dry the infant; wrap in prewarmed, dry blankets; cover the infant's head with a wool or polyethylene cap; and use specially designed bags, skin-to-skin care, TransWarmer mattresses, radiant warmers, and thermal blankets to keep the infant warm. EB/EBN: *These methods can help keep the vulnerable newborn warm in the delivery room (McCall et al, 2018; Trevisanuto et al, 2018). See care plan for Neonatal* ***Hypothermia****.*

- Avoid bathing neonates for at least 12 to 24 hours after birth when temperature stability is achieved; perform immersion bathing rather than sponge bathing for newborns and swaddled bathing for premature neonates; avoid removing the vernix caseosa and allow it to wear off with normal activity and handling; grossly contaminated vernix caseosa may be gently removed. EBN: *Early bathing of a neonate can result in hypothermia; the vernix caseosa protects and moisturizes the skin (Johnson & Hunt, 2019). See care plan for Neonatal* ***Hypothermia***.
- Targeted hypothermia to 34°C (93.2°F) for 72 hours may be implemented in the treatment of neonates with hypoxic-ischemic encephalopathy (HIE). EB: *Cooling may be achieved by selective head cooling or whole body cooling with a cooling blanket (Benedetti & Silverstein, 2018; Schump, 2018). See care plan for Neonatal* ***Hypothermia***.
- Measure the temperature of the neonate undergoing therapeutic hypothermia for HIE with a rectal or esophageal probe. EB: *Although rectal and esophageal temperatures accurately reflect the core body temperature of neonates undergoing targeted hypothermia, axillary temperature measurements do not (Schump, 2018). See care plan for Neonatal* ***Hypothermia***.

Geriatric

- Normal aging often includes changes in touch-related sensations, making it harder to differentiate cool and cold. *Decreased temperature sensitivity increases the risk of hypothermia in the older adult (Martin, 2016).*
- Recognize that older adults can develop hypothermia even from exposure to mildly cold temperatures of 15.5°C to 18.3°C (60°F–65°F).
  - Set the room temperature to 20°C to 21.1°C (68°F–70°F).
  - Instruct client to wear warm clothes as appropriate (long underwear, socks, slippers, and a cap or hat) and to use a blanket to keep shoulders and legs warm while indoors.
  - Instruct client to dress in loose layers and wear a hat, scarf, and gloves or mittens when going outside during cold weather.
  - Instruct client to maintain adequate calorie intake.

  EB: *Clients present with vague complaints of mental and/or other skill deterioration (Hypothermia and Older Adults, 2016).*
- Assess neurological signs frequently, watching for confusion and decreased level of consciousness. CEB: *Mechanisms to control body temperature decrease with age, coupled with a slower counterregulatory response, lower rate of metabolism, and less effective vascular response, making hypothermia less obvious (Danzl, 2012).*

Home Care

- Hypothermia is not a symptom that appears in the normal course of home care, but when it occurs it is a clinical emergency, and the client/family should access emergency medical services immediately.
- Some of the interventions described earlier may be adapted for home care use.
- Before a medical crisis occurs, confirm that the client or family has a thermometer that registers accurately, and the client or family can read it.
- Instruct the client or family to take the temperature when the client displays cyanosis, pallor, or shivering.

▲ Monitor temperature every hour, as noted previously; if the temperature of the client begins dropping below the normal range, apply layers of clothing or blankets, or adjust environmental heat to the comfort level, being careful to not overheat the client. Passive rewarming is the only method of rewarming that is appropriate for home care under normal circumstances.

▲ If temperature continues to drop, activate the emergency system and notify a health care provider. Hypothermia is a clinically acute condition that cannot be managed safely in the home.

▲ If the client is in hospice care or is terminally ill, follow advance directives, client wishes, and the health care provider's orders; keep the client free of pain. The goal of terminal care is to provide dignity and comfort during the dying process.

Client/Family Teaching and Discharge Planning

- Teach the client and family signs of hypothermia and the method of taking the temperature (age appropriate).
- Teach the client methods to prevent hypothermia: wearing adequate clothing, including a hat and mittens; heating the environment to a minimum of 20°C (68°F); and ingesting adequate food and fluid. EB: *Simple*

measures such as layering clothes, wearing a hat, and avoiding extremes in temperature prevent significant heat loss (Hypothermia and Older Adults, 2016).

- ● Teach clients who engage in cold weather outdoor activities the importance of appropriate clothing, survival skills, and emergency planning.
- ▲ Teach the client and family about medications such as sedatives, opioids, and anxiolytics that predispose the client to hypothermia (as appropriate). **EB:** *If the client has had hypothermia in the past, using alternative medications is an option if there is no contraindication (Danzl, 2012).*

REFERENCES

Ahtiala, M., Laitio, R., & Soppi, E. (2018). Therapeutic hypothermia and pressure ulcer risk in critically ill intensive care patients: A retrospective study. *Intensive and Critical Care Nursing, 46*, 80–85. https://doi.org/10.1016/j.iccn.2018.02.008.

Armahizer, M. J., Strein, M., & Pajoumand, M. (2020). Control of shivering during targeted temperature management. *Critical Care Nursing Quarterly, 43*(2), 251–266. https://doi.org/10.1097/CNQ.0000000000000305.

Benedetti, G. M., & Silverstein, F. S. (2018). Targeted temperature management in pediatric neurocritical care. *Pediatric Neurology, 88*, 12–24. https://doi.org/10.1016/j.pediatrneurol.2018.07.004.

Calabró, L., Bougouin, W., Cariou, A., et al. (2019). Effect of different methods of cooling for targeted temperature management on outcome after cardiac arrest: A systematic review and meta-analysis. *Critical Care, 23*(1), 285. https://doi.org/10.1186/s13054-019-2567-6.

Cook, C. J. (2017). Induced hypothermia in neurocritical care: A review. *Journal of Neuroscience Nursing, 49*(1), 5–11. https://doi.org/10.1097/JNN.0000000000000215.

Danzl, D. F. (2012). Hypothermia and frostbite. In D. L. Longo, A. S. Fauci, D. L. Kasper, S. L. Hauser, J. L. Jameson, & J. Loscalzo (Eds.), *Harrison's principles of internal medicine* (18th ed.) (pp. 165–170). New York: McGraw-Hill.

Donnino, M. W., Andersen, L. W., Berg, K. M., & The ILCOR ALS Task Force., et al. (2016). Temperature management after cardiac arrest: An advisory statement by the Advanced Life Support Task Force of the International Liaison Committee on Resuscitation and the American Heart Association Emergency Cardiovascular Care Committee and the Council on Cardiopulmonary, Critical Care, Perioperative and Resuscitation. *Resuscitation, 98*, 97–104. https://doi.org/10.1016/j.resuscitation.2015.09.396.

Dow, J., Giesbrecht, G. G., Danzl, D. F., et al. (2019). Wilderness medical Society clinical practice guidelines for the out-of-hospital evaluation and treatment of accidental hypothermia: 2019 update. *Wilderness and Environmental Medicine, 30*(4S), S47–S69. https://doi.org/10.1016/j.wem.2019.10.002.

Geocadin, R. G., Armstrong, M. J., Damian, M., et al. (2017). Practice guideline summary: Reducing brain injury following cardiopulmonary resuscitation: Report of the Guideline Development, Dissemination, and Implementation Subcommittee of the American Academy of Neurology. *Neurology, 88*(22), 2141–2149. https://doi.org/10.1212/WNL.0000000000003966.

Hypothermia and older adults. (2016). *Home Healthcare Now, 34*(1), 9.

Johnson, E., & Hunt, R. (2019). Infant skin care: Updates and recommendations. *Current Opinion in Pediatrics, 31*(4), 476–481. https://doi.org/10.1097/MOP.0000000000000791.

Makic, M. B. F., VonRueden, K. T., Rauen, C. A., & Chadwick, J. (2011). Evidence-based practice habits: Putting more sacred cows out to pasture. *Critical Care Nurse, 31*(2), 38–62. https://doi.org/10.4037/ccn2011908.

Martin, J. (2016). Aging changes in the senses. *MedlinePlus*. National Library of Medicine. Retrieved from https://medlineplus.gov/ency/article/004013.htm. Accessed 6 July 2021.

McCall, E. M., Alderdice, F., Halliday, H. L., Vohra, S., & Johnston, L. (2018). Interventions to prevent hypothermia at birth in preterm and/or low birth weight infants. *Cochrane Database of Systematic Reviews, 2*, CD004210. https://doi.org/10.1002/14651858.CD004210.pub5.

Paal, P., Gordon, L., Strapazzon, G., et al. (2016). Accidental hypothermia—an update: The content of this review is endorsed by the International Commission for Mountain Emergency Medicine (ICAR MEDCOM). *Scandinavian Journal of Trauma, Resuscitation and Emergency Medicine, 24*(1), 111. https://doi.org/10.1186/s13049-016-0303-7.

Pasquier, M., Blancher, M., Buse, S., et al. (2019). Intra-patient potassium variability after hypothermic cardiac arrest: A multicentre, prospective study. *Scandinavian Journal of Trauma, Resuscitation and Emergency Medicine, 27*(1), 113. https://doi.org/10.1186/s13049-019-0694-3.

Rathjen, N. A., Shahbodaghi, S. D., & Brown, J. A. (2019). Hypothermia and cold weather injuries. *American Family Physician, 100*(11), 680–686.

Rischall, M. L., & Rowland-Fisher, A. (2016). Evidence-based management of accidental hypothermia in the emergency department. *Emergency Medicine Practice, 18*(1), 1–18.

Schump, E. A. (2018). Neonatal encephalopathy: Current management and future trends. *Critical Care Nursing Clinics of North America, 30*(4), 509–521. https://doi.org/10.1016/j.cnc.2018.07.007.

Sgro, M., Campbell, D. M., & Gandhi, N. (2016). Nontherapeutic neonatal hypothermia. *Paediatrics and Child Health, 21*(4), 178–180. https://doi.org/10.1093/pch/21.4.178.

Shah, A., & Madhok, M. (2019). Management of pediatric hypothermia and peripheral cold injuries in the emergency department. *Pediatric Emergency Medicine Practice, 16*(1), 1–16.

Taccone, F. S., Picetti, E., & Vincent, J. L. (2020). High quality targeted temperature management (TTM) after cardiac arrest. *Critical Care, 24*(1), 6. https://doi.org/10.1186/s13054-019-2721-1.

Trevisanuto, D., Testoni, D., & Fernanda de Almeida, M. (2018). Maintaining normothermia: Why and how? *Seminars in Fetal and Neonatal Medicine, 23*(5), 333–339. https://doi.org/10.1016/j.siny.2018.03.009.

Walker, A. C., & Johnson, N. J. (2019). Targeted temperature management and postcardiac arrest care. *Emergency Medicine Clinics of North America, 37*(3), 381–393. https://doi.org/10.1016/j.emc.2019.03.002.

Wright, S., Peralta, S., & Ranasinghe, L. (2020). A review of adverse effects of targeted temperature management for post-cardiac arrest patients. *American Journal of Biomedical Science & Research, 9*(1). https://doi.org/10.34297/AJBSR.2020.09.001349.

Zafren, K. (2017). Out-of-hospital evaluation and treatment of accidental hypothermia. *Emergency Medicine Clinics of North America, 35*(2), 261–279. https://doi.org/10.1016/j.emc.2017.01.003.

H

Risk for Hypothermia Domain 11 Safety/protection Class 6 Thermoregulation

Rosemary Timmerman, DNP, APRN, CCNS, CCRN-CSC-CMC

NANDA-I

Definition

Susceptible to a failure of thermoregulation that may result in a core body temperature below the normal diurnal range, in individuals >28 days of life, which may compromise health.

Risk Factors

Alcohol consumption; excessive conductive heat transfer; excessive convective heat transfer; excessive evaporative heat transfer; excessive radiative heat transfer; inactivity; inadequate caregiver knowledge of hypothermia prevention; inadequate clothing; low environmental temperature; malnutrition

At-Risk Population

Economically disadvantaged individuals; individuals at extremes of age; individuals at extremes of weight

Associated Conditions

Damage to hypothalamus; decreased metabolic rate; pharmaceutical preparations; radiotherapy; trauma

NIC, NOC, Client Outcomes, Nursing Interventions and *Rationales,* Client/Family Teaching and Discharge Planning, and References

Refer to care plan for **Hypothermia**.

Neonatal Hypothermia Domain 11 Safety/protection Class 6 Thermoregulation

Barbara Reyna, PhD, RN, NNP-BC

Definition

Core body temperature of an infant below the normal diurnal range.

Defining Characteristics

Acrocyanosis; bradycardia; decreased blood glucose level; decreased metabolic rate; decreased peripheral perfusion; decreased ventilation; hypertension; hypoglycemia; hypoxia; increased oxygen demand; insufficient energy to maintain sucking; irritability; metabolic acidosis; pallor; peripheral vasoconstriction; respiratory distress; skin cool to touch; slow capillary refill; tachycardia; weight gain <30 g/day

Related Factors

Delayed breastfeeding; early bathing of newborn; excessive conductive heat transfer; excessive convective heat transfer; excessive evaporative heat transfer; excessive radiative heat transfer; inadequate caregiver knowledge of hypothermia prevention; inadequate clothing; malnutrition

At-Risk Population

Low birth weight neonates; neonates aged 0-28 days; neonates born by cesarean delivery; neonates born to an adolescent mother; neonates born to economically disadvantaged families; Neonates exposed to low environmental temperatures; Neonates with high-risk out-of-hospital birth; neonates with inadequate subcutaneous fat; neonates with increased body surface area to weight ratio; neonates with unplanned out-of-hospital birth; premature neonates

Associated Conditions

Damage to hypothalamus; immature stratum corneum; increased pulmonary vascular resistance; ineffective vascular control; inefficient nonshivering thermogenesis; low Appearance, Pulse, Grimace, Activity, & Respiration (APGAR) scores; pharmaceutical preparations

NOC (Nursing Outcomes Classification)

Suggested NOC Outcomes

Thermoregulation; Thermoregulation: Newborn

Example NOC Outcome with Indicators

Thermoregulation as evidenced by the following indicators: Increased skin temperature/Decreased skin temperature/Skin color changes/Dehydration/Hypothermia. (Rate the outcome and indicators of **Thermoregulation:** 1 = severe, 2 = substantial, 3 = moderate, 4 = mild, 5 = none

Client Outcomes

Client Will (Specify Time Frame)

- Maintain a body temperature of 36.5°C to 37.5°C (97.7°F–99.5°F)
- Identify risk factors of hypothermia
- State measures to prevent hypothermia
- Identify symptoms of hypothermia and actions to take when hypothermia is present

H

NIC (Nursing Interventions Classification)

Suggested NIC Interventions

Hypothermia Treatment; Temperature Regulation: Monitor Skin Color and Temperature

Example NIC Activities

Promote delayed bathing; Remove wet clothing; Promote adequate fluid and nutritional intake; Monitor vital signs associated with hypothermia in infants

Nursing Interventions and *Rationales*

- At delivery, neonates should be maintained at a temperature of 36.5°C to 37.5°C (97.7°F–99.5°F). Room temperature should be increased to 23°C to 25°C (74°F–77°F). EB: *Increasing the temperature of the delivery room can reduce the incidence of neonatal hypothermia (Duryea, 2016; American Academy of Pediatrics & American Heart Association, 2021).*
- Monitor infants at risk for hypothermia and cold stress. EB: *Infants at risk for hypothermia include late preterm and preterm infants and small-for-gestational-age infants (Bartal et al, 2021).* CEB: *Late preterm infants are at high risk for developing medical complications during hospitalization (Medoff-Cooper et al, 2012).*
- Monitor temperature by skin or axillary measurements using digital/electronic thermometers. EB: *Skin temperature changes are an early indication of cold stress (Fanaroff & Klaus, 2013).*
- Reduce risk of hypothermia by avoiding exposure to sources of heat loss, such as exposing wet skin to the air; direct contact with a cold surface; or placing close to a window or cold wall or near open doors or air conditioner vents. EB: *Newborns lose heat from the body surface to the environment through convection, radiation, evaporation, and conduction (Trevisanuto et al, 2018).*
- Infants with mild hypothermia (36°C–36.4°C [96.8°F–97.5°F]) can be warmed by being placed skin-to-skin with mother in a warm room. EB: *Infants exposed to early skin-to-skin care have improved temperatures and maintain thermal control (WHO, 1997; Nimbalkar et al, 2014).*
- Infants with moderate (32°C–35.9°C [89.6°F–96.6°F]) or severe (<32°C [<89.6°F]) hypothermia should be placed on a radiant warmer or a preheated, double-walled incubator set at 35°C to 36°C (95°F–96.8°F). EB: *Physiological alterations occur that result in adverse metabolic events if hypothermia is not corrected (WHO, 1997).*
- Bathing or weighing the infant should be delayed if evidence of cold stress or hypothermia exists. EB: *Bathing can cause a drop in the infant's temperature and should be delayed for at least 6 hours after birth (WHO, 1997).* EBN: *Delayed bathing for up to 24 hours after birth can reduce the risk of cold stress and hypoglycemia (Chamberlain et al, 2019).*

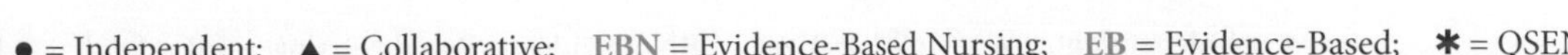

- Monitor the cold-stressed or hypothermic infant for respiratory distress (grunting, tachypnea, retractions) and hypoglycemia. EBN: *Signs of hypothermia can be nonspecific and affect multiple body systems (Vilinsky & Sheridan, 2014).*

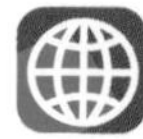

Multicultural

- An occlusive plastic wrap or bag at birth can be used in resource-limited settings. EB: *Hypothermia can be reduced as compared with standard thermoregulation care without resulting in hyperthermia (Belsches et al, 2013; Leadford et al, 2013).*

REFERENCES

American Academy of Pediatrics & American Heart Association. (2021). *Textbook of neonatal resuscitation* (8th ed.). G. M. Weiner (Ed.). American Academy of Pediatrics.

Bartal, M. F., Chen, H. Y., Blackwell, S. C., Chauhan, S. P., & Sibai, B. M. (2021). Neonatal morbidity in late preterm small for gestational age neonates. *Journal of Maternal-Fetal and Neonatal Medicine, 32*(19), 3208–3213. https://doi.org/10.1080/14767058.2019.1680630.

Belsches, T. C., Tilly, A. E., Miller, T. R., et al. (2013). Randomized trial of plastic bags to prevent term neonatal hypothermia in a resource-poor setting. *Pediatrics, 132*(3), e656–e661. https://doi.org/10.1542/peds.2013-0172.

Chamberlain, J., McCarty, S., Source, J., et al. (2019). Impact on delayed newborn bathing on exclusive breastfeeding rates, glucose and temperature stability, and weight loss. *Journal of Neonatal Nursing, 25*(2), 74–77. https://doi.org/10.1016/j.jnn.2018.11.001.

Duryea, E. L., Nelson, D. B., Wyckoff, M. H., et al. (2016). The impact of ambient operating room temperature on neonatal and maternal hypothermia and associated morbidities: A randomized controlled trial. *American Journal of Obstetrics and Gynecology, 214*(4), 505.e1–505.e7. https://doi.org/10.1016/j.ajog.2016.01.190.

Fanaroff, A., & Klaus, M. (2013). The physical environment. In A. A. Fanaroff, & J. M. Fanaroff (Eds.), *Klaus & Fanaroff's care of the high-risk neonate* (6th ed.) (pp. 132–150). Philadelphia: Elsevier.

Leadford, A. E., Warren, J. B., Manasyan, A., et al. (2013). Plastic bags for prevention of hypothermia in preterm and low birth weight infants. *Pediatrics, 132*(1), e128–e134. https://doi.org/10.1542/peds.2012-2030.

Medoff-Cooper, B., Holditch-Davis, D., Verklan, M. T., et al. (2012). Newborn clinical outcomes of the AWHONN late preterm infant research-based practice project. *Journal of Obstetric, Gynecologic, and Neonatal Nursing: Journal of Obstetric, Gynecologic, and Neonatal Nursing, 41*(6), 774–785. https://doi.org/10.1111/j.1552-6909.2012.01401.x.

Nimbalkar, S. M., Patel, V. K., Patel, D. V., Nimbalkar, A. S., Sethi, A., & Phatak, A. (2014). Effect of early skin-to-skin contact following normal delivery on incidence of hypothermia in neonates more than 1800 g: Randomized control trial. *Journal of Perinatology, 34*(5), 364–368. https://doi.org/10.1038/jp.2014.15.

Trevisanuto, D., Testoni, D., & Fernanda B de Almeida, M. (2018). Maintaining normothermia: Why and how? *Seminar in Fetal and Neonatal Medicine, 23*(5), 333–339. https://doi.org/10.1016/j.siny.2018.03.009.

Vilinsky, A., & Sheridan, A. (2014). Hypothermia in the newborn: An exploration of its cause, effect and prevention. *British Journal of Midwivery, 22*(8).

World Health Organization (WHO). (1997). *Thermal protection of the newborn: A practical guide.* Maternal and Newborn Health/ Safe Motherhood Unit, Division of Reproductive Health. Geneva, Switzerland: WHO.

H

Risk for Neonatal Hypothermia

Domain 11 Safety/protection Class 6 Thermoregulation

Mary Beth Flynn Makic, PhD, RN, CCRN-K, CCNS, FAAN, FNAP, FCNS

NANDA-I

Definition

Susceptibility of an infant to a core body temperature below the normal diurnal range, which may compromise health.

Risk Factors

Delayed breastfeeding; early bathing of newborn; excessive conductive heat transfer; excessive convective heat transfer; excessive evaporative heat transfer; excessive radiative heat transfer; inadequate caregiver knowledge of hypothermia prevention; inadequate clothing; malnutrition

At-Risk Population

Low birth weight neonates; neonates aged 0-28 days; neonates born by cesarean delivery; neonates born to an adolescent mother; neonates born to economically disadvantaged families; neonates exposed to low environmental temperatures; neonates with high-risk out-of-hospital birth; neonates with inadequate subcutaneous fat; neonates with increased body surface area to weight ratio; neonates with unplanned out-of- hospital birth; premature neonates

Associated Conditions

Damage to hypothalamus; immature stratum corneum; increased pulmonary vascular resistance; ineffective vascular control; inefficient nonshivering thermogenesis; low Appearance, Pulse, Grimace, Activity, & Respiration (APGAR) scores; pharmaceutical preparations

NOC, NIC, Client Outcomes, Nursing Interventions and *Rationales,* and References

Refer to care plan for Neonatal **Hypothermia**.

Risk for Perioperative Hypothermia

Domain 11 Safety/protection Class 6 Thermoregulation

Kristen A. Oster, DNP, APRN, ACNS-BC, CNOR, CNS-CP

H

NANDA-I

Definition

Susceptible to an inadvertent drop in core body temperature below 36°C/96.8°F occurring one hour before to 24 hours after surgery, which may compromise health.

Risk Factors

Anxiety; body mass index below normal range for age and gender; environmental temperature <21°C/69.8°F; inadequate availability of appropriate warming equipment; wound area uncovered

At-Risk Population

Individuals aged ≥60 years; individuals in environment with laminar air flow; individuals receiving anesthesia for a period >2 hours; individuals undergoing long induction time; individuals undergoing open surgery; individuals undergoing surgical procedure >2 hours; individuals with American Society of Anesthesiologists (ASA) Physical Status classification score >1; individuals with high Model for End-Stage Liver Disease (MELD) score; individuals with increased intraoperative blood loss; individuals with intraoperative diastolic arterial blood pressure <60 mm Hg; individuals with intraoperative systolic blood pressure <140 mm Hg; individuals with low body surface area; neonates <37 weeks gestational age; women

Associated Conditions

Acute hepatic failure; anemia; burns; cardiovascular complications; chronic renal impairment; combined regional and general anesthesia; neurological disorder; pharmaceutical preparations; trauma

NOC (Nursing Outcomes Classification)

Suggested NOC Outcome

Thermoregulation

Example NOC Outcome with Indicators

Thermoregulation as evidenced by the following indicators: Increased skin temperature/Decreased skin temperature/Skin color changes/Dehydration/Hypothermia. (Rate the outcome and indicators of **Thermoregulation:** 1 = severe, 2 = substantial, 3 = moderate, 4 = mild, 5 = none [see Section I].)

Client Outcomes

Client Will (Specify Time Frame)

- Maintain body temperature within normal range

- Identify risk factors of hypothermia
- State measures to prevent hypothermia
- Identify symptoms of hypothermia and actions to take when hypothermia is present
- Be free of surgical site infection

NIC (Nursing Interventions Classification)

Suggested NIC Interventions

Hypothermia Treatment; Temperature Regulation; Temperature Regulation: Intraoperative; Vital Signs Monitoring

Example NIC Activities—Temperature Regulation

Institute use of a continuous core temperature-monitoring device, as appropriate; Promote adequate fluid and nutritional intake

H

Nursing Interventions and *Rationales*

Temperature Measurement

- ✱ Recognize perioperative hypothermia as a drop in core body temperature below 36°C (96.8°F). Hypothermia can be divided into mild (36°C–34°C [96.8°F–93.2°F]), moderate (33°C–28°C [91.4°F–82.4°F]), and severe (≤28°C [<82.4°F]) (Granum et al, 2019; Centers for Disease Control and Prevention [CDC], 2020; Nordgren et al, 2020).
- ● Measure the client's temperature frequently, at least every 15 minutes, while the client is undergoing general anesthesia and with changes in client condition (e.g., chills, change in mental status); if more than mild hypothermia is present (temperature lower than 36°C [96.8°F]), use a continuous temperature-monitoring device. Two modes of temperature monitoring may be indicated. Continuous temperature monitoring using an indwelling method of temperature measurement is usually indicated to monitor effectiveness of treating body alterations in core body temperature. EBN: *Hypothermia can be a life-threatening crisis that requires accurate temperature measurement. Core temperature is obtained by a pulmonary artery catheter or less invasively from sublingual, the distal esophagus, nasopharyngeal, or direct tympanic sites (Atallah et al, 2020; Aykanat, Broadbent, & Peyton, 2021). Near core temperature measurement sites include oral, bladder, rectal, and temporal artery, and peripheral measurements are obtained by skin surface measurements and in the axilla (Atallah et al, 2020; Shetti & Singla, 2020; Aykanat, Broadbent, & Peyton, 2021). Research is limited on the accuracy of temporal artery, carotid artery, and "zero heat flux" measurements outside normal ranges; however, recent research is demonstrating improved accuracy and reliability (Evron et al, 2017; Morettini et al, 2020; Shetti & Singla, 2020). Axillary temperature is accurate in neonates, but it is not well supported in adults; tympanic membrane measurements and chemical dot thermometers are least accurate and should be avoided in caring for the acutely ill adult client (Mahmoudi et al, 2020; Olasinde et al, 2020). As technology improves, the accuracy and reliability of noninvasive temperature monitoring will make the use of these measures an acceptable choice.*
- ● Use the same site and method (device) for temperature measurement for a given client so that temperature trends are assessed accurately, and record site of temperature measurement. EB: *There are differences in temperature depending on the site (esophageal, oral, bladder, rectal, axillary, or temporal artery); however, differences should not be greater than half a degree (Torossian et al, 2016).*
- ● Bladder temperature may be used because an indwelling urinary catheter is often inserted in the management of hypothermia to monitor diuresis. EBN: *Bladder temperature probes have been shown to be accurate during states of increased diuresis, but measurements may be less accurate when urine volume is low (low rate of diuresis). Temperatures obtained by this method may lag up to 20 minutes during targeted temperature hypothermia interventions (Burlingame & Conner, 2019).*

Unintentional Perioperative Hypothermia

- ● Keep the client warm throughout the perioperative period (preoperatively, intraoperatively, and postoperatively) to prevent unintentional perioperative hypothermia. EB: *Initiating warming interventions preoperatively has been found to assist with normothermia and client comfort (Grote et al, 2020).*

- Factors that increase the risk of perioperative hypothermia include anesthetic agents, ambient room air temperature, intravenous (IV) fluid infusion, cavity solution irrigation, blood product administration, duration and type of surgical procedure, anemia, extremes of age, neurological disorders, cachexia, minimal covering during surgery, and preexisting conditions (e.g., peripheral vascular disease, endocrine disease, pregnancy, burns, open wounds) (Brodshaug, Tettum, & Raeder, 2019; Bu et al, 2019; Link, 2020; American Society of PeriAnesthesia Nurses [ASPAN], 2021).
- Closely monitoring and preventing unintentional perioperative hypothermia is necessary to prevent adverse client outcomes. **CEB:** *Adverse outcomes include client discomfort, shivering, cardiac events (e.g., arrhythmias), increased catecholamine release, impaired coagulation, altered drug metabolism, impaired wound healing, and impaired immune function (Collins et al, 2019; Grote et al, 2020; ASPAN, 2021).*
- Several interventions should be implemented to prevent unintentional perioperative hypothermia:
  - Use warming booties perioperatively
  - Use warming blankets over and under the client perioperatively
  - Use warming blankets under the client on the operating table
  - Use of reflective blankets
  - Adjust environmental room controls to maintain ambient room temperature between 20°C (68°F) and 25°C (77°F)
  - Use humidified heated breathing circuit
  - Use warmed forced-air blankets preoperatively, during surgery, and in the postanesthesia care unit
  - Use circulating-water mattress
  - Use warmed IV fluids and irrigation solutions
  - Designate responsibility and accountability for thermoregulation

  EBN/EB: *Maintaining the client's temperature during the surgical procedure has been found to be essential in preventing surgical complications, especially surgical site infections. Maintaining normothermia also enhances client comfort (Institute for Healthcare Improvement [IHI], 2012a; Riley & Andrzejowski, 2018; Bu et al, 2019; CDC, 2020; ASPAN, 2021). Preoperative warming should be initiated for any client with a core temperature below 36°C (96.8°F) before induction of anesthesia, whereas preoperative warming for at least 30 minutes for any client may prevent the client from developing hypothermia and positively affect the client to maintain normothermia (Honkavuo & Koivusalo Loe, 2020; Nordgren et al, 2020). Results from previous investigations have shown that a 2°C decrease (approximately 3.6°F) in core temperature triples the incidence of surgical site infection and increases the length of hospital stay by 20% (de Brito Poveda, Oliviera, & Galvão, 2020).*
- Using warmed IV fluids and irrigation solutions during the operative period may assist with reducing the client's risk of unintentional perioperative hypothermia. **EB:** *Researchers found that warmed IV fluids and irrigation solutions assisted with clients' ability to maintain a higher body temperature and reduced the risk for intraoperative hypothermia and postoperative shivering (Giuliano & Hendricks, 2017; Lindahl, 2020).*
- Active warming interventions include the use of warm blankets and forced-air warming devices. **EBN:** *Blankets used for warming clients quickly lose heat. To prevent rapid heat loss from blankets, warming cabinets should be set at 93.3°C (200°F), and reapply blankets frequently (Kelly et al, 2017).* **EBN:** *Actively warming clients with forced-air warming is the most effective method to prevent hypothermia and offers a clinically important reduction in time to achieve normothermia in postoperative clients (Sumida et al, 2019; Nordgren et al, 2020; Özsaban, & Acaroğlu, 2020).*
- A heated humidified breathing circuit can be used intraoperatively to decrease hypothermia. **EB:** *Heated humidified breathing circuits have decreased the severity of hypothermia in clients undergoing thyroid surgery (Park et al, 2017).*
- Watch the client for signs of hypothermia: shivering, slurred speech, confusion, clumsy movements, fatigue, and dehydration. Shivering increases oxygen consumption by about 40%. As hypothermia progresses, the skin becomes pale, muscles are tense, fatigue and weakness progress, breathing is decreased, and pulmonary congestion is present, compromising oxygenation. Pulses are decreased and blood pressure and heart rate decrease, progressing to lethal arrhythmias (e.g., ventricular fibrillation) (Torossian et al, 2016; Danzl, 2018).

▲ Administer oxygen as ordered. **EB:** *Oxygenation is hampered by the change in the oxyhemoglobin curve caused by hypothermia (Danzl, 2018).*

- ▲ Attach electrodes and a cardiac monitor. Watch for dysrhythmias. EB: *With hypothermia, the client is prone to dysrhythmias because of the cold myocardium; dysrhythmias may include atrial fibrillation, ventricular fibrillation, or asystole (Danzl, 2018; Jandu et al, 2020).*
- ▲ Monitor for signs of coagulopathy (e.g., oozing of blood from any open areas or from intravascular catheter sites or mucous membranes). Also note results of clotting studies as available. EB: *Coagulopathy is a common occurrence during hypothermia (Rösli et al, 2020; ASPAN, 2021).*
- ▲ Monitor for signs of surgical site infection (e.g., increased incisional pain, drainage, poor healing, poor incision approximation). EB: *Unintentional perioperative hypothermia has been associated with increased risk of surgical site infections (IHI, 2012a; CDC, 2020 ASPAN, 2021).*
- • See care plans for Ineffective **Thermoregulation** and **Hypothermia** as appropriate.

Pediatric

- • Interventions implemented in the care of adult clients are similar when providing care to pediatric clients to prevent hypothermia. EB: *Keep the head covered, use warm blankets, or force warm air to keep the client warm; maintain normal ambient room temperature in the perioperative units and use warmed IV fluids (IHI, 2012b).* EBN: *Children lose their body core temperature at a faster rate than adults. Children with a lower preoperative body temperature are more likely to develop hypothermia during the intraoperative and postoperative periods (Beedle et al, 2017; Lai et al, 2019).*

H

Home Care

- ▲ Hypothermia is not a symptom that appears in the normal course of postoperative home care. If the client continues to complain of chills or feeling cold after discharge home from a surgical procedure, provide the client with warm blankets and, if the client is allowed to drink, provide warm fluids by mouth.
- ▲ Monitor temperature every hour, as noted previously. If the temperature of the client begins dropping below the normal range, apply layers of clothing or blankets, or adjust environmental heat to the comfort level. Do not overheat. Contact a health care provider. EB: *Passive rewarming is the only method of rewarming that is appropriate for home care under normal circumstances (Connelly et al, 2017).*
- ▲ If temperature continues to drop, activate the emergency system and notify a health care provider. EB: *Hypothermia is a clinically acute condition that cannot be managed safely in the home.*

Client/Family Teaching and Discharge Planning

- ✱ Teach the client/family signs of hypothermia and the method of taking the temperature (age appropriate).
- ▲ Teach the client and family about medications such as sedatives, opioids, and anxiolytics that predispose the client to hypothermia (as appropriate). If the client has had hypothermia in the past, using alternative medications is an option if there is no contraindication (Danzl, 2018).

REFERENCES

American Society of PeriAnesthesia Nurses (ASPAN). (2021). Normothermia clinical guideline. In *2021-2022 Perianesthesia Nursing Standards: Practice Recommendations and Interpretive Statements*. Cherry Hill, NJ: ASPAN.

Atallah, L., Ciuhu, C., Paulussen, I., et al. (2020). Perioperative measurement of core body temperature using an unobtrusive passive heat flow sensor. *Journal of Clinical Monitoring and Computing, 34*(6), 1351–1359. https://doi.org/10.1007/s10877-019-00446-1.

Aykanat, V. M., Broadbent, E., & Peyton, P. J. (2021). Reliability of alternative devices for postoperative patient temperature measurement: Two prospective, observational studies. *Anaesthesia, 76*(4), 514–519. https://doi.org/10.1111/anae.15248.

Beedle, S. E., Phillips, A., Wiggins, S., & Struwe, L. (2017). Preventing unplanned perioperative hypothermia in children. *AORN Journal, 105*(2), 170–183. https://doi.org/10.1016/j.aorn.2016.12.002.

Brodshaug, I., Tettum, B., & Raeder, J. (2019). Thermal suit or forced air warming in prevention of perioperative hypothermia: A randomized controlled trial. *Journal of PeriAnesthesia Nursing, 34*(5), 1006–1015. https://doi.org/10.1016/j.jopan.2019.03.002.

Bu, N., Zhao, E., Gao, Y., et al. (2019). Association between perioperative hypothermia and surgical site infection. A meta-analysis. *Medicine, 98*(6), e14392. https://doi.org/10.1097/MD.0000000000014392.

Burlingame, B. L., & Conner, R. (2019). Guideline for prevention of hypothermia. In R. Connor (Ed.), *Guidelines for perioperative practice (2020 ed.)* (pp. 327–356). Denver: AORN.

Centers for Disease Control and Prevention (CDC). (2020). *Surgical site infection event*. Retrieved from https://www.cdc.gov/nhsn/PDFs/pscManual/9pscSSIcurrent.pdf. Accessed 6 July 2021.

Collins, S., Budds, M., Raines, C., & Hooper, V. (2019). Risk factors for perioperative hypothermia: A literature review. *Journal of PeriAnesthesia Nursing, 34*(2), 338–346. https://doi.org/10.1016/j.jopan.2018.06.003.

Connelly, L., Cramer, E., DeMott, Q., et al. (2017). The optimal time and method for surgical prewarming: A comprehensive review of the literature. *Journal of PeriAnesthesia Nursing, 32*(3), 199–209. https://doi.org/10.1016/j.jopan.2015.11.010.

Danzl, D. F. (2018). Hypothermia and peripheral cold injuries. In J. L. Jameson, A. S. Fauci, D. L. Kasper, S. L. Hauser, D. L. Longo, & J. Loscalzo (Eds.), *Harrison's principles of internal medicine* (20th ed.). New York: McGraw-Hill.

de Brito Poveda, V., Oliveria, R. A., & Galvão, C. M. (2020). Perioperative body temperature maintenance and occurrence of surgical site infection: A systematic review with meta-analysis. *American Journal of Infection Control, 48*(10), 1248–1254. https://doi.org/10.1016/j.ajic.2020.01.002.

Evron, S., Weissman, A., Toivis, V., et al. (2017). Evaluation of the temple touch pro, a novel noninvasive core-temperature monitoring system. *Anesthesia & Analgesia, 125*(1), 103–109. https://doi.org/10.1213/ane.0000000000001695.

Giuliano, K. K., & Hendricks, J. (2017). Inadvertent perioperative hypothermia: Current nursing knowledge. *AORN Journal, 105*(5), 453–463. https://doi.org/10.1016/j.aorn.2017.03.003.

Granum, M. N., Kaasby, K., Skou, S. T., & Grønkjaer, M. (2019). Preventing inadvertent hypothermia in patients undergoing major spinal surgery: A nonrandomized controlled study of two different methods of preoperative and intraoperative warming. *Journal of PeriAnesthesia Nursing, 34*(5), 999–1005.

Grote, R., Wetz, A., Bräuer, A., & Menzel, M. (2020). Short interruptions between pre-warming and intraoperative warming are associated with low intraoperative hypothermia rates. *Acta Anaesthesiologica Scandinavica, 64*(4), 489–493. https://doi.org/10.1111/aas.13521.

Honkavuo, L., & Koivusalo Loe, S. A. (2020). Nurse anesthetists' and operating theater nurses' experiences with inadvertent hypothermia in clinical perioperative nursing care. *Journal of PeriAnesthesia Nursing, 35*(6), 676–681. https://doi.org/10.1016/j.jopan.2020.03.011.

Institute for Healthcare Improvement (IHI). (2012a). *How-to-guide: Prevent surgical site infections*. Cambridge, MA: IHI. Retrieved from www.ihi.org. Accessed 6 July 2021.

Institute for Healthcare Improvement (IHI). (2012b). *How-to guide: Prevent surgical site infections, pediatric supplement*. Cambridge, MA: IHI. Retrieved from www.ihi.org. Accessed 6 July 2021.

Jandu, S., Sefa, N., Sawyer, K. N., & Swor, R. (2020). Electrocardiographic changes in patients undergoing targeted temperature management. *Journal of the American College of Emergency Physicians Open, 1*(4), 327–332. https://doi.org/10.1002/emp2.12104.

Kelly, P. A., Morse, E. C., Swanfeldt, J. V., et al. (2017). Safety of rolled and folded cotton blankets warmed in 130°F and 200°F cabinets. *Journal of PeriAnesthesia Nursing, 32*(6), 600–608. https://doi.org/10.1016/j.jopan.2016.03.013.

Lai, L. L., See, M. H., Rampal, S., Ng, K. S., & Chan, L. (2019). Significant factors influencing inadvertent hypothermia in pediatric anesthesia. *Journal of Clinical Monitoring and Computing, 33*(6), 1105–1112. https://doi.org/10.1007/s10877-019-00259-2.

Lindahl, S. B. (2020). Intraoperative irrigation: Fluid administration and management amidst conflicting evidence. *AORN Journal, 111*(5), 495–507. https://doi.org/10.1002/aorn.13010.

Link, T. (2020). Guidelines in practice: Hypothermia prevention. *AORN Journal, 111*(6), 653–666. https://doi.org/10.1002/aorn.13038.

Mahmoudi, Z., Jahanpour, F., Azodi, P., & Ostovar, A. (2020). Comparison of the specificity and sensitivity of the infrared temporal artery and digital axillary body temperature measurements with nasopharyngeal method in adult patients. *Journal of Clinical Care and Skills, 1*(3), 147–151.

Morettini, E., Turchini, F., Tofani, L., Villa, G., Ricci, Z., & Romagnoli, S. (2020). Intraoperative core temperature monitoring: Accuracy and precision of zero-heat flux heated controlled servo sensor compared with esophageal temperature during major surgery; the ESOSPOT study. *Journal of Clinical Monitoring and Computing, 34*(5), 1111–1119. https://doi.org/10.1007/s10877-019-00410-z.

Nordgren, M., Herborg, O., Hamberg, Sandström, E., Larsson, G., & Söderström, L. (2020). The effectiveness of four intervention methods for preventing inadvertent perioperative hypothermia during total knee or total hip arthroplasty. *AORN Journal, 111*(3), 303–312. https://doi.org/10.1002/aorn.12961.

Olasinde, Y., Ernest, M., Popoola, G., Adesiyun, O., & Ernest, K. (2020). Temperature measurements in neonates: Assessing the agreement of two methods. *Open Journal of Pediatrics, 10*(1), 224–230. https://doi.org/10.4236/ojped.2020.101022.

Özsaban, A., & Acaroğlu, R. (2020). The effect of active warming on postoperative hypothermia on body temperature and thermal comfort: A randomized controlled trial. *Journal of PeriAnesthesia Nursing, 35*(4), 423–429. https://doi.org/10.1016/j.jopan.2019.12.006.

Park, H. J., Moon, H. S., Moon, S. H., et al. (2017). The effect of humidified heated breathing circuit on core body temperature in perioperative hypothermia during thyroid surgery. *International Journal of Medical Sciences, 14*(8), 791–797. https://doi.org/10.7150/ijms.19318.

Riley, C., & Andrzejowski, J. (2018). Inadvertent perioperative hypothermia. *BJA Education, 18*(8), 227–233. https://doi.org/10.1016/j.bjae.2018.05.003.

Rösli, D., Schnüriger, B., Candinas, D., & Haltmeier, T. (2020). The impact of accidental hypothermia on mortality in trauma patients overall and patients with traumatic brain injury specifically: A systematic review and meta-analysis. *World Journal of Surgery, 44*(12), 4106–4117. https://doi.org/10.1007/s00268-020-05750-5.

Shetti, A. N., & Singla, B. (2020). Correlation of nasopharyngeal temperature with transcutaneous carotid artery temperature of adult patients under general anesthesia in rural tertiary care hospital. *Anesthesia, Pain, and Intensive Care, 24*(3), 302–307. https://doi.org/10.35975/apic.v24i3.1284.

Sumida, H., Sugino, S., Kuratani, N., Konno, D., Hasegawa, J. I., & Yamauchi, M. (2019). Effect of forced-air warming by an underbody blanket on end-of-surgery hypothermia: A propensity score-matched analysis of 5063 patients. *BMC Anesthesiology, 19*(1), 50. https://doi.org/10.1186/s12871-019-0724-8.

Torossian, A., Van Gerven, E., Geertsen, K., Horn, B., Van de Velde, M., & Raeder, J. (2016). Active perioperative patient warming using a self-warming blanket (BARRIER EasyWarm) is superior to passive thermal insulation: A multinational, multicenter, randomized trial. *Journal of Clinical Anesthesia, 34*, 547–554. https://doi.org/10.1016/j.jclinane.2016.06.030.

Disturbed Family Identity Syndrome

Domain 7 Role relationship Class 2 Family relationships

Stacey M. Carroll, PhD, APRN-BC

I

NANDA-I

Definition

Inability to maintain an ongoing interactive, communicative process of creating and maintaining a shared collective sense of the meaning of the family.

Defining Characteristics

Decisional conflict (00083); disabled family coping (00073); disturbed personal identity (00121); dysfunctional family processes (00063); impaired resilience (00210); ineffective childbearing process (00221); ineffective relationship (00223); ineffective sexuality pattern (00065); interrupted family processes (00060)

Related Factors

Ambivalent family relations; different coping styles among family members; disrupted family rituals; disrupted family roles; excessive stress; inadequate social support; ineffective coping strategies; ineffective family communication; perceived social discrimination; sexual dysfunction; unaddressed domestic violence; unrealistic expectations; values incongruent with cultural norms

At-Risk Population

Blended families; economically disadvantaged families; families experiencing infertility; families with history of domestic violence; families with incarcerated member; families with member experiencing alteration in health status; families with member experiencing developmental crisis; families with member living far from relatives; families with member with history of adoption; families with member with intimacy dysfunction; families with unemployed member; infertility treatment regimen

NOC (Nursing Outcomes Classification)

Suggested NOC Outcomes

Family Social Climate; Family Integrity; Family Coping; Family Functioning

Example NOC Outcome with Indicators

Family Social Climate as evidenced by the following indicators: Works cooperatively to meet family goals/Promotes cohesion. (Rate the outcome and indicators of **Family Social Climate:** 1 = never demonstrated, 2 = rarely demonstrated, 3 = sometimes demonstrated, 4 = often demonstrated, 5 = consistently demonstrated [see Section I].)

Client Outcomes

Client Will (Specify Time Frame)

- Identify communication strategies that family members can use to facilitate an improved sense of family identity
- Express feelings and share collective experiences
- Meet physical, psychosocial, and spiritual needs of members
- Support one another and family goals
- Work cooperatively to solve problems

NIC (Nursing Interventions Classification)

Suggested NIC Interventions

Family Integrity Promotion; Family Process Maintenance; Family Support

Example NIC Activities—Family Integrity Promotion

Collaborate with family in problem solving and decision-making; Facilitate open communication among family members; Identify typical family coping mechanisms

Nursing Interventions and *Rationales*

- Provide family-centered care in all nursing settings to alleviate disturbed family identity. EB: *Family members of clients in the intensive care unit (ICU) had depression, anxiety, and posttraumatic stress during the ICU stay, and many had symptoms persisting months later (Harlan et al, 2020).*
- Include family assessment as part of comprehensive nursing assessment to guide appropriate interventions. EBN: *Family assessment was a component of implementing a family-centered care approach in acute care (Eustace et al, 2015).*
- ✱ Assess for clients' self-reports of family dysfunction, particularly noting any reports of abuse or self-injury. EB: *Family dysfunction in a community corrections sample was associated with higher suicide risk (Clark et al, 2016).*
- Apply theoretical models to understand family dynamics and communication patterns. EB: *The Family Communication Pattern Theory (FCPT) was used to show that a family climate of free conversation combined with stressing homogeneous beliefs is passed on intergenerationally (Rauscher et al, 2020).* EB: *Using the Family Adjustment and Adaptation Model to study home-front mothers in military families showed that finding benefits to service can be a positive factor in improving family functioning (Kritikos et al, 2020).*
- Ascertain client's own meaning of family. EB: *Gay adoptive parents view family in a way that is socially and culturally constructed and may not follow heteronormative views of family and parenting (Zhang & Chen, 2020).*
- Use established instruments to assess for family communication and functioning. EB: *The Revised Family Communication Patterns Scale (RFCP), with three items omitted, was used to measure family members' perception of their family communication patterns (Rauscher et al, 2020).* EB: *The Family Coping Questionnaire for Eating Disorders (FCQ-ED) is brief and has good psychometric qualities (Fiorillo et al, 2015).*
- ▲ Involve families, with client consent, in decision-making processes to facilitate family harmony. EBN: *Supporting family involvement in decision-making in cancer care assisted in the adjustment process for the client (Lim & Shon, 2016).* EBN: *Families who were aware of clients' end-of-life wishes experienced less decisional conflict (Jeon et al, 2018).*
- ▲ Consider novel family therapy interventions aimed at coping and reducing relational conflict during periods of extended isolation. EB: *A program called Reaching Up, Down, In, and Around is proposed as a unique way for families to foster coping and resilience during the coronavirus pandemic (Fraenkel & Cho, 2020).*
- ▲ Include early identification of family dysfunction in a comprehensive chronic pain treatment program. EB: *Clients with chronic widespread pain had poorer family functioning than those with chronic localized pain (Hayaki et al, 2016).*

Pediatric

- Encourage families to maintain and develop family rituals and traditions. EB: *Research suggests that family rituals have a positive impact on child behaviors (Bao et al, 2019).*
- Encourage and support the family to have frequent and regular family meals. EB: *Findings from a systematic review of protective factors for disordered eating suggest that family meals promote a healthy family environment around eating (Langdon-Daly & Serpell, 2017).*

Geriatric

- Encourage intergenerational communication among family members. EB: *Shared family identity can be fostered by encouraging grandchild-grandparent interactions (Fowler, 2015).*
- Incorporate family interventions for early-onset Alzheimer's disease. EB: *Family satisfaction and communication contributed to increased quality of life in clients with early-onset Alzheimer's disease (Lima et al, 2020).*

- • Conduct family life review with older adults as they transition to new environments to enhance family relations. EB: *Family life review among older adults relocating to assisted living enhanced family relationships during the transition (O'Hora & Roberto, 2019).*
- ▲ Explore alternative means for family interaction if in-person visits are restricted or not feasible, to maintain connections. EB: *Increased phone and email contact with family members resulted in more positive emotions among clients in long-term care who could not receive in-person visits during the coronavirus pandemic (Monin et al, 2020).*

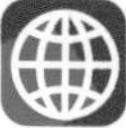

Multicultural

- ▲ Incorporate multicultural considerations into family therapy. EB: *Among families of incarcerated individuals of color, incorporating multicultural family therapy is essential (Tadros et al, 2019).*
- • Consider cultural factors in assessing family identity. EB: *Culture influenced family identity in the context of severe mental illness (Acero et al, 2017).* EB: *Battered women in Ghana often stayed in relationships because of the importance of preserving family social image (Adjei, 2017).*
- ▲ Be aware of cultural considerations when using instruments to assess family functioning. EBN: *The Decisional Conflict Scale in nursing home placement decisions of Chinese family caregivers may not fully capture cultural considerations (Chang et al, 2017).*
- • Incorporate faith tenets, as relevant, to strengthen family dynamics. EB: *Accessing spiritual and religious values is proposed as a way for families to cope during the coronavirus pandemic (Fraenkel & Cho, 2020).* EB: *Family members of clients who had a stroke experienced less burden when they had higher religious coping scores (Kes & Yildirim, 2020).*
- • Encourage cultural rituals to enhance expression of family identity. EB: *Quinceanera was theorized as a way for Hispanic families to embrace family identity amidst various social contexts (Verdin & Camacho, 2019).*

I

Home Care

- ▲ Refer clients with chronic pain and their families for occupational therapy (OT) interventions. EB: *OTs can use assertiveness training and occupation-centered interventions to facilitate family communication (Swift et al, 2019).*
- • Be sensitive about timing of a family coping intervention. EB: Many families of clients in palliative home care declined a nurse-led family coping home care intervention, citing the intervention as being offered too soon in the process (*Ammari et al, 2015*).

Client/Family Teaching and Discharge Planning

- ▲ Refer families experiencing substance use disorder for family counseling. EBN: *Positive family communication patterns led to reduced drug cravings in the client (Badie et al, 2020).* EB: *Family cohesion positively influenced family communication in young adults, even when family opioid misuse was present (Alhussain et al, 2019).*
- ▲ Refer couples to relationship education that includes family social supports in its curriculum. EB: *Social support influenced family functioning outcomes in low-income couples attending relationship education (Carlson et al, 2020).*
- ▲ Refer couples with infertility for specialist consultation. EB: *Decisional conflict scores of couples, individually, decreased after a consultation with an infertility specialist (Anguzu et al, 2020).*

REFERENCES

Acero, A. R., Cano-Prous, A., Castellanos, G., Martín-Lanas, R., & Canga-Armayor, A. (2017). Family identity and severe mental illness: A thematic synthesis of qualitative studies. *European Journal of Social Psychology*, *47*(5), 611–627. https://doi.org/10.1002/ejsp.2240.

Adjei, S. B. (2017). Entrapment of victims of spousal abuse in Ghana: A discursive analysis of family identity and agency of battered women. *Journal of Interpersonal Violence*, *32*(5), 730–754. https://doi.org/10.1177/0886260515586375.

Alhussain, K., Shah, D., Thornton, J. D., & Kelly, K. M. (2019). Familial opioid misuse and family cohesion: Impact on family communication and well-being. *Addictive Disorders & Their Treatment*, *18*(4), 194–204. https://doi.org/10.1097/ADT.0000000000000165.

Ammari, A. B. H., Hendriksen, C., & Rydahl-Hansen, S. (2015). Recruitment and reasons for non-participation in a family-coping-oriented palliative home care trial (FamCope). *Journal of Psychosocial Oncology*, *33*(6), 655–674. https://doi.org/10.1080/07347332.2015.1082168.

Anguzu, R., Cusatis, R., Fergestrom, N., et al. (2020). Decisional conflict among couples seeking specialty treatment for infertility in the USA: A longitudinal exploratory study. *Human Reproduction*, *35*(3), 573–582. https://doi.org/10.1093/humrep/dez292.

Badie, A., Makvandi, B., Bakhtiarpour, S., & Pasha, R. (2020). Drug cravings and its relationship with family communication patterns and resiliency through the mediatory role of difficult in cognitive emotion regulation. *Journal of Client-Centered Nursing Care, 6*(2), 125–134. https://doi.org/10.32598/JCCNC.6.2.329.1.

Bao, J., Gudmunson, C. G., Greder, K., & Smith, S. R. (2019). The impact of family rituals and maternal depressive symptoms on child externalizing behaviors: An urban–rural comparison. *Child and Youth Care Forum, 48*, 935–953. https://doi.org/10.1007/s10566-019-09512-w.

Carlson, R. G., Wheeler, N. J., Liu, X., Hipp, C., & Daire, A. P. (2020). The relationship between social support and family relationships among low-income couples attending relationship education. *Family Process, 59*(4), 1498–1516. https://doi.org/10.1111/famp.12499.

Chang, Y. P., Sessanna, L., & Schneider, J. K. (2017). The applicability of the decisional conflict Scale in nursing home placement decision among Chinese family caregivers: A mixed methods approach. *Asian Pacific Island Nursing Journal, 2*(3), 110–120. https://doi.org/10.9741/23736658.1064.

Clark, C. B., Li, Y., & Cropsey, K. L. (2016). Family dysfunction and suicide risk in a community corrections sample. *Crisis, 37*(6), 454–460. https://doi.org/10.1027/0227-5910/a000406.

Eustace, R. W., Gray, B., & Curry, D. M. (2015). The meaning of family nursing intervention: What do acute care nurses think? *Research and Theory for Nursing Practice: International Journal, 29*(2), 125–142. https://doi.org/10.1891/1541-6577.29.2.125.

Fiorillo, A., Sampogna, G., Del Vecchio, V., et al. (2015). Development and validation of the Family Coping Questionnaire for Eating Disorders. *International Journal of Eating Disorders, 48*(3), 298–304. https://doi.org/10.1002/eat.22367.

Fowler, C. (2015). The role of shared family identity and future time perspective in shaping the outcomes of grandparents' positive and negative social behaviors. *Journal of Family Communication, 15*(1), 20–40. https://doi.org/10.1080/15267431.2014.980822.

Fraenkel, P., & Cho, W. L. (2020). Reaching up, down, in, and around: Couple and family coping during the coronavirus pandemic. *Family Process, 59*(3), 847–864. https://doi.org/10.111/famp.12570.

Harlan, E. A., Miller, J., Costa, D. K., et al. (2020). Emotional experiences and coping strategies of family members of critically ill patients. *Chest, 158*(4), 1464–1472. https://doi.org/10.1016/j.chest.2020.05.535.

Hayaki, C., Anno, K., Shibata, M., et al. (2016). Family dysfunction: A comparison of chronic widespread pain and chronic localized pain. *Medicine, 95*(49), e5495. https://doi.org/10.1097/MD.0000000000005495.

Jeon, B. M., Kim, S. H., & Lee, S. J. (2018). Decisional conflict in end-of-life cancer treatment among family surrogates: A cross-sectional survey. *Nursing and Health Sciences, 20*(4), 472–478. https://doi.org/10.1111/nhs.12537.

Kes, D., & Yildirim, T. A. (2020). The relationship of religious coping strategies and family harmony with caregiver burden for family members of patients with stroke. *Brain Injury, 34*(11), 1461–1466. https://doi.org/10.1080/02699052.2020.1810317.

Kritikos, T. K., DeVoe, E. R., Spencer, R., et al. (2020). Finding meaning in times of family stress: A mixed methods study of benefits and challenges amongst home-front parents in military families. *Military Psychology, 32*(4), 287–299. https://doi.org/10.1080/08995605.2020.1754122.

Langdon-Daly, J., & Serpell, L. (2017). Protective factors against disordered eating in family systems: A systematic review of research. *Journal of Eating Disorders, 5*, 12. https://doi.org/10.1186/s40337-017-0141-7.

Lim, J. W., & Shon, E. J. (2016). Decisional conflict: Relationships between and among family context variables in cancer survivors. *Oncology Nursing Forum, 43*(4), 480–488. https://doi.org/10.1188/16.ONF.480-488.

Lima, S., Sevilha, S., & Pereira, M. G. (2020). Quality of life in early-stage Alzheimer's disease: The moderator role of family variables and coping strategies from the patients' perspective. *Psychogeriatrics, 20*(5), 557–567. https://doi.org/10.1111/psyg.12544.

Monin, J. K., Ali, T., Syed, S., et al. (2020). Family communication in long-term care during a pandemic: Lessons for enhancing emotional experiences. *American Journal of Geriatric Psychiatry, 28*(12), 1299–1307. https://doi.org/1.1016/j.jagp.2020.09.008.

O'Hora, K. A., & Roberto, K. A. (2019). Navigating emotions and relationship dynamics: Family life review as a clinical tool for older adults during a relocation transition into an assisted living facility. *Aging & Mental Health, 23*(4), 404–410. https://doi.org/10.1080/13607863.2017.1423028.

Rauscher, E. A., Schrodt, P., Campbell-Salome, G., & Freytag, J. (2020). The intergenerational transmission of family communication patterns: (In)consistencies in conversation and conformity orientations across two generations of family. *Journal of Family Communication, 20*(2), 97–113. https://doi.org/10.1080/15267431.2019.1683563.

Swift, C., Hocking, C., Dickinson, A., & Jones, M. (2019). Facilitating open family communication when a parent has chronic pain: A scoping review. *Scandinavian Journal of Occupational Therapy, 26*(2), 103–120. https://doi.org/10.1080/11038128.2018.1486885.

Tadros, E., Fye, J. M., McCrone, C. L., & Finney, N. (2019). Incorporating multicultural couple and family therapy into incarcerated settings. *International Journal of Offender Therapy and Comparative Criminology, 63*(4), 641–658. https://doi.org/10.1177/0306624X18823442.

Verdin, A., & Camacho, J. (2019). Changing family identity through the quinceanera ritual. *Hispanic Journal of Behavioral Sciences, 41*(2), 185–196. https://doi.org/10.1177/0739986319837266.

Zhang, D., & Chen, Y. W. (2020). "We are the unusual factor": Queering family communication norms with gay adoptive parents. *Journal of Family Communication, 20*(3), 206–220. https://doi.org/10.1080/15267431.2020.1767621.

I

Risk for Disturbed Family Identity Syndrome

Domain 7 Role relationship Class 2 Family relationships

Marina Martinez-Kratz, MS, RN, CNE

NANDA-I

Definition

Susceptible to an inability to maintain an ongoing interactive, communicative process of creating and maintaining a shared collective sense of the meaning of the family, which may compromise family members' health

Risk Factors

Ambivalent family relations; different coping styles among family members; disrupted family rituals; disrupted family roles; excessive stress; inadequate social support; ineffective coping strategies; ineffective family communication; perceived social discrimination; sexual dysfunction; unaddressed domestic violence; unrealistic expectations; values incongruent with cultural norm

At-Risk Population

Blended families; economically disadvantaged families; families experiencing infertility; families with history of domestic violence; families with incarcerated member; families with member experiencing alteration in health status; families with member experiencing developmental crisis; families with member living far from relatives; families with member with history of adoption; families with member with intimacy dysfunction; families with unemployed member

Associated Conditions

Infertility treatment regimen

NIC, NOC, Client Outcomes, Nursing Interventions and *Rationales,* Client/Family Teaching, and References

Refer to care plan for Disturbed **Family** Identity Syndrome.

Disturbed Personal Identity Domain 6 Self-perception Class 1 Self-concept

Ruth A. Wittmann-Price, PhD, RN, CNS, CNE, CNEcl, CHSE, ANEF, FAAN

NANDA-I

Definition

Inability to maintain an integrated and complete perception of self.

Defining Characteristics

Altered body image; confusion about cultural values; confusion about goals; confusion about ideological values; delusional description of self; expresses feeling of emptiness; expresses feeling of strangeness; fluctuating feelings about self; impaired ability to distinguish between internal and external stimuli; inadequate interpersonal relations; inadequate role performance; inconsistent behavior; ineffective coping strategies; reports social discrimination

Related Factors

Altered social role; cult indoctrination; dysfunctional family processes; gender conflict; low self-esteem; perceived social discrimination; values incongruent with cultural norms

At-Risk Population

Individuals experiencing developmental transition; individuals experiencing situational crisis; individuals exposed to toxic chemical

Associated Conditions

Dissociative identity disorder; mental disorders; neurocognitive disorders; pharmaceutical preparations

NOC (Nursing Outcomes Classification)

Suggested NOC Outcomes

Anxiety Self-Control; Abuse Recovery (Emotional, Physical, Sexual); Body Image; Decision-Making; Distorted Thought Self-Control; Identity; Mutilation; Suicide/Self-Restraint

Example NOC Outcome with Indicators

Identity as evidenced by the following indicators: Verbalizes affirmations of personal identity/Exhibits congruent verbal and nonverbal behavior about self/Differentiates self from environment and other human beings. (Rate the outcome and indicators of **Identity:** 1 = never demonstrated, 2 = rarely demonstrated, 3 = sometimes demonstrated, 4 = often demonstrated, 5 = consistently demonstrated [see Section I].)

Client Outcomes

Client Will (Specify Time Frame)

- Demonstrate new purposes for life
- Show interests in surroundings
- Perform self-care and self-control activities appropriate for age
- Acknowledge personal strengths
- Engage in interpersonal relationships

NIC (Nursing Interventions Classification)

Suggested NIC Interventions

Decision-Making Support; Mutual Goal Setting; Self-Awareness Enhancement; Self-Esteem Enhancement; Sexual Counseling; Substance Use Prevention

Example NIC Activities—Self-Esteem Enhancement

Monitor client's statements of self-worth; Encourage client to identify strengths

I

Nursing Interventions and *Rationales*

- ● Assess and support family strengths of commitment, appreciation, and affection toward each other; positive communication; time together; a sense of spiritual well-being; and the ability to cope with stress and crisis. EB: *Hayes, Maliski, and Warner (2017) discovered through a qualitative study that family is an important support for clients but found that clients are less likely to disclose sensitive health issues when family members are present.* EB: *Jagtiani et al (2019) studied family belonging (family meal frequency, strength of family support, and personal identity) and its relationships between the amount of time spent on social networking sites in young adults (n = 2229) and well-being. Well-being was lower for heavy social networking users and those families who had fewer family meals.*
- ▲ Assess for suicidal ideation and make appropriate referral for clients dealing with mental illness or other risk factors. EB: *Dutta et al (2017) completed a large quantitative study about the genetics of suicidal ideation with twins (n = 3906 twins) and nontwins (n = 2016) and found that suicidal ideation was 13.0% for men, 21.8% for women, and no difference between twins and nontwins.* EB: *Eikelenboom et al (2019) completed a 6-year longitudinal study assessing predictors of suicide and found the highest risk was for clients with major depressive disorder (MDD), along with younger age, lower education, unemployment, insomnia, antidepressant use, a previous suicide attempt, and current suicidal thoughts predicted a future suicide attempt.*
- ▲ Assess clients with mood disorders and make appropriate referrals for treatment. EB: *Verhoeven et al (2017) compared the Mini International Neuropsychiatric Interview (MINI) with clinical diagnosis for mood disorders and anxiety differentiation and found that agreement between the MINI and clinical diagnoses was moderate but increased for clients with just one diagnosis.* EB: *Researchers (Sumiyana & Sriwidharmanely, 2020) examined how proactive personality (confront and transform) mitigated technostress and found that participants who identified as proactive were better able to endure technostress.*
- ▲ Assess and make appropriate referrals for clients with physical or mental disabilities. EB: *A study compared mental health and physical health participants (n = 701) attending an exercise referral program over a 12-month period and found that the mental health participants were more likely to drop out than those with physical health problems, indicating that better referral decisions can be made (Tobi, Kemp, & Schmidt, 2017).* EB: *Sultan et al (2020) examined the effects of personality traits and the relationship between religiosity and mental health of university students (n = 372). The results demonstrated that openness to experience and agreeableness as personal traits moderated the relationship between religiosity and mental health.*

- ▲ Assess clients for substance misuse or addictive behaviors and make appropriate referrals. EB: *Nandrino and Gandolphe (2017) studied clients with alcohol use disorder (n = 27) and their self-defining memories (SDMs). Their SDMs disrupt positive memories and negatively affect personal identity and personal goals.* EB: *Fenton-O'Creevy and Furnham (2020) studied the relationship between demographic, personality, and attitude and impulsive buying. Results demonstrated that people who were neurotic and extroverts and had low conscientiousness were more likely to be impulse buyers and materialism was akin to their personal identity.*
- ● Use empathetic communication and encourage the client and family to verbalize fears, express emotions, and set goals. EBN: *Families (n = 612) were provided interventions with emphasis on five positive psychology themes, namely, gratitude, flow, happiness, health, and savoring, in a "kitchen project." Results demonstrated that family communication time and frequency of family meal preparation increased with sustainable effects (Ho et al, 2017).* EB: *Szwimer et al (2020) used a phenomenological exploratory approach to study female adolescent clients (n = 8) with chronic pain. The participants reported that having engaging hobbies, accepting the incurability of chronic pain, and envisioning a fulfilling future were factors that improved their quality of life.*
- ● Be present for clients physically or by telephone. EBN: *Barrett (2017) completed a grounded theory study about the use of teleconsultation by nurses (n = 17) and found that nursing presence was the core category identified and subcategories of nursing presence were operational, clinical, therapeutic, and social, indicating that nurses provided presence during teleconsultation.* EB: *Lindo and Ceballos (2020) studied children's and adolescents' self-expression and career exploration. Using art interventions in case studies, the researchers spent time with the children to assist them with integration of personal identity and career identity variables.*
- ● Encourage expression of positive thoughts and emotions. EBN: *Hughes, Williams, and Shaw (2017) did a literature review (n = 6) about psychological issues faced by teenagers and young adults during cancer treatment, and analysis identified the following themes: anxieties about treatment, concerns regarding the impact on life (feeling restricted and different, the benefits of being sick, facing uncertainty), and coping strategies (positive thinking and problem-solving, support).* EB: *Dang et al (2020) used the Multidimensional Perfectionism Scale, Perfectionistic Self-Presentation Scale, Attitudes Towards Seeking Professional Help Scale, and Thoughts About Psychotherapy Survey on 376 community individuals and university students and found that perfectionistic behavior may be an important factor that interferes with seeking and obtaining psychological help when needed.*
- ● Encourage the client to use coping mechanisms. EBN: *Nursing researchers used a cross-sectional study to better understand family satisfaction with health care of their child by measuring support, family quality of life, expressive family functioning, coping strategies, and health care satisfaction in parents (159 mothers and 60 fathers). Results for mothers demonstrated that satisfaction with health care was predicted by family support and their coping strategies, whereas for fathers, satisfaction was predicted by perceived family support, family quality of life, and whether the child had been hospitalized before (Sigurdardottir, Garwick, & Svavarsdottir, 2017).* EB: *Bürger Lazar and Musek (2020) investigated how personal parental identity (n = 99) and coping affected the quality of life of children with cancer. Parents with emotion-focused coping skills had a negative effect on the child's well-being.*
- ● Help clients with serious and chronic conditions to maintain social support networks or assist in building new ones. EBN: *Hagedoorn et al (2017) descriptively studied family caregiving of elderly clients (n = 62) with one or more chronic conditions, and themes identified were addressing the clients' social network, which included "social network structure" and "social network support," and addressing coordination of care issues.* EB: *Arroyo-Anlló et al (2020) studied clients with Alzheimer's disease and the effect on self-consciousness, because emotions are an integral part of personal identity and "self." The researchers used sensory stimulation such as familiar smells, taste, music, and visuals to promote recall of autobiographical events with positive effects on memory, affective state, and personal identity.*
- ▲ Refer women facing diagnostic and curative breast cancer surgery for psychosocial support. EB: *A literature review (n = 190) about breast cancer treatment for African women found that breast tumors are diagnosed at earlier ages and later stages than in high-income countries, and there is a higher prevalence of triple-negative cancers. Lack of nursing care, inadequate access to radiotherapy and surgery, and poor availability of systemic therapies produce poor survival rates (Vanderpuye et al, 2017).* EB: *Rochefort et al (2019) looked at personal traits and identity associated with health and well-being in women with breast cancer (n = 55). The researchers found that higher conscientiousness and lower neuroticism were associated with better health behaviors and health.*

- Refer for cognitive behavioral therapy (CBT). EBN: *Choi, Lee, and Cho (2017) used CBT with clients (*n *= 76) who had panic disorder and found that it was useful and produced greater positive effects in the acute treatment phase than those they experienced when receiving only routine treatment.* EB: *Domhardt et al (2020) completed a meta-analysis of adults with panic attacks or agoraphobia and found 16 studies eligible for evaluation. The conclusion of the meta-analysis lent credence to the use of Internet and mobile-based interventions (IMIs) in adults with diagnosed panic disorder and/or agoraphobia. IMI as a CBT decreased symptoms for clients with panic disorder and/or agoraphobia.*
- ▲ Refer clients with borderline personality disorder (BPD) and dual-diagnosed BPD and substance misuse for dialectical behavior therapy (DBT) and psychoanalytical-orientated day-hospital therapy. EB: *Stepp and Lazarus (2017) did a study to identify dimensions of children (*n *= 2450) with temperament and psychopathology symptoms that predict future BPD. Researchers found that parent and teacher ratings of emotionality predicted BPD; therefore early detection may increase care for children with BPD.* EBN: *Eckerström et al (2020) competed an interventional qualitative study for clients (*n *= 15) diagnosed with BPD. The intervention was a "brief admission" (BA) and provided a timeout, in situations of increased stress and threat, in order to foster self-management in a safe environment. The qualitative interviews of the clients experiencing the BA produced four themes: (1) a timeout when life is tough, (2) it is comforting to know that help exists, (3) encouraged to take personal responsibility, and (4) it is helpful to see the problems from a different perspective.*
- ▲ Refer to the care plans for Readiness for Enhanced **Communication** and Readiness for Enhanced **Spiritual** Well-Being.

Pediatric

- Encourage adolescents to promote positive self-esteem, to enhance coping, and to prevent behavioral and psychological problems. EB: *Zhang, Huebner, and Tian (2020) studied the association of cyberbullying and personality characteristics of early adolescent participants (*n *= 3961). The researchers discovered that neuroticism and depression were related personality attributes and that neuroticism predicted cyberbullying victimization and depression predicted both cyberbullying perpetration and victimization.* EBN: *Ruhl and Lordly (2017) found that students who are a part of a competitive educational program display a negative effect on personal identity, learning motivation, student collaboration, participation in academic opportunities, and student relationships with faculty.*
- ▲ Evaluate and refer children and adolescents for eating disorder prevention programs that include medical care, nutritional intervention, and mental health treatment and care coordination. EBN: *Kendal et al (2017) qualitatively studied eating disorders and social media (400 messages) and found the following online discussion themes: taking on the role of mentor, the online discussion forum as a safe space, friendship within the online forum, flexible help, and peer support for recovery and relapse prevention.* EB: *Tsotsi et al (2019) studied maternal anxiety and stress as related to 4-year-olds' (*n *= 391) self-regulation. The researchers found a direct correlation between increased maternal anxiety and external behavioral problems.*
- Use computer-mediated support groups to enhance identity formation. EBN: *Jackson and Mixer (2017) used Apple iPads in a pilot study for pediatric clients and families who spoke Spanish and found it assisted in bedside communication, and the results assisted in developing a larger-scale communication interface.* EB: *Strøm et al (2019) completed a study that examined Internet support groups (ISGs) for clients who experienced lumbar spine fusion (*n *= 48). ISGs qualitative analysis identified the following thematic categories: social recognition, experience of pain, experience of physical activity, psychosocial well-being, exploring the ISG, and employment, which correlated with reports of anxiety and depression.*

Geriatric

- Evaluate the effectiveness of nursing interventions used to promote positive self-identify in older adults. EBN: *A descriptive study about applying a therapeutic relationship to people (*n *= 112) with a common mental disorder found that the nursing therapeutic relationship in mental health transcends the area of specialty and builds client coping strategies and helps clients make changes in daily life (Nóbrega et al, 2017).* EB: *Steenhaut et al (2020) studied psychological flexibility and its relation to well-being in young (less than 60 years old) and older (more than 60 years old) participants. The results demonstrated that psychological flexibility (being open minded and having the ability to make flexible choices) was associated with well-being.*
- Encourage clients to discuss their "life histories." Life history–based interventions and self-esteem and life-satisfaction questionnaires may be used to reinforce personal identity and foster hope. EBN: *Tamura-Lis (2017) used reminiscing as an effective evidence-based tool in understanding and treating older adults.*

Reminiscing has demonstrated that it improves communication and socialization. EB: *Hausknecht et al (2019) used digital storytelling to provide older adults with an opportunity to tell their life history. Results from the focus group interviews demonstrated social and emotional benefits, including social connectedness through shared experience and story, reminiscence and reflecting on life, and creating a legacy.*

- ▲ Refer the older client to support groups. EB: *Canata Becker et al (2017) studied telephone support for diabetic control in elderly clients compared with clients in a group with written materials and found the telephone group had better metabolic results in glucose level and blood pressure.* EB: *Wiles et al (2019) explored qualitatively older adults' (n = 76) experiences of a befriending service, among service users and non–service users, drawing on interviews and focus groups. Results suggest that befriending services helped alleviate social isolation and loneliness and connect them to needed support services.*
- ▲ Refer the client with Alzheimer's disease who is terminally ill to hospice. EBN: *Schaustz Bom, Chaves Sá, and da Silva Serejo Cardoso (2017) studied overload in caregivers (n = 53) of the elderly and found that 45.3% of the caregivers presented with moderate overload, 13.2% presented with moderate to severe overload, 3.8% presented with severe overload, and 32.1% presented with no overload, indicating the need for supportive care.* EB: *Saari et al (2020) studied the reporting of memory loss symptoms between clients (n = 3198) with dementia and their informant. The results revealed that informant information only captured the more visible symptoms of Alzheimer's disease and did not often report the hopelessness and worthlessness reported by many Alzheimer clients.*

I

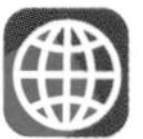

Multicultural

- ● Assess an individual's sociocultural background in teaching self-management and self-regulation as a means of supporting hope and coping. EB: *Meca et al (2017) qualitatively studied recent Hispanic adolescent immigrants (n = 302) in the United States and found that personal identity associated with the United States predicted positivism and decreased antisocial behavior.*
- ● Decrease discrimination to promote positive ethnic identity. EB: *Researchers studied ethnic identity development of East Asian adolescents (n = 13) and found that five themes emerged in their qualitative study: ethnic/cultural identity and socialization, bicultural living, racial context–racism and stereotypes, family context–parental expectation, and peer context–friendship/dating. Participants experienced hurtful racial discrimination but experienced ethnic identity at home (Yoon et al, 2017).*
- ● Refer to care plan for Ineffective **Coping.**

Home Care

- ● The interventions described previously may be adapted for home care use.
- ● Provide an Internet-based health coach to encourage self-management for clients with chronic conditions such as depression, impaired mobility, and chronic pain. Use computer-mediated support groups to enhance identity formation. EB: *Researchers studied using the Internet to treat social anxiety disorder (SAD) in participants (n = 42) randomized into two groups. One group had therapy support. Both groups decreased symptoms of SAD, and the group with the therapist interventions had a lower attrition rate (Gershkovich et al, 2017).*
- ▲ Refer the client to mutual health support groups. Participating in mutual health support groups led to enhanced coping by improving psychological and social functioning. EB: *Urbanoski, van Mierlo, and Cunningham (2017) used social network analysis to examine online support groups for clients with drinking addictions (n = 711) and found that active members were older and after 5 years the online support group was cohesive and stable.*
- ▲ Refer cancer clients and their spouses to family programs that include family-based interventions for communication, hope, coping, uncertainty, and symptom management. EB: *A qualitative study explored the role of family members (n = 41) with cancer clients in the communication process, and all clients and family members preferred open communication with physicians. The study discussed the importance of family for physical and psychological care and discovered that there needed to be a balance between client autonomy and relatives' desire to be protective (Datta et al, 2017).* EB: *Oyibo and Vassileva (2019) studied personality traits on users' susceptibility to social influence (n = 350). The results demonstrated that neuroticism is the most consistent determinant of users' susceptibility to social influence, followed by openness and conscientiousness.*
- ● Refer combat veterans and service members directly involved in combat, as well as those providing support to combatants, including nurses, for mental health services. EB: *Gould et al (2017) developed*

a telephone-based program for older veterans to reduce loneliness and qualitatively found that it benefited socialization, which included connectedness, learning from others, being active despite limitations, and distraction from limitations.

Client/Family Teaching and Discharge Planning

- Teach the client about available community resources (e.g., therapists, ministers, counselors, self-help groups, family education groups). EBN: *Kangovi et al (2017) examined whether community health worker interventions improved outcomes in a low-income population (*n = 302*) with multiple chronic conditions. They found that using a standardized intervention improved chronic disease control, mental health, and quality of care.*
- Teach coping skills to family caregivers of cancer clients. EB: *Blanco et al (2017) studied family environment (*n = 50*) in relation to childhood and found that families with obese children had higher trait anxiety, criticism and overprotectiveness, and maladaptive coping skills.*

REFERENCES

Refer to Ineffective **Coping** for additional references.

Arroyo-Anlló, E. M., Sánchez, J. C., & Gil, R. (2020). Could self-consciousness be enhanced in Alzheimer's disease? An approach from emotional sensorial stimulation. *Journal of Alzheimer's Disease, 77*(2), 505–521. https://doi.org/10.3233/JAD-200408.

Barrett, D. (2017). Rethinking presence: A grounded theory of nurses and teleconsultation. *Journal of Clinical Nursing, 26*(19–20), 3088–3098. https://doi.org/10.1111/jocn.13656.

Blanco, M., Sepulveda, A. R., Lacruz, T., et al. (2017). Examining maternal psychopathology, family functioning and coping skills in childhood obesity: A case-control study. *European Eating Disorders Review, 25*(5), 359–365. https://doi.org/10.1002/erv.2527.

Bürger Lazar, M., & Musek, J. (2020). Well-being in parents of children with cancer: The impact of parental personality, coping, and the child's quality of life. *Scandinavian Journal of Psychology, 61*(5), 652–662. https://doi.org/10.1111/sjop.12653.

Canata Becker, T. A., de Souza Teixeira, C. R., Zanetti, M. L., Pace, A. E., Araújo Almeida, F., & da Costa Gonçalves Torquato, M. T. (2017). Effects of supportive telephone counseling in the metabolic control of elderly people with diabetes mellitus. *Revista Brasileira de Enfermagem, 70*(4), 704–710. https://doi.org/10.1590/0034-7167-2017-0089.

Choi, Y. S., Lee, E. J., & Cho, Y. (2017). The effect of Korean-group cognitive behavioural therapy among patients with panic disorder in clinic settings. *Journal of Psychiatric and Mental Health Nursing, 24*(1), 28–40. https://doi.org/10.1111/jpm.12337.

Dang, S. S., Quesnel, D. A., Hewitt, P. L., Flett, G. L., & Deng, X. (2020). Perfectionistic traits and self-presentation are associated with negative attitudes and concerns about seeking professional psychological help. *Clinical Psychology & Psychotherapy, 27*(5), 621–629. https://doi.org/10.1002/cpp.2450.

Datta, S. S., Tripathi, L., Varghese, R., et al. (2017). Pivotal role of families in doctor-patient communication in oncology: A qualitative study of patients, their relatives and cancer clinicians. *European Journal of Cancer Care, 26*(5), 1–8. https://doi.org/10.1111/ecc.1254.

Domhardt, M., Letsch, J., Kybelka, J., Koenigbauer, J., Doebler, P., & Baumeister, H. (2020). Are internet- and mobile-based interventions effective in adults with diagnosed panic disorder and/or agoraphobia? A systematic review and meta-analysis. *Journal of Affective Disorders, 276*, 169–182. https://doi.org/10.1016/j.jad.2020.06.059.

Dutta, R., Ball, H. A., Siribaddana, S. H., et al. (2017). Genetic and other risk factors for suicidal ideation and the relationship with depression. *Psychological Medicine, 47*(14), 2438–2449. https://doi.org/10.1017/S0033291717000940.

Eckerström, J., Flyckt, L., Carlborg, A., Jayaram-Lindström, N., & Perseius, K. I. (2020). Brief admission for patients with emotional instability and self–harm: A qualitative analysis of patients' experiences during crisis. *International Journal of Mental Health Nursing, 29*(5), 962–971. https://doi.org/10.1111/inm.12736.

Eikelenboom, M., Beekman, A. T. F., Penninx, B. W. J. H., & Smit, J. H. (2019). A 6-year longitudinal study of predictors for suicide attempts in major depressive disorder. *Psychological Medicine, 49*(6), 911–921. https://doi.org/10.1017/S0033291718001423.

Fenton-O'Creevy, M., & Furnham, A. (2020). Money attitudes, personality and chronic impulse buying. *Applied Psychology: International Review, 69*(4), 1557–1572. https://doi.org/1572.10.1111/apps.12215.

Gershkovich, M., Herbert, J. D., Forman, E. M., Schumacher, L. M., & Fischer, L. E. (2017). Internet-delivered acceptance-based cognitive-behavioral intervention for social anxiety disorder with and without therapist support: A randomized trial. *Behavior Modification, 41*(5), 583–608. https://doi.org/10.1177/0145445517694457.

Gould, C., Shah, S., Brunskill, S. R., et al. (2017). Resolv: Development of a telephone-based program designed to increase socialization in older veterans. *Educational Gerontology, 43*(8), 379–392. https://doi.org/10.1080/03601277.2017.1299522.

Hagedoorn, E. I., Paans, W., Jaarsma, T., Keers, J. C., van der Schans, C., & Luttik, M. L. (2017). Aspects of family caregiving as addressed in planned discussions between nurses, patients with chronic diseases and family caregivers: A qualitative content analysis. *BMC Nursing, 16*, 37. https://doi.org/10.1186/s12912-017-0231-5.

Hausknecht, S., Vanchu-Orosco, M., & Kaufman, D. (2019). Digitising the wisdom of our elders: Connectedness through digital storytelling. *Ageing and Society, 39*(12), 2714–2734. https://doi.org/10.1017/S0144686X18000739.

Hayes, A., Maliski, R., & Warner, B. (2017). Analyzing the effects of family communication patterns on the decision to disclose a health issue to a parent: The benefits of conversation and dangers of conformity. *Health Communication, 32*(7), 837–844. https://doi.org/10.1080/10410236.2016.1177898.

Ho, H. C. Y., Mui, M., Wan, A., et al. (2017). Happy family kitchen: Behavioral outcomes of a brief community-based family intervention in Hong Kong. *Journal of Child and Family Studies, 26*(10), 2852–2864. http://dx.doi.org/10.1007/s10826-017-0788-3.

Hughes, N., Williams, J., & Shaw, C. (2017). Supporting the psychological needs of teenagers and young adults during cancer treatment: A literature review. *British Journal of Nursing, 26*(4), S4–S10. https://doi.org/10.12968/bjon.2017.26.4.S4.

Jackson, K. H., & Mixer, S. J. (2017). Using an iPad for basic communication between Spanish-speaking families and nurses in pediatric acute care: A feasibility pilot study. *Computers, Informatics, Nursing, 35*(8), 401–407. https://doi.org/10.1097/CIN.0000000000000354.

I

Jagtiani, M. R., Kelly, Y., Fancourt, D., Shelton, N., & Scholes, S. (2019). Family meal frequency moderates the association between time on social networking sites and well-being among U.K. young adults. *Cyberpsychology, Behavior, and Social Networking, 22*(12), 753–760. https://doi.org/10.1089/cyber.2019.0338.

Kangovi, S., Mitra, N., Grande, D., Huo, H., Smith, R. A., & Long, J. A. (2017). Community health worker support for disadvantaged patients with multiple chronic diseases: A randomized clinical trial. *American Journal of Public Health, 107*(10), 1660–1667. https://doi.org/10.2105/AJPH.2017.303985.

Kendal, S., Kirk, S., Elvey, R., Catchpole, R., & Pryjmachuk, S. (2017). How a moderated online discussion forum facilitates support for young people with eating disorders. *Health Expectations, 20*(1), 98–111. https://doi.org/10.1111/hex.12439.

Lindo, N. A., & Ceballos, P. (2020). Child and adolescent career construction: An expressive arts group intervention. *Journal of Creativity in Mental Health, 15*(3), 364–377. https://doi.org/10.1080/15401383.2019.1685923.

Meca, A., Sabet, R. F., Farrelly, C. M., et al. (2017). Personal and cultural identity development in recently immigrated Hispanic adolescents: Links with psychosocial functioning. *Cultural Diversity and Ethnic Minority Psychology, 23*(3), 348–361. https://doi.org/10.1037/cdp0000129.

Nandrino, J. L., & Gandolphe, M. C. (2017). Characterization of self-defining memories in individuals with severe alcohol use disorders after mid-term abstinence: The impact of the emotional valence of memories. *Alcoholism: Clinical and Experimental Research, 41*(8), 1484–1491. http://doi.org/10.1111/acer.13424.

Nóbrega, M. D. P. S.S., Trigo Fernandes, M. F., & de Freitas Silva, P. (2017). Application of the therapeutic relationship to people with common mental disorder. *Revista Gaucha de Enfermagem, 38*(1), e63562. http://dx.doi.org/10.1590/1983-1447.2017.01.63562.

Oyibo, K., & Vassileva, J. (2019). The relationship between personality traits and susceptibility to social influence. *Computers in Human Behavior, 98*, 174–188. https://doi.org/10.1016/j.chb.2019.01.032.

Rochefort, C., Hoerger, M., Turiano, N. A., & Duberstein, P. (2019). Big Five personality and health in adults with and without cancer. *Journal of Health Psychology, 24*(11), 1494–1504. https://doi.org/10.1177/1359105317753714.

Ruhl, I., & Lordly, D. (2017). The nature of competition in dietetics education: A narrative review. *Canadian Journal of Dietetic Practice and Research, 78*(3), 129–136. https://doi.org/10.3148/cjdpr-2017-004.

Saari, T. T., Hallikainen, I., Hintsa, T., & Koivisto, A. M. (2020). Network structures and temporal stability of self- and informant-rated affective symptoms in Alzheimer's disease. *Journal of Affective Disorders, 276*, 1084–1092. https://doi.org/10.1016/j.jad.2020.07.100.

Schaustz Bom, F., Chaves Sá, S. P., & da Silva Serejo Cardoso, R. (2017). Overload in caregivers of the elderly. *Journal of Nursing UFPE, 11*(1), 160–164. https://doi.org/10.5205/reuol.9978-88449-6-1101201719.

Sigurdardottir, A. O., Garwick, A. W., & Svavarsdottir, E. K. (2017). The importance of family support in pediatrics and its impact on healthcare satisfaction. *Scandinavian Journal of Caring Sciences, 31*(2), 241–252. https://doi.org/10.1111/scs.12336.

Steenhaut, P., Rossi, G., Demeyer, I., & De Raedt, R. (2020). Flexibility as a mediator between personality and well-being in older and younger adults: Findings from questionnaire data and a behavioral task. *Experimental Aging Research, 46*(5), 446–468. https://doi.org/10.1080/0361073X.2020.1805935.

Stepp, S. D., & Lazarus, S. A. (2017). Identifying a borderline personality disorder prodrome: Implications for community screening. *Personality and Mental Health, 11*(3), 195–205. https://doi.org/10.1002/pmh.1389.

Strøm, J., Høybye, M. T., Laursen, M., Jørgensen, L. B., & Nielsen, C. V. (2019). Lumbar spine fusion patients' use of an internet support Group: Mixed methods study. *Journal of Medical Internet Research, 21*(7), e9805. https://doi.org/10.2196/jmir.9805.

Sultan, S., Kanwal, F., & Hussain, I. (2020). Moderating effects of personality traits in relationship between religious practices and mental health of university students. *Journal of Religion and Health, 59*(5), 2458–2468. https://doi.org/10.1007/s10943-019-00875-x.

Sumiyana, S., & Sriwidharmanely, S. (2020). Mitigating the harmful effects of technostress: Inducing chaos theory in an experimental setting. *Behaviour & Information Technology, 39*(10), 1079–1093. https://doi.org/10.1080/0144929X.2019.1641229.

Szwimer, R., Widjaja, M., Ingelmo, P., & Hovey, R. B. (2020). A phenomenological exploration of the personal implications of female adolescents living with chronic pain. *Journal of Pediatric Health Care, 34*(5), 470–477. https://doi.org/10.1016/j.pedhc.2020.05.004.

Tamura-Lis, W. (2017). Reminiscing—a tool for excellent elder care and improved quality of life. *Urologic Nursing, 37*(3), 151–156. https://doi.org/10.7257/1053-816X.2017.37.3.151.

Tobi, P., Kemp, P., & Schmidt, E. (2017). Cohort differences in exercise adherence among primary care patients referred for mental health versus physical health conditions. *Primary Health Care Research & Development, 18*(5), 463–471. https://doi.org/10.1017/S1463423617000214.

Tsotsi, S., Broekman, B. F. P., Sim, L. W., et al. (2019). Maternal anxiety, parenting stress, and preschoolers' behavior problems: The role of child self-regulation. *Journal of Developmental and Behavioral Pediatrics, 40*(9), 696–705. https://doi.org/10.1097/DBP.0000000000000737.

Urbanoski, K., van Mierlo, T., & Cunningham, J. (2017). Investigating patterns of participation in an online support group for problem drinking: A social network analysis. *International Journal of Behavioral Medicine, 24*(5), 703–712. https://doi.org/10.1007/s12529-016-9591-6.

Vanderpuye, V., Grover, S., Hammad, N., et al. (2017). An update on the management of breast cancer in Africa. *Infectious Agents and Cancer, 12*, 13. https://doi.org/10.1186/s13027-017-0124-y.

Verhoeven, F. E. A., Swaab, L. S. M. A., Carlier, I. ,V. E., et al. (2017). Agreement between clinical and MINI diagnoses in outpatients with mood and anxiety disorders. *Journal of Affective Disorders, 221*, 268–274. https://doi.org/10.1016/j.jad.2017.06.041.

Wiles, J., Morgan, T., Moeke-Maxwell, T., et al. (2019). Befriending services for culturally diverse older people. *Journal of Gerontological Social Work, 62*(7), 776–793. https://doi.org/10.1080/01634372.2019.1640333.

Yoon, E., Adams, K., Clawson, A., Chang, H., Surya, S., & Jérémie-Brink, G. (2017). East Asian adolescents' ethnic identity development and cultural integration: A qualitative investigation. *Journal of Counseling Psychology, 64*(1), 65–79. https://doi.org/10.1037/cou0000181.

Zhang, D., Huebner, E. S., & Tian, L. (2020). Longitudinal associations among neuroticism, depression, and cyberbullying in early adolescents. *Computers in Human Behavior, 112*, 106475. https://doi.org/10.1016/j.chb.2020.106475.

Risk for Disturbed Personal Identity

Domain 6 Self-perception Class 1 Self-concept

Marina Martinez-Kratz, MS, RN, CNE

NANDA-I

Definition

Susceptible to the inability to maintain an integrated and complete perception of self, which may compromise health.

Risk Factors

Altered social role; cult indoctrination; dysfunctional family processes; gender conflict; low self-esteem; perceived social discrimination; values incongruent with cultural norms

At-Risk Population

Individuals experiencing developmental transition; individuals experiencing situational crisis; individuals exposed to toxic chemicals

Associated Conditions

Dissociative identity disorder; mental disorders; neurocognitive disorders; pharmaceutical preparations

NOC, NIC, Client Outcomes, Nursing Interventions and *Rationales,* Client/Family Teaching and Discharge Planning, and References

Refer to care plan for Disturbed Personal **Identity**.

Risk for Complicated Immigration Transition

Domain 9 Coping/stress tolerance Class 1 Post-trauma responses

Nadia Ali Muhammad Ali Charania, PhD, RN

NANDA-I

Definition

Susceptible to experiencing negative feelings (loneliness, fear, anxiety) in response to unsatisfactory consequences and cultural barriers to one's immigration transition, which may compromise health.

Related Factors

Abusive landlord; available work below educational preparation; communication barriers; cultural barriers; inadequate knowledge about accessing resources; inadequate social support; non-related persons within household; overcrowded housing; overt social discrimination; parent-child conflicts related to enculturation; unsanitary housing

At-Risk Population

Individuals experiencing forced migration; individuals experiencing labor exploitation; individuals experiencing precarious economic situation; individuals exposed to hazardous work conditions with inadequate training; individuals living far from significant others; individuals with undocumented immigration status; individuals with unfulfilled expectations of immigration

NOC (Nursing Outcomes Classification)

Suggested NOC Outcomes

Relocation Adaptation, Anxiety Level; Fear Level; Loneliness Severity; Coping

Example NOC Outcome with Indicators

Relocation Adaptation as evidenced by the following indicators: Participates in decision-making in new environment/Expresses satisfaction with daily routine/Fear/Loneliness/Anxiety. (Rate the outcome and indicators of **Relocation Adaptation:** 1 = never demonstrated; 2 = rarely demonstrated, 3 = sometimes demonstrated, 4 = often demonstrated, 5 = consistently demonstrated [see Section I].)

Client Outcomes

Client Will (Specify Time Frame)

- Participate in community activities
- State satisfaction with social relationships, living arrangements, and social integration
- State satisfaction with health status and access to health care
- Demonstrate actions that are congruent with expressed feelings and thoughts
- State sense of belonging
- Accept strengths and limitations of new environment

NIC (Nursing Interventions Classification)

Suggested NIC Interventions

Support System Enhancement; Socialization Enhancement; Values Clarification

Example NIC Activities—Risk for Complicated Immigration Transition

Encourage patience in developing relationships; Encourage social and community activities

Nursing Interventions and *Rationales*

- Understand immigrants' perspectives/stories about their health maintenance and illness management. CEB: *Nurses are concerned with the life experiences of people and how these life experiences may affect their health and responses to illness. Furthermore, to diagnose and treat immigrants who are ill, we must be able to put their responses within the context of their lives; otherwise, our understanding and interpretation of their responses to illness will be limited (Meleis, 2010).*
- Assess for use of acculturation strategies. EB: *The Multicultural Adolescents Panel Study identified four acculturation strategies: marginalization, separation, assimilation, and integration. A one-way analysis of variance showed that life satisfaction was highest for integration and decreased for assimilation, separation, and marginalization (Yoo, 2021).*
- Focus on providing holistic (physical, emotional, psychological, social, and spiritual) care while caring for immigrants. When appropriate, integrate the use of complementary and alternative approaches. EBN: *A small study of Indian immigrants in the United States found that participants preferred complementary and alternative medicine home remedies to address their health needs (Joseph et al, 2019).*
- Assess for intergenerational conflict and parental stress. EB: *A study of older immigrant parents found that higher parental stress was found among those with greater intergenerational conflict (Mitchell, Wister, & Zdaniuk, 2019).*
- Assist clients to identify coping strategies and sources of social support. EB: *A study of international students found that social support and coping were partial mediators of the relationship between acculturation and acculturative stress (Ra & Trusty, 2017).*
- Obtain a professional translator to enhance cross-cultural communication. EB: *Culturally competent verbal and nonverbal communication skills should also identify the need for interpretation and translation (Purnell, 2018).*
- Demonstrate cultural humility to achieve cultural competence to offer individualized discharge services to immigrant mothers with their preterm babies from the neonatal intensive care unit. EB: *Regardless of the number of years of being in the migrated country, at discharge, immigrant mothers tend to have less discharge readiness; have poor perceptions of infant well-being; have less comfort to be able to care for their preterm babies after discharge in areas such as infant development, sleep, nutrition, and meeting overall medical needs; and struggled with their well-being, including mental health (McGowan et al, 2019).*
- Health care professionals need to identify risks and obstacles that migrant women transitioning to motherhood may be faced with, including poverty, language barriers, loneliness, and limited access to health

care, which can contribute to mental health concerns such as stress, anxiety, depression, and social isolation. EB: *It was argued that the outlined efforts would enhance migrant mothers' engagement in and benefit from health care services (Aydın, Körükcü, & Kabukçuoğlu, 2017).*

- Nurses working with immigrant clients in psychiatric units need to (1) assess for posttraumatic stress syndrome and associated symptoms, (2) employ compassionate and trauma-informed care, (3) educate about early recognition of mental illness, (4) share information about psychiatric services, (5) use family-oriented and interpreter services often and as needed, and (6) create trusting relationship in the psychiatric community care. EB: *The finding of the qualitative study involving nurses' experiences of caring for immigrant clients pointed toward the need for integrating areas identified above; suggested determining care-related challenges and their manifestations of working with such populations; and suggested offering support to nurses in their efforts toward maintaining professional well-being to be able to provide compassionate and needed care (Kallakorpi, Haatainen, & Kankkunen, 2018).*
- Actively engage in policy-driven solutions to mitigate structural racism. Such macrolevel factors shape the health of racial and ethnic minorities. EB: *The finding of the study that aimed to understand the influence of a transition from unlawful to lawful status on the psychological well-being of Latino immigrant young adults suggests that well-being is linked to positive and complete social integration (Patler & Pirtle, 2018).*
- Explore immigrant women's experience of menopause and self-management strategies for menopausal symptoms to be able to provide culturally relevant care and enhance their satisfaction with the specific care they received. EB: *The systematic review of the limited available literature indicated that compared with nonimmigrant women, immigrant women reported more physical symptoms (e.g., vasomotor symptoms) and poorer mental health. Moreover, immigrant women were mostly not satisfied with the menopause-specific care that they had received (Stanzel, Hammarberg, & Fisher, 2018).*

I

Pediatric

- Promote self-efficacy of the newly migrated adolescents by supporting their effort to learn and use the language of the migrated country. EB: *Evidence suggests that newly migrated adolescents initially have lower levels of self-efficacy than more experienced adolescent immigrants. Language use was found to be imperative in the adaptation process of newly migrated adolescents contributing to their self-efficacy (Titzmann & Jugert, 2017).*
- Assess for mental health consequences among youth from the ethnic and racial minorities of trauma experienced across the migration process (including before, during, and after migration) through the use of culturally sensitive diagnostic tools, and offer treatment services to facilitate a positive transition to healthy adulthood. EB: *Evidence suggests that the trauma experienced by Latino youth at different migration stages seemed to be linked with their current mental health symptoms, including anxiety, depression, and posttraumatic stress disorder (Cleary et al, 2018).*
- Recognize and address the specific needs of both immigrant youths with disabilities transitioning to adulthood (e.g., autonomy) and their caregivers' needs (e.g., information about their youths' condition and of available health services). EB: *The research with immigrant youths with disabilities and caregivers from the Middle East suggests providing culturally sensitive care focused on offering support and health care– and health management–specific information in their language (Björquist et al, 2017).*

Home Care

- Educate and encourage immigrants' family members to use available home care–specific support services as needed. EB: *It is critical to recognize that the immigrated family is faced with both health care system barriers (e.g., discrimination within the health care system and complex bureaucracies) and individual barriers (e.g., limited communication ability, lack of financial resources, and the experience of shame or stigma) when in need of accessing care (Hacker et al, 2015).*

REFERENCES

Aydın, R., Körükcü, Ö., & Kabukçuoğlu, K. (2017). Transition to motherhood as an immigrant: Risks and obstacles. *Current Approaches in Psychiatry*, *9*(3), 250–262. https://doi.org/10.18863/pgy.285927.

Björquist, E., Nordmark, E., Almasri, N. A., & Hallström, I. (2017). Immigrant youths with disabilities and caregivers from the Middle-East—Challenges and needs during transition to adulthood. *Research in Health Science*, *2*(4), 363–384. http://dx.doi.org/10.22158/rhs.v2n4p363.

Cleary, S. D., Snead, R., Dietz-Chavez, D., Rivera, I., & Edberg, M. C. (2018). Immigrant trauma and mental health outcomes among Latino youth. *Journal of Immigrant and Minority Health*, *20*(5), 1053–1059. https://doi.org/10.1007/s10903-017-0673-6.

Hacker, K., Anies, M., Folb, B. L., & Zallman, L. (2015). Barriers to health care for undocumented immigrants: A literature review. *Risk Management and Healthcare Policy*, *8*, 175–183. https://doi.org/10.1097/CNJ.0000000000000546.

Joseph, R., Fernandes, S., Derstine, S., & McSpadden, M. (2019). Complementary medicine & spirituality: Health-seeking behaviors of Indian immigrants in the United States. *Journal of Christian Nursing*, *36*(3), 190–195.

Kallakorpi, S., Haatainen, K., & Kankkunen, P. (2018). Nurses' experiences caring for immigrant patients in psychiatric units. *International Journal of Caring Sciences*, *11*(3), 1802–1811.

McGowan, E. C., Abdulla, L. S., Hawes, K. K., Tucker, R., & Vohr, B. R. (2019). Maternal immigrant status and readiness to transition to home from the NICU. *Pediatrics*, *143*(5) e20182657. https://doi.org/10.1542/peds.2018-2657.

Meleis, A. I. (2010). Immigrant transitions and health care: An action plan. In A. I. Meleis (Ed.), *Transition theory* (pp. 241–242). New York: Springer.

Mitchell, B. A., Wister, A. V., & Zdaniuk, B. (2019). Are the parents all right? Parental stress, ethnic culture and intergenerational relations in aging families. *Journal of Comparative Family Studies*, *50*(1), 51–74. https://doi.org/10.3138/jcfs.037-2018.

Patler, C., & Pirtle, W. L. (2018). From undocumented to lawfully present: Do changes to legal status impact psychological wellbeing among Latino immigrant young adults? *Social Science & Medicine*, *199*, 39–48. http://dx.doi.org/10.1016/j.socscimed.2017.03.009.

Purnell, L. (2018). Cross cultural communication: Verbal and non-verbal communication, interpretation and translation. In M. Douglas, D. Pacquiao, & L. Purnell (Eds.), *Global applications of culturally competent health care: Guidelines for practice*. New York: Springer. https://doi.org/10.1007/978-3-319-69332-3_14.

Ra, Y. A., & Trusty, J. (2017). Impact of social support and coping on acculturation and acculturative stress of East Asian international students. *Journal of Multicultural Counseling and Development*, *45*(4), 276–291. https://doi.org/10.1002/jmcd.12078.

Stanzel, K. A., Hammarberg, K., & Fisher, J. (2018). Experiences of menopause, self-management strategies for menopausal symptoms and perceptions of health care among immigrant women: A systematic review. *Climacteric*, *21*(2), 101–110. https://doi.org/10.1080/13697137.2017.1421922.

Titzmann, P. F., & Jugert, P. (2017). Transition to a new country: Acculturative and developmental predictors for changes in self-efficacy among adolescent immigrants. *Journal of Youth and Adolescence*, *46*(10), 2143–2156. doi:10.1007/s10964-017-0665-9.

Yoo, C. (2021). Acculturation strategies of multi-cultural family adolescents in South Korea: Marginalization, separation, assimilation, and integration. *International Journal of Intercultural Relations*, *81*, 9–19. https://doi.org/10.1016/j.ijintrel.2020.12.011.

Ineffective Impulse Control Domain 5 Perception/cognition Class 4 Cognition

Marina Martinez-Kratz, MS, RN, CNE

NANDA-I

Definition

A pattern of performing rapid, unplanned reactions to internal or external stimuli without regard for the negative consequences of these reactions to the impulsive individual or to others.

Defining Characteristics

Acting without thinking; asking personal questions despite discomfort of others; dangerous behavior; gambling addiction; impaired ability to regulate finances; inappropriate sharing of personal details; irritable mood; overly familiar with strangers; sensation seeking; sexual promiscuity; temper outbursts

Related Factors

Hopelessness; mood disorder; neurobehavioral manifestations; smoking; substance misuse

Associated Conditions

Altered development; developmental disabilities; neurocognitive disorders; personality disorders

NOC (Nursing Outcomes Classification)

Suggested NOC Outcome

Impulse Self-Control

Example NOC Outcome with Indicators

Impulse Self-Control as evidenced by the following indicators: Identifies harmful impulsive behaviors/Identifies feelings that lead to impulsive actions/Avoids high-risk situations/Controls impulses/Maintains self-control without supervision. (Rate the outcome and indicators of **Impulse Self-Control:** 1 = never demonstrated, 2 = rarely demonstrated, 3 = sometimes demonstrated, 4 = often demonstrated, 5 = continually demonstrated [see Section I].)

Client Outcomes

Client Will (Specify Time Frame)

- Be free from harm
- Cooperate with behavioral modification plan
- Verbalize adaptive ways to cope with stress by means other than impulsive behaviors
- Delay gratification and use adaptive coping strategies in response to stress
- Verbalize understanding that behavior is unacceptable
- Accept responsibility for own behavior

NIC (Nursing Interventions Classification)

Suggested NIC Intervention

Impulse Control Training

Example NIC Activities—Impulse Control Training

Use a behavior modification plan, as appropriate, to reinforce the problem-solving strategy that is being taught; Teach client to cue himself/herself to "stop and think" before acting impulsively

I

Nursing Interventions and *Rationales*

- Refer to mental health treatment for cognitive behavioral therapy (CBT). **EB:** *A review identified the efficacy of CBT for treatment of impulse control symptoms in Parkinson's disease (Koychev & Okai, 2017).*
- Assess individuals with impulsive behaviors for exposure to trauma and referral for mental health evaluation. **EB:** *Research indicates that impulsivity is associated with trauma exposure and posttraumatic stress disorder (PTSD) (Netto et al, 2016).*
- Implement motivational interviewing for clients with impulse control disorders. **EB:** *This research review found motivational interviewing helps individuals with gambling addictions work through ambivalence and commit to change (Choi et al, 2017).*
- Teach client mindfulness meditation techniques. Mindfulness meditation includes observing experiences in the present moment, describing those experiences without judgments or evaluations, and participating fully in one's current context. **EB:** *This study showed that developing mindfulness was an effective way of diminishing binge eating, eating psychopathology, and depression and increasing quality of life in women with obesity (Pinto-Gouveia et al, 2016).*
- Refer to self-help groups such as Gambler's Anonymous. **EB:** *This research review found that Gambler's Anonymous is helpful as an adjunct therapy for individuals with gambling addictions (Choi et al, 2017).*
- Use a brief intervention model to screen and provide information and referral to services for clients that may experience at-risk gambling. **EB:** *A pilot study found that when trained, primary care staff were able to screen clients at routine visits for at-risk gambling behavior by using the brief intervention model (Nehlin et al, 2016).*
- Teach clients to use urge surfing techniques when impulses or urges are triggered. **EB:** *This study demonstrated that the mindfulness coping skill of urge surfing was an effective intervention when used by teens experiencing urges to use alcohol (Harris, Stewart, & Stanton, 2017).*
- Teach client to use cue avoidance techniques to reduce impulsive behaviors. **EB:** *This study shows that cue avoidance techniques were successful in reducing alcohol consumption (Di Lemma & Field, 2017).*

Pediatric

- Assess children for environmental lead exposure. **EB:** *This research shows that a 1 mcg/dL increase in average childhood blood lead level significantly predicts a 0.37 (95% confidence interval [CI] = 0.11, 0.64) point increase in adolescent impulsivity (Winter & Sampson, 2017).*
- ▲ Refer to mental health treatment for CBT. **EB:** *CBT has been beneficial in treating impulse control disorders in pediatric populations (Farrell et al, 2016).*

▲ Refer adolescent clients with impulsive symptoms at risk of self-harm to Dialectical Behavioral Therapy for Adolescents (DBT-A). EB: *A systematic review found that behavioral impulsivity is related to self-harm and negative affect. DBT-A includes distress tolerance and problem-solving skills directed toward impulsivity and self-harm (Lockwood et al, 2017).*

Geriatric

- Assess for impulsive symptoms and maintain increased surveillance of the client whenever the use of dopamine agonists has been initiated. EB: *Dopamine agonist therapy is related to the development of impulse control disorders in clients with Parkinson's disease (Voon et al, 2017).*
- Implement fall risk screening and precautions for geriatric clients with inattention and impulse control symptoms. EBN: *The Marianjoy Fall Risk Assessment tool has internal validity and reliability and includes impulsive behavior as one of the fall risk indicators (Ruroede, Pilkington, & Guernon, 2016).*
- Monitor caregivers for evidence of caregiver burden. EB: *A study found that mild behavioral impairment was common in memory clinic clients without dementia and was associated with greater caregiver burden (Sheikh et al, 2018).*

Client/Family Teaching and Discharge Planning

- Families should be encouraged to use practical measures to manage behavior such as limiting access to credit cards and restricting and monitoring Internet access gambling and casino websites, checking medication compliance, reporting behavior typical of impulse control disorders, and transferring control of financial affairs to a partner or other family members. EB: *This review showed effective management of impulsive behaviors through client and caregiver education (Zhang et al, 2016).*

I

REFERENCES

Choi, S. W., Shin, Y. C., Kim, D. J., et al. (2017). Treatment modalities for patients with gambling disorder. *Annals of General Psychiatry*, *16*, 23. https://doi.org/10.1007/s00213-017-4639-0.

Di Lemma, L. C. G., & Field, M. (2017). Cue avoidance training and inhibitory control training for the reduction of alcohol consumption: A comparison of effectiveness and investigation of their mechanisms of action. *Psychopharmacology*, *234*(16), 2489–2498. https://doi.org/10.1007/s00213-017-4639-0.

Farrell, L. J., Oar, E. L., Waters, A. M., et al. (2016). Brief intensive CBT for pediatric OCD with E-therapy maintenance. *Journal of Anxiety Disorders*, *42*, 85–94. doi:10.1016/j.janxdis.2016.06.005.

Harris, J. S., Stewart, D. G., & Stanton, B. C. (2017). Urge surfing as aftercare in adolescent alcohol use: A randomized control trial. *Mindfulness*, *8*(1), 144–149. https://doi.org/10.1007/s12671-016-0588-7.

Koychev, I., & Okai, D. (2017). Cognitive-behavioural therapy for non-motor symptoms of Parkinson's disease: A clinical review. *Evidence-Based Mental Health*, *20*(1), 15–20. https://doi.org/10.1136/eb-2016-102574.

Lockwood, J., Daley, D., Townsend, E., & Sayal, K. (2017). Impulsivity and self-harm in adolescence: A systematic review. *European Child & Adolescent Psychiatry*, *26*(4), 387–402. https://doi.org/10.1007/s00787-016-0915-5.

Nehlin, C., Nyberg, F., & Jess, K. (2016). Brief intervention within primary care for at-risk gambling: A pilot study. *Journal of Gambling Studies*, *32*(4), 1327–1335. https://doi.org/10.1007/s10899-016-9610-1.

Netto, L. R., Pereira, J. L., Nogueira, J. F., et al. (2016). Impulsivity is relevant for trauma exposure and PTSD symptoms in a non-clinical population. *Psychiatry Research*, *239*, 204–211.

Pinto-Gouveia, J., Carvalho, S. A., Palmeira, L., et al. (2016). Incorporating psychoeducation, mindfulness and self-compassion in a new programme for binge eating (BEfree): Exploring processes of change. *Journal of Health Psychology*, *24*(4), 466–479.

Ruroede, K., Pilkington, D., & Guernon, A. (2016). Validation study of the Marianjoy fall risk assessment tool. *Journal of Nursing Care Quality*, *31*(2), 146–152.

Sheikh, F., Ismail, Z., Mortby, M. E., et al. (2018). Prevalence of mild behavioral impairment in mild cognitive impairment and subjective cognitive decline, and its association with caregiver burden. *International Psychogeriatrics*, *30*(2), 233–244. https://doi.org/10.1017/S104161021700151X.

Voon, V., Napier, T. C., Frank, M. J., et al. (2017). Impulse control disorders and levodopa-induced dyskinesias in Parkinson's disease: An update. *The Lancet Neurology*, *16*(3), 238–250. https://doi.org/10.1016/S1474-4422(17)30004-2.

Winter, A. S., & Sampson, R. J. (2017). From lead exposure in early childhood to adolescent health: A Chicago birth cohort. *American Journal of Public Health*, *107*(9), 1496–1501. https://doi.org/10.2105/AJPH.2017.303903.

Zhang, S., Dissanayaka, N. N., Dawson, A., et al. (2016). Management of impulse control disorders in Parkinson's disease. *International Psychogeriatrics*, *28*(10), 1597–1614. https://doi.org/10.1017/S104161021600096X.

Disability-Associated Urinary Incontinence

Domain 3 Elimination and exchange Class 1 Urinary function

Amanda Andrews, BSc (Hons), MA and Bernie St Aubyn, BSc (Hons), MSc

NANDA-I

Definition

Involuntary loss of urine not associated with any pathology or problem related to the urinary system.

Defining Characteristics

Adaptive behaviors to avoid others' recognition of urinary incontinence; mapping routes to public bathrooms prior to leaving home; time required to reach toilet is too long after sensation of urge; use of techniques to prevent urination; voiding prior to reaching toilet

Related Factors

Avoidance of non-hygienic toilet use; caregiver inappropriately implements bladder training techniques; difficulty finding the bathroom; difficulty obtaining timely assistance to bathroom; embarrassment regarding toilet use in social situations; environmental constraints that interfere with continence; habitually suppresses urge to urinate; impaired physical mobility; impaired postural balance; inadequate motivation to maintain continence; increased fluid intake; neurobehavioral manifestations; pelvic floor disorders

At-Risk Population

Children; older adults

Associated Conditions

Heart diseases; impaired coordination; impaired hand dexterity; intellectual disability; neuromuscular diseases; osteoarticular diseases; pharmaceutical preparations; psychological disorder; vision disorders

NOC (Nursing Outcomes Classification)

Suggested NOC Outcomes

Urinary Continence; Urinary Elimination

Example NOC Outcome with Indicators

Urinary Continence as evidenced by the following indicators: Recognizes urge to void/Responds to urge in timely manner/Voids in appropriate receptacle/Underclothing remains dry during day/Underclothing or bedding remains dry during night. (Rate the outcome and indicators of **Urinary Continence:** 1 = never demonstrated, 2 = rarely demonstrated, 3 = sometimes demonstrated, 4 = often demonstrated, 5 = consistently demonstrated [see Section I].)

Client Outcomes

Client Will (Specify Time Frame)

- Eliminate or reduce incontinent episodes on a daily basis
- Eliminate or overcome environmental barriers to toileting on a daily basis
- Use adaptive equipment to reduce or eliminate incontinence related to impaired mobility or dexterity on a daily basis
- Use portable urinary collection devices or urine containment devices when access to the toilet is not feasible on a daily basis

NIC (Nursing Interventions Classification)

Suggested NIC Interventions

Urinary Habit Training; Urinary Incontinence Care

Example NIC Activities—Urinary Habit Training

Keep a continence-specification record for 3 days to establish voiding pattern; Establish interval for toileting of preferably not less than 2 hours

Nursing Interventions and *Rationales*

- Introduce yourself to the client and anyone accompanying him or her and inform them of your role. EB: *Introducing yourself to a client helps establish and develop a therapeutic relationship that recognizes the person within the client and forms the basis for building trust on which to base the provision of care (Ellis et al, 2020).*
- Gain consent to provide care before proceeding further with the assessment. For clients unable to give consent, discuss permission with relevant health care professionals and/or family members. EB: *Clients have the right of autonomy both legally and morally and therefore should be fully involved in the decision-making process (Griffith & Tengnah, 2020).*
- Wash hands using a recognized technique. EB: *Evidence shows that strict hand hygiene regimens significantly reduce the incidence of methicillin-resistant* Staphylococcus aureus *and* Clostridioides (Clostridium) difficile *infection (Goldberg, 2017).*
- Assess usual pattern of bladder management and establish the extent of the problem to include a detailed and accurate assessment of the client.
- Evaluate the client's bladder habits:
  - Episodes of incontinence during the day and night
  - Alleviating and aggravating factors
- Current management strategies include containing/collection devices, restriction of fluid intake, and avoidance of fluid/food groups that cause bladder irritation. EB: *Several types of incontinence exist and since the treatments will vary, it is important that the assessment, also known as "diagnostic evaluation," establishes which type is present. The authors recognize that guidelines should be adapted to individual clients' needs (Nambiar et al, 2018).*
- Complete a Lifestyle and Risk Assessment that includes assessment of toilet access and ability to use, including the following:
  - Distance of the toilet from the bed, chair, and living quarters
  - Characteristics of the bed, including presence of side rails and distance of the bed from the floor
  - Characteristics of the pathway to the toilet, including barriers such as stairs, loose rugs on the floor, and inadequate lighting
  - Characteristics of the bathroom, including patterns of use, lighting, height of the toilet from the floor, the presence of handrails to assist transfers to the toilet, and breadth of the door and its accessibility for a wheelchair, walker, or other assistive devices

  EB: *When assessing different client groups, relevant assessment factors should be considered because standard assessment and treatment pathways may not be appropriate. Examples include older people with cognitive impairment (dementia is strongly associated with urinary incontinence), people with reduced mobility, and women who are pregnant, because the standard assessment and treatment pathways might not be appropriate for them (Stewart, 2018).*
- Assess the client's physical and mental abilities:
  - Ability to rise from chair and bed, transfer to the toilet, and ambulate and the need for physical assistive devices such as a cane, walker, or wheelchair. EB: *A study carried out in a nursing home care setting identified a significant association between impaired mobility and urinary incontinence in nursing home residents (Jachan et al, 2019).*
  - Ability to manipulate buttons, hooks, and zippers as needed to remove clothing. EB: *It is important to ensure the client is assessed for motor capability as this is integral to the client's ability to maintain continence (Keenan et al, 2018).*
  - Functional and cognitive status assessment should be done using a tool such as the Mini-Mental Status Examination for the older client with functional incontinence. EB: *A dementia diagnosis (or severe cognitive impairment) is associated with a higher prevalence of incontinence compared with people without such a diagnosis (Gove et al, 2017). An association has also been observed between incontinence and more severe cognitive impairment and mobility problems (Jerez-Roig et al, 2016).*

I

  - ❍ Daily fluid intake, including amount and types of fluids consumed.
  - ❍ Risk of falls caused by dizziness, impaired vision, and hearing.
  - ❍ Functional ability declines secondary to comorbidities (e.g., cerebrovascular incidents, amputation).
- • Discuss quality-of-life issues relating to socialization and family events. EB: *The impact on the client's quality of life should not be underestimated. One of the key consequences of urinary incontinence is loss of self-confidence and social isolation (Pizzol et al, 2021).*
- • Review the client's medical history:
  - ❍ Obstetrical/gynecological/urological history and surgeries
  - ❍ Relevant comorbidities such as cardiac, respiratory, renal, or neurological
  - ❍ Recurrent urinary tract infections

  EB: *Reviewing the client's medical history, considering any significant medical, surgical, obstetric, or genitourinary history, is essential as any identified conditions may affect an individual's ability to maintain continence (Bardsley, 2016).*
- • Teach the client, the client's care providers, or the family to complete a bladder diary. Each 24-hour period should be subdivided into 1- to 2-hour periods and include number of urinations occurring in the toilet, actual episodes of incontinence and amount of urine leaked, reasons for episode of incontinence, type and amount of liquid intake, number of bowel movements, and incontinence pads or other products used. EB: *Bladder diaries provide accurate data and are more reliable than clients recollections of symptoms. In addition to being inexpensive and low risk, clients view diaries as easy to complete and helpful for their care (Dixon & Nakib, 2016).*
- • Consult with the health care provider and complete a medication review relating to side effects and contraindications. EB: *Health professionals should review the use of any medication that could affect a client's urine production. Side effects for consideration should include sedation, impaired cognition, or a change in sensation and muscle tone (Bardsley, 2016).*
- • Ensure that an appropriate, safe urinary receptacle such as a three-in-one commode, female or male handheld urinal, no-spill urinal, or containment device when toileting access is limited by immobility or environmental barriers is available to assist the client with elimination needs while other interventions are being implemented. EB: *Containment is important for people with urinary incontinence and should be considered when active treatment does not cure the problem, when it is not available or not possible, or if the risks of treatment outweigh the benefits to the client (Nambiar et al, 2018). A useful resource for health care professionals and clients can be found at www.continenceproductadvisor.org.*
- ▲ Refer to occupational therapy for help in obtaining assistive devices and adapting the home for optimal toilet accessibility. EB: *Occupational therapists are needed to assist clients with dexterity and mobility issues that may be contributing to incontinence (Spencer, McManus, & Sabourin, 2017).*
- • Provide advice to clients relating to loose-fitting clothing with stretch waistbands rather than buttoned or zippered waist; minimize buttons, snaps, and multilayered clothing; and substitute a loop-and-pile closure or other easily loosened systems such as Velcro for buttons, hooks, and zippers in existing clothing. EB: *Clients with impaired dexterity or weakness may benefit from clothing that has been modified or is without buttons and zippers (Leaver, 2017).*
- • Work with the client on retraining the bladder by regularly timed toileting regimens (every 2 hours). For the older client in the home or a long-term care facility who has functional incontinence and dementia:
  - ❍ Determine the frequency of current urination using an alarm system or check-and-change device.
  - ❍ Record urinary elimination and incontinent patterns in a bladder log to use as a baseline for assessment and evaluation of treatment efficacy.
  - ❍ Begin a prompted toileting program based on the results of this program; toileting frequency may vary from every 1.5 to 2 hours to every 4 hours.
  - ❍ Provide positive reinforcement.

  EB: *Bladder retraining aims to increase the time in between trips to the toilet by encouraging the clients to "hold on" when they need to go. This aims to improve the client's control of their bladder and this can reduce symptoms of urinary frequency, urinary urgency, and nocturia (Stewart, 2018).*
- • Monitor older clients in a long-term care facility, acute care facility, or home for dehydration. EB: *Clients may have anxiety about incontinence and intentionally reduce fluid intake as a personal strategy to manage the problem. Such clients need to be monitored regularly as the onset of dehydration has the potential to develop slowly over time (Cook et al, 2019).*
- • Inspect the perineal and perianal skin for evidence of incontinence-associated dermatitis, including inflammation, vesicles in skin exposed to urinary leakage, and especially skinfolds or denudation of the

skin, particularly when incontinence is managed by absorptive pads or containment briefs. EB: *Skinfolds and the perineal skin are at risk for dermatitis and fungal or bacterial infections (Beeckman, 2017).*

- Begin a preventive skin care regimen for all clients with urinary incontinence and treat clients with incontinence-associated dermatitis or related skin damage. EB: *Minimizing exposure to urine; gentle cleansing; moisture protection, preferably with an emollient; and application of a skin protectant are the necessary components of a skin protection program (Beeckman, 2017).*
- Advise the client about the advantages of using disposable or reusable insert pads, pad-pant systems, or replacement briefs specifically designed for urinary incontinence as indicated for short-term/long-term use, including social events. EB: *A systematic review identified that the use of incontinence pads is the main conservative behavioral approach to managing continence. They are preferred to invasive management strategies (e.g., catheterization) (Roe, Flanagan, & Maden, 2015).*
- Consider the use of an indwelling catheter for continuous drainage in the client who is both homebound and bedbound and is receiving palliative or end-of-life care (requires a health care provider's order). At end of life, they may be the best choice. EB: *Catheters provided relief when mobility was a challenge for clients and getting out of bed was painful. The insertion of an indwelling catheter will not cure incontinence but aligns with the objective of managing symptoms at end of life (Smith et al, 2019).*
- When an indwelling urinary catheter is in place, follow prescribed maintenance protocols for managing the catheter, taping and replacing the catheter, the drainage bag, and care of perineal skin and urethral meatus. Teach infection control measures adapted to the home care setting. EB: *Proper care reduces the risk of catheter-associated urinary tract infection (Centers for Disease Control and Prevention, 2021).*
- Assist the client in adapting to the catheter. Encourage discussion of the client's response to the catheter. Research has consistently shown that indwelling catheter users need to be given more information, but some clients still feel poorly informed. EB: *Nurses are in a good position to find out what people know and what they need and to ensure that clients have contact phone numbers for further information and details of reliable websites and support organizations (Prinjha et al, 2016).*
- Provide clients with comprehensive written information about the management of continence-related problems. EB: *Client information materials and decision aids are essential tools for helping clients to make informed decisions and share in the decision-making process about their care (Posch et al, 2020).*
- Document all care and advice given in a factual and comprehensive manner. EB: *Good record keeping is an integral part of nursing practice and is essential to the provision of safe and effective care (Andrews & St Aubyn, 2015).*

REFERENCES

Andrews, A., & St Aubyn, B. (2015). If it's not written down—It didn't happen. *Journal of Community Nursing, 29*(5), 20–22.

Bardsley, A. (2016). An overview of urinary incontinence. *British Journal of Nursing, 25*(18), S14–S21.

Beeckman, D. (2017). A decade of research on incontinence-associated dermatitis (IAD): Evidence, knowledge gaps and next steps. *Journal of Tissue Viability, 26*(1), 47–56. http://dx.doi.org/10.1016/j.jtv.2016.02.004.

Centers for Disease Control and Prevention. (2021). *Urinary tract infection (catheter-associated urinary tract infection [CAUTI] and non-catheter-associated urinary tract infection [UTI]) and other urinary system infection [USI]) events.* National Healthcare Safety Network. Retrieved from http://www.cdc.gov/nhsn/PDFs/pscManual/7pscCAUTIcurrent.pdf. [Accessed July 6, 2021].

Cook, G., Hodgson, P., Hope, C., Thompson, J., & Shaw, L. (2019). Hydration practices in residential and nursing care homes for older people. *Journal of Clinical Nursing, 28*(7–8), 1205–1215.

Dixon, C. A., & Nakib, N. A. (2016). Are bladder diaries helpful in management of overactive bladder? *Current Bladder Dysfunction Reports, 11*(1), 14–17.

Ellis, P., Standing, M., & Roberts, S. (2020). *Patient assessment and care planning in nursing (Transforming nursing practice series)* (3rd ed.). London: Sage Publications.

Goldberg, J. L. (2017). Guideline implementation: Hand hygiene. *AORN Journal, 105*(2), 203–212.

Gove, D., Scerri, A., Georges, J., et al. (2017). Continence care for people with dementia living at home in Europe: A review of literature with a focus on problems and challenges. *Journal of Clinical Nursing, 26*(3–4), 356–365.

Griffith, R., & Tengnah, C. (2020). *Law and professional issues in nursing (transforming nursing practice series)* (5th ed.). London: Sage Publications.

Jachan, D., Müller-Werdan, U., & Lahmann, N. A. (2019). Impaired mobility and urinary incontinence in nursing home residents: A multicenter study. *Journal of Wound, Ostomy and Continence Nursing, 46*(6), 524–529.

Jerez-Roig, J., Santos, M. M., Souza, D. L. B., Amaral, F. L. J. S., & Lima, K. C. (2016). Prevalence of urinary incontinence and associated factors in nursing home residents. *Neurourology and Urodynamics, 35*(1), 102–107.

Keenan, P. M., Fleming, S., Horan, P. F., et al. (2018). Urinary continence promotion and people with an intellectual disability. *Learning Disability Practice.*

Leaver, R. (2017). Assessing patients with urinary incontinence: The basics. *Journal of Community Nursing, 31*(1), 40–46.

Nambiar, A. K., Bosch, R., Cruz, F., et al. (2018). EAU guidelines on assessment and nonsurgical management of urinary incontinence. *European Urology, 73*(4), 596–609.

Pizzol, D., Demurtas, J., Celotto, S., et al. (2021). Urinary incontinence and quality of life: A systematic review and meta-analysis. *Aging Clinical and Experimental Research, 33*(1), 25–35.

Posch, N., Horvath, K., Wratschko, L., Plath, J., Brodnig, R., & Siebenhofer, A. (2020). Written patient information materials used in general practices fail to meet expectable quality standards. *BMC Family Practice*, *21*(1), 23.

Prinjha, S., Chapple, A., Feneley, R., & Mangnall, J. (2016). Exploring the information needs of people living with a long-term indwelling urinary catheter: A qualitative study. *Journal of Advanced Nursing*, *72*(6), 1335–1346.

Roe, B., Flanagan, L., & Maden, M. (2015). Systematic review of systematic reviews for the management of urinary incontinence and promotion of continence using conservative behavioural approaches in older people in care homes. *Journal of Advanced Nursing*, *71*(7), 1464–1483.

Smith, N., Hunter, K., Rajabali, S., Fainsinger, R., & Wagg, A. (2019). Preferences for continence care experienced at end of life: A qualitative study. *Journal of Pain and Symptom Management*, *57*(6), 1099–1105.e3.

Spencer, M., McManus, K., & Sabourin, J. (2017). Incontinence in the older adult: The role of the geriatric multidisciplinary team. *British Columbia Medical Journal*, *59*(2), 99–105.

Stewart, E. (2018). Assessment and management of urinary incontinence in women. *Nursing Standard*, *33*(2), 75–81.

Mixed Urinary Incontinence

Domain 3 Elimination and exchange Class 1 Urinary function

Amanda Andrews, BSc (Hons), MA and Bernie St Aubyn, BSc (Hons), MSc

NANDA-I

Definition

Involuntary loss of urine in combination with or following a strong sensation or urgency to void, and also with activities that increase intra-abdominal pressure.

Defining Characteristics

Expresses incomplete bladder emptying; involuntary loss of urine upon coughing; involuntary loss of urine upon effort; involuntary loss of urine upon laughing; involuntary loss of urine upon physical exertion; involuntary loss of urine upon sneezing; nocturia; urinary urgency

Related Factors

Incompetence of the bladder neck; incompetence of the urethral sphincter; overweight; pelvic organ prolapse; skeletal muscular atrophy; smoking; weak anterior wall of the vagina

At-Risk Population

Individuals with chronic cough; individuals with one type of urinary incontinence; multiparous women; older adults; women experiencing menopause; women giving birth vaginally

Associated Conditions

Diabetes mellitus; estrogen deficiency; motor disorders; pelvic floor disorders; prolonged urinary incontinence; surgery for stress urinary incontinence; urethral sphincter injury

NOC (Nursing Outcomes Classification)

Suggested NOC Outcomes

Urinary Continence; Urinary Elimination

Example NOC Outcome with Indicators

Urinary Continence as evidenced by the following indicators: Absence of urinary leakage between catheterizations or containment of micturition by condom catheter and drainage bag/Absence of symptomatic urinary tract infection (absence of leukocytes and absence of bacterial growth or >100,000 colony-forming units/mL)/Underclothing dry during day/Underclothing or bedding dry during night. (Rate the outcome and indicators of **Urinary Continence:** 1 = never demonstrated, 2 = rarely demonstrated, 3 = sometimes demonstrated, 4 = often demonstrated, 5 = consistently demonstrated [see Section I].)

Client Outcomes

Client Will (Specify Time Frame)

- Follow prescribed schedule for bladder emptying on a daily basis

- Have intact perineal skin on a daily basis
- Remain clear of symptomatic urinary tract infection on a daily basis
- Demonstrate how to apply containment device or insert intermittent catheter or be able to provide caregiver with instructions for performing these procedures as per individual needs on a daily basis

NIC (Nursing Interventions Classification)

Suggested NIC Interventions

Urinary Catheterization: Intermittent; Urinary Elimination Management; Urinary Incontinence Care

Example NIC Activities—Urinary Elimination Management

Monitor urinary elimination including frequency, consistency, odor, volume, and color as appropriate; Teach client signs and symptoms of urinary tract infection

Nursing Interventions and *Rationales*

- Introduce yourself to the client and anyone accompanying him or her and inform them of your role. **EB:** *Introducing yourself to a client helps establish and develop a therapeutic relationship that recognizes the person within the client and forms the basis for building trust on which to base the provision of care (Ellis et al, 2020).*
- Gain consent to provide care before proceeding further with the assessment. **EB:** *Clients have the right of autonomy both legally and morally and therefore should be fully involved in the decision-making process (Griffith & Tengnah, 2020).*
- Wash hands using a recognized technique. **EB:** *Evidence shows that strict hand hygiene regimens significantly reduce the incidence of methicillin-resistant* Staphylococcus aureus *and* Clostridioides (Clostridium) difficile *infection (Goldberg, 2017).*
- Assess the usual pattern of bladder management and establish the extent of the problem. **EB:** *Several types of incontinence exist and since the treatments will vary, it is important that the assessment, also known as "diagnostic evaluation," establishes which type is present. The authors recognize that guidelines should be adapted to individual clients' needs (Nambiar et al, 2018).*
- Ask the client to complete a bladder diary/log to determine the pattern of urine elimination, any incontinence episodes, and current bladder management program. An electronic voiding diary may be kept whenever feasible. **EB:** *Bladder diaries provide accurate data and are more reliable than clients' recollections of symptoms. In addition to being inexpensive and low risk, clients view diaries as easy to complete and helpful for their care (Dixon & Nakib, 2016).*
- ▲ Consult with the health care provider concerning current bladder function and the potential of the bladder to produce hydronephrosis, vesicoureteral reflux, febrile urinary tract infection, or compromised renal function. **EB:** *Early diagnosis of a urinary tract infection, along with adequate management and new infection prevention, is key to reducing the risk of further compromised renal function leading to hospitalization and increased mortality rates from urinary tracts infections (Gomes De Medeiros Jr et al, 2020).*
- ▲ Consult with the health care provider and physical therapist concerning the neuromuscular ability to perform bladder management. The type of neurological disorder, as well as the level of neurological impairment and the ability to use the hands effectively, determines the method of urine management in reflex incontinence. **EB:** *An individual's function and experience of disability needs to be considered in relation to their underpinning pathology. Any resulting impairment, both personal and environmental, needs to be analyzed and assessed in relation to the implementation of a rehabilitation plan (Stevenson & Playford, 2016).*
- Inspect the perineal and perigenital skin for signs of incontinence-associated dermatitis and pressure ulcers. **EB:** *Standardizing skin care routines and making them an integrated part of essential care for incontinence clients will improve client care in specialized areas, which helps reduce the incidence of incontinence-associated dermatitis (Beeckman, 2017).*
- ▲ In consultation with the rehabilitation team, counsel the client and family concerning the merits and potential risks associated with each possible bladder management program, including spontaneous voiding, intermittent self-catheterization (ISC), and reflex voiding with condom catheter containment and in some cases, indwelling suprapubic catheterization. **EB:** *A systematic review of the literature suggests that indwelling suprapubic catheterization is favorable to indwelling urethral catheterization because there is a reduction in both the rate of recatheterization and asymptomatic infection. However, suprapubic*

catheterization is also associated with a higher rate of hematuria generally following the catheter's insertion. Intermittent catheterization is favored over indwelling catheterization in relation to a reduction in symptomatic urinary tract infections (Li et al, 2019).

- Ensure the client is aware of when and how to report any problems and/or complications of reflex incontinence care when at home. EB: *Clients should be routinely asked about how they are adjusting to and managing ISC. The use of regular reviews provides clients with opportunities to report any problems, complications, or concerns in a timely manner (Lake, 2018).*
- Provide clients with comprehensive written information about the management of continence-related problems. EB: *Client information materials and decision aids are essential tools for helping clients to make informed decisions and share in the decision-making process about their care (Posch et al, 2020).*
- Assist the family with arranging care in a way that allows the client to participate in family or favorite activities without embarrassment. Elicit discussion of the client's concerns about the social or emotional burden of incontinence. EB: *Urinary incontinence can have a negative effect on the quality of life for clients and their families. Effective communication, support, and reassurance are essential to help clients and families make the lifestyle adjustments required for continence management (Collins, 2019).*
- Teach the client to ensure good hydration. EB: *Clients may have anxiety about incontinence and intentionally reduce fluid intake as a personal strategy to manage the problem. Such clients need to be monitored regularly as the onset of dehydration has the potential to develop slowly over time (Cook et al, 2019).*
- Teach the client with a spinal injury the signs of autonomic dysreflexia, its relationship to bladder fullness, and management of the condition. Refer to the care plan for **Autonomic Dysreflexia.**

I

Intermittent Self-Catheterization

- Begin intermittent catheterization as ordered using sterile technique; the client may be taught to use clean technique in the home situation. EB: *Clean ISC has recently been advocated as a safe and simple technique to teach clients who are experiencing voiding dysfunction (Lake, 2018).*
- Adopt a person-centered ISC approach to motivate and schedule the frequency of intermittent catheterization based on the frequency/volume records of previous catheterizations, functional bladder capacity, and the impact of catheterization on the quality of the client's life. EB: *Adopting an individualized approach to ISC management should be reflective of the client's lifestyle, fitting ISC into existing routines (Nørager et al, 2019). The use of previous drainage regimens will help develop the client's new individual voiding regimen (Hillery, 2020).*
- Teach the client to recognize signs of symptomatic urinary tract infection and to seek care promptly when these signs occur. The signs of symptomatic infection include the following:
  - Discomfort over the bladder or during urination
  - Acute onset of urinary incontinence
  - Fever
  - Markedly increased spasticity of muscles below the level of the spinal lesion
  - Malaise, lethargy
  - Hematuria
  - Autonomic dysreflexia (hyperreflexia) symptoms

  EB: *Clients need the skills and knowledge to identify signs of symptomatic urinary tract infections. In order for clients to maintain adherence to ISC regimens they need to know how to manage any urinary tract infections by liaising with appropriate health professionals (Nørager et al, 2019).*
- Recognize that intermittent catheterization is typically associated with asymptomatic bacteriuria, and the indwelling catheter is routinely associated with asymptomatic colonization. EB: *There is a clinical need to refine the management of asymptomatic infection in association with bacteriuria. Effective strategies should include minimizing inappropriate antimicrobial use unless a symptomatic infection is detected (Nicolle, 2016).*
- Teach intermittent catheterization as the client approaches discharge as per operational guidelines and best practices. Instruct the client and at least one family member in the performance of catheterization. Teach the client with quadriplegia how to instruct others to perform this procedure. EB: *Intermittent catheterization is a safe and effective bladder management strategy for persons with reflex urinary incontinence. More and more clients are advised to perform intermittent catheterization. Quality-of-life studies show that intermittent catheterization has a great impact on daily life (Cobussen-Boekhorst et al, 2016).*
- Clients using ISC may experience bladder spasms that hinder the insertion process. EB: *Clients need to be educated about the use and side effects (constipation, dry mouth, and dizziness) of antispasmodic*

(parasympathetic) medications as prescribed by the health care provider. Antispasmodic medication is useful when clients are experiencing incomplete emptying, leading to an overactive bladder. In such cases antispasmodic medication can be prescribed to reduce involuntary bladder contractions (Diokno, 2019).

Condom Catheter/Sheath System

- For a male client with reflex incontinence who does not have urinary retention and cannot manage the condition effectively with spontaneous voiding, who does not choose to perform intermittent catheterization, or who cannot perform catheterization, teach the client and his family to obtain, select, and apply an external collective device and urinary drainage system. Assist the client and family to choose a product that adheres to the glans penis or penile shaft without allowing seepage of urine onto surrounding skin or clothing, which avoids provoking hypersensitivity reactions on the skin, and that includes a urinary drainage reservoir that is easily concealed under the clothing and does not cause irritation to the skin of the thigh. EB: *When considering the use of an external continence device, it is vital that the correct size is measured and fitted to eliminate many of the problems associated with leakage and the sheath falling off (Woodward, 2015).*
- Teach the client whose incontinence is managed by a condom catheter to routinely inspect the skin with each catheter change for evidence of lesions caused by pressure from the containment device or by exposure to urine, to cleanse the penis thoroughly, and to reapply a new device daily or every other day. EB: *A well-fitted sheath reduces the risk of skin irritation or ulceration. The sheath should always be fitted leaving a space between the tip of the penis and the shaft allowing urine to flow without the sheath "ballooning" (Woodward, 2015).*
- Document all care and advice given in a factual and comprehensive manner. EB: *Good record keeping is an integral part of nursing practice and is essential to the provision of safe and effective care (Andrews & St Aubyn, 2015).*

REFERENCES

Andrews, A., & St Aubyn, B. (2015). If it's not written down—it didn't happen. *Journal of Community Nursing, 29*(5), 20–22.

Beeckman, D. (2017). A decade of research on incontinence-associated dermatitis (IAD): Evidence, knowledge gaps and next steps. *Journal of Tissue Viability, 26*(1), 47–56. http://dx.doi.org/10.1016/j.jtv.2016.02.004.

Cobussen-Boekhorst, H., Hermeling, E., Heesakkers, J., & van Gaal, B. (2016). Patients' experience with intermittent catheterisation in everyday life. *Journal of Clinical Nursing, 25*(9–10), 1253–1261.

Collins, L. (2019). Intermittent self-catheterisation: Good patient education and support are key. *British Journal of Nursing, 28*(15), 964–966.

Cook, G., Hodgson, P., Hope, C., Thompson, J., & Shaw, L. (2019). Hydration practices in residential and nursing care homes for older people. *Journal of Clinical Nursing, 28*(7–8), 1205–1215.

Diokno, A. C. (2019). Legends in urology. *The Canadian Journal of Urology, 26*(4), 9803–9805.

Dixon, C. A., & Nakib, N. A. (2016). Are bladder diaries helpful in management of overactive bladder? *Current Bladder Dysfunction Reports, 11*(1), 14–17.

Ellis, P., Standing, M., & Roberts, S. (2020). *Patient assessment and care planning in nursing (transforming nursing practice series)* (3rd ed.). London: Sage Publications.

Goldberg, J. L. (2017). Guideline implementation: Hand hygiene. *AORN Journal, 105*(2), 203–212.

Gomes De Medeiros, W. L., Jr., Desmore, C. C., Peres Mazaro, L., et al. (2020). Urinary tract infection in patients with multiple sclerosis: An overview. *Multiple Sclerosis and Related Disorders, 46*, 102462.

Griffith, R., & Tengnah, C. (2020). *Law and professional issues in nursing (transforming nursing practice series)* (5th ed.). London: Sage Publications.

Hillery, S. (2020). Intermittent self-catheterisation: A person-centred approach. *British Journal of Nursing, 29*(15), 858–860.

Lake, H. (2018). Intermittent self-catheterisation: Patients' perceptions and experience. *British Journal of Nursing, 27*(18), S4–S6.

Li, M., Yao, L., Han, C., et al. (2019). The incidence of urinary tract infection of different routes of catheterization following gynecologic surgery: A systematic review and meta-analysis of randomized control trials. *The International Urogynecology Journal, 30*(4), 523–535.

Nambiar, A. K., Bosch, R., Cruz, F., et al. (2018). EAU guidelines on assessment and nonsurgical management of urinary incontinence. *European Urology, 73*(4), 596–609.

Nicolle, L. E. (2016). Asymptomatic bacteriuria in older adults. *Current Geriatrics Reports, 5*, 1–8.

Nørager, R., Bøgebjerg, C., Plate, I., & Lemaitre, S. (2019). Supporting better adherence among patients engaged in intermittent self-catheterisation. *British Journal of Nursing, 28*(2), 90–95.

Posch, N., Horvath, K., Wratschko, L., Plath, J., Brodnig, R., & Siebenhofer, A. (2020). Written patient information materials used in general practices fail to meet expectable quality standards. *BMC Family Practice, 21*(1), 23.

Stevenson, V. L., & Playford, D. (2016). Neurologic rehabilitation and the management of spasticity. *Medicine, 44*(9). https://doi.org/10.1016/j.mpmed.2016.06.002. Retrieved from https://ur.booksc.eu/book/60251815/4d4095.

Woodward, S. (2015). Selecting and fitting a penile sheath. *British Journal of Nursing, 25*(5), 290–292.

Stress Urinary Incontinence

Domain 3 Elimination and exchange Class 1 Urinary function

Amanda Andrews, BSc (Hons), MA and Bernie St Aubyn, BSc (Hons), MSc

NANDA-I

Definition

Involuntary loss of urine with activities that increase intra-abdominal pressure, which is not associated with urgency to void.

Defining Characteristics

Involuntary loss of urine in the absence of detrusor contraction; involuntary loss of urine the absence of overdistended bladder; involuntary loss of urine upon coughing; involuntary loss of urine upon effort; involuntary loss of urine upon laughing; involuntary loss of urine upon physical exertion; involuntary loss of urine upon sneezing

Related Factors

Overweight; pelvic floor disorders; pelvic organ prolapse

At-Risk Population

Individuals who perform high-intensity physical exercise; multiparous women; pregnant women; women experiencing menopause; women giving birth vaginally

Associated Conditions

Damaged pelvic floor muscles; degenerative changes in pelvic floor muscles; intrinsic urethral sphincter deficiency; nervous system diseases; prostatectomy; urethral sphincter injury

NOC (Nursing Outcomes Classification)

Suggested NOC Outcomes

Urinary Continence; Urinary Elimination

Example NOC Outcome with Indicators

Urinary Continence as evidenced by the following indicators: Experiences no urine leakage with increased abdominal pressure (e.g., sneezing, laughing, lifting)/Voids in appropriate receptacle/Able to move to toilet after strong desire to urinate is perceived/Underclothing remains dry during day/Underclothing or bedding remains dry during night. (Rate the outcome and indicators of **Urinary Continence:** 1 = never demonstrated, 2 = rarely demonstrated, 3 = sometimes demonstrated, 4 = often demonstrated, 5 = consistently demonstrated [see Section I].)

Client Outcomes

Client Will (Specify Time Frame)

- Report no stress incontinence episodes and/or a decrease in the severity of urine loss over a 24-hour period
- Experience no episodes of urinary incontinence as recorded on voiding diary (bladder log) over a 24-hour period
- Identify containment devices that assist in management of stress incontinence over a 24-hour period

NIC (Nursing Interventions Classification)

Suggested NIC Interventions

Pelvic Muscle Exercises; Urinary Incontinence Care

Example NIC Activities—Urinary Incontinence Care

Explain etiology of problem and rationale for actions; Modify clothing and environment to provide easy access to toilet

Nursing Interventions and *Rationales*

- Introduce yourself to the client and anyone accompanying him or her and inform them of your role. EB: *Introducing yourself to a client helps establish and develop a therapeutic relationship that recognizes the person within the client and forms the basis for building trust on which to base the provision of care (Ellis et al, 2020).*
- Gain consent to provide care before proceeding further with the assessment. For clients unable to give consent, discuss permission with relevant health care professionals and/or family members. EB: *Clients have the right of autonomy both legally and morally and therefore should be fully involved in the decision-making process (Griffith & Tengnah, 2020).*
- Wash hands using a recognized technique. EB: *Evidence shows that strict hand hygiene regimens significantly reduce the incidence of methicillin-resistant* Staphylococcus aureus *and* Clostridioides (Clostridium) difficile *infection (Goldberg, 2017).*
- Assess usual pattern of bladder management to understand the extent of the problem and establish pattern of bladder management. Explore factors provoking urine loss (diuretics, bladder irritants, alcohol), focusing on the differential diagnosis of stress, urge or mixed stress, and urge urinary symptoms. Consider using a symptom questionnaire that elicits relevant lower urinary tract symptoms and provides differentiation between stress and urge incontinence symptoms. EB: *Several types of incontinence exist and since the treatments will vary, it is important that the assessment, also known as "diagnostic evaluation," establishes which type is present. The authors recognize that guidelines should be adapted to individual clients' needs (Nambiar et al, 2018).*
- Review the client's medical history to identify possible risk factors for stress incontinence (i.e., pregnancy, parity, large babies, forceps or breech deliveries, obesity, chronic cough, physical activity, previous urinary tract or gynecological surgery, smoking history). EB: *Reviewing the client's medical history, considering any significant medical, surgical, obstetric, or genitourinary history, is essential as any identified conditions may affect an individual's ability to maintain continence (Bardsley, 2016).*
- Review the client's medication list (e.g., diuretics, lithium, adrenergic blockers, diabetes medications) to see what may exacerbate the client's urinary urgency. EB: *Health professionals should review the use of any medication that could affect a client's urine production. Side effects for consideration should include sedation, impaired cognition, or a change in sensation and muscle tone (Bardsley, 2016).*
- Review the client's bladder habits:
  - Onset and duration of urinary leakage
  - Related lower urinary tract symptoms, including voiding frequency (day/night) and urgency, severity (small, moderate, large amounts) of urinary leakage
- Assess for mixed urinary incontinence (a combination of stress and urge incontinence) by asking the client:
  - Can you delay urination for a 2-hour movie or car ride?
  - How often do you wake/arise at night to urinate?
  - When you have the urge to urinate, can you reach the toilet without leaking?

  EB: *The assessment is enhanced by the use of a questionnaire. This questionnaire needs to be a validated incontinence-specific quality of life questionnaire (Bardsley, 2016) to capture the possibility of mixed urinary incontinence.*
- Complete a lifestyle assessment to understand the effect of stress urinary incontinence on an individual's lifestyle. Inquire about incontinence pad use and change in daily, social, or recreational activities, as well as emotional impact. EB: *The impact of urinary incontinence on the quality of life is well recognized and includes a negative effect on psychological well-being, social interactions and activities, and sexual and interpersonal relationships (Minassian et al, 2015).*
- Inspect the perineal skin for evidence of incontinence-associated dermatitis, including inflammation, vesicles in skin exposed to urinary leakage, and especially skinfolds or denudation of the skin, particularly when incontinence is managed by absorptive pads or containment briefs. EB: *Ammonia produced from the breakdown of urea in urine causes an increase in skin pH, which increases the permeability of the skin; excess moisture and damage to the acid mantle further increases permeability and vulnerability to bacterial and*

I

fungal infections (Beeckman, 2017). Skin exposed to urine or stool will become bright red, and the surface may appear shiny because of serous exudate; inflamed areas of individuals with darker skin tones may be a duller red or hypopigmented when compared with adjacent skin. Inspect the skin for a maculopapular red rash typical of candidiasis (Beeckman, 2017).

▲ Refer client for specific testing to confirm incontinence etiology and diagnosis. If trained to do so, perform the cough stress test and request a 24-hour pad test (if appropriate) and urodynamic studies (including urine speed and flow, postvoid residual measurement, leak point pressure, and pressure flow study). EB: *A greater agreement rating was found between cough stress test and urodynamics than between 24-hour pad test and urodynamics in the assessment of stress incontinence (Minassian et al, 2015).*

• Establish with the client the current use of containment devices, for example, a well-fitted sheath; evaluate the devices for their ability to adequately contain urine loss, protect clothing, and control odor. Assist the client in identifying containment devices specifically designed to contain urinary leakage and not to use sanitary pads. EB: *A well-fitted sheath reduces the risk of skin irritation or ulceration. The sheath should always be fitted leaving a space between the tip of the penis and the shaft allowing urine to flow without the sheath "ballooning" (Woodward, 2015).*

• Teach the client to complete a bladder diary by recording voiding frequency, the frequency and degree of urinary incontinence episodes, association with urgency (a sudden and strong desire to urinate that is difficult to defer), fluid intake, and pad usage over a 3- to 7-day period. An electronic voiding diary may be kept whenever feasible. EB: *Use of a bladder diary may reduce client discrepancies in recall and is a valuable tool for assessment; the short (24-hour) duration of the bladder diary may yield inadequate data, and excessive diary duration reduces compliance (Dixon & Nakib, 2016).*

I

▲ With the client and in close consultation with the health care provider, review treatment options, including behavioral management; drug therapy; use of a pessary, vaginal device, or urethral insert; and surgery. Outline the potential benefits, efficacy, and side effects of each treatment option. CEB: *A 10-year review of the literature identified that there are two common conservative treatments recommended to treat stress urinary incontinence in women: strengthening pelvic floor muscles including biofeedback and weighted vaginal cones, and the use of intravaginal devices such as pessaries (McIntosh, Andersen, & Reekie, 2015).*

• Teach the client how to carry out pelvic floor muscle training. Teach the client to identify, contract, and relax the pelvic floor muscles without contracting distal muscle groups (e.g., abdominal muscles or gluteus muscles) using verbal feedback based on vaginal or anal palpation, biofeedback, or electrical stimulation and the assistance of an incontinence specialist or health care provider as necessary. EB: *A study carried out by Al Belushi et al (2020) concluded that a home-based pelvic floor muscle training program was effective in decreasing the severity of symptoms and improving the quality of life among women with stress urinary incontinence.*

• Incorporate principles of exercise physiology into a pelvic muscle training program using the following strategies:
  ❍ Begin a graded exercise program, usually starting with 5 to 10 repetitions and advancing gradually to no more than 35 to 50 repetitions every day or every other day based on baseline and ongoing evaluation of maximal strength and endurance.
  ❍ Continue exercise sessions over a period of 3 to 6 months.
  ❍ Integrate muscle training into activities of daily living.
  ❍ Assess progress every 2 weeks during the first month and every 4 to 6 weeks thereafter.

  EB: *Pelvic floor muscle exercises are carried out repetitively contracting and relaxing specific pelvic floor muscles. The contraction of the periurethral muscles leads to improved efficiency of the supportive functions for the urethra. Pelvic floor muscle exercises are therefore considered as the first-line intervention of prevention and treatment for stress urinary incontinence (Sangsawang & Sangsawang, 2016).*

• Work with the client on retraining the bladder by regularly timed toileting regimens (every 2 hours). For the older client in the home or a long-term care facility who has functional incontinence and dementia:
  ❍ Determine the frequency of current urination using an alarm system or check-and-change device.
  ❍ Record urinary elimination and incontinent patterns in a bladder log to use as a baseline for assessment and evaluation of treatment efficacy.
  ❍ Begin a prompted toileting program based on the results of this program; toileting frequency may vary from every 1.5 to 2 hours to every 4 hours.
  ❍ Provide positive reinforcement.

  EB: *Bladder retraining aims to increase the time in between trips to the toilet by encouraging the client to "hold on" when they need to go. This aims to improve the client's control of their bladder and this can reduce symptoms of urinary frequency, urinary urgency, and nocturia (Stewart, 2018).*

▲ Teach the client to self-administer duloxetine as ordered by the consulting health care provider and to monitor for adverse side effects. EB: *Duloxetine is a serotonin-norepinephrine reuptake inhibitor approved for treatment of stress urinary incontinence. A systematic review carried out by Rodrigues-Amorim et al (2020) identified that in the studies evaluated duloxetine was found to be safe and tolerable in over 70% of clients studied.*

▲ Teach the client to self-administer topical (vaginal) estrogens as directed and to monitor for adverse side effects. EB: *The use of local estrogens has been found to be safe and effective in improving the urinary symptoms in postmenopausal clients with urinary incontinence (Bodner-Adler et al, 2020).*

- Refer the female client with stress urinary incontinence and pelvic organ prolapse who wishes to use a pessary to manage stress incontinence to a nurse specialist or gynecologist with expertise in the placement and maintenance of these devices. EB: *The use of vaginal pessaries is an effective nonsurgical option for women experiencing stress urinary incontinence. The satisfaction rate with pessary use is high, and vaginal pessaries provide an adequate control of stress urinary incontinence if they are fit properly and managed by frequent replacements and regular checkups (Al-Shaikh et al, 2018).*
- Discuss potentially reversible or controllable risk factors, such as weight loss, with the client with stress incontinence, and assist the client to formulate a strategy to eliminate these conditions. EB: *Clinical studies have found that increased intraabdominal pressure due to obesity adversely stresses the pelvic floor and contributes to the development of stress urinary incontinence (Fuselier et al, 2018).*
- Refer the client with persistent stress incontinence to a continence service, health care provider, or nurse who specializes in the management of this condition. EB: *All clients presenting with incontinence should be offered an initial assessment by an individual who specializes in management of continence disorders. Continence specialists can provide expert knowledge, for example, around products and management (Kumah & McGlashan, 2019).*
- Teach the client to ensure good hydration. EB: *Clients may have anxiety about incontinence and intentionally reduce fluid intake as a personal strategy to manage the problem. Such clients need to be monitored regularly as the onset of dehydration has the potential to develop slowly over time (Cook et al, 2019).*
- Provide client with comprehensive written information about bladder care and how to access relevant support resources (e.g., national associations). EB: *Client information materials and decision aids are essential tools for helping clients to make informed decisions and share in the decision-making process about their care (Posch et al, 2020).*
- Encourage a program of self-care management. EB: *Addressing self-care activities through exercise, diet, fluid intake, and protective devices helps the client exercise control over incontinence and may reduce the substantial care provider burden affecting a significant proportion of spouse, partner, or familial care providers.*
- Assist the family with arranging care in a way that allows the client to participate in family or favorite activities without embarrassment. Elicit discussion of the client's concerns about the social or emotional burden of incontinence. EB: *Urinary incontinence can have a negative effect on the quality of life for clients and their families. Effective communication, support, and reassurance are essential to help clients and families make the lifestyle adjustments required for continence management (Collins, 2019).*
- Document all care and advice given in a factual and comprehensive manner. EBN: *Good record keeping is an integral part of nursing practice and is essential to the provision of safe and effective care (Andrews & St Aubyn, 2015).*
- Refer to the Disability-Associated Urinary **Incontinence** care plan.

REFERENCES

Al Belushi, Z. I., Al Kiyumi, M. H., Al-Mazrui, A. A., Jaju, S., Alrawahi, A. H., & Al Mahrezi, A. M. (2020). Effects of home-based pelvic floor muscle training on decreasing symptoms of stress urinary incontinence and improving the quality of life of urban adult Omani women: A randomized- controlled single blind study. *Neurourology and Urodynamics*, *39*(5), 1557–1566.

Al-Shaikh, G., Syed, S., Osman, S., Bogis, A., & Al-Badr, A. (2018). Pessary use in stress urinary incontinence: A review of advantages, complications, patient satisfaction, and quality of life. *International Journal of Women's Health*, *10*, 195–201.

Andrews, A., & St Aubyn, B. (2015). If it's not written down—it didn't happen. *Journal of Community Nursing*, *29*(5), 20–22.

Bardsley, A. (2016). An overview of urinary incontinence. *British Journal of Nursing*, *25*(18), S14–S21.

Beeckman, D. (2017). A decade of research on incontinence-associated dermatitis (IAD): Evidence, knowledge gaps and next steps. *Journal of Tissue Viability*, *26*(1), 47–56. doi:10.1016/j.jtv.2016.02.004.

Bodner-Adler, B., Alarab, M., Ruiz-Zapata, A., & Latthe, P. (2020). Effectiveness of hormones in postmenopausal pelvic floor disfunction—international Urogynecological Association research and development-committee opinion. *International Urogynecological Journal*, *31*(8), 1577–1582.

Collins, L. (2019). Intermittent self-catheterisation: Good patient education and support are key. *British Journal of Nursing*, *28*(15), 964–966.

Cook, G., Hodgson, P., Hope, C., Thompson, J., & Shaw, L. (2019). Hydration practices in residential and nursing care homes for older people. *Journal of Clinical Nursing, 28*(7–8), 1205–1215.

Dixon, C. A., & Nakib, N. A. (2016). Are bladder diaries helpful in management of overactive bladder? *Current Bladder Dysfunction Reports, 11*(1), 14–17.

Ellis, P., Standing, M., & Roberts, S. (2020). *Patient assessment and care planning in nursing (transforming nursing practice series)* (3rd ed.). London: Sage Publications.

Fuselier, A., Hanberry, J., Lovin, J. M., & Gomelsky, A. (2018). Obesity and stress urinary incontinence: Impact on pathophysiology and treatment. *Current Urology Reports, 19*(1), 10.

Goldberg, J. L. (2017). Guideline implementation: Hand hygiene. *AORN Journal, 105*(2), 203–212.

Griffith, R., & Tengnah, C. (2020). *Law and professional issues in nursing (transforming nursing practice series)* (5th ed.). London: Sage Publications.

Kumah, C., & McGlashan, D. (2019). Benefits of nurse–led continence prescription services for effective stock management and streamlined prescribing. *British Journal of Community Nursing, 24*(9), 424–431.

McIntosh, L., Andersen, E., & Reekie, M. (2015). Conservative treatment of stress incontinence in women: A 10-year (2004–2013) scoping review of the literature. *Urologic Nursing, 35*(4), 179–186, 203.

Minassian, V. A., Sun, H., Yan, X. S., Clarke, D. N., & Stewart, W. F. (2015). The interaction of stress and urgency urinary incontinence and its effect on quality of life. *International Urogynecology Journal, 26*(2), 269–276.

Nambiar, A. K., Bosch, R., Cruz, F., et al. (2018). EAU guidelines on assessment and nonsurgical management of urinary incontinence. *European Urology, 73*(4), 596–609.

Posch, N., Horvath, K., Wratschko, L., Plath, J., Brodnig, R., & Siebenhofer, A. (2020). Written patient information materials used in general practices fail to meet expectable quality standards. *BMC Family Practice, 21*(1), 23.

Rodrigues-Amorim, D., Olivares, J. M., Spuch, C., & Rivera-Baltanás, T. (2020). A systematic review of efficacy, safety and tolerability of duloxetine. *Frontiers in Psychiatry, 11*, 554899.

Sangsawang, B., & Sangsawang, N. (2016). Is a 6-week supervised pelvic floor muscle exercise programme effective in preventing stress urinary incontinence in late pregnancy in primigravida women? A randomized controlled trial. *European Journal of Obstetrics & Gynecology and Reproductive Biology, 197*, 103–110.

Stewart, E. (2018). Assessment and management of urinary incontinence in women. *Nursing Standard, 33*(2), 75–81.

Woodward, S. (2015). Selecting and fitting a penile sheath. *British Journal of Nursing, 25*(5), 290–292.

Urge Urinary Incontinence

Domain 3 Elimination and exchange Class 1 Urinary function

Amanda Andrews, BSc (Hons), MA and Bernie St Aubyn, BSc (Hons), MSc

NANDA-I

Definition

Involuntary loss of urine in combination with or following a strong sensation or urgency to void.

Defining Characteristics

Decreased bladder capacity; feeling of urgency with triggered stimulus; increased urinary frequency; involuntary loss of urine before reaching toilet; involuntary loss of urine with bladder contractions; involuntary loss of urine with bladder spasms; involuntary loss of varying volumes of urine between voids, with urgency; nocturia

Related Factors

Alcohol consumption; anxiety; caffeine consumption; carbonated beverage consumption; fecal impaction; ineffective toileting habits; involuntary sphincter relaxation; overweight; pelvic floor disorders; pelvic organ prolapse

At-Risk Population

Individuals exposed to abuse; individuals with history of urinary urgency during childhood; older adults; women; women experiencing menopause

Associated Conditions

Atrophic vaginitis; bladder outlet obstruction; depression; diabetes mellitus; nervous system diseases; nervous system trauma; overactive pelvic floor; pharmaceutical preparations; treatment regimen; urologic diseases

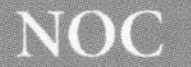

NOC (Nursing Outcomes Classification)

Suggested NOC Outcomes

Tissue Integrity: Skin and Mucous Membranes; Urinary Continence; Urinary Elimination

Example NOC Outcome with Indicators

Urinary Continence as evidenced by the following indicators: Responds in timely manner to urge/Voids in appropriate receptacle/Has adequate time to reach toilet between urge and evacuation of urine/Underclothing remains dry during day/Underclothing or bedding remains dry during night. (Rate the outcome and indicators of **Urinary Continence:** 1 = never demonstrated, 2 = rarely demonstrated, 3 = sometimes demonstrated, 4 = often demonstrated, 5 = consistently demonstrated [see Section I].)

Client Outcomes

Client Will (Specify Time Frame)

- Report relief from urge urinary incontinence or a decrease in the frequency of incontinent episodes on a daily basis
- Identify containment devices that assist in the management of urge urinary incontinence on a daily basis

NIC (Nursing Interventions Classification)

Suggested NIC Interventions

Urinary Habit Training; Urinary Incontinence Care

I

Example NIC Activities—Urinary Habit Training

Keep a continence specification record for 3 days to establish voiding pattern; Establish interval for toileting of preferably not less than 2 hours

Nursing Interventions and *Rationales*

- Introduce yourself to the client and anyone accompanying him or her and inform them of your role. EB: *Introducing yourself to a client helps establish and develop a therapeutic relationship that recognizes the person within the client and forms the basis for building trust on which to base the provision of care (Ellis et al, 2020).*
- Gain consent to perform care before proceeding further with the assessment. EB: *Clients have the right of autonomy both legally and morally and therefore should be fully involved in the decision-making process (Griffith & Tengnah, 2020).*
- Wash hands using a recognized technique. EB: *Evidence shows that strict hand hygiene regimens significantly reduce the incidence of methicillin-resistant* Staphylococcus aureus *and* Clostridioides (Clostridium) difficile *infection (Goldberg, 2017).*
- Assess the usual pattern of bladder management and establish the pattern of bladder management and extent of the problem. EB: *Several types of incontinence exist and since the treatments will vary, it is important that the assessment, also known as "diagnostic evaluation," establishes which type is present. The authors recognize that guidelines should be adapted to individual clients' needs (Nambiar et al, 2018).*
- Assess bladder habits and quality-of-life issues:
  - Diurnal frequency (voiding more than once every 2 hours while awake)
  - Urgency, daytime frequency, and nocturia
  - Involuntary leakage and leakage accompanied by or preceded by urgency
  - Amount of urine loss, moderate or large volume
  - Severity of symptoms
  - Alleviating and aggravating factors
  - Effect on quality of life

  EB: *Incontinence is distressing and may contribute to decreased quality of life. This includes a negative effect on psychological well-being, social interactions and activities, and sexual and interpersonal relationships (Minassian et al, 2015).*
- Ask specific questions relating to urge presentation:
  - Can you delay urination for a 2-hour movie or car ride?
  - How often do you wake at night to urinate?
  - When you have the urge to urinate, can you reach the toilet without leaking?

  EB: *This questionnaire needs to be a validated incontinence-specific quality-of-life questionnaire (Bardsley, 2016) to capture the possibility of mixed urinary incontinence.*

- Assess the severity of incontinence and the effect on the individual's lifestyle; inquire about incontinence pad use and change in daily, social, or recreational activities, and emotional impact. EB: *Incontinence is distressing and may contribute to decreased quality of life, especially for women with mixed incontinence (Bardsley, 2016).*
- ▲ Perform a focused physical assessment, in close consultation with a health care practitioner or advanced practice nurse, including the following:
  - Bladder palpation after voiding to check for retention
  - Bladder scanning for postvoid residual
  - Inspection of the perineal skin
  - Vaginal examination to determine hypoestrogenic changes in the mucosa (may contribute to urge incontinence)
  - Pelvic examination to determine the presence, location, and severity of vaginal wall prolapse, and reproduction of stress urinary incontinence with the cough test
- Anal tone and constipation should be assessed. EB: *A thorough abdominal and pelvic examination must be completed to accurately assess incontinence. Identification of "red flag" symptoms (e.g., nocturia, hematuria) needs referral to the appropriate consultant (NICE, 2015).*
- Inspect the perineal and perianal skin for evidence of incontinence-associated dermatitis, including inflammation, vesicles in skin exposed to urinary leakage, and especially skinfolds or denudation of the skin, particularly when incontinence is managed by absorptive pads or containment briefs. EB: *Ammonia produced from the breakdown of urea in urine causes an increase in skin pH, which increases the permeability of the skin; excess moisture and damage to the acid mantle further increase permeability and vulnerability to bacterial and fungal infections (Beeckman, 2017). Skin exposed to urine or stool will become bright red, and the surface may appear shiny because of serous exudate; inflamed areas of individuals with darker skin tones may be a duller red or hypopigmented when compared with adjacent skin. Inspect the skin for a maculopapular red rash typical of candidiasis (Beeckman, 2017).*
- Teach the client to complete a bladder diary by recording voiding frequency, the frequency and degree of urinary incontinence episodes, their association with urgency (a sudden and strong desire to urinate that is difficult to defer), fluid intake, and pad usage over a 3- to 7-day period. An electronic voiding diary may be kept whenever feasible. In addition to these parameters, the client may be asked to record voided volume and fluid intake. EB: *Use of a bladder diary may reduce client discrepancies in recall and is a valuable tool for assessment; short (24-hour) duration of the bladder diary may yield inadequate data, and excessive diary duration reduces compliance (Dixon & Nakib, 2016).*
- Review all medications the client is receiving, paying particular attention to sedatives, opioid analgesics, diuretics, antidepressants, psychotropic drugs, and cholinergics. Consult the health care practitioner or nurse practitioner about altering or eliminating these medications if they are suspected of affecting incontinence. EB: *Health professionals should review the use of any medication that could affect a client's urine production. Side effects for consideration should include sedation, impaired cognition, or a change in sensation and muscle tone (Bardsley, 2016).*
- Assess the client for urinary retention (see the care plan for **Urinary Retention**).
- Assess the client for functional limitations (environmental barriers, limited mobility or dexterity, and impaired cognitive function). EB: *Clients with impaired dexterity or weakness may benefit from clothing that has been modified or is without buttons and zippers (Leaver, 2017).*
- Consult the health care practitioner concerning diabetic management or pharmacotherapy for urinary tract infection when indicated. In specific cases, urgency and an increased risk of urge incontinence may be related to bacteriuria or urinary tract infection. EB: *Studies have found that clients with urge incontinence and the coexistence of recurrent urinary tract infections have diverse urinary microbiota. This suggests that persistent bladder colonization augments the pathology of clients' incontinence (Chen et al, 2018).*
- ▲ Assess for signs and symptoms of atrophic vaginal changes in the perimenopausal or postmenopausal woman, including vaginal dryness, tenderness to touch, mucosal dryness, friability, and discomfort with gentle palpation. Specifically query the woman with atrophic vaginitis concerning associated lower urinary tract symptoms (usually voiding frequency, urgency, and dysuria). Refer the woman with atrophic vaginal changes and bothersome lower urinary tract symptoms to a gynecologist, urologist, or women's health nurse practitioner for further evaluation and management. EB: *The use of local estrogens has been found to be safe and effective in improving the urinary symptoms in postmenopausal clients with urinary incontinence (Bodner-Adler et al, 2020).*

Pelvic Floor Training Program

- Teach the client how to carry out pelvic floor muscle training. Teach the client to identify, contract, and relax the pelvic floor muscles without contracting distal muscle groups (e.g., abdominal muscles or gluteus muscles) using verbal feedback based on vaginal or anal palpation, biofeedback, or electrical stimulation and the assistance of an incontinence specialist or health care provider as necessary. **EB:** *A study carried out by Al Belushi et al (2020) concluded that a home-based pelvic floor muscle training program was effective in decreasing the severity of symptoms and improving the quality of life among women with stress urinary incontinence.*
- Incorporate principles of exercise physiology into a pelvic muscle training program using the following strategies:
  - Begin a graded exercise program, usually starting with 5 to 10 repetitions and advancing gradually to no more than 35 to 50 repetitions every day or every other day based on baseline and ongoing evaluation of maximal strength and endurance.
  - Continue exercise sessions over a period of 3 to 6 months.
  - Integrate muscle training into activities of daily living.
  - Assess progress every 2 weeks during the first month and every 4 to 6 weeks thereafter.

  EB: *Pelvic floor muscle exercises are carried out repetitively contracting and relaxing specific pelvic floor muscles. The contraction of the periurethral muscles leads to improved efficiency of the supportive functions for the urethra. Pelvic floor muscle exercises are therefore considered the first-line intervention of prevention and treatment for stress urinary incontinence (Sangsawang & Sangsawang, 2016).*

I

Bladder Training Program

- Assist the client in completing a voiding diary over a period of a minimum of 3 days or up to 7 days.
- Review the results with the client, determining typical voiding frequency and establishing goals for voiding frequency based on the longest time interval between voids that is comfortable for the client.
- Using baseline voiding frequency, as determined by the diary, teach the client to void first thing in the morning, every time the predetermined voiding interval passes, and before going to bed at night.
- Encourage adherence to the program with timing devices and verbal encouragement and support, and address individual reasons for schedule interruption.
- Teach distraction and urge suppression techniques (see later discussion) to control urgency while the client postpones urination.
- Gradually increase the time between urinations to the negotiated goal. Time intervals between voiding are typically increased in increments of 15 to 30 minutes for clients with a baseline frequency of less than every 60 minutes and increments of 25 to 30 minutes for clients with a baseline frequency of more than every 60 minutes. The voiding interval should be increased by 15 to 30 minutes each week (based on the client's tolerance) until a voiding interval of 3 to 4 hours is achieved. Use a bladder diary to monitor progress. **EB:** *Bladder training involves adjusting your habits and developing a schedule to void even if the client does not have an urge to void. Gradually increase the time intervals between urination, allowing the bladder to fill more fully and providing more control over the urge to urinate (Mayo Clinic Staff, 2020).*
- Review with the client the types of beverages consumed, focusing on the intake of caffeine, which is associated with a transient effect on lower urinary tract symptoms. Advise all clients to reduce or eliminate intake of caffeinated beverages or over-the-counter medications of dietary aids containing caffeine. Identify and counsel the client to eliminate other bladder irritants that may exacerbate incontinence, such as smoking, carbonated beverages, citrus, sugar substitutes, and tomato products. **EB:** *Caffeine is a diuretic and a bladder irritant, increases detrusor pressure, and is a risk factor for detrusor instability; reducing caffeine may decrease both stress and urge incontinence. Decrease caffeine gradually to avoid caffeine withdrawal. Carbonated beverages, citrus fruits, sugar substitutes, and tomato products may be bladder irritants (Mayo Clinic Staff, 2020).*
- Teach the client to ensure good hydration. **EB:** *Clients may have anxiety about incontinence and intentionally reduce fluid intake as a personal strategy to manage the problem. Such clients need to be monitored regularly as the onset of dehydration has the potential to develop slowly over time (Cook et al, 2019).*
- Teach the client methods to avoid constipation such as increasing dietary fiber, moderately increasing fluid intake, exercising, and establishing a routine defecation schedule.

Urge Suppression

- Urge suppression skills are essential in helping clients learn a new way of responding to the sense of urgency. EB: *Rushing to the toilet increases physical pressure on the bladder, enhances the sensation of fullness, exposes the client to visual cues that can trigger incontinence, and exacerbates urgency.*
- Teach the client the following techniques:
  - When a strong or precipitous urge to urinate is perceived, teach the client to avoid running to the toilet.
  - Pause, sit down, and relax the entire body.
  - Perform repeated, rapid pelvic muscle contractions until the urge is relieved.
  - Use distraction: count backward from 100 by sevens; recite a poem; write a letter; balance a checkbook; do handwork such as knitting; and take five deep breaths, focusing on breathing.
  - Relief is followed by micturition within 5 to 15 minutes, using nonhurried movements when locating a toilet and voiding.
  - Use urge suppression strategies on waking during the night. If the urge subsides, the client should be encouraged to go back to sleep. If after a minute or two the urge does not subside, clients should be instructed to get up to void to avoid sleep interruption.

  EB: *Behavioral therapy is considered first-line therapy due to its effectiveness and minimal risk to the client. A key factor in bladder training is the use of timed voiding incorporated with pelvic muscle exercises (Raju & Linder, 2020).*
- Teach the client to self-administer antimuscarinic (anticholinergic) drugs as directed. Teach dosage side effects and administration of the medication and the importance of combining pharmacotherapy with scheduled voiding, adequate fluid intake, restriction of bladder irritants, and urge suppression techniques. EB: *Numerous antimuscarinic medications are available (e.g., oxybutynin and tolterodine). When adequate symptom control is achieved, an attempt to manage side effects should be made (e.g., the use of oral lubricants to aid dry mouth) (Raju & Linder, 2020).*
- Assist the client in selecting, obtaining, and applying a containment device for urine loss as indicated. EB: *Containment is important for people with urinary incontinence and should be considered when active treatment does not cure the problem, when it is not available or not possible, or if the risks of treatment outweigh the benefits to the client. A useful resource for health care professionals and clients can be found at* www.continenceproductadvisor.org *(Nambiar et al, 2018).*
- Provide client with comprehensive written information about bladder care and how to access relevant support resources (e.g., national associations). EB: *Client information materials and decision aids are essential tools for helping clients to make informed decisions and share in the decision-making process about their care (Posch et al, 2020).*
- Assess the functional and cognitive status of all clients with urge incontinence; use interventions to improve mobility. EB: *Clients with severe cognitive impairments (dementia) and functional mobility problems have an increased likelihood of developing urge incontinence (Jerez-Roig et al, 2016).*
- Refer client for occupational therapy for help in obtaining assistive devices and adapting the home for optimal toilet accessibility. EB: *Occupational therapists are needed to assist clients with dexterity and mobility issues that may be contributing to incontinence (Spencer, McManus, & Sabourin, 2017).*
- Encourage the client to develop an action plan for self-care management of incontinence. Making an action plan facilitates behavior change.
- Document all care and advice given in a factual and comprehensive manner. EBN: *Good record keeping is an integral part of nursing practice and is essential to the provision of safe and effective care (Andrews & St Aubyn, 2015).*
- Refer to Functional Urinary **Incontinence** care plan.

I

REFERENCES

Al Belushi, Z. I., Al Kiyumi, M. H., Al-Mazrui, A. A., Jaju, S., Alrawahi, A. H., & Al Mahrezi, A. M. (2020). Effects of home-based pelvic floor muscle training on decreasing symptoms of stress urinary incontinence and improving the quality of life of urban adult Omani women: A randomized- controlled single blind study. *Neurourology and Urodynamics, 39*(5), 1557–1566.

Andrews, A., & St Aubyn, B. (2015). If it's not written down—it didn't happen. *Journal of Community Nursing, 29*(5), 20–22.

Bardsley, A. (2016). An overview of urinary incontinence. *British Journal of Nursing, 25*(18), S14–S21.

Beeckman, D. (2017). A decade of research on incontinence-associated dermatitis (IAD): Evidence, knowledge gaps and next steps. *Journal of Tissue Viability, 26*(1), 47–56. doi:10.1016/j.jtv.2016.02.004.

Bodner-Adler, B., Alarab, M., Ruiz-Zapata, A., & Latthe, P. (2020). Effectiveness of hormones in postmenopausal pelvic floor disfunction—International Urogynecological Association research and development-committee opinion. *International Urogynecological Journal, 31*(8), 1577–1582.

Chen, Z., Phan, M. D., Bates, L. J., et al. (2018). The urinary microbiome in patients with refractory urge incontinence and recurrent urinary

tract infection. *International Urogynecology Journal, 29*(12), 1775–1782.
Cook, G., Hodgson, P., Hope, C., Thompson, J., & Shaw, L. (2019). Hydration practices in residential and nursing care homes for older people. *Journal of Clinical Nursing, 28*(7–8), 1205–1215.
Dixon, C. A., & Nakib, N. A. (2016). Are bladder diaries helpful in management of overactive bladder? *Current Bladder Dysfunction Reports, 11*(1), 14–17.
Ellis, P., Standing, M., & Roberts, S. (2020). *Patient assessment and care planning in nursing (transforming nursing practice series)* (3rd ed.). London: Sage Publications.
Goldberg, J. L. (2017). Guideline implementation: Hand hygiene. *AORN Journal, 105*(2), 203–212.
Griffith, R., & Tengnah, C. (2020). *Law and professional issues in nursing (transforming nursing practice series)* (5th ed.). London: Sage Publications.
Jerez-Roig, J., Santos, M. M., Souza, D. L. B., Amaral, F. L. J. S., & Lima, K. C. (2016). Prevalence of urinary incontinence and associated factors in nursing home residents. *Neurourology and Urodynamics, 35*(1), 102–107.
Leaver, R. (2017). Assessing patients with urinary incontinence: The basics. *Journal of Community Nursing, 31*(1), 40–46.
Mayo Clinic Staff. (2020). *Bladder control: Lifestyle strategies ease problems.* Retrieved from https://www.mayoclinic.org/diseases-conditions/urinary-incontinence/in-depth/bladder-control-problem/ART-20046597?p=1. Accessed July 7, 2021.
Minassian, V. A., Sun, H., Yan, X. S., Clarke, D. N., & Stewart, W. F. (2015). The interaction of stress and urgency urinary incontinence and its effect on quality of life. *International Urogynecology Journal, 26*(2), 269–276.
Nambiar, A. K., Bosch, R., Cruz, F., et al. (2018). EAU guidelines on assessment and nonsurgical management of urinary incontinence. *European Urology, 73*(4), 596–609.
National Institute for Health and Care Excellence (NICE). (2015). *Suspected cancer: Recognition and referral.* Retrieved from https://www.nice.org.uk/guidance/ng12. Accessed July 7, 2021.
Posch, N., Horvath, K., Wratschko, L., Plath, J., Brodnig, R., & Siebenhofer, A. (2020). Written patient information materials used in general practices fail to meet expectable quality standards. *BMC Family Practice, 21*(1), 23.
Raju, R., & Linder, B. (2020). Evaluation and treatment of overactive bladder in women. *Mayo Clinic Proceedings, 95*(2), 370–377.
Sangsawang, B., & Sangsawang, N. (2016). Is a 6-week supervised pelvic floor muscle exercise programme effective in preventing stress urinary incontinence in late pregnancy in primigravida women? A randomized controlled trial. *European Journal of Obstetrics & Gynecology and Reproductive Biology, 197*, 103–110.
Spencer, M., McManus, K., & Sabourin, J. (2017). Incontinence in the older adult: The role of the geriatric multidisciplinary team. *British Columbia Medical Journal, 59*(2), 99–105.

Risk for Urge Urinary Incontinence

Domain 3 Elimination and exchange Class 1 Urinary function

Mary Beth Flynn Makic, PhD, RN, CCNS, CCRN-K, FAAN, FNAP, FCNS

NANDA-I

Definition

Susceptible to involuntary passage of urine occurring soon after a strong sensation or urgency to void, which may compromise health.

Risk Factors

Alcohol consumption; anxiety; caffeine consumption; carbonated beverage consumption; fecal impaction; ineffective toileting habits; involuntary sphincter relaxation; overweight; pelvic floor disorders; pelvic organ prolapse

At-Risk Population

Individuals exposed to abuse; individuals with history of urinary urgency during childhood; older adults; women; women experiencing menopause

Associated Conditions

Atrophic vaginitis; bladder outlet obstruction; depression; diabetes mellitus; nervous system diseases; nervous system trauma; overactive pelvic floor; pharmaceutical preparations; treatment regimen; urologic disease

NIC, NOC, Client Outcomes, Nursing Interventions and *Rationales,* Client/Family Teaching and Discharge Planning, and References

Refer to care plan for Urge Urinary **Incontinence**.

Disorganized Infant Behavior

Domain 9 Coping/stress tolerance Class 3 Neurobehavioral stress

Margaret Quinn, DNP, CPNP, CNE

NANDA-I

Definition

Disintegration of the physiological and neurobehavioral systems of functioning.

Defining Characteristics

Attention-Interaction System

Impaired response to sensory stimuli

Motor System

Altered primitive reflexes; exaggerated startle response; fidgeting; finger splaying; fisting; hands to face behavior; hyperextension of extremities; impaired motor tone; maintains hands to face position; tremor; twitching; uncoordinated movement

Physiological

Abnormal skin color; arrhythmia; bradycardia; inability to tolerate rate of feedings; inability to tolerate volume of feedings; oxygen desaturation; tachycardia; time-out signals

Regulatory Problems

Impaired ability to inhibit startle reflex; irritable mood

State-Organization System

Active-awake state; diffuse alpha electroencephalogram (EEG) activity with eyes closed; irritable crying; quiet-awake state; state oscillation

Related Factors

Caregiver misreading infant cues; environmental overstimulation; feeding intolerance; inadequate caregiver knowledge of behavioral cues; inadequate containment within environment; inadequate physical environment; insufficient environmental sensory stimulation; malnutrition; pain; sensory deprivation; sensory overstimulation

At-Risk Population

Infants exposed to teratogen in utero; infants with low postmenstrual age; premature infants

Associated Conditions

Congenital disorders; immature neurological functioning; impaired infant motor functioning; inborn genetic diseases; invasive procedure; oral impairment

NOC (Nursing Outcomes Classification)

Suggested NOC Outcomes

Child Development; Neurological Status; Newborn Adaptation; Preterm Infant Organization; Sleep; Thermoregulation: Newborn; Infant Nutritional Status

Example NOC Outcome with Indicators

Preterm Infant Organization as evidenced by the following indicators: O_2 saturation >85%/ Thermoregulation/Sleep-awake state organization/Smooth transition between states/Ability to attend to visual and auditory stimuli/Habituation. (Rate the outcome and indicators of **Preterm Infant Organization:** 1 = severely compromised, 2 = substantially compromised, 3 = moderately compromised, 4 = mildly compromised, 5 = not compromised [see Section I].)

Client Outcomes

Client Will (Specify Time Frame)

Infant/Child

- Display physiological/autonomic stability: cardiopulmonary, digestive functioning
- Display signs of organized motor system
- Display signs of organized state system: ability to achieve and maintain a state and transition smoothly between states
- Demonstrate progress toward effective self-regulation
- Demonstrate progress toward or ability to maintain calm attention
- Demonstrate progress or ability to engage in positive interactions
- Demonstrate ability to respond to sensory information (visual, auditory, tactile) in an adaptive way

Parent/Significant Other

- Recognize infant/child behaviors as a complex communication system that expresses specific needs and wants (e.g., hunger, pain, stress, desire to engage or disengage)
- Educate parents/caregivers to recognize infant's avenues of neurobehavioral communication: autonomic/physiological, motor, state, attention/interaction
- Recognize how infants respond to environmental sensory input through stress/avoidance and approach/engagement behaviors
- Recognize and support infant's self-regulatory, coping behaviors used to regain or maintain homeostasis
- Teach parents to "tune in" to their own interactive style and how that affects their infant's behavior
- Teach parents ways to adapt their interactive style in response to infant's style of communication appropriate for developmental stage and gestational age
- Identify appropriate positioning and handling techniques that will enhance normal motor development
- Promote infant/child's attention capabilities that support visual and auditory development
- Engage parents in pleasurable parent–infant interactions that encourage bonding and attachment
- Structure and modify the environment in response to infant/child's behavior and personal needs; personalize their bed space
- Identify available community resources that provide early intervention services, emotional support, community health nursing, and parenting classes
- Communicate the infant's medical, nursing, and developmental needs to the family in a culturally sensitive and appropriate way that is understandable

I

NIC (Nursing Interventions Classification)

Suggested NIC Interventions

Physiological and Autonomic Stability; Developmental Enhancement; Infant Care; Environmental Management; Kangaroo Care; Nonnutritive Sucking; Parent Education: Infant; Positioning and Handling; Sleep and Awake Stability; Teaching: Infant Stimulation 0-4 months; Bonding and Attachment

Example NIC Activities—Developmental Enhancement, Infant

Provide information to parent about child development and child rearing; Promote and facilitate family bonding and attachment with infant

Nursing Interventions and *Rationales*

- Sensitive nursing care must be implemented at the infant's admission to the neonatal intensive care unit (NICU), continued during the stay, and continued past discharge as the family adjusts to transitioning home and into the community. **EBN:** *"Learning the principles of neurodevelopment and understanding the meaning of preterm behavioral cues make it possible for NICU caregivers and parents to provide individualized developmentally appropriate, neuroprotective care to each infant" (Altimier & Phillips, 2016).*
- Assess the neurobehavior systems through which infants communicate organized and/or disorganized stress behaviors within the subsystems of functioning (i.e., physiological/autonomic, motor, states, attention/interactional, self-regulatory). **EBN:** *The stress responses of hospitalized preterm infants vary and are measured in all stress exposures (Nist et al, 2020).*

- Recognize and educate parents to recognize the behavior cues infants use to communicate stress/avoidance and approach/engagement. EB: *Mothers of preterm infants were as able as the mothers of full-term infants in configural processing of their own infant's face. Preterm mothers made comparable use of configural processing for the body and face of both familiar and unfamiliar infants, in keeping with the pattern of performance of the full-term mothers who had similarly low levels of maternal sensitivity (Butti et al, 2018).*
- Provide high-quality individualized developmental care for low-birth-weight preterm infants in a family-centered care environment that promotes normal neurological, physical, and emotional developmental and prevents disabilities. EB: *A study focused on changing NICU "to family-integrated care where parents are intimately involved in baby's care for as many hours a day" and changed the unit's name to newborn intensive parenting unit (NIPU), leading to improved outcomes for NIPU babies (Hall et al, 2017).*
- Identify and manage pain using appropriate pain management techniques during invasive procedures (e.g., tube insertion, heel sticks, intravenous lines). EBN: *Breastfeeding or oral sucrose and holding and swaddling reduce pain during procedures (Yilmaz & Inal, 2020).* EB: *The skin-to-skin method reduces procedural pain (Johnston et al, 2017).*
- Provide care that supports development state organization, such as the ability to achieve and maintain quiet sleep and awake states and transition smoothly between states. EBN: *Promote sleep by timing care and avoiding unnecessary procedures that disrupt sleep (Altimier & Phillips, 2016).* EBN: *A study found methods to reduce NICU noise are necessary and achievable (Reeves-Messner & Spilker, 2017).*
- Encourage parents to speak slowly and/or sing to their babies during visits. EB: *Maternal voice demonstrates increased stability in preterm infants (Filippa et al, 2017).*
- Provide infants several opportunities for nonnutritive sucking (NNS). EB: Infants receiving NNS during tube feedings showed reduced time transitioning to full oral feedings and decreased the length of hospital stay (*Foster, Psaila, & Patterson, 2016*).
- Provide parents opportunities to experience physical closeness through loving touch, massage, cuddling, and skin-to-skin contact (kangaroo care), which enhances parent–infant attachment. EB: *Premature infants receiving kangaroo mother care, compared with those who did not, have better neurodevelopmental performance between 36 and 41 weeks of postconceptual age (Gurgel de Castro Silva et al, 2016).*
- Teach parents to use calming interventions that mimic the sensory environment in the womb such as swaddling, side position, sound (white noise), swinging, and sucking (5 S's). EBN: *The 5 S's technique is teachable, learnable, useful, and effective in calming crying infants, and it can boost mothers' parental self-efficacy (Botha et al, 2020).*
- Encourage parental engagement and early interactions in the NICU to set the foundation for parent–infant attachment and social relationships. EB: *Parents' emotional closeness to NICU infants may be crucial for developing an affective parent–infant relationship (Stefana & Lavelli, 2017).*
- Support effective and pleasurable feeding practices, such as breast, bottle, or combination, as essential for healthy nutrition/calories, for mother–baby bonding and attachment, and for setting the foundation for successful feeding/eating patterns. EBN: *Support breastfeeding for successful oral feedings (Altimier & Phillips, 2016).* EB: *Full or partial breastfeeding for the first few months is protective against sudden infant death syndrome (SIDS) risk (Thompson, et al, 2017).*
- Provide infants with positive sensory experiences (e.g., visual, auditory, tactile, olfactory, vestibular, proprioceptive) to enhance development of sensory pathways and avoid overstimulation of sensory systems. EB: *Auditory: Music activities provide multisensory neurological stimulation (Standley & Gutierrez, 2020).* EBN: *Gustatory: Position infant allowing finger/fist sucking.* EBN: *Tactile: Skin-to-skin contact is a positive sensory experience for both mothers and babies (Baley & Committee on Fetus and Newborn, 2015).* EB: *Olfactory: Exposure of breast milk odor can reduce need for O_2 therapy (Karbandi et al, 2015).* EBN: *Visual: Provide stable lighting, shield eyes from bright lights, and monitor visual stimulation until 37 weeks' gestation (Altimier & Phillips, 2016).* EBN: *Vestibular: Change position every 4 hours (Altimier & Phillips, 2016). Vestibular stimulation (movement in space such as rocking, being carried while an adult is walking, being held while the infant sways) is critical for neurodevelopment (Standley & Gutierrez, 2020).*
- Incorporate parents as coparticipants of infant care by communicating daily progress of their infant's condition. EBN: *Parents would rather speak with a physician or nurse they are already familiar with versus outside sources for education and support* (*Wigert & Bry, 2018*).
- Provide social support to parents including all members of the family. EB: *Implement parent-to-parent support as an effective way for NICU parents to gain confidence, improve mental health, and prepare for discharge (Hall et al, 2017).*

I

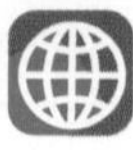

Multicultural

- Identify cultural beliefs, norms, and values of family's perceptions of infant/child behavior. EB: *Additional cultural perspectives would complement research guided by attachment theory and could shed new light on this phenomenon (Bader & Fouts, 2019).*
- Recognize and support positive mother–infant interactive behaviors and be sensitive to cultural and ethnic backgrounds. EB: *In a systematic literature review, it was noted that cultural factors influence what parents expect in regard to their emotional displays and how parents will respond. Research methods suggest that perception of infant emotion is complex (Bader & Fouts, 2019).*

Client/Family Teaching and Discharge Planning

- Perform a family assessment to understand the family's specific needs and circumstances. EB: *A family assessment will complement the discharge readiness assessment and should be a standard part of the discharge process (Smith, 2019).*
- Assess for any sociodemographic risks within the family. EB: *Global maternal insensitivity was associated with higher attachment disorganization for infants of mothers with higher sociodemographic risk, but not for those of mothers with lower sociodemographic risk (Gedaly & Leeks, 2016).*
- Educate parents on safe "back-to-sleep" practice before NICU discharge. EBN: *Parental knowledge of safe sleep recommendations and compliance with safe sleep practices were both significantly higher after written and verbal education. The results supported previous findings that providing current written material along with modeling safe sleep practices in the hospital before discharge to home can help further reduce the incidence of SIDS (Dufer & Godfrey, 2017).*
- ▲ Provide information or refer to community-based follow-up programs for preterm/at-risk infants and their families. EBN: *Strategies may include support groups, home nurse visiting programs, psychotherapy, parent-to-parent support activities, wellness coaching, and online parent community connections (Mosher, 2017).*
- ▲ Refer and support transition to early intervention services on discharge. EBN: *Initiating NICU discharge planning earlier by a trusted health care professional may influence participation (Koldoff, 2018).*

Home Care

- Assess for domestic violence risks in the home environment. EB: *Infants and toddlers who witness violence in their homes or community show excessive irritability, immature behavior, sleep disturbances, emotional distress, fear of being alone, and regression in toileting and language (Hagan, Shaw, & Duncan, 2017).*
- Listening to fears, answering questions, and giving time to practice new skills before discharge may increase parents' confidence for NICU discharge. EB: *Some parents will have difficulty bonding with their infant, may be less responsive to infant cues, and may be less aware of their infant's development (Mosher, 2017).*
- Encourage parents to use home visitation whenever possible because it enhances neonatal progress and parental support. EBN: *Home visitation is effective for education and support for infants and families after NICU discharge (Parker, Warmuskerken, & Sinclair, 2015).*
- Encourage families to teach extended family and support persons to recognize and respond appropriately to the infant's behavioral cues; supportive help may be most appreciated doing physical tasks. EB: *Early relationship between infants and their primary caregivers is critical to future child mental health and well-being; the development of secure and organized infant attachment depends on caregiving and parenting behaviors characterized by high sensitivity, responsivity, and nurturance (Erickson, Julian, & Muzik, 2019).*
- Provide education on positioning and handling that supports optimal infant growth and development. EB: *Encourage the importance of tummy time when awake and supervised (Hewitt et al, 2020).*
- Suggest babywearing. Babywearing holds babies in a kangaroo position to support caregivers and promote positive health outcomes after NICU discharge. EBN: *The themes identified indicate that babywearing has the potential to address harms—such as stress, fear, depression, anxiety, and posttraumatic stress disorder—that may be experienced by caregivers of infants discharged from the NICU (Miller et al, 2020).*
- Encourage home visitors to recognize maternal depression resulting from the NICU or new parent experiences. EB: *Mothers who are at risk for depression in their infants' early lives may be hampered in their capacity to respond appropriately to their infants' mental states. Infants with mothers who have difficulty responding appropriately to their mental states, as suggested by low appropriate mind-mindedness, may feel less known and recognized by their mothers, a key theme in the origins of disorganized attachment (Bigelow et al, 2018).*
- Provide families with information about community resources, developmental follow-up services, and parent-to-parent support programs, and request primary health care providers to follow developmental

progress with parent-friendly developmental questionnaires. EBN: *The validated Premature and Young Infant Development Assessment Tool (PYIDAT) is designed for premature infants from 34 weeks' gestation to 5 months adjusted age, and is a validated tool that offers a comprehensive assessment of premature infants (DeWys et al, 2016).*

REFERENCES

Altimier, L., & Phillips, R. (2016). The neonatal integrative developmental care model: Advanced clinical applications of the seven core measures for neuroprotective family-centered developmental care. *Newborn and Infant Nursing Reviews, 16*(4), 230–244. https://doi.org/10.1053/j.nainr.2016.09.030.

Bader, L. R., & Fouts, H. N. (2019). Parents' perceptions about infant emotions: A narrative cross-disciplinary systematic literature review. *Developmental Review, 51*, 1–30. https://doi.org/10.1016/j.dr.2018.11.003.

Baley, J., & Committee on Fetus and Newborn. (2015). Skin-to-skin care for term and preterm infants in the neonatal NICU. *Pediatrics, 136*(3), 596–599. https://doi.org/10.1542/peds.2015-2335.

Bigelow, A. E., Beebe, B., Power, M., et al. (2018). Longitudinal relations among maternal depressive symptoms, maternal mind-mindedness, and infant attachment behavior. *Infant Behavioral Development, 51*, 33–44. https://doi.org/10.1016/j.infbeh.2018.02.006.

Botha, E., Helminen, M., Kaunonen, M., Lubbe, W., & Joronen, K. (2020). The effects of an infant calming intervention on mothers' parenting self-efficacy and satisfaction during the postpartum period: A randomized controlled trial. *Journal of Perinatal and Neonatal Nursing, 34*(4), 300–310. https://doi.org/10.1097/JPN.0000000000000510.

Butti, M., Montirosso, R., Borgatti, R., & Urgesi, C. (2018). Maternal sensitivity is associated with configural processing of infant's cues in preterm and full-term mothers. *Early Human Development, 125*, 35–45. https://doi.org/10.1016/j.earlhumdev.2018.08.018.

DeWys, M., Mlynarczyk, S., Anderson, K., et al. (2016). *Reliability and validity of the premature & Young infant assessment tool (PYIDAT).* Milwaukee: Grand Valley State University, presentation, 40th Annual Midwest Nursing Research Conference.

Dufer, H., & Godfrey, K. (2017). Integration of safe sleep and sudden infant death syndrome (SIDS) education among parents of preterm infants in the neonatal intensive care unit (NICU). *Journal of Neonatal Nursing, 23*(2), 103–108. https://doi.org/10.1016/j.jnn.2016.09.001.

Erickson, N., Julian, M., & Muzik, M. (2019). Perinatal depression, PTSD, and trauma: Impact on mother–infant attachment and interventions to mitigate the transmission of risk. *International Review of Psychiatry, 31*(3), 245–263. https://doi.org/10.1080/09540261.2018.1563529.

Filippa, M., Panza, C., Ferrari, F., et al. (2017). Systematic review of maternal voice interventions demonstrates increased stability in preterm infants. *Acta Paediatrica, 106*(8), 1220–1229. https://doi.org/10.1111/apa.13832.

Foster, J. P., Psaila, K., & Patterson, T. (2016). Non-nutritive sucking for increasing physiologic stability and nutrition in preterm infants. *Cochrane Database of Systematic Reviews, 10*, CD001071. https://doi.org/10.1002/14651858.

Gedaly, L. R., & Leeks, E. M. (2016). The role of sociodemographic risk and maternal behavior in the prediction of infant attachment disorganization. *Attachment & Human Development, 18*(6), 554–569. https://doi.org/10.1080/14616734.2016.1213306.

Gurgel de Castro Silva, M., Carvalho de Moraes Barros, M., Lima Pessoa, Ú. M., & Guinsburg, R. (2016). Kangaroo-mother care method and neurobehavior of preterm infants. *Early Human Development, 95*, 55–59. https://doi-org.proxy.libraries.rutgers.edu/10.1016/j.earlhumdev.2016.02.004.

Hagan, J. F., Shaw, J. S., & Duncan, P. M. (Eds.). (2017). *Bright futures: Guidelines for health supervision of infants, children, and adolescents* (4th ed.). Itasca, IL: American Academy of Pediatrics.

Hall, S. L., Hynan, M. T., Phillips, R., et al. (2017). The neonatal intensive parenting unit: An introduction. *Journal of Perinatology, 37*(12), 1259–1264. https://doi.org/10.1038/jp.2017.108.

Hewitt, L., Kerr, E., Stanley, R. M., & Okely, A. D. (2020). Tummy time and infant health outcomes: A systematic review. *Pediatrics, 145*(6), e20192168.

Johnston, C., Campbell-Yeo, M., Disher, T., et al. (2017). Skin-to-skin care for procedural pain in neonates. *Cochrane Database of Systematic Reviews, 2*, CD008435. https://doi.org/10.1002/14651858.CD008435.pub3.

Karbandi, S., Dehghanian, S., Pourarian, S., & Salari, M. (2015). The effect of breast milk odor on concentration percentage of oxygen saturation and respiratory rate in premature infants. *Evidence-Based Care, 5*(1), 25–34.

Koldoff, E. (2018). *Transition to early intervention for infants with very low birth weight.* Oklahoma City: University of Oklahoma Health Sciences Center, 10787184. [Doctoral dissertation].

Miller, R. R., Bedwell, S., Laubach, L. L., & Tow, J. (2020). What is the experience of babywearing a NICU graduate? *Nursing for Women's Health, 24*(3), 175–184.

Mosher, S. L. (2017). Comprehensive NICU parental education: Beyond baby basics. *Neonatal Network, 36*(1), 18–25. https://doi-org/10.1891/0730-0832.36.1.18.

Nist, M. D., Harrison, T. M., Pickler, R. H., & Shoben, A. B. (2020). Measures of stress exposure for hospitalized preterm infants. *Nursing Research, 69*(5S Suppl. 1), S3–S10. https://doi.org/10.1097/NNR.0000000000000444.

Parker, C., Warmuskerken, G., & Sinclair, L. (2015). Enhancing neonatal wellness with home visitation. *Nursing for Women's Health, 19*(1), 37–41. https://doi.org/10.1111/1751-486X.12174.

Reeves-Messner, T., & Spilker, A. (2017). Shh…babies growing: A clinical practice guideline for reducing noise level in the neonatal intensive care unit. *Journal of Neonatal Nursing, 23*(4), 199–203. https://doi.org/10.1016/j.jnn.2017.02.006.

Smith, V. C. (2019). From the National Perinatal association: NICU discharge preparation and transition planning. *Neonatology Today, 14*(6), 51–53. https://pediatrics.aappublications.org/content/143/6/e20182915.abstract.

Standley, M. J., & Gutierrez, C. (2020). Benefits of a comprehensive evidence-based NICU-MT program: Family-centered, neurodevelopmental music therapy for premature infants. *Pediatric Nursing, 46*(1), 40–46.

Stefana, A., & Lavelli, M. (2017). Parental engagement and early interactions with preterm infants during the stay in the neonatal intensive care unit: Protocol of a mixed-method and longitudinal study. *BMJ Open, 7*(2), e013824.

Thompson, J. M. D., Tanabe, K., Moon, R. Y., et al. (2017). Duration of breastfeeding and risk of SIDS: An individual participant data meta-analysis. *Pediatrics, 140*(5), e20171324. https://doi.org/10.1542/peds.2017-1324.

Wigert, H., & Bry, K. (2018). Dealing with parents' existential issues in neonatal intensive care. *Journal of Neonatal Nursing, 24*(4), 213–217. http://doi.org/10.1016/jnn.2017.09.002.

Yilmaz, D., & Inal, S. (2020). Effects of three different methods used during heel lance procedures on pain level in term neonates. *Japan Journal of Nursing Science, 17*(4), e12338. https://doi-org.proxy.libraries.rutgers.edu/10.1111/jjns.12338.

I

Readiness for Enhanced Organized Infant Behavior

Domain 9 Coping/stress tolerance Class 3 Neurobehavioral stress

Marina Martinez-Kratz, MS, RN, CNE

NANDA-I

Definition

An integrated pattern of modulation of the physiological and neurobehavioral systems of functioning, which can be strengthened.

Defining Characteristics

Primary caregiver expresses desire to enhance cue recognition; primary caregiver expresses desire to enhance environmental conditions; primary caregiver expresses desire to enhance recognition of infant's self-regulatory behaviors

NOC, NIC, Client Outcomes, Nursing Interventions and *Rationales,* Client/Family Teaching and Discharge Planning, and References

Refer to care plans for Disorganized **Infant** Behavior and Risk for Disorganized **Infant** Behavior.

Risk for Disorganized Infant Behavior

Domain 9 Coping/stress tolerance Class 3 Neurobehavioral stress

Marina Martinez-Kratz, MS, RN, CNE

NANDA-I

Definition

Susceptible to disintegration in the pattern of modulation of the physiological and neurobehavioral systems of functioning, which may compromise health.

Risk Factors

Caregiver misreading infant cues; environmental overstimulation; feeding intolerance; inadequate caregiver knowledge of behavioral cues; inadequate containment within environment; inadequate physical environment; insufficient environmental sensory stimulation; malnutrition; pain; sensory deprivation; sensory overstimulation

At-Risk Population

Infants exposed to teratogen in utero; infants with low postmenstrual age; premature infants

Associated Conditions

Congenital disorders; immature neurological functioning; impaired infant motor functioning; inborn genetic diseases; invasive procedure; oral impairment

NOC, NIC, Client Outcomes, Nursing Interventions and *Rationales,* Client/Family Teaching and Discharge Planning, and References

Refer to Disorganized **Infant** Behavior.

Risk for Infection Domain 11 Safety/protection Class 1 Infection

Teri Hulett, RN, BSN, CIC, FAPIC

NANDA-I

Definition

Susceptible to invasion and multiplication of pathogenic organisms, which may compromise health.

Risk Factors

Difficulty managing long-term invasive devices; difficulty managing wound care; dysfunctional gastrointestinal motility; exclusive formula feeding; impaired skin integrity; inadequate access to individual protective equipment; inadequate adherence to public health recommendations; inadequate environmental hygiene; inadequate health literacy; inadequate hygiene; inadequate knowledge to avoid exposure to pathogens; inadequate oral hygiene habits; inadequate vaccination; malnutrition; mixed breastfeeding; obesity; smoking; stasis of body fluid

At-Risk Population

Economically disadvantaged individuals; individuals exposed to disease outbreak; individuals exposed to increased environmental pathogens; individuals with low level of education; infants who are not breastfed

Associated Conditions

Altered pH of secretion; anemia; chronic illness; decrease in ciliary action; immunosuppression; invasive procedure; leukopenia; premature rupture of amniotic membrane; prolonged rupture of amniotic membrane; suppressed inflammatory response

NOC (Nursing Outcomes Classification)

Suggested NOC Outcomes

Risk Control: Infectious Process; Immune Status

Example NOC Outcome with Indicators

Risk Control: Infectious Process: Identifies signs and symptoms of infection/Maintains a clean environment/ Practices infection control strategies: universal precautions, hand sanitization. (Rate the outcome and indicators of **Risk Control: Infectious Process:** 1 = never demonstrated, 2 = rarely demonstrated, 3 = sometimes demonstrated, 4 = often demonstrated, 5 = consistently demonstrated [see Section I].)

Client Outcomes

Client Will (Specify Time Frame)

- Remain free from symptoms of infection during contact with health care providers
- State symptoms of infection before initiating a health care–related procedure
- Demonstrate appropriate care of infection-prone sites within 48 hours of instruction
- Maintain white blood cell count and differential within normal limits within 48 hours of treatment initiation
- Demonstrate appropriate hygienic measures such as handwashing, oral care, and perineal care within 24 hours of instruction

NIC (Nursing Interventions Classification)

Suggested NIC Interventions

Immunization/Vaccination Management; Infection Control; Infection Protection

Example NIC Activities—Infection Protection and Control

Wash hands before and after each client contact; Ensure aseptic handling of all intravenous lines; Ensure appropriate wound care technique; Teach client and family members how to avoid infections

Nursing Interventions and *Rationales*

- Maintain open communication with the infection prevention (IP) department. Inquire about facility-specific targeted multidrug-resistant organism (MDRO) surveillance. Learn which MDROs are of significant importance at your facility. Acquire a basic understanding of antibiotic stewardship through collaboration with IP and pharmacy. EB: *Active surveillance for targeted MDROs is an integral component of infection prevention and control, allowing for early detection of colonized clients. Early detection provides the ability for early implementation of evidence-based best practices to prevent transmission in health care settings (Bastiaens et al, 2020). Antibiotic stewardship ensures that clients get the right antibiotics at the right time for the right duration. Data support that at least 1 in 3 antibiotic prescriptions, or 47 million prescriptions per year, prescribed in doctors' offices and emergency departments are unnecessary (US Task Force for Combating Antibiotic-Resistant Bacteria, 2017).*
- Obtain a travel history and history of any overnight stay in a hospital in a foreign country from clients presenting to the health care site (e.g., emergency department, clinic). EB: *MDROs pose a global threat. Carbapenem-resistant Enterobacteriaceae (CRE) is a worldwide urgent public health problem. Antibiotic misuse, genetic mobile elements, international travel, and ineffective infection control measures are the main predisposing factors for the emergence of resistance. Often clients are asymptomatic due to colonization versus an active infection (European Centre for Disease Prevention and Control, 2018; Alotaibi, 2019).*
- Antimicrobial resistance and health care–associated infections (HAIs) are global health problems that increase social and economic burden and are associated with higher mortality and increased hospital stays. Inappropriate antimicrobial use is estimated to be at 20% to 50% and is believed to be a key contributor to antimicrobial resistance. The Centers for Disease Control and Prevention (CDC) and the American Nurses Association (ANA) identify staff nurses as critical players in antibiotic stewardship (AS) work. Nurses play a key role in ensuring client safety and quality (Olans et al, 2017; Jeffs et al, 2018; CDC, 2019a; Monsees et al, 2020). EB: *Nurses are key to driving AS interventions directly at the point of care. Review microbiology laboratory culture and sensitivity reports. Actively participate in AS, including AS rounds. Facilitate discussion on antibiotic time-outs, appropriateness of switching from IV to oral antibiotic administration, and monitoring and reporting of possible antibiotic-related adverse events* (Olans et al, 2017; Jeffs et al, 2018; Monsees et al, 2020).
- Sepsis is the body's overwhelming and life-threatening response to infection that can lead to tissue damage, organ failure, and death. Sepsis and septic shock are leading causes of death worldwide. Early identification and aggressive treatment are integral to sepsis survival. Nurses play a significant role in early identification of sepsis. Monitor vital signs and mental status. EB: *Implement nurse-led sepsis screening interventions to improve early recognition of sepsis (Kleinpell, 2017). Monitor the client for signs and/or symptoms of sepsis (confusion or disorientation, high or low blood pressure, fever, shivering, or feeling very cold, shortness of breath, extreme pain or discomfort, clammy or sweaty skin) and notify providers immediately (CDC, 2020; Sepsis Alliance, 2020).*
- Assess temperature of neutropenic clients; report a single temperature of greater than 38°C (100.5°F). EB: *Fever is often the first sign of an infection (Klastersky et al, 2016).* EB: *Clients with depressed immune function are unable to mount the usual immune responses to the onset of infection; abnormal temperature (high or low) may be the only sign of infection. A neutropenic client with abnormal temperature (high or low) represents an absolute medical emergency. Febrile neutropenia is a medical emergency that requires urgent evaluation, the timely administration of empiric broad-spectrum antimicrobials, and careful monitoring to optimize client outcomes and mitigate the risk of complications (Braga et al, 2019).*
- Oral, rectal, tympanic, temporal artery, or axillary thermometers may be used to assess temperature in adults and infants. EBN: *The use of axillary in addition to oral, tympanic, and temporal artery temperature measurement is supported (Bland, Conner, & Messenger, 2020). Rectal and oral temperature measurements are more accurate than other methods of temperature measurement, such as temporal or axillary measurement (Bland, Conner, & Messenger, 2020).*

▲ Note and report laboratory values (e.g., white blood cell count and differential, serum protein, serum albumin, cultures). EBN: *Although the white blood cell count may be in the normal range, an increased number of immature bands may be present (Shi et al, 2015).* EBN: *A neutropenic client with fever represents an absolute medical emergency (Braga et al, 2019).*

- Assess skin for color, moisture, texture, and turgor (elasticity). Keep accurate, ongoing documentation of changes. EB: *A number of instruments have been developed to assess for risk of pressure ulcers, including the Braden, Norton, and Waterlow scales. All three scales include items related to activity mobility, nutritional status, incontinence, and cognition (Balzar & Kottner, 2015).*

- Carefully wash and pat dry skin, including skinfold areas. Use hydration and moisturization on all at-risk surfaces. EBN: *Moisturizers result in an increase of skin hydration and restoration of the skin barrier function and play a prominent role in the long-term management of atopic dermatitis (Mayo Clinic Staff, 2020a).* EB: *Applying moisturizer improves skin barrier repair and maintains skin's integrity and appearance by acting as humectants, emollients, and occlusives, each with its own mechanism of action and enhancing skin barrier function. Moisturizers improve skin hydration and increase stratum corneum water content (Purnamawati et al, 2017). Refer to care plan for Risk for Impaired* ***Skin*** *Integrity.*
- ▲ Monitor client's vitamin D level. EB: *Vitamin D deficiency has been correlated with increased risk and greater severity of infection, particularly of the respiratory tract. Vitamin D influences the body's immune system by influencing the production of endogenous antimicrobial peptides and regulating the inflammatory cascade (Dankers et al, 2017). Refer to care plan Readiness for Enhanced* ***Nutrition*** *for additional interventions.*
- Use strategies to prevent health care–acquired pneumonia: implement an evidence-based pneumonia prevention bundle, aggressive mobilization, assess client risk for aspiration and request swallow evaluation as necessary, position client in an upright position for all meals, and provide aggressive oral care at least twice per day (Tablan et al, 2004; Gupta et al. 2019; Naik et al, 2019). Implementation of an evidence-based ventilator-associated pneumonia (VAP) bundle should be followed. Management of ventilated clients should include avoidance of benzodiazepines to manage agitation, daily interruption of sedation (sedation vacation), daily assessment of readiness to extubate (spontaneous breathing trials), use of endotracheal (ET) tubes that accommodate subglottic suctioning, and maintaining head of bed (HOB) at 30 to 45 degrees (Tablan et al, 2004; Klompas et al, 2014). EB: *All-cause mortality associated with VAP has been reported to range from 20% to 50% and attributed mortality estimated to be 13%. VAP also adds an estimated cost of $40,000 to a typical hospital admission (Kalil et al, 2016).*
- Encourage fluid intake. EB: *Fluid intake helps thin secretions and replace fluid lost during fever (Mayo Clinic Staff, 2020b).*
- Use appropriate hand hygiene (i.e., handwashing or use of alcohol-based hand rubs). EBN: *Meticulous infection prevention precautions are required to prevent HAI, with particular attention to hand hygiene and standard precautions (Boyce et al, 2002).* CEB: *Handwashing is currently the recommended strategy for reducing transmission of Clostridioides (Clostridium) difficile. Alcohol gels do not inactivate C. difficile spores (World Health Organization [WHO], 2009).*
- When using an alcohol-based hand rub, apply an ample amount of product to the palm of one hand and rub hands together, covering all surfaces of hands and fingers, until hands are dry. Note that the volume needed to reduce the number of bacteria on hands varies by product. EB: *Adequate hand antisepsis reduces infection rates. The use of alcohol-based hand rubs is particularly effective; in contrast to handwashing, hand rubs kill susceptible bacteria more rapidly and to a greater extent and are less time-consuming. Also, skin health is better preserved when moisturizers are added (Boyce et al, 2002).*
- Follow standard precautions and wear gloves during any contact with blood, mucous membranes, nonintact skin, or any body substance except sweat. Use goggles and gowns when appropriate. Standard precautions apply to all clients. You must assume all clients are carrying blood-borne pathogens (Siegel et al, 2007). EB: *Hands of health care workers are a common cause of HAIs. Evidence supports decreased HAIs with increased handwashing frequency among hospital staff (Boyce et al, 2002).*
- Implement respiratory hygiene/cough etiquette. CEB: *Providing control measures (tissues and masks) and accessibility to hand hygiene materials reduces risks of transmission of respiratory illness (Siegel, 2007).*
- Follow transmission-based precautions for airborne-, droplet-, and contact-transmitted microorganisms:
  - **Airborne:** Isolate the client in a room with monitored negative air pressure, with the room door closed and the client remaining in the room. Always wear appropriate respiratory protection when you enter the room. Limit the movement and transport of the client from the room to essential purposes only. Have the client wear a surgical mask during transport.
  - **Droplet:** Keep the client in a private room, if possible. If not possible, maintain a spatial separation of 3 feet from other beds or visitors. The door may remain open. Wear a surgical mask when you must come within 3 feet of the client. Some hospitals may choose to implement a mask requirement for droplet precautions for anyone entering the room. Limit transport to essential purposes and have the client wear a mask, if possible.
  - **Contact:** Place the client in a private room, if possible, or with someone (cohorting) who has an active infection from the same microorganism. Wear clean, nonsterile gloves when entering the room. When providing care, change gloves after contact with any infective material such as wound drainage. Remove

I

the gloves and clean your hands before leaving the room and take care not to touch any potentially infectious items or surfaces on the way out. Wear a gown before entering the contact precaution room. Remove the gown before leaving the room. Limit transport of the client to essential purposes and take care that the client does not contact other environmental surfaces along the way. Dedicate the use of noncritical client care equipment to a single client. CEB: *If use of common equipment is unavoidable, adequately clean and disinfect equipment before use with other clients (Siegel et al, 2007).*

- ▲ Use alternatives to indwelling catheters whenever possible (external catheters, incontinence pads, and bladder control techniques). EB: *It is estimated that catheter-associated urinary tract infections (CAUTIs) increase length of stay by 0.5 to 1 day and increase costs between $1200 and $4700 (2009 dollars) (Brusch, 2021).*
- ● If a urinary catheter is necessary, follow catheter management practices. All indwelling catheters should be connected to a sterile, closed drainage system (i.e., not broken), except for good clinical reasons. Cleanse the perineum and meatus twice daily using soap and water. EBN: *A nurse-driven protocol CAUTI reduction process and protocol can significantly reduce catheter use and duration, as well as CAUTIs and hospital length of stay (Johnson et al, 2016).* EB: *Significant rates of inappropriate urinary catheter use underscore the importance of establishing guidelines and implementing policy for appropriate use of urinary catheters (Agency for Healthcare Research and Quality [AHRQ], 2015).*
- ● Use evidence-based practices and educate personnel in care of peripheral catheters: use aseptic technique for insertion and care, label insertion sites and all tubing with date and time of insertion, inspect every 8 hours for signs of infection, record, and report. EB: *Use of chlorhexidine gluconate for vascular catheter site care reduces catheter-related bloodstream infections and catheter colonization (O'Grady et al, 2011).*
- ● Use sterile technique wherever there is a loss of skin integrity. EBN: *Skin and soft tissue infections arise when skin integrity is broken by treatments associated with trauma, surgery, burns, and so forth (Stevens et al, 2014).*
- ● Good personal hygiene is essential for skin health but it also has an important role in maintaining self-esteem and quality of life. Supporting clients to maintain personal hygiene is a fundamental aspect of nursing care. Personal hygiene includes hair, skin, nails, mouth, perineal areas, and facial shaving (Lawton & Shepherd, 2019). Ensure the client's daily personal needs are met by either the client, family, or nurse. EBN: *Daily showers or baths can reduce skin pathogen bioburden. Use evidence-based bathing protocols including chlorhexidine bathing to reduce skin pathogen burden for clients with indwelling devices (Donskey & Deshpande, 2016).*
- ● Recommend responsible use of antibiotics; use antibiotics sparingly. EB: *Use and misuse of antibiotics diminishes their therapeutic benefit and facilitates the development of MDROs and* C. difficile*–associated disease and increases health care costs. Antibiotic stewardship is essential in reducing current and future resistance in bacteria (Barlam et al, 2016; CDC, 2019a).*

Pediatric

Note: Many of the preceding interventions are appropriate for the pediatric client.

- ● Follow meticulous hand hygiene when working with children. EB: *Keep nails short; prohibit false fingernails, and limit wearing jewelry because it interferes with effective hand hygiene (American Academy of Pediatrics & The American College of Obstetricians and Gynecologists, 2017).*
- ● Encourage early enteral feeding with human milk. *Human milk enhances immune defenses of the infant (Praveen et al, 2015).*
- ▲ Monitor recurrent antibiotic use in children.
- ● Instruct parents on appropriate indicators for medical visits and the risks associated with overuse of antibiotics. EB: *Guidelines addressing treatment of asthma in children state that antibiotics should not be used as part of chronic asthma therapy or for acute exacerbations, with the exception of clients with comorbid bacterial infections such as pneumonia or sinusitis (Leung et al, 2021).*

Geriatric

- ▲ Suspect pneumonia when the client has symptoms of disorientation, confusion, respiratory rate of 30 or higher, and fever above 37.8°C (100°F). Offer clients influenza and pneumococcal vaccinations per national guidelines (CDC, 2019b). Assess response to treatment, especially antibiotic therapy. EB: *Pneumonia is a leading cause of hospitalization and death among the elderly (US Department of Health and Human Services, 2021). Together, influenza and pneumonia are the eighth leading cause of mortality among adults in the United States. Community-acquired pneumonia (CAP) disproportionately affects the elderly, with an annual incidence of 9.2 to 33 per 1000 person-years (Kaysin & Viera, 2016).*

- ● Most clients develop health care–associated pneumonia (HCAP) by either aspirating contaminated substances or inhaling airborne particles. Refer to care plan for Risk for **Aspiration.**
- ▲ Carefully screen older women with incontinence for urinary tract infections. CEB: *Consider alternatives to chronic indwelling catheters, such as intermittent catheterization. CAUTI has been associated with increased morbidity, mortality, hospital cost, and length of stay (Gould et al, 2009).*
- ● Observe and report if the client has a low-grade fever or new onset of confusion. EB: *Immunosenescence is the weakening of the immune system in the elderly. Immunosenescence leaves the elderly client with a decreased ability to mount strong immune responses and therefore at increased risk of infections. Those caring for elderly clients must be alert to the potential presence of infection when even low-grade temperature elevations appear for short periods due to the client's inability to mount a strong immune response (Ventura et al, 2017).*
- ● Recognize that chronically ill geriatric clients have an increased susceptibility to *C. difficile* infection; practice meticulous hand hygiene and monitor antibiotic response to antibiotics. EB: *The incidence of* C. difficile *illness (CDI) is increasing with the greatest impact in persons older than 65 years. More than 90% of deaths from CDI have occurred in this population (CDC, 2019a).*

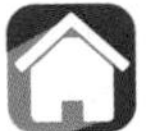

Home Care

I

- ● Adapt the previously mentioned interventions for home care as needed.
- ● Assess and treat wounds in the home. EBN: *Promotion of wound healing is a nursing priority. Managing wounds and promoting healing of wounds requires a set of interventions that when used together can speed healing and help to maintain overall health. Families can be taught wound care/management with nurses evaluating the client at regular intervals for management of care. Families must be educated on the triad of wound care—nutrition, technique, and infection prevention—to manage their loved ones at home (Berden, 2021).*
- ● Review standards for surveillance of infections in home care. EB: *Infection surveillance in the home care setting poses unique challenges for home care providers and clients. The lack of standard definitions and surveillance methods for home care–acquired infections hinders efforts to collect and analyze valid data on infection rates, which hampers efforts to analyze risk factors that lead to effective control efforts. Other obstacles include insufficient infrastructure to meaningfully capture numerator and denominator data (Carpenter et al, 2017).*
- ● Maintain infection-prevention standards of practice. EBN: *The increasing care complexity of clients in the home, ineffective care coordination, and communication challenges present significant safety issues, including infections (Carpenter et al, 2017).*
- ● Refer for nutritional evaluation; implement dietary changes to support recovery and maintain health. EB: *Evidence supports that individual medical nutrition therapy has strong effects on clinical outcomes, reinforcing the aim to practice "evidence-based medical nutrition" (EBMN), especially with the vulnerable malnourished population. EBMN incorporates combining clinical judgment, client preferences, and the most current scientific evidence. Such an approach may be helpful to improve clinical outcomes in the vulnerable population (Kaegi-Braun et al, 2020).*

Client/Family Teaching and Discharge Planning

- ● Teach the client risk factors contributing to surgical wound infection. EB: *The risk of infection is influenced by characteristics of the client such as age, obesity, and nutritional status (Carpenter et al, 2017).*
- ● Teach the client and family the importance of hand hygiene in preventing postoperative infections. CEB: Two-thirds of wound infections occur after discharge. Using good hand hygiene practices is effective for preventing these infections (*Siegel et al, 2007*).
- ▲ Encourage high-risk persons, including health care workers, to get vaccinated (CDC, 2019b; CDC, 2021).
- ▲ Influenza: Teach symptoms of influenza and the importance of vaccination for influenza. Provide client education using the CDC Vaccine Information Sheets (VISs). EB: *Influenza can be associated with serious illness, hospitalization, and death, particularly among the very young, the elderly, pregnant women, and persons of all ages with certain chronic medical conditions. Routine annual influenza vaccination is recommended for all persons age ≥6 months who do not have contraindications (Grohskopf et al, 2020).*

REFERENCES

Agency for Healthcare Research and Quality (AHRQ). (2015). Appendix M: Example of a nurse-driven protocol for catheter removal. In *Toolkit for reducing catheter-associated urinary tract infections in hospital units: Implementation guide*. Rockville, MD: AHRQ.

Alotaibi, F. (2019). Carbapenem-resistant Enterobacteriaceae: An update narrative review from Saudi Arabia. *Journal of Infection and Public Health, 12*(4), 465–471. https://doi.org/10.1016/j.jih.2019.03.024.

American Academy of Pediatrics, & The American College of Obstetricians and Gynecologists. (2017). Infection control. In S. J. Kilpatrick, & L. A. Papile (Eds.), *Guidelines for perinatal care* (8th ed.) (pp. 559–580). Elk Grove Village, IL: American Academy of Pediatrics.

Balzer, K., & Kottner, J. (2015). Evidence-based practices in pressure ulcer prevention: Lost in implementation? *International Journal of Nursing Studies, 52*(11), 1655–1658. https://doi.org/10.1016/j.ijnurstu.2015.08.006

Barlam, T. F., Cosgrove, S. E., Abbo, L. M., et al. (2016). Implementing an antibiotic stewardship program: Guidelines by the infectious diseases Society of America and the Society for healthcare Epidemiology of America. *Clinical Infectious Diseases, 62*(10), e51–e77. https://doi.org/10.1093/cid/ciw118.

Bastiaens, G. J. H., Baarslag, T., Pelgrum, C., & Mascini, E. M. (2020). Active surveillance for highly resistant microorganisms in patients with prolonged hospitalization. *Antimicrobial Resistance and Infection Control, 9*(1), 8. doi:10.1186/s13756-019-0670-8.

Berden, J. (2021). Managing wounds in the home. *RN Journal*. Retrieved from http://rn-journal.com/journal-of-nursing/managing-wounds-in-the-home#google_vignette. [Accessed 8 July 2021].

Bland, W., Conner, H. M., & Messenger, D. (2020). *Fever temperatures: Accuracy and comparison*. Retrieved from https://www.uofmhealth.org/health-library/tw9223. [Accessed 8 July 2021].

Boyce, J. M., & Pittet, D. (2002). Healthcare infection control practices Advisory Committee, HICPAC/SHEA/APIC/IDSA hand hygiene Task Force. Guideline for hand hygiene in health-care settings: recommendations of the Healthcare Infection Control Practices Advisory Committee and the HICPAC/SHEA/APIC/IDSA Hand Hygiene Task Force *Morbidity and Mortality Weekly Report Recommendations and Reports, 51*(RR–16), 1–45.

Braga, C. C., Taplitz, R. A., & Flowers, C. R. (2019). Clinical implications of febrile neutropenia guidelines in the cancer patient population. *Journal of Oncology Practice, 15*(1), 25–26. doi:10.1200/jop.18.00718.

Brusch, J. L. (2021). *Catheter-related urinary tract infection (UTI)*. Medscape [website]. Retrieved from https://emedicine.medscape.com/article/2040035-overview. [Accessed 8 July 2021].

Carpenter, D., Famolaro, T., Hassell, S., et al. (2017). *Patient safety in the home: Assessment of issues, challenges, and opportunities*. Cambridge, MA: Institute for Healthcare Improvement and National Patient Safety Foundation. Retrieved from https://homecarenh.org/wp-content/uploads/2018/07/PatientSafetyInTheHome_2017.pdf. [Accessed 8 July 2021].

Centers for Disease Control and Prevention (CDC). (2019a). *Core elements of hospital antibiotic stewardship programs*. Retrieved from https://www.cdc.gov/antibiotic-use/healthcare/pdfs/hospital-core-elements-H.pdf. [Accessed 30 September 2021].

Centers for Disease Control and Prevention (CDC). (2019b). *Vaccine information statement (VIS): Influenza*. https://www.cdc.gov/vaccines/hcp/vis/. [Accessed 8 July 2021].

Centers for Disease Control and Prevention (CDC). (2020). *Sepsis*. Retrieved from https://www.cdc.gov/sepsis/clinicaltools/index.html. [Accessed 8 July 2021].

Centers for Disease Control and Prevention (CDC). (2021). *Prevent seasonal flu*. Retrieved from www.CDC.gov/flu/protect/vaccine. [Accessed 8 July 2021].

Dankers, W., Colin, E. M., van Hamburg, J. P., & Lubberts, E. (2017). Vitamin D in autoimmunity: Molecular mechanisms and therapeutic potential. *Frontiers in Immunology, 7*, 697.

Donskey, C. J., & Deshpande, A. (2016). Effect of chlorhexidine bathing in preventing infections and reducing skin burden and environmental contamination: A review of the literature. *American Journal of Infection Control, 44*(Suppl. 5), e17–e21. https://doi.org/10.1016/ajic.2016.02.024.

European Centre for Disease Prevention and Control (ECDC). (2018). *Rapid risk assessment: Carbapenem-resistant Enterobacteriaceae—first update. 7 June 2018*. Stockholm: ECDC. Retrieved from https://www.ecdc.europa.eu/en/publications-data/rapid-risk-assessment-carbapenem-resistant-enterobacteriaceae-first-update. [Accessed 8 July 2021].

Gould, C. V., Umscheid, C. A., Agarwal, R. K., Kuntz, G., Pegues, D. A., & Healthcare Infection Control Practices Advisory Committee. (2009). *Healthcare infection control practices Advisory Committee: Guideline for prevention of catheter-associated urinary tract infections*. Retrieved from http://www.cdc.gov/hicpac/pdf/CAUTI/CAUTIguideline2009final.pdf. [Accessed 30 September 2021].

Grohskopf, L. A., Alyanak, E., Broder, K. R., et al. (2020). Prevention and control of seasonal influenza with vaccines: Recommendations of the Advisory Committee on Immunization practices—United States, 2020-21 influenza season. *Morbidity and Mortality Weekly Report Recommendations and Reports, 69*(8), 1–24. http://dx.doi.org10.15585/mmwr.rr6908a1.

Gupta, N. M., Lindenauer, P. K., Yu, P. C., Imrey, P. B., Haessler, S., Deshpande, A., et al. (2019). Association between alcohol use disorders and outcomes of patients hospitalized with community-acquired pneumonia. *JAMA Network Open, 2*(6), e195172. https://doi.org/10.1001/jamanetworkopen.2019.5172

Jeffs, L., Law, M. P., Zahradnik, M., et al. (2018). Engaging nurses in optimizing antimicrobial use in ICUs: A qualitative study. *Journal of Nursing Care Quality, 33*(2), 173–179. doi:10.1097/NCQ.0000000000000281.

Johnson, P., Gilman, A., Lintner, A., & Buckner, E. (2016). Nurse-driven catheter-associated urinary tract infection reduction process and protocol: Development through an academic-practice partnership. *Critical Care Nursing Quarterly, 39*(4), 352–362. doi:10.1097/CNQ.0000000000000129.

Kaegi-Braun, N., Baumgartner, A., Gomes, F., Stanga, Z., Deutz, N. E., & Schuetz, P. (2020). Evidence-based medical nutrition—A difficult journey, but worth the effort. *Clinical Nutrition, 39*(10), 3014–3018. https://doi.org/10.1016/j.clnu.2020.01.023.

Kalil, A. C., Metersky, M. L., Klompas, M., et al. (2016). Management of adults with hospital-acquired and ventilator-associated pneumonia: 2016 clinical practice guidelines by the Infectious Diseases Society of America and the American Thoracic Society. *Clinical Infectious Diseases, 63*(5), e61–e111. https://doi.org/10.1093/cid/ciw353.

Kaysin, A., & Viera, A. J. (2016). Community-acquired pneumonia in adults: Diagnosis and management. *American Family Physician, 94*(9), 698–706. PMID:27929242.

Klastersky, J., de Naurois, J., Rolston, K., et al. (2016). Management of febrile neutropaenia: ESMO clinical practice guidelines. *Annals of Oncology, 27*(Suppl. 5), v111–v118.

Kleinpell, R. (2017). Promoting early identification of sepsis in hospitalized patients with nurse-led protocols. *Critical Care, 21*(1), 10. https://doi.org/10.1186/s13054-016-1590-0.

Klompas, M., Branson, R., Eichenwald, E., et al. (2014). Strategies to prevent ventilator-associated pneumonia in acute care hospitals: 2014 update. *Infection Control and Hospital Epidemiology, 35*(8), 915–936. doi:10.1086/677144.

Lawton, S., & Shepherd, E. (2019). The underlying principles and procedure for bed bathing patients. *Nursing Times* [online], *115*(5), 45–47.

Leung, D. Y., Akdis, C. A., Bacharier, L. B., Cunningham-Rundles, C., Sicherer, S., & Sampson, H. (Eds.). (2021). *Pediatric allergy: Principles and practice* (4th ed.). St. Louis: Elsevier.

Mayo Clinic Staff. (2020a). *Atopic dermatis (eczema)*. Retrieved from https://www.mayoclinic.org/diseases-conditions/atopic-dermatitis-eczema/diagnosis-treatment/drc-20353279. [Accessed 8 July 2021].

Mayo Clinic Staff. (2020b). *Dehydration*. Retrieved from https://www.mayoclinic.org/diseases-conditions/dehydration/diagnosis-treatment/drc-20354092. [Accessed 8 July 2021].

Monsees, E., Lee, B., Wirtz, A., & Goldman, J. (2020). Implementation of a nurse-driven antibiotic engagement tool in 3 hospitals. *American Journal of Infection Control*, *48*(12), 1415–1421.

Naik, S., Lucerne, C., Kevorkova, Y., et al. (2019). Significant reduction of non-ventilator hospital acquired pneumonia (HAP) with a prevention bundle and clinical and leadership feedback in a large integrated healthcare system. *Open Forum Infectious Diseases*, *6*(Suppl. 2), S423. https://doi.org/10.1093/ofid/ofz360.1044.

O'Grady, N. P., Alexander, M., Burns, L. A., et al. (2011). *Guidelines for the prevention of intravascular catheter-related infections, 2011*. Centers for Disease Control and Prevention (Updated 2017). Retrieved from https://www.cdc.gov/infectioncontrol/pdf/guidelines/bsi-guidelines-H.pdf. [Accessed 8 July 2021].

Olans, R. D., Olans, R. N., & Witt, D. J. (2017). Good nursing is good antibiotic stewardship. *American Journal of Nursing*, *117*(8), 58–63. doi:10.1097/01.NAJ.0000521974.76835.e0.

Praveen, P., Jordon, F., Priami, C., & Morine, M. J. (2015). The role of breast-feeding in infant immune system: A systems perspective on the intestinal microbiome. *Microbiome*, *3*, 41. Retrieved from https://microbiomejournal.biomedcentral.com/articles/10.1186/s40168-015-0104-7. [Accessed 17 February 2022.]

Purnamawati, S., Indrastuti, N., Danarti, R., & Saefudin, T. (2017). The role of moisturizers in addressing various kinds of dermatitis: A review. *Clinical Medicine & Research*, *15*(3–4), 75–87. https://doi.org/10.3121/cmr.2017.1363.

Sepsis Alliance. (2020). *Symptoms*. Retrieved from https://www.sepsis.org/sepsis-basics/symptoms/. [Accessed 8 July 2021].

Shi, E., Vilke, G. M., Coyne, C. J., Oyama, L. C., & Castillo, E. M. (2015). Clinical outcomes of ED patients with bandemia. *American Journal of Emergency Medicine*, *33*(7), 876–881. https://doi.org/10.1016/j.ajem.2015.03.035.

Siegel, J. D., Rhinehart, E., Jackson, M., Chiarello, L., & & Health Care Infection Control Practices Advisory Committee. (2007). Guideline for isolation precautions: Preventing transmission of infectious agents in health care settings. *American Journal of Infection Control*, *35*(10 Suppl. 2), S65–S164.

Stevens, D. L., Bisno, A. L., Chambers, H. F., et al. (2014). Practice guidelines for the diagnosis and management of skin and soft tissue infections: 2014 update by the Infectious Diseases Society of America. *Clinical Infectious Diseases*, *59*(2), 147–159. (Updated 2015). https://doi.org/10.1093/cid/ciu444.

Tablan, O. C., Anderson, L. J., Besser, R., et al. (2004). Guidelines for preventing health-care–associated pneumonia, 2003: Recommendations of CDC and the healthcare infection control practices Advisory Committee. *Morbidity and Mortality Weekly Report Recommendations and Reports*, *53*(RR-3), 1–36. (Reviewed 2015).

US Department of Health and Human Services, Office of Disease Prevention and Health Promotion. (2021). *Healthy People 2030*. Retrieved from: https://health.gov/healthypeople/objectives-and-data/browse-objectives/respiratory-disease/reduce-rate-hospital--admissions-pneumonia-among-older-adults-oa-06. [Accessed July 8, 2021].

US Task Force for Combating Antibiotic-Resistant Bacteria. (2017). *National action plan for combating antibiotic-resistant bacteria: Progress report for years 1 and 2*. US Department of Health and Human Services, Office of the Assistant Secretary for Planning and Evaluation. Retrieved from https://aspe.hhs.gov/system/files/pdf/258516/ProgressYears1and2CARBNationalActionPlan.pdf. [Accessed 8 July 2021].

Ventura, M. T., Casciaro, M., Gangemi, S., & Buquicchio, R. (2017). Immunosenescence in aging: Between immune cells depletion and cytokines up-regulation. *Clinical and Molecular Allergy*, *15*, 21. https://doi.org/10.1186/s12948-017-0077-0.

World Health Organization (WHO). (2009). Appendix 2: Guide to appropriate hand hygiene in connection with *Clostridium difficile* spread. In *WHO guidelines on hand hygiene in health care: First global patient safety challenge—Clean care is safer care*. Geneva: WHO.

I

Risk for Surgical Site Infection

Domain 11 Safety/protection Class 1 Infection

Teri Hulett, RN, BSN, CIC, FAPIC

NANDA-I

Definition

Susceptible to invasion of pathogenic organisms at surgical site, which may compromise health.

Risk Factors

Alcoholism, obesity, smoking

At-Risk Population

Individuals exposed to excessive number of personnel during surgical procedure; individuals exposed to increased environmental pathogens; individuals with American Society of Anesthesiologists (ASA) Physical health status score ≥ 2

Associated Conditions

Diabetes mellitus; extensive surgical procedures; general anesthesia; hypertension; immunosuppression; inadequate antibiotic prophylaxis; ineffective antibiotic prophylaxis; infections at other surgical sites; invasive procedure; post-traumatic osteoarthritis; prolonged duration of surgical procedure; prothesis; rheumatoid arthritis; significant comorbidity; surgical implant; surgical wound contamination

NOC (Nursing Outcomes Classification)

Suggested NOC Outcomes

Risk Control: Infectious Process, Immune Status

Example NOC Outcome with Indicators

Risk Control: Infectious Process. Personal actions to understand, prevent, eliminate, or reduce the threat of acquiring an infection as evidenced by client demonstrating the following indicators: Identifies risk factors for infection/Acknowledges personal risk factors for infection/Acknowledges behaviors associated with risk for infection/Monitors personal behaviors for factors associated with infection/Maintains a clean environment/Practices hand sanitization. (Rate the outcome and indicators of **Risk Control: Infectious Process:** 1 = never demonstrated, 2 = rarely demonstrated, 3 = sometimes demonstrated, 4 = often demonstrated, 5 = consistently demonstrated [see Section I].)

I

Client Outcomes

Client Will (Specify Time Frame)

- Remain free from symptoms of surgical site infections (SSIs)
- Identify personal risk factors associated with increased SSI risk
- Modify personal behaviors that increase SSI risk
- Demonstrate appropriate hygienic practices to reduce infection risk such as handwashing

NIC (Nursing Interventions Classification)

Suggested NOC Outcomes

Infection Control, Infection Control: Intraoperative, Infection Protection, Teaching: Individual, Preoperative

Example NIC Activities—Risk for Surgical Site Infection

Verify that prophylactic antibiotics have been ordered and administered as appropriate; Monitor and maintain client normothermia (temperature of 35.5°C [95.9°F] or above) during the perioperative period

Nursing Interventions and *Rationales*

- ▲ The number of surgical procedures performed in the United States continues to rise, and surgical clients often have comorbidities that increase the complexity. It is estimated that approximately half of SSIs are deemed preventable using evidence-based strategies (World Health Organization [WHO], 2018). SSIs are a complication of surgical care and are associated with significant morbidity, mortality, and cost (Preas, O'Hara, & Thom, 2017).
- ▲ Optimizing the client's medical condition before surgery and eliminating or even diminishing modifiable risk factors for infection can lower the risk of SSIs (Hutzler & Williams, 2017). EB: *Modifiable risk factors include current or history of orthopedic infection, rheumatoid arthritis, poor oral health, urinary tract infection, obesity, methicillin-resistant* Staphylococcus aureus *(MRSA), preoperative and anticipated postoperative anemia, smoking, malnutrition, diabetes, and HIV (Hutzler & Williams, 2017). The American College of Surgeons (ACS) identifies additional modifiable risk factors as poor glycemic control and diabetic status, dyspnea, alcohol and smoking history, preoperative albumin level (<3.5 mg/dL), total bilirubin greater than 1.0 mg/dL, obesity, and immunosuppression (Ban et al, 2017).*
- ▲ SSI prevention, known as surgical care bundles, consists of evidence-based interventions that, when implemented together, can reduce the risk of infection. There are different surgical care bundles for specific high-risk surgical procedures, for example, colorectal surgery bundle, pediatric spinal surgery bundle, total joint arthroplasty surgery bundle, and cardiothoracic surgery bundle. EB: *Aspects of each*

surgical care bundle that are universal for all surgical procedures include prehospital preoperative bathing, smoking cessation, and glucose control. Hospital-focused bundle interventions include perioperative blood glucose monitoring, surgical site hair-removal technique, surgical site skin preparation, surgical hand scrub, antibiotic prophylaxis, intraoperative normothermia, and supplemental oxygen delivery for clients undergoing general anesthesia (intubated clients) (Anderson et al, 2017; Ban et al, 2017).

▲ SSIs can occur because of either client-related (endogenous) or procedure-related (exogenous) risk factors. Risk factors are further stratified into preoperative, intraoperative, and postoperative risk.

• Review endogenous client-related risk factors. EB: *Review client history with client before surgical procedure to identify modifiable risk factors that can be addressed preoperatively (Anderson et al, 2017; Kahn et al, 2020).*

Compromised Host Defenses

• Age: Extremes of ages and advanced age increase client risk. EB: *Relationship to increased risk of SSI may be secondary to more comorbidities, impaired immune response to infectious agents, or inferior nutritional status (Triantafyllopoulos et al, 2015).*

• Wound: A wound classification scoring system is used to identify the degree of surgical site skin integrity at the time of surgery. Assess and document skin integrity during the preoperative period to identify classification of surgical site. EB: *The Centers for Disease Control and Prevention (CDC) recommends assessing surgical wounds and determining the probability of SSI by using a classification that consists of four types of surgical wounds: clean (sterile body site), clean-contaminated, contaminated, and dirty (heavily contaminated site) wounds (Onyekwelu et al, 2017).* EB: *The method of wound classification has been adopted by the ACS and has been effectively used for more than 40 years to stratify the client's risk for SSI. The traditional wound classification system of categorizing procedures into risk groups is based on the degree of microbial contamination (Allen, Apisarnthanarak, & Archer, 2017).*

• Smoking: The nicotine in tobacco products results in microvascular vasoconstriction, in addition to tissue hypoxia, which can contribute to the development of SSI. Surgical complications, such as SSI, can be decreased by 50% in clients who successfully stop smoking before surgery (Anderson et al, 2017). EB: *The increased risk of SSI in clients who smoke is partially related to vasoconstriction of vessels in the surgical bed, which leads to tissue hypovolemia and hypoxia. Poor tissue perfusion affects the transport of nutrients and alters the immune response, which affects healing (Ban et al, 2017). Smoking cessation before surgery is critical to optimally preparing clients for surgery. To be effective, smoking cessation needs to occur 4 to 8 weeks before surgery. Smoking cessation of less than 4 weeks does not affect risk of SSI (Anderson et al, 2017).*

▲ Assess client's smoking status and offer smoking cessation information to the receptive client. Seek nicotine patch order for client use during hospital admission.

▲ Educate the client on smoking risks using the CDC Fact Sheet on Health Effects of Cigarette Smoking (CDC, 2020).

• Nutrition status: Assess the client's nutrition status. Preoperative risk factors include albumin less than 3.5 mg/dL or total bilirubin greater than 1.0 mg/dL (Ban et al, 2017; Tsantes et al, 2020). Malnutrition leads to less competent immune response and increased risk of acquiring infections (Tsantes et al, 2020). EBN: *Clients who are malnourished and have low albumin levels are more likely to develop SSIs (Tsantes et al, 2020). Review preoperative laboratory tests and monitor postoperative laboratory values to assess for malnourishment. Provide nutritional consultation and support as needed. Anticipate the malnourished client to receive total parenteral nutrition (TPN) in addition to oral nutrition during the initial postoperative period. Consider the administration of oral nutritional supplements (e.g., protein shakes, high-protein snacks) as recommended by the registered dietitian after dietary consultation.*

• Immunocompromised/immunosuppression: Clients who are immunocompromised or who have immunosuppression are at increased risk of developing infection because of their weakened immune system and inability to mount a defense against pathogenic organisms. Clients who may be immunocompromised or immunosuppressed include clients receiving cancer treatment, organ transplant recipients, clients taking steroids, and clients with HIV. EBN: *Determine the use of chronic medications such as steroids and immunosuppressives. These medications have been shown to increase SSI rates and negatively affect wound healing. There is no recommendation to taper or discontinue systemic steroid use (when medically permissible) before elective surgery (Triantafyllapoulos et al, 2015; Berríos-Torres et al, 2017).*

• Review the client's medical history and current medications. Medications that compromise the client's immune response may increase the risk of SSI.

- Diabetes mellitus: Monitor blood glucose levels with the goal to maintain normoglycemia in the perioperative period. Educate the client of the increased risk for SSI with episodes of hyperglycemia. When available, coordinate referral to a diabetic educator as part of the discharge education. EB: *Due to the disruption of the vascular system in clients with diabetes, SSIs are increased. Clients with diabetes have been shown to have worse client-reported outcomes up to 2 years after spine surgery. It is recommended that hemoglobin A1C values be measured during the perioperative period. Clients with a hemoglobin A1C less than 7 had a 0% infection rate, whereas clients with hemoglobin AIC values greater than 7 had infection rates of 35.3%. Improved glycemic management can restore white blood cell function and reduce risk of infection (Anderson et al, 2017).*
- Preexisting infection: Be aware of all preoperative laboratory work, positive cultures, and actions taken to treat the infection (e.g., was the client started on oral antibiotics). EBN: *Remote infections should be identified and treated following evidence-based guidelines before surgical procedure (Triantafyllopoulos et al, 2015).*
- Obesity: Obesity is defined as a body mass index (BMI) greater than 30 kg/m^2. Obese clients are at significant risk for SSI, more surgical blood loss, and a longer operation time. EB: *Obese clients have excessive subcutaneous fat tissue, which predisposes these clients to impaired healing, low regional perfusion, and low oxygen tension at the surgical site. Longer operation times and increased blood loss greater than 1 L are significant predictors of postoperative wound infections. The obese client is also likely to have more comorbidities, such as diabetes, than nonobese clients, increasing the risk of SSI (Tjeertes et al, 2015; Anderson et al, 2017). Provide discharge teaching for signs and symptoms of poor wound healing and SSI.*

I

Procedure-Related Risk Factors—Exogenous

- SSI pathogenic microbes may originate from exogenous sources such as the operating room environment, members of the surgical team, and instruments and material brought within the surgical field during the procedure (Kahn et al, 2020). Observe clients identified as being at increased risk for SSI because of modifiable risk factors for signs and/or symptoms of postoperative SSI.
- Extended procedure time may increase SSI risk. EB: *Prolonged operations that increase the length of time that tissues are exposed increase the risk of exogenous contamination of the surgical site (Triantafyllopoulos et al, 2015; Anderson et al, 2017; Ban et al, 2017).*
- Estimated blood loss greater than 1 L requiring blood transfusion increases the risk of SSI. EB: *Allogeneic (donor) blood transfusion is an independent risk factor for SSI. Transfusion of allogeneic blood is considered to induce immunomodulation to the recipient, due to the presence of white blood cells (WBCs) above a critical level (Triantafyllopoulos et al, 2015). The use of allogeneic (donor) blood transfusions is associated with increased length of stay and induces immunomodulation that can lead to increased risk for infection at the surgical site (Huntzler & Williams, 2017).*
- Suboptimal timing of prophylactic antibiotic places the client at increased risk of SSI. EB: *Administer preoperative prophylactic antimicrobial agent(s) as prescribed (Berríos-Torres et al, 2017). Surgical antibiotic prophylaxis (SAP) should be administered within 1 hour before incision or within 2 hours for vancomycin or fluoroquinolones. This allows for maximal antibiotic concentration circulating in the blood serum and tissue at the time of surgical incision (Ban et al, 2017). Evidence shows that the administration of SAP after the incision causes a significant increase of SSI risk compared with administration of the SAP before incision (WHO, 2018).*
- Preoperative infections place the client at increased risk of SSI before elective surgery. EB: *Appropriately identify and treat infections (e.g., urinary tract infection) before surgical procedures. Do not routinely treat urinary tract colonization or contamination in the absence of clinical urinary tract infection symptoms (urgency, costovertebral angle pain, flank pain, pain with urination, and fever). Obtaining urine cultures when not clinically indicated, including for routine screening, promotes inappropriate antimicrobial use. Given the potential negative societal consequence of antimicrobial resistance, the Infectious Diseases Society of America (IDSA) guideline committee felt that screening for bacteriuria and treatment of asymptomatic bacteriuria (ASB) should be discouraged unless there is evidence to support a benefit of treatment for a defined population (Nicolle et al, 2019).*
- Preoperative interventions: Establish a protocol for procedure-specific preoperative testing to detect medical conditions that increase the risk of SSI. The protocol should focus on nutritional counseling, glycemic control, smoking cessation, preadmission infections, and reconciling medications with adjustments before surgery as indicated (Anderson et al, 2017; Kahn et al, 2020).

- ❍ Identify high risks: diabetes, history of transplant, chemotherapy, immunosuppressed or immunocompromised, elderly, poor dentition, obese, and malnourished. Clients having a high-risk procedure with an extended surgical procedure time (e.g., cardiac surgery, joint replacement, major abdominal surgery) are at increased risk of SSI. **EB:** *Identifying high-risk clients through screening and electronic medical record alerts should be used to inform all members of the perioperative team of the client's high-risk condition(s) (Anderson et al, 2017; Kahn et al, 2020).*
- ❍ Maintain glycemic control for clients with and without diabetes. **EB:** *Elevated blood glucose levels greater than 200 mg/dL cause the release of proinflammatory cytokines that depress the immune system, increasing susceptibility to SSIs (Berríos-Torres et al, 2017). Hyperglycemia in the immediate preoperative period is associated with an increased risk of SSI (Ban et al, 2017).*
- ❍ *Staphylococcus aureus* (SA) is the most frequent pathogen causing about 50% of SSIs. MRSA accounts for up to 35% of SA infections in primary cases and up to 48% in revision surgery. Studies show that 18% to 25% of clients undergoing elective spine and orthopedic surgery are colonized with methicillin-sensitive SA (MSSA) and 3% to 5% are MRSA carriers. Carriers of MSSA are 2 to 3 times and MRSA 8 to 10 times more likely to have an SSI. Perform SA intranasal decolonization by using cotton-tipped applicators to apply a 2% mupirocin ointment in each nostril and with 2% chlorhexidine gluconate (CHG) showers for up to 5 days before surgery (Anderson et al, 2017). **EB:** *Screen for SA (MSSA and MRSA) colonization and decolonize surgical clients before high-risk procedures, including some orthopedic and cardiothoracic procedures (Anderson et al, 2017).*
- ❍ Provide education on preoperative bathing with soap (antimicrobial or nonantimicrobial) or an antiseptic agent on at least the night before and morning of the day of surgical intervention. **EB:** *It is good clinical practice for the client to bathe or shower before surgery to ensure that the skin is as clean as possible and to reduce the bacterial load, especially at the site of incision (WHO, 2018). Instruct the client to bathe, at a minimum, the night before and morning of the surgical procedure using liquid soap, clean washcloth, and clean towel each time. Instruct the client to wear freshly laundered pajamas after showering the night before the surgical procedure and freshly laundered clothes the morning of the procedure. This process of using liquid soap and clean washcloths, towels, and clothes prevents recontamination with shed epithelial cells from previously used bar soap, washcloths/towels, and clothes.*
- ❍ Address preexisting dental and nutritional status. **EB:** *Periodontal clients have higher risk of bacteremia than those with healthy periodontium (Mirzashahi et al, 2019).* **EBN:** *Preoperative dental screenings are needed to evaluate for the presence of tooth decay, inflammatory gum disease/gingivitis, periodontitis, or dental abscesses, which lead to seeding of bacteria (Mirzashahi et al, 2019). Encourage the client to seek oral and dental examinations before high-risk surgical procedures. Educate the client on the need for good oral hygiene to decrease the risk of developing SSI. Provide the client with oral hygiene products while in the hospital. Perform oral hygiene for the client if unable to perform independently.*
- ❍ Nutrition consultation as needed.
- ❍ Prepare the surgical site using an alcohol-based antiseptic agent unless contraindicated to reduce SSI risk. **EB:** *Alcohol-based antiseptic solutions for surgical site skin preparation are more effective compared with aqueous solutions in reducing SSIs (WHO, 2018; Berríos-Torres et al, 2017).* **EB:** *Overall, there is evidence that alcohol-based preparations are more effective in reducing SSIs than aqueous preparations and should be used unless contraindications exist (Ban et al, 2017).*
- ❍ Proper hair removal. **EB:** *Shaving causes microscopic cuts and abrasions, resulting in disruption of the skin's barrier defense against microorganisms. When hair removal at the operative site is necessary, removal should be done using clippers (Ban et al, 2017).* **EB:** *Do not remove hair at the operative site unless the presence of hair will interfere with the operation. Do not use razors. If hair removal is necessary, remove hair outside the operating room using clippers or a depilatory agent (Ban et al, 2017). Shaving causes microscopic cuts and abrasions, resulting in disruption of the skin's barrier defense against microorganisms (Ban et al, 2017).*

- ● If possible, educate the client preoperatively on the risk of shaving the surgical site, or the area near in which the surgical incision will be, because of the risk for microscopic cuts and abrasions. These cuts and abrasions increase the risk of developing an SSI. For example, for breast surgery, instruct the client not to shave underarms because the underarm is potentially in close proximity to the surgical site. Another example is instructing the client having a total knee replacement not to shave the leg involved in the surgery.
- ● Intraoperative interventions:

I

- ❍ Maintain glycemic control. EB: *Implement perioperative glycemic control and use blood glucose target levels less than 200 mg/dL in clients with and without diabetes clients (Berríos-Torres et al, 2017). Short-term glucose control can be more impactful in decreasing SSIs than long-term control of hemoglobin (Hgb) A1C (Ban et al, 2017).*
- ❍ Maintain normothermia (temperature of 35.5°C [95.9°F] or above) during the perioperative period in surgical clients who have an anesthesia duration of at least 60 minutes (Anderson et al, 2017). WHO defines hypothermia as a core temperature less than 36°C (WHO, 2018). EB: *Hypothermia can trigger subcutaneous vasoconstriction and subsequent tissue hypoxia and increase blood loss that may lead to wound hematomas or need for transfusion, both of which can increase SSI rates (Anderson et al, 2017).*
- ❍ Provide supplemental oxygenation, during surgery for intubated clients and in the immediate postoperative period for 2 to 6 hours via a nonrebreathing mask for procedures performed under general anesthesia to ensure Hgb saturation of greater than 95% is maintained. EB: *Studies have found that perioperative hyperoxygenation led to a 25% decrease in SSIs (WHO, 2018; Anderson et al, 2017).* EB: *For clients with normal pulmonary function undergoing general anesthesia with endotracheal intubation, administer increased FiO_2 intraoperatively and postextubation in the immediate postoperative period (Berríos-Torres et al, 2017). The administration of supplemental oxygen is recommended in the immediate postoperative period after surgery performed under general anesthesia (Ban et al, 2017).*

- Postoperative interventions:
  - ❍ Discharge instructions: Teach the client postoperative self-care after discharge. Provide written instructions that include information on how and when to contact the provider, date and time for the scheduled follow-up visit, and signs and symptoms of infection. EB: *Educational materials should be provided in multiple languages based on the population served (Anderson et al, 2017).*
  - ❍ Wound care: Wound care instructions will be based on the type of surgical wound closure. EB: *Protect primarily closed incisions with a sterile dressing for 24 to 48 hours postoperatively (Berríos-Torres et al, 2017). Instruct the client to keep the surgical wound clean and dry. Teach the client signs and symptoms that would indicate an SSI, such as fever, redness, drainage, swelling, pain, and foul odor at the surgical site. Stress to the client and family that any of these signs and symptoms should be promptly reported to their provider. Assess whether the client and family know how to read a thermometer and provide instructions as necessary. Provide written wound care instructions on the prevention of SSI.*
  - ❍ Nutrition follow-up: For the malnourished and obese clients, provide written dietary instructions by the registered dietitian, if appropriate. Encourage a diet that supports wound healing (high protein) and glycemic control. If appropriate, provide written information on community nutrition support group options and contact information.
  - ❍ Bathing/showering instructions: Review instructions with client and family on timing to shower and if/when the client can take a bath. Explain to the client that taking a bath is generally discouraged, at a minimum, for the first week after surgery. *Submerging a fresh surgical wound in warm bath water and allowing it to soak is not advised because this provides an environment that potentially exposes the surgical wound to pathogenic organisms, increasing the risk for surgical wound infection.*
  - ❍ Physical therapy (PT): For clients prescribed PT after discharge, review options to access services, provide contact phone numbers to call and schedule therapy, and review options for transportation to PT appointments (e.g., spouse, family, friend, senior center transport, cab, Uber, Lyft). Work with the discharge coordinator for client assistance with transport options as needed.
  - ❍ Medications: Review discharge medication prescription(s). Provide written instructions on medication(s) ordered, how often to take them, and side effects of the prescribed medication(s). Reinforce with client and family that client should not be driving if taking prescription narcotic medications. Review with client and family pain relief expectations, explaining that 100% postoperative pain relief is not realistic, but adequate pain relief should allow the client to function, to ambulate, and to perform activities of daily living (ADLs) with minimal pain.

Pediatric

- SSI prevention measures deemed effective in adults are also indicated in the pediatric surgical population (Berríos-Torres et al, 2017).

Geriatric

- The most common cause of postoperative complication in the frail elderly is delirium (Ersan & Schwer, 2021). *Delirium will affect the ability to provide postoperative education in this population.*

- For the frail, elder client who lived independently in a private home before surgical procedure, work with the discharge coordinator to assess appropriate client placement in the immediate postoperative period. Explore independent living, acute rehabilitation facility, or skilled nursing facility.
- For the cognitively impaired client being discharged back to independent living (private home or home with a family member), identify a key contact person who will participate in discharge education. Assess for any need of community services (e.g., food assistance, meal prep, transport, home health care) at time of discharge.
- Nutritional deficiencies can be common in elderly clients. Monitor laboratory tests; an albumin level less than 3.2 mg/dL and a cholesterol level of less than 160 mg/dL in the frail elderly are indicators for increased mortality. EB: *A BMI of less than 20 kg/m² is a marker for increased risk of wound healing. A dietary consultation should be initiated, and nutritional supplements should be provided (Ersan & Schwer. 2021).*
- As part of the discharge process, ask the client how they will be obtaining groceries: Will they be cooking? Will they need assistance with meal prep? Do they have someone (friend or family member) who can come into the home to assist with cooking? Does the client need to have a food service (i.e., Meals on Wheels) set up for the immediate postdischarge period? Refer client to community services as necessary.

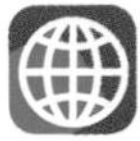

Multicultural

- Consider race and ethnicity as a key factor when developing the client's plan of care. EBN: *Nurses should use culturally competent verbal and nonverbal communication skills to identify clients' values, beliefs, practices, perceptions, and unique health care needs. Effective cultural communication demonstrates respect, dignity, and the preservation of human rights (Douglas et al, 2014).*
- In the case of a language barrier, use a qualified interpreter rather than family members, unless as a last resort, to communicate with the non–English-speaking client. The use of family members to translate health care–specific information may risk client privacy issues and interpretation bias. Nurses must be attentive to nonverbal cues, such as effective listening, attentive body language, and use of eye contact.
- Cultural nonverbal communication may also include values of modesty, touch, silence, and provider gender (Douglas et al, 2014). Identify the need for an interpreter at time of admission and schedule an interpreter to be available, either by phone or in person, for discussions with providers and for education sessions.
- Identify and accommodate the client who prefers same-gender providers. Effective communication may be affected in the client assigned opposite-gender caregivers, which may negatively affect recovery.

Home Care

- Previously listed interventions appropriately pertain to home care.
- Coordinate with discharge planner, as necessary, for assessment of the client's home care situation that suggests potential safety and mobility concerns.
- Clients discharged back to independent living with new use of walker, crutches, wheelchair, oxygen, and so forth should have egress access evaluated, and bathing/showering options and potential need for grab bars.

REFERENCES

Allen, V., Apisarnthanarak, A., & Archer, J. (2017). Prevention measures for healthcare-associated infections. In *APIC text of infection control and epidemiology* [online version]. Retrieved from http://text.apic.org/. [Accessed January 15, 2021].

Anderson, P. A., Savage, J. W., Vaccaro, A. R., et al. (2017). Prevention of surgical site infection in spine surgery. *Neurosurgery*, *80*(3S), S114–S123. https://doi.org/10.1093/neuros/nyw066.

Ban, K. A., Minei, J. P., Laronga, C., et al. (2017). American College of Surgeons and surgical infection society: Surgical site infection guidelines, 2016 update. *Journal of the American College of Surgeons*, *224*(1), 59–74.

Berríos-Torres, S. I., Umscheid, C. A., Bratzler, D. W., et al. (2017). Centers for Disease Control and Prevention guideline for the prevention of surgical site infection, 2017. *JAMA Surgery*, *152*(8), 784–791.

Centers for Disease Control and Prevention (CDC). (2020). *Health effects of cigarette smoking*. Retrieved from https://www.cdc.gov/tobacco/data_statistics/fact_sheets/health_effects/effects_cig_smoking/index.htm. Accessed July 8, 2021.

Douglas, M. K., Rosenkoetter, M., Pacquiao, D. F., et al. (2014). Guidelines for implementing culturally competent nursing care. *Journal of Transcultural Nursing*, *25*(2), 109–121.

Ersan, T., & Schwer, W. A. (2021). *Perioperative management of the geriatric patient*. Medscape [website]. Retrieved from https://emedicine.medscape.com/article/285433-overview#a2. [Accessed July 8, 2021].

Hutzler, L., & Williams, J. (2017). Decreasing the incidence of surgical site infections following joint replacement surgery. *Bulletin of the Hospital for Joint Diseases*, *75*(4), 268–273.

Khan, F. U., Khan, Z., Ahmed, N., & Rehman, A. U. (2020). A general overview of incidence, associated risk factors, and treatment outcomes of surgical site infections. *Indian Journal of Surgery*, *82*(4), 449–459. https://doi.org/10.1007/s12262-020-02071-8.

Mirzashahi, B., Tonkaboni, A., Chehrassan, M., Doosti, R., & Kharazifard, M. J. (2019). The role of poor oral health in surgical site infection following elective spinal surgery. *Musculoskeletal Surgery*, *103*(2), 167–171. https://doi.org/10.1007/s12306-018-0568-2.

Nicolle, L. E., Gupta, K., Bradley, S. F., et al. (2019). Clinical practice guideline for the management of asymptomatic bacteriuria: 2019 update by the Infectious Diseases Society of America. *Clinical Infectious Diseases*, *68*(10), e83–e110. doi:10.1093/cid/ciy1121.

Onyekwelu, I., Yakkanti, R., Protzer, L., Pinkston, C. M., Tucker, C., & Seligson, D. (2017). Surgical wound classification and surgical site infections in the orthopaedic patient. *Journal of the American Academy of Orthopaedic Surgeons: Global Research and Reviews*, *1*(3) e022. doi:10.5435/JAAOSGlobal-D-17-00022.

Preas, M. A., O'Hara, L., & Thom, K. (2017). *2017 HICPAC-CDC guideline for prevention of surgical site infection: What the IP needs to know. Prevention Strategist. Fall 2017*, 69–72. Retrieved from https://apic.org/Resource_/TinyMceFileManager/Periodical_images/SSI_2017_Fall_PS.pdf. [Accessed July 8, 2021].

Tjeertes, E. K. M., Hoeks, S. E., Beks, S. B. J. C., Valentijn, T. M., Hoofwijk, A. G. M., & Stolker, R. J. (2015). Obesity—a risk factor for postoperative complications in general surgery? *BMC Anesthesiology*, *15*, 112.

Triantafyllopoulos, G., Stundner, O., Memtsoudis, S., & Poultsides, L. A. (2015). Patient, surgery, and hospital related risk factors for surgical site infections following total hip arthroplasty. *The Scientific World Journal*, *2015*, 979560. https://doi.org/10.1155/2105/979560.

Tsantes, A. G., Papadopoulos, D. V., Lytras, T., et al. (2020). Association of malnutrition with surgical site infection following spinal surgery: Systematic review and meta-analysis. *Journal of Hospital Infection*, *104*(1), 111–119. https://doi.org/10.1016/j.jhin.2019.09.015.

World Health Organization (WHO). (2018). *Global guidelines for the prevention of surgical site infection*. Geneva: WHO Press. Retrieved from https://www.who.int/publications/i/item/global-guidelines-for-the-prevention-of-surgical-site-infection-2nd-ed. [Accessed November 11, 2021].

I

Risk for Injury Domain 11 Safety/protection Class 2 Physical injury

Julianne E. Doubet, BSN, RN, EMT-B

NANDA-I

Definition

Susceptible to physical damage due to environmental conditions interacting with the individual's adaptive and defensive resources, which may compromise health.

Risk Factors

Exposure to toxic chemicals; immunization level within community; inadequate knowledge of modifiable factors; malnutrition; neurobehavioral manifestations; nosocomial agent; pathogen exposure; physical barrier; tainted nutritional source; unsafe mode of transport

Associated Conditions

Altered psychomotor performance; autoimmune diseases; biochemical dysfunction; effector dysfunction; hypoxia; immune system diseases; impaired primary defense mechanisms; sensation disorders; sensory integration dysfunction

NOC (Nursing Outcomes Classification)

Suggested NOC Outcomes

Personal Safety Behavior; Risk Control; Safe Home Environment; Knowledge: Fall Prevention

Example NOC Outcome with Indicators

Risk Control as evidenced by the following indicators: Monitors environmental risk factors/Develops effective risk control strategies/Follows selected risk control strategies. (Rate the outcome and indicators of **Risk Control:** 1 = never demonstrated, 2 = rarely demonstrated, 3 = sometimes demonstrated, 4 = often demonstrated, 5 = consistently demonstrated [see Section I].)

Client Outcomes

Client Will (Specify Time Frame)

- Remain free of injuries
- Explain methods to prevent injuries
- Demonstrate behaviors that decrease the risk for injury

NIC (Nursing Interventions Classification)

Suggested NIC Interventions

Health Education; Environmental Management; Fall Prevention

Example NIC Activities—Health Education

Identify internal or external factors that may enhance or reduce motivation for healthy behavior; Determine current health knowledge and lifestyle behaviors of individual, family, or target group

Nursing Interventions and *Rationales*

- Prevent iatrogenic harm to the hospitalized client by following the National Patient Safety Goals.
- Accuracy of client identification:
  - Use at least two methods (e.g., client's name and medical record number or birth date) to identify the client on initial entrance to a client's room and before administering medications, blood products, treatments, or procedures.
- Effectiveness of communication among care staff:
  - Get important test results to the right staff person on time.
- Medication safety:
  - Before a procedure, label medications that are not labeled. For example, medicines in syringes, cups, and basins.
  - Take extra care with clients who take medications to thin their blood.
  - Record and pass along correct information about a client's medications. Find out what medications the client is taking. Compare those medications to new medications given to the client.
  - Give the client written information about the medicines they need to take.
  - Tell the client it is important to bring their up-to-date list of medicines every time they visit a health care provider.
- Alarm safety:
  - Make improvements to ensure that alarms on medical equipment are heard and responded to on time.
- Infection control:
  - Use the hand cleaning guidelines from the Centers for Disease Control and Prevention (2020) or the World Health Organization. Set goals for improving hand cleaning. Use the goals to improve hand cleaning.
- Identify clients with safety risks:
  - Identify which clients are at risk for suicidal behavior.
- Prevent errors in surgery:
  - Make sure that the correct surgery is done on the correct client and at the correct place on the client's body.
  - Mark the correct place on the client's body where the surgery is to be done.
  - Pause before the surgery to make sure that a mistake is not being made.

  EB: *These actions have been shown to increase client safety and are required actions for accreditation by The Joint Commission (2021).*
- See care plans for Risk for **Falls,** Risk for **Suicidal** Behavior, and Risk for **Poisoning.**
- Avoid use of physical and chemical restraints, if possible. Restraint free is now the standard of care for hospitals and long-term care facilities. Obtain a health care provider's order if restraints are necessary. EBN: *The use of restraints has been associated with serious client injuries and at present there is no satisfactory evidence to confirm that the use of restraints is beneficial in reducing falls and preventing injuries (Rahn et al, 2017).*
- Consider providing individualized music of the client's choice if a client is agitated. EBN: *In their study of the utilization of music as a complementary treatment, researchers discovered that many nurses currently employ music therapy in their client's therapy; it was found that music assists in the alleviation of anxiety, helps to stabilize vital signs, and aids in pain management (Ciğerci et al, 2019).*
- Review drug profile for potential side effects and interactions that may increase risk of injury. EBN: *Interventions to reduce polypharmacy are considered critical strategies to prevent disabilities in older adults (Lee et al, 2020).*

- Provide a safe environment:
  - ❍ Use one-fourth– to one-half–length side rails only and maintain bed in a low position. Ensure that wheels are locked on bed and commode. Keep dim light in room at night.
  - ❍ Remove all possible hazards in environment such as razors, medications, room clutter, wet floors, and matches.

  EBN: *The Joint Commission (2021), a national organization devoted to the health and well-being of those clients who are admitted to a hospital, directs that health care institutions must evaluate the client for fall risks using an effective and consistently dependable fall risk evaluation tool and then institute environmental interventions to establish a safe, client-centered milieu (West et al, 2018).*
- If the client has a new onset of confusion (delirium), refer to the care plan for Acute **Confusion.** If the client has chronic confusion, see the care plan for Chronic **Confusion.**

▲ Refer the client for physical therapy for strengthening as needed.

- Use nonphysical forms of behavior management for the agitated client with psychosis disorder. EB: *Educating staff in how to deal with a disturbed client should be a primary goal, particularly in the use of verbal communication to defuse a tense encounter (Fernández-Costa et al, 2020).*

Pediatric

I

- Teach parents the need for close supervision of young children playing near water. EB: *Most drowning victims age 6 years or less drown in swimming pools, even though adults were close by but engaged in other activities. Dynamic adult management of children near water requires "attention, proximity, and continuity" (Cohen et al, 2020).*
- Assess the client's socioeconomic status because financial hardship may correlate with increased rates of injury. EB: *In their review of the literature regarding children's socioeconomic status (SES) and injury, Mahboob et al (2019) found that most of the studies evaluated established an association between low SES and additional risk for injury.*
- Never leave young children unsupervised around cooking or open flames. EB: *Lack of adult supervision is often cited as a major factor for thermal trauma in children: the danger of burn injury is strongly associated with lack of parental awareness of risk (Juškausikienė & Raškelienė, 2018).*
- Teach parents and children the need to maintain safety for the physically active child, including wearing helmets when biking and skateboarding. EB: *Although this study by Axelsson & Stigson (2019) indicated that bicycle helmets successfully aided in reducing head and facial injuries, parents will want to consider additional measures to reduce other types of injuries connected to bicycle use.* EB: *In their analysis of skateboarding injuries seen in emergency departments over a 10-year span, Partiali et al (2020) established that there is further need for skateboarding injury prevention programs and the necessity of increasing parental awareness concerning injury protective helmet use.*
- Encourage parents to insist on safety precautions in all phases of participation in sports involving children. EB: *Parents and youth athletes should be aware that there are increased risks of injury caused by sports specialization and the intense volume of participation the child is subject to when involved in many sports (Post et al, 2017).*
- Provide parents of children with traumatic brain injury with written instruction and emergency phone numbers. Ensure that instructions are understood before the child is discharged from a health care setting. Instruct parents to observe for the following symptoms: nausea, mild headache, dizziness, irritability, lethargy, poor concentration, loss of appetite, and insomnia. EBN: *The nurse plays a pivotal part in educating the client, family, school, and perhaps coaches on the necessity of lifestyle modifications based on the client's condition (Gillooly, 2016).*
- Teach both parents and children the need for gun safety. EBN: *The position statement published by the American Academy of Pediatrics (2018) and endorsed by other professional organizations, including the American College of Nursing and the Emergency Nurses Association, advocate for child gun safety by educating both gun owners and children about firearm safety measures, including lock boxes, trigger locks, and high-pressure trigger mechanisms (Beal, 2019).*
- Educate parents regarding proper car safety seat use. EBN: *Webb (2019), in her doctoral thesis on parental knowledge of car seat safety, affirms that many children (and adolescent) deaths and injuries from motor vehicle accidents continue today due to deficiencies in the use of safety restraints; parental education on height, weight, age, and transition guidelines for car seats and booster seats remains a critical intervention.*

Geriatric

- Encourage the client to wear glasses and hearing aids and to use walking aids, including nonslip footwear when ambulating. **EBN:** *Providing community-dwelling older adults with techniques to avoid falls may allow them to live on their own longer in a secure, safe environment (Minnier et al, 2019).*
- Assess for orthostatic hypotension when getting up, and teach methods to decrease dizziness, such as rising slowly, remaining seated several minutes before standing, flexing feet upward several times while sitting, sitting down immediately if feeling dizzy, and trying to have someone present when standing. **EBN:** *In a study by Nazarko (2015), it was found that addressing physiological risk factors for falls improves functional capability, a feeling of well-being, and improvement in the quality of life.*
- Discourage driving at night. **EB:** *Elderly drivers cannot always distinguish or will not admit to a decline in their driving skills; as a result, they may well create dangerous situations for themselves and others (Albert et al, 2018).*

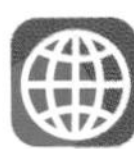

Multicultural

- Evaluate the influence of culture on the client's perceptions of risk for injury. **EB:** *Sael (2019), in his master's thesis concerning the increase in occupational accidents of foreign employees, found that the largest safety barrier for multicultural/multilingual workers is disparity in language and that this problem must be addressed in some way to maintain the employees' safekeeping.*
- Evaluate whether exposure to community violence is a contributor to a client's risk for injury. **EB:** *Researchers, in their study of male youth caught up in the criminal justice system, concluded that there is an association between psychological distress and gun possession, most likely triggered by previously experiencing or witnessing violence (Reid et al, 2017).*
- Use culturally relevant injury prevention programs when possible. Validate the client's feelings and concerns related to environmental risks. **EB:** *Chicago youth residing in high-crime areas explained to researchers that they have created environs of safety within dangerous neighborhoods and use certain strategies to keep themselves safe; some of these approaches may incorporate circumvention, "hypervigilance," self-protection, and emotional control (DaVieria et al, 2020).*

Home Care and Client/Family Teaching and Discharge Planning

- Previous interventions can be adapted for home care use.
- See Risk for Physical **Trauma** for Nursing Interventions and *Rationales.*

I

REFERENCES

Albert, G., Lotan, T., Weiss, P., & Shiftan, Y. (2018). The challenge of safe driving among elderly drivers. *Healthcare Technology Letters, 5*(1), 45–48. https://doi.org/10.1049/htl.2017.0002.

Axelsson, A., & Stigson, H. (2019). Characteristics of bicycle crashes among children and the effect of bicycle helmets. *Traffic Injury Prevention, 20*(Suppl. 3), 21–26. http://doi.org/10.1080/15389588.2019.1694666.

Beal, J. A. (2019). Children and gun safety: A call to action for nurses. *American Journal of Maternal/Child Nursing, 44*(3), 171. https//doi.org/10.1097/NMC.0000000000000522.

Centers for Disease Control and Prevention (CDC). (2020). *Hand hygiene guidance*. Retrieved from https://www.cdc.gov/handhygiene/providers/guideline.html. [Accessed 8 July 2021].

Ciğerci, A., Kisacik, Ö. G., Özyürek, P., & Çevik, C. (2019). Nursing music intervention: A systematic mapping study. *Complimentary Therapies in Clinical Practice, 35*, 109–120. https://doi.org/10.1016/j.ctcp.2019.02.007.

Cohen, N., Scolnik, D., Rimon, A., Balla, U., & Glatstein, M. (2020). Childhood drowning: Review of patients presenting to the emergency department of 2 large tertiary care pediatric hospitals near and distant from the sea coast. *Pediatric Emergency Care, 36*(5), e258–e262. https//doi:10.1097/PEC.0000000000001394.

DaViera, A. L., Roy, A. L., Uriostegui, M., & Fiesta, D. (2020). Safe spaces embedded in dangerous contexts: How Chicago youth navigate daily life and demonstrate resilience in high–crime neighborhoods. *American Journal of Community Psychology, 66*(1–2), 65–80. https://doi.org/10.1002/ajcp.12434.

Fernández-Costa, D., Gómez-Salgado, J., Fagundo-Rivera, J., Martín-Pereira, J., Prieto-Callejero, B., & García-Iglesias, J. J. (2020). Alternatives to the use of mechanical restraints in the management of agitation or aggressions of psychiatric patients: A scoping review. *Journal of Clinical Medicine, 9*(9), 2791. https://doi.org/jcm9092791.

Gillooly, D. (2016). Current recommendations on management of pediatric concussions. *Pediatric Nursing, 42*(5), 217–220. PMID:29406639.

The Joint Commission. (2021). *Hospital national patient safety goals*. Retrieved from https://www.jointcommission.org/-/media/tjc/documents/standards/national-patient-safety-goals/2021/simplified-2021-hap-npsg-goals-final-11420.pdf. [Accessed 8 July 2021].

Juškausikienė, E., & Raškelienė, V. (2018). *Parent's knowledge about burns prevention of their children* (Vol. 168). University Research Publication. Retrieved from https://hdl.handle.net/20.500.12512/97314. [Accessed 8 July 2021].

Lee, E. A., Brettler, J. W., Kanter, M. H., et al. (2020). Refining the definition of polypharmacy and its link to disability in older adults: Conceptualizing necessary polypharmacy, unnecessary polypharmacy, and polypharmacy of unclear benefit. *The Permanente Journal, 24*(18), 212. https//doi.org/10.7812/TPP/18.212.

Mahboob, A., Richmond, S. A., Harkins, J. P., & Macpherson, A. K. (2019). Childhood unintentional injury: The impact of family income, education level, occupation status, and other measures of socioeconomic status. A systematic review. *Paediatrics and Child Health, 26*(1), e39–e45. https://doi.org/10.1093/pch/pxz145.

Minnier, W., Leggett, M., Persaud, I., & Breda, K. (2019). Four smart steps: Fall prevention for community-dwelling older adults. *Creative Nursing, 25*(2), 169–175. https//doi.org/10.1891/1078-4535.25.2169.

Nazarko, L. (2015). Modifiable risk factors for falls and minimizing the risk of harm. *Nurse Prescribing, 13*(4), 192–198. https://doi.org/10.12968/npre.2015.13.4.192.

Partiali, B., Oska, S., Barbat, A., Sneij, J., & Folbe, A. (2020). Injuries to the head and face from skateboarding: A 10-year analysis from National Electronic Injury Surveillance System Hospitals. *Journal of Oral and Maxillofacial Surgery, 78*(9), 1590–1594. https://doi.org/10.1016/j.joms.2020.04.039.

Post, E. G., Trigsted, S. M., Riekena, J. W., et al. (2017). The association of sport specialization and training volume with injury history in youth athletes. *American Journal of Sports Medicine, 45*(6), 1405–1412. https://doi.org/10.1177/0363546517690848.

Rahn, A. C., Behncke, A., Buhl, A., & Köpke, S. (2017). Implementation of a guideline-based programme on physical restraint reduction in home care and nursing homes in northern Germany—Multi-centre before-after study. *BMC Nursing, 16*, 4–11. https://doi.org/10.1093/geroni/igx004.1560.

Reid, J. A., Richards, T. N., Loughran, T. A., & Mulvey, E. P. (2017). The relationships among exposure to violence, psychological distress, and gun carrying among male adolescents found guilty of serious legal offenses: A longitudinal cohort study. *Annals of Internal Medicine, 166*(6), 412–418. https://www.acpjournals.org/doi/pdf/10.7326/M16-1648.

Sael, J. (2019). *A risk-based study of safety barriers in multicultural work environments.* [Master's thesis]. Faculty of Science and Technology, University of Stavanger, Stavanger, Norway. Retrieved from https://uis.brage.unit.no/uis-xmlui/bitstream/handle/11250/2628711/Sael_Javeed.pdf?sequence=1&isAllowed=y. [Accessed 8 July 2021].

Webb, B. P. (2019). Parental knowledge of car seat safety. *DNP Projects, 293*. Retrieved from https://uknowledge.uky.edu/dnp_etds/293. [Accessed 8 July 2021]. https://doi.org/10.1093/geroni/igx004.1560.

West, G. F., Rose, T., & Throop, M. D. (2018). Assessing nursing interventions to reduce patient falls. *Nursing2018, 48*(8), 59–60. https://doi: 10.1097/01.NURSE.0000541404.79920.4e.

Risk for Corneal Injury Domain 11 Safety/protection Class 2 Physical injury

Rachel Klompmaker, BScN, NP-PHC, MScN

NANDA-I

Definition

Susceptible to infection or inflammatory lesion in the corneal tissue that can affect superficial or deep layers, which may compromise health.

Risk Factors

Exposure of the eyeball; inadequate knowledge of modifiable factors

At-Risk Population

Individuals experiencing prolonged hospitalization

Associated Conditions

Artificial respiration; Blinking <5 times per minute; Glasgow Coma Scale score <6; oxygen therapy; periorbital edema; pharmaceutical preparations; tracheostomy

NOC (Nursing Outcomes Classification)

Suggested NOC Outcomes (Visual)

Sensory Function: Vision; Vision Compensation Behavior

Example NOC Outcome with Indicators

Vision Compensation Behavior as evidenced by the following indicators: Wears protective eye wear for prevention/Eye discomfort improves daily with healing. (Rate each indicator of **Vision Compensation Behavior:** 1 = never demonstrated, 2 = rarely demonstrated, 3 = sometimes demonstrated, 4 = often demonstrated, 5 = consistently demonstrated [see Section I].)

Client Outcomes

Client Will (Specify Time Frame)

- Demonstrate relaxed facial expressions and grimacing reduction
- Remain as independent as possible

- Remain free of physical harm resulting from vision injury risk
- Demonstrate improvement in visual acuity

NIC (Nursing Interventions Classification)

Suggested NIC Interventions

Visual Deficit; Environmental Management

Example NIC Activities—Communication Enhancement: Visual Deficit

Clearly identify yourself when you enter the client's space; Build on client's remaining vision, as appropriate

Nursing Interventions and *Rationales*

Emergency Department Visit or Primary Care Office Visit

- ▲ Perform a standard ophthalmic examination or examine eye with a slit lamp using fluorescein stain to optimize visualization of the abrasion injury if available.
- ● Attempt visual acuity measuring using the Snellen eye chart (corrected with glasses).
- ● Ensure immunization status is current, namely tetanus-diphtheria-pertussis status (every 10 years).
- ● Teach the client that foreign body corneal abrasions are one of the most common eye injuries and are at risk for complications (Zimmerman et al, 2019). EB: *The Cochrane systematic review of 12 randomized controlled trials (RCTs) with 1080 participants suggested that treating simple corneal abrasions with a patch may not improve healing rate or reduce pain. Application of an eye patch decreases oxygen delivery and results in higher risk of infection due to moisture. Furthermore, people receiving an eye patch may be less likely to have a healed corneal abrasion after 24 to 72 hours. Additionally, corneal abrasions in people patched probably take slightly longer to heal. Lastly, using eye patches may lead to more pain at 24 hours (Lim, Turner, & Lim, 2016; Thiel, Sarau, & Ng, 2017).*
- ● Topical anesthetics such as tetracaine may be used to provide pain relief for corneal abrasions (Fusco et al, 2019).
- ▲ Clients will require topical antibiotics to reduce the risk of infection (Thiel, Sarau, & Ng, 2017; Fusco et al, 2019). Nonsteroidal antiinflammatory drugs (NSAIDs) may be prescribed to facilitate healing and reduce pain. EB: *According to the Cureus systematic review of 10 RCTs, the use of topical NSAIDs decreases pain symptoms in clients with corneal abrasions and does not complicate wound healing. The use of NSAID drops also reduces the need for oral pain medication. This is important because of the absence of gastrointestinal side effects and a decreased need for narcotics (Thiel, Sarau, & Ng, 2017).*
- ● Injuries that penetrate the cornea are more serious. The outcome depends on the specific injury. Corneal abrasions usually heal quickly and without vision concerns. Even after the original injury is healed, however, the surface of the cornea is sometimes not as smooth as before. EB: *Clients who have had a corneal abrasion may notice that the eye feels irritated for a while after the abrasion heals (Cleveland Clinic, 2015).*

Hospitalization

- ● Traumatic corneal abrasions are common ophthalmic injuries, accounting for 8% of emergency department visits, with fingernail-induced corneal abrasions being common (Gotekar, 2017; Wakai et al, 2017).
- ● Perioperative corneal abrasions typically heal within 72 hours. Risk factors include advanced age, prominent eyes (proptosis, exophthalmos), ocular surface abnormalities (dry eye, recurrent erosion syndrome), surgery greater than 60 to 90 minutes, prone/lateral and Trendelenburg positions, operations on the head and neck body regions, intraoperative hypotension, and preoperative anemia. Potential sources of corneal injury in the surgical client are after induction (laryngoscope, name badge, watch band), before incision (surgical preparation, gauze/sponges/drapes), during the procedure (instruments, chemical solutions, heat sources, pressure on globe, eye shields), and awakening/recovery (oxygen face mask, fingernails) (Malafa et al, 2016; Kaye et al, 2019).
- ▲ All surgical clients should have eyelids secured in the closed position immediately after induction. A strip of tape is generally sufficient; however, in high-risk cases with Trendelenburg position clients may benefit from use of transparent bio-occlusive dressing, which can span the entire lid and provide strong uniform closure, minimizing tear evaporation and acting as a barrier to trauma (Malafa et al, 2016).

I

- Ocular lubricants support surface moisture, but studies comparing different types of lubricants fail to demonstrate differences in efficacy. However, preservative-free methylcellulose-based ointments are preferred because they are retained in the eye longer than aqueous solutions. Paraffin-based (petroleum) ointments disrupt tear film stability, carry a higher risk of eye irritation, and are flammable (Malafa et al, 2016).
- Assess for corneal abrasion and eye dryness, which are common problems in clients in the intensive care unit. Eye dryness is the main risk factor for the development of corneal abrasions. EB: *Sedated clients or clients in induced comas may experience ineffective eye closure, presenting higher risk for corneal injury (Kaye et al, 2019).* EBN: *Eye care and eye assessment should be essential parts of nursing care for clients in intensive care. To prevent corneal abrasions, use eye lubricants, which are more effective than closing eyes with adhesive tapes (Ebadi et al, 2017; French Society for Anaesthesia and Intensive Care et al, 2017).*

Client/Family Teaching and Discharge Planning

- ▲ First-aid principles should be reinforced in the event of an eye injury. Clients should not attempt to remove any object in the eye; reserve this for the provider. A referral to an ophthalmologist may be required (Jacobs, 2021).
- Teach clients to use caution when using household cleaners. Many household products contain strong acids, alkalis, or other chemicals. Drain and oven cleaners are particularly dangerous and can lead to blindness if not used correctly.
- If chemical exposure has occurred, flush the eye immediately with clean water for 10 minutes. Seek prompt health care attention.
- Wear safety goggles at all times when using hand or power tools or chemicals, during high-impact sports, or in other situations when eye injury is more likely.
- Most fingernail injuries to the cornea are preventable, and health teaching should be provided about the importance of supervision in children (Gotekar, 2017).
- Wear sunglasses that screen ultraviolet light when outdoors, even in winter.
- Pain is usually improved within 3 days. If pain becomes intolerable, an analgesic may be prescribed short term. Seek medical attention if pain is not resolving.
- Driving should be restricted for safety until client's visual acuity is evaluated.

REFERENCES

Cleveland Clinic. (2015). Corneal abrasion. Retrieved from http://my.clevelandclinic.org/services/cole-eye/diseases-conditions/hic-corneal-abrasion. Accessed July 8, 2021.

Ebadi, A., Saeid, Y., Ashrafi, S., & Taheri-Kharameh, Z. (2017). Development and psychometric evaluation of a questionnaire on nurse's clinical competence eye care in intensive care unit patients. *Nursing in Critical Care*, *22*(3), 169–175. http://doi-org.libproxy.wlu.ca/10.1111/nicc.12113.

French Society for Anaesthesia and Intensive Care (SFAR), French Ophthalmology Society (SFO), French-speaking Intensive Care Society (SRLF), et al. (2017). Eye protection in anaesthesia and intensive care. *Anaesthesia Critical Care & Pain Medicine*, *36*(6), 411–418. https://doi.org/10.1016/j.accpm.2017.08.001.

Fusco, N., Stead, T. G., Lebowitz, D., & Ganti, L. (2019). Traumatic corneal abrasion. *Cureus*, *11*(4), e4396. https://doi.org/10.7759/cureus.4396.

Gotekar, R. B. (2017). A clinical study of accidental fingernail injuries to the cornea in Alquwayiah General Hospital, Riyadh, Region, KSA. *Journal of Evolution of Medical and Dental Sciences*, *6*(62), 4526. Retrieved from https://link.gale.com/apps/doc/A504623361/AONE?u=wate1800&sid=AONE&xid=91c29a58. [Accessed February 17, 2022].

Jacobs, D. S. (2021). Corneal abrasions and corneal foreign bodies: Management. UpToDate [website], M. F. Gardiner, R. G. Bachur, & J. F. Wiley (Eds.). Waltham, MA: UpToDate. Retrieved from http://www.uptodate.com/contents/corneal-abrasions-and-corneal-foreign-bodies-management?source=see_link. Accessed July 8, 2021.

Kaye, A. D., Renschler, J. S., Cramer, K. D., et al. (2019). Postoperative management of corneal abrasions and clinical implications: A comprehensive review. *Current Pain and Headache Reports*, *23*(7), 48. https://doi.org/10.1007/s11916-019-0784-y.

Lim, C. H. L., Turner, A., & Lim, B. X. (2016). Patching for corneal abrasion. *Cochrane Database of Systematic Reviews*, *7*, CD004764.

Malafa, M. M., Coleman, J. E., Bowman, R. W., & Rohrich, R. J. (2016). Perioperative corneal abrasion: Updated guidelines for prevention and management. *Plastic and Reconstructive Surgery*, *137*(5), 790e–798e.

Thiel, B., Sarau, A., & Ng, D. (2017). Efficacy of topical analgesics in pain control for corneal abrasions: A systematic review. *Cureus*, *9*(3), e1121. https://doi.org/10.7759/cureus.1121.

Wakai, A., Lawrenson, J. G., Lawrenson, A. L., et al. (2017). Topical non-steroidal anti-inflammatory drugs for analgesia in traumatic corneal abrasions. *Cochrane Database of Systematic Reviews*, *5*, CD009781.

Zimmerman, D. R., Shneor, E., Millodot, M., & Gordon-Shaag, A. (2019). Corneal and conjunctival injury seen in urgent care centres in Israel. *Ophthalmic and Physiological Optics*, *39*(1), 46–52. https://doi-org-libproxy.wlu.ca/10.1111/opo.12600.

Risk for Occupational Injury

Domain 11 Safety/projection Class 4 Environmental hazards

Patrick Luna, MSN, RN, CEN, NRP

NANDA-I

Definition

Susceptible to a work-related accident or illness, which may compromise health.

Risk Factors

Individual

Distraction from interpersonal relations; excessive stress; improper use of personal protective equipment; inadequate knowledge; inadequate time management skills; ineffective coping strategies; misinterpretation of information; psychological distress; unhealthy habits; unsafe work behaviors

Unmodified Environmental Factors

Environmental constraints; exposure to biological agents; exposure to chemical agents; exposure to noise; exposure to radiotherapy; exposure to teratogenic agents; exposure to vibration; inadequate access to individual protective equipment; inadequate physical environment; labor relationships; night shift work rotating to day shift work; occupational burnout; physical workload; shift work

I

At-Risk Population

Individuals exposed to environmental temperature extremes

NOC (Nursing Outcomes Classification)

Suggested NOC Outcomes

Personal Health and Safety Behaviors; Risk Control; Adequate Training

Example NOC Outcome with Indicators

Occupational Health as evidenced by the following indicators: Knowledge and compliance with health and safety policies and procedures/Demonstration of personal health-promoting behaviors/Knowledge and self-management of a healthy lifestyle. (Rate the outcome and indicators of **Occupational Health:** 1 = never demonstrated, 2 = rarely demonstrated, 3 = sometimes demonstrated, 4 = often demonstrated, 5 = consistently demonstrated [see Section I].)

Client Outcomes

Client Will (Specify Time Frame)

- Attend and participate in all required health and safety training activities
- Demonstrate safe and healthy work behaviors to reduce the risk of occupational injuries and illnesses
- Comply with the organization's health and safety policies and procedures
- Report to management any work hazards, such as facility, tools, and equipment that needs to be repaired
- Demonstrate healthy personal habits, such as healthy nutritional choices, regular exercise, smoking cessation, and effective sleep patterns

NIC (Nursing Interventions Classification)

Suggested NIC Interventions

Health Coaching; Health Education; Health Screening; Risk Identification

Example NIC Activities—Risk for Occupational Injury

Encourage early reporting of signs and symptoms related to health and safety hazard exposures

Nursing Interventions and *Rationales*

- Interventions to reduce the risks of occupational injury focus on providing resources for safe work and education to the individual to know safety rules and procedures. Occupational safety requires the individual to engage in safe acts, proper use of equipment (including personal protective equipment [PPE]), cognitive focus during work, and self-identification of stressors that may adversely affect the individual's personal safety during work.
- Encourage employee compliance with safety policies and procedures to reduce the opportunity for slips, trips, and falls; breaks in skin integrity through chemical exposure, mechanical means (trauma, friction, pressure), physical exposure (heat, cold, radiation), and exposure to biological elements (viruses, bacteria, fungi); musculoskeletal injuries; and misuse of equipment and tools. **EB:** *Workers who have a positive interpretation of their occupational safety culture are more likely to follow safety policies and avoid injury (Mazzetti et al, 2020). Initiatives to improve compliance with health and safety policies include training, posters and notices in workplaces, and use and availability of PPE (Gómez La-Rotta et al, 2020).*
- Enforce compliance with organizational and regulatory health and safety policies and procedures, demonstrating at least adequate training and the proper use of appropriate tools, equipment, and PPE to reduce risk of injury and illness and ensure that the client receives appropriate training and education on occupational tasks and equipment. **EB:** *Equipment, parts, materials, and hand tools were the major cause of injury to mechanical contractors resulting in 55% of total injuries (Shrestha et al, 2018). To increase compliance with the use of PPE, training should focus on the benefits of PPE to prevent personal injury and illness (Wright et al, 2019).*
- Assist the client in reduction of personal and work stress to increase coping skills, improve interpersonal relationships, and avoid burnout. **EBN:** *Work-related burnout is characterized by symptoms of exhaustion that are related to the client's work. Factors that decrease work-related burnout include social support, sense of community, job satisfaction, and degree of freedom at work (Ilić et al, 2017).*
- Educate clients to engage in active coping strategies to reduce work-related stress. **CEB:** *Recommendations include reducing psychological strain, work overload, and role confusion through the adoption of job redesign techniques and organizational support of counseling and stress reduction workshops (Dar et al, 2011).*
- Promote good sleep hygiene, which will result in increased alertness and decreased occupational injuries and illnesses. **EB:** *The two most common sleep disorders affecting the workplace are insomnia and obstructive sleep apnea, which can negatively affect quality of life and increase work-related injuries (Judd, 2017).*
- Educate client on the detrimental effects of shift work, atypical working time, and nonstandard work schedules. **EB:** *To prevent injuries resulting from shift work, educational strategies and safety policies aimed at developing awareness of the harmful effects of shift work are recommended (Alali et al, 2018).*
- Provide medical screening, surveillance, and postexposure testing for symptomatic employees to identify exposure and control effects that can lead to illness and injury. **CEB:** *The Occupational Safety and Health Administration (OSHA) requires that exposures to specific hazards require a medical surveillance program to identify adverse effects related to those exposures. OSHA Standards provide the opportunity to monitor exposure to health hazards from inhalation, ingestion, or skin absorption from chemical, biological agent, or radiological exposures. The fundamental purpose of screening is early diagnosis and treatment with a clinical focus, whereas surveillance is to detect and eliminate the underlying causes providing a prevention focus (US Department of Labor, OSHA, 2000).*
- Assist in the integration of personal health behaviors that promote total worker health and safety for the employee, which translates to a more productive worker generating better quality products, resulting in fewer occupational injuries and illnesses for the workers. **EB:** *Studies have shown that health education activities and materials should address prevention topics for modifiable behaviors observed to be injury risk factors, such as overuse of alcohol and drugs, stress, tobacco use, and poor sleep habits (Schuh-Renner et al, 2018).*
- Identify client risk factors that can lead to occupational injury and address them with health coaching techniques. **EBN:** *Health coaching is the use of evidence-based skillful conversation, clinical strategies, and interventions to actively and safely engage clients in health behavior change to better self-manage their health, health risks, and acute or chronic health conditions, resulting in optimal wellness, improved health outcomes, lowered health risk, and decreased health care costs (Huffman, 2016).*
- Provide resources to assist with smoking/vaping cessation. **EB:** *According to the American Lung Association (2020a), smoking is the leading cause of preventable death in the United States, causing more than 438,000 deaths per year and worsening preexisting conditions including cardiovascular disease. The process of using an e-cigarette is called "vaping" rather than smoking. The US Food and Drug Administration (FDA)*

describes an e-cigarette as a battery-operated device that turns nicotine, formaldehyde, flavorings (diacetyl that causes popcorn lung), and other chemicals into a vapor that can be inhaled. American Lung Association (2020b) provides information about smoking and smoking cessation programs that can be helpful when counseling employees as to the adverse effects of smoking and vaping.

- Implement environmental and behavioral strategies to aid workers in maintaining a healthy weight. EBN: *A multicomponent approach of environmental (standing workstations, on-site walking routes, access to an onsite wellness center, access to healthy meals) and behavioral (meeting with dietitians, counseling sessions, trainer-led exercise, incentivized goal setting) strategies were successful in improving weight-related outcomes (Upadhyaya et al, 2020).*
- Promote a drug-free workplace through education, training, policy development, and evaluation. EBN: *A drug-free workplace program seeks to modify behaviors of employees who misuse drugs and prevents the use of illicit substances through educational programs and workplace policy (Betcher et al, 2020).*
- Identify high-risk work areas and environmental hazards by conducting periodic walkthroughs of the workplace for unsafe acts and conditions. Possible risks include excessive noise, poorly maintained equipment, lack of PPE, uneven or poorly designed workspaces, inadequate lighting, environmental toxins, and lack of safety training. CEB: *Identifying hazards in the work environment is the first step to maintaining a safe workplace. This information is used to establish priorities for intervention (Brnich & Mallett 2003).*
- Ensure that appropriate respiratory protection is available and used when workers can be potentially exposed to transmissible respiratory infections. EB: *Medical masks are recommended when in close contact with potentially infected individuals for routine interaction and care. N95 respirators are recommended for aerosol-generating medical procedures such as endotracheal intubation, extubation, noninvasive ventilation, and exposure to aerosols in an open circuit (Bartoszko et al, 2020).*
- Ensure that infection prevention and control policies and procedures are enforced. Blood-borne pathogen risks are inherent when providing nursing care in health care facilities for injured or ill employees, and appropriate measures must be taken to avoid contact with and spread of infectious organisms. EB: *Compliance with policies and procedures to prevent blood-borne pathogen exposure increased with continuous and regular training, posters and notices in the work area, and increased qualifications for workers (Gómez La-Rotta et al, 2020).*
- Implement measures to prevent occupational back pain, which can be prevented or limited in its severity. EB: *Discouraging bed rest, promoting early return to work with modified job tasks, implementing accommodations to avoid back injury risk factors, individualized interventions, and follow-up monitoring is encouraged as part of a rehabilitation program to prevent and treat occupational back pain (Al-Otaibi, 2015).*
- Ensure workers have access to and use PPE to reduce noise exposure. Engineering and administrative controls should be considered before the use of PPE. CEB: *A United Auto Workers/General Motors–funded study that assessed the effects of noise on blood pressure and heart rate demonstrated a significant positive relationship between acute noise exposure and both diastolic and systolic blood pressure and heart rate. In assessing the effect of chronic noise exposure, workers who used hearing protection had lower blood pressure and heart rate than workers without hearing protection (McCauley, 2012).*
- Health professionals should understand potential interruptions and cognitive distractions to adopt a task-design–oriented approach that focuses on aspects of the work environment that can be observed, measured, and controlled. EB: *Using signs, no-interruptions zones, personal electronics policies, and available technologies to promote attention-keeping and limit cognitive distractions can be implemented by organizations to maintain safe environments (Cohen et al, 2017).*
- Provide multiprofessional collaboration to reduce occupational risks to health and safety. CEB: *According to Wachs (2005), teamwork is beneficial to American business and industry because of its strength through diversity when a variety of multiprofessional health and safety professionals offer solutions to complex problems.*
- Implement an early reporting system that allows workers to safely report injuries or illness. EB: *OSHA requires a mechanism that identifies to whom the employees report injuries and illnesses and that they are encouraged to do so as early as possible. Educating employees on the signs and symptoms of occupational disease is critical to stop and reverse the process before disability results. Early reporting of signs and symptoms related to health hazard exposures provides for the best outcomes (US Department of Labor, OSHA, 2016).*
- Ensure appropriate medical referrals and communication with health care providers to achieve safe work environment goals and include follow-up assessment to ensure that the worker is not further injured by the accommodated work situation. EB: *Providing appropriate medical referrals and multiprofessional collaboration can reduce occupational risks to health and safety (US Department of Labor, OSHA, 2000).*

- Provide accurate and legal documentation for medical and exposure records with adverse health effects from health and safety exposures, maintaining confidentiality of personal medical issues. Legal requirements for documentation ensure correct communication of all aspects of the injury or illness and protects the nurse in case of litigation. **CEB:** *OSHA documentation specifics include medical, exposure, and training records that must be retained for at least 30 years. The documentation provides a history of the employee's exposure to hazards, assessment and treatment received, and any worksite hazard abatements or reduction to exposures and any outcomes of exposure and treatments (US Department of Labor, OSHA, 2020).*

Geriatric

- Consider the physiological changes in the aging population. **EB:** *The aging workforce typically has experienced changes in their physical systems that require attention to physical needs. These changes may include slower reaction times, predisposing factors to developing musculoskeletal disorders, a compromised cardiovascular system, less acute hearing and vision, and impaired cognition (Algarni et al, 2015).*
- Although older clients may experience fewer occupational injuries and illnesses, the aging workforce may take longer to heal and return to work. **EB:** *A review of current best practices by Delloiacono (2015) found that the extent of age-related physical changes in older workers is significantly influenced by chronic illnesses. However, improving lifestyles could reduce organizational costs, and reducing costs is important because although older worker statistics report lower work-related injury rates, their recovery is slower and lost work time is longer.*

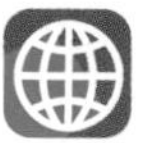

Multicultural

- Address differences in cultures that affect attitudes toward health care professionals and treatment modalities. **EB:** *Understanding the written and verbal language can significantly affect the instructions and training given to workers.*
- According to the Centers for Disease Control and Prevention (CDC, 2021), young workers have high rates of job-related injury. These injuries are often the result of the many hazards present in the places they typically work, such as sharp knives and slippery floors in restaurants. Limited or no prior work experience and a lack of safety training also contribute to high injury rates. Middle and high school workers may be at increased risk for injury because they may not have the strength or cognitive ability needed to perform certain job duties. **EB:** *In 2016 there were about 19.3 million workers under the age of 24. These workers represented 13% of the total workforce, and in 2015, 403 workers under the age of 24 died from work-related injuries (CDC, 2018).*
- The US workforce is becoming more diverse (National Center for Public Policy and Higher Education, 2005). Baby boomers are remaining in the workforce past traditional retirement age because their health is better, and they need or want additional income (Bureau of Labor Statistics, 2008).
- The size of the minority workforce is growing, and more women are entering the workforce (Thompson & Wachs, 2012). There is greater diversity in the workplace, and people from different backgrounds and cultures are working alongside each other, often speaking different languages with different educational and literacy backgrounds. **CEB:** *As the minority workforce continues to grow, especially the Hispanic workforce, businesses must recognize the unique needs and contributions of this workforce in terms of language, customs, culture, and values (Thompson & Wachs, 2012). It is recommended that occupational health nurses promote health and prevent injuries among vulnerable workers at both the individual and system levels (Burgel, Nelson, & White, 2015).*
- Depending on the setting, comprehensive health care, including, for example, smoking cessation and early diagnosis and treatment of depression, could be provided to high-risk populations using culturally sensitive outreach and motivational interviewing strategies. **EB:** *Because of underreporting, active case findings for occupational injuries are needed when day laborers access any health care system. To ensure the provision of health and safety training and PPE for day laborers at the system level, occupational health nurses can advocate for comprehensive occupational health and safety legal protections for all contingent workers. Reporting health complaints and injuries, in addition to providing rest breaks, deserves further study in this population. In addition to targeted hearing conservation and respiratory protection programs for this high-risk group, the risk of falls from heights is a serious hazard facing day laborers, and this phenomenon also deserves further investigation (Burgel, Nelson, & White, 2015).*

- The Americans with Disabilities Act (ADA) requires that public buildings be designed to accommodate wheelchairs and other accommodations and that jobs be modified if accommodation is reasonable so that people with disabilities can gain access to buildings and jobs (see https://www.ada.gov/ada_req_ta.htm).

REFERENCES

Al-Otaibi, S. T. (2015). Prevention of occupational back pain. *Journal of Family Community Medicine*, *22*(2), 73–77.

Alali, H., Braeckman, L., Van Hecke, T., & Abdel Wahab, M. (2018). Shift work and occupational accident absence in Belgium: Findings from the Sixth European working condition survey. *International Journal of Environmental Research and Public Health*, *15*(9), 1811. doi:10.3390/ijerph15091811.

Algarni, F. S., Gross, D. P., Senthilselvan, A., & Battié, M. C. (2015). Ageing workers with work-related musculoskeletal injuries. *Occupational Medicine*, *65*(3), 229–237.

American Lung Association. (2020a). *Smoking facts*. Retrieved from https://www.lung.org/quit-smoking/smoking-facts. Accessed July 12, 2021.

American Lung Association. (2020b). *Quit smoking*. Retrieved from https://www.lung.org/quit-smoking. Accessed July 12, 2021.

Americans with Disabilities Act. (n.d.). ADA requirements and technical assistance. Retrieved from https://www.ada.gov/ada_req_ta.htm. Accessed July 12, 2021.

Bartoszko, J. J., Farooqi, M. A. M., Alhazzani, W., & Loeb, M. (2020). Medical masks vs N95 respirators for preventing COVID–19 in healthcare workers: A systematic review and meta-analysis of randomized trials. *Influenza and Other Respiratory Viruses*, *14*(4), 365–373. https://doi.org/10.1111/irv.12745.

Betcher, C. A., Standish, M. D., & Gillespie, G. L. (2020). Need and capacity of a toolkit for occupational health nurses to promote a new or enhanced drug-free workplace program. *Workplace Health & Safety*, *68*(6), 263–271. https://doi.org/10.1177/2165079920911550.

Brnich, M. J., & Mallett, L. G. (2003). *Focus on prevention: Conducting a hazard risk assessment*. Retrieved from http://www.cdc.gov/niosh/mining/UserFiles/works/pdfs/2003-139.pdf. Accessed September 29, 2021.

Bureau of Labor Statistics. (2008). More seniors working fulltime. *TED: The Economics Daily*. Retrieved from https://www.bls.gov/opub/ted/2008/aug/wk1/art03.htm. Accessed July 12, 2021.

Burgel, B. J., Nelson, R. W., Jr., & White, M. C. (2015). Work-related health complaints and injuries, and health and safety perceptions of Latino day laborers. *Workplace Health & Safety*, *63*(8), 350–361.

Centers for Disease Control and Prevention (CDC). (2021). *Traumatic occupational injuries*. Retrieved from https://www.cdc.gov/niosh/injury/fastfacts.html. Accessed September 29, 2021.

Cohen, J., LaRue, C., & Cohen, H. H. (2017). Attention interrupted: Cognitive distraction & workplace safety. *Professional Safety 2017* (11), 28–34. Retrieved from https://aeasseincludes.assp.org/professionalsafety/pastissues/062/11/F1_1117.pdf. Accessed July 12, 2021.

Dar, L., Akmal, A., Naseem, M. A., & Din Khan, K. U. (2011). Impact of stress on employees job performance in business sector of Pakistan. *Global Journal of Management and Business Research*, *11*(6) Retrieved from https://globaljournals.org/GJMBR_Volume11/1-Impact-of-Stress-on-Employees-Job-Performance.pdf. Accessed July 12, 2021.

Delloiacono, N. (2015). Musculoskeletal safety for older adults in the workplace review of current best practice evidence. *Workplace Health & Safety*, *63*(2), 48–53.

Gómez La-Rotta, E. I., Garcia, C. S., Pertuz, C. M., et al. (2020). Knowledge and compliance as factors associated with needlestick injuries contaminated with biological material: Brazil and Colombia. *Ciência & Saúde Coletiva*, *25*(2), 715–727.

Huffman, M. H. (2016). Advancing the practice of health coaching: Differentiation from wellness coaching. *Workplace Health & Safety*, *64*(9), 400–403.

Ilić, I. M., Arandjelović, M. Ž., Jovanović, J. M., & Nešić, M. M. (2017). Relationships of work-related psychosocial risks, stress, individual factors and burnout—Questionnaire survey among emergency physicians and nurses. *Medycyna Pracy*, *68*(2), 167–178. https://doi.org/10.13075/mp.5893.00516.

Judd, S. R. (2017). Uncovering common sleep disorders and their impacts on occupational performance. *Workplace Health & Safety*, *65*(5), 232.

Mazzetti, G., Valente, E., Guglielmi, D., & Vignoli, M. (2020). Safety doesn't happen by accident: A longitudinal investigation on the antecedents of safety behavior. *International Journal of Environmental Research and Public Health*, *17*(12), 4332.

McCauley, L. A. (2012). Research to practice in occupational health nursing. *Workplace Health & Safety*, *60*(4), 183–190.

National Center for Public Policy and Higher Education. (2005). *Income of U.S. workforce projected to decline if education doesn't improve*. Retrieved from http://www.highereducation.org/reports/pa_decline/index.shtml. Accessed July 12, 2021.

Schuh-Renner, A., Canham-Chervak, M., Hearn, D. W., Loveless, P. A., & Jones, B. H. (2018). Factors associated with injury among employees at a U.S. Army hospital. *Workplace Health & Safety*, *66*(7), 322–330. https://doi.org/10.1177/2165079917736069.

Shrestha, P. P., Shrestha, K., & Becerra, E. (2018). Types and factors affecting injury rates of mechanical contractors. *Work (Reading, Mass.)*, *61*(1), 135–148.

Thompson, M. C., & Wachs, J. E. (2012). Occupational health nursing in the United States. *Workplace Health & Safety*, *60*(3), 127–133.

United States US Department of Labor, Occupational Safety and Health Administration (OSHA). (2000). *Medical screening and surveillance*. Retrieved from https://www.osha.gov/SLTC/medicalsurveillance/index.html. Accessed July 12, 2021.

US United States Department of Labor, Occupational Safety and Health Administration (OSHA). (2016). *Recommended practices for safety and health programs*. Retrieved from https://www.osha.gov/shpguidelines/docs/OSHA_SHP_Recommended_Practices.pdf. Accessed July 12, 2021.

US United States Department of Labor, Occupational Safety and Health Administration (OSHA). (2020). *Access to medical and exposure records*. Retrieved from https://www.osha.gov/Publications/osha3110.pdf. Accessed July 12, 2021.

Upadhyaya, M., Sharma, S., Pompeii, L. A., Sianez, M., & Morgan, R. O. (2020). Obesity prevention worksite wellness interventions for health care workers: A narrative review. *Workplace Health & Safety*, *68*(1), 32–49. https://doi.org/10.1177/2165079919863082.

Wachs, J. E. (2005). Building the occupational health team keys to successful interdisciplinary collaboration. *AAOHN Journal*, *53*(4), 166–171.

Wright, T., Adhikari, A., Yin, J., Vogel, R., Smallwood, S., & Shah, G. (2019). Issue of compliance with use of personal protective equipment among wastewater workers across the southeast region of the United States. *International Journal of Environmental Research and Public Health*, *16*(11), 2009.

Nipple-Areolar Complex Injury Domain 11 Safety/protection Class 2 Physical injury

Nichol Chesser, RN, CNM, DNP

NANDA-I

Definition

Localized damage to nipple-areolar complex as a result of the breastfeeding process.

Defining Characteristics

Abraded skin; altered skin color; altered thickness of nipple-areolar complex; blistered skin; discolored skin patches; disrupted skin surface; ecchymosis; eroded skin; erythema; expresses pain; hematoma; macerated skin; scabbed skin; skin fissure; skin ulceration; skin vesicles; swelling; tissue exposure below the epidermis

Related Factors

Breast engorgement; hardened areola; improper use of milk pump; inadequate latching on; inappropriate maternal hand support of breast; inappropriate positioning of the infant during breastfeeding; inappropriate positioning of the mother during breastfeeding; ineffective infant sucking reflex; ineffective non-nutritive sucking; mastitis; maternal anxiety about breastfeeding; maternal impatience with the breastfeeding process; mother does not wait for the infant to spontaneously release the nipple; mother withdraws infant from breast without breaking the suction; nipple confusion due to use of artificial nipple; postprocedural pain; prolonged exposure to moisture; supplementary feeding; use of products that remove the natural protection of the nipple

At-Risk Population

Primiparous women; sole mother; women aged < 19 years; women breastfeeding for the first time; women with depigmented nipple areolar complex; women with history of inadequate nipple-areolar preparation during prenatal care; women with history of nipple trauma in breastfeeding; women with non-protruding nipples; women with pink nipple-areolar complex

Associated Conditions

Ankyloglossia; maxillofacial abnormalities

NOC (Nursing Outcomes Classification)

Suggested NOC Outcome

Breastfeeding Establishment: Maternal

Example NOC Outcome with Indicators

Breastfeeding Establishment: Maternal: Suction broken before removing infant from breast. (Rate outcome and indicators of **Breastfeeding Establishment: Maternal:** 1 = not adequate, 2 = slightly adequate 3 = moderately adequate, 4 = substantially adequate, 5 = totally adequate [see Section I].

Client Outcomes

Client Will (Specify Time Frame)

- Avoid artificial nipple use with infant
- Use techniques to prevent nipple tenderness
- Establish a position of comfort during nursing
- Recognize infant swallowing

NIC (Nursing Interventions Classification)

Suggested NIC Intervention

Pain Management: Acute

Example NIC Activities—Pain Management: Acute

Question client regarding the level of pain that allows a state of comfort and appropriate function and attempt to keep pain at or lower than identified level

Nursing Interventions and *Rationales*

- Nipple trauma and sore nipples are common complaints among breastfeeding women and are a leading cause of breastfeeding discontinuation. EB: *Nipple soreness usually occurs between the first 3 and 7 days after childbirth and can last for at least 6 weeks. About 90% of lactating women experience some sort of nipple soreness, with up to 26% of women experiencing painful nipple fissures (As'adi et al, 2017).*
- Identify clients at risk for nipple trauma. EB: *The most common causes of nipple trauma are incorrect latch and incorrect nipple suckling (Ghaheri et al, 2017; Niazi et al, 2018). Other causes of nipple trauma may include nipple infection, the infant having a short frenulum, strong or weak suckling, and washing the nipple with a harsh soap (Niazi et al, 2018). Awareness of a woman's breastfeeding technique including latch and baby positioning during breastfeeding can help prevent nipple trauma (Gianni et al, 2019).*
- Evaluate the nipple for five signs of nipple trauma in order to help reduce pain and further trauma and to promote continuation of breastfeeding. EB: *Erythema and swelling are the first signs of nipple trauma, followed by blistering, fissures, and scabbing (Nakamura et al, 2018). Nipple piercing seems to not interfere with lactation but may interfere with a correct latch and potentially may increase risk of infection if the piercing was obtained within the past 6 to 12 months (National Library of Medicine, 2021).*
- Use a valid and reliable tool for assessing nipple trauma associated with breastfeeding. EB: *Assessing pain by client self-report is the most accurate and reliable method of obtaining information on pain experienced by the client (Karcioglu, 2018). The numeric rating scale (NRS) of 0 to 10 is easily documented, easily interpreted, and meets regulatory guidelines for assessing and documenting pain (Karcioglu, 2018). The NRS can be used in conjunction with observed characteristics of nipple trauma in order to facilitate appropriate interventions.*
- Help to correct any factors that may be contributing to nipple trauma. EB: *Assess for correct infant mouth attachment to nipple, strong suckling of the infant and/or frequent suckling, use of the breast pump, nipple vasoconstriction, engorgement, clogged ducts, or infection (Spencer, 2021).*
- Offer options to promote healing. EB: *There are numerous options to promote healing, including herbal, medicinal, and nonmedicinal therapies (As'adi et al, 2017). Remedies such as lanolin, hydrogel, LED lights, and tea bag or hot water compresses are easy to use and can be initiated at home as needed (Niazi et al, 2018). Another holistic remedy includes putting breast milk on the area of trauma. This may be beneficial as topical human milk has antiinflammatory properties, which can promote healing and reduce recovery time (Amiri-Farahani et al, 2020). Aloe vera has been shown to reduce pain from cracked nipples if applied to the area 3 times per day after an episode of breastfeeding (Hekmatpou et al, 2019). LED therapy is a novel treatment for nipple trauma that can control pain and accelerate the healing process of nipple fissures/cracks (Campos et al, 2018).*
- Offer instruction on latch in order to promote effective milk transfer and decrease potential nipple trauma. EB: *The LATCH scoring system for infant latch during breastfeeding can help ensure adequate latch to decrease nipple trauma (Westerfield et al, 2018). The LATCH scoring system refers to latch, audible swallowing, type of nipple, comfort of the mother, help required (Westerfield, 2018).*
- Usage of a breast pump to express milk can be beneficial to promote feeding an infant breast milk when feeding at the breast is causing nipple trauma. EB: *Over one-quarter of women who start pumping while still in hospital postpartum cite problems with latch as the reason (Weisband et al, 2017).*
- Assist the client in alternative feeding methods if nipple trauma is severe in order to promote healing and prevent further damage. EB: *Breast milk is found to be the best nutrition for infants; however, not all infants are able to feed at the breast (Becker et al, 2016).*

Home Care

- Assess availability of and refer client to lactation support if nursing interventions and self-management are not alleviating the nipple trauma. EB: *Lactation consultations can improve nipple latch and decrease nipple pain and trauma (Patel & Patel, 2016).*
- Refer client to pediatrician to assess if the infant has an upper, anterior, or submucosal tongue and/or lip-tie. EB: *Infant tongue and/or lip tie can be a main cause of nipple trauma (Ghaheri et al, 2017). Frenotomy, when indicated, can improve breastfeeding success and decrease nipple trauma (Ghaheri et al, 2017).*

I

- Assess clients' emotional state as nipple trauma can lead to inefficient breastfeeding, which can account for unstable mood and postpartum depression. EB: *Studies have shown a link between health problems in the early postpartum period and depression (Cooklin et al, 2018). Breast problems, which can contribute to poor mood postpartum and an increase in physical discomfort, can be ameliorated by appropriate clinical care and support (Cooklin et al, 2018).*
- Encourage family participation and provide information to the father as appropriate in order to support the breastfeeding mother. EB: *Many women perceive their partner as playing a role in the breastfeeding process (Lok et al, 2017). Providing information to the partner to support the breastfeeding woman can encourage continuation of breastfeeding (Lok et al, 2017).*

REFERENCES

Amiri-Farahani, L., Sharifi-Heris, Z., & Mojab, F. (2020). The anti-inflammatory properties of the topical application of human milk in dermal and optical diseases. *Evidence-Based Complementary and Alternative Medicine*, *2020*, 4578153. https://doi.org/10.1155/2020/4578153.

As'adi, N., Kariman, N., Mojab, F., & Pourhoseingholi, M. A. (2017). The effect of Saqez *(Pistacia atlantica)* ointment on the treatment of nipple fissures and nipple pain in breastfeeding women. *Electronic Physician*, *9*(8), 4952–4960.

Becker, G. E., Smith, H. A., & Cooney, F. (2016). Methods of milk expression for lactating women. *Cochrane Database of Systematic Reviews*, *9*, CD006170. https://doi.org/10.1002/14651858.CD006170.pub5.

Campos, T. M., Dos Santos Traverzim, M. A., Sobral, A. P. T., et al. (2018). Effect of LED therapy for the treatment nipple fissures: Study protocol for randomized controlled trial. *Medicine (Baltimore)*, *97*(41), e12322. https://doi.org/10.1097/MD.0000000000012322.

Cooklin, A. R., Amir, L. H., Ngyuen, C. D., et al. (2018). Physical health, breastfeeding problems and maternal mood in the early postpartum: A prospective cohort study. *Archives of Women's Mental Health*, *21*(3), 365–374.

Ghaheri, B. A., Cole, M., Fausel, S. C., Chuop, M., & Mace, J. (2017). Breastfeeding improvement following tongue-tie and lip-tie release: A prospective cohort study. *The Laryngoscope*, *127*(5), 1217–1223.

Gianni, M. L., Bettinelli, M. E., Manfra, P., et al. (2019). Breastfeeding difficulties and risk for early breastfeeding cessation. *Nutrients*, *11*(10), 2266. https://doi.org/10.3390/nu11102266.

Hekmatpou, D., Mehrabi, F., Rahzani, K., & Aminiyan, A. (2019). The effect of aloe vera clinical trials on prevention and healing of skin wound: A systemic review. *Iran Journal of Medical Sciences*, *44*(1), 1–9.

Karcioglu, O., Topacoglu, H., Dikme, O., & Dikme, O. (2018). A systematic review of the pain scales in adults: Which to use? *The American Journal of Emergency Medicine*, *36*(4), 707–714. https://doi.org/10.1016/j.ajem.2018.01.008.

Lok, K. Y. W., Bai, D. L., & Tarrant, M. (2017). Family member's infant feeding preferences, maternal breastfeeding exposures and exclusive breastfeeding intentions. *Midwifery*, *53*, 49–54.

Nakamura, M., Asaka, Y., Ogawara, T., & Yorozu, Y. (2018). Nipple skin trauma in breastfeeding women during postpartum week one. *Breastfeeding Medicine*, *13*(7), 479–484.

National Library of Medicine. (2021). Drugs and Lactation Database (LactMed) [Internet]. Bethesda, MD: National Library of Medicine (US); 2006. *Nipple piercing*. [Updated 2021 Jun 21]. Retrieved from https://www.ncbi.nlm.nih.gov/sites/books/NBK500564/. [Accessed September 29, 2021].

Niazi, A., Rahimi, V. B., Soheili-Far, S., et al. (2018). A systemic review of prevention and treatment of nipple pain and fissure: Are they curable? *Journal of Pharmacopuncture*, *21*(3), 139–150.

Patel, S., & Patel, S. (2016). The effectiveness of lactation consultants and lactation counselors on breastfeeding outcomes. *Journal of Human Lactation*, *32*(3), 530–541.

Spencer, J. (2021). Common problems of breastfeeding and weaning. UpToDate [website], S. A. Abrams, J. E. Drutz, & A. G. Hoppin (Eds.). Waltham, MA: UpToDate. Retrieved from https://www.uptodate.com/contents/common-problems-of-breastfeeding-and-weaning?search=common%20problems%20of%20breastfeeding%20and%20weaning&source=search_result&selectedTitle=1~150&usage_type=default&display_rank=1. [Accessed July 12, 2021].

Weisband, Y. L., Keim, S. A., Keder, L. M., Geraghty, S. R., & Gallo, M. F. (2017). Early breast milk pumping intentions among postpartum women. *Breastfeeding Medicine*, *12*(1), 28–32.

Westerfield, K. L., Koenig, K., & Oh, R. (2018). Breastfeeding: Common questions and answers. *American Family Physician*, *98*(6), 368–373.

Risk for Nipple-Areolar Complex Injury

Domain 11 Safety/protection Class 2 Physical injury

Mary Beth Flynn Makic, PhD, RN, CCNS, CCRN-K, FAAN, FNAP, FCNS

NANDA-I

Definition

Susceptible to localized damage to nipple-areolar complex as a result of the breastfeeding process.

Related Factors

Breast engorgement; hardened areola; improper use of milk pump; inadequate latching on; inadequate nipple-areolar preparation during prenatal care; inappropriate maternal hand support of breast; inappropriate positioning of the infant during breastfeeding; inappropriate positioning of the mother during breastfeeding; ineffective infant sucking reflex; ineffective non-nutritive sucking; mastitis; maternal anxiety about breastfeeding; maternal impatience with the breastfeeding process; mother does not wait for the infant to spontaneously release the nipple; mother withdraws infant from breast without breaking the suction; nipple confusion due to use of artificial nipple; postprocedural pain; prolonged exposure to moisture; supplementary feeding; use of products that remove the natural protection of the nipple

At-Risk Population

Primiparous women; sole mother; women aged < 19 years; women breastfeeding for the first time; women with depigmented nipple areolar complex; women with history of nipple trauma in breastfeeding; women with non-protruding nipples; women with pink nipple-areolar complex

Associated Conditions

Ankyloglossia; maxillofacial abnormalities

NOC, NIC, Client Outcomes, Nursing Interventions and *Rationales,* and References

Refer to care plan for Nipple-Areolar Complex **Injury**.

Risk for Urinary Tract Injury Domain 11 Safety/protection Class 2 Physical injury

Tammy Spencer, DNP, RN, CNE, ACNS-BC, CCNS

I

NANDA-I

Definition

Susceptible to damage of the urinary tract structures from use of catheters, which may compromise health.

Risk Factors

Confusion; inadequate caregiver knowledge regarding urinary catheter care; inadequate knowledge regarding urinary catheter care; neurobehavioral manifestations; obesity

At-Risk Population

Individuals at extremes of age

Associated Conditions

Anatomical variation in the pelvic organs; condition preventing ability to secure catheter; detrusor sphincter dyssynergia; latex allergy; long-term use of urinary catheter; medullary injury; prostatic hyperplasia; repetitive catheterizations; retention balloon inflated to ≥30 mL; use of large caliber urinary catheter

NOC (Nursing Outcomes Classification)

Suggested NOC Outcomes

Urinary Elimination; Knowledge: Infection Management; Treatment Regimen; Treatment Procedure, Tissue Integrity: Skin and Mucous Membranes, Risk Control: Infectious Process, Risk Detection

Example NOC Outcome with Indicators

Urinary Elimination as evidenced by the following indicators: Urine clarity/Urine odor, Urine volume, fluid intake, pain with urination. (Rate the outcome and indicators of **Urinary Elimination:** 1 = severely compromised 2 = substantially compromised, 3 = moderately compromised, 4 = mildly compromised, 5 = not compromised [see Section I].)

Client Outcomes

Client Will (Specify Time Frame)

- Remain free of urinary tract injury
- State absence of pain with catheter care and during urination
- Experience unobstructed urination after removal of catheter

- Identify signs and symptoms of urinary obstruction and urinary tract injury after removal of catheter
- Identify interventions to prevent catheter-associated urinary tract infection (CAUTI)
- Maintain adequate urine volume (0.5–1.0 mL/kg/h for adult); urine without odor; urine clear
- Maintain adequate fluid intake considering client age and comorbidities

NIC (Nursing Interventions Classification)

Suggested NIC Intervention

Urinary Elimination Management

Example NIC Activities—Urinary Elimination Management

Monitor urinary elimination, including frequency, consistency, odor, volume, and color, as appropriate; Assess client for pain and increased temperature associated with catheter

Nursing Interventions and *Rationales*

I

- Monitor urinary elimination, including frequency, consistency, odor, volume, and color, as appropriate.
- Teach the client and caregiver signs and symptoms of urinary tract infection and CAUTI. EB: *Clients may be asymptomatic or have a range of symptoms that may include a persistent and frequent urge to urinate, burning or painful sensation during urination, cloudy and/or strong-smelling urine, blood-tinged urine, fever, flank pain, suprapubic tenderness, delirium, inability to perform activities of daily living, and fatigue (Blodgett et al, 2015; Gbinigie et al, 2018).*
- Assess for appropriate use of an indwelling urinary catheter. Insert urinary catheters only when indicated and leave in only as long as clinically necessary. EB: *To prevent trauma to the urinary tract structure, as well as infections (e.g., CAUTI and urosepsis), use urinary catheters only as indicated (Gould et al, 2019; Kranz et al, 2020). Approximately 80% of all health care–associated urinary tract infections are caused by urinary catheterization; infection represents the most significant adverse event following urinary catheter use (Gould et al, 2019). CAUTIs are linked to increased mortality, morbidity, hospital cost, antibiotic use, and length of stay (Gould et al, 2019). Health care providers need to have written guidelines for the use, insertion, and maintenance of urinary catheters (Agency for Healthcare Research and Quality [AHRQ], 2015; Saint et al, 2016).*
- To prevent injury, educate the client and family and/or caregiver regarding the use of an indwelling urinary catheter (AHRQ, 2015; Mody et al, 2017). EB: *Accidental or improper removal of catheter can cause urethral injury. Urinary catheters are used in up to 16% of adult hospital inpatients (Gould et al, 2019).*
- Assess clinical indications for urinary catheter use daily. EB: *It is important for providers to understand the appropriate and inappropriate indications for use of urinary catheters to decrease the risk of CAUTI (Meddings et al, 2015; Gould et al, 2019). Minimize urinary catheter use in all clients, especially those at risk for CAUTIs such as women, the elderly, and immunocompromised clients (Gould et al, 2019; Kranz et al, 2020). Urinary catheter use is inappropriate in several client situations, including when used as a substitute for nursing care of the incontinent client, when obtaining a urine culture for the client who can void, and for prolonged periods after surgery without appropriate indications (AHRQ, 2015; Meddings et al, 2015). There is a 3% to 7% daily risk of bacteriuria when an indwelling urinary catheter remains in place (Gould et al, 2019). Decreasing the number of days the catheter is in place and avoiding unnecessary catheterization are the primary interventions to decrease CAUTI and unintended client harm (Meddings et al, 2015; Kranz et al, 2020).*
- To avoid catheterizations, evaluate alternative strategies for managing urine output for the client. EB: *Using alternative strategies decreases the risk for infection and immobility complications (AHRQ, 2015). Developing toileting schedules and scheduled nursing staff rounding can reduce urgency and incontinence episodes (Meddings et al, 2015; Saint et al, 2016). Consider using external catheters, straight catheters, bedside commode, incontinent garments, barrier creams, or intermittent catheterization in appropriate clients (AHRQ, 2015; Meddings et al, 2015). Use bladder scanner to assess for urinary retention before inserting urinary catheter (Meddings et al, 2015; Gould et al, 2019).*
- If an indwelling urinary catheter is determined to be clinically indicated in the care of a client, proper selection of the right catheter, technique during insertion, and evidence-based care management are needed to reduce infection and injury to the urinary tract structures.
  - Perform hand hygiene and use Standard Precautions before and after insertion of the urinary catheter and any time the catheter, catheter site, or collection system is accessed (AHRQ, 2015; Gould et al, 2019).

- ❍ Ensure that only properly trained personnel familiar with appropriate catheter care techniques are used for inserting and maintaining the catheter (AHRQ, 2015; Gould et al, 2019). EB: *Periodic in-service training helps personnel to maintain proper catheter care techniques (Gould et al, 2019; Narula et al, 2019).*
- Selecting the smallest catheter size (e.g., smaller than 18 French) reduces irritation and inflammation of the urethra and reduces infection risk (Gould et al, 2019).
- Insert the catheter using aseptic technique in the acute care setting. Wash hands and use sterile technique when opening the catheterization kit and cleansing the urethral meatus and perineal area with an antiseptic solution. Insert the catheter using a no-touch technique (AHRQ, 2015; Gould et al, 2019). EB: *In the nonacute care setting, nonsterile technique may be used for intermittent catheterization (Gould et al, 2019). Using a no-touch technique may reduce the risk of infection.*
- If a urine sample is needed from the urinary collection system sampling port, disinfect the sampling port and allow disinfectant to dry before accessing the port. EB: *Disinfecting the sampling port decreases the introduction of pathogens into the urinary collection system (AHRQ, 2015).*
- Provide routine hygiene care; once a urinary catheter is placed, optimal management includes care of the urethral meatus according to "routine hygiene" (e.g., daily cleansing of the meatal surface during bathing with soap and water and as needed, such as following a bowel movement) (AHRQ, 2015; Gould et al, 2019). EB: *In recent studies, no definitive method has been found for cleaning or disinfecting the external urethral orifice (Kranz et al, 2020). Do not clean the periurethral area with antiseptics while the catheter is in place (Gould et al, 2019).*
- Secure the catheter after placement to reduce friction and pain from movement *(Gould et al, 2019; Kranz et al, 2020).*
  - ❍ Disruptions in aseptic technique, disconnection, or leakage require the catheter and collection system to be replaced using aseptic technique and sterile equipment (AHRQ, 2015; Gould et al, 2019). EB: *Risk factors for CAUTI include not maintaining a closed drainage system (Gould et al, 2019).*
  - ❍ Maintain unobstructed urine flow; maintain the catheter and collecting tube below the level of the bladder and free of kinks. Do not rest the collection bag on the floor. EB: *Keeping the collection bag off the floor prevents contamination. Maintaining the urine collection bag below the level of the bladder and the catheter without kinks minimizes reflux into the catheter itself, preventing retrograde flow of urine and risk for infection (AHRQ, 2015; Gould et al, 2019).*
- Establish workflow protocols to routinely empty the drainage bag frequently and before transport to reduce urine reflux and opportunities for infection. EB: *Use a separate, clean collecting container for each client when emptying the collection bag; avoid splashing, and prevent contact of the drainage spout with a nonsterile container (AHRQ, 2015; Gould et al, 2019). The collection bag of a bacteriuric client is a reservoir for organisms that may be transmitted by the hands of health care personnel to other clients (AHRQ, 2015).*
- Change urinary catheters and drainage systems based on clinical indications such as infection, obstruction, or when the drainage system is not adequately maintained. EB: *Changing indwelling catheters or drainage bags at a routine time interval is not recommended because it opens a closed drainage system and predisposes the client to infection (AHRQ, 2015; Gould et al, 2019).*
- Monitor the client with an indwelling urinary catheter for increased temperature (>38°C; 100.4°F), suprapubic pain, frequency, urgency, and flank pain; monitor the skin around the catheter for redness, drainage, or swelling. EB: *The most common clinical presentation for CAUTI is fever with a positive urine culture (Lo et al, 2014).* EB: *Monitor the client for CAUTI symptoms caused by localized or systemic inflammatory response (Blodgett et al, 2015; Gbinigie et al, 2018).*
- Consider an ultrasound scanner for clients who require intermittent catheterization to assess urine volume and reduce unnecessary catheter insertion (Gould et al, 2019; Meddings et al, 2015).

▲ Implement systemwide quality improvement programs, including the following interventions to decrease CAUTI:
  - ❍ Establish health care provider alerts or reminders for all clients with catheters regarding the need for continued catheterization. EB/EBN: *Health care providers frequently forget that the catheter is in place, increasing the risk for CAUTI. Studies have shown that the rate of CAUTI was decreased with the use of daily checklists, catheter reminders, developing competencies for providers, and stop orders (Saint et al, 2016; Narula et al, 2019).*
  - ❍ Provide performance feedback and education to personnel responsible for catheter care (Gould et al, 2019; Mody et al, 2017). EB: *Implementing safety teams; engaging family, organizational leadership, and staff; and setting goals can decrease CAUTI (Mody et al, 2017).*

I

- ❍ Establish evidence-based "bladder bundles" as part of a multimodal approach to preventing CAUTI. "Bladder bundles" may include educational interventions aimed at health care providers for appropriate use of urinary catheters, use of appropriately trained personnel to insert and care for the catheter, catheter restriction and removal protocols, and the use of bladder ultrasound to assess urine volume (Saint et al, 2016; Mody et al, 2017). **EB/EBN:** *Evidence-based "bundles" of interventions, when implemented simultaneously, decrease the risk of CAUTI (AHRQ, 2015; Durant, 2017; Gould et al, 2019).*

Home Care and Client/Family Teaching and Discharge Planning

- Teach the client and family discharged with an indwelling urinary catheter or performing intermittent catheterization at home techniques for care of urinary catheter and collection bag using the interventions listed above (AHRQ, 2015).
- Ensure client has adequate supplies at home for catheter insertion and care.
- Teach the client and family to contact the health care provider regarding symptoms of CAUTI, including increased temperature (>38°C; 104°F), suprapubic pain, frequency, urgency, and flank pain; no drainage of urine in the collection bag; inability to perform activities of daily living; delirium; and foul-smelling, cloudy, or bloody urine (Blodgett et al, 2015; Gbinigie et al, 2018; Shah, 2019).
- Teach client and family to monitor for signs of obstruction such as decreased urine output after catheter is removed.

REFERENCES

Agency for Healthcare Research and Quality (AHRQ). (2015). *Toolkit for reducing catheter-associated urinary tract infections in hospital units: Implementation guide.* AHRQ Pub No. 15-0013-2-EF. Retrieved from https://www.ahrq.gov/hai/cauti-tools/impl-guide/index.html. Accessed 12 July 2021.

Blodgett, T. J., Gardner, S. E., Blodgett, N. P., Peterson, L. V., & Pietraszak, M. (2015). A tool to assess the signs and symptoms of catheter associated urinary tract infection: Development and reliability. *Clinical Nursing Research, 24*(4), 341–356.

Durant, D. J. (2017). Nurse driven protocols and the prevention of CAUTI: A systematic review. *American Journal of Infection Control, 45*(12), 1331–1341.

Gbinigie, O. A., Ordóñez-Mena, J. M., Fanshawe, T. R., Plüddemann, A., & Heneghan, C. (2018). Diagnostic value of symptoms and signs for identifying urinary tract infection in older adult outpatients: Systematic review and meta-analysis. *Journal of Infection, 77*(5), 379–390.

Gould, C. V., Umscheid, C. A., Agarwal, R. K., Kuntz, G., Pegues, D. A., & Healthcare Infection Control Practices Advisory Committee. (2019). *Guideline for prevention of catheter-associated urinary tract infections 2009.* Retrieved from https://www.cdc.gov/infectioncontrol/guidelines/cauti/. Accessed 12 July 2021.

Kranz, J., Schmidt, S., Wagenlehner, F., & Schneidewind, L. (2020). Catheter associated urinary tract infections in adult patients. *Deutsches Aerzteblatt International, 117*(6), 83–88.

Lo, E., Nicolle, L. E., Coffin, S. E., et al. (2014). Strategies to prevent catheter-associated urinary tract infections in acute care hospitals: 2014 update. *Infection Control and Hospital Epidemiology, 35*(Suppl. 2), S32–S47. https://doi.org/10.1086/675718.

Meddings, J., Saint, S., Fowler, K. E., et al. (2015). The Ann Arbor criteria for appropriate urinary catheter use in hospitalized medical patients: Results obtained by using the RAND/UCLA Appropriateness method. *Annals of Internal Medicine, 162*(Suppl. 9), S1–S34.

Mody, L., Greene, M. T., Meddings, J., et al. (2017). A national implementation project to prevent catheter-associated urinary tract infection in nursing home residents. *JAMA Internal Medicine, 177*(8), 1154–1162.

Narula, N., Lillemoe, H. A., Caudle, A. S., et al. (2019). Postoperative urinary tract infection quality assessment and improvement: The S.T.O.P. UTI program and its impact on hospitalwide CAUTI rates. *Joint Commission Journal on Quality and Patient Safety, 45*(10), 686–693.

Saint, S., Greene, M. T., Krein, S. L., et al. (2016). A program to prevent catheter-associated urinary tract infection in acute care. *New England Journal of Medicine, 374*(22), 2111–2119.

Shah, S. M. (2019). *Indwelling catheter care.* Medline Plus [website]. Retrieved from https://medlineplus.gov/ency/patientinstructions/000140.htm. Accessed 12 July 2021.

Insomnia **Domain 4 Activity/rest Class 1 Sleep/rest**

Judith Ann Floyd, PhD, RN, FNAP, FAAN

NANDA-I

Definition

Inability to initiate or maintain sleep, which impairs functioning.

Defining Characteristics

Altered affect; altered attention; altered mood; early awakening; expresses dissatisfaction with quality of life; expresses dissatisfaction with sleep; expresses forgetfulness; expresses need for frequent naps during the day; impaired health status; increased absenteeism; increased accidents; insufficient physical endurance; nonrestorative sleep-wake cycle

Related Factors

Anxiety; average daily physical activity is less than recommended for age and gender; caffeine consumption; caregiver role strain; consumption of sugar-sweetened beverages; depressive symptoms; discomfort; dysfunctional sleep beliefs; environmental disturbances; fear; frequent naps during the day; inadequate sleep hygiene; lifestyle incongruent with normal circadian rhythms; low psychological resilience; obesity; stressors; substance misuse; use of interactive electronic devices

At-Risk Population

Adolescents; economically disadvantaged individuals; grieving individuals; individuals undergoing changes in marital status; night shift workers; older adults; pregnant women in third trimester; rotating shift workers; women

Associated Conditions

Chronic disease; hormonal change; pharmaceutical preparations

NOC (Nursing Outcomes Classification)

Suggested NOC Outcomes

Comfort Level; Pain Level; Personal Well-Being; Psychosocial Adjustment: Life Change; Quality of Life; Rest; Sleep

Example NOC Outcome with Indicators

Sleep as evidenced by the following indicators: Hours of sleep/Sleep pattern/Sleep quality/Sleep efficiency/Feels rejuvenated after sleep/Sleeps consistently through the night. (Rate the outcome and indicators of **Sleep:** 1 = severely compromised, 2 = substantially compromised, 3 = moderately compromised, 4 = mildly compromised, 5 = not compromised [see Section I].)

Client Outcomes

Client Will (Specify Time Frame)

- Verbalize plan to implement sleep-promoting routines
- Fall asleep with less difficulty a minimum of four nights out of seven
- Wake up less frequently during night a minimum of four nights out of seven
- Sleep a minimum of 6 hours most nights and more if needed to meet next stated outcome
- Awaken refreshed and not be fatigued during day most of the time

NIC (Nursing Interventions Classification)

Suggested NIC Intervention

Sleep Enhancement

Example NIC Activities—Sleep Enhancement

Monitor/record client's sleep pattern and number of sleep hours; Encourage client to establish a bedtime routine to facilitate transition from wakefulness to sleep

Nursing Interventions and *Rationales*

- Obtain a sleep history including amount of time needed to initiate sleep, duration of any awakenings after sleep onset, total nighttime sleep amounts, and dissatisfaction with daytime energy levels and alertness. EB: *Inability to drift off to sleep at bedtime or during the night if awakened can lead to short sleep and poor daytime functioning, as well as negatively affect physical and mental health (Khurshid, 2015).*
- From the history, assess client's current ability to initiate and maintain sleep and the short-term versus chronic nature of inability to initiate and maintain sleep. EB: *Adults can be considered to have insomnia*

if they report daytime tiredness or sleepiness due to shortened nighttime sleep three or more nights per week. Insomnia is considered chronic if the inability to initiate and/or maintain sleep continues beyond 3 months (Khurshid, 2015).

For Short-Term Insomnia

- For clients historically able to initiate and maintain sleep but unable to do so in the current situation: (1) minimize sleep disruptions (see Nursing Interventions and *Rationales* for Disturbed **Sleep** Pattern) and (2) promote sleep hygiene practices (see Nursing Interventions and *Rationales* for Readiness for Enhanced **Sleep**). EB: *Inability to initiate and maintain sleep is common in new sleep environments, especially during times of stress or worry (Honkavuo, 2018).*
- Also attend to the following factors often associated with short-term insomnia:
  - ❍ Assess pain medication use and, when feasible, advocate for pain medications that promote rather than interfere with sleep. (See Nursing Interventions and *Rationales* for Acute **Pain** and Chronic **Pain.**) EB: *Some pain medications also promote sleep, whereas others promote alertness and thus interfere with falling and staying asleep (Dean et al, 2017; Tan et al, 2019).*
  - ❍ Assess level of tension and encourage use of relaxation techniques as needed. EBN: *A review of evidence from nine intervention studies suggested that relaxation, meditation, guided imagery, or combinations of these strategies resulted in better sleep and less fatigue in heart-failure clients (Kwekkeboom & Bratzke, 2016).* EBN: *A clinical pilot study (n = 12) found that client-controlled relaxation and/or imagery interventions may improve sleep for hospitalized clients (Nooner et al, 2016).*
  - ❍ Assess level of distress and use therapeutic communication to increase comfort. (See further Nursing Interventions and *Rationales* for Readiness for Enhanced **Comfort.**) CEB: *A qualitative study of 10 clients' experiences with sleep during hospitalization identified several themes that promote clients' comfort, increase clients' ability to initiate and maintain sleep, and support the nurse's ability to co-create a safe sleep environment with the client (Gellerstedt et al, 2014).* EBN: *A qualitative study of how experienced nurses promote sleep in hospitals (n = 8) identified caring conversation as one of four sleep-promoting nursing strategies (Salzmann-Erikson et al, 2016).*
- ▲ Assess for signs of overactive bladder. CEB: *A descriptive study (n = 24) found that subjects with overactive bladder syndrome (OAB), but no formal insomnia diagnosis, awakened during sleep as often as insomniacs; however, waking durations were shorter in OAB subjects than those with diagnosed insomnia (Preud'homme et al, 2013).* EB: *Among 51 subjects diagnosed with OAB, incontinence and OAB symptoms were associated with sleep disturbance and daytime fatigue (Ge et al, 2017).*

For Chronic Insomnia

- ▲ Rule out and/or address any disorders and syndromes associated with chronic insomnia (e.g., addiction to alcohol or other psychoactive substances, anxiety and depressive disorders, chronic pain syndrome, or other sleep disorders). EB: *Coexisting medical conditions, mental disorders, and sleep disorders are interactive and bidirectional (Khurshid, 2015).*
- Monitor for uncomfortable sensations in legs and involuntary leg movements during sleep. CEB: *In a sleep laboratory study of urban, community-based participants (n = 592), symptoms of insomnia were significantly higher in individuals with periodic limb movements during sleep (PLMS), although African Americans were less likely to have elevated PLMS than other participants (Scofield et al, 2008).*
- Be aware that clients diagnosed with chronic insomnia may have a low pain threshold. CEB: *In a laboratory study (n = 34), subjects with shortened sleep caused by chronic insomnia were twice as likely to report experiencing spontaneous pain as healthy controls with no sleep loss; they also had lower pain thresholds during applications of heat and pressure than healthy controls (Haack et al, 2012).*
- Encourage use of the following stimulus control strategies in addition to any relaxation and sleep hygiene interventions recommended for short-term insomnia that the client finds helpful; (1) if feasible, have client arise from bed to participate in calming activities whenever anxious about failure to fall asleep; (2) if not feasible for client to get out of bed when unable to sleep, encourage sitting up in bed to engage in calming activities or simply resting in bed without attempting to fall asleep; (3) avoid a focus on what time it is and subsequent worry about amount of sleep time lost to sleeplessness; and (4) distract from sleeplessness with a focus on positive aspects of life. EB: *A meta-analysis of 37 comparative effectiveness studies found medium to large improvements in the ability to initiate and maintain sleep when a combination of stimulus control, relaxation, and sleep hygiene strategies was used to treat insomnia in clients with comorbid medical and psychiatric conditions (Wu et al, 2015).*

- Consider use of warm foot baths. EBN: *A review of evidence from 31 papers found that passive body heating via foot baths often relaxed and improved quality of sleep in insomnia clients (Talebi et al, 2016).*
- For clients whose chronic inability to initiate and maintain sleep has led to sleep deprivation, see Nursing Interventions and *Rationales* for **Sleep** Deprivation.
- For clients with unremitting chronic insomnia, refer to a nurse practitioner trained in cognitive behavioral therapies for insomnia (CBT-I). EB: *A meta-analysis of 37 comparative effectiveness studies found chronic insomnia clients with comorbid medical and psychiatric conditions improved their ability to initiate and maintain sleep after completion of multicomponent CBT-I programs (Wu et al, 2015).*
- Assist clients diagnosed with chronic insomnia who have been treated with CBT-I to limit use of sleeping medications and to select intermittent nights for sleeping pill use if complete discontinuance of sleeping pills is not feasible. EB: *An updated review of evidence supported the ability of clients treated with CBT-I to reduce or even eliminate their dependence on sleeping pills (Winkelman, Benca, & Eichler, 2021).*
- Supplement other interventions with teaching about sleep and sleep promotion. (See further Nursing Interventions and Rationales for Readiness for Enhanced **Sleep.**)

Geriatric

- Most interventions discussed above may be used with geriatric clients. In addition, see the Geriatric section of Nursing Interventions and *Rationales* for (1) Readiness for Enhanced **Sleep** and (2) Disturbed **Sleep**, and **Sleep** Deprivation.
- Note that it is especially helpful for the elderly client with short-term or chronic insomnia to engage in routine exercise unless contraindicated by health status. EB: *In an evidence review of 34 research reports, exercise increased sleep efficiency and duration in healthy older adults regardless of the mode and intensity of activity, and even more so in the elderly with sleep disorders (Dolezal et al, 2017).*

I

Home Care

- Assessments and interventions discussed previously can all be adapted for use in home care.
- In addition, see the Home Care section of Nursing Interventions and *Rationales* for Readiness for Enhanced **Sleep.**

Client/Family Teaching

- Teach family about normal sleep and promote adoption of behaviors that enhance it. See Nursing Interventions and *Rationales* for Readiness for Enhanced **Sleep.**
- Teach family about sleep deprivation and how to avoid it. See Nursing Interventions and *Rationales* for **Sleep** Deprivation.
- Advise family of importance of not disrupting sleep of others unnecessarily. See Nursing Interventions and *Rationales* for Disturbed **Sleep** Pattern.
- Advise family about the importance of minimizing noise and light, including light from electronic devices, in the sleep environment. See Nursing Interventions and *Rationales* for Disturbed **Sleep** Pattern.
- Help family members understand the difference between the two major precursors of sleep deprivation, that is, insomnia versus externally caused sleep disruptions. EB: *Insomnia is defined as persistent difficulty with sleep initiation, duration, consolidation, or quality—that occurs despite adequate opportunity and circumstances for sleep—and results in daytime impairment (Tan et al, 2019).*

REFERENCES

Dean, G. E., Weiss, C., Morris, J. L., & Chasens, E. R. (2017). Impaired sleep: A multifaceted geriatric syndrome. *Nursing Clinics of North America, 5*(2 Suppl. 3), 387–404. https://doi.org/10.1016/j.cnur.2017.04.009.

Dolezal, B. A., Neufeld, E. V., Boland, D. M., Martin, J. L., & Cooper, C. B. (2017). Interrelationship between sleep and exercise: A systematic review. *Advances in Preventive Medicine, 2017*, 1364387. https://doi.org/10.1155/2017/1364387.

Ge, T. J., Vetter, J., & Lai, H. H. (2017). Sleep disturbance and fatigue are associated with more severe urinary incontinence and overactive bladder symptoms. *Urology, 109*, 67–73. https://doi.org/10.1016/j.urology.2017.07.039 67 0090-4295.

Gellerstedt, L., Medin, J., & Karlsson, M. R. (2014). Patients' experiences of sleep in hospital: A qualitative interview study. *Journal of Research in Nursing, 19*(3), 176–188. https://doi.org/10.1177/1744987113490415.

Haack, M., Scott-Sutherland, J., Santangelo, G., Simpson, N. S., Sethna, N., & Mullington, J. M. (2012). Pain sensitivity and modulation in primary insomnia. *European Journal of Pain, 16*(4), 522–533. https://doi.org/10.1016/j.ejpain.2011.07.007.

Honkavuo, L. (2018). Nurses' experiences of supporting sleep in hospitals—a hermeneutical study. *International Journal of Caring Sciences, 11*(1), 4–11. Retrieved from www.internationaljournalofcaringsciences.org.

Khurshid, K. A. (2015). A review of changes in DSM-5 sleep-wake disorders. *Psychiatric Times, 32*(9), 1–3. https://doi.org/10.1016/j.patbio.2014.07.002.

Kwekkeboom, K. L., & Bratzke, L. C. (2016). A systematic review of relaxation, meditation, and guided imagery strategies for symptom management in heart failure. *Journal of Cardiovascular Nursing, 31*(5), 457–468. https://doi.org/10.1097/JCN.0000000000000274.

Nooner, A. K., Dwyer, K., DeShea, L., & Yeo, T. P. (2016). Using relaxation and guided imagery to address pain, fatigue, and sleep disturbances: A pilot study. *Clinical Journal of Oncology Nursing, 20*(5), 547–552. https://doi.org/10.1188/16.CJON.547-552.

Preud'homme, X. A., Amundsen, C. L., Webster, G. D., & Krystal, A. D. (2013). Comparison of diary-derived bladder and sleep measurements across OAB individuals, primary insomniacs, and healthy controls. *International Urogynecological Journal, 24*(3), 501–508. https://doi.org/10.1007/s00192-012-1890-0.

Salzmann-Erikson, M., Lagerqvist, L., & Pousette, S. (2016). Keep calm and have a good night: Nurses' strategies to promote inpatients' sleep in the hospital environment. *Scandinavian Journal of Caring Science, 30*(2), 356–364. https://doi.org/doi:10.1111/scs.12255.

Scofield, H., Roth, T., & Drake, C. (2008). Periodic limb movements during sleep: Population prevalence, clinical correlates, and racial differences. *Sleep, 31*(9), 1221–1227. Retrieved from https://www.ncbi.nlm.nih.gov/pmc/articles/PMC2542977/.

Talebi, H., Heydari-Gorji, M. A., & Hadinejad, Z. (2016). The impact of passive body heating on quality of sleep: A review study. *Journal of Sleep Science, 1*(4), 176–181. Retrieved from https://jss.tums.ac.ir/index.php/jss/article/view/39.

Tan, X., van Egmond, L., Partinen, M., Lange, T., & Benedict, C. (2019). A narrative review of interventions for improving sleep and reducing circadian disruption in medical inpatients. *Sleep Medicine, 59*, 42–50. https://doi.org/10.1016/j.sleep.2018.08.007.

Winkelman, J. W., Benca, R., & Eichler, A. F. (2021). *Overview of the treatment of insomnia in adults*. UpToDate. Topic 97867, version 16.0. Retrieved from https://www-uptodate-com.proxy.hsl.ucdenver.edu/contents/overview-of-the-treatment-of-insomnia-in-adults.

Wu, J. Q., Appleman, E. R., Salazar, R. D., & Ong, J. C. (2015). Cognitive behavioral therapy for insomnia co-morbid with psychiatric and medical conditions: A meta-analysis. *JAMA Internal Medicine, 175*(9), 1461–1472. https://doi.org/10.1001/jamainternmed.2015.3006.

Deficient Knowledge **Domain 5 Perception/cognition Class 4 Cognition**

Lauren McAlister, MSN, FNP-BC, DNP and Kathaleen C. Bloom, PhD, CNM

K

NANDA-I

Definition

Absence of cognitive information related to a specific topic, or its acquisition.

Defining Characteristics

Inaccurate follow-through of instruction; inaccurate performance on a test; inaccurate statements about a topic; inappropriate behavior

Related Factors

Anxiety; depressive symptoms; inadequate access to resources; inadequate awareness of resources; inadequate commitment to learning; inadequate information; inadequate interest in learning; inadequate knowledge of resources; inadequate participation in care planning; inadequate trust in health care professional; low self efficacy; misinformation; neurobehavioral manifestations

At-Risk Population

Economically disadvantaged individuals; illiterate individuals; individuals with low educational level

Associated Conditions

Depression; developmental disabilities; neurocognitive disorders

NOC (Nursing Outcomes Classification)

Suggested NOC Outcomes

Knowledge: Disease Process; Energy Conservation; Health Behavior; Health Resources; Healthy Diet; Infection Management; Medication; Personal Safety; Prescribed Activity; Substance Use Control; Treatment Procedure(s); Treatment Regimen

Example NOC Outcome with Indicators

Knowledge: Health Behavior as evidenced by the following indicators: Healthy nutritional practices/Benefits of regular exercise/Safe use of prescribed and nonprescribed medication. (Rate the outcome and indicators of **Knowledge: Health Behavior:** 1 = no knowledge, 2 = limited knowledge, 3 = moderate knowledge, 4 = substantial knowledge, 5 = extensive knowledge [see Section I].)

Client Outcomes

Client Will (Specify Time Frame)

- Explain disease state, recognize need for medications, and understand treatments
- Describe the rationale for therapy/treatment options
- Incorporate knowledge of health regimen into lifestyle
- State confidence in one's ability to manage health situation and remain in control of life
- Demonstrate how to perform health-related procedure(s) satisfactorily
- Identify resources that can be used for more information or support after discharge

NIC (Nursing Interventions Classification)

Suggested NIC Interventions

Teaching: Disease Process, Individual; Learning Facilitation

Example NIC Activities—Teaching: Disease Process

Discuss therapy/treatment options; Describe rationale behind management/therapy/treatment recommendations

Nursing Interventions and Rationales

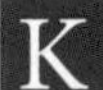

- Health care providers who are nonjudgmental and supportive can assist clients to be involved in planning individual intervention strategies that can increase compliance. EBN: *Health care providers need to improve their therapeutic relationships and compliance and address not only clients' assessment needs but also their health beliefs, their lifestyle and social networks, and their individualism (Chitambira, 2019).*
- Consider the health literacy and the readiness to learn for all clients and caregivers (e.g., mental acuity, ability to see or hear, existing pain, emotional readiness, motivation, previous knowledge). EBN: *A systematic review by McCleary-Jones (2016) discussed the importance of nursing curricula to include information on health literacy to enhance new nurses' awareness that clients' limited health literacy can have an effect on client outcomes, and therefore strategies would be used to make sure they know if their clients are understanding and if they are providing appropriate information for their clients (McCleary-Jones, 2016).* EBN: *A study looking at a new tool, the Newest Vital Sign (NVS), was used to measure clients' health literacy. Findings showed that this tool is efficient to administer and could help identify low health literacy clients (McCune, Lee, & Pohl, 2016).*
- Focus on the nature of spoken and written communication when teaching clients and caregivers, especially those who may have health literacy needs. EBN: *A recent study by Hommes et al (2018) focused on the importance of improving health care and health promotion for the deaf community by improving communication, health literacy, and client empowerment by holding health care staff and organizations accountable for ensuring adequate staffing of ASL interpreters and communication resources in order to reduce health disparities.* EBN: *A qualitative study explored the relationship between health literacy and effective communication. One of the overarching themes was that building trust and relationships with the older adults to achieve effective communication can then be applied to meet the individual health literacy needs of the client (Brooks et al, 2017).*
- Consider the context, timing, and order of how information is presented. EBN: *The ability to personalize written health information to reinforce key health messages, instructions, medication information, or discharge instructions for clients has been shown to be an effective way to improve the knowledge of the consumer (Johnson, 2016).*
- Use person-centered approaches that engage clients and caregivers as active versus passive learners. EBN: *In a study by Rushton et al (2017), the reduction of hospital readmission in postoperative clients with complications during a recovery period after coronary artery bypass graft can be decreased by using person-centered education with individualized education programs to meet each individual client's needs.*
- Reinforce learning through frequent repetition and follow-up sessions. EBN: *In a qualitative study with semistructured interviews, it was discovered that clients who were in the intensive care unit (ICU) and who attended a follow-up session were better able to process their feelings and emotions. The findings from this*

study supported the hypothesis that the follow-up session for an ICU client can aid in processing the illness after the fact (Haraldsson et al, 2015).

- Use electronic methods for delivery of information when appropriate. **EBN:** *A recent study by Wang et al (2020) concluded that the use of smart phones as a clinical platform for diabetes nurses for educational purposes can be an effective way to provide personalized coaching and care to clients remotely.*
- Help the client and caregivers locate appropriate postdischarge groups and resources. **EBN:** *A systematic review concluded that the use of postdischarge support for clients with chronic obstructive pulmonary disease (COPD) significantly reduced the readmission rates within 30 days and had an effect up to 180 days (Pedersen et al, 2017).*
- Encourage clients and caregivers to maintain and/or expand supportive social networks as self-care learning resources when appropriate. **CEB:** *In a longitudinal study of 300 clients with long-term chronic health conditions, those who had sustained or expanded community networks were more likely to sustain self-care management, maintain behavioral change and treatment regimens, and access voluntary caregiving over formal caregiving (Reeves et al, 2014).*

Pediatric

- Use family-centered approaches when teaching children and adolescents. **EBN:** *According to Manente et al (2017), when families are educated about the client and know what to expect during the transition out of the ICU, their fears and anxieties are decreased, which can promote healing for the client.*
- Guide children and adolescents to credible information about their condition. **EBN:** *A mixed methods study showed that the best way to inform adolescents about HIV and sexual/reproductive health is via radio, television, mass media, and social media (Adams et al, 2017).*

K

Geriatric

✱ Educate all older clients on safety issues, including fall prevention and medication management. **CEB:** *In a meta-analysis of 19 studies, clients receiving targeted fall prevention education face to face or through multimedia methods had decrease in falls from those either receiving no formal education or written education (Lee et al, 2014).*

- Use multiprofessional teams to enhance client education. **EBN:** *A qualitative study exploring medication management in people with dementia showed potential positive benefits of a community pharmacist working in a multiprofessional environment outside the pharmacy and can improve medication management (Maidment et al, 2017).*
- Consider using teaching methods and materials appropriate for older adults, especially those with cognitive challenges. **EBN:** *A study concluded that screening for cognitive impairment in the elderly population and including the family and caregivers in the discharge education has the potential to minimize the risk of readmission (Agarwal et al, 2016).*
- Assess readiness of older adults for use of technological resources. **EBN:** *In a descriptive study, the utilization of technology for the aging population solely depended on the ease of use, affordability, and convenience, and barriers included a breach in privacy or security (Depatie & Bigbee, 2015).*

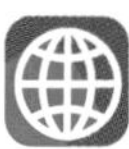

Multicultural

- Use educational interventions that are culturally tailored to the health literacy needs of the client. **CEB:** *A Cochrane review of 33 randomized controlled trials focusing on diabetes type 2 found that culturally appropriate health education improved blood sugar control among participants, compared with those receiving the "usual" care, at 3, 6, 12, and 24 months after the intervention (Attridge et al, 2014).*
- Assess for cultural/ethnic self-care practices. **EB:** *The use of simulated clients can be an effective way to help foster cultural competence in nursing education. It can allow nurses to learn how to improve their knowledge, skills, and attitudes with regard to providing culturally congruent nursing care (Ozkara San, 2020).*
- Consider the potential influence of medical interpreters in information sharing and decision-making and of the possible difficulties for clients when using medical interpreters. **EBN:** *The use of medical interpreters can help bridge the culture and language gap, allowing clients to feel more comfortable expressing themselves (Rorie, 2015).*
- Consider involving bilingual members of a community who are considered outside the traditional health care system who may assist in the teaching of community health issues. **EBN:** *A cross-sectional design study examined challenges associated with migrant and English-speaking cancer clients and found that the*

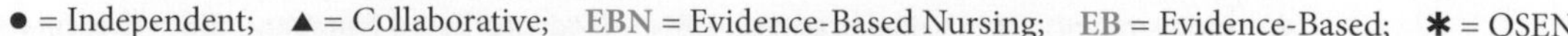
● = Independent; ▲ = Collaborative; EBN = Evidence-Based Nursing; EB = Evidence-Based; ✱ = QSEN

majority of participants in all migrant groups reported difficulty communicating with the health care providers and team in English (Hyatt et al, 2017).

Home Care

- All of the previously mentioned interventions are applicable to the home setting.
- Use telehealth and technology-enhanced practices as appropriate. EBN: *A review of 11 studies looking at the role of telehealth in diabetic foot ulcer management found that telehealth was well received by clients and providers; assessments via the telehealth modalities were congruent with face-to-face assessment (Singh et al, 2016).*

REFERENCES

Adams, R. M., Riess, H., Massey, P. M., et al. (2017). Understanding where and why Senegalese adolescents and young adults access health information: A mixed methods study examining contextual and personal influences on health information seeking. *Journal of Communication in Healthcare, 10*(2), 116–148. https://doi.org/10.1080/17538068.2017.1313627.

Agarwal, K. S., Kazim, R., Xu, J., Borson, S., & Taffet, G. E. (2016). Unrecognized cognitive impairment and its effect on heart failure readmissions of elderly adults. *Journal of the American Geriatrics Society, 64*(11), 2296–2301. https://doi.org/10.1111/jgs.14471.

Attridge, M., Creamer, J., Ramsden, M., Cannings-John, R., & Hawthorne, K. (2014). Culturally appropriate health education for people in ethnic minority groups with type 2 diabetes mellitus. *Cochrane Database of Systematic Reviews, 9*, CD006424. https://doi.org/10.1002/14651858.CD006424.pub3.

Brooks, C., Ballinger, C., Nutbeam, D., & Adams, J. (2017). The importance of building trust and tailoring interactions when meeting older adults' health literacy needs. *Disability & Rehabilitation, 39*(23), 2428–2435. https://doi.org/10.1080/09638288.2016.1231849.

Chitambira, F. (2019). Patient perspectives: Explaining low rates of compliance to compression therapy. *Wound Practice & Research, 27*(4), 168–174. https://doi.org/10.33235/wpr.27.4.168-174.

Depatie, A., & Bigbee, J. L. (2015). Rural older adult readiness to adopt mobile health technology: A descriptive study. *Online Journal of Rural Nursing and Health Care, 15*(1), 150–184. https://doi.org/10.14574/ojrnhc.v15i1.346.

Haraldsson, L., Christensson, L., Conlon, L., & Henricson, M. (2015). The experiences of ICU patients during follow up sessions—a qualitative study. *Intensive and Critical Care Nursing, 31*(4), 223–231. https://doi.org/10.1016/j.iccn.2015.01.002.

Hommes, R. E., Borash, A. I., Hartwig, K., & DeGracia, D. (2018). American sign language interpreter's perceptions of barriers to healthcare communication in deaf and hard of hearing patients. *Journal of Community Health, 43*(5), 956–961. https://doi.org/10.1007/s10900-018-0511-3.

Hyatt, A., Lipson-Smith, R., Schofield, P., et al. (2017). Communication challenges experienced by migrants with cancer: A comparison of migrant and English-speaking Australian-born cancer patients. *Health Expectations, 20*(5), 886–895. https://doi.org/10.1111/hex.12529.

Johnson, A. (2016). Health literacy: How nurses can make a difference. *Australian Journal of Advanced Nursing, 33*(2), 20–27.

Lee, D. C. A., Pritchard, E., McDermott, F., & Haines, T. P. (2014). Falls prevention education for older adults during and after hospitalization: A systematic review and meta-analysis. *Health Education Journal, 73*(5), 530–544. https://doi.org/10.1177/0017896913499266.

Maidment, I. D., Aston, L., Moutela, T., Fox, C. G., & Hilton, A. (2017). A qualitative study exploring medication management in people with dementia living in the community and the potential role of the community pharmacist. *Health Expectations, 20*(5), 929–942. https://doi.org/10.1111/hex.12534.

Manente, L., McCluskey, T., & Shaw, R. (2017). Transitioning patients from the intensive care unit to the general pediatric unit: A piece of the puzzle in family-centered care. *Pediatric Nursing, 43*(2), 77–95.

McCleary-Jones, V. (2016). A systematic review of literature on health literacy in nursing education. *Nurse Educator, 41*(2), 93–97. https://doi.org/10.1097/NNE.0000000000000204.

McCune, R. L., Lee, H., & Pohl, J. M. (2016). Assessing health literacy in safety net primary care practices. *Applied Nursing Research, 29*, 188–194. https://doi.org/10.1016/j.apnr.2015.04.004.

Ozkara San, E. (2020). The influence of the oncology-focused transgender-simulated patient simulation nursing students' cultural competence development. *Nursing Forum, 55*(4), 621–630. https://doi.org/10.1111/nuf.12478.

Pedersen, P. U., Ersgard, K. B., Soerensen, T. B., & Larsen, P. (2017). Effectiveness of structured planned post discharge support to patients with chronic obstructive pulmonary disease for reducing readmission rates: A systematic review. *JBI Database of Systematic Reviews and Implementation Reports, 15*(8), 2060–2086. https://doi.org/10.11124/JBISRIR-2016-003045.

Reeves, D., Blickem, C., Vassilev, I., et al. (2014). The contribution of social networks to the health and self-management of patients with long-term conditions: A longitudinal study. *PLoS One, 9*(6), e98340. https://doi.org/10.1371/journal.pone.0098340.

Rorie, S. (2015). Using medical interpreters to provide culturally competent care. *AORN Journal, 101*(2), P7–P9. https://doi.org/10.1016/S0001-2092(14)01420-3.

Rushton, M., Howarth, M., Grant, M. J., & Astin, F. (2017). Person-centered discharge education following coronary artery bypass graft: A critical review. *Journal of Clinical Nursing, 26*(23–24), 5206–5215. https://doi.org/10.1111/jcon.14071.

Singh, T. P., Vangaveti, V. N., Kennedy, R. L., & Malabu, U. H. (2016). Role of telehealth in diabetic foot ulcer management: A systematic review. *Australian Journal of Rural Health, 24*(4), 224–229. https://doi.org/10.1111/ajr.12284.

Wang, W., Cheng, M. T. M., Leong, F. L., Goh, A. W. L., Lim, S. T., & Jiang, Y. (2020). The development and testing of a nurse led smartphone-based self-management programme for diabetes patients with poor glycemic control. *Journal of Advanced Nursing, 76*(11), 3179–3189. https://doi.org/10.1111/jan.14519.

Readiness for Enhanced Knowledge

Domain 5 Perception/cognition Class 4 Cognition

Lauren McAlister, MSN, FNP-BC, DNP and Kathaleen C. Bloom, PhD, CNM

NANDA-I

Definition

A pattern of cognitive information related to a specific topic, or its acquisition, which can be strengthened.

Defining Characteristics

Expresses desire to enhance learning

NOC (Nursing Outcomes Classification)

Suggested NOC Outcome

Knowledge: Health Promotion

Example NOC Outcome with Indicators

Knowledge: Health Promotion as evidenced by the following indicators: Behaviors that promote health/ Reputable health care resources. (Rate the outcome and indicators of **Knowledge: Health Promotion:** 1 = no knowledge, 2 = limited knowledge, 3 = moderate knowledge, 4 = substantial knowledge, 5 = extensive knowledge [see Section I].)

K

Client Outcomes

Client Will (Specify Time Frame)

- Meet personal health-related goals
- Explain how to incorporate new health regimen into lifestyle
- List sources to obtain information

NIC (Nursing Interventions Classification)

Suggested NIC Interventions

Health Education; Health System Guidance

Example NIC Activities—Health Education

Prioritize identified learner needs based on client preference, skills of nurse, resources available, and likelihood of successful goal attainment

Nursing Interventions and *Rationales*

- Assume a facilitator role versus an authority role when engaging clients seeking health-related knowledge. EBN: *Educators in all disciplines must practice multiprofessional education experiences in order to provide due diligence in educating both clients and the future health care workforce in order to understand expectations and role responsibilities within the profession and that of others (Furr et al, 2020).* EBN: *According to Stacey and Légaré (2015), by assuming a facilitator role, nurses are able to provide balanced evidence on options, understand what is most important to the client, and advocate for the client's preferences. All of this facilitates shared decision-making and enables the opportunity to determine best practice.*
- Consider "health coaching" and motivational interviewing techniques when focusing on health-related goals, priorities, and preferences. EBN: *A study by Chang et al (2019) found that motivational interviewing enhanced knowledge and confidence and the care of older adults.* EBN: *In a randomized controlled trial (RCT) by Benzo et al (2017), health coaching, using motivational interviewing, significantly improved disease-specific quality of life compared with the control group.*

- Seek teachable moments for those with chronic conditions to enhance their knowledge of health promotion. EB: *Findings from a 2015 study indicated that using cancer diagnosis as the teachable moment for health promotion efforts should be tailored and targeted at specific comorbidities (Highland et al, 2015).*
- Refer clients to interactive and Web-based technological resources as appropriate. EB: *In a qualitative study by van der Gugten et al (2016), 70% of adults reported that they seek health-related information through Internet resources.*
- Refer to Deficient **Knowledge** care plan.

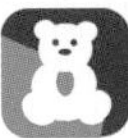

Pediatric

- Consider the use of mobile text messaging as a resource for delivery of health promotion information. EB: *A systematic review of 16 studies indicated that multimedia technologies and mobile messaging are viable adjuncts that can help engage adolescents in disease prevention and health promotion (Geckle, 2016).*
- Involve children and especially adolescents in designing health promotion programs and teaching methods. EBN: *In a systematic review of eight qualitative studies, when the health care professional ensures children receive education and information appropriate to their health literacy, children are apt to be more involved in their decision-making (Davies & Randall, 2015).*
- Refer to Deficient **Knowledge** care plan.

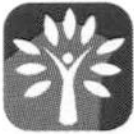

Geriatric

- Discuss healthy lifestyle changes that promote safety, health promotion, and health maintenance for older clients. EB: *A study by Hsu et al (2016) indicated that elderly individuals with poor health status were more apt to receive a health examination for their diseases. Early detection via health promotion and disease prevention of the potential health risks would reduce the severity of diseases in the prognosis.*
- Consider involving bilingual members of a community who are considered outside the traditional health care system who may assist in the teaching of community health issues.

K

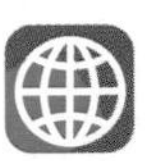

Multicultural

- Refer to Geriatric interventions.
- Refer to Deficient **Knowledge** care plan.

REFERENCES

Benzo, R., Kirsch, J. L., Hathaway, J. C., McEvoy, C. E., & Vickers, K. S. (2017). Health coaching in severe COPD after a hospitalization: A qualitative analysis of a large randomized study. *Respiratory Care, 62*(11), 1403–1411. https://doi.org/10.4187/respcare.05574.

Chang, Y., Cassalia, J., Warunek, M., & Scherer, Y. (2019). Motivational interviewing training with standardized patient simulation for prescription opioid abuse among older adults. *Perspectives in Psychiatric Care, 55*(4), 681–689. https://doi.org/10.1111/ppc.12402.

Davies, A., & Randall, D. (2015). Perceptions of children's participation in their healthcare: A critical review. *Issues in Comprehensive Pediatric Nursing, 38*(3), 202–221. https://doi.org/10.3109/01460862.2015.1063740.

Furr, S., Lane, S. H., Martin, D., & Brackney, D. E. (2020). Understanding roles in health care through interprofessional educational experiences. *British Journal of Nursing, 29*(6), 364–372. https://doi.org/10.12968/bjon.2020.29.6.364.

Geckle, J. (2016). Use of multimedia or mobile devices by adolescents for health promotion and disease prevention: A literature review. *Pediatric Nursing, 42*(4), 163–167.

Highland, K. B., Hurtado-de-Mendoza, A., Stanton, C. A., Dash, C., & Sheppard, V. B. (2015). Risk-reduction opportunities in breast cancer survivors: Capitalizing on teachable moments. *Supportive Care in Cancer, 23*(4), 933–941. https://doi.org/10.1007/s00520-014-2441-7.

Hsu, H. C., Chang, W. C., Luh, D. L., & Pan, L. Y. (2016). Health, healthy lifestyles, and health examinations among the older people in Taiwan. *Australasian Journal on Ageing, 35*(3), 161–166. https://doi.org/10.1111/ajag.12249.

Stacey, D., & Légaré, F. (2015). Engaging patients using an interprofessional approach to shared decision making. *Canadian Oncology Nursing Journal, 25*(4), 455–461.

van der Gugten, A. C., de Leeuw, R. J. R. J., Verheij, T. J. M., van der Ent, C. K., & Kars, M. C. (2016). E-Health and health care behaviour of parents of young children: A qualitative study. *Scandinavian Journal of Primary Health Care, 34*(2), 135–142. https://doi.org/10.3109/02813432.2016.1160627.

Risk for Latex Allergy Reaction

Domain 11 Safety/protection Class 5 Defensive processes

Gail B. Ladwig, MSN, RN and Julianne E. Doubet, BSN, RN, EMT-B

NANDA-I

Definition

Susceptible to a hypersensitive reaction to natural latex rubber products or latex reactive foods, which may compromise health.

Risk Factors

Inadequate knowledge about avoidance of relevant allergens; inattentive to potential environmental latex exposure; inattentive to potential exposure to latex reactive foods

At-Risk Population

Individuals frequently exposed to latex product; individuals receiving repetitive injections from rubber topped bottles; individuals with family history of atopic dermatitis; individuals with history of latex reaction; infants undergoing numerous operations beginning soon after birth

Associated Conditions

Asthma; atopy; food allergy; hypersensitivity to natural latex rubber protein; multiple surgical procedures; poinsettia plant allergy; urinary bladder diseases

NOC (Nursing Outcomes Classification)

L

Suggested NOC Outcomes

Allergic Response: Systemic; Immune Hypersensitivity Response; Risk Control; Risk Detection; Tissue Integrity: Skin and Mucous Membranes

Example NOC Outcome with Indicators

Immune Hypersensitivity Response as evidenced by the following indicators: Respiratory, cardiac, gastrointestinal, renal, and neurological function status IER/Free of allergic reactions. (Rate the outcome and indicators of **Immune Hypersensitivity Response:** 1 = not controlled, 2 = slightly controlled, 3 = moderately controlled, 4 = well controlled, 5 = very well controlled [see Section I].)

IER, In expected range.

Client Outcomes

Client Will (Specify Time Frame)

- State risk factors for natural rubber latex (NRL) allergy
- Request latex-free environment
- Demonstrate knowledge of plan to treat NRL allergic reaction

NIC Interventions (Nursing Interventions Classification)

Suggested NIC Interventions

Allergy Management; Latex Precautions; Environmental Risk Protection

Example NIC Activities—Latex Precautions

Question client or appropriate other about history of systemic reaction to NRL (e.g., facial or scleral edema, tearing eyes, urticaria, rhinitis, and wheezing); Place an allergy band on client

Nursing Interventions and *Rationales*

- Clients at high risk for NRL allergy need to be identified. EB: *Allergy to NRL remains a serious public health problem, especially in health care workers and others who are "at risk": rubber industry workers, hairdressers, and hotel/motel housekeepers (Nucera et al, 2020).*
- Clients with spina bifida are a high-risk group for NRL allergy and should remain latex free from the first day of life. EB: *In their research, Gold and Salsberg (2017) found that as many as 50% of those who have spina bifida may have a latex allergy probably caused by their multiple surgeries, intermittent catheterization, and condition-related susceptibility.*
- Assess for NRL allergy in clients who are exposed to "hidden" latex. EB: *The usual vulcanization and purification processes used in the manufacturing of latex can leave up to 2% to 3% surplus of free proteins in the finished product (Meneses et al, 2020).*
- Assess for NRL allergy in clients with a history of multiple surgeries or other latex-exposing procedures. EB: *According to Stinkens et al (2019), certain clients who describe a latex allergy reaction had a history of multiple surgical procedures.*
- Assess for NRL allergy in atopic individuals (persons with a tendency to have multiple allergic conditions, including allergies to certain food products). EB: *In his study of occupational food allergies, Fukutomi (2019) found that latex-food syndrome is relatively common among health care workers.* EBN: *Latex allergy related fruits and nuts include Kiwifruit, banana, chestnut, and avocado (Kajiwara et al, 2018).*
- Assess persons who have an ongoing occupational exposure to NRL. EB: *Latex can not only trigger occupational allergies among health care workers but could conceivably act as an allergen to produce allergic symptoms in those in the same environment (Kartel et al, 2020).*
- Assess for latex sensitization in older adults. EB: *The incidence of allergic disease, and anaphylaxis, in the elderly becomes more common as lifespan increases (González-de-Olano et al, 2016).*
- Obtain a thorough history of the client at risk before performing procedures that may involve latex products, such as urinary catheter insertion or venipuncture. EBN: *Liberatore (2019) states that one of the most important question to ask a new client is, "Are you allergic to latex?"*
- Have management protocols in place for treating anaphylaxis. EB: *A report from the World Allergy Organization (Kowalski et al, 2016) advised that safety measures such as continuous supervision, specific emergency equipment, and quick access to emergency services should be readily available during at-risk testing procedures.* EB: *As overseeing the increase in allergic clients is becoming more problematic, a systematic approach was developed by Flokstra-de Blok et al (2017) to make available for the primary care physicians a plan of action "allergy management support system" (AMAS) for diagnosis and management of allergic clients.*
- Question the client about associated symptoms of itching, swelling, and redness after contact with rubber products such as rubber gloves, balloons, and barrier contraceptives, or swelling of the tongue and lips after dental examinations. EBN: *The chance of hidden latex in the health care setting presents a threat to clients' safety, especially in the utilization of equipment, supplies, and procedures (Liberatore, 2019).*
- Treat all latex-sensitive clients as if they have NRL allergy. EB: *If it is established that a client is at risk for latex allergy, avoidance of any latex exposure is critical (Nguyen & Kohli, 2020).*
- Clients with spina bifida and others with a positive history of NRL sensitivity or NRL allergy should have all medical/surgical/dental procedures performed in a latex-controlled environment. EBN: *According to Méndez et al (2018), most existing surgical protocols concur that latex-sensitive clients' elective surgery should be slated as the first case of the day in an operating suite that has had no prior activity for 12 hours.*
- In select high-risk atopic individuals, a specific immunotherapy regimen should be discussed with their health care provider. EB: *Currently, allergen-specific immunotherapy (AIT) remains the only conclusive treatment able to mitigate the natural course of allergic disorders (Nucera et al, 2020).*
- ▲ If latex gloves are chosen for protection from blood or body fluids, a reduced-protein, powder-free glove should be selected. EB: *According to a study by Baid and Agarwal (2017), powdered gloves have been shown to have greater NRL proteins compared with nonpowdered gloves. These substances could cause life-threatening reactions in sensitized clients and present a risk to health care workers.*
- Ensure that the client has a medical plan if a latex response develops. EB: *Prompt treatment of anaphylactic symptoms decreases the probability of a life-threatening situation. Sicherer and Simons (2017) stress the importance of client, family, and community education in the recognition and immediate management of anaphylaxis.*
- Note client history and environmental assessment.

L

Client Family Teaching and Discharge Planning

- ▲ Instruct the client to inform health care professionals if he or she has an NRL allergy, particularly if the client is scheduled for surgery. **EBN:** *It is crucial that, as part of preassessment activity before surgery, clients who have elevated risk factors for latex sensitivity are detected (European Operating Room Nurses Association [EORNA], 2020).*
- ● Provide the client with written information about latex allergy and sensitivity. **EB:** *All latex-sensitive clients should be provided a list of substitute latex-safe products for hospital and home use, and should also include identification of cross-reacting fruits, and hidden sources of NRL (Nucera et al, 2020).*
- ● Teach clients that the most effective approach to preventing NRL anaphylaxis is complete latex avoidance. **EB:** *After identifying "at-risk" clients for NRL, prevention of exposure becomes critical (Nguyen & Kohli, 2020).*
- ▲ Teach clients that materials and items that contain NRL must be identified and latex-free alternatives must be substituted. **EB:** *The substitution of nonlatex materials and the identification of latex-derived products are valuable in the successful control of health risks linked to NRL (Quirce & Fiandor, 2016).*
- ● Health care workers should avoid the use of latex gloves and seek alternatives such as unpowdered gloves made from nitrile. **EB:** *According to a study by Baid and Agarwal (2017), powdered gloves have been shown to have greater NRL proteins in contrast to unpowdered gloves: these substances could cause life-threatening reactions in sensitized clients and they present a risk to health care workers.*
- ● Institute measures that reduce or completely avoid any latex exposure to clients. **EB:** *Any latex-sensitive individual who has experienced an allergic reaction during surgical or medical procedures should wear a Medic Alert bracelet or necklace and carry autoinjectable epinephrine and sterile nonlatex gloves if needed in an emergency. Discuss latex allergy with all health care and community providers; the concept of "latex safe" would seem a practical and complementary strategy for prevention of serious reactions in those who are latex sensitive (Nucera et al, 2020).*
- ● Health care institutions should develop prevention programs and establish latex-safe areas in their facilities. **EBN:** *According to Liberatore and Kelley (2018), it is essential that all health care staff maintain strict attention to the avoidance of latex products for clients with a history of latex allergy.*

L

Home Care

- ● Assess the home environment for presence of NRL products (e.g., balloons, condoms, gloves, and products of related allergies, such as bananas, avocados, and poinsettia plants). **EB:** *According to Wu et al (2016), latex-derived products are still in use universally and latex allergy remains a widespread health risk for many occupations and for the general populace.*
- ● Ensure that the client has a medical plan if a response develops. **EB:** *Prompt treatment of anaphylactic symptoms decreases the probability of a life-threatening situation. Sicherer & Simons (2017) stress the importance of client, family, and community education in the recognition and immediate management of anaphylaxis.*
- ● Note client history and environmental assessment.

REFERENCES

Baid, R., & Agarwal, R. (2017). Powdered gloves: Time to bid adieu. *Journal of Postgraduate Medicine, 63*(3), 206. Retrieved from www.eorna.eu. [Accessed September 5, 2020].

European Operating Room Nurses Association (EORNA). (2020). *EORNA best practice for perioperative care* (2nd ed.). Brussels, Belgium: EORNA. Retrieved from https://eorna.eu/wp-content/uploads/2020/09/EORNA-Best-Practice-for-Perioperative-Care-Edition-2020.pdf. [Accessed July 12, 2021].

Flokstra-de Blok, B. M. J., van der Molen, T., Christoffers, W. A., et al. (2017). Development of an allergy management support system in primary care. *Journal of Asthma and Allergy, 10*, 57–65. https://doi.org/10.2147/JAA.S123260.

Fukutomi, Y. (2019). Occupational food allergy. *Current Opinion in Allergy and Clinical Immunology, 19*(3), 243–248. https://doi:10.10.1097/ACI.0000000000000530.

Gold, J. T., & Salsberg, D. H. (2017). Pediatric disorders: Cerebral palsy and spina bifida. In A. Moroz, S. R. Flanagan, & H. Zaretsky (Eds.), *Medical aspects of disability for the rehabilitation professional* (5th ed.) (p. 327). New York: Springer Publishing.

González-de-Olano, D., Lombardo, C., & González-Mancebo, E. (2016). The difficult management of anaphylaxis in the elderly. *Current Opinion in Allergy and Clinical Immunology, 16*(4), 352–360. https://doi.org/10.1097/ACI.0000000000000280.

Kajiwara, E., Iino, H., & Ono, S. (2018). *Matching of the latex-fruit syndrome and daily rubber products survey to Japanese nursing students. Presented at the 29th International Nursing research Congress.* July 19-23, 2018 Melbourne, Australia: Innovative Global Nursing Practice and Education Through Research and Evidence-based Practice. Retrieved from http://hdl.handle.net/10755/624513. [Accessed July 12, 2021].

Kartel, Ö., Ayetekin, G., Aydoğan, Ü., Sari, O., Yeşilik, S., & Demirel, F. (2020). Symptoms and awareness of latex allergy among healthcare workers. *Asthma Allergy Immunology, 18*(2), 73–81. https://doi:10.21911/aai.511.

Kowalski, M. L., Ansotegui, I., Aberer, W., et al. (2016). Risk and safety requirements for diagnostic and therapeutic procedures in allergology: World Allergy Organization statement. *World Allergy Organization Journal, 9*(1), 33. https://doi.org/10.1186/s40413-016-0122-3.

Liberatore, K. (2019). Protecting patients with latex allergies. *American Journal of Nursing, 119*(1), 60–63. https://doi.org/10.1097/01.NAJ.0000552616.96652.72.

Liberatore, K., & Kelly, K. J. (2018). Latex allergies risks live on. *The Journal of Allergy and Immunology in Practice, 6*(6), 1877–1878. https:// doi.org/10.106/j.jaip.2018.08.007.

Méndez, C., Martínez, E., Lopez, E., et al. (2018). Analysis of environmental conditions in the operating room for latex-allergic patients' safety. *Journal of PeriAnesthesia Nursing*, *33*(4), 490–498. https://doi.org/10.1016/j.jopan.2015.12.017.

Meneses, V., Parenti, S., Burns, H., & Adams, R. (2020). Latex allergy guidelines for people with spina bifida. *Journal of Pediatric Rehabilitation Medicine*, *13*(4), 601–609. https://doi.10.3233/PRM-200741.

Nguyen, K., & Kohli, A. (2020). *Latex allergy.* StatPearls. Treasure Island, FL: StatPearls Publishing. Retrieved from https://europepmc.org/article/NBK545164. [Accessed September 4, 2020].

Nucera, E., Aruanno, A., Rizzi, A., & Centrone, M. (2020). Latex allergy: Current status and future perspectives. *Journal of Asthma and Allergy*, *13*, 385–398. https://doi.10.2147/JAA.S242058.

Quirce, S., & Fiandor, A. (2016). How should occupational anaphylaxis be investigated and managed? *Current Opinion in Allergy and Clinical Immunology*, *16*(2), 86–92. https://doi.org/10.1097/ACI.0000000000000241.

Sicherer, S. H., & Simons, F. E. R. (2017). Epinephrine for first-aid management of anaphylaxis. *Pediatrics*, *139*(3), e20164006. https://doi.org/10.1542/peds.2016-4006.

Stinkens, R., Verbeke, N., Van de Velde, M., et al. (2019). Safety of a powder-free latex allergy protocol in the operating theatre: A prospective observational cohort study. *European Journal of Anaesthesiology*, *36*(4), 312–313. https://doi.101097/EJA.0000000000000953.

Wu, M., McIntosh, J., & Liu, J. (2016). Current prevalence rate of latex allergy: Why it remains a problem? *Journal of Occupational Health*, *58*(2), 138–144. https://doi.org/10.1539/joh.15-0275-RA.

Readiness for Enhanced Health Literacy

Domain 1 Health promotion Class 1 Health awareness

Kathaleen C. Bloom, PhD, CNM

NANDA-I

Definition

A pattern of using and developing a set of skills and competencies (literacy, knowledge, motivation, culture and language) to find, comprehend, evaluate and use health information and concepts to make daily health decisions to promote and maintain health, decrease health risks and improve overall quality of life, which can be strengthened.

Defining Characteristics

Expresses desire to enhance ability to read, write, speak and interpret numbers for everyday health needs; expresses desire to enhance awareness of civic and/or government processes that impact public health; expresses desire to enhance health communication with health care providers; expresses desire to enhance knowledge of current determinants of health on social and physical environments; expresses desire to enhance personal health care decision-making; expresses desire to enhance social support for health; expresses desire to enhance understanding of customs and beliefs to make health care decisions; expresses desire to enhance understanding of health information to make health care choices; expresses desire to obtain sufficient information to navigate the health care system

NOC (Nursing Outcomes Classification)

Suggested NOC Outcomes

Health Beliefs: Perceived Resources; Health-Promoting Behavior; Health-Seeking Behavior

Example NOC Outcome with Indicators

Health-Seeking Behavior as evidenced by the following indicators: Completes health-related tasks/Performs self-screening/Obtains assistance from health professional/Uses reputable heath information. (Rate the outcome and indicators of **Health-Seeking Behavior:** 1 = never demonstrated, 2 = rarely demonstrated, 3 = sometimes demonstrated, 4 = often demonstrated, 5 = consistently demonstrated [see Section I].)

Client Outcomes

Client Will (Specify Time Frame)

- Use reputable information sources
- Seek information from health care providers
- Communicate with health care provider about understanding of information provided

L

NIC (Nursing Interventions Classification)

Suggested NIC Interventions

Health Literacy Enhancement; Health Education; Health System Guidance

Example NIC Activities—Health Literacy Enhancement

Create a health care environment in which a client with impaired literacy can seek help without feeling ashamed or stigmatized; Provide understandable health information; Use strategies to enhance understanding

Nursing Interventions and *Rationales*

- ▲ Work collaboratively with multiprofessional groups to create and maintain health-literate health care organizations. EB: *A scoping review of 106 studies found that interventions focusing on support for clients, support for staff, and support for governance are all important to achieve a health-literate health care organization (Zanobini et al, 2020).*
- • Use a standard tool to identify the level of health literacy. EB: *A variety of tools have been developed to measure individuals' health-related reading comprehension (Agency for Healthcare Research and Quality [AHRQ], 2016).*
- • Identify and take into consideration factors affecting health literacy such as age, ethnicity, education, and cognitive function. EBN: *Improved health literacy is associated with positive outcomes, including increased health promotion (Chahardah-Cherik et al, 2018) and adherence to medical treatments (Miller, 2016).*
- • Implement health literacy universal precautions: assume that all clients may have difficulty understanding health information. EB: *Less than 15% of adults possess the level of health literacy needed to navigate the health care system (AHRQ, 2017). All clients need health information that is accurate, accessible, and understandable (French, 2015).*
- • Tailor health teaching and educational materials to accommodate the needs of those with low health literacy. EBN: *A systematic review and meta-analysis of diabetes self-management interventions (n = 13 studies) found that health literacy–sensitive interventions focused on communication (both written and spoken) and empowerment in the context of language and cultural considerations were the most effective for self-care and health outcomes, including reduction of hemoglobin (Hb) A1C (Kim & Lee, 2016).*
- • Modify health teaching and educational materials to client preferences. EB: *Individuals who have lower health literacy prefer, understand, and correctly interpret pictures and icons that are familiar, contextual, and less complex (van Beusekom et al, 2015; Arcia et al, 2016; van Beusekom et al, 2017). Individuals with low health literacy prefer to be supported with reliable, understandable information and interactions with health care providers and others experiencing similar medical issues (Visscher et al, 2020).*
- • Use empowerment to enhance health literacy and improve client outcomes. EBN: *A study with 295 individuals with type 2 diabetes found empowerment directly leading to health literacy, which then influenced self-efficacy, self-care behaviors, and finally HbA1C levels (Lee et al, 2016).* EB: *A meta-analysis of 61 studies determined that health literacy was directly associated with diabetes knowledge, self-care, and glycemic control (Marciano et al, 2019).*

Geriatric

- • The above interventions may be adapted for geriatric use.
- • Assess health literacy as it relates to health perceptions in older adults. EB: *Health literacy has been found to have a substantial effect on older adults' perceptions of the importance of their overall health and, to a lesser extent, their self-awareness of health and their health locus of control (Deniz et al, 2018).*
- • Use simple educational materials targeted at health-promoting behaviors. EB: *Older adults with good health literacy are more likely to have mammography, to exercise, and to eat nutritiously and are less likely to perform monthly breast examinations or to smoke (Fernandez et al, 2016; Geboers et al, 2016).*

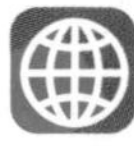

Multicultural

- • Take the client's culture into account when designing teaching and educational materials. EB: *Higher levels of health literacy challenge are associated with being from a culturally diverse background and/or not speaking English (Jessup et al, 2017).* **EB:** *A scoping review of 27 studies revealed three consistent barriers to health care services access: cultural differences between providers and clients, language barriers, and information barriers (Kalich et al, 2016).*

- Use educational strategies targeted at both the individual and the community. **EBN:** *Targeting both individuals and communities allows for improvement in functional health literacy as well as improvement in knowledge (Fernández-Gutiérrez et al, 2018).*

Client/Family Teaching and Discharge Planning

- Promote shared decision-making. **EB:** *Increasing health literacy has the potential to enhance clients' engagement in health care and their participation in decision-making about their care (Wigfall & Tanner, 2018).*

REFERENCES

Agency for Healthcare Research and Quality (AHRQ). (2016). *Health literacy measurement tools (revised).* Rockville, MD: AHRQ. Retrieved from http://www.ahrq.gov/professionals/quality-patient-safety/quality-resources/tools/literacy/index.html. [Accessed July 13, 2021].

Agency for Healthcare Research and Quality (AHRQ). (2017). *AHRQ health literacy universal precautions toolkit* (2nd ed.). Rockville, MD: AHRQ. Retrieved from https://www.ahrq.gov/health-literacy/improve/precautions/index.html. [Accessed July 13, 2021].

Arcia, A., Suero-Tejeda, N., Bales, M. E., et al. (2016). Sometimes more is more: Iterative participatory design of infographics for engagement of community members with varying levels of health literacy. *Journal of the American Medical Informatics Association, 23*(1), 174–183. https://doi.org/10.1093/jamia/ocv079.

Chahardah-Cherik, S., Gheibizadeh, M., Jahani, S., & Cheraghian, B. (2018). The relationship between health literacy and health promoting behaviors in patients with type 2 diabetes. *International Journal of Community Based Nursing and Midwifery, 6*(1), 65–75.

Deniz, S. Ş., Özer, Ö., & Songür, C. (2018). Effect of health literacy on health perception: An application in individuals at age 65 and older. *Social Work in Public Health, 33*(2), 85–95. https://doi.org/10.1080/19371918.2017.1409680.

Fernandez, D. M., Larson, J. L., & Zikmund-Fisher, B. J. (2016). Associations between health literacy and preventive health behaviors among older adults: Findings from the Health and Retirement Study. *BMC Public Health, 16*, 596. https://doi.org/10.1186/s12889-016-3267-7.

Fernández-Gutiérrez, M., Bas-Sarmiento, P., Albar-Marín, M. J., Paloma-Castro, O., & Romero-Sánchez, J. M. (2018). Health literacy interventions for immigrant populations: A systematic review. *International Nursing Review, 65*(1), 54–64. https://doi.org/10.1111/inr.12373.

French, K. S. (2015). Transforming nursing care through health literacy ACTS. *Nursing Clinics of North America, 50*(1), 87–98. https://doi.org/10.1016/j.cnur.2014.10.007.

Geboers, B., Reijneveld, S. A., Jansen, C. J. M., & de Winter, A. F. (2016). Health literacy is associated with health behaviors and social factors among older adults: Results from the LifeLines Cohort Study. *Journal of Health Communication, 21*(Suppl. 2), 45–53. https://doi.org/10.1080/10810730.2016.1201174.

Jessup, R. L., Osborne, R. H., Beauchamp, A., Bourne, A., & Buchbinder, R. (2017). Health literacy of recently hospitalised patients: A cross-sectional survey using the Health Literacy Questionnaire (HLQ). *BMC Health Services Research, 17*(1), 52. https://doi.org/10.1186/s12913-016-1973-6.

Kalich, A., Heinemann, L., & Ghahari, S. (2016). A scoping review of immigrant experience of health care access barriers in Canada. *Journal of Immigration and Minority Health, 18*(3), 697–709. https://doi.org/10.1007/s10903-015-0237-6.

Kim, S. H., & Lee, A. (2016). Health-literacy-sensitive diabetes self-management interventions: A systematic review and meta-analysis. *Worldviews on Evidence-Based Nursing, 13*(4), 324–333. https://doi.org/10.1111/wvn.12157.

Lee, Y. J., Shin, S. J., Wang, R. H., Lin, K. D., Lee, Y. L., & Wang, Y. H. (2016). Pathways of empowerment perceptions, health literacy, self-efficacy, and self-care behaviors to glycemic control in patients with type 2 diabetes mellitus. *Patient Education and Counseling, 99*(2), 287–294. https://doi.org/10.1016/j.pec.2015.08.021.

Marciano, L., Camerini, A. L., & Schulz, P. J. (2019). The role of health literacy in diabetes knowledge, self-care, and glycemic control: A meta-analysis. *Journal of General Internal Medicine, 34*(6), 1007–1017. https://doi.org/10.1007/s11606-019-04832-y.

Miller, T. A. (2016). Health literacy and adherence to medical treatment in chronic and acute illness: A meta-analysis. *Patient Education and Counseling, 99*(7), 1079–1086. https://doi.org/10.1016/j.pec.2016.01.020.

van Beusekom, M., Bos, M., Wolterbeek, R., Guchelaar, H. J., & van den Broek, J. (2015). Patients' preferences for visuals: Differences in the preferred level of detail, type of background and type of frame of icons depicting organs between literate and low-literate people. *Patient Education and Counseling, 98*(2), 226–233. https://doi.org/10.1016/j.pec.2014.10.023.

van Beusekom, M. M., Land-Zandstra, A. M., Bos, M. J. W., van den Broek, J. M., & Guchelaar, H. J. (2017). Pharmaceutical pictograms for low-literate patients: Understanding, risk of false confidence, and evidence-based design strategies. *Patient Education and Counseling, 100*(5), 966–973. https://doi.org/10.1016/j.pec.2016.12.015.

Visscher, B. B., Steunenberg, B., Heerdink, E. R., & Rademakers, J. (2020). Medication self-management support for people with diabetes and low health literacy: A needs assessment. *PLoS One, 15*(4), e0232022. https://doi.org/10.1371/journal.pone.0232022.

Wigfall, L. T., & Tanner, A. H. (2018). Health literacy and health-care engagement as predictors of shared decision-making among adult information seekers in the USA: A secondary data analysis of the health information national trends survey. *Journal of Cancer Education, 33*(1), 67–73. https://doi.org/10.1007/s13187-016-1052-z.

Zanobini, P., Lorini, C., Baldasseroni, A., Dellisanti, C., & Bonaccorsi, G. (2020). A scoping review on how to make hospitals health literate healthcare organizations. *International Journal of Environmental Research and Public Health, 17*(3), 1036. https://doi.org/10.3390/ijerph17031036.

Risk for Impaired Liver Function

Domain 2 Nutrition Class 4 Metabolism

Janelle M. Tipton, DNP, APRN-CNS, AOCN

NANDA-I

Definition

Susceptible to a decrease in liver function, which may compromise health.

Risk Factors

Substance misuse

Associated Conditions

Human immunodeficiency virus (HIV) coinfection; pharmaceutical preparations; viral infection

NOC (Nursing Outcomes Classification)

Suggested NOC Outcomes

Knowledge: Health Behavior; Liver Function

Example NOC Outcome with Indicators

Knowledge: Health Behavior as evidenced by the following indicators: Safe use of prescription drugs/Adverse health effects of alcohol misuse/Adverse health effects of recreational drug use/Healthy nutritional practices/Self-screening techniques. (Rate the outcome and indicators of **Knowledge: Health Behavior:** 1 = no knowledge, 2 = limited knowledge, 3 = moderate knowledge, 4 = substantial knowledge, 5 = extensive knowledge [see Section I].)

L

Client Outcomes

Client Will (Specify Time Frame)

- State the upper limit of the amount of acetaminophen safely taken per day
- Verbalize understanding that over-the-counter (OTC) medications may contain acetaminophen (e.g., OTC cold medicines)
- Have normal liver enzymes, serum and urinary bilirubin levels, white blood cell count, and red blood cell count
- Be free of unexplained weight loss, jaundice, pruritus, bruising, petechiae, gastrointestinal bleeding, and hemorrhage
- Be free of abdominal tenderness/pain, increased abdominal girth, and have normal-colored stool and urine
- Be able to eat frequent small meals per day without nausea and/or vomiting
- If alcohol abuse is factor, state relationship between abuse and worsening gastrointestinal and liver disease

NIC (Nursing Interventions Classification)

Suggested NIC Interventions

Teaching: Disease Process; Substance Use Treatment

Example NIC Activities—Teaching Disease Process

Appraise the client's current level of knowledge related to specific disease process; Discuss lifestyle changes that may be required to prevent future complications and/or control the disease process

Nursing Interventions and *Rationales*

▲ Assess for signs of liver dysfunction including fatigue, nausea, jaundice of the eyes or skin, pruritus, gastrointestinal bleeding, coagulopathy, infections, increasing abdominal girth, fluid overload, shortness of breath, mental status changes, light-colored stools, dark urine, and increased serum and urinary bilirubin levels. EB: *These are symptoms and laboratory results associated with liver disorders (Ghany et al, 2015; Lee, Divens, & Fowler, 2017).*

- ▲ Evaluate liver function tests. Standard liver panels include the serum enzymes aspartate transaminase (AST), alanine transaminase (ALT), alkaline phosphatase, and γ-glutamyl transferase; total, direct, and indirect serum bilirubin; and serum albumin. EB: *Hepatitis C is often asymptomatic early in the disease state (Kwo, Cohen, & Lim, 2017) and may be found during a routine examination when liver function test results are elevated (Kelly & Wattacheril, 2019). It is recommended that all people should be screened for hepatitis C at least once when above age 18 (Centers for Disease Control and Prevention [CDC], 2020). In immunotherapy-related hepatitis, there may be an elevation in AST and ALT without an increased bilirubin (Lleo et al, 2019).*
- ▲ Discuss with the client/family preparations for other diagnostic studies, such as ultrasound, computed tomography, and magnetic resonance imaging (MRI) examinations. EB: *Although costly, MRI has the best quantification of steatosis (Cassard, Gérard, & Perlemuter, 2017). A noninvasive tool to assess liver stiffness is through a vibration-controlled transient elastography scan. The scan detects steatosis and fibrosis, providing scored assessments (Kelly & Wattacheril, 2019).*
- ▲ Evaluate coagulation studies such as international normalized ratio, prothrombin time, and partial thromboplastin time, especially when there is bleeding of the mouth or gums. Prolonged prothrombin time and decreased production of clotting factors can result in bleeding.
- ● Monitor for signs of hemorrhage, especially in the upper gastrointestinal tract, because it is the most frequent site. EB: *Synthesis of coagulation factors is affected with liver impairment (McGinnis & Hays, 2018). Management may include volume replacement and pharmacologic interventions with vitamin K to promote synthesis of coagulation proteins and vasopressin analogue to reduce portal pressures and minimize bleeding.*
- ● Obtain a list of all medications, including OTC nonsteroidal antiinflammatory drugs, acetaminophen, herbal remedies, and dietary supplements. Review risk of drug-induced liver disease. The list includes some antibiotics, anticonvulsants, antidepressants, antiinflammatory drugs, antiplatelets, antihypertensives, calcium channel blockers, cyclosporine, lipid-lowering drugs, chemotherapy drugs, immunotherapy drugs, oral hypoglycemics, proton pump inhibitors, inhaled anesthetics, and tranquilizers, among others (Hamilton, Collins-Yoder, & Collins, 2016; Suzman et al, 2018). If client is taking either OTC medications or herbals, discuss signs and symptoms of toxic hepatitis. EB: *Toxic hepatitis is caused by direct toxins, drugs, herbs, and industrial chemicals. The risk of toxicity with aspirin, ibuprofen, naproxen sodium, and acetaminophen increases with frequency and in combination with use of alcohol (Hamilton, Collins-Yoder, & Collins, 2016).*
- ▲ For clients receiving drugs associated with liver injury, review risk factors to prevent potentially severe drug reactions. EB: *Drug-induced liver disease accounts for about 50% of hepatitis cases. The most common risk factors are advanced age, female gender, alcohol use with associated infection, and genetic predisposition (Hamilton, Collins-Yoder, & Collins, 2016). Cancer clients are at higher risk for developing liver dysfunction due to complex medication regimens, treatment such as radiation therapy, and disease involvement to the liver. Due to significant morbidity and mortality associated with chemotherapy drugs, drug-induced liver injury is of concern. Consultation with an oncology clinical pharmacist may be indicated (Wen et al, 2020).*
- ▲ Determine the total amount of acetaminophen the client is taking per day. The amount of acetaminophen ingested should not exceed 3.25 g/day, or even lower in the client with chronic alcohol intake (Hamilton, Collins-Yoder, & Collins, 2016). EB: *It is common for clients to take multiple pain medications, all containing acetaminophen. Acetaminophen is the most common cause of drug-induced liver injury, and approximately 46% of all people with acute liver failure in the United States have liver damage caused by acetaminophen (Ortega-Alonso et al, 2016).*
- ▲ Evaluation of acetaminophen-associated drug-induced liver injury is done by client history of ingestion, time, and doses of the medication per weight calculation and serum level of acetaminophen. EB: *One of the tools most commonly used for decision-making in the use of* N-*acetylcysteine is the Rumack-Matthew nomogram for drug overdose. Prompt intervention with* N-*acetylcysteine has reduced mortality to 0.7% for those clients who overdosed on acetaminophen (Hamilton, Collins-Yoder, & Collins, 2016).*
- ▲ If the client is on statin medications, ensure that liver enzyme testing is done at intervals. Liver enzymes can become elevated from taking statin medications; it is rare but possible for statins to cause actual liver damage (Hamilton, Collins-Yoder, & Collins, 2016).
- ▲ If the client is an alcoholic, refer to a cessation program. It is essential the client stop drinking as soon as possible to allow the liver to heal. Alcoholism is associated with malnutrition, which is harmful to the liver

L

(Fabrellas, 2017). Alcoholism is also associated with increased plasma endotoxins and disruption of the gut barrier, which cause inflammation and resultant damage to the liver (Cassard, Gérard, & Perlemuter, 2017). See care plans for Ineffective **Denial** and Dysfunctional **Family** Processes.

- ▲ Provide frequent smaller meals for easier digestion. Provide diet with optimal carbohydrates, proteins, and fats. Consult with a registered dietitian to discuss best nutritional support. EB: *Proteins can be increased as tolerated and serum protein, albumin levels, and bilirubin levels indicate improved liver function. The goals of nutrition therapy are to provide adequate nutrition, support growth, preserve lean body mass, and prevent micronutrient deficiencies (Leon & Lerret, 2017).*
- ▲ Recognize that severe malnutrition may result in acute liver failure, which is reversible with improved nutrition.
- ▲ Review medical history with the client, recognizing that obesity and type 2 diabetes, along with hypertriglyceridemia and polycystic ovarian syndrome, are major risk factors in the development of liver disease, specifically nonalcoholic fatty liver disease. EB: *For those clients showing signs of fatty liver involvement, sound nutritional support can reduce the severity and mitigate the already existing secondary malnutrition (Kelly & Wattacheril, 2019).*
- • Encourage vaccinations for hepatitis A and B for all ages. EB: *Hepatitis A can affect anyone in the United States. Vaccination can prevent hepatitis A and B, which at times can cause liver failure (CDC, 2020).*
- • Measure abdominal girth if individual presents with abdominal distention and pain. EB: *Increasing abdominal distention and pain are signs of impending portal hypertension with the presence of fluid shifts, resulting in ascites. Increasing leg edema may also result, causing a significant effect on quality of life in those with cirrhosis (Ghany et al, 2015; Fabrellas et al, 2020).*
- • Assess for tenderness and/or pain level in the right upper quadrant. Tenderness in this area is a symptom of biliary, liver, and/or pancreatic problems. EB: *This pain, along with a palpable mass and weight loss, is a classic triad for malignancies (Kelly & Wattacheril, 2019).*
- • Use standard precautions for handling of blood and body fluids. Review sterile techniques when giving intravenous solution and/or medications. EB: *This is imperative to decrease the incidence of infection with hepatitis B and hepatitis C viruses. The viruses have been spread in health care settings when injection equipment and intravenous solutions were mishandled and became contaminated (CDC, 2020).*
- ▲ Observe for signs and symptoms of mental status changes such as confusion from encephalopathy. EB: *The symptoms can fluctuate in severity within hours. Increased ammonia levels greater than 100 μg/dL have been shown to be a risk factor for developing high-grade hepatic encephalopathy. The most commonly used medical treatment is lactulose, orally or rectally, because it has a prebiotic effect, lowers the pH in the colon, and binds to ammonia, and excretion is promoted by this laxative effect (Bager, 2017; McGinnis & Hays, 2018).*

L

Pediatric/Parents

- ▲ Prescreen pregnant women for hepatitis B surface antigens. If found, recommend nursing case management during pregnancy. EB: *Despite advances in prevention of hepatitis B transmission, approximately half of the infections are caused by mother-to-child transmission. Efforts to prevent transmission are an essential element of perinatal maternal and infant care (Pokorska-Śpiewak et al, 2017).*
- ▲ Recommend implementation of postexposure prophylaxis, including the hepatitis B virus vaccine for an infant born to a hepatitis B surface antigen–positive woman (CDC, 2020).
- • Encourage vaccinations for hepatitis A and B for all ages. EB: *Children should be vaccinated between ages 12 and 23 months for hepatitis A (CDC, 2020).*
- ▲ Recognize that children can develop fatty liver disease, which can result in liver failure. Most children are asymptomatic, but others complain of malaise, fatigue, or vague recurrent abdominal pain. The development of NAFLD may be affected by perinatal and in utero stressors, with increased sensitivity to environmental and genetic factors (Goldner & Lavine, 2020).
- ▲ During a well-baby visit, assess for signs of potential liver problems. Observe for prolonged jaundice, pale stools, and urine that is anything other than colorless. Consult with health care provider to order a split bilirubin as needed (CDC, 2020).

Home Care

- • Encourage rest, optimal nutrition (high carbohydrates, sufficient protein, and essential vitamins and minerals) during initial inflammatory processes of the liver.

- The COVID-19 pandemic has increased the need for home care, telemedicine, and telephone visits for clients with chronic liver disease. Prioritization of client care is indicated, including transplantation, diagnostic evaluations, and hospitalization, with consideration for clients with NAFLD or NASH at higher risk for severity related to COVID-19 infections due to comorbidities (Boettler et al, 2020).
- Consider referral to palliative care for clients with end-stage liver disease. EB: *Increased symptom burden, poor quality of life, and higher health care costs emphasize the need for early integration of palliative care, including advanced care planning and discussion of goals of care (Rakoski & Volk, 2019).*

Client/Family Teaching and Discharge Planning

- Teach the client and family to examine all medications the client is taking, looking for acetaminophen as an ingredient, and reinforce the 3.25-g upper limit of intake of acetaminophen to protect liver function (Hamilton, Collins-Yoder, & Collins, 2016).
- For the caregiver or client with hepatitis A, B, or C, teach the need for careful handwashing, use of gloves, and other precautions to prevent spread of any of these diseases.
- Teach avoidance of high-risk behaviors that cause hepatitis and ways to avoid those behaviors.
- For clients with chronic liver disease, provide education and support on lifestyle changes to prevent or delay disease progression. Structured follow-up may minimize readmission to the hospital (Hjorth et al, 2018).
- Educate clients and their caregivers about treatment options and interventions for hepatitis. Recommend other informational support: risk factors, side effects of the different treatment options, and dietary advice.
- Recommend psychological support if possible during education sessions. EBN: *Hepatitis can result in liver inflammation and chronic liver disease and is a common reason for a liver transplant. The client may not have an understanding of liver disease or its complications, may be elderly, or may have mental health issues or additions that affect the need for nursing intervention. Developing a plan and/or services to support and to give person-centered care can provide better support to the client in dealing with liver disease (Greenslade, 2017).*
- Assess for adherence to antiviral therapies for the treatment of hepatitis and institute nursing interventions such as client education, communication, and reminder tools to assist clients in medication adherence. EB: *Adherence to antiviral therapies is imperative to help suppress viral load and to reduce progressive liver disease (Polis et al, 2017).*
- For those clients with mental health problems, collaborate with outreach programs to teach signs/symptoms of hepatitis, risk factors, and factors that increase transmission. EBN: *These clients have higher potential for substance use and injected-drug use, and increased chances of transmission because of homelessness and living conditions in night shelters. Protocols have proven to be successful in developing an effective approach to meeting the needs of clients with or at risk for infection with hepatitis A, B, and C virus and severe mental health problems. Culturally sensitive, nurse-led interventions, such as counseling and bringing vaccinations to the community through mobile services, are valuable health promotion strategies in high-risk populations (Nyamathi et al, 2015; Fabrellas, 2017).*

REFERENCES

Bager, P. (2017). The assessment and care of patients with hepatic encephalopathy. *British Journal of Nursing, 26*(13), 724–729.

Boettler, T., Newsome, P. N., Mondelli, M. U., et al. (2020). Care of patients with liver disease during the COVID-19 pandemic: EASL-ESCMID position paper. *JHEP Reports, 2*(3), 100113. https://doi.org/10.1016/j.jhepr.2020.100113.

Cassard, A. M., Gérard, P., & Perlemuter, G. (2017). Microbiota, liver diseases, and alcohol. *Microbiology Spectrum, 5*(4).

Centers for Disease Control and Prevention (CDC). (2020). *The ABCs of hepatitis*. Retrieved from https://www.cdc.gov/hepatitis/resources/professionals/pdfs/abctable.pdf. [Accessed July 13, 2021].

Fabrellas, N. (2017). Research about nursing care for persons with liver disease: A step in the right direction. *Nursing Research, 66*(6), 419–420.

Fabrellas, N., Carol, M., Palacio, E., et al. (2020). Nursing care of patients with cirrhosis: The LiverHope nursing Project. *Hepatology, 71*(3), 1106–1116. https://doi.org/10.1002/hep.31117.

Ghany, M., Hoofnagle, J., et al. (2015). Approach to the patient with liver disease. In D. Kasper, A. Fauci, S. Houser, et al. (Eds.), *Harrison's principles of internal medicine* (19th ed.). New York: McGraw-Hill.

Goldner, D., & Lavine, J. E. (2020). Nonalcoholic fatty liver disease in children: Unique considerations and challenges. *Gastroenterology, 158*(7), 1967–1983.e1. https://doi.org/10.1053/j.gastro.2020.01.048.

Greenslade, L. (2017). Providing high-quality care for patients with liver disease. *British Journal of Nursing, 26*(13), 739.

Hamilton, L. A., Collins-Yoder, A., & Collins, R. E. (2016). Drug-induced liver injury. *AACN Critical Care, 27*(4), 430–440.

Hjorth, M., Sjöberg, D., Svanberg, A., Kaminsky, E., Langenskiöld, S., & Rorsman, F. (2018). Nurse-led clinic for patients with liver cirrhosis—effects on health-related quality of life: Study protocol of a pragmatic multicentre randomized controlled trial. *BMJ Open, 8*(10), e023064. https://doi.org/10.1136/bmjopen-2018-023064.

Kelly, N., & Wattacheril, J. (2019). Nonalcoholic fatty liver disease: Evidence-based management and early recognition of nonalcoholic

steatohepatitis. *The Journal for Nurse Practitioners, 15*(9), 622–626. https://doi.org/10.1016/j.nurpra.2019.06.008.
Kwo, P. Y., Cohen, S. M., & Lim, J. K. (2017). ACG clinical guideline: Evaluation of abnormal liver chemistries. *American Journal of Gastroenterology, 112*(1), 18–35.
Lee, S., Divens, L., & Fowler, L. H. (2017). The role of liver function in the setting of cirrhosis with chronic infection and critical illness. *Critical Care Nursing Clinics of North America, 29*(1), 37–50.
Leon, C. D. G., & Lerret, S. M. (2017). Role of nutrition and feeding for the chronically ill pediatric liver patient awaiting liver transplant. *Gastroenterology Nursing, 40*(2), 109–116.
Lleo, A., Rimassa, L., & Colombo, M. (2019). Hepatotoxicity of immune check point inhibitors: Approach and management. *Digestive and Liver Disease, 51*(8), 1074–1078. https://doi.org/10.1016/j.dld.2019.05.006.
McGinnis, C. W., & Hays, S. M. (2018). Adults with liver failure in the intensive care unit: A transplant primer for nurses. *Critical Care Nursing Clinics of North America, 30*(1), 137–148. https://doi.org/10.1016/j.cnc.2017.10.012.
Nyamathi, A., Salem, B. E., Zhang, S., et al. (2015). Nursing case management, peer coaching, and hepatitis A and B vaccine completion among homeless men and recently released on parole: Randomized clinical trial. *Nursing Research, 64*(3), 177–189.
Ortega-Alonso, A., Stephens, C., Lucena, M. I., & Andrade, R. J. (2016). Case characterization, clinical features and risk factors in drug-induced liver injury. *International Journal of Molecular Science, 17*(5), 714.
Pokorska-Śpiewak, M., Kowalik-Mikołajewska, B., Aniszewska, M., Pluta, M., Walewska-Zielecka, B., & Marczyńska, M. (2017). Liver steatosis in children with chronic hepatitis B and C: Prevalence, predictors, and impact on disease progression. *Medicine, 96*(3), e5832. https://doi.org/10.1097/MD.0000000000005832.
Polis, S., Zablotska-Manos, I., Zekry, A., & Maher, L. (2017). Adherence to hepatitis B antiviral therapy: A qualitative study. *Gastroenterology Nursing, 40*(3), 239–246.
Rakoski, M. O., & Volk, M. L. (2019). Palliative care and end-stage liver disease: A critical review of current knowledge. *Current Opinion in Gastroenterology, 35*(3), 155–160. https://doi.org/10.1097/MOG.0000000000000530.
Suzman, D. L., Pelosof, L., Rosenberg, A., & Avigan, M. I. (2018). Hepatotoxicity of immune checkpoint inhibitors: An evolving picture of risk associated with a vital class of immunotherapy agents. *Liver International, 38*(6), 976–987. https://doi.org/10.1111/liv.13746.
Wen, H., Ge, M., Yao, D., & Liu, L. (2020). A simple method to identify undiagnosed drug-induced liver injury (DILI) and its application in oncology pharmacy practice. *Journal of Oncology Pharmacy Practice, 26*(5), 1060–1069. https://doi.org/10.1177/1078155219880604.

Risk for Loneliness Domain 12 Comfort Class 3 Social comfort

Marina Martinez-Kratz, MS, RN, CNE

NANDA-I

Definition

Susceptible to experiencing discomfort associated with a desire or need for more contact with others, which may compromise health.

Risk Factors

Affectional deprivation; emotional deprivation; physical isolation; social isolation

NOC (Nursing Outcomes Classification)

Suggested NOC Outcomes

Loneliness Severity; Social Interaction Skills; Social Involvement; Social Support

Example NOC Outcome with Indicators

Loneliness Severity as evidenced by the following indicators: Sense of social isolation/Difficulty in establishing contact with others. (Rate the outcome and indicators of **Loneliness Severity:** 1 = severe, 2 = substantial, 3 = moderate, 4 = mild, 5 = none [see Section I].)

Client Outcomes

Client Will (Specify Time Frame)

- Maintain one or more meaningful relationships (growth-enhancing versus codependent or abusive in nature)
- Sustain relationships that allow self-disclosure and demonstrate a balance between emotional dependence and independence
- Participate in personally meaningful activities and interactions that are ongoing, positive, and relevant socially
- Demonstrate positive use of time alone when socialization is not possible

NIC (Nursing Interventions Classification)

Suggested NIC Interventions

Family Integrity Promotion; Socialization Enhancement; Visitation Facilitation

Example NIC Activities—Socialization Enhancement

Encourage enhanced involvement in already established relationships; Help client increase awareness of strengths and limitations in communicating with others

Nursing Interventions and *Rationales*

- Assess the client's perception of loneliness. (Is the person alone by choice, or are there other factors that contribute to the feelings of loneliness? Is the client in one of the at-risk populations for loneliness?) **EBN:** *Nyatanga (2017) stated that loneliness can be a consequence of hardship, discrimination, inequality, loss of control, decrease in independence, and lack of options.*
- Assess the client's needs through mapping to assess existing networks, current activities, and the impact on well-being. **EB:** *Mapping allows nurse and client to examine the quality of existing relationships and activities to identify where intervention is needed (Mann et al, 2017).*
- Assess the client for signs of emotional distress. **EB:** *Research found that loneliness was the strongest overall predictor of mental distress and strong social connections are needed to prevent emotional distress (McIntyre et al, 2018).*
- ▲ Assess the bereaved client for risk of suicide and make appropriate referrals as necessary. **EB:** *A study by Stickley and Koyanagi (2016) found that there is a connection between loneliness and suicidal ideation; therefore efforts to reduce loneliness may play a significant part in decreasing its detrimental effects on the client's health and well-being.*
- Evaluate the client's desire for social interaction. **EB:** *Nurses and other health professionals must have an awareness of the client's social disconnectedness so that they can offer assistance in making and perpetuating social connections (Dinkins, 2017).*
- Teach the client problem-focused coping strategies. **EB:** *Findings from a systematic review suggest that learning how to use problem-focused coping strategies could target loneliness (Deckx et al, 2018).*

L

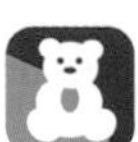

Pediatric

- Evaluate peer relationships. **EB:** *Peer relationships have been shown to play a significant role in self-esteem development across adolescence and also to remain influential throughout adulthood (Gruenenfelder-Steiger, Harris, & Fend, 2016).*
- Encourage relationships with peers and involvement with groups and organizations. **EB:** *According to Choukas-Bradley et al (2015), researchers have reported that peer influence is not intrinsically detrimental and that attempts to fashion one's own attitude to match that of peers could be seen as a healthy, constructive growth pattern.*
- Encourage organized activity (OA) participation for adolescent clients with a diagnosis of autism spectrum disorder. **EB:** *Research indicated that OA involvement was associated with fewer depressive symptoms and less feelings of loneliness (Bohnert, Lieb, & Arola, 2019).*
- ▲ Refer parents of disabled or seriously ill children to support groups. **EB:** *Participation in a family-oriented support group provides community support and possible solutions to common problems in a caring and trusting environment (Mitwalli, Rabaia, & Kienzler, 2018).*

Geriatric

- Identify risk factors for loneliness in older persons. **EB:** *In their study of aging and loneliness, Brittain et al (2017) stated that recognized risks factors for loneliness include widowhood, living alone, depression, and being female.*
- Practice laughter therapy with the client through laughter exercises or other humorous activities. **EB:** *A systematic review reported significant decreases in loneliness following interventions with laughter therapy (Quan et al, 2020).*

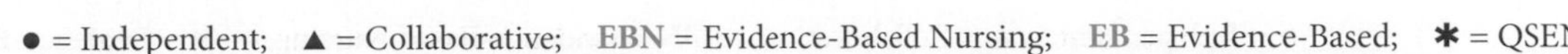

- Consider use of technology, such as computers, video conferencing, the Internet, and apps to alleviate or reduce loneliness or social isolation among older adults. **EB:** *An integrative review found that use of these technologies reduced isolation in older adults (Gardiner, Geldenhuys, & Gott, 2018).*
- Engage the client in positive reminiscence. **EB:** *A systematic review reported significant decreases in loneliness following interventions with reminiscence therapy (Quan et al, 2020).*
- Consider telephone outreach for isolated older individuals. **EB:** *The Yale Geriatrics Student Interest Group implemented the Telephone Outreach in the COVID-19 Outbreak Program at three nursing homes with initial success. Nursing home residents report looking forward to their weekly phone calls and gratitude for social connectedness (van Dyck et al, 2020).*
- ▲ Refer client to horticulture therapy. **EB:** *A systematic review reported significant decreases in loneliness following interventions with horticulture therapy (Quan et al, 2020).*
- ▲ Refer client to pet therapy or consider pet ownership if feasible. **EB:** *An integrative review found that individual pet therapy reduced isolation in older adults (Gardiner, Geldenhuys, & Gott, 2018).*
- Encourage support for the client when the decision to stop driving must be made. **EB:** *The nurse should direct the client toward community support systems and alternate methods of transportation when it is no longer feasible for them to continue driving (Pachana, 2016).*

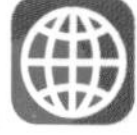

Multicultural

- The preceding interventions may be adapted for diverse clients. Refer to the care plan for **Social** Isolation. Use a person-centered, biopsychosocial, health-focused approach to incorporate and address social determinants of health. **EBN:** *A study found that the nurse's ability to use a person-centered approach to address social determinants of health resulted in a significant reduction of self-reported loneliness in a diverse population (Sadarangani et al, 2019).*

L

Home Care

- ▲ The preceding interventions may be adapted for home care use.
- ▲ Assess for depression with the lonely older client and make appropriate referrals. **EBN:** *The heightened prevalence of depressive symptoms and their relationship to the associated factors (gender, age group, schooling, marital status, and place of residence) of depression in the elderly affirm the necessity to implement means for the advancement of public policies and prioritize strategies that can best guarantee health care for the elderly population (Carréra Campos Leal et al, 2015).*
- If the client has unexplained somatic complaints, evaluate these complaints to ensure that the client's physical needs are being met and assess for a possible relationship between somatic complaints and loneliness. **EB:** *"Our bodies manifest emotions physically when we cannot effectively express them" (Spencer, 2016).* **EBN:** *In their study, Zimmerman et al (2016) confirmed that the nurse can, in collaboration with the client's physician, competently support self-management of clients with psychosomatic symptoms and their psychosocial needs.*
- Assist clients to interact with neighbors in the community when they move to supported housing. **EB:** *Those clients transferring to supported housing will be placed in an unfamiliar environment that necessitates the need to develop skills to successfully adapt to their new surroundings (Kirchen & Hersch, 2015).*
- Refer to the care plan for **Social** Isolation.

Client/Family Teaching and Discharge Planning

- Provide appropriate education for clients and their support persons about disease transmission and treatment if applicable. **EBN:** *Pandur (2015), in her study of infections in home care settings, concluded that home health clients are cared for in a totally unconstrained environment innate with infection possibilities.*
- Refer to the care plan for **Social** Isolation for additional interventions.

REFERENCES

Bohnert, A., Lieb, R., & Arola, N. (2019). More than leisure: Organized activity participation and socio-emotional adjustment among adolescents with autism spectrum disorder. *Journal of Autism and Developmental Disorders, 49*(7), 2637–2652. https://doi.org/10.1007/s10803-016-2783-8

Brittain, K., Kingston, A., Davies, K., et al. (2017). An investigation into the patterns of loneliness and loss in the oldest old—Newcastle 85+ study. *Ageing and Society, 37*(1), 39–62.

Carréra Campos Leal, M., Alves Apóstolo, J. L., Oliveira Cruz Mendes, A. M., & de Oliveira Marques, A. P. (2015). Depression among the elderly in the community, in day care centers, and in geriatric homes. *Journal of Nursing UFPE Online, 9*(4), 7383–7390.

Choukas-Bradley, S., Giletta, M., Cohen, G. L., & Prinstein, M. J. (2015). Peer influence, peer status, and prosocial behavior: An experimental investigation of peer socialization and adolescents' intentions to volunteer. *Journal of Youth and Adolescence, 44*(12), 2197–2210.

Deckx, L., van den Akker, M., Buntinx, F., & van Driel, M. (2018). A systematic literature review on the association between loneliness and coping strategies. *Psychology Health & Medicine, 23*(8), 899–916. https://doi.org/10.1080/13548506.2018.1446096
Dinkins, C. S. (2017). Seeing oneself in the face of the other: The value and challenge of human connectedness for older adults. *Journal of Psychosocial Nursing & Mental Health Services, 55*(7), 13–17.
van Dyck, L. I., Wilkins, K. M., Ouellet, J., Ouellet, G. M., & Conroy, M. L. (2020). Combating heightened social isolation of nursing home elders: The telephone outreach in the COVID-19 outbreak program. *American Journal of Geriatric Psychiatry, 28*(9), 989–992. https://doi.org/10.1016/j.jagp.2020.05.026
Gardiner, C., Geldenhuys, G., & Gott, M. (2018). Interventions to reduce social isolation and loneliness among older people: An integrative review. *Health and Social Care in the Community, 26*(2), 147–157. https://doi.org/10.1111/hsc.12367
Gruenenfelder-Steiger, A. E., Harris, M. A., & Fend, H. A. (2016). Subjective and objective peer approval evaluation and self-esteem development: A test of reciprocal, prospective, and long-term effects. *Developmental Psychology, 52*(10), 1563–1577.
Kirchen, T., & Hersch, G. (2015). Understanding person and environment factors that facilitate veteran adaptation to long-term care. *Physical & Occupational Therapy in Geriatrics, 33*(3), 204–219.
Mann, F., Bone, J. K., Lloyd-Evans, B., et al. (2017). A life less lonely: The state of the art in interventions to reduce loneliness in people with mental health problems. *Social Psychiatry and Psychiatric Epidemiology, 52*(6), 627–638. https://doi.org/10.1007/s00127-017-1392-y
McIntyre, J. C., Worsley, J., Corcoran, R., Woods, P. H., & Bentall, R. P. (2018). Academic and non-academic predictors of student psychological distress: The role of social identity and loneliness. *Journal of Mental Health, 27*(3), 230–239. https://doi.org/10.1080/09638237.2018.1437608
Mitwalli, S., Rabaia, Y., & Kienzler, H. (2018). Support groups for mothers of children with a handicap: A quantitative and qualitative study. *The Lancet, 391*(Suppl. 2), S47. https://doi.org/10.1016/S0140-6736(18)30413-6
Nyatanga, B. (2017). Being lonely and isolated: Challenges for palliative care. *British Journal of Community Nursing, 22*(7), 360.
Pachana, N. A. (2016). Driving, space, and access to activity. *The Journal of Gerontology B Psychological Sciences & Social Sciences, 71*(1), 69–70.
Pandur, R. A. (2015). Infection surveillance in the home healthcare setting. *Australian Nursing and Midwifery Journal, 23*(3), 43.
Quan, N. G., Lohman, M. C., Resciniti, N. V., & Friedman, D. B. (2020). A systematic review of interventions for loneliness among older adults living in long-term care facilities. *Aging & Mental Health, 24*(12), 1945–1955. https://doi.org/10.1080/13607863.2019.1673311
Sadarangani, T., Missaelides, L., Eilertsen, E., Jaganathan, H., & Wu, B. (2019). A mixed-methods evaluation of a nurse-led community-based health home for ethnically diverse older adults with multimorbidity in the adult day health setting. *Policy, Politics, & Nursing Practice, 20*(3), 131–144. https://doi.org/10.1177/1527154419864301
Spencer, D. (2016). Managing psychosomatic symptoms. *The Brown University Child and Adolescent Behavior Letter, 32*(8), 1–7. https://doi.org/10.1002/cbl.30142
Stickley, A., & Koyanagi, A. (2016). Loneliness, common mental disorders and suicidal behavior: Findings from a general population survey. *Journal of Affective Disorders, 197*, 81–87.
Zimmerman, T., Puschmann, E., van den Bussche, H., et al. (2016). Collaborative nurse-led self-management support for primary care patients with anxiety, depressive or somatic problems: Cluster-randomised controlled trial (findings of the SMADS study). *International Journal of Nursing Studies, 63*, 101–111.

L

Ineffective Lymphedema Self-Management
Domain 4 Activity/rest Class 4 Cardiovascular/pulmonary responses

Morgan Nestingen, MSN, APRN, AGCNS-BC, OCN, ONN-CG

NANDA-I

Definition

Unsatisfactory management of symptoms, treatment regimen, physical, psychosocial, and spiritual consequences and lifestyle changes inherent in living with edema related to obstruction or disorders of lymph vessels or nodes.

Defining Characteristics

Lymphedema Signs

Fibrosis in affected limb; recurring infections; swelling in affected limb

Lymphedema Symptoms

Expresses dissatisfaction with quality of life; reports feeling of discomfort in affected limb; reports feeling of heaviness in affected limb; reports feeling of tightness in affected limb

Behaviors

Average daily physical activity is less than recommended for age and gender; inadequate manual lymph drainage; inadequate protection of affected area; inappropriate application of nighttime bandaging;

inappropriate diet; inappropriate skin care; inappropriate use of compression garments; inattentive to carrying heavy objects; inattentive to extreme temperatures; inattentive to lymphedema signs; inattentive to lymphedema symptoms; inattentive to sunlight exposure; reduced range of motion of affected limb; refuses to apply night-time bandages; refuses to use compression garments

Related Factors

Competing demands; competing lifestyle preferences; conflict between health behaviors and social norms; decreased perceived quality of life; difficulty accessing community resources; difficulty managing complex treatment regimen; difficulty navigating complex health care systems; difficulty with decision-making; inadequate commitment to a plan of action; inadequate health literacy; inadequate knowledge of treatment regimen; inadequate number of cues to action; inadequate role models; inadequate social support; limited ability to perform aspects of treatment regimen; low self efficacy; negative feelings toward treatment regimen; neurobehavioral manifestations; nonacceptance of condition; perceived barrier to treatment regimen; perceived social stigma associated with condition; unrealistic perception of seriousness of condition; unrealistic perception of susceptibility to sequelae; unrealistic perception of treatment benefit

At-Risk Population

Adolescents; children; economically disadvantaged individuals; individuals with history of ineffective health self-management; individuals with limited decision making experience; individuals with low educational level; older adults

Associated Conditions

Chemotherapy; chronic venous insufficiency; developmental disabilities; infections; invasive procedure; major surgery; neoplasms; obesity; radiotherapy; removal of lymph nodes; trauma

L

NOC Outcomes (Nursing Outcomes Classification)

Suggested NOC Outcome

Lymphedema severity: Severity of adverse physical, emotional, and social responses due to lymphedema

Example NOC Outcome with Indicators

Lymphedema Severity: Identifies area of edema and impact on health as evidenced by limited physical function or mobility. (Rate outcome and indicators 1 = severe 2 = substantial 3 = moderate, 4 = mild 5 = none)

Client Outcomes

Client Will (Specify Time Frame)

- Monitor skin firmness of affected area
- Report numbness of affected area
- Report redness of affected area
- Report pain
- Report feelings of anxiety and/or depression

NIC Interventions (Nursing Interventions Classification)

Suggested NIC Intervention

Lymphedema severity: Assist the client with understanding and minimize the side effects of radiation treatment

Example NIC Activities

Promote activities to modify the identified risk factors that may lead to lymphedema

Nursing Interventions and *Rationales*

- Recognize individual client risk factors for development of immediate or delayed lymphedema and assess at-risk clients at each visit to promote early identification. EB: *Lymphedema may be primary (i.e., congenital) or secondary to illness or treatment (e.g., cancer related). Older age, obesity, inflammatory conditions, malignancy, and surgical or radiation treatment affecting the lymph node system are key risk factors for both immediate and delayed onset lymphedema. Certain specific treatments increase the risk of local lymphedema (e.g., axillary lymph node dissection and upper limb lymphedema). Early detection is key to treating and potentially reversing low-stage lymphedema; progressive stages are less amenable to treatment (National Comprehensive Cancer Network [NCCN], 2021). Isolated hand edema in breast cancer survivors may be a prognostic indicator for subsequent edema progression in the at-risk limb (Brunelle et al, 2018).*
- At each visit, ask clients if they are experiencing any early symptoms of lymphedema, including swelling or a sense of heaviness, fullness, tightness, or pain in the at-risk limb. Assess signs of lymphedema, including observation of swelling, pitting, or fibrosis. EB: *The NCCN recommends routine screening and assessment of lymphedema in at-risk survivors of cancer to ensure early identification and treatment (NCCN, 2021).*
- Perform detailed medication reconciliation, consider medications that may exacerbate lymphedema symptoms, and review concerning medications with client and ordering provider. EB: *Many commonly used medications may exacerbate or mask lymphedema symptoms, complicating early diagnosis and treatment (Tesar & Armer, 2018).*
- Assess the client's skin and understanding of skin self-care regimen. Demonstrate and instruct the client in meticulous skin care in the at-risk limb. EB: *A systematic review found that lymphedema self-care regimens including hygiene were associated with improved outcomes, including volume reduction and improved quality of life (Douglass et al, 2016). Assessment of the client's understanding of self-care can help to identify gaps and promote effective self-care.*
- Review the client's dietary habits and encourage a healthy diet. EB: *A healthy diet supports healthy weight maintenance and combats inflammatory processes to reduce the lymphedema risk and reduces fluid shifting; dietary consultation may assist in determining client's specific dietary needs (Cavezzi et al, 2019; Vafa et al, 2020).*
- If the client has experienced symptoms of lymphedema, assess the frequency, severity, and impact on activities of daily living, pain, range of motion, and strength. Inspect the at-risk limb for signs or symptoms of infection. EB: *Thorough assessment of related factors and limitations supports determination of lymphedema severity (NCCN, 2021).*
- Refer the client with lymphedema to a trained lymphedema specialist, if available. EB: *The NCCN recommends referral to a trained lymphedema specialist to ensure accuracy in volume measurements, recommendation of additional diagnostics, specialized therapeutic techniques, and expert education (NCCN, 2021).*
- When possible, assist the client in establishing baseline limb measurements for comparison with subsequent posttreatment and interval measures. Advocate for client access to a trained lymphedema specialist, if available. EB: *Limb measurements are an inexpensive, accessible way to evaluate lymphedema severity, particularly when measured by a trained specialist. Lymphedema specialists may perform a detailed examination of limb volume, range of motion, muscle function, circulation, sensation, hemodynamics, and mobility (NCCN, 2021).*
- Assess the client for psychosocial distress, including anxiety, depression, fear of cancer recurrence, body image disturbance, difficulty coping, financial challenges, and changes in sexuality. In cancer clients and survivors, use of a validated psychosocial screening tool may facilitate screening and assessment. EB: *Cancer survivors with lymphedema often face psychosocial challenges, including age-related, sexuality, body image, and relational challenges, requiring intervention (Eaton et al, 2020).*
- Connect the client with appropriate, individualized resources and referrals for any psychosocial distress identified. For example, a client struggling to cope with adherence to self-management may benefit from motivational interviewing, whereas a client suffering from lymphedema-related body image disturbance may wish to connect with a lymphedema support group. EB: *A recent systematic review found an association between lymphedema and lower quality of life and poor physical, psychosocial, relational, and financial functioning; lymphedema symptoms and severity were associated with a lower quality of life (Bowman et al, 2020). A phenomenological study described the supportive care needs of women with breast cancer–related lymphedema, including physical (e.g., difficulties with chores and self-care), psychosocial (e.g., uncertainty and social needs), health care systems and information (e.g., educational), and financial supportive care*

needs; these were alleviated by support from family members and health care professionals (Arikan Dönmez et al, 2021).

- Explore any client beliefs, priorities, support, and financial resources that may affect client's adherence to lymphedema self-management plan. **EB:** *Cultural beliefs may affect client's adherence to lymphedema self-management plan and should be assessed and proactively addressed to support effective self-management (Anderson & Armer, 2021).*
- Provide individualized lymphedema teaching, including basic explanation of the lymphatic system, personal risk factors, signs and symptoms of lymphedema, self-management, treatments, and potential psychosocial concerns. **EB:** *There is no clear consensus on what constitutes effective lymphedema self-management teaching; thus education varies widely and teaching may be inadequate with regard to self-care and exercise (Hurren & Yates, 2019). However, a systematic review found that self-management education was associated with improvement in lymphedema symptoms and quality of life (Howell et al, 2017).*
- Confirm fit and demonstrate donning/doffing of compression garments and devices, when applicable. Assist the client with obtaining ordered compression garments and devices and connect client with referrals and resources to address client financial responsibility. **EB:** *The Oncology Nursing Society (ONS) recommends preventive use in clients at risk for extremity, truncal, or head and neck edema, based on low-level evidence (Armer et al, 2020).*
- Demonstrate self-massage and exercises (typically a combination of resistance and strength training) to promote lymphatic drainage, as instructed by a provider or lymphedema specialist. In postoperative clients at risk for lymphedema, delay start of exercises for 7 days or until cleared by the surgeon and lymphedema specialist. **EB:** *The ONS recommends self-massage of postoperative scar tissue in clients at risk for extremity, truncal, or head and neck edema, as instructed by a surgical or lymphedema specialist and as tolerated by the client (Armer et al, 2020). Exercise is associated with decreased lymphedema symptoms in at-risk, postsurgical clients (Ali et al, 2019).*
- Provide dietary teaching. **EB:** *Dietary teaching supports maintenance of a healthy diet to reduce lymphedema risk factors (Cavezzi et al, 2019; Vafa et al, 2020).*
- Assess impact of lymphedema on client's physiological, functional, and occupational status. Consider limitations in activities of daily living and work limitations, when appropriate. **EB:** *Studies show that lymphedema can affect work through changes in physical and emotional functioning at work, work disruption for treatment, and introduction of work challenges and complicate personal factors involved in returning to work (Sun et al, 2020; Vignes et al, 2020).*
- If lymphedema symptoms worsen or fail to improve with intervention, assess client's understanding of and adherence to treatment plan. Consider approaches to improve client adherence to self-management and health-promoting behaviors (e.g., motivational interviewing). **EB:** *A recent meta-analysis found that using motivation–behavioral skills approach and teaching mindfulness skills may play in improving client adherence by supporting health-promoting behaviors (Sala et al., 2020).*
- Support client-provider interactions to identify some form of appropriate, active lymphedema treatment plan (e.g., complete decongestive therapy, resistance training, surgery) in addition to self-management if lymphedema cannot be managed by self-care alone. **EBN:** *The ONS recommends active treatment of lymphedema in addition to self-management, based on low-level evidence (Armer et al, 2020). Decongestive lymphatic therapy has been shown to significantly decrease limb volume despite previous treatment, suggesting that subsequent treatment in recurrent or refractory lymphedema may be warranted (Bozkurt et al, 2017). A recent systematic review found surgery to be associated with improved quality of life (Coriddi et al, 2020).*

Pediatrics and Adolescents

- Support caregivers of children and adolescents with lymphedema by teaching self-management techniques to both the child and caregiver, using flexible and individualized approaches, and addressing caregiver fears and anxiety over the child's health condition. **EB:** *Parents and caregivers may struggle to balance children's ability to self-manage with rigid teaching approaches provided by clinicians, while coping with fear and anxiety (Moffat et al, 2019a, 2019b).*

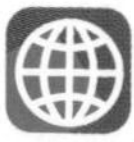

Multicultural

- In Latina cancer survivors, family involvement, peer-mentoring, culturally competent education, and self-care skills are important additions to the client's lymphedema self-management plan. **EB:** *A literature* *review of factors affecting management of breast cancer–related lymphedema in Latina survivors demonstrated the importance of these additional factors (Anderson & Armer, 2021).*

ClientFamily Teaching and Discharge Planning

- Encourage the client to inform health care providers of any history of lymphedema, procedures that increase lymphedema risk, and contraindications against venipuncture or blood pressure in the at-risk/affected limb. EB: *Limited observational data suggest that air travel, venipuncture of the at-risk/affected limb, and blood pressures taken on the at-risk/affected limb are safe; however, when possible the NCCN recommends avoiding the at-risk/affected limb because this limb may be used in case of urgent medical need (NCCN, 2021).*
- Instruct the client to take medication only as ordered and review all medications with health care providers. EB: *Medications may exacerbate lymphedema or complicate diagnosis and should be reviewed with a provider (Tesar & Armer, 2018).*
- Teach the client to self-monitor and report early signs or symptoms of lymphedema (e.g., swelling, fullness, tightness, heaviness, or pain in the at-risk limb). EB: *Early-stage lymphedema is often reversible, whereas late-stage lymphedema is less responsive to treatment (NCCN, 2021). Breast cancer clients with lymphedema experience specific, timely informational needs and benefit from private education sessions provided by clinicians or social networks (Dorri et al, 2020; Arikan Dönmez et al, 2021).*
- Instruct the client to observe the at-risk limb for signs of infection, including fever, warmth, redness, or swelling, and immediately report these to a health care provider if they occur. EB: *Lymphedema and increased risk for lymphedema are associated with potentially serious localized infections and may require hospitalization and treatment with intravenous antibiotics (NCCN, 2021).*
- Teach meticulous skin care in the at-risk limb, including keeping skin clean and dry; applying lotion; using an electric razor versus a razor blade to shave; avoiding exposure of the limb to excessive heat, cold, or direct sunlight; and protecting skin from injury. EB: *A systematic review of lymphedema self-care regimens found that regimens including hygiene were commonly associated with improved outcomes, including volume reduction and improved quality of life (Douglass et al, 2016). Additionally, meticulous skin care is critical to preventing and identifying lymphedema-related infections quickly (NCCN, 2021).*
- Emphasize the importance of regular exercise in reducing lymphedema risk and severity. EB: *Exercise is associated with prevention, delayed onset, and decreased severity of lymphedema symptoms in at-risk clients (Ali et al, 2019).*
- Encourage the client to discuss any psychosocial concerns related to lymphedema, including anxiety, depression, body image disturbance, difficulty coping, financial challenges, and changes in sexuality. EB: *A recent literature review found that breast cancer survivors with lymphedema often faced age-related, sexuality, body image, and relational challenges, requiring psychosocial intervention (Eaton et al, 2020).*

L

REFERENCES

Ali, J. S., Gamal, L. M., & El-saidy, T. M. K. (2019). Effect of prophylactic physical activities on reducing lymphedema among women post mastectomy. *Journal of Health, Medicine and Nursing, 61*, 95–113.

Anderson, E. A., & Armer, J. M. (2021). Factors impacting management of breast cancer-related lymphedema (BCRL) in Hispanic/Latina breast cancer survivors: A literature review. *Hispanic Health Care International: The Official Journal of the National Association of Hispanic Nurses, 19*(3), 190–202. https://doi.org/10.1177/1540415321990621.

Arikan Dönmez, A., Kuru Alici, N., & Borman, P. (2021). Lived experiences for supportive care needs of women with breast cancer-related lymphedema: A phenomenological study. *Clinical Nursing Research, 30*(6), 799–808.

Armer, J. M., Ostby, P. L., Ginex, P. K., et al. (2020). ONS Guidelines™ for cancer treatment-related lymphedema. *Oncology Nursing Forum, 47*(5), 518–538.

Bowman, C., Piedalue, K. A., Baydoun, M., & Carlson, L. E. (2020). The quality of life and psychosocial implications of cancer-related lower-extremity lymphedema: A systematic review of the literature. *Journal of Clinical Medicine, 9*(10), 3200.

Bozkurt, M., Palmer, L. J., & Guo, Y. (2017). Effectiveness of decongestive lymphatic therapy in patients with lymphedema resulting from breast cancer treatment regardless of previous lymphedema treatment. *Breast Journal, 23*(2), 154–158.

Brunelle, C. L., Swaroop, M. N., Skolny, M. N., Asdourian, M. S., Sayegh, H. E., & Taghian, A. G. (2018). Hand edema in patients at risk of breast cancer–related lymphedema: Health professionals should take notice. *Physical Therapy, 98*(6), 510–517.

Cavezzi, A., Urso, S. U., Ambrosini, L., Croci, S., Campana, F., & Mosti, G. (2019). Lymphedema and nutrition: A review. *Veins and Lymphatics, 8*(1).

Coriddi, M., Dayan, J., Sobti, N., et al. (2020). Systematic review of patient-reported outcomes following surgical treatment of lymphedema. *Cancers, 12*(3), 565.

Dorri, S., Olfatbakhsh, A., & Asadi, F. (2020). Informational needs in patients with breast cancer with lymphedema: Is it important? *Breast Cancer: Basic and Clinical Research, 14*, 1178223420911033.

Douglass, J., Graves, P., & Gordon, S. (2016). Self-care for management of secondary lymphedema: A systematic review. *PLoS Neglected Tropical Diseases, 10*(6), e0004740. https://doi.org/10.1371/journal.pntd.0004740.

Eaton, L., Narkthong, N., & Hulett, J. (2020). Psychosocial Issues associated with breast cancer-related lymphedema: A literature review. *Current Breast Cancer Reports*. [Online ahead of print].

Howell, D., Harth, T., Brown, J., Bennett, C., & Boyko, S. (2017). Self-management education interventions for patients with cancer: A systematic review. *Supportive Care in Cancer*, *25*(4), 1323–1355.

Hurren, S. J., & Yates, K. (2019). At what point can I lift things? Women's satisfaction with lymphoedema prevention information after breast cancer surgery. *Collegian Journal of the Royal College of Nursing Australia*, *26*(3), 335–340.

Moffatt, C., Aubeeluck, A., Stasi, E., et al. (2019a). A study to explore the parental impact and challenges of self-management in children and adolescents suffering with lymphedema. *Lymphatic Research and Biology*, *17*(2), 245–252.

Moffatt, C., Aubeeluck, A., Stasi, E., et al. (2019b). A study using visual art methods to explore the perceptions and barriers of self-management in children and adolescents with lymphedema. *Lymphatic Research and Biology*, *17*(2), 231–244.

National Comprehensive Cancer Network (NCCN). (2021). Survivorship (version 1.2021). Retrieved from https://www.nccn.org/professionals/physician_gls/pdf/survivorship.pdf.

Sala, M., Rochefort, C., Lui, P. P., & Baldwin, A. S. (2020). Trait mindfulness and health behaviours: A meta-analysis. *Health Psychology Review*, *14*(3), 345–393. https://doi.org/10.1080/17437199.2019.1650290.

Sun, Y., Shigaki, C. L., & Armer, J. M. (2020). The influence of breast cancer related lymphedema on women's return-to-work. *Women's Health (London, England)*, *16*, 1745506520905720. https://doi.org/10.1177/1745506520905720.

Tesar, E., & Armer, J. M. (2018). Effect of common medications on breast cancer-related lymphedema. *Rehabilitation Oncology*, *36*(1), 7–12.

Vafa, S., Zarrati, M., Malakootinejad, M., et al. (2020). Calorie restriction and synbiotics effect on quality of life and edema reduction in breast cancer-related lymphedema, a clinical trial. *The Breast*, *54*, 37–45.

Vignes, S., Fau-Prudhomot, P., Simon, L., Sanchez-Bréchot, M. L., Arrault, M., & Locher, F. (2020). Impact of breast cancer–related lymphedema on working women. *Supportive Care in Cancer*, *28*(1), 79–85.

Risk for Ineffective Lymphedema Self-Management

Domain 4 Activity/rest

Class 4 Cardiovascular/pulmonary responses

Mary Beth Flynn Makic, PhD, RN, CCNS, CCRN-K, FAAN, FNAP, FCNS

NANDA-I

Definition

Susceptible to unsatisfactory management of symptoms, treatment regimen, physical, psychosocial, and spiritual consequences and lifestyle changes inherent in living with edema related to obstruction or disorders of lymph vessels or nodes which may compromise health.

Related Factors

Competing demands; competing lifestyle preferences; conflict between health behaviors and social norms; decreased perceived quality of life; difficulty accessing community resources; difficulty managing complex treatment regimen; difficulty navigating complex health care systems; difficulty with decision-making; inadequate commitment to a plan of action; inadequate health literacy; inadequate knowledge of treatment regimen; inadequate number of cues to action; inadequate role models; inadequate social support; limited ability to perform aspects of treatment regimen; low self efficacy; negative feelings toward treatment regimen; neurobehavioral manifestations; nonacceptance of condition; perceived barrier to treatment regimen; perceived social stigma associated with condition; unrealistic perception of seriousness of condition; unrealistic perception of susceptibility to sequelae; unrealistic perception of treatment benefit

At-Risk Population

Adolescents; children; economically disadvantaged individuals; individuals with history of ineffective health self-management; individuals with limited decision making experience; individuals with low educational level; older adults

Associated Conditions

Chemotherapy; chronic venous insufficiency; developmental disabilities; infections; invasive procedure; major surgery; neoplasms; obesity; radiotherapy; removal of lymph nodes; trauma

NOC, NIC, Client Outcomes, Nursing Interventions and *Rationales,* and References

Refer to care plan for Ineffective **Lymphedema** Self-Management.

Risk for Disturbed Maternal–Fetal Dyad

Domain 8 Sexuality Class 3 Reproduction

Dianne F. Hayward, RN, MSN, WHNP

NANDA-I

Definition

Susceptible to a disruption of the symbiotic motherfetal relationship as a result of comorbid or pregnancy-related conditions, which may compromise health.

Risk Factors

Inadequate prenatal care; substance misuse; unaddressed abuse

Associated Conditions

Compromised fetal oxygen transport; glucose metabolism disorders; pregnancy complication; treatment regimen

NOC (Nursing Outcomes Classification)

Suggested NOC Outcomes

Fetal Status: Antepartum; Maternal Status: Antepartum, Intrapartum; Depression Level; Blood Glucose Level; Family Resiliency; Knowledge: Self-Management; Nausea and Vomiting Severity; Social Support; Spiritual Support, Parent-Infant Attachment

Example NOC Outcome with Indicators

Maternal Status: Antepartum as evidenced by the following indicators: Emotional attachment to fetus/Coping with discomforts of pregnancy/Mood lability/Blood pressure/Blood glucose/Hemoglobin. (Rate the outcome and indicators of **Maternal Status: Antepartum:** 1 = Severe deviation from normal range, 2 = Substantial deviation from normal range, 3 = Moderate deviation from normal range, 4 = Mild deviation from normal range, 5 = No deviation from normal range [see Section I].)

Client Outcomes

Client Will (Specify Time Frame)

During Pregnancy

- Attend all scheduled prenatal visits and attend prenatal education either virtual or in person with significant other or involved family member
- Cope with fears and discomforts of high-risk pregnancy until delivery of baby
- Demonstrate emotional attachment to fetus during pregnancy
- Adhere to prescribed regimens to maintain homeostasis during pregnancy

NIC (Nursing Interventions Classification)

Suggested NIC Interventions

High-Risk Pregnancy Care; Intrapartal Care: High-Risk Delivery

Example NIC Activities—High-Risk Pregnancy Care

Determine the presence of medical factors that are related to poor pregnancy outcome (e.g., diabetes, hypertension, lupus erythematosus, herpes, hepatitis, HIV, multiple gestation, substance abuse, epilepsy, infection); Provide educational materials that address the risk factors and usual surveillance tests and procedures.

M

Nursing Interventions and *Rationales*

Prenatal

- Encourage early prenatal care and regular prenatal visits. EB: *Prenatal care is crucial for a good pregnancy outcome for mothers and infants. Many women in the United States receive late (starting in third trimester) or no prenatal care, resulting in avoidable adverse health outcomes (Oghogho & Beck-Sagué, 2020). The World Health Organization (WHO) guidelines for prenatal care include a minimum of eight contacts to reduce perinatal mortality and improve women's experience of care, counseling about a healthy lifestyle, and keeping physically active during pregnancy (World Health Organization, 2016).*
- Determine the presence of medical factors that are related to poor pregnancy outcome (e.g., diabetes, hypertension, lupus erythematosus, herpes, hepatitis, HIV, multiple gestation, substance abuse, epilepsy, infection); provide educational materials that address the risk factors and usual surveillance tests and procedures. EB: *Early identification of at-risk mothers can ensure interventions either to control the risk-causing factor or delivery of timely and appropriate care as and when needed (Chaudhry et al, 2019).*
- Assess the antenatal client for fear related to high-risk pregnancy and fetal outcomes. EBN: *An Istanbul study found that pregnant women with a poor level of psychosocial adaptation showed more depressive symptoms (Fiskin et al, 2017).*
- Assess antepartum clients for depression using a culturally competent tool that evaluates the bio-psycho-social-spiritual dimensions. EBN: *Susser et al (2016) reported that nearly 20% of women in pregnancy and in the postpartum period are affected with depression. There is a high risk of morbidity and mortality when a woman is affected with perinatal depression, and this may have long-term consequences on child development.*
- Focus on the abilities of a pregnant woman with disabilities by encouraging identification of support systems, resources, and need for environmental modification. EBN: *In a recent study of pregnant women with disabilities, the women reported a lack of knowledge, awareness, sensitivity, and respect, as well as stereotyping, as issues that contributed to compromised perinatal care (Smeltzer et al, 2016).*
- Assess for lack of social support system, loneliness, depression, lack of confidence, maternal powerlessness, domestic violence, and socioeconomic problems. EBN: *Screening should include significant risk factors to detect at-risk women (Ruyak et al, 2017).*
- Identify patterns of intimate partner violence in all pregnant and postpartum women. EBN: *Violence during pregnancy can result in poor maternal, neonatal, and early childhood outcomes; routine screening and assessment may interrupt further abuse and promote positive outcomes (Bianchi et al, 2016).* EBN: *Nurses play a vital role in the identification and support of women who experience violence (Bianchi, 2016).*
- Perform accurate blood pressure readings at each client's clinic encounter. EB: *As hypertension is one of the most common medical disorders complicating pregnancy, good control of blood pressure during pregnancy helps prevent adverse maternal–fetal outcomes (Bello et al, 2018).*
- Provide educational materials and support for personal autonomy about genetic counseling and testing options before pregnancy with preimplantation genetic testing or during pregnancy with fetal nuchal translucency ultrasound, quadruple screen, and cystic fibrosis screening. EBN: *Nurses can advocate, understand the perceptions of, and assist clients in their reproductive decision-making (Shiroff & Nemeth, 2015).*
- Ensure that pregnant clients have an adequate diet and take multimicronutrient supplements containing at least 400 μg of folic acid, especially during early pregnancy. EB: *Nutritional information can be found at* choosemyplate.gov. *which presents healthy choices from each food group needed for a healthy pregnancy (U.S. Department of Agriculture [USDA], 2020).* EB: *The US Preventive Services Task Force (USPSTF) has updated its recommendation that all women who are planning or capable of pregnancy take a daily supplement containing 0.4 to 0.8 mg (400–800 μg) of folic acid to prevent neural tube defects (Bibbins-Domingo et al, 2017).*
- Provide pregnant women diagnosed with gestational diabetes with education about management and treatment. EBN: *Good control of blood glucose is important during delivery to reduce the risk of neonatal hypoglycemia (King, 2017).*
- Assess use of tobacco and, if positive for use, offer a tobacco cessation program and explain the health risks to the unborn fetus and mother. EBN *Many women who do stop smoking during their pregnancies relapse in the postpartum period. Smoking is a major cause of adverse pregnancy and birth outcomes (Fallin-Bennett et al, 2019). A free and helpful website for quitting smoking is available at https://women.smokefree.gov/tools-tips-women/text-programs/smokefreemom (U.S. Department of Health and Human Services, n.d.).*

M

- Assess for alcohol misuse and counsel women to stop drinking during pregnancy. Provide appropriate referral for treatment as needed. EB: *There is no safe time to drink alcohol during pregnancy, and drinking during pregnancy can result in fetal alcohol spectrum disorder (FASD). FASD is a range of physical, mental, behavioral, and/or learning disabilities with potential lifelong implications that occur after exposure to alcohol in utero (Association of Women's Health, Obstetric and Neonatal Nurses [AWHONN], 2019).*
- Screen for current illicit drug use. Emphasize the risks of drug exposure to the fetus/newborn and the potential for withdrawal. EB: *Pregnancy is an opportune time to identify substance misuse dependence, facilitate conversion to maintenance treatment, and coordinate comprehensive prenatal care with specialists in addiction medicine, behavioral health, and social services (Krans et al, 2015).*
- Refer clients who self-report drug misuse or have positive toxicology screens to a comprehensive treatment program designed for the pregnant woman. EBN: *Untreated addiction can lead to poor maternal and fetal health outcomes. Neonates born to women receiving treatment may have withdrawal symptoms and require additional treatment (Keough & Fantasia, 2017).*
- Encourage pregnant women to use digital resources, such as Text4Baby (see https://www.text4baby.org) or https://www.whattoexpect.com, to track pregnancy progress and provide education and motivation to make healthy lifestyle choices. EBN: *Multiple digital sources of health-related information are available, and women may need help to identify those that are most reputable and useful (Lowe & Hartley, 2018).*

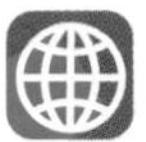

Multicultural

Prenatal

- Assess the client's beliefs and concerns about pregnancy. EB: *Continuity of supportive care and sensitivity to the mother's cultural, religious, and individual beliefs and values reduce the risk of psychological trauma and enhance women's trust in their caregivers, their experiences of childbearing, and their willingness to accept care and to seek it in the future (LaLonde et al, 2019).*

M

REFERENCES

Association of Women's Health, Obstetric and Neonatal Nurses (AWHONN). (2019). Optimizing outcomes for women with substance use disorders in pregnancy and the postpartum period. *Journal of Obstetric Gynecologic & Neonatal Nursing*, *48*(5), 583–585. https://doi.org/10.1016/j.jogn.2019.06.001

Bello, N. A., Woolley, J. J., Cleary, K. L., et al. (2018). Accuracy of blood pressure measurement devices in pregnancy: A systematic review of validation studies. *Hypertension*, *71*(2), 326–335. https://doi.org/10.1161/hypertensionaha.117.10295

Bianchi, A. L. (2016). Intimate partner violence during the childbearing years. *Journal of Obstetric Gynecologic & Neonatal Nursing*, *45*(4), 577–578. https://doi.org/10.1016/j.jogn.2016.03.140

Bianchi, A. L., Cesario, S. K., & McFarlane, J. (2016). Interrupting intimate partner violence during pregnancy with an effective screening and assessment program. *Journal of Obstetric Gynecologic & Neonatal Nursing*, *45*(4), 579–591. https://doi.org/10.1016/j.jogn.2016.02.012

Bibbins-Domingo, K., Grossman, D. C., Curry, S. J., et al. (2017). Folic acid supplementation for the prevention of neural tube defects: US preventive services task force recommendation Statement. *The Journal of the American Medical Association*, *317*(2), 183–189. https://doi.org/10.1001/jama.2016.19438

Chaudhry, M., Patil, K., Swamy, M. K., & Khandelwal, S. (2019). Antepartum risk assessment for pregnant women visiting a tertiary care university teaching hospital in Southern India. *Indian Obstetrics and Gynaecology*, *9*(1), 19–25. https://pubmed.ncbi.nlm.nih.gov/32747874/.

Fallin-Bennett, A., Scott, T., Fallin-Bennett, K., & Ashford, K. (2019). Call to action to reduce tobacco use during pregnancy. *Journal of Obstetric Gynecologic & Neonatal Nursing*, *48*(5), 563–567. https://doi.org/10.1016/jogn.2019.02.009

Fiskin, F., Kaydirak, M. M., & Oskay, U. Y. (2017). Psychosocial adaptation and depressive manifestations in high-risk pregnant women: Implications for clinical practice. *Worldviews on Evidence-Based Nursing*, *14*(1), 55–64. https://doi.org/10.1111/wvn.12186

Keough, L., & Fantasia, H. C. (2017). Pharmacologic treatment of opioid addiction during pregnancy. *Nursing for Women's Health*, *21*(1), 34–44. https://doi.org/10.1016/j.nwh.2016.12.010

King, P. (2017). Gestational diabetes: A practical guide. *Journal of Diabetes Nursing*, *21*(3), 84–89.

Krans, E. E., Cochran, G., & Bogen, D. L. (2015). Caring for opioid-dependent pregnant women: Prenatal and postpartum care considerations. *Clinical Obstetrics and Gynecology*, *58*(2), 370–379. https://doi.org/10.1097/GRF.0000000000000098

Lalonde, A., Herschderfer, K., Pascali-Bonaro, D., Hanson, C., Fuchtner, C., & Visser, G. H. A. (2019). The International Childbirth Initiative: 12 steps to safe and respectful MotherBaby–family maternity care. *International Journal of Gynecology & Obstetrics*, *146*(1), 65–73. https://doi.org/10.1002/ijgo.12844

Lowe, N. K., & Hartley, A. K. (2018). The evolving landscape of mHealth apps. *Journal of Obstetric Gynecologic & Neonatal Nursing*, *47*(6), 725–727. https://doi.org/10.1016/j.jogn.2018.10.001

Oghogho, E. S., & Beck-Sagué, C. (2020). Effect of Medicaid expansion status on risk of late or no prenatal care in black and white US mothers: Analysis of US natality data, 2010-17. *Lancet Global Health*, *8*(Suppl. 1), S27. https://doi.org/10.1016/s2214-109x(20)30168-6

Ruyak, S. L., Flores-Montoya, A., & Boursaw, B. (2017). Antepartum services and symptoms of postpartum depression in at-risk women. *Journal of Obstetric Gynecologic & Neonatal Nursing*, *46*(5), 696–708. https://doi.org/10.1016/j.jogn.2017.07.006

Shiroff, J. J., & Nemeth, L. S. (2015). Public perceptions of recessive carrier testing in the preconception and prenatal periods. *Journal of Obstetric Gynecologic & Neonatal Nursing*, *44*(6), 717–725. https://doi.org/10.1111/1552-6909.12764

Smeltzer, S. C., Mitra, M., Iezzoni, L. I., Long-Bellil, L., & Smith, L. D. (2016). Perinatal experiences of women with physical disabilities and their recommendations for clinicians. *Journal of Obstetric Gynecologic & Neonatal Nursing, 45*(6), 781–789. https://doi.org/10.1016/j.jogn.2016.07.007

Susser, L. C., Sansone, S. A., & Hermann, A. D. (2016). Selective serotonin reuptake inhibitors for depression in pregnancy. *American Journal of Obstetrics and Gynecology, 215*(6), 722–730. https://doi.org/10.1016/j.ajog.2016.07.011

U.S. Department of Agriculture. (2020). MyPlate. Choosemyplate.gov.

U.S. Department of Health and Human Services. (n.d.). SmokefreeMOM. https://women.smokefree.gov/tools-tips-women/text-programs/smokefreemom.

World Health Organization (WHO). (2016). *New guidelines on antenatal care for a positive pregnancy experience.* Retrieved from https://www.who.int/reproductivehealth/news/antenatal-care/en. Accessed July 13, 2021.

Impaired Memory Domain 5 Perception/cognition Class 4 Cognition

Olga F. Jarrín, PhD, RN, Nishat S. Poppy, BSN, RN, and Linda J. Hassler, DNP, RN, GCNS-BC, FGNLA

NANDA-I

Definition

Persistent inability to remember or recall bits of information or skills, while maintaining the capacity to independently perform activities of daily living.

Defining Characteristics

Consistently forgets to perform a behavior at the scheduled time; difficulty acquiring a new skill; difficulty acquiring new information; difficulty recalling events; difficulty recalling factual information; difficulty recalling familiar names; difficulty recalling familiar objects; difficulty recalling familiar words; difficulty recalling if a behavior was performed; difficulty retaining a new skill; difficulty retaining new information

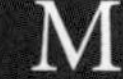

Related Factors

Depressive symptoms; inadequate intellectual stimulation; inadequate motivation; inadequate social support; social isolation; water-electrolyte imbalance

At-Risk Population

Economically disadvantaged individuals; individuals aged 60 years; individuals with low educational level

Associated Conditions

Anemia; brain hypoxia; cognition disorders

NOC (Nursing Outcomes Classification)

Suggested NOC Outcomes

Cognitive Orientation; Memory; Neurological Status: Consciousness

Example NOC Outcome with Indicators

Memory as evidenced by the following indicators: Recalls immediate information accurately/Recalls recent information accurately/Recalls remote information accurately. (Rate each indicator of **Memory:** 1 = severely compromised, 2 = substantially compromised, 3 = moderately compromised, 4 = mildly compromised, 5 = not compromised [see Section I].)

Client Outcomes

Client Will (Specify Time Frame)

- Demonstrate use of techniques to help with memory loss
- State he or she has improved memory for everyday concerns

NIC (Nursing Interventions Classification)

Suggested NIC Interventions

Memory Training; Dementia Management; Reality Orientation

Example NIC Activities—Memory Training

Discuss with client/family any practical memory problems experienced; Implement appropriate memory techniques, such as visual imagery, mnemonic devices, memory games, memory cues, association techniques, making lists, using computers, using name tags, or rehearsing information; Structure the teaching methods according to client's organization of information; Refer to occupational therapy, as appropriate; Monitor changes in memory with training

Nursing Interventions and *Rationales*

- Determine whether onset of memory loss is gradual or sudden; if sudden, screen for delirium using the Confusion Assessment Method (CAM) (see digital resources). EB: *The CAM is a standardized tool that enables non–psychiatrically trained clinicians to identify and recognize delirium quickly and accurately (Inouye, 2018).*
- Assess overall cognitive function and memory. A brief screening instrument such as the short Montreal Cognitive Assessment (s-MoCA) or Revised Metamemory in Adulthood (MIA) Questionnaire (MIA-Revised) is useful as a first level of evaluation. EB: *The s-MoCA is valid across neurological disorders and can be administered in approximately 5 minutes to determine whether the client has cognitive impairment and needs to be referred for further evaluation and treatment (Roalf et al, 2016, 2017).* EBN: *The 20-item (2-factor) version of the metamemory in adulthood questionnaire has strong internal reliability and validity for change and capacity subscales (McDonough et al, 2020).*
- Assess risk of B-vitamin deficiencies, including thiamine (vitamin B_1), associated with aging, chronic alcohol abuse, cancer, or bariatric surgery, and encourage a diet plan with adequate B vitamins. EB: *Low B-vitamin status is associated with cognitive dysfunction during the aging process, and supplementation with folic acid (vitamin B_9) or B-complex may improve global cognition, memory, and visuospatial skills (McGrattan et al, 2018).*
- Assess risk of vitamin D deficiency associated with history of inadequate exposure to sunlight and associated with depression and impaired cognitive function in older adults. EBN: *Vitamin D supplementation has a role in improving cognitive performance for those who are deficient in vitamin D (Ombech, 2020).*
- Determine the client's sleep quality and patterns; if sleep quantity and quality are insufficient and client shows symptoms of daytime sleepiness, or symptoms of sleep apnea are present, report to physician/primary care provider and refer to the care plan for Disturbed **Sleep** Pattern. EB: *Sleep-disordered breathing is associated with an increased risk of cognitive impairment and a small worsening of executive function (Leng et al, 2017).*
- Teach clients, including those with cognitive disorders, to use memory techniques such as concentrating and attending, repeating information, making mental associations, and placing items in strategic places so that they will not be forgotten. EBN: *A systemic review of memory-strategy training interventions found improvements in perceived memory ability, memory self-efficacy, strategy use, memory-related affect, psychological well-being, and quality of life (Yang et al, 2018; Hudes et al, 2019).*
- Encourage the client to incorporate daily meditation such as multimodal Kirtan Kriya or other mind-body interventions to improve memory functioning and health. EB: *A 12-week Kirtan Kriya meditation program (30-minute training, followed by 12-minute daily practice) resulted in significant improvement in memory, psychological well-being, mood, and sleep in community-dwelling older adults with early memory loss (Innes et al, 2016).* EB: *The Dejian Mind-Body Intervention (DMBI) delivered once a week for 10 weeks improved memory and subjective physical and psychological health of older adults with subjective memory complaints (Chan et al, 2017a).*

▲ Where available, refer for access to computer-based cognitive training or socially assistive robots. EB: *Computerized cognitive training (including commercially available Cogmed and Lumosity) and socially assistive robots are effective tools for improving cognition and memory (Alnajiar et al, 2019; Pang et al, 2021).*

▲ Where available and of interest to client, refer for regular yoga training and practice. EB: *A weekly yoga education program and self-practice improved community-dwelling older adults' scores on the Mini-Mental State Examination (MMSE) and Rivermead Behavioral Memory Test–Third Edition (RBMT-3) (Pandya, 2020).* EBN: *Octogenarians were able to improve their memory performance when they challenged their limits, used appropriate strategies, practiced yoga, and invested energy and time in learning novel memory techniques (McDougall et al, 2015).*

▲ Where available and of interest to client, refer for participation in calligraphy classes. EB: *An 8-week Chinese calligraphy writing training significantly improved working memory in clients with early mild cognitive impairment (Chan et al, 2017b).*

▲ Refer the client for participation in a multicomponent cognitive rehabilitation program that includes stress and relaxation training, physical activity, structured learning, and social interaction. EB: *Meditation interventions, cognitive training, cognitive rehabilitation, and exercise were the most effective interventions for adult non–central nervous system cancer clients to manage cancer-related cognitive impairment (Zeng et al, 2020).* EBN: *Cognitive rehabilitation in the form of memory skills training, compensatory memory strategies, and use of assistive devices may be helpful for managing the memory deficits associated with stroke or brain injury (Pamaiahgari, 2020).*

- For clients with memory impairments associated with dementia, also see care plan for Chronic **Confusion.**

Geriatric

- All interventions are appropriate for geriatric clients.
- Assess for signs and symptoms of depression using an age-appropriate screening tool such as the Geriatric Depression Scale, and notify provider of results. EBN: *Depression is often associated with memory loss in older adults; however, cognitive behavior therapy, competitive memory training, reminiscence group therapy, problem-adaptation therapy, and problem-solving therapy are all effective interventions to reduce depressive symptoms (Apóstolo et al, 2016).*

M

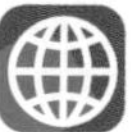

Multicultural

- When using cognitive assessments translated into other languages, refer to translation-specific scoring instructions and any recommended adjustment for low levels of education. EB: *Although cognitive assessments such as the MoCA and MMSE have been translated and validated in many languages, there is wide variation in published cutoff scores, and not correcting for educational bias may result in inappropriate referral or diagnosis (Rosli et al, 2016; Delgado, Araneda, & Behrens, 2019).*
- Visitation facilitation: stigma may result in social isolation, and older adults with memory impairment may need assistance to rebuild and strengthen their social network. EB: *Social network quality and emotional closeness are positively associated with cognitive functioning among older Chinese adults (Li & Dong, 2018).*

Home Care

- The previously mentioned interventions may be adapted for home care use.
- Assist clients to select and use cuing strategies or assistive technology, such as a smart watch, smart phone, pill box, calendar, alarm clock, microwave oven, whistling tea kettle, sign, or written list, to cue behaviors at designated times. EB: *Cues and assistive technology are positively associated with individuals' abilities to perform daily tasks regardless of age or cognitive disease (Leopold et al, 2015).*

Client Family Teaching and Discharge Planning

- Evaluate the need for skilled home health care (skilled nursing, occupational therapy).
- Discuss and assist with use of assistive technology to support client and caregiver with discharge plan: memory aids (e.g., medication reminders, pill box, timers, lists); orientation aids (e.g., electronic clocks and calendars, voice assistant, built-in "Remember This" feature); safety devices (e.g., nightlights, personal alarms); communication aids (e.g., easy-to-use landline and mobile phones, speed dialing, voice-activated dialing, or photo dialing); other devices (e.g., easy-to-use TV remote controls, microwave oven, whistling tea kettle).
- Clarify instructions for medications, treatments, and exercises in writing.

- Assist with developing schedule/chart and reminder system for scheduled and as-needed medications and use of nonpharmacological strategies.

REFERENCES

Alnajiar, F., Khalid, S., Vogan, A. A., Shimoda, S., Nouchi, R., & Kawashima, R. (2019). Emerging cognitive intervention technologies to meet the needs of an aging population: A systematic review. *Frontiers in Aging Neuroscience, 11*, 291. https://doi.org/10.3389/fnagi.2019.00291.

Apóstolo, J., Bobrowicz-Campos, E., Rodrigues, M., Castro, I., & Cardoso, D. (2016). The effectiveness of non-pharmacological interventions in older adults with depressive disorders: A systematic review. *International Journal of Nursing Studies, 58*, 59–70. https://doi.org/10.1016/j.ijnurstu.2016.02.006.

Chan, A. S., Cheung, W. K., Yeung, M. K., et al. (2017a). A Chinese Chan-based Mind-Body Intervention improves memory of older adults. *Frontiers in Aging Neuroscience, 9*, 190. https://doi.org/10.3389/fnagi.2017.00190.

Chan, S. C. C., Chan, C. C. H., Derbie, A. Y., et al. (2017b). Chinese calligraphy writing for augmenting attentional control and working memory of older adults at risk of mild cognitive impairment: A randomized controlled trial. *Journal of Alzheimer's Disease, 58*(3), 735–746. https://doi.org/10.3233/JAD-170024.

Delgado, C., Araneda, A., & Behrens, M. I. (2019). Validation of the Spanish-language version of the Montreal Cognitive Assessment test in adults older than 60 years. *Neurologia, 34*(6), 376–385. https://doi.org/10.1016/j.nrl.2017.01.013.

Hudes, R., Rich, J. B., Troyer, A. K., Yusupov, I., & Vandermorris, S. (2019). The impact of memory-strategy training interventions on participant-reported outcomes in healthy older adults: A systematic review and meta-analysis. *Psychology and Aging, 34*(4), 587–5973. https://doi.org/10.1037/pag0000340.

Innes, K. E., Selfe, T. K., Khalsa, D. S., & Kandati, S. (2016). Effects of meditation versus music listening on perceived stress, mood, sleep, and quality of life in adults with early memory loss: A pilot randomized controlled trial. *Journal of Alzheimer's Disease, 52*(4), 1277–1298. https://doi.org/10.3233/JAD-151106.

Inouye, S. K. (2018). Delirium—a framework to improve acute care for older persons. *Journal of the American Geriatrics Society, 66*(3), 446–451. https://doi.org/10.1111/jgs.15296.

Leng, Y., McEvoy, C. T., Allen, I. E., & Yaffe, K. (2017). Association of sleep-disordered breathing with cognitive function and risk of cognitive impairment: A systematic review and meta-analysis. *JAMA Neurology, 74*(10), 1237–1245. https://doi.org/10.1001/jamaneurol.2017.2180.

Leopold, A., Lourie, A., Petras, H., & Elias, E. (2015). The use of assistive technology for cognition to support the performance of daily activities for individuals with cognitive disabilities due to traumatic brain injury: The current state of the research. *NeuroRehabilitation, 37*(3), 359–378. https://doi.org/10.3233/NRE-151267.

Li, M., & Dong, X. (2018). Is social network a protective factor for cognitive impairment in US Chinese older adults? Findings from the PINE study. *Gerontology, 64*, 246–256. https://doi.org/10.1159/000485616.

McDonough, I. M., McDougall, G. J., LaRocca, M., Dalmida, S. G., & Arheart, K. L. (2020). Refining the metamemory in adulthood questionnaire: A 20-item version of change and capacity designed for research and clinical settings. *Aging & Mental Health, 24*(7), 1054–1063. https://doi.org/10.1080/13607863.2019.1594160.

McDougall, G. J., Jr., Vance, D. E., Wayde, E., Ford, K., & Ross, J. (2015). Memory training plus yoga for older adults. *Journal of Neuroscience Nursing, 47*(3), 178–188. https://doi.org/10.1097/JNN.0000000000000133.

McGrattan, A. M., McEvoy, C. T., McGuinness, B., McKinley, M. C., & Woodside, J. V. (2018). Effect of dietary interventions in mild cognitive impairment: A systematic review. *British Journal of Nutrition, 120*(12), 1388–1405. https://doi.org/10.1017/S0007114518002945.

Ombech, E. A. (2020). *Vitamin D supplementation: Cognitive function [evidence summary]*. Joanna Briggs Institute EBP Database. Retrieved from http://joannabriggs.org.

Pamaiahgari, P. (2020). *Stroke: Cognitive rehabilitation for memory deficits [evidence summary]*. Joanna Briggs Institute EBP Database. Retrieved from http://joannabriggs.org.

Pandya, S. P. (2020). Yoga education program for improving memory in older adults: A multicity 5-year follow-up study. *Journal of Applied Gerontology, 39*(6), 576–587. https://doi.org/10.1177/0733464818794153.

Pang, S. H., Lim, S. F., & Siah, C. J. (2021). Online memory training intervention for early-stage dementia: A systematic review and meta-analysis. *Journal of Advanced Nursing, 77*(3), 1141–1154. https://doi.org/10.1111/jan.14664.

Roalf, D. R., Moore, T. M., Mechanic-Hamilton, D., et al. (2017). Bridging cognitive screening tests in neurologic disorders: A crosswalk between the short montreal cognitive assessment and Mini-Mental State Examination. *Alzheimer's and Dementia, 13*(8), 947–952. https://doi.org/10.1016/j.jalz.2017.01.015.

Roalf, D. R., Moore, T. M., Wolk, D. A., et al. (2016). Defining and validating a short form Montreal Cognitive Assessment (s-MoCA) for use in neurodegenerative disease. *Journal of Neurology Neurosurgery and Psychiatry, 87*(12), 1303–1310. https://doi.org/10.1136/jnnp-2015-312723.

Rosli, R., Tan, M. P., Gray, W. K., Subramanian, P., & Chin, A. V. (2016). Cognitive assessment tools in Asia: A systematic review. *International Psychogeriatrics, 28*(2), 189–210. https://doi.org/10.1017/S1041610215001635.

Yang, H. L., Chan, P. T., Chang, P. C., et al. (2018). Memory-focused interventions for people with cognitive disorders: A systematic review and meta-analysis of randomized controlled studies. *International Journal of Nursing Studies, 78*, 44–51. https://doi.org/10.1016/j.ijnurstu.2017.08.005.

Zeng, Y., Dong, J., Huang, M., et al. (2020). Nonpharmacological interventions for cancer-related cognitive impairment in adult cancer patients: A network meta-analysis. *International Journal of Nursing Studies, 104*, 103514. https://doi.org/10.1016/j.ijnurstu.2019.103514.

M

Risk for Metabolic Syndrome

Domain 2 Nutrition Class 4 Metabolism

Marina Martinez-Kratz, MS, RN, CNE

NANDA-I

Definition

Susceptible to developing a cluster of symptoms that increase risk of cardiovascular disease and type 2 diabetes mellitus, which may compromise health.

Risk Factors

Absence of interest in improving health behaviors; average daily physical activity is less than recommended for age and gender; body mass index above normal range for age and gender; excessive accumulation of fat for age and gender; excessive alcohol intake; excessive stress; inadequate dietary habits; inadequate knowledge of modifiable factors; inattentive to second-hand smoke; smoking

At-Risk Population

Individuals aged >30 years; individuals with family history of diabetes mellitus; individuals with family history of dyslipidemia; individuals with family history of hypertension; individuals with family history of metabolic syndrome; individuals with family history of obesity; individuals with family history of unstable blood pressure

Associated Conditions

Hyperuricemia; insulin resistance; polycystic ovary syndrome

NOC (Nursing Outcomes Classification)

Suggested NOC Outcomes

Weight Loss Behavior; Blood Glucose Level; Circulation Status; Exercise Participation; Hypertension Severity; Knowledge: Lipid Disorder Management; Knowledge: Hypertension Management; Knowledge: Prescribed Diet; Knowledge: Prescribed Activity; Knowledge: Weight Management; Metabolic Function; Nutritional Status: Nutrient Intake; Risk Control: Obesity; Risk Control: Lipid Disorder; Risk Control: Hypertension

Example NOC Outcome with Indicators

Risk Control: Lipid Disorder as evidenced by the following indicators: Seeks current information about lipid disorders/Identifies risk factors for lipid disorders/Modifies lifestyle to reduce risk/Develops effective risk control strategies/Maintains recommended body weight. (Rate the outcome and indicators of **Risk Control: Lipid Disorder:** 1 = severe deviation from normal range, 2 = substantial deviation from normal range, 3 = moderate deviation from normal range, 4 = mild deviation from normal range, 5 = no deviation from normal range [see Section I].)

Client Outcomes

Client Will (Specify Time Frame)

- Maintain blood glucose within normal limits
- Explain actions and precautions to decrease cardiovascular risk
- Maintain waist circumference of less than 102 cm (40 inches) in men, or less than 88 cm (35 inches) in women
- Explain the risk factors associated with lipid disorders
- Maintain normal laboratory results, specifically high-sensitivity C-reactive protein, triglycerides, fasting blood glucose, and high-density lipoprotein (HDL) cholesterol
- Design lifestyle modifications to meet individual long-term goal of health, using effective risk control strategies
- Maintain weight within normal range for height and age
- Develop a system of self-management for improved dietary intake and physical activity

NIC (Nursing Interventions Classification)

Suggested NIC Interventions

Cardiac Risk Management; Exercise Promotion; Health Screening; Hyperglycemia Management; Hyperlipidemia Management; Nutritional Counseling; Teaching: Disease Process

Example NIC Activities—Cardiac Risk Management

Screen client for risk behaviors associated with adverse cardiac events; Prioritize areas for risk reduction in collaboration with client and family

Nursing Interventions and *Rationales*

- Assess for risk factors associated with metabolic syndrome. Risk factors for metabolic syndrome include central obesity, dyslipidemia, insulin resistance, and increased blood pressure. CEB: *Metabolic syndrome is a clustering of metabolic abnormalities associated with subsequent cardiovascular disease and mortality (Grundy et al, 2005).*
- Assess clients for elevated waist circumference measures; greater than 102 cm/40 inches or more in men, or greater than 88 cm/35 inches or more in women. EB: *An elevated waist circumference reflects central obesity, and metabolic syndrome screening is recommended in the effort to combat cardiovascular disease and type 2 diabetes mellitus (Cheong et al, 2015).*
- Assess clients for problematic eating behaviors and relationship with food. EB: *Logistic regression found that endorsement of problematic eating behaviors at an average age of 35 years was associated with metabolic syndrome and diabetes (Yoon et al, 2019).*
- Assess for metabolic syndrome in adults with intellectual disabilities. EB: *Individuals with intellectual disability and behavior problems showed a 46% prevalence of metabolic syndrome (Room, Timmermans, & Roodbol, 2016).*
- Examine the client's skin for acanthosis nigricans, acrochordons, keratosis pilaris, hyperandrogenism, and hirsutism, which are skin diseases associated with insulin resistance and obesity. EB: *Early recognition of insulin resistance and obesity-associated skin diseases may facilitate an earlier metabolic syndrome diagnosis and therapy initiation (Uzuncakmak et al, 2018).*

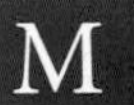

- Assess and report abnormal laboratory results, specifically high-sensitivity C-reactive protein, triglycerides, fasting blood glucose, and HDL cholesterol. EB: *A recent study found that high-sensitivity C-reactive protein, triglycerides, fasting blood glucose, and HDL cholesterol were factors associated with metabolic syndrome (Tayefi et al, 2018).*
- Screen clients who are prescribed antipsychotic medications for metabolic syndrome during routine health treatment. EBN: *A recent study found that despite an increased awareness of comorbid physical health issues among mental health consumers, guidelines and policy directives to clinical practice to address this disparity remain low (Ward et al, 2018).*
- Screen clients with a family history of polycystic ovary syndrome for metabolic syndrome. EB: *A recent meta-analysis suggests that mothers, fathers, sisters, and brothers of women with polycystic ovary syndrome have an increased risk of metabolic syndrome, hypertension, and dyslipidemia when compared with parents and siblings of women without polycystic ovary syndrome (Yilmaz et al, 2018).*
- Assist obese clients to develop a system of self-management, which may include self-monitoring of weight, body mass index (BMI), realistic goal setting, planning, and action planning for improved dietary intake and physical activity; problem-solving; and tracking dietary intake and exercise. EB: *A key component of successful weight loss and maintenance is regular self-monitoring (Thomason et al, 2016).*
- Encourage strength training for the client to address modifiable risk factors of metabolic syndrome. EBN: *A 2017 study of a 12-week strength training protocol demonstrated a significant reduction in C-reactive protein level, a positive trend in other biomarkers, and increased functional outcomes of premenopausal women with moderate cardiovascular risk (Flandez et al, 2017).*
- Provide nutritional teaching targeted at reducing daily energy, fat intakes, and sugar intakes, and increasing the frequency of eating two portions of vegetables during each meal. EB: *A randomized controlled trial demonstrated a reduction in metabolic syndrome risk factors after the implementation of lifestyle modifications focused on dietary intake and physical activity (Watanabe et al, 2017). A study of clients with metabolic*

syndrome showed that consumption of added sugar decreased after 1 year with American Heart Association dietary counseling (Zhang et al, 2018).

- Encourage the client to engage in vigorous-intensity physical activity for at least 150 minutes weekly or moderate-intensity physical activity for at least 300 minutes weekly to improve cardiorespiratory fitness and influence body shape and weight. EB: *A recent study indicated that being highly fit increased the likelihood of lower metabolic risk approximately 2 and 2.5 times independently of central adiposity compared with average and low fitness, respectively (Lätt et al, 2018).*
- Counsel clients to slow the pace of their eating during meals. EB: *A Japanese study found that a fast eating speed was associated with obesity and future prevalence of metabolic syndrome (Yamaji et al, 2018).*
- Provide teaching about reducing intake of ultra-processed foods and increasing intake of minimally processed foods. EB: *A study divided foods into ultra-processed, processed, and minimally processed. Ultra-processed foods consisted mainly of fast foods, snacks, sausage, nuts, sweets, and liquor, whereas minimally processed foods consisted mostly of fruits, vegetables, legumes, breads, cheeses, and eggs. Participants in the highest quartile of the "minimally processed/processed" pattern had significantly lower odds for metabolic syndrome (Nasreddine et al, 2018).*
- Encourage once or more weekly consumption of lean fish. EB: *A Norwegian study found that lean fish consumption once a week or more was significantly associated with decreased future metabolic score, decreased triglycerides, and increased HDL cholesterol in both men and women. In addition, men also showed decreased waist circumference and decreased blood pressure (Tørris et al, 2017).*
- Use social media for communication with clients to implement social support and share information about lifestyle modifications. EB: *A study using social media to augment the delivery of, and provide support for, a weight management program delivered to overweight and obese individuals during a 24-week intervention found that the Facebook group reported a 4.8% reduction in initial weight and numerically greater improvements in BMI, waist circumference, fat mass, lean mass, and energy intake (Monica et al, 2017).*
- Refer clients with Class II and III obesity and diabetes for bariatric surgery consideration. EB: *A recent review found that metabolic surgery is highly effective in obtaining significant and durable weight loss, enhancing glycemic control, and achieving diabetes remission (Pareek et al, 2018).*

M

Pediatric

- Assess adolescent clients for vitamin D deficiency with additional screening for prediabetes if deficiencies are found. EBN: *A recent study found an association of vitamin D deficiency with an increased risk of elevated fasting blood glucose levels (Kim et al, 2018).*
- Assess and report uric acid levels in at-risk children. EB: *A systematic review and meta-analysis found a significant association between serum uric acid levels and metabolic syndrome components in at-risk children (Goli et al, 2020).*
- Provide preventive interventions for obesity during early childhood. EBN: *A meta-analysis found that overweight or obesity in early childhood was associated with a higher risk of adult metabolic syndrome compared with the controls (Kim et al, 2017).*

Geriatric

Note: Many of the preceding interventions also apply.

- Encourage strength training for older women. EB: *A recent study found that women who participated in a 12-week resistance training program showed decreased C-reactive protein concentrations, reduced blood glucose levels, decreased waist circumference, and lowered systolic blood pressure regardless of diet (Tomeleri et al, 2018).*
- Encourage Tai chi training for older adults. EB: *Recent research found that the practice of Tai chi exercise was associated with a statistically significant decrease in hemoglobin (Hb) A1C concentration and oxidative stress score in a group of older adults (Mendoza-Núñez et al, 2018).*

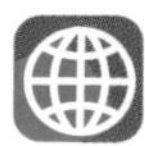

Multicultural

- Use criteria in addition to overweight and obesity when screening for cardiometabolic abnormalities in racial/ethnic minority populations. EB: *A cross-sectional study with participants from several U.S. racial/ethnic groups found that nearly a third of the participants with normal weight had cardiometabolic abnormalities (Gujral et al, 2017).*
- Provide African American women with community-based prevention education targeted toward improving knowledge, reducing clinical risk profiles, adoption of heart-healthy lifestyles, reducing inflammatory

burden, and decreasing cardiometabolic risk. EB: *A 4-month precardiovascular/postcardiovascular disease preventive educational intervention found that compared with baseline, there was a 60% reduction ($p < 0.05$) in the number of participants who met diagnostic criteria for metabolic syndrome (Villablanca et al, 2016).*

- Provide Hispanic clients at risk of metabolic syndrome with cultural and language appropriate teaching and cooking demonstrations. EB: *A cultural- and language-appropriate intervention included a Spanish-language lecture on metabolic syndrome and healthy nutrition and an interactive cooking demonstration for the participants and their significant others. Participants showed reductions in BMI, blood pressure, lipid levels, and HbA1C, and increased nutrition knowledge (Marks, 2016).*

Home Care

- Previously discussed interventions may be adapted for home care use.
- Screen clients who are cancer caregivers for signs and symptoms of metabolic syndrome. EB: *A prospective study of advanced cancer caregivers had higher rates of metabolic syndrome than had the general population (Steel et al, 2019).*

Client/Family Teaching and Discharge Planning

- Many of the preceding interventions involve teaching.
- Work with the family members regarding information on how to identify and reduce risk factors related to metabolic syndrome.

REFERENCES

Cheong, K. C., Ghazali, S. M., Hock, L. K., et al. (2015). The discriminative ability of waist circumference, body mass index and waist-to-hip ratio in identifying metabolic syndrome: Variations by age, sex and race. *Diabetes and Metabolic Syndrome Clinical Research & Reviews*, *9*(2), 74–78. https://doi.org/10.1016/j.dsx.2015.02.006.

Flandez, J., Belando, N., Gargallo, P., et al. (2017). Metabolic and functional profile of premenopausal women with metabolic syndrome after training with elastics as compared to free weights. *Biological Research For Nursing*, *19*(2), 190–197. https://doi.org/10.1177/1099800416674307.

Goli, P., Riahi, R., Daniali, S. S., Pourmirzaei, M., & Kelishadi, R. (2020). Association of serum uric acid concentration with components of pediatric metabolic syndrome: A systematic review and meta-analysis. *Journal of Research in Medical Sciences*, *25*, 43. https://doi.org/10.4103/jrms.JRMS_733_19O.

Grundy, S. M., Cleeman, J. I., Daniels, S. R., et al. (2005). Diagnosis and management of the metabolic syndrome: An American Heart Association/National Heart, Lung, and Blood Institute scientific statement. *Circulation*, *112*(17), 2735–2752. https://doi.org/10.1161/CIRCULATIONAHA.105.169404.

Gujral, U. P., Vittinghoff, E., Mongraw-Chaffin, M., et al. (2017). Cardiometabolic abnormalities among normal-weight persons from five racial/ethnic groups in the United States: A cross-sectional analysis of two cohort studies. *Annals of Internal Medicine*, *166*, 628–636. https://doi.org/10.7326/M16-1895.

Kim, Y. S., Hwang, J. H., & Song, M. R. (2018). The association between vitamin D deficiency and metabolic syndrome in Korean adolescents. *Journal of Pediatric Nursing*, *38*, e7–e11. https://doi.org/10.1016/j.pedn.2017.11.005.

Kim, J., Lee, I., & Lim, S. (2017). Overweight or obesity in children aged 0 to 6 and the risk of adult metabolic syndrome: A systematic review and meta-analysis. *Journal of Clinical Nursing*, *26*(23–24), 3869–3880. https://doi.org/10.1111/jocn.13802.

Lätt, E., Jürimäe, J., Harro, J., Loit, H. M., & Mäestu, J. (2018). Low fitness is associated with metabolic risk independently of central adiposity in a cohort of 18-year-olds. *Scandinavian Journal of Medicine & Science in Sports*, *28*(3), 1084–1091. https://doi.org/10.1111/sms.13002.

Marks, S. (2016). Culturally sensitive education can decrease hispanic workers' risk of metabolic syndrome. *Workplace Health & Safety*, *64*(11), 543–549. https://doi.org/10.1177/2165079916634712O.

Mendoza-Núñez, V. M., Arista-Ugalde, T. L., Rosado-Pérez, J., Ruiz-Ramos, M., & Santiago-Osorio, E. (2018). Hypoglycemic and antioxidant effect of Tai chi exercise training in older adults with metabolic syndrome. *Clinical Interventions in Aging*, *13*, 523–531. https://doi.org/10.2147/CIA.S157584.

Monica, J., Hagger, M., Foster, J., Ho, S., Kane, R., & Pal, S. (2017). Effects of a weight management program delivered by social media on weight and metabolic syndrome risk factors in overweight and obese adults: A randomised controlled trial. *PLoS One*, *12*(6), e0178326. https://doi.org/10.1371/journal.pone.0178326.

Nasreddine, L., Tamim, H., Itani, L., et al. (2018). A minimally processed dietary pattern is associated with lower odds of metabolic syndrome among Lebanese adults. *Public Health Nutrition*, *21*(1), 160–171. https://doi.org/10.1017/S1368980017002130.

Pareek, M., Schauer, P. R., Kaplan, L. M., Leiter, L. A., Fubino, F., & Bhatt, D. L. (2018). Metabolic surgery: Weight loss, diabetes, and beyond. *Journal of the American College of Cardiology*, *71*(6), 670–687. https://doi.org/10.1016/j.jacc.2017.12.014.

Room, B., Timmermans, O., & Roodbol, P. (2016). The prevalence and risk factors of the metabolic syndrome in inpatients with intellectual disability. *Journal of Intellectual Disability Research*, *60*(6), 594–605. https://doi.org/10.1111/jir.12282.

Steel, J. L., Cheng, H., Pathak, R., et al. (2019). Psychosocial and behavioral pathways of metabolic syndrome in cancer caregivers. *Psycho-Oncology*, *28*(8), 1735–1742. https://doi.org/10.1002/pon.5147.

Tayefi, M., Saberi-Karimian, M., Esmaeili, H., et al. (2018). Evaluating of associated risk factors of metabolic syndrome by using decision tree. *Comparative Clinical Pathology*, *27*, 215–223. https://doi.org/10.1007/s00580-017-2580-6.

Thomason, D. L., Lukkahatai, N., Kawi, J., Connelly, K., & Inouye, J. (2016). A systematic review of adolescent self-management and weight loss. *Journal of Pediatric Health Care*, *30*(6), 569–582. https://doi.org/10.1016/j.pedhc.2015.11.016.

M

Tomeleri, C. M., Souza, M. F., Burini, R. C., et al. (2018). Resistance training reduces metabolic syndrome and inflammatory markers in older women: A randomized controlled trial. *Journal of Diabetes*, *10*(4), 328–337. https://doi.org/10.1111/1753-0407.12614.

Tørris, C., Molin, M., & Småstuen, M. C. (2017). Lean fish consumption is associated with beneficial changes in the metabolic syndrome components: A 13-year follow-up study from the Norwegian Tromsø study. *Nutrients*, *9*(3), 247. https://doi.org/10.3390/nu9030247.

Uzuncakmak, T. K., Akdeniz, N., & Karadag, A. S. (2018). Cutaneous manifestations of obesity and the metabolic syndrome. *Clinics in Dermatology*, *36*(1), 81–88. https://doi.org/10.1016/j.clindermatol.2017.09.014.

Villablanca, A. C., Warford, C., & Wheeler, K. (2016). Inflammation and cardiometabolic risk in African American women is reduced by a pilot community-based educational intervention. *Journal of Women's Health*, *25*(2), 188–199. https://doi.org/10.1089/jwh.2014.5109.

Ward, T., Wynaden, D., & Heslop, K. (2018). Who is responsible for metabolic screening for mental health clients taking antipsychotic medications? *International Journal of Mental Health Nursing*, *27*(1), 196–203. https://doi.org/10.1111/inm.12309.

Watanabe, M., Yokotsuka, M., Yamaoka, K., Adachi, M., Nemoto, A., & Tango, T. (2017). Effects of a lifestyle modification programme to reduce the number of risk factors for metabolic syndrome: A randomized controlled trial. *Public Health Nutrition*, *20*(1), 142–153. https://doi.org/10.1017/S1368980016001920.

Yamaji, T., Mikami, S., Kobatake, H., Kobayashi, K., Tanaka, H., & Tanaka, K. (2018). Does eating fast cause obesity and metabolic syndrome? *Journal of the American College of Cardiology*, *71*(11), A1846. https://doi.org/10.1016/S0735-1097(18)32387-8.

Yilmaz, B., Vellanki, P., Ata, B., & Yildiz, B. O. (2018). Metabolic syndrome, hypertension, and hyperlipidemia in mothers, fathers, sisters, and brothers of women with polycystic ovary syndrome: A systematic review and meta-analysis. *Fertility and Sterility*, *109*(2), 356–364.e32. https://doi.org/10.1016/j.fertnstert.2017.10.018.

Yoon, C., Jacobs, D. R., Jr., Duprez, D. A., Neumark-Sztainer, D., Steffen, L. M., & Mason, S. M. (2019). Problematic eating behaviors and attitudes predict long-term incident metabolic syndrome and diabetes: The Coronary Artery Risk Development in Young Adults Study. *International Journal of Eating Disorders*, *52*(3), 304–308. https://doi.org/10.1002/eat.23020.

Zhang, L., Pagoto, S., May, C., et al. (2018). Effect of AHA dietary counselling on added sugar intake among participants with metabolic syndrome. *European Journal of Nutrition*, *57*(3), 1073–1082. https://doi.org/10.1007/s00394-017-1390-6.

Impaired Bed Mobility **Domain 4 Activity/rest Class 2 Activity/exercise**

Wendie A. Howland, MN, RN-BC, CRRN, CCM, CNLCP, LNCC

NANDA-I

Definition

Limitation in independent movement from one bed position to another.

Defining Characteristics

Difficulty moving between long sitting and supine positions; difficulty moving between prone and supine positions; difficulty moving between sitting and supine positions; difficulty reaching objects on the bed; difficulty repositing self in bed; difficulty returning to the bed; difficulty rolling on the bed; difficulty sitting on edge of bed; difficulty turning from side to side

Related Factors

Decreased flexibility; environmental constraints; impaired postural balance; inadequate angle of headboard; inadequate knowledge of mobility strategies; insufficient muscle strength; obesity; pain; physical deconditioning

At-Risk Population

Children; individuals experiencing prolonged bed rest; individuals in the early postoperative period; older adults

Associated Conditions

Artificial respiration; critical illness; dementia; drain tubes; musculoskeletal impairment; neurodegenerative disorders; neuromuscular diseases; Parkinson's disease; pharmaceutical preparations; sedation

NOC (Nursing Outcomes Classification)

Suggested NOC Outcomes

Immobility Consequences: Physiological; Mobility; Self-Care: Activities of Daily Living (ADLs)

Example NOC Outcome with Indicators

Immobility Consequences: Physiological as evidenced by the following indicators: Pressure sores/Constipation/Hypoactive bowel/Paralytic ileus/Urinary calculi/Contracted joints/Venous thrombosis/Pneumonia. (Rate the outcome and indicators of **Immobility Consequences: Physiological:** 1 = severely compromised, 2 = substantially compromised,
3 = moderately compromised, 4 = mildly compromised, 5 = not compromised [see Section I].)

Client Outcomes

Client Will (Specify Time Frame)

- Demonstrate optimal independence in positioning, exercising, and performing functional activities in bed
- Demonstrate ability to direct others on how to do bed positioning, exercising, and functional activities

NIC (Nursing Interventions Classification)

Suggested NIC Intervention

Bed Rest Care

Example NIC Activities—Best Rest Care

Position in proper body alignment; Teach bed exercises, as appropriate

Nursing Interventions and *Rationales*

- ▲ Normal bed mobility includes rolling, bridging, scooting, long sitting, and sitting upright. Begin with the client supine, flat in bed. Promote normal movements that are bilateral, segmental, and well-timed, with set positions using weight-bearing and trunk centering. Consult a physical therapist (PT) for individualized instructions and mobility strategies.
- Choose therapeutic beds and positions based on client's history and risk profile.
  - ❍ Advocate for specialty beds for bedbound clients incorporating low-air-loss pressure relief, shear reduction with position changes, turn assist, and moisture management.
  - ❍ Use devices such as trapeze, friction-reducing slide sheets, mechanical lateral transfer aids, or ceiling-mounted or floor lifts to move (rather than drag) clients in bed to prevent injury to caregivers.
  - ❍ Use a special bed and equipment, such as mattress overlay, sliding/roller board, trapeze, and stirrup with pulley attached to overhead traction system (holds one leg up during peri care).
- Place clients in free-standing or ceiling-mounted lifts with padded slings while changing bed linen. EB: *Turn-assist features in beds greatly decreased spine loading and pull forces for nurses turning and lateral repositioning in clients of both normal and obese weight, thus decreasing injury potential to staff (Wiggerman, 2016). Staff should use lifting/transfer equipment and devices, ergonomic assessments, no-lift policies, and education to decrease risk of injury (Choi & Brings, 2016; Olinsky & Norton, 2017). Only about one-third of nurses with available lifting equipment use it (Lee & Lee, 2017). A sliding sheet is preferable over a regular cotton sheet to decrease musculoskeletal load for caregivers (Weiner et al, 2017).*
- Many clients can benefit from a high sitting position to potentially minimize orthostatic intolerance *(Khan et al., 2002).*
- Assess to determine whether positioning for one condition may negatively affect another; use critical thinking skills for risk–benefit analysis. Use critical thinking to determine when specialty bed surfaces will help protect clients from tissue injury if frequent turning is contraindicated by client instability.
- Elevate head of bed (HOB) to 30 to 45 degrees unless contraindicated, and elevate HOB to 90 degrees during oral intake of fluids, solids, and oral medications. EB: *Elevation of HOB to at least 30 degrees is an effective, low-cost, and low-risk intervention associated with a decreased incidence of aspiration and ventilator-associated pneumonia (Agency for Healthcare Research and Quality [AHRQ], 2017).*

- Raise HOB to 30 degrees for clients with acute increased intracranial pressure and brain injury. Refer to care plan for Decreased **Intracranial** Adaptive Capacity.
- ▲ Consult health care provider for HOB elevation for acute stroke and monitor response. Refer to care plan for Decreased **Intracranial** Adaptive Capacity.
- Raise HOB as close to 45 degrees as possible for critically ill ventilated clients to prevent pneumonia (this height may place clients at higher risk for pressure ulcers). EB: *Elevating the HOB decreases regurgitation and risk for aspiration of gastric contents (Green et al, 2016).*
- Assist client with dysphagia to sit as upright as possible for oral intake, including solids, fluids, and oral medications. Refer to care plan for Impaired **Swallowing.**
- Periodically sit client upright as tolerated in bed; dangle client, if vital signs and oxygen saturation levels remain stable. EB: *Placing a client who is generally immobilized in an upright position is beneficial, using adaptive equipment if necessary (Green et al, 2016). Being vertical has many physiological and psychological benefits (Green et al, 2016).*
- To decrease risk of pressure injury, maintain HOB at lowest elevation that is medically possible and raise the foot of the bed to prevent shear-related injury. Assess the client's sacrum, ischial tuberosities, and heels at least every 2 hours. EB: *Shear results when external friction stretches the top layers of the skin as it slides against underlying layers and as internal tissues slide over deeper muscle and bone. These forces increase over the ischial tuberosities and sacrum when the backrest of the bed is elevated and result in tissue damage. Raising the foot of the bed in proportion to the HOB to distribute weight brings the body into maximum contact with the supporting surface, helping to eliminate shear. Placing a client who is generally immobilized in a recliner is a good alternative to the bed only if shear- and pressure-reducing bed surfaces cannot be obtained (Martin et al, 2017). Use critical thinking and consult with a nurse specialist in pressure injury harm reduction to determine when advocating for specialty bed surfaces will help protect clients from tissue injury.*
- Try periods of prone positioning for clients and monitor their tolerance/response. EB: *Prone positioning after both above the knee and below the knee amputations promotes extension, preventing flexor contractions (Monaro, West, & Gullick, 2017). Prone positioning improves oxygenation in respiratory failure (Lucchini et al, 2020).*
- Assess client's risk for falls using a valid fall risk assessment tool, such as the Morse Fall Scale (Morse, Tylko, & Dixon, 1987; Dykes, 2020) and implement specific measures to mitigate identified risk factors. EB: *Establish individualized fall prevention strategies and perform postfall assessment to further refine fall prevention interventions. Self-reported fear of falling has been shown to be a significantly more sensitive predictor for fall risk than the STRATIFY fall risk assessment tool (Strupeit, Buss, & Wolf-Ostermann, 2016).*
- Beds should be kept locked and in the lowest position when occupied.
- ▲ Although placing all four bed rails up is considered a form of restraint and requires a provider's prescription, two and even three rails up can be a support for bed mobility (Zhao et al, 2019).
- Place frequently used items within client's reach; demonstrate use of call bell (Zhao et al, 2019).
- Use a formalized screening tool to identify clients who are at high risk for deep venous thrombosis (e.g., obesity, cancer diagnosis, pelvic surgery, immobility, prior history of deep vein thrombosis). EB: *Best clinical practice encourages adherence to a clinical decision tool for deep venous thrombosis risk and prescribed therapy (Elder et al, 2016).*
- ▲ Assess for injury associated with thromboembolism prophylaxis and other prescribed treatment (e.g., anticoagulants, compression stockings, elastic leg wraps, sequential compression devices, feet/ankle exercises, and hydration). Refer to care plan for Ineffective Peripheral **Tissue Perfusion.**
- Use a valid and reliable tool to assess a client's risk for pressure injury. EB: *Routine assessment of risk factors is crucial in planning individualized interventions to diminish the risk of hospital-acquired pressure injury occurrences (Moyse et al, 2017).*
- Implement interventions to prevent pressure ulcers and complications of immobility. EB: *Delay in using an upgraded support surface for clients has been associated with greater numbers of pressure injuries in the critically ill (Bly et al, 2016).*
- Refer to care plan for Risk for Impaired **Skin** Integrity.
- Explain importance of avoiding breath-holding (Valsalva maneuver) and straining during bed mobility.
- Reassess pain level, especially before movement and/or exercising, and accept clients' pain ratings and levels they think are appropriate for comfort. Administer analgesics based on clients' pain rating. Refer to Acute **Pain** or Chronic **Pain.**

M

Exercise

- Test strength in bilateral grips, arms at elbow flexion and extension, bilateral arm abduction and adduction, bilateral leg or thigh raise (one at a time in bed or chair), and quadriceps and hamstring strength to extend and flex at knee to assess baseline and interval strength gains.
- Perform passive range of motion (ROM) of three repetitions, at least twice a day, to immobile joints. Perform ROM slowly and rhythmically. Do not range beyond point of pain. Range only to point of resistance in those with loss of sensation and mentation. Fast, jerky ROM increases pain and tone. Slow, rhythmical movements relax/lengthen spastic muscles so they can be ranged further. For clients with neuromuscular conditions, consult with physical therapy for ROM exercises.
- Range or move a hemiplegic arm with the shoulder slightly externally rotated (hand up).
- ▲ Encourage client's practice of exercises taught by therapists (muscle setting, strengthening, contraction against resistance, and weight lifting). *Exercises and weight lifting help maintain muscle tone, strength, and lengthening.*

Bed Positioning

- Incorporate the following measures to promote normal tone and prevent complications in clients with neurological impairment:
  - Use a flat head pillow when clients are supine. Use a small pillow behind the head and/or between shoulder blades if neck extension occurs to prevent contractures of the cervical spine and abnormal tone of the neck.
  - Abduct the shoulders of clients with high paraplegia or quadriplegia horizontally to 90 degrees briefly two to three times a day while client is supine.
  - Position a hemiplegic shoulder fairly close to the client's body.
- Tilt hemiplegics onto both unaffected and affected sides with the affected shoulder slightly forward (e.g., move/lift the affected shoulder, not the forearm/hand).
- ▲ Elevate a client's paralyzed forearms on a pillow when client is supine. Elevate edematous legs on a pillow supporting the knees to prevent hyperextension. Apply resting wrist, hand, and foot/ankle splints and pressure garments or other devices as prescribed. Range joints before applying splints. Adhere to on/off schedule as prescribed by the PT. Remove splints and compression garments or devices to check underlying tissues for signs of pressure/poor circulation every 2 hours or more often if client resists or manipulates them.

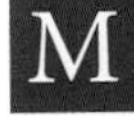

Geriatric

- Assess caregiver's strength, health history, and cognitive status to predict ability/risk for assisting bed-bound clients at home. Explore alternatives if risk is too high. Caregivers are often frail older adults with chronic health problems who cannot physically help loved ones. Refer to care plan for **Caregiver** Role Strain.
- Assess the client's stamina and energy level during bed activities/exercises; if limited, spread out activities and allow rest breaks.

Home Care

- ▲ Collaborate with nurse case managers, care coordinators, social workers, visiting nurses, and physical/occupational therapists to assess home support systems and needs and to provide for home safety and access modifications, durable medical equipment as needed for condition (e.g., bariatric), handling equipment (e.g., friction pads, slide boards, lifts) needed for safe bed mobility, exercise, toileting, and bathing, ramps, rails, assistive technology, and home health follow-up.
- Encourage use of the client's own bed unless contraindicated. Raise HOB with commercial blocks or grooved-out pieces of wood under legs; set bed against walls in a corner. Emotionally, clients may benefit from sleeping in their own beds with familiar partners.
- Stress psychological/physical benefits of clients being as self-sufficient as possible with bed mobility/care even though it may be time-consuming. Allowing independence and autonomy may help prevent disuse syndromes and feelings of helplessness and low self-esteem.
- Offer emotional support and help client identify usual coping responses to help with adjustment and loss issues. The home environment may trigger the reality of lost function and disability.
- Discuss support systems available for caregivers to help them cope. Refer to care plan for **Caregiver** Role Strain.

- ▲ Institute case management for frail older adults to support continued independent living as much as possible or as desired by the client.
- • Refer to the home care interventions in the care plan for Impaired Physical **Mobility.**

Client/Family Teaching and Discharge Planning

- • Teach client/caregivers correct ROM, exercises, positioning, self-care activities, and use of devices. Assess readiness and learning styles, which vary but may be enhanced with visual/auditory/tactile/cognitive stimuli such as the following:
  - ❍ Demonstrations, sketches, online resources (e.g., YouTube), written directions/schedules, notes
  - ❍ Verbal instructions, recorded audiotapes, timers, reading written directions aloud, and self-talk during activities
  - ❍ Motor task practice/repetition, return demonstrations, note taking, manual guidance, or staff's-hand-on-client's-hand technique
  - ❍ Referral to community group activities, support groups, parish nursing, adaptive recreation, or other out-of-the-home resources
- ▲ Schedule time with family/caregivers for education and practice for nursing, physical therapy, and occupational therapy. Suggest family come prepared with questions and wear comfortable, safe clothing/shoes. Practice provides opportunity for learning; repetition helps memory retention.
- ▲ Teach safe approaches for caregivers/home care staff and reinforce an adequate number of people to decrease risk of injury *(Olinsky & Norton, 2017).*

REFERENCES

Agency for Healthcare Research and Quality (AHRQ). (2017). *Head of bed elevation or semirecumbent positioning literature review.* Rockville, MD: Agency for Healthcare Research and Quality. Retrieved from http://www.ahrq.gov/professionals/quality-patient-safety/hais/tools/mvp/modules/technical/head-bed-elevation-litreview.html. [Accessed 15 July 2021].

Bly, D., Schallom, M., Sona, C., & Klinkenberg, D. (2016). A model of pressure, oxygenation, and perfusion risk factors for pressure ulcers in the intensive care unit. *American Journal of Critical Care, 25*(2), 156–164. https://doi.org/10.4037/ajcc2016840.

Choi, S. D., & Brings, K. (2016). Work-related musculoskeletal risks associated with nurses and nursing assistants handling overweight and obese patients: A literature review. *Work (Reading, MA), 53*(2), 439–448.

Dykes, P. C. (2020). *Using fall risk assessment tools in care planning.* Center for Patient Safety Research and Practice, Center for Nursing Excellence, Brigham and Women's Hospital. Retrieved from https://www.ahrq.gov/sites/default/files/wysiwyg/professionals/systems/hospital/fallprevention-training/webinars/webinar4_falls_usingriskassttools.pdf. [Accessed 15 July 2021].

Elder, S., Hobson, D. B., Rand, C. S., et al. (2016). Hidden barriers to delivery of pharmacological venous thromboembolism prophylaxis: the role of nursing beliefs and practices. *Journal of Patient Safety, 12*(2), 63–68. https://doi.org/10.1097/PTS.0000000000000086.

Green, M., Marzano, V., Leditschke, I. A., Mitchell, I., & Bissett, B. (2016). Mobilization of intensive care patients: A multidisciplinary practical guide for clinicians. *Journal of Multidisciplinary Healthcare, 9*, 247–256.

Khan, M. H., Kunselman, A. R., Leuenberger, U. A., et al. (2002). Attenuated sympathetic nerve responses after 24 hours of bed rest. *American Journal of Physiology, Heart and Circulatory Physiology, 282*(6), H2210–H2215.

Lee, S. J., & Lee, J. H. (2017). Safe patient handling behaviors and lift use among hospital nurses: A cross-sectional study. *International Journal of Nursing Studies, 74*, 53–60.

Lucchini, A., Bambi, S., Mattiusi, E., et al. (2020). Prone position in acute respiratory distress syndrome patients: A retrospective analysis of complications. *Dimensions of Critical Care Nursing, 39*(1), 39–46.

Martin, D., Albensi, L., Van Haute, S., et al. (2017). Healthy skin wins: A glowing pressure ulcer prevention program that can guide evidence-based practice. *Worldviews on Evidence-based Nursing, 14*(6), 473–483.

Monaro, S., West, S., & Gullick, J. (2017). Patient outcomes following lower leg major amputations for peripheral arterial disease: A series review. *Journal of Vascular Nursing, 35*(2), 49–56. https://doi.org/10.1016/j.jvn.2016.10.003.

Morse, J. M., Tylko, S. J., & Dixon, H. A. (1987). Characteristics of the fall-prone patient. *The Gerontologist, 27*(4), 516–522.

Moyse, T., Bates, J., Karafa, M., Whitman, A., & Albert, N. M. (2017). Validation of a model for predicting pressure injury risk in patients with vascular diseases. *Journal of Wound, Ostomy & Continence Nursing, 44*(2), 118–122.

Olinsky, C., & Norton, C. E. (2017). Implementation of a safe patient handling program in a multihospital health system from inception to sustainability: Successes over 8 years and ongoing challenges. *Workplace Health and Safety, 65*(11), 546–559. https://doi.org/10.1177/2165079917704670.

Strupeit, S., Buss, A., & Wolf-Ostermann, K. (2016). Assessing risk of falling in older adults—A comparison of three methods. *Worldviews on Evidence-Based Nursing, 13*(5), 349–355. https://doi.org/10.1111/wvn.12174.

Weiner, C., Kalichman, L., Ribak, J., & Alperovitch-Najenson, D. (2017). Repositioning a passive patient in bed: Choosing an ergonomically advantageous assistive device. *Applied Ergonomics, 60*, 22–29. https://doi.org/10.1177/0018720815612625.

Wiggerman, N. (2016). Biomechanical evaluation of a bed feature to assist in turning and laterally repositioning patients. *Human Factors, 58*(5), 748–757.

Zhao, Y. L., Bott, M., He, J., Kim, H., Park, S. H., & Dunton, N. (2019). Evidence on fall and injurious fall prevention in acute care hospitals. *Journal of Nursing Administration, 49*(2), 86–92.

M

Impaired Physical Mobility Domain 4 Activity/rest Class 2 Activity/exercise

Wendie A. Howland, MN, RN-BC, CRRN, CCM, CNLCP, LNCC

NANDA-I

Definition

Limitation in independent, purposeful movement of the body or of one or more extremities.

Defining Characteristics

Altered gait; decreased fine motor skills; decreased gross motor skills; decreased range of motion; difficulty turning; engages in substitutions for movement; expresses discomfort; movement-induced tremor; postural instability; prolonged reaction time; slowed movement; spastic movement; uncoordinated movement

Related Factors

Anxiety; body mass index >75th percentile appropriate for age and gender; cultural belief regarding acceptable activity; decreased activity tolerance; decreased muscle control; decreased muscle strength; disuse; inadequate environmental support; inadequate knowledge of value of physical activity; insufficient muscle mass; insufficient physical endurance; joint stiffness; malnutrition; neurobehavioral manifestations; pain; physical deconditioning; reluctance to initiate movement; sedentary lifestyle

Associated Conditions

Altered bone structure integrity; contractures; depression; developmental disabilities; impaired metabolism; musculoskeletal impairment; neuromuscular diseases; pharmaceutical preparations; prescribed movement restrictions; sensory-perceptual impairment

NOC (Nursing Outcomes Classification)

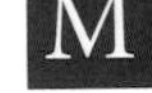

Suggested NOC Outcomes

Ambulation; Ambulation: Wheelchair; Mobility; Self-Care: Activities of Daily Living (ADLs); Instrumental Activities of Daily Living (IADLs); Transfer Performance

Example NOC Outcome with Indicators

Ambulation as evidenced by the following indicators: Walks with effective gait/Walks at moderate pace/Walks up and down steps/Walks moderate distance. (Rate the outcome and indicators of **Ambulation:** 1 = severely compromised, 2 = substantially compromised, 3 = moderately compromised, 4 = mildly compromised, 5 = not compromised [see Section I].)

Client Outcomes

Client Will (Specify Time Frame)

- Meet mutually defined goals of increased ambulation and exercise that include individual choice, preference, and enjoyment in the exercise prescription
- Describe feeling stronger and more mobile
- Describe less fear of falling and pain with physical activity
- Demonstrate use of adaptive equipment (e.g., wheelchairs, walkers, gait belts, weighted walking vests) to increase mobility
- Increase exercise to 20 minutes/day for those who were previously sedentary (less than 150 minutes/week). Note: Light to moderate intensity exercise may be beneficial in deconditioned persons. In very deconditioned individuals exercise bouts of less than 10 minutes are beneficial
- Increase pedometer step counts with a daily goal for most healthy adults of at least 4400 steps per day (Harvard Women's Health Watch, 2019)
- Perform resistance exercises that involve all major muscle groups (legs, hips, back, chest, abdomen, shoulders, and arms) performed 2 or 3 days/week

- Perform flexibility exercise (stretching) for each of the major muscle-tendon groups 2 days/week for 10 to 60 seconds to improve joint range of motion (ROM); greatest gains occur with daily exercise
- Engage in neuromotor exercise 20 to 30 minutes/day including motor skills (e.g., balance, agility, coordination, gait), proprioceptive exercise training, and multifaceted activities (e.g., Tai chi, yoga) to improve and maintain physical function and reduce falls in those at risk for falling (older persons)
- Engage in purposeful moderate-intensity cardiorespiratory (aerobic) exercise for 30 to 60 minutes/day at least 5 days/week for a total of 2 hours and 30 minutes (150 minutes) per week

NIC (Nursing Interventions Classification)

Suggested NIC Interventions

Exercise Therapy: Ambulation; Joint Mobility; Positioning

Example NIC Activities—Exercise Therapy

Assist the client to use footwear that facilitates walking and prevents injury; Instruct in use of assistive devices, if appropriate

Nursing Interventions and *Rationales*

- Adults should be as physically active as their abilities allow and avoid inactivity. Use "start low and go slow" approach for intensity and duration of physical activity if client is deconditioned, functionally limited, or has chronic conditions affecting performance of physical tasks. When progressing client's activities, use an individualized and tailored approach based on client's tolerance and preferences (US Department of Health and Human Services, 2018).
- Screen for mobility skills in the following order: (1) bed mobility; (2) dangling and supported and unsupported sitting; (3) weight-bearing for sit to stand, transfer to chair; (4) standing and walking with assistance; and (5) walking independently. EBN: *Use a structured tool to assess and determine the client's highest activity level and guide planning exercise progression toward independence (Jackman et al, 2016).*
- Assess muscle strength and other factors affecting balance, mobility, and endurance. Immobility can affect tissue perfusion and increase risk of postural hypotension; shortness of breath decreases endurance and increases fear; bowel or bladder incontinence can decrease motivation to be mobile; cognitive and neuromuscular deficits, including side effects of medications that affect balance, coordination, and movement; and pain, fear, or sick role because expectations can decrease willingness to be mobile. EBN: *Assess for mobility impairment and hazards of limited mobility, and plan care to mitigate complications (Crawford & Harris, 2016).*
- Assess for fear of falling. EBN: *Self-reported fear of falling has been shown to be a significantly more sensitive predictor for fall risk than the STRATIFY fall risk assessment tool (Strupeit, Buss, & Wolf-Ostermann, 2016).*

▲ Consult physical therapist (PT) for recommendations for assistive devices, such as gait belt, weighted vest, walker, cane, crutches, wheelchair, shower chairs; lifts; lateral transfer devices.

- Refer to care plans for Risk for **Falls,** Acute **Pain,** Chronic **Pain,** Ineffective **Coping,** or **Hopelessness.**
- Increase activity tolerance with graded increases in self-care (function-focused care [FFC]), such as bathing, walking to the bathroom instead of using a bedpan/urinal, and ROM. EBN: *A study of FFC in older adults hospitalized after trauma found greater improvement in function, less fear of falling, and better physical resilience than controls at discharge and 30 days after (Resnick et al, 2016b).*

▲ Before activity, observe for and, if possible, treat pain with massage, heat pack to affected area, or medication. EB: *Pain limits mobility and if exacerbated by specific movements should be temporarily avoided (American College of Sports Medicine [ACSM], 2018).*

- Monitor and record the client's response to activity, such as pulse rate, blood pressure, dyspnea, skin color, subjective report. Refer to the care plan for Decreased **Activity** Tolerance. Intolerance. EB: *Use valid and reliable screening procedures and tools to assess the client's preparticipation in exercise health screening and risk stratification for exercise testing (low, moderate, or high risk) (ACSM, 2018).*

Special Considerations: Immobility

- Refer to the care plan for Impaired Bed **Mobility.**
- Help the client achieve mobility and start walking as soon as possible if not contraindicated. EB: *Older clients who are hospitalized for medical illness often leave the hospital with increased disability in*

M

activities of daily living, even when the condition that led to admission is successfully treated (Covinsky, 2017). EB: *Early mobilization after hip replacement surgery resulted in decreased time until readiness for discharge (Okamoto et al, 2016).*

- Initiate a "no lift" policy where appropriate assistive devices are used for manual lifting. Refer to the care plan for Impaired Bed **Mobility**.

Other Clinical Conditions

- ▲ Osteoarthritis or rheumatoid arthritis: Consult with a physical therapist on ways to integrate aerobic exercise, resistance exercise, and flexibility exercise (stretching) into care.
- ▲ Cerebrovascular accident (CVA) with hemiparesis: Consult with physical therapist on constraint-induced movement therapy, in which the functional extremity is purposely constrained and the client is forced to use the involved extremity (Wattchow, McDonnell, & Hillier, 2018) or graded motor mirror therapy (Mekonen, 2019). EB: *These noninvasive therapeutic approaches produced significant positive effects in improving arm function after stroke.*
- If the client does not feed or groom self, sit side by side with the client, put your hand over the client's hand, support the client's elbow with your other hand, and help the client complete these simple movements.

Geriatric

- Assess ability to move using valid and reliable criterion-referenced standards for fitness testing that can predict the level of capacity associated with maintaining physical independence into later years of life (e.g., Get Up and Go test).
- Help the mostly immobile client achieve mobility as soon as possible, depending on physical condition. EB: *A meta-analysis found exercise beneficial in increasing gait speed and improving balance and ADL performance (Lipardo et al, 2017). Mobilization should occur at least three times daily, mobilization should be progressive and scaled, and assessment should take place within 24 hours of admission (Liu et al, 2017).*
- Use the FFC rehabilitative philosophy of care in older adults to prevent avoidable functional decline. EBN: *Mood, satisfaction with staff and activities, and social support for exercise were directly associated with time spent in physical activity (Holmes, Galik, & Resnick, 2017).*
- If the client will have elective surgery that will result in immobility, initiate a rehabilitation program with warm-up, aerobic activity, strength, flexibility, neuromotor, and functional task work. EBN: *The risk of declines in functional status when older adults are hospitalized requires using evidence-based strategies to reduce the incidence and effect of decreased mobility, pressure ulcers, pain, dehydration, malnutrition, and sequelae of invasive treatments (Resnick et al, 2016a).*
- Use gestures and nonverbal cues when helping clients move if they are anxious or have difficulty understanding and following verbal instructions. Nonverbal gestures are part of a universal language that can be understood when the client is having difficulty with communication.
- Recognize that wheelchairs are not a good mobility device and often serve as a mobility restraint.
- Ensure that chairs fit clients. Chair seat should be 3 inches above the height of the knee. Provide a raised toilet seat if needed. Raising the height of a chair can dramatically improve the ability of many older clients to stand up. Low, deep, soft seats with armrests that are far apart reduce a person's ability to get up and down without help.
- If the client is mainly immobile, provide opportunities for socialization and sensory stimulation. Refer to the care plan for Deficient **Diversional** Activity.
- Recognize that immobility and a lack of social support and sensory input may result in confusion or depression in older adults. Refer to nursing interventions for Acute **Confusion** or **Hopelessness** as appropriate.

Home Care

- All preceding interventions should be applied and used for home care.
- ▲ Begin discharge planning as soon as possible with a personal health navigator (e.g., nurse care coordinator or case manager) to assess need for and arrange home support systems, assistive devices, community or home health services, and provider follow-up. EB: *Nurses are often the first health care providers to assess the client on admission; this creates the opportunity for early discharge planning (McNeil, 2016).*
- ▲ Assess home environment for factors that create barriers to physical mobility. Refer to occupational therapy for home safety evaluation and adaptive technology. EB: *Use the Home Safety Self-Assessment Tool to identify fall risk, prevent falls, and improve mobility and function (Horowitz, Almonte, & Vasil, 2016).*

- ▲ Refer to home health services to support the client and family through changing levels of mobility. Reinforce need to promote independence in mobility as tolerated. EB: *Providing unnecessary assistance with transfers, bathing, and dressing activities may promote dependence and a loss of mobility rather than optimizing a person's underlying physical capability. Such attentive care may actually prevent older adults from using their remaining abilities (Resnick et al, 2016b).*
- ▲ Refer to home physical therapy for evaluation, gait training, strengthening, and balance training. EB: *Physical therapists can provide direct interventions and assess need for assistive devices (e.g., cane, walker) (Miller, Sabol, & Pastva, 2017).*
- ● Assess skin condition at every visit. Establish a skin care program that enhances circulation and maximizes position changes. Impaired mobility decreases circulation to dependent areas. Decreased circulation and shearing place the client at risk for skin breakdown.
- ● Once the client is able to walk independently, suggest that the client enter an exercise program or walk with a friend. EB: *Nurse practitioners providing primary care should prescribe regular physical activity to minimize progressive impaired mobility (Miller, Sabol, & Pastva, 2017).*
- ● Provide support to the client and family/caregivers during long-term impaired mobility. Long-term impaired mobility may necessitate role changes within the family and precipitate caregiver stress. Refer to the care plan for **Caregiver** Role Strain.

Client/Family Teaching and Discharge Planning

- ● Consider using motivational interviewing techniques to increase a client's activity. Refer to the care plan for **Sedentary** Lifestyle or Motivational Interviewing.
- ● Teach the client and caregivers processes and tools used during care to use at home to assess fall risk and promote progressive mobility. Involve them in planning for these activities at home. EBN: *Few studies have investigated the point of view of older clients on prevention of this decline. This study shows that participants are sensitive to the risk of functional decline but have internal and external barriers to implementing preventive strategies to maintain physical abilities and good spirits, keep a clear mind, and foster nutrition and sleep. Older hospitalized clients would benefit from more helpful nursing strategies (Lafrenière et al, 2017).*

REFERENCES

American College of Sports Medicine (ACSM). (2018). In *American College of Sports Medicine's guidelines for exercise testing and prescription* (10th ed.). Philadelphia: Lippincott Williams & Wilkins.

Covinsky, K. E. (2017). Hospital-acquired disability: An overview. *Innovation in Aging, 1*(Suppl. 1), 963. https://doi.org/10.1093/geroni/igx004.3474.

Crawford, A., & Harris, H. (2016). Caring for adults with impaired physical mobility. *Nursing, 46*(12), 36–41.

Harvard Women's Health Watch. (2019). Do you really need to take 10,000 steps a day for better health? Retrieved from https://www.health.harvard.edu/staying-healthy/do-you-really-need-to-take-10000-steps-a-day-for-better-health. Accessed July 15, 2021.

Holmes, S., Galik, E., & Resnick, B. (2017). Factors that influence physical activity among residents in assisted living. *Journal of Gerontological Social Work, 60*(2), 120–137.

Horowitz, B., Almonte, T., & Vasil, A. (2016). Use of the Home Safety Self-Assessment Tool (HSSAT) within community health education to improve home safety. *Occupational Therapy in Health Care, 30*(4), 356–372.

Jackman, C., Gammon, H., Kane, P., et al. (2016). A reliable mobility assessment tool for multidisciplinary use. *Journal of Physical Medicine Rehabilitation and Disabilities, 2*, 009.

Lafrenière, S., Folch, N., Dubois, S., Bédard, L., & Ducharme, F. (2017). Strategies used by older patients to prevent functional decline during hospitalization. *Clinical Nursing Research, 26*(1), 6–26.

Lipardo, D. S., Aseron, A. M. C., Kwan, M. M., & Tsang, W. W. (2017). Effect of exercise and cognitive training on falls and fall-related factors in older adults with mild cognitive impairment: A systematic review. *Archives of Physical Medicine and Rehabilitation, 98*(10), 2079–2096.

Liu, B., Moore, J., Khan, S., Chan, W., Harris, C., & Straus, S. E. (2017). Sustainability and spread of move on: A mobilization initiative two years after implementation. *Innovation in Aging, 1*(Suppl. 1), 652–653.

McNeil, A. (2016). Using evidence to structure discharge planning. *Nursing Management, 47*(5), 22–23.

Mekonen, C. (2019). Graded motor imagery to address pain and motor dysfunction from phantom limb pain, complex regional pain syndrome, chronic musculoskeletal pain, and stroke. *Journal of Nurse Life Care Planning, 19*(3), 45–51.

Miller, J. M., Sabol, V. K., & Pastva, A. M. (2017). Promoting older adult physical activity throughout care transitions using and interprofessional approach. *The Journal for Nurse Practitioners, 13*(1), 64–71.

Okamoto, T., Ridley, R. J., Edmondston, S. J., Visser, M., Headford, J., & Yates, P. J. (2016). Day-of-surgery mobilization reduces the length of stay after elective hip arthroplasty. *Journal of Arthroplasty, 31*(10), 2227–2230.

Resnick, R., Galik, E., Vigne, E., & Carew, A. P. (2016b). Dissemination and implementation of function focused care for assisted living. *Health Education & Behavior, 43*(3), 296–304.

Resnick, B., Wells, C., Galik, E., et al. (2016a). Feasibility and efficacy of function-focused care for orthopedic trauma patients. *Journal of Trauma Nursing, 23*(3), 144–155.

Strupeit, S., Buss, A., & Wolf-Ostermann, K. (2016). Assessing risk of falling: A comparison of three different methods. *Worldviews on Evidence-Based Nursing, 13*(5), 349–355. https://doi.org/10.1111/wvn.12174.

US Department of Health and Human Services. (2018). Physical activity guidelines for Americans. In *President's Council on Sports, Fitness, and Nutrition* (2nd ed.). Washington, DC: USDHHS. Retrieved from https://health.gov/our-work/physical-activity/current-guidelines. Accessed July 15, 2021.

Wattchow, K. A., McDonnell, M. N., & Hillier, S. L. (2018). Rehabilitation interventions for upper limb function in the first four weeks following stroke: A systematic review and meta-analysis of the evidence. *Archives of Physical Medicine and Rehabilitation, 99*(2), 367–382. https://doi.org/10.1016/j.apmr.2017.06.014.

Impaired Wheelchair Mobility Domain 4 Activity/rest Class 2 Activity/exercise

Wendie A. Howland, MN, RN-BC, CRRN, CCM, CNLCP, LNCC

NANDA-I

Definition

Limitation of independent operation of wheelchair within environment.

Defining Characteristics

Difficulty bending forward to pick up object from the floor; difficulty folding or unfolding wheelchair; difficulty leaning forward to reach for something above head; difficulty locking brakes on manual wheelchair; difficulty maneuvering wheelchair sideways; difficulty moving wheelchair out of an elevator; difficulty navigating through hinged door; difficulty operating battery charger of power wheelchair; difficulty operating power wheelchair on a decline; difficulty operating power wheelchair on an incline; difficulty operating power wheelchair on curbs; difficulty operating power wheelchair on even surface; difficulty operating power wheelchair on uneven surface; difficulty operating wheelchair backwards; difficulty operating wheelchair forward; difficulty operating wheelchair in corners; difficulty operating wheelchair motors; difficulty operating wheelchair on a decline; difficulty operating wheelchair on an incline; difficulty operating wheelchair on curbs; difficulty operating wheelchair on even surface; difficulty operating wheelchair on stairs; difficulty operating wheelchair on uneven surface; difficulty operating wheelchair while carrying an object; difficulty performing pressure relief; difficulty performing stationary wheelie position; difficulty putting feet on the footplates of the wheelchair; difficulty rolling across side-slope while in wheelchair; difficulty selecting drive mode on power wheelchair; difficulty selecting speed on power wheelchair; difficulty shifting weight; difficulty sitting on wheelchair without losing balance; difficulty stopping wheelchair before bumping something; difficulty transferring from wheelchair; difficulty transferring to wheelchair; difficulty turning in place while on wheelie position

M

Related Factors

Altered mood; environmental constraints; inadequate adjustment to wheelchair size; inadequate knowledge of wheelchair use; insufficient muscle strength; insufficient physical endurance; neurobehavioral manifestations; obesity; pain; physical deconditioning; substance misuse; unaddressed inadequate vision

At-Risk Population

Individuals using wheelchair for short time; individuals with history of fall from wheelchair; older adults

Associated Conditions

Musculoskeletal impairment; neuromuscular diseases; vision disorders

NOC (Nursing Outcomes Classification)

Suggested NOC Outcome

Ambulation: Wheelchair

Example NOC Outcome with Indicators

Ambulation: Wheelchair as evidenced by the following indicators: Propels wheelchair safely/Transfers to and from wheelchair/Maneuvers curbs, doorways, ramps. (Rate the outcome and indicators of **Ambulation: Wheelchair:** 1 = severely compromised, 2 = substantially compromised, 3 = moderately compromised, 4 = mildly compromised, 5 = not compromised [see Section I].)

Client Outcomes

Client Will (Specify Time Frame)

- Demonstrate independence in operating and moving a wheelchair or other wheeled device
- Demonstrate ability to direct others in operating and moving a wheelchair or other device

- Demonstrate therapeutic positioning, pressure relief, and safety principles while operating and moving a wheelchair or other wheeled device

NIC (Nursing Interventions Classification)

Suggested NIC Interventions

Exercise Therapy: Muscle Control; Positioning: Wheelchair

Example NIC Activities—Positioning

Wheelchair

Collaborate with occupational therapist [OT]/physical therapist [PT] to select the appropriate wheelchair for the client: standard adult, semi-reclining/fully reclining/tilt-in-space, amputees; Monitor client's ability to maintain correct positioning in wheelchair

Nursing Interventions and *Rationales*

- Assess the client's coccyx and encourage frequent repositioning. EB: *Deep tissue pressure injury (DTPI) begins in muscles closest to bone and may not be visible early on. They are most common over coccyx, sacrum, buttocks, and heels (Preston et al, 2017).*
- ▲ Refer to physical and occupational therapy or wheelchair seating clinic. EB: *Seating for wheelchair-dependent clients should be assessed by health care specialists, not vendors, in conjunction with client/caregiver education on weight-shift maneuvers (Howland & McMahon, 2015). There are many pressure-relieving cushions. Several commonly used are the ROHO cushion, Varilite Evolution, and Invacare Matrix cushions.* Refer to care plan for Risk for Adult **Pressure Injury**; Risk for Child **Pressure Injury.**
- ▲ Support surfaces on chairs and beds should redistribute pressure and be used for at-risk clients as an adjunct to reduce risk of pressure injury. EB: *Current clinical practices for pressure injury prevention include the use of pressure distribution systems; frequent monitoring of skin integrity, moisture, and temperature; use of low-friction textiles and dressings; and continuous repositioning of clients (Kottner et al, 2019).*
- Tilt-in-space chairs are effective at off-loading pressure areas. EB: *Cell deformation from shear is more important that tissue ischemia in the development of tissue necrosis and pressure injury. Frequent small adjustments in tilt-in-space and recline angle might be important for preventing cell deformation and any associated cell necrosis. Larger angles of tilt-in-space and recline seem to support blood flow returning to the tissues, which is likely to play a positive role in healing damaged tissue (Zemp et al, 2019).*
- Intervene to maintain continence or use air-permeable absorbent underpads or diapers to help prevent skin breakdown caused by excessive moisture and macerated skin. Some wheelchair cushions have moisture-wicking characteristics.
- Assess client's sitting posture frequently and reposition for alignment. Document specific measures to allow for reproducibility. EB: *Pressure mapping alone insufficiently describes tissue health (National Pressure Ulcer Advisory Panel, 2016; Slayton et al, 2017).*
- Implement use of friction-coated projection hand rims and leather gloves for clients to propel manual wheelchairs. Friction-coated projection rims are less invasive and slippery than aluminum rims; gloves absorb forces of propulsion and help prevent nerve damage/carpal tunnel injury.
- Manually guide or explain to the client to push forward on both wheel rims to move ahead, push the right rim to turn left and vice versa, and pull backward on both wheel rims to back up.
- Recommend that clients back wheelchair into an elevator. If entering face first, instruct them to turn chairs around to face the elevator doors and controls.
- ▲ In conjunction with physical therapy for teaching and assessment, reinforce principle of descending a curb backward ("popping a wheelie") if balance, trunk control, strength, and timing are adequate. Backward descent carries less risk of clients losing control and falling forward out of the wheelchair.
- Ascend curbs in a forward position by popping a wheelie or having someone aid in tilting the chair back, place front wheels over curb, and roll chair up. If surface is muddy or sandy, ascend backward. Front casters will not roll on soft surfaces; a backward approach requires less energy and prevents getting stuck or falling forward.
- During assisted wheelies, helper must hold wheelchair until all four wheels are back on the ground and client has control of wheelchair. Releasing one's grip too soon may alter client's balance and cause injury.

M

- ▲ Follow therapist's recommendations for how clients should propel manual wheelchairs to prevent upper extremity pain and joint degeneration.
- • Recognize that ultra-lightweight, push rim–activated, power-assisted, or powered wheelchairs may be indicated. Striking the balance between optimum independence and preventing injury (e.g., rotator cuff injury from years of manual propulsion) is a consideration. Consider push rim–activated power-assisted wheelchairs (manual wheelchairs with a motor linked to the push rim in each rear hub) because they reduce energy needed for propulsion and reserve energy for uneven terrain or obstacle negotiation. Recommend antirollback devices for inclined planes to decrease stress on shoulders. EB: *Manual wheelchair users rely on their upper limbs to provide independent mobility, which leads to high muscular demand on their upper extremities and often results in shoulder pain and injury (Walford et al, 2019). If the client does not have sufficient strength or motor control of the extremities to propel a standard wheelchair, the client should be evaluated for a power chair.*
- ▲ Reduce floor clutter and establish safety rules for drivers of electric/power mobility devices; make referrals to physical or occupational therapy for driver reevaluations if accidents occur or client's health deteriorates.
- • Request and receive client's permission before moving an unoccupied wheelchair. Wheelchair-dependent clients may view the chair as part of their identity and independence.
- • Reinforce compensatory strategies for unilateral neglect and agnosia (e.g., visual scanning, self-talk, self-questioning as to what could be wrong) as clients propel wheelchair through doorways and around obstacles. Too often nurses physically move the wheelchair or obstacle instead of cueing the client to detect and solve problems. Refer to care plan for **Unilateral Neglect.**
- • Offer support to help clients cope with issues related to physical disability. Depression and anxiety may occur with physical loss. Refer to care plan for Ineffective **Role** Performance.
- • Provide information on support group and reliable Internet resource options.
- • Provide information about advocacy, accessibility, assistive technology, and issues under the Americans with Disabilities Act as Amended (2008) (U.S. Department of Justice, Civil Rights Division, 2020).
- ▲ Make social service or wheelchair clinic referral to educate clients on financial coverage/regulations of third-party payers and Health Care Financing Association for wheelchairs. It is wise to recognize cost, advantages, and durability of different wheelchair models before purchasing one.
- • Recommend that clients test-drive wheelchairs and try out cushions/postural supports with the advice of a qualified seating professional, not a vendor, before purchasing. If a specialty chair is indicated, for example, for sports or outdoor use, having clients test-drive the wheelchair is especially important. Equipment is expensive, and different models have different advantages and disadvantages.
- • Optimize nutrition and hydration for skin and tissue health.

Pediatric

- • Consult physical or occupational therapist for special considerations for wheelchair fitting and positioning for pediatric client EB: *In children with cerebral palsy, poor trunk control can lead to spinal deformity and pulmonary compromise. Evidence links posture and pulmonary function; special techniques for measuring these may be necessary (Barks & Shaw, 2011).*
- • Help client/family transition from a manual to a powered wheelchair/scooter if disability is severe. EB: *Wheelchairs are essential for maximizing mobility and function. Power wheelchairs can enhance independence for children who are able to use them with hand, head, or mouth mechanisms but may prompt grief in parents when introduced (Paguinto et al, 2020).*

Geriatric

- • Avoid using restraints on fidgeting clients who slide down in a wheelchair. Instead, assess for deformities; spinal curvatures; abnormal tone; limited joint range; discomfort from clothing, pressure, or constriction areas; social isolation; and toileting needs.
- • Ensure proper seat depth/leg positioning and use custom footrests (not elevated leg rests) to prevent older adults from sliding down in wheelchairs.
- ▲ Assess for side effects of medications and potential need for dosage readjustments to increase wheelchair tolerance. Give prescribed hydration and medications to treat orthostatic hypotension. Consider leg wraps. Assist client to perform warm-up bed exercises if possible. Cerebral hypoperfusion and prolonged bed rest are common causes of orthostatic intolerance and hypotension. Refer to the care plan for Impaired Bed **Mobility**.

- Allow client to control speed to propel wheelchair independently if possible. Older adults may move slowly because of diminished range of motion/strength, stiff/sore joints, and cardiopulmonary compromise. Observe carefully for fatigue, shoulder pain, or other signs of activity intolerance.
- Assess the client's ability to safely maneuver independently using a wheelchair. **EB:** *Use an evidence-based tool to assess the client's skill and physical ability to safely use a wheelchair (AHRQ, 2017).*

Home Care

▲ Establish a support system for emergency and contingency care (e.g., remote monitoring, emergency call system, alert local emergency medical system, smart speaker). Wheelchair dependence may be life-threatening during a crisis (e.g., fall, fire, or other environmental emergency).

- Recommend the following changes to the home to accommodate the use of a wheelchair: *Refer to the Easter Seals Summary on Home Accessibility* (see http://www.easterseals.com/shared-components/document-library/easy_access_housing.pdf).
  - Arrange traffic patterns so they are wide enough to maneuver a wheelchair.
  - Recognize that a 5-foot turning space is necessary to maneuver wheelchairs, doorways need to have 32 to 36 inches clear width, and entrance ramps/path slope should be assessed before permanent ramps are installed because standardized slopes may not be appropriate. Temporary ramps are cost-effective and easier to adjust.
  - Replace door hardware with fold-back hinges, remove doorway encasements (if too narrow), remove/replace thresholds (if too high), hang wall-mounted sinks/handrails, grade floors in showers for roll-in chairs, and use nonskid/nonslip floor coverings (e.g., nonwaxed wood, linoleum, or Berber carpet).
  - Rearrange room functions, furniture, and storage so that toileting, sleeping, bathing, and preparing/eating meals can safely take place on one level of the home.

▲ Request physical and occupational therapy referrals to evaluate wheelchair fitting, skills, safety, and maintenance. Suggest community resources for servicing and tuning up wheelchairs and/or locating parts so clients can service their own chairs; an annual tune-up is recommended.

M

Client/Family Teaching and Discharge Planning

▲ Assess pain levels of long-term wheelchair users and make referrals to therapists or wheelchair clinics for modifications as needed. Have client check warranty information for servicing options.

- Instruct and have client return demonstrate reinflation of pneumatic tires; encourage client to monitor tire pressure every 2 to 3 weeks.
- Instruct family/clients to remove large wheelchair parts (leg rests, armrests) when lifting wheelchair into car for transport; when reassembling, check that all parts are fastened securely and temperature is tepid. This reduces weight that needs to be lifted; locked parts and a safe temperature prevent injury/thermal injury.
- Teach the critical importance of using seatbelts and secure chair tie-downs when riding in motor vehicles in a wheelchair. Never transport a client in an unsecured wheelchair in any kind of vehicle or allow this to occur with any method of transport. Teach users and family to check safe tie-downs in any transport vehicle.
- For further information, refer to care plan for Impaired **Transfer** Ability.

REFERENCES

Agency for Healthcare Research and Quality (AHRQ). (2017). Appendix B7: Wheelchair seating assessment. In *The falls Management Program: A quality improvement initiative for nursing facilities*. Rockville, MD: AHRQ. Retrieved from https://www.ahrq.gov/professionals/systems/long-term-care/resources/injuries/fallspx/fallspxmanapb4.html. [Accessed July 15, 2021].

Barks, L., & Shaw, P. (2011). Wheelchair positioning and breathing in children with cerebral palsy: Study methods and lessons learned. *Rehabilitation Nursing*, *36*(4), 146–152 174.

Howland, W. A., & McMahon, J. K. (2015). Spinal cord injury. In D. J. Apuna, & W. A. Howland (Eds.), *A core curriculum for nurse life care planning*. Salt Lake City: American Association of Nurse Life Care Planning (AANLCP).

Kottner, J., Cuddigan, K., Carville, K., et al. (2019). Prevention and treatment of pressure ulcers/injuries: The protocol for the second update of the international clinical practice guideline 2019. *Journal of Tissue Viability*, *28*(2), 51–58.

National Pressure Ulcer Advisory Panel. (2016). *National Pressure Ulcer Advisory Panel (NPUAP) announces a change in terminology from pressure ulcer to pressure injury and updates the stages of pressure injury*. Washington, DC: NPUAP. Retrieved from https://cdn.ymaws.com/npiap.com/resource/resmgr/online_store/npiap_pressure_injury_stages.pdf. [Accessed October 31, 2021].

Paguinto, S. G., Kasparian, N. A., Bray, B., & Farrar, M. (2020). *Multidisciplinary perspectives and practices of wheelchair prescription for children with neuromuscular conditions. Disability and Rehabilitation: Assistive Technology.* [Online ahead of print]. https://doi.org/10.1080/17483107.2020.1839793.

Preston, A., Rao, A., Strauss, R., Stamm, R., & Zalman, D. (2017). Deep tissue pressure injury: A clinical review. *American*

Journal of Nursing, *117*(5), 50–57. https://doi.org/10.1097/01.NAJ.0000516273.66604.c7.

Slayton, S., Morris, P., & Brinkley, J. (2017). Pressure mapping of a standard hospital recliner and select cushions with healthy adults: A comparative study. *The Journal of Wound, Ostomy and Continence Nursing*, *44*(3), 228–235.

U.S. Department of Justice, Civil Rights Division. (2020). *A guide to disability rights laws*. Retrieved from https://www.ada.gov/cguide.htm. [Accessed July 15, 2021].

Walford, S. L., Requejo, P. S., Mulroy, S. J., & Neptune, R. R. (2019). Predictors of shoulder pain in manual wheelchair users. *Clinical Biomechanics*, *65*, 1–12. https://doi.org/10.1016/j.clinbiomech.2019.03.003.

Zemp, R., Rhiner, J., Plüss, S., Togni, R., Plock, J. A., & Taylor, W. R. (2019). Wheelchair tilt-in-space and recline functions: Influence on sitting interface pressure and ischial blood flow in an elderly population. *BioMed Research International*, 2019, 4027976. https://doi.org/10.1155/2019/4027976.

Impaired Mood Regulation

Domain 9 Coping/stress tolerance Class 2 Coping response

Friso Raemaekers, B Health, RN, CEN and Helen I. de Graaf-Waar, MSc, RN

NANDA-I

Definition

A mental state characterized by shifts in mood or affect and which is comprised of a constellation of affective, cognitive, somatic, and/or physiologic manifestations varying from mild to severe.

Defining Characteristics

Altered verbal behavior; appetite change; disinhibition; dysphoria; excessive guilt; excessive self-awareness; flight of thoughts; hopelessness; impaired attention; irritable mood; psychomotor agitation; psychomotor retardation; sad affect; self-blame; social alienation

Related Factors

Altered sleep-wake cycle; anxiety; difficulty functioning socially; external factors influencing self-concept; hypervigilance; loneliness; pain; recurrent thoughts of death; recurrent thoughts of suicide; social isolation; substance misuse; weight change

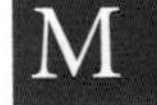

Associated Conditions

Chronic disease; functional impairment; psychosis

NOC (Nursing Outcomes Classification)

Suggested NOC Outcomes

Agitation Level; Hope; Symptom Control; Mood Equilibrium; Comfort Status: Psychospiritual; Concentration; Symptom Severity; Self-Esteem

Example NOC Outcome with Indicators

Mood Equilibrium as evidenced by the following indicators: Exhibits affect that fits situation/Exhibits impulse control/Shows interest in surroundings. (Rate the outcome and indicators of **Mood Equilibrium:** 1 = never demonstrated, 2 = rarely demonstrated, 3 = sometimes demonstrated, 4 = often demonstrated, 5 = consistently demonstrated [see Section I].)

Client Outcomes

Client Will (Specify Time Frame)

- State feelings related to changes in mood
- Follow exercise plan
- Have no attempts at self-harm
- Attention during activities
- Have a regular sleep-wake cycle
- Have sense of self-efficacy
- Achieve a mindfulness-based awareness

NIC (Nursing Interventions Classification)

Suggested NIC Interventions

Activity Therapy; Aromatherapy; Art Therapy; Cognitive Restructuring; Emotional Support; Environmental Management; Forgiveness Facilitation; Hope Inspiration; Milieu Therapy; Presence; Mood Management; Suicide Prevention; Exercise Promotion; Health Education

Nursing Interventions and *Rationales*

- Monitor the client's mood with a rating scale. **EB:** *Daily recording of mood symptoms such as through a mood diary or a self-rating scale can help identify early warning signs of relapse, as well as outline relationships between mood and treatment or lifestyle factors such as diet, exercise, or stress (Yatham et al, 2018).*
- Enable the client to express his or her feelings and try to support the client emotionally if necessary. **EBN:** *A nurse-led psychological intervention program designed to provide emotional support found significantly lower mood disturbance, anxiety, and depression in the intervention group (Kim et al, 2018).*
- Promote the self-efficacy of the client. **EB:** *A study of clients discharged from cardiac rehabilitation found self-efficacy was negatively correlated with anxiety (r = −0.4009) and depression (Madueño Caro et al, 2017).*
- Instill hopefulness in client about regaining his or her health. **EBN:** *A qualitative study of clients waiting for day surgery found that regardless of mood, feeling hope about regaining health may help clients to balance their mood (Svensson, Nilsson, & Svantesson, 2016).*
- Encourage physical activities. **EBN:** *Findings from the meta-analysis suggest that physical activity interventions can improve adolescents' mental health, but additional studies are needed to confirm the effects of physical activity on children's mental health. Findings from observational studies suggest that promoting physical activity and decreasing sedentary behavior might protect mental health in children and adolescents (Rodriguez-Ayllon et al, 2019).*
- Encourage regular physical exercise to increase physical mobility and independence in daily activities. **EB:** *Kobylańska et al (2018) found that improvement in mobility and independence in daily activities positively correlated with mood improvement in the rehabilitation process after stroke.*
- Inform clients about the negative effects associated with excessive mobile phone and social media use. **EB:** *A large-scale cross-sectional study of Korean adolescents found that smartphone usage time was positively associated with depressive symptoms, suicidal thoughts, and suicide attempts (Kim et al, 2020).* **EB:** *A review of observational studies about the links between mobile phone use and mental health found associations between depressive symptoms and sleep problems (Thomée, 2018).*
- Avoid circadian rhythm disturbances. **EB:** *Molecular mechanisms linking the circadian clock with neurological functions have been uncovered, suggesting that disruption of the clock may be critically involved in the development of mood disorders (Albrecht, 2017).*
- Encourage the client to practice dance therapy. **EBN:** *Dance therapy is beneficial in improving executive function, including mood, for adults with Parkinson's disease (Zhang et al, 2019).*
- Encourage the client to listen to music when in a negative mood. **EB:** *Findings of a meta-analysis indicate that music therapy provides short-term beneficial effects for people with depression (Aalbers et al, 2017).*
- ▲ Refer to aromatherapy massage. **EBN:** *Participants in an aromatherapy massage intervention reported multiple positive effects including improvement of mood (Ho et al, 2017).*
- ▲ Refer to cognitive behavior therapy. **EBN:** *A nurse-delivered, cognitive behavioral therapy intervention for adherence and depression among antiretroviral therapy users with depression in South Africa found improvements in mood and adherence (Andersen et al, 2018).*

M

REFERENCES

Aalbers, S., Fusar-Poli, L., Freeman, R. E., et al. (2017). Music therapy for depression. *Cochrane Database of Systematic Reviews, 11*, CD004517. https://doi.org/10.1002/14651858.CD004517.pub3.

Albrecht, U. (2017). Molecular mechanisms in mood regulation involving the circadian clock. *Frontiers in Neurology, 8*(30). https://doi.org/10.3389/fneur.2017.00030.

Andersen, L. S., Magidson, J. F., O'Cleirigh, C., et al. (2018). A pilot study of a nurse-delivered cognitive behavioral therapy intervention (Ziphamandla) for adherence and depression in HIV in South Africa. *Journal of Health Psychology, 23*(6), 776–787. https://doi.org/10.1177/1359105316643375.

Ho, S. S. M., Kwong, A. N. L., Wan, K. W. S., Ho, R. M. L., & Chow, K. M. (2017). Experiences of aromatherapy massage among adult female cancer patients: A qualitative study. *Journal of Clinical Nursing, 26*(23–24), 4519–4526. https://doi.org/10.1111/jocn.13784.

Kim, H., Cho, M. K., Ko, H., Yoo, J. E., & Song, Y. M. (2020). Association between smartphone usage and mental health in South Korean adolescents: The 2017 Korea youth risk behavior web-based survey. *Korean Journal of Family Medicine, 41*(2), 98–104. https://doi.org/10.4082/kjfm.18.0108.

Kim, Y. H., Choi, K. S., Han, K., & Kim, H. W. (2018). A psychological intervention program for patients with breast cancer under chemotherapy and at a high risk of depression: A randomised clinical trial. *Journal of Clinical Nursing*, *27*(3–4), 572–581. https://doi.org/10.1111/jocn.13910.

Kobylańska, M., Kowalska, J., Neustein, J., et al. (2018). The role of biopsychosocial factors in the rehabilitation process of individuals with a stroke. *Work*, *61*(4), 523–535. https://doi.org/10.3233/WOR-162823.

Madueño Caro, A. J., Mellado Fernández, M. L., Delgado Pacheco, J., Muñoz Ayllon, M., Pardos Lafarga, M., & Saez García, L. (2017). Perceived self-efficacy, personality and bioethics before a heart rehabilitation program in primary health care. *Enfermeria Clinica*, *27*(6), 346–351. https://doi.org/10.1016/j.enfcli.2017.04.004.

Rodriguez-Ayllon, M., Cadenas-Sánchez, C., Estévez-López, F., et al. (2019). Role of physical activity and sedentary behavior in the mental health of preschoolers, children and adolescents: A systematic review and meta-analysis. *Sports Medicine*, *49*(9), 1383–1410. https://doi.org/10.1007/s40279-019-01099-5.

Svensson, M., Nilsson, U., & Svantesson, M. (2016). Patients' experience of mood while waiting for day surgery. *Journal of Clinical Nursing*, *25*(17–18), 2600–2608. https://doi.org/10.1111/jocn.13304.

Thomée, S. (2018). Mobile phone use and mental health. A review of the research that takes a psychological perspective on exposure. *International Journal of Environmental Research and Public Health*, *15*(12), 2692. https://doi.org/10.3390/ijerph15122692.

Yatham, L. N., Kennedy, S. H., Parikh, S. V., et al. (2018). Canadian Network for Mood And Anxiety Treatments (CANMAT) and International Society for Bipolar disorders (ISBD) 2018 guidelines for the management of patients with bipolar disorder. *Bipolar Disorders*, *20*(2), 97–170. https://doi.org/10.1111/bdi.12609.

Zhang, Q., Hu, J., Wei, L., Jia, Y., & Jin, Y. (2019). Effects of dance therapy on cognitive and mood symptoms in people with Parkinson's disease: A systematic review and meta-analysis. *Complementary Therapies in Clinical Practice*, *36*, 12–17. https://doi.org/10.1016/j.ctcp.2019.04.005.

Moral Distress Domain 10 Life principles Class 3 Value/belief/action congruence

Ruth A. Wittmann-Price, PhD, RN, CNS, CNE, CNEcl, CHSE, ANEF, FAAN

NANDA-I

Definition

Response to the inability to carry out one's chosen ethical or moral decision and/or action.

Defining Characteristics

Reports anguish about acting on one's moral choice

Related Factors

Conflict among decision-makers; difficulty making end-of-life decisions; difficulty making treatment decision; information available for decision making conflicts; time constraint for decision-making; values incongruent with cultural norms

At-Risk Population

Individuals experiencing loss of personal autonomy; individuals physically distant of decision-maker

NOC (Nursing Outcomes Classification)

Suggested NOC Outcomes

Personal Autonomy; Client Satisfaction; Protection of Rights

Example NOC Outcomes with Indicators

Client Satisfaction: Protection of Rights as evidenced by the following indicators: Requests respected/Included in decisions about care/Care consistent with religious and spiritual needs. (Rate the outcome and indicators of **Client Satisfaction: Protection of Rights:** 1 = not at all satisfied, 2 = somewhat satisfied, 3 = moderately satisfied, 4 = very satisfied, 5 = completely satisfied [see Section I].)

Client Outcomes

Client Will (Specify Time Frame)

- Be able to act in accordance with values, goals, and beliefs
- Regain confidence in the ability to make decisions and/or act in accord with values, goals, and beliefs
- Express satisfaction with the ability to make decisions consistent with values, goals, and beliefs
- Have choices respected

M

NIC (Nursing Interventions Classification)

Suggested NIC Interventions

Patient Rights Protection; Emotional Support

Example NIC Activities—Patient Rights Protection

Provide environment conducive for private conversations between client, family, and health care professionals

Nursing Interventions and *Rationales*

- Assess if moral distress is present and its relationship to intrinsic or extrinsic factors. EBN: *Meghani and Lalani (2020) completed a literature review about front-line nurses working during the COVID-19 pandemic and found that they experienced fear, anxiety, depression, posttraumatic symptoms, spiritual distress, and moral distress related to extrinsic factors such as lack of staff, lack of personal protective equipment, limited knowledge regarding standard infection control practices, isolation protocols, lack of administrative support, transportation, accommodation, and child care facility.*
- Affirm the distress, commitment "to take care of yourself," and your obligations. Validate feelings and perceptions with others. EB: *Hjelle et al (2017) qualitatively studied reablement (a home-based, intensive, goal-oriented rehabilitation intervention for older adults) using semistructured interviews with eight clients, and four main themes emerged: "My willpower is needed," "Being with my stuff and my people," "The home-trainers are essential," and "Training is physical exercises, not everyday activities."* EBN: *McAdam and Erikson (2020) found that critical care nurses who provide end-of-life care are at high risk for frequent moral distress, compassion fatigue, and burnout. Using a case study approach, the researchers incorporated self-care into what critical care nurses normally do on the job to assist in maintaining health and well-being.*
- Implement strategies to change situations causing moral distress. EBN: *Karagozoglu et al (2017) studied the use of a moral distress tool in another country to evaluate the moral distress of nurses (n = 200) in an intensive care unit (ICU) by descriptive and cross-sectional design. The results concluded that the tool was reliable and valid, and the study identified communication as key to decreasing moral distress.* EB: *Halper et al (2020) surveyed pediatric medical residents who were experiencing moral distress during half-day pediatric intensive care (PICU) rotations. Handing off PICU client care was producing moral distress, which was alleviated by keeping the same provider on the PICU for a full day.*
- Assess sources and severity of distress. EBN: *Young, Froggatt, and Brearley (2017) studied moral distress in nursing home clinicians (n = 16) with clients who are near the end of life using an interpretive descriptive design and found participants described holding "good dying" values that influenced their practice, including advocating, caring, communicating, and relating with residents, and were found to influence interactions with residents, relatives, general practitioners, and colleagues. Moral distress was described when the right thing could not be done and a "bad death" incurred because of a feeling of powerlessness.* EB: *Ross and Clayton (2019) and the research team on the BabySeq genetic identification project experienced moral distress when an adult-onset condition was identified. The team changed the study protocol due to knowing information that was not requested, but important enough that they felt obligated to disclose.*
- Give voice/recognition to moral distress and express concerns about constraints to supportive individuals. EBN: *Researchers explored moral distress in Chief Nursing Officers (CNOs) (n = 20) using interviews and found six themes: lacking psychological safety, feeling a sense of powerlessness, seeking to maintain moral compass, drawing strength from networking, moral residue, and living with the consequences. This research demonstrated that CNOs experience moral distress but are pressed to show moral courage (Prestia, Sherman, & Demezier, 2017).* EB: *Griffin et al (2020) completed an exploratory study about the experience of moral distress among veteran students (n = 498) and the associated psychological, social, and religious or spiritual consequences. Themes identified by the participants (1) troubled by what they witnessed, (2) troubled by what they did, (3) troubled by what they failed to do, (4) betrayed by military leaders, or (5) betrayed by fellow service members. The study suggests that understanding the events that led up to moral distress can help health care providers and educators develop individual plans of study and appropriate referrals.*
- Engage in healthy problem-solving. EBN: *Authors studied strategies to decrease nurses' moral distress and provide better client care and strategies including legitimizing the experience, mentoring and empowering one*

another, allocating a safe haven, and improving the ethical climate of organizations (Forozeiya et al, 2017). **EBN:** *Lachance (2017) completed a review of moral courage and how it emerges to offset moral distress and found that it encompasses building safe, collaborative client- and family-centered teams.*

- Engage in multiprofessional problem-solving forums, including family meeting and/or multiprofessional rounds. **EB:** Helmers et al (2020) *explored the experience of health care providers in a PICU related to moral distress to identify attributes of moral resilience. Participants relayed that moral resilience can be assisted by strategies for positive adaptation including active, reflective, and structured supports.*
- Identify/use a support system. **EBN:** *Ramdinmawii (2017) completed a descriptive study to understand the level of stress, social support, and life satisfaction among parents (n = 60) who have a child with autism spectrum disorder (ASD). Results showed that parents have moderate stress, moderate social support, and a neutral life satisfaction, and social support is correlated inversely to stress and positively with life satisfaction.* **EB:** *Barimani et al (2017) qualitatively studied the transition to parenthood. The elements that helped the transition to parenthood included perceiving parenthood as normal, enjoying the child's growth, being prepared, having knowledge, and having social support.*
- Initiate an ethics consultation or ethics committee review. **EBN:** *Ohnishi et al (2020) studied nurses' moral distress in Japan and provided an online mental health consultant. Nurses who used the mental health consultant online provided the researchers with positive feedback and assisted in improving client care, managing nurses' moral distress, and building ethics into decision-making.*

Pediatric

- Consider the developmental age of children when evaluating decisions and conflict. **EB:** *Malas et al (2017) studied somatic symptom disorder (SSD) in children who present disproportionate or inconsistent physical manifestations with history, physical examination, laboratory, and other assessment findings and made recommendations on how to evaluate and assist parents and children who exhibit manifestations and their underlying cause.* **EBN:** *Mooney-Doyle and Ulrich (2020) completed a dimensional analysis to describe family moral distress in serious pediatric conditions. Three themes emerged from the literature surrounding parent moral distress: an intrapersonal dimension, an interpersonal dimension, and a spiritual/existential dimension. Therefore moral distress is present for families facing severe pediatric illnesses and needs to be assessed and addressed by nurses.*

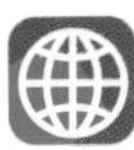

Multicultural

- Acknowledge and understand cultural differences that may influence a client's moral choices. **EBN:** *Bressler, Hanna, and Smith (2017) qualitatively studied moral distress in a nursing care unit with elderly Orthodox Jewish clients at the end of life to better understand the cultural complexity and differences in expectations for client care between nurses and families. Interviews revealed the incongruence of perspectives indicating there is needed educational strategies, clinical interventions, and research to address moral distress and cultural complexity.* **EB:** *Welles and Cervantes* (2019) *studied care providers of undocumented immigrants who have end-stage renal disease and receive emergency-only hemodialysis. The treatment is not optimal and therefore produces moral distress and negatively affects the clients' quality of life.*

Geriatric and Home Care

- Previous interventions may be adapted for geriatric or home care use.
- Assess for the effect of functional independence. **EB:** *Harigane et al (2017) explored the relationship between psychological distress and degree of functional independence among elderly adults (n = 20,282) and found that psychological distress was significantly associated with decreased independence in all activities of daily living.*
- Refer to a palliative care team as needed. **EBN:** *Koch and Grier (2020) used a case study method to identify moral distress in a situation of community palliative care involving a pregnant mother who was carrying a fetus with a life-threatening genetic disease. The palliative care team used five assumptions to decrease moral distress: (1) identification of biases, (2) utilization of a culturally safe approach, (3) effective communication, (4) assessment and support, and (5) knowledge of community resources.*

REFERENCES

Barimani, M., Vikström, A., Rosander, M., Frykedal, K. F., & Berlin, A. (2017). Facilitating and inhibiting factors in transition to parenthood—Ways in which health professionals can support parents. *Scandinavian Journal of Caring Sciences*, *31*(3), 537–546. https://doi:org/fmarion.idm.oclc.org/10.1111/scs.12367.

Bressler, T., Hanna, D. R., & Smith, E. (2017). Making sense of moral distress within cultural complexity. *Journal of Hospice and Palliative Nursing*, *19*(1), 7–14. https://doi.org/10.1097/NJH.0000000000000308.

Forozeiya, D., Vanderspank-Wright, B., Fothergill-Bourbonnais, F., Wright, D., & Moreau, D. (2017). Searching for answers: Strategies for supporting nurses who experience moral distress [abstract]. *Canadian Journal of Critical Care Nursing*, *28*(2), 34–35.

Griffin, B. J., Williams, C. L., Shaler, L., et al. (2020). Profiles of moral distress and associated outcomes among student veterans. *Psychological Trauma: Theory, Research, Practice & Policy*, *12*(7), 669–677. https://doi.org/10.1037/tra0000584.

Halper, J., Aguilera, A., Petras, L., Price, L., Slaven, J., & Swinger, N. (2020). Promoting resident wellness: A novel clinic scheduling model during pediatric intensive care unit rotations. *Academic Pediatrics*, *20*(7), e3–e4. https://doi.org/10.1016/j.acap.2020.06.022.

Harigane, M., Suzuki, Y., Yasumura, S., et al. (2017). The relationship between functional independence and psychological distress in elderly adults following the Fukushima Daiichi nuclear power plant accident: The Fukushima health management survey. *Asia-Pacific Journal of Public Health*, *29*(Suppl. 2), 120S–130S. https://doi:org.fmarion.idm.oclc.org/10.1177/1010539516683498.

Helmers, A., Palmer, K. D., & Greenberg, R. A. (2020). Moral distress: Developing strategies from experience. *Nursing Ethics*, *27*(4), 1147–1156. https://doi.org/10.1177/0969733020906593.

Hjelle, K. M., Tuntland, H., Førland, O., & Alvsvåg, H. (2017). Driving forces for home-based reablement; A qualitative study of older adults' experiences. *Health and Social Care in the Community*, *25*(5), 1581–1589. https://doi:org.fmarion.idm.oclc.org/10.1111/hsc.12324.

Karagozoglu, S., Yildirim, G., Ozden, D., & Çinar, Z. (2017). Moral distress in Turkish intensive care nurses. *Nursing Ethics*, *24*(2), 209–221. https://doi:org.fmarion.idm.oclc.org/10.1177/0969733015593408.

Koch, A., & Grier, K. (2020). Communication and cultural sensitivity for families and children with life-limiting diseases: An informed decision-making ethical case in community-based palliative care. *Journal of Hospice and Palliative Nursing*, *22*(4), 270–275. https://doi.org/10.1097/NJH.0000000000000654.

Lachance, C. (2017). Tough decisions, lots of uncertainties: Moral courage as a strategy to ease moral distress [Abstract]. *Canadian Journal of Critical Care Nursing*, *28*(2), 37.

Malas, N., Ortiz-Aguayo, R., Giles, L., & Ibeziako, P. (2017). Pediatric somatic symptom disorders. *Current Psychiatry Reports*, *19*(2), 11. https://doi.org/10.1007/s11920-017-0760-3.

McAdam, J. L., & Erikson, A. (2020). Self-care in the bereavement process. *Critical Care Nursing Clinics of North America*, *32*(3), 421–437. https://doi.org/10.1016/j.cnc.2020.05.005.

Meghani, S., & Lalani, N. (2020). Critical care nurses as frontline warriors during COVID-19 in Pakistan. *Connect: The World of Critical Care Nursing*, *13*(4), 196–201. https://doi.org/10.1891/WFCCN-D-20-00009.

Mooney-Doyle, K., & Ulrich, C. M. (2020). Parent moral distress in serious pediatric illness: A dimensional analysis. *Nursing Ethics*, *27*(3), 821–837. https://doi.org/10.1177/0969733019878838.

Ohnishi, K., Stone, T. E., Yoshiike, T., & Kitaoka, K. (2020). The role of online ethics consultation on mental health. *Nursing Ethics*, *27*(5), 1261–1269. https://doi.org/10.1177/0969733020906596.

Prestia, A. S., Sherman, R. O., & Demezier, C. (2017). Chief nursing officers' experiences with moral distress. *The Journal of Nursing Administration*, *47*(2), 101–107. https://doi.org/10.1097/NNA.0000000000000447.

Ramdinmawii, K. R. (2017). A descriptive study to assess the level of stress, social support and life satisfaction among parents of children with autism spectrum disorder at selected centres in Delhi. *International Journal of Nursing Education*, *9*(2), 172–177. https://doi.org/10.5958/0974-9357.2017.00058.7.

Ross, L. F., & Clayton, E. W. (2019). Ethical issues in newborn sequencing research: The case study of BabySeq. *Pediatrics*, *144*(6), e20191031.

Welles, C. C., & Cervantes, L. (2019). Hemodialysis care for undocumented immigrants with end-stage renal disease in the United States. *Current Opinion in Nephrology and Hypertension*, *28*(6), 615–620. https://doi.org/10.1097/MNH.0000000000000543.

Young, A., Froggatt, K., & Brearley, S. G. (2017). "Powerlessness" or "doing the right thing"—moral distress among nursing home staff caring for residents at the end of life: An interpretive descriptive study. *Palliative Medicine*, *31*(9), 853–860. https://doi.org/10.1177/0269216316682894.

M

Risk for Dry Mouth **Domain 11 Safety/protection Class 2 Physical injury**

Katherine Foss, MSN, RN

NANDA-I

Definition

Susceptible to discomfort or damage to the oral mucosa due to reduced quantity or quality of saliva to moisten the mucosa, which may compromise health.

Risk Factors

Dehydration; depressive symptoms; excessive stress; excitement; smoking

At-Risk Population

Pregnant women

Associated Conditions

Chemotherapy; depression; fluid restriction; inability to feed orally; oxygen therapy; pharmaceutical preparations; radiotherapy to the head and neck; systemic diseases

NOC (Nursing Outcomes Classification)

Suggested NOC Outcomes

Oral Health; Self-Care: Oral Hygiene; Tissue Integrity: Skin and Mucous Membranes

Example NOC Outcome with Indicators

Oral Health as evidenced by the following indicators: Cleanliness of mouth and teeth/Moisture of oral mucosa and tongue/Color of mucous membranes/Oral mucosa/Tongue/Gum integrity. (Rate the outcome and indicators of **Oral Health:** 1 = severely compromised, 2 = substantially compromised, 3 = moderately compromised, 4 = mildly compromised, 5 = not compromised [see Section I].)

Client Outcomes

Client Will (Specify Time Frame)

- Maintain intact, moist oral mucous membranes that are free of ulceration, inflammation, infection, and debris
- Demonstrate measures to maintain or regain oral health
- Demonstrate oral hygiene knowledge and skills to maintain moisture within the mouth
- Be free of halitosis and oral discomfort
- State tolerable to no changes in taste sensation (dysgeusia)

NIC (Nursing Interventions Classification)

Suggested NIC Intervention

Oral Health Restoration

Example NIC Activities—Oral Health Restoration

Monitor condition of client's mouth including character of abnormalities; Instruct client to perform regular oral hygiene measures

M

Nursing Interventions and *Rationales*

- Perform a comprehensive extraoral and intraoral examination for associated conditions and risk factors that reduce quantity or quality of saliva and client complaints of oral dryness and difficulty speaking, eating, or swallowing. EB: *Inspection is a critical assessment and diagnostic tool that can lead to identification of current oral health and impending problems (van der Waal, 2015).*
- Assess for symptoms of dry mouth. EB: *Observe for atrophic and erythematous oral mucosa, loss of papillae on the tongue, and lips that peel and crack. Traumatic lesions may be visible on the buccal mucosa and the lateral borders of the tongue (Plemons, Al-Hashimi, & Marek, 2014).*
- Inspecting and palpating major salivary glands and lymph nodes for masses, enlargement, tenderness, purulent discharge, or absence of salivary pooling/secretions are components of a comprehensive head and neck examination to differentiate between salivary and nonsalivary causes of dry mouth (Plemons, Al-Hashimi, & Marek, 2014).
- Inspect nasal turbinates for enlargement, swelling, polyps, and nasal flow because nasal blockages increase mouth breathing, which may exacerbate oral dryness symptoms.
- Assess client for oral candidiasis, dental caries, and gingival recession (Plemons, Al-Hashimi, & Marek, 2014). Oral candidiasis may suggest the client is immunocompromised or on a treatment that increases the risk of fungal infection, which can lead to additional health care concerns.
- Assess client for dental caries and gingival recession EB: *Clinical signs of hyposalivation also include increased incidence of tooth decay at the gingival margin and nonspecific gingival inflammation (Plemons, Al-Hashimi, & Marek, 2014).*
- Assess client for difficulty chewing, swallowing (dysphagia), or speaking. EB: *Dry mouth may cause difficulties with chewing and swallowing, which may place the client at risk of choking and/or malnutrition (Plemons, Al-Hashimi, & Marek, 2014; American Academy of Oral Medicine [AAOM], 2016).*

- Assess client for mouth breathing caused by functional impairment of the upper airway and/or presence of nasal, endotracheal, or orogastric tubes that may prevent mouth closure or irritate oral mucosa, which may contribute to an increase in dry mouth symptoms experienced by clients.
- Assess client hydration status. A dry tongue and mucous membranes are symptoms of decreased hydration status. Decreased hydration status can worsen symptoms of dry mouth.
- Assess fluid status because dehydration will also affect salivary flow *(Plemons, Al-Hashimi, & Marek, 2014).* Consider fluid loss associated with fever, cachexia, vomiting, or diarrhea. Recognize that dehydration is prevalent in older adults and may affect salivary flow (Plemons, Al-Hashimi, & Marek, 2014).

▲ Dry mouth, mouth dryness, or oral dryness (xerostomia) is a dryness of the oral cavity resulting from insufficient or complete lack of saliva secretion. Although dry mouth is a common symptom of salivary gland hyposecretion, there is a distinction between dryness caused by malfunction of the salivary glands and the client's subjective report of oral dryness despite normal salivary gland function (Tanasiewicz, Hildebrandt, & Obersztyn, 2016). **EB:** *In a review summary of 90 articles, clinical application to the etiology, diagnosis, and treatment of dry mouth requires an interdisciplinary approach to symptom assessment, clinical examination, functional and cognitive assessment, and identifying goals of care. The management of dry mouth begins with a thorough history of symptoms; review of medical, dental, and medication use history; clinical examination; salivary flow rate measurements; salivary imaging studies; and biopsies and laboratory analysis (Han, Suarez-Durall, & Mulligan, 2015).*

▲ The client may require a dental referral to evaluate salivary flow rate as a tool to monitor dry mouth symptoms (Plemons, Al-Hashimi, & Marek, 2014).

▲ Consider use of oral screening, client self-report tool, and/or subjective questioning regarding dry mouth symptoms to assess client oral health and to predict need for dental intervention and degree of salivary hypofunction. **CEB:** *One validated screening tool, for use by nondental professionals, to assess client oral health and identification of need for a dental examination is the Oral Health Assessment Tool (OHAT) and can be used to monitor client progress during an oral hygiene plan of care (State of Victoria, Health and Human Services, 2018).* **EB:** *A study comparing oral health assessments by nurses with oral health interventionists found that with proper training nurses using the OHAT implemented interventions that improved oral care of hospitalized older adults* (p <0.001) *(Gibney et al, 2019).*

M

▲ Use client self-report to measure symptoms of dry mouth. **EB:** *The Xerostomia Inventory (XI) questionnaire, developed in Australia during the 1990s and validated in international studies, provided a summative rating of client's xerostomia symptoms (Thomson, 2015).* **EB:** *A Cochrane review found that a change in XI score of 6 or more points is likely to be meaningful, and the tools measure the severity of dry mouth and act as a responsive measure to interventions for dry mouth (Furness et al, 2013).*

- Ask the client about symptoms of hyposalivation. **CEB/EB:** *A study of subjective oral dryness compared with salivary flow reports that certain complaints were highly predictive of impaired salivary flow. Positive responses to any of the following complaints are associated with significant hyposalivation: oral dryness when eating, need to sip fluids to swallow dry foods, difficulty swallowing, and the perception of too little saliva (Fox, Busch, & Baum, 1987).* **EB:** *Ask the client to describe symptoms, triggers, and treatments that exacerbate or help oral discomfort associated with hyposalivation (Epstein & Beier Jensen, 2015).*

▲ Review client medication usage for dry mouth as a side effect of medication. If symptoms are present consult with provider, or refer client to see a dentist or specialist. **EB:** *Assess the client's use of xerostomic medications or medications that are known to directly inhibit saliva flow (Plemons, Al-Hashimi, & Marek, 2014). Anticholinergic and antihypertensive drugs (angiotensin-converting enzyme inhibitors, angiotensin receptor blockers, α- and β-adrenergic blockers, and diuretics), antihistamines, opioids, antidepressants, immunostimulants, and antipsychotic and skeletal muscle relaxant drugs are identified as common causes of dry mouth.* **EBN:** *Consult with a pharmacist regarding timing of medications and possible drug substitutions. Most medications do not cause damage to salivary glands but can reduce salivary flow (Plemons, Al-Hashimi, & Marek, 2014; Tanasiewicz, Hildebrandt, & Obersztyn, 2016).*

▲ Administer pilocarpine and cevimeline as prescribed because these medications are considered first-line therapy in Sjögren's syndrome and head and neck cancer clients with radiotherapy-induced dry mouth and hyposalivation. **EB:** *A systematic review and meta-analysis of 1732 clients in 20 studies indicated that both cevimeline and pilocarpine can reduce dry mouth symptoms and increase salivary flow compared with placebo (Mercadante et al, 2017).*

▲ The American Dental Association (ADA) Council on Scientific Affairs report identifies that pilocarpine and cevimeline have US Food and Drug Administration approval for treating dry mouth caused by Sjögren's syndrome or radiation therapy (Plemons, Al-Hashimi, & Marek, 2014).

- Teach clients about conditions that can exacerbate dry mouth symptoms:
  - Avoidance of low-humidity environments
  - Avoidance of oral irritants: acidic fluids such as carbonated beverages and juices, caffeine, alcohol, tobacco
  - Avoidance of salty, spicy, acidic, or high-sucrose content foods
  - Avoidance of dry, hard, and sticky foods
  - Referral of client to smoking and/or alcohol cessation program
    EB: *Avoiding conditions that can worsen dry mouth can facilitate client self-management of the symptom severity (Plemons, Al-Hashimi, & Marek, 2014; Cohen et al, 2016).*
- Teach the client good oral hygiene:
  - Twice daily toothbrushing with regular topical fluoride toothpaste.
  - Use of soft bristle toothbrush. EB: *Twice daily use of a soft bristle toothbrush is an accepted standard of care by the ADA to maintain and promote oral health and dentition (ADA, 2020).*
  - Daily use of dental floss or another interdental cleaner. EB: *Daily use of dental floss or interdental cleaner is an accepted standard of care to maintain and promote oral health and dentition (ADA, 2020).*
  - Daily use of alcohol-free mouth rinse. EB: *Systematic review by an expert panel recommends regular use of fluoride toothpastes or mouth rinses as highly effective in preventing caries in dry mouth (Zero et al, 2016).*
  - Recommend use of prescription-strength fluoride toothpastes for severe salivary hypofunction. EB: *Use 1.1% neutral sodium fluoride, or fluoride gel in custom-fit oral tray, or 0.09% fluoride mouth rinse daily (Plemons, Al-Hashimi, & Marek, 2014; ADA, 2021).*
- Provide instruction regarding cleaning, and assist with care of dental prosthesis as needed. Daily cleansing of a dental prosthetic is an accepted standard of care to maintain and promote oral health and dentition (ADA, 2020).

▲ Provide instruction on candidiasis prevention and control. Administer antifungal topical treatments as prescribed using available suspensions, pastilles, and lozenges for uncomplicated oral candidiasis. Systemic antifungal agents may be prescribed for complicated candidiasis mucosal infection (*Baer & Sankar, 2020*).

▲ Soak partial or complete dental prosthesis overnight in 0.2% chlorhexidine HCl. EB: *A literature review of treatment of dry mouth and other nonocular sicca symptoms in Sjögren's syndrome identified that oral candidiasis mucosal infection is common in clients with salivary gland hypofunction. Administer prescribed antifungal rinses, ointments, or lozenges. Include daily partial or complete denture antifungal treatment; soak dentures overnight in 0.2% chlorhexidine HCl (Baer & Sankar, 2020).*

▲ Recommend professional dental oral examination every 3 to 6 months. Recommend professional teeth cleaning at least every 6 months. EB: *ADA Council of Scientific Affairs identifies preventive oral health care for clients with hyposalivation as essential. This includes more frequent dental visits and associated management of secondary infections (Plemons, Al-Hashimi, & Marek, 2014).*

- Discuss selection and use of salivary substitutes with client and health care provider to assist in maintaining mouth moisture. EB: *A Cochrane review of nonpharmacological topical treatments for dry mouth that included salivary substitutes of sugar-free gums, mints, lozenges, sprays, gels, oils, and toothpastes indicated lack of strong evidence that topical therapies are effective in improving salivary flow. Many saliva substitutes are available without prescription and contain a mix of components such as carboxymethylcellulose, polyethylene glycol, sorbitol, and electrolytes. These products typically provide more viscosity and lubrication than water. A saliva spray that contains oxygenated glycerol trimester (OGT) is more effective than a water-based electrolyte spray (McMillan et al, 2016).* EB: *A review of the primary aspects of saliva preparations, including biological properties and antimicrobial effect, identified that saliva substitutes reduce symptoms of dry mouth albeit temporarily. The data on saliva substitutes that try to mimic human saliva with antimicrobial substances and remineralization properties are "ambiguous." For oral lubrication, mucin-based preparations are better than those with carboxymethylcellulose (Łysik et al, 2019).*
- Teach the client that any topical product that is acidic or contains sugar, or noted as sugarless with high fructose, should be avoided. EB: *Citrus-flavored sugar-free tablets or oral drops with malic acid may stimulate salivary flow. Additional nonpharmacological management of dry mouth using gel-releasing devices worn in the mouth requires more research. Client preference also appears to have a significant effect in the acceptance and attribution of topical agent efficacy (Furness et al, 2013; Treister, Villa, & Thompson, 2020).* EB: *A predesign and postdesign study of 118 elderly clients using an edible oral moisturizing jelly (OMJ) examined the efficacy of OMJ with results of reduced symptoms of dry mouth and prevention of decline of*

M

saliva pH, but further study is needed with a larger population and randomized-controlled study design (Dalodom et al, 2016).

- Encourage the client to try several products, based on client preference, to find a suitable saliva substitute. Clients reported that use of saliva substitutes may be more helpful before sleep because of diurnal variation on reduction in salivary flow at night. It is also suggested that clients mix and match salivary agents based on their daily schedules or activities such as eating or public speaking (Baer & Sankar, 2020). CEB/EB: *A literature review through September 2017 of treatment of dry mouth and other nonocular sicca symptoms in Sjögren's syndrome that use saliva substitutes is supported by several randomized trials and studies that show benefit when compared with placebo in relieving symptoms of dry mouth, burning tongue, and difficulties with chewing and swallowing (Wu, 2008; National Institute of Dental and Craniofacial Research, 2018).* EB: *A systematic review of the effects of acupuncture on dry mouth and hyposalivation concluded absence of significant effect on saliva production or dry mouth symptoms in Sjögren's syndrome (Assy & Brand, 2018) with the recommendation that additional, well-designed studies are needed to determine the benefit of acupuncture, and current cost of acupuncture does not justify use outside of clinical trials.*
- Lubricate lips every 2 hours, while awake, and as needed. Apply moisturizer (e.g., lanolin) to dry lips every 2 hours, as needed to assist with dryness.
- Teach clients preventive measures to reduce oral dryness:
  - Maintain adequate oral hydration by sipping water regularly and/or sucking on ice chips (AAOM, 2016).
  - While eating, drink fluids carefully.
  - Maintain an oral intake log.
  - Rinse with normal saline or clean water as a part of daily oral care to prevent dry mouth, or sodium bicarbonate solution (1 teaspoon salt and 1 teaspoon baking soda to 1 L of water). EB: *Oral rinses with clean water or normal saline every 2 hours while awake promote a moist oral mucosa, neutralize oral pH, and are readily available with minimal side effects and are inexpensive (AAOM, 2016; ADA, 2020).*

M

- Encourage the client to use sugar-free gum or sugar-free candy to promote salivary flow. EB: *A Cochrane review of nonpharmacological topical treatments for dry mouth included salivary substitutes of sugar-free gum and candy. Although mastication increases saliva production, the evidence is not conclusive that sugar-free chewing gum is better or worse than other saliva substitutes for symptom management of dry mouth, but the use of these interventions also was supported by extensive clinical experience (Furness et al, 2013).* EB: *A randomized phase III trial using customized sugar-free gum to alleviate radiation-induced xerostomia confirmed an immediate stimulating effect of salivary flow and viscosity after 5 minutes of chewing. However, changes in flow and viscosity between the intervention group (chewing gum) and standard care (control) was not significant over time. The subjective feeling of xerostomia was reduced in the intervention group in spite of objective assessment of hyposalivation. "This finding emphasizes the importance of talking with clients about symptom burdens, as subjective and objective assessment do not always correlate" (Kaae et al, 2020).*
- Encourage the client to use saline nasal sprays to maintain open nasal passages. EB: *Maintenance of open nasal passage to avoid mouth breathing includes saline nasal sprays or gentle nasal lavage to remove dried secretions (AAOM, 2016; Baer & Sankar, 2020).*
- The client may find the use of a humidifier during sleep at night helpful in reducing symptoms.
- ▲ Discuss with the client the use of acupuncture, electrical nerve stimulation, and powered versus manual toothbrushes to assist in maintaining mouth moisture. CEB: *In a systematic review, nonpharmacological therapies using acupuncture, transcutaneous electrical nerve stimulation, and powered versus manual toothbrushing were reported as insufficient or low-quality evidence to determine effects of these interventions on dry mouth or saliva production but continued to be studied as alternatives for symptom relief (Furness et al, 2013; Simcock et al, 2013).*
- ▲ Encourage the client to discuss the use of emerging preventive treatments with the health care provider such as gene therapy, tissue engineering, stem cell therapy, and growth factors for etiologies associated with dry mouth. EB: *Current research of Sjögren's syndrome and head and neck radiation etiologies associated with salivary hypofunction reported that future approaches to treatment and/or prevention of the feeling of dry mouth include gene therapy, stem cell therapy, and tissue engineering (Quock, 2016).* EB: *In a review of 90 articles with clinical application, there are emerging therapies for radiation-induced salivary hypofunction, but the most efficacious with cost-effectiveness are not identified (Han, Suarez-Durall, & Mulligan, 2015). Emerging therapies also include use of hyperbaric oxygen after head and neck radiation (Millsop et al, 2017).*

▲ Discuss use of bethanechol HCl saliva stimulant in head and neck cancer clients with radiotherapy-induced dry mouth and hyposalivation with the client and health care provider. EB: *Clinical application of bethanechol HCl to treat dry mouth in clients with radiotherapy-induced dry mouth and salivation is not supported because further research is needed to determine optimal dosing, frequency of use, long-term efficacy, and safety (Han, Suarez-Durall, & Mulligan, 2015; McMillan et al, 2016).*

Geriatric

- Recognize that symptoms of dry mouth are more common in menopausal women and geriatric clients. CEB/EB: *Symptoms of dry mouth are more common in menopausal women and almost 50% of the elderly population because of an age-related increase of systemic disease occurrence and disease treatment, including medications (Turner & Ship, 2007; Thomson, 2015; Dalodom et al, 2016).* EB: *Composition of saliva changes with age, including decreased sodium and potassium ions, IgA, lactoferrin and lysozyme, and proline-rich proteins, including reduced antimicrobial factors in the saliva. Xerostomia in the elderly can be severe with the addition of missing teeth and use of dentures (Łysik et al, 2019).*
- Age-associated increase of systemic disease and subsequent disease treatment are the primary causes of dry mouth. EB: *Older adults experience increased incidence of xerostomia, hyposalivation, and oral health disorders because of the high prevalence of polypharmacy. Daily oral assessment and interventions to reduce severity of oral dryness are needed to improve oral health, address nutritional concerns, and prevent cavities. The most commonly prescribed pharmaceutical treatment options are pilocarpine (a parasympathomimetic agent with potent muscarinic, cholinergic, salivation-stimulating properties) and cevimeline (a quinuclidine analog with therapeutic and side effects similar to those of pilocarpine) (Barbe, 2018).*
- Older adults are at risk of xerostomia from a variety of etiologies. EB: *In a narrative review of systemic disease in older adults and review of the literature of xerostomia caused by various etiologies, it is recommended to assess the client for dehydration, nutritional alteration manifested by weight loss, decreased appetite, increased thirst, and any changes in food or beverage preferences. Oral symptoms of malnutrition, such as sore tongue, burning mouth, and gingivitis, may be caused by iron, vitamin B_1, B_2, B_6, and B_{12} or vitamin C deficiencies (Tanasiewicz, Hildebrandt, & Obersztyn, 2016; Critchlow, 2017).*
- Review client medication list routinely. EB: *In a cross-sectional study to examine the relationship between nutrition, oral health, and drug use among adults age 75 and older, it was found that excessive polypharmacy, the use of particular drug groups, and depressive symptoms were associated with xerostomia, supporting the need for a multiprofessional approach to care (Thomson, 2015; Viljakainen et al, 2016).*

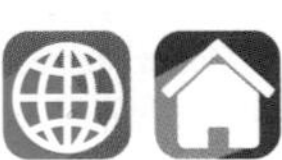

Multicultural and Home Care Considerations

- The previously mentioned nursing interventions and client teaching may be adapted for multicultural and home care considerations. See care plan on Impaired **Oral Mucous Membrane** Integrity.

M

REFERENCES

American Academy of Oral Medicine. (2016). AAOM clinical practice Statement. Subject: Clinical management of cancer therapy-induced salivary gland hypofunction and xerostomia. *Oral Surgery Oral Medicine Oral Pathology Oral Radiology*, *122*(3), 310–312. https://doi/10.1016/j.oooo.2016.04.015.

American Dental Association (ADA). (2020). *Home oral care*. Retrieved from https://www.ada.org/en/member-center/oral-health-topics/home-care. [Accessed July 19, 2021].

American Dental Association (ADA). (2021). *Xerostomia (dry mouth)*. Retrieved from http://www.ada.org/en/member-center/oral-health-topics/xerostomia. [Accessed July 19, 2021].

Assy, Z., & Brand, H. S. (2018). A systematic review of the effects of acupuncture on xerostomia and hyposalivation. *BMC Complementary and Alternative Medicine*, *18*(1), 57. https://doi.org/10.1186/s12906-018 2124-x.

Baer, A. N., & Sankar, V. (2020). Treatment of dry mouth and other non-ocular sicca symptoms in Sjögren's syndrome. In R. Fox, & P. L. Romain (Eds.), *UpToDate*. Waltham, MA: UpToDate. Retrieved from https://www.uptodate.com/contents/treatment-of-dry-mouth-and-other-non-ocular-sicca-symptoms-in-sjogrens-syndrome. [Accessed July 19, 2021].

Barbe, A. G. (2018). Medication-induced xerostomia and hyposalivation in the elderly: Culprits, complications, and management. *Drugs & Aging*, *35*(10), 877–885. https://doi.org/10.1007/s40266-018-0588-5.

Cohen, E. E. W., LaMonte, S. J., Erb, N. L., et al. (2016). American Cancer Society head and neck cancer survivorship care guideline. *CA Cancer Journal for Clinicians*, *66*(3), 203–239.

Critchlow, D. (2017). Part 3: Impact of systemic conditions and medication on oral health. *British Journal of Community Nursing*, *22*(4), 181–190.

Dalodom, S., Lam-Ubol, A., Jeanmaneechotechai, S., et al. (2016). Influence of oral moisturizing jelly as a saliva substitute for the relief of xerostomia in elderly patients with hypertension and diabetes mellitus. *Geriatric Nursing*, *37*(2), 101–109. https://doi.org/10.1016/j.gerinurse.2015.10.014.

Epstein, J. B., & Beier Jensen, S. (2015). Management of hyposalivation and xerostomia: Criteria for treatment strategies. *Compendium of Continuing Education in Dentistry*, *36*(8), 600–603.

Fox, P. C., Busch, K. A., & Baum, B. J. (1987). Subjective reports of xerostomia and objective measures of salivary gland performance. *Journal of the American Dental Association*, *115*(4), 581–584.

Furness, S., Bryan, G., McMillan, R., Birchenough, S., & Worthington, H. V. (2013). Interventions for the management of dry mouth: Non-pharmacological interventions. *Cochrane Database of Systematic Reviews, 9*, CD009603. https://doi.org/10.1002/14651858.CD009603.pub3.

Gibney, J. M., Wright, F. A., D'Souza, M., & Naganathan, V. (2019). Improving the oral health of older people in hospital. *Australasian Journal on Ageing, 38*(1), 33–38. https://doi.org/10.1111/ajag.12588.

Han, P., Suarez-Durall, P., & Mulligan, R. (2015). Dry mouth: A critical topic for older adult patients. *Journal of Prosthodontic Research, 59*(1), 6–19. https://doi.org/10.1016/j.jpor.2014.11.001.

Kaae, J. K., Stenfeldt, L., Hyrup, B., Brink, C., & Eriksen, J. G. (2020). A randomized phase III trial for alleviating radiation-induced xerostomia with chewing gum. *Radiotherapy & Oncology, 142*, 72–78. https://doi.org/10.1016/j.radonc.2019.09.013.

Łysik, D., Niemirowicz-Laskowska, K., Bucki, R., Tokajuk, G., & Mystkowska, J. (2019). Artificial saliva: Challenges and future perspectives for the treatment of xerostomia. *International Journal of Molecular Sciences, 20*(13), 3199. https://doi.org/10.3390/ijms20133199.

McMillan, R., Forssell, H., Buchanan, J. A. G., Glenny, A. M., Weldon, J. C., & Zakrzewska, J. M. (2016). Interventions for treating burning mouth syndrome. *Cochrane Database of Systematic Reviews, 11*, CD002779. https://doi.org/10.1002/14651858.CD002779.pub3.

Mercadante, V., Al Hamad, A., Lodi, G., Porter, S., & Fedele, S. (2017). Interventions for the management of radiotherapy-induced xerostomia and hyposalivation: A systematic review and meta-analysis. *Oral Oncology, 66*, 64–74. Retrieved from https://www.ncbi.nlm.nih.ov/pubmed/28249650.1.

Millsop, J. W., Wang, E. A., & Fazel, N. (2017). Etiology, evaluation, and management of xerostomia. *Clinics in Dermatology, 35*(5), 468–476. https://doi.org/10.1016/j.clindermatol.2017.06.010.

National Institute of Dental and Craniofacial Research. (2018). Dry mouth. Retrieved from https://www.nidcr.nih.gov/OralHealth/Topics/DryMouth/DryMouth.htm#. [Accessed July 19, 2021].

Plemons, J. M., Al-Hashimi, I., & Marek, C. L. (2014). Managing xerostomia and salivary gland hypofunction: Executive summary of a report from the American Dental Association Council on Scientific Affairs. *Journal of the American Dental Association, 145*(8), 867–873. https://doi.org/10.14219/jada.archive.2007.0358.

Quock, R. L. (2016). Xerostomia: Current streams of investigation. *Oral Surgery Oral Medicine Oral Pathology Oral Radiology, 122*(1), 53–60. https://doi.org/10.1016/j.oooo.2016.03.002.

Simcock, R., Fallowfield, L., Monson, K., et al. (2013). Arix: A randomised trial of acupuncture v oral care sessions in patients with chronic xerostomia following treatment of head and neck cancer. *Annals of Oncology, 24*(3), 776–783. https://doi-org.proxy.hsl.ucdenver.edu/10.1093/annonc/mds515.

State of Victoria, Health and Human Services. (2018). Oral and dental hygine standardized care process. Retrieved from https://www.health.vic.gov.au/sites/default/files/migrated/files/collections/factsheets/s/scp-oral-and-dental-hygiene-pdf.pdf.

Tanasiewicz, M., Hildebrandt, T., & Obersztyn, I. (2016). Xerostomia of various etiologies: A review of the literature. *Advances in Clinical and Experimental Medicine, 25*(1), 199–206.

Thomson, W. M. (2015). Dry mouth and older people. *Australian Dental Journal, 60*(Suppl. 1), 54–63. https://doi.org/10.1111/adj.12284. doi:10.17219/acem/29375.

Treister, N. S., Villa, A., & Thompson, L. (2020). Palliative care: Overview of mouth care at the end of life. In E. Bruera, & J. Given (Eds.), *UpToDate.* Waltham, MA: UpToDate. Retrieved from https://www.uptodate.com/contents/palliative-care-overview-of-mouth-care-at-the-end-of-life/print. [Accessed July 19, 2021].

Turner, M. D., & Ship, J. A. (2007). Dry mouth and its effects on the oral health of elderly people. *Journal of the American Dental Association, 138*(Suppl. l), 15S–20S.

Viljakainen, S., Nykänen, I., Ahonen, R., et al. (2016). Xerostomia among older home care clients. *Community Dentistry and Oral Epidemiology, 44*(3), 232–238.

van der Waal, I. (2015). Oral leukoplakia: The ongoing discussion on definition and terminology. *Medicina Oral, Patología Oral Y Cirugía Bucal, 20*(6), e685–e692. https://doi.org/10.4317/medoral.21007.

Wu, A. J. (2008). Optimizing dry mouth treatment for individuals with Sjögren's syndrome. *Rheumatic Disease Clinics of North America, 34*(4), 1001–1010.

Zero, D. T., Brennan, M. T., Daniels, T. E., et al. (2016). Clinical practice guidelines for oral management of Sjögren disease: Dental caries prevention. *Journal of the American Dental Association, 147*(4), 295–305.

M

Nausea Domain 12 Comfort Class 1 Physical comfort

Janelle M. Tipton, DNP, APRN-CNS, AOCN

NANDA-I

Definition

A subjective phenomenon of an unpleasant feeling in the back of the throat and stomach, which may or may not result in vomiting.

Defining Characteristics

Food aversion; gagging sensation; increased salivation; increased swallowing; sour taste

Related Factors

Anxiety; exposure to toxin; fear; noxious taste; unpleasant sensory stimuli

At-Risk Population

Pregnant women

Associated Conditions

Abdominal neoplasms; altered biochemical phenomenon; esophageal disease; gastric distention; gastrointestinal irritation; intracranial hypertension; labyrinthitis; liver capsule stretch; localized tumor; Ménière's disease; meningitis; motion sickness; pancreatic diseases; pharmaceutical preparations; psychological disorder; splenetic capsule stretch; treatment regimen

NOC (Nursing Outcomes Classification)

Suggested NOC Outcomes

Comfort Level; Hydration; Nausea and Vomiting Severity; Nutritional Status: Food and Fluid Intake; Nutrient Intake

Example NOC Outcome with Indicators

Nausea and Vomiting Severity as evidenced by the following indicators: Frequency of nausea/Intensity of nausea/Distress of nausea. (Rate the outcome and indicators of **Nausea and Vomiting Severity:** 1 = severe, 2 = substantial, 3 = moderate, 4 = mild, 5 = none [see Section I].)

Client Outcomes

Client Will (Specify Time Frame)

- State relief of nausea
- Explain methods clients can use to decrease nausea and vomiting (N&V)

NIC (Nursing Interventions Classification)

Suggested NIC Interventions

Distraction; Medication Administration; Progressive Muscle Relaxation; Simple Guided Imagery; Therapeutic Touch

Example NIC Activities—Distraction

Encourage the individual to choose the distraction techniques desired, such as music, engaging in conversation or telling a detailed account of event or story, guided imagery, or humor; Advise client to practice the distraction technique before the time needed, if possible

Nursing Interventions and *Rationales*

- ▲ Determine cause or risk for N&V (e.g., medication effects, infectious causes [viral and bacterial gastroenteritis], disorders of the gut and peritoneum [mechanical obstruction, motility disorders, or other intraabdominal causes], central nervous system causes [including anxiety], endocrine and metabolic causes [including pregnancy], postoperative-related status). EB: *Because N&V are clinically identifiable symptoms, it is important for the cause to be determined and appropriate plan and interventions to be developed. Review the client's medication record, alcohol history, and electrolytes as appropriate for early identification of cause of nausea (Koth & Kolesar, 2017).* EB: *Prophylactic interventions given before chemotherapy have proven to be most successful in preventing N&V. Client expectancy of nausea after chemotherapy is predictive of that treatment-related side effect (Oncology Nursing Society, 2019; Patel et al, 2017).*
- ▲ Evaluate and document the client's history of N&V, with attention to onset, duration, timing, volume of emesis, frequency of pattern, setting, associated factors, aggravating factors, and medical and social histories. EB: *The onset and duration of N&V may be distinctly associated with specific events and may be treated differently (Dranitsaris et al, 2017).*
- • Document each episode of nausea and/or vomiting separately and the effectiveness of interventions. Consider an assessment tool for consistency of evaluation. EB: *A systematic approach can provide consistency, accuracy, and measurement needed to direct care. It is important to recognize that nausea is a subjective experience (Dranitsaris et al, 2017).*

- Identify and eliminate contributing causative factors. This may include eliminating unpleasant odors or medications that may be contributing to nausea. These interventions are theory based; however, there is no research evidence to support these interventions outside of expert opinion.
- ▲ Implement appropriate dietary measures such as nothing by mouth (NPO) status as appropriate; small, frequent meals; and low-fat, high-protein meals. It may be helpful to avoid foods that are spicy, fatty, or highly salty. Reverting to previous practices when ill in the past and consuming "comfort foods" may also be helpful at this time. EB: *Expert opinion consensus recommends these interventions, with no research data available (Marx et al, 2016).*
- ▲ Recognize and implement interventions and monitor complications associated with N&V. This may include administration of intravenous fluids and electrolytes. EB: *Recognition of complications of N&V is critical to prevent and manage complications of dehydration, electrolyte imbalance, and malnourishment. Adequate hydration corrects imbalances and reduces further emesis (Tilleman et al, 2018).*
- ▲ Administer appropriate antiemetics, according to guidelines, with consideration to emetic cause, most effective route, and side effects of the medication, and with attention to and coverage for the time frames in which the nausea is anticipated. EB: *Antiemetic medications are effective at different receptor sites and treat different causes of N&V. A combination of agents may be more effective than a single agent (Koth & Kolesar, 2017; Razvi et al, 2019).*
- Consider nonpharmacological interventions such as acupressure, acupuncture, music therapy, distraction, and slow, deliberate movements. EB: *Nonpharmacological interventions can augment pharmacological interventions because they predominantly affect the higher cortical centers that trigger N&V. Nonpharmacological interventions are often low cost, relatively easy to use, and have few adverse events. The nonpharmacological interventions most likely to be effective include progressive muscle relaxation, hypnosis for anticipatory chemotherapy-induced N&V (CINV), and managing client expectations. Effectiveness has not been established for several other nonpharmacological interventions, primarily because of study limitations, lack of effect in small studies, and inconsistent results (Oncology Nursing Society, 2019; Patel et al, 2017).*
- Provide oral care after the client vomits. Oral care helps remove the taste and smell of vomitus, reducing the stimulus for further vomiting.

N

Nausea in Pregnancy

- Early recognition and conservative measures are recommended to successfully manage nausea in pregnancy and to prevent progression to hyperemesis gravidarum. Dietary and lifestyle modifications should be implemented before pharmacological interventions. Avoidance of any aversive odors or foods is recommended. Eating multiple small meals per day is also recommended to have some food in the stomach at all times, avoiding hypoglycemia and gastric overdistention. Foods with higher protein (before bedtime) and carbohydrate and lower fat content are helpful (between meals and before getting out of bed early in the morning). Drinking smaller volumes of liquids at multiple times throughout the day is recommended. EB: *These are traditional strategies for alleviating nausea during pregnancy, and there is limited evidence supporting the effectiveness of dietary changes in minimizing N&V with pregnancy symptoms (Campbell et al, 2016; Argenbright, 2017).*
- Recognize that certain maternal characteristics may be at higher risk for nausea and vomiting in pregnancy and hyperemesis gravidarum. EB: *Young mothers, women of black and Asian ethnic origin, those from lower socioeconomic status, and women with multiple pregnancies are more likely to be affected (Fiaschi et al, 2019).*
- ▲ It is well established that *Helicobacter pylori* infection is associated with hyperemesis gravidarum. EB: *It may also be recommended to test for* H. pylori *if there are persistent symptoms of nausea with pregnancy, prolonged symptoms of gastroesophageal reflux disease (GERD), or a previous history of* H. pylori *infection.* H. pylori *is an independent risk factor for vomiting in pregnancy, and in women with daily vomiting there is an association of adverse birth outcomes such as reduced birth weight (Grooten et al, 2017).*
- ▲ Coexisting psychosocial factors may also influence the severity of N&V with pregnancy. Symptoms of anxiety and depression can occur in early pregnancy, especially when N&V is severe and can make the treatment of the N&V more challenging and even ineffective. EB: *Timely diagnosis and treatment is recommended (Argenbright, 2017).*
- ▲ The American College of Obstetricians and Gynecologists (ACOG) currently recommends converting the prenatal vitamin to folic acid only if nausea persists. Pharmacological options include a combination

of oral pyridoxine hydrochloride (vitamin B_6, 10–25 mg) and doxylamine succinate (antihistamine 12.5 mg) to be used three to four times a day as first-line treatment for N&V of pregnancy after failure of pyridoxine alone. This combination agent of pyridoxine and doxylamine (Diclegis) is the only US Food and Drug Administration pregnancy Category A approved therapy for N&V of pregnancy. There are, however, several pharmacological treatments outlined by the ACOG. EB: *A stepwise, cost-effective strategy may be helpful in approaching N&V. Considerable N&V with associated dehydration may require intravenous antiemetics, hydration, and/or parenteral nutrition (Campbell et al, 2016; ACOG, 2018).*

▲ Nonpharmacological interventions that are recommended include P6 acupressure with wrist bands and ginger capsules, 250 mg four times a day. EB: *These interventions have been shown to be safe and beneficial for the treatment of N&V with pregnancy (Campbell et al, 2016; ACOG, 2018). Mindfulness-based cognitive therapy may also be a helpful adjunct to pyridoxine therapy (Campbell et al, 2016).*

Nausea After Surgery

▲ Evaluate for risk factors for postoperative N&V (PONV). EB: *Strong evidence suggests that client-related risk factors such as female gender, age group (<50 years), history of PONV, history of motion sickness, nonsmoking behavior, and environmental risk factors such as postoperative opioid use, emetogenic surgery (type and duration), and volatile anesthetics may increase the risk for PONV. It is important to determine this risk in the preoperative period to better plan strategies to reduce baseline risk (Smith & Ruth-Sahd, 2016). Childhood risk factors include surgery duration of more than 30 minutes, age older than 3 years, strabismus surgery, and a history of postoperative vomiting or a relative with PONV (Simon, 2020). PONV in children is twice as common as it is in adults, with the occurrence of 13% to 42% in all pediatric cases (Matthews, 2017).*

▲ Reduction of risk factors associated with PONV is beneficial for both adults and children. EB: *Avoidance of the use of general anesthesia by the use of regional anesthesia has been associated with a decreased incidence of PONV. The avoidance of both nitrous oxide and volatile anesthetics has also minimized PONV. Decreased and minimal use of intraoperative and postoperative opioids has demonstrated reduction in PONV. Adequate hydration is also an intervention to decrease the risk of PONV (Matthews, 2017; Simon, 2020).*

▲ Medicate the client prophylactically for nausea as ordered, throughout the period of risk. EB: *Antiemetic medications can reduce the incidence of PONV and use of combination treatment such as 5-HT3 antagonist plus dexamethasone is more effective than monotherapy. This recommendation is for clients at moderate or high risk for PONV. Other antiemetics, such as the neurokinin (NK-1) receptor antagonists, may have a role, particularly in preventing vomiting and severity 24 to 48 hours after surgery. Antihistamines may be helpful in those with previous motion sickness or after ear surgery (Matthews, 2017).*

▲ Alleviate postoperative pain using ordered analgesic agents (refer to the care plan for Acute **Pain**). Pain is known to be a factor in the development of PONV (Bruderer et al, 2017).

• Consider the use of nonpharmacological techniques, such as P6 acupoint stimulation, as an adjunct for controlling PONV, which has been shown to be effective in reducing PONV by 30%. Acupoint pressure is noninvasive, is inexpensive, and has no side effects; thus it is part of a combined approach with antiemetic medication. EB: *Acupuncture and acustimulation have been studied with the most consistent results, similarly effective across methods of stimulation (acupuncture or acupressure or wristlike electrical stimulation) (Matthews, 2017). Aromatherapy may be a modality that can be considered as treatment for adult PONV. Additional research should be conducted for support (Asay et al, 2019).*

• Include client education on the management of PONV for all outpatients and discuss key assessment criteria.

Nausea After Chemotherapy

• Perform risk assessment before chemotherapy administration. Risk factors include female gender, younger age, history of low alcohol consumption, history of morning sickness during pregnancy, anxiety, previous history of chemotherapy, client expectancy of nausea, and emetic potential of the regimen. EB: *It is important to recognize the many risk factors individual clients may have and tailor the antiemetic strategy accordingly. N&V continues to be among the most feared side effects of cancer treatment and can significantly affect quality of life and other complications. Poor control of N&V also has an economic impact, with increased costs related to increased emergency department visits, hospitalizations, and outpatient visits (Koth & Kolesar, 2017).*

▲ Initiate antiemetic strategy prophylactically or when N&V occurs in accordance with evidence-based guidelines. EB: *Preventing N&V is important; one failure in antiemetic therapy can result in anticipatory*

N

nausea for the remainder of the client's treatments, and interventions are less likely to be effective (Tageja & Groninger, 2016).

- ▲ Drug classes that are recommended for practice include serotonin receptor antagonists, NK-1 receptor antagonists, and cannabinoids. **EB:** *Triple-drug regimens including serotonin receptor antagonists, NK-1 receptor antagonists, and dexamethasone are recommended for adults receiving highly emetogenic chemotherapy. Recently, olanzapine has been used for highly emetogenic chemotherapy (Razvi et al, 2019).*
- ▲ Consider the use of the following integrative therapies that are likely to be effective in reducing N&V: hypnosis with anticipatory N&V, and progressive muscle relaxation and guided imagery with antiemetics. Ginger may be effective for acute N&V and showed significant efficacy in a recent meta-analysis. **EB:** *There has been benefit associated with these interventions; however, further data are warranted (Chang & Peng, 2019; Oncology Nursing Society, 2019).*
- ● Consider managing client expectations about CINV. **EBN:** *Education and discussion are interventions that may minimize negative expectations. This intervention is based on the idea that if a client expects to experience a problem, he or she is more likely to do so. If a client believes that an intervention will be effective for symptoms, it is more likely to be effective (Oncology Nursing Society, 2019).*

Geriatric

- ● There are no specific guidelines that address the prophylaxis of CINV in older adults. Risk still needs to be assessed, although many older clients are often treated with less emetic chemotherapy. Chemotherapy, however, can cause increased toxicity caused by age-related decreases in organ function, comorbidities, and drug–drug interactions secondary to polypharmacy. Additionally, adherence may be an issue because of cognitive decline, impaired senses, and economic issues. **EB:** *Increased caution is warranted in this population because of increased safety concerns. Some drugs, such as olanzapine, are recommended to be given at lower doses in the elderly due to increased sedation (Clemons, 2018; Razvi et al, 2019).*

Pediatric

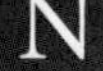

- ● Interventions for CINV should be implemented before and after chemotherapy. **EB:** *Despite the extensive use of antiemetics, it is estimated that nausea occurs in 40% to 70% of children treated for cancer (Hockenberry & Rodgers, 2015).*
- ● Use of a validated nausea tool in pediatrics for estimating incidence and severity of CINV is useful in clinical trials and standard practice. Examples include the PeNAT and pictorial scales (Sherani, Boston, & Mba, 2019).
- ● Relatively few systematic reviews exist examining the antiemetic medications used for CINV in children. It appears that a triple-drug regimen, including 5-HT3 antagonists, combined with dexamethasone and aprepitant, is recommended in children receiving highly emetogenic chemotherapy (Sherani, Boston, & Mba, 2019).
- ● Integrative therapies for control of nausea in children with cancer have not yet been studied as adequately as they have with adults. Some integrative therapies with potential include cognitive distraction, hypnosis, and acupressure (Momani & Berry, 2017).

Home Care

- ● Previously mentioned interventions may be adapted for home care use.
- ▲ In palliative care and hospice care clients, N&V is common and can considerably affect quality of life. Assessment is relevant in the management of N&V and should include history, physical examination, and evaluation of reversible causes. **EB:** *There can be multiple causes of nausea in clients with advanced cancer, and the causes may be treatment related or nontreatment related. The causes may be obstructive; examples include increased intracranial pressure and bowel obstruction. Metabolic causes may be related to hypercalcemia, hyponatremia, or opioids (Walsh et al, 2017).* **EBN:** *Nausea can effectively be controlled if a cause can be identified. An N&V protocol (e.g., Horvitz Center for Palliative Medicine N&V Protocol) can be used to identify and resolve any reversible causes of nausea, such as metabolic abnormalities or medications (Gupta et al, 2013). If none are found and symptoms persist, a flat-plate radiograph of the abdomen is done to evaluate for obstruction or constipation. Appropriate medications can then be used to treat central nervous system causes and obstructive or nonobstructive causes (Moorthy & Letizia, 2018).*

- Assist the client and family with identifying and avoiding irritants in the home that exacerbate nausea (e.g., strong odors from food, plants, perfume, and room deodorizers). All medications except antiemetics should be given after meals to minimize the risk of nausea. EB: *Nausea triggered by odors is related to altered chemoreceptors and pathology (Moorthy & Letizia, 2018).*

Client/Family Teaching and Discharge Planning

- Teach the client techniques to use before and after chemotherapy, including antiemetics/medication management schedules and dietary approaches, such as eating smaller meals, avoiding spicy and fatty foods, and avoiding an empty stomach before chemotherapy (Marx et al, 2016).

REFERENCES

American College of Obstetricians and Gynecologists (ACOG). (2018). ACOG practice Bulletin No. 189 summary: Nausea and vomiting of pregnancy. *ACOG Practice Bulletin*, *131*(1), 190–193.

Argenbright, C. A. (2017). Complementary approaches to pregnancy induced nausea and vomiting. *International Journal of Childbirth Education*, *32*(1), 6–9.

Asay, K., Olson, C., Donnelly, J., & Perlman, E. (2019). The use of aromatherapy in postoperative nausea and vomiting: A systematic review. *Journal of PeriAnesthesia Nursing*, *34*(3), 502–516. https://doi.org/10.1016/j.jopan.2018.08.006.

Bruderer, U., Fisler, A., Steurer, P., Steurer, M., & Dullenkopf, A. (2017). Post-discharge nausea and vomiting after total intravenous anaesthesia and standardized PONV prophylaxis for ambulatory surgery. *Acta Anaesthesiologica Scandinavica*, *61*(7), 758–766.

Campbell, K., Rowe, H., Azzam, H., & Lane, C. A. (2016). The management of nausea and vomiting of pregnancy. *Journal of Obstetrics and Gynaecology Canada*, *38*(12), 1127–1137.

Chang, W. P., & Peng, Y. X. (2019). Does the oral administration of ginger reduce chemotherapy-induced nausea and vomiting? A meta-analysis of 10 randomized controlled trials. *Cancer Nursing*, *42*(6), E14–E23. https://doi.org/10.1097/NCC.0000000000000648.

Clemons, M. (2018). Guidelines versus individualized care for the management of CINV. *Supportive Care in Cancer*, *26*(Suppl. 1), S11–S17. https://doi.org/10.1007/s00520-018-4115-3.

Dranitsaris, G., Molassiotis, A., Clemons, M., et al. (2017). The development of a prediction tool to identify cancer patients at high risk for chemotherapy-induced nausea and vomiting. *Annals of Oncology*, *28*(6), 1260–1267. https://doi.org/10.1093/annonc/mdx100.

Fiaschi, L., Nelson-Piercy, C., Deb, S., King, R., & Tata, L. J. (2019). Clinical management of nausea and vomiting in pregnancy and hyperemesis gravidarum across primary and secondary care: A population-based study. *British Journal of Obstetrics and Gynaecology*, *126*(10), 1201–1211. https://doi.org/10.1111/1471-0528.15662.

Grooten, I. J., Den Hollander, W. J., Roseboom, T. J., et al. (2017). *Helicobacter pylori* infection: A predictor of vomiting severity in pregnancy and adverse birth outcome. *American Journal of Obstetrics and Gynecology*, *216*(5), 512.e1–512.e9.

Gupta, M., Davis, M., LeGrand, S., Walsh, D., & Lagman, R. (2013). Nausea and vomiting in advanced cancer: The Cleveland Clinic protocol. *Journal of Supportive Oncology*, *11*(1), 8–13. https://doi.org/10.1016/j.suponc.2012.10.002.

Hockenberry, M. J., & Rodgers, C. C. (2015). Nausea, vomiting, anorexia, and fatigue. In L. S. Wiener, M. Pao, A. E. Kazak, et al. (Eds.), *Pediatric psycho-oncology: A quick reference on psychosocial dimensions of cancer symptom management* (pp. 79–104). New York: Oxford University Press.

Koth, S. M., & Kolesar, J. (2017). New options and controversies in the management of chemotherapy-induced nausea and vomiting. *American Journal of Health System Pharmacists*, *74*(11), 812–819.

Marx, W., Kiss, N., McCarthy, A. L., McKavanagh, D., & Isenring, L. (2016). Chemotherapy-induced nausea and vomiting: A narrative review to inform dietetics practice. *Journal of the Academy of Nutrition and Dietetics*, *116*(5), 819–827. https://doi.org/10.1016/j.jand.2015.10.020.

Matthews, C. (2017). A review of nausea and vomiting in the anaesthetic and post anaesthetic environment. *Journal of Perioperative Practice*, *27*(10), 224–227.

Momani, T. G., & Berry, D. L. (2017). Integrative therapeutic approaches for the management and control of nausea in children undergoing cancer treatment: A systematic review. *Journal of Pediatric Oncology Nursing*, *34*(3), 173–184.

Moorthy, G. S., & Letizia, M. (2018). The management of nausea at the end of life. *Journal of Hospice and Palliative Nursing*, *20*(5), 442–449. https://doi.org/10.1097/NJH.0000000000000453.

Oncology Nursing Society. (2019). Putting evidence into practice for chemotherapy-induced nausea and vomiting—Adult. Retrieved from https://www.ons.org/pep/chemotherapy-induced-nausea-and-vomiting-adult. [Accessed November 2, 2021].

Patel, P., Robinson, P. D., Thackray, J., et al. (2017). Guideline for the prevention of acute chemotherapy-induced nausea and vomiting in pediatric cancer patients: A focused update. *Pediatric Blood and Cancer*, *64*(10), e26542. https://doi.org/10.1002/pbc.26542.

Razvi, Y., Chan, S., McFarlane, T., et al. (2019). ASCO, NCCN, MASCC/ESMO: A comparison of antiemetic guidelines for the treatment of chemotherapy-induced nausea and vomiting in adult patients. *Supportive Care in Cancer*, *27*(1), 87–95. https://doi.org/10.1007/s00520-018-4464-y.

Sherani, F., Boston, C., & Mba, N. (2019). Latest update on prevention of acute chemotherapy-induced nausea and vomiting in pediatric cancer patients. *Current Oncology Reports*, *21*(10), 88–89. https://doi.org/10.1007/s11912-019-0840-0.

Simon, R. W. (2020). Pediatric postoperative nausea and vomiting: Assessing the impact of evidence-based practice change. *AANA Journal*, *88*(4), 264–271.

Smith, C. A., & Ruth-Sahd, L. (2016). Reducing the incidence of postoperative nausea and vomiting begins with risk screening: An evaluation of the evidence. *Journal of PeriAnesthesia Nursing*, *31*(2), 158–171.

Tageja, N., & Groninger, H. (2016). Chemotherapy-induced nausea and vomiting: An overview and comparison of three consensus guidelines. *Postgraduate Medicine*, *92*(1083), 34–40.

Tilleman, J. A., Pick, A., DeSimone, E. M., Price, S., & Runia-Bade, L. (2018). Chemotherapy-induced nausea and vomiting. *U.S. Pharmacist*, *43*(2), 2–5.

Walsh, D., Davis, M., Ripamonti, C., Bruera, E., Davies, A., & Molassiotis, A. (2017). 2016 Updated MASCC/ESMO consensus recommendations: Management of nausea and vomiting in advanced cancer. *Supportive Care in Cancer*, *25*(1), 333–340.

N

Neonatal Abstinence Syndrome

Domain 9 Coping/stress tolerance Class 3 Neurobehavioral stress

Patricia Hindin, PhD, CNM and Marina Martinez-Kratz, MS, RN, CNE

NANDA-I

Definition

A constellation of withdrawal symptoms observed in newborns as a result of in-utero exposure to addicting substances, or as a consequence of postnatal pharmacological pain management.

Defining Characteristics

Diarrhea (00013); disorganized infant behavior (00116); disturbed sleep pattern (00198); impaired comfort (00214); ineffective feeding pattern (00107); neurobehavioral stress; risk for aspiration (00039); risk for impaired attachment (00058); risk for impaired skin integrity (00047); risk for ineffective thermoregulation (00274); risk for injury (00035)

Related Factors

To be developed

At-Risk Population

Neonates exposed to maternal substance misuse in utero; neonates iatrogenically exposed to substance for pain control; premature neonates

NOC (Nursing Outcomes Classification)

Suggested NOC Outcomes

Comfort Status: Physical; Breastfeeding Establishment: Infant; Bottle Feeding Establishment: Infant; Parent-Infant Attachment; Stress Level; Sleep; Thermoregulation: Newborn; Tissue Integrity: Skin and Mucous Membranes; Newborn Adaptation; Risk Control; Bowel Elimination; Risk Control: Aspiration

N

Example NOC Outcome with Indicators

Parent-Infant Attachment as evidenced by the following indicators: Holds infant close/Uses eye contact/Infant looks at parent/Consoles infant/Responds to infant cues. (Rate the outcome and indicators of **Parent-Infant Attachment:** 1 = never demonstrated, 2 = rarely demonstrated, 3 = sometimes demonstrated, 4 = often demonstrated, 5 = consistently demonstrated range [see Section I].)

Client Outcomes

Client Will (Specify Time Frame)

- Tolerate small frequent formula feedings or frequent breastfeedings
- Maintain weight and readjust feedings frequency as necessary for appropriate growth
- Provide calorie-dense formula, which is appropriate for weight gain
- Maintain proper hydration with elastic skin turgor and moist mucous membranes
- Maintain adequate nutrition, which will promote adequate growth
- Preserve skin integrity in perianal area

NIC (Nursing Interventions Classification)

Suggested NIC Interventions

Diarrhea Management; Bottle Feeding; Infant Care: Newborn; Developmental Enhancement: Infant; Feeding

Example NIC Activities—Diarrhea Management

Monitor for signs and symptoms of diarrhea; Observe skin turgor regularly; Monitor skin in perianal area for irritation and ulceration; Weigh client regularly

Nursing Interventions and *Rationales*

- Provide supportive nonpharmacological care with formula feeding as prescribed. **EBN:** *A randomized controlled trial (N = 49) assessed the early initiation of feeding infants with a high-calorie formula compared with feeding with standard-calorie formula. The authors concluded that high-calorie feeding might be advantageous for weight gain (Bogen et al, 2018).*
- Encourage breastfeeding for nutrition and nonpharmacological supportive care. **EB:** *A retrospective cohort study of neonatal abstinence syndrome (NAS) neonates (N = 3725) indicated that there is an association between breastfeeding and a 9.4% decrease in length of stay when compared with nonbreastfed neonates (Short, Gannon, & Abatemarco, 2016).*
- Use nursing skills to provide supportive nonpharmacological care. **EBN:** *An ethnographic study described the culture of care provided by 12 full-time registered nurses to infants with NAS in an intensive care unit (ICU). The six themes point to the direction for the culture of care practice: learn the baby, team relationships, role satisfaction, grief, making a difference, and educate and care for the mother (Nelson, 2016).*
- Use vibrotactile stimulation (VS) as a nonpharmacological supportive care option. **EB:** *A prospective study was conducted on 26 opioid-exposed newborns to determine whether exposure to a specially constructed mattress that delivered a dose of stochastic (randomly determined) VS would affect symptoms. The results indicated a 35% reduction in movement with a significant increase in normal breathing and heart rate (Zuzarte et al, 2017).*
- Practice supportive nursing interventions with an understanding of the levels of evidence. **EB:** *Ryan et al (2019) reviewed research papers on NAS from the years 2000 and 2017. The author's goal was to substantiate the efficacy of supportive interventions for the treatment of NAS. The authors determined that level I to III evidence (experimental studies) exists for breastfeeding, swaddling, rooming-in, skin to skin, and environmental control for NAS infants.* **EBN:** *A systematic review performed by MacMullen, Dulski, and Blobaum (2014) evaluated supportive nursing care with NAS infants. The authors found level IV evidence (expert opinion, case reports, and descriptive studies) for interventions such as swaddling, gentle awaking, quiet environment, and nonnutritive sucking.*
- Provide pharmacological treatment as indicated for symptoms. **EB:** *A double-blind, randomized control trial assigned term infants who had been exposed to opioids in utero to either a sublingual buprenorphine treatment group or an oral morphine treatment group. The authors noted that the infants treated with sublingual buprenorphine experienced a shorter duration of treatment (15 days versus 28 days) and a shorter length of hospital stay (21 days versus 33 days) (Kraft et al, 2017).* **EB:** *Streetz, Gildon, and Thompson (2016) engaged in a systematic review of clonidine as treatment for NAS. There is limited evidence that clonidine as a single therapy or in combination with other therapies can be effective with limited adverse reactions and a shorter treatment time.*
- Use of nonpharmacological and complementary therapy to comfort infants and provide relief of symptoms. **EB:** *A prospective, cohort, pilot study was conducted with a sample of infants who were given a one-dose, 30-minute Reiki massage session. The authors found the treatment to be safe for the infants and acceptable to the mothers (Radziewicz et al, 2018).*
- Use of rooming-in and promotion of maternal–infant bonding for mother–infant dyad. **EB:** *A systematic review and meta-analysis were conducted on 549 infants with NAS. MacMillan et al (2018) concluded that rooming-in was associated with a reduction in pharmacological treatment and earlier discharge when compared with infants treated in the ICU.* **EB:** *Howard et al (2017) performed a retrospective, single cohort study with 86 mother–infant dyads. Infants with NAS were treated with pharmacological modalities and the rooming-in model of care. The presence of the parents was associated with decreased NAS scores and reduction in opioid treatment days.* **EB:** *Boucher (2017) reviewed eight studies on the rooming-in model of care and the use of acupuncture for NAS infants. The author established that the rooming-in model might decrease use of opioids and length of stay and that acupuncture is safe for infants.*
- Provide compassionate care, free of judgment, to substance-abusing mothers. **EBN:** *A qualitative study was conducted with 15 mothers with substance abuse disorders. The judgmental attitudes and behaviors of health care professionals served to retraumatize them during their hospitalization. The importance of nursing care with the empathic approach is essential in the care of these women (Cleveland, Bonugli, & McGlothen, 2016).* **EBN:** *The use of a structured communication tool based on the organization of the concepts of knowledge creates circumstances for reflection, teaching, and support (ACTS). The ACTS was an implementation to assist neonatal ICU (NICU) nurses in developing positive strategies to change negative attitudes among their peers toward substance-abusing mothers (Marcellus & Poag, 2016).*

N

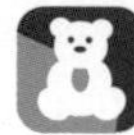

Pediatric

- When available, consider professional, supportive programs for infants with a history of NAS. EB: *Beckwith and Burke (2015) followed the development of 28 infants exposed to prenatal drugs over a 3-year period and determined that the exposed infants have a limitation in language and cognition.*
- Refer children and adolescents with a diagnostic history of NAS to educational supports and resources. EB: *A diagnostic code of NAS is strongly associated with poor school performance. Children and adolescents with a history of NAS must be identified early and provided with support to minimize the consequences of poor educational outcomes (Oei et al, 2017).*

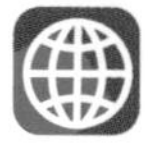

Multicultural

- Identify specific rural areas that are high risk for NAS. EB: *Brown, Goodin, and Talbert (2018) reviewed data in Kentucky and determined that rural Appalachian counties in Kentucky experienced NAS rate per 1000 births that are 2 to 2.5 times greater than urban and non-Appalachian counties in the state.* EB: *The authors evaluated NAS admissions from the Uniform Billing data from the West Virginia Health Care Authority. They found that the NAS rate in rural West Virginia increased from 7.74 to 31.5 per live births per year, indicating an increased need for services for this growing health problem (Stabler et al, 2017).*

Client/Family Teaching and Discharge Planning

- Develop plans of safe care for opioid-exposed mother–infant dyads before discharge. EB: *Safe discharge planning will include home visiting programs, maternal opioid use disorder treatment, parenting education, support for breastfeeding, and postdischarge follow-up with the baby's provider (Whalen, Holmes, & Blythe, 2019).*
- Provide parenting education before discharge that includes infant signs of hunger, infant feeding, ways to calm a fussy baby, the importance of never shaking a baby, safe sleep practices (including safe swaddling), and the importance of not co-sleeping. EB: *Safe discharge planning includes parental education that enhances the safe transition from hospital to the home setting (Whalen, Holmes, & Blythe, 2019).*

Home Care

- Consider alternative models of care for treatment for infants with NAS. EB: *A review article by Whalen, Holmes, and, Blythe concluded that models of care for NAS that are baby-centered and function-based, provide nonpharmacological care, and have the mother as the primary means of treatment may be more effective in reducing length of treatment and length of stay than models focused on specific medications, protocol standardization, or home-based pharmacotherapy (Whalen, Holmes, & Blythe, 2019).* CEB: *Belcher et al (2005) reported on three community programs implemented in Baltimore to provide services to substance-abusing mothers and their infants. The Early Transition Center provided 24-hour on-call services for newly discharged mother and infant dyads. The Home-U-Go-Safely program used community nurses to provide supportive care, health monitoring of the infant, and education to mothers.*

REFERENCES

Beckwith, A. M., & Burke, S. A. (2015). Identification of early developmental deficit in infants with prenatal heroin, methadone, and other opioid exposure. *Clinical Pediatrics, 54*(4), 328–335. https://doi.org/10.1177/0009922814549545.

Belcher, H. E., Butz, A. M., Wallace, P., et al. (2005). Spectrum of early intervention services for children with intrauterine drug exposure. *Infants & Young Children, 18*(1), 2–15.

Bogen, D. L., Hanusa, B. H., Baker, R., Medoff-Cooper, B., & Cohlan, B. (2018). Randomized clinical trial of standard- versus high-calorie formula for methadone-exposed infants: A feasibility study. *Hospital Pediatrics, 8*(1), 7–14. https://doi.org/10.1542/hpeds.2017-0114.

Boucher, A. M. (2017). Nonopioid management of neonatal abstinence syndrome. *Advances in Neonatal Care, 17*(2), 84–90. https://doi.org/10.1097/anc.0000000000000371.

Brown, J. D., Goodin, A. J., & Talbert, J. C. (2018). Rural and Appalachian disparities in neonatal abstinence syndrome incidence and access to opioid abuse treatment. *The Journal of Rural Health, 34*(1), 6–13.

Cleveland, L. M., Bonugli, R. J., & McGlothen, K. S. (2016). The mothering experiences of women with substance use disorders. *Advances in Nursing Science, 39*(2), 119–129. https://doi.org/10.1097/ANS.0000000000000118.

Howard, M. B., Schiff, D. M., Penwill, N., et al. (2017). Impact of parental presence at infants' bedside on neonatal abstinence syndrome. *Hospital Pediatrics, 7*(2), 63–69.

Kraft, W. K., Adeniyi-Jones, S. C., Chervoneva, I., et al. (2017). Buprenorphine for the treatment of the neonatal abstinence syndrome. *New England Journal of Medicine, 376*(24), 2341–2348. https://doi.org/10.1056/NEJMoa1614835.

MacMillan, K. D., Rendon, C. P., Verma, K., Riblet, N., Washer, D. B., & Holmes, A. V. (2018). Association of rooming-in with outcomes for neonatal abstinence syndrome: A systematic review and meta-analysis. *JAMA Pediatrics, 172*(4), 345–351. https://doi.org/10.1001/jamapediatrics.2017.5195.

MacMullen, N. J., Dulski, L. A., & Blobaum, P. (2014). Evidenced-based interventions for neonatal abstinence syndrome. *Pediatric Nursing, 40*(4), 165–172.

Marcellus, L., & Poag, E. (2016). Adding to our practice toolkit: Using the ACTS script to address stigmatizing peer behaviors in the context of maternal substance use. *Neonatal Network*, *35*(5), 327–331. https://doi.org/10.1891/0730-0832.35.5.327.

Nelson, M. M. (2016). NICU culture of care for infants with neonatal abstinence syndrome: A focused ethnography. *Neonatal Network*, *35*(5), 287–296. https://doi.org/10.1891/0730-0832.35.5.287.

Oei, J. L., Melhuish, E., Uebel, H., et al. (2017). Neonatal abstinence syndrome and high school performance. *Pediatrics*, *139*(2), e20162651. https://doi.org/10.1542/peds.2016-2651.

Radziewicz, R. M., Wright-Esber, S., Zupancic, J., Gargiulo, D., & Woodall, P. (2018). Safety of Reiki therapy for newborns at risk for neonatal abstinence syndrome. *Holistic Nursing Practice*, *32*(2), 63–70. https://doi.org/10.1097/HNP.0000000000000251.

Ryan, G., Dooley, J., Finn, G., & Kelly, L. (2019). Nonpharmacological management of neonatal abstinence syndrome: A review of the literature. *Journal of Maternal-Fetal and Neonatal Medicine*, *32*(10), 1735–1740. https://doi.org/10.1080/14767058.2017.1414180.

Short, V. L., Gannon, M., & Abatemarco, D. J. (2016). The association between breastfeeding and length of stay among infants diagnosed with neonatal abstinence syndrome: A population-based study of in-hospital births. *Breastfeeding Medicine*, *11*, 343–349. https://doi.org/10.1089/bfm.2016.0084.

Stabler, M. E., Long, D., Chetok, I. R. A., Giacobbi, P. R., Jr., Pilkerton, C., & Lander, L. R. (2017). Neonatal abstinence syndrome in West Virginia substate regions, 2007–2013. *The Journal of Rural Health*, *33*(1), 92–101.

Streetz, V. N., Gildon, B. L., & Thompson, D. F. (2016). Role of clonidine in neonatal abstinence syndrome: A systematic review. *The Annals of Pharmacotherapy*, *50*(4), 301–310. https://doi.org/10.1177/1060028015626438.

Whalen, B. L., Holmes, A. V., & Blythe, S. (2019). Models of care for neonatal abstinence syndrome: What works? *Seminars in Fetal and Neonatal Medicine*, *24*(2), 121–132. https://doi.org/10.1016/j.siny.2019.01.004.

Zuzarte, I., Indic, P., Barton, B., Paydarfar, D., Bednarek, F., & Bloch-Salisbury, E. (2017). Vibrotactile stimulation: A non-pharmacological intervention for opioid-exposed newborns. *PLoS One*, *12*(4), e0175981. https://doi.org/10.1371/journal.pone.0175981.

Readiness for Enhanced Nutrition

Domain 2 Nutrition Class 1 Ingestion

Marina Martinez-Kratz, MS, RN, CNE

NANDA-I

Definition

A pattern of nutrient intake, which can be strengthened.

Defining Characteristics

Expresses desire to enhance nutrition

NOC (Nursing Outcomes Classification)

Suggested NOC Outcomes

Nutritional Status; Nutritional Status: Food and Fluid Intake; Nutrient Intake; Weight Control

Example NOC Outcome with Indicators

Nutritional Status as evidenced by the following indicators: Food and fluid intake/Hydration/Body mass index/Weight-height ratio/Hematocrit. (Rate the outcome and indicators of **Nutritional Status:** 1 = severe deviation from normal range, 2 = substantial deviation from normal range, 3 = moderate deviation from normal range, 4 = mild deviation from normal range, 5 = no deviation from normal range [see Section I].)

Client Outcomes

Client Will (Specify Time Frame)

- Explain how to eat according to the US Dietary Guidelines
- Design dietary modifications to meet individual long-term goal of health, using principles of variety, balance, and moderation
- Maintain weight within normal range for height and age

NIC (Nursing Interventions Classification)

Suggested NIC Interventions

Nutrition Management; Nutritional Counseling; Weight Reduction Assistance

N

Example NIC Activities—Nutrition Management

Determine the client's motivation for changing eating habits; Develop with the client a method to keep a daily record of intake

Nursing Interventions and *Rationales*

- Assess the meaning and importance of food in the client's life. EB: *Recent research found strong associations between the different domains of food meanings and behavioral outcomes (Arbit et al, 2017).*
- Assess client readiness to determine whether he or she is ready to discuss enhanced nutrition and/or would like nutrition information. EB: *Client motivation is a key component of success in a weight loss program and a prerequisite for weight loss therapy* (Raynor & Champagne, 2016).
- Use a motivational interviewing technique when working with clients to promote healthy eating and improved nutrition. EB: *Research shows significant weight loss for clients when motivational interviewing techniques were used (Barnes et al, 2018).*
- Counsel the client to measure regularly consumed foods periodically. Help the client learn usual portion sizes. Measuring food alerts the client to normal portion sizes. Estimating amounts can be extremely inaccurate. EB: *A randomized controlled trial of 278 overweight and obese participants was conducted to increase portion size awareness with results that demonstrated that the intervention improved portion control behavior and in turn influenced body mass index (BMI) (Poelman et al, 2015).*
- Assist the client to develop a system of self-management, which may include self-monitoring of weight and BMI; realistic goal setting, planning, and action planning for improved dietary intake and physical activity; problem-solving; and tracking dietary intake and exercise. EB: *A key component of successful weight loss and maintenance is regular self-monitoring (Thomason et al, 2016).*
- Document the client's height and weight and teach the significance of his or her BMI in relation to current nutritional health. Use a chart or a website such as http://www.cdc.gov/healthyweight/assessing/bmi/index.html (Centers for Disease Control and Prevention [CDC], 2020a). EB: *Successful enhancement of nutrition in adults requires adoption and maintenance of effective self-monitoring (Raynor & Champagne, 2016).*
- Recommend that the client avoid eating in fast-food restaurants. EB: *A study found that fast-food consumption was the most frequent risk factor for adiposity found in 61.67% of study participants (Popa et al, 2020).*
- Assist the client to reframe slips in nutrition or physical activity behavior as lapses that are a single event and not a full return to previous unhealthy behaviors. Relapse prevention strategies include managing lapses in healthy behavior, identifying high-risk situations for relapses, self-monitoring, providing social support, enhancing skills for coping, and increasing self-efficacy for avoiding relapse. EB: *A study of a weight maintenance intervention, delivered primarily by telephone, modestly slowed the rate of weight regain (Voils et al, 2017).*
- Assist clients to engage their social support systems either digitally or face to face in ways that facilitate healthy eating and physical activity behavior change. EB: *Significant others, family, friends, and coworkers can facilitate or hinder weight loss success (Romo, 2018).*
- Assist the client to implement informal and formal mindfulness-based interventions (MBIs). Informal MBIs include mindful eating, increasing awareness of hunger and satiety cues, taste satisfaction, and decreasing impulsive tendencies to overeat when experiencing negative emotions. Meditation practice is a formal MBI. EB: *Results of a research review suggest that a combination of formal and informal MBIs are effective in reducing weight and improving obesity-related eating behaviors among individuals with overweight and obesity (Carrière et al, 2018).*
- Assist the client to develop stimulus control techniques designed to reduce environmental cues associated with eating behaviors. Specifically, clients should be taught to limit the presence of high-calorie/high-fat foods in the home; to reduce the visibility of unhealthy food choices in the home; to limit where and when they eat; to avoid distractions like reading, using the computer, or watching television when eating; and to eat more slowly. EB: *Stimulus control strategies are the keys to healthy eating (Butryn et al, 2017).*
- Encourage 7.5 to 8.5 hours of sleep nightly. EB: *Evidence suggests that weight management is hindered when attempted in the context of sleep restriction because there is an upregulation of reward, pleasure, and salience networks in response to food stimuli (St-Onge, 2017).*

- Recommend the CDC behavior modification approach "reflect, replace, and reinforce" to improve eating habits. EB: *Reflect, replace, and reinforce consists of the following: (1) Reflect about intake through food journals, listing food habits, and identification of eating cues. (2) Replace habits identified during reflection with new and healthier behaviors, such as eating more slowly or planning meals ahead of time. (3) Reinforce changes made and having patience with the process (CDC, 2020b).*

Pediatric

- Offer obese or overweight adolescents healthy methods for weight loss. EB: *A study showed statistically significant health behavior improvements after implementing a developmentally informed intervention to increase positive health diet and exercise behaviors (Issner et al, 2017).*
- Offer families of obese or overweight children prejudice-free, individually accepting, and supportive interventions to address weight loss. EB: *A review summarized recent evidence on weight stigma and found that it is highly prevalent among youth with high body weight, who are targets of weight-based victimization from peers, parents, and teachers (Puhl & Lessard, 2020).*
- Recommend that families eat together for at least one meal per day. EB: *A large Korean study found that the frequency of family meals was strongly an inverse association with childhood overweight or obesity (Lee, Lee, & Park, 2016).*
- Recommend involving the family in planning meals and food preparation. Children can learn about nutrition as they help plan and make meals. EB: *The Healthy Home Offerings via the Mealtime Environment Plus program showed increased cooking skills among the children participating (Fulkerson et al, 2018).*
- Assist parents at being good role models of healthy eating. EB: *The Healthy Home Offerings via the Mealtime Environment Plus program showed significantly improved parental self-efficacy for identifying appropriate portion sizes (Fulkerson et al, 2018).*
- Recommend that the family try new foods, either a new food or recipe every week. EB: *The Healthy Home Offerings via the Mealtime Environment Plus program showed decreasing child neophobia scores over time that were developmentally appropriate (Fulkerson et al, 2018).*

Geriatric

- Observe for social, psychological, and economic factors that influence diet quality. EB: *An exploratory study of diet quality influences in community-dwelling older individuals revealed the following influences: food experiences, retirement, bereavement, medical conditions, food environment, food-related habits, social engagement, personal/psychological factors, and transportation (Bloom et al, 2017).*

N

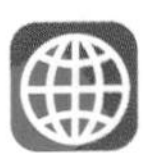

Multicultural

- Tailor nutritional interventions to be consistent with cultural beliefs, norms, and values. EB: *A systemic review of culturally tailored interventions for Hispanic women included literacy modification, Hispanic foods/recipes, cultural diabetes beliefs, family/friend participation, structured community input, and innovative experiential learning (McCurley et al, 2016).*
- Offer tailored lifestyle counseling via the telephone. EBN: *Investigators have included biweekly and/or monthly health coach calls for African American participants with significant weight gain prevention (Goode et al, 2017).*
- Integrate weight loss and weight maintenance interventions with church faith-based supports for cultural congruence with African American clients. EB: *Recent research found that a church-based weight loss intervention using automated text messages was well-received by African American participants and resulted in significant weight loss (Newton et al, 2018).*

Client/Family Teaching and Discharge Planning

- The majority of the preceding interventions involve teaching.
- Work with the family members regarding information on how to support and promote enhanced nutritional choices and healthy intakes.

REFERENCES

Arbit, N., Ruby, M., & Rozin, P. (2017). Development and validation of the meaning of food in life questionnaire (MFLQ): Evidence for a new construct to explain eating behavior. *Food Quality and Preference, 59*, 35–45. https://doi.org/10.1016/j.foodqual.2017.02.002.

Barnes, R. D., Ivezaj, V., Martino, S., Pittman, B. P., Paris, M., & Grilo, C. M. (2018). Examining motivational interviewing plus nutrition psychoeducation for weight loss in primary care. *Journal of*

Psychosomatic Research, *104*, 101–107. https://doi.org/10.1016/j.jpsychores.2017.11.013.

Bloom, I., Lawrence, W., Barker, M., et al. (2017). What influences diet quality in older people? A qualitative study among community-dwelling older adults from the Hertfordshire Cohort Study, UK. *Public Health Nutrition*, *20*(15), 2685–2693. https://doi.org/10.1017/S1368980017001203.

Butryn, M. L., Forman, E. M., Lowe, M. R., Gorin, A. A., Zhang, F., & Schaumberg, K. (2017). Efficacy of environmental and acceptance-based enhancements to behavioral weight loss treatment: The ENACT trial. *Obesity*, *25*(5), 866–872. https://doi.org/10.1002/oby.21813.

Carrière, K., Khoury, B., Günak, M. M., & Knäuper, B. (2018). Mindfulness-based interventions for weight loss: A systematic review and meta-analysis. *Obesity Reviews*, *19*(2), 164–177. https://doi.org/10.1111/obr.12623.

Centers for Disease Control and Prevention (CDC). (2020a). *Body mass index (BMI)*. Retrieved from https://www.cdc.gov/healthyweight/assessing/bmi/index.html. Accessed 19 July 2021.

Centers for Disease Control and Prevention (CDC). (2020b). *Improving your eating habits*. Division of Nutrition, Physical Activity, and Obesity, National Center for Chronic Disease Prevention and Health Promotion. Retrieved from https://www.cdc.gov/healthyweight/losing_weight/eating_habits.html. Accessed 19 July 2021.

Fulkerson, J. A., Friend, S., Horning, M., et al. (2018). Family home food environment and nutrition-related parent and child personal and behavioral outcomes of the Healthy Home Offerings via the Mealtime Environment (HOME) Plus program: A randomized controlled trial. *Journal of the Academy of Nutrition and Dietetics*, *118*(2), 240–251. https://doi.org/10.1016/j.jand.2017.04.006.

Goode, R. W., Styn, M. A., Mendez, D. D., & Gary-Webb, T. L. (2017). African Americans in standard behavioral treatment for obesity, 2001–2015: What have we learned? *Western Journal of Nursing Research*, *39*(8), 1045–1069. https://doi.org/10.1177/0193945917692115.

Issner, J. H., Mucka, L. E., & Barnett, D. (2017). Increasing positive health behaviors in adolescents with nutritional goals and exercise. *Journal of Child and Family Studies*, *26*(2), 548–558. https://doi.org/10.1007/s10826-016-0585-4.

Lee, H. J., Lee, S. Y., & Park, E. C. (2016). Do family meals affect childhood overweight or obesity? Nationwide survey 2008–2012. *Pediatric Obesity*, *11*(3), 161–165. https://doi.org/10.1111/ijpo.12035.

McCurley, J. L., Gutierrez, A. P., & Gallo, L. C. (2016). Diabetes prevention in U.S. Hispanic adults: A systematic review of culturally tailored interventions. *American Journal of Preventive Medicine*, *52*(4), 519–529. https://doi.org/10.1016/j.amepre.2016.10.028.

Newton, R. L., Jr., Carter, L. A., Johnson, W., et al. (2018). A church-based weight loss intervention in African American adults using text messages (LEAN Study): Cluster randomized controlled trial. *Journal of Medical Internet Research*, *20*(8), e256. https://doi.org/10.2196/jmir.9816.

Poelman, M. P., de Vet, E., Velema, E., de Boer, M. R., Seidell, J. C., & Steenhuis, I. H. M. (2015). PortionControl@HOME: Results of a randomized controlled trial evaluating the effect of a multi-component portion size intervention on portion control behavior and body mass index. *Annals of Behavioral Medicine*, *49*(1), 18–28. https://doi.org/10.1007/s12160-014-9637-4.

Popa, A. R., Fratila, O., Rus, M., et al. (2020). Risk factors for adiposity in the urban population and influence on the prevalence of overweight and obesity. *Experimental and Therapeutic Medicine*, *20*(1), 129–133. https://doi.org/10.3892/etm.2020.8662.

Puhl, R. M., & Lessard, L. M. (2020). Weight stigma in youth: prevalence, consequences, and considerations for clinical practice. *Current Obesity Reports*, *9*(4), 402–411. https://doi.org/10.1007/s13679-020-00408-8.

Raynor, H. A., & Champagne, C. M. (2016). Position of the Academy of Nutrition and Dietetics: Interventions for the treatment of overweight and obesity in adults. *Journal of the Academy of Nutrition and Dietetics*, *116*(1), 129–147. https://doi.org/10.1016/j.jand.2015.10.031.

Romo, L. K. (2018). An examination of how people who have lost weight communicatively negotiate interpersonal challenges to weight management, health communication. *Health Communication*, *33*(4), 469–477. https://doi.org/10.1080/10410236.2016.1278497.

St-Onge, M. P. (2017). Sleep-obesity relation: Underlying mechanisms and consequences for treatment. *Obesity Reviews*, *18*(Suppl. 1), 34–39. https://doi.org/10.1111/obr.12499.

Thomason, D. L., Lukkahatai, N., Kawi, J., Connelly, K., & Inouye, J. (2016). A systematic review of adolescent self-management and weight loss. *Journal of Pediatric Health Care*, *30*(6), 569–582. https://doi.org/10.1016/j.pedhc.2015.11.016.

Voils, C. I., Olsen, M. K., Gierisch, J. M., et al. (2017). Maintenance of weight loss after initiation of nutrition training: A randomized trial. *Annals of Internal Medicine*, *166*(7), 463–471. https://doi.org/10.7326/M16-2160.

Imbalanced Nutrition: Less Than Body Requirements

Domain 2 Nutrition Class 1 Ingestion

Jody L. Vogelzang, PhD, RDN, CHES, FAND

NANDA-I

Definition

Intake of nutrients insufficient to meet metabolic needs.

Defining Characteristics

Abdominal cramping, abdominal pain; body weight below ideal weight range for age and gender; capillary fragility; constipation; delayed wound healing; diarrhea; excessive hair loss; food intake less than recommended daily allowance (RDA); hyperactive bowel sounds; hypoglycemia; inadequate head circumference growth for age and gender; inadequate height increase for age and gender; lethargy; muscle hypotonia; neonatal weight gain < 30 g per day; pale mucous membranes; weight loss with adequate food intake

Related Factors

Altered taste perception; depressive symptoms; difficulty swallowing; food aversion; inaccurate information; inadequate food supply; inadequate interest in food; inadequate knowledge of nutrient requirements; injured buccal cavity; insufficient breast milk production; interrupted breastfeeding; misperception about ability to ingest food; satiety immediately upon ingesting food; sore buccal cavity; weakened muscles required for swallowing; weakened of muscles required for mastication

At-Risk Population

Competitive athletes; displaced individuals; economically disadvantaged individuals; individuals with low educational level; premature infants

Associated Conditions

Body dysmorphic disorders; digestive system diseases; immunosuppression; kwashiorkor; malabsorption syndromes; mental disorders; neoplasms; neurocognitive disorders; parasitic disorders

NOC (Nursing Outcomes Classification)

Suggested NOC Outcomes

Nutritional Status; Food and Fluid Intake; Nutrient Intake; Weight Control

Example NOC Outcome with Indicators

Nutritional Status as evidenced by the following indicators: Food and fluid intake/Body mass index/ Weight-height ratio/Hematocrit. (Rate the outcome and indicators of **Nutritional Status:** 1 = severe deviation from normal range, 2 = substantial deviation from normal range, 3 = moderate deviation from normal range, 4 = mild deviation from normal range, 5 = no deviation from normal range [see Section I].)

Client Outcomes

Client Will (Specify Time Frame)

- Promote weight gain of 5% to 10% of body weight
- Receive feeding assistance and texture modification as needed
- Identify factors contributing to being underweight
- Identify nutritional requirements based on specific client needs
- Increase overall intake
- Minimize further decline of weight status
- Be free of signs and symptoms of malnutrition

NIC (Nursing Interventions Classification)

Suggested NIC Interventions

Feeding; Nutrition Management; Nutrition Therapy; Weight Gain Assistance

Example NIC Activities—Nutrition Management

Ascertain the client's food preferences; Provide the client with high-protein, high-calorie, nutritious finger foods and drinks that can be readily consumed, as appropriate

Nursing Interventions and *Rationales*

- Conduct a nutrition screen on all clients within 24 hours of admission and refer to a dietitian as deemed necessary. EB: *Clients who received malnutrition screening and subsequent nutritional therapy is a prerequisite to beginning an evidence-based nutritional therapy (Eglseer et al, 2017). A study showed that malnutrition at admission and poor food intake early during hospitalization were associated with prolonged length of stay, suggesting that prompt nutrition intervention and monitoring should be performed when clients are admitted to the hospital (Allard et al, 2016).*

N

- The screening tool should be based on the unique characteristics of the client population and the validity and reliability of the screening tool. EB: *Screening is the starting point of high-quality nutritional care, which needs to be completed using a valid screening tool that fits the population (Eglseer et al, 2017).*
- Recognize the importance of rescreening and monitoring oral intake in hospitalized individuals to help facilitate the early identification and prevention of nutritional decline. EB: *Poor food intake during hospitalization is common and can lead to or perpetuate malnutrition; insufficient (i.e., ≤50%) food intake, regardless of nutritional state, is an independent predictor of length of stay (McCullough et al, 2017).*
- Recognize the characteristics that classify individuals as malnourished and refer to a dietitian for a complex nutritional assessment and intervention. CEB: *According to the Academy of Nutrition and Dietetics and the American Society of Parenteral and Enteral Nutrition, two or more of the following characteristics are recommended to support the diagnosis of malnutrition: insufficient energy intake, weight loss, loss of muscle mass, loss of subcutaneous fat, localized or generalized fluid accumulation, and/or decreased functional status (White, Guenter, & Jensen, 2012).* EB: *Dietetic consultations for adults in primary care settings appear to be effective for improvement in diet quality, diabetes outcomes (including blood glucose and glycated hemoglobin values), and weight loss outcomes (e.g., changes in weight and waist circumference) and to limit gestational weight gain (Mitchell et al, 2017).*
- Recognize clients who are likely to experience malnutrition in the context of social or environmental circumstances, characterized by cachexia without the presence of an inflammatory process (chronic disease-related malnutrition: those with organ failure, pancreatic cancer, rheumatoid arthritis, sarcopenic obesity, acute disease, or injury-related malnutrition; those with major infection, burns, trauma, or closed-head injuries accompanied by a marked inflammatory response). EB: *Mortality during admission was increased 10-fold in malnourished complex clients with chronic needs, and a clear influence of malnutrition on mortality at 5 months was observed (Burgos et al, 2020).* EB: *Clients who were identified with preexisting malnutrition had more days of ventilator support and a longer hospital stay than those who were not preburn malnutrition (Rosenfeld et al, 2019).*

▲ Note laboratory values cautiously; decrease in albumin and prealbumin may be indicators of the inflammatory response that often accompanies acute malnutrition, but it should not be used to diagnose malnutrition. Other potential indicators of inflammatory response include C-reactive protein, white blood cell count, and blood glucose values.

N

- Weigh the client daily in acute care and weekly to monthly in extended care at the same time (usually before breakfast) with same amount of clothing.
- Observe for potential barriers to eating such as willingness, ability, and appetite. EB: *Research findings provide evidence to support the positive impact of using visual assistance and full physical assistance to improve residents' pace of food intake and thus potentially improve the amount of food and fluid consumption (Liu et al, 2019).*
- If the client is unable to feed self, refer to Feeding **Self-Care** Deficit. If the client has difficulty swallowing, refer to Nursing Interventions for Impaired **Swallowing.** If the client is receiving tube feedings, refer to the Nursing Interventions for Risk for **Aspiration.**
- Advocate for the implementation of a feeding protocol, if not already in place, to avoid unnecessary and/or prolonged nothing by mouth/clear liquid diet (NPO/CLD) status in hospitalized clients. EB: *A study found that, on average, clients with unjustified NPO or CLD orders spent 3 days on an NPO or CLD diet, which corresponded to a mean of 10 missed meals (Gallinger et al, 2017).*
- For the client with anorexia nervosa, consider offering high-calorie foods and snacks often. EB: *Evidence supports a switch in current care practices for refeeding from a conservative approach to higher calorie refeeding, although this should only occur in a hospital setting (Bargiacchi et al, 2019).*
- For the client who is able to eat but has a decreased appetite, try the following activities:
  - Offer oral nutritional supplements (ONSs) based on client preference and indication of need. EB: *The use of high-protein ONSs (>20% energy from protein) reduces complications and readmissions with no impact on normal food intake (Loman et al, 2019).*
  - Avoid interruptions during mealtimes and offer companionship; meals should be eaten in a calm and peaceful environment. EB: *The average number and length of interruptions decreased and the average length of mealtime assistance provided to clients increased when the protected mealtime policy was implemented, resulting in a slight increase in energy and protein consumption (Goarley et al, 2020).*
  - Allow for access to meals or snacks during "off times" if the client is not available at time of meal delivery, monitor food and ONS intake, and communicate with dietitian/health provider. EB: *According to*

a study conducted in an adult setting, interruption of mealtimes and not receiving food when a meal was missed were obstacles to poor food intake in clients (Keller et al, 2015).

- ❍ If the client lacks endurance, schedule rest periods before meals, and open packages and cut up food for the client. EB: *Residents who receive physical help more often during mealtimes have more calories and protein intake, whereas those who receive physical help intermittently have less intake (Keller et al, 2017).*

- ● For the client who has had a stroke, repeat nutritional screenings weekly and provide timely interventions for those at risk or who may already be malnourished. EB: *A systematic review revealed that malnutrition was present in up to 49% of clients after stroke and the incidence increased during rehabilitation (Sakai et al, 2019).*
- ● Monitor state of oral cavity (gums, tongue, mucosa, and teeth). Provide good oral hygiene before each meal. EB: *Xerostomia showed an association with incident malnutrition in edentulous people; hyposalivation can reduce the retention of the dentures as well as the comfort of wearing dentures, which may explain the interaction between xerostomia and dental status with regard to malnutrition (Kiesswetter et al, 2019).*
- ▲ Administer antiemetics and pain medications as ordered and needed before meals. *The presence of nausea or pain decreases the appetite.*
- ● If client is nauseated, remove cover of food tray before bringing it into the client's room. *The sudden, concentrated food odors that come when the cover is removed in front of the client can trigger nausea.*
- ● Work with the client to develop a plan for increased activity. *Immobility leads to negative nitrogen balance, which fosters anorexia.*

Critical Care

- ● Recognize the need to begin enteral feeding within 24 to 48 hours of admission to the critical care environment, once the client is free of hemodynamic compromise, if the client is unable to eat. EB: *Provision of early enteral nutrition was associated with a significant reduction in mortality and infectious morbidity, compared with withholding early enteral nutrition (delayed enteral nutrition or standard therapy) (McClave et al, 2016).*
- ● Recognize that it is important to administer feedings to the client and that frequently checking for gastric residual and fasting clients for procedures can be a limiting factor to adequate nutrition in the tube-fed client. EB: *Several studies have challenged the usefulness of residual gastric volume monitoring by gastric suction, showing that it led to reduced caloric intake without any benefits in terms of reducing the occurrence of vomiting or incidence of ventilator-associated pneumonia (Bouvet et al, 2020).*
- ● Refer to care plan for Risk for **Aspiration.**

Pediatric

- ▲ Use a nutritional screening tool designed for nurses such as the Subjective Global Nutrition Assessment (SGNA), and if the child's malnutrition is identified as moderate or severe, refer to a dietitian.
- ● Watch for symptoms of malnutrition in the child, including short stature; thin arms and legs; poor condition of skin and hair; visible vertebrae and rib cage; wasted buttocks; wasted facial appearance; lethargy; and, in extreme cases, edema.
- ● Weigh and measure the length (height) of the child and use a growth chart to help determine growth pattern, which reflects nutrition. Age-related growth charts are available from https://www.cdc.gov/growthcharts/.
- ▲ Refer to a health provider and a dietitian a child who is underweight for any reason. EB: *Good nutrition is extremely important for children to ensure sufficient growth and development of all body system (Pearson et al, 2018).*
- ● Work with the child and parent to develop an appropriate weight gain plan. *The goal for a child is sometimes to maintain existing weight as the body grows taller.*
- ● Recognize that a large percentage of girls and teenagers are dieting, which can result in nutritional problems.

Geriatric

- ● Screen for malnutrition in older clients. EB: *To find out which clients need a dietitian and further nutritional interventions, the nutritional status of each client must be routinely screened when they are admitted to the hospital and each week if they stay in hospital for a longer time period (Eglseer, 2017).*
- ● Screen for dysphagia in all older clients. EB: *Clients with impaired nutritional status (risk of malnutrition, malnutrition, and sarcopenia) is very high among clients with oropharyngeal dysphagia associated with*

either chronic diseases or aging and those with community-acquired pneumonia (Carrión et al, 2017). See the care plan for Impaired **Swallowing.**

- ● Recognize that geriatric clients with moderate or severe cognition impairment have a significant risk for developing malnutrition. EBN: *Dementia is one of the factors most consistently associated with poor nutrition (Liu et al, 2019).*
- ▲ Interpret laboratory findings cautiously. Watch the color of urine for an indication of fluid balance; darker urine demonstrates dehydration. Low axillary moisture could indicate mild to moderate dehydration. EB: *Because urine color is correlated with urine specific gravity and urine osmolality, observing urine color is a low-cost method of monitoring dehydration (Kostelnik et al, 2021).*
- ● Consider using dining assistants and trained nonnursing staff, to provide feeding assistance care in extended care facilities to ensure adequate time for feeding clients as needed. EB: *A study found that when trained volunteers were able to deliver mealtime assistance on a large scale, nursing staff could complete clinical tasks (Roberts et al, 2017).*
- ● Encourage high-protein foods for the older client unless medically contraindicated by organ failure. EB: *Higher dietary protein intake was associated with a lower risk of becoming dependent in functional tasks requiring strength and endurance (Mustafa et al, 2018).*
- ● Recognize the implications of malnutrition on client strength and mobility. EB: *Dietary protein and/or amino acid intake combined with resistance exercise can stimulate muscle protein synthesis and slow breakdown (resulting in positive net protein balance) despite advancing age (Mustafa et al, 2018).*
- ● Monitor for onset of depression. EB: *Depression and eating styles contributed independently to poorer diet quality and higher intake of sweets and snacks/fast foods (Paans et al, 2019).*
- ● If the client is unable to feed self, refer to Nursing Interventions and *Rationales* for Feeding **Self-Care** Deficit. If client has impaired physical function, malnutrition, depression, or cognitive impairment, refer to care plan for **Frail Elderly** Syndrome.
- ● Emphasize the importance of good oral care in the older client.
- ● Initiate multiprofessional approach if the client is at high risk for pressure ulcers or has a pressure ulcer. EB: *This study suggests that it might be cost effective to provide basic preventive pressure injury care to all hospitalized clients; however, hospitals still need to invest in treatment technologies and skilled practitioners that enhance these preventive efforts (Padula et al, 2019).*

Home Care

- ● The preceding interventions may be adapted for home care use.
- ● Monitor food intake. Instruct the client in the intake of small frequent meals of foods with increased calories and protein.
- ● Assess the client's willingness and ability to eat. EB: *Poor intake among older adults has been found to be associated with lack of self-feeding ability, poor dining environment, inadequate time to eat, poor sensory properties of the food, and lack of choice and variety of the food (Keller et al, 2015).*
- ● Consider social factors that may interfere with nutrition (e.g., lack of transportation, inadequate income, lack of social support).
- ● Continue to encourage intake of oral nutritional support to help optimize oral intake. EB: *Consumption of oral nutrition supplements in hospitalized older adults in postdischarge settings improves overall nutrient intake (Loman et al, 2019).*
- ▲ Recognize that the client on home parenteral nutrition requires regularly scheduled laboratory work for electrolyte monitoring, increased risk of catheter-related complication, parenteral nutrition–associated liver disease (PNALD), and metabolic bone disease.

Client Family Teaching and Discharge Planning

- ● Develop a client-centered nutrition plan with measurable goals.
- ● Amplify the identified strengths in the client/family's food habits. Select appropriate teaching aids for the client/family's background and educational level.
- ● Review food safety guidelines and hand hygiene when working with food.
- ● Implement instructional follow-up to answer the client/family's questions.
- ● Recommend that clients discuss with their primary health provider before taking any supplements such as vitamins, minerals, and botanicals.
- ● Suggest community resources for home-delivered or congregate meals.

- Encourage socialization at meal time.
- Teach the client and family how to manage tube feedings or parenteral therapy at home as needed.

REFERENCES

Allard, J. P., Keller, H., Jeejeebhoy, K. N., et al. (2016). Malnutrition at hospital admission—contributors and effect on length of stay: A prospective cohort study from the Canadian malnutrition task force. *Journal of Parenteral and Enteral Nutrition*, *40*(4), 487–497. https://doi.org/10.1177/0148607114567902.

Bargiacchi, A., Clarke, J., Paulsen, A., & Leger, J. (2019). Refeeding in anorexia nervosa. *European Journal of Pediatrics*, *178*(3), 413–422. https://doi.org/10.1007/s00431-018-3295-7.

Bouvet, L., Zieleskiewicz, L., Loubradou, E., et al. (2020). Reliability of gastric suctioning compared with ultrasound assessment of residual gastric volume: A prospective multicentre cohort study. *Anaesthesia*, *75*(3), 323–330. https://doi.org/10.1111/anae.14915.

Burgos, R., Joaquín, C., Blay, C., & Vaqué, C. (2020). Disease-related malnutrition in hospitalized chronic patients with complex needs. *Clinical Nutrition*, *39*(5), 1447–1453. https://doi.org/10.1016/j.clnu.2019.06.006.

Carrión, S., Roca, M., Costa, A., et al. (2017). Nutritional status of older patients with oropharyngeal dysphagia in a chronic versus an acute clinical situation. *Clinical Nutrition*, *36*(4), 1110–1116. https://doi.org/10.1016/j.clnu.2016.07.009.

Eglseer, D., Halfens, R. J. G., & Lohrmann, C. (2017). Is the presence of a validated malnutrition screening tool associated with better nutritional care in hospitalized patients? *Nutrition*, *37*, 104–111. https://doi.org/10.1016/j.nut.2016.12.016.

Gallinger, Z. R., Rumman, A., Pivovarov, K., Fortinsky, K. J., Steinhart, A. H., & Weizman, A. V. (2017). Frequency and variables associated with fasting orders in inpatients with ulcerative colitis: The Audit of Diet Orders—Ulcerative Colitis (ADORE-UC) study. *Inflammatory Bowel Disease*, *23*(10), 1790–1795. https://doi.org/10.1097/MIB.0000000000001244.

Goarley, A., El Hassan, D. A., & Ahmadi, L. (2020). Effect of a protected mealtime pilot on energy and protein intake in a Canadian hospital. *Canadian Journal of Dietetic Practice and Research*, *81*(2), 94–96. https://doi.org/10.3148/cjdpr-2019.

Keller, H., Allard, J., Vesnaver, E., et al. (2015). Barriers to food intake in acute care hospitals: A report of the Canadian malnutrition task force. *Journal of Human Nutrition and Dietetics*, *28*(6), 546–557. https://doi.org/10.1111/jhn.12314.

Keller, H. H., Carrier, N., Slaughter, S. E., et al. (2017). Prevalence and determinants of poor food intake of residents living in long-term care. *Journal of the American Medical Directors Association*, *18*(11), 941–947. https://doi.org/10.1016/j.jamda.2017.05.003.

Kiesswetter, E., Hengeveld, L. M., Keijser, B. J., Volkert, D., & Visser, M. (2019). Oral health determinants of incident malnutrition in community-dwelling older adults. *Journal of Dentistry*, *85*, 73–80. https://doi.org/10.1016/j.jdent.2019.05.017.

Kostelnik, S. B., Davy, K. P., Hedrick, V. E., Thomas, D. T., & Davy, B. M. (2021). The validity of urine color as a hydration biomarker within the general adult population and athletes: A systematic review. *Journal of the American College of Nutrition*, *40*(2), 172–179. https://doi.org/10.1080/07315724.2020.1750073.

Liu, W., Jao, Y. L., & Williams, K. (2019). Factors influencing the pace of food intake for nursing home residents with dementia: Resident characteristics, staff mealtime assistance. *Nursing Open*, *6*(3), 772–782. https://doi.org/10.1002/nop2.250.

Loman, B. R., Luo, M., Baggs, G. E., et al. (2019). Specialized high–protein oral nutrition supplement improves home nutrient intake of malnourished older adults without decreasing usual food intake. *Journal of Parenteral and Enteral Nutrition*, *43*(6), 794–802. https://doi.org/10.1002/jpen.1467.

McClave, S. A., Taylor, B. E., Martindale, R. G., et al. (2016). Guidelines for the provision and assessment of nutrition support therapy in the adult critically ill patient: Society of Critical Care Medicine (SCCM) and American Society for Parenteral and Enteral Nutrition (A.S.P.E.N). *Journal of Parenteral and Enteral Nutrition*, *40*(2), 159–211. https://doi.org/10.1177/0148607115621863.

McCullough, J., Marcus, H., & Keller, H. (2017). The Mealtime Audit Tool (MAT)—Inter-rater reliability testing of a novel tool for the monitoring and assessment of food intake barriers in acute care hospital patients. *The Journal of Nutrition, Health & Aging*, *21*(9), 962–970. https://doi.org/10.1007/s12603-017-0890-7.

Mitchell, L. J., Ball, L. E., Ross, L. J., Barnes, K. A., & Williams, L. T. (2017). Effectiveness of dietetic consultations in primary health care: A systematic review of randomized controlled trials. *Journal of the Academy of Nutrition and Dietetics*, *117*(12), 1941–1962. https://doi.org/10.1016/j.jand.2017.06.364.

Mustafa, J., Ellison, C. R., Singer, M. R., et al. (2018). Dietary protein and preservation of physical functioning among middle-aged and older adults in the Framingham offspring study. *American Journal of Epidemiology*, *187*(7), 1411–1419. https://doi.org/10.1093/aje/kwy014.

Paans, N. P. G., Gibson-Smith, D., Bot, M., et al. (2019). Depression and eating styles are independently associated with dietary intake. *Appetite*, *134*, 103–110. https://doi.org/10.1016/j.appet.2018.12.030.

Padula, W. V., Pronovost, P. J., Makic, M. B. F., et al. (2019). Value of hospital resources for effective pressure injury prevention: A cost-effectiveness analysis. *BMJ Quality and Safety*, *28*(2), 132–141. https://doi.org/10.1136/bmjqs-2017-007505.

Pearson, R., Killedar, M., Petravic, J., et al. (2018). Optima nutrition: An allocative efficiency tool to reduce childhood stunting by better targeting of nutrition-related interventions. *BMC Public Health*, *18*(1), 384. https://doi.org/10.1186/s12889-018-5294-z.

Roberts, H. C., Pilgrim, A. L., Jameson, K. A., Cooper, C., Sayer, A. A., & Robinson, S. (2017). The impact of trained volunteer mealtime assistants on the dietary intake of older female in-patients: The Southampton Mealtime Assistance Study. *Journal of Nutrition, Health & Aging*, *21*(3), 320–328. https://doi.org/10.1007/s12603-016-0791-1.

Rosenfeld, J., Rabbitts, A., & Bessey, P. Q. (2019). Pre-burn malnutrition: Does it make a difference? *Journal of Burn Care and Research*, *40*(Suppl. 1), S178. https://doi-org.ezproxy.gvsu.edu/10.1093/jbcr/irz013.311.

Sakai, K., Kinoshita, S., Tsuboi, M., Fukui, R., Momosaki, R., & Wakabayashi, H. (2019). Effects of nutrition therapy in older stroke patients undergoing rehabilitation: A systematic review and meta-analysis. *The Journal of Nutrition, Health & Aging*, *23*(1), 21–26. https://doi.org/10.1007/s12603-018-1095-4.

White, J. V., Guenter, P., Jensen, G., et al. (2012). Consensus statement of the Academy of Nutrition and Dietetics/American Society for Parenteral and Enteral Nutrition: Characteristics recommended for the identification and documentation of adult malnutrition (undernutrition). *Journal of the Academy of Nutrition and Dietetics*, *112*(5), 730–738. https://doi.org/10.1016/j.jand.2012.03.012.

Impaired Oral Mucous Membrane Integrity

Domain 11 Safety/protection Class 2 Physical injury

Morgan Nestingen, MSN, APRN, AGCNS-BC, OCN, ONN-CG

NANDA-I

Definition

Injury to the lips, soft tissue, buccal cavity, and/or oropharynx.

Defining Characteristics

Bad taste in mouth; bleeding; cheilitis; coated tongue; decreased taste perception; desquamation; difficulty eating; difficulty swallowing; dysphonia; enlarged tonsils; geographic tongue; gingival hyperplasia; gingival pallor; gingival pocketing deeper than 4 mm; gingival recession; halitosis; hyperemia; macroplasia; mucosal denudation; oral discomfort; oral edema; oral fissure; oral lesion; oral mucosal pallor; oral nodule; oral pain; oral papule; oral ulcer; oral vesicles; pathogen exposure; presence of mass; purulent oral-nasal drainage; purulent oral-nasal exudates; smooth atrophic tongue; spongy patches in mouth; stomatitis; white patches in mouth; white plaque in mouth; white, curd-like oral exudate; xerostomia

Related Factors

Alcohol consumption; decreased salivation; dehydration; depressive symptoms; difficulty performing oral self-care; inadequate access to dental care; inadequate knowledge of oral hygiene; inadequate oral hygiene habits; inappropriate use of chemical agent; malnutrition; mouth breathing; smoking; stressors

At-Risk Population

Economically disadvantaged individuals

Associated Conditions

Allergies; autosomal disorder; behavioral disorder; chemotherapy; decreased female hormone levels; decreased platelets; depression; immune system diseases; immunosuppression; infections; loss of oral support structure; mechanical factor; nil per os (NPO) >24 hours; oral trauma; radiotherapy; Sjögren's syndrome; surgical procedures; trauma; treatment regimen

O

NOC (Nursing Outcomes Classification)

Suggested NOC Outcomes

Oral Health; Oral Hygiene; Tissue Integrity: Skin and Mucous Membranes

Example NOC Outcome with Indicators

Oral Health as evidenced by the following indicators: Cleanliness of mouth and teeth/Moisture of oral mucosa and tongue/Color of mucous membranes/Oral mucosa/tongue/gum integrity. (Rate the outcome and indicators of **Oral Health:** 1 = severely compromised, 2 = substantially compromised, 3 = moderately compromised, 4 = mildly compromised, 5 = not compromised [see Section I].)

Client Outcomes

Client Will (Specify Time Frame)

- Maintain intact, moist oral mucous membranes that are free of ulceration, inflammation, infection, and debris
- Demonstrate measures to maintain or regain intact oral mucous membranes
- Demonstrate oral hygiene knowledge and skills

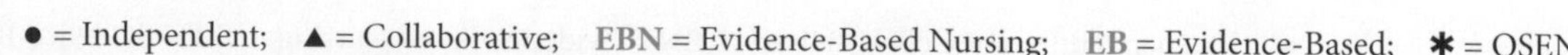

NIC (Nursing Interventions Classification)

Suggested NIC Intervention

Oral Health Restoration

Example NIC Activities—Oral Health Restoration

Monitor condition of client's mouth including character of abnormalities; Instruct client to avoid commercial mouthwashes

Nursing Interventions and *Rationales*

- ▲ Inspect the oral cavity/teeth/gingiva at least once daily and note any discoloration; presence of debris; amount of plaque buildup; presence of lesions such as white lesions or patches, edema, or bleeding; and intactness of teeth. Refer to a dentist or periodontist as appropriate. EB: *Inspection is a critical diagnostic tool; observations can identify impending problems. Leukoplakia is the presence of uncharacterized white lesions, which can be a precursor to squamous cell carcinoma. If leukoplakia is observed, prompt referral for diagnosis and potential biopsy is indicated (Lingen et al, 2017; Abadeh et al, 2019).*
- • If the client is free of bleeding disorders and able to swallow, encourage toothbrushing with a soft toothbrush using fluoride-containing toothpaste at least two times per day. EB: *The toothbrush is the most effective method for reducing plaque and controlling periodontal disease (Brignardello-Petersen, 2019).*
- • Recommend the use of a power, rotation-oscillation toothbrush for removal of dental plaque and prevention of gingivitis. EB: *Two systematic reviews found the powered/oscillating toothbrush to be safe for use on both hard and soft dental tissues and more effective in cleaning teeth (Adam, Erb, & Grender, 2020; Elkerbout et al, 2020).*
- • Use foam sticks to moisten the oral mucous membranes, clean out debris, and swab out the mouth of the edentulous client. Do not use foam sticks to clean the teeth unless the platelet count is very low and the client is prone to bleeding gums. EB: *Use of swabs is not an adequate substitute for toothbrushing but may be used to improve oral cleanliness and appearance (Onubogu et al, 2019). Adequate cleaning with toothbrush and fluoride toothpaste helps to reduce biofilm and prevent secondary infection of mucosal ulcers; if thrombocytopenia is severe, swabs with saline may reduce mucosal trauma to damaged tissues (Madeswaran et al, 2019).*
- • Avoid lemon-glycerin swabs for oral care. EB: *Lemon-glycerin swabs are no longer recommended for use in tooth cleaning, prevention of ventilator-associated pneumonia, or treating xerostomia because they may cause disturbances in the pH and microbial balance within the oral cavity, decalcification, and worsening of xerostomia (Lavigne & Lavigne, 2019).*
- • If the client does not have a bleeding disorder, encourage the client to perform interdental hygiene by flossing or cleaning between teeth with interdental brushes, woodsticks, or oral irrigation. If the client is unable to floss, assist with flossing or encourage the use of an oral irrigator (i.e., "water flossing"). EB: *A Cochrane review determined that all forms of interdental cleaning performed in addition to toothbrushing are associated with decreased gingivitis; no specific method of interdental cleaning was found to be superior (Worthington et al, 2019). Some interdental cleaning techniques may also assist with interdental plaque removal, but current findings are inconsistent (Ng & Lim, 2019; Slot, Valkenburg, & Van der Weijden, 2020).*
- • Over-the-counter mouthwashes containing mint or essential oils may be used in combination with toothbrushing and interdental cleaning to maintain oral health. Avoid routine use of hydrogen peroxide, chlorhexidine, or alcohol-based mouthwashes. EB: *Mint and essential oil mouthwashes have been shown to exert an antimicrobial effect on biofilm, reduce loss of mineralization, and improve halitosis when used with toothbrushing and interdental cleaning with minimal discomfort and other adverse effects (Alaee et al, 2017; Albuquerque et al, 2018; Kulaksiz et al, 2018).*
- • Provide oral hygiene if the client is unable to care for himself or herself. The nursing diagnosis Bathing **Self-Care** Deficit is then applicable.
- • If the client is unable to brush own teeth, follow this procedure:
  - ❍ Position the client sitting upright or on side.
  - ❍ Use a soft bristle toothbrush.
  - ❍ Use fluoride toothpaste and tap water or saline as a solution.
  - ❍ Brush teeth in an up-and-down manner.
  - ❍ Suction as needed.

O

EB: *Each client must receive oral care including toothbrushing two times every day to maintain healthy teeth and mouth and to prevent complications associated with periodontitis (the advanced form of gum disease that can cause tooth loss), which is associated with health problems, such as cardiovascular disease, stroke, and bacterial pneumonia (American Dental Association [ADA], 2020).*

- ● Monitor the client's nutritional and fluid status to determine whether it is adequate. Dehydration and malnutrition predispose clients to impaired oral mucous membranes. Refer to the care plan for Deficient **Fluid** Volume or Imbalanced **Nutrition:** Less Than Body Requirements if applicable.
- ● Encourage fluid intake of up to 3000 mL/day if not contraindicated by the client's medical condition. Fluids help increase moisture in the mouth, which protects the mucous membranes from damage.
- ▲ Determine the client's usual method of oral care and address any concerns regarding oral hygiene. If the client has a dry mouth (xerostomia):
  - ❍ Recognize that more than 50 classes of medications may cause xerostomia, which is often exacerbated by polypharmacy. When feasible, medications can be discontinued or replaced to increase the client's comfort (Marcott et al, 2020).
  - ❍ Provide saliva substitutes as ordered. **EB:** *Saliva substitutes are helpful to decrease the discomfort of dry mouth and may help prevent stomatitis (Vinke et al, 2020).*
  - ❍ Suggest the client chew sugarless gum or sugarless sour candy to promote salivary flow. **EB:** *Both sugarless gum and candy stimulate the formation of saliva (Hemalatha et al, 2019).*
  - ❍ Examine the oral cavity for signs of caries, dental plaque, infection, mucositis ulceration, and oral candidiasis. **EB:** *Untreated xerostomia may result in these conditions (Hemalatha et al, 2019; Kurapati et al, 2020).*
- ● Recommend that the client decrease or preferably stop intake of soft drinks. Sugar-containing soft drinks can cause cavities, and the low pH of the drink can cause erosion in teeth. **EB:** *Diets high in sugar are strongly associated with formation of caries in adults and children (Laniado et al, 2020).*
- ● If client has halitosis, review good oral care with the client including brushing teeth, using floss, and brushing the tongue. **EB:** *Halitosis can be a beginning sign of gingivitis and can be eradicated by a good program of dental hygiene (Raghu Ram, 2019).*
- ● Instruct the client with halitosis to clean the tongue when performing oral hygiene; brush tongue with tongue scraper or toothbrush and follow with a mouth rinse. **EB:** *A Cochrane review found limited evidence that tongue cleaning, chewing gum, systemic deodorizing agents, topical agents, and specialized toothpastes/mouth rinses were effective in controlling halitosis; toothbrushing combined with tongue cleaning and mouthwash has been identified as the most effective method of control (Van der Sluijs et al, 2018; Nagraj et al, 2019).*
- ▲ Assess the client for underlying medical conditions that may be causing halitosis. Causes of halitosis can be subdivided into three categories: oral origin, in which good mouth care can help prevent halitosis; halitosis from the upper respiratory tract, including the sinuses and nose; and halitosis from systemic diseases that are blood-borne, volatilized in the lungs, and expelled from the lower respiratory tract. Potential sources of blood-borne halitosis are some systemic diseases, metabolic disorders, medication, and certain foods such as onions and garlic (*Raghu Ram, 2019*).
- ● Keep the lips well lubricated using a water-based or aloe-based lip balm. **EB:** *This is a comfort measure (Kurapati et al, 2020).*

O

Client Receiving Chemotherapy and/or Radiation

- ● Ensure that the client receives a comprehensive oral examination before initiation of chemotherapy or radiation, with aggressive preventive dental care given as needed. **EB:** *Baseline assessment is necessary to identify posttreatment changes to oral health (Hong et al, 2019; Quinn et al, 2020b).*
- ● Provide both verbal and written instruction about the need for and method of providing frequent oral care to the client before radiation therapy or chemotherapy. Assess the condition of the oral cavity daily in the client receiving radiation or chemotherapy. **EB:** *Ongoing reassessment supports early identification and management of treatment-related changes to oral health (Hong et al, 2019; Quinn et al, 2020b).*
- ● For measurement of presence or severity of mucositis, use the Oral Mucositis Assessment Scale (OMAS). **EBN:** *This is an instrument that has two components: clinician's assessment of presence and severity of mucositis and client report about pain, difficulty swallowing, and ability to eat. Scores indicating the presence of a more severe oral mucositis are associated with decreased quality of life (Franco et al, 2017; Minhas et al, 2021).*

- Use a protocol to prevent/treat mucositis that includes the following:
  - Use a soft toothbrush that is replaced on a regular basis; brush teeth at least two times a day and for at least 90 seconds. Continue to floss teeth daily.
  - Use a bland, alcohol-free rinse to remove debris and moisten the oral cavity. Rinse the mouth often (every 2 hours while awake) if the client has mouth sores.
  - Avoid tobacco, alcohol, and irritating foods (hot, rough, acidic, or spicy).
  - Use a valid and reliable pain assessment tool and treatment of pain as needed.

  EB: *Use of an oral care protocol helps to decrease oral mucositis in clients receiving treatment for cancer (Hong et al, 2019; Naibaho et al, 2020).*
- Help the client use a mouth rinse of normal saline or salt and soda every 1 to 2 hours for prevention and treatment of stomatitis. A typical mixture is 1 teaspoon of salt or sodium bicarbonate per pint of water. Clients are directed to take a tablespoon of the rinse and swish it in the mouth for 30 seconds, then expectorate. EB: *Rinses are helpful to remove debris and hydrate the oral mucous membranes; sodium bicarbonate can discourage yeast colonization (Hong et al, 2019; Naibaho et al, 2020).*
- ▲ If the mouth is severely inflamed and it is painful to swallow, contact the health care provider for a topical anesthetic or analgesic order. Modification of oral intake (e.g., soft or liquid diet) may also be necessary to prevent friction trauma. *The nursing diagnosis Imbalanced* ***Nutrition:*** *Less Than Body Requirements may apply.*
- If the client's platelet count is lower than 50,000/mm^3 or the client has a bleeding disorder, use a soft toothbrush or a toothette that is not soaked in glycerin or flavorings; if the client cannot tolerate a toothbrush or a toothette, a piece of gauze wrapped around a finger can be used to remove plaque and debris. EB: *Use of toothettes is not an adequate substitute for toothbrushing but may be used to improve oral cleanliness and appearance (Onubogu et al, 2019). Adequate cleaning with toothbrush and fluoride toothpaste helps to reduce biofilm and prevent secondary infection of mucosal ulcers; if thrombocytopenia is severe, toothettes with saline may reduce mucosal trauma to damaged tissues (Madeswaran et al, 2019).*

Critical Care—Client on a Ventilator

- Use a soft toothbrush to brush teeth to clean the client's teeth at least every 12 hours; use suction to remove secretions. Provide oral moisturizer to oral mucosa and lips every 4 hours. Recognize that good oral care is paramount in the prevention of ventilator-associated events (VAEs) and ventilator-associated pneumonia (VAP). EBN: *Increased plaque on the teeth is associated with increased contamination of the mouth and incidence of VAP (Takahama et al, 2021). An integrative review of the literature found that consistently performing frequent oral care along with other interventions (e.g., head of bed >30 degrees, adequate endotracheal tube cuff pressure to reduce aspiration, daily evaluation of client's readiness for extubation) and oral moisturizing reduced VAP and decreased overall health care expenses (Quinn et al, 2020a).*
- ▲ Apply chlorhexidine gluconate mouthwash or gel in the oral cavity after performing tooth brushing, which may reduce the risk of the client developing VAEs and VAP. EB: *Routine oral care with chlorhexidine gluconate in the care of ventilated clients is associated with reduced risk of VAEs and VAP (Quinn et al, 2020a).*

Geriatric

- Determine the functional ability of the client to provide his or her own oral care. Interventions must be directed toward both treatment of the functional loss and care of oral health.
- Provide appropriate oral care to older adults with a self-care deficit, brushing the teeth after breakfast and in the evening. EB: *The ADA recommends toothbrushing twice daily in addition to interdental cleaning (ADA, 2021). Numerous references have found oral care effective in preventing new-onset pneumonia, although heterogeneity in interventions weakens the level and consistency of evidence (Mitchell et al, 2019; Quinn et al, 2020a; Satheeshkumar, Papatheodorou, & Sonis, 2020).*
- If the client has dementia or delirium and exhibits care-resistant behavior, such as fighting, biting, or refusing care, use the following method:
  - Ensure client is in a quiet environment such as own bathroom, sitting or standing at the sink to prime memory for appropriate actions.
  - Approach the client at eye level within his or her range of vision.
  - Approach with a smile and begin conversation with a touch of the hand and gradually move up.
  - Use mirror–mirror technique, standing behind the client, and brush and floss teeth.

O

- Use respectful adult speech. Avoid "elderspeak," a style of speech characterized by short phrases and questions uttered in a sing-song voice and use of collective pronouns and intimate terms (e.g., first name, nicknames, "deary" or "honey"). EB: *Elderspeak is perceived as demeaning and is a documented trigger for care-resistant behavior (Schnabel et al, 2020; Zhang, Zhao, & Meng, 2020).*
- Promote self-care in which client brushes own teeth if possible.
- Use distractors when needed: talking, reminiscing, singing. EBN: *Use of specific techniques can decrease resistance to nursing care and increase the effectiveness of nurses providing oral care to older clients (National Institute for Health and Care Excellence [NICE], 2016).*

- Carefully observe the oral cavity and lips for abnormal lesions such as white or red patches, masses, ulcerations with an indurated margin, or a raised granular lesion. EB: *Malignant lesions are more common in older adults than in younger persons, especially if there is a history of smoking or alcohol use. Suspicious lesions identified on inspections should be referred for potential biopsy and diagnosis (Lingen et al, 2017; Abadeh et al, 2019).*
- Ensure that dentures are removed and cleaned regularly, preferably after every meal and before bedtime. Dentures left in the mouth at night may impede circulation to the palate and predispose the client to oral lesions.

Home Care

- The interventions described previously may be adapted for home care use.
- Instruct the client in ways to soothe the oral cavity (e.g., cool beverages, popsicles, viscous lidocaine).
- ▲ If necessary, refer for home health aide services to support the family in oral care and observation of the oral cavity.

Client/Family Teaching and Discharge Planning

- Teach the client how to inspect the oral cavity and monitor for signs and symptoms of infection or complications and when to call the health care provider. EB: *Education is key to supporting clients' understanding of their oral health and thus their self-care behaviors (Albano et al, 2019).*
- Recommend the client not smoke, use chewing tobacco, or drink excessive amounts of alcohol. EB: *Tobacco use, alcohol consumption, human papillomavirus, and poor oral hygiene are all independently associated with the development of squamous cell carcinomas of the head, neck, and oral cavity (Ganly et al, 2019); use of alcohol and tobacco may synergistically increase overall risk (Mello et al, 2019).*
- Teach the client and family, if necessary, how to perform appropriate mouth care. Use the motivational interviewing technique. EB: *Recent systematic reviews have demonstrated an association between motivational interviewing with improved adherence to oral hygiene self-care and may decrease gingival bleeding times and plaque scores; results are more significant among high-risk groups (Carra et al, 2020; Carrinconde Colvara et al, 2021). See Appendix C on Evolve for motivational interviewing.*

O

REFERENCES

Abadeh, A., Ali, A. A., Bradley, G., & Magalhaes, M. A. (2019). Increase in detection of oral cancer and precursor lesions by dentists: Evidence from an oral and maxillofacial pathology service. *Journal of the American Dental Association, 150*(6), 531–539.

Adam, R., Erb, J., & Grender, J. (2020). Randomized controlled trial assessing plaque removal of an oscillating-rotating electric toothbrush with micro-vibrations. *International Dental Journal, 70*(Suppl. 1), S22–S27.

Alaee, A., Aghayan, S., Kamalinejad, M., & Arezoomand, M. (2017). The comparison of mint mouthwash effect on microbial plaque with chlorhexidine, and acceptance of persons. *Journal of Research in Dental Sciences, 14*(2), 97–102.

Albano, M. G., d'Ivernois, J. F., de Andrade, V., & Levy, G. (2019). Patient education in dental medicine: A review of the literature. *European Journal of Dental Education, 23*(2), 110–118.

Albuquerque, Y. E., Danelon, M., Salvador, M. J., et al. (2018). Mouthwash containing *Croton doctoris* essential oil: In vitro study using a validated model of caries induction. *Future Microbiology, 13*, 631–643.

American Dental Association (ADA). (2020). *Oral health topics: Home oral care*. Retrieved from https://www.ada.org/en/member-center/oral-health-topics/home-care. Accessed 21 July 2021.

American Dental Association (ADA). (2021). *Oral health topics: Aging and dental health*. Retrieved from https://www.ada.org/en/member-center/oral-health-topics/aging-and-dental-health. Accessed 21 July 2021.

Brignardello-Petersen, R. (2019). Very small differences in caries, periodontal parameters, and tooth loss between powered and manual toothbrushing after 11 years. *Journal of the American Dental Association, 150*(11), e176.

Carra, M. C., Detzen, L., Kitzmann, J., Woelber, J. P., Ramseier, C. A., & Bouchard, P. (2020). Promoting behavioural changes to improve oral hygiene in patients with periodontal diseases: A systematic review. *Journal of Clinical Periodontology, 47*(Suppl. 22), 72–89.

Carrinconde Colvara, B., Faustino-Silva, D. D., Meyer, E., Neves Hugo, F., Celeste, R. K., & Balbinot Hilgert, J. (2021). Motivational interviewing for preventing early childhood caries: A systematic review and meta-analysis. *Community Dentistry and Oral Epidemiology*, *49*(1), 10–16.

Elkerbout, T. A., Slot, D. E., Rosema, N. M., & Van der Weijden, G. A. (2020). How effective is a powered toothbrush as compared to a manual toothbrush? A systematic review and meta-analysis of single brushing exercises. *International Journal of Dental Hygiene*, *18*(1), 17–26.

Franco, P., Martini, S., Di Muzio, J., et al. (2017). Prospective assessment of oral mucositis and its impact on quality of life and patient-reported outcomes during radiotherapy for head and neck cancer. *Medical Oncology*, *34*(5), 81.

Ganly, I., Yang, L., Giese, R. A., et al. (2019). Periodontal pathogens are a risk factor of oral cavity squamous cell carcinoma, independent of tobacco and alcohol and human papillomavirus. *International Journal of Cancer*, *145*(3), 775–784.

Hemalatha, V. T., Julius, A., Kishore Kumar, S. P., Thangam Periyasamy, T., & Mani Sundar, N. (2019). Xerostomia: A current update for practitioners. *Drug Invention Today*, *12*(3), 388–392.

Hong, C. H. L., Alcino Gueiros, L., Fulton, J. S., et al. (2019). Systematic review of basic oral care for the management of oral mucositis in cancer patients and clinical practice guidelines. *Supportive Care in Cancer*, *27*(10), 3949–3967.

Kulaksiz, B., Sevda, E., Üstündağ-Okur, N., & Saltan-İşcan, G. (2018). Investigation of antimicrobial activities of some herbs containing essential oils and their mouthwash formulations. *Turkish Journal of Pharmaceutical Sciences*, *15*(3), 370–375.

Kurapati, M., Pradusha, R., Rao, D. ,B., Sajjan, M. C. S., Ramaraju, A. V., & Nair, K. C. (2020). Management of xerostomia: An overview. *Trends in Prosthodontics and Dental Implantology*, *10*(1 & 2), 20–23.

Laniado, N., Sanders, A. E., Godfrey, E. M., Salazar, C. R., & Badner, V. M. (2020). Sugar-sweetened beverage consumption and caries experience: An examination of children and adults in the United States, National Health and Nutrition Examination Survey 2011-2014. *The Journal of the American Dental Association*, *151*(10), 782–789.

Lavigne, M. C., & Lavigne, M. C. (2019). A performance summary of agents used in oral care for non-ventilated and mechanically-ventilated patients. *Anna Pul and Crit Car Med*, *2*(2), 1–34.

Lingen, M. W., Abt, E., Agrawal, N., et al. (2017). Evidence-based clinical practice guideline for the evaluation of potentially malignant disorders in the oral cavity: A report of the American dental association. *Journal of the American Dental Association*, *148*(10), 712–727.e710.

Madeswaran, S., Saravanan, D., Rethinam, S., & Muthu, K. (2019). Oral mucositis: Role of the dentist. *Journal of Oral Health and Community Dentistry*, *13*(3), 106–111.

Marcott, S., Dewan, K., Kwan, M., Baik, F., Lee, Y. J., & Sirjani, D. (2020). Where dysphagia begins: Polypharmacy and xerostomia. *Federal Practitioner*, *37*(5), 234–241.

Mello, F. W., Melo, G., Pasetto, J. J., Barcellos Silva, C. A., Warnakulasuriya, S., & Correa Rivero, E. R. (2019). The synergistic effect of tobacco and alcohol consumption on oral squamous cell carcinoma: A systematic review and meta-analysis. *Clinical Oral Investigations*, *23*(7), 2849–2859.

Minhas, S., Sajjad, A., Mushtaq Chaudhry, R., Zahid, H., Shahid, A., & Kashif, M. (2021). Assessment and prevalence of concomitant chemo-radiotherapy-induced oral mucositis in patients with oral squamous cell carcinoma. *Turkish Journal of Medical Sciences*, *51*(2), 675–684.

Mitchell, B. G., Russo, P. L., Cheng, A. C., et al. (2019). Strategies to reduce non-ventilator-associated hospital-acquired pneumonia: A systematic review. *Infection, Disease & Health*, *24*(4), 229–239.

Nagraj, S. K., Eachempati, P., Uma, E., Singh, V. P., Ismail, N. M., & Varghese, E. (2019). Interventions for managing halitosis. *Cochrane Database of Systematic Reviews*, *12*, CD012213.

Naibaho, E. N., Dharmajaya, R., & Harahap, I. A. (2020). Effectiveness of oral care using normal saline and baking soda towards pain and comfort in mucositis patients undergoing chemotherapy. *Indian Journal of Public Health Research & Development*, *11*(10), 222–228.

National Institute for Health and Care Excellence (NICE). (2016). *Oral health for adults in care homes*. NICE guideline [NG48]. Retrieved from https://www.nice.org.uk/guidance/ng48. Accessed 21 July 2021.

Ng, E., & Lim, L. P. (2019). An Overview of different interdental cleaning aids and their effectiveness. *Dentistry Journal*, *7*(2), 56.

Onubogu, U., Mansfield, W. M., & Ozbek, I. N. (2019). Oral healthcare measures to improve overall health in older adults. *Journal of Comprehensive Nursing Research and Care*, *4*, 156.

Quinn, B., Giuliano, K. K., & Baker, D. (2020a). Non-ventilator health care-associated pneumonia (NV-HAP): Best practices for prevention of NV-HAP. *American Journal of Infection Control*, *48*(Suppl. 5), A23–A27.

Quinn, B. G., Campbell, F., Fulman, L., et al. (2020b). Oral care of patients in the cancer setting. *Cancer Nursing Practice*, *19*(5), 35–42.

Raghu Ram, S. S. R. (2019). Halitosis-bad breath: Etiology, diagnosis, treatment. *Indian Journal of Public Health Research & Development*, *10*(11), 917–920.

Satheeshkumar, P. S., Papatheodorou, S., & Sonis, S. (2020). Enhanced oral hygiene interventions as a risk mitigation strategy for the prevention of non-ventilator-associated pneumonia: A systematic review and meta-analysis. *British Dental Journal*, *228*(8), 615–622.

Schnabel, E. L., Wahl, H. W., Streib, C., & Schmidt, T. (2020). Elderspeak in Acute hospitals? The role of context, cognitive and functional impairment. *Research on Aging* [Online ahead of print].

Slot, D. E., Valkenburg, C., & Van der Weijden, G. A. F. (2020). Mechanical plaque removal of periodontal maintenance patients: A systematic review and network meta-analysis. *Journal of Clinical Periodontology*, *47*(Suppl. 22), 107–124.

Takahama, A., Jr., de Sousa, V. I., Tanaka, E. E., et al. (2021). Analysis of oral risk-factors for ventilator-associated pneumonia in critically ill patients. *Clinical Oral Investigations*, *25*(3), 1217–1222.

Van der Sluijs, E., Van der Weijden, G. A., Hennequin-Hoenderdos, N. L., & Slot, D. E. (2018). The effect of a tooth/tongue gel and mouthwash regimen on morning oral malodour: A 3-week single-blind randomized clinical trial. *International Journal of Dental Hygiene*, *16*(1), 92–102.

Vinke, J., Kaper, H. J., Vissink, A., & Sharma, P. K. (2020). Dry mouth: Saliva substitutes which adsorb and modify existing salivary condition films improve oral lubrication. *Clinical Oral Investigations*, *24*(11), 4019–4030.

Worthington, H. V., MacDonald, L., Pericic, T. P., et al. (2019). Home use of interdental cleaning devices, in addition to toothbrushing, for preventing and controlling periodontal diseases and dental caries. *Cochrane Database of Systematic Reviews*, *4*, CD012018.

Zhang, M., Zhao, H., & Meng, F. P. (2020). Elderspeak to resident dementia patients increases resistiveness to care in health care profession. *Inquiry*, *57*, 0046958020948668.

Risk for Impaired Oral Mucous Membrane Integrity Domain 11 Safety/protection Class 2 Physical injury

Mary Beth Flynn Makic, PhD, RN, CCNS, CCRN-K, FAAN, FNAP, FCNS

NANDA-I

Definition

Susceptible to injury to the lips, soft tissues, buccal cavity, and/or oropharynx, which may compromise health.

Risk Factors

Alcohol consumption; decreased salivation; dehydration; depressive symptoms; difficulty performing oral self-care; inadequate access to dental care; inadequate knowledge of oral hygiene; inadequate oral hygiene habits; inappropriate use of chemical agent; malnutrition; mouth breathing; smoking; stressors

At-Risk Population

Economically disadvantaged individuals

Associated Conditions

Allergies; autosomal disorder; behavioral disorder; chemotherapy; decreased female hormone levels; decreased platelets; depression; immune system diseases; immunosuppression; infections; loss of oral support structure; mechanical factor; nil per os (NPO) >24 hours; oral trauma; radiotherapy; Sjögren's syndrome; surgical procedures; trauma; treatment regimen

NIC, NOC, Client Outcomes, Nursing Interventions and *Rationales,* Client/Family Teaching, and References

Refer to care plan for Impaired **Oral Mucous Membrane** Integrity.

O

Obesity Domain 2 Nutrition Class 1 Ingestion

Marina Martinez-Kratz, MS, RN, CNE

NANDA-I

Definition

A condition in which an individual accumulates excessive fat for age and gender that exceeds overweight.

Defining Characteristics

Adult: Body mass index >30 kg/m^2; Child 2 to 18 years: body mass index >30 kg/m^2 or >95th percentile or 30 kg/m^2 for age and gender; Child <2 years: term not used with children at this age

Related Factors

Abnormal eating behavior patterns; abnormal eating perception patterns; average daily physical activity is less than recommended for age and gender; consumption of sugar-sweetened beverages; dyssomnias; energy expenditure below energy intake based on standard assessment; excessive alcohol consumption; fear regarding lack of food supply; frequent snacking; high frequency of restaurant or fried food; insufficient dietary calcium intake by children; portion sizes larger than recommended; sedentary behavior occurring for ≥2 hours/day; shortened sleep time; solid foods as major food source at <5 months of age

At-Risk Population

Economically disadvantaged individuals; individuals who experienced premature pubarche; individuals who experienced rapid weight gain during childhood; individuals who experienced rapid weight gain during infancy; individuals who inherit interrelated factors; individuals who were not exclusively breastfed; individuals who were overweight during infancy; individuals whose mothers had gestational diabetes; individuals whose mothers have diabetes; individuals whose mothers smoke during childhood; individuals whose mothers smoke during pregnancy; individuals with high disinhibition and restraint eating behavior score; individuals with parents who are obese neonates whose mothers had gestational diabetes

Associated Conditions

Inborn genetic diseases

NOC (Nursing Outcomes Classification)

Suggested NOC Outcomes

Nutritional Status; Nutritional Status: Food and Fluid Intake; Nutrient Intake; Weight Control

Example NOC Outcome with Indicators

Nutritional Status as evidenced by the following indicators: Food and fluid intake/Hydration/Body mass index/Weight-height ratio/Hematocrit. (Rate the outcome and indicators of **Nutritional Status:** 1 = severe deviation from normal range, 2 = substantial deviation from normal range, 3 = moderate deviation from normal range, 4 = mild deviation from normal range, 5 = no deviation from normal range [see Section I].)

Client Outcomes

Client Will (Specify Time Frame)

- Explain how to eat according to the US Dietary Guidelines
- Design dietary modifications to meet individual long-term goal of health, using principles of variety, balance, and moderation
- Maintain weight within normal range for height and age

NIC (Nursing Interventions Classification)

Suggested NIC Interventions

Nutrition Management; Nutritional Counseling; Weight Reduction Assistance

Example NIC Activities—Nutrition Management

Determine the client's motivation for changing eating habits; Develop with the client a method to keep a daily record of intake

Nursing Interventions and *Rationales*

- Assess the meaning and importance of food in the client's life. EB: *Research found strong associations between the different domains of food meanings and behavioral outcomes (Arbit et al, 2017).*
- Assess client readiness to determine whether the client is ready to discuss weight loss and/or would like weight loss information. EB: *Client motivation is a key component of success in a weight loss program and a prerequisite for weight loss therapy (Raynor & Champagne, 2016).*
- Use a motivational interviewing technique when working with clients to promote healthy eating and weight loss. EB: *Research shows significant weight loss for clients when motivational interviewing techniques were used (Barnes et al, 2018).*
- Counsel the client to measure regularly consumed foods periodically. Help the client learn usual portion sizes. Measuring food alerts the client to normal portion sizes. Estimating amounts can be extremely inaccurate. EB: *A randomized controlled trial of 278 overweight and obese participants was conducted to increase portion size awareness with results that demonstrated the intervention improved portion control behavior and in turn influenced body mass index (BMI) (Poelman et al, 2015).*
- Assist the client to develop a system of self-management, which may include self-monitoring of weight and BMI; realistic goal setting, planning, and action planning for improved dietary intake and physical

activity; problem-solving; and tracking dietary intake and exercise. EB: *A key component of successful weight loss and maintenance is regular self-monitoring (Thomason et al, 2016).*

- Encourage the client to adopt dietary as well as physical activity changes. EB: *A research review found that aerobic exercise without additional dietary changes achieves only a 3% to 5% weight loss in clients with obesity (McCafferty, Hill, & Gunn, 2020).*
- Document the client's height and weight and teach the significance of his or her BMI in relationship to current health. Use a chart or a website such as http://www.cdc.gov/healthyweight/assessing/bmi/index.html (Centers for Disease Control and Prevention [CDC], 2020a). EB: *Successful treatment of overweight and obesity in adults requires adoption and maintenance of effective self-monitoring (Raynor & Champagne, 2016).*
- Encourage the client to engage in moderate- to vigorous-intensity physical activity for at least 200 to 300 minutes weekly for weight loss. EB: *There is strong evidence to demonstrate that clients who engage in moderate- to vigorous-intensity physical activity for greater amounts of time decrease weight gain (Jakicic et al, 2019).*
- Recommend that the client limit fast food and take-out meals. EB: *A study found that fast-food consumption was the most frequent risk factor for adiposity found in 61.67% of study participants (Popa et al, 2020).*
- Assist the client to reframe slips in weight loss or physical activity behavior as lapses that are a single event and not a full return to previous unhealthy behaviors. Relapse prevention strategies (Centers for Disease Control and Prevention, 2020a) include managing lapses in healthy behavior, identifying high-risk situations for relapses, self-monitoring, providing social support, enhancing skills for coping, and increasing self-efficacy for avoiding relapse. EB: *A study of a weight maintenance intervention, delivered primarily by telephone, modestly slowed the rate of weight regain (Voils et al, 2017).*
- Assist clients to engage their social support systems either digitally or face to face in ways that facilitate weight loss, healthy eating, and physical activity behavior change. EB: *Significant others, family, friends, and coworkers can facilitate or hinder weight loss success (Romo, 2018).*
- Assist the client to reframe the goal from a focus on outcome (weight loss) to a focus on process (weight-loss behaviors) for weight loss. EB: *A study found that the self-monitoring behaviors of self-weigh-in, daily steps, high-intensity activity, and persistent food logging were significant predictors of weight loss during a 6-month intervention (Painter et al, 2017).*
- Assist the client to implement informal and formal mindfulness-based interventions (MBIs). Informal MBIs include mindful eating, increasing awareness of hunger and satiety cues, taste satisfaction, and decreasing impulsive tendencies to overeat when experiencing negative emotions. Meditation practice is a formal MBI. EB: *Results of a research review suggested that a combination of formal and informal MBIs are effective in reducing weight and improving obesity-related eating behaviors among individuals with overweight and obesity (Carrière et al, 2018).*
- Assist the client to develop stimulus control techniques designed to reduce environmental cues associated with eating behaviors. Specifically, clients should be taught to limit the presence of high-calorie/high-fat foods in the home; to reduce the visibility of unhealthy food choices in the home; to limit where and when they eat; to avoid distractions (Newton et al, 2018) such as reading, using the computer, or watching television when eating; and to eat more slowly. EB: *Stimulus control strategies are a key to successful weight loss and weight maintenance in conjunction with other weight-loss strategies (Butryn et al, 2017).*
- Encourage 7.5 to 8.5 hours of sleep nightly. EB: *Evidence suggests that weight management is hindered when attempted in the context of sleep restriction because there is an upregulation of reward, pleasure, and salience networks in response to food stimuli (St-Onge, 2017).*
- Refer the client to a weight loss–related therapy group. EBN: *A study found significant changes in BMI, waist circumference, body fat percentage, and strength of the lower limbs for weight-loss group therapy participants (Ferrari et al, 2017).*
- Recommend that clients use dietary supplements such as vitamins and minerals after consulting with their primary health care provider. EB: *Research shows that micronutrient deficits are prevalent in weight-loss plans, especially vitamin B_{12}, calcium, and vitamin D (Engel et al, 2018).*
- Recommend the CDC behavior modification approach "reflect, replace, and reinforce" to improve eating habits. EB: *Reflect, replace, and reinforce consists of the following: (1) Reflect about intake through food journals, listing food habits, and identification of eating cues. (2) Replace habits identified during reflection with new and healthier behaviors, such as eating more slowly or planning meals ahead of time. (3) Reinforce changes made and having patience with the process (CDC, 2020b).*

- Incorporate the following recommendations from the Academy of Nutrition and Dietetics "Interventions for the Treatment of Overweight and Obesity in Adults" (Raynor & Champagne, 2016):
  - Assess food- and nutrition-related history; anthropometric measures; biochemical data, medical tests, and procedures; nutrition-focused physical findings; and client history.
  - Assess the energy intake and nutrient content of the diet.
  - Use height and weight to calculate BMI; use waist circumference to determine risk of cardiovascular disease, type 2 diabetes, and all-cause mortality.
  - Use a measured resting metabolic rate to determine energy needs.
  - Set a realistic weight-loss goal such as one of the following: up to 2 pounds/week, up to 10% of baseline body weight, or a total of 3% to 5% of baseline weight if cardiovascular risk factors (hypertension, hyperlipidemia, and hyperglycemia) are present.
  - To achieve weight loss, use an individualized diet, including client preferences and health status, to achieve and maintain nutrient adequacy and reduce caloric intake, based on one of the following caloric reduction strategies: 1200 to 1500 kcal/day for women and 1500 to 1800 kcal/day for men, with an energy deficit of approximately 500 or 750 kcal/day.
- ▲ Refer for medical management of obesity. **EB:** *Pharmacological intervention for clients with obesity is indicated for individuals with a BMI of >30 kg/m², or ≥27 kg/m² with obesity-related comorbidities (McCafferty, Hill, & Gunn, 2020).*

Pediatric

- Offer obese or overweight adolescents healthy methods for weight loss. **EB:** *A recent study showed statistically significant health behavior improvements after implementing a developmentally informed intervention to increase positive health diet and exercise behaviors (Issner et al, 2017).*
- Offer families of obese or overweight children prejudice-free, individually accepting, and supportive interventions to address weight loss. **EB:** *A review summarized recent evidence on weight stigma and found that it is highly prevalent among youth with high body weight, who are targets of weight-based victimization from peers, parents, and teachers (Puhl & Lessard, 2020).*
- Recommend that families eat together for at least one meal per day. **EB:** *A large Korean study found that the frequency of family meals was inversely associated with childhood overweight or obesity (Lee, Lee, & Park, 2016).*
- Recommend involving the family in planning meals and food preparation. Children can learn about nutrition as they help plan and make meals. **EB:** *The Healthy Home Offerings via the Mealtime Environment Plus program showed increased cooking skills among the children participating (Fulkerson et al, 2018).*
- Assist parents at being good role models of healthy eating. **EB:** *The Healthy Home Offerings via the Mealtime Environment Plus program showed significantly improved parental self-efficacy for identifying appropriate portion sizes (Fulkerson et al, 2018).*
- Recommend that the family try new foods, either a new food or recipe every week. **EB:** *The Healthy Home Offerings via the Mealtime Environment Plus program showed decreasing child neophobia scores over time that were developmentally appropriate (Fulkerson et al, 2018).*

Geriatric

- Determine the risks and benefits of weight loss in the older client. A BMI greater than 30 in the older client suggests a moderate weight-loss approach. **EB:** *Recommendations for treating obesity in the elderly include ensuring a balanced and appropriately distributed intake of high-quality nutrients, particularly of high-quality protein (i.e., 1.2 to 1.5 g/kg of body weight), limiting the intake of simple carbohydrates and saturated fats, and providing sufficient intake of calcium and vitamin D_3 (Blaž, 2016).*
- Observe for social, psychological, and economic factors that influence diet quality. **EB:** *An exploratory study of diet quality influences in community-dwelling older individuals revealed the following influences: food experiences, retirement, bereavement, medical conditions, food environment, food-related habits, social engagement, personal/psychological factors, and transportation (Bloom et al, 2017).*

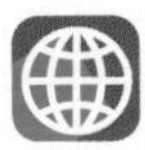

Multicultural

- Tailor nutritional interventions to be consistent with cultural beliefs, norms, and values. **EB:** *A systemic review of culturally tailored interventions for Hispanic women included literacy modification, Hispanic foods/recipes, cultural diabetes beliefs, family/friend participation, structured community input, and innovative experiential learning (McCurley et al, 2017).*

- Offer tailored lifestyle counseling via the telephone. **EBN:** *Investigators have included biweekly and/or monthly health coach calls for African American participants with significant weight gain prevention (Goode et al, 2017).*
- Integrate weight loss and weight maintenance interventions with church faith–based supports for African American clients. **EB:** *Recent research found a church-based weight loss intervention using automated text messages was well-received by African American participants and resulted in significant weight loss (Newton, 2018).*

Client/Family Teaching and Discharge Planning

- The majority of the preceding interventions involve teaching.
- Work with the family members regarding information on how to support and promote weight loss and healthy intakes.

REFERENCES

Arbit, N., Ruby, M., & Rozin, P. (2017). Development and validation of the meaning of food in life questionnaire (MFLQ): Evidence for a new construct to explain eating behavior. *Food Quality and Preference*, *59*, 35–45. https://doi.org/10.1016/j.foodqual.2017.02.002.

Barnes, R. D., Ivezaj, V., Martino, S., Pittman, B. P., Paris, M., & Grilo, C. M. (2018). Examining motivational interviewing plus nutrition psychoeducation for weight loss in primary care. *Journal of Psychosomatic Research*, *104*, 101–107. http://doi.org.proxy/10.1016/j.jpsychores.2017.11.013.

Blaž, M. K. (2016). Obesity in the elderly, weight loss yes or no? [Abstract]. *Clinical Nutrition ESPEN*, *14*, 56. https://doi.org/10.1016/j.clnesp.2016.04.025.

Bloom, I., Lawrence, W., Barker, M., et al. (2017). What influences diet quality in older people? A qualitative study among community-dwelling older adults from the Hertfordshire Cohort study, UK. *Public Health Nutrition*, *20*(15), 2685–2693. https://doi.org/10.1017/S1368980017001203.

Butryn, M. L., Forman, E. M., Lowe, M. R., Gorin, A. A., Zhang, F., & Schaumberg, K. (2017). Efficacy of environmental and acceptance-based enhancements to behavioral weight loss treatment: The ENACT trial. *Obesity*, *25*(5), 866–872. https://doi.org/10.1002/oby.21813.

Carrière, K., Khoury, B., Günak, M. M., & Knäuper, B. (2018). Mindfulness-based interventions for weight loss: A systematic review and meta-analysis. *Obesity Reviews*, *19*(2), 164–177. https://doi.org/10.1111/obr.12623.

Centers for Disease Control and Prevention (CDC). (2020a). *Body Mass Index (BMI): How do I interpret body mass index information?* Retrieved from http://www.cdc.gov/healthyweight/assessing/bmi/index.html. Accessed 21 July 2021.

Centers for Disease Control and Prevention (CDC). (2020b). *Improving your eating habits*. Division of Nutrition, Physical Activity, and Obesity, National Center for Chronic Disease Prevention and Health Promotion. Retrieved from https://www.cdc.gov/healthyweight/losing_weight/eating_habits.html. Accessed July 21, 2021.

Engel, M. G., Kern, H. J., Brenna, J. T., & Mitmesser, S. H. (2018). Micronutrient gaps in three commercial weight-loss diet plans. *Nutrients*, *10*(1), 108. https://doi.org/10.3390/nu10010108.

Ferrari, G. D., Azevedo, M., Medeiros, L., et al. (2017). A multidisciplinary weight-loss program: The importance of psychological group therapy. *Motriz: Revista de Educacao Fisica*, *23*(1), 47–52. https://doi.org/10.1590/s1980-6574201700010007.

Fulkerson, J. A., Friend, S., Horning, M., et al. (2018). Family home food environment and nutrition-related parent and child personal and behavioral outcomes of the Healthy Home Offerings via the Mealtime Environment (Home) Plus program: A randomized controlled trial. *Journal of the Academy of Nutrition and Dietetics*, *118*(2), 240–251. https://doi.org/10.1016/j.jand.2017.04.006.

Goode, R. W., Styn, M. A., Mendez, D. D., & Gary-Webb, T. L. (2017). African Americans in standard behavioral treatment for obesity, 2001–2015: What have we learned? *Western Journal of Nursing Research*, *39*(8), 1045–1069. https://doi.org/10.1177/0193945917692115.

Issner, J. H., Mucka, L. E., & Barnett, D. (2017). Increasing positive health behaviors in adolescents with nutritional goals and exercise. *Journal of Child and Family Studies*, *26*(2), 548–558. https://doi.org/10.1007/s10826-016-0585-4.

Jakicic, J. M., Powell, K. E., Campbell, W. W., et al. (2019). Physical activity and the prevention of weight gain in adults: A systematic review. *Medicine & Science in Sports & Exercise*, *51*(6), 1262–1269. https://doi.org/10.1249/MSS.0000000000001938.

Lee, H. J., Lee, S. Y., & Park, E. C. (2016). Do family meals affect childhood overweight or obesity? Nationwide survey 2008–2012. *Pediatric Obesity*, *11*(3), 161–165. https://doi.org/10.1111/ijpo.12035.

McCafferty, B. J., Hill, J. O., & Gunn, A. J. (2020). Obesity: Scope, lifestyle interventions, and medical management. *Techniques in Vascular and Interventional Radiology*, *23*(1), 100653. https://doi.org/10.1016/j.tvir.2020.100653.

McCurley, J. L., Gutierrez, A. P., & Gallo, L. C. (2017). Diabetes prevention in U.S. Hispanic adults: A systematic review of culturally tailored interventions. *American Journal of Preventive Medicine*, *52*(4), 519–529. https://doi.org/10.1016/j.amepre.2016.10.028.

Newton, R. L., Jr., Carter, L. A., Johnson, W., et al. (2018). A church-based weight loss intervention in African American adults using text messages (LEAN study): Cluster randomized controlled trial. *Journal of Medical Internet Research*, *20*(8), e256. https://doi.org/10.2196/jmir.9816.

Painter, S. L., Ahmed, R., Hill, J. O., et al. (2017). What matters in weight loss? An in-depth analysis of self-monitoring. *Journal of Medical Internet Research*, *19*(5), e160. https://doi.org10.2196/jmir.7457.

Poelman, M. P., de Vet, E., Velema, E., de Boer, M. R., Seidell, J. C., & Steenhuis, I. H. M. (2015). PortionControl@HOME: Results of a randomized controlled trial evaluating the effect of a multi-component portion size intervention on portion control behavior and body mass index. *Annals of Behavioral Medicine*, *49*(1), 18–28. https://doi.org/10.1007/s12160-014-9637-4.

Popa, A. R., Fratila, O., Rus, M., et al. (2020). Risk factors for adiposity in the urban population and influence on the prevalence of overweight and obesity. *Experimental and Therapeutic Medicine*, *20*(1), 129–133. https://doi.org/10.3892/etm.2020.8662.

Puhl, R. M., & Lessard, L. M. (2020). Weight stigma in youth: Prevalence, consequences, and considerations for clinical practice. *Current Obesity Reports*, *9*(4), 402–411. https://doi.org/10.1007/s13679-020-00408-8.

Raynor, H. A., & Champagne, C. M. (2016). Position of the academy of nutrition and dietetics: Interventions for the treatment of overweight

O

and obesity in adults. *Journal of the Academy of Nutrition and Dietetics, 116*(1), 129–147. https://doi.org/10.1016/j.jand.2015.10.031.

Romo, L. K. (2018). An examination of how people who have lost weight communicatively negotiate interpersonal challenges to weight management, health communication. *Health Communication, 33*(4), 469–477. https://doi.org/10.1080/10410236.2016.1278497.

St-Onge, M. P. (2017). Sleep-obesity relation: Underlying mechanisms and consequences for treatment. *Obesity Reviews, 18*(Suppl. 1), 34–39. https://doi.org/10.1111/obr.12499.

Thomason, D. L., Lukkahatai, N., Kawi, J., Connelly, K., & Inouye, J. (2016). A systematic review of adolescent self-management and weight loss. *Journal of Pediatric Health Care, 30*(6), 569–582. https://doi.org/10.1016/j.pedhc.2015.11.016.

Voils, C. I., Olsen, M. K., Gierisch, J. M., et al. (2017). Maintenance of weight loss after initiation of nutrition training: A randomized trial. *Annals of Internal Medicine, 166*(7), 463–471. https://doi.org/10.7326/M16-2160.

Overweight Domain 2 Nutrition Class 1 Ingestion

Marina Martinez-Kratz, MS, RN, CNE

NANDA-I

Definition

A condition in which an individual accumulates abnormal or excessive fat for age and gender.

Defining Characteristics

Adult: Body mass index >25 kg/m^2; Child 2 to 18 years: Body mass index >85th percentile or 25 kg/m^2 but <95th percentile or 30 kg/m^2 for age and gender; Child <2 years: Weight-for-length >95th percentile

Related Factors

Abnormal eating behavior patterns; abnormal eating perception patterns; average daily physical activity is less than recommended for age and gender; consumption of sugar-sweetened beverages; dyssomnias; energy expenditure below energy intake based on standard assessment; excessive alcohol consumption; fear regarding lack of food supply; frequent snacking; high frequency of restaurant or fried food; inadequate knowledge of modifiable factors; insufficient dietary calcium intake by children; portion sizes larger than recommended; sedentary behavior occurring for ≥ 2 hours/day; shortened sleep time; solid foods as major food source at < 5 months of age

At-Risk Population

ADULT: Body mass index approaching 25 kg/m^2; CHILD 2 to 18 years: Body mass index approaching 85th percentile or 25 kg/m^2; CHILD < 2 years: Weight-for-length approaching 95th percentile; children with body mass index crossing percentiles upward; children with high body mass index percentiles for age and gender; economically disadvantaged individuals; individuals who experienced premature pubarche; individuals who experienced rapid weight gain during childhood; individuals who experienced rapid weight gain during infancy; individuals who inherit interrelated factors; individuals who were not exclusively breastfed; individuals who were obese during childhood; individuals whose mothers have diabetes; individuals whose mothers smoke during childhood; individuals whose mothers smoke during pregnancy; individuals with high disinhibition and restraint eating behavior score; individuals with parents who are obese

Associated Conditions

Inborn genetic disorders

NOC (Nursing Outcomes Classification)

Suggested NOC Outcomes

Nutritional Status; Nutritional Status: Food and Fluid Intake; Nutrient Intake; Weight Control

Example NOC Outcome with Indicators

Nutritional Status as evidenced by the following indicators: Food and fluid intake/Hydration/Body mass index/Weight-height ratio/Hematocrit. (Rate the outcome and indicators of **Nutritional Status:** 1 = severe deviation from normal range, 2 = substantial deviation from normal range, 3 = moderate deviation from normal range, 4 = mild deviation from normal range, 5 = no deviation from normal range [see Section I].)

Client Outcomes

Client Will (Specify Time Frame)

- Explain how to eat according to the US Dietary Guidelines
- Design dietary modifications to meet individual long-term goal of health, using principles of variety, balance, and moderation
- Maintain weight within normal range for height and age

NIC (Nursing Interventions Classification)

Suggested NIC Interventions

Nutrition Management; Nutritional Counseling; Weight Reduction Assistance

Example NIC Activities—Nutrition Management

Determine the client's motivation for changing eating habits; Develop with the client a method to keep a daily record of intake

Nursing Interventions and *Rationales*

- Assess the meaning and importance of food in the client's life. **EB:** *Research found strong associations between the different domains of food meanings and behavioral outcomes (Arbit et al, 2017).*
- Assess client readiness to determine whether the client is ready to discuss weight loss and/or would like weight-loss information. **EB:** *Client motivation is a key component of success in a weight-loss program and a prerequisite for weight-loss therapy (Raynor & Champagne, 2016).*
- Use a motivational interviewing technique when working with clients to promote healthy eating and weight loss. **EB:** *Research shows significant weight loss for clients when motivational interviewing techniques were used (Barnes et al, 2018).*
- Counsel the client to measure regularly consumed foods periodically. Help the client learn usual portion sizes. Measuring food alerts the client to normal portion sizes. Estimating amounts can be extremely inaccurate. **EB:** *A randomized controlled trial of 278 overweight and obese participants was conducted to increase portion size awareness with results that demonstrated the intervention improved portion control behavior and in turn influenced body mass index (BMI) (Poelman et al, 2015).*
- Assist the client to develop a system of self-management, which may include self-monitoring of weight and BMI; realistic goal setting, planning, and action planning for improved dietary intake and physical activity; problem-solving; and tracking dietary intake and exercise. **EB:** *A key component of successful weight loss and maintenance is regular self-monitoring (Thomason et al, 2016).*
- Document the client's height and weight and teach the significance of his or her BMI in relationship to current health. Use a chart or a website such as http://www.cdc.gov/healthyweight/assessing/bmi/index.html (Centers for Disease Control and Prevention [CDC], 2020a). **EB:** *Successful treatment of overweight and obesity in adults requires the adoption and maintenance of effective self-monitoring (Raynor & Champagne, 2016).*
- Encourage the client to engage in vigorous-intensity physical activity for at least 150 minutes weekly or moderate-intensity physical activity for at least 300 minutes weekly. **EB:** *Research evidence suggests that regular physical activity is critical for weight loss and weight-loss maintenance (Ostendorf et al, 2018).*
- Recommend the client avoid eating in fast-food restaurants. **EB:** *A study found that fast-food consumption was the most frequent risk factor for adiposity found in 61.67% of study participants (Popa et al, 2020).*
- Assist the client to reframe slips in weight loss or physical activity behavior as lapses that are a single event and not a full return to previous unhealthy behaviors. Relapse prevention strategies include managing lapses in healthy behavior, identifying high-risk situations for relapses, self-monitoring, providing social

O

support, enhancing skills for coping, and increasing self-efficacy for avoiding relapse. **EB:** *A study of a weight maintenance intervention, delivered primarily by telephone, modestly slowed the rate of weight regain (Voils et al, 2017).*

- Assist clients to engage their social support systems either digitally or face to face in ways that facilitate weight loss, healthy eating, and physical activity behavior change. **EB:** *Significant others, family, friends, and coworkers can facilitate or hinder weight-loss success (Romo, 2018).*
- Assist the client to reframe the goal from a focus on outcome (weight loss) to a focus on process (eating behaviors) for weight loss. **EB:** *A study found that the self-monitoring behaviors of self-weigh-in, daily steps, high-intensity activity, and persistent food logging were significant predictors of weight loss during a 6-month intervention (Painter et al, 2017).*
- Assist the client to implement informal and formal mindfulness-based interventions (MBIs). Informal MBIs include mindful eating, increasing awareness of hunger and satiety cues, taste satisfaction, and decreasing impulsive tendencies to overeat when experiencing negative emotions. Meditation practice is a formal MBI. **EB:** *Results of a research review suggest that a combination of formal and informal MBIs are effective in reducing weight and improving obesity-related eating behaviors among individuals with overweight and obesity (Carrière et al, 2018).*
- Assist the client to develop stimulus control techniques designed to reduce environmental cues associated with eating behaviors. Specifically, clients should be taught to limit the presence of high-calorie/high-fat foods in the home; to reduce the visibility of unhealthy food choices in the home; to limit where and when they eat; to avoid distractions such as reading, using the computer, or watching television when eating; and to eat more slowly. **EB:** *Stimulus control strategies are the key to successful weight loss and weight maintenance in conjunction with other weight-loss strategies (Butryn et al, 2017).*
- Encourage 7.5 to 8.5 hours of sleep nightly. **EB:** *Evidence suggests that weight management is hindered when attempted in the context of sleep restriction because there is an upregulation of reward, pleasure, and salience networks in response to food stimuli (St-Onge, 2017).*
- Refer the client to a weight loss–related therapy group. **EBN:** *A study found significant changes in BMI, waist circumference, body fat percentage, and strength of the lower limbs for weight-loss group therapy participants (Ferrari et al, 2017).*
- Recommend that clients use dietary supplements such as vitamins and minerals after consulting with their primary health care provider. **EB:** *Research shows that micronutrient deficits are prevalent in weight-loss plans, especially vitamin B_{12}, calcium, and vitamin D (Engel et al, 2018).*
- Recommend the CDC behavior modification approach "reflect, replace, and reinforce" to improve eating habits. **EB:** *Reflect, replace, and reinforce consists of the following: (1) Reflect about intake through food journals, listing food habits, and identification of eating cues. (2) Replace habits identified during reflection with new and healthier behaviors, such as eating more slowly or planning meals ahead of time. (3) Reinforce changes made and having patience with the process (CDC, 2020b).*
- Incorporate the following recommendations from the Academy of Nutrition and Dietetics "Interventions for the Treatment of Overweight and Obesity in Adults" (Raynor & Champagne, 2016):
  - Assess food- and nutrition-related history; anthropometric measures; biochemical data, medical tests, and procedures; nutrition-focused physical findings; and client history.
  - Assess the energy intake and nutrient content of the diet.
  - Use height and weight to calculate BMI and waist circumference to determine risk of cardiovascular disease, type 2 diabetes, and all-cause mortality.
  - Use a measured resting metabolic rate to determine energy needs.
  - Set a realistic weight-loss goal such as one of the following: up to 2 pounds/week, up to 10% of baseline body weight, or a total of 3% to 5% of baseline weight if cardiovascular risk factors (hypertension, hyperlipidemia, and hyperglycemia) are present.
  - To achieve weight loss, use an individualized diet, including client preferences and health status, to achieve and maintain nutrient adequacy and reduce caloric intake, based on one of the following caloric reduction strategies: 1200 to 1500 kcal/day for women and 1500 to 1800 kcal/day for men, and energy deficit of approximately 500 or 750 kcal/day.

Pediatric

- Offer obese or overweight adolescents healthy methods for weight loss. **EB:** *A study showed statistically significant health behavior improvements after implementing a developmentally informed intervention to increase positive health diet and exercise behaviors (Issner et al, 2017).*

- Offer families of obese or overweight children prejudice-free, individually accepting, and supportive interventions to address weight loss. EB: *A review summarized recent evidence on weight stigma and found that it is highly prevalent among youth with high body weight, who are targets of weight-based victimization from peers, parents, and teachers (Puhl & Lessard, 2020).*
- Recommend that families eat together for at least one meal per day. EB: *A large Korean study found that the frequency of family meals was inversely associated with childhood overweight or obesity (Lee, Lee, & Park, 2016).*
- Recommend involving the family in planning meals and food preparation. Children can learn about nutrition as they help plan and make meals. EB: *The Healthy Home Offerings via the Mealtime Environment Plus program showed increased cooking skills among the children participating (Fulkerson et al, 2018).*
- Assist parents at being good role models of healthy eating. EB: *The Healthy Home Offerings via the Mealtime Environment Plus program showed significantly improved parental self-efficacy for identifying appropriate portion sizes (Fulkerson et al, 2018).*
- Recommend that the family try new foods, either a new food or recipe every week. EB: *The Healthy Home Offerings via the Mealtime Environment Plus program showed decreasing child neophobia scores over time that were developmentally appropriate (Fulkerson et al, 2018).*

Geriatric

- Determine the risks and benefits of weight loss in the older client. A BMI greater than 30 in the older client suggests a moderate weight-loss approach. EB: *Recommendations for treating obesity in the elderly include ensuring a balanced and appropriately distributed intake of high-quality nutrients, particularly of high-quality protein (i.e., 1.2 to 1.5 g/kg of body weight), limiting the intake of simple carbohydrates and saturated fats, and providing sufficient intake of calcium and vitamin D_3 (Blaž, 2016).*
- Observe for social, psychological, and economic factors that influence diet quality. EB: *An exploratory study of diet quality influences in community-dwelling older individuals revealed the following influences: food experiences, retirement, bereavement, medical conditions, food environment, food-related habits, social engagement, personal/psychological factors, and transportation (Bloom et al, 2017).*

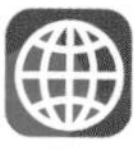

Multicultural

O

- Tailor nutritional interventions to be consistent with cultural beliefs, norms, and values. EB: *A systemic review of culturally tailored interventions for Hispanic women included literacy modification, Hispanic foods/recipes, cultural diabetes beliefs, family/friend participation, structured community input, and innovative experiential learning (McCurley et al, 2017).*
- Offer tailored lifestyle counseling via the telephone. EBN: *Investigators have included biweekly and/or monthly health coach calls for African American participants with significant weight gain prevention (Goode et al, 2017).*
- Integrate weight loss and weight maintenance interventions with church faith-based supports for African American clients. EB: *Recent research found that a church-based weight loss intervention using automated text messages was well-received by African American participants and resulted in significant weight loss (Newton, 2018).*

Client/Family Teaching and Discharge Planning

- The majority of the preceding interventions involve teaching.
- Work with the family members regarding information on how to support and promote weight loss and healthy intakes.

REFERENCES

Arbit, N., Ruby, M., & Rozin, P. (2017). Development and validation of the meaning of food in life questionnaire (MFLQ): Evidence for a new construct to explain eating behavior. *Food Quality and Preference*, *59*, 35–45. https://doi.org/10.1016/j.foodqual.2017.02.002.

Barnes, R. D., Ivezaj, V., Martino, S., Pittman, B. P., Paris, M., & Grilo, C. M. (2018). Examining motivational interviewing plus nutrition psychoeducation for weight loss in primary care. *Journal of Psychosomatic Research*, *104*, 101–107. https://doi.org/10.1016/j.jpsychores.2017.11.013.

Blaž, M. K. (2016). Obesity in the elderly, weight loss yes or no? [Abstract]. *Clinical Nutrition ESPEN*, *14*, 56. https://doi.org/10.1016/j.clnesp.2016.04.025.

Bloom, I., Lawrence, W., Barker, M., et al. (2017). What influences diet quality in older people? A qualitative study among community-dwelling older adults from the Hertfordshire Cohort Study, UK.

Public Health Nutrition, *20*(15), 2685–2693. https://doi.org/10.1017/S1368980017001203.

Butryn, M. L., Forman, E. M., Lowe, M. R., Gorin, A. A., Zhang, F., & Schaumberg, K. (2017). Efficacy of environmental and acceptance-based enhancements to behavioral weight loss treatment: The ENACT trial. *Obesity*, *25*(5), 866–872. https://doi.org/10.1002/oby.21813.

Carrière, K., Khoury, B., Günak, M. M., & Knäuper, B. (2018). Mindfulness-based interventions for weight loss: A systematic review and meta-analysis. *Obesity Reviews*, *19*(2), 164–177. https://doi.org/10.1111/obr.12623.

Centers for Disease Control and Prevention (CDC). (2020a). *Body mass index (BMI): How do I interpret body mass index information?* Retrieved from http://www.cdc.gov/healthyweight/assessing/bmi/index.html. [Accessed July 21, 2021].

Centers for Disease Control and Prevention (CDC). (2020b). *Improving your eating habits. Division of Nutrition, Physical Activity, and Obesity.* National Center for Chronic Disease Prevention and Health Promotion. Retrieved from https://www.cdc.gov/healthyweight/losing_weight/eating_habits.html. [Accessed July 21, 2021].

Engel, M. G., Kern, H. J., Brenna, J. T., & Mitmesser, S. H. (2018). Micronutrient gaps in three commercial weight-loss diet plans. *Nutrients*, *10*(1), 108. https://doi.org/10.3390/nu10010108.

Ferrari, G. D., Azevedo, M., Medeiros, L., et al. (2017). A multidisciplinary weight-loss program: The importance of psychological group therapy. *Motriz Revista de Educacao Fisica*, *23*(1), 47–52. https://doi.org/10.1590/s1980-6574201700010007.

Fulkerson, J. A., Friend, S., Horning, M., et al. (2018). Family home food environment and nutrition-related parent and child personal and behavioral outcomes of the healthy Home Offerings via the Mealtime Environment (Home) Plus program: A randomized controlled trial. *Journal of the Academy of Nutrition and Dietetics*, *118*(2), 240–251. https://doi.org/10.1016/j.jand.2017.04.006.

Goode, R. W., Styn, M. A., Mendez, D. D., & Gary-Webb, T. L. (2017). African Americans in standard behavioral treatment for obesity, 2001–2015: What have we learned? *Western Journal of Nursing Research*, *39*(8), 1045–1069. https://doi.org/10.1177/0193945917692115.

Issner, J. H., Mucka, L. E., & Barnett, D. (2017). Increasing positive health behaviors in adolescents with nutritional goals and exercise. *Journal of Child and Family Studies*, *26*(2), 548–558. https://doi.org/10.1007/s10826-016-0585-4.

Lee, H. J., Lee, S. Y., & Park, E. C. (2016). Do family meals affect childhood overweight or obesity? Nationwide survey 2008–2012. *Pediatric Obesity*, *11*(3), 161–165. https://doi.org/10.1111/ijpo.12035.

McCafferty, B. J., Hill, J. O., & Gunn, A. J. (2020). Obesity: Scope, lifestyle interventions, and medical management. *Techniques in Vascular and Interventional Radiology*, *23*(1), 100653. https://doi.org/10.1016/j.tvir.2020.100653.

McCurley, J. L., Gutierrez, A. P., & Gallo, L. C. (2017). Diabetes prevention in U.S. Hispanic adults: A systematic review of culturally tailored interventions. *American Journal of Preventive Medicine*, *52*(4), 519–529. https://doi.org/10.1016/j.amepre.2016.10.028.

Newton, R. L., Jr., Carter, L. A., Johnson, W., et al. (2018). A church-based weight loss intervention in African American adults using text messages (LEAN study): Cluster randomized controlled trial. *Journal of Medical Internet Research*, *20*(8), e256. https://doi.org/10.2196/jmir.9816.

Ostendorf, D. M., Lyden, K., Pan, Z., et al. (2018). Objectively measured physical activity and sedentary behavior in successful weight loss maintainers. *Obesity*, *26*(1), 53–60. https://doi.org/10.1002/oby.22052.

Painter, S. L., Ahmed, R., Hill, J. O., et al. (2017). What matters in weight loss? An in-depth analysis of self-monitoring. *Journal of Medical Internet Research*, *19*(5), e160. https://doi.org/10.2196/jmir.7457.

Poelman, M. P., de Vet, E., Velema, E., de Boer, M. R., Seidell, J. C., & Steenhuis, I. H. M. (2015). PortionControl@HOME: Results of a randomized controlled trial evaluating the effect of a multi-component portion size intervention on portion control behavior and body mass index. *Annals of Behavioral Medicine*, *49*(1), 18–28. https://doi.org/10.1007/s12160-014-9637-4.

Popa, A. R., Fratila, O., Rus, M., et al. (2020). Risk factors for adiposity in the urban population and influence on the prevalence of overweight and obesity. *Experimental and Therapeutic Medicine*, *20*(1), 129–133. https://doi.org/10.3892/etm.2020.8662.

Puhl, R. M., & Lessard, L. M. (2020). Weight stigma in youth: Prevalence, consequences, and considerations for clinical practice. *Current Obesity Reports*, *9*(4), 402–411. https://doi.org/10.1007/s13679-020-00408-8.

Raynor, H. A., & Champagne, C. M. (2016). Position of the academy of nutrition and dietetics: Interventions for the treatment of overweight and obesity in adults. *Journal of the Academy of Nutrition and Dietetics*, *116*(1), 129–147. https://doi.org/10.1016/j.jand.2015.10.031.

Romo, L. K. (2018). An examination of how people who have lost weight communicatively negotiate interpersonal challenges to weight management, health communication. *Health Communication*, *33*(4), 469–477. https://doi.org/10.1080/10410236.2016.1278497.

St-Onge, M. P. (2017). Sleep-obesity relation: Underlying mechanisms and consequences for treatment. *Obesity Reviews*, *18*(Suppl. 1), 34–39. https://doi.org/10.1111/obr.12499.

Thomason, D. L., Lukkahatai, N., Kawi, J., Connelly, K., & Inouye, J. (2016). A systematic review of adolescent self-management and weight loss. *Journal of Pediatric Health Care*, *30*(6), 569–582. https://doi.org/10.1016/j.pedhc.2015.11.016.

Voils, C. I., Olsen, M. K., Gierisch, J. M., et al. (2017). Maintenance of weight loss after initiation of nutrition training: A randomized trial. *Annals of Internal Medicine*, *166*(7), 463–471. https://doi.org/10.7326/M16-2160.

Risk for Overweight

Domain 2 Nutrition Class 1 Ingestion

Marina Martinez-Kratz, MS, RN, CNE

NANDA-I

Definition

Susceptible to excessive fat accumulation for age and gender, which may compromise health.

Risk Factors

Abnormal eating behavior patterns; abnormal eating perception patterns; average daily physical activity is less than recommended for age and gender; consumption of sugar-sweetened beverages; dyssomnias;

energy expenditure below energy intake based on standard assessment; excessive alcohol consumption; fear regarding lack of food supply; frequent snacking; high frequency of restaurant or fried food; inadequate knowledge of modifiable factors; insufficient dietary calcium intake by children; portion sizes larger than recommended; sedentary behavior occurring for ≥ 2 hours/day; shortened sleep time; solid foods as major food source at < 5 months of age

At-Risk Population

ADULT: Body mass index approaching 25 kg/m²; CHILD 2-18 years: Body mass index approaching 85th percentile or 25 kg/m²; CHILD < 2 years: Weight-for-length approaching 95th percentile; children with body mass index crossing percentiles upward; children with high body mass index percentiles for age and gender; economically disadvantaged individuals; individuals who experienced premature pubarche; individuals who experienced rapid weight gain during childhood; individuals who experienced rapid weight gain during infancy; individuals who inherit interrelated factors; individuals who were not exclusively breastfed; individuals who were obese during childhood; individuals whose mothers have diabetes; individuals whose mothers smoke during childhood; individuals whose mothers smoke during pregnancy; individuals with high disinhibition and restraint eating behavior score; individuals with parents who are obese

Associated Conditions

Inborn genetic diseases

NOC (Nursing Outcomes Classification)

Suggested NOC Outcomes

Nutritional Status; Nutritional Status: Food and Fluid Intake; Nutrient Intake; Weight Control

Example NOC Outcome With Indicators

Nutritional Status as evidenced by the following indicators: Food and fluid intake/Hydration/Body mass index/Weight-height ratio/Hematocrit. (Rate the outcome and indicators of **Nutritional Status:** 1 = severe deviation from normal range, 2 = substantial deviation from normal range, 3 = moderate deviation from normal range, 4 = mild deviation from normal range, 5 = no deviation from normal range [see Section I].)

O

Client Outcomes

Client Will (Specify Time Frame)

- Explain how to eat according to the US Dietary Guidelines
- Design dietary modifications to meet individual long-term goal of health, using principles of variety, balance, and moderation
- Maintain weight within normal range for height and age

NIC (Nursing Interventions Classification)

Suggested NIC Interventions

Nutrition Management; Nutritional Counseling; Weight Reduction Assistance

Example NIC Activities—Nutrition Management

Determine the client's motivation for changing eating habits; Develop with the client a method to keep a daily record of intake

Nursing Interventions and *Rationales*

- Assess the meaning and importance of food in the client's life. EB: *Recent research found strong associations between the different domains of food meanings and behavioral outcomes (Arbit et al, 2017).*
- Assess client readiness to determine whether the client is ready to discuss weight loss and/or would like weight-loss information. EB: *Client motivation is a key component of success in a weight-loss program and a prerequisite for weight-loss therapy (Raynor & Champagne, 2016).*

- Use a motivational interviewing technique when working with clients to promote healthy eating and weight loss. **EB:** *Research shows significant weight loss for clients when motivational interviewing techniques were used (Barnes et al, 2018).*
- Counsel the client to measure regularly consumed foods periodically. Help the client learn usual portion sizes. Measuring food alerts the client to normal portion sizes. Estimating amounts can be extremely inaccurate. **EB:** *A randomized controlled trial of 278 overweight and obese participants was conducted to increase portion size awareness with results that demonstrated the intervention improved portion control behavior and in turn influenced body mass index (BMI) (Poelman et al, 2015).*
- Assist the client to develop a system of self-management, which may include self-monitoring of weight and BMI; realistic goal setting, planning, and action planning for improved dietary intake and physical activity; problem-solving; and tracking dietary intake and exercise. **EB:** *A key component of successful weight loss and maintenance is regular self-monitoring (Thomason et al, 2016).*
- Document the client's height and weight and teach significance of his or her BMI in relationship to current health. Use a chart or a website such as http://www.cdc.gov/healthyweight/assessing/bmi/index.html (Centers for Disease Control and Prevention [CDC], 2020a). **EB:** *Successful treatment of overweight and obesity in adults requires adoption and maintenance of effective self-monitoring (Raynor & Champagne, 2016).*
- Encourage the client to engage in moderate-intensity physical activity (at least 150 minutes/week of moderate physical activity) to prevent weight gain. **EB:** *Research evidence suggests that regular physical activity is critical for weight loss and weight-loss maintenance (McCafferty, Hill, & Gunn, 2020).*
- Recommend that the client avoid eating in fast-food restaurants. **EB:** *A study found that fast-food consumption was the most frequent risk factor for adiposity found in 61.67% of study participants (Popa et al, 2020).*
- Assist the client to reframe slips in weight loss or physical activity behavior as lapses that are a single event and not a full return to previous unhealthy behaviors. Relapse prevention strategies include managing lapses in healthy behavior, identifying high-risk situations for relapses, self-monitoring, providing social support, enhancing skills for coping, and increasing self-efficacy for avoiding relapse. **EB:** *A study of a weight maintenance intervention, delivered primarily by telephone, modestly slowed the rate of weight regain (Voils et al, 2017).*
- Assist clients to engage their social support systems either digitally or face to face in ways that facilitate weight loss, healthy eating, and physical activity behavior change. **EB:** *Significant others, family, friends, and coworkers can facilitate or hinder weight-loss success (Romo, 2018).*
- Assist the client to reframe the goal from a focus on outcome (weight loss) to a focus on process (eating behaviors) for weight loss. **EB:** *A study found the self-monitoring behaviors of self-weigh-in, daily steps, high-intensity activity, and persistent food logging were significant predictors of weight loss during a 6-month intervention (Painter et al, 2017).*
- Assist the client to implement informal and formal mindfulness-based interventions (MBIs). Informal MBIs include mindful eating, increasing awareness of hunger and satiety cues, taste satisfaction, and decreasing impulsive tendencies to overeat when experiencing negative emotions. Meditation practice is a formal MBI. **EB:** *Results of a research review suggested that a combination of formal and informal MBIs are effective in reducing weight and improving obesity-related eating behaviors among individuals with overweight and obesity (Carrière et al, 2018).*
- Assist the client to develop stimulus control techniques designed to reduce environmental cues associated with eating behaviors. Specifically, clients should be taught to limit the presence of high-calorie/high-fat foods in the home; to reduce the visibility of unhealthy food choices in the home; to limit where and when they eat; to avoid distractions such as reading, using the computer, or watching television when eating; and to eat more slowly. **EB:** *Stimulus control strategies are a key to successful weight loss and weight maintenance in conjunction with other weight-loss strategies (Butryn et al, 2017).*
- Encourage 7.5 to 8.5 hours of sleep nightly. **EB:** *Evidence suggests that weight management is hindered when attempted in the context of sleep restriction because there is an upregulation of reward, pleasure, and salience networks in response to food stimuli (St-Onge, 2017).*
- Refer the client to a weight loss–related therapy group. **EBN:** *A study found significant changes in BMI, waist circumference, body fat percentage, and strength of the lower limbs for weight-loss group therapy participants (Ferrari et al, 2017).*
- Recommend that clients use dietary supplements such as vitamins and minerals after consulting with their primary health care provider. **EB:** *Research shows that micronutrient deficits are prevalent in weight-loss plans, especially vitamin B_{12}, calcium, and vitamin D (Engel et al, 2018).*

O

- Recommend the CDC behavior modification approach "reflect, replace, and reinforce" to improve eating habits. EB: *Reflect, replace, and reinforce consists of the following: (1) Reflect about intake through food journals, listing food habits, and identification of eating cues. (2) Replace habits identified during reflection with new and healthier behaviors, such as eating more slowly or planning meals ahead of time. (3) Reinforce changes made and having patience with the process (CDC, 2020b).*
- Incorporate the following recommendations from the Academy of Nutrition and Dietetics "Interventions for the Treatment of Overweight and Obesity in Adults" (Raynor & Champagne, 2016):
  - Assess food- and nutrition-related history; anthropometric measures; biochemical data, medical tests, and procedures; nutrition-focused physical findings; and client history.
  - Assess the energy intake and nutrient content of the diet.
  - Use height and weight to calculate BMI and waist circumference to determine risk of cardiovascular disease, type 2 diabetes, and all-cause mortality.
  - Use a measured resting metabolic rate to determine energy needs.
  - Set a realistic weight-loss goal such as one of the following: up to 2 pounds/week, up to 10% of baseline body weight, or a total of 3% to 5% of baseline weight if cardiovascular risk factors (hypertension, hyperlipidemia, and hyperglycemia) are present.
  - To achieve weight loss, use an individualized diet, including client preferences and health status, to achieve and maintain nutrient adequacy and reduce caloric intake, based on one of the following caloric reduction strategies: 1200 to 1500 kcal/day for women and 1500 to 1800 kcal/day for men and energy deficit of approximately 500 or 750 kcal/day.

Pediatric

- Offer obese or overweight adolescents healthy methods for weight loss. EB: *A study showed statistically significant health behavior improvements after implementing a developmentally informed intervention to increase positive health diet and exercise behaviors (Issner et al, 2017).*
- Offer families of obese or overweight children prejudice-free, individually accepting, and supportive interventions to address weight loss. EB: *A review summarized recent evidence on weight stigma and found that it is highly prevalent among youth with high body weight, who are targets of weight-based victimization from peers, parents, and teachers (Puhl & Lessard, 2020).*
- Recommend that families eat together for at least one meal per day. EB: *A large Korean study found that the frequency of family meals was inversely associated with childhood overweight or obesity (Lee, Lee, & Park, 2016).*
- Recommend involving the family in planning meals and food preparation. Children can learn about nutrition as they help plan and make meals. EB: *The Healthy Home Offerings via the Mealtime Environment Plus program showed increased cooking skills among the children participating (Fulkerson et al, 2018).*
- Assist parents at being good role models of healthy eating. EB: *The Healthy Home Offerings via the Mealtime Environment Plus program showed significantly improved parental self-efficacy for identifying appropriate portion sizes (Fulkerson et al, 2018).*
- Recommend that the family try new foods, either a new food or recipe every week. EB: *The Healthy Home Offerings via the Mealtime Environment Plus program showed decreasing child neophobia scores over time that were developmentally appropriate (Fulkerson et al, 2018).*

O

Geriatric

- Determine the risks and benefits of weight loss in the older client. A BMI greater than 30 in the older client suggests a moderate weight-loss approach. EB: *Recommendations for treating obesity in the elderly include ensuring a balanced and appropriately distributed intake of high-quality nutrients, particularly of high-quality protein (i.e., 1.2 to 1.5 g/kg of body weight), limiting the intake of simple carbohydrates and saturated fats, and providing sufficient intake of calcium and vitamin D_3 (Blaž, 2016).*
- Observe for social, psychological, and economic factors that influence diet quality. EB: *An exploratory study of diet quality influences in community-dwelling older individuals revealed the following influences: food experiences, retirement, bereavement, medical conditions, food environment, food-related habits, social engagement, personal/psychological factors, and transportation (Bloom et al, 2017).*

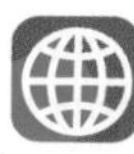

Multicultural

- Tailor nutritional interventions to be consistent with cultural beliefs, norms, and values. EB: *A systemic review of culturally tailored interventions for Hispanic women included literacy modification, Hispanic foods/recipes, cultural diabetes beliefs, family/friend participation, structured community input, and innovative experiential learning (McCurley et al, 2017).*

- Offer tailored lifestyle counseling via the telephone. EBN: *Investigators have included biweekly and/or monthly health coach calls for African American participants with significant weight gain prevention (Goode et al, 2017).*
- Integrate weight loss and weight maintenance interventions with church faith–based supports for African American clients. EB: *Recent research found a church-based weight loss intervention using automated SMS text messages was well-received by African American participants and resulted in significant weight loss (Newton et al, 2018).*

Client/Family Teaching and Discharge Planning

- The majority of the preceding interventions involve teaching.
- Work with the family members regarding information on how to support and promote weight loss and healthy intakes.

REFERENCES

Arbit, N., Ruby, M., & Rozin, P. (2017). Development and validation of the meaning of food in life questionnaire (MFLQ): Evidence for a new construct to explain eating behavior. *Food Quality and Preference*, *59*, 35–45. https://doi.org/10.1016/j.foodqual.2017.02.002.

Barnes, R. D., Ivezaj, V., Martino, S., Pittman, B. P., Paris, M., & Grilo, C. M. (2018). Examining motivational interviewing plus nutrition psychoeducation for weight loss in primary care. *Journal of Psychosomatic Research*, *104*, 101–107. https://doi.org.proxy/10.1016/j.jpsychores.2017.11.013.

Blaž, M. K. (2016). Obesity in the elderly, weight loss yes or no? [Abstract]. *Clinical Nutrition ESPEN*, *14*, 56. https://doi.org/10.1016/j.clnesp.2016.04.025.

Bloom, I., Lawrence, W., Barker, M., et al. (2017). What influences diet quality in older people? A qualitative study among community-dwelling older adults from the Hertfordshire Cohort Study, UK. *Public Health Nutrition*, *20*(15), 2685–2693. https://doi.org/10.1017/S1368980017001203.

Butryn, M. L., Forman, E. M., Lowe, M. R., Gorin, A. A., Zhang, F., & Schaumberg, K. (2017). Efficacy of environmental and acceptance-based enhancements to behavioral weight loss treatment: The ENACT trial. *Obesity*, *25*(5), 866–872. https://doi.org/10.1002/oby.21813.

Carrière, K., Khoury, B., Günak, M. M., & Knäuper, B. (2018). Mindfulness-based interventions for weight loss: A systematic review and meta-analysis. *Obesity Reviews*, *19*(2), 164–177. https://doi.org/10.1111/obr.12623.

Centers for Disease Control and Prevention (CDC). (2020a). *Body mass index (BMI): How do I interpret body mass index information?* Retrieved from http://www.cdc.gov/healthyweight/assessing/bmi/index.html Accessed July 21, 2021.

Centers for Disease Control and Prevention (CDC). (2020b). *Improving your eating habits*. Division of Nutrition, Physical Activity, and Obesity, National Center for Chronic Disease Prevention and Health Promotion. Retrieved from https://www.cdc.gov/healthyweight/losing_weight/eating_habits.html. Accessed July 21, 2021.

Engel, M. G., Kern, H. J., Brenna, J. T., & Mitmesser, S. H. (2018). Micronutrient gaps in three commercial weight-loss diet plans. *Nutrients*, *10*(1), 108. https://doi.org/10.3390/nu10010108.

Ferrari, G. D., Azevedo, M., Medeiros, L., et al. (2017). A multidisciplinary weight-loss program: The importance of psychological group therapy. *Motriz: Revista de Educacao Fisica*, *23*(1), 47–52. https://doi.org/10.1590/s1980-6574201700010007.

Fulkerson, J. A., Friend, S., Horning, M., et al. (2018). Family home food environment and nutrition-related parent and child personal and behavioral outcomes of the Healthy Home Offerings via the Mealtime Environment (Home) Plus Program: A randomized controlled trial. *Journal of the Academy of Nutrition and Dietetics*, *118*(2), 240–251. https://doi.org/10.1016/j.jand.2017.04.006.

Goode, R. W., Styn, M. A., Mendez, D. D., & Gary-Webb, T. L. (2017). African Americans in standard behavioral treatment for obesity, 2001–2015: What have we learned? *Western Journal of Nursing Research*, *39*(8), 1045–1069. https://doi.org/10.1177/0193945917692115.

Issner, J. H., Mucka, L. E., & Barnett, D. (2017). Increasing positive health behaviors in adolescents with nutritional goals and exercise. *Journal of Child and Family Studies*, *26*(2), 548–558. https://doi.org/10.1007/s10826-016-0585-4.

Lee, H. J., Lee, S. Y., & Park, E. C. (2016). Do family meals affect childhood overweight or obesity? Nationwide survey 2008–2012. *Pediatric Obesity*, *11*(3), 161–165. https://doi.org/10.1111/ijpo.12035.

McCafferty, B. J., Hill, J. O., & Gunn, A. J. (2020). Obesity: Scope, lifestyle interventions, and medical management. *Techniques in Vascular and Interventional Radiology*, *23*(1), 100653. https://doi.org/10.1016/j.tvir.2020.100653.

McCurley, J. L., Gutierrez, A. P., & Gallo, L. C. (2017). Diabetes prevention in U.S. Hispanic adults: A systematic review of culturally tailored interventions. *American Journal of Preventive Medicine*, *52*(4), 519–529. https://doi.org/10.1016/j.amepre.2016.10.028.

Newton, R. L., Jr., Carter, L. A., Johnson, W., et al. (2018). A church-based weight loss intervention in African American adults using text messages (LEAN study): Cluster randomized controlled trial. *Journal of Medical Internet Research*, *20*(8), e256. https://doi.org/10.2196/jmir.9816.

Painter, S. L., Ahmed, R., Hill, J. O., et al. (2017). What matters in weight loss? An in-depth analysis of self-monitoring. *Journal of Medical Internet Research*, *19*(5), e160. https://doi.org/10.2196/jmir.7457.

Poelman, M. P., de Vet, E., Velema, E., de Boer, M. R., Seidell, J. C., & Steenhuis, I. H. M. (2015). PortionControl@HOME: Results of a randomized controlled trial evaluating the effect of a multi-component portion size intervention on portion control behavior and body mass index. *Annals of Behavioral Medicine*, *49*(1), 18–28. https://doi.org/10.1007/s12160-014-9637-4.

Popa, A. R., Fratila, O., Rus, M., et al. (2020). Risk factors for adiposity in the urban population and influence on the prevalence of overweight and obesity. *Experimental and Therapeutic Medicine*, *20*(1), 129–133. https://doi.org/10.3892/etm.2020.8662.

Puhl, R. M., & Lessard, L. M. (2020). Weight stigma in youth: Prevalence, consequences, and considerations for clinical practice. *Current Obesity Reports*, *9*(4), 402–411. https://doi.org/10.1007/s13679-020-00408-8.

Raynor, H. A., & Champagne, C. M. (2016). Position of the academy of nutrition and dietetics: Interventions for the treatment of overweight

O

and obesity in adults. *Journal of the Academy of Nutrition and Dietetics*, *116*(1), 129–147. https://doi.org/10.1016/j.jand.2015.10.031.

Romo, L. K. (2018). An examination of how people who have lost weight communicatively negotiate interpersonal challenges to weight management, health communication. *Health Communication*, *33*(4), 469–477. https://doi.org/10.1080/10410236.2016.1278497.

St-Onge, M. P. (2017). Sleep-obesity relation: Underlying mechanisms and consequences for treatment. *Obesity Reviews*, *18*, 34–39. https://doi.org/10.1111/obr.12499. Suppl 1.

Thomason, D. L., Lukkahatai, N., Kawi, J., Connelly, K., & Inouye, J. (2016). A systematic review of adolescent self-management and weight loss. *Journal of Pediatric Health Care*, *30*(6), 569–582. https://doi.org/10.1016/j.pedhc.2015.11.016.

Voils, C. I., Olsen, M. K., Gierisch, J. M., et al. (2017). Maintenance of weight loss after initiation of nutrition training: A randomized trial. *Annals of Internal Medicine*, *166*(7), 463–471. https://doi.org/10.7326/M16-2160.

Acute Pain **Domain 12 Comfort Class 1 Physical comfort**

Denise Sullivan, MSN, ANP-BC, ACHPN, AP-PMN and Maureen F. Cooney, DNP, FNP-BC, ACHPN, AP-PMN

NANDA-I

Definition

Unpleasant sensory and emotional experience associated with actual or potential tissue damage, or described in terms of such damage (International Association for the Study of Pain); sudden or slow onset of any intensity from mild to severe with an anticipated or predictable end, and with a duration of less than 3 months.

Defining Characteristics

Altered physiological parameter; appetite change; diaphoresis; distraction behavior; evidence of pain using standardized pain behavior checklist for those unable to communicate verbally; expressive behavior; facial expression of pain; guarding behavior; hopelessness; narrow focus; positioning to ease pain; protective behavior; proxy report of activity changes; proxy report of pain behavior; pupil dilation; reports intensity using standardized pain scale; reports pain characteristics using standardized pain instrument; self-focused

O

Related Factors

Biological injury agent; inappropriate use of chemical agent; physical injury agent

NOC (Nursing Outcomes Classification)

Suggested NOC Outcomes

Pain Control; Pain Level; Pain: Adverse Psychological Response

Example NOC Outcome

Pain Level as evidenced by severity of observed or reported pain

Note: **Pain Level** is the NOC Outcome label; this text recommends use of the self-report numerical pain rating scale in place of the NOC indicator scales because of the amount of research supporting its use.

Client Outcomes

Client Will (Specify Time Frame)

For the Client Who Is Able to Provide a Self-Report

- Use a self-report pain tool to identify current pain intensity level and establish a comfort-function goal
- Report that the pain management regimen achieves comfort-function goal without side effects
- Notify member of the health care team promptly for pain intensity level that is consistently greater than the comfort-function goal, or occurrence of side effects
- Describe nonpharmacological methods that can be used to help achieve comfort-function goal
- Perform activities of recovery or activities of daily living (ADLs) easily
- Describe how unrelieved pain will be managed
- State ability to obtain sufficient amounts of rest and sleep

For the Client Who Is Unable to Provide a Self-Report

- Decrease in pain-related behaviors
- Perform activities of recovery or ADLs easily as determined by client condition
- Demonstrate the absence of side effects of analgesics
- No pain-related behaviors will be evident in the client who is completely unresponsive; demonstrate a reasonable absence of side effects related to the prescribed pain treatment plan

NIC (Nursing Interventions Classification)

Suggested NIC Interventions

Analgesic Administration; Pain Management; Client-Controlled Analgesia (PCA) Assistance

Example NIC Activities—Pain Management

Ensure client-attentive analgesic care; Perform a comprehensive assessment of pain to include location, characteristics, onset/duration, frequency, quality, intensity or severity of pain, and precipitating factors

Nursing Interventions and *Rationales*

- During the initial assessment and interview, if the client is experiencing pain, or when pain first occurs, conduct and document a comprehensive pain assessment, using appropriate pain assessment tools. CEB/EBN: *Determining location, quality, onset/duration, temporal aspects, pain intensity, characteristics, and the effect of pain on function and quality of life are critical to determine the underlying cause of pain and effectiveness of treatment (McCaffery, 1968; Drew & Peltier, 2018). The initial assessment includes all pain information that the client can provide for the development of the individualized pain management plan (Drew & Peltier, 2018; Raja et al, 2020).*
- Assess if the client is able to provide a self-report of pain intensity, and if so, assess pain intensity level using a valid and reliable self-report pain tool. EB: *Acute pain should be regularly and routinely assessed both at rest (important for comfort) and during movement (important for function and decreased client risk for cardiopulmonary and thromboembolic events) and with interventions or procedures likely to cause pain (Chou et al, 2016; Drew & Peltier, 2018; Raja et al, 2020).*
- Ask the client to describe prior experiences with pain, effectiveness of pain management interventions, responses to analgesic medications (including occurrence of side effects), and concerns about pain and its treatment (e.g., fear about addiction, worries, anxiety). EBN: *Obtaining an individualized pain history helps identify potential factors that may influence the client's willingness to report pain, as well as factors that may influence pain intensity, the client's response to pain, anxiety, and response to analgesic interventions (Drew & Peltier, 2018).* EB: *Anxiety and fear may intensify pain, and pain may trigger emotional responses such as fear and anxiety (Zhuo, 2016).*
- Using a self-report pain tool, ask the client to identify a comfort-function goal that will allow the client to perform necessary or desired activities easily. EBN: *The comfort-function goal provides the basis for individualized pain management plans and assists in determining effectiveness of pain management interventions (Arnstein et al, 2019).*
- Use the Hierarchy of Pain Measures as a framework for pain assessment: (1) consider the client's condition and search for possible causes of pain (e.g., presence of tissue injury, pathological conditions, exposure to procedures/interventions that are thought to result in pain); (2) attempt to obtain the client's self-report of pain; (3) observe for behaviors that may indicate pain presence (e.g., facial expressions, crying, restlessness, changes in activity); (4) speak with the client's significant others (i.e., parent, spouse, health care provider) about the client's customary behavioral responses to pain; and (5) conduct an analgesic trial. EBN: *When a client is unable to use a self-report tool (e.g., developmental age, intellectual disability, advanced dementia, critical illness/unconscious, anesthetized or sedated), the presence of pain may be assessed by observing specific client behaviors using a valid and reliable behavioral tool (e.g., Critical Care Observation Tool in the critically ill or Checklist of Nonverbal Pain Indicators in cognitively impaired older adults) (Herr et al, 2019).*
- Vital signs should not be used to determine or validate the presence or absence of pain. EBN: *Vital signs do not provide strong evidence for the presence of pain, particularly in the neurosurgical intensive care unit client, but may be used as cues for the presence of pain when behavioral indicators are not validated in*

P

unconscious clients (Erden et al, 2018). **EB:** *Vital signs do not reflect or substantiate self-reported acute pain in clients in the emergency department (Daoust et al, 2016).*

- ● Assume that pain is present if the client is unable to provide a self-report and has tissue injury, has a pathological condition, or has undergone a procedure that is thought to produce pain, and conduct an analgesic trial. **EBN:** *Pain is associated with actual or potential tissue damage such as pathological conditions (e.g., cancer) and procedures (e.g., surgery or trauma, fractures). In the absence of self-report (e.g., anesthetized, critically ill, or cognitively impaired client), the health care provider should use clinical judgment and assume pain is present, and then implement pain management interventions accordingly (Herr et al, 2019).*
- ✱ Obtain and review an accurate and complete list of medications the client is taking or has taken. **EB:** *Accurate medication reconciliation can guide analgesic plan development and prevent errors associated with incorrect medications, dosages, omission of components of the home medication regimen, drug–drug interactions, and toxicity that can occur when incompatible drugs are combined or when allergies are present (Rungvivatjarus et al, 2020).*
- ▲ Recognize the adverse effects of unrelieved pain. **EB:** *Unrelieved acute pain can have harmful effects that facilitate negative client outcomes such as increased morbidity, decreased quality of life, functional impairment, and prolonged recovery time and duration of opioid use and may lead to the development of chronic pain (Gan, 2017).*
- ▲ Explain to the client the pain management approach, including pharmacological and nonpharmacological interventions, the assessment and reassessment process, potential side effects, and the importance of prompt reporting of unrelieved pain. **EBN:** *Clients who receive education interventions preoperatively have been shown to readily report medication side effects and use more nonpharmacological methods for pain control compared to those who do not receive preoperative educational interventions (O'Donnell, 2018).*
- ▲ Reassure the client that pain will be regularly assessed and treated and that they will be observed for medication side effects and signs of opioid use disorder (OUD). **CEB:** *Cogan et al (2014) reported that among 379 clients scheduled for cardiac surgery, 31% stated that it is easy to become addicted to pain medication, 20% report that "good clients" do not talk about their pain, and 35% believe that pain medication should be "saved in case the pain worsens."*
- ● Teach the client about pain and pharmacological and nonpharmacological interventions when pain is relatively well controlled. **EB:** *Pain causes cognitive impairment (Baker et al, 2017).*
- ▲ Regularly reassess the client for the presence of pain and response to pain management interventions, including effectiveness and the presence of adverse effects related to pain management interventions. Review the client's pain flow sheet and medication administration record to evaluate effectiveness of pain relief, previous 24-hour opioid requirements, and occurrence of side effects. **EBN:** *Systematic tracking of pain is an important factor in improving pain management and making adjustments to the pain management regimen (Eksterowicz & DiMaggio, 2018).*
- ▲ Advocate for and manage acute pain using a multimodal, opioid-sparing approach. **EB:** *A multimodal approach (combining two or more drugs that act by different mechanisms for providing analgesia) enhances pain relief and allows the lowest effective dose of each drug to be administered, resulting in fewer or less severe side effects, such as nausea, sedation, and respiratory depression (Sullivan et al, 2016; Polomano et al, 2017).*
- ▲ Select the route for administration of analgesics based on client condition and pain characteristics. **EB:** *Routes have different rates of onset and duration. The oral route is preferred because of its convenience and the resulting relatively steady blood levels; the rectal route may be used when the oral route is not feasible; the intravenous (IV) route is preferred for rapid control of severe pain and would therefore not generally be used for chronic pain; and intramuscular (IM) injections are avoided because of variable absorption and the potential for nerve injury and tissue damage (Chou et al, 2016).*
- ▲ Support the use of perineural infusions and intraspinal analgesia when appropriate and available. **EB:** *Regional analgesia techniques offer the advantages of reduced opioid use, improved satisfaction, early mobility, and prevention of chronic postoperative surgical pain (Hassell & Stimpson, 2019).*
- ▲ Use diverse analgesic delivery methods such as PCA to improve postoperative pain control and increase clients' satisfaction with pain management. **EB:** *In a systematic review of the use of PCA for postoperative pain, moderate- to low-quality evidence was found that PCA provided better pain control and increased client satisfaction compared with non–client-controlled approaches (McNicol et al, 2015).*
- ▲ Administer a nonopioid analgesic for mild to moderate pain and add an opioid analgesic if indicated for moderate to severe acute pain. **EB:** *Nonopioids, such as acetaminophen and nonsteroidal antiinflammatory*

P

drugs, are first-line analgesics for the treatment of mild and some moderate acute pain, whereas opioids are included for the treatment of moderate to severe acute pain (Chou et al, 2016).

- • Avoid administering analgesics based solely on a client's pain intensity rating. EB: *Administering opioid doses based solely on pain intensity disregards the other essential elements of the pain assessment and may contribute to adverse client outcomes such as excessive sedation and respiratory depression as a result of overmedication or result in poorly controlled pain from undermedication (Pasero et al, 2016).*
- • Administer nonopioid analgesics around the clock for acute postoperative pain and if necessary opioid analgesics for intermittent or breakthrough pain. EB: *Postoperative pain is often constant during the first 24 hours after surgery, therefore necessitating the use of around-the-clock analgesics (Chou et al, 2016).*
- • Prevent pain by administering analgesia before painful procedures whenever possible (e.g., endotracheal suctioning, wound care, heel puncture, venipunctures, and peripherally inserted IV catheters). CEB: *Adult clients in the intensive care setting experience numerous sources of procedural pain, and chest tube removal, wound drain removal, and arterial line insertion are identified as the most painful procedures (Puntillo et al, 2014).*
- • Perform nursing care during the peak effect of analgesics to optimize client comfort and participation in care. EB: *Providing care such as mobilization and bathing should be performed when analgesics have reached peak effect: oral medications peak in 60 minutes, subcutaneous opioids in 30 minutes, and IV analgesics in 15 to 30 minutes (Eksterowicz & DiMaggio, 2018).*
- • Advocate for the use of "as needed" opioid range orders to provide effective and appropriate pain relief. EB: *Correctly prescribed range orders for the delivery of IV opioids give nurses the flexibility needed to treat clients' pain in a timely manner while allowing for differences in client response to pain and to analgesia (Drew et al, 2018).*
- • Choose analgesic and dose based on orders that reflect the client's report of pain severity and response to the previous dose in terms of pain relief, occurrence of side effects, and ability to perform the activities of recovery or ADLs. EB: *Safe and effective pain management requires opioid dose adjustment based on individualized adequate pain and sedation assessment, opioid administration, and evaluation of the response to treatment (Drew et al, 2018).*
- ▲ When converting opioids from parenteral doses to oral doses (the preferred route when the client can tolerate and absorb oral medications), use equianalgesic dosing charts and carefully monitor the client's response to the new medication route and dose. EB: *Equianalgesic dosing calculations should be used cautiously to guide dose conversion of an opioid from one route to another to avoid the toxicity associated with overdosing and the inadequate pain control caused by underdosing (Fudin et al, 2017).*
- ▲ Although all clients who are receiving opioids for acute pain are at risk for serious opioid-related adverse effects such as advancing sedation and respiratory depression, some are at even higher risk. Clients should have frequent respiratory assessment (rate, rhythm, noisiness, and depth) and systematic assessment of sedation level using a sedation scale. EB: *Opioid-induced respiratory depression occurs with the greatest frequency in postoperative clients during the first 24 hours after surgery, and factors contributing to postoperative respiratory depression include opioid dosage, administrative route, client-specific factors, concurrent administration of other sedating medications, and inadequate nursing assessments of sedation and respiratory status (Gupta et al, 2018; Jungquist et al, 2020).*
- ▲ When opioids are included in the multimodal analgesic plan, clients need regular assessment for common side effects such as constipation, nausea, pruritus, lack of appetite, and changes in rest and sleep, and preventive measures are implemented when possible.
- • Monitor frequency of bowel movements and alert the opioid prescriber when frequency is reduced. EB: *Opioid-induced constipation significantly affects quality of life. There is controversy as to the most effective prevention and treatment. Opioid reduction strategies and use of nonopioid analgesics are recommended to reduce risk (Müller-Lissner et al, 2017).*
- ▲ Support the client's use of nonpharmacological methods to supplement pharmacological analgesic approaches to help control pain, such as distraction, imagery, music therapy, simple massage, relaxation, and application of heat and cold. EBN: *Although more evidence is needed to conclude effectiveness, nonpharmacological methods (which are low cost and low risk) can be used to complement pharmacological treatment of pain (dos Santos Felix et al, 2019).* EBN: *Evidence suggests efficacy and satisfaction when complementary therapies are integrated into pain treatment plans of older adults (Bruckenthal et al, 2016).*
- ▲ Assist client to identify resources for coping with psychological impact of pain. EB: *Cognitive behavioral (mind–body) strategies can restore the client's sense of self-control, personal efficacy, and active participation in his or her own care.* EB: *Nurses should advocate for cognitive behavioral therapy as first-line therapy and*

P

especially when medications are contraindicated, not well tolerated, or refused and when clients are exhibiting ineffective coping skills (O'Connor-Von & Heck, 2018).

Pediatric

- Assess for the presence of pain using a valid and reliable pain scale based on age, cognitive development, and the child's ability to provide a self-report. Pain intensity scales should be used in conjunction with valid and reliable tools that assess the impact of pain on the child's quality of life (Manworren & Stinson, 2016). EB: *The Face, Legs, Activity, Cry, Consolability (FLACC) Scale demonstrated strong reliability in clients ages 6 months to 5 years in the pediatric emergency department (Kochman et al, 2017).* EB: *Whenever possible, a child's report of pain should be obtained. In a study of children ages 3 to 7.5 years with acute pain in the emergency department, there was no agreement between child's self-report and caregiver report of pain (Lawson et al, 2019).*
- ▲ Administer prescribed analgesics using a multimodal approach to treat pain in children, infants, and neonates. EB: *Multimodal analgesia improves pain and reduces opioid requirements in postoperative pediatric clients (Manworren et al, 2016).* EB: *Multimodal analgesia, including nonpharmacological and pharmacological approaches, reduces procedural pain and anxiety in pediatric acute care (Olsen & Weinberg, 2017).*
- Prevent procedural pain in neonates, infants, and children by using analgesics and sedatives as indicated. EB: *The use of intranasal fentanyl and midazolam when administered alone or in combination can provide effective pain and anxiety relief for pediatric clients undergoing minor procedures in the pediatric urgent care setting (Williams et al, 2020; Young, 2017).*
- Use a topical local anesthetic treatment or other nonpharmacological treatment before performing venipuncture in neonates, infants, and children. EBN: *Nonpharmacological methods can be used to reduce pain and fear in children during painful procedures. Mechanical vibration with use of the Buzzy System has been shown to be more effective than the ShotBlocker or bubble blowing in children undergoing IM injections in the emergency department (Yilmaz & Alemdar, 2019).*
- For the neonate, use oral sucrose and nonnutritional sucking (NNS) or human milk for pain of short duration such as heel stick or venipuncture. Neonates, especially preterm neonates, are more sensitive to pain than older children. CEB: *In an integrated literature review, Naughton (2013) found that the combination of oral sucrose and NNS is a safe and effective method of relieving pain in neonates and increases the calming effect in infants undergoing painful procedures.* EBN: *In a randomized control trial involving newborns undergoing heel stick, the use of either breastfeeding, oral sucrose, NNS, or skin-to-skin contact decreased pain when compared with the control group (Chang et al, 2020).*
- As with adults, use nonpharmacological analgesic interventions to supplement, not replace, pharmacological interventions in pediatric clients. EB: *Infants who underwent upper limb massage before venipuncture had significantly less pain with venipuncture than when massage was not used (Chik et al, 2017). Pain and distress in children receiving immunizations were significantly reduced when live music therapy was used during the immunization procedure (Sundar et al, 2016).*

P

Geriatric

- Refer to the Nursing Interventions and *Rationales* in the care plan for Chronic **Pain.**

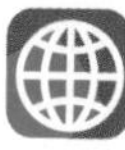

Multicultural

- Refer to the Nursing Interventions and *Rationales* in the care plan for Chronic **Pain.**

Home Care

- ▲ Develop the treatment plan with the client and caregivers. EB: *Client education and motivation play important roles in self-management of clients with pain. Self-management is influenced by client–provider communication (Drake & Williams, 2017; Haverfield et al, 2018).*
- ✱ Assess the client's full medication profile, including medications prescribed by all health care providers and all over-the-counter (OTC) medications for drug interactions, and educate the client about the need to discuss use of all medications, including OTC medications, with the health care provider. EB: *A medication safety improvement project using an evidence-based medication management software system was used to address the need for accurate identification of medications taken by clients, early identification of medication-related problems, identification of drug duplication, and identification of problems with medication self-management, with the goal of improving medication safety in home health care (LeBlanc & Choi, 2015).*

▲ Assess the client/family's knowledge of side effects and safety precautions associated with pain medications. EB: *Educational activities related to pain medications are necessary to ensure that clients are knowledgeable about opioid side effects and safety. McCarthy et al (2015) found that clients who read a one-page information sheet they were given about hydrocodone-acetaminophen safety had better knowledge of precautions related to acetaminophen dosing, and they were less likely to drive a car within 6 hours of taking the medication than those who did not receive this educational intervention.*

• If medication is administered using highly technological methods, assess the home for the necessary resources (e.g., electricity) and ensure that there will be responsible caregivers available to assist the client with administration. EB: *The use of advanced medical technologies is part of the technical nursing process, and nurses have a key role supporting clients and family care providers in their safe use (Ten Haker et al, 2018).*

• Assess the knowledge base of the client and family regarding highly technological medication administration and provide necessary education, including the procedure to follow if analgesia is unsatisfactory. EB: *With appropriate education and training, the use of PCA in home care has been shown to be a safe and effective analgesic modality for children and young adults with cancer (Anghelescu et al, 2015).*

Client/Family Teaching and Discharge Planning

Note: To avoid the negative connotations associated with the words "drugs" and "narcotics," use the term "pain medicine" when teaching clients.

• Discuss the various discomforts encompassed by the word "pain" and ask the client to give examples of previously experienced pain. Explain the pain assessment process and the purpose of the pain rating scale. EB: *It is often difficult for clients to understand the concept of pain and describe their pain experience. Using alternative words and providing a complete description of the assessment process, including the use of scales, ensures that an accurate treatment plan is developed (Drew & Peltier, 2018).*

• Teach the client to use the self-report pain tool to rate the intensity of past or current pain. Ask the client to set a comfort-function goal by selecting a pain level on the self-report tool that will allow performance of desired or necessary activities of recovery with relative ease (e.g., turn, cough, deep breathe, ambulate, participate in physical therapy). If the pain level is consistently above the comfort-function goal, the client should take action that decreases pain or notify a member of the health care team so that effective pain management interventions may be implemented promptly. EB: *The use of comfort-function goals provides the basis for the direction and modification of the treatment plan (Eksterowicz & DiMaggio, 2018).*

• Provide written educational materials on various aspects of pain control to improve client understanding of pain and pain-related interventions. EB: *Written materials and other educational tools assist in improving clients' knowledge related to pain management. In knee replacement clients, the use of a simple educational pain management card was associated with reduced opioid use without compromising pain satisfaction in pain relief or participation in rehabilitation therapy. The education card listed scheduled and as-needed (PRN) analgesic medications, the indication and frequency of availability, and a pain rating scale (Yajnik et al, 2019).*

• Discuss and evaluate the client's understanding of the total plan for pharmacological and nonpharmacological treatment, including the medications prescribed and their indication, proper dosing schedule, and adverse events and what to do should they occur. EB: *Appropriate instruction increases the accuracy and safety of medication administration (Drew & Peltier, 2018).*

• Teach basic principles of pain management using a variety of educational strategies, and evaluate learning. EB: *Client educational strategies that have been shown to increase knowledge, decrease anxiety, and increase satisfaction include the use of computer technology, audiotapes and videotapes, written materials, and demonstrations, or combinations of these strategies (Curtiss & Wrona, 2018).*

▲ Reinforce the importance of taking pain medications to maintain the comfort-function goal. EB: *Teaching clients to stay on top of their pain and prevent it from getting out of control will improve the ability to accomplish the goals of recovery (Eksterowicz & DiMaggio, 2018).*

▲ Reinforce that short-term use of opioids for acute pain relief is an appropriate part of their multimodal pain treatment plan. EB: *Taking opioids only as directed, avoiding alcohol, and talking with the health care provider when pain is poorly controlled are strategies that will lessen the risks for OUD or major opioid-related adverse effects such as respiratory depression and arrest (Costello, 2015).*

▲ Reinforce the importance of safe storage of opioid medications out of the reach of others, and teach clients how to responsibly dispose of any unused opioids. EBN: *Perianesthesia nurses have a responsibility to educate their clients on discharge from ambulatory surgery about safe opioid use, storage, and disposal (Odom-Forren et al, 2019).*

P

* ✱ Client education by nurses in the emergency department setting related to the use, storage, and disposal of pain medications may increase client knowledge and promote safety (Waszak et al, 2018).
* ▲ Demonstrate the use of appropriate nonpharmacological approaches in addition to pharmacological approaches to help control pain, such as application of heat and/or cold, distraction techniques, relaxation breathing, visualization, rocking, stroking, listening to music, and watching television. **EB:** *Nonpharmacological interventions are used to complement, not replace, pharmacological interventions (Bruckenthal et al, 2016).*

REFERENCES

Anghelescu, D. L., Zhang, K., Faughnan, L. G., & Pei, D. (2015). The safety and effectiveness of patient-controlled analgesia in outpatient children and young adults with cancer: A retrospective study. *Journal of Pediatric Hematology, 37*(5), 378–382.

Arnstein, P., Gentile, D., & Wilson, M. (2019). Validating the functional pain scale for hospitalized adults. *Pain Management Nursing, 20*(5), 418–424.

Baker, K. S., Georgiou-Karistianis, N., Gibson, S. J., & Giummarra, M. J. (2017). Optimizing cognitive function in persons with chronic pain. *The Clinical Journal of Pain, 33*(5), 462–472.

Bruckenthal, P., Marino, M. A., & Snelling, L. (2016). Complementary and integrative therapies for persistent pain management in older adults: A review. *Journal of Gerontological Nursing, 42*(12), 40–48.

Chang, J., Filoteo, L., & Nasr, A. S. (2020). Comparing the analgesic effects of 4 nonpharmacologic interventions on term newborns undergoing heel lance: A randomized controlled trial. *Journal of Perinatal and Neonatal Nursing, 34*(4), 338–345.

Chik, Y. M., Ip, W. Y., & Choi, K. C. (2017). The effect of upper limb massage on infants' venipuncture pain. *Pain Management Nursing, 18*(1), 50–57.

Chou, R., Gordon, D. B., de Leon-Casasola, O. A., et al. (2016). Management of postoperative pain: A clinical practice guideline from the American Pain Society, the American Society of Regional Analgesia and Pain Medicine, and the American Society of Anesthesiologists' Committee on Regional Anesthesia, Executive Committee, and Administrative Council. *Journal of Pain, 17*(2), 131–157.

Cogan, J., Ouimette, M. F., Vargas-Schaffer, G., Yegin, Z., Deschamps, A., & Denault, A. (2014). Patient attitudes and beliefs regarding pain medication after cardiac surgery: Barriers to adequate pain management. *Pain Management Nursing, 15*(3), 574–579.

Costello, M. (2015). Prescription opioid analgesics: Promoting patient safety with better patient education. *American Journal of Nursing, 115*(11), 50–56.

Curtiss, C. P., & Wrona, S. (2018). Pain management education. In M. L. Czarnecki, & H. N. Turner (Eds.), *Core curriculum for pain management nursing* (3rd ed.) (pp. 589–601). St. Louis: Elsevier.

Daoust, R., Paquet, J., Bailey, B., et al. (2016). Vital signs are not associated with self-reported acute pain intensity in the emergency department. *Canadian Journal of Emergency Medicine, 18*(1), 19–27.

Drake, G., & Williams, A. C. D. C. (2017). Nursing education interventions for managing acute pain in hospital settings: A systematic review of clinical outcomes and teaching methods. *Pain Management Nursing, 18*(1), 3–15.

Drew, D. J., Gordon, D. B., Morgan, B., & Manworren, R. C. B. (2018). "As-needed" range orders for opioid analgesics in the management of pain: A consensus statement of the American Society for Pain Management Nursing and the American Pain Society. *Pain Management Nursing, 19*(3), 207–210.

Drew, D. J., & Peltier, C. H. (2018). Pain assessment. In M. L. Czarnecki, & H. N. Turner (Eds.), *Core curriculum for pain management nursing* (3rd ed.) (pp. 218–237). St Louis: Elsevier.

dos Santos Felix, M. M., Guimarães Ferreira, M. B., Falcão da Cruz, L., & Barbosa, M. H. (2019). Relaxation therapy with guided imagery for postoperative pain management: An integrative review. *Pain Management Nursing, 20*(1), 3–9.

Eksterowicz, N., & DiMaggio, T. J. (2018). Acute pain management. In M. L. Czarnecki, & H. N. Turner (Eds.), *Core curriculum for pain management nursing* (3rd ed.) (pp. 238–278). St. Louis: Elsevier.

Erden, S., Demir, N., Ugras, G. A., Arslan, U., & Arslan, S. (2018). Vital signs: Valid indicators to assess pain in intensive care unit patients? An observational, descriptive study. *Nursing and Health Sciences, 20*(4), 502–508.

Fudin, J., Raouf, M., & Wegrzyn, E. L. (2017). *Opioid dosing policy: Pharmacological considerations regarding equianalgesic dosing.* Lenexa, KS: American Academy of Integrative Pain Management.

Gan, T. J. (2017). Poorly controlled postoperative pain: Prevalence, consequences, and prevention. *Journal of Pain Research, 10*, 2287–2298.

Gupta, K., Prasad, A., Nagappa, M., Wong, J., Abrahamyan, L., & Chung, F. F. (2018). Risk factors for opioid-induced respiratory depression and failure to rescue: A review. *Current Opinion in Anaesthesiology, 31*(1), 110–119.

Hassell, P., & Stimpson, J. (2019). The role of regional anaesthesia in the management of acute pain. *Anaesthesia and Intensive Care Medicine, 20*(8), 436–439.

Haverfield, M. C., Giannitrapani, K., Timko, C., & Lorenz, K. (2018). Patient-centered pain management communication from the patient perspective. *Journal of General Internal Medicine, 33*(8), 1374–1380.

Herr, K., Coyne, P. J., Ely, E., Gélinas, C., & Manworren, R. C. B. (2019). Pain assessment in the patient unable to self-report: Clinical practice recommendations in support of the ASPMN 2019 position statement. *Pain Management Nursing, 20*(5), 404–417.

Jungquist, C. R., Quinlan-Colwell, A., Vallerand, A., et al. (2020). American Society for pain management nursing guidelines on monitoring for opioid-induced advancing sedation and respiratory depression: Revisions. *Pain Management Nursing, 21*(1), 7–25.

Kochman, A., Howell, J., Sheridan, M., et al. (2017). Reliability of the faces, legs, activity, cry, and consolability scale in assessing acute pain in the pediatric emergency department. *Pediatric Emergency Care, 33*(1), 14–17.

Lawson, S. L., Hogg, M. M., Moore, C. G., et al. (2019). Pediatric pain assessment in the emergency department: Patient and caregiver agreement using the Wong-Baker FACES® and the Faces Pain Scale-Revised. *Pediatric Emergency Care*, 2019. [Online ahead of print]. https://doi.org/10.1097/PEC.0000000000001837.

LeBlanc, R. G., & Choi, J. (2015). Optimizing medication safety in the home. *Home Healthcare Now, 33*(6), 313–319.

Manworren, R. C. B., McElligott, C. D., Deraska, P. V., et al. (2016). Efficacy of analgesic treatments to manage children's postoperative pain after laparoscopic appendectomy: Retrospective medical record review. *AORN Journal, 103*(3), 317.e1–317.e11.

Manworren, R. C. B., & Stinson, J. (2016). Pediatric pain measurement, assessment, and evaluation. *Seminars in Pediatric Neurology, 23*(3), 189–200. https://doi.org/10.1016/j.spen.2016.10.001

McCaffery, M. (1968). *Nursing practice theories related to cognition, bodily pain, and man environment interactions.* Los Angeles: University of California at Los Angeles Students' Store.

P

McCarthy, D. M., Wolf, M. S., McConnell, R., et al. (2015). Improving patient knowledge and safe use of opioids: A randomized controlled trial. *Academic Emergency Medicine, 22*(3), 331–339.

McNicol, E. D., Ferguson, M. C., & Hudcova, J. (2015). Patient controlled opioid analgesia versus non-patient controlled opioid analgesia for postoperative pain. *Cochrane Database of Systematic Reviews, 6*, CD003348.

Müller-Lissner, S., Bassotti, G., Coffin, B., et al. (2017). Opioid-induced constipation and bowel dysfunction: A clinical guideline. *Pain Medicine, 18*(10), 1837–1863.

Naughton, K. A. (2013). The combined use of sucrose and nonnutritive sucking for procedural pain in both term and preterm neonates: An integrative review of the literature. *Advances in Neonatal Care, 13*(1), 9–19.

O'Connor-Von, S. K., & Heck, C. R. (2018). Complementary and integrative therapies for pain management. In M. L. Czarnecki, & H. N. Turner (Eds.), *Core curriculum for pain management nursing* (3rd ed.) (pp. 505–532). St. Louis: Elsevier.

Odom-Forren, J., Brady, J., Rayens, M. K., & Sloan, P. (2019). Perianesthesia nurses' knowledge and promotion of safe use, storage, and disposal of opioids. *Journal of PeriAnesthesia Nursing, 34*(6), 1156–1168.

O'Donnell, K. F. (2018). Preoperative pain management education: An evidence-based practice project. *Journal of PeriAnesthesia Nursing, 33*(6), 956–963.

Olsen, K., & Weinberg, E. (2017). Pain-less practice: Techniques to reduce procedural pain and anxiety in pediatric acute care. *Clinical Pediatric Emergency Medicine, 18*(1), 32–41.

Pasero, C., Quinlan-Colwell, A., Rae, D., Broglio, K., & Drew, D. (2016). American Society for Pain Management Nursing position statement: Prescribing and administering opioid doses based solely on pain intensity. *Pain Management Nursing, 17*(3), 170–180.

Polomano, R. C., Fillman, M., Giordano, N. A., Vallerand, A. H., Nicely, K. L. W., & Jungquist, C. R. (2017). Multimodal analgesia for acute postoperative and trauma-related pain. *American Journal of Nursing, 117*(3 Suppl. 1), S12–S26.

Puntillo, K. A., Max, A., Timsit, J. F., et al. (2014). Determinants of procedural pain intensity in the intensive care unit. The European study. *American Journal of Respiratory and Critical Care Medicine, 189*(1), 39–47.

Raja, S., Carr, D. B., Cohen, M., et al. (2020). The revised International Association for the Study of Pain definition of pain: Concepts, challenges, and compromises. *Pain, 161*(9), 1976–1982.

Rungvivatjarus, T., Kuelbs, C. L., Miller, L., et al. (2020). Medication reconciliation improvement utilizing process redesign and clinical decision support. *Joint Commission Journal on Quality and Patient Safety, 46*(1), 27–36.

Sullivan, D., Lyons, M., Montgomery, R., & Quinlan-Colwell, A. (2016). Exploring opioid-sparing multimodal analgesia options in trauma: A nursing perspective. *Journal of Trauma Nursing, 23*(6), 361–375.

Sundar, S., Ramesh, B., Dixit, P. B., Venkatesh, S., Das, P., & Gunasekaran, D. (2016). Live music therapy as an active focus of attention for pain and behavioral symptoms of distress during pediatric immunization. *Clinical Pediatrics, 55*(8), 745–748.

Ten Haken, I., Allouch, S. B., & van Harten, W. H. (2018). The use of advanced medical technologies at home: A systematic review of the literature. *BMC Public Health, 18*(1), 284.

Waszak, D. L., Mitchell, A. M., Ren, D., & Fennimore, L. A. (2018). A quality improvement project to improve education provided by nurses to ED patients prescribed opioid analgesics at discharge. *Journal of Emergency Nursing, 44*(4), 336–344.

Williams, J. M., Schuman, S., Regen, R., et al. (2020). Intranasal fentanyl and midazolam for procedural analgesia and anxiolysis in pediatric urgent care centers. *Pediatric Emergency Care, 36*(9), e494–e499.

Yajnik, M., Hill, J. N., Hunter, O. O., et al. (2019). Patient education and engagement in postoperative pain management decreases opioid use following knee replacement surgery. *Patient Education and Counseling, 102*(2), 383–387.

Yilmaz, G., & Alemdar, D. K. (2019). Using Buzzy, Shotblocker, and bubble blowing in a pediatric emergency department to reduce the pain and fear caused by intramuscular injection: A randomized controlled trial. *Journal of Emergency Nursing, 45*(5), 502–511.

Young, V. B. (2017). Effective management of pain and anxiety for the pediatric patient in the emergency department. *Critical Care Nursing Clinics of North America, 29*(2), 205–216.

Zhuo, M. (2016). Neural mechanisms underlying anxiety-chronic pain interactions. *Trends in Neurosciences, 39*(3), 136–145.

Chronic Pain Domain 12 Comfort Class 1 Physical comfort

Maureen F. Cooney, DNP, FNP-BC, ACHPN, AP-PMN and Denise Sullivan, MSN, ANP-BC, ACHPN, AP-PMN

NANDA-I

Definition

Unpleasant sensory and emotional experience associated with actual or potential tissue damage, or described in terms of such damage (International Association for the Study of Pain); sudden or slow onset of any intensity from mild to severe, constant or recurring without an anticipated or predictable end, and a duration of greater than 3 months.

Defining Characteristics

Altered ability to continue activities; anorexia; evidence of pain using standardized pain behavior checklist for those unable to communicate verbally; expresses fatigue; facial expression of pain; proxy report of activity changes; proxy report of pain behavior; reports altered sleep-wake cycle; reports intensity using standardized pain scale; reports pain characteristics using standardized pain instrument; self-focused

Related Factors

Body mass index above normal range for age and gender; fatigue; ineffective sexuality pattern; injury agent; malnutrition; prolonged computer use; psychological distress; repeated handling of heavy loads; social isolation; whole-body vibration

At-Risk Population

Individuals aged >50 years; individuals with history of being abused; individuals with a history of genital mutilation; individuals with history of over indebtedness; individuals with history of static work postures; individuals with history of substance misuse; individuals with history of vigorous exercise; women

Associated Conditions

Bone fractures; central nervous system sensitization; chronic musculoskeletal diseases; contusion; crush syndrome; imbalance of neurotransmitters, neuromodulators, and receptors; immune system diseases; impaired metabolism; inborn genetic diseases; ischemia; neoplasms; nerve compression syndromes; nervous system diseases; post-trauma related condition; prolonged increase in cortisol level; soft tissue injuries; spinal cord injuries

NOC (Nursing Outcomes Classification)

Suggested NOC Outcomes

Comfort Level; Pain Control; Pain: Disruptive Effects; Pain Level

Example NOC Outcome with Indicators

Pain Level as evidenced by use of a numerical pain rating scale (NRS), asking the client to rate the level of pain from 0 to 10. Self-report is considered the single most reliable indicator of pain presence and intensity (American Pain Society [APS], 2016)

Note: **Pain Level** is the NOC Outcome label; this text recommends use of the self-report NRS in place of the NOC indicator scales because of the amount of research supporting its use.

Client Outcomes

Client Will (Specify Time Frame)

For the Client Who Is Able to Provide a Self-Report

- Provide a description of the pain experience including physical, social, emotional, and spiritual aspects
- Use a self-report pain tool to identify current pain level and establish a comfort-function goal
- Report that the pain management regimen achieves comfort-function goal without the occurrence of side effects
- Describe nonpharmacological methods that can be used to supplement, or enhance, pharmacological interventions and help achieve the comfort-function goal
- Perform necessary or desired activities at a pain level less than or equal to the comfort-function goal
- Demonstrate the ability to pace activity, taking rest breaks before they are needed
- Describe how unrelieved pain will be managed
- State the ability to obtain sufficient amounts of rest and sleep
- Notify a member of the health care team for pain level consistently greater than the comfort-function goal or occurrence of side effect

For the Client Who Is Unable to Provide a Self-Report

- Demonstrate decrease or resolved pain-related behaviors
- Perform desired activities as determined by client condition
- Demonstrate the absence of side effects
- No pain-related behaviors will be evident in the client who is completely unresponsive; a reasonable outcome is to demonstrate the absence of side effects related to the prescribed pain treatment plan

NIC (Nursing Interventions Classification)

Suggested NIC Interventions

Analgesic Administration; Pain Management

Example NIC Activities—Pain Management

Ensure that the client receives attentive analgesic care; Perform comprehensive assessment of pain, including location, characteristics, onset and duration, frequency, quality, intensity or severity, and precipitating factors

Nursing Interventions and *Rationales*

- ▲ During the initial assessment and interview, if the client is experiencing pain, conduct and document a comprehensive pain assessment, using appropriate pain assessment tools. CEB/EBN: *Determining location, temporal aspects, pain intensity, characteristics, and the effect of pain on function and quality of life is critical to determine the underlying cause of pain and effectiveness of treatment (McCaffery, 1968; Turk et al, 2016).* EB: *The initial assessment includes all pain information that the client can provide for the development of the individualized pain management plan (Stanos et al, 2016).*
- ▲ Determine the quality of the pain and whether the pain has persisted beyond the usual duration for tissue healing. EB: *Chronic pain is persistent, lasting beyond the expected time or usual time of tissue healing (usually 3 months). Descriptors such as "sharp," "shooting," or "burning" assist in discriminating neuropathic pain from nociceptive pain (Treede et al, 2019).* Refer to the care plan for Acute **Pain** and discussion of the Hierarchy of Pain Measures for assessment approach in clients who are unable to provide self-report of pain.
- ▲ Perform a pain assessment using a reliable self-report pain tool. EB: *Tools such as the 0 to 10 Numerical Rating Scale (NRS) or Faces Pain Scale (FPS) and the Wong-Baker FACES Pain Rating Scale assess pain intensity. Multidimensional tools such as the Brief Pain Inventory (BPI), the McGill Pain Questionnaire (MPQ), the Pain Relief Scale (PRS), or the Chronic Pain Grade Scale (CPGS) provide a comprehensive evaluation of the client with persistent pain assessing the characteristics and quality of pain; satisfaction with pain control; and how pain affects mood, activity, sleep, and diet (Fillingim et al, 2016).* EBN: *Assessment of function, using a functional pain assessment tool, allows clients to describe how pain affects their daily behaviors, including physical and cognitive abilities (Halm et al, 2019).*
- ▲ Ask the client to describe prior experiences with pain, effectiveness of pain management interventions, responses to analgesic medications (including occurrence of side effects), and concerns about pain and its treatment (e.g., fear about addiction, worries, anxiety) and informational needs. EBN: *Obtaining an individualized pain history helps identify potential factors that may influence the client's willingness to report pain, as well as factors that may influence pain intensity, the client's response to pain, anxiety, and pharmacokinetics of analgesics (Drew & Peltier, 2018; Raja et al, 2020).*
- • Using a self-report tool, ask the client to identify a comfort-function goal that will allow the client to perform necessary or desired activities easily. EBN: *The comfort-function goal provides the basis for individualized pain management plans and assists in determining effectiveness of pain management interventions (Boswell & Hall, 2017).*
- ▲ Assess chronic pain regularly, including the impact of chronic pain on activity; sleep; eating habits; and social conditions, including relationships, finances, and employment. EB: *Regular assessment of clients with chronic pain is critical because changes in the underlying pain condition, presence of comorbidities, and changes in psychosocial circumstances can affect pain intensity and characteristics and require revision of the pain management plan (Turk et al, 2016).* EB: *Sleep disturbance and decreased physical activity are adverse effects of people with chronic pain. In a study of clients with chronic pain, those who participated in a 4-week multiprofessional program that included psychoeducation and training related to pain, sleep, exercise, and activity training had improvement in sleep quality and pain intensity (de la Vega et al, 2019).*
- ▲ Assess the client for the presence of psychiatric conditions, including anxiety and depression. EB: *Among clients with chronic pain, there is an increased incidence of mental health disorders, including major depression and personality disorders, which increase the risks for suicidality (Pergolizzi et al, 2018). Among clients who receive specialized care for chronic pain, the prevalence of depression is as high as 68% (Works & Culmer, 2020).*

- ▲ If opioid therapy is considered, assist the provider with aspects of an opioid risk assessment, which includes a comprehensive client interview and examination with a pain focus, mental health screening, use of an opioid risk assessment tool, examination of prescription drug monitoring program results, and urine drug screening. **EB:** *Although prevalence rates vary, there is evidence of opioid misuse and opioid use disorder (OUD) among those who are prescribed opioids for chronic pain; thus to reduce risk and optimize safe opioid use, risk assessment and stratification are recommended (Cheatle et al, 2019).*
- ▲ For the client who is receiving outpatient opioid therapy, at each visit, assess effect of opioids on pain status, function, goal achievement, and presence of side effects, including sleep disturbance and sexual dysfunction; assessment for signs of misuse and OUD should be included, which may involve the use of random urine drug toxicology screening, pill counts, and review of prescription monitoring database. **EB:** *Opioid therapy is associated with risk for misuse and OUD and overdose, whereas the evidence for the long-term use of opioid therapy in chronic pain is inconclusive. To minimize risk, a number of risk mitigation practices, including careful assessment of the client response to opioid therapy, are recommended (Dowell et al, 2016).*
- ● Ask the client to maintain a diary (if able) of pain ratings, timing, precipitating events, medications, and effectiveness of pain management interventions. **EB:** *Systematic tracking of pain has been demonstrated to be an important factor in improving pain management (Fillingim et al, 2016). In a study of a smartphone-based pain app with two-way messaging option for clients with cancer and noncancer chronic pain, clients and providers found the app to be easy to use, and with two-way messaging, there was an increase in the frequency of daily pain assessments and client perception of beneficial connection to the health care providers (Jamison et al, 2017).*
- ▲ Obtain and review an accurate and complete list of medications the client is taking or has taken. **EBN:** *In a study using the "Brown Bag Medication Tool" developed by the Agency for Healthcare Research and Quality, clients cared for at a low-income clinic were asked to bring their medications, including empty bottles and discontinued bottles, in a brown bag to their clinic appointment, and health providers compared the bottles of medications and amount of remaining medication with their medical record to assess compliance with medication prescriptions, identify barriers to adherence, errors, safety concerns, and opportunities for improved adherence (Murtha et al, 2020).*
- ✱ Medication review has been found to improve the quality of medication interventions, including client adherence, and outcomes (Rose et al, 2015).
- ▲ Explain to the client the pain management approach that has been ordered or revised, including therapies, medication administration, side effects, and complications. **EB:** *One of the most important steps toward improved control of pain is a better client understanding of the nature of pain, its treatment, pain management goals, and the role the client needs to play in pain control (Curtiss & Wrona, 2018).*
- ● Discuss the client's fears of undertreated pain, side effects, OUD, and overdose and reassure the client that there will be regular assessment and treatment of pain and assessment for side effects and signs of OUD. **EBN:** *St. Marie (2016), in a qualitative study of clients with chronic pain who receive opioid therapy, reported that clients fear OUD or relapse, loss of access to opioids, and undertreated pain.*
- ▲ Manage chronic pain using an individualized, multimodal nonopioid or opioid-sparing approach. **EB:** *A multimodal approach (combining two or more drugs that act by different mechanisms for providing analgesia) such as acetaminophen, an anticonvulsant, an antidepressant, and an opioid in chronic pain enhances pain relief and allows the lowest effective dose of each drug to be administered, resulting in fewer or less severe side effects such as nausea, sedation, and respiratory depression. Nonopioid therapy is the treatment of choice in chronic noncancer pain. Opioids may be considered when all other reasonable attempts at analgesia have failed; however, evidence for long-term effectiveness is not clear (Dowell et al, 2016; Jungquist et al, 2016).*
- ▲ When chronic pain has a neuropathic component, treat with adjuvant analgesics, such as anticonvulsants, antidepressants, and topical local anesthetics. **EB:** *First-line analgesics for neuropathic pain belong to the adjuvant analgesic group and include anticonvulsants, antidepressants, and some topical local anesthetics. Analgesic efficacy with opioids in chronic neuropathic pain is inconclusive (Dowell et al, 2016; Fornasari, 2017).*
- ▲ Administer a nonopioid analgesic for mild to moderate chronic pain and as a component of the treatment for all levels of pain for clients with cancer pain. **CEB:** *Nonopioids, such as acetaminophen and nonsteroidal antiinflammatory drugs (NSAIDs), are first-line analgesics for the treatment of mild and moderate pain conditions (e.g., osteoarthritis pain) (Dowell et al, 2016). Consider adding nonopioid analgesics such as acetaminophen and NSAIDs for cancer pain, provided comorbidities and other risks do not prevent the use of these analgesics; NSAIDs are used cautiously, especially when used chronically, because many cancer*

P

clients may be at high risk for renal, gastrointestinal (GI), or cardiac toxicities; thrombocytopenia; or bleeding problems (National Comprehensive Cancer Network [NCCN], 2017).

- ▲ Recognize that opioid therapy may be indicated for some clients experiencing chronic pain. **EB:** *Opioids are often used in the management of moderate to severe chronic cancer pain. Opioid initiation for chronic, noncancer pain is controversial because of the limited data on long-term efficacy and safety. Opioid therapy may be considered with careful client selection when the benefits for pain control and function outweigh client risk (Dowell et al, 2016; Busse et al, 2018).*
- ▲ Administer analgesics around the clock for continuous pain and as needed (PRN) for intermittent or breakthrough pain as may be experienced by clients with cancer pain. **EB:** *The use of immediate-release opioids for clients with advanced cancer who have adequately controlled background pain are necessary to provide adequate relief for breakthrough pain episodes (Vellucci et al, 2017; Azhar et al, 2019).*
- ▲ Long-acting or extended-release opioids may be indicated for clients with cancer pain if clients require the regular use of short-acting opioids and receive adequate relief with them. **EB:** *Controlled-release preparations are helpful because the long duration lessens the severity of end-of-dose pain and decreases analgesic gaps (Swarm et al, 2019).*
- ▲ At regular intervals, assess inpatient clients with chronic pain for opioid-related adverse events and include frequent assessment of pain level, assessment of respiratory status (including rate, rhythm, noisiness, and depth), and systematic assessment of sedation level using a sedation scale. **EB:** *Tolerance to opioid-induced respiratory depression usually develops within a week of regular daily opioid dosing, making this side effect less likely to occur in those who are opioid tolerant than those who are not tolerant; however, opioid-tolerant clients are at similar risk for respiratory depression when they misuse opioids, are admitted to the hospital for surgery, or receive more than their usual opioid dose to treat an acute condition, or receive concomitant sedating medications (Jungquist et al, 2016).*
- ▲ During outpatient follow-up, assess clients receiving opioids for risk factors that may increase opioid-related harm. **EB:** *Clients who are receiving higher opioid doses, prescribed concurrent benzodiazepines, have cognitive impairment that could lead to accidental ingestion of excess opioids, mental health disorders that place a client at greater risk for suicide, or a history of OUDare at greater risk for opioid overdose. Take-home naloxone for the treatment of opioid-induced respiratory depression is recommended by numerous federal, state, and professional organizations (Coe & Walsh, 2015).*
- ▲ Provide the client with a bowel regimen, including adequate hydration, fiber, and laxatives to prevent/treat opioid-related constipation. Ask about other opioid-related side effects including nausea, pruritus, lack of appetite, and changes in rest and sleep. **EB:** *Although clients may develop tolerance to nausea, pruritus, and other opioid side effects, they do not develop tolerance to opioid-induced constipation (Nelson & Camilleri, 2016).*
- ▲ In addition to administering analgesics, support the client's use of nonpharmacological methods to help control pain, such as distraction, imagery, relaxation, and application of heat and cold. **EBN:** *Evidence suggested efficacy and satisfaction when complementary therapies are integrated into pain treatment plans of older adults (Bruckenthal et al, 2016).*
- ▲ Cognitive behavioral techniques have been shown to be useful in the management of chronic pain. **EBN:** *In a review of 35 studies involving the use of cognitive behavioral therapy (CBT) in the management of chronic pain, CBT was found to reduce pain intensity in 43% of the trials (Knoerl et al, 2016).* **EB:** *Motivational interviewing, a counseling method that aims to resolve a client's ambivalence about behavior change, may improve chronic pain treatment adherence, but more study is needed to determine whether it will improve pain intensity and function (Alperstein & Sharpe, 2016).* **EB:** *Multiprofessional outpatient rehabilitation using physical therapy, occupational therapy, and CBT can significantly improve function in people with chronic pain (Kurklinsky et al, 2016).*
- ▲ Encourage the client to plan activities around periods of greatest comfort whenever possible. **EB:** *Some literature supported the use of pacing (a CBT strategy), which is an active self-management strategy in which individuals learn to balance activity and rest for the purpose of increasing function (Racine et al, 2018).*
- ▲ Explore appropriate resources for long-term management of chronic pain (e.g., hospice, pain care center). **EB:** *Outpatient pain management resources must be identified to ensure appropriate chronic pain management. In a study involving a multisite telehealth group model for chronic pain management in rural/remote settings, when compared with face-to-face programs, clients experienced similar improvements in pain acceptance and pain interference, as well as improvements in overall function, mood, and physical activity (Scriven et al, 2019).*

▲ If the client has progressive cancer pain, assist the client and family with handling issues related to death and dying and provide access to palliative care programs and hospice services. **CEB:** *In a study by Temel et al (2010), clients with non–small cell lung cancer who received early palliative care intervention had significant improvements in quality of life and mood, less aggressive care at the end of life, and longer survival.*

Pediatric

● Assess for the presence of pain using a valid and reliable pain scale based on age, cognitive development, and the child's ability to provide a self-report. **EB:** *Pain intensity scales should be used in conjunction with other valid and reliable tools that assess the impact of pain on the child's quality of life (Manworren & Stinson, 2016).* **CEB:** *Behavioral tools such as the Face, Legs, Activity, Cry, Consolability (FLACC) Scale may be used to assess pain in infants and children who cannot provide a self-report (Crellin et al, 2015).*

▲ Manage chronic pain children, infants, and neonates with an interdisciplinary and multimodal approach. **EB:** *There is a lack of randomized controlled trials among pediatric clients to identify the best approach to the treatment of pain in this age group. Expert consensus recommends treatment using a multiprofessional approach, including physical therapies and CBT, and when pharmacological approaches are needed, a multimodal pharmacological approach, using medications from a variety of classes, is recommended (Mathew et al, 2016; Bruce et al, 2017).*

● Use a variety of nonpharmacological analgesic interventions to address chronic pain in pediatric clients. **EBN:** *Complementary therapies such as cognitive behavioral strategies, mindfulness-based approaches, and other nonpharmacological approaches may play an important role in chronic pain management in children and adolescents (Bruce et al, 2017).* **EB:** *In a study of children ages 9 to 14 years with functional abdominal pain, the use of tailored CBT compared with standard medical treatment showed greater improvements in pain-related disability but not pain levels, and greater improvements in anxiety symptoms compared with usual medical treatment (Cunningham et al, 2021).*

Geriatric

▲ An older client's report of pain should be taken seriously and assessed and treated. **EB:** *Chronic pain in the elderly is associated with an increase in physical, social, and psychological frailty (Coelho et al, 2017).* **EBN:** *Among the elderly, the presence of severe daily pain is positively correlated with the presence of depression and the frequency of falls and fatigue (Crowe et al, 2017).*

● When assessing pain, speak clearly, slowly, and loudly enough for the client to hear; ensure hearing aids and glasses are in place as appropriate; enlarge pain scales and written materials; and repeat information as needed. **EB:** *Older clients often have multiple sensory deficits, including vision and hearing difficulties, which can affect cognition, lead to loneliness and isolation, and contribute to declines in social interactions and relationships (Humes & Young, 2016; Stephan et al, 2017).*

● Handle the client's body gently and allow the client to move at his or her own speed. **EB:** *Older adults are particularly susceptible to injury during care activities. Age-related skeletal muscle changes result in weakness and muscle loss, placing clients at risk for injuries. Slow walking and turns may preserve muscle mass and strength in the trunk and limbs, which may enable continued independence (Araki et al, 2017).*

▲ Use nonpharmacological approaches including physical therapy, exercise, or other movement-based programs as the core components to persistent pain management in the older adult. **EB:** *In a randomized controlled trial of older adults with chronic pain, when compared with a control group, those who participated in an 8-week physical activity and education program had lower pain intensity and frailty and improved physical performance after participation and at 3 months after the program (Otones et al, 2020).*

▲ When pharmacological measures are needed to address chronic pain in the elderly, use a multimodal approach, including nonopioid analgesics for mild to moderate pain. **CEB:** *Acetaminophen (maximum dosage 3000 mg/day) is preferred and recommended, unless contraindicated, as first-line therapy for older persons with persistent pain; NSAIDs (preferably in topical form because there is less system absorption than in the oral form) should be used short term and with extreme caution because of the higher GI, cardiovascular, and renal adverse effects; if a systemic NSAID is needed, naproxen has the safest cardiac profile (Mehta et al, 2019).*

▲ Use opioids cautiously in the older client with chronic pain. **EB:** *In a systematic review consisting of seven studies of the use of opioids for the treatment of chronic noncancer pain in community-dwelling older adults, the majority of people experienced continued pain despite the use of opioids, and the results in terms of social engagement and participation in activities daily living were mixed; There was limited evidence to support the long-term use of opioids in this client population (O'Brien & Wand, 2020).*

P

▲ Monitor for signs of depression in older clients and refer to specialists with relevant expertise. EB: *Both depression and pain are common in older clients and have a bidirectional relationship. Pharmacological treatment of each condition may provide better outcomes than the treatment of one of these conditions. There is increasing evidence to support the role of neuroinflammation in the development of depression and pain (Zis et al, 2017).*

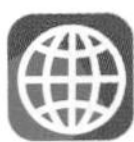

Multicultural

▲ Assess for and identify the presence of pain disparities among clients and work to develop opportunities for equal care. EB: *Ethnicity, culture, race, gender, and socioeconomic status are among factors that place clients at greater risk for disparities in pain treatment, and nurses have an obligation to raise attention to these disparities and take action to eliminate them (Vallerand, 2018).*

▲ Assess for the influence of cultural beliefs, norms, and values on the client's perception and experience of pain. EB: *The large variations in chronic back pain prevalence and prognosis across different countries may be influenced by culturally determined health beliefs (Henschke et al, 2016).*

▲ Social support should be facilitated as it has a positive impact on the client's ability to cope with chronic pain. EB: *In a study of the effect of social support on the attendance and participation in treatment sessions of clients with chronic back pain, social support provided a significant positive impact on treatment adherence and disability (Oraison & Kennedy, 2021).*

▲ Use culturally relevant pain scales to assess pain in the client. CEB: *Clients from minority cultures may express pain differently than clients from the majority culture. The FPS-Revised was shown to be preferred over other self-report pain rating tools in older minority adults (Ware et al, 2006) and in Chinese adults (Li et al, 2009). A later study demonstrated that the Iowa Pain Thermometer was the preferred tool in older Chinese adults (Li et al, 2009).*

Home Care

● The interventions previously described may be adapted for home care use. Refer to the Nursing Interventions and *Rationales* in the care plan for Acute **Pain.**

Client Family Teaching and Discharge Planning

Note: To avoid the negative connotations associated with the words "drugs" and "narcotics," use the term "pain medicine" when teaching clients.

● Discuss the various discomforts encompassed by the word "pain" and ask the client to give examples of previously experienced pain. Explain the pain assessment process and the purpose of the pain rating scale. EB: *It is often difficult for clients to understand the concept of pain and describe their pain experience. Using alternative words and providing a complete description of the assessment process, including the use of scales, ensures that an accurate treatment plan is developed (Drew & Peltier, 2018; Raja et al, 2020).*

● Teach the client that if the pain level is consistently above the comfort-function goal, the client should take action that decreases pain or should notify a member of the health care team so that effective pain management interventions may be implemented promptly. (See information on teaching clients to use the pain rating scale.) EB: *The use of comfort-function goals provides direction for the treatment plan. Changes are made according to the client's response and achievement of the goals of recovery or rehabilitation (Boswell & Hall, 2017).*

● Provide educational materials on various aspects of pain control to improve client understanding of pain and pain-related interventions. EBN: *In a pilot study of the use of a guided Internet-based program for clients with chronic pain, Internet delivery of client education and evidence-based therapies, along with content in audio, video, and text formats, increased client access to these therapies; the pilot study identified benefits of this approach and informed the need for further intervention refinement, content development, and research (Perry et al, 2017).*

● Discuss and evaluate the client's understanding of the total plan for pharmacological and nonpharmacological treatment, including the medication plan, the maintenance of a pain diary, and the use of supplies and equipment. EBN: *In a study of 279 clients with chronic pain, those who received comprehensive nurse-led intervention on healthy lifestyle, self-esteem, pain awareness, communication, and relaxation techniques noted improvement in quality of life, pain intensity, and mental health compared with those who received usual care (Morales-Fernández et al, 2021).*

▲ Reinforce that opioids, when prescribed for chronic pain, may be an appropriate component of multimodal pain treatment plan, but clients require knowledge of safe opioid use and potential adverse effects.

P

EB: *Taking opioids only as directed, avoiding alcohol, and talking with the health care provider when pain is poorly controlled are strategies that will lessen the risks for OUD or major opioid-related adverse effects such as respiratory depression and arrest (Denenberg & Curtiss, 2016).*

- ▲ Reinforce the importance of safe storage of opioid medications out of the reach of others and to responsibly dispose of any unused opioids. **EB:** *Community medication "take back" days and drop boxes are becoming increasingly popular. Encourage clients/families to check community resources (Hawk et al, 2015).*
- • Demonstrate the use of appropriate nonpharmacological approaches in addition to pharmacological approaches for helping control pain, such as application of heat and/or cold, distraction techniques, relaxation breathing, visualization, rocking, stroking, listening to music, and watching television. Teach these methods when pain is relatively well controlled, because pain interferes with cognition. **EBN:** *In an integrative review, evidence suggests that when nurses educate clients on nonpharmacological modalities for the management of chronic noncancer pain, they may be more motivated to try these modalities, which may lead to improved outcomes (Andrews-Cooper & Kozachik, 2020).*
- ▲ Emphasize to the client the importance of participating in a structured, individualized pacing activity and taking rest breaks before they are needed to reduce fatigue, reduce joint stiffness, and maintain physical activity. **EB:** *In a systematic review that included seven studies involving the use of pacing as a strategy to assist with chronic pain management, a learned pacing intervention reduced fatigue interference, joint stiffness, and variability in physical activity but did not reduce pain severity (Guy et al, 2019).*
- • Teach nonpharmacological methods when pain is relatively well controlled. **EB:** *Pain interferes with cognition (Baker et al, 2017).*

REFERENCES

Alperstein, D., & Sharpe, L. (2016). The efficacy of motivational interviewing in adults with chronic pain: A meta-analysis and systematic review. *The Journal of Pain, 17*(4), 393–403.

American Pain Society (APS). (2016). *Principles of analgesic use* (7th ed.). Chicago: American Pain Society.

Andrews-Cooper, I. N., & Kozachik, S. L. (2020). How patient education influences utilization of nonpharmacological modalities for persistent pain management: An integrative review. *Pain Management Nursing, 21*(2), 157–164.

Araki, M., Hatamoto, Y., Higaki, Y., & Tanaka, H. (2017). "Slow walking with turns" increases quadriceps and erector spinae muscle activity. *Journal of Physical Therapy Science, 29*(3), 419–424.

Azhar, A., Kim, Y. J., Haider, A., et al. (2019). Response to oral immediate-release opioids for breakthrough pain in patients with advanced cancer with adequately controlled background pain. *The Oncologist, 24*(1), 125–131.

Baker, K. S., Georgiou-Karistianis, N., Gibson, S. J., & Giummarra, M. J. (2017). Optimizing cognitive function in persons with chronic pain. *The Clinical Journal of Pain, 33*(5), 462–472.

Boswell, C., & Hall, M. (2017). Engaging the patient through comfort-function levels. *Nursing, 47*(10), 68–69.

Bruce, B. K., Ale, C. M., Harrison, T. E., et al. (2017). Getting back to living: Further evidence for the efficacy of an interdisciplinary pediatric pain treatment program. *The Clinical Journal of Pain, 33*(6), 535–542.

Bruckenthal, P., Marino, M. A., & Snelling, L. (2016). Complementary and integrative therapies for persistent pain management in older adults: A review. *Journal of Gerontological Nursing, 42*(12), 40–48.

Busse, J. W., Wang, L., Kameleldin, M., et al. (2018). Opioids for chronic noncancer pain: A systemic review and meta-analysis. *JAMA, 320*(23), 2448–2460.

Cheatle, M. D., Compton, P. A., Dhingra, L., Wasser, T. E., & O'Brien, C. P. (2019). Development of the revised opioid risk tool to predict opioid use disorder in patients with chronic nonmalignant pain. *The Journal of Pain, 20*(7), 842–851.

Coe, M. A., & Walsh, S. L. (2015). Distribution of naloxone for overdose prevention to chronic pain patients. *Preventive Medicine, 80*, 41–43.

Coelho, T., Paúl, C., Gobbens, R. J. J., & Fernandes, L. (2017). Multidimensional frailty and pain in community dwelling elderly. *Pain Medicine, 18*(4), 693–701.

Crellin, D. J., Harrison, D., Santamaria, N., & Babl, F. E. (2015). Systematic review of the face, legs, activity, cry, and consolability scale for assessing pain in infants and children: Is it reliable, valid and feasible for use? *Pain, 156*(11), 2132–2151.

Crowe, M., Jordan, J., Gillon, D., McCall, C., Frampton, C., & Jamieson, H. (2017). The prevalence of pain and its relationship to falls, fatigue and depression in a cohort of older people living in the community. *Journal of Advanced Nursing, 73*(11), 2642–2651.

Cunningham, N., Kalomiros, A., Peugh, J., et al. (2021). Cognitive behavior therapy tailored to anxiety symptoms improves pediatric functional abdominal pain outcomes: A randomized clinical trial. *The Journal of Pediatrics, 230*, 62–70.e3. https://doi.org/10.1016/j.peds.2020.10.060.

Curtiss, C. P., & Wrona, S. (2018). Pain management education. In M. L. Czarnecki, & H. N. Turner (Eds.), *Core curriculum for pain management nursing* (3rd ed.) (pp. 589–601). St. Louis: Elsevier.

Denenberg, R., & Curtiss, C. P. (2016). CE: Appropriate use of opioids in managing chronic pain. *American Journal of Nursing, 116*(7), 26–38.

Dowell, D., Haegerich, T. M., & Chou, R. (2016). CDC guideline for prescribing opioids for chronic pain—United States, 2016. *Journal of the American Medical Association, 315*(15), 1624–1645.

Drew, D. J., & Peltier, C. H. (2018). Pain assessment. In M. L. Czarnecki, & H. N. Turner (Eds.), *Core curriculum for pain management nursing* (3rd ed.) (pp. 218–237). St. Louis: Elsevier.

Fillingim, R. B., Loeser, J. D., Baron, R., & Edwards, R. R. (2016). Assessment of chronic pain: Domains, methods, and mechanisms. *The Journal of Pain, 17*(9 Suppl. l), T10–T20.

Fornasari, D. (2017). Pharmacotherapy for neuropathic pain: A review. *Pain and Therapy, 6*(Suppl. 1), 25–33.

Guy, L., McKinstry, C., & Bruce, C. (2019). Effectiveness of pacing as a learned strategy for people with chronic pain: A systematic review. *American Journal of Occupational Therapy, 73*(3) 7303205060p1-7303205060p10.

Halm, M., Bailey, C., St Pierre, J., et al. (2019). Pilot evaluation of a functional pain assessment scale. *Clinical Nurse Specialist*, *33*(1), 12–21.

Hawk, K. F., Vaca, F. E., & D'Onofrio, G. (2015). Focus: Addiction: Reducing fatal opioid overdose: Prevention, treatment and harm reduction strategies. *Yale Journal of Biology & Medicine*, *88*(3), 235–245.

Henschke, N., Lorenz, E., Pokora, R., Michaleff, Z. A., Quartey, J. N. A., & Oliveira, V. C. (2016). Understanding cultural influences on back pain and back pain research. Best Practice & Research. *Clinical Rheumatology*, *30*(6), 1037–1049.

Humes, L. E., & Young, L. A. (2016). Sensory–cognitive interactions in older adults. *Ear and Hearing*, *37*(Suppl. 1), 52S–61S.

Jamison, R. N., Jurcik, D. C., Edwards, R. R., Huang, C. C., & Ross, E. L. (2017). A pilot comparison of a smartphone app with or without 2-way messaging among chronic pain patients: Who benefits from a pain app? *The Clinical Journal of Pain*, *33*(8), 676–686.

Jungquist, C. R., Correll, D. J., Fleisher, L. A., et al. (2016). Avoiding adverse events secondary to opioid-induced respiratory depression: Implications for nurse executives and patient safety. *The Journal of Nursing Administration*, *46*(2), 87–94.

Knoerl, R., Lavoie Smith, E. M., & Weisberg, J. (2016). Chronic pain and cognitive behavioral therapy: An integrative review. *Western Journal of Nursing Research*, *38*(5), 596–628.

Kurklinsky, S., Perez, R. B., Lacayo, E. R., & Sletten, C. D. (2016). The efficacy of interdisciplinary rehabilitation for improving function in people with chronic pain. *Pain Research and Treatment*, *2016*, 7217684. https://doi.org/10.1155/2016/7217684.

Li, L., Herr, K., & Chen, P. (2009). Postoperative pain assessment with three intensity scales in Chinese elders. *Journal of Nursing Scholarship*, *41*(3), 241–249.

Manworren, R. C. B., & Stinson, J. (2016). Pediatric pain measurement, assessment, and evaluation. *Seminars in Pediatric Neurology*, *23*(3), 189–200. https://doi.org/10.1016/j.spen.2016.10.001.

Mathew, E., Kim, E., & Zempsky, W. (2016). Pharmacologic treatment of pain. *Seminars in Pediatric Neurology*, *23*(3), 209–219.

McCaffery, M. (1968). *Nursing practice theories related to cognition, bodily pain, and man—Environment interactions*. Los Angeles: University of California at Los Angeles Students' Store.

Mehta, S. S., Ayers, E. R., & Reid, M. C. (2019). Effective approaches for pain relief in older adults. In G. A. Cordts, & P. J. Christo (Eds.), *Effective treatments for pain in the older patient* (pp. 1–11). New York: Springer.

Morales-Fernández, Á., Jimenez-Martín, J. M., Morales-Asencio, J. M., et al. (2021). Impact of a nurse-led intervention on quality of life in patients with chronic non-malignant pain: An open randomized controlled trial. *Journal of Advanced Nursing*, *77*(1), 255–265. https://doi.org/10.1111/jan.14608.

Murtha, E., Elder, B., & Faragher, M. (2020). Brown bag medication review: Using AHRQ's brown bag medication tool. *Journal of Nursing Care Quality*, *35*(1), 58–62.

National Comprehensive Cancer Network. (2017). *NCCN clinical practice guidelines in oncology. Adult cancer pain. Version 2.2017*.

Nelson, A. D., & Camilleri, M. (2016). Opioid-induced constipation: Advances and clinical guidance. *Therapeutic Advances in Chronic Disease*, *7*(2), 121–134.

O'Brien, M. D. C., & Wand, A. P. F. (2020). A systematic review of the evidence for the efficacy of opioids for chronic non-cancer pain in community-dwelling older adults. *Age and Ageing*, *49*(2), 175–183.

Oraison, H. M., & Kennedy, G. A. (2021). The effect of social support in chronic back pain: Number of treatment sessions and reported level of disability. *Disability & Rehabilitation*, *43*(11), 1526–1531.

Otones, P., García, E., Sanz, T., & Pedraz, A. (2020). A physical activity program versus usual care in the management of quality of life for pre-frail older adults with chronic pain: Randomized controlled trial. *BMC Geriatrics*, *20*(1), 396.

Pergolizzi, J. V., Jr., Passik, S., LeQuang, J. A., et al. (2018). The risk of suicide in chronic pain patients. *Nursing and Palliative Care*, *3*(3), 2–11. https://doi.org/10.15761/NPC.1000189.

Perry, J., VanDenKerkhof, E. G., Wilson, R., & Tripp, D. A. (2017). Development of a guided internet-based psycho-education intervention using cognitive behavioral therapy and self-management for individuals with chronic pain. *Pain Management Nursing*, *18*(2), 90–101.

Racine, M., Galán, S., de la Vega, R., et al. (2018). Pain-related activity management patterns and function in patients with fibromyalgia syndrome. *The Clinical Journal of Pain*, *34*(2), 122–129. https://doi.org/10.1097/AJP.0000000000000526.

Raja, S., Carr, D. B., Cohen, M., et al. (2020). The revised International Association for the Study of Pain definition of pain: Concepts, challenges, and compromises. *Pain*, *161*(9), 1976–1982.

Rose, O., Schaffert, C., Czarnecki, K., et al. (2015). Effect evaluation of an interprofessional medication therapy management approach for multimorbid patients in primary care: A cluster-randomized controlled trial in community care (WestGem study protocol). *BMC Family Practice*, *16*, 84.

Scriven, H., Doherty, D. P., & Ward, E. C. (2019). Evaluation of a multisite telehealth group model for persistent pain management for rural/remote participants. *Rural and Remote Health*, *19*(1), 4710. https://doi.org/10.22605/RRH4710.

Stanos, S., Brodsky, M., Argoff, C., et al. (2016). Rethinking chronic pain in a primary care setting. *Postgraduate Medicine*, *128*(5), 502–515.

Stephan, Y., Sutin, A. R., Bosselut, G., & Terracciano, A. (2017). Sensory functioning and personality development among older adults. *Psychology and Aging*, *32*(2), 139–147.

St Marie, B. (2016). Primary care experiences of people who live with chronic pain and receive opioids to manage pain: A qualitative methodology. *Journal of the American Association of Nurse Practitioners*, *28*(8), 429–435.

Swarm, R. A., Paice, J. A., Anghelescu, D. L., et al. (2019). Adult cancer pain, version 3.2019, NCCN clinical practice guidelines in oncology. *Journal of the National Comprehensive Cancer Network*, *17*(8), 977–1007.

Temel, J. S., Greer, J. A., Muzikansky, M. A., et al. (2010). Early palliative care for patients with metastatic non-small-cell lung cancer. *New England Journal of Medicine*, *363*(8), 733–742.

Treede, R. D., Rief, W., Barke, A., et al. (2019). Chronic pain as a symptom or a disease: The IASP classification of chronic pain for the International Classification of Diseases (ICD-11). *Pain*, *160*(1), 19–27.

Turk, D., Fillingim, R., Ohrbach, R., & Patel, K. V. (2016). Assessment of psychosocial and functional impact of chronic pain. *The Journal of Pain*, *17*(9 Suppl. l), T21–T49.

Vallerand, A. H. (2018). Pain-related disparities: Are they something nurses should care about? *Pain Management Nursing*, *19*(1), 1–2.

de la Vega, R., Racine, M., Castarlenas, E., et al. (2019). The role of sleep quality and fatigue on the benefits of an interdisciplinary treatment for adults with chronic pain. *Pain Practice*, *19*(4), 354–362.

Vellucci, R., Mediati, R. D., Gasperoni, S., Mammucari, M., Marinangeli, F., & Romualdi, P. (2017). Assessment and treatment of breakthrough cancer pain: From theory to clinical practice. *Journal of Pain Research*, *10*, 2147–2155.

Ware, L. J., Epps, C. D., Herr, K., & Packard, A. (2006). Evaluation of the revised faces pain scale, verbal descriptor scale, numeric rating scale, and Iowa pain thermometer in older minority adults. *Pain Management Nursing*, *7*(3), 117–125.

Works, C., & Culmer, K. F. (2020). What is the prevalence of depression in patients with chronic pain? *Evidenced-Based Practice*, *23*(11), 43–44.

Zis, P., Daskalaki, A., Bountouni, I., Sykioti, P., Varrassi, G., & Paladini, A. (2017). Depression and chronic pain in the elderly: Links and management challenges. *Clinical Interventions in Aging*, *12*, 709–720.

P

Chronic Pain Syndrome Domain 12 Comfort Class 1 Physical comfort

Mary Beth Flynn Makic, PhD, RN, CCNS, CCRN-K, FAAN, FNAP, FCNS

NANDA-I

Definition

Recurrent or persistent pain that has lasted at least 3 months and that significantly affects daily functioning or well-being.

Defining Characteristics

Anxiety (00146); constipation (00011); disturbed sleep pattern (00198); fatigue (00093); fear (00148); impaired mood regulation (00241); impaired physical mobility (00085); insomnia (00095); social isolation (00053); stress overload (00177)

Related Factors

Body mass index above normal range for age and gender; fear of pain; fear-avoidance beliefs; inadequate knowledge of pain management behaviors; negative affect; sleep disturbances

NIC, NOC, Client Outcomes, Nursing Interventions and *Rationales,* Client/Family Teaching and Discharge Planning, and References

Refer to care plan for Acute **Pain** and Chronic **Pain.**

Labor Pain Domain 12 Comfort Class 1 Physical comfort

Nichol Chesser, RN, CNM, DNP

P

NANDA-I

Definition

Sensory and emotional experience that varies from pleasant to unpleasant, associated with labor and childbirth.

Defining Characteristics

Altered blood pressure; altered heart rate; altered muscle tension; altered neuroendocrine functioning; altered respiratory rate; altered urinary functioning; anxiety; appetite change; diaphoresis; distraction behavior; expressive behavior; facial expression of pain; narrow focus; nausea; perineal pressure; positioning to ease pain; protective behavior; pupil dilation; reports altered sleep-wake cycle; self-focused; uterine contraction; vomiting

Related Factors

Behavioral Factors

Insufficient fluid intake; supine position

Cognitive Factors

Fear of childbirth; inadequate knowledge about childbirth; inadequate preparation to deal with labor pain; low self efficacy; perception of labor pain as nonproductive; perception of labor pain as negative; perception of labor pain as threatening; perception of labor pain as unnatural; perception of pain as meaningful

Social Factors

Interference in decision-making; unsupportive companionship

Unmodified Environmental Factors

Noisy delivery room; overcrowded delivery room; turbulent environment

At-Risk Population

Women experiencing emergency situation during labor; women from cultures with negative perspective of labor pain; women giving birth in a disease based health care system; women whose mothers have a high level of education; women with history of pre-pregnancy dysmenorrhea; women with history of sexual abuse during childhood; women without supportive companion

Associated Conditions

Cervical dilation; depression; fetal expulsion; high maternal trait anxiety; prescribed mobility restriction; prolonged duration of labor

NOC (Nursing Outcomes Classification)

Suggested NOC Outcomes

Client Satisfaction: Pain Management, Comfort Status; Knowledge: Pain Management, Pain Control, Pain Level

Example NOC Outcomes with Indicators

Labor Pain management as evidenced by the following indicators: Recognizes pain onset/Discusses pain treatment options with health care professional/Monitors therapeutic effects of analgesic/Uses effective coping strategies/Reports changes in pain symptoms to health care provider. (Rate the outcome and indicators of **Labor Pain:** 1 = never demonstrated, 2 = rarely demonstrated, 3 = sometimes demonstrated, 4 = often demonstrated, 5 = consistently demonstrated [see Section I].)

Client Outcomes

Client Will (Specify Time Frame)

- Recognize pharmacological and nonpharmacological interventions to address labor pain
- Demonstrate coping strategies to address labor pain
- Verbalize pain relief effectiveness throughout the labor process

NIC (Nursing Intervention Classification)

Suggested NIC Interventions

Acute, Analgesic Administration: Intraspinal, Analgesic Administration, Aromatherapy, Dance Therapy, Distraction, Environmental Management: Comfort, Guided Imagery, Massage, Medication Administration: Intraspinal, Meditation Facilitation, Relaxation Therapy, Transcutaneous Electrical Nerve Stimulation

Example NIC Activity—Acute Pain Management

Explore the client's knowledge and beliefs about labor pain including cultural influences; Monitor pain using a valid and reliable rating tool

Nursing Intervention and *Rationales*

- Initial assessment and interview, if the client is experiencing pain, conduct and document a comprehensive pain assessment, using appropriate pain assessment tools. EB: *A pain assessment tool consists of obtaining all the information that a client can provide to help individualize a pain management plan of care. This includes presence of pain and pain treatment (Karcioglu et al, 2018). Information includes loca tion, intensity, characteristics, quality, ability to cope, and desire for pharmacological or nonpharmacological interventions. Pain level, as evidenced by client self-report of coping or not coping with pain from labor contractions, is considered the best indicator of pain presence and intensity. The pain level a client experiences can be seen by behavioral indices such as facial expressions, verbal expressions, tone of voice, body movement, ability to relax, and breathing rate (Asl et al, 2018). Use an evidence-based coping algorithm to help the client find the best means available to cope well with labor pain (Fairchild et al, 2017). The Coping with Labor Algorithm (CWLA) is especially useful for nurses as it allows them to look for specific cues from the client to determine how well they are coping with pain (Fairchild et al, 2017).*

- Observe for nonverbal pain assessment such as grimacing, lackluster eyes, and fixed or scattered movements.
- Assess pain on pain level tool such as the 0 to 10 numerical pain rating scale (NRS) if appropriate or the CWLA (Fairchild et al, 2017). Discuss with client the desire for pain management for this labor, past experiences with labor and effectiveness of pain management techniques employed at that time, concerns about pain and its treatment, and information needs (e.g., pain coping techniques that are both analgesic and nonpharmaceutical). **EBN:** *Obtaining individualized history and goals for coping with pain during labor and birth helps identify how to better guide a client through childbirth and increase client satisfaction with the process. Women's satisfaction with the childbirth process is not directly correlated with pharmacological pain relief, but it is greatly enhanced by continuity of care and care provider presence (Van der Gucht & Lewis, 2015).*
- Goal is for the client to manage labor pain from admission until delivery of infant with either natural childbirth and associated pain management techniques or pharmaceutical measures to reduce pain experience. **EB:** *For the client who is able to self-report, when using a self-report pain tool, caution must be used because a high or low score is not always associated with lack of coping or suffering when used for labor pain (Caughey & Tilden, 2021).*
- Based on the client's ability to cope with labor pain, discuss with client pain management options, including pharmacological and nonpharmacological interventions. Coping strategies women may implement include being still or rocking, focusing on breathing, relaxing muscles, changing position, listening to soothing music, making noises, and being in water (ACNM, 2020). **EB:** *Implement strategies or request orders to help client cope with labor pain. This may include massage, movement (such as rocking or swaying, sitting on birthing ball, and position changes), rhythmic breathing, relaxation techniques, aromatherapy, intradermal water blocks, intravenous (IV) narcotics, transcutaneous electrical nerve stimulation (TENS), nitrous oxide, hydrotherapy, and neuraxial anesthesia (Gilbert, 2020).* **EBN:** *Self-identified nonpharmacological coping strategies, such as relaxation techniques, movement, distraction, imagery, breathing techniques, and making noises, can assist with labor pain (ACNM, 2020).*
- Based on the client's ability to cope and their perception of labor pain, assess the physiological-natural process of labor, physical environment, and emotional/psychosocial dynamics and behaviors (Asl et al, 2018). **CEB:** *Labor pain is a combination of physiological and psychosocial process (Koyyalamudi et al, 2016). The best way to help a laboring woman cope includes continuous support, creating a safe environment, and helping to relieve feelings of fear and vulnerability (Van der Gucht & Lewis, 2015). Being present with a laboring woman and observing indicators of pain can also help a laboring woman cope (Van der Gucht & Lewis, 2015; Asl et al, 2018).*
- Based on the client's ability to cope, offer intervention (either nonpharmacological or pharmacological). **EBN:** *Nonpharmacological pain interventions are low cost and low risk. They are also directed at increasing comfort during labor, preventing suffering, and allowing women to cope with labor pain (Caughey & Tilden, 2021). Nonpharmacological pain measures can be used by themselves or in combination with pharmacological intervention during labor. If the client is unable to cope with labor by using nonpharmacological pain relief measures, offering pharmacological pain relief measures is appropriate. A client may be able to proceed through labor and delivery without pain medication but should never be denied medication if she requests it (Caughey & Tilden, 2021).*
- Nonpharmacological pain relief measures are low-risk and low-resource interventions (Caughey & Tilden, 2021). These approaches can encompass the physical sensation of pain and the psychoemotional and spiritual components of care. By addressing all aspects of client needs (physical, emotional, and spiritual), suffering can be reduced during labor (Caughey & Tilden, 2021).
  - Ambulation/rocking/swaying is a safe and effective coping measure for labor pain. This is usually a client-initiated response to labor pain; however, caregivers can encourage women to ambulate or change position to ease pain or allow clients to cope better with labor pain.
  - Hydrotherapy either as immersion in water or bathing can be used to promote relaxation, decrease acute anxiety, help cope with pain, promote greater maternal movement, reduce the need for pharmacological pain relief measures, and promote normal physiological labor (Shaw-Battista, 2017; Sidebottom et al, 2020). **EBN:** *Water labor may be indicated for women to help with relaxation during labor.*

P

This may enable the client to proceed through labor without pharmacological intervention because it may reduce anxiety around labor and contraction pain (Shaw-Battista, 2017).

- TENS is a small, handheld device that transmits low-voltage electrical impulses to the skin (Caughey & Tilden, 2021). The device suppresses the conduction of pain through pain fibers by using small electrical impulses (Shahoei et al, 2017). **EBN:** *The use of this device is controlled by the client herself and can vary the pattern and intensity of the cutaneous electrical impulse depending on the contraction pattern and pain (Caughey & Tilden, 2021). The use of TENS has no adverse side effects and can improve overall satisfaction with the labor and birth experience when used correctly (Shahoei et al, 2017).*

- Pharmacological measures for pain relief are high resource and high risk; they require professional training for administration, incur cost, and have a greater risk to mother and baby (Caughey & Tilden, 2021).
- Nitrous oxide is a blend of 50% nitrous oxide with 50% oxygen. The use of nitrous oxide may not alleviate pain, but it may help with satisfaction of the birth experience (Richardson et al, 2019). **EBN:** *Nitrous should be avoided in clients with vitamin B_{12} deficiency or MHFR mutation/deficiency (Hays, 2020). Most common side effects of nitrous oxide are nausea and dizziness (Richardson et al, 2019). Correct usage of nitrous is needed for optimum efficacy; it must be initiated before contraction pain because the peak onset is 50 seconds from initial inhalation (Collins et al, 2018).*
- IV medications for pain management are an alternative for some women who do not desire an epidural; IV medications are generally opioids. **EBN:** *These are advantageous because they are easy to administer, are widely available, and are less invasive than neuraxial techniques of pain relief (i.e., an epidural). Side effects are common and include nausea, vomiting, and drowsiness (Collins et al, 2018).*
- Epidural, combined spinal-epidural (CSE), and dural puncture epidural (DPE) are appropriate for laboring women when requested by the client (unless there is a contraindication). **EB:** *Contraindications to neuraxial anesthesia may include cardiac disease, hematologic disorders, spinal muscular or neurologic disease, and/or hepatic or renal disease (American College of Obstetricians and Gynecologists' Committee on Practice Bulletins—Obstetrics, 2016).* **EBN:** *During placement of neuraxial anesthesia maternal oxygen saturation and heart rate should be measured continuously. Blood pressure should be measured every 5 minutes, and fetal heart rate should be monitored at least before and after administration according to institution guidelines. Continue to monitor maternal blood pressure, pain control, motor function, and sensory levels at regular intervals to make sure the anesthesia is working properly. Also, continue to document client's vital signs and pain assessment (Collins et al, 2018).*
- Account for clients' abilities to cope with labor pain regarding their psychosocial, cultural, and spiritual backgrounds. A woman's positive perceptions of how she will be able to cope with labor are associated with reduced anxiety, pain, and intervention during labor (Van der Gucht & Lewis, 2015; Caughey & Tilden, 2021). **EB:** *Coping has many facets, including cognitive, behavioral, and emotional aspects (Van der Gucht & Lewis, 2015). How a woman copes with pain during labor includes factors such as personality traits, type of stress, religious thoughts and beliefs, confidence in ability to cope, support available, and attitude toward pain; coping methods encompass physiological, psychological, cognitive, and spiritual methods (Van der Gucht & Lewis, 2015). Each method of coping is an individual decision and greatly influenced by personality traits. Culturally learned values and attitudes as well as personality traits and emotional behavior may greatly influence how women cope with acute labor pain (Segerstrom & Smith, 2019).*
- Document pain assessment through direct observation. Also document interventions to facilitate labor pain management through the continuum of the women's labor experience (Van der Gucht & Lewis, 2015).

REFERENCES

American College of Nurse-Midwives (ACNM). (2020). Coping with labor pain. *Journal of Midwifery & Women's Health*, *65*(3), 435–436.

American College of Obstetricians and Gynecologists' Committee on Practice Bulletins—Obstetrics. (2016). Practice bulletin no. 171: Management of preterm labor. *Obstetrics & Gynecology*, *128*(4), e155–e164. https://doi.org/10.1097/AOG.0000000000001711

Asl, B. M. H., Vatanchi, A., Golmakani, N., & Najafi, A. (2018). Relationship between behavioral indices of pain during labor pain with pain intensity and duration of delivery. *Electronic Physician*, *10*(1), 6240–6248.

Caughey, A. B., & Tilden, E. (2021). *Nonpharmacologic approaches to management of labor pain*. UpToDate. C. J. Lockwood, & K. Eckler (Eds.). Waltham, MA: UpToDate. Retrieved from https://www.uptodate.com/contents/nonpharmacologic-approaches-to-management-of-labor-pain. Accessed July 22, 2021.

Collins, M. R., Starr, S. A., Bishop, J. T., & Baysinger, C. L. (2012). Nitrous oxide for labor analgesia: Expanding analgesic options for women in the United States. *Reviews in Obstetrics & Gynecology*, *5*(3–4), e126–e131.

Fairchild, E., Roberts, L., Zelman, K., Michelli, S., & Hastings-Tolsma, M. (2017). Implementation of Robert's Coping with Labor Algorithm© in a large tertiary care facility. *Midwifery*, *50*, 208–218.

Gilbert, G. J. (2020). *Pharmacologic management of pain during labor and delivery*. UpToDate. D. L. Hepner, V. Berghella, & M. Crowley (Eds.).

Waltham, MA: UpToDate. Retrieved from https://www.uptodate.com/contents/pharmacologic-management-of-pain-during-labor-and-delivery. Accessed July 22, 2021.

Hays, S. R. (2020). *Inhalation anesthetic agents: Clinical effects and uses.* UpToDate. G. P. Joshi, & N. A. Nussmeier (Eds.). Waltham, MA: UpToDate. Retrieved from https://www.uptodate.com/contents/inhalation-anesthetic-agents-clinical-effects-and-uses. Accessed July 22, 2021.

Karcioglu, O., Topacoglu, H., Dikme, O., & Dikme, O. (2018). A systematic review of the pain scales in adults: Which to use? *American Journal of Emergency Medicine, 36*(4), 707–714.

Koyyalamudi, V., Sidhu, G., Cornett, E. M., et al. (2016). New labor pain treatment options. *Current Pain and Headache Reports, 20*(2), 11.

Richardson, M. G., Raymond, B. L., Baysinger, C. L., Kook, B. T., & Chestnut, D. H. (2019). A qualitative analysis of parturients' experiences using nitrous oxide for labor analgesia: It is not just about pain relief. *Birth, 46*(1), 97–104.

Segerstrom, S. C., & Smith, G. T. (2019). Personality and coping: Individual differences in responses to emotion. *Annual Review of Psychology, 70*, 651–671.

Shahoei, R., Shahghebi, S., Rezaei, M., & Naqshbandi, S. (2017). The effect of transcutaneous electrical nerve stimulation on the severity of labor pain among nulliparous women: A clinical trial. *Complementary Therapies in Clinical Practice, 28*, 176–180.

Shaw-Battista, J. (2017). Systemic review of hydrotherapy research: Does a warm bath in labor promote normal physiologic childbirth? *Journal of Perinatal and Neonatal Nursing, 31*(4), 303–316.

Sidebottom, A., Vacquier, M., Simon, K., et al. (2020). Maternal and neonatal outcomes in hospital-based deliveries with water immersion. *Obstetrics & Gynecology, 136*(4), 707–715.

Van der Gucht, N., & Lewis, K. (2015). Women's experience of coping with pain during childbirth: A critical review of qualitative research. *Midwifery, 31*(3), 349–358.

Impaired Parenting

Domain 7 Role relationship Class 1 Caregiving roles

Marina Martinez Kratz, MS, RN, CNE

NANDA-I

Definition

Limitation of primary caregiver to nurture, protect, and promote optimal growth and development of the child, through a consistent, empathic exercise of authority and appropriate behavior in response to the child's needs.

Defining Characteristics

Parental Externalizing Symptoms

Hostile parenting behaviors; impulsive behaviors; intrusive behaviors; negative communication

Parental Internalizing Symptoms

Decreased engagement in parent-child relations; decreased positive temperament; decreased subjective attention quality; extreme mood swings; failure to provide safe home environment; inadequate response to infant behavioral cues; inappropriate child-care arrangements; rejects child; social alienation

Infant or Child

Anxiety; conduct problems; delayed cognitive development; depressive symptoms; difficulty establishing healthy intimate interpersonal relations; difficulty functioning socially; difficulty regulating emotion; extreme mood alterations; low academic performance; obesity; role reversal; somatic complaints; substance misuse

Related Factors

Altered parental role; decreased emotion recognition abilities; depressive symptoms; difficulty managing complex treatment regimen; dysfunctional family processes; emotional vacillation; high use of internet-connected devices; inadequate knowledge about child development; inadequate knowledge about child health maintenance; inadequate parental role model; inadequate problem-solving skills; inadequate social support; inadequate transportation; inattentive to child's needs; increased anxiety symptoms; low self efficacy; marital conflict; nonrestorative sleep-wake cycle; perceived economic strain; social isolation; substance misuse; unaddressed intimate partner violence

At-Risk Population

Parent

Adolescents; economically disadvantaged individuals; homeless individuals; individuals experiencing family substance misuse; individuals experiencing situational crisis; individuals with family history of post-traumatic shock; individuals with history of being abused; individuals with history of being abusive; individuals with history of being neglected; individuals with history of exposure to violence; individuals with history of inadequate prenatal care; individuals with history of prenatal stress; individuals with low educational level; sole parents

Infant or Child

Children experiencing prolonged separation from parent; children with difficult temperament; children with gender other than that desired by parent; children with history of hospitalization in neonatal intensive care; premature infants

Associated Conditions

Parent

Depression; mental disorders

Infant or Child

Behavioral disorder; complex treatment regimen; emotional disorder; neurodevelopmental disabilities

NOC (Nursing Outcomes Classification)

Suggested NOC Outcomes

Abuse Cessation; Abuse Protection; Abuse Recovery: Abusive Behavior Self-Restraint; Child Development (all); Coping; Family Functioning; Family Social Climate; Knowledge: Child Physical Safety; Neglect Recovery; Parent-Infant Attachment; Parenting Performance; Psychosocial Safety; Role Performance; Social Support

Example NOC Outcome with Indicators

Parenting Performance: Psychosocial Safety as evidenced by the following indicators: Fosters open communication/Recognizes risks for abuse/Uses strategies to eliminate risks for abuse/Selects appropriate supplemental caregivers/Uses strategies to prevent high-risk social behaviors/Provides required level of supervision/Sets clear rules for behavior/Maintains structure and daily routine in child's life. (Rate the outcome and indicators of **Parenting Performance: Psychosocial Safety:** 1 = never demonstrated, 2 = rarely demonstrated, 3 = sometimes demonstrated, 4 = often demonstrated, 5 = consistently demonstrated [see Section I].)

P

Client Outcomes

Client Will (Specify Time Frame)

- Initiate appropriate measures to develop a safe, nurturing environment
- Acquire and display attentive, supportive parenting behaviors and child supervision
- Identify appropriate strategies to manage a child's inappropriate behaviors
- Identify strategies to protect child from harm and/or neglect and initiate action when indicated

NIC (Nursing Interventions Classification)

Suggested NIC Interventions

Abuse Protection Support: Child; Attachment Promotion; Caregiver Support; Developmental Enhancement: Adolescent, Child; Environmental Management: Family Integrity Promotion; Impulse Control Training; Infant Care; Parent Education: Adolescent, Childrearing Family, Infant; Parenting Promotion; Role Enhancement; Substance Use Prevention, Treatment; Teaching: Infant Stimulation; Toddler Nutrition; Toddler Safety

Example NIC Activities—Family Integrity Promotion

Identify typical family coping mechanisms; Determine typical family relationships for each family; Counsel family members on additional effective coping skills for their own use; Assist family with conflict resolution; Monitor current family relationships; Facilitate a tone of togetherness within and among the family; Encourage family to maintain positive relationships; Refer for family therapy, as indicated

Nursing Interventions and *Rationales*

- Use the Parenting Sense of Competence (PSOC) scale to measure parental self-efficacy. EB: *The PSOC contains three useful factors that reflect satisfaction with the parental role, parenting efficacy, and interest in parenting. Mothers and fathers will differ in parenting of their children and their sense of competence* (*Karp et al, 2015*).
- Determine parent/family sources of stress, using the Parental Stress Scale. CEB: *The Parental Stress Scale is a valid and reliable self-report scale that contains 18 items representing pleasure or positive themes of parenthood* (*Berry & Jones, 1995*).
- Use family-centered care and role modeling for holistic care of families. EBN: *Incorporating family-centered care helps enhance the parents' role in caring for their child (Cady et al, 2015).*
- Assess for the following signs of parental burnout: exhaustion in one's parental role, contrast with previous parental self, feelings of being fed up with one's parental role, and emotional distancing from one's children. EB: *A study to measure parental burnout identified the four dimensions of parental burnout syndrome as exhaustion in one's parental role, contrast with previous parental self, feelings of being fed up with one's parental role, and emotional distancing from one's children (Roskam, Brianda, & Mikoljczak, 2018).*
- ▲ Institute abuse/neglect protection measures if evidence exists of an inability to cope with family stressors or crises, signs of parental substance abuse are observed, or a significant level of social isolation is apparent. EBN: *Encouraging parents to be involved with social networking can help reduce stressors and assist with coping in a crisis (Bennett et al, 2017).*
- Evaluate the family's perceived strength of its social support system. Encourage the family to use social support. EB: *A study of African American mothers found that social support moderated the relationship between parental stress and child behavior* (*Royal et al, 2017*).
- Support parents' competence in appraising their infant's behavior and responses and aim supportive interventions to minimize parents' experiences of strain or stress. EBN: *Encourage and support the presence of the parents with the care of the infant (Ottosson & Lantz, 2017).*
- ▲ Refer to parenting training programs. EB: *For parents of young children with neurodevelopmental disabilities, a systematic review found that parental participation in parent training programs significantly increased parental self-efficacy levels (Hohlfeld et al, 2018).*
- Refer to Readiness for Enhanced **Parenting** for additional interventions.

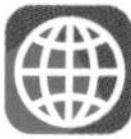

Multicultural

P

- Acknowledge racial/ethnic differences at the onset of care. EBN: *Providing culturally competent care is important to health care equality and is important for nurses to understand the importance of identifying the cultural differences that their clients will require* (*Dzubaty, 2016*).
- Assess for the influence of stigma related to parent help-seeking behaviors. EB: *A study found that self-stigma was the strongest predictor of help-seeking among African American parents (Dempster et al, 2015).*
- Assess for the influence of cultural beliefs, norms, and values on the client's perceptions of the parental role. EBN: *Understanding the cultures and beliefs of parents can enhance the interactions between nurse and family and assist the nurse to better care for the child and the family* (*Xiong et al, 2016*).
- Acknowledge that value conflicts arising from acculturation stresses may contribute to increased anxiety and significant conflict with the parental role. EB: *Study results suggest that lower acculturation conflict is associated with higher perceptions of general parenting competence for both Asian and Latin American parents (Kiang, Glatz, & Buchanan, 2017).*
- Refer parents of young children in specific cultural communities to support programs. EBN: *Parents and children benefit when a support group is incorporated into the care (Thomson-Salo et al, 2017).*

Home Care

- The interventions previously described may be adapted for home care use.

Client/Family Teaching and Discharge Planning

- Encourage children and parent involvement in bereavement support groups, as an adjunct to grief therapy. EB: *A systematic review found that online support groups may be a useful adjunct to, but not an alternative to, grief therapy or counseling* (*Robinson & Pond, 2019*).

- ▲ Refer to a parenting program to facilitate learning of parenting skills. EBN: *A study of foster parents showed that participation in parenting programs increased levels of skills and knowledge following training than did those in the control group (Solomon, Niec, & Schoonover, 2017).*
- ● Teach the client about available community resources (e.g., therapists, ministers, counselors, self-help groups). EBN: *Community-based resources can support caregivers and ensure that they can identify needed services (Tallon et al, 2017).*
- ● Teach parents the importance of involvement with and monitoring of child/adolescent technology usage, social media presence, and online activities for digital safety. EB: *A study found that parents' parental involvement was associated with a change in adolescent online risk-taking behavior through co-viewing, discussion of content viewed, and joint decision making regarding online activities (Wang & Xing, 2018).*
- ● Promotion of better-quality relationships between parents and children is an effective strategy that can lead to enhanced learning. Good-quality parenting leads to improved cognitive and social skills for children. EBN: *Parents have a positive effect on their children, which can lead to improved self-confidence and a stronger parent–child relationship (Kim et al, 2015).*

REFERENCES

Bennett, C. T., Buchan, J. L., Letourneau, N., et al. (2017). A realist synthesis of social connectivity interventions during transition to parenthood: The value of relationships. *Applied Nursing Research, 34*, 12–23. https://doi.org/10.1016/j.apnr.2016.11.004.

Berry, J. O., & Jones, W. H. (1995). The parental stress scale: Initial psychometric evidence. *Journal of Social and Personal Relationships, 12*(3), 463–472. https://doi.org/10.1177/0265407595123009.

Cady, R. G., Looman, W. S., Lindeke, L. L., et al. (2015). Pediatric care coordination: Lessons learned and future priorities. *Online Journal of Issues in Nursing, 20*(3), 3. https://doi.org//10.3912/OJIN.Vol20No03Man03.

Dempster, R., Davis, D. W., Jones, V. F., Keating, A., & Wildman, B. (2015). The role of stigma in parental help-seeking for perceived child behavior problems in urban, low-income African American parents. *Journal of Clinical Psychology in Medical Settings, 22*(4), 265–278. https://doi.org/10.1007/s10880-015-9433-8.

Dzubaty, D. R. (2016). Providing family-centered care in maternal-newborn settings: A case study. *Newborn and Infant Nursing Reviews, 16*(2), 55–57. https://doi.org/10.1053/j.nainr.2016.03.006.

Hohlfeld, A. S. J., Harty, M., & Engel, M. E. (2018). Parents of children with disabilities: A systematic review of parenting interventions and self-efficacy. *African Journal of Disability, 7*, 437. https://doi.org/10.4102/ajod.v7i0.437.

Karp, S. M., Lutenbacher, M., & Wallston, K. A. (2015). Evaluation of the parenting sense of competence scale in mothers of infants. *Journal of Child and Family Studies, 24*(11), 3474–3481. https://doi.org/10.1007/s10826-015-0149-z.

Kiang, L., Glatz, T., & Buchanan, C. M. (2017). Acculturation conflict, cultural parenting self-efficacy, and perceived parenting competence in Asian American and Latino/a families. *Family Process, 56*(4), 943–961. https://doi.org/10.1111/famp.12266.

Kim, J., Thompson, E. A., Walsh, E. M., & Schepp, K. G. (2015). Trajectories of parent–adolescent relationship quality among at-risk youth: Parental depression and adolescent developmental outcomes. *Archives of Psychiatric Nursing, 29*(6), 434–440. https://doi.org/10.1016/j.apnu.2015.07.001.

Ottosson, C., & Lantz, B. (2017). Parental participation in neonatal care. *Journal of Neonatal Nursing, 23*(3), 112–118. https://doi.org/10.1016/j.jnn.2016.11.001.

Robinson, C., & Pond, R. (2019). Do online support groups for grief benefit the bereaved? Systematic review of the quantitative and qualitative literature. *Computers in Human Behavior, 100*, 48–59. https://doi.org/10.1016/j.chb.2019.06.011.

Roskam, I., Brianda, M. E., & Mikolajczak, M. (2018). A step forward in the conceptualization and measurement of parental burnout: The parental burnout assessment (PBA). *Frontiers in Psychology, 9*, 758. https://doi.org/10.3389/fpsyg.2018.00758.

Royal, K. J., Eaton, S. C., Smith, N., Cliette, G., & Livingston, J. N. (2017). The impact of parental stress and social support on behavioral outcomes of children in African American single-mother households. *Journal of Black Sexuality and Relationships, 3*(4), 17–33. https://doi.org/10.1353/bsr.2017.0011.

Solomon, D. T., Niec, L. N., & Schoonover, C. E. (2017). The impact of foster parent training on parenting skills and child disruptive behavior: A meta-analysis. *Child Maltreatment, 22*(1), 3–13. https://doi.org/10.1177/1077559516679514.

Tallon, M. M., Kendall, G. E., Priddis, L., Newall, F., & Young, J. (2017). Barriers to addressing social determinants of health in pediatric nursing practice: An integrative review. *Journal of Pediatric Nursing, 37*, 51–56. https://doi.org/10.1016/j.pedn.2017.06.009.

Thomson-Salo, F., Kuschel, C. A., Kamlin, O. F., & Cuzilla, R. (2017). A fathers' group in NICU: Recognising and responding to paternal stress, utilising peer support. *Journal of Neonatal Nursing, 23*(6), 294–298. https://doi.org/10.1016/j.jnn.2017.04.001.

Wang, X., & Xing, W. (2018). Exploring the influence of parental involvement and socioeconomic status on teen digital citizenship: A path modeling approach. *Journal of Educational Technology & Society, 21*(1), 186–199. http://www.jstor.org/stable/26273879.

Xiong, S., Degroote, N., Byington, H., Harder, J., Kaminski, K., & Haglund, K. (2016). Engaging in culturally informed nursing care with Hmong children and their families. *Journal of Pediatric Nursing, 31*(1), 102–106. https://doi.org/10.1016/j.pedn.2015.08.008.

Readiness for Enhanced Parenting

Domain 7 Role relationship Class 1 Caregiving roles

Marina Martinez Kratz, MS, RN, CNE

NANDA-I

Definition

A pattern of primary caregiver to nurture, protect, and promote optimal growth and development of the child, through a consistent, empathic exercise of authority and appropriate behavior in response to the child's needs, which can be strengthened.

Defining Characteristics

Expresses desire to enhance acceptance of child; expresses desire to enhance attention quality; expresses desire to enhance child health maintenance; expresses desire to enhance childcare arrangements; expresses desire to enhance engagement with child; expresses desire to enhance home environmental safety; expresses desire to enhance mood stability; expresses desire to enhance parent-child relations; expresses desire to enhance patience; expresses desire to enhance positive communication; expresses desire to enhance positive parenting behaviors; expresses desire to enhance positive temperament; expresses desire to enhance response to infant behavioral cues

NOC (Nursing Outcomes Classification)

Suggested NOC Outcomes

Child Development; Knowledge: Child Physical Safety; Parenting Performance; Parenting: Psychosocial Safety

Example NOC Outcome with Indicators

Parenting Performance as evidenced by the following indicators: Provides preventive and episodic health care/Stimulates cognitive and social development/Stimulates emotional and spiritual growth/Empathizes with child/Expresses satisfaction with parental role/Expresses positive self-esteem. (Rate the outcome and indicators of **Parenting Performance:** 1 = never demonstrated, 2 = rarely demonstrated, 3 = sometimes demonstrated, 4 = often demonstrated, 5 = consistently demonstrated [see Section I].)

Client Outcomes

Client/Family Will (Specify Time Frame)

- Affirm desire to improve parenting skills to further support growth and development of children
- Demonstrate loving relationship with children
- Provide a safe, nurturing environment
- Assess risks in home/environment and take steps to prevent possibility of harm to children
- Meet physical, psychosocial, and spiritual needs or seek appropriate assistance

NIC (Nursing Interventions Classification)

Suggested NIC Interventions

Anticipatory Guidance; Attachment Promotion; Developmental Enhancement: Adolescent; Child; Family Integrity Promotion: Childbearing Family; Infant Care; Newborn Care; Parent Education: Adolescent, Childrearing Family, Infant; Parenting Promotion; Teaching: Infant Stimulation

Example NIC Activities—Parenting Promotion

Assist parents to have realistic expectations appropriate to developmental and ability level of child; Assist parents with role transition and expectations of parenthood

Nursing Interventions and *Rationales*

- Use family-centered care and role modeling for holistic care of families. EBN: *Incorporating family-centered care helps enhance the parents' role in caring for their child (Cady et al, 2015).*
- Use cell phone technology to enhance parenting interventions. EB: *A study found that a cellular phone–supported version of a parent–child interactions intervention promoted intervention retention and improved children's behavior (Lefever et al, 2017).*
- Promote low-technology interventions, such as massage and multisensory interventions (maternal voice, eye-to-eye contact, and rocking) and music, to reduce maternal and infant stress and improve mother–infant relationship. EB: *When mothers sing to their infants it can calm the infants and make them feel safe (de l'Etoile et al, 2017).*
- Promote mindful parenting techniques such as being fully present during interactions, maintaining freedom from distractions or judgment, and responding with an open mind. EB: *A study of parent–adolescent recurrent conflict found that higher levels of mindful parenting were significantly related to lower levels of recurrent conflict 2 to 3 months later and lower levels of recurrent conflict were significantly related to lower levels of externalizing problems and internalizing problems 1 year later (Park et al, 2020).*
- Support skin-to-skin care for infants at risk at birth; maintain infants in an upright position during skin-to-skin contact. EB: *Skin-to-skin care helps the mother and infant bond and assists in the infant's growth and development (Gavhane, Eklare, & Mohammad, 2016).*
- Encourage family meals and rituals. EB: *Study findings suggest that dinnertime rituals can potentially moderate the effects of parenting stress on child outcomes (Yoon et al, 2015).*
  - Refer to parenting training programs. EB: *For parents of young children with neurodevelopmental disabilities, a systematic review found that parental participation in parent training programs significantly increased parental self-efficacy levels (Hohlfeld et al, 2018).*
  - Refer to the care plan for Impaired **Parenting** for additional interventions.

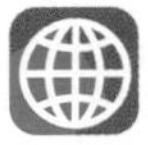

Multicultural

- Understand and incorporate cultural differences into interventions to enhance the impact of interventions. EB: *Tailoring interventions to the customs, beliefs, preferences, and strengths of specific groups may increase effectiveness (McCalman et al, 2017).*
- Support programs for parents of young children in specific cultural communities. EBN: *Parents and children benefit when a support group is incorporated into the care (Thomson-Salo et al, 2017).*
- Acknowledge and praise parenting strengths noted. EBN: *Parents see what they are doing right and are encouraged to continue the behavior (Ludmer et al, 2017).*

P

Home Care

- The nursing interventions previously described should be used in the home environment with adaptations as necessary. EB: *Clinicians should help educate parents on the care the child will need at home and modify to meet the family's needs (Thrasher et al, 2018).*
- ▲ Refer to a parenting program to facilitate learning of parenting skills. EBN: *A study of foster parents showed that participation in parenting programs increased levels of skills and knowledge following training more than did those in the control group (Solomon, Niec, & Schoonover, 2017).*

Client/Family Teaching and Discharge Planning

- Refer to Client/Family Teaching and Discharge Planning for Impaired **Parenting** for suggestions that may be used with minor adaptations.
- Teach parents home safety: reduction of hot water temperature, proper poison storage, use of smoke alarms, and installation of safety gates for stairs. EB: *Participation in a parent training program that emphasized home safety found significant reductions in home hazards after program participation (Rostad et al, 2017).*
- Provide parent teaching about supportive emotion communication practices such as listening and connection, labeling feelings, and providing emotional support. EB: *The Let's Connect program is an emotion-focused parenting intervention that showed significant increases in supportive emotion communication practices as well as significant reductions in unsupportive emotion communication in a pilot study (Shaffer et al, 2019).*

- ▲ Refer mothers of children with type 1 diabetes for community support in babysitting, child care, or respite. EB: *Families raising children with diabetes need to have support and interventions to assist with the care of the child to help reduce the burden of care on the parents (Kobos & Imiela, 2015).*
- ▲ Refer parents of sexual minority adolescents to supportive parenting resources and programs. EB: *The Parent Resource for Increasing Sexual Minority Support (PRISMS) is an interactive online intervention designed to promote parental self-efficacy and behavioral intentions for supporting a sexual minority child. Participation in PRISMS appears to be effective for parents who were highly distressed about their child's sexual orientation (Goodman & Israel, 2020).*
- • Teach parents the importance of involvement with and monitoring of child/adolescent technology usage, social media presence, and online activities for digital safety. EB: *A study found that parental involvement was associated with a change in adolescent online risk-taking behavior through co-viewing, discussion of content viewed, and joint decision-making regarding online activities (Wang & Xing, 2018).*
- • Promotion of better-quality relationships between parents and children is an effective strategy that can lead to enhanced learning. Good-quality parenting leads to improved cognitive and social skills for children. EBN: *Parents have a positive effect on their children, which can lead to improved self-confidence and a stronger parent–child relationship (Kim et al, 2015).*

REFERENCES

See Impaired **Parenting** for additional references.

Cady, R. G., Looman, W. S., Lindeke, L. L., et al. (2015). Pediatric care coordination: Lessons learned and future priorities. *Online Journal of Issues in Nursing*, *20*(3), 3. https://doi.org/10.3912/OJIN.Vol20No03Man03.

de l'Etoile, S., Behura, S., & Zopluoglu, C. (2017). Acoustic parameters of infant-directed singing in mothers of infants with down syndrome. *Infant Behavior and Development*, *49*, 151–160. https://doi.org/10.1016/j.infbeh.2017.09.001

Gavhane, S., Eklare, D., & Mohammad, H. (2016). Long term outcomes of kangaroo mother care in very low birth weight infants. *Journal of Clinical and Diagnostic Research*, *10*(12), SC13–SC15. https://doi.org/10.7860/JCDR/2016/23855.9006

Goodman, J. A., & Israel, T. (2020). An online intervention to promote predictors of supportive parenting for sexual minority youth. *Journal of Family Psychology*, *34*(1), 90–100. https://doi.org/10.1037/fam0000614

Hohlfeld, A. S. J., Harty, M., & Engel, M. E. (2018). Parents of children with disabilities: A systematic review of parenting interventions and self-efficacy. *African Journal of Disability*, *7*, 437. https://doi.org/10.4102/ajod.v7i0.437

Kim, J., Thompson, E. A., Walsh, E. M., & Schepp, K. G. (2015). Trajectories of parent–adolescent relationship quality among at-risk youth: Parental depression and adolescent developmental outcomes. *Archives of Psychiatric Nursing*, *29*(6), 434–440. https://doi.org/10.1016/j.apnu.2015.07.001

Kobos, E., & Imiela, J. (2015). Factors affecting the level of burden of caregivers of children with type 1 diabetes. *Applied Nursing Research*, *28*(2), 142–149. https://doi.org/10.1016/j.apnr.2014.09.008

Lefever, J. E. B., Bigelow, K. M., Carta, J. J., et al. (2017). Long-term impact of a cell phone–enhanced parenting intervention. *Child Maltreatment*, *22*(4), 305–314. https://doi.org/10.1177/1077559517723125

Ludmer, J. A., Salsbury, D., Suarez, J., & Andrade, B. F. (2017). Accounting for the impact of parent internalizing symptoms on parent training benefits: The role of positive parenting. *Behaviour Research and Therapy*, *97*, 252–258. https://doi.org/10.1016/j.brat.2017.08.012

McCalman, J., Heyeres, M., Campbell, S., et al. (2017). Family-centred interventions by primary healthcare services for Indigenous early childhood well-being in Australia, Canada, New Zealand, and the United States: A systematic scoping review. *BMC Pregnancy and Childbirth*, *17*(1), 71. https://doi.org/10.1186/s12884-017-1247-2

Park, Y. R., Nix, R. L., Duncan, L. G., Coatsworth, J. D., & Greenberg, M. T. (2020). Unfolding relations among mindful parenting, recurrent conflict, and adolescents' externalizing and internalizing problems. *Family Process*, *59*(4), 1690–1705. https://doi.org/10.1111/famp.12498

Rostad, W. L., McFry, E. A., Self-Brown, S., Damashek, A., & Whitaker, D. J. (2017). Reducing safety hazards in the home through the use of an evidence-based parenting program. *Journal of Child and Family Studies*, *26*, 2602–2609. https://doi.org/10.1007/s10826-017-0756-y

Shaffer, A., Fitzgerald, M. M., Shipman, K., & Torres, M. (2019). Let's connect: A developmentally-driven emotion-focused parenting intervention. *Journal of Applied Developmental Psychology*, *63*, 33–41. https://doi.org/10.1016/j.brat.2017.08.012

Solomon, D. T., Niec, L. N., & Schoonover, C. E. (2017). The impact of foster parent training on parenting skills and child disruptive behavior: A meta-analysis. *Child Maltreatment*, *22*(1), 3–13. https://doi.org/10.1177/1077559516679514

Thomson-Salo, F., Kuschel, C. A., Kamlin, O. F., & Cuzilla, R. (2017). A fathers' group in NICU: Recognising and responding to paternal stress, utilising peer support. *Journal of Neonatal Nursing*, *23*(6), 294–298. https://doi.org/10.1016/j.jnn.2017.04.001

Thrasher, J., Baker, J., Ventre, K. M., et al. (2018). Hospital to home: A quality improvement initiative to implement high-fidelity simulation training for caregivers of children requiring long-term mechanical ventilation. *Journal of Pediatric Nursing*, *38*, 114–121. https://doi.org/10.1016/j.pedn.2017.08.028

Wang, X., & Xing, W. (2018). Exploring the influence of parental involvement and socioeconomic status on teen digital citizenship: A path modeling approach. *Journal of Educational Technology & Society*, *21*(1), 186–199. http://www.jstor.org/stable/26273879.

Yoon, Y., Newkirk, K., & Perry-Jenkins, M. (2015). Parenting stress, dinnertime rituals, and child and child well-being in working-class families. *Family Relations*, *64*(1), 93–107. https://doi.org/10.1111/fare.12107

Risk for Impaired Parenting

Domain 7 Role relationship Class 1 Caregiving roles

Marina Martinez-Kratz, MS, RN, CNE

NANDA-I

Definition

Primary caregiver susceptible to a limitation to nurture, protect, and promote optimal growth and development of the child, through a consistent, empathic exercise of authority and appropriate behavior in response to the child's needs.

Risk Factors

Altered parental role; decreased emotion recognition abilities; depressive symptoms; difficulty managing complex treatment regimen; dysfunctional family processes; emotional vacillation; high use of Internet-connected devices; inadequate knowledge about child development; inadequate knowledge about child health maintenance; inadequate parental role model; inadequate problem-solving skills; inadequate social support; inadequate transportation; inattentive to child's needs; increased anxiety symptoms; low self efficacy; marital conflict; nonrestorative sleep-wake cycle; perceived economic strain; social isolation; substance misuse; unaddressed intimate partner violence

At-Risk Population

Parent

Adolescents; economically disadvantaged individuals; homeless individuals; individuals experiencing family substance misuse; individuals experiencing situational crisis; individuals with family history of post-traumatic shock; individuals with history of being abused; individuals with history of being abusive; individuals with history of being neglected; individuals with history of exposure to violence; individuals with history of inadequate prenatal care; individuals with history of prenatal stress; individuals with low educational level; sole parents

Infant or Child

Children experiencing prolonged separation from parent; children with difficult temperament; children with gender other than that desired by parent; children with history of hospitalization in neonatal intensive care; premature infants

Associated Conditions

Parent

Depression; mental disorders

Infant or Child

Behavioral disorder; complex treatment regimen; emotional disorder; neurodevelopmental disabilities

NOC, NIC, Client Outcomes, Nursing Interventions and *Rationales,* Client/Family Teaching and Discharge Planning, and References

Refer to care plans for Readiness for Enhanced **Parenting** and Impaired **Parenting**.

Risk for Perioperative Positioning Injury

Domain 11 Safety/protection Class 2 Physical injury

Kristen A. Oster, DNP, APRN, ACNS-BC, CNOR, CNS-CP

NANDA-I

Definition

Susceptible to inadvertent anatomical and physical changes as a result of posture or positioning equipment used during an invasive/surgical procedure, which may compromise health.

P

Risk Factors

Decreased muscle strength; dehydration; factors identified by standardized, validated screening tool; inadequate access to appropriate equipment; inadequate access to appropriate support surfaces; inadequate availability of equipment for individuals with obesity; malnutrition; obesity; prolonged non-anatomic positioning of limbs; rigid support surface

At-Risk Population

Individuals at extremes of age; individuals in lateral position; individuals in lithotomy position; individuals in prone position; individuals in Trendelenburg position; individuals undergoing surgical procedure >1 hour

Associated Conditions

Diabetes mellitus; edema; emaciation; general anesthesia; immobilization; neuropathy; sensoriperceptual disturbance from anesthesia; vascular diseases

NOC (Nursing Outcomes Classification)

Suggested NOC Outcomes

Circulation Status; Immobility Consequences: Physiological; Joint Movement; Neurological Status; Respiratory Status; Risk Control; Sensory Function; Skeletal Function; Tissue Integrity: Skin and Mucous Membranes; Tissue Perfusion: Peripheral

Example NOC Outcome with Indicators

Tissue Perfusion: Peripheral as evidenced by the following indicators: Peripheral edema/Localized extremity pain/Skin breakdown/Muscle cramps/Peripheral pulses/Numbness/Tingling/Necrosis. (Rate the outcome and indicators of **Tissue Perfusion: Peripheral:** 1 = severe, 2 = substantial, 3 = moderate, 4 = mild, 5 = none [see Section I].)

Client Outcomes

Client Will (Specify Time Frame)

- Demonstrate unchanged skin condition, with exception of the incision, throughout the perioperative experience
- Demonstrate resolution of redness of the skin at points of pressure within 30 minutes after pressure is eliminated
- Remain injury-free related to surgical positioning, including intact skin and absence of pain and/or numbness associated with surgical positioning
- Demonstrate unchanged or improved physical mobility from preoperative status
- Demonstrate unchanged or improved peripheral sensory integrity from preoperative status

NIC (Nursing Interventions Classification)

Suggested NIC Interventions

Circulatory Precautions; Fall Prevention; Neurological Monitoring; Peripheral Sensation Management; Positioning: Intraoperative; Pressure Ulcer Prevention; Risk Identification; Skin Surveillance; Surgical Precautions

Example NIC Activities—Positioning: Intraoperative

Use an adequate number of personnel to transfer client; Maintain client's proper body alignment

Nursing Interventions and *Rationales*

General Interventions for Any Surgical Client

▲ Positioning of the client during a surgical procedure is the responsibility of all members of the perioperative team, including registered nurse, surgical technologist, surgeon, and anesthesia professional (Spruce, 2018).

- Assess the client's skin integrity throughout the perioperative process to avoid skin breakdown during surgical/invasive procedures. Continuous evaluation of clinical changes in the client is necessary to assess outcomes and effects of nursing interventions for surgical positioning (Bjorkland-Lima et al, 2019). EB: *Developing skin breakdown manifested as a skin tear, pressure ulcer, deep tissue injury, or burn is a significant client complication affected by the duration of surgery and client positioning (National Pressure Injury Advisory Panel [NPIAP] & European Pressure Ulcer Advisory Panel [EPUAP], 2019; Van Wicklin, 2019).*
- Recognize that surgery increases a client's risk for skin injury because of the time the client is immobile for the procedure (Park, Park, & Hwang, 2019).
- An operating room–related pressure injury is any pressure injury that develops within 48 to 72 hours intraoperatively, interoperatively, or postoperatively of a surgical procedure (Khong et al, 2020).

Prevention of Pressure Injuries

- Complete a preoperative assessment to identify client factors that will increase a client's risk for pressure injuries. This includes physical alterations that may require additional precautions for procedure-specific positioning and to identify specific procedural positioning needs, type of anesthesia, and so on. EBN: *Factors to consider when assessing the surgical client to plan for proper positioning are preexisting conditions such as vascular disease or diabetes, range of motion, presence of prostheses and/or fractures, skin condition, advanced age, nutritional status, weight, American Society of Anesthesiologists (ASA) physical status classification, and the presence of moisture (Spruce, 2017; Van Wicklin, 2019).*
- Identify procedure risk factors such as length and type of surgery, potential for intraoperative hypotensive episodes, low core temperatures, and decreased mobility on postoperative day 1. EB: *Assess the client for additional risk factors, including the duration of immobilization before and during the surgical procedure, client severity of illness, preoperative nutritional status, position for the procedure, and type of anesthesia (NPIAP & EPUAP, 2019; Van Wicklin, 2019). Increased length of surgery has been identified as an intraoperative-specific risk factor to pressure injury development (Miller et al, 2020). Surgeries lasting more than 3 hours provide a significant risk for pressure ulcer development, with continued risk for development increasing every hour (Riemenschneider, 2018).* EB: *Recent studies have identified the use of vasopressor as a significant risk for pressure ulcer development (NPIAP & EPUAP, 2019). Additional review showed the number of surgeries a client has during his or her hospital inpatient stay and the length of surgery (over 1 hour), body mass index, Braden score, mortality risk, and history of diabetes are also risk factors for pressure ulcer development (Tschannen & Anderson, 2020).*
- Recognize that all surgical clients should be considered at high risk for pressure ulcer development, because pressure ulcers can develop in as little as 20 minutes in the operating room. EBN: *Operating room mattresses, the client support surface, should be chosen for their pressure redistribution (Spruce, 2017). Support surfaces that redistribute pressure are recommended. Alternating pressure overlays may improve outcomes in regard to pressure injuries, including clients deemed at high risk for pressure injury development during surgery (Joseph et al, 2019).*
- Remove all client jewelry and accessories. EBN: *Jewelry and accessories, such as body piercings and hair devices, can get caught and torn out, causing skin injury; the client can lie on them and develop a pressure injury; or the client can experience a burn from cautery equipment (Van Wicklin, 2019).*
- Protect the heels during surgery by elevating the heels completely. EB: *Ensure that the heels are free of the surface of the operating table (NPIAP & EPUAP, 2019). Heel pressure ulcers are one of the most common sites for pressure injury during surgery. Traditional devices such as egg crates, booties, and heel pads do not decrease the pressure. It is recommended that a device be used to elevate the heels and distribute the weight of the client's leg along the calf (Van Wicklin, 2019).*
- Use pressure-reducing devices and pressure-relieving mattresses as necessary to prevent pressure injury. EB: *Use a high-specification reactive or alternating pressure support surface on the operating table for all individuals identified as being at risk for pressure ulcer development (NPIAP & EPUAP, 2019). Additional support surfaces may be indicated to offload pressure points on the face and body when the client is placed in a prone position (NPIAP & EPUAP, 2019; Van Wicklin, 2019). Support surfaces may be made of foam, gel, air, fluid, or a combination of these surfaces. The goal is to have pressure distributed over the largest area possible. This is accomplished by having the surface envelop the client (Van Wicklin, 2019). Assess for shearing forces that may cause tissue injury when placing the client in the Trendelenburg position for selected robotic surgical procedures (Das et al, 2019).*
- Avoid using rolled sheets and towels as positioning devices because they tend to produce high and inconsistent pressures. Special positioning devices are available that redistribute pressure. EBN: *Towels and*

P

rolled sheets contribute to friction injuries and increase pressure on the client. Pillows are an acceptable alternative when other positioning devices are unavailable (Van Wicklin, 2019).

- Avoid covering positioning devices or placing extra blankets on top of a pressure-reducing surface. **EB:** *Adding material to a pressure-reduction surface actually increases the pressure, producing a negative result (Van Wicklin, 2019). Use of rolled sheets and towels beneath overlays decreases the overlays' effectiveness and causes pressure (Van Wicklin, 2019).*
- The nurse should demonstrate knowledge not only of the equipment but also of anatomy and the application of physiological principles to properly position the client. **EBN:** *Preplanning ensures that the correct positioning devices are available and in good working condition, and that appropriate numbers of personnel are available to position the client safely and appropriately. High-specification reactive foam mattresses should be used for clients at high risk for pressure injury (Van Wicklin, 2019).*
- Monitor client position and pressure being applied to the client intraoperatively by staff, equipment, and/or instruments. *Clients may move slightly or shift during surgery, especially during long procedures or when new equipment is introduced, requiring that the client be repositioned to avoid pressure or nerve injury (Van Wicklin, 2019).*
- Use additional pressure-redistributing padding on all bony prominences. **EB:** *Additional padding increases client comfort, helps redistribute pressure, and decreases the chance for development of pressure or nerve injuries (Van Wicklin, 2019). Some positioning devices are solid and can increase pressure over bony prominences (Bjøro et al, 2020).*
- Recognize that reddened areas or areas injured by pressure should not be massaged. **EB:** *Rubbing causes friction that can lead to damage to skin/tissue (NPIAP & EPUAP, 2019; Van Wicklin, 2019).*
- Implement measures to prevent inadvertent hypothermia. *Anesthesia can compromise perfusion by causing hypotension and hypothermia. When coupled with the client being immobile on a noncompliant surface for an extended time period, hypothermia increases vulnerability for pressure ulcer development during surgery.*
- Many surgical clients have medical devices placed as a part of the surgical procedure. Avoid positioning the client on the medical device and perform frequent assessments of the skin under and around the device (NPIAP & EPUAP, 2019; Cooper et al, 2020). **EB:** *If a medical device is used for a prolonged period of time it can create pressure or edema and cause friction/shearing resulting in reduced sensation, circulation, and alteration in the microclimate (Cooper et al, 2020).*

Positioning the Perioperative Client

- Ensure linens on the operating room table are free of wrinkles. **EBN:** *Wrinkles may cause pressure/injury to the skin if the client is unable to move for prolonged periods of time. Layers of linens or blankets between the client and the support surface decrease the pressure-redistributing effect of the support surface (Van Wicklin, 2019).*
- Lock the operating room table, cart, or bed and stabilize the mattress before transfering/positioning the client. Monitor the client while on the operating room table at all times. **EBN:** *Studies showed that a lack of clear communication about who should be watching the client has contributed to falls (Van Wicklin, 2019).*
- Lift rather than pull or slide the client when positioning to reduce the incidence of skin injury from shearing and/or friction. **EB/EBN:** *Sliding or pulling the client can cause shearing force and/or friction (NPIAP & EPUAP, 2019; Van Wicklin, 2019).*
- Ensure that appropriate numbers of personnel are present to assist in positioning the client. **EBN:** *A minimum of two people should assist an awake client to transfer from a cart/bed to the operating room table: one person on the stretcher side to assist the client onto the table and a second person on the far side of the table to prevent the client from falling off. A minimum of four persons are necessary when transferring/positioning an anesthetized, unconscious, obese, or weak client (Van Wicklin, 2019).*
- Recognize that, optimally, clients (especially those with limited range of motion/mobility) should be asked to position themselves under the nurse's guidance before induction of anesthesia so that the nurse can verify that a position of comfort has been obtained.
- Ensure that nerves are protected by positioning extremities carefully. **EB/EBN:** *Nerves can be injured by stretching and compression, which is caused by a loss of protective muscle tone and pressure between two fixed points. Careful attention to proper body alignment and padding is necessary to prevent peripheral nerve injury (Van Wicklin, 2019; Bjøro et al, 2020).*
- Use slow and smooth movements during positioning *to allow the circulatory system to readjust.*
- Reassess the client after positioning and periodically during the procedure to maintain proper alignment and skin integrity. **EBN:** *Changes in position can expose or injure body parts (e.g., shearing, friction,*

P

compression) that were originally protected, and the safety strap can shift and apply increased pressure. If possible, after 3 or 4 hours of surgery, the client should be checked, under the drapes, to make sure the client remains in alignment (Van Wicklin, 2019).

- Frequently assess the eyes and/or monitor intraocular pressure, especially when client is in the prone, Trendelenburg, or knee-chest position. EBN: *The cornea can easily be injured during surgery because of a decrease in lacrimation, failure of the eyes to fully close and/or improperly applied face masks, or prolonged prone positioning (Van Wicklin, 2019).*
- Position hips in proper alignment with knees flexed. Unaligned hips can cause pressure to the low back and hip joints. EBN: *Proper body alignment needs to be maintained to prevent nerve and pressure injuries (Van Wicklin, 2019).*
- Position the arms extended on arm boards so that they do not extend beyond a 90-degree angle. The arms should be at the level of the bed and should not be allowed to hang off the bed. Do not position arms at sides unless surgically necessary. EBN: *Positioning at less than a 90-degree angle, with elbows slightly flexed and hands supine, decreases the risk of a stretching injury to the brachial plexus and possible compression or occlusion injury to the subclavian and axillary arteries. When positioning arms at the sides is necessary, place the arms beneath the sheet and bring the sheet over the top of the arm and then tuck the sheet beneath the mattress so that the arm cannot fall off the mattress and hang over the metal edge of the table, where the surgical team could lean against it (Van Wicklin, 2019).*
- Protect the client's skin surfaces from injury by preventing pooling of preparative solutions, blood, irrigation, urine, and feces. EBN: *Prep solutions may change the pH of the skin and remove protective oils, making the skin more susceptible to pressure and friction. Pooling also increases the risk of maceration (Van Wicklin, 2019).*
- Keep the client appropriately covered and limit traffic in the room during the procedure. EBN:*Reducing unnecessary exposure provides privacy and dignity for the client during positioning and helps prevent hypothermia (Van Wicklin, 2019).*
- When positioning the client prone, care should be taken to ensure the head and neck are properly positioned. In addition, 5- to 10-degree reverse Trendelenburg should be used, if possible, to reduce intraocular pressure and decrease facial edema. EB/EBN: *Inappropriate positioning of the head and neck in the prone position can lead to vertebral artery obstruction and possible stroke. Standard foam prone pillows should be used because they stabilize the neck in neutral, and the endotracheal tube can be positioned away from the face to decrease excessive pressure (Spruce, 2017; Van Wicklin, 2019).*
- Recognize that clients positioned in the lithotomy position should be kept in this position for as short a time as possible. EBN: *One research review suggested that the client's legs be removed from lithotomy positioning devices every 2 hours when the procedure is expected to last 4 hours or longer. Reported complications from extended time in this position include muscle contusion, compartment syndrome, and acute renal failure (Van Wicklin, 2019).*
- The lowest heel position should be used in the lithotomy position. EBN: *When possible, the legs should be at or lower than the level of the heart to prevent complications (Van Wicklin, 2019).*
- Maintain normal body alignment. EBN: *Misalignment, flexion, extension, and rotation may cause muscle and nerve damage and airway interference; pressure on the carotid sinus can cause arrhythmias; and restricted venous outflow can occur with extreme rotation of the head (Van Wicklin, 2019).*
- When applying body supports and restraint straps (safety belt), apply loosely and secure over waist or midthigh at least 2 inches above the knees, avoiding bony prominences by placing a blanket between the strap and the client. EBN: *Belts positioned directly over the knees cause compression of the peroneal nerve against the fibula (Van Wicklin, 2019).*
- Assess the client's skin integrity immediately postoperatively. EB: *Assess and document postoperative skin/tissue integrity focusing on areas with constant pressure during the procedure and limb function for nerve damage (Celik, Karayurt, & Ogce, 2019; NPIAP & EPUAP, 2019).*
- Ensure that complete, concise, accurate documentation of client assessment and use of positioning devices is in the client's medical record.

Geriatric

- Common age-related diseases include cardiovascular, diabetes, lung, renal, musculoskeletal, and neurodegenerative diseases. Progression of these diseases can lead to impaired systems and organs, leading to complications including anemia, malnutrition, and recurrent infection (Jaul et al, 2018).
- The skin of older adults (i.e., ≥65 years) is fragile and prone to shear injuries as the skin is less elastic; the dermis is thin and has less collagen, muscle, and adipose tissue than the skin of younger adults (Van

P

Wicklin, 2019). These changes leave the older adult's skin more susceptible to pressure, bruising, skin tears, infection, impaired thermoregulation, and slow healing (Van Wicklin, 2019). **EBN:** *Use of prophylactic dressings to bony prominences or other areas subjected to pressure, friction, and shear may be beneficial. Use of prophylactic dressings reduces the amount of shear delivered to skin through displacement and absorption of shearing forces (Van Wicklin, 2019).*

Pediatric

- Pressure injury sites in the pediatric client differ from those in the adult population due to differences in anatomic structure. **EBN:** *The occipital region is at increased risk for injury in infants and toddlers in the supine position due to disproportionately large head size (Van Wicklin, 2019).*
- Neonates are vulnerable to skin and pressure injuries because of an immature and underdeveloped epidermis and dermis (Broom, Dunk, & Mohamed, 2019). **EBN:** *The skin of children may be more resilient to normal and shear pressures than the skin of older adults because it is supported with sufficient collagen and elastin (Van Wicklin, 2019).*
- Neonates and children are at higher risk for nutritional deficiencies as a result of smaller appetites and dietary intake in combination with increased nutritional requirement necessary to meet growth needs (Van Wicklin, 2019).
- Use of pediatric- and neonatal-specific pressure injury risk assessment tools accounts for age-specific indicators. **EBN:** *Tools include the Braden Q Scale, Braden Q+P Scale, Glamorgan Scale, and Neonatal Skin Risk Assessment Scale (Van Wicklin, 2019).*

Client/Family Teaching and Discharge Planning

- Teach the client/family signs and symptoms of pressure injury, extremity nerve damage, compartment syndrome, and ocular injury based on surgical positioning. Early detection and treatment is beneficial.

REFERENCES

Bjorkland-Lima, L., Müller-Staub, M., Cardoso e Cardozo, M., de Souza Bernardes, D., & Rabelo-Silva, E. R. (2019). Clinical indicators of nursing outcomes classification for patient with risk for perioperative positioning injury: A cohort study. *Journal of Clinical Nursing, 28*(23–24), 4367–4378. https://doi.org/10.1111/jocn.15019.

Bjøro, B., Mykkeltveit, I., Rustøen, T., Altinbas, B. C., Røise, O., & Bentsen, S. B. (2020). Intraoperative peripheral nerve injury related to lithotomy positioning with steep Trendelenburg in patients undergoing robotic-assisted laparoscopic surgery—A systematic review. *Journal of Advanced Nursing, 76*(2), 490–503. https://doi.org/10.1111/jan.14271.

Broom, M., Dunk, A. M., & Mohamed, A. L. E. (2019). Predicting neonatal skin injury: The first step to reducing skin injuries in neonates. *Health Services Insights, 12*, 1178632919845630. https://doi.org/10.1177/1178632919845630.

Celik, B., Karayurt, O., & Ogce, F. (2019). The effect of selected risk factors on perioperative pressure injury development. *AORN Journal, 110*(1), 29–38. https://doi.org/10.1002/aorn.12725.

Cooper, K. D., McQueen, K. M., Halm, M. A., & Flayter, R. (2020). Prevention and treatment of device-related hospital-acquired pressure injuries. *American Journal of Critical Care, 29*(2), 150–154. https://doi.org/10.4037/ajcc2020167.

Das, D., Propst, K., Wechter, M. E., & Kho, R. M. (2019). Evaluation of positioning devices for optimization of outcomes in laparoscopic and robotic-assisted gynecologic surgery. *Journal of Minimally Invasive Gynecology, 26*(2), 244–252.e1. https://doi.org/10.1016/j.jmig.2018.08.027.

Jaul, E., Barron, J., Rosenweig, J. P., & Menczel, J. (2018). An overview of co-morbidities and the development of pressure ulcers among older adults. *BMC Geriatrics, 18*(1), 305. https://doi.org/10.1186/s12877-018-0997-7.

Joseph, J., McLaughlin, D., Darian, V., Hayes, L., & Siddiqui, A. (2019). Alternating pressure overlay for prevention of intraoperative pressure injury. *The Journal of Wound, Ostomy and Continence Nursing, 46*(1), 13–17. https://doi.org/10.1097/WON.0000000000000497.

Khong, B. P. C., Goh, B. C., Phang, L. Y., & David, T. (2020). Operating room nurses' self-reported knowledge and attitude on perioperative pressure injury. *International Wound Journal, 17*(2), 455–465. https://doi.org/10.1111/iwj.13295.

Miller, M. W., Emeny, R. T., Snide, J. A., & Freed, G. L. (2020). Patient-specific factors associated with pressure injuries revealed by electronic health record analyses. *Health Informatics Journal, 26*(1), 474–485. https://doi.org/10.1177/1460458219832053.

National Pressure Injury Advisory Panel (NPIAP) and European Pressure Ulcer Advisory Panel (EPUAP). (2019). In E. Haesler (Ed.), *Prevention and treatment of pressure ulcers*. Perth, Australia: Cambridge Media.

Park, S., Park, H., & Hwang, H. (2019). Development and comparison of predictive models for pressure injuries in surgical patients. *The Journal of Wound, Ostomy and Continence Nursing, 46*(4), 291–297. https://doi.org/10.1097/WON.0000000000000544.

Riemenschneider, K. J. (2018). Prevention of pressure injuries in the operating room: A quality improvement project. *The Journal of Wound, Ostomy and Continence Nursing, 45*(2), 141–145. https://doi.org/10.1097/WON.0000000000000410.

Spruce, L. (2017). Back to basics: Preventing perioperative pressure injuries. *AORN Journal, 105*(1), 92–99. https://doi.org/10.1016/j.aorn.2016.10.018.

Spruce, L. (2018). Back to basics: Orthopedic positioning. *AORN Journal, 107*(3), 355–367 doi.org/10.1002/aorn.12071.

Tschannen, D., & Anderson, C. (2020). The pressure injury predictive model: A framework for hospital-acquired pressure injuries. *Journal of Clinical Nursing, 29*(7–8), 1398–1421. https://doi.org/10.1111/jocn.15171.

Van Wicklin, S. A. (2019). *Guideline for positioning the patient*. Retrieved from http://aornguidelines.org/guidelines/content?sectionid=173734066&view=book#173734066. [Accessed 28 September 2020].

Risk for Peripheral Neurovascular Dysfunction

Domain 11 Safety/projection Class 2 Physical injury

Krystal Chamberlain Tenure, MS, RN, CCRN, SCRN

NANDA-I

Definition

Susceptible to disruption in the circulation, sensation, and motion of an extremity, which may compromise health.

Risk Factors

To be developed

Associated Conditions

Bone fractures; burns; immobilization; mechanical compression; orthopedic surgery; trauma; vascular obstruction

NOC (Nursing Outcomes Classification)

Suggested NOC Outcomes

Circulation Status; Neurological Status: Spinal Sensorimotor Function; Tissue Perfusion: Peripheral

Example NOC Outcome with Indicators

Tissue Perfusion: Peripheral as evidenced by the following indicators: Radial or pedal pulse strength/Capillary refill in fingers or toes/Extremity skin temperature/Localized extremity pain/Numbness/Tingling/Skin color/Muscle strength/Skin integrity/Peripheral edema. (Rate the outcome and indicators of **Tissue Perfusion: Peripheral:** 1 = severe deviation from normal range, 2 = substantial deviation from normal range, 3 = moderate deviation from normal range, 4 = mild deviation from normal range, 5 = no deviation from normal range [see Section I].)

Client Outcomes

Client Will (Specify Time Frame)

- Maintain circulation, sensation, and movement of an extremity within client's own normal limits
- Explain signs of neurovascular compromise

P

NIC (Nursing Interventions Classification)

Suggested NIC Interventions

Exercise Therapy: Joint Mobility; Peripheral Sensation Management

Example NIC Activities—Peripheral Sensation Management

Monitor for paresthesia: numbness, tingling, hyperesthesia, and hypoesthesia; Monitor for thrombophlebitis and deep vein thrombosis

Nursing Interventions and *Rationales*

- Recognize the risk factors that may result in peripheral neurovascular dysfunction. EB: *Conditions that diminish limb perfusion (e.g., tight-fitting dressings, casts, intraoperative positioning, edema, burns, trauma, snake or insect bites) could result in peripheral neurovascular dysfunction and/or compartment syndrome, an elevation of pressure within a compartment, leading to decreased tissue perfusion and cell death (Oak & Abrams, 2016; Schreiber, 2016). The nurse's proficient and timely assessment is critical in ensuring a positive client outcome (Schreiber, 2016).*

- Assess for the early onset of neurovascular dysfunction or compartment syndrome by performing the neurovascular assessment as ordered or as indicated by the client's condition, and report abnormal findings to the provider promptly. **EB:** *Early recognition of neurovascular dysfunction will minimize tissue necrosis and functional loss (Oak & Abrams, 2016). Historically, the "five Ps" of assessment, as outlined in the following list, have been used to identify compartment syndrome. However, pain is the most reliable finding and the other findings may be absent or late signs of compartment syndrome though may be helpful in the identification of vascular injury (Maher, 2016; Oak & Abrams, 2016).*
  - Pain: Assess severity (using an appropriate pain scale), quality, radiation, and relief by medications. **EB:** *Pain out of proportion to the injury that does not respond to opiates, and elicited with passive stretching of the compartment, is the earliest indicator and most reliable sign of compartment syndrome (Maher, 2016).*
  - Pulses: Assess the pulses distal to the injury and compare with the unaffected limb; use a 0-to-4 point scale (0 = absent and 4 = strong/bounding). **EB:** *Inequality of pulses is an abnormal finding that can indicate poor perfusion; pulses could still be present in the setting of compartment syndrome (Oak & Abrams, 2016; Schreiber, 2016).*
  - Pallor: Assess skin color and temperature changes below the injury site and compare with unaffected limb; assess capillary refill. **EB:** *Changes in temperature or color could indicate poor perfusion; consider the client's baseline skin tone. Skin that is shiny and pale suggests building pressure. Capillary refill time greater than 3 seconds can indicate abnormal perfusion (Schreiber, 2016).*
  - Paresthesia (change in sensation): Assess by lightly touching the skin proximal and distal to the injury; ask if the client has any unusual sensations such as hypersensitivity, tingling, prickling, decreased feeling, or numbness. **EB:** *Abnormal sensory findings may be related to nerve compression, compromised blood flow, and/or tissue ischemia (Maher, 2016; Schreiber, 2016).*
  - Paralysis: Ask the client to perform appropriate range-of-motion exercises in the unaffected and then the affected extremity. **EB:** *Loss of movement (paralysis) is a late sign of neurovascular dysfunction (Schreiber, 2016).*
  - In addition to the five Ps, assess for swelling or increase in compartment pressure by feeling the extremity; note new onset of firmness of the extremity. Intracompartmental pressures may also be measured with proprietary monitoring devices. **EB:** *Edema can contribute to neurovascular compromise, leading to muscle and nerve damage due to decreased perfusion and ischemia (Oak & Abrams, 2016; Schreiber, 2016).*
- Monitor appropriate application and function of corrective device (e.g., cast, splint, traction) as needed. **EB:** *Neurovascular compromise can result from restrictive pressure from devices or swelling of injured tissue (Oak & Abrams, 2016; Schreiber, 2016). After immobilization (casting or splinting), if pain worsens or there is any tingling or numbness, swelling, delayed capillary refill, or change in color of exposed digits, immediate evaluation is needed.*
- For prevention of deep vein thrombosis (DVT), nursing care of DVT, and pulmonary embolism, refer to the interventions on DVT prevention and treatment in the care plan for Ineffective Peripheral **Tissue** Perfusion.

P

REFERENCES

Maher, A. B. (2016). Neurological assessment. *International Journal of Orthopaedic and Trauma Nursing, 22*, 44–53. https://doi.org/10.1016/j.ijotn.2016.01.002.

Oak, N. R., & Abrams, R. A. (2016). Compartment syndrome of the hand. *Orthopedic Clinics of North America, 47*(3), 609–616. https://doi.org/10.1016/j.ocl.2016.03.006.

Schreiber, M. L. (2016). Neurovascular assessment: An essential nursing focus. *Medsurg Nursing, 25*(1), 55–57.

Risk for Poisoning Domain 11 Safety/protection Class 4 Environmental hazards

Marina Martinez-Kratz, MS, RN, CNE

NANDA-I

Definition

Susceptible to accidental exposure to, or ingestion of, drugs or dangerous products in sufficient doses, which may compromise health.

Risk Factors

External

Access to dangerous product; access to illicit drugs potentially contaminated by poisonous additives; access to pharmaceutical preparations; occupational setting without adequate safeguards

Internal

Excessive emotional disturbance; inadequate knowledge of pharmaceutical preparations; inadequate knowledge of poisoning prevention; inadequate precautions against poisoning; neurobehavioral manifestations; unaddressed inadequate vision

NOC (Nursing Outcomes Classification)

Suggested NOC Outcomes

Knowledge: Child Physical Safety, Medication, Personal Safety; Parenting Performance; Risk Control; Risk Control: Alcohol Use, Drug Use; Risk Detection; Safe Home Environment

Example NOC Outcome with Indicators

Knowledge: Child Physical Safety as evidenced by the following indicators: Appropriate activities for child's developmental level/Strategies to prevent medication misuse/Strategies to prevent exposure to toxic chemicals or substances. (Rate the outcome and indicators of **Knowledge: Child Physical Safety:** 1 = no knowledge, 2 = limited knowledge, 3 = moderate knowledge, 4 = substantial knowledge, 5 = extensive knowledge [see Section I].)

P

Client Outcomes

Client Will (Specify Time Frame)

- Prevent inadvertent ingestion of or exposure to toxins or poisonous substances
- Explain and undertake appropriate safety measures to prevent ingestion of or exposure to toxins or poisonous substances
- Verbalize appropriate response to apparent or suspected toxic ingestion or poisoning

NIC (Nursing Interventions Classification)

Suggested NIC Interventions

Environmental Management: Safety, First Aid; Health Education; Medication Management; Surveillance; Surveillance: Safety

Example NIC Activities—Environmental Management: Safety

Identify safety hazards in the environment (e.g., physical, biological, chemical); Remove hazards from the environment, when possible

Nursing Interventions and *Rationales*

- When a client presents with possible/actual poisoning, follow the ABCs (airway, breathing and circulation) and administer oxygen if needed. EB: *Poisoning is a major cause of morbidity/mortality worldwide.*

Initial evaluation should include vital signs, mental status, pupil size, oxygenation, finger-stick glucose, and cardiac monitoring. Management is geared to supportive care, prevention of poison absorption, antidote use, and enhancement of elimination techniques (Chandran, 2019).

- ▲ When a client presents with possible poisoning, call the poison control center. EB: *The poison control hotline is 1-800-222-1222 or can be reached by texting POISON to 484848. Poison centers are a valuable tool for medical consultations. They are staffed by nurses, pharmacists, toxicologists, and other specialists in poisons and toxins who can recommend treatment advice (American Association of Poison Control Centers, 2021).*
- • Obtain a thorough history of what was ingested, how much, and when, and ask to look at the containers. Note the client's age, weight, medications, medical conditions, and any history of vomiting, choking, coughing, or change in mental status. Also take note of any interventions performed before seeking treatment. EB: *The history is needed to confirm the diagnosis and is often unreliable when provided by clients with intentional ingestion. Additional information should be obtained from paramedics, police, family, and friends when possible (Chandran, 2019).*
- ▲ Note results of toxicology screens, arterial blood gases, blood glucose levels, and other ordered laboratory tests. EB: *When ingestion information is incomplete or inaccurate, laboratory tests may be needed to determine treatment (Chandran, 2019).*
- • For suspected acetaminophen poisoning, obtain an accurate history of the time(s) of acetaminophen ingestion, the quantity, and the formulation of acetaminophen ingested. EB: *Acetaminophen poisoning is the most common cause of liver failure. Data collected will inform the timing of the serum acetaminophen level and hepatotoxicity risk. Treatment will include supportive care, prevention of absorption, and treatment with N-acetylcysteine (Saccomano, 2019).*
- ▲ Initiate prescribed treatment for poisoning promptly. The poison control center will specify any treatment or medications that need to be administered. EB: *Some poisoning deaths may be preventable. Substances ingested in preventable deaths have delayed gastrointestinal absorption or require metabolic activation to produce severe toxicity. This allows a time frame for recognition and successful intervention. Early poison center consultation may improve outcomes and decrease deaths (Srisuma et al, 2016).*
- ▲ Ensure that recommendations from the poison control center are clearly documented and readily accessible in the client's chart. EB: *The poison control center expertise provides specialized medical toxicology information needed to manage more serious exposures (Gummin et al, 2019).*
- • Follow the "five rights" as guidelines when administering medications. EB: *The five traditional rights of medication administration are identified as the right client, the right drug, the right route, the right time, and the right dose (Hanson & Haddad, 2020).*
- • Use a bar code scanning system for client identification whenever possible. EBN: *The implementation of the barcode administration showed statistically significant reduction in wrong medication, administration omission, wrong dose, and wrong order of administration errors (Macias et al, 2018).*
- • Standardize use of abbreviations, acronyms, symbols, and dose designations and eliminate those that are prone to cause errors. EB: *The Institute for Safe Medication Practices (2021) has a list of Error-Prone Abbreviations (see https://www.ismp.org/recommendations/error-prone-abbreviations-list).*
- • Be aware of the medications that look/sound alike and ensure that the correct medication is ordered and administered. EB: *The Institute for Safe Medication Practices (2019) has a list of Confused Drug Names containing look-alike and sound-alike (LASA) name pairs (see https://www.ismp.org/recommendations/confused-drug-names-list).*
- • Identify all the client's current medications on admission to a health care facility and compare the list with the current ordered medications. Reconcile any differences in medications. Use the expertise of the pharmacy department if there is any uncertainty regarding the accuracy of the client's medications. Reconcile the list of medications if the client is transferred from one unit to another, when there is a handoff to the next provider of care, and when the client is discharged. EB: *Medication reconciliation is an important safety issue because of the number of people taking multiple medications and involves determining what medications the person should be taking, medications they are actually taking, and resolving discrepancies (Aronson, 2017).*
- • Assess for possible interactions and adverse effects among prescribed medications and over-the-counter products with a computerized drug interaction checker. EBN: *A study found that drug interactions were minimized with tools to support nurses' clinical decision-making (Bueno et al, 2020).*

Pediatric

- ▲ Evaluate lead exposure risk and consult the health care provider regarding lead screening measures as indicated (public/ambulatory health). EB: *High levels of lead can cause anemia, multiorgan damage,*

P

seizures, and death in children. Chronic low lead levels can result in physical, cognitive, and neurobehavioral impairment. Sources of lead exposure include lead industries, leaded gasoline, lead-based paint, water pipes, paint, dust, soil, and water. Children at risk for lead exposure include those living in deteriorating or renovated older homes with lead-based paint, living in areas with lead-based industry, and socioeconomic disadvantage (Nussbaumer-Streit et al, 2016).

- Provide multifaceted medication teaching to parents that includes an easy-to-read dosing handout, a teaching session, a teach-back method, and a standardized dosing device for liquid medications. EB: *A randomized controlled trial of parents in the emergency department found a 58% increase in reported safe dosing in the experimental group after a medication teaching intervention (Li et al, 2020).*
- Provide guidance for parents and caregivers regarding age-related safety measures, including the following (Safe Kids Worldwide, 2021):
  - Store household products safely out of child's reach and sight to prevent poisoning.
  - Keep all household cleaning products in their original containers. Shop for child-resistant containers.
  - Read and follow product labels.
  - Check home for products such as cleaning supplies, liquid laundry packets, personal care products, plants, pesticides, alcohol, and medicine.
  - Post Poison Help number in phone and visibly at home: 1-800-222-1222.

  EB: *Pediatric poisoning deaths most commonly come from ingestion of opioids, other analgesics, cardiovascular medications, antihistamines, and sedatives (Tadros et al, 2016).* EB: *A multicenter case-control study found that there were increased odds of poisoning in children ages 0 to 4 years when medicines were not locked away or stored out of reach and household products and medicines were not put away immediately after use (Kendrick et al, 2017).*
- Advise families that syrup of ipecac is no longer recommended to be kept and used in the home. EB: *The American Academy of Clinical Toxicology (AACT), the European Association of Poison Centres and Clinical Toxicologists (EAPCCT), and the American Academy of Pediatrics (AAP) do not recommend the use of ipecac syrup (Benzoni & Gibson, 2020).*
- Advise families that over-the-counter cough and cold suppressant medications are not recommended and are no longer considered safe for children 2 or younger. EB: *A study found that since the US Food and Drug Administration advised against the use of cough/cold medicines in children younger than 2 in 2008, there has been a decline in physician prescriptions of cough and cold medicines (Horton et al, 2019).*
- Recognize that some children may have been exposed to methamphetamines or the components used to make methamphetamines. EB: *Home-based methamphetamine manufacturing may represent significant hazards and exposures to those who manufacture the drug but also to others living in the home. Children are most susceptible to these hazards and these exposures may result in immediate and long-term adverse health effects (Wright, Edwards, & Walker, 2016).*
- Advise families to safely dispose of unused medications. EB: *A study found that most families do not practice all recommended safe management strategies for controlled medications (Engster et al, 2019).*

P

Geriatric

- Caution the client and family to avoid storing medications with similar appearances close to one another (e.g., nitroglycerin ointment near toothpaste or denture creams). Confusion and visual impairment can place the older person at risk of incorrectly identifying the contents. Place medications in a medication organizer that indicates when they are to be taken. Failing eyesight, the use of multiple drugs, and difficulty in remembering whether a medication was taken are among the causes of accidental poisoning in older persons. EB: *For both sexes, poisoning is a common, self-inflicted injury in clients admitted to hospital. Among seniors, there is concern regarding the recognition of intentional harm by self-induced poisoning (Skinner et al, 2016).*
- Perform medication reconciliation in all older clients entering the health care system and on discharge. EB: *A study evaluated the prevalence and nature of potentially inappropriate medications and found increased safety in older clients through reduction of the number of drugs prescribed (Aiezza et al, 2021).*
- Use the Screening Tool of Older People's Prescriptions (STOPP) and the Screening Tool to Alert Right Treatment (START) to promote safety, avoid omissions, and prevent inappropriateness in prescriptions. EB: *The STOPP criteria for frail older persons (>65 years) is largely associated with adverse drug events and recommends against taking medications to treat symptoms unassociated with selected illnesses (Nwadiugwu, 2020).*

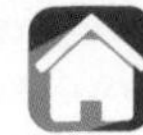

Home Care

- The previous interventions may be adapted for home care use.
- Provide the client and/or family with information about the free poison control application webPOISONCONTROL. EB: *A study found that the webPOISONCONTROL application augmented traditional poison control services by providing automated, accurate online access to case-specific triage and first aid guidance for poison ingestions (Litovitz et al, 2016).*
- Identify poisonous substances in the immediate surroundings of the home, such as a garage or barn, including paints and thinners, fertilizers, rodent and bug control substances, animal medications, gasoline, and oil. Label with the name, a poison warning sign, and a poison control center number. Lock out of the reach of children. EB: *A hospital-based cross-sectional study found that household chemicals were involved in 54.25% of poisoning cases and 11.8% of poisoning cases occurred in the home surroundings (Saikia et al, 2020).*
- Identify the risk of toxicity from environmental activities such as spraying trees or roadside shrubs. Contact local departments of agriculture or transportation to obtain material safety data sheets or to prevent the activity in desired areas. EB: *Very young children, women who are of childbearing age or who are pregnant, and older adults are at greatest risk of poisoning (Ashgur et al, 2016).*
- To prevent carbon monoxide poisoning, instruct the client and family in the importance of using a carbon monoxide detector in the home and changing it every 6 months, having the home heating system serviced every year by a qualified technician, and ensuring proper installation and venting of all combustion equipment. Carbon monoxide results from fumes produced by portable generators, stoves, lanterns, gas ranges, running vehicles, or burning charcoal and wood, which can build up in enclosed or partially enclosed spaces and result in harm or death for people and animals exposed. EB: *Carbon monoxide poisoning may not be readily identified because many of the effects are similar to various childhood illnesses (Chang et al, 2017).*

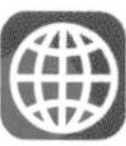

Multicultural

- Prompt caregivers to take action to prevent lead poisoning. EB: *Lead knowledge in urban youth is limited and includes misinformation. Some youth demonstrated awareness of specific sources including paint, dust, and water but had limited awareness of prevention strategies (Bogar et al, 2017).*
- If children live in a high-lead environment, teach the need for handwashing before each meal, annual blood testing for lead levels, and avoidance of high-lead areas. EB: *Lead industries, leaded petrol, lead-based paint, water pipes, paint, dust, soil, and water are all sources of lead exposure for children (Nussbaumer-Streit et al, 2016).*

P

Client/Family Teaching and Discharge Planning

- The previous interventions may be adapted for teaching needs and discharge planning.
- Counsel the client and family members regarding the following points of medication safety:
  - Avoid sharing prescriptions.
  - Always use good light when preparing medication. Do not dispense medication during the night without a light on.
  - Read the label before you open the bottle, after you remove a dose, and again before you give it.
  - Always use child-resistant caps and lock all medications away from your child or confused older adult.
  - Give the correct dose. *Never* guess.
  - Do not increase or decrease the dose without calling the health care provider.
  - Always follow the weight and age recommendations on the label.
  - Avoid making conversions. If the label calls for 2 teaspoons and you have a dosing cup labeled only with ounces, do not use it.
  - Be sure the health care provider knows if you are taking more than one medication at a time.
  - Never let young children take medication by themselves.
  - Read and follow labeling instructions on all products; adjust dosage for age.
  - Avoid excessive amounts and/or frequency of doses. ("If a little does some good, a lot should do more.")

  EB: *Data from the Nationwide Emergency Department Sample (NEDS) from 2006 to 2012 show that there were 21,928 pediatric emergency department visits for prescription opioid poisonings. An increase in adult prescription opioid abuse contributes to unintentional ingestion of medications in children (Tadros et al, 2016).*

EB: *Unintentional poisoning is the fastest growing cause of childhood fatal injury. Per the Centers for Disease and Prevention (CDC), most of this increase is linked to the inappropriate use of prescription opioids (CDC, 2021).* **EB:** *Poisoning in children is common and places a significant burden on health care. Parents of poisoned children were more likely to not have safely stored or locked medicines (Kendrick et al, 2017).*

REFERENCES

Aiezza, M., Bresciani, A., Guglielmi, G., et al. (2021). Medication review versus usual care to improve drug therapies in hospitalised older patients admitted to internal medicine wards. *European Journal of Hospital Pharmacy*, *28*, 160–164. https://doi.org/10.1136/ejhpharm-2019-002072.

American Association of Poison Control Centers. (2021). *Health care providers*. Retrieved from http://www.aapcc.org/. [Accessed 22 July 2021].

Aronson, J. (2017). Medication reconciliation. *BMJ*, *356*, i5336. https://doi.org/10.1136/bmj.i5336.

Asghar, U., Malik, M. F., & Javed, A. (2016). Pesticide exposure and human health: A review. *Journal of Ecosystem & Ecography*, *S5*, 005. https://doi.org/10.4172/2157-7625.

Benzoni, T., & Gibson, J. G. (2020). Ipecac. In: *StatPearls* [Internet]. Treasure Island, FL: StatPearls Publishing.

Bogar, S., Szabo, A., Woodruff, S., & Johnson, S. (2017). Urban youth knowledge and attitudes regarding lead poisoning. *Journal of Community Health*, *42*(6), 1255–1266. https://doi.org/10.1007/s10900-017-0378-8.

Bueno, B., Aline, A., Caldas, P., et al. (2020). Patient safety: Potential drug-drug interactions caused by the overlapping of medications agreed by the nurse. *Revista de Enfermagem Referência*, *3*, 1–6.

Centers for Disease Control and Prevention (CDC). (2021). *Carbon monoxide (CO) poisoning prevention*. Retrieved from https://www.cdc.gov/nceh/features/copoisoning/. [Accessed 22 July 2021].

Chandran, J., & Krishna, B. (2019). Initial management of poisoned patient. *Indian Journal of Critical Care Medicine: Peer-Reviewed, Official Publication of Indian Society of Critical Care Medicine*, *23*(Suppl. 4), S234–S240. https://doi.org/10.5005/jp-journals-10071-23307.

Chang, Y. C., Lee, H. Y., Huang, J. L., Chiu, C. H., Chen, C. L., & Wu, C. T. (2017). Risk factors and outcome analysis in children with carbon monoxide poisoning. *Pediatrics and Neonatology*, *58*(2), 171–177.

Engster, S. A., Bogen, D. L., & Molina, B. S. G. (2019). Adolescent and parent management of controlled prescription medications. *Substance Use & Misuse*, *54*(14), 2264–2274. https://doi.org/10.1080/10826084.2019.1645176.

Gummin, D. D., Mowry, J. B., Spyker, D. A., et al. (2019). 2018 annual report of the American Association of Poison Control Centers' National Poison Data System (NPDS): 36th annual report. *Clinical Toxicology*, *57*(12), 1220–1413. https://doi.org/10.1080/15563650.2019.1677022.

Hanson, A., & Haddad, L. M. (2020). Nursing rights of medication administration. In: *StatPearls* [Internet]. Treasure Island, FL: StatPearls Publishing. https://www.ncbi.nlm.nih.gov/books/NBK560654/.

Horton, D. B., Gerhard, T., & Strom, B. L. (2019). Trends in cough and cold medicine recommendations for children in the United States, 2002-2015. *JAMA Pediatrics*, *173*(9), 885–887. https://doi.org/10.1001/jamapediatrics.2019.2252.

Institute for Safe Medication Practices (ISMP). (2019). *List of confused drug names*. Retrieved from https://www.ismp.org/recommendations/confused-drug-names-list. [Accessed 22 July 2021].

Institute for Safe Medication Practices (ISMP). (2021). *List of error-prone abbreviations*. Retrieved from https://www.ismp.org/recommendations/error-prone-abbreviations-list. [Accessed 22 July 2021].

Kendrick, D., Majsak-Newman, G., Benford, P., et al. (2017). Poison prevention practices and medically attended poisoning in young children: Multicentre case-control study. *Injury Prevention*, *23*(2), 93–101. https://doi.org/10.1136/injuryprev-2015-041828.

Li, C. N., Camargo, C. A., Jr., Faridi, M., et al. (2020). Medication education for dosing safety: A randomized controlled trial. *Annals of Emergency Medicine*, *76*(5), 637–645. https://doi.org/10.1016/j.annemergmed.2020.07.007.

Litovitz, T., Benson, B. E., & Smolinske, S. (2016). webPOISONCONTROL: can poison control be automated? *American Journal of Emergency Medicine*, *34*(8), 1614–1619. https://doi.org/10.1016/j.ajem.2016.06.018.

Macias, M., Bernabeu-Andreu, F. A., Arribas, I., Navarro, F., & Baldominos, G. (2018). Impact of a barcode medication administration system on patient safety. *Oncology Nursing Forum*, *45*(1), E1–E13. https://doi.org/10.1188/18.ONF.E1-E13.

Nussbaumer-Streit, B., Yeoh, B., Griebler, U., et al. (2016). Household interventions for preventing domestic lead exposure in children. *Cochrane Database of Systematic Reviews*, *10*, CD006047. https://doi.org/10.1002/14651858.CD006047.pub5.

Nwadiugwu, M. C. (2020). Frailty and the risk of polypharmacy in the older person: Enabling and preventative approaches. *Journal of Aging Research*, *2020*, 6759521. https://doi.org/10.1155/2020/6759521.

Saccomano, S. J. (2019). Acute acetaminophen toxicity in adults. *Nursing in Critical Care*, *14*(5), 10–17. https://doi.org/10.1097/01.CCN.0000578816.14164.9f.

Safe Kids Worldwide. (2021). *Poison*. Retrieved from https://www.safekids.org/poisonsafety. [Accessed 22 July 2021].

Saikia, D., Sharma, R. K., & Janardhan, K. V. (2020). Clinical profile of poisoning due to various poisons in children of age 0–12 years. *Journal of Family Medicine and Primary Care*, *9*(5), 2291–2296. https://doi.org/10.4103/jfmpc.jfmpc_365_20.

Skinner, R., McFaull, S., Draca, J., et al. (2016). Suicide and self-inflicted injury hospitalizations in Canada (1979 to 2014/15). Health promotion and chronic disease prevention in Canada: Research. *Policy and Practice*, *36*(11), 243–251. https://doi.org/10.24095/hpcdp.36.11.02.

Srisuma, S., Cao, D., Kleinschmidt, K., Heffner, A. C., & Lavonas, E. J. (2016). Missed opportunities? An evaluation of potentially preventable poisoning deaths. *Clinical Toxicology*, *54*(5), 441–446. https://doi.org/10.3109/15563650.2016.1157721.

Tadros, A., Layman, S. M., Davis, S. M., Bozeman, R., & Davidov, D. M. (2016). Emergency department visits by pediatric patients for poisoning by prescription opioids. *The American Journal of Drug and Alcohol Abuse*, *42*(5), 550–555. https://doi.org/10.1080/00952990.2016.1194851.

Wright, J., Edwards, J., & Walker, S. (2016). Exposures associated with clandestine methamphetamine drug laboratories in Australia. *Reviews on Environmental Health*, *31*(3), 329–352. https://doi.org/10.1515/reveh-2016-0017.

P

Post-Trauma Syndrome
Domain 9 Coping/stress tolerance Class 1 Post-trauma responses

Gail B. Ladwig, MSN, RN and Julianne E. Doubet, BSN, RN, EMT-B

NANDA-I

Definition

Sustained maladaptive response to a traumatic, overwhelming event.

Defining Characteristics

Aggressive behaviors; alienation; altered attention; altered mood; anxiety (00146); avoidance behaviors; compulsive behavior; denial; depressive symptoms; dissociative amnesia; enuresis; exaggerated startle response; expresses anger; expresses numbness; expresses shame; fear (00148); flashbacks; gastrointestinal irritation; headache; heart palpitations; hopelessness (00124); horror; hypervigilance; individuals with history of detachment; intrusive dreams; intrusive thoughts; irritable mood; neurosensory irritability; nightmares; panic attacks; rage; reports feeling guilty; repression; substance misuse

Related Factors

Diminished ego strength: environment not conducive to needs; exaggerated sense of responsibility; inadequate social support; perceives event as traumatic; self-injurious behavior; survivor role

At-Risk Population

Individuals displaced from home; individuals experiencing prolonged duration of traumatic event; individuals exposed to disaster; individuals exposed to epidemic; individuals exposed to event involving multiple deaths; Individuals exposed to event outside the range of usual human experience; individuals exposed to serious accident; individuals exposed to war; individuals in human service occupations; individuals suffering serious threat; individuals who witnessed mutilation; individuals who witnessed violent death; individuals whose loved ones suffered serious injuries; individuals whose loved ones suffered serious threats; individuals with destructed home; individuals with history of being a prisoner of war; individuals with history of being abused; individuals with history of criminal victimization; individuals with history of torture

Associated Conditions

Depression

P

NOC (Nursing Outcomes Classification)

Suggested NOC Outcomes

Abuse Cessation; Abuse Protection; Abuse Recovery: Emotional, Aggression Self-Control, Anxiety Self-Control, Grief Resolution, Impulse Self-Control; Self-Mutilation Restraint; Sleep

Example NOC Outcome with Indicators

Abuse Recovery: Emotional as evidenced by the following indicators: Trauma-induced psychoneurotic behaviors, conduct disorders, and learning difficulties. (Rate outcome and indicators of **Abuse Recovery: Emotional:** 1 = extensive, 2 = substantial, 3 = moderate, 4 = limited, 5 = none [see Section I].)

Client Outcomes

Client Will (Specify Time Frame)

- Return to pretrauma level of functioning as quickly as possible
- Acknowledge traumatic event and begin to work with the trauma by talking about the experience and expressing feelings of fear, anger, anxiety, guilt, and helplessness
- Identify support systems and available resources and be able to connect with them
- Return to and strengthen coping mechanisms used in previous traumatic event
- Acknowledge event and perceive it without distortions
- Assimilate event and move forward to set and pursue life goals

NIC (Nursing Interventions Classification)

Suggested NIC Interventions

Counseling; Support System Enhancement

Example NIC Activities—Counseling

Encourage expression of feelings; Assist client to identify strengths and reinforce them

Nursing Interventions and *Rationales*

- Observe for a reaction to a traumatic event in all clients regardless of age or sex. EBN: *Treatment, after a traumatic incident, is usually concentrated on stabilizing the client physically; what is not always addressed is the emotional and/or psychological damage that can follow a traumatizing event (Frank, Schroeter, & Shaw, 2017).*
- Use a trauma-informed approach with survivors. EBN: *Trauma-informed care addresses medical, legal, and psychosocial needs while acknowledging the connection between presenting symptoms and the individual's past trauma history. A trauma-informed framework emphasizes safety; trustworthiness and transparency; peer support; collaboration and mutuality; empowerment, voice, and choice; and cultural, historical, and gender issues (Emergency Nurses Association & International Association of Forensic Nurses, 2017).*
- After a traumatic event, assess for intrusive memories, avoidance and numbing, and hyperarousal. EB: *According to a study by Ellis and Zaretsky (2018), untreated posttraumatic stress disorder (PTSD) will impose lasting impairments for the client; these may include avoidance, vocational and social dysfunction, and other negative manifestations.*
- Use an open and nonthreatening body positioning and posture. EBN: *The use of nonthreatening body positioning and posture will help prevent the threat detection areas of the client's brain from taking over (Fleishman, Kamsky, & Sundborg, 2019).*
- Remain with the client and provide support during periods of overwhelming emotions. EBN: *Nurses must be approachable and prepared to listen to clients as they attempt to convey their feelings, even if they are negative in nature (Kukkonen & Sharifullin, 2017).*
- Help the individual to comprehend the trauma if possible. EBN: *Laughon and Lewis-O'Connor (2019) stress that as a nurse investigating client trauma, there is a need for a comprehensive approach that will give clients the opportunity to disclose only what information they choose, in a secure and supportive setting.*
- Use touch with the client's permission (e.g., a hand on the shoulder, holding a hand). EBN: *"Asking permission before you touch clients gives them a choice and empowers them to have control over their body and physical space," state Fleishman et al (2019) in their report regarding trauma-informed care.*
- Help the client regain previous sleeping and eating habits. EB: *In their pilot study of postdeployed US veterans with PTSD symptoms, Walters et al (2020) observed that the utilization of evidence-based sleep treatment should be included for full PTSD rehabilitation.*
- ▲ Provide the client pain medication if he or she has physical pain. EB: *In their study examining the link between PTSD and chronic pain, Fishbain et al (2017) found evidence that though the degree of PTSD may vary between types of chronic pain, there is a connection between the two.*
- ▲ Assess the need for pharmacotherapy and refer as needed. EB: *Health care providers may use medications for symptom relief in PTSD, including appropriate antidepressants and anxiolytics (Johnson, 2017).* EBN: *According to Kukkonen and Sharifullin (2017), nurses, in addition to the capability to propose psychotherapies and pharmacotherapies, must first generate trust and communication with their clients.*
- ▲ Refer for appropriate psychotherapy: cognitive therapy, exposure therapy, eye movement desensitization and reprocessing (EMDR), and cognitive-behavioral therapy (CBT). EB: *Shapiro and Brown (2019) found that EMDR and related treatments are beneficial, advanced, evidence-based therapies for PTSD.*
- Help the client use positive cognitive restructuring to reestablish feelings of self-worth. EBN: *Cognitive restructuring is another psychotherapeutic strategy that has been found useful in communicating to clients that adverse thoughts are a result of negative thinking (Kukkonen & Sharifullin, 2017).*
- Provide the means for the client to express feelings through therapeutic drawing. EB: *Because traumatic events are many times too difficult to describe in words, art therapy gives victims another avenue by which they can project their emotions (Ramirez, 2016).*

P

- Encourage the client to return to his or her normal routine as quickly as possible. EB: *According to Kendrick et al (2017), it is well documented that physical, psychological, and financial well-being develop when a client returns to work after an unintentional trauma.*
- Talk to and assess the client's social support after a traumatic event. EBN: *Nasirian et al (2018) found that the support of family, social, and work circles and their medical networks were most important to the physical and psychological recovery of trauma survivors.*

Pediatric

- Refer to nursing care plan Risk for **Post-Trauma** Syndrome.
- ▲ Carefully assess children exposed to disasters and trauma. Note behavior specific to developmental age. Refer for therapy as needed. EB: *According to Broaddus-Shea et al (2021), a medical history obtained from children and adolescent victims of trauma should be taken employing language personalized to their age and comprehension, which will aid in establishing trust and convey empathy; alliance with other protection agencies (e.g., child welfare, legal services, law enforcement) is also essential to the future well-being of the child or adolescent.*

Geriatric

- Carefully screen older adults for signs of PTSD, especially after a disaster. EB: *Older persons who have undergone an earlier in life trauma may react in a different manner than younger persons to a disaster; age alone does not presage psychological outcomes (Cherry et al, 2015).*
- Consider using the Impact of Event Scale—Revised (IES-R), which is an appropriate instrument to measure the subjective response to stress in the older population. EBN: *The use of the IES-R, although not diagnostic for PTSD, is an appropriate means of assessing an older adult client's response to a specific traumatic event (McCabe, 2019).*
- ▲ Monitor the client for clinical signs of depression and anxiety; refer to a health care provider for medication if appropriate. EBN: *In their review of articles concerning the nursing care of the institutionalized elderly with anxiety and depression, Manungkalit & Purnama Sari (2020) found that stress, especially PTSD, is frequently comorbid with depression and unresolved physical symptoms (somatization disorder).*
- Instill hope. EB: *The quality of hope has shown a significant correlation to the moderation of mental health problems (Sahranavard et al, 2018).*

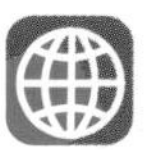

Multicultural

- Assess the influence of cultural beliefs, norms, and values on the client's ability to cope with a traumatic experience. EBN: *Cultural sensitivity is the awareness of what is required to understand cultural diversity and in what ways culture may affect clients' values, beliefs, and attitudes (Brooks et al, 2019).*
- Acknowledge racial and ethnic differences at the onset of care. EBN: *In her study of cognitive assessment tools that were initially established for use within specific cultures, Sluder (2020) found that the use of these tools is not appropriate for all cultural groups and may lead to a false diagnosis.*
- ▲ Carefully assess refugees for PTSD and refer for treatment as appropriate. EB: *Countless refugees have been exposed to traumatic incidents, both in their homeland and again during their flight; this then results in an increased probability for the development of trauma-related syndromes (Hecker et al, 2018).*
- Use a family-centered approach when working with Latin, Asian, African American, and Native American clients. EBN: *Chauhan et al (2020), in their review of the literature concerning the health care of ethnic minorities, determined that client well-being can be augmented by developing cooperation with those family and friends who are supportive and will take a role in the client care process.*
- When working with Asian American clients, provide opportunities by which the family can save face. EB: *Understanding Asian American beliefs concerning the basis of mental illnesses can assist health care professionals in recognizing the feelings of shame and stigma that prevent this group from seeking mental health treatment (Bignall, Jacquez, & Vaughn, 2015).* EBN: *Health care providers must recognize common cultural practices and agree to the use of the recommended strategies that address the challenges of providing culturally appropriate, person-centered support for ailing South Asian clients and their families (Khosla et al, 2017).*
- Incorporate cultural traditions as appropriate. EBN: *Alegría et al (2016), in their research relating to the health care of ethnic-minority clients, found that the introduction of culturally mediated interventions resulted in the progressive improvement of health care for this diverse population.*

Home Care

- ▲ Assess family support and the response to the client's coping mechanisms. Refer the family for medical social services or other counseling, as necessary. **EBN:** *The hospitalization of a loved one after a traumatic event, plus the emerging responsibilities of caregiving, can be acutely stressful, often triggering a family crisis and serving as the basis of psychological distress (Newcomb & Hymes, 2017).*
- • Assess the effect of the trauma on family and significant others and provide empathy and caring to them. **EBN:** *Donaldson-Andersen (2017) affirmed that nurses must continuously assess and reevaluate the needs of clients, and the client's loved ones, during a traumatic event and provide essential emotional and social support as needed.*

Client/Family Teaching and Discharge Planning

- • Teach positive coping skills and avoidance of negative coping skills. **EB:** *Contractor et al (2020) found that previous research suggests that those with PTSD symptoms will present with deficits in positive internal experiences.* **EB:** *Mattson et al (2018), in their study of veterans with PTSD, propose that coping adapted clinical mediation could ease PTSD symptoms and advance positive growth after a traumatic experience.*
- • Teach mindfulness strategies and encourage use when intrusive thoughts or flashbacks occur. **EB:** *The use of mindfulness has been linked with decreased symptoms in those experiencing PTSD. Acting with awareness and nonreactivity were the characteristics of mindfulness most commonly associated with the moderation of PTSD markers (Stephenson et al, 2017).*
- • Refer the client to peer support groups. **EB:** *In a review of successful therapies for PTSD, Drebing et al (2018) observed that peer support groups, in combination with clinical treatments, resulted in better outcomes than either alone.*
- • Consider the use of complementary and alternative therapies. **EB:** *Complementary and alternative medicine (CAM) for the treatment of PTSD is accepted internationally; CAM can include a variety of therapies (e.g., yoga, acupuncture, neurostimulation) (Song et al, 2020).*

REFERENCES

Alegría, M., Alvarez, K., Ishikawa, R. Z., DiMarzio, K., & McPeck, S. (2016). Removing obstacles to eliminating racial and ethnic disparities in behavioral health care. *Health Affairs, 35*(6), 991–999. https://doi.org/10.377/hthhaff206.0029.

Bignall, W. J. R., Jacquez, F., & Vaughn, L. M. (2015). Attributions of mental illness: An ethnically diverse community perspective. *Community Mental Health Journal, 51*(5), 540–545. https://doi.org/10.1007/s10597-014-9820-x.

Broaddus-Shea, E. T., Scott, K., Reijnders, M., & Amin, A. (2021). A review of the literature in good practice considerations for initial health system response to child and adolescent sexual abuse. *Child Abuse & Neglect, 116*(Pt 1), 104225. https://doi.org/10.1016/j.chiabu.2019.104225.

Brooks, L. A., Manias, E., & Bloomer, M. J. (2019). Culturally sensitive communication in healthcare: A concept analysis. *Collegian, 26*(3), 383–391. https://doi.org/10.1016/j.colegn.2018.09.007.

Chauhan, A., Walton, M., Manias, E., et al. (2020). The safety of health care for ethnic minority patients: A systematic review. *International Journal for Equity in Health, 19*(1), 118. https://doi.org/10.1186/s12939-020-01223-2.

Cherry, K. E., Sampson, L., Nezat, P. F., Cacamo, A., Marks, L. D., & Galea, S. (2015). Long-term psychological outcomes in older adults after disaster: Relationships to religiosity and social support. *Aging & Mental Health, 19*(5), 430–443.

Contractor, A. A., Weiss, N. H., Forkus, S. R., & Keegan, F. (2020). Positive internal experiences in PTSD interventions: A critical review. Trauma: Violence & Abuse. [Online ahead of print]. https://doi:10.1177/1524838020925784.

Donaldson-Andersen, J. (2017). The nurse's role in supporting patients and family in sharing personal accounts of traumatic events: Personal experience. *Journal of Trauma Nursing, 24*(2), 134–140. https://doi.org/10.1097/JTN.0000000000000276.

Drebing, C. E., Reilly, E., Henze, K. T., et al. (2018). Using peer support groups to enhance community integration of veterans in transition. *Psychological Services, 15*(2), 135–145. https://doi.org/10.1037/ser0000178.

Ellis, J., & Zaretsky, A. (2018). Assessment and management of posttraumatic stress disorder. *Continuum, 24*(3), 873–892. https//:doi.org/10.1212/CON.0000000000000610.

Emergency Nurses Association & International Association of Forensic Nurses. (2017). Joint position statement: Adult and adolescent sexual assault patients in the emergency care setting. *Journal of Forensic Nursing* (13)2, 91–93.

Fishbain, D. A., Pulikal, A., Lewis, J. E., & Gao, J. (2017). Chronic pain types differ in their reported prevalence of post-traumatic stress disorder (PTSD) and there is consistent evidence that chronic pain is associated with PTSD: An evidence-based, structured systematic review. *Pain Medicine, 18*(4), 711–735. https://doi.org/10.1093/pm/pnw065.

Fleishman, J., Kamsky, H., & Sundborg, S. (2019). Trauma-informed nursing practice. *Online Journal of Issues in Nursing, 24*(2), 3. https://doi.org/10.3912/OJIN.Vol24No02Man03.

Frank, C. A., Schroeter, K., & Shaw, C. (2017). Addressing traumatic stress in the acute traumatically injured patient. *Journal of Trauma Nursing, 24*(2), 78–84. https://doi.org/10.1097/JTN.0000000000000270.

Hecker, T., Huber, S., Maier, T., & Maercker, A. (2018). Differential associations among PTSD and complex PTSD symptoms and traumatic experiences and postmigration difficulties in a culturally diverse refugee sample. *Journal of Traumatic Stress, 31*(6), 795–804. https://doi.org/10.1002/jts.22342.

Johnson, K. (2017). The DMS-5 definition of PTSD. *Journal of Legal Nurse Consulting, 28*(3), 25–29.

Kendrick, D., Dhiman, P., Kellezi, B., et al. (2017). Psychological morbidity and return to work after injury: Multicentre cohort study.

P

British Journal of General Practice, 67(661), e555–e564. https://doi.org/10.3399/bjgp17X69167.

Khosla, N., Washington, K. T., Shaunfield, S., & Aslakson, R. (2017). Communication challenges and strategies of U.S. health professionals caring for seriously ill South Asian patients and their families. *Journal of Palliative Medicine, 20*(6), 611–617. https://doi.org/10.1089/jpm.2016.0167.

Kukkonen, N., & Sharifullin, R. (2017). *Nursing interventions for post-traumatic stress disorder: A narrative literature review. [Thesis]*. Lahti, Finland: Lahti University of Applied Sciences. Retrieved from https://www.theseus.fi/bitstream/handle/10024/127457/Kukkonen_Nina.pdf?sequence=2. [Accessed 23 July 2021].

Laughon, K., & Lewis-O'Connor, A. (2019). Trauma-informed nursing improves equity. *Journal of Forensic Nursing, 15*(4), 195–196. https://doi.org/10.1097/JFN.0000000000000270.

Manungkalit, M., & Purnama Sari, N. P. W. (2020). The influence of anxiety and stress toward depression in institutionalized elderly. *Journal of Educational, Health and Community Psychology, 9*(1), 65–76. Retrieved from https://core.ac.uk/download/pdf/296309806.pdf. [Accessed 13 December 2021].

Mattson, E., James, L., & Engdahl, B. (2018). Personality factors and their impact on PTSD and post-traumatic growth is mediated by coping style among OIF/OEF veterans. *Military Medicine, 183*(9–10), e475–e480. https://doi.org/10.1093/milmed/usx201.

McCabe, D. (2019). The Impact of event Scale—Revised (IES-R). *Try this: Best practices in nursing care to older adults, 19*. Retrieved from https://hign.org/sites/default/files/2020-06/Try_This_General_Assessment_19.pdf. [Accessed 23 July 2021].

Nasirian, S., Fagevik Olsén, M., & Engström, M. (2018). Patients' experiences of their recovery process after minor physical trauma. *Journal of Trauma Nursing, 25*(4), 233–241. https://doi.org/10.1097/JTN.0000000000000378.

Newcomb, A. B., & Hymes, R. A. (2017). Life interrupted: The trauma caregiver experience. *Journal of Trauma Nursing, 24*(2), 125–133. https://doi.org/10.1097/JTN.0000000000000278.

Ramirez, J. (2016). A review of art therapy among military service members and veterans with post-traumatic stress disorder. *Journal of Military and Veterans' Health, 24*(2), 40–51. Retrieved from jmvh.org/article/a-review-of-art-therapy-among-military-service-members-and-veterans-with-post-traumatic-stress-disorder/ . [Accessed 23 July 2021].

Sahranavard, S., Esmaeili, A., Dastjerdi, R., & Salehiniya, H. (2018). The effectiveness of stress-management-based cognitive-behavioral treatments on anxiety sensitivity, positive and negative affect and hope. *Biomedicine, 8*(4), 23. https://doi:10.1051/bmdcn/2018080423.

Shapiro, R., & Brown, L. S. (2019). Eye movement desensitization and reprocessing therapy and related treatments for trauma: An innovative, integrative trauma treatment. *Practice Innovations, 4*(3), 139–155. Retrieved from https://psycnet.apa.org/buy/2019-33965-002. [Accessed 23 July 2021].

Sluder, K. M. (2020). Acknowledging disparities in dementia care for increasingly diverse ethnoracial patient populations. *Federal Practioner, 37*(2), 69–71. Retrieved from https://www.ncbi.nlm.nih.gov/pmc/articles/PMC7138339. [Accessed 23 September 2020].

Song, K., Xiong, F., Ding, N., Huang, A., & Zhang, H. (2020). Complementary and alternative therapies for post-traumatic stress disorder: A protocol for systematic review and network meta-analysis. *Medicine (Baltimore), 99*(28), e21142. https://doi.org/10.1097/MD.0000000000021142.

Stephenson, K. R., Simpson, T. L., Martinez, M. E., & Kearney, D. J. (2017). Changes in mindfulness and posttraumatic stress disorder symptoms among veterans enrolled in mindfulness-based stress reduction. *Clinical Psychology, 73*(3), 201–217. https://doi.org/10.1002/jclp.22323.

Walters, E. M., Jenkins, M. M., Nappi, C. M., et al. (2020). The impact of prolonged exposure on sleep and enhancing treatment outcomes with evidence-based sleep interventions: A pilot study. *Psychological Trauma, Theory, Research, Practice and Policy, 12*(2), 175–185. https://doi.org/10.1037/tra0000478.

P

Risk for Post-Trauma Syndrome

Domain 9 Coping/stress tolerance Class 1 Post-trauma responses

Gail B. Ladwig, MSN, RN and Julianne E. Doubet, BSN, RN, EMT-B

NANDA-I

Definition

Susceptible to sustained maladaptive response to a traumatic, overwhelming event, which may compromise health.

Risk Factors

Diminished ego strength; environment not conducive to needs; exaggerated sense of responsibility; inadequate social support; perceives event as traumatic; self-injurious behavior; survivor role

At-Risk Population

Individuals displaced from home; individuals experiencing prolonged duration of traumatic event; individuals exposed to disaster; individuals exposed to epidemic; individuals exposed to event involving multiple deaths; individuals exposed to event outside the range of usual human experience; individuals exposed to serious accident; individuals exposed to war; individuals in human service occupations; individuals suffering serious threat; individuals who witnessed mutilation; individuals who witnessed violent death; individuals whose loved ones suffered serious injuries; individuals whose loved ones suffered serious threats; individuals with destructed home; individuals with history of being a prisoner of war; individuals with history of being abused; individuals with history of criminal victimization; individuals with history of torture

Associated Conditions

Depression

NOC (Nursing Outcomes Classification)

Refer to the care plan for **Post-Trauma** Syndrome for suggested NOC outcomes

Example NOC Outcome with Indicators

Risk Detection as evidenced by the following indicators: Recognizes signs and symptoms that indicate risk/Uses health care services congruent with need. (Rate the outcome and indicators of **Risk Detection:** 1 = never demonstrated, 2 = rarely demonstrated, 3 = sometimes demonstrated, 4 = often demonstrated, 5 = consistently demonstrated [see Section I].)

Client Outcomes

Client Will (Specify Time Frame)

- Identify symptoms associated with posttraumatic stress disorder (PTSD) and seek help
- Acknowledge event and perceive it without distortions
- Identify support systems and available resources and be able to connect with them
- State that he/she is not to blame for the event

NIC (Nursing Interventions Classification)

Refer to the care plan for **Post-Trauma** Syndrome for suggested NIC interventions.

Nursing Interventions and *Rationales*

- Assess for PTSD in a client who has chronic/critical illness, anxiety, or personality disorder; was a witness to severe injury or death; or experienced sexual molestation. EBN: *Current literature validates that early identification and intervention in the treatment of traumatic stress is essential to optimal recovery for trauma clients (Frank, Schroeter, & Shaw, 2017).*
- Consider the use of a self-reported screening questionnaire. EB: *PTSD self-screens are questionnaires that may help to identify those who could have PTSD; positive responses might signal that a referral to a mental health professional is warranted (National Center for PTSD, 2017).*
- Assess for ongoing symptoms of posttraumatic stress such as dissociation, avoidance behavior, hypervigilance, and reexperiencing. EB: *The symptoms for individuals with PTSD can vary considerably, but they generally fall into these categories: reexperience, avoidance, negative changes in beliefs and/or feelings, and increased arousal (National Center for PTSD, 2017).*
- Assess for past experiences with traumatic events. EBN: *In their study of rural women with a history of trauma, Handley et al (2015) found that these clients may have other psychological and social repercussions, along with the development of PTSD.*
- Consider screening for PTSD in a client who is a high user of medical care. EB: *Prins et al (2016) found that PTSD is linked to greater health care use, medical debility, and tobacco and alcohol dependence.*
- ▲ Provide deployed combat veterans with previous history of low mental or physical health status before deployment with appropriate referral after deployment. EB: *Yang and Burr (2016), in their study of the well-being of older veterans exposed to combat, cited a previous study done of identical and fraternal twin combat veterans. It was surmised in that study that both environmental and genetic components played a role in combat veterans' negative mental and physical health outcomes.*
- Provide peer support to contact coworkers experiencing trauma to remind them that others in the organization are concerned about their welfare. EB: *A study by Bartone et al (2019) determined that there are lasting benefits in furnishing peer support; these may include the enhanced development of personal growth and a renewed positive awareness of the meaning of life.*
- Provide posttrauma debriefings. Effective posttrauma coping skills are taught, and each participant creates a plan for his or her recovery. EB: *Findings by Richins et al (2020) in their study implied that immediate posttrauma interventions can be successful in organizations if they are directed in accordance with evidence-based criteria and incorporated into the organizational system.*
- Provide posttrauma counseling and debriefings. EB: *In their study of veterans' health and wellness, Oster et al (2017) established a link between mental, physical, and social health and consequently encouraged a combined clinical approach to the veterans' problems.*

- Consider exposure therapy for civilian trauma survivors after an assault or motor vehicle crash. EB: *According to Weisman and Rodebaugh (2018), exposure therapy is typically looked on as the benchmark for behavioral intercessions and clinical anxiety.*
- ▲ Assess for a history of life-threatening illness such as cancer and provide appropriate counseling. EBN: *Clients who are confronted by a critical illness often exhibit signs of apprehension and anxiety (Ford, 2016).*
- Children with cancer should continue to be assessed for PTSD into adulthood. EBN: *The mental and emotional distress caused by a child's cancer can linger and many of these clients, though cured, will continue to have problems involving neurological, physical, and social issues (Katzman & John, 2018).*
- Provide protection for a child who has witnessed violence or who has had traumatic injuries. Help the child acknowledge the event and express grief over the event. EBN: *Many asylum-seeking children have experienced past trauma, hospitalization, and health care encounters that may trigger traumatic memories and cause further distress (Flood & Coyne, 2019).*
- Assess for a medical history of anxiety disorders. EBN: *Evaluate the client for events that trigger anxiety and distress and help the client recognize and control these situations (Braga Mendonça et al, 2020).*
- ▲ Assess children of deployed parents for PTSD and provide appropriate referrals. EB: *Lucier-Greer et al (2016) found in their research that multiple parental deployments are a powerful indicator of detrimental outcomes for adolescents in military families.*
- Consider implementation of a school-based program for children to decrease PTSD after catastrophic events. EBN: *According to Cogan et al (2019), there is a demand for programs that guide the selection of evidence-based safety plans that reflect the developmental and the mental health needs of the school community.*

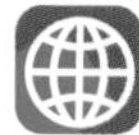

Geriatric and Multicultural

- Refer to the care plan for **Post-Trauma** Syndrome.

Home Care

- ▲ Evaluate the client's response to a traumatic or critical event. If screening warrants, refer to a therapist for counseling/treatment. EB: *Osofsky et al (2017) found that addressing life stressors is an important function in integrated client care.*
- Refer to the care plan for **Post-Trauma** Syndrome.

Client Family Teaching and Discharge Planning

- Provide education to explain that acute stress disorder symptoms may be common when preparing combatants for their role in deployment. Provide referrals if the symptoms persist. EB: *Because US military forces have been engaged in overseas conflicts since 2001, servicemen and servicewomen have faced stressors related to combat and long deployments. Most manage this stress successfully, but others struggle with mental health problems (Farmer et al, 2015).*

P

REFERENCES

Bartone, P. T., Bartone, J. V., Violanti, J. M., & Gileno, Z. M. (2019). Peer support services for bereaved survivors; a systematic review. *Omega, 80*(1), 137–166. https://doi.org/10.1177/0030222817728204.

Braga Mendonça, A., Ramos Pereira, E., Magnago, C., Costa Rosa Andrade Silva, R. M., & de Oliveira Martins, A. (2020). Nursing process for a patient with needle phobia: A case study. *Revista Brasileira de Enfermagem, 73*(4), e20190095. https://doi.org/10.1590/0034-7167-2019-0095.

Cogan, R., Nickitas, D. M., Mazyck, D., & Hallowell, S. G. (2019). School nurses share their voices, trauma, and solutions by sounding the alarm on gun violence. *Current Trauma Reports, 5*, 178–186. https://doi.org/10.1007/s40719-019-00179-1.

Farmer, C. M., Vaughan, C. A., Garnett, J., & Weinick, R. M. (2015). Pre-deployment stress, mental health, and help-seeking behaviors among Marines. *Rand Health Quarterly, 5*(1), 23. Retrieved from https://www.rand.org/pubs/periodicals/health-quarterly/issues/v5/n1/23.html. [Accessed December 13, 2021].

Flood, C., & Coyne, I. (2019). A literature review of the psychological status of asylum-seeking: Children: Implications for nursing practice. *British Journal of Nursing, 28*(7), 461–466. https://doi.org/10.12968/bjon.2019.28.7.461.

Ford, J. A. (2016). The complexity of assessment and treatment for anxiety in patients with a terminal illness. *Journal of Hospice and Palliative Nursing, 18*(2), 131–138. https://doi.org/10.1097/NJH.0000000000000223.

Frank, C. A., Schroeter, K., & Shaw, C. (2017). Addressing traumatic stress in the acute traumatically injured patient. *Journal of Trauma Nursing, 24*(2), 78–84. https://doi.org/10.1097/JTN.0000000000000270.

Handley, T. E., Kelly, B. J., Lewin, T. J., et al. (2015). Long-term effects on lifetime trauma exposure in a rural community sample. *BMC Public Health, 15*, 1176. https://doi.org/10.1186/s12889-015-2490-y.

Katzman, B. I., & John, R. (2018). Adolescent cancer survivors: A literature review of psychological effects following remission. *Clinical Journal of Oncology Nursing, 22*(5), 507–515. https://doi.org/10.1188/.CJON.507-515.

Lucier-Greer, M., Arnold, A. L., Grimsley, R. N., Ford, J. L., Bryant, C., & Mancini, J. A. (2016). Parental military service and adolescent well-being: Mental health, social connections and coping among youth in the USA. *Child & Family Social Work, 21*(4), 421–432. https://doi.org/10.1111/cfs.12158.

National Center for PTSD. (2021). Primary care PTSD screen for DSM-5 (PC-PTSD-5). Retrieved from https://www.ptsd.va.gov/professional/assessment/screens/pc-ptsd.asp. [Accessed December 13, 2021].

Osofsky, H. J., Weems, C. F., Hansel, T. C., et al. (2017). Identifying trajectories of change to improve understanding of integrated health care outcomes on PTSD symptoms post disaster. *Families, Systems & Health, 35*(2), 155–166. https://doi.org/10.1037/fsh0000274.

Oster, C., Morello, A., Venning, A., Redpath, P., & Lawn, S. (2017). The health and wellbeing needs of veterans: A rapid review. *BMC Psychiatry, 17*(1), 414. https://doi.org/10.1186/s12888-017-1547-0.

Prins, A., Bovin, M. J., Smolenski, D. J., et al. (2016). The primary care PTSD screen for DSM-5 (PC-PTSD-5): Development and evaluation within a veteran primary care sample. *Journal of General Internal Medicine, 31*(10), 1206–12011. https://doi.org/10.1017/s1606-016-3703-5.

Richins, M. T., Gauntlett, L., Tehrani, N., et al. (2020). Early post-trauma interventions in organizations: A scoping review. *Frontiers in Psychology, 11*, 1176. https://doi.org/10.3389/fpsyg.2020.01176.

Weisman, J. S., & Rodebaugh, T. L. (2018). Exposure therapy augmentation: A review and extension of techniques informed by an inhibitory learning approach. *Clinical Psychology Review, 59*, 41–51. https://doi.org/10.1016/j.cpr.2017.10.010.

Yang, M. S., & Burr, J. A. (2016). Combat exposure, social relationships, and subjective well-being among middle-aged and older veterans. *Aging & Mental Health, 20*(6), 637–646. https://doi.org/10.1080/13607863.2015.1033679.

Readiness for Enhanced Power

Domain 9 Coping/stress tolerance Class 2 Coping responses

Marina Martinez-Kratz, MS, RN, CNE

NANDA-I

Definition

A pattern of participating knowingly in change for well-being, which can be strengthened.

Defining Characteristics

Expresses desire to enhance awareness of possible changes; expresses desire to enhance decisions that could lead to changes; expresses desire to enhance independence by taking action for change; expresses desire to enhance involvement in change; expresses desire to enhance knowledge for participation in change; expresses desire to enhance participation in choices for daily living; expresses desire to enhance participation in choices for health; expresses desire to enhance power

NOC (Nursing Outcomes Classification)

Suggested NOC Outcomes

Health Beliefs: Perceived Control; Participation in Health Care Decisions; Personal Autonomy

Example NOC Outcome with Indicators

Health Beliefs: Perceived Control as evidenced by the following indicators: Belief that own actions and decisions control health outcomes/Perceived responsibility for health decisions/Efforts at gathering information. (Rate the outcome and indicators of **Health Beliefs: Perceived Control** as 1 = very weak, 2 = weak, 3 = moderate, 4 = strong, 5 = very strong [see Section I].)

Client Outcomes

Client Will (Specify Time Frame)

- Describe power resources
- Identify realistic perceptions of control
- Develop a plan of action based on power resources
- Seek assistance as needed

NIC (Nursing Interventions Classification)

Suggested NIC Interventions

Mutual Goal Setting; Self-Esteem Enhancement; Self-Responsibility Facilitation

P

Example NIC Activities—Mutual Goal Setting

Encourage the identification of specific life values; Identify with client the goals of care; Assist client in examining available resources to meet goals

Nursing Interventions and *Rationales*

- Assess the meaning of the event to the person. EBN: *Assessing meaning gives a voice to clients and makes it more likely that solutions reached will have meaning and be useful to the individual (Holmberg et al, 2019).*
- Establish a trusting relationship with the client. EBN: *A systematic review and synthesis of 61 studies revealed that individualized relational work by nursing staff could mitigate feelings of powerlessness in older hospitalized clients (Bridges et al, 2020).*
- Assist and encourage the client to identify sources of emotional support. EBN: *A study of parents found that gaining emotional support from others was a successful coping strategy to deal with feelings of powerlessness (Stevens & O'Connor-Von, 2016).*
- Provide support for client families to identify the balance between client care responsibilities and self-care. EBN: *A study found that by supporting client families and considering them as resources, family feelings of powerlessness can be reduced (Lindgren, Söderberg, & Skär, 2016).*
- Initiate and facilitate family health conversations between the client and their family. EBN: *Research findings showed that participation in family health conversations mediated consolation, helped identify family members' problems and suffering, and assisted in identifying their family's resources and strengths (Dorell & Sundin, 2016).*
- Provide the client with information and regular updates regarding their care. EBN: *A study found that powerlessness was a major component of client dissatisfaction that could be addressed by nursing rounds and continuous updates (Forsgärde, From Attebring, & Elmqvist, 2016).*
- Refer client to an empowerment support group. EBN: *A randomized controlled trial found that clients who participated in an empowerment support group showed significant increases in levels of empowerment and self-care behaviors (Hsiao et al, 2016).*

Pediatric

- Provide empowerment-based education for parents that includes a focus on caregiving knowledge, caring behaviors, self-efficacy, and indicators of the child's recovery. EBN: *A study of an empowerment-based health education program for parents caring for children with a congenital heart defect after corrective surgery showed parental improvement in caregiving knowledge, caring behaviors, and self-efficacy (Ni, Chao, & Xue, 2016).*
- Initiate problem-solving opportunities, empowering discussions, and reflection to help families take action to manage their child's illness. EBN: *A randomized clinical trial found that implementation of an asthma family empowerment program decreased parental stress, improved family functioning, and increased children's pulmonary function (Yeh et al, 2016).*
- Provide teaching so chronically ill children can learn about their illness, recommendations, identify their limitations, and adapt by changing their routines. EB: *A systematic review found that children with congenital heart disease gained a sense of control by learning to adapt to their limitations (Chong et al, 2018).*

Geriatric

- The preceding interventions may be adapted for use with older adults.
- Provide health education for older individuals that is tailored, interactive, structured, and continuous and incorporates motivational and encouragement techniques. EB: *A systematic review of the literature showed that use of specific educational interventions for older nursing home residents was an empowering strategy that increased self-efficacy and self-care (Shoberer et al, 2016).*

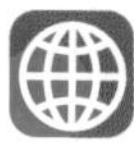

Multicultural

- The preceding interventions may be adapted for use with diverse clients.
- Provide support and educational interventions that are culturally tailored. EB: *A randomized control trial found that Latino families assigned to a culturally sensitive, cognitive-behavioral group intervention reported lower neuropsychiatric symptoms in their relative, less caregiver distress, a greater sense of caregiver self-efficacy, and less depressive symptoms over time (Gonyea, López, & Velásquez, 2016).*

P

Home Care

- The preceding interventions may be adapted for use in home care.
- Provide caregivers with support, listen to their concerns, and advocate for their needs. EBN: *A qualitative study found that when nurses acted as advocates through dialogues and interactions, the family caregivers' feelings of powerlessness were decreased (Høgsnes et al, 2019).*

REFERENCES

Bridges, J., Collins, P., Flatley, M., Hope, J., & Young, A. (2020). Older people's experiences in acute care settings: Systematic review and synthesis of qualitative studies. *International Journal of Nursing Studies, 102*, 103469. https://doi.org/10.1016/j.ijnurstu.2019.103469.

Chong, L. S. H., Fitzgerald, D. A., Craig, J. C., et al. (2018). Children's experiences of congenital heart disease: A systematic review of qualitative studies. *European Journal of Pediatrics, 177*(3), 319–336. https://doi.org/10.1007/s00431-017-3081-y.

Dorell, Å., & Sundin, K. (2016). Becoming visible—experiences from families participating in Family Health Conversations at residential homes for older people. *Geriatric Nursing, 37*(4), 260–265. https://doi.org/10.1016/j.gerinurse.2016.02.015.

Forsgärde, E. S., Attebring, M., & Elmqvist, C. (2016). Powerlessness: Dissatisfied patients' and relatives' experience of their emergency department visit. *International Emergency Nursing, 25*, 32–36. https://doi-org.ezproxy.jccmi.edu/10.1016/j.ienj.2015.07.004.

Gonyea, J. G., López, L. M., & Velásquez, E. H. (2016). The effectiveness of a culturally sensitive cognitive behavioral group intervention for Latino Alzheimer's caregivers. *The Gerontologist, 56*(2), 292–302. https://doi.org/10.1093/geront/gnu045.

Høgsnes, L., Norbergh, K. G., & Melin-Johansson, C. (2019). "Being in between": Nurses' experiences when caring for individuals with dementia and encountering family caregivers' existential life situations. *Research in Gerontological Nursing, 12*(2), 91–98. https://doi.org/10.3928/19404921-20190207-01.

Holmberg, B., Hellström, I., Norberg, A., & Österlind, J. (2019). Assenting to exposedness—Meanings of receiving assisted bodily care in a nursing home as narrated by older persons. *Scandinavian Journal of Caring Sciences, 33*(4), 868–877. https://doi.org/10.1111/scs.12683.

Hsiao, C. Y., Lin, L. W., Su, Y. W., Yeh, S. H., Lee, L. N., & Tsai, F. M. (2016). The effects of an empowerment intervention on renal transplant recipients: A randomized controlled trial. *Journal of Nursing Research, 24*(3), 201–210.

Lindgren, E., Söderberg, S., & Skär, L. (2016). Being a parent to a young adult with mental illness in transition to adulthood. *Issues in Mental Health Nursing, 37*(2), 98–105. https://doi.org/10.3109/01612840.2015.1092621.

Ni, Z., Chao, Y., & Xue, X. (2016). An empowerment health education program for children undergoing surgery for congenital heart diseases. *Journal of Child Health Care, 20*(3), 354–364.

Shoberer, D., Leino-Kilpi, H., Breimaier, H. E., Halfens, R. J., & Lohrmann, C. (2016). Educational interventions to empower nursing home residents: A systematic literature review. *Clinical Interventions in Aging, 11*, 1351–1363. https://doi.org/10.2147/CIA.S114068.

Stevens, M. S., & O'Connor-Von, S. (2016). Parent coping with adolescent trichotillomania. *Journal of School Nursing, 32*(6), 423–435. https://doi.org/10.1177/1059840516658332.

Yeh, H. Y., Ma, W. F., Huang, J. L., Hsueh, K. C., & Chiang, L. C. (2016). Evaluating the effectiveness of a family empowerment program on family function and pulmonary function of children with asthma: A randomized control trial. *International Journal of Nursing Studies, 60*, 133–144. https://doi.org/10.1016/j.ijnurstu.2016.04.013.

Powerlessness Domain 9 Coping/stress tolerance Class 2 Coping responses

Marina Martinez-Kratz, MS, RN, CNE

NANDA-I

Definition

A state of actual or perceived loss of control or influence over factors or events that affect one's well-being, personal life, or the society (adapted from American Psychology Association).

Defining Characteristics

Delayed recovery; depressive symptoms; expresses doubt about role performance; expresses frustration about inability to perform previous activities; expresses lack of purpose in life; expresses shame; fatigue; loss of independence; reports inadequate sense of control; social alienation

Related Factors

Anxiety; caregiver role strain; dysfunctional institutional environment; impaired physical mobility; inadequate interest in improving one's situation; inadequate interpersonal relations; inadequate knowledge to manage a situation; inadequate motivation to improve one's situation; inadequate participation in treatment regimen; inadequate social support; ineffective coping strategies; low self-esteem; pain; perceived complexity of treatment regimen; perceived social stigma; social marginalization

At-Risk Population

Economically disadvantaged individuals; individuals exposed to traumatic events

Associated Conditions

Cerebrovascular disorders; cognition disorders; critical illness; progressive illness; unpredictability of illness trajectory

NOC (Nursing Outcomes Classification)

Suggested NOC Outcomes

Depression Self-Control; Health Beliefs; Health Beliefs: Perceived Ability to Perform, Perceived Control, Perceived Resources; Participation in Health Care Decisions

Example NOC Outcome with Indicators

Health Beliefs: Perceived Control as evidenced by the following indicators: Perceived responsibility for health decisions/Beliefs that own decisions and actions control health outcomes. (Rate the outcome and indicators of **Health Beliefs: Perceived Control:** 1 = very weak belief, 2 = weak belief, 3 = moderately strong belief, 4 = strong belief, 5 = very strong belief [see Section I].)

Client Outcomes

Client Will (Specify Time Frame)

- State feelings of powerlessness and other feelings related to powerlessness (e.g., anger, sadness, hopelessness)
- Identify factors that are uncontrollable
- Participate in planning and implementing care; make decisions regarding care and treatment when possible
- Ask questions about care and treatment
- Verbalize hope for the future and sense of participation in planning and implementing care

P

NIC (Nursing Interventions Classification)

Suggested NIC Interventions

Cognitive Restructuring; Complex Relationship Building; Mutual Goal Setting; Self-Esteem Enhancement; Self-Responsibility Facilitation

Example NIC Activities—Self-Responsibility Facilitation

Encourage independence but assist client when unable to perform; Assist client to identify areas in which they could readily assume more responsibility

Nursing Interventions and *Rationales*

Note: Before implementation of interventions in the face of client powerlessness, nurses should examine their own philosophies of care to ensure that control issues or lack of faith in client capabilities will not bias the ability to intervene sincerely and effectively.

- Assess powerlessness with tools that are available for general and specific client groups:
  - Measure of Powerlessness for Adult Patients (de Almeida Lopes Monteiro da Cruz & Braga, 2006)
  - Personal Progress Scale–Revised, tested with women (Johnson, Worell, & Chandler, 2005)
  - Life Situation Questionnaire–Powerlessness subscale, tested with stroke caregivers (Larson et al, 2005)
  - Making Decisions Scale, tested in clients with mental illness (Hansson & Björkman, 2005)
  - Family Empowerment Scale, tested on parents of children with emotional disorders (Koren, DeChillo, & Friesen, 1992)

- Establish a trusting relationship with the client. EBN: *A systematic review and synthesis of 61 studies revealed that individualized relational work by nursing staff could mitigate feelings of powerlessness in older hospitalized clients (Bridges et al, 2020).*
- Assist and encourage the client to identify sources of emotional support. EBN: *A study of parents found that gaining emotional support from others was a successful coping strategy to deal with feelings of powerlessness (Stevens & O'Connor-Von, 2016).*
- Engage with clients using respectful listening and questioning to develop an awareness of clients' most important concerns. EB: *Engaging clients will integrate clinician expertise with client needs and can diminish feelings of powerlessness (Sheridan et al, 2015).*
- Provide clients with a collaborative decision-making process. EB: *A study revealed that clients felt their choices were limited, due to the nature of their illness or pressure from other people, and described feeling powerless to influence decisions about their care (Morant et al, 2018).*
- Provide support for client families to identify the balance between client care responsibilities and self-care. EBN: *A study found that by supporting client families and considering them as resources, family feelings of powerlessness can be reduced (Lindgren, Söderberg, & Skär, 2016).*
- Use a rehabilitative behavioral learning model that assists clients to understand how the mechanisms of habit and ritual work to reinforce powerlessness in their lives. EB: *For clients with addiction, understanding the learning processes and mechanisms of powerlessness is an important part of recovery (Butler et al, 2015).*
- Provide the client with information and regular updates regarding their care. EBN: *A study found that powerlessness was a major component of client dissatisfaction that could be addressed by nursing rounds and continuous updates (Forsgärde, From Attebring, & Elmqvist, 2016).*
- Refer client to an empowerment support group. EBN: *A randomized controlled trial found that clients who participated in an empowerment support group showed significant increases in levels of empowerment and self-care behaviors (Hsiao et al, 2016).*
- Refer to the care plans for **Hopelessness** and **Spiritual** Distress.

Pediatric

- Provided empowerment-based educational preparation for parents that includes a focus on caregiving knowledge, caring behaviors, self-efficacy, and indicators of the child's recovery. EBN: *A study of an empowerment-based health education program for parents caring for children with a congenital heart defect after corrective surgery showed parental improvement in caregiving knowledge, caring behaviors, and self-efficacy (Ni, Chao, & Xue, 2016).*
- Initiate problem-solving opportunities, empowering discussions, and reflection to help families take action to manage their child's illness. EBN: *A randomized clinical trial found that implementation of an asthma family empowerment program decreased parental stress, improved family functioning, and increased children's pulmonary function (Yeh et al, 2016).*
- Provide teaching so chronically ill children can learn about their illness, recommendations, identify their limitations, and adapt by changing their routines. EB: *A systematic review found that children with congenital heart disease gained a sense of control by learning to adapt to their limitations (Chong et al, 2018).*

Geriatric

- The preceding interventions may be adapted for use with older adults.
- Initiate and facilitate family health conversations between older clients and their family. EBN: *Research findings showed that participation in family health conversations mediated consolation, helped identify family members' problems and suffering, and assisted in identifying their family's resources and strengths (Dorell & Sundin, 2016).*
- Provide health education for older individuals that is tailored, interactive, structured, and continuous and incorporates motivational and encouragement techniques. EB: *A systematic review of the literature showed that use of specific educational interventions for older nursing home residents was an empowering strategy that increased self-efficacy and self-care (Shoberer et al, 2016).*

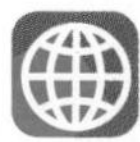

Multicultural

- The preceding interventions may be adapted for use with diverse clients.

P

- Provide support and educational interventions that are culturally tailored. **EB:** *A randomized control trial found that Latino families assigned to a culturally sensitive, cognitive-behavioral group intervention reported lower neuropsychiatric symptoms in their relative, less caregiver distress, a greater sense of caregiver self-efficacy, and less depressive symptoms over time (Gonyea, López, & Velásquez, 2016).*

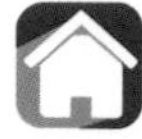

Home Care

- The preceding interventions may be adapted for use in home care.
- Provide caregivers with support, listen to their concerns, and advocate for their needs. **EBN:** *A qualitative study found that when nurses acted as advocates through dialogues and interactions, the family caregivers' feelings of powerlessness were decreased (Høgsnes et al, 2019).*

Client Family Teaching and Discharge Planning

- The preceding interventions may be adapted for teaching and discharge planning.

REFERENCES

Bridges, J., Collins, P., Flatley, M., Hope, J., & Young, A. (2020). Older people's experiences in acute care settings: Systematic review and synthesis of qualitative studies. *International Journal of Nursing Studies, 102*, 103469. https://doi.org/10.1016/j.ijnurstu.2019.103469.

Butler, M. H., Meloy, K. C., & Call, M. L. (2015). Dismantling powerlessness in addiction: Empowering recovery through rehabilitating behavioral learning. *Sexual Addiction & Compulsivity, 22*(1), 26–58.

Chong, L. S. H., Fitzgerald, D. A., Craig, J. C., et al. (2018). Children's experiences of congenital heart disease: A systematic review of qualitative studies. *European Journal of Pediatrics, 177*(3), 319–336. https://doi.org/10.1007/s00431-017-3081-y.

de Almeida Lopes Monteiro da Cruz, D., & Braga, C. G. (2006). Construction and validation of an instrument to assess powerlessness [Abstract]. *International Journal of Nursing Terminologies and Classifications, 17*(1), 67.

Dorell, Å., & Sundin, K. (2016). Becoming visible—experiences from families participating in Family Health Conversations at residential homes for older people. *Geriatric Nursing, 37*(4), 260–265. https://doi.org/10.1016/j.gerinurse.2016.02.015.

Forsgärde, E. S., Attebring, M., & Elmqvist, C. (2016). Powerlessness: Dissatisfied patients' and relatives' experience of their emergency department visit. *International Emergency Nursing, 25*, 32–36. https://doi.org/10.1016/j.ienj.2015.07.004.

Gonyea, J. G., López, L. M., & Velásquez, E. H. (2016). The effectiveness of a culturally sensitive cognitive behavioral group intervention for Latino Alzheimer's caregivers. *The Gerontologist, 56*(2), 292–302. https://doi.org/10.1093/geront/gnu045.

Hansson, L., & Björkman, T. (2005). Empowerment in people with a mental illness: Reliability and validity of the Swedish version of an empowerment scale. *Scandinavian Journal of Caring Sciences, 19*(1), 32–38.

Høgsnes, L., Norbergh, K. G., & Melin-Johansson, C. (2019). "Being in between": Nurses' experiences when caring for individuals with dementia and encountering family caregivers' existential life situations. *Research in Gerontological Nursing, 12*(2), 91–98. https://doi.org/10.3928/19404921-20190207-01.

Hsiao, C. Y., Lin, L. W., Su, Y. W., Yeh, S. H., Lee, L. N., & Tsai, F. M. (2016). The effects of an empowerment intervention on renal transplant recipients: A randomized controlled trial. *Journal of Nursing Research, 24*(3), 201–210.

Johnson, D. M., Worell, J., & Chandler, R. K. (2005). Assessing psychological health and empowerment in women: The personal progress scale revised. *Women & Health, 41*(1), 109–129.

Koren, P. E., DeChillo, N., & Friesen, B. J. (1992). Measuring empowerment in families whose children have emotional disabilities: A brief questionnaire. *Rehabilitation Psychology, 37*(4), 305–321. https://doi.org/10.1037/h0079106.

Larson, J., Franzén-Dahlin, A., Billing, E., Murray, V., & Wredling, R. (2005). Spouse's life situation after partner's stroke: Psychometric testing of a questionnaire. *Journal of Advanced Nursing, 52*(3), 300–306.

Lindgren, E., Söderberg, S., & Skär, L. (2016). Being a parent to a young adult with mental illness in transition to adulthood. *Issues in Mental Health Nursing, 37*(2), 98–105. https://doi.org/10.3109/01612840.2015.1092621.

Morant, N., Azam, K., Johnson, S., & Moncrieff, J. (2018). The least worst option: User experiences of antipsychotic medication and lack of involvement in medication decisions in a UK community sample. *Journal of Mental Health, 27*(4), 322–328. https://doi.org/10.1080/09638237.2017.1370637.

Ni, Z., Chao, Y., & Xue, X. (2016). An empowerment health education program for children undergoing surgery for congenital heart diseases. *Journal of Child Health Care, 20*(3), 354–364. https://doi.org/10.1177/1367493515587057.

Sheridan, N. F., Kenealy, T. W., Kidd, J. D., et al. (2015). Patients' engagement in primary care: Powerlessness and compounding jeopardy. A qualitative study. *Health Expectations, 18*(1), 32–43.

Shoberer, D., Leino-Kilpi, H., Breimaier, H. E., Halfens, R. J., & Lohrmann, C. (2016). Educational interventions to empower nursing home residents: A systematic literature review. *Clinical Interventions in Aging, 11*, 1351–1363. https://doi.org/10.2147/CIA.S114068.

Stevens, M. S., & O'Connor-Von, S. (2016). Parent coping with adolescent trichotillomania. *The Journal of School Nursing, 32*(6), 423–435. https://doi.org/10.1177/1059840516658332.

Yeh, H. Y., Ma, W. F., Huang, J. L., Hsueh, K. C., & Chiang, L. C. (2016). Evaluating the effectiveness of a family empowerment program on family function and pulmonary function of children with asthma: A randomized control trial. *International Journal of Nursing Studies, 60*, 133–144. https://doi.org/10.1016/j.ijnurstu.2016.04.013.

Risk for Powerlessness

Domain 9 Coping/stress tolerance Class 2 Coping responses

Marina Martinez-Kratz, MS, RN, CNE

NANDA-I

Definition

Susceptible to a state of actual or perceived loss of control or influence over factors or events that affect one's well-being, personal life, or the society, which may compromise health (adapted from American Psychology Association).

Risk Factors

Anxiety; caregiver role strain; dysfunctional institutional environment; impaired physical mobility; inadequate interest in improving one's situation; inadequate interpersonal relations; inadequate knowledge to manage a situation; inadequate motivation to improve one's situation; inadequate participation in treatment regimen; inadequate social support; ineffective coping strategies; low self-esteem; pain; perceived complexity of treatment regimen; perceived social stigma; social marginalization

At-Risk Population

Economically disadvantaged; individuals exposed to traumatic events

Associated Conditions

Cerebrovascular disorders, cognition disorders; critical illness; progressive illness; unpredictability of illness trajectory

NOC, NIC, Client Outcomes, Nursing Interventions and *Rationales,* Client/Family Teaching and Discharge Planning, and References

See the care plan for **Powerlessness.**

Adult Pressure Injury

Domain 11 Safety/protection Class 2 Physical injury

JoAnn Coar, MSN, RN-BC, A-GNP-C, CWOCN

P

NANDA-I

Definition

Localized damage to the skin and/or underlying tissue of an adult, as a result of pressure, or pressure in combination with shear (European Pressure Ulcer Advisory Panel, 2019).

Defining Characteristics

Blood-filled blister; erythema; full thickness tissue loss; full thickness tissue loss with exposed bone; full thickness tissue loss with exposed muscle; full thickness tissue loss with exposed tendon; localized heat in relation to surrounding tissue; pain at pressure points; partial thickness loss of dermis; purple localized area of discolored intact skin; ulcer is covered by eschar; ulcer is covered by slough

Related Factors

External Factors

Altered microclimate between skin and supporting surface; excessive moisture; inadequate access to appropriate equipment; inadequate access to appropriate health services; inadequate availability of equipment for individuals with obesity; inadequate caregiver knowledge of pressure injury prevention strategies; increased magnitude of mechanical load; pressure over bony prominence; shearing forces; surface friction; sustained mechanical load; use of linen with insufficient moisture wicking property

Internal Factors

Decreased physical activity; decreased physical mobility; dehydration; dry skin; hyperthermia; inadequate adherence to incontinence treatment regimen; inadequate adherence to pressure injury prevention plan; inadequate knowledge of pressure injury prevention strategies; protein-energy malnutrition; smoking; substance misuse

Other Factors

Factors identified by standardized, validated screening tool

At-Risk Population

Individuals in aged care settings; individuals in intensive care units; individuals in palliative care settings; individuals in rehabilitation settings; individuals in transit to or between clinical care settings; individuals receiving home-based care; individuals with American Society of Anesthesiologists (ASA) Physical health status score ≥3; individuals with body mass index above normal range for age and gender; individuals with body mass index below normal range for age and gender; individuals with history of pressure injury; individuals with physical disability; older adults

Associated Conditions

Anemia; cardiovascular diseases; chronic neurological conditions; critical illness; decreased serum albumin level; decreased tissue oxygenation; decreased tissue perfusion; diabetes mellitus; edema; elevated C-reactive protein; hemodynamic instability; hip fracture; immobilization; impaired circulation; intellectual disability; medical devices; peripheral neuropathy; pharmaceutical preparations; physical trauma; prolonged duration of surgical procedure; sensation disorders; spinal cord injuries

NOC (Nursing Outcomes Classification)

Suggested NOC Outcomes

Tissue Integrity: Skin and Mucous Membranes

Example NOC Outcome with Indicators

Intact Tissue Integrity: Skin and Mucous Membranes as evidenced by the following indicators: Skin intactness/Skin lesions absent/Tissue perfusion/Skin temperature. (Rate the outcome and indicators of **Tissue Integrity: Skin and Mucous Membranes:** 1 = severely compromised, 2 = substantially compromised, 3 = moderately compromised, 4 = mildly compromised, 5 = not compromised [see Section I].)

P

Client Outcomes

Client Will (Specify Time Frame)

- Report any altered sensation or pain at site of tissue impairment
- Skin, without redness over bony prominences and capillary refill of less than 6 seconds over areas of redness
- Be repositioned off of bony prominences frequently if risk for pressure injuries is high (e.g., Braden Scale score ≤18)
- Demonstrate understanding of plan to reduce pressure injury risk
- Describe measures to protect the skin

NIC (Nursing Interventions Classification)

Suggested NIC Interventions

Pain Management; Pressure Injury Care; Pressure Injury Prevention; Risk Identification; Skin Care: Topical Treatments; Skin Surveillance

Example NIC Activities—Pressure Injury Care

Monitor color of skin, temperature, edema, erythema, moisture, and appearance of surrounding skin; Note characteristics of skin over bony prominences or under/in contact with medical devices

Nursing Interventions and *Rationales*

▲ The National Pressure Ulcer Advisory Panel (NPUAP) redefined the definition of a pressure ulcer, which is now referred to as pressure injuries, during the NPUAP 2016 Staging Consensus Conference in 2016. The new definitions more accurately define alterations in tissue integrity from pressure. Classify pressure injuries (NPUAP & European Pressure Ulcer Advisory Panel [EPUAP], 2016) using national guidelines and definitions (see http://www.npuap.org/resources/educational-and-clinical-resources/npuap-pressure-injury-stages/).

- **Pressure Injury:** A pressure injury is localized damage to the skin and underlying soft tissue usually over a bony prominence or related to a medical or other device. The injury can present as intact skin or an open ulcer and may be painful. The injury occurs as a result of intense and/or prolonged pressure or pressure in combination with shear. The tolerance of soft tissue for pressure and shear may also be affected by microclimate, nutrition, perfusion, comorbidities, and condition of the soft tissue (NPUAP & EPUAP, 2016).
- **Stage 1 Pressure Injury:** Nonblanchable erythema of intact skin. Area of localized nonblanchable erythema that may appear differently in darkly pigmented skin, and changes in sensation, temperature, or firmness may precede visual changes. Color changes do not include purple or maroon discoloration, which is more likely to indicate deep tissue pressure injury (NPUAP & EPUAP, 2016).
- **Stage 2 Pressure Injury:** Partial-thickness skin loss with exposed dermis. Partial-thickness skin loss with exposed dermis in which the wound bed is pink/red and moist and adipose (fat) and deeper tissues are not visible. Granulation tissue, slough, and eschar are not present. A stage 2 pressure injury may also present as an intact or ruptured blister. These injuries commonly result from adverse microclimate and shear in the skin over the pelvis and shear in the heel. This stage should not be used to describe moisture-associated skin damage (MASD) including incontinence-associated dermatitis (IAD), intertriginous dermatitis (ITD), medical adhesive–related skin injury (MARSI), or traumatic wounds (skin tears, burns, and abrasions) (NPUAP & EPUAP, 2016).
- **Stage 3 Pressure Injury:** Full-thickness skin loss. Full-thickness loss of skin, in which adipose is visible and granulation tissue and epibole (rolled wound edges) are often present and undermining/tunneling may occur. Slough and/or eschar may also be visible. Fascia, muscle, tendon, ligament, cartilage, and/or bone are not exposed. The depth of tissue damage varies by anatomical location, and areas of significant adiposity can develop deep wounds. If slough or eschar obscures the extent of tissue loss, this is an unstageable pressure injury (NPUAP & EPUAP, 2016).
- **Stage 4 Pressure Injury:** Full-thickness skin and tissue loss. Full-thickness skin and tissue loss with exposed or directly palpable fascia, muscle, tendon, ligament, cartilage, or bone, and slough and/or eschar may be visible. Epibole, undermining, and/or tunneling often occur and depth varies by anatomical location. If slough or eschar obscures the extent of tissue loss, this is an unstageable pressure injury (NPUAP & EPUAP, 2016).
- **Deep Tissue Pressure Injury:** Persistent nonblanchable deep red, maroon, or purple discoloration. Intact or nonintact skin with localized area of persistent nonblanchable deep red, maroon, or purple discoloration or epidermal separation revealing a dark wound bed or blood-filled blister. Pain and temperature change often precedes skin color changes. Discoloration may appear differently in darkly pigmented skin. This injury results from intense and/or prolonged pressure and shear forces at the bone–muscle interface. The wound may evolve rapidly to reveal the actual extent of tissue injury, or it may resolve without tissue loss. If necrotic tissue, subcutaneous tissue, granulation tissue, fascia, muscle, or other underlying structures are visible, this indicates a full-thickness pressure injury (unstageable, stage 3, or stage 4). Do not use deep tissue pressure injury to describe vascular, traumatic, neuropathic, or dermatological conditions (NPUAP & EPUAP, 2016).
- **Unstageable Pressure Injury:** Obscured full-thickness skin and tissue loss. Full-thickness skin and tissue loss in which the extent of tissue damage within the ulcer cannot be confirmed because it is obscured by slough or eschar. If slough or eschar is removed, a stage 3 or stage 4 pressure injury will

P

be revealed. Stable eschar (i.e., dry, adherent, intact without erythema or fluctuance) on the heel or ischemic limb should not be softened or removed (NPUAP & EPUAP, 2016).

- Routinely assess clients for risk of pressure injuries using a valid and reliable risk assessment tool (National Pressure Injury Advisory Panel [NPIAP] & European Pressure Injury Advisory Panel [EPIAP], 2019). A validated risk-assessment tool such as the Norton scale or Braden scale should be used to identify clients at risk for pressure-related skin breakdown (NPIAP & EPIAP, 2019). **EB:** *Targeting variables (e.g., Braden scale risk subscale categories, age, severity of illness) can focus assessment on particular risk factors (e.g., pressure, immobility, perfusion) and help guide the plan of prevention and care (Ratliff et al, 2017; NPIAP/EPIAP, 2019).*
- Pressure injury risk assessment should be completed on admission, daily, and after procedures or changes in the client's condition (Baranoski & Ayello, 2016; NPIAP & EPIAP, 2019).
- Inspect the skin daily, especially bony prominences and dependent areas, for pallor, redness, and breakdown. In addition to assessing pressure injury risk, client-specific interventions should be implemented to prevent tissue injury. Implement the following interventions to prevent tissue breakdown:
  - Turn and reposition all individuals at risk for pressure injury, unless contraindicated because of medical condition or medical treatments.
  - Position client properly; use pressure-redistributing surfaces based on the individual's needs (e.g., pillows, gel or foam cushions, reactive/nonreactive foam mattresses, alternating pressure mattress, air-fluidized surface) if indicated. Continue to turn and reposition the individual regardless of the support surface in use. Establish turning frequency based on the characteristics of the support surface and the individual's response (NPIAP & EPIAP, 2019).
  - Lift and move client carefully using a turn sheet and adequate assistance; keep bed linens dry and wrinkle-free.
  - Perform actions to keep client from sliding down in bed (e.g., bend knees slightly when head of bed is elevated 30 degrees or higher) to reduce the risk of skin surface abrasion and shearing. Use the 30-degree tilted side-lying position (alternately, right side, back, left side). Maintain the head of the bed as flat as possible. Avoid extended use of prone positioning unless the individual can tolerate this and his or her medical condition allows (NPIAP & EPIAP, 2019).
  - Select a seated posture that is acceptable for the individual and minimizes the pressure and shear exerted on the skin and soft tissues. Limit time in seated position and encourage pressure relieving maneuvers (NPIAP & EPIAP, 2019).
  - Keep client's skin clean. Thoroughly dry skin after bathing and as often as needed, paying special attention to skinfolds and opposing skin surfaces (e.g., axillae, perineum, beneath breasts). Pat skin dry rather than rub and use a mild soap for bathing. Avoid alkaline soaps and cleansers. Apply moisturizing lotion at least once a day (NPIAP & EPIAP, 2019).
  - Protect the skin from contact with urine and feces (e.g., keep perineal area clean and dry, apply a protective ointment or cream to perineal area).
  - Provide and encourage adequate daily fluid intake for hydration for an individual assessed to be at risk of or with a pressure injury (NPUAP & EPUAP, 2016). Adjust protein intake for individuals with or at risk for pressure injuries. This must be consistent with the individual's comorbid conditions and goals (NPIAP & EPIAP, 2019).
  - If the individual cannot be moved or is positioned with the head of the bed elevated over 30 degrees, place a polyurethane foam dressing on the sacrum (NPUAP & EPUAP, 2016). Use heel offloading device or polyurethane foam dressings on individuals at high risk for heel ulcers (NPUAP & EPUAP, 2016).
  - Consult with nutrition/dietary specialist to evaluate client's nutritional status.
  - Increase activity as allowed.

  EB: *Pressure injuries result in additional pain and treatment for the client and additional health care services and costs. A comprehensive assessment of the client's risk for pressure injuries and proactive interventions is necessary to reduce the risk for tissue injury (NPUAP & EPUAP, 2016; NPIAP & EPIAP, 2019).*
- Medical device–related pressure injuries (MDRPIs) result from the use of devices designed and applied for diagnostic or therapeutic purposes. The resultant pressure injury generally conforms to the pattern or shape of the device. The injury should be staged using the NPUAP pressure injury staging system and the etiology of the pressure injury noted to be caused by the device (NPUAP & EPUAP, 2016).
  - Assess the skin around and under medical devices routinely to identify signs of pressure-related injuries (NPIAP & EPIAP, 2019).

P

- ❍ Common devices associated with pressure-related tissue injury include oxygen delivery and monitoring devices (e.g., face mask, nasal cannula, pulse oximetry, bilevel positive airway pressure [BiPAP] mask), feeding tubes (e.g., nasogastric, gastric, jejunal tubes), endotracheal devices (oral and/or nasal endotracheal tubes, tracheostomy tubes), urinary and bowel elimination equipment (indwelling urinary catheter, fecal containment catheter), and musculoskeletal appliances (cervical collar, splints, braces).
- ❍ Assess and evaluate the purpose and function of the medical device. Remove medical devices as soon as medically feasible (NPIAP & EPIAP, 2019).
- ❍ Assess proper fit of the medical device and securement to prevent tension, and assess the skin under the device regularly for pressure-related injury (NPIAP & EPIAP, 2019).
- ❍ Protect the skin below and around the device to reduce pressure. Use a prophylactic dressing under the medical device to protect skin (NPIAP & EPIAP, 2019).

EB: *Incorporate daily and frequent skin inspection around and under the medical device. See the NPIAP Best Practice flyer to help provide education about medical device–related pressure injuries (NPIAP & EPIAP, 2019).*

- **Mucosal Membrane Pressure Injury:** Mucosal membrane pressure injury is found on mucous membranes with a history of a medical device in use at the location of the injury. Due to the anatomy of the tissue these ulcers cannot be staged (NPUAP & EPUAP, 2016).
- Critically ill clients are at increased risk for pressure ulcers, often requiring frequent skin risk assessment and preventive interventions. EB: *Reposition all individuals with or at risk for pressure injuries on an individualized schedule unless contraindicated (NPIAP & EPIAP, 2019). Reposition in such a way that pressure is optimally removed from bony prominences and maximal pressure redistribution is achieved (NPIAP & EPIAP, 2019).*
- Efforts must be taken to disseminate evidence-based guidelines and ensure that health care providers, in all settings, are making every effort to identify individuals who are at risk for pressure injuries and implement preventive and treatment interventions (Ratliff et al, 2017). EB: *Consider optimizing work procedures at a professional level through the introduction of tailored staff education, and assess and maximize workforce characteristics to reduce pressure injury incidence (NPIAP & EPIAP, 2019).*
- A client at risk for skin, wound, and related complications can benefit from the expert knowledge and skill set of a certified wound, ostomy, continence nurse (Berke et al, 2019). See care plan for Impaired **Skin** Integrity for additional interventions if a pressure ulcer occurs.

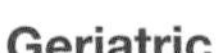

Geriatric

- Consider the older client's cognitive status when assessing the skin and in developing a comprehensive plan of care to prevent pressure injuries (NPUAP & EPUAP, 2016; NPIAP & EPIAP, 2019).
- Aging skin, medications (e.g., steroids), and moisture place the older client at increased risk for pressure-associated skin breakdown. EB: *Assess the client for pressure injury (NPUAP & EPUAP, 2016) risk, skin tear, and moisture-associated skin breakdown. It is important to differentiate the cause of the older client's skin breakdown to effectively implement prevention and treatment strategies. An individual with continence-related issues is always at risk for skin or pressure-related injuries (Berke et al, 2019).*
- Clients over age 65 years are at higher risk for pressure injuries because they have reduced subcutaneous fat and capillary blood flow, as well as physiological skin changes, including decreased cohesion of the dermis and epidermis and reduced sensory function (Podd, 2018).
- Use atraumatic wound dressings to prevent and treat pressure injuries (NPUAP & EPUAP, 2016) to reduce further injury to a frail older client's skin (NPIAP & EPIAP, 2019).
- For older clients with continence concerns, develop and implement an individualized continence management program (NPIAP & EPIAP, 2019). EB: *Use skin barrier products and moisture wicking pads to reduce moisture-associated skin irritation that increases the risk for pressure injury development (NPUAP & EPUAP, 2016); use high-absorbency incontinence products to protect the skin; avoid the use of diapers except when the client is ambulating (NPIAP & EPIAP, 2019).*
- Regularly reposition the older client who is unable to reposition independently. Consider pressure redistribution support surface for clients assessed to be at high risk for pressure injuries (NPUAP & EPUAP, 2016; NPIAP & EPIAP, 2019).

Home Care

- The interventions described previously may be adapted for home care use.

- Instruct and assist the client and caregivers in how to assess the skin for excessive pressure. Provide written instructions for actions they can implement to reduce the risk of pressure injury development (NPUAP & EPUAP, 2016).
- Educate client and caregivers on proper nutrition and when to call the agency and/or health care provider with concerns.
- ▲ It may be beneficial to initiate a consultation in a case assignment with a wound, ostomy, continence nurse (or wounds specialist) to establish a comprehensive plan for pressure ulcer risk reduction for clients at high risk for skin breakdown.

REFERENCES

Baranoski, S., & Ayello, E. A. (Eds.). (2016). *Wound care essentials: Practice principles* (4th ed.) Ambler, PA: Lippincott Williams & Wilkins.

Berke, C., Conley, M. J., Netsch, D., et al. (2019). Role of the wound, ostomy and continence nurse in continence care: 2018 update. *Journal of Wound, Ostomy and Continence Nursing*, *46*(3), 221–225.

National Pressure ulcer Advisory Panel (NPUAP) and European pressure ulcer Advisory Panel (EPUAP). (2016). *Pressure injury stages*. Retrieved from http://www.npuap.org/resources/educational-and-clinical-resources/npuap-pressure-injury-stages/. Accessed November 16, 2020.

National Pressure injury Advisory Panel (NPIAP) and European pressure injury Advisory Panel (EPIAP). (2019). *Prevention and treatment of pressure ulcers*. Perth, Australia: Cambridge Media.

Podd, D. (2018). Beyond skin deep, managing pressure injuries. *Journal of the American Academy of Physician Assistants*, *31*(4), 10–17.

Ratliff, C. R., Droste, L. R., Bonham, P., Wound, Ostomy and Continence Nurses Society–Wound Guidelines Task Force, et al. (2017). WOCN 2016 guidelines for prevention and management of pressure injuries (ulcers). An executive summary. *Journal of Wound Ostomy and Continence Nursing*, *44*(3), 241–246.

Risk for Adult Pressure Injury

Domain 11 Safety/protection Class 2 Physical injury

Mary Beth Flynn Makic, PhD, RN, CCNS, CCRN-K, FAAN, FNAP, FCNS

NANDA-I

Definition

P

Adult susceptible to localized damage to the skin and/or underlying tissue, as a result of pressure, or pressure in combination with shear, which may compromise health (European Pressure Ulcer Advisory Panel, 2019).

Risk Factors

External Factors

Altered microclimate between skin and supporting surface; excessive moisture; inadequate access to appropriate equipment; inadequate access to appropriate health services; inadequate availability of equipment for individuals with obesity; inadequate caregiver knowledge of pressure injury prevention strategies; increased magnitude of mechanical load; pressure over bony prominence; shearing forces; surface friction; sustained mechanical load; use of linen with insufficient moisture wicking property

Internal Factors

Decreased physical activity; decreased physical mobility; dehydration; dry skin; hyperthermia; inadequate adherence to incontinence treatment regimen; inadequate adherence to pressure injury prevention plan; inadequate knowledge of pressure injury prevention strategies; protein-energy malnutrition; smoking; substance misuse

Other Factors

Factors identified by standardized, validated screening tool

At-Risk Population

Individuals in aged care settings; individuals in intensive care units; individuals in palliative care settings; individuals in rehabilitation settings; individuals in transit to or between clinical care settings; individuals receiving home-based care; individuals with American Society of Anesthesiologists (ASA) physical health status score ≥3; individuals with body mass index above normal range for age and gender; individuals with body mass index below normal range for age and gender; individuals with history of pressure injury; individuals with physical disability; older adults

Associated Conditions

Anemia; cardiovascular diseases; chronic neurological conditions; critical illness; decreased serum albumin level; decreased tissue oxygenation; decreased tissue perfusion; diabetes mellitus; edema; elevated C-reactive protein; hemodynamic instability; hip fracture; immobilization; impaired circulation; intellectual disability; medical devices; peripheral neuropathy; pharmaceutical preparations; physical trauma; prolonged duration of surgical procedure; sensation disorders; spinal cord injuries

NIC, NOC, Client Outcomes, Nursing Interventions and *Rationales*, Client/Family Teaching and Discharge Planning, and References

See the care plan for Adult **Pressure** Injury.

Child Pressure Injury Domain 11 Safety/protection Class 2 Physical injury

JoAnn Coar, MSN, RN-BC, A-GNP-C, CWOCN

NANDA-I

Definition

Localized damage to the skin and/or underlying tissue of a child or adolescent, as a result of pressure, or pressure in combination with shear (European Pressure Ulcer Advisory Panel, 2019).

Defining Characteristics

Blood-filled blister; erythema; full thickness tissue loss; full thickness tissue loss with exposed bone; full thickness tissue loss with exposed muscle; full thickness tissue loss with exposed tendon; localized heat in relation to surrounding tissue; pain at pressure points; partial thickness loss of dermis; purple localized area of discolored intact skin; ulcer is covered by eschar; ulcer is covered by slough

P

Related Factors

External Factors

Altered microclimate between skin and supporting surface; difficulty for caregiver to lift client completely off bed; excessive moisture; inadequate access to appropriate equipment; inadequate access to appropriate health services; inadequate access to appropriate supplies; inadequate access to equipment for children with obesity; inadequate caregiver knowledge of appropriate methods for removing adhesive materials; inadequate caregiver knowledge of appropriate methods for stabilizing devices; inadequate caregiver knowledge of modifiable factors; inadequate caregiver knowledge of pressure injury prevention strategies; increased magnitude of mechanical load; pressure over bony prominence; shearing forces; surface friction; sustained mechanical load; use of linen with insufficient moisture wicking property

Internal Factors

Decreased physical activity; decreased physical mobility; dehydration; difficulty assisting caregiver with moving self; difficulty maintaining position in bed; difficulty maintaining position in chair; dry skin; hyperthermia; inadequate adherence to incontinence treatment regimen; inadequate adherence to pressure injury prevention plan; inadequate knowledge of appropriate methods for removing adhesive materials; inadequate knowledge of appropriate methods for stabilizing devices; protein-energy malnutrition; water-electrolyte imbalance

Other Factors

Factors identified by standardized, validated screening tool

At-Risk Population

Children in intensive care units; children in long-term care facilities; children in palliative care settings; children in rehabilitation settings; children in transit to or between clinical care settings; children receiving home-based care; children with body mass index above normal range for age and gender; children with body mass index below normal range for age and gender; children with developmental issues; children with growth issues; children with large head circumference; children with large skin surface area

Associated Conditions

Alkaline skin pH; altered cutaneous structure; anemia; cardiovascular diseases; decreased level of consciousness; decreased serum albumin level; decreased tissue oxygenation; decreased tissue perfusion; diabetes mellitus; edema; elevated C-reactive protein; frequent invasive procedures; hemodynamic instability; immobilization; impaired circulation; intellectual disability; medical devices; pharmaceutical preparations; physical trauma; prolonged duration of surgical procedure; sensation disorders; spinal cord injuries

NOC (Nursing Outcomes Classification)

Suggested NOC Outcomes

Tissue Integrity: Skin and Mucous Membranes

Example NOC Outcome with Indicators

Intact Tissue Integrity: Skin and Mucous Membranes as evidenced by the following indicators: Skin intactness/Skin lesions absent/Tissue perfusion/Skin temperature. (Rate the outcome and indicators of **Tissue Integrity: Skin and Mucous Membranes:** 1 = severely compromised, 2 = substantially compromised, 3 = moderately compromised, 4 = mildly compromised, 5 = not compromised [see Section I].)

Client Outcomes

Client Will (Specify Time Frame)

- Report any altered sensation or pain at site of tissue impairment
- Skin, without redness over bony prominences and capillary refill of less than 6 seconds over areas of redness
- Be repositioned off of bony prominences frequently if risk for pressure injuries is high (e.g., Braden QD or Glamorgan scale score)
- Family/caregiver will demonstrate understanding of plan to reduce pressure injury risk
- Describe measures to protect the skin

P

NIC (Nursing Interventions Classification)

Suggested NIC Interventions

Pain Management; Pressure Injury Care; Pressure Injury Prevention; Risk Identification; Skin Care: Topical Treatments; Skin Surveillance

Example NIC Activities—Pressure Injury Care

Monitor color of skin, temperature, edema, erythema, moisture, and appearance of surrounding skin; Note characteristics of skin over bony prominences or under/in contact with medical devices

Nursing Interventions and *Rationales*

- Consider the impact of skin maturity, perfusion, and oxygenation and medical devices related to risk for pressure injury development in neonates and children (National Pressure Injury Advisory Panel [NPIAP] & European Pressure Injury Advisory Panel [EPIAP], 2019).
- Perform an age-appropriate pressure injury (National Pressure Ulcer Advisory Panel [NPUAP] & European Pressure Ulcer Advisory Panel [EPUAP], 2016) risk assessment using a valid and reliable tool. EB/EB: *The Braden QD and Glamorgan pediatric pressure ulcer risk assessment scales have been found to be*

reliable and predictive in assessing pediatric-specific pressure injury risk assessment to assist with identification of pressure-related injury risk in the population from preterm to 21 years of age, in the acute care setting (Willock et al, 2016; Freundlich, 2017; Chamblee et al, 2018; Curley et al, 2018).

- • Pressure injury risk assessment should be completed on admission, daily, and after procedures or changes in the client's condition (Baranoski & Ayello, 2016; Freundlich, 2017; NPIAP & EPIAP, 2019).
- ▲ NPUAP redefined the definition of a "pressure ulcer," which is now referred to as "pressure injuries," during the NPUAP 2016 Staging Consensus Conference in 2016. The new definitions more accurately define alterations in tissue integrity from pressure. Classify pressure injuries (NPUAP & EPUAP, 2016) using national guidelines and definitions (see http://www.npuap.org/resources/educational-and-clinical-resources/npuap-pressure-injury-stages/).
  - ❍ **Pressure Injury:** A pressure injury is localized damage to the skin and underlying soft tissue usually over a bony prominence or related to a medical or other device. The injury can present as intact skin or an open ulcer and may be painful. The injury occurs as a result of intense and/or prolonged pressure or pressure in combination with shear. The tolerance of soft tissue for pressure and shear may also be affected by microclimate, nutrition, perfusion, comorbidities, and condition of the soft tissue (NPUAP & EPUAP, 2016).
  - ❍ **Stage 1 Pressure Injury:** Nonblanchable erythema of intact skin. Area of localized nonblanchable erythema that may appear differently in darkly pigmented skin, and changes in sensation, temperature, or firmness may precede visual changes. Color changes do not include purple or maroon discoloration, which is more likely to indicate deep tissue pressure injury (NPUAP & EPUAP, 2016).
  - ❍ **Stage 2 Pressure Injury:** Partial-thickness skin loss with exposed dermis. Partial-thickness skin loss with exposed dermis in which the wound bed is pink/red and moist and adipose (fat) and deeper tissues are not visible. Granulation tissue, slough, and eschar are not present. A stage 2 pressure injury may also present as an intact or ruptured blister. These injuries commonly result from adverse microclimate and shear in the skin over the pelvis and shear in the heel. This stage should not be used to describe moisture-associated skin damage (MASD) including incontinence-associated dermatitis (IAD), intertriginous dermatitis (ITD), medical adhesive–related skin injury (MARSI), or traumatic wounds (skin tears, burns, and abrasions) (NPUAP & EPUAP, 2016).
  - ❍ **Stage 3 Pressure Injury:** Full-thickness skin loss. Full-thickness loss of skin, in which adipose is visible and granulation tissue and epibole (rolled wound edges) are often present and undermining/tunneling may occur. Slough and/or eschar may also be visible. Fascia, muscle, tendon, ligament, cartilage, and/or bone are not exposed. The depth of tissue damage varies by anatomical location, and areas of significant adiposity can develop deep wounds. If slough or eschar obscures the extent of tissue loss, this is an unstageable pressure injury (NPUAP & EPUAP, 2016).
  - ❍ **Stage 4 Pressure Injury:** Full-thickness skin and tissue loss. Full-thickness skin and tissue loss with exposed or directly palpable fascia, muscle, tendon, ligament, cartilage, or bone, and slough and/or eschar may be visible. Epibole, undermining, and/or tunneling often occur and depth varies by anatomical location. If slough or eschar obscures the extent of tissue loss, this is an unstageable pressure injury (NPUAP & EPUAP, 2016).
  - ❍ **Deep Tissue Pressure Injury:** Persistent nonblanchable deep red, maroon, or purple discoloration. Intact or nonintact skin with localized area of persistent nonblanchable deep red, maroon, or purple discoloration or epidermal separation revealing a dark wound bed or blood-filled blister. Pain and temperature change often precedes skin color changes. Discoloration may appear differently in darkly pigmented skin. This injury results from intense and/or prolonged pressure and shear forces at the bone–muscle interface. The wound may evolve rapidly to reveal the actual extent of tissue injury, or it may resolve without tissue loss. If necrotic tissue, subcutaneous tissue, granulation tissue, fascia, muscle, or other underlying structures are visible, this indicates a full-thickness pressure injury (unstageable, stage 3, or stage 4). Do not use deep tissue pressure injury to describe vascular, traumatic, neuropathic, or dermatological conditions (NPUAP & EPUAP, 2016).
  - ❍ **Unstageable Pressure Injury:** Obscured full-thickness skin and tissue loss. Full-thickness skin and tissue loss in which the extent of tissue damage within the ulcer cannot be confirmed because it is obscured by slough or eschar. If slough or eschar is removed, a stage 3 or stage 4 pressure injury will be revealed. Stable eschar (i.e., dry, adherent, intact without erythema or fluctuance) on the heel or ischemic limb should not be softened or removed (NPUAP & EPUAP, 2016).
- • Routinely assess clients for risk of pressure injuries using a valid and reliable risk assessment tool (NPIAP & EPIAP, 2019). A validated risk-assessment tool such as the Norton Scale or Braden Scale should be used

P

to identify clients at risk for pressure-related skin breakdown (NPIAP & EPIAP, 2019). **EB:** *Targeting variables (e.g., Braden scale risk subscale categories, age, severity of illness) can focus assessment on particular risk factors (e.g., pressure, immobility, perfusion) and help guide the plan of prevention and care (Ratliff et al, 2017; NPIAP & EPIAP, 2019).*

- Inspect the skin daily, especially bony prominences and dependent areas, for pallor, redness, and breakdown. In addition to assessing pressure injury risk, client-specific interventions should be implemented to prevent tissue injury. Implement the following interventions to prevent tissue breakdown:
  - Turn and reposition all individuals at risk for pressure injury, unless contraindicated because of medical condition or medical treatments.
  - Position client properly; use pressure-redistributing surfaces based on the individual's needs (e.g., pillows, gel or foam cushions, reactive/nonreactive foam mattresses, alternating pressure mattress, air-fluidized surface) if indicated. Continue to turn and reposition the individual regardless of the support surface in use. Establish turning frequency based on the characteristics of the support surface and the individual's response (NPIAP & EPIAP, 2019).
  - Lift and move client carefully using a turn sheet and adequate assistance; keep bed linens dry and wrinkle-free.
  - Perform actions to keep client from sliding down in bed (e.g., bend knees slightly when head of bed is elevated 30 degrees or higher) to reduce the risk of skin surface abrasion and shearing. Use the 30-degree tilted side-lying position (alternately, right side, back, left side). Maintain the head of the bed as flat as possible (NPIAP & EPIAP, 2019).
  - Select a seated posture that is acceptable for the individual and minimizes the pressure and shear exerted on the skin and soft tissues. Limit time in seated position and encourage pressure-relieving maneuvers (NPIAP & EPIAP, 2019).
  - Keep client's skin clean and moisturized. Thoroughly dry skin after bathing and as often as needed, paying special attention to skinfolds and opposing skin surfaces (e.g., axillae, perineum). Pat skin dry rather than rub and use a mild soap for bathing. Avoid alkaline soaps and cleansers. Apply moisturizing lotion at least once a day (NPIAP & EPIAP, 2019).
  - Protect the skin from contact with urine and feces (e.g., keep perineal area clean and dry, apply a protective ointment or cream to perineal area). Avoid diapers when possible. Apply skin protectant cream with each episode of cleansing skin of urine and feces (NPIAP & EPIAP, 2019).
  - Provide and encourage adequate daily fluid intake for hydration for an individual assessed to be at risk of or with a pressure injury (NPUAP & EPUAP, 2016). Adjust protein intake for individuals with or at risk for pressure injuries. This must be consistent with the individual's comorbid conditions and goals (NPIAP & EPIAP, 2019).
  - If the individual cannot be moved or is positioned with the head of the bed elevated over 30 degrees, place a pressure reduction pillow under the occiput and if appropriate a polyurethane foam dressing on the sacrum (NPUAP & EPUAP, 2016).
  - Implement automated nutrition/dietary specialist consultations to evaluate client's nutritional status.
  - Increase activity as allowed.

    EB: *Pressure injuries result in additional pain and treatment for the client and additional health care services and costs. A comprehensive assessment of the client's risk for pressure injuries and proactive interventions is necessary to reduce the risk for tissue injury (NPUAP & EPUAP, 2016; NPIAP & EPIAP, 2019).*
- Evaluate high-risk areas for pressure injury. Changes in growth influences at risk areas of the body for pressure injury areas. **EB:** *Body proportions also change as children grow. In younger infants and children, the occiput is the largest bony prominence and site of greatest risk for pressure injury. Ears are also a high-risk area for pressure injury (Freundlich, 2017).*
- Select an age-appropriate support surface for premature neonates and pediatric clients at high risk for pressure ulcers. **CEBN:** *A longitudinal study found that the use of continuous and reactive low-pressure mattresses reduced the observed incidence of pressure ulcers (García-Molina et al, 2012). Select a support surface to prevent occipital pressure ulcers for at-risk clients (NPIAP & EPIAP, 2019).*
- Medical device–related pressure injuries (MDRPIs) result from the use of devices designed and applied for diagnostic or therapeutic purposes. The resultant pressure injury generally conforms to the pattern or shape of the device. The injury should be staged using the NPUAP pressure injury staging system and the etiology of the pressure injury noted to be caused by the device (NPUAP & EPUAP, 2016).

- ❍ Assess the skin around and under medical devices routinely to identify signs of pressure-related injuries (NPIAP & EPIAP, 2019).
- ❍ Common devices associated with pressure-related tissue injury include oxygen delivery and monitoring devices (e.g., face mask, nasal cannula, pulse oximetry), feeding tubes (e.g., nasogastric, gastric, jejunal tubes), endotracheal devices (oral and/or nasal endotracheal tubes, tracheostomy tubes), urinary and bowel elimination equipment (indwelling urinary catheter, fecal containment catheter), and musculoskeletal appliances (cervical collar, splints, braces). EB: *Children are at greatest risk of pressure injury associated with medical devices from oxygen devices, tracheostomy tubes and ties, and casts/immobilization devices (Freundlich, 2017; Cummins et al, 2019).*
- ❍ Assess and evaluate the purpose and function of the medical device. Remove medical devices as soon as medically feasible (NPIAP & EPIAP, 2019).
- ❍ Assess proper fit of the medical device and securement to prevent tension, and assess the skin under the device regularly for pressure-related injury (NPIAP & EPIAP, 2019).
- ❍ Protect the skin below and around the device to reduce pressure. Use a prophylactic dressing under the medical device to protect skin (NPIAP & EPIAP, 2019). EB: *Incorporate daily and frequent skin inspection around and under the medical device. See the NPIAP Best Practice flyer to help provide education about medical device–related pressure injuries (NPIAP & EPIAP, 2019)*

- ● **Mucosal Membrane Pressure Injury:** Mucosal membrane pressure injury is found on mucous membranes with a history of a medical device in use at the location of the injury. Due to the anatomy of the tissue these ulcers cannot be staged (NPUAP & EPUAP, 2016).
- ● Critically ill children are at increased risk for pressure injury, often requiring frequent skin risk assessment and preventive interventions. EB: *Reposition all individuals with or at risk for pressure injuries on an individualized schedule unless contraindicated (NPIAP & EPIAP, 2019). Reposition in such a way that pressure is optimally removed from bony prominences and maximal pressure redistribution is achieved (NPIAP & EPIAP, 2019).*
- ● Review evidence-based practice interventions to assess and implement nursing interventions to reduce pressure injury risk. EB: *Efforts must be taken to disseminate evidence-based guidelines and ensure that health care providers, in all settings, are making every effort to identify individuals who are at risk for pressure injuries and implement preventive and treatment interventions (Ratliff et al, 2017; Cummins et al, 2019).*
- ● Involve family/caregiver in education focused on reducing risks and management strategies for pressure injuries. EB: *Consider optimizing family/caregiver engagement and education aligned and taught by expert clinicians/wound, ostomy, continence nurse (Berke et al, 2019). Involving family/caregiver early in the presentation and management of pressure injury prevention is necessary in preparation of discharge planning (Nie, 2020).*
- ● Select an age-appropriate support surface for premature neonates and pediatric clients at high risk for pressure ulcers. CEBN: *A longitudinal study found that the use of continuous and reactive low-pressure mattresses reduced the observed incidence of pressure ulcers (García-Molina et al, 2012). Select a support surface to prevent occipital pressure ulcers for at-risk clients (NPIAP & EPIAP, 2019).*
- ● Engage the client/family/legal guardian in the development of a client-specific plan of care to reduce pressure-related risk for skin breakdown (NPIAP & EPIAP, 2019).
- ● Document risk assessment and interventions implemented to reduce the client's risk for pressure injury development (NPUAP & EPUAP, 2016).

Home Care

- ● The interventions described previously may be adapted for home care use.
- ● Instruct and assist the client and caregivers in how to assess the skin for excessive pressure. Provide written instructions for actions they can implement to reduce the risk of pressure injury development (NPUAP & EPUAP, 2016).
- ● Educate family/caregivers and client (age-appropriate instruction) on proper nutrition and when to call the agency and/or health care provider with concerns.
- ▲ Initiate a consultation in a case assignment with a wound, ostomy, continence nurse (or wounds specialist) to establish a comprehensive plan for pressure ulcer risk reduction for clients at high risk for skin breakdown.

P

REFERENCES

Baranoski, S., & Ayello, E. A. (Eds.). (2016). *Wound care essentials: Practice principles* (4th ed.) Ambler, PA: Lippincott Williams & Wilkins.

Berke, C., Conley, M. J., Netsch, D., et al. (2019). Role of the wound, ostomy and continence nurse in continence care: 2018 update. *The Journal of Wound, Ostomy and Continence Nursing, 46*(3), 221–225.

Chamblee, T. B., Pasek, T. A., Caillouette, C. N., Stellar, J. J., Quigley, S. M., & Curley, M. A. Q. (2018). How to predict pediatric pressure injury risk with the Braden QD Scale. *American Journal of Nursing, 118*(11), 34–43.

Cummins, K. A., Watters, R., & Leming-Lee, T. (2019). Reducing pressure injuries in the pediatric intensive care unit. *Nursing Clinics of North America, 54*(1), 127–140. https://doi.org/10.1016/j.cnur.2018.10.005.

Curley, M. A. Q., Hasbani, N. R., Quigley, S. M., et al. (2018). Predicting pressure injury risk in pediatric patients: The Braden QD scale. *The Journal of Pediatrics, 192*, 189–195.e2. https://doi.org/10.1016/j.jpeds.2017.09.045.

Freundlich, K. (2017). Pressure injuries in medically complex children: A review. *Children, 4*(4), 25. https://doi.org/10.3390/children4040025.

García-Molina, P., Balaguer-López, E., Enric Torra I Bou, J., Alvarez-Ordiales, A., Quesada-Ramos, C., & Verdú-Soriano, J. (2012). A prospective, longitudinal study to assess use of continuous and reactive low-pressure mattresses to reduce pressure ulcer incidence in a pediatric intensive care unit. *Ostomy/Wound Management, 58*(7), 32–39.

National Pressure Injury Advisory Panel (NPIAP) & European Pressure Injury Advisory Panel (EPIAP). (2019). *Prevention and treatment of pressure ulcers*. Perth, Australia: Cambridge Media.

National Pressure Ulcer Advisory Panel (NPUAP) & European Pressure Ulcer Advisory Panel (EPUAP). (2016). *Pressure injury stages*. Retrieved from http://www.npuap.org/resources/educational-and-clinical-resources/npuap-pressure-injury-stages/. Accessed 16 November 2020.

Nie, A. M. (2020). Creating a pediatric and neonatal pressure injury prevention program when evidence was sparse or absent: A view from here. *The Journal of Wound, Ostomy and Continence Nursing, 47*(4), 353–355. https://doi.org/10.1097/WON.0000000000000676.

Ratliff, C. R., Droste, L. R., Bonham, P., Wound, Ostomy and Continence Nurses Society–Wound Guidelines Task Force, et al. (2017). WOCN 2016 guidelines for prevention and management of pressure injuries (ulcers). An executive summary. *Journal of Wound, Ostomy and Continence Nursing, 44*(3), 241–246.

Willock, J., Habiballah, L., Long, D., Palmer, K., & Anthony, D. (2016). A comparison of the performance of the Braden Q and the Glamorgan paediatric pressure ulcer risk assessment scales in general and intensive care paediatric and neonatal units. *Journal of Tissue Viability, 25*(2), 119–126. https://doi.org/10.1016/j.jtv.2016.03.001.

Risk for Child Pressure Injury

Domain 11 Safety/protection Class 2 Physical injury

Mary Beth Flynn Makic, PhD, RN, CCNS, CCRN-K, FAAN, FNAP, FCNS

NANDA-I

Definition

Child or adolescent susceptible to localized damage to the skin and/or underlying tissue, as a result of pressure, or pressure in combination with shear, which may compromise health (European Pressure Ulcer Advisory Panel, 2019).

P

Risk Factors

External Factors

Altered microclimate between skin and supporting surface; difficulty for caregiver to lift patient completely off bed; excessive moisture; inadequate access to appropriate equipment; inadequate access to appropriate health services; inadequate access to appropriate supplies; inadequate access to equipment for children with obesity; inadequate caregiver knowledge of appropriate methods for removing adhesive materials; inadequate caregiver knowledge of appropriate methods for stabilizing devices; inadequate caregiver knowledge of modifiable factors; inadequate caregiver knowledge of pressure injury prevention strategies; increased magnitude of mechanical load; pressure over bony prominence; shearing forces; surface friction; sustained mechanical load; use of linen with insufficient moisture wicking property

Internal Factors

Decreased physical activity; decreased physical mobility; dehydration; difficulty assisting caregiver with moving self; difficulty maintaining position in bed; difficulty maintaining position in chair; dry skin; hyperthermia; inadequate adherence to incontinence treatment regimen; inadequate adherence to pressure injury prevention plan; inadequate knowledge of appropriate methods for removing adhesive materials; inadequate knowledge of appropriate methods for stabilizing devices; protein-energy malnutrition; water-electrolyte imbalance

Other Factors

Factors identified by standardized, validated screening tool

At-Risk Population

Children in intensive care units; children in long-term care facilities; children in palliative care settings; children in rehabilitation settings; children in transit to or between clinical care settings; children receiving home-based care; children with body mass index above normal range for age and gender; children with body mass index below normal range for age and gender; children with developmental issues; children with growth issues; children with large head circumference; children with large skin surface area

Associated Conditions

Alkaline skin pH; altered cutaneous structure; anemia; cardiovascular diseases; decreased level of consciousness; decreased serum albumin level; decreased tissue oxygenation; decreased tissue perfusion; diabetes mellitus; edema; elevated C-reactive protein; frequent invasive procedures; hemodynamic instability; immobilization; impaired circulation; intellectual disability; medical devices; pharmaceutical preparations; physical trauma; prolonged duration of surgical procedure; sensation disorders; spinal cord injuries

NIC, NOC, Client Outcomes, Nursing Interventions and *Rationales,* Client/Family Teaching and Discharge Planning, and References

See the care plan for Child **Pressure** Injury.

Neonatal Pressure Injury Domain 11 Safety/protection Class 2 Physical injury

JoAnn Coar, MSN, RN-BC, A-GNP-C, CWOCN

NANDA-I

Definition

Localized damage to the skin and/or underlying tissue of a neonate, as a result of pressure, or pressure in combination with shear (European Pressure Ulcer Advisory Panel, 2019).

Defining Characteristics

Blood-filled blister; erythema; full thickness tissue loss; full thickness tissue loss with exposed bone; full thickness tissue loss with exposed muscle; full thickness tissue loss with exposed tendon; localized heat in relation to surrounding tissue; maroon localized area of discolored intact skin; partial thickness loss of dermis; purple localized area of discolored intact skin; skin ulceration; ulcer is covered by eschar; ulcer is covered by slough

Related Factors

External Factors

Altered microclimate between skin and supporting surface; excessive moisture; inadequate access to appropriate equipment; inadequate access to appropriate health services; inadequate access to appropriate supplies; inadequate caregiver knowledge of appropriate methods for removing adhesive materials; inadequate caregiver knowledge of appropriate methods for stabilizing devices; inadequate caregiver knowledge of modifiable factors; inadequate caregiver knowledge of pressure injury prevention strategies; increased magnitude of mechanical load; pressure over bony prominence; shearing forces; surface friction; sustained mechanical load; use of linen with insufficient moisture wicking property

Internal Factors

Decreased physical mobility; dehydration; dry skin; hyperthermia; water-electrolyte imbalance

Other Factors

Factors identified by standardized, validated screening tool

P

At-Risk Population

Low birth weight neonates; neonates <32 weeks gestation; neonates experiencing prolonged intensive care unit stay; neonates in intensive care units

Associated Conditions

Anemia; decreased serum albumin level; decreased tissue oxygenation; decreased tissue perfusion; edema; immature skin integrity; immature skin texture; immature stratum corneum; immobilization; medical devices; nutritional deficiencies related to prematurity; pharmaceutical preparations; prolonged duration of surgical procedure; significant comorbidity

NOC (Nursing Outcomes Classification)

Suggested NOC Outcomes

Tissue Integrity: Skin and Mucous Membranes

Example NOC Outcome with Indicators

Intact Tissue Integrity: Skin and Mucous Membranes as evidenced by the following indicators: Skin intactness/Skin lesions absent/Tissue perfusion/Skin temperature. (Rate the outcome and indicators of **Tissue Integrity: Skin and Mucous Membranes:** 1 = severely compromised, 2 = substantially compromised, 3 = moderately compromised, 4 = mildly compromised, 5 = not compromised [see Section I].)

Client Outcomes

Client Will (Specify Time Frame)

- Intact skin; prevention of skin alterations
- Report any altered sensation or pain at site of tissue impairment
- Skin, without redness over bony prominences and capillary refill of less than 6 seconds over areas of redness
- Be repositioned off of bony prominences frequently if risk for pressure injuries is high
- Family/caregiver will demonstrate understanding of plan to reduce pressure injury risk
- Family/caregiver will describe measures to protect the skin

NIC (Nursing Interventions Classification)

Suggested NIC Interventions

Pain Management; Pressure Injury Care; Pressure Injury Prevention; Risk Identification; Skin Care: Topical Treatments; Skin Surveillance

Example NIC Activities—Pressure Injury Care

Monitor color of skin, temperature, edema, erythema, moisture, and appearance of surrounding skin; Note characteristics of skin over bony prominences or under/in contact with medical devices

Nursing Interventions and *Rationales*

- Gestational age influences the development of the skin and its function as a barrier. Epidermal maturation is complete at 34 weeks of age. Prematurely or critically ill infants are at a higher risk of skin alterations related to intrinsic and extrinsic factors (Broom et al, 2019). EB: *Consider the impact of skin maturity, perfusion, and oxygenation (National Pressure Injury Advisory Panel [NPIAP] & European Pressure Injury Advisory Panel [EPIAP], 2019). Intrinsic factors that increase the risk for skin injury include gestation, birth weight, skin integrity, immobility, impaired skin integrity, sepsis, and malnutrition (Broom et al, 2019).*
- Assess the presence of a medical device and pressure injury risk as well as illness severity and need for critical care in neonates and children (NPIAP & EPIAP, 2019). EB: *Medical devices account for a large percent of pressure injuries (Delmore et al, 2019).*

- Select medical devices that minimize tissue injury. Apply according to the manufacturer's recommendations, ensuring correct sizing and shape. Reposition devices regularly and remove as soon as they are no longer medically necessary. Apply prophylactic dressings under devices to reduce the risk of pressure injuries (NPIAP & EPIAP, 2019).
- Protect neonates against toxicity due to topical agents, including iodine, isopropyl ethyl and methyl alcohol, infection, and injury until the stratum corneum has reached maturity (Delmore et al, 2019).
- Routine skin assessment is essential as a lower gestational age is at a higher risk for skin injury (Broom et al, 2019).
- Assess for excessive moisture, especially in between skinfolds and dependent areas. EB: *Neonates skin may not be able to tolerate excessive moisture and is more likely to macerate and develop pressure injury (Broom et al, 2019; Johnson & Hunt, 2019).* EB: *Use of zinc oxide or petroleum-based products is recommended for prevention or alterations due to excess moisture (Delmore et al, 2019).*
- Risk assessment tools for high-risk neonates are limited; however, current best evidence has found the Braden QD and Glamorgan to be valid and reliable with assessing pressure injury risk in children and neonates. Clinicians should routinely perform an age-appropriate pressure injury (National Pressure Ulcer Advisory Panel [NPUAP] & European Pressure Ulcer Advisory Panel [EPUAP], 2016) risk assessment using a valid and reliable tool. EB/EBN: *The Braden QD and Glamorgan pediatric pressure ulcer risk assessment scales have been found to be reliable and predictive in assessing neonate- and pediatric-specific pressure injury risk assessment to assist with identification of pressure-related injury risk in the population from preterm to 21 years of age, in the acute care setting (Willock et al, 2016; Freundlich, 2017; Chamblee et al, 2018; Curley et al, 2018).*
- Avoid daily bathing of the skin, which can disrupt normal barrier function. EB: *Daily bathing can dry the skin, increasing the risk of injury* (Delmore et al, 2019).
- Avoid adhesives and products that increase adhesion, which may result in increased epidermal stripping (Delmore et al, 2019).
- Use support surfaces to alleviate poor tissue tolerance and shear and improve microclimate. EB: *Muscle and fat tissue structures are softer in neonates than in children and adults, increasing the risk of deformation injuries in the neonate (Delmore et al, 2019). Support surfaces do not take the place of regular turning and repositioning (NPIAP & EPIAP, 2019).*
- Involve family/caregiver in education focused on reducing risks and management strategies for pressure injuries. EB: *Involving family/caregiver early in the presentation and management of pressure injury prevention is necessary in preparation of discharge planning (Nie, 2020).*

Home Care

- The interventions described previously may be adapted for home care use.
- Instruct and assist the client and caregivers in how to assess the skin for excessive pressure. Provide written instructions for actions they can implement to reduce the risk of pressure injury development (NPIAP & EPIAP, 2019).
- Educate client and caregivers on proper nutrition and when to call the agency and/or health care provider with concerns.
- ▲ Initiate a consultation in a case assignment with a wound, ostomy, continence nurse (or wound specialist) to establish a comprehensive plan for pressure ulcer risk reduction for clients at high risk for skin breakdown (Berke et al, 2019).
- ▲ Collaboration with health care professionals, including medical, nursing, nutrition, and industry stakeholders, is imperative to improve outcomes in pressure injury prevention (Delmore et al, 2019; NPIAP & EPIAP, 2019).

REFERENCES

Berke, C., Conley, M. J., Netsch, D., et al. (2019). Role of the wound, ostomy and continence nurse in continence care: 2018 update. *Journal of Wound Ostomy and Continence Nursing, 46*(3), 221–225. https://doi.org/10.1097/WON.0000000000000529.

Broom, M., Dunk, A. M., & Mohamed, A. L. E. (2019). Predicting neonatal skin injury: The first step to reducing skin injuries in neonates. *Health Services Insights, 12*, 1178632919845630.

Chamblee, T. B., Pasek, T. A., Cailloutte, C. N., Stellar, J. J., Quigley, S. M., & Curley, M. A. Q. (2018). How to predict pediatric pressure injury risk with the Braden QD Scale. *American Journal of Nursing, 118*(11), 34–43.

Curley, M. A. Q., Hasbani, N. R., Quigley, S. M., et al. (2018). Predicting pressure injury risk in pediatric patients: The Braden QD Scale. *Journal of Pediatrics, 192*, 189–195.e2. https://doi.org/10.1016/j.jpeds.2017.09.045.

Delmore, B., Deppisch, M., Sylvia, C., Luna-Anderson, C., & Nie, A. M. (2019). Pressure injuries in the pediatric population: A National pressure ulcer Advisory Panel white paper. *Advances in*

Skin & Wound Care, 32(9), 394–408. https://doi.org/10.1097/01.ASW.0000577804.72042.f7.
Freundlich, K. (2017). Pressure injuries in medically complex children: A review. *Children, 4*(4), 25. https://doi.org/10.3390/children4040025.
Johnson, E., & Hunt, R. (2019). Infant skin care: Updates and recommendations. *Current Opinion in Pediatrics, 31*(4), 476–481. https://doi.org/10.1097/MOP.0000000000000791.
National Pressure Injury Advisory Panel (NPIAP) & European Pressure Injury Advisory Panel (EPIAP). (2019). *Prevention and treatment of pressure ulcers*. Perth, Australia: Cambridge Media.
National Pressure Ulcer Advisory Panel (NPUAP) & European Pressure Ulcer Advisory Panel (EPUAP). (2016). *Pressure injury stages*. Retrieved from http://www.npuap.org/resources/educational-and-clinical-resources/npuap-pressure-injury-stages/. Accessed November 16, 2020.
Nie, A. M. (2020). Creating a pediatric and neonatal pressure injury prevention program when evidence was sparse or absent: A view from here. *Journal of Wound, Ostomy and Continence Nursing, 47*(4), 353–355. https://doi.org/10.1097/WON.0000000000000676.
Willock, J., Habiballah, L., Long, D., Palmer, K., & Anthony, D. (2016). A comparison of the performance of the Braden Q and the Glamorgan paediatric pressure ulcer risk assessment scales in general and intensive care paediatric and neonatal units. *Journal of Tissue Viability, 25*(2), 119–126. https://doi.org/10.1016/j.jtv.2016.03.001.

Risk for Neonatal Pressure Injury

Domain 11 Safety/protection Class 2 Physical injury

Mary Beth Flynn Makic, PhD, RN, CCNS, CCRN-K, FAAN, FNAP, FCNS

NANDA-I

Definition

Neonate susceptible to localized damage to the skin and/or underlying tissue, as a result of pressure, or pressure in combination with shear, which may compromise health (European Pressure Ulcer Advisory Panel, 2019).

Risk Factors

External Factors

Altered microclimate between skin and supporting surface; excessive moisture; inadequate access to appropriate equipment; inadequate access to appropriate health services; inadequate access to appropriate supplies; inadequate caregiver knowledge of appropriate methods for removing adhesive materials; inadequate caregiver knowledge of appropriate methods for stabilizing devices; inadequate caregiver knowledge of modifiable factors; inadequate caregiver knowledge of pressure injury prevention strategies; increased magnitude of mechanical load; pressure over bony prominence; shearing forces; surface friction; sustained mechanical load; use of linen with insufficient moisture wicking property

P

Internal Factors

Decreased physical mobility; dehydration; dry skin; hyperthermia; water-electrolyte imbalance

Other Factors

Factors identified by standardized, validated screening tool

At-Risk Population

Low birth weight neonates; neonates <32 weeks gestation; neonates experiencing prolonged intensive care unit stay; neonates in intensive care units

Associated Conditions

Anemia; decreased serum albumin level; decreased tissue oxygenation; decreased tissue perfusion; edema; immature skin integrity; immature skin texture; immature stratum corneum; immobilization; medical devices; nutritional deficiencies related to prematurity; pharmaceutical preparations; prolonged duration of surgical procedure; significant comorbidity

NIC, NOC, Client Outcomes, Nursing Interventions and *Rationales,* Client/Family Teaching and Discharge Planning, and References

See the care plan for Neonatal **Pressure** Injury.

Ineffective Protection

Domain 1 Health promotion Class 2 Health management

Teri Hulett, RN, BSN, CIC, FAPIC

NANDA-I

Definition

Decrease in the ability to guard self from internal or external threats such as illness or injury.

Defining Characteristics

Altered sweating; anorexia; chilling; coughing; disorientation; dyspnea; expresses itching, fatigue; impaired physical mobility; impaired tissue healing; insomnia; leukopenia; low serum hemoglobin level; maladaptive stress response; neurosensory impairment; pressure injury; psychomotor agitation; thrombocytopenia; weakness

Related Factors

Depressive symptoms; difficulty managing complex treatment regimen; hopelessness; inadequate vaccination; ineffective health self-management; low self- efficacy; malnutrition; physical deconditioning; substance misuse

Associated Conditions

Blood coagulation disorders; immune system diseases; neoplasms; pharmaceutical preparations; treatment regimen

NOC (Nursing Outcomes Classification)

Suggested NOC Outcomes

Health-Promoting Behavior; Blood Coagulation; Endurance; Immune Status

Example NOC Outcome with Indicators

Immune Status as evidenced by the following indicators: Recurrent infections/Tumors/Weight loss. (Rate the outcome and indicators of **Immune Status:** 1 = severe, 2 = substantial, 3 = moderate, 4 = mild, 5 = none [see Section I].)

P

Client Outcomes

Client Will (Specify Time Frame)

- Remain free of infection while in contact during contact with health care
- Remain free of any evidence of new bleeding as evident by stable vital signs
- Explain precautions to take to prevent infection including hand hygiene
- Explain precautions to take to prevent bleeding including fall prevention

NIC (Nursing Interventions Classification)

Suggested NIC Interventions

Bleeding Precautions; Infection Prevention; Infection Protection

Example NIC Activities—Infection Protection

Monitor for systemic and localized signs and symptoms of infection; Inspect skin and mucous membranes for redness, extreme warmth, or drainage

Nursing Interventions and *Rationales*

- Take temperature, pulse, and blood pressure (e.g., every 1–4 hours). EBN: *Changes in vital signs can indicate the onset of bleeding or infection. Temperatures taken by the tympanic and forehead methods have the highest and lowest accuracy for measuring body temperature, respectively. It is recommended to use the tympanic method for assessing a client's body temperature in the intensive care unit (ICU) because of high accuracy and acceptable precision (Asadian et al, 2016).*

- ▲ Observe nutritional status (e.g., weight, serum protein and albumin levels, muscle mass, and usual food intake). Work with the dietitian to improve nutritional status if needed. EB: *Clients diagnosed with asthma, repeated respiratory infections, cancer, and/or immunocompromise should have a nutritional assessment.* EB: *Vitamin D influences the body's immune system by influencing the production of endogenous antimicrobial peptides and regulating the inflammatory cascade (Martineau et al, 2017).*
- • Observe the client's sleep pattern; if altered, see Nursing Interventions and *Rationales* for Disturbed **Sleep** Pattern.
- • Identify stressors in the client's life; stress can negatively affect the immune system. If stress is uncontrollable, see Nursing Interventions and *Rationales* for Ineffective **Coping.** EB: *Delirium is the most common surgical complication among older adults, with an incidence of 15% to 25% after major elective surgery and 50% after high-risk procedures such as hip-fracture repair and cardiac surgery. Among clients undergoing mechanical ventilation in the ICU, the cumulative incidence of delirium, when combined with stupor and coma, exceeds 75%. Delirium is present in 10% to 15% of older adults in the emergency department. The prevalence of delirium at the end of life approaches 85% in palliative care settings (Marcantonio, 2017).*

Prevention of Infection

- ▲ Monitor for and report any signs of infection (e.g., fever, chills, flushed skin, drainage, edema, redness, abnormal laboratory values, pain) and notify the health care provider promptly. EBN: *Although the white blood cell count may be in the normal range, an increased number of immature bands may be present (Shi et al, 2015).* EBN: *A neutropenic client with fever represents an absolute medical emergency (Klastersky et al, 2016). If the client's immune system is depressed, notify the health care provider of abnormal (high or low) temperature, even in the absence of other symptoms of infection.* EB: *Clients with depressed immune function are unable to mount the usual immune responses to the onset of infection; abnormal temperature (high or low) may be the only sign of infection. A neutropenic client with abnormal temperature (high or low) represents an absolute medical emergency.* EBN: *Febrile neutropenia is a medical emergency that requires urgent evaluation, the timely administration of empirical broad-spectrum antimicrobials, and careful monitoring to optimize client outcomes and mitigate the risk of complications (Braga et al, 2019).*
- • If white blood cell count is severely decreased (i.e., absolute neutrophil count of less than 1000/mm^3), initiate the following precautions:
  - ❍ Take vital signs every 2 to 4 hours.
  - ❍ Complete a head-to-toe assessment twice daily, including inspection of oral mucosa, invasive sites, wounds, urine, and stool; monitor for onset of new reports of pain.
- ▲ Avoid any invasive procedures, including catheterization, injections, or rectal or vaginal procedures, unless absolutely necessary. EBN: *Immunocompromised clients are susceptible to bacterial, fungal, viral, and parasitic infections that healthy immune systems usually overcome. They are also more susceptible to complications from common infections (Bula-Rudas, 2020).*
  - ❍ Consider warming the client before elective surgery. *Normothermia is associated with low postoperative infection rates (Moucha, 2016).*
- ▲ Administer granulocyte growth factor as ordered. EB: *Clients most likely to benefit from therapy are identified in the clinical guidelines for the use of granulocyte transfusions with indications to include clients with severe neutropenia meeting specific criteria per the guidelines. Clients who should not receive granulocyte therapy are identified, as well, in the guidelines (Estcourt et al. 2016).* EB: *Granulocyte macrophage colony-stimulating factor is mostly well tolerated, although some cancer and kidney disease clients have demonstrated significant complications such as leukopenia (McDowell, 2018).*
  - ❍ Take meticulous care of all invasive sites; use chlorhexidine gluconate for cleansing. EB: *Use of chlorhexidine gluconate for vascular catheter site care reduces catheter-related bloodstream infections and catheter colonization (O'Grady et al, 2011).*
  - ❍ Provide frequent oral care and nutritional evaluation. EBN: *The effects of chemotherapy or radiation can cause changes in taste and smell. Self-reported taste and smell alterations are prevalent in up to 86% of cancer clients. In some clients, taste and smell alterations may continue well after their cancer treatment has been completed. Such disorders can increase distress, reduce appetite, and contribute toward poor nutritional status. Both adult and child cancer clients should be referred for nutritional consultation (Cohen et al, 2016).*

- ❍ Follow standard precautions, especially performing hand hygiene, to prevent health care–associated infections. **EBN:** *Hands of health care workers are the most common cause of health care–associated infections (Boyce et al, 2011).*

▲ Refer for appropriate prophylactic antifungal treatment and avoid pathogen exposure (through air filtration, regular hand hygiene, and avoidance of plants and flowers). **CEB:** *Practical measures can be taken to avoid exposing the client to respiratory pathogens (Siegel et al, 2007).* **EB:** *Viruses are the second most common cause of severe respiratory infections in the immunocompromised client. Invasive fungal infections (*Aspergillus, Mucorales, *and* Pneumocystis jirovecii*) account for about 15% of severe respiratory infections. Parasites rarely cause severe acute infections in the immunocompromised client (Azoulay et al, 2020).*

- ❍ Have the client wear a mask when leaving the room. **EB:** *Hospital construction and renovation activities are an ever-constant phenomenon in health care facilities, causing dust contamination and possible dispersal of fungal spores. Fungal outbreaks still occur in health care settings, especially among clients with hematological malignancies and those who are immunocompromised. The causative pathogens of these outbreaks are usually* Aspergillus *species, but* Zygomycetes *and other fungi were occasionally reported. The overall mortality of construction/renovation-associated fungal infection was approximately 50%. Protective measures include relocating high-risk clients away from construction areas (Kanamori et al, 2015). To prevent health care–acquired pulmonary aspergillosis during hospital construction, at risk (neutropenic) clients should wear N-95 (fit-tested) protective masks if it is necessary to transport them through or near to the construction zone (Aspergillosis Subcommittee of the Health Protection Surveillance Centre Scientific Advisory Committee, 2018). Limit and screen visitors to minimize exposure to contagion.*
- ❍ Help the client bathe daily.
- ❍ Practice food safety: a neutropenic diet may not be necessary. **EBN:** *The rationale behind the neutropenic diet is to limit the bacterial load delivered to the gut. Fresh fruits and vegetables harbor organisms, and the ingestion of contaminated foods is believed to serve as a source of pathogenic bacteria, which may cause potentially life-threatening infections. Cooking foods destroys bacteria, rendering the cooked foods safe. Multiple studies have been done that do not support the benefit of the neutropenic diet. The inefficacy of the neutropenic diet may be attributed to the fact that the organisms on fresh fruits and vegetables are part of the normal gut flora. Unnecessary dietary restrictions can place clients at further risk of inadequate intake and malnutrition. Maintaining nutrition in this client population is already a challenge, and the restriction of a wide variety of food items (fresh fruits, vegetables, dairy, certain meats, and eggs) can cause malnutrition, low client satisfaction, and poor quality of life (Wolfe et al, 2018).*
- ❍ Ensure that the client is well nourished. Provide food with protein and consider vitamin supplements. If appetite is suppressed, institute a dietary referral. Keep track of serum albumin levels and transferrin and prealbumin levels. **EB:** *Initiate a dietitian-driven comprehensive nutrition assessment, including a food and nutrition-related history, anthropometric measurements, biochemical data, medical tests and procedures, nutrition-focused physical assessment, medical history, and treatment plan, which will be used to develop interventions (National Cancer Institute, 2021).*
- ❍ Help the client cough and practice deep breathing regularly. Maintain an appropriate activity level.
- ❍ Obtain a private room for the client. Use high-energy particulate air filters if available and appropriate. **EB:** *Published data support placing allogeneic hematopoietic stem cell transplant (HSCT) clients in a protective environment. Communicate with infection prevention and facilities management to ensure appropriate environmental controls are in place, on, and functioning to confirm the client is in a protective environment (Siegel et al, 2007).*

▲ Nurses play a pivotal role in the early identification and management of sepsis. Early identification is key to survival. Identifying abnormal vital signs is the first step in early sepsis recognition. If early signs of sepsis are identified, immediately notify the health care provider. **EB:** *Elevated heart rate, hypotension, increased respiratory rate, and elevated temperature are early sepsis indicators (Kleinpell et al, 2019).*

- Refer to care plan for Risk for **Infection**.
- Refer to care plan for Readiness for Enhanced **Nutrition** for additional interventions.

Pediatric

- Skin-to-skin contact (SSC) is the practice of placing a diapered infant onto the bare chest of the mother so that the mother and infant are in direct SSC contact with each other. In resource-rich countries, SSC has been motivated by a push to humanize a process that has become a medical experience. SSC has been a process to facilitate infant transition to extrauterine life. **EB:** *Evidence supports the benefit of SSC for preterm infants (<37 weeks gestation) targeted at temperature regulation and increased cardiorespiratory*

P

stability. Evidence supports the benefit to the breastfeeding mother with increased maternal milk volume and promoting exclusive breastfeeding and duration in the preterm infant (Campbell-Yeo et al, 2015). **EBN:** *In reviewing the entire hospitalization, SSC is associated with decreased likelihood of infection, severe illness, and death. Additional evidence supports homeostasis (temperature regulation, cardiorespiratory stability), and positive effects on sleep, neurodevelopment, and growth (Campbell-Yeo et al, 2015).*

- ● Assess postoperative fever in pediatric oncology clients promptly. **EB:** *Fever is a common sign that suggests infection in children. Signs and symptoms are often absent or minimized in the child with cancer because of inability to evoke an inflammatory response. Chemotherapy agents and radiation therapy cause myelosuppression. When the myelosuppressive effect is severe enough, the child becomes predisposed to infection. Because of high mortality rates associated with untreated infection, all febrile children with cancer should be evaluated immediately for neutropenia. If neutropenic, the child is at risk for a life-threatening infection until proven otherwise (Texas Children's Hospital EBOC, 2016).*

Geriatric

- ▲ If not contraindicated, encourage exercise to promote improved quality of life in older adults. **EB:** *A study of healthy adults women over 60 years and older suggested that the effects of resistance-type exercise training can counteract the loss of muscle mass and strength with aging (Braverman, 2019). Give older clients with imbalanced nutrition a vitamin D supplement to reduce risk of fracture.* **EB:** *Vitamin D deficiency has been correlated with increased risk and greater severity of infection, particularly of the respiratory tract. Vitamin D influences the body's immune system by influencing the production of endogenous antimicrobial peptides and regulating the inflammatory cascade (Dankers et al, 2017).*

Prevention of Bleeding

- ▲ Immune thrombocytopenia (ITP), previously known as idiopathic thrombocytopenic purpura, is an autoimmune disorder characterized by a severe reduction in peripheral blood platelet count. Bleeding events are often unpredictable, and clients with ITP may not exhibit bleeding beyond bruising and petechiae. However, more serious mucosal bleeding may occur, including menorrhagia, epistaxis, gastrointestinal hemorrhage, hematuria, or intracranial hemorrhage (Khan et al, 2017; Neunert et al, 2019). Monitor the client's risk for bleeding; evaluate results of clotting studies and platelet counts. **EB:** *Laboratory studies give a good indication of the seriousness of the bleeding disorder.*
- ● Watch for hematuria, melena, hematemesis, hemoptysis, epistaxis, bleeding from mucosa, petechiae, and ecchymoses. **EBN:** *Severe bleeding is reported in 9.5% of adults and 20.2% of children. Adults with ITP had a 1.3- to 2.2-fold higher mortality rate than the general population due to cardiovascular disease, infection, and bleeding (Neunert et al, 2019).*
- ▲ Give medications orally or intravenously only; avoid giving intramuscularly, subcutaneously, or rectally.
- ● Apply pressure for a longer time than usual to invasive sites, such as venipuncture or injection sites. Additional pressure is needed to stop bleeding of invasive sites in clients with bleeding disorders.
- ● Take vital signs often; watch for changes associated with fluid volume loss. **EB:** *Excessive bleeding causes decreased blood pressure and increased pulse and respiratory rates (Johnson & Burns, 2020).*
- ● Monitor menstrual flow if relevant; have the client use pads instead of tampons. **EB:** *Menstruation can be excessive in clients with bleeding disorders. Adolescents presenting with heavy menstrual bleeding at or near menarche assessment should include bleeding disorders (Adeyemi-Fowode et al, 2019).*
- ● Have the client use a moistened toothette or a very soft child's toothbrush instead of an adult toothbrush. Follow the dentist's recommendation for flossing and appropriate rinses to use. Control gum bleeding by applying pressure to gums with gauze pad soaked in ice water. **EB:** *These actions help prevent trauma to the oral mucosa, which could result in bleeding (National Institute of Dental and Craniofacial Research [NIDCR], 2018).*
- ▲ To decrease risk of bleeding, avoid administering salicylates or nonsteroidal antiinflammatory drugs (NSAIDs) if possible. **CEB:** *Gastrointestinal bleeding caused by NSAIDs, acetylsalicylic acid, or warfarin was the most common adverse drug reaction (ADR) that resulted in hospital admission and represented 40% of all ADRs (12 of 30), according to the World Health Organization (WHO) causality criteria (Tennant, 2015).*

Home Care

- ● Some of the interventions previously described may be adapted for home care use.
- ▲ The Patient-Centered Medical Home (PCMH) model facilitates a team-based approach to care, wherein providers coordinate care across all elements of the larger health care system (Frasso et al, 2017). Consider using

P

a nurse-led PCMH for monitoring high-need, high-cost clients (Breland et al, 2016). EBN: *The PCMH model supports team-based coordination of care and client self-management capacity in an effort to improve quality of care and associated health outcomes. Nurse-led practices have shown promise in alleviating the US demand for primary care and have been identified as practice models for improving quality of care. Nurse-led centers emphasize the holistic model of care and integrate an understanding of the social determinants of health. Additionally, nurse-led centers often use the client–provider team approach to care, which promotes client autonomy and supports shared decision-making—all key constructs in the PCMH model (Frasso et al, 2017).*

- End-of-life (EOL) care is defined as care that helps those with advanced, progressive, incurable, and serious illness to live as well as possible until they die. EOL care in the United States is provided through palliative and hospice medicine. Both hospice and palliative care focus on ensuring the best possible quality of life for individuals with serious illness and their families by providing support, symptom management, and comfort care. Palliative care need depends on the psychosocial, spiritual, and physical necessities of each client rather than the diagnosis. Caution should be used when assessing need for palliative care; the diagnosis should not be the primary trigger but instead use of a provider tool consisting of three elements: nutritional decline, disease progression, and functional decline. Building trust and shared decision making among the health care team, client, and family are pivotal in all palliative care conversations. Seriously ill clients have a high symptom burden, depending on their diagnosis (Cruz-Oliver, 2017). EB: *Develop with the client, family, and health care providers a multiprofessional plan of care to address immediate and anticipated needs of the client, including nausea, pain, fatigue, anorexia, breathlessness, and spiritual needs (Cruz-Oliver, 2017).*

Client/Family Teaching and Discharge Planning

Depressed Immune Function

- Discharge planning should start at admission. Key elements to focus on when providing discharge teaching to clients and their families to promote a successful transition from acute care to self-management at home are to develop health knowledge, provide resources, and promote self-efficacy. Identify clients' needs to provide tailored, individual support and education. Teach the client and family how and when to take the client's temperature and provide temperature parameters so the client/family knows when to call the provider (Pollack et al, 2016). EBN: *Identify clients' needs to provide client-specific, tailored individual support. Assess the client's ability to effectively participate in discharge teaching. Provide client-specific parameters, including when the client/family should notify provider. Provide discharge instruction in writing and provide community resource and follow-up contact information to client and family (Pollock et al, 2016).*
- Teach precautions to use to decrease the chance of infection. Teach/reinforce appropriate self-care, including good hand hygiene, personal hygiene, and ensuring a safe environment. Teach the client to avoid crowds and contact with persons who have infections. Teach the need for good nutrition, avoidance of stress, and adequate rest to maintain immune system function. CEBN: *Approaches to avoiding infection at home for the client with neutropenia include good hand hygiene and careful management of food, drink, and the client's environment (Braga et al, 2019; Bula-Rudas, 2020).*

P

Bleeding Disorder

- Teach the client to wear a medical alert bracelet and to notify all health care personnel of the bleeding disorder. CEB: *Emergency identification schemes such as medical alert bracelets use emblems that alert health care professionals to potential problems and can ensure appropriate and prompt treatment (National Hemophilia Foundation, Medical and Scientific Advisory Council [MASAC], 2019).*
- Teach the client and family the signs of bleeding, precautions to take to prevent bleeding, and action to take if bleeding begins. Caution the client to avoid taking over-the-counter medications without the permission of the health care provider. Medications containing salicylates can increase bleeding.
- Teach the client to wear loose-fitting clothes and avoid physical activity that might cause trauma.

REFERENCES

Adeyemi-Fowode, O., Simms-Cendan, J., & American College of Obstetricians and Gynecologists' Committee on Adolescent Health Care. (2019). Screening and management of bleeding disorders in adolescents with heavy menstrual bleeding: ACOG Committee Opinion, number 785. *Obstetrics & Gynecology*, *134*(3), e71–e83. Retrieved from https://www.acog.org/-/media/project/acog/acogorg/clinical/files/committee-opinion/articles/2019/09/screening-and-management-of-bleeding-disorders-in-adolescents-with-heavy-m.pdf. [Accessed 13 December 2021].

Asadian, S., Khatony, A., Moradi, G., Abdi, A., & Rezaei, M. (2016). Accuracy and precision of four common peripheral temperature measurement methods in intensive care patients. *Medical Devices (Auckland, N.Z.)*, *9*, 301–308. https://doi.org/10.2147/MDER.S109904.

Aspergillosis Subcommittee of the Health Protection Surveillance Centre Scientific Advisory Committee. (2018). *National guidelines for the prevention of nosocomial aspergillus*. Dublin: Health Protection Surveillance Center.

Azoulay, E., Russell, L., Van de Louw, A., et al. (2020). Diagnosis of severe respiratory infections in immunocompromised patients. *Intensive Care Medicine, 46*(2), 298–314. https://doi.org/10.1007/s00134-019-05906-5.

Boyce, J. M., Pittet, D., & Healthcare Infection Control Practices Advisory Committee, HICPAC/SHEA/APIC/IDSA Hand Hygiene Task Force. (2011). Guideline for hand hygiene in health-care settings. Recommendations of the Healthcare Infection Control Practices Advisory Committee and the HICPAC/SHEA/APIC/IDSA Hand Hygiene Task Force. Society for Healthcare Epidemiology of America/Association for Professionals in Infection Control/ Infectious Diseases Society of America. *MMWR: Recommendations and Reports, 51*(RR–16), 1–45.

Braga, C. C., Taplitz, R. A., & Flowers, C. R. (2019). Clinical implications of febrile neutropenia guidelines in the cancer patient population. *Journal of Oncology Practice, 15*(1), 25–26. https://doi.org/10.1200/jop.18.00718.

Braverman, J. (2019). *Strength training for women over 60*. Livestrong.com [website]. Retrieved from https://www.livestrong.com/article/452842-strength-training-for-women-over-60-years-old/. [Accessed 23 July 2021].

Breland, J. Y., Asch, S. M., Slightam, C., Wong, A., & Zulman, D. M. (2016). Key ingredients for implementing intensive outpatient programs within patient-centered medical homes: A literature review and qualitative analysis. *Healthcare (Amsterdam, Netherlands), 4*(1), 22–29. https://doi.org/10.1016/j.hjdsi.2015.12.005.

Bula-Rudas, F. J. (2020). *Infections in the immunocompromised host*. Medscape [website]. Retrieved from https://emedicine.medscape.com/article/973120-overview. [Accessed 23 July 2021].

Campbell-Yeo, M. L., Disher, T. C., Benoit, B. L., & Johnston, C. C. (2015). Understanding kangaroo care and its benefits to preterm infants. *Pediatric Health, Medicine and Therapeutics, 6*, 15–32. https://doi.org/10.2147/PHMT.S51869.

Cohen, J., Wakefield, C. E., & Laing, D. G. (2016). Smell and taste disorders resulting from cancer and chemotherapy. *Current Pharmaceutical Designs, 22*(15), 2253–2263. https://doi.org/10.2174/1381612822666160216150812.

P

Cruz-Oliver, D. M. (2017). Palliative care: An update. *Missouri Medicine, 114*(2), 110–115.

Dankers, W., Colin, E. M., van Hamburg, J. P., & Lubberts, E. (2017). Vitamin D in autoimmunity: Molecular mechanisms and therapeutic potential. *Frontiers in Immunology, 7*, 697.

Estcourt, L. J., Stanworth, S. J., Hopewell, S., Doree, C., Trivella, M., & Massey, E. (2016). Granulocyte transfusions for treating infections in people with neutropenia or neutrophil dysfunction. *Cochrane Database of Systematic Reviews, 4*, CD005339. https://doi.org/10.1002/14651858.CD005339.pub2.

Frasso, R., Golinkoff, A., Klusaritz, H., et al. (2017). How nurse-led practices perceive implementation of the patient-centered medical home. *Applied Nursing Research, 34*, 34–39. https://doi:10.1016/j.apnr.2017.02.005.

Johnson, A. B., & Burns, B. (2020). *Hemorrhage*. StatPearls [Internet] Treasure Island, FL: StatPearls Publishing. Retrieved from https://www.ncbi.nlm.nih.gov/books/NBK542273/.

Kanamori, H., Rutala, W. A., Sickbert-Bennet, E. E., & Weber, D. J. (2015). Review of fungal outbreaks and infection prevention in healthcare settings during construction and renovation. *Clinical Infectious Diseases, 61*(3), 433–444. https://doi.org/10.1093/cid/civ297.

Khan, A. M., Mydra, H., & Nevarez, A. (2017). Clinical practice updates in the management of immune thrombocytopenia. *P and T, 42*(12), 756–763.

Klastersky, J., de Naurois, J., Rolston, K., et al. (2016). Management of febrile neutropaenia: ESMO clinical practice guidelines. *Annals of Oncology, 27*(Suppl. 5), v111–v118.

Kleinpell, R., Blot, S., Boulanger, C., Fulbrook, P., & Blackwood, B. (2019). International critical care nursing considerations and quality indicators for the 2017 surviving sepsis campaign guidelines. *Intensive Care Medicine, 45*(11), 1663–1666. https://doi.org/10.1007/s00134-019-05780-1.

Marcantonio, E. R. (2017). Delirium in hospitalized older adults. *New England Journal of Medicine, 377*(15), 1456–1466. https://doi.org/10.1056/NEJMcp1605501.

Martineau, A. R., Jolliffe, D. A., Hooper, R. L., et al. (2017). Vitamin D supplementation to prevent acute respiratory tract infections: Systematic review and meta-analysis of individual participant data. *British Medical Journal, 356*, i6583. https://doi.org/10.1136/bmj.i6583.

McDowell, S. (2018). *What is leukopenia?* Healthline [website]. Retrieved from https://www.healthline.com/health/leukopenia. [Accessed 23 July 2021].

Moucha, C. S. (2016). *Patient warming and surgical site infections: A critical analysis of the data*. Medscape [website]. Retrieved from https://www.medscape.org/viewarticle/862135. [Accessed 23 July 2021].

National Cancer Institute. (2021). *Nutrition in cancer care (PDQ®)—Health professional version*. Bethesda, MD: National Cancer Institute. Retrieved from https://www.ncbi.nlm.nih.gov/books/NBK65854/. [Accessed 23 July 2021].

National Hemophilia Foundation, Medical and Scientific Advisory Council. (2019). *Guidelines for emergency department management of individuals with hemophilia and other bleeding disorders*. MASAC document 257. Retrieved from https://www.hemophilia.org/sites/default/files/document/files/257.pdf. [Accessed 23 July 2021].

National Institute of Dental and Craniofacial Research (NIDCR). (2018). *Cancer treatments & oral health*. Retrieved from https://www.nidcr.nih.gov/health-info/cancer-treatments/more-info. [Accessed 23 July 2021].

Neunert, C., Terrel, D. R., Arnold, D. M., et al. (2019). American Society of Hematology 2019 guidelines for immune thrombocytopenia. *Blood Advances, 3*(23), 3829–3866. https://doi.org/10.1182bloodadbances.2019000966.

O'Grady, N. P., Alexander, M., Burns, L. A., et al. (2011). Guidelines for the prevention of intravascular catheter-related infections. *Clinical Infectious Diseases, 52*(9), e162–e193.

Pollack, A. H., Backonja, U., Miller, A. D., et al. (2016). Closing the gap: Supporting patients' transition to self-management after hospitalization. Proceedings of the SIGCHI Conference on human factors in Computing systems. *CHI Conference, 2016*, 5324–5336. https://doi.org/10.1145/2858240.

Shi, E., Vilke, G. M., Coyne, C. J., Oyama, L. C., & Castillo, E. M. (2015). Clinical outcomes of ED patients with bandemia. *The American Journal of Emergency Medicine, 33*(7), 876–881. https://doi.org/10.1016/j.ajem.2015.03.035.

Siegel, J. D., Rhinehart, E., Jackson, M., Chiarello, L., & Healthcare Infection Control Practices Advisory Committee. (2007). 2007 guideline for isolation precautions: Preventing transmission of infectious agents in healthcare settings. *American Journal of Infection Control, 35*(10 Suppl. 2), S65–S164. Retrieved from https://www.cdc.gov/infectioncontrol/guidelines/isolation/index.html. [Accessed 13 December 2021].

Tennant, F. (2015). *GI bleeding and NSAIDs*. Practical Pain Management [website]. Retrieved from https://www.practicalpainmanagement.com/patient/treatments/medications/gi-bleeding-nsaids. [Accessed 23 July 2021].

Texas Children's Hospital Evidence-Based Outcomes Center. (2016). *Fever and neutropenia in children receiving cancer treatment or with blood disorders: Evidence-based guideline*. Retrieved from https://www.texaschildrens.org/sites/default/files/uploads/documents/outcomes/standards/FN_042117.pdf. [Accessed 23 July 2021].

Wolfe, H. R., Sadeghi, N., Agrawal, D., Johnson, D. H., & Gupta, A. (2018). Things we do for no good reason: Neutropenic diet. *Journal of Hospital Medicine, 13*(8), 573–576.

Rape-Trauma Syndrome

Domain 9 Coping/stress tolerance Class 1 Post-trauma responses

Marina Martinez-Kratz, MS, RN, CNE

NANDA-I

Definition

Sustained maladaptive response to a forced, violent, sexual penetration against the victim's will and consent.

Defining Characteristics

Aggressive behaviors; altered interpersonal relations; anger behaviors; anxiety (00146); cardiogenic shock; confusion; denial; depressive symptoms; difficulty with decision-making; disordered thinking; expresses anger; expresses embarrassment; expresses shame; fear (00148); humiliation; hypervigilance; loss of independence; low self-esteem; mood variability; muscle spasm; muscle tension; nightmares; paranoia; perceived vulnerability; phobic disorders; physical trauma; powerlessness (00125); psychomotor agitation; reports altered sleep-wake cycle; reports feeling guilty; self-blame; sexual dysfunction (00059); substance misuse; thoughts of revenge

Related Factors

To be developed

At-Risk Population

Individuals who experienced rape; individuals with history of suicide attempt

Associated Conditions

Depression; dissociative identity disorder

NOC (Nursing Outcomes Classification)

Suggested NOC Outcomes

Abuse Cessation; Abuse Protection; Abuse Recovery: Emotional, Sexual, Coping; Impulse Self-Control; Self-Mutilation Restraint

Example NOC Outcome with Indicators

Abuse Recovery: Sexual as evidenced by the following indicators: Acknowledgment of right to disclose abusive situation/Expression of right to have been protected from abuse. (Rate the outcome and indicators of **Abuse Recovery: Sexual:** 1 = none, 2 = limited, 3 = moderate, 4 = substantial, 5 = extensive [see Section I].)

R

Client Outcomes

Client Will (Specify Time Frame)

- Share feelings, concerns, and fears
- Recognize that the rape or attempt was not client's own fault
- State that, no matter what the situation, no one has the right to assault another
- Describe medical/legal treatment procedures and reasons for treatment
- Report absence of physical complications or pain
- Identify support resources and attend psychotherapy/group assistance in coping with the trauma and effects of the traumatic experience
- Function at same level as before crisis, including sexual functioning
- Recognize that it is normal for full recovery to take a minimum of 1 year

NIC (Nursing Interventions Classification)

Suggested NIC Interventions

Abuse Protection Support; Counseling; Crisis Intervention; Sexual Counseling; Infection Protection; Rape-Trauma Treatment

Example NIC Activities—Rape-Trauma Treatment

Explain rape protocol and obtain consent to proceed through protocol; Implement crisis intervention counseling

Nursing Interventions and *Rationales*

- Use a trauma-informed approach with survivors of sexual assault. **EBN:** *Trauma-informed care addresses medical, legal, and psychosocial needs while acknowledging the connection between presenting symptoms and the individual's past trauma history. A trauma-informed framework emphasizes safety; trustworthiness and transparency; peer support; collaboration and mutuality; empowerment, voice, and choice; and cultural, historical, and gender issues (Emergency Nurses Association & International Association of Forensic Nurses, 2017).*
- Introduce yourself and your role in all interactions. **EBN:** *The client's understanding of who the nurse is and the nurse's role in their care can make the client feel empowered and more actively engaged (Fleishman, Kamsky, & Sundborg, 2019).*
- Escort the client to a treatment room immediately on arrival to the emergency department. Stay with the client and provide access to a community-based advocate. **EB:** *Timely care will assist survivors of sexual assault to feel safe, avoid anxiety, and avoid retraumatizing (Menschner & Maul, 2016).*
- Assure the client of confidentiality. **EB:** *According to Ogunwale and Oshiname (2017), rape is a traumatic experience, which has known physical and psychosocial destructive effects, but survivors rarely seek support to escape being stigmatized.*
- Provide a sexual assault response team (SART), if available, that includes a sexual assault nurse examiner (SANE), rape counseling advocate, and representative of law enforcement for best possible outcomes. **EB:** *According to a study by Patterson and Tringali (2015), a team of forensic nurses and survivor advocates partner together to provide treatment not only for the necessary physical and medical requirements of sexual assault survivors but also for dealing with the complex legal and mental health needs that necessitate follow-up.*
- Use an open and nonthreatening body positioning and posture. **EBN:** The use of nonthreatening body positioning and posture will help prevent the threat detection areas of the client's brain from taking over (*Fleishman, Kamsky, & Sundborg, 2019*).
- Use open-ended questions to document the client's chief complaint and request an event history of the sexual assault in his or her own words. **EBN:** *Participants felt cared for and emotionally supported when they were probed about what had happened to them (Selenga & Jooste, 2015).*
- Use the sexual assault evidence collection kits that have been reviewed by the SART members and provided by your state to collect adequate and accurate evidence for analysis by a forensic laboratory. **EB:** *The health care provider who examines survivors of sexual assault must be responsible for acting in accordance with state and local statutory or policy requirements for the use of evidence-gathering kits (American College of Obstetrics and Gynecology [ACOG], 2019).*
- Before proceeding with a medical forensic examination, consent for the medical evaluation and for evidence collection and release must be obtained from the sexual assault client. **EB:** *Consent is a legal need that is a critical component of the forensic examination as the client's clothing may be kept for evidential purposes and photographs may be taken to document the client's injuries (ACOG, 2019).*
- Ask permission before you touch the client. **EBN:** *Asking a client for permission before touching provides choice and empowers them to have control over their body and physical space (Fleishman, Kamsky, & Sundborg, 2019).*
- Provide anticipatory guidance by explaining every step of the physical examination and nursing care to the client before performing and check for understanding. **EBN:** *Sexual assault clients should receive consistent, objective, immediate care, and information about the collection of evidence and protocols for evidence collection (Emergency Nurses Association & International Association of Forensic Nurses, 2017).*

- Observe for signs of physical injury. CEB: *Locations to assess for genital injuries would include tears or abrasions of the posterior labia, abrasion or bruising of the labia minora and fossa navicularis, and ecchymosis or tears of the hymen; document these injuries as evidence for any future legal proceedings (Linden, 2011).*
- Inform client of the risk of pregnancy and sexually transmitted infections (STIs) and offer available treatments. EB: *Survivors of sexual assault should be advised that they are at risk for pregnancy and STIs; as survivors of sexual assault, they should be monitored and offered emergency contraception and STI prophylaxis (ACOG, 2019).*
- Assess sexual assault clients for health problems related to human sex trafficking: infectious diseases; noninfectious diseases (malnutrition, dental problems, and skin problems); reproductive health problems; substance abuse; mental health problems; and violence. EB: *Nurses are positioned to recognize the health problems associated with sex trafficking and can assist clients to access appropriate care (Roney & Villano, 2020).*
- Provide reassurance that the sexual violence was not the client's fault. EB: *Shortly after a sexual assault, clients need acknowledgment from care providers that the violence was real and not their fault (Hutschemaekers et al, 2019).*
- Emphasize the client's resilience and strengths. EB: *The skills and strategies the client has used previously can facilitate coping (Machtinger et al, 2019).*
- Encourage the client to verbalize his or her feelings. EBN: *Research by Thomas, Tilley, and Esquibel (2015) indicated that survivors want nonjudgmental attitudes from health care providers, acknowledgment of the violence they have suffered, and acknowledgment that their stories are heard and believed.*
- Assess to determine whether physically abused women are also survivors of sexual assault. EBN: *According to a study by Santos de Oliveira et al (2016), there is a need for primary care professionals to focus on women who are involved in relationships in which they experience sexual violence.*
- ▲ Encourage the client to report the sexual assault to a law enforcement agency. EB: *Sexual assault survivors often feel apprehensive about involvement in the criminal justice system; therefore many do not report their sexual assault to law enforcement (Patterson & Tringali, 2015).*
- ▲ Refer the client for cognitive behavioral therapy (CBT). EB: *A randomized clinical trial of a CBT-based, telepsychology-delivered interactive program for rape survivors showed a large reduction in post-test posttraumatic stress disorder (PTSD) symptoms (Littleton & Grills, 2019).*
- ▲ Stress the necessity of follow-up care with counselors, mental health specialists, and medical subspecialists as appropriate. EB: *Follow-up with appropriate referrals is crucial in physical and emotional healing (Hovelson, Scheiman, & Pearlman, 2016).*

Male Rape

- Some of the interventions described previously may be adapted for use with male clients.
- Assist male survivors of sexual assault to identify and verbalize their victimization experiences as rape. EB: *Male survivors are less likely to conceptualize their victimization experiences as rape than women, which may impede their recovery (Reed et al, 2020).*

Geriatric

- Some of the interventions described previously may be adapted for use with older clients.
- Build a trusting relationship with the client. EBN: *A person-centered communication style by the nurse can have positive outcomes in the client–nurse relationship (Selenga & Jooste, 2015).*
- All examinations should be done on older adults as they would be done on any adult client after sexual assault, with modifications for comfort if necessary. EB: *All sexual assault clients should receive consistent, objective, immediate medical care, as well as options for the collection of evidence by emergency nurses and physicians knowledgeable of jurisdictional guidelines and protocols for evidence collection (Emergency Nurses Association & International Association of Forensic Nurses, 2017).*
- Assess for mobility limitations and cognitive impairment. EB: *Providing support is complicated by challenges associated with aging bodies and cognitive impairments (Bows, 2018).*
- Explain and encourage the client to report sexual abuse. EBN: *It is of the utmost importance that the client's wishes, feelings, and beliefs are taken into consideration before any action is taken (Andrews, 2017).*
- Observe for psychosocial distress. EBN: *The elderly are often isolated and mistreated, leaving them insecure and vulnerable and without support of family and/or friends (Carvalho Sena Damasceno, de Sousa, & Batista Moura, 2016).*

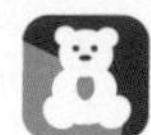

Pediatric

- Some of the interventions described previously may be adapted for use with child and adolescent populations.
- For minors, follow state-mandated reporting laws and report to Child Protective Services. EBN: *Minors who present with sexual assault injuries may also be experiencing neglect, as well as physical, sexual, or emotional abuse (Roney & Villano, 2020).*
- Use language that is tailored to the age and abilities of the child or adolescent. EB: *It is necessary to obtain medical history and information in ways that avoid retraumatizing the individual (Broaddus-Shea et al, 2021).*
- Assess adolescent sexual assault clients for health problems related to human sex trafficking: infectious diseases; noninfectious diseases (malnutrition, dental problems, and skin problems); reproductive health problems; substance abuse; mental health problems; and violence. EB: *Minor clients being trafficked may not openly identify themselves as victims; therefore nurses and other health care professionals must be aware of the signs and symptoms of trafficking (Roney & Villano, 2020).*

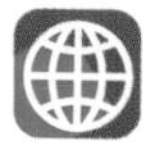

Multicultural

- Some of the interventions described previously may be adapted for use with diverse clients.
- Assess how an individual's culture affects how they perceive trauma, safety, and privacy. EB: *A safe environment will promote client engagement (Menschner & Maul, 2016).*
- Provide information and referrals for follow-up care that recognize and address the unique needs of sexual and gender minority clients. EB: *Integrated and coordinated follow-up services are the goal for all sexual assault survivors (Hendriks et al, 2018).*

Home Care

- Some of the interventions described previously may be adapted for home care use.
- Assist the client with assessing the home setting for safety and/or selecting a safe living environment. EB: *Survivors of sex trafficking identified the need for a safe place away from their pimp so that they can work through the immediate impact of their experiences (Rajaram & Tidball, 2018).*
- ▲ Ensure that the client has systems in place for long-term support. EBN: *When treating a survivor of sexual assault, the health care provider should not only treat the survivor's physical injuries but understand and support the emotional needs of the survivor and follow up with them during the period of recovery (Dos Reis, Baena de Moraes Lopes, & Duarte Osis, 2017).*
- ▲ Assess for other client vulnerabilities, such as mental health issues or addiction, and refer the client to social agencies for implementation of a therapeutic regimen. EB: *Those who have the dual diagnosis of addiction and mental illness are highly prone to sexual victimization, and actions should be taken to reduce their vulnerability (de Waal, Decker, & Goudriaan, 2017).*

Client/Family Teaching and Discharge Planning

- Provide teaching about the emotional and physical aftermath of sexual trauma. EBN: *Initial reactions may include generalized physical pain, disturbances in eating and sleeping patterns, and feelings of shame, fear, anxiety, or anger. Later responses may include phobias, flashbacks, nightmares, physical symptoms, and PTSD (Wisner, 2019).*
- Screen the client for suicide risk and refer to appropriate services. EBN: *Study results indicated that it was valuable to screen all sexual assault clients for suicide risk as it promoted client safety and promoted the emotional healing process (Cochran, 2019).*

REFERENCES

American College of Obstetrics and Gynecology (ACOG), Committee on Health Care for Underserved Women. (2019). ACOG Committee Opinion No. 777: Sexual assault. *Obstetrics and Gynecology, 133*(4), e296–e302.

Andrews, J. (2017). Abuse of older people: The responsibilities of community nurses. *British Journal of Community Nursing, 22*(5), 224–225.

Bows, H. (2018). Practitioner views on the impacts, challenges, and barriers in supporting older survivors of sexual violence. *Violence Against Women, 24*(9), 1070–1090. https://doi.org/10.1177/1077801217732348.

Broaddus-Shea, E. T., Scott, K., Reijnders, M., & Amin, A. (2021). A review of the literature on good practice considerations for initial health system response to child and adolescent sexual abuse. *Child Abuse & Neglect, 116*(Pt 1), 104225. https://doi.org/10.1016/j.chiabu.2019.104225.

Carvalho Sena Damasceno, C. K., de Sousa, M., & Batista Moura, M. E. (2016). Violence against older people registered in specialized police station for security and protection to elderly. *Journal of Nursing UFPE, 10*(3), 949–957. https://doi.org/10.5205/reuol.8702-76273-4-SM.1003201602.

Cochran, C. B. (2019). An evidence-based approach to suicide risk assessment after sexual assault. *Journal of Forensic Nursing, 15*(2), 84–92. https://doi.org/10.1097/JFN.0000000000000241.
Dos Reis, M. J., Baena de Moraes Lopes, M. H., & Duarte Osis, M. J. (2017). "It's much worse than dying": The experience of female victims of sexual violence. *Journal of Clinical Nursing, 25*(15–16), 2353–2361.
Emergency Nurses Association & International Association of Forensic Nurses. (2017). Joint position statement: Adult and adolescent sexual assault patients in the emergency care setting. *Journal of Forensic Nursing, 13*(2), 91–93.
Fleishman, J., Kamsky, H., & Sundborg, S. (2019). Trauma-informed nursing practice. *OJIN Online Journal of Issues in Nursing, 24*(2), 3. https://doi.org/10.3912/OJIN.Vol24No02Man03.
Hendriks, B., Vandenberghe, A. M. J. A., Peeters, L., Roelens, K., & Keygnaert, I. (2018). Towards a more integrated and gender-sensitive care delivery for victims of sexual assault: Key findings and recommendations from the Belgian sexual assault care centre feasibility study. *International Journal for Equity in Health, 17*(1), 152. https://doi.org/10.1186/s12939-018-0864-3.
Hovelson, S., Scheiman, L., & Pearlman, M. (2016). After a sexual assault: A guide for the OB/GYN. Contemporary OB/GYN, 61(12), 17–49. Retrieved from https://www.contemporaryobgyn.net/view/after-sexual-assault-guide-obgyn. [Accessed July 23, 2021].
Hutschemaekers, G. J. M., Zijlstra, E., de Bree, C., Wong, S. L. F., & Lagro-Janssen, A. (2019). Similar yet unique: The victim's journey after acute sexual assault and the importance of continuity of care. *Scandinavian Journal of Caring Sciences, 33*(4), 949–958. https://doi.org/10.1111/scs.12693.
Linden, J. A. (2011). Clinical practice. Care of the adult patient after sexual assault. *New England Journal of Medicine, 365*(9), 834–841.
Littleton, H., & Grills, A. (2019). Changes in coping and negative cognitions as mechanisms of change in online treatment for rape-related posttraumatic stress disorder. *Journal of Traumatic Stress, 32*(6), 927–935. https://doi.org/10.1002/jts.22447.
Machtinger, E. L., Davis, K. B., Kimberg, L. S., et al. (2019). From treatment to healing: Inquiry and response to recent and past trauma in adult health care. *Women's Health Issues, 29*(2), 97–102. https://doi.org/10.1016/j.whi.2018.11.003.
Menschner, C., & Maul, A. (2016). *Issue brief. Key ingredients for successful trauma-informed care implementation*. Center for Health Care Strategies. Retrieved from http://www.chcs.org/media/ATC-whitepaper-040616-rev.pdf. [Accessed July 23, 2021].
Ogunwale, A. O., & Oshiname, F. O. (2017). A qualitative exploration of date rape survivors' physical and psycho-social experiences in a Nigerian university. *Journal of Interpersonal Violence, 32*(2), 227–248.
Patterson, D., & Tringali, B. (2015). Understanding how advocates can affect sexual assault victim engagement in the criminal justice process. *Journal of Interpersonal Violence, 30*(12), 1987–1997.
Rajaram, S. S., & Tidball, S. (2018). Survivors' voices—complex needs of sex trafficking survivors in the Midwest. *Behavioral Medicine, 44*(3), 189–198. https://doi.org/10.1080/08964289.2017.1399101.
Reed, R. A., Pamlanye, J. T., Truex, H. R., et al. (2020). Higher rates of unacknowledged rape among men: The role of rape myth acceptance. *Psychology of Men & Masculinities, 21*(1), 162–167. https://doi.org/10.1037/men0000230.
Roney, L. N., & Villano, C. E. (2020). Recognizing victims of a hidden crime: Human trafficking victims in your pediatric trauma bay. *Journal of Trauma Nursing, 27*(1), 37–41. https://doi.org/10.1097/JTN.0000000000000480.
Santos de Oliveira, P., Palmarella Rodrigues, V., Laise Gomez Leite Morais, R., & Costa Machado, J. (2016). Health professionals' assistance to women in situation of sexual violence: An integrated review. *Journal of Nursing UFPE, 10*(5), 1828–1839. https://doi.org/10.5205/reuol.9003-78704-1-SM.1005201632.
Selenga, M., & Jooste, K. (2015). The experience of youth victims of physical violence attending a community health centre: A phenomenological study. *Africa Journal of Nursing and Midwifery, 17*(Suppl. 1), S529–S542.
Thomas, L., Tilley, D. S., & Esquibel, K. (2015). Sexual assault: Where are mid-life women in this research? *Perspectives in Psychiatric Care, 51*(2), 86–97.
de Waal, M. M., Dekker, J. J. M., & Goudriaan, A. (2017). Prevalence of victimization in patients with dual diagnosis. *Journal of Dual Diagnosis, 13*(2), 119–123.
Wisner, K. (2019). Sexual assault: What do perinatal nurses need to know? *MCN The American Journal of Maternal Child Nursing, 44*(5), 296. https://doi.org/10.1097/NMC.0000000000000553.

Ineffective Relationship Domain 7 Role relationship Class 3 Role performance

Mary Beth Flynn Makic, PhD, RN, CCNS, CCRN-K, FAAN, FNAP, FCNS

R

NANDA-I

Definition

A pattern of mutual partnership that is insufficient to provide for each other's needs.

Defining Characteristics

Delayed attainment of developmental goals appropriate for family life-cycle stage; expresses dissatisfaction with complementary interpersonal relations between partners; expresses dissatisfaction with emotional need fulfillment between partners; expresses dissatisfaction with idea sharing between partners; expresses dissatisfaction with information sharing between partners; expresses dissatisfaction with physical need fulfillment between partners; imbalance in autonomy between partners; imbalance in collaboration between partners; inadequate mutual respect between partners; inadequate mutual support in daily activities between partners; inadequate understanding of partner's compromised functioning; partner not identified as support person; reports unsatisfactory communication with partner

Related Factors

Ineffective communication skills; stressors; substance misuse; unrealistic expectations

At-Risk Population

Individuals experiencing developmental crisis; individuals with history of domestic violence; individuals with incarcerated intimate partner

Associated Conditions

Cognitive dysfunction in one partner.

NOC (Nursing Outcomes Classification)

Suggested NOC Outcomes

Coping; Family Functioning/Integrity; Role Performance; Social Support

Example NOC Outcome with Indicators

Family Integrity as evidenced by the following indicators: Members share thoughts, feelings, interests, concerns/Members communicate openly and honestly with one another/Members encourage individual autonomy and independence/Members assist one another in performing roles and daily tasks. (Rate the outcome and indicators of **Family Integrity:** 1 = never demonstrated, 2 = rarely demonstrated, 3 = sometimes demonstrated, 4 = often demonstrated, 5 = consistently demonstrated [see Section I].)

Client Outcomes

Family/Client Will (Specify Time Frame)

- Share thoughts and feelings with each other
- Communicate openly with each other
- Assist in performing family roles and tasks
- Provide support for each other
- Obtain appropriate assistance

NIC (Nursing Interventions Classification)

Suggested NIC Interventions

Coping Enhancement; Family Integrity Promotion; Role Enhancement

Example NIC Activities—Family Integrity Promotion

Facilitate a tone of togetherness within/among the family; Encourage family to maintain positive relationships; Facilitate open communication among family members

R

Nursing Interventions and *Rationales*

- Assess communication patterns concerning role and satisfaction within the relationship, including elements associated with intimacy. EB: *A recent study found that underlying chronic pain was a predominant factor that adversely affected communication and family roles between partners (Signs & Woods, 2020).*
- Assess relationship quality using the Relationship Flourishing Scale. EB: *The Relationship Flourishing Scale is a 12-item measure of eudaimonic relationship quality that assesses meaning, personal growth, relational giving, and goal sharing (Fowers et al, 2016).*
- Focus on helping couples maintain or develop marital closeness, especially during times of extreme stress. EB: *A review found that marital closeness and verbalization of stress were protective factors that may prevent relationship breakdown (Albuquerque, Pereira, & Narciso, 2016).*
- Assess the presence of stressors; physical, emotional, and behavioral health; and physical health status of the couple. EB: *The biobehavioral family model suggests that there is an interactive synergy between a partnership and family associated with family emotional climate, biobehavioral reactivity, and disease activity.*

How individuals react to each dynamic can positively or adversely influence the perceived satisfaction in the relationship (Priest, 2019).

- Explore the couple's perceptions of the impact of illness on the relationship. EB: *A study that explored psychophysiological variables on the relationship, including intimacy, found that depressive symptoms, anxiety, and diseases with chronic inflammation adversely affected the relationship; however, severity of illness appeared to strengthen the partnership* (Priest, Roberson, & Woods, 2019).
- Assist couples to identify sources of their own perceived dyadic empathy in the relationship. EB: *A study exploring empathy among partners found that for new parents who reported greater dyadic empathy, both partners reported higher sexual satisfaction and relationship adjustment* (Rosen, Mooney, & Muise, 2017).
- Assist clients to identify sources of gratitude in their relationships. EB: *Sharing feelings of gratitude was predictive of both one's own and one's spouse's relationship satisfaction* (Hogan & Gordon, 2020).
- Encourage couples to engage in reappraisal of conflict in their relationship. EB: *Reappraisal of conflict has been found to protect partners against declines in marital quality over time (Finkel et al, 2013).*
- Encourage the use of positive relational humor and humor evaluation between partners. EB: *Relational humor, which is created and shared between partners, and humor evaluation, which is one partner's judgment of the other partner's sense of humor, were both strongly associated with relationship satisfaction in a meta-analysis* (Hall, 2017).
- Provide support resources to provide military members and their families with assistance in preparation for deployments and education about the importance of maintaining communication during deployment. EBN: *Veterans who have been deployed report that dedicated resources are needed to successfully reestablish their social connections with family and reclaim their place within the family* (Messecar, 2017).
- Provide resources to military family members with posttraumatic stress disorder (PTSD). EB: *A study of combat veterans found that PTSD symptoms interfere with relationship functioning, specifically communication, intimacy, problem solving, and low self-esteem in the relationship. Involving the partner in PTSD therapy was found to improve the relationship (Malaktaris et al, 2019).*
- Encourage couples to participate together in leisure activities. EB: *A study of persons with physical disabilities found that social and physical activities improved communication and coping skills (Han et al, 2019).* EB: *A study of cancer survivors and their partners found that light-intensity ballroom dancing intervention improved the quality of life and the relationship with loved ones (Pisu et al, 2017).*
- Openly explore communication and satisfaction in the same-sex relationship without bias. EB: *Research is demonstrating that the elements of satisfaction in relationships are similar between opposite- and same-sex partners. The Rainbow Couples Relationship Standards Scale (Rainbow CRSS) measures elements that bond couples such as expression of love, caring, intimacy, family relationships, and harmony and religion (Baker & Halford, 2020).*
- Refer to care plans Readiness for Enhanced **Relationship**, Readiness for Enhanced **Family** Processes, and Readiness for Enhanced Family **Coping.**

Geriatric

- Assess geriatric spousal caregivers for positive and negative consequences of providing medical care. EB: *A study found that spouses who assist with more health-related tasks feel they are directly benefitting their partner, which further enhances perceptions of gains and promotes positive feelings among spousal caregivers (Park, 2017).*
- Assess intimacy and sexuality of older adults EB: *A study of older adults found that intimacy evolved with aging but remained important with overall quality of life and satisfaction in the relationship. Intimate behaviors were not limited to intercourse but more frequently included kissing, cuddling, and touch (Skalacka & Germyski, 2019).*
- Facilitate and increase opportunities for social connectedness for older individuals through the use of technology training. EBN: *A study demonstrated that computer training at a senior citizens club helped participants build group cohesion and form tiered connections with partners, family, and friends with whom they no longer live (Burmeister et al, 2016).*

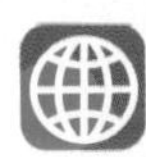

Multicultural

- Assess relationship dynamics without bias as to race, gender identity, or ethnicity. EB: *A study of Asian Americans found that this population values primacy of family goals over individual wishes and is more likely to engage in intimate/sexual relationship within the context of marriage. Asian Americans reported being more reluctant to obtain sexual and reproductive care associated with cultural beliefs (Okazaki, 2002).*

R

- Use culturally tailored cognitive behavioral techniques to promote communication, problem solving, self-disclosure, empathic response skills, and sexual education and counseling. EB: *A review of 39 studies found that interventions to promote communication, problem solving, self-disclosure, empathic responses, and sexual education could enhance marital intimacy and strengthen family bonds and stability. Health care providers need to individualize interventions that are appropriate to the couple's characteristics and their relationship (Kardan-Souraki et al, 2016).*

REFERENCES

Albuquerque, S., Pereira, M., & Narciso, I. (2016). Couple's relationship after the death of a child: A systematic review. *Journal of Child and Family Studies*, *25*(1), 30–53. https://doi:10.1007/s10826-015-0219-2.

Baker, N. A., & Halford, W. K. (2020). Assessment of couple relationships standards in same-sex attracted adults. *Family Process*, *59*(2), 537–555. https://doi.org/10.1111/famp.12447.

Burmeister, O. K., Bernoth, M., Dietsch, E., & Cleary, M. (2016). Enhancing connectedness through peer training for community-dwelling older people: A person centred approach. *Issues in Mental Health Nursing*, *37*(6), 406–411. https://doi:10.3109/01612840.2016.1142623.

Finkel, E. J., Slotter, E. B., Luchies, L. B., Walton, G. M., & Gross, J. J. (2013). A brief intervention to promote conflict reappraisal preserves marital quality over time. *Psychological Science*, *24*(8), 1595–1601. https://doi:10.1177/0956797612474938.

Fowers, B. J., Laurenceau, J. P., Penfield, R. D., et al. (2016). Enhancing relationship quality measurement: The development of the Relationship Flourishing Scale. *Journal of Family Psychology*, *30*(8), 997–1007. https://doi:10.1037/fam0000263.

Hall, J. A. (2017). Humor in romantic relationships: A meta-analysis. *Personal Relationships*, *24*(2), 306–322. https://doi:10.1111/pere.12183.

Han, A., Kim, J., & Kim, J. (2019). Coping strategies, social support, leisure activities, and physical disabilities. *American Journal of Health Behavior*, *43*(5), 937–949. https://doi.org/10.5993/AJHB.43.5.6.

Hogan, J. N., & Gordon, C. L. (2020). Six of one, half a dozen of another" or do mindfulness and gratitude each add unique value to relationship functioning? *Contemporary Family Therapy: An International Journal*, *42*(3), 299–304. https://doi.org/10.1007/s10591-020-09534-w.

Kardan-Souraki, M., Hamzehgardeshi, Z., Asadpour, I., Mohammadpour, R. A., & Khani, S. (2016). A review of marital intimacy-enhancing interventions among married individuals. *Global Journal of Health Science*, *8*(8), 53109. https://doi:10.5539/gjhs.v8n8p74.

Malaktaris, A. L., Buzzella, B. A., Siegel, M. E., et al. (2019). OEF/OIF/OND Veterans seeking PTSD treatment: perceptions of partner involvement in trauma-focused treatment. *Military Medicine*, *184*(3-4), e263–e270. https://doi.org/10.1093/milmed/usy231.

Messecar, D. C. (2017). Finding their way back in: Family reintegration following guard deployment. *Military Medicine*, *182*(S1), 266–273. https://doi:10.7205/MILMED-D-16-00109.

Okazaki, S. (2002). Influences of culture on Asian Americans' sexuality. *Journal of Sex Research*, *39*(1), 34–41. https://doi.org/10.1080/00224490209552117.

Park, M. (2017). In sickness and in health: Spousal caregivers and the correlates of caregiver outcomes. *American Journal of Geriatric Psychiatry*, *25*(10), 1094–1096. https://doi:10.1016/j.jagp.2017.05.001.

Pisu, M., Demark-Wahnefried, W., Kenzik, K. M., et al. (2017). A dance intervention for cancer survivors and their partners (RHYTHM). *Journal of Cancer Survivorship*, *11*(3), 350–359. https://doi:10.2196/resprot.6489.

Priest, J. B. (2019). Examining differentiation of self as a mediator in the biobehavioral family model. *Journal of Marital and Family Therapy*, *45*(1), 161–175. https://doi.org/10.1111/jmft.12301.

Priest, J. B., Roberson, P. N. E., & Woods, S. B. (2019). In our lives and under our skin: An investigation of specific psychobiological mediators linking family relationships and health using the biobehavioral family model. *Family Process*, *58*(1), 79–99. https://doi.org/10.1111/famp.12357.

Rosen, N. O., Mooney, K., & Muise, A. (2017). Dyadic empathy predicts sexual and relationship well-being in couples transitioning to parenthood. *Journal of Sex & Marital Therapy*, *43*(6), 543–559. https://doi.org/10.1080/0092623X.2016.1208698.

Signs, T. L., & Woods, S. B. (2020). Linking family and intimate partner relationships to chronic pain: An application of the biobehavioral family model. *Families, Systems & Health*, *38*(1), 38–50. https://doi.org/10.1037/fsh0000459.

Skałacka, K., & Gerymski, R. (2019). Sexual activity and life satisfaction in older adults. *Psychogeriatrics*, *19*(3), 195–201. https://doi.org/10.1111/psyg.12381.

R

Readiness for Enhanced Relationship Domain 7 Role relationship Class 3 Role performance

Marina Martinez-Kratz, MS, RN, CNE

NANDA-I

Definition

A pattern of mutual partnership to provide for each other's needs, which can be strengthened.

Defining Characteristics

Expresses desire to enhance autonomy between partners; expresses desire to enhance collaboration between partners; expresses desire to enhance communication between partners; expresses desire to enhance emotional need fulfillment for each partner; expresses desire to enhance mutual respect between partners; expresses desire to enhance satisfaction with complementary interpersonal relationship between partners; expresses desire to enhance satisfaction with emotional need fulfillment for each partner; expresses desire to enhance satisfaction with idea sharing between partners; expresses desire to enhance satisfaction with information sharing between partners; expresses desire to enhance satisfaction with physical need fulfillment for each partner; expresses desire to enhance understanding of partner's functional impairment

NOC (Nursing Outcomes Classification)

Suggested NOC Outcomes

Coping; Family Functioning/Integrity; Role Performance; Social Support

Example NOC Outcome with Indicators

Family Integrity as evidenced by the following indicators: Members share thoughts, feelings, interests, concerns/Members communicate openly and honestly with one another/Members encourage individual autonomy and independence/Members assist one another in performing roles and daily tasks. (Rate the outcome and indicators of **Family Integrity:** 1 = never demonstrated, 2 = rarely demonstrated, 3 = sometimes demonstrated, 4 = often demonstrated, 5 = consistently demonstrated [see Section I].)

Client Outcomes

Family/Client Will (Specify Time Frame)

- Share thoughts and feelings with each other
- Communicate openly with each other
- Assist in performing family roles and tasks
- Provide support for each other
- Obtain appropriate assistance

NIC (Nursing Interventions Classification)

Suggested NIC Interventions

Coping Enhancement; Family Integrity Promotion; Role Enhancement

Example NIC Activities—Family Integrity Promotion

Facilitate a tone of togetherness within/among the family; Encourage family to maintain positive relationships; Facilitate open communication among family members

Nursing Interventions and *Rationales*

- Assess the ways in which the relationship has been altered (e.g., communication, sexuality, intimacy) from both partner's perspective. **EB:** *A review found that when involving both partners in marital interventions, it is necessary to assess both views of the relationship (Albuquerque, Pereira, & Narciso, 2016).*
- Assess relationship quality using the Relationship Flourishing Scale. **EB:** *The Relationship Flourishing Scale is a 12-item measure of eudaimonic relationship quality that assesses meaning, personal growth, relational giving, and goal sharing (Fowers et al, 2016).*
- Focus on helping couples maintain or develop marital closeness. **EB:** *A review found that marital closeness is a protective factor that may prevent relationship breakdown (Albuquerque, Pereira, & Narciso, 2016).*
- Assist couples to identify sources of their own perceived dyadic empathy in the relationship. **EB:** *A study found that for new parents who reported greater dyadic empathy, both partners reported higher sexual satisfaction and relationship adjustment (Rosen, Mooney, & Muise, 2017).*
- Assist clients to identify sources of gratitude in their relationships. **EB:** *A study found that individual gratitude was predictive of both one's own and one's spouse's relationship satisfaction (Hogan & Gordon, 2020).*
- Encourage couples to engage in reappraisal of conflict in their relationship. **EB:** *A study demonstrated that a reappraisal of conflict in their marriages protected participants against declines in marital quality over time (Finkel et al, 2013).*

- Encourage the use of positive relational humor and humor evaluation between partners. EB: *Relational humor, which is created and shared between partners, and humor evaluation, which is one partner's judgment of the other partner's sense of humor, were both strongly associated with relationship satisfaction in a meta-analysis (Hall, 2017).*
- Provide support resources to provide military members and their families with assistance in preparation for deployments and education about the importance of maintaining communication during deployment. EBN: *Veterans who have been deployed report that dedicated resources are needed to successfully reestablish their social connections with family and reclaim their place within the family (Messecar, 2017).*
- Encourage couples to participate together in leisure activities such as dance. EB: *This study demonstrated that a light-intensity ballroom dancing intervention improved the life of cancer survivors and the relationship with loved ones (Pisu, Demark-Wahnefried, & Kenzik, 2017).*
- Refer to care plans Readiness for Enhanced **Family** Processes and Readiness for Enhanced Family **Coping.**

Pediatric

- Encourage guidance and information on communication for parents of seriously ill children. EBN: The findings of this study suggested that parents are an important focus of care, and enhancing couples' communication is a way to address changes in marital relationships (Machado Silva-Rodrigues et al, 2016).
- Encourage young children to express gratitude. EB: *A study found that expressions of gratitude positively affected preschool children's prosocial behavior (Shoshani et al, 2020).*

Geriatric

- Assess geriatric spousal caregivers for positive and negative consequences of providing medical care. EB: *A study found that more medical/nursing tasks were linked to greater caregiving gains. Spouses who assist with more medical/nursing tasks feel they are directly benefitting their partner, which further enhances perceptions of gains and promotes positive feelings among spousal caregivers (Park, 2017).*
- Assess sexuality needs and support consensual sexual expression. EB: *Older adult participants in an Australian study made suggestions related to the visibility and normalization of sex in later life, cultural representations of sex and older people, and the need to provide sex-positive aged care and retirement home facilities (Fileborn et al, 2017).*
- Facilitate and increase opportunities for social connectedness for older individuals through the use of technology training. EBN: *A study demonstrated that computer training at a senior citizens club helped participants build group cohesion and form tiered connections with partners, family, and friends with whom they no longer live (Burmeister et al, 2016).*

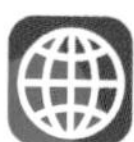

Multicultural

- Provide a relationship-focused intervention to enhance communication for multicultural couples. EB: *A Korean study found that a relationship-focused communication intervention improved couples' abilities to communicate effectively and to resolve conflicts, and it enhanced intimacy (Kim et al, 2016).*
- Use culturally tailored cognitive behavioral techniques to promote communication, problem-solving, self-disclosure, empathic response skills, and sexual education and counseling. EB: *A review of 39 studies found that interventions to promote communication, problem-solving, self-disclosure, empathic responses, and sexual education could enhance marital intimacy and strengthen family bonds and stability. Health care providers need to individualize interventions that are appropriate to the couple characteristics and their relationship (Kardan-Souraki et al, 2016).*

R

REFERENCES

Albuquerque, S., Pereira, M., & Narciso, I. (2016). Couple's relationship after the death of a child: A systematic review. *Journal of Child and Family Studies*, *25*(1), 30–53. https://doi:10.1007/s10826-015-0219-2.

Burmeister, O. K., Bernoth, M., Dietsch, E., & Cleary, M. (2016). Enhancing connectedness through peer training for community-dwelling older people: A person centred approach. *Issues in Mental Health Nursing*, *37*(6), 406–411. https://doi:10.3109/01612840.2016.1142623.

Fileborn, B., Lyons, A., Hinchliff, S., et al. (2017). Improving the sexual lives of older Australians: Perspectives from a qualitative study. *Australasian Journal on Ageing*, *36*, E36–E42. https://doi:10.1111/ajag.12405.

Finkel, E. J., Slotter, E. B., Luchies, L. B., Walton, G. M., & Gross, J. J. (2013). A brief intervention to promote conflict reappraisal preserves marital quality over time. *Psychological Science*, *24*(8), 1595–1601. https://doi:10.1177/0956797612474938.

Fowers, B. J., Laurenceau, J. P., Penfield, R. D., et al. (2016). Enhancing relationship quality measurement: The development of the Relationship Flourishing Scale. *Journal of Family Psychology*, *30*(8), 997–1007. https://doi:10.1037/fam0000263.

Hall, J. A. (2017). Humor in romantic relationships: A meta-analysis. *Personal Relationships*, *24*(2), 306–322. https://doi:10.1111/pere.12183.

Hogan, J. N., & Gordon, C. L. (2020). "Six of one, half a dozen of another" or do mindfulness and gratitude each add unique value to relationship functioning? *Contemporary Family Therapy: International Journal*, *42*(3), 299–304. https://doi.org/10.1007/s10591-020-09534-w.

Kardan-Souraki, M., Hamzehgardeshi, Z., Asadpour, I., Mohammadpour, R. A., & Khani, S. (2016). A review of marital intimacy-enhancing interventions among married individuals. *Global Journal of Health Science*, *8*(8), 53109. https://doi:10.5539/gjhs.v8n8p74.

Kim, G. H., Lee, Y. S., & Ishii, H. (2016). Relationship-focused intervention to enhance marriage communication for multicultural couples. *Korean Journal of Family Relations*, *21*(2), 97–127. https://doi:10.21321/jfr.21.2.97.

Machado Silva-Rodrigues, F., Pan, R., Mota Pacciulio Sposito, A., de Andrade Alvarenga, W., & Castanheira Nascimento, L. (2016). Childhood cancer: Impact on parents' marital dynamics. *European Journal of Oncology Nursing*, *23*, 34–42. https://doi:10.1016/j.ejon.2016.03.002.

Messecar, D. C. (2017). Finding their way back in: Family reintegration following guard deployment. *Military Medicine*, *182*(S1), 266–273. https://doi:10.7205/MILMED-D-16-00109.

Park, M. (2017). In sickness and in health: Spousal caregivers and the correlates of caregiver outcomes. *American Journal of Geriatric Psychiatry*, *25*(10), 1094–1096. https://doi:10.1016/j.jagp.2017.05.001.

Pisu, M., Demark-Wahnefried, W., Kenzik, K. M., et al. (2017). A dance intervention for cancer survivors and their partners (RHYTHM). *Journal of Cancer Survivorship*, *11*(3), 350–359. https://doi:10.2196/resprot.6489.

Rosen, N. O., Mooney, K., & Muise, A. (2017). Dyadic empathy predicts sexual and relationship well-being in couples transitioning to parenthood. *Journal of Sex & Marital Therapy*, *43*(6), 543–559. https://doi.org/10.1080/0092623X.2016.1208698.

Shoshani, A., De-Leon Lendner, K., Nissensohn, A., Lazarovich, G., & Aharon-Dvir, O. (2020). Grateful and kind: The prosocial function of gratitude in young children's relationships. *Developmental Psychology*, *56*(6), 1135–1148. https://doi.org/0.1037/dev0000922.

Risk for Ineffective Relationship

Domain 7 Role relationship Class 3 Role performance

Mary Beth Flynn Makic, PhD, RN, CCNS, CCRN-K, FAAN, FNAP, FCNS

NANDA-I

Definition

Susceptible to developing a pattern that is insufficient for providing a mutual partnership to provide for each other's needs.

Risk Factors

Inadequate communication skills; stressors; substance misuse; unrealistic expectations

At-Risk Population

Individuals experiencing developmental crisis; individuals with history of domestic violence; individuals with incarcerated intimate partner

Associated Conditions

Cognitive dysfunction in one partner

NOC, NIC, Client Outcomes, Nursing Interventions and *Rationales,* and References

Refer to care plan for Ineffective **Relationship**.

R

Impaired Religiosity

Domain 10 Life Principles Class 3 Value/belief/action congruence

Barbara Baele Vincensi, PhD, RN, FNP-BC and Mary E. Desmond, PhD, RN, MA, MSN, AHN-BC

NANDA-I

Definition

Impaired ability to exercise reliance on beliefs and/or participate in rituals of a particular faith tradition.

Defining Characteristics

Desires to reconnect with belief pattern; desires to reconnect with customs; difficulty adhering to prescribed religious beliefs; difficulty adhering to prescribed religious rituals; expresses distress about separation from faith community; questions religious beliefs; questions religious customs

Related Factors

Anxiety; cultural barrier to practicing religion; depressive symptoms; environmental constraints; fear of death; inadequate social support; inadequate sociocultural interaction; inadequate transportation; ineffective caregiving; ineffective coping strategies; insecurity; pain; spiritual distress

At-Risk Population

Hospitalized individuals; individuals experiencing end of life crisis; individuals experiencing life transition; individuals experiencing personal crisis; individuals experiencing spiritual crisis; individuals with history of religious manipulation; older adults

Associated Conditions

Depression; impaired health status

NOC (Nursing Outcomes Classification)

Suggested NOC Outcomes

Client Satisfaction: Cultural Needs Fulfillment

Example NOC Outcome with Indicators

Client Satisfaction: Cultural Needs Fulfillment as evidenced by the following indicators: Respect for religious beliefs/Respect for cultural health behaviors/Incorporation of cultural beliefs in health teaching/Respect for personal values. (Rate each indicator of **Client Satisfaction: Cultural Needs Fulfillment:** 1 = not at all satisfied, 2 = somewhat satisfied, 3 = moderately satisfied, 4 = very satisfied, 5 = completely satisfied [see Section I].)

R

Client Outcomes

Client Will (Specify Time Frame)

- Express satisfaction with the ability to express religious practices
- Express satisfaction with access to religious materials and rituals
- Demonstrate balance between religious practices and healthy lifestyles
- Avoid high-risk, controlling religious relationships that inflict physical, sexual, or emotional harm and/or exploitation

NIC (Nursing Interventions Classification)

Suggested NIC Interventions

Religious Ritual Enhancement; Culture Brokerage; Religious Addiction Prevention

Example NIC Activities—Religious Ritual Enhancement

Encourage the use of and participation in usual religious rituals that are not detrimental to health

Nursing Interventions and *Rationales*

Adults

- Recognize when clients integrate religious practices into their life. EB: *In a prospective study of 110 clients before, during, and after chemotherapy Kaliampos and Roussi (2017) found that use of religious coping significantly predicted a positive affect 7 months later.*
- Assist clients to work around or overcome barriers to participating in their usual religious rituals or practices that support coping. EBN: *In a cross-sectional descriptive study (Akgül & Karadağ, 2016) fecal ostomies were found to be a barrier to incorporating specific religious practices of salat, fasting, and pilgrimage in the lives of 150 Muslims postoperatively, providing an opportunity for nurses to assist clients in meeting their religious needs through adaptation or facilitation around this barrier.*
- Encourage the use of prayer or meditation as appropriate. EBN: *In a qualitative study by Woods-Giscombé and Gaylord (2014) with 15 African American participants who had mindfulness meditation experience mindfulness meditation was helpful in managing stress and it also had several concepts in common with African American religious concepts, suggesting that this type of meditation could be used within a religious framework with this population.*
- Promote family coping using religious practices to help cope with loss, as appropriate. EBN: *In a longitudinal qualitative study by Nilmanat et al (2015) of 15 Thai clients dying of cancer, three themes emerged to help cope with the dying process: surrounded by love from family, moving beyond suffering, and reconnecting to religious faith to counter suffering.*
- Refer to a religious leader, professional counseling, or support group as needed. EB: *A cross-sectional survey by Ghesquiere et al (2015) of 591 hospices in the United States found that complicated grief or depression related to death can be assessed and managed by most hospices in varying degrees with the use of multiprofessional teams, support groups, individual counseling, or group therapy.* EBN: *In a descriptive study by Brelsford et al (2016) of 52 neonatal intensive care unit (NICU) parents, family cohesiveness decreased with the use of negative religious and spiritual coping, providing an indicator to nurses of a need for potential referral or support.*

End-of-Life Care

- Refer to a religious leader, professional counseling, or support group as needed. EB: *A cross-sectional survey by Ghesquiere et al (2015) of 591 hospices in the United States found that complicated grief or depression related to death can be assessed and managed by most hospices in varying degrees with the use of multiprofessional teams, support groups, individual counseling, or group therapy.*

✱ Implement QSEN competencies and evidence-based practice in providing end-of-life (EOL) care. EBN: *Using mixed methods, Lindemulder et al (2018) evaluated BSN students' incorporation of QSEN competencies related to teamwork, collaboration, person-centered care, spiritual/religious care, professionalism, and safety during an EOL simulation scenario and found significantly improved students pre– to post–self-assessment scores on all the above items.*

Maternal–Child Health

- Provide support for pregnant client's religiosity to promote health-seeking behaviors. EBN: *Cyphers et al (2017) found significant correlations between pregnant women and their use of religiosity to promote health-seeking behaviors during pregnancy.*

Sexual Minority Individuals (Lesbian, Gay, Bisexual, Transgender, Queer)

- Provide support using religiosity with caution. EB: *Brewster et al (2016) found that religious coping strategies may or may not promote psychological well-being or relieve psychological symptoms of distress caused by internalization of specific thoughts and experiences in a sample of self-identified sexual minority participants (n = 143), in which sexual discrimination and harassment had occurred within and outside of the religious/church establishment; therefore, promotion of religious coping or practices for this minority should be approached carefully.*

Pediatric

- Provide spiritual care for children based on developmental level. EB: *When nurses are comfortable providing spiritual care, they can implement numerous spiritual care activities and intervention to meet the spiritual needs of the child and family. After determining the child's spiritual beliefs and spiritual needs, a plan of care is developed based on the child's developmental age (Fowler, 1987).*

R

- **Parents:** Incorporate religious traditions and faith practices for parents with hospitalized and chronically ill children. EB: *A qualitative study indicated that religion was a positive coping mechanism for parents with infants in the neonatal intensive care unit (NICU) (Huenink & Porterfield, 2017).* EBN: *In a quantitative descriptive study, parents of children with cancer demonstrated an increase in their religious faith (Wiener et al, 2016).* EBN: *Additional relevant research can be found in Wang et al (2019).*

Geriatric

- Promote established religious practices in older adults. EB: *In a systematic review by Agli et al (2015), encouraging spiritual and religious practices in older adults with dementia increased positive coping strategies, cognitive function, and quality of life.* EBN: *Using a pre-post control group with 66 older clients admitted to an ICU, Elham et al (2015) found a significant inverse relationship between groups regarding spiritual well-being and anxiety when client concerns were met after an adequate assessment of spiritual/religious needs was completed and interventions implemented by nurses.*

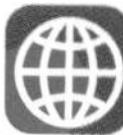

Multicultural

Promote religious practices that are culturally appropriate:

- **African American.** EB: *Salas-Wright et al (2015) found an inverse relationship between religious involvement and violent and nonviolent antisocial behaviors in adolescent African American females living in high-risk communities.* EB: *In a cross-sectional survey of 1013 African American women, Ludema et al (2015) found that those who highly identified with organized religion, nonorganized religion, and spirituality had less risky sexual behaviors for potential HIV exposure than those who had no affiliation.* EBN: *Additional relevant research can be found in Woods-Giscombé and Gaylord (2014).*
- **Hispanic.** EB: *Rivera-Hernandez (2016)* found a positive relationship between religiosity with diabetes care and blood sugar control in a sample of 2216 Hispanic individuals 50 years and older living in Mexico.
- **Jordanian.** EBN: *Using a cross-sectional and correlational design, Musa et al (2016) found that spiritual well-being and religiosity had a positive correlation with self-rated health in a convenience sample of 340 Jordanian Arab Christians who make up only 3% of the population of this country.*
- **Muslim.** EBN: *In a cross-sectional descriptive study (Akgül & Karadağ, 2016) fecal ostomies were found to be a barrier to incorporating specific religious practices of salat, fasting, and pilgrimage in the lives of 150 Muslims postoperatively, providing an opportunity for nurses to assist clients in meeting their religious needs through adaptation or facilitation around this barrier.*

Multiprofessional

- Refer to a religious leader, professional counseling, or support group as needed. EB: *A cross-sectional survey by Ghesquiere et al (2015) of 591 hospices in the United States found that complicated grief or depression related to death can be assessed and managed by most hospices in varying degrees with the use of transdisciplinary teams, support groups, individual counseling, or group therapy.*

R

REFERENCES

Agli, O., Bailly, N., & Ferrand, C. (2015). Spirituality and religion in older adults with dementia: A systematic review. *International Psychogeriatrics*, *27*(5), 715–725. https://doi.org/10.1017/S1041610214001665.

Akgül, B., & Karadağ, A. (2016). The effect of colostomy and ileostomy on acts of worship in the Islamic faith. *Journal of Wound, Ostomy, and Continence Nursing*, *43*(4), 392–397. https://doi.org/10.1097/WON.0000000000000237.

Brelsford, B., Ramirez, J., Veneman, K., & Doheny, K. K. (2016). Religious and secular coping and family relationships in the neonatal intensive care unit. *Advances in Neonatal Care*, *16*(4), 315–322. https://doi.org/10.1097/ANC.0000000000000263.

Brewster, M. E., Velez, B. L., Foster, A., Esposito, J., & Robinson, M. A. (2016). Minority stress and the moderating role of religious coping among religious and spiritual sexual minority individuals. *Journal of Counseling Psychology*, *63*(1), 119–126. https://doi.org/10.1037/cou0000121.

Cyphers, N. A., Clements, A. D., & Lindseth, G. (2017). The relationship between religiosity and health promoting behaviors in pregnant women. *Western Journal of Nursing Research*, *39*(11), 1429–1446. https://doi.org/10.1177/01930459166779623.

Elham, H., Hazrati, M., Momennasab, M., & Sareh, K. (2015). The effect of need-based spiritual/religious intervention on spiritual well-being and anxiety of elderly people. *Holistic Nursing Practice*, *29*(3), 136–143. https://doi.org/10.1097/HNP.0000000000000083.

Fowler, J. W. (1987). *Faith development and pastoral care*. Philadelphia: Fortress Press.

Ghesquiere, A. R., Aldridge, M. D., Johnson-Hürzeler, R., Kaplan, D., Bruce, M. L., & Bradley, E. (2015). Hospice services for complicated grief and depression: Results from a national survey. *Journal of the American Geriatric Society*, *63*(10), 2173–2180. https://doi.org/10.1111/jgs.13656.

Huenink, E., & Porterfield, S. (2017). Parent support programs and coping mechanisms in NICU parents. *Advances in Neonatal Care, 17*(2), E10–E18. https://doi.org/10.1097/ANC.0000000000000359.

Kaliampos, A., & Roussi, P. (2017). Religious beliefs, coping, and psychological well-being among Greek cancer patients. *Journal of Health Psychology, 22*(6), 754–764. https://doi.org/10.1177/13591053156114995.

Lindemulder, L., Gouwens, S., & Stefo, K. (2018). Using QSEN competencies to assess nursing student end-of-life care in simulation. *Nursing, 48*(4), 60–65. https://doi.org/10.1097/01.NURSE.0000531006.94600.28.

Ludema, C., Doherty, I. A., White, B. L., et al. (2015). Religiosity, spirituality, and HIV risk behaviors among African American women from four rural counties in the Southeastern U.S. *Journal of Health Care for the Poor and Underserved, 26*(1), 168–181. https://doi.org/10.1353/hpu.2015.0005.

Musa, A. S., Pevalin, D. J., & Shahin, F. I. (2016). Impact of spiritual well-being, spiritual perspective, and religiosity on the self-rated health of Jordanian Arab Christians. *Journal of Transcultural Nursing, 27*(6), 550–557. https://doi.org/10.1177/1043659615587590.

Nilmanat, K., Promnoi, C., Phungrassami, T., et al. (2015). Moving beyond suffering: The experiences of Thai persons with advanced cancer. *Cancer Nursing, 38*(3), 224–231. https://doi.org/10.1097/NCC.0000000000000169.

Rivera-Hernandez, M. (2016). Religiosity, social support and care associated with health in older Mexicans with diabetes. *Journal of Religion and Health, 55*(4), 1394–1410. https://doi.org/10.1007/s10943-015-0150-7.

Salas-Wright, C. P., Tirmazi, T., Lombe, M., & Nebbitt, V. E. (2015). Religiosity and antisocial behavior: Evidence from young African American women in public housing communities. *Social Work Research, 39*(2), 82–93. https://doi.org/10.1093/swr/svv010.

Wang, S. C., Wu, L. M., Yang, Y. M., & Sheen, J. M. (2019). The experience of parents living with a child with cancer at the end of life. *European Journal of Cancer Care, 28*(4), e13061. https://doi.org/10.1111/ecc.13061.

Wiener, L., Viola, A., Kearney, J., et al. (2016). Impact of caregiving for a child with cancer on parental health behaviors, relationship quality, and spiritual faith: Do lone parents fare worse? *Journal of Pediatric Oncology Nursing, 33*(5), 378–386. https://doi.org/10.1177/1043454215616610.

Woods-Giscombé, C. L., & Gaylord, S. A. (2014). The cultural relevance of mindfulness meditation as a health intervention for African Americans: Implications for reducing stress-related health disparities. *Journal of Holistic Nursing, 32*(3), 147–160. https://doi.org/10.1177/0898010113519010.

Readiness for Enhanced Religiosity **Domain 10 Life principles Class 3 Value/belief/action congruence**

Barbara Baele Vincensi, PhD, RN, FNP-BC and Mary E. Desmond, PhD, RN, MA, MSN, AHN-BC

NANDA-I

Definition

A pattern of reliance on religious beliefs and/or participation in rituals of a particular faith tradition, which can be strengthened.

Defining Characteristics

Expresses desire to enhance connection with a religious leader; Expresses desire to enhance forgiveness; Expresses desire to enhance participation in religious experiences; Expresses desire to enhance participation in religious practices; Expresses desire to enhance religious options; Expresses desire to enhance use of religious material; Expresses desire to reestablish belief patterns; Expresses desire to reestablish religious customs

R

NOC (Nursing Outcomes Classification)

Suggested NOC Outcomes

Client Satisfaction: Cultural Needs Fulfillment

Example NOC Outcome with Indicators

Client Satisfaction: Cultural Needs Fulfillment as evidenced by the following indicators: Respect for religious beliefs/Respect for cultural health behaviors/Incorporation of cultural beliefs in health teaching/Respect for personal values. (Rate each indicator of **Client Satisfaction: Cultural Needs Fulfillment:** 1 = not at all satisfied, 2 = somewhat satisfied, 3 = moderately satisfied, 4 = very satisfied, 5 = completely satisfied [see Section I].)

Client Outcomes

Client Will (Specify Time Frame)

- Express satisfaction with the ability to express religious practices
- Express satisfaction with access to religious materials and rituals
- Demonstrate balance between religious practices and healthy lifestyles
- Avoid high-risk, controlling religious relationships that inflict physical, sexual, or emotional harm and/or exploitation

NIC (Nursing Interventions Classification)

Suggested NIC Interventions

Religious Ritual Enhancement; Culture Brokerage; Religious Addiction Prevention

Example NIC Activities—Religious Ritual Enhancement

Encourage the use of and participation in usual religious rituals that are not detrimental to health

Nursing Interventions and *Rationales*

Adults

- Encourage centering prayer or other forms of meditation to promote mental and spiritual health. **EB:** *In a small sample, centering prayer demonstrated positive effects on emotional and spiritual health (Fox et al, 2016).* **EB:** *A prospective study found religious coping, including prayer used during chemotherapy, predicted a positive affect 7 months later (Kaliampos & Roussi, 2017).*

Disabled

- Use prayer as a coping mechanism for those with disabilities. **EB:** *Hodge and Reynolds (2019) found, in a cross-sectional exploratory study, that those with disabilities are more likely to pray several times a day as compared to those without disabilities.*

Maternal–Child Health

- Provide support for pregnant client's religiosity to promote health-seeking behaviors. **EBN:** *Cyphers et al (2017) found significant correlations between pregnant women and their use of religiosity to promote health-seeking behaviors during pregnancy.*

Sexual Minority Individuals (Lesbian, Gay, Bisexual, Transgender, Queer)

- Encourage the use of religion to decrease stigma and improve quality of life (QOL) for HIV-positive men. **EBN:** *A cross-sectional observational study of men having sex with men (MSM) by Desyani et al (2019) found a negative relationship* ($p = 0.007$) *between stigma and QOL and a positive relationship* ($p = 0.000$) *between religiosity and QOL, indicating the potential use of religiosity to improve QOL in MSM who are HIV positive.*

Uninsured/Low Income

- Explore the use of a faith community nurse to provide wellness services and care monitoring. **EB:** *Faith Community Nursing is a nursing specialty focusing on integration of faith and health while providing wellness care within faith communities and outreach into the surrounding community (Morris, 2015; Young et al, 2015).*

Veterans

- Encourage the use of religion to help decrease sleep disturbances in veterans. **EB:** *A cross-sectional study on combat casualty exposed veterans found that religious salience and attendance was a buffering element to sleep disturbances (White et al, 2018).*

End-of-Life Care

✱ Implement QSEN competencies and evidence-based practice in providing end-of-life (EOL) care. **EBN:** *Using mixed methods,* Lindemulder et al (2018) *evaluated BSN students' incorporation of QSEN*

R

competencies related to teamwork, collaboration, person-centered care, spiritual/religious care, professionalism, and safety during an EOL simulation scenario and found significantly improved students pre- to post-self-assessments scores on all the above items.

- ▲ Refer to a religious leader, professional counseling, or support group as needed. **EB:** *A cross-sectional survey by* Ghesuiere et al (2015) *of 591 hospices in the United States found that complicated grief or depression related to death can be assessed and managed by most hospices in varying degrees with the use of a multiprofessional team, support groups, individual counseling, or group therapy.*

Pediatric

- Provide spiritual care for children based on developmental level. **EB:** *When nurses are comfortable providing spiritual care, they can implement numerous spiritual care activities and intervention to meet the spiritual needs of the child and family. After determining the child's spiritual beliefs and spiritual needs, a plan of care is developed based on the child's developmental age (Fowler, 1987).* **EBN:** *In a meta-synthesis on children living with chronic disease by Bakker et al (2018), children ages 0 to 18 found comfort and strength in their relationship with God, used their religious beliefs to cope, and reported their spiritual experiences using religious terminology.*
- **Parents:** Incorporate religious traditions and faith practices for parents with hospitalized and chronically ill children. **EB:** *A qualitative study indicated that religion was a positive coping mechanism for parents with infants in the neonatal intensive care unit (NICU) (Huenink & Porterfield, 2017).* **EBN:** *In a quantitative descriptive study, parents of children with cancer demonstrated an increase in their religious faith (Wiener et al, 2016).* **EBN:** *Additional relevant research can be found in Wang et al (2019).*
- **School-Age Children:** Encourage faith community involvement and religious attendance with parent(s). **EBN:** *In a meta-synthesis by Bakker et al (2018) on children living with chronic disease, children ages 0–18 found comfort and strength in their relationship with God, used their religious beliefs to cope, and described spiritual experiences using religious terminology.*
- **School-Age Children:** Encourage children to participate in faith community health programs. **EBN:** *An ethnographic study indicated that faith communities provide a forum for healthy nutrition as part of the faith culture (Opalinski et al, 2017).*
- **African American Children:** Incorporate faith traditions in coping with chronic disease. **EBN:** *In an ethnographic study of African American parents of children with autism, religious faith in God was a positive theme and can support culturally congruent health care (Burkett et al, 2017).*
- **Latino Children:** Incorporate faith traditions among clients and families in pediatric settings. **EBN:** *In an ethno-nursing study with Latino families and providers of care on a medical-surgical unit, a culturally competent model was developed with findings indicating five care factors as most valuable: family, faith, communication, care integration, and meeting basic needs (Mixer et al, 2015).*
- **Adolescents:** Encourage prayer, particularly within the African American community. **EBN:** *Qualitative research indicates that urban African American youth have multifaceted dimensions of their spirituality, including the role of prayer in their lives, an unwavering faith in a higher power, and the importance of giving back to their communities (Dill, 2017).*
- **Adolescents/Young Adults:** Encourage religious coping in the adolescent/young adult population. **EB:** *A secondary analysis using a national database found a significant difference ($p = 0.001$) between females' and males' risk perception scores of marijuana use and total religiosity scores, suggesting that religiosity has an indirect effect on marijuana use; females were more religious with a higher risk perception score than males, and less likely to use the drug (Hai et al, 2018).*

Geriatric

- Encourage listening to religious music. **EB:** *A national quantitative study found that frequency of listening to religious music was associated with decreases in death anxiety and increases in life satisfaction, self-esteem, and sense of control (Bradshaw et al, 2015).*

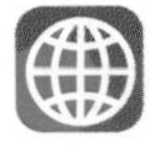

Multicultural

- **African American:** Collaborate with faith communities to promote wellness. Also, incorporate faith traditions in coping with chronic disease. **EB:** *In a qualitative participatory action study with church leaders, findings indicated feelings of distrust of the medical system with a preference for self-management and suggested incorporating a religious orientation to rebuild trust within the African American community (Lew* *et al, 2015).* **EBN:** *In an ethnographic study of African American parents of children with autism, religious faith in God was a positive theme and can support culturally congruent health care (Burkett et al, 2017).*

- **Latino:** Incorporate faith traditions among clients and families in pediatric settings. **EBN:** *In an ethnonursing study with Latino families and providers of care on a medical-surgical unit, a culturally competent model was developed with findings indicating five care factors as most valuable: family, faith, communication, care integration, and meeting basic needs (Mixer et al, 2015). Collaborate with faith communities to promote wellness. A cross-sectional study by Sanchez et al (2019) identified the importance of religious capital, which promoted health through social support, as useful in decreasing immigration stress, especially among undocumented immigrants.*
- **Thai:** Encourage both religious and spiritual coping strategies to help cope. **EBN:** *The Thai people were found to be both religious and spiritual, using coping strategies from both areas to help manage concerns and to explain the development of kidney disease in a qualitative study by Yodchai et al (2017).*

Multiprofessional

▲ Chaplain referral when individuals engage in religious coping mechanisms. **EB:** *When individuals engage in religious coping, additional religious struggles follow, which may benefit from chaplain expertise to promote well-being (Fox et al, 2016).* **EB:** *A cross-sectional survey by Ghesuiere et al (2015) of 591 hospices in the United States found that complicated grief or depression related to death can be assessed and managed by most hospices in varying degrees with the use of a multiprofessional team, support groups, individual counseling, or group therapy.*

REFERENCES

Bakker, A. A. D., van Leeuwen, R. R. R., & Roodbol, P. F. P. (2018). The spirituality of children with chronic conditions: A qualitative meta-synthesis. *Journal of Pediatric Nursing, 43*, e106–e113. https://doi.org/10,1016/j.pedn.2018.08.003.

Bradshaw, M., Ellison, C. G., Fang, Q., & Mueller, C. (2015). Listening to religious music and mental health in later life. *The Gerontologist, 55*(6), 961–971. https://doi.org/10.1093/geront/gnu020.

Burkett, K., Morris, E., Anthony, J., Shambley-Ebron, D., & Manning-Courtney, P. (2017). Parenting African American children with autism: The influence of respect and faith in mother, father, single-, and two-parent care. *Journal of Transcultural Nursing, 28*(5), 496–504. https://doi.org/10.1177/1043659616662316.

Cyphers, N. A., Clements, A. D., & Lindseth, G. (2017). The relationship between religiosity and health promoting behaviors in pregnant women. *Western Journal of Nursing Research, 39*(11), 1429–1446. https://doi.org/10.1177/01930459166779623.

Desyani, N. L. J., Waluyo, A., & Yona, S. (2019). The relationship between stigma, religiosity, and the quality of life of HIV-positive MSM in Medan, Indonesia. *Enfermería Clínica, 29*(Suppl 2), 510–514. https://doi.org/10.1016/j.enfcli.2019.04.077.

Dill, L. J. (2017). "Wearing my spiritual jacket": The role of spirituality as a coping mechanism among African American youth. *Health Education & Behavior, 44*(5), 696–704. https://doi.org/10.1177/1090198117729398.

Fowler, J. W. (1987). *Faith development and pastoral care*. Philadelphia: Fortress Press.

Fox, J., Gutierrez, D., Haas, J., & Durnford, S. (2016). Centering prayer's effects on psycho spiritual outcomes: A pilot outcome study. *Mental Health, Religion & Culture, 19*(4), 379–392. https://doi.org/10.1080/13674676.2016.1203299.

Ghesquiere, A. R., Aldridge, M. D., Johnson-Hürzeler, R., Kaplan, D., Bruce, M. L., & Bradley, E. (2015). Hospice services for complicated grief and depression: Results from a national survey. *Journal of the American Geriatric Society, 63*(10), 2173–2180.

Hai, A. H., Currin-McCulloch, J., Franklin, C., & Cole, A. H., Jr. (2018). Spirituality/religiosity's influence on college students' adjustment to bereavement: A systematic review. *Death Studies, 42*(8), 513–520. https://doi.org/10.1080/07481187.2017.1390503.

Hodge, D. R., & Reynolds, C. (2019). Spirituality among people with disabilities: A nationally representative study of spiritual and religious profiles. *Health and Social Work, 44*(2), 75–86. https://doi.org/10.1093/hsw/hly035.

Huenink, E., & Porterfield, S. (2017). Parent support programs and coping mechanisms in NICU parents. *Advances in Neonatal Care, 17*(2), E10–E18. https://doi.org/10.1097/ANC.0000000000000359.

Kaliampos, A., & Roussi, P. (2017). Religious beliefs, coping, and psychological well-being among Greek cancer patients. *Journal of Health Psychology, 22*(6), 754–764. https://doi.org/10.1177/1359105315614995.

Lew, K. N., Arbauh, N., Banach, P., & Melkus, G. (2015). Diabetes: Christian worldview, medical distrust and self-management. *Journal of Religion and Health, 54*(3), 1157–1172. https://doi.org/10.1007/s10943-015-0022-9.

Lindemulder, L., Gouwens, S., & Stefo, K. (2018). Using QSEN competencies to assess nursing student end-of-life care in simulation. *Nursing, 48*(4), 60–65. https://doi.org/10.1097/01.NURSE.0000531006.94600.28.

Mixer, S. J., Carson, E., & McArthur, P. M. (2015). Nurses in action: A response to cultural care challenges in a pediatric acute care setting. *Journal of Pediatric Nursing, 30*(6), 896–907. https://doi.org/10.1016/j.pedn.2015.05.001.

Morris, G. S. (2015). Holistic health care for the medically uninsured: The church health center of Memphis. *Ethnicity & Disease, 25*(4), 507–510. https://doi.org/10.18865/ed.25.4.507.

Opalinski, A. S., Dyess, S. M., & Gropper, S. S. (2017). Food culture of faith communities and potential impact on childhood obesity. *Public Health Nursing, 34*(5), 437–443. https://doi.org/10.1111/phn.12340.

Sanchez, M., Diez, S., Fava, N. M., et al. (2019). Immigration stress among recent Latino immigrants: The protective role of social support and religious social capital. *Social Work in Public Health, 34*(4), 279–292. https://doi.org/10.1080/19371918.2019.1606749.

Wang, S. C., Wu, L. M., Yang, Y. M., & Sheen, J. M. (2019). The experience of parents living with a child with cancer at the end of life. *European Journal of Cancer Care, 28*(4), e13061. https://doi.org/10.1111/ecc.13061.

White, J., Xu, X., Ellison, C. G., DeAngelis, R. T., & Sunil, T. (2018). Religion, combat casualty exposure, and sleep disturbance in the US

Military. *Journal of Religion and Health, 57*(6), 2362–2377. https://doi.org/10.1007/s10943-018-0596-0.
Wiener, L., Viola, A., Kearney, J., et al. (2016). Impact of caregiving for a child with cancer on parental health behaviors, relationship quality, and spiritual faith: Do lone parents fare worse? *Journal of Pediatric Oncology Nursing, 33*(5), 378–386. https://doi.org/10.1177/1043454215616610.
Yodchai, K., Dunning, T., Savage, S., & Hutchinson, A. M. (2017). The role or religion and spirituality in coping with kidney disease and haemodialysis in Thailand. *Scandinavian Journal of Caring Science, 31*(2), 359–367. https://doi.org/10.1111/scs.12355.
Young, S., Patterson, L., Wolff, M., Greer, Y., & Wynne, N. (2015). Empowerment, leadership, and sustainability in a faith-based partnership to improve health. *Journal of Religion and Health, 54*(6), 2086–2098. https://doi.org/10.1007/s10943-014-9911-6.

Risk for Impaired Religiosity

Domain 10 Life principles Class 3 Value/belief/action congruence

Mary Beth Flynn Makic, PhD, RN, CCNS, CCRN-K, FAAN, FNAP, FCNS

NANDA-I

Definition

Susceptible to an impaired ability to exercise reliance on religious beliefs and/or participate in rituals of a particular faith tradition, which may compromise health.

Risk Factors

Anxiety; cultural barrier to practicing religion; depressive symptoms; environmental constraints; fear of death; inadequate social support; inadequate sociocultural interaction; inadequate transportation; ineffective caregiving; ineffective coping strategies; insecurity; pain; spiritual distress

At-Risk Population

Hospitalized individuals; individuals experiencing end of life crisis; individuals experiencing life transition; individuals experiencing personal crisis; individuals experiencing spiritual crisis; Individuals with history of religious manipulation; older adults

Associated Conditions

Depression; impaired health status

NOC, NIC, Client Outcomes, Nursing Interventions and *Rationales,* and References

Refer to care plan for Impaired **Religiosity.**

R

Relocation Stress Syndrome

Domain 9 Coping/stress tolerance Class 1 Post-trauma responses

Margaret M. Egan-Touw, DNP, RN, CNE

NANDA-I

Definition

Physiological and/or psychosocial disturbance following transfer from one environment to another.

Defining Characteristics

Anger behaviors; anxiety (00146); decreased self concept; depressive symptoms; expresses anger; expresses frustration; fear (00148); increased morbidity; increased physical symptoms; increased verbalization of needs; loss of identity; loss of independence; low self-esteem; pessimism; preoccupation; reports altered sleep-wake cycle; reports concern about relocation; reports feeling alone; reports feeling insecure; reports feeling lonely; social alienation; unwillingness to move

Related Factors

Communication barriers; inadequate control over environment; inadequate predeparture counseling; inadequate social support; ineffective coping strategies; powerlessness; situational challenge to self-worth; social isolation

At-Risk Population

Individuals facing unpredictability of experience; individuals who move from one environment to another; individuals with history of loss

Associated Conditions

Depression; diminished mental competency; impaired health status; impaired psychosocial functioning

NOC (Nursing Outcomes Classification)

Suggested NOC Outcomes

Relocation Adaptation; Anxiety Self-Control; Child Adaptation to Hospitalization; Coping; Depression Level; Depression Self-Control; Loneliness Severity; Psychosocial Adjustment: Life Change, Quality of Life; Stress Level

Example NOC Outcome with Indicators

Relocation Adaptation as evidenced by the following indicators: Recognizes reason for change in living environment/Participates in decision-making in new environment/Expresses satisfaction with daily routine/Expresses satisfaction with level of independence/Compares care needs with available resources/Expresses satisfaction with social relationships/Expresses satisfaction with variety of food/Expresses satisfaction with food preparation/Expresses satisfaction with retained personal belongings/Expresses satisfaction with living arrangements/Exhibits positive mood/Appears content/Respects others' rights/Maintains positive relationships with family/Maintains positive relationships with friends/Maintains positive relationships with others in new environment/Participates in social activities/Seeks information to reduce anxiety/Plans coping strategies for stressful situations/Uses effective coping strategies/Uses relaxation techniques to reduce anxiety/Maintains social relationships/Maintains adequate sleep/Controls anxiety response. (Rate the outcome and indicators of **Relocation Adaptation:** 1 = never demonstrated, 2 = rarely demonstrated, 3 = sometimes demonstrated, 4 = often demonstrated, 5 = consistently demonstrated [see Section I].)

Client Outcomes

Client Will (Specify Time Frame)

- Recognize and know the name of at least one staff member or new neighbor within 1 week of relocating
- Engage at least one staff member of new neighbor in a conversation within 2 weeks of relocating
- Express concern about move when encouraged to do so during individual contacts within 24 hours of awareness of impending relocation
- Perform activities of daily living (ADLs) in safe manner
- Proactively ask for assistance with ADLs
- Maintain previous mental and physical health status (e.g., nutrition, elimination, sleep, social interaction, physical activity) within 2 months of relocating

NIC (Nursing Interventions Classification)

Suggested NIC Interventions

Anxiety Reduction; Coping Enhancement; Discharge Planning; Hope Instillation; Self-Responsibility Facilitation; Animal-Assisted Therapy; Art Therapy; Music Therapy; Massage; Mood Management; Active Listening

Example NIC Activities—Anxiety Reduction

Stay with client to promote safety and reduce fear; Provide objects that symbolize safeness to the client; Orient to the new setting and personnel daily; Encourage sharing life experiences with peers and staff; Promote autonomy.

Nursing Interventions and *Rationales*

- Orientation to the new environment is a proactive means that alleviates anxiety and increases confidence. EBN: *Orientation before the move can serve as a means to reduce fear and anxiety associated with the newness of the move (Luo, Chen, & Lian, 2020). The authors proposed guidelines to facilitate optimal adjustment and autonomy inclusive for structured and free-style exploration by the resident to familiarize oneself with the new setting.*
- Be aware that relocation to retirement communities may be a positive change. EBN: *The elderly, when facing moving from the marital home into a structured residential facility, verbalized and demonstrated confidence and self-satisfaction when identified as the primary decision-maker regarding the move. This was reinforced on arrival at the facility. A cross-sectional study of older individuals relocating to retirement communities found older individuals experienced less stress when they had a greater role in the decision-making associated with the relocation, positive cognitions, and adjustment resources (Peck & Jacob, 2019).*
- Begin relocation planning as early in the decision-making process as possible. EBN: *Having a well-organized proactive plan for the move with support and advocacy through the planning and decision-making process may reduce anxiety and alleviate fear(s) (Peck & Jacob, 2019; Luo, Chen, & Lian, 2020).*
- Obtain a history, including the reason for the move, the client's usual coping mechanisms, history of losses, and family and financial support for the client. EBN: *A complete history helps the nurse determine the type of support needed and appropriate interventions to reduce relocation stress. Getting to know the resident's premove lifestyle will help identify quality of life and safety concerns that will enable to receiving facility to plan accordingly (Ryman et al, 2018; Luo, Chen, & Lian, 2020).*
- Identify to what extent the client can participate in the relocation decision-making process and advocate for this participation. EBN: *As the population of those over 60 increases, one can anticipate nursing taking a more proactive role in the planning and education of individuals facing moving into continuing care facilities (Ryman et al, 2018). Engaging older adults in the decision-making process is likely to enhance the level of adjustment after the relocation and promote psychological well-being (Hertz et al, 2016; Peck & Jacob, 2019).* EB: *A study of highly dependent older adults who were relocated found that the subjects had a higher use of new antidepressant agents and new antibiotic orders, suggesting the need for vigilant planning to reduce the stress of the move (Mello & O'Connor, 2016).*
- Assess client's readiness to relocate and relocation self-efficacy. EB: *Relocation is a complex process that requires careful consideration and planning before the move (prelocation) and adjustment to the new home after the move (postrelocation) to promote the older client's adjustment (Hertz et al, 2016; Ryman et al, 2018; Luo, Chen, & Lian, 2020).*
- Consult an evidence-based practice guide for relocation. EBN: *Researchers compiled the latest findings to develop a protocol to assist in relocating older adults (Hertz et al, 2016; Luo, Chen, & Lian, 2020).*
- Assess family members' perceptions of client's ability to participate in relocation decisions. Particularly in incidences of neurocognitive impairment such as dementia, be attentive to health care workers' involvement in making the decision to relocate. They may need support and encouragement through the process. EB: *Health care workers were found to be highly stressed during the relocation decision-making process and "walking a tightrope" between the older adult's needs and those of the person's family members (Canham et al, 2018).*
- Consider the cultural and ethnic values of the client and family as much as possible when choosing roommates, foods, and other aspects of care. EB: *Inclusion of culturally and ethnically sensitive foods during meals and leisure activities where snacks are an expectation can promote inclusion and thereby facilitate adjustment to the new facility. Nurses need to be aware of the differences in values and practices of different cultures and ensure that they provide culturally appropriate care that is respectful of individual and familial caregivers' beliefs (Lee et al, 2017; Lin & Yen, 2018; Shekriladze, Javakhishvili, & Tchanturia, 2019; Luo, Chen, & Lian, 2020).*
- Promote clear communication between all participants involved in the relocation process. EB: *A narrative study exploring older client's transitions found that communication and exploring unspoken fears helped reduce concerns of loss of control and uncertainty (Lee et al, 2017; Lin & Yen, 2018; Luo, Chen, & Lian, 2020).*
- Observe the following procedures if the client is being transferred to an extended care or assisted living facility:
  - Facilitate the client's participation in decisions and choice of placement, and arrange a preadmission visit if possible.
  - If the client cannot visit the new facility, arrange for a visit or telephone call by a member of the staff to welcome the client and show a videotape or at least provide pictures of the new care facility.

R

- Have a familiar person accompany the client to the new facility. This lessens client and family anxiety, confusion, and dissatisfaction.
- Encourage the resident and/or caregiver to write a journal regarding thoughts and feelings about the relocation.
- Continue to assess caregiver psychological distress during a 6-month period after relocation. Caregivers experience guilt and distress because of the responsibility of moving their loved one.

EB: *The adjustment period for the resident as well as the caregiver is usually 3 to 6 months after relocation. Caregivers may begin to identify conflicted feelings and work on resolution during this time and need support* (*Lee et al, 2017*).

- Identify previous routines for ADLs. Try to maintain as much continuity with the previous schedule as possible. EB: *Continuity of client's everyday personal care by care aides that is both empathetic and nurturing is perceived as supportive and compassionate and eases relocation stress (Andersen & Spiers, 2016).*
- Bring in familiar items from home (e.g., pictures, clocks, afghans). EB: *Familiarity eases transition, reinforces one's identity, and symbolizes safeness* (*Wiles et al, 2012; Iecovich, 2014*).
- Establish the way the client would like to be addressed (Mr., Mrs., Miss, first name, or calling name/nickname). EB: *Calling clients by their desired name shows respect and acknowledgement of their individuality.*
- Thoroughly orient the client and the family to the new environment and routines; repeat directions as needed. EB: *Providing honest answers to client questions and supporting the individual adjustment to the new location will be necessary for at least 6 months until the client feels at home* (*Hertz et al, 2016; Luo, Chen, & Lian, 2020*).
- Spend one-to-one time with the client. Allow the client to express feelings and convey acceptance of them; emphasize that the client's feelings are real and individual and that it is acceptable to be sad or angry about moving. EB: *Interventions should recognize personal values; allow adequate time to listen to and respect the views and needs of the older adult* (*Hertz et al, 2016; Luo, Chen, & Lian, 2020*).
- Allocate an attentive staff member to help the client adjust to the move. Assign the same staff members to the client for care if the therapeutic relationship is compatible with client needs; maintain consistency in the staffing personnel with whom the client interacts on a daily basis.
- Encourage the client to verbalize one positive aspect of the new living situation each day. Helping the client to focus on the positive aspects of the move can facilitate adaptation and adjustment by reframing one's attitude in a positive fashion. EBN: *Assisting clients to focus on positive thinking has been found to promote their ability to manage daily activities and adapt to change. Clients with greater resourcefulness have been found to be able to adapt to challenging situations in a more constructive and successful manner (Luo, Chen, & Lian, 2020).*
- Ask the client to verbalize one positive aspect of the new living situation each day. EB: *Helping the client focus on the positive aspects of the move can help change attitude and reframe the situation in a positive fashion (Hertz et al, 2016).*
- Monitor the client's well-being and provide appropriate interventions for problems with social interaction, nutrition, sleep, new onset of infection, or elimination problems. EB: *Older clients and lower socioeconomic status are associated with greater risk of maladjustment after relocation (Hertz et al, 2016). A study found a significant increase in morbidity before and after transfer. Residents who transferred had increased rates of illness and greater antibiotic and antidepressant medication prescription rates in the months before and after relocation (Mello & O'Connor, 2016; Costlow & Parmelee, 2019).*
- If the client is being transferred within a facility, have staff members from the new unit visit the client and the family, if possible, before transfer.
- Work with the caregivers and family members, helping them work with and adjust to the stages of "making the best of it," "making the move," and "making it better." EBN: *Provide opportunities for family to visit, encourage engagement in facility social events, and provide electronic access for the client to maintain ties with loved ones and friends (Hertz et al, 2016; Lee et al, 2017).*
- If a client is being transferred from the intensive care unit (ICU), have previous staff make occasional visits until the client is comfortable in the new surroundings. Ensure that the family is told relevant information. EB: *Providing an individualized transfer plan from the ICU to the medical-surgical unit that addresses client and family questions before transfer reduces relocation stress (Dale et al, 2020; Won & Son, 2020).*
- Watch for coping problems (e.g., withdrawal, regression, angry behavior, impaired sleeping, refusal to eat, flat affect, anxiety) and intervene immediately. EB: *Loss of independence with transfer to a nursing home may manifest in anxiety, anger, and depression (Dale et al, 2020; Won & Son, 2020).*

R

- Encourage the client to express grief for the loss of former residence and of interpersonal relationships and explain that it is normal to feel sadness over change and loss. EB: *Acknowledging and verbalizing feelings of grief can help alleviate the heartache and promote healing (Costlow & Parmelee, 2019).*
- Assess the client's psychological needs along with physiological needs. EB: *Although physical care needs may predicate the relocation, meeting psychosocial care needs must be individualized via thorough assessment (Hertz et al, 2016; Luo, Chen, & Lian, 2020).*
- Encourage clients to take a proactive role in their care as much as is possible inclusive of autonomous decision-making (e.g., arrangement of the furniture in the residence, choice of roommate, bathing routines). EB: *Autonomy facilitates making choices that help prevent feelings of powerlessness that may lead to depression (Hertz et al, 2016; Peck & Jacob, 2019).*

Pediatric

- Assess family history and contact information from children relocated to rescue shelters. EB: *Efforts have been made to develop systematic processes to reunite children who are separated from families during disasters. Current guidelines established by the Federal Emergency Management Agency (FEMA), the Red Cross, the Centers for Disease Control and Prevention (CDC), and the National Center for Missing and Exploited Children focus on providing effective, efficient action through the following:*
  - *A shared understanding of local and national resources and capabilities*
  - *Collaboration, coordination, effective communication for children with disabilities and other access and functional needs, and needs assessments during disasters*
  - *Shared operational procedures and technologies (FEMA et al, 2013; Miller et al, 2019)*
- Be aware that community relocation may be beneficial for children and assess community and academic resources of new location (Miller et al, 2019).
- Provide support for a child and family who must relocate to be near a higher acuity health care facility such as a transplant center (Søndergaard et al, 2016).
- In situations of familial discord such as divorce, recommend alternative dispute resolution versus traditional litigated settlement. EBN: *This nonadversarial approach may mitigate some of the loss of trust and trauma experienced by children of divorce (Søndergaard et al, 2016).*
- Assess presence of allergies before and after relocation.
  - If the client is an adolescent, try to avoid a move in the middle of the school year, find a newcomers' club for the adolescent to join, and refer for counseling if needed. EB: *Most adolescents who relocate suffer a brief period of loss of companionship and intimacy with close friends (McBride, 2015; Miller et al, 2019).*
- Assess adolescents' perceptions of their acceptance by peers. EB: *Poor perceptions of peer acceptance have been related to less initiation of social interactions in new settings (McBride, 2015).*
- Help parents recognize that relocation stress syndrome may persist for prolonged periods (e.g., 2 years), especially in adolescents. EB: *Adolescents were found to commonly express their ideology of the relocation (McBride, 2015).*
- Be aware that adolescents may cope with the transition by exerting control in particular domains. EBN: *Adolescents may be at risk of developing eating disorders after a major transition (McBride, 2015).*
- The effects of frequent relocation may not manifest immediately and may have long-term effects on physical and mental health. EBN: *Longitudinal analysis found that frequent relocation in adolescence was associated with higher rates of stress and physical exhaustion in adulthood (McBride, 2015; Søndergaard et al, 2016).*

Geriatric

- Monitor the need for transfer and relocate only when medically or psychologically necessary. EB: *Older adults often experience loss of physical and psychological well-being following relocation (Lee et al, 2017).*
- Implement discharge planning early and engage the older adult in the planning and decision-making process about relocation. EB: *Engaging the older adult in decision-making is key to successful relocation (Hertz et al, 2016; Luo, Chen, & Lian, 2020).*
- Use technologies, such as sensing devices, to measure average in-home gait speed (AIGS) as a predictor of fall risk. EBN: *AIGS was found to be a more reliable and valid predictor of fall risk than traditional physical performance assessments (Stone et al, 2015).*
- Implement a registered nurse (RN) care coordination care planning model to restore older adults' health, maintain their independence, and reduce care costs. EBN: *RN care coordination was found to significantly*

and positively affect older adult outcome variables and to result in lesser costs of care (Lee et al, 2017; Dale et al, 2020).

- After the transfer, assess the client's mental status. Document and observe for any new onset of confusion. Confusion can follow relocation because of the overwhelming stress and sensory overload. **EB:** *Elderly women are more at risk for experiencing moderate to severe anxiety when compounded with loneliness. Many have outlived their spouses and friends, which highlights the sense of isolation (Wiyono, Sukartini, & Mundakir, 2018).*
- Facilitate visits from companion animals. **EB:** *Pet therapy has been found to improve depressive symptoms and cognitive function in residents of long-term care facilities with mental illness (Ambrosi et al, 2019)*

Client/Family Teaching and Discharge Planning

- Teach family members about symptoms of relocation stress syndrome. Encourage them to monitor for signs of the syndrome.
- Help significant others learn how to support the client in the relocation process by setting up social engagements such as a schedule of visits, arranging for holidays, bringing familiar items from home, and establishing a system for contact when the client needs support. **EBN:** *Social support of family and friends was significantly related to relocation adjustment (Hertz et al, 2016).*
- Assist family members and the relocating older adult to use Internet/webcam technology for interaction to supplement in-person visits. **EB:** *When older adults in a care facility have less than one visitor per week, interaction can be supplemented with technological "visits" (Hertz, 2016).*

REFERENCES

Ambrosi, C., Zaiontz, C., Peragine, G., Sarchi, S., & Bona, F. (2019). Randomized controlled study on the effectiveness of animal-assisted therapy on depression, anxiety, and illness perception in institutionalized elderly. *Psychogeriatrics: The Official Journal of the Japanese Psychogeriatric Society*, *19*(1), 55–64. https://doi.org/10.1111/psyg.12367.

Andersen, E. A., & Spiers, J. (2016). Care aides' relational practices and caring contributions. *Journal of Gerontological Nursing*, *42*(11), 24–30. https://doi.org/10.3928/00989134-20160901-03.

Canham, S. L., Fang, M. L., Battersby, L., Woolrych, R., Sixsmith, J., Ren, T. H., & Sixsmith, A. (2018). Contextual factors for aging well: Creating socially engaging spaces through the use of deliberative dialogues. *Gerontologist*, *58*(1), 140–148. https://doi.org/10.1093/geront/gnx121.

Costlow, K., & Parmelee, P. A. (2019). The impact of relocation stress on cognitively impaired and cognitively unimpaired long-term care residents. *Aging and Mental Health*, *24*(10), 1589–1595. https://doi.org/10.1080/13607863.2019.1660855.

Dale, C. M., Carbone, S., Istanboulian, L., et al. (2020). Support needs and health-related quality of life of family caregivers of patients requiring prolonged mechanical ventilation and admission to a specialized weaning center: A qualitative longitudinal interview study. *Intensive & Critical Care Nursing*, *58*, 102808. https://doi.org/10.1016/j.iccn.2020.102808.

Federal Emergency Management Agency (FEMA), National Center for Missing & Exploited Children (NCMEC), United States Department of Health and Human Services (HHS), & American Red Cross (ARC). (2013). Post-disaster reunification of children: a nationwide approach. Retrieved from https://nationalmasscarestrategy.org/new-release-post-disaster-reunification-of-children-a-nationwide-approach/. Accessed 26 July 2021.

Hertz, J. E., Koren, M. E., Rossetti, J., & Tibbits, K. (2016). Evidence-based practice guideline: management of relocation in cognitively intact older adults. *Journal of Gerontological Nursing*, *42*(11), 14–23.

Iecovich, E. (2014). Aging in place: From theory to practice. *Anthropological Notebooks*, *20*(1), 21–33.

Lee, S., Oh, H., Suh, Y., & Seo, W. (2017). A tailored relocation stress intervention programme for family caregivers of patients transferred from a surgical intensive care unit to a general ward. *Journal of Clinical Nursing*, *26*(5–6), 784–794. https://doi.org/10.1111/jocn.13568.

Lin, L. J., & Yen, H. Y. (2018). The benefits of continuous leisure participation in relocation adjustment among residents of long-term care facilities. *Journal of Nursing Research*, *26*(6), 427–437.

Luo, Y. Z., Chen, W., & Lian, Y. (2020). Correlations among relocation stress, health conditions and life adjustment of the elderly in long-term care institutions. *Revista de Cercetare si Interventie Sociala*, *69*, 69–78.

McBride, M. E. (2015). Beyond butterflies: Generalized anxiety disorder in adolescents. *The Nurse Practitioner*, *40*(3), 28–37.

Mello, S., & O'Connor, K. A. (2016). Morbidity and mortality following relocation of highly dependent long-term care residents: A retrospective analytical study. *Journal of Gerontological Nursing*, *42*(11), 34–38. https://doi.org/10.3928/00989134-20160908-01.

Miller, K. K., Brown, C. R., Shramko, M., & Svetaz, M. V. (2019). Applying trauma-informed practices to the care of refugee and immigrant youth: 10 clinical pearls. *Children*, *6*(8), 94. https://doi.org/doi.org/10.3390/children6080094.

Peck, H., & Jacob, A. (2019). Relocation to/within a retirement community: older adults' perceived satisfaction with transitioning. *Journal of Baccalaureate Social Work*, *24*(1), 167–181.

Ryman, F. V. M., Erisman, J. C., Darvey, L. M., Osborne, J., Swartzsenburg, E., & Syurina, E. V. (2018). Health effects of the relocation of patients with dementia: A scoping review to inform medical and policy decision-making. *The Gerontologist*, *59*(6), e674–e682. https://doi.org/10.1093/geront/gny031.

Shekriladze, I., Javakhishvili, N., & Tchanturia, K. (2019). Culture change and eating patterns: A study of Georgian women. *Frontiers in Psychiatry*, *10*, 619. https://doi.org/10.3389/fpsyt.2019.00619.

Søndergaard, S., Robertson, K., Silfversten, E., et al. (2016). *Families support to transition: A systematic review of the evidence.* Santa Monica, CA: RAND Corporation. Retrieved from https://www.rand.org/pubs/research_reports/RR1511.html. Accessed 26 July 2021.

Stone, E., Skubic, M., Rantz, M., Abbott, C., & Miller, S. (2015). Average in-home gait speed: Investigation of a new metric for mobility and fall risk assessment of elders. *Gait and Posture*, *41*(1), 57–62.

R

Wiles, J. L., Leibing, A., Guberman, N., Reeve, J., & Allen, R. E. S. (2012). The meaning of "aging in place" to older people. *The Gerontologist, 52*(3), 357–366.

Wiyono, H., Sukartini, T., & Mundakir (2018). *An overview of loneliness, anxiety and depression level of elderly suspected relocation stress syndrome*. Nurses at the Forefront in Transforming Care, Science and Research, 9th International Nursing Conference.

Won, M. H., & Son, Y. J. (2020). Development and psychometric evaluation of the Relocation Stress Syndrome Scale–Short Form for patients transferred from adult intensive care units to general wards. *Intensive & Critical Care Nursing, 58*, 102800. https://doi.org/10.1016/j.iccn.2020.102800.

Risk for Relocation Stress Syndrome

Domain 9 Coping/stress tolerance Class 1 Post-trauma responses

Marina Martinez-Kratz, MS, RN, CNE

NANDA-I

Definition

Susceptible to physiological and/or psychosocial disturbance following transfer from one environment to another, which may compromise health.

Risk Factors

Communication barriers; inadequate control over environment; inadequate predeparture counseling; inadequate social support; ineffective coping strategies; powerlessness; situational challenge to self-worth; social isolation

At-Risk Population

Individuals facing unpredictability of experience; individuals who move from one environment to another; individuals with history of loss

Associated Conditions

Diminished mental competency; impaired health status; impaired psychosocial functioning

NIC, NOC, Client Outcomes, Nursing Interventions and *Rationales,* Client/Family Teaching and Discharge Planning, and References

Refer to care plan for **Relocation** Stress Syndrome.

R

Impaired Resilience

Domain 9 Coping/stress tolerance Class 2 Coping responses

Gail B. Ladwig, MSN, RN and Julianne E. Doubet, BSN, RN, EMT-B

NANDA-I

Definition

Decreased ability to recover from perceived adverse or changing situations, through a dynamic process of adaptation.

Defining Characteristics

Decreased interest in academic activities; decreased interest in vocational activities; depressive symptoms; expresses shame; impaired health status; inadequate sense of control; ineffective coping strategies; ineffective integration; low self-esteem; renewed elevation of distress; reports feeling guilty; social isolation

Related Factors

Altered family relations; community violence; disrupted family rituals; disrupted family roles; dysfunctional family processes; inadequate health resources; inadequate social support; inconsistent parenting; ineffective family adaptation; multiple coexisting adverse situations; perceived vulnerability; substance misuse

At-Risk Population

Economically disadvantaged individuals; individuals experiencing a new crisis; individuals experiencing chronic crisis; individuals exposed to violence; individuals who are members of an ethnic minority; individuals whose parents have mental disorders; individuals with history of exposure to violence; individuals with large families; mothers with low educational level; women

Associated Conditions

Intellectual disability; psychological disorder

NOC (Nursing Outcomes Classification)

Suggested NOC Outcomes

Personal Resiliency; Coping; Decision-Making; Self-Esteem

Example NOC Outcome with Indicators

Personal Resiliency as evidenced by the following indicators: Adapts to adversities as challenges. (Rate the outcome and indicators of **Personal Resiliency:** 1 = never demonstrated, 2 = rarely demonstrated, 3 = sometimes demonstrated, 4 = often demonstrated, 5 = consistently demonstrated [see Section I].)

Client Outcomes

Client Will (Specify Time Frame)

- Demonstrate reduced or cessation of drug and alcohol usage
- State effective life events on feelings about self
- Seek help when necessary
- Verbalize or demonstrate cessation of abuse
- Adapt to unexpected crises or challenges
- Verbalize positive outlook on illness, family, situation, and life
- Use available resources to meet coping needs
- Identify role models
- Identify available assets and resources
- Be able to verbalize meaning of one's life

R

NIC (Nursing Interventions Classification)

Suggested NIC Interventions

Resiliency Promotion; Coping Enhancement; Counseling; Emotional Support; Self-Esteem Enhancement; Support Group; Support System Enhancement

Example NIC Activities—Resiliency Promotion

Encourage positive health-seeking behaviors; Facilitate family communication

Nursing Interventions and *Rationales*

- Encourage positive, health-seeking behaviors. EB: *Johansson et al (2016) concluded, in their study of diabetic health, that caregivers should establish an atmosphere of open learning that generates interactions in a climate that establishes and encourages contemplation to promote health and well-being.*
- Ensure access to biological, psychological, and spiritual resources. EB: *Tay and Lin (2020) characterize psychological resistance as an evolving response to stress that is adaptable, is durable, and can be fostered and maintained by the influence of "biological, psychological, spiritual, and social factors."*

- Foster cognitive skills in decision-making. EB: *Client's comprehension of pertinent information is an essential part of the standard that allows for informed decisions (Gerstenecker et al, 2015).*
- Assist client in cognitive restructuring of negative thought processes. EB: *Ayoningtyas et al (2019) found that group counseling, with exercises in both cognitive restructuring and self-instruction techniques, strengthened career decision-making capabilities.*
- Facilitate supportive family environments and communication. EBN: *Family caregivers of clients with cancer may find themselves subjected to struggles with physical, mental, and spiritual problems, which if ignored could put strain on the whole family (Borji et al, 2017).*
- Promote engagement in positive social activities. EB: *In their study of persons with learning disabilities, Howarth et al (2016) ascertained that taking part in various social activities provided a key opportunity for individuals to expand their social connections.*
- Assist client to identify strengths and reinforce these. EBN: *According to Strandis and Bonds (2017), a positive nurse–client relationship aids the client in recognizing their innate ability to maintain their own health and well-being.*
- Help the client identify positive emotions during adverse situations. EBN: *Terrill et al (2017) found that a concentration on positive emotions can introduce strength-based processes in end-of-life care.*
- Build on supportive counseling and therapy. EBN: *Education and counseling are important interventions in client care, but clients can also gain a feeling of well-being and control using their own inner strengths and methods of coping (Sadruddin et al, 2017).*
- Identify protective factors such as assets and resources to enhance coping. EBN: *The reinforcement of beneficial protective influences can improve the resilience of elderly people and facilitate their abilities to deal with possible crises quickly and productively (Yang-Tzu et al, 2019).*
- Provide positive reinforcement and emotional support during the learning process. EBN: *Families caring for family members with dementia face a multitude of problems; dementia specialists found that by using video diaries provided by caregivers, they were able to evaluate and then provide personalized care counseling (Sohyun et al, 2019).*
- Encourage mindfulness, a conscious attention, and awareness of self. EBN: *Key elements that promote the alleviation of stress and encourage resilience are mindfulness and meditation (Savel & Munro, 2017).*
- Educate and encourage the use of stress-reduction techniques. EB: *The use of stress reduction interventions such as relaxation music, mindful meditation, and other relaxation techniques has been accepted and considered valuable as related treatments (Hwang & Bunt, 2020).*
- Enhance knowledge and use of self-care strategies. EBN: *In their study of heart failure clients and self-care, Awoke et al (2019) found that nurses have distinctive skills required to direct educational programs that advance positive health effects.*

Pediatric

- The preceding interventions may be adapted for the pediatric client.
- Promote nurturing, supportive relationships with family. EB: *According to the National Scientific Council on the Developing Child (2015), "Supportive relationships with adults help children develop resilience, or the set of skills needed to respond to adversity and thrive."*
- Facilitate health and well-being opportunities. EB: *Fostering resilience in pediatric clients is an opportunity to cultivate the health and welfare of succeeding generations and subsequently enrich national productivity (Traub & Boynton-Jarrett, 2017).*
- Promote the development of positive mentor relationships. EB: *DeWit et al (2016) found, in their study of supported mentoring, that girls and boys involved in long-term, supported mentoring connections experienced beneficial outcomes.*

▲ Consider referral to appropriate community resource for children who have had adverse childhood experiences. EB: *Curtis (2018), in his study of strength in families, found that the data he collected support counseling programs that concentrate on positive family dynamics to foster strengths.*

REFERENCES

Awoke, M. S., Baptiste, D., Davidson, P., et al. (2019). A quasi-experimental study examining a nurse-led education program to improve knowledge, self-care and reduce readmission for individuals with heart failure. *Contemporary Nurse*, *55*(1), 15–26. https://doi:.org/10.1080/10376178-2019.

Ayoningtyas, I. P. I., Wibowo, M. E., & Purante, E. (2019). Group counseling with self—instruction and cognitive restructuring using techniques to improve decision making. *Jurnal Bimbingan Konseling*, *8*(3), 14–19.

Borji, M., Nourmohammadi, H., Otaghi, M., etal, (2017). Positive effects of cognitive behavioral therapy on depression, anxiety and stress of family caregivers of patients with prostate cancer: a randomized clinical trial. *Asian Pacific Journal of Cancer Prevention, 18*(2), 3207-3212. https://doi:10.22034/APJCP.2017.18.12.3207.

Curtis, A. (2018). *Strengthening families: The relationships between hope, spirituality, resilience and attachments among parents following adverse childhood experiences.* Dissertation PDF. Repository at TWU. Retrieved from https://hdl.handle.net/11274/11018.

DeWit, D., DuBois, D., Erdem, G., Larose, S., & Lipman, E. L. (2016). The role of program-supported mentoring relationships in promoting youth mental health, behavioral and developmental outcomes. *Prevention Science, 17*(5), 646–657. https://doi.org/10.1016/j.iccn.2020.102800.

Gerstenecker, A., Meneses, K., Duff, K., Fiveash, J. B., Marson, D. C., & Triebel, K. L. (2015). Cognitive predictors of understanding treatment decisions in patients with newly diagnosed brain metastasis. *Cancer, 121*(12), 2013–2019. https://doi.org/10.1002/cncr.29326.

Howarth, S., Morris, D., Newlin, M., & Webber, M. (2016). Health and social care interventions which promote social participation for adults with learning disabilities: A review. *British Journal of Learning Disabilities, 44*(1), 3–15. https://doi.org/10.1111/bld.12100.

Hwang, M. H., & Bunt, L. (2020). Relaxation music (RM) mindfulness (MM) and relaxation techniques (RT) on healthcare: A qualitative study of practices in the UK and South Korea. *Approaches: An Interdisciplinary Journal of Music Therapy*. Retrieved from https://uwe-repository.worktribe.com/preview/669115/preview/6691159/Approaches_FirstView-a20200822-hwang.pdf.

Johansson, K., Österberg, S. A., Leskell, J., & Berglund, M. (2016). Patients' experiences of support for learning to live with diabetes to promote health and well-being: A lifeworld phenomenological study. *International Journal of Qualitative Studies on Health and Well-Being, 11*, 31330. https://.doi.org/10.3402/ghw.v11.31330.

National Scientific Council on the Developing Child. (2015). *Supportive relationships and active skill-building strengthen the foundations of resilience: Working paper no. 13*. Retrieved from www.developingchild.harvard.edu. Accessed July 26, 2021.

Sadruddin, S., Rafat, J., Jabber, A. A., Nanji, K., & Name, A. T. (2017). Patient education and mind diversion in supportive care. *British Journal of Nursing, 26*(10), S14–S19. https://doi.org/10.12968/bjon.2017.26.10.S14.

Savel, R. H., & Munro, C. L. (2017). Quiet the mind: Mindfulness, meditation, and the search for inner peace. *American Journal of Critical Care, 26*(6), 433–436. https://doi.org/10.4037/ajcc2017914.

Sohyun, K., Shaw, C., Williams, K. N., et al. (2019). Typology of technology-supported dementia care interventions from an in-home telehealth trial. *Western Journal of Nursing Research, 41*(12), 1724–1746. https://doi.org/10.1177/0193945919825861.

Strandas, M., & Bondas, T. (2018). The nurse–patient relationship as a story of health enhancement in community care: A meta-ethnography. *Journal of Advanced Nursing, 74*(1), 11–22. https://doi.org/10.1161/jan.13389.

Tay, P. K. C., & Lim, K. K. (2020). Psychological resilience as an emergent characteristic for well-being: A pragmatic view. *Gerontology, 66*(5), 476–483. https://doi.org/10.1159/000509210.

Terrill, A. L., Ellington, L., John, K. K., et al. (2018). Positive emotion communication: Fostering well-being at end of life. *Patient Education and Counseling, 101*(4), 631–638. https://doi.org/10.1016/j.pec.2017.11.018.

Traub, F., & Boynton-Jarrett, R. (2017). Modifiable resilience factors to childhood adversity for clinical pediatric practice. *Pediatrics, 139*(5), e20162569. https://doi.org/10.1542/peds.2016-2569.

Yang-Tzu, L., & Tao,-Hsin, T. (2020). Effects of protective factors on depressive status of elderly people in Taiwan. *Medicine (Baltimore), 99*(1), e18461. https:// doi:10.1097/MD.0000000000018461.

Readiness for Enhanced Resilience

Domain 9 Coping/stress tolerance Class 2 Coping responses

Gail B. Ladwig, MSN, RN and Julianne E. Doubet, BSN, RN, EMT-B

R

NANDA-I

Definition

A pattern of ability to recover from perceived adverse or changing situations, through a dynamic process of adaptation, which can be strengthened.

Defining Characteristics

Expresses desire to enhance available resources; expresses desire to enhance communication skills; expresses desire to enhance environmental safety; expresses desire to enhance goal setting; expresses desire to enhance interpersonal relations; expresses desire to enhance involvement in activities; expresses desire to enhance own responsibility for action; expresses desire to enhance positive outlook; expresses desire to enhance progress toward goal; expresses desire to enhance psychological resilience; expresses desire to enhance self-esteem; expresses desire to enhance sense of control; expresses desire to enhance support system; expresses desire to enhance use of conflict management strategies; expresses desire to enhance use of coping skills; expresses desire to enhance use of resources

NOC (Nursing Outcomes Classification)

Suggested NOC Outcomes

Personal Resiliency; Family Resiliency; Quality of Life

Example NOC Outcome with Indicators

Personal Resiliency as evidenced by the following indicator: Adapts to adversities and challenges. (Rate the outcome and indicators of **Personal Resiliency:** 1 = never demonstrated, 2 = rarely demonstrated, 3 = sometimes demonstrated, 4 = often demonstrated, 5 = consistently demonstrated [see Section I].)

Client Outcomes

Client Will (Specify Time Frame)

- Adapt to adversities and challenges
- Communicate clearly and appropriately for age
- Take responsibility for own actions
- Make progress towards goals
- Use effective coping strategies
- Express emotions

NIC (Nursing Interventions Classification)

Suggested NIC Interventions

Resiliency Promotion; Self-Efficacy Enhancement; Counseling; Emotional Support

Example NIC Activities—Self-Efficacy Enhancement

Explore individual's perception of his or her capability to perform the desired behavior

Nursing Interventions and *Rationales*

- Listen to and encourage expressions of feelings and beliefs. EBN: *Listening is the skill of demonstrating interest and sensitivity to another but understanding that wanting to be listened to is also a universal desire (Duarte-Quilao, 2019).*
- Establish a therapeutic relationship based on trust and respect. EBN: *A vital element of nursing practice is the formation of a positive and trusting therapeutic relationship that paves the way for effective client care (Fao et al, 2017).*
- Assist client in rating current level of resilience. EBN: *Maurović and colleagues (2020) link family resilience to the philosophies of individual resilience and community resilience; this connection may pose not only challenges but also solutions.*
- Facilitate supportive family environments and communication. EB: *A study by Waters (2020) suggests that introducing positive practices in family interactions, with the goal of change in family relationship dynamics, may help modify divisive family elements.*
- Assist client to identify and reinforce strengths. EBN: *A sound nurse–client relationship has the potential to identify the client's personal strengths and to encourage their use in the management of the client's own health care (Strandås & Bondas, 2018).*
- Enhance skills associated with social and executive functioning. EB: *Executive functioning is a term used to describe high-level intellectual activities that may include "planning, working memory, inhibition, mental flexibility." These functions facilitate the manner in which people control and adjust their goal-targeted activities (Cropley et al, 2016).*
- Provide positive reinforcement and emotional support during implementation of nursing care. EBN: *In their study concerning the introduction of self-care guidelines for clients who have had a permanent pacemaker placed, researchers found that the guidelines had beneficial effects not only in enhancing the clients' self-care management but also in augmenting all aspects of nursing sensitive clients' outcomes (Ebada et al, 2017).*
- ▲ Facilitate the engagement with mentorship and volunteer opportunities. EB: *Volunteering is consistently recognized as a positive factor in enriching one's sense of purpose and meaning (Johnson, 2017).*
- Determine how family behavior affects the client. EBN: *As the family is usually the most dedicated support system for clients, it is essential that the nurse evaluate the family's circumstances and then subsidize the family's decision-making abilities (Judha, 2019).* EB: *Family can be instrumental in fostering resilience when faced with adverse difficulties (Theiss, 2018).*

R

- Promote use of mindfulness and other stress-reduction techniques. EB: *In their study of the use of mindfulness-based stress reduction (MBSR) in Parkinson's disease, McClean et al (2017) noted that the use of MBSR as an intervention has increased and improved outcomes in a mix of long-term conditions, including stress and depression.*

Pediatric

- The preceding interventions may be adapted for the pediatric client.
- Encourage the promotion of protective factors by fostering the seeking of opportunities to improve cognitive abilities, such as tutoring and other resources; the development of positive and supportive relations such as family, community members, or mentors; and the improvement of general health. EB: *According to Lehrer et al (2017), adolescents who experience positive emotions and receive social support will develop an increased sense of well-being.*

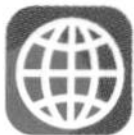

Multicultural

- Use teaching strategies that are culturally and age appropriate. EBN: *Lee et al (2020), in their study of nurses' cultural competence capabilities, realized that it is necessary for nurses to distinguish cultural variances and utilize unique communication skills to deliver client-centered nursing care to those from diverse backgrounds.*

REFERENCES

Cropley, M., Zijlstra, F. R. H., Querstret, D., & Beck, S. (2016). Is work-related rumination associated with deficits in executive functioning? *Frontiers in Psychology, 7*, 1524. https://doi.org/10.3389/fpsyg.2016.01524.

Duarte-Quilao, T. (2019). *A living experience of being listened to: A parsesciencing inquiry [Dissertation]*. New York: CUNY University of New York. Retrieved from academicworks.cuny.edu/gc_etds/3166. [Accessed 26 July 2021].

Ebada, R. A., El Senousy, T. A., Mohamed, S. Y., & Abdelatief, D. A. (2017). Effects of self-care management on nursing-sensitive patients' outcomes after permanent pacemaker implantation. *Egyptian Journal of Health Care, 8*(1), 294–313. https://doi.10.21608/EJHC.2017.23165.

Fao, R., Rasmussen, P., Wiechula, R., Conroy, T., & Kitson, A. (2017). Developing effective and caring nurse-patient relationships. *Nursing Standard, 31*(28), 54–63. https://doi.org/10.7748/ns.2017.e10735.

Johnson, S. S. (2017). The art of health promotion ideas for improving health outcomes. *American Journal of Health Promotion, 31*(2), 163–164. https://doi.org/10.1177/0890117117691705.

Judha, M. (2019). Family perception in readiness accepting discharge planning determined by nursing advocacy program. *Indonesian Journal of Education and Clinic, 4*(2). http://doi.org/10.24990/injec.v4i2.268.

Lee, Y. H., Lin, S. C., Wang, P. Y., & Lin, M. H. (2020). Objective structural clinical examination for evaluating learning efficacy of Cultural Competence Cultivation Programme for nurses. *BMC Nursing, 19*(1), 114. https://doi.org/10.21203/rs.3.rs-55953/v1.

Lehrer, H. M., Janus, K. C., Gloria, C. T., & Steinhardt, M. A. (2017). Personal and environmental resources mediate the positivity-emotional dysfunction relationship. *American Journal of Health Behavior, 41*(2), 186–193. https://doi.org/10.5993/AJHB.41.2.10.

Maurović, I., Liebenberg, L., & Ferić, M. (2020). A review of family resilience: Understanding the concept and operationalization challenges to inform research and practice. *Child Care in Practice, 26*(4), 337–357. https://doi.org/10.1080/13575279.2020.1792838.

McClean, G., Lawrence, M., Simpson, R., & Mercer, S. W. (2017). Mindfulness-based stress reduction in Parkinson's disease: A systematic review. *BMC Neurology, 17*(1), 92. https://doi.org/10.1186/s12883-017-0876-4.

Strandås, M., & Bondas, T. (2018). The nurse-patient relationship as a story of health enhancement in community care: A meta ethnography. *Journal of Advanced Nursing, 74*(1), 11–22. https://doi.org/10.1111/jan.13389.

Theiss, J. A. (2018). Family communication and resilience. *Journal of Applied Communication Research, 46*(1), 10–13. https//doi.org/10.1080/00909882.2018.1426706.

Waters, L. (2020). Using positive psychology interventions to strengthen family happiness: A family systems approach. *The Journal of Positive Psychology, 15*(5), 645–652. https://doi.org/10.1080/17439760.2020.1789704.

R

Risk for Impaired Resilience

Domain 9 Coping/stress tolerance Class 2 Coping responses

Gail B. Ladwig, MSN, RN and Julianne E. Doubet, BSN, RN, EMT-B

NANDA-I

Definition

Susceptible to decreased ability to recover from perceived adverse or changing situations, through a dynamic process of adaptation, which may compromise health.

Risk Factors

Altered family relations; community violence; disrupted family rituals; disrupted family roles; dysfunctional family processes; inadequate health resources; inadequate social support; inconsistent parenting; ineffective family adaptation; multiple coexisting adverse situations; perceived vulnerability; substance misuse

At-Risk Population

Economically disadvantaged individuals; individuals experiencing a new crisis; individuals experiencing chronic crisis; individuals exposed to violence; individuals who are members of an ethnic minority; individuals whose parents have mental disorders; individuals with history of exposure to violence; individuals with large families; mothers with low educational level; women

Associated Conditions

Intellectual disability; psychological disorder

NOC (Nursing Outcomes Classification)

Suggested NOC Outcomes

Personal Resiliency; Family Resiliency; Knowledge: Health Resources

Example NOC Outcome with Indicators

Personal Resiliency as evidenced by the following indicator: Takes responsibility for own actions. (Rate the outcome and indicators of **Personal Resiliency:** 1 = never demonstrated, 2 = rarely demonstrated, 3 = sometimes demonstrated, 4 = often demonstrated, 5 = consistently demonstrated [see Section I].)

Client Outcomes

Client Will (Specify Time Frame)

- Identify available community resources
- Propose practical, constructive solutions for disputes
- Identify and access community resources for assistance
- Accept assistance with activities of daily living from family and friends
- Verbalize an enhanced sense of control
- Verbalize meaningfulness of one's life

NIC (Nursing Interventions Classification)

Suggested NIC Interventions

Resiliency Promotion; Assertiveness Training; Values Clarification; Parenting Promotion

Example NIC Activities—Resiliency Promotion

Encourage family involvement with child's schoolwork and activities; Assist family in providing atmosphere conducive to learning

Nursing Interventions and *Rationales*

- Determine how family behavior affects client. EBN: *The model of resilience is based on the presupposition that individuals and families are connected to each other and their community and have collective strengths, which will help them compensate for their adversity (Deist & Greeff, 2015).*
- Help the client to identify personal rights, responsibilities, and conflicting norms. EBN: *According to Salmond and Echevarria (2017), in their study of nursing in a rapidly shifting health care milieu, the end results of comprehensive health care are subject to a series of considerations beyond that of the clinical, such as environment, social and economic conditions, and the client's own health maintenance behaviors.*

R

- Encourage consideration of values underlying choices and consequences of the choice. EBN: *A study found that acceptance of responsibility must take place before one can make lifestyle choices and/or feel satisfaction for these choices (Finderup et al, 2016).*
- Help the client practice conversational and social skills. EBN: *When it is evident that a client's active participation in self-care is diminished, the next step is to incorporate a facilitator in the process (du Pon et al, 2019).*
- Assist client to prioritize values. EBN: *Evidence-based practice merges cutting-edge research with clinical proficiency and client values to implement objective interventions for favorable client outcomes and improvement in quality of life (Butcher, 2016).*
- Foster an accepting, nonjudgmental atmosphere. EB: *The results of a study by Usaite and Cameron (2015) found that active participation in pleasurable but structured pastimes can enrich the lives of children and their families by promoting "a positive sense of self, constructive relationships, roles, routines and responsibilities."*
- Help to identify self-defeating thoughts. EBN: *McRae (2016) writes, in her article concerning emotional regulation, that a commonly used approach to help manage a client's emotional insecurity is cognitive appraisal; this strategy involves shifting the manner in which the client envisages a past stressful situation and then generates a positive modification to the negative stressor.*

▲ Refer to community resources/social services as appropriate. EB: *Social support is assistance provided by others in the community that promotes and maintains a client's well-being and resilience (Fuentes-Peláez et al, 2016).*

▲ Help clarify problem areas in interpersonal relationships. EB: *It is well established that appropriate communications are not only connective but also indispensable in interpersonal relationships: communication competencies are key to the construction of social connections (Trancă & Neagoe, 2018).*

▲ Promote a sense of an individual's autonomy and control over choices to be made in one's environment. EBN: Meeting one's psychological needs and goals is thought to contribute to a sense of well-being and to support autonomy, especially in the selection of beneficial options that can influence "value, self-respect, and dignity" (*Liu et al, 2020*).

▲ Identify and enroll high-risk families in follow-up programs. EBN: Programs aimed at community health are offered by local agencies to assist in the adjustment of attitudes toward culture and relationships and by fostering affirmative means of communication in schools, peer groups, and families (*Horner, 2017*).

REFERENCES

Butcher, H. K. (2016). Development and use of gerontological evidence-based practice guidelines. *Journal of Gerontological Nursing*, *42*(7), 25–32. https://doi.org/10.3928/00989134-20160613-02.

Deist, M., & Greeff, A. P. (2015). Resilience in family members caring for a family member diagnosed with dementia. *Educational Gerontology*, *41*(2), 93–105. https://doi.org/10.1080/03601277.2014.942146.

du Pon, E., Wildeboer, A. T., van Dooren, A. A., Bilo, H. J. G., Kleefstra, N., & van Dulmen, S. (2019). Active participation of patients with type 2 diabetes in consultations with their primary care practice nurses—what helps and what hinders: A qualitative study. *BMC Health Services Research*, *19*(1), 814. https://doi.org/10.1186/s12913-019-4572-5.

Finderup, J., Bjerre, T., Soendergaard, A., Nielsen, M. E., & Zoffmann, V. (2016). Developing life skills in haemodialysis using the guided self-determination method: A qualitative study. *Journal of Renal Care*, *42*(2), 83–92. https://doi.org/10.1111/jorc.12146.

Fuentes-Peláez, N., Balsells, M. À., Fernández, J., Vaquero, E., & Amorós, P. (2016). The social support in kinship foster care: A way to enhance resilience. *Child & Family Social Work*, *21*(4), 581–590. https://doi.org/10.1111/cfs.12182.

Horner, G. (2017). Resilience. *Journal of Pediatric Health*, *31*(3), 384–390. https://doi.org/10.1016/j.pedhc.2016.09.005.

Liu, L. H., Kao, C. C., & Ying, J. C. (2020). Functional capacity and life satisfaction in older adult residents living in long-term care facilities: The mediator of autonomy. *Journal of Nursing Research*, *28*(4), e102. https://doi: 10.1097/JNR.0000000000000362.

McRae, K. (2016). Cognitive emotion regulation: A review of theory and scientific findings. *Current Opinion in Behavioral Sciences*, *10*, 119–124. https://doi.org/10.1016/j.cobeha.2016.06.004.

Salmond, S. W., & Echevarria, M. (2017). Healthcare transformation and changing roles for nursing. *Orthopedic Nursing*, *36*(1), 12–25. https://doi.1097/NOR.0000000000000308.

Trancă, L. M., & Neagoe, A. (2018). The importance of positive language for the quality of interpersonal relationships. *Agora Psycho-Pragmatica*, *12*(1), 69–77.

Usaite, K., & Cameron, J. (2015). Participation in enjoyable activities can promote resilience in young people [Abstract]. *British Journal of Occupational Therapy*, *78*(8 Suppl. l), 2–3.

R

Parental Role Conflict Domain 7 Role relationship Class 3 Role performance

Marina Martinez-Kratz, MS, RN, CNE

NANDA-I

Definition

Parental experience of role confusion and conflict in response to crisis.

Defining Characteristics

Anxiety; disrupted caregiver routines; expresses fear; expresses frustration; perceived inadequacy to provide for child's needs; perceived loss of control over decisions relating to child; reluctance to participate in usual caregiver activities; reports concern about change in parental role; reports concern about family; reports feeling guilty

Related Factors

Interruptions in family life due to home treatment regimen; intimidated by invasive modalities; intimidation by restrictive modalities; parent–child separation

At-Risk Population

Individuals living in nontraditional setting; individuals undergoing changes in marital status; parents with child requiring home care for special needs

NOC (Nursing Outcomes Classification)

Suggested NOC Outcomes

Caregiver Emotional Health; Caregiver Well-Being; Caregiver Lifestyle Disruption; Coping; Parenting Performance; Role Performance; Family Coping

Example NOC Outcome with Indicators

Family Coping as evidenced by the following indicators: Establishes role flexibility/Manages family problems/Uses family-centered stress reduction activities. (Rate the outcome and indicators of **Family Coping:** 1 = never demonstrated, 2 = rarely demonstrated, 3 = sometimes demonstrated, 4 = often demonstrated, 5 = consistently demonstrated [see Section I].)

Client Outcomes

Client Will (Specify Time Frame)

- Express feelings and perceptions regarding effects of illness, disability, and/or hospitalization on parental role
- Participate in hospital and home care as much as able given the availability of resources and support systems
- Exhibit assertiveness and responsibility in active family decision-making regarding care of the child
- Describe and select available resources to support parental management of the needs of the child and family

NIC (Nursing Interventions Classification)

Suggested NIC Interventions

Caregiver Support; Counseling; Decision-Making Support; Family Process Maintenance; Family Therapy; Parenting Promotion; Role Enhancement

Example NIC Activities—Role Enhancement

Teach new behaviors needed by client/parent to fulfill a role; Serve as role model for learning new behaviors as appropriate

R

Nursing Interventions and *Rationales*

- Assess and support parent's previous coping behaviors. EBN: *Understanding what experience a parent has with coping will enable the nurse to support the parents in the current situation (Senger et al, 2016).*
- Assess for the following signs of parental burnout: exhaustion in one's parental role, contrast with previous parental self, feelings of being fed up with one's parental role, and emotional distancing from one's children. EB: *A study to measure parental burnout identified the four dimensions of parental burnout syndrome as exhaustion in one's parental role, contrast with previous parental self, feelings of being fed up with one's parental role, and emotional distancing from one's children (Roskam, Brianda, & Mikoljczak, 2018).*
- Determine parent/family sources of stress, using the Parental Stress Scale. CEB: *The Parental Stress Scale is a valid and reliable self-report scale that contains 18 items representing pleasure or positive themes of parenthood (Berry & Jones, 1995).*
- Evaluate the family's perceived strength of its social support system. Encourage the family to use social support. EB: *A study of African American mothers found that social support moderated the relationship between parental stress and child behavior (Royal et al, 2017).*
- Determine the older childbearing woman's support systems and expectations for motherhood. EBN: *Supporting mothers during their transition into parenthood can assist with the bonding of the mother and the infant (Gilmer et al, 2016).*
- Use family-centered care and role modeling for holistic care of families. EBN: *Incorporating family-centered care helps enhance the parents' role in caring for their child (Cady et al, 2015).*
- ▲ Maintain parental involvement in shared decision-making regarding care by using the following steps: incorporate parents' information concerning the child's typical routines, behaviors, fears, likes, and dislikes; provide clear and direct firsthand information concerning the child's condition and progress; normalize the home/hospital environment as much as possible; and collaborate in care by providing choices when possible. EB: *A study found that parental involvement in decision-making was related to clinician communication and information sharing (Links et al, 2020).*
- Seek and support parental participation in care. EBN: *Nurses can support parents' participation in their child's care through a family-friendly environment, counseling, and good communication (Palomaa, Korhonen, & Pölkki, 2016).*
- ▲ Inform parents of financial resources, respite care, and home support to assist them in maintaining sufficient energy and personal resources to continue caregiving responsibilities. EB: *There can be a financial burden on parents of children with chronic illness and a need to help the family identify their resources (Stewart et al, 2016).*
- Provide family-centered care: allow parents to touch and talk to the child, and assist in the handling of medical equipment; offer open visiting hours; promote family presence at the bedside; promote open communication; provide for privacy. EBN: *Family-centered care can support family involvement with a child's care and decrease the stress associated with a child's hospitalization (Coats et al, 2018).*
- Refer parents to available telephone and/or Internet support groups. EB: *A study found that peer support meetings moderated by resource parents provided a unique and useful means to support NICU parents (Dahan et al, 2020).*
- Involve new mother's partner or parents in clinical encounters and invite family members to discuss their expectations and parenting experiences. EBN: *Health care providers realize the importance of family-centered care of the infant to help the mother and her partner care for the infant (Dzubaty, 2016).*

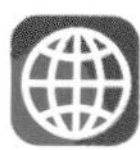

Multicultural

- Acknowledge racial/ethnic differences at the onset of care. EBN: *Providing culturally competent care is important to health care equality, and it is important for nurses to understand the importance of identifying the cultural differences that their clients will require (Dzubaty, 2016).*
- Assess for the influence of cultural beliefs, norms, and values on the client's perceptions of the parental role. EBN: *Understanding the cultures and beliefs of parents can enhance the interactions between nurse and family and assist the nurse to better care for the child and their family (Xiong et al, 2016).*
- Acknowledge that value conflicts arising from acculturation stresses may contribute to increased anxiety and significant conflict with the parental role. EB: *Study results suggest that lower acculturation conflict is associated with higher perceptions of general parenting competence for both Asian and Latin American parents (Kiang, Glatz, & Buchanan, 2017).*

▲ Refer parents of young children in specific cultural communities to support programs. EBN: *Parents and children benefit when a support group is incorporated into the care (Thomson-Salo et al, 2017).*

Home Care

- The interventions described previously may be adapted for home care use.
- Assess family preference for prenatal and postpartum visits; assist new parents to renegotiate parenting roles and responsibilities with coparenting. EB: *A cross-sectional survey of postpartum clients found that current prenatal and postpartum care delivery does not match clients' preferences for the number of visits or between-visit contacts. Clients also expressed openness to alternative models of prenatal care, including remote monitoring (Peahl et al, 2020).*

Client/Family Teaching and Discharge Planning

- Offer family-led education interventions to improve participants' knowledge about their condition and its treatment and decrease their information needs. EBN: *A study of caregivers found an association between the Stress-related Vulnerability Scale (SVS) and the perception of the usefulness of health care education (Di Stasio et al, 2020).*
- Encourage children and parent involvement in bereavement support groups, as an adjunct to grief therapy. EB: *A systematic review found that online support groups may be a useful adjunct to, but not an alternative to, grief therapy or counseling (Robinson & Pond, 2019).*

▲ Refer to a parenting program to facilitate learning of parenting skills. EBN: *A study of foster parents showed that participation in parenting programs increased levels of skills and knowledge following training than did those in the control group (Solomon, Niec, & Schoonover, 2017).*

- Teach the client about available community resources (e.g., therapists, ministers, counselors, self-help groups). EBN: *Community-based resources can support caregivers and ensure that they can identify needed services (Tallon et al, 2017).*

REFERENCES

Berry, J. O., & Jones, W. H. (1995). The parental stress scale: Initial psychometric evidence. *Journal of Social and Personal Relationships, 12*(3), 463–472. https://doi.org/10.1177/0265407595123009.

Cady, R. G., Looman, W. S., Lindeke, L. L., et al. (2015). Pediatric care coordination: Lessons learned and future priorities. *Online Journal of Issues in Nursing, 20*(3), 30. https://doi.org//10.3912/OJIN.Vol20No03Man03.

Coats, H., Bourget, E., Starks, H., et al. (2018). Nurses' reflections on benefits and challenges of implementing family-centered care in pediatric intensive care units. *American Journal of Critical Care, 27*(1), 52–58. https://doi.org/10.4037/ajcc2018353.

Dahan, S., Bourque, C. J., Reichherzer, M., et al. (2020). Peer support groups for families in neonatology: Why and how to get started? *Acta Paediatrica, 109*, 2525–2531. https://doi.org/10.1111/apa.15312.

Di Stasio, E., Di Simone, E., & Galeti, A. (2020). Stress-related vulnerability and usefulness of healthcare education in Parkinson's disease: The perception of a group of family caregivers, a cross-sectional study. *Applied Nursing Research, 51*, 151186. https://doi.org/10.1016/j.apnr.2019.151186.

Dzubaty, D. R. (2016). Providing family-centered care in maternal-newborn settings: A case study. *Newborn and Infant Nursing Reviews, 16*(2), 55–57. https://doi.org/10.1053/j.nainr.2016.03.006.

Gilmer, C., Buchan, J. L., Letourneau, N., et al. (2016). Parent education interventions designed to support the transition to parenthood: A realist review. *International Journal of Nursing Studies, 59*(Suppl. C), 118–133. https://doi.org/10.1016/j.ijnurstu.2016.03.015.

Kiang, L., Glatz, T., & Buchanan, C.M. (2017). Acculturation conflict, cultural parenting self-efficacy, and perceived parenting competence in Asian American and Latino/a families. *Family Process, 56*(4), 943-961.

Links, A.R., Callon, W. Wasserman, C., et al. (2020). Parental role in decision-making for pediatric surgery: Perceptions of involvement in consultations for tonsillectomy. *Patient Education and Counseling, 103*(5), 944-951. https://doi.org/10.1111/famp.12266.

Palomaa, A. K., Korhonen, A., & Pölkki, T. (2016). Factors influencing parental participation in neonatal pain alleviation. *Journal of Pediatric Nursing, 31*(5), 519–527. https://doi.org/10.1016/j.pedn.2016.05.004.

Peahl, A. F., Novara, A., Heisler, M., Dalton, V. K., Moniz, M. H., & Smith, R. D. (2020). Patient preferences for prenatal and postpartum care delivery. *Obstetrics & Gynecology, 135*(5), 1038–1046. https://doi.org/10.1097/AOG.0000000000003731.

Robinson, C., & Pond, R. (2019). Do online support groups for grief benefit the bereaved? Systematic review of the quantitative and qualitative literature. *Computers in Human Behavior, 100*, 48–59. https://doi.org/10.1016/j.chb.2019.06.011.

Roskam, I., Brianda, M. E., & Mikolajczak, M. (2018). A step forward in the conceptualization and measurement of parental burnout: The Parental Burnout Assessment (PBA). *Frontiers in Psychology, 9*, 758. https://doi.org/10.3389/fpsyg.2018.00758.

Royal, K. J., Eaton, S. C., Smith, N., Cliette, G., & Livingston, J. N. (2017). The impact of parental stress and social support on behavioral outcomes of children in African American single-mother households. *Journal of Black Sexuality and Relationships, 3*(4), 17–33. https://doi.org/10.1353/bsr.2017.0011.

Senger, B. A., Ward, L. D., Barbosa-Leiker, C., & Bindler, R. C. (2016). Stress and coping of parents caring for a child with mitochondrial disease. *Applied Nursing Research, 29*(Suppl. C), 195–201. https://doi.org/10.1016/j.apnr.2015.03.010.

Solomon, D. T., Niec, L. N., & Schoonover, C. E. (2017). The impact of foster parent training on parenting skills and child disruptive behavior: A meta-analysis. *Child Maltreatment, 22*(1), 3–13. https://doi.org/10.1177/1077559516679514.

Stewart, M., Evans, J., Letourneau, N., Masuda, J., Almond, A., & Edey, J. (2016). Low-income children, adolescents, and caregivers facing

R

respiratory problems: Support needs and preferences. *Journal of Pediatric Nursing, 31*(3), 319–329. https://doi.org/10.1016/j.pedn.2015.11.013.

Tallon, M. M., Kendall, G. E., Priddis, L., Newall, F., & Young, J. (2017). Barriers to addressing social determinants of health in pediatric nursing practice: An integrative review. *Journal of Pediatric Nursing, 37*(Suppl. C), 51–56. https://doi.org/10.1016/j.pedn.2017.06.009.

Thomson-Salo, F., Kuschel, C. A., Kamlin, O. F., & Cuzzilla, R. (2017). A fathers' group in NICU: Recognising and responding to paternal stress, utilising peer support. *Journal of Neonatal Nursing, 23*(6), 294–298. https://doi.org/10.1016/j.jnn.2017.04.001.

Xiong, S., Degroote, N., Byington, H., Harder, J., Kaminski, K., & Haglund, K. (2016). Engaging in culturally informed nursing care with Hmong children and their families. *Journal of Pediatric Nursing, 31*(1), 102–106. https://doi.org/10.1016/j.pedn.2015.08.008.

Ineffective Role Performance

Domain 7 Role relationship Class 3 Role performance

Marina Martinez-Kratz, MS, RN, CNE

NANDA-I

Definition

A pattern of behavior and self-expression that does not match the environmental context, norms, and expectations.

Defining Characteristics

Altered pattern of responsibility; altered perception of role by others; altered role perception; altered role resumption; anxiety; depressive symptoms; domestic violence; harassment; inadequate confidence; inadequate external support for role enactment; inadequate knowledge of role requirements; inadequate motivation; inadequate opportunity for role enactment; inadequate self-management; inadequate skills; inappropriate developmental expectations; ineffective adaptation to change; ineffective coping strategies; ineffective role performance; perceived social discrimination; pessimism; powerlessness; reports social discrimination; role ambivalence; role denial; role dissatisfaction; system conflict; uncertainty

Related Factors

Altered body image; conflict; fatigue; inadequate health resources; inadequate psychosocial support system; inadequate rewards; inadequate role models; inadequate role preparation; inadequate role socialization; inappropriate linkage with the health care system; low self-esteem; pain; role conflict; role confusion; role strain; stressors; substance misuse; unaddressed domestic violence; unrealistic role expectations

R

At-Risk Population

Economically disadvantaged individuals; individuals with developmental level inappropriate for role expectation; individuals with high demand job role; individuals with low educational level

Associated Conditions

Depression; neurological defect; personality disorders; physical illness; psychosis

NOC (Nursing Outcomes Classification)

Suggested NOC Outcomes

Coping; Psychosocial Adjustment: Life Change; Role Performance

Example NOC Outcome with Indicators

Role Performance as evidenced by the following indicators: Knowledge of role transition periods/Reported comfort with role changes. (Rate the outcome and indicators of **Role Performance:** 1 = not adequate, 2 = slightly adequate, 3 = moderately adequate, 4 = substantially adequate, 5 = totally adequate [see Section I].)

Client Outcomes

Client Will (Specify Time Frame)

- Identify realistic perception of role
- State personal strengths
- Acknowledge problems contributing to inability to perform usual role
- Accept physical limitations regarding role responsibility and consider ways to change lifestyle to accomplish goals associated with role performance
- Demonstrate knowledge of appropriate behaviors associated with new or changed role
- State knowledge of change in responsibility and new behaviors associated with new responsibility
- Verbalize acceptance of new responsibility

NIC (Nursing Interventions Classification)

Suggested NIC Intervention

Role Enhancement

Example NIC Activities—Role Enhancement

Assist client to identify behaviors needed for role development; Assist client to identify positive strategies for managing role changes

Nursing Interventions and *Rationales*

- Assess the client's level of resilience and implement nursing actions that increase client resilience and sense of coherence. EBN: *A study of individuals with chronic obstructive pulmonary disease indicated that high levels of a sense of coherence and resilience were negatively associated with symptoms of anxiety and depression and perceived illness-specific disability (Keil et al, 2017).*
- Assess the effect of uncertainty on the client's role and provide support and education. EBN: *A study of caregivers with hospitalized children showed that levels of uncertainty and stress decreased and role performance improved after an educational intervention (Jeong & Kwon, 2017).*
- Assess the client's social support system. EB: *A study showed that clients with good social support are more likely to change their lifestyle and make more changes (Clementi et al, 2016).*
- Assess for the presence of shame related to current health situation. EBN: *A Greek study of intensive care unit (ICU) families found that family members who live with the client and have low educational levels are prone to feel shame, which could interfere with coping and caregiving (Koulouras et al, 2017).*
- Assess for the characteristics of role stress. EB: *A study showed that a lack of role clarity was significantly linked to emotional exhaustion (Portoghese et al, 2017).*
- Assess male military members for gender role stressors with the Male Gender Role Stressor Inventory (MGRSI). EB: *Research piloting the MGRSI found that honor, strength, and achievement were the most commonly reported sources of male gender role stress and may be associated with suicidal behaviors (Sterling et al, 2017).*
- Ask the client what they need to feel prepared for the tasks and demands of their role. EBN: *A study of family caregivers found the need for services to address emotional needs and resources to mitigate the stress of caregiving (Muliira, Kizza, & Nakitende, 2019).*
- Support the client's spirituality practices. EB: *Spiritual care was found to reduce care strain in caregivers of elderly clients with Alzheimer's disease (Mahdavi et al, 2017).*
- Refer to the care plans for Readiness for Enhanced Family **Coping,** Readiness for Enhanced **Decision-Making,** Ineffective **Home** Maintenance Behaviors, Impaired **Parenting,** Risk for **Loneliness,** Readiness for Enhanced Community **Coping,** Readiness for Enhanced **Self-Care,** and Ineffective **Sexuality** Pattern.

Pediatric

▲ Provide parents of disabled children with information about and referrals to educational and social resources available to assist their child. EB: *A longitudinal study found that parents' educational expectations shape academic development and changes in self-concept among young people with different types of disabilities (McCoy et al, 2016).*

R

- Provide parents with information about mindfulness-based interventions (MBIs) to enhance coping when the role change is associated with a critically and chronically ill child. EB: *Research found that MBI is a culturally adaptable, acceptable, and effective method to improve quality of life and positive stress reappraisal coping in parents of children with autism spectrum disorder (Rayun & Ahmad, 2016).*

Geriatric

- Assess older adults' choices regarding their care and enable them to live as they wish and receive the help they want by carefully listening to their stories. EB: *A study found that complementing standardized assessment data with informal interviews provided information that older adults and their families believed was important to their care (Lafortune et al, 2017).*
- Assess older adults for a sense of competence in their daily life. EB: *A French study showed that increased competence was associated with a decrease in depressive symptoms and apathy (Souesme et al, 2016).*
- Provide support and practice for older adults to use technology. EB: *A study found that participants used information and communication technology (ICT) to connect with friends and family. ICT use predicted higher well-being across outcomes (Sims et al, 2017).*
- Support the client's spiritual beliefs and activities and provide appropriate spiritual support persons. EB: *Spiritual care was found to reduce care strain in caregivers of elderly clients with Alzheimer's disease (Mahdavi et al, 2017).*

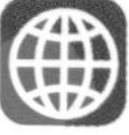

Multicultural

- Assess for the influence of cultural beliefs, norms, values, and expectations on the individual's role. CEB: *The individual's role may be based on cultural perceptions (Leininger & McFarland, 2002).*
- Negotiate with the client regarding the aspects of their role that can be modified and still honor cultural beliefs. CEB: *Give-and-take with the client will lead to culturally congruent care (Leininger & McFarland, 2002).*
- Identify perceived barriers to family to use support groups or other service programs to assist with role changes. EB: *A systematic review identified that assessment for support resources, home care, or community assistance was needed before discharge and at routine intervals throughout the care situation (Greenwood et al, 2015).*
- The preceding interventions may be adapted for home care use.

Client/Family Teaching and Discharge Planning

- ▲ Refer client to comprehensive services to assist with transition needs at discharge. EB: *A study found no 30-day rehospitalizations for participants in the Kentucky Care Coordination for Community Transitions (KCT-T-3) program, which provided access to medical, social, and environmental services to support community transitions (Kitzman et al, 2017).*
- Provide educational materials to family members on client behavior management plus caregiver stress-coping management. EB: *Research has identified that multiple components to provide education, support, counseling, care continuity, and linkage to community resources to ease transitions can improve caregiver health and coping (Naylor et al, 2017).*
- Help the client identify resources for assistance in caring for a disabled or aging parent (e.g., adult day care, nursing home placement). EB: *A systematic review identified that assessment for support resources, home care, or community assistance was needed before discharge and at routine intervals throughout the care situation (Greenwood et al, 2015).*

REFERENCES

Clementi, S., Ernandez, E., Barile, G. P., Rivera, S., & Gonella, M. (2016). The role of psychosocial status in the change of lifestyles in patients with colorectal cancer in follow up. *Annals of Oncology*, *27*(Suppl. 4), iv81. https://doi:10.1093/annonc/mdw339.06.

Greenwood, N., Habibi, R., Smith, R., & Manthorpe, J. (2015). Barriers to access and minority ethnic carers' satisfaction with social care services in the community: A systematic review of qualitative and quantitative literature. *Health and Social Care in the Community*, *23*(1), 64–78. https://doi:10.1111/hsc.12116.

Jeong, E., & Kwon, I. S. (2017). Effect of caregiver's role improvement program on the uncertainty, stress, and role performance of caregivers with hospitalized children. *Child Health Nursing Research*, *23*(1), 70–80. https://doi:10.4094/chnr.2017.23.1.70.

Keil, D. C., Vaske, I., Kenn, K., Rief, W., & Stenzel, N. M. (2017). With the strength to carry on: The role of sense of coherence and resilience for anxiety, depression and disability in chronic obstructive pulmonary disease. *Chronic Respiratory Disease*, *14*(1), 11–21. https://doi:10.1177/1479972316654286.

Kitzman, P., Hudson, K., Sylvia, V., Feltner, F., & Lovins, J. (2017). Care coordination for community transitions for individuals post-stroke returning to low-resource rural communities. *Journal*

R

of Community Health, 42(3), 565–572. https://doi:10.1007/s10900-016-0289-0.

Koulouras, V., Konstanti, Z., Lepida, D., Papathanakos, G., & Gouva, M. (2017). Shame feeling in the intensive care unit patient's family members. *Intensive and Critical Care Nursing*, *41*, 84–89. https://doi:10.1016/j.iccn.2017.03.011.

Lafortune, C., Elliott, J., Egan, M. Y., & Stolee, P. (2017). The rest of the story: A qualitative study of complementing standardized assessment data with informal interviews with older patients and families. *The Patient—Patient-Centered Outcomes Research*, *10*(2), 215–224. https://doi:10.1007/s40271-016-0193-9.

Leininger, M. M., & McFarland, M. R. (2002). *Transcultural nursing: Concepts, theories, research and practices* (3rd ed.). New York: McGraw-Hill.

Mahdavi, B., Fallahi-Khoshknab, M., Mohammadi, F., Hosseini, M. A., & Haghi, M. (2017). Effects of spiritual group therapy on caregiver strain in home caregivers of the elderly with Alzheimer's disease. *Archives of Psychiatric Nursing*, *31*(3), 269–273. https://doi.org/10.1016/j.apnu.2016.12.003.

McCoy, S., Maître, B., Watson, D., & Banks, J. (2016). The role of parental expectations in understanding social and academic well-being among children with disabilities in Ireland. *European Journal of Special Needs Education*, *31*(4), 535–552. https://doi:10.1080/08856257.2016.1199607.

Muliira, J. K., Kizza, I. B., & Nakitende, G. (2019). Roles of family caregivers and perceived burden when caring for hospitalized adult cancer patients: Perspective from a low-income country. *Cancer Nursing*, *42*(3), 208–217. https://doi.org/10.1097/NCC.0000000000000591.

Naylor, M. D., Shaid, E. C., Carpenter, D., et al. (2017). Components of comprehensive and effective transitional care. *Journal of the American Geriatrics Society*, *65*(6), 1119–1125. https://doi:10.1111/jgs.14782.

Portoghese, I., Galletta, M., Burdorf, A., Cocco, P. ,D., Aloja, E., & Campagna, M. (2017). Role stress and emotional exhaustion among health care workers: The buffering effect of supportive coworker climate in a multilevel perspective. *Journal of Occupational and Environmental Medicine*, *59*(10), e187–e193. https://doi:10.1097/JOM.0000000000001122.

Rayun, A., & Ahmad, M. (2016). Effectiveness of mindfulness-based interventions on quality of life and positive reappraisal coping among parents of children with autism spectrum disorder. *Research in Developmental Disabilities*, *55*, 185–196. https://doi:10.1016/j.ridd.2016.04.002.

Sims, T., Reed, A. E., & Carr, D. C. (2017). Information and communication technology use is related to higher well-being among the oldest-old. *Journals of Gerontology Series B: Psychological Sciences and Social Sciences*, *72*(5), 761–770. https://doi:10.1093/geronb/gbw130.

Souesme, G., Martinent, G., & Ferrand, C. (2016). Perceived autonomy support, psychological needs satisfaction, depressive symptoms and apathy in French hospitalized older people. *Archives of Gerontology and Geriatrics*, *65*, 70–78. https://doi:10.1016/j.archger.2016.03.001.

Sterling, A.G., 4th, Bakalar, J.L., Perera, K.U., et al. (2017). Perspectives of suicide bereaved individuals on military suicide decedents' life stressors and male gender role stress. *Archives of Suicide Research*, *21*(1), 155–168. https://doi:10.1080/13811118.2016.1166087.

Sedentary Lifestyle

Domain 1 Health promotion Class 1 Health awareness

Marina Martinez-Kratz, MS, RN, CNE

NANDA-I

Definition

An acquired mode of behavior that is characterized by waking hour activities that require low energy expenditure.

Defining Characteristics

Average daily physical activity is less than recommended for age and gender; chooses a daily routine lacking physical exercise; does not exercise during leisure time; expresses preference for low physical activity; performs majority of tasks in a reclining posture; performs majority of tasks in a sitting posture; physical deconditioning

Related Factors

Conflict between cultural beliefs and health practices; decreased activity tolerance; difficulty adapting areas for physical activity; exceeds screen time recommendations for age; impaired physical mobility; inadequate interest in physical activity; inadequate knowledge of consequences of sedentarism; inadequate knowledge of health benefits associated with physical activity; inadequate motivation for physical activity; inadequate resources for physical activity; inadequate role models; inadequate social support; inadequate time management skills; inadequate training for physical exercise; low self-efficacy; low self-esteem; negative affect toward physical activity; pain; parenting practices that inhibit child's physical activity; perceived physical disability; perceived safety risk

At-Risk Population

Adolescents; individuals aged ≥ 60 years; individuals living in urban areas; individuals living with a partner; individuals with high educational level; individuals with high socioeconomic status; individuals with significant time constraints; married individuals; women

NOC (Nursing Outcomes Classification)

Suggested NOC Outcomes

Ambulation; Activity Tolerance; Endurance; Exercise Participation; Health Promoting Behavior; Lifestyle Balance; Personal Health Status; Physical Fitness; Exercise Promotion

Example NOC Outcome with Indicators

Ambulation as evidenced by the following indicators: Walks with effective gait/Walks at moderate pace/ Walks up and down steps/Walks moderate distance. (Rate the outcome and indicators of **Ambulation:** 1 = severely compromised, 2 = substantially compromised, 3 = moderately compromised, 4 = mildly compromised, 5 = not compromised [see Section I].)

Client Outcomes

Client Will (Specify Time Frame)

- Engage in purposeful moderate-intensity cardiorespiratory (aerobic) exercise for 30 to 60 minutes/day on 5 or more days per week for a total of 2 hours and 30 minutes (150 minutes) per week
- Increase exercise to 20 minutes/day (>150 minutes/week); light to moderate intensity exercise may be beneficial in deconditioned persons
- Increase pedometer step counts by 1000 steps per day every 2 weeks to reach a daily step count of at least 7000 steps per day, with a daily goal for most healthy adults of 10,000 steps per day
- Perform resistance exercises that involve all major muscle groups (legs, hips, back, chest, abdomen, shoulders, and arms) performed 2 to 3 days/week
- Perform flexibility exercise (stretching) for each of the major muscle-tendon groups 2 days/week for 10 to 60 seconds to improve joint range of motion; greatest gains occur with daily exercise
- Engage in neuromotor exercise 20 to 30 minutes/day including motor skills (e.g., balance, agility, coordination, and gait), proprioceptive exercise training, and multifaceted activities (e.g., Tai chi and yoga) to improve and maintain physical function and reduce falls in those at risk for falling (older persons)

NIC (Nursing Interventions Classification)

Suggested NIC Interventions

Exercise Therapy: Ambulation; Joint Mobility; Positioning; Exercise Promotion; Activity Therapy; Energy Management

S

Example NIC Activities—Exercise Therapy: Ambulation

Assist the client to use footwear that facilitates walking and prevents injury; Instruct in availability of assistive devices, if appropriate

Nursing Interventions and *Rationales*

- Assess the client with the American College of Sports Medicine (ACSM, 2018) guidelines for exercise preparticipation health screening before implementing physical activity interventions. EB: *The ACSM exercise guidelines focus on assessing (1) the individual's current level of physical activity; (2) presence of signs or symptoms of and/or known cardiovascular, metabolic, or renal disease; and (3) desired exercise intensity. The ACSM algorithm referred a smaller proportion of adults for preparticipation medical clearance than previously used screening tools. This lower referral proportion may mitigate the barrier of medical clearance from exercise participation (Whitfield et al, 2017).*

- Observe the client for sedentary behaviors such as prolonged sitting, physical inactivity, and prolonged sleep. EB: *Prolonged sitting, physical inactivity, and prolonged sleep were identified as lifestyle health risk behaviors in an Australian study (Ding et al, 2015).*
- Recommend the client enter an exercise program with an active person who supports exercise behavior (e.g., friend or exercise buddy). EB: *A 12-week pilot controlled trial of a physical activity buddy program found that the active buddy group (p = 0.005) showed significantly higher step changes than the inactive buddy group (Choi, 2017).*
- Recommend the client use a mobile fitness application for customizing, cueing, tracking, and analyzing an exercise program. EB: *A 3-year university community engagement study reported that a combination of coaching and wrist-worn activity tracker reduced general sitting time (Kiessling et al, 2017).*
- Encourage prescriptive resistance exercise of each major muscle group (hips, thighs, legs, back, chest, shoulders, and abdomen) using a variety of exercise equipment. EB: *Equipment such as free weights, bands, stair climbing, or machines should be used 2 to 3 days/week. Involve the major muscle groups for 8 to 12 repetitions to improve strength and power in most adults, 10 to 15 repetitions to improve strength in middle-aged and older persons starting exercise, and 15 to 20 repetitions to improve muscular endurance. Intensity should be between moderate (5 to 6) and hard (7 to 8) on a scale of 0 to 10 (ACSM, 2018).*
- Encourage gradual progression of greater resistance, more repetitions per set, and/or increasing frequency. EB: *A study found that a global progressive resistance strength training program was effective for improving the functional capacity of clients with rheumatoid arthritis (Lourenzi et al, 2015).*
- Encourage pregnant clients to engage in regular physical activity. EB: *A study reported that pregnant women spend the majority of their day engaged in sedentary behaviors with more sedentary behaviors on weekdays and during evening hours (Odabasic et al, 2018).*

▲ Assess the client for depression and refer for counseling and follow-up as appropriate. EB: *A study reported data indicating that depression may be a barrier to health-promoting behavior in middle-aged and older women with hypertension or heart disease (Cramer et al, 2020).*

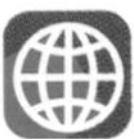

Multicultural

- Assess for reasons why the client would be unable to participate in regular physical activity; address reasons and refer to resources as needed. EB: *A systematic integrative literature review to identify barriers to physical activity among African American women found intrapersonal barriers (lack of time, knowledge, and motivation; physical appearance concerns; health concerns; monetary cost of exercise facilities; and tiredness/fatigue), interpersonal barriers (family/caregiving responsibilities; lack of social support; and lack of a physical activity partner), and environmental barriers (safety concerns; lack of facilities; weather concerns; lack of sidewalks; and lack of physically active African American role models) (Joseph et al, 2015).*
- Assess for clients' perceptions of the neighborhood they reside in. EB: *A study found that negative neighborhood environment perceptions were associated with greater sedentary time for individuals living in lower socioeconomic areas (Ahuja et al, 2017).*
- Encourage and support spiritual practices. EB: *A study by Silfee et al (2017) found that Latino adults who are more spiritual are also less sedentary, and this association was stronger in men than women.*
- Encourage participation in group physical activity programs. EBN: *Results of a physical activity study suggest that a team-based exercise training program may assist in overcoming sedentary behavior for African American women (Piacentine et al, 2018).*

S

Pediatric

- Assess the child's current activity status using the Pediatric Inactivity Triad (Faigenbaum et al, 2018). EB: *Components of the Pediatric Inactivity Triad include (1) exercise deficit disorder (less than 60 minutes of recommended physical activity daily), (2) pediatric dynapenia (decreased muscle strength and power), and (3) physical illiteracy (low competence and confidence). Addressing these components collectively will enhance effective change (Faigenbaum et al, 2018).*
- Assess parent's perceptions of children's screen time and active play. EB: *A study identified that parental perceptions of the benefits and risks of screen time and active play were not always consistent with current research (Hinkley & McCann, 2018).*
- Children and adolescents should participate in 60 minutes (1 hour) or more of physical activity daily.
  - Aerobic: Sixty or more minutes a day should be either moderate-intensity or vigorous-intensity aerobic physical activity and should include vigorous-intensity physical activity at least 3 days a week.

- Muscle-strengthening: As part of daily physical activity, children and adolescents should include muscle-strengthening physical activity on at least 3 days of the week.
- Bone strengthening: As part of daily physical activity, children and adolescents should include bone-strengthening physical activity on at least 3 days of the week.
- Providing activities that are age appropriate, are enjoyable, and offer variety will encourage young people to participate in physical activities (U.S. Department of Health and Human Services, 2018).

- Assist families to develop family-based interventions to increase child physical activity. EB: *A meta-analysis of family-based interventions found a small effect on physical activity when interventions were tailored to the ethnicity, motivation, and time constraints of the family; combined goal-setting and reinforcement techniques were used; educational strategies were used to increase knowledge as needed; and consideration of the family psychosocial environment (Brown et al, 2016).*
- Encourage parents and caregivers to adhere to the following American Academy of Pediatrics guidelines for children's media use (Chassiakos et al, 2016):
  - For children younger than 18 months, avoid use of screen media other than video-chatting.
  - Parents of children 18 to 24 months of age who want to introduce digital media should choose high-quality programming and watch it with their children to help them understand what they are seeing.
  - For children ages 2 to 5 years, limit screen use to 1 hour/day of high-quality programs. Parents should co-view media with children to help them understand what they are seeing and apply it to the world around them.
  - For children ages 6 and older, place consistent limits on the time spent using media, and the types of media, and make sure media does not take the place of adequate sleep, physical activity, and other behaviors essential to health.
  - Designate media-free times together, such as dinner or driving, and media-free locations at home, such as bedrooms.
  - Have ongoing communication about online citizenship and safety, including treating others with respect online and off-line.
  - Encourage parents and caregivers to create their personalized family media plan (see https://www.healthychildren.org/English/media/Pages/default.aspx) (American Academy of Pediatrics, 2021).

Geriatric

- Use valid and reliable criterion-referenced standards for fitness testing (e.g., Senior Fitness Test) designed for older adults that can predict the level of capacity associated with maintaining physical independence into later years of life (e.g., get up and go test). EB: *Interventions can subsequently be designed to target weak areas and therefore help reduce the risk of immobility and dependence (Bhattacharya, Deka, & Roy, 2016).*
- Recommend the client begin a regular exercise program, even if generally active. EB: *A meta-analysis of the association between time in sedentary behavior and hospitalizations, mortality, cardiovascular disease, cancer, and diabetes found prolonged sedentary time associated as an independent risk factor for poor health outcomes despite engagement in physical activity (Biswas et al, 2015).*
- Implement progressive resistance training plus balance exercise for older adults as indicated. EB: *A cluster randomized controlled trial showed that the Sunbeam Program of progressive resistance training in conjunction with balance exercise significantly reduced the rate of falls and improved physical performance in clients of residential care (Hewitt et al, 2018).*
- Before surgery, refer clients to a personalized "prehabilitation" program that includes a warm-up followed by aerobic, strength, flexibility, neuromotor, and functional task work. EB: *A study of major surgery clients assigned to personalized prehabilitation programs showed enhanced aerobic capacity and reduction in post-operative complications by 51% (Barbaren-Garcia et al, 2018).*

S

Home Care

- The preceding interventions may be adapted for home care use.
- ▲ Assess home environment for factors that create barriers to mobility. Refer to physical and occupational therapy services if needed to assist the client in restructuring home environment and daily living patterns.

Client/Family Teaching and Discharge Planning

- Provide teaching to clients and family to increase awareness of the health benefits of reducing sedentary behavior. EB: *A qualitative study found that clients placed little importance on reducing sedentary behavior, were unconvinced of the health benefits of reducing sedentary behavior, did not perceive themselves to be sedentary, and did not associate nonsedentary behaviors with enjoyment and relaxation (Biswas et al, 2018).*

- Consider using motivational interviewing techniques when working with both children and adult clients to increase their activity. **EB:** *A study to increase physical activity among clients with rheumatoid arthritis found that at posttreatment and 6-months follow-up, significantly more clients met current physical activity recommendations (Knittle et al, 2015).*

REFERENCES

Ahuja, C., Ayers, C., Hartz, J., et al. (2017). Unfavorable perceptions of neighborhood environment are associated with greater sedentary time—Data from the Washington, D.C. Cardiovascular Health and Needs Assessment [abstract]. *Circulation, 135*(Suppl. 1). Retrieved from http://circ.ahajournals.org/content/135/Suppl_1/AMP025. Accessed July 26, 2021.

American Academy of Pediatrics. (2021). *Family media plan.* Healthychildren.org. Retrieved from https://www.healthychildren.org/English/media/Pages/default.aspx. Accessed July 26, 2021.

American College of Sports Medicine (ACSM). (2018). *American College of Sports Medicine's guidelines for exercise testing and prescription* (10th ed.). Philadelphia: Lippincott Williams & Wilkins.

Barbaren-Garcia, A., Ubré, M., Roca, J., et al. (2018). Personalised prehabilitation in high-risk patients undergoing elective major abdominal surgery: A randomized blinded controlled trial. *Annals of Surgery, 267*(1), 50–56. https://doi.org/10.1097/SLA.0000000000002293.

Bhattacharya, P. K., Deka, K., & Roy, A. (2016). Assessment of inter-rater variability of the senior fitness test in the geriatric population: A community based study. *International Journal of Biomedical and Advance Research, 7*(5), 208–212. https://doi.org/10.7439/ijbar.

Biswas, A., Faulkner, G. E., Oh, P. I., & Alter, D. A. (2018). Patient and practitioner perspectives on reducing sedentary behavior at an exercise-based cardiac rehabilitation program. *Disability & Rehabilitation, 40*(19), 2267–2274. https://doi.org/10.1080/09638288.2017.1334232.

Biswas, A., Oh, P. I., Faulkner, G. E., et al. (2015). Sedentary time and its association with risk for disease incidence, mortality, and hospitalization in adults. *Annals of Internal Medicine, 162*(2), 123–132.

Brown, H. E., Atkin, A. J., Panter, J., Wong, G., Chinapaw, M. J. M., & van Sluijs, E. M. F. (2016). Family-based interventions to increase physical activity in children: A systematic review, meta-analysis and realist synthesis. *Obesity Reviews: An Official Journal of the International Association for the Study of Obesity, 17*(4), 345–360. https://doi.org/10.1111/obr.12362.

Chassiakos, Y. L. R., Radesky, J., Christakis, D., Moreno, M. A., Cross, C., & Council on Communications and Media. (2016). Children and adolescents and digital media. *Pediatrics, 138*(5), e1–e18. https://doi.org/10.1542/peds.2016-2593.

Choi, J. (2017). Active exercise buddies help women with young children improve physical activity [Abstract]. *Circulation, 135*(Suppl. 1). Retrieved from https://www.ahajournals.org/doi/10.1161/circ.135.suppl_1.mp002 Accessed July 26, 2021.

Cramer, H., Lauche, R., Adams, J., Frawley, J., Broom, A., & Sibbritt, D. (2020). Is depression associated with unhealthy behaviors among middle-aged and older women with hypertension or heart disease? *Women's Health Issues, 30*(1), 35–40. https://doi.org/doi:10.1016/j.whi.2019.09.003.

Ding, D., Rogers, K., van der Ploeg, H., Stamatakis, E., & Bauman, A. E. (2015). Traditional and emerging lifestyle risk behaviors and all-cause mortality in middle-aged and older adults: Evidence from a large population-based Australian cohort. *PLoS Medicine, 12*(12), e1001917.

Faigenbaum, A. D., Rebullido, T. R., & MacDonald, J. P. (2018). Pediatric inactivity triad: A risky pit. *Current Sports Medicine Reports, 17*(2), 45–47. https://doi.org/10.1249/JSR.0000000000000450.

Hewitt, J., Goodall, S., Clemson, L., Henwood, T., & Refshauge, K. (2018). Progressive resistance and balance training for falls prevention in long-term residential aged care: A cluster randomized trial of the Sunbeam program. *Journal of the American Medical Directors Association, 19*(4), 361–369. https://doi.org/10.1016/j.jamda.2017.12.014.

Hinkley, T., & McCann, J. R. (2018). Mothers' and father's perceptions of the risks and benefits of screen time and physical activity during early childhood: A qualitative study. *BMC Public Health, 18*(1), 1271. https://doi.org/10.1186/s12889-018-6199-6.

Joseph, R. P., Ainsworth, B. E., Keller, C., & Dodgson, J. E. (2015). Barriers to physical activity among African American women: An integrative review of the literature. *Women & Health, 55*(6), 679–699. https://doi.org/10.1080/03630242.2015.1039184.

Kiessling, P. B., Kennedy-Armbruster, C., Deinhart, M., et al. (2017). Move more, sit less? Analysis of an employer activity tracker workplace wellness program. *Medicine & Science in Sports & Exercise, 49*(Suppl. 5), 493. https://doi.org/10.1249/01.mss.0000518250.55130.00.

Knittle, K., De Gucht, V., Hurkmans, E., et al. (2015). Targeting motivation and self-regulation to increase physical activity among patients with rheumatoid arthritis: A randomised controlled trial. *Clinical Rheumatology, 34*(2), 231–238. https://doi.org/10.1007/s10067-013-2425-x.

Lourenzi, F. M., Jones, A., Pereira, D. F., dos Santos, J. H. C. A., & Natour, J. (2015). FRI0611-HPR global progressive resistance training improved functional capacity in patients with rheumatoid arthritis. *Annals of the Rheumatic Diseases, 74*, 1323. https://doi.org/10.1136/annrheumdis-2015-eular.2451.

Odabasic, A., Baruth, M., Schlaff, R. A., & Deere, S. J. (2018). Patterns of sedentary behavior in pregnant women. *Medicine & Science in Sports & Exercise, 50*(Suppl. 5), 711–712. https://doi.org/10.1249/01.mss.0000538345.80211.a5.

Piacentine, L. B., Robinson, K. M., Waltke, L. J., Tjoe, J. A., & Ng, A. V. (2018). Promoting team-based exercise among African American breast cancer survivors. *Western Journal of Nursing Research, 40*(12), 1885–1902. https://doi.org/10.1177/0193945918795313.

Silfee, V. J., Haughton, C. F., Lemon, S. C., Lora, V., & Rosal, M. C. (2017). Spirituality and physical activity and sedentary behavior among Latino men and women in Massachusetts. *Ethnicity & Disease, 27*(1), 3–10. https://doi.org/10.18865/ed.27.1.3.

U.S. Department of Health and Human Services. (2018). *Physical activity guidelines for Americans: Youth physical activity recommendations.* Washington, DC: US Department of Health and Human Services.

Whitfield, G. P., Riebe, D., Magal, M., & Liguori, G. (2017). Applying the ACSM preparticipation screening algorithm to U.S. adults. *Medicine & Science in Sports & Exercise, 49*(10), 2056–2063. https://doi.org/10.1249/MSS.0000000000001331.

S

Readiness for Enhanced Self-Care

Domain 4 Activity/rest Class 5 Self-care

Ruth A. Wittmann-Price, PhD, RN, CNS, CNE, CNEcl, CHSE, ANEF, FAAN

NANDA-I

Definition

A pattern of performing activities for oneself to meet health-related goals, which can be strengthened.

Defining Characteristics

Expresses desire to enhance independence with health; expresses desire to enhance independence with life; expresses desire to enhance independence with personal development; expresses desire to enhance independence with well-being; expresses desire to enhance knowledge of self-care strategies; expresses desire to enhance self-care

NOC (Nursing Outcomes Classification)

Suggested NOC Outcomes

Adherence Behavior; Health-Seeking Behavior; Self-Care Status

Example NOC Outcome with Indicators

Health-Seeking Behavior as evidenced by the following indicators: Completes health-related tasks/Performs self-screening/Obtains assistance from health professionals. (Rate the outcome and indicators of **Health-Seeking Behavior:** 1 = never demonstrated, 2 = rarely demonstrated, 3 = sometimes demonstrated, 4 = often demonstrated, 5 = consistently demonstrated [see Section I].)

Client Outcomes

Client Will (Specify Time Frame)

- Evaluate current levels of self-care as optimum for abilities
- Express the need or desire to continue to enhance levels of self-care
- Seek health-related information as needed
- Identify strategies to enhance self-care
- Perform appropriate interventions as needed
- Monitor level of self-care
- Evaluate the effectiveness of self-care interventions at regular intervals

NIC (Nursing Interventions Classification)

S

Suggested NIC Interventions

Coping Enhancement; Energy Management; Learning Facilitation; Multidisciplinary Care Conference; Mutual Goal Setting; Self-Care Assistance

Example NIC Activity—Self-Care Assistance

Encourage person to perform normal activities of daily living to level of ability

Nursing Interventions and *Rationales*

- For assessment of self-care, use a valid and reliable screening tool if available for specific characteristics of the person, such as arthritis, diabetes, stroke, heart failure (HF), or dementia. EBN: *Bryant (2017) developed a Self-Care to Success toolkit that supports nurse practitioners to empower clients with HF and promote self-care behaviors (SCBs) successfully.* EBN: *Powell and Deroche (2020) researched how clients (n = 500) with chronic illnesses used electronic health care portals to assist with self-care and found overall low usage among registered users. Clients were more likely to use the electronic portal if they had HF and were located a distance from their provider's practice.*

- Support the person's awareness that enhanced self-care is an achievable, desirable, and positive life goal. EBN: *Kauric-Klein, Peters, and Yarandi (2017) examined how educational sessions and individual counseling affected blood pressure self-efficacy and self-care outcomes in adults (n = 118) receiving hemodialysis and found that self-efficacy was related to SCBs such as decreased salt intake, lower weight gain, increased adherence to medications, and fewer missed appointments.* EB: *Fletcher et al (2020) studied partners' awareness of self-care needs when the new mothers of their babies had severe mental illness (SMI). The researchers provided text information to partners about self-care, baby care, and partner care. The results demonstrated that partners of new mothers with SMI increased in knowledge and awareness about caring for themselves and their family's needs.*
- Show respect for the person, regardless of characteristics and/or background. EBN: *Marzband and Zakayi (2017) explored the concept of self-care in Islamic texts and found that self-care is participating in responsible activities to God for health promotion, preventive disease, and treatment. Self-care included physical, mental, spiritual, and social dimensions.* EB: *By conducting a cross-sectional descriptive correlational study, Miano et al (2020) investigated how adolescents and young adults (AYA) with cancer view self-care in relation to decision-making. Most AYA clients preferred an "active collaborative" role (39%) or a "shared decision-making" role (34%).*
- Promote trust and enhanced communication between the person and health care providers. EBN: *Chen (2020) studied the effects of low literacy on the health-seeking behaviors of older adults and found that it delayed treatment, had negative effects on client–provider communication, and decreased the use of preventive services.* EBN: *Researchers studied the client–provider relationships (communication, integration, collaboration, and empowerment) in pregnant clients (n = 139) in relation to better client self-care and women's perceptions of better communication, collaboration, and empowerment from their midwives, which were associated with more frequent SCBs (Nicoloro-Santa Barbara et al, 2017).*
- Promote opportunities for spiritual care and growth. EBN: *Salamizadeh, Mirzaei, and Ravari (2017) studied the effects of a spiritual care educational intervention with caretakers (n = 60) of Alzheimer's clients using a random group pretest–posttest method and concluded that spiritual care enhanced the self-efficacy of the caregivers.* EB: *Agarwal et al (2020) used interpretive phenomenological analysis to understand the effects of a spiritually focused meditation practice on clients with breast cancer. The research discovered that the self-care practice promoted a positive state of mind, self-awareness, awareness of God's healing power, spiritual support, and spiritual growth.*
- Promote social support through facilitation of family involvement. EB: *Morgan et al (2017) performed a literature review regarding social support for self-management for clients to manage their chronic condition(s) and found the two elements that were most important for self-care were commitment and empowerment.*
- Provide opportunities for ongoing group support through establishment of self-help groups on the Internet. EB: *A mixed-methods study was conducted by Bradley et al (2020) about homeless families (n = 15) with children ages 2 to 11. They used a peer-teaching program that increased parenting knowledge and practices and improved child behavioral difficulties. The program did not change social support perceptions but improved family self-care.*
- Help the person identify and reduce the barriers to self-care. EB: *Lim et al (2020) used a mixed-method study to identify the barriers and the facilitators to regular physical exercise for prediabetic clients (n = 433). Barriers to physical exercise self-care were lack of knowledge, medical conditions, lack of family participation, extended sitting, and lack of time.* EB: *Novak et al (2020) studied the barriers that diabetic clients have to self-care. The researchers studied the clients' lived experience of managing diabetes and how the work of self-care is embedded in the other routines of everyday living. The researchers found that everyday objects and spaces were instrumental in the incorporation of diabetic self-care into daily routines.*
- Provide literacy-appropriate education for self-care activities. EBN: *Lelorain et al (2017) studied health care professionals' perception of therapeutic client education for promoting self-care and found that nurses often lack skills and knowledge and are disillusioned about the effectiveness of therapeutic client education, and that person-centered care is needed in many places to promote education that can increase self-care.* EBN: *Hu et al (2020) examined the reliability and validity of the Spoken Knowledge in Low Literacy in Diabetes (SKILLD) scale in measuring diabetes knowledge among Hispanics with type 2 diabetes (T2DM) and found that it was reliable and valid for T2DM Spanish-speaking patents with low literacy ability.*
- Facilitate self-efficacy by ensuring the adequacy of self-care education. EBN: *Researchers used a correlation (a descriptive design to examine the relationship between glycemic control and SCBs in clients with type 2 diabetes) and found that clients with poor glycemic control had poorer self-efficacy and SCBs (D'Souza*

S

et al, 2017). EBN: *Rhee et al (2020) examined the relationship of three measures of self-efficacy in asthmatic adolescent clients (n = 371). The researchers compared the three measures to variables of self-care (quality of life, medication adherence, asthma control, asthma knowledge, and attitudes) and found that the Asthma Self-Efficacy scale (ASE) was the best scale to evaluate self-efficacy for this population.*

- Provide alternative mind–body therapies such as reiki, guided imagery, yoga, and self-hypnosis. EBN: *Orellana-Rios et al (2017) piloted an "on the job" mindfulness and compassion-oriented meditation training for multiprofessional team members (n = 27) designed to reduce distress, foster resilience, and strengthen a prosocial motivation in the clinical encounter. Improvements were realized in two burnout components (emotional exhaustion and personal accomplishment) and overall improvement of self-care.* EB: *Researchers used cognitive behavioral therapy and adherence counseling with HIV clients. Depressive symptoms were unchanged, but adherence to therapy improved at both 4 and 8 months after treatment (Safren et al, 2020).*
- Promote the person's hope to maintain self-care. EB: *Anderson, Turner, and Clyne (2017) developed a self-management intervention called the Help to Overcome Problems Effectively (HOPE: MS) to improve the physical and psychological well-being of people living with multiple sclerosis (MS) and found that the HOPE: MS was helpful and useful to clients living with MS and covered the parameters needed to identify self-care needs.* EBN: *Armstrong and Murtaugh (2020) studied clients with traumatic brain injury (TBI) and found that throughout their care (trauma, intensive, acute, and rehabilitation) that the multiprofessional team played a pivotal role in providing hope through specific individualized interventions.*

Pediatric

- Assess and evaluate a child's level of self-care and adjust strategies as needed. EBN: *Burgess et al (2020) completed a longitudinal study of children (n = 71) with cerebral palsy (CP) and their self-care trajectories. The study demonstrated that self-care for many levels increased in children 8 to 12 years old, but it was very dependent on the level of functioning of the child with CP and actually decreased in children who had more limited functioning.* EB: *Burns-Nader, Joe, and Pinion (2017) studied using computer tablets with children who were burned during treatments, and nurses reported significantly less pain and anxiety for the tablet distraction group compared with the control group.*
- Assist families to engage in and maintain social support networks. EB: *Pumar-Méndez et al (2017) interviewed stakeholders (n = 90) in six countries about the support for self-care for clients with chronic illness (SSSC) and investigated the stakeholders' roles. The stakeholders described the ideal SSSC as inclusive, interdependent, and person-centered and needed support was from clients, governments, health care professionals, associations, private companies, and the media. The recommendations were to continue to promote SSSC with stakeholders and health professionals to improve care.* EBN: *Murfield et al (2020) completed an integrative review about family caregivers of older adults and focused on self-compassion. They noted that self-compassion as a part of self-care increased with the caregivers' ability to cope.*
- Encourage activities that support or enhance spiritual care. EBN: *O'Shea et al (2017) completed a qualitative descriptive study about meeting the physical, emotional, and spiritual needs of parents with seriously ill children and found there was a need among providers to enhance both basic education and advanced skills in pediatric palliative and end-of-life care education statewide.* EB: *Jenkins et al (2020) completed a qualitative analysis of participants (n = 6) in leadership roles and revealed, through focus group interviews, themes that permeate leadership roles. The themes included taking responsibility for others; taking responsibility for self-care; addressing stigma in the workplace; and having a spiritual calling to help.*

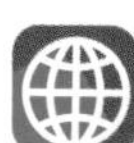

Multicultural

- Identify cultural beliefs, values, lifestyle practices, and problem-solving strategies when assessing the client's level of self-care. EBN: *Chen et al (2020) studied Taiwanese clients (n = 62) with HF for readiness to participate in self-care. The researchers implemented a predischarge educational program and followed up 1 year after discharge to examine self-care behaviors, readmission, sleep quality, and depression in clients with HF. The results demonstrated a significant increase in self-care 1 year after discharge by instituting a predischarge educational program.* EBN: *Researchers studied the COM-B model (consisting of capability, opportunity, and motivation) to explore SCBs and examine the self-care confidence on Chinese clients (n = 321) with chronic HF and found that Chinese clients have poor SCBs caused by lack of confidence, functional capacity, knowledge, and health literacy (Zou et al, 2017).*
- Recognize the effect of culture on SCBs. EB: *Researchers studied the elements that affect self-care in HF clients (n = 226) in Jordan by looking at knowledge, sociodemographics, and SCBs. Results revealed that*

knowledge, income, and educational levels; shorter duration of disease; fewer people living at home; older age; and being unemployed were significant predictors of low self-care scores (Tawalbeh et al, 2017). EBN: *Dehghani, Khoramkish, and Isfahani (2019) used content analysis from interviews to study Iranian clients with MS (n = 14) and their self-care abilities. The Iranian participants with MS identified the following self-care challenges: (1) confrontation to physical, emotional, psychological, and behavioral changes; (2) fear of becoming crippled; (3) tolerance of financial burden of the disease; and (4) confrontation to cultural social beliefs.*

- Provide culturally competent care. EBN: *Labore et al (2017) culturally explored the meaning of transition to self-care in sickle cell disease clients using an existential framework, and meaning was found in lived time, space, body, and human relationship.* EBN: *Kes and Gökdoğan (2020) developed a Turkish version of the Hypertension Self-Care Profile and examined its reliability and validity. The nurse researchers studied the tool with 200 people to determine whether the translation of the scale remained valid and reliable to use with the Turkish population.*
- Support independent self-care activities. EBN: *Teppala et al (2017) studied postacute rehabilitation for clients with hip fracture by examining the variation in mobility and self-care using a retrospective cohort study and found variation in discharge mobility and self-care related to health care organization differences.* EBN: *Mackintosh et al (2020) completed a descriptive analysis of women's (n = 632) use and experiences of digital resources for self-diagnosis and help seeking and found that over half the participants experienced concerns about themselves or their baby and accessed online information, noting that digital self-monitoring is increasingly integral to women's self-care during pregnancy.*

Home Care

- The nursing interventions described previously may also be used in home care settings. Provide clients with information about digital resources and health applications. EBN: *Göransson et al (2020) investigated a home care electronic application (app) among older persons (n = 17) to help maintain their health. The results demonstrated that the app provided a sense of security about self-care but without maintaining the app's educational information it decreased afterward.*
- Assist individuals and families to identify self-care activities for prevention of exacerbations of chronic illness symptoms to avoid rehospitalization. EB: *Toukhsati et al (2019) completed a meta-analysis study about self-care activity for HF clients in relation to rehospitalizations. The researchers found a variety of educational and behavioral interventions developed by health care providers to encourage and support client self-care.*
- Use educational guidelines for stroke survivors. EB: *Atler et al (2017) completed a study about yoga as an intervention in poststroke clients (n = 13), and five themes were identified from qualitative analysis: (1) improved abilities, (2) gained new knowledge, (3) enhanced engagement in activities, (4) improved relaxation, and (5) increased confidence.* EBN: *Wales, Dunford, and Davis (2020) studied children who had strokes and their ability for self-care. The researchers found that rehabilitation therapy was important for gaining self-care independence.*
- Ensure appropriate multiprofessional communication to support client safety. EB: *Weiss, Robertson, and Goebel (2019) completed a pilot project to develop a self-management tool for elderly clients in the community in order for them to understand when they needed to "take action" and call a provider. An multiprofessional palliative care team developed the tool and participants rated the tool as easy to understand and helpful in recognizing and reporting symptoms.*
- For public safety, health care professionals and consumers should participate in decision-making when managing reflux-related symptoms in the self-care setting. EB: *Johnson et al (2017) explored the consensus of an expert panel related to over-the-counter (OTC) proton pump inhibitors (PPIs) for gastroesophageal reflux disease and found that although OTC PPIs would probably not mask gastric cancer or affect bone density,* Clostridioides difficile *infection, or cardiovascular adverse events, they may be associated with slightly increased risks for infectious diarrhea, certain idiosyncratic reactions, and cirrhosis-related spontaneous bacterial peritonitis.*
- Enhance individual and family coping with chronic illnesses. EBN: *Kim and Kim (2017) studied elements that affected health-related quality of life (HRQOL) in elderly clients (n = 365) with diabetes and found that gender (male) and depression were negatively correlated with diabetic self-care.* EB: *Currow et al (2020) surveyed a large population of clients (n = 2883) in the community with shortness of breath and found that chronic breathlessness was iteratively associated with lower mobility, interference with daily activities, and worse pain/discomfort. Decreased self-care and increased anxiety/depression were connected to the most*

S

severe breathlessness. Respondents who had chronic breathlessness for 2 to 6 years had the worst self-care scores.

- Encourage participation in a community care management program. **EBN:** *Merius and Rohan (2017) completed a literature review (n = 14) related to adult attrition from community programs on diabetes self-care and found that barriers for retention included transportation, family obligations, and scheduling conflicts.* **EB:** *Williamson and Ennals (2020) studied young people with mental illness in the community to focus on self-regulation. Qualitatively the researchers discovered that self-care for the young people and their families was dependent on the following themes: (1) knowing yourself; (2) understanding the "why": developing shared reasons for engaging in sensory modulation; (3) creating comfort; (4) creating connection; and (5) constantly learning.*

Client/Family Teaching and Discharge Planning

- Teach clients how to regularly assess their level of self-care.
- Instruct clients that a variety of interventions may be needed to enhance self-care.
- Help clients to understand that enhanced self-care is an achievable goal.
- Empower clients.
- Teach clients about the decision-making process and self-care activities needed to manage their illness state and promote well-being.
- Continuously stress that all self-care activities must be regularly evaluated to ensure that enhanced levels of self-care can be maintained.

REFERENCES

Agarwal, K., Fortune, L., Heintzman, J. C., & Kelly, L. L. (2020). Spiritual experiences of long-term meditation practitioners diagnosed with breast cancer: An interpretative phenomenological analysis pilot study. *Journal of Religion and Health*, *59*(5), 2364–2380. https://doi.org/10.1007/s10943-020-00995-9.

Anderson, J. K., Turner, A., & Clyne, W. (2017). Development and feasibility of the Help to Overcome Problems Effectively (HOPE) self-management intervention for people living with multiple sclerosis. *Disability & Rehabilitation*, *39*(11), 1114–1121. https://doi.org/10.1080/09638288.2016.1181211.

Armstrong, T., & Murtaugh, B. M. (2020). Hope after TBI begins with rehabilitation. *Journal of Christian Nursing*, *37*(3), 144–152. https://doi.org/10.1097/CNJ.0000000000000734.

Atler, K. E., Van Puymbroeck, M., Portz, J. D., & Schmid, A. A. (2017). Participant-perceived outcomes of merging yoga and occupational therapy: Self-management intervention for people post stroke. *British Journal of Occupational Therapy*, *80*(5), 294–301. https://doi.org/10.1177/0308022617690536.

Bradley, C., Day, C., Penney, C., & Michelson, D. (2020). "Every day is hard, being outside, but you have to do it for your child": Mixed-methods formative evaluation of a peer-led parenting intervention for homeless families. *Clinical Child Psychology and Psychiatry*, *25*(4), 860–876. https://doi.org/10.1177/1359104520926247.

Bryant, R. (2017). Heart failure: Self-care to success: Development and evaluation of a program toolkit. *The Nurse Practitioner*, *42*(8), 1–8. https://doi.org/10.1097/01.NPR.0000520833.22030.d0.

Burgess, A., Boyd, R. N., Chatfield, M. D., Ziviani, J., & Sakzewski, L. (2020). Self-care performance in children with cerebral palsy: A longitudinal study. *Developmental Medicine and Child Neurology*, *62*(9), 1061–1067. https://doi.org/10.1111/dmcn.14561.

Burns-Nader, S., Joe, L., & Pinion, K. (2017). Computer tablet distraction reduces pain and anxiety in pediatric burn patients undergoing hydrotherapy: A randomized trial. *Burns*, *43*(6), 1203–1211. https://doi.org/10.1016/j.burns.2017.02.015.

Chen, S. Y. C. (2020). Self-care and medical treatment-seeking behaviors of older adults in rural areas of Taiwan: Coping with low literacy. *The International Quarterly of Community Health Education*, *41*(1), 69–75. https://doi.org/10.1177/0272684X20908846.

Chen, H. M., Wang, S. T., Wu, S. J., Lee, C. S., Fetzer, S. J., & Tsai, L. M. (2020). Effects of predischarge patient education combined with postdischarge follow-ups on self-care, readmission, sleep, and depression in patients with heart failure. *Journal of Nursing Research*, *28*(5), e112. https://doi.org/10.1097/JNR.0000000000000395.

Currow, D. C., Chang, S., Dal Grande, E., et al. (2020). Quality of life changes with duration of chronic breathlessness: A random sample of community-dwelling people. *Journal of Pain and Symptom Management*, *60*(4), 818-818. https://doi.org/10.1016/j.jpainsymman.2020.05.015.

Dehghani, A., Khoramkish, M., & Isfahani, S. S. (2019). Challenges in the daily living activities of patients with multiple sclerosis: A qualitative content analysis. *International Journal of Community Based Nursing & Midwifery*, *7*(3), 201–210. https://doi.org/10.30476/IJCBNM.2019.44995.

D'Souza, M. S., Karkada, S. N., Parahoo, K., Venkatesaperumal, R., Achora, S., & Cayaban, A. R. R. (2017). Self-efficacy and self-care behaviours among adults with type 2 diabetes. *Applied Nursing Research*, *36*, 25–32. https://doi.org/10.1016/j.apnr.2017.05.004.

Fletcher, R., St George, J. M., Rawlinson, C., Baldwin, A., Lanning, P., & Hoehn, E. (2020). Supporting partners of mothers with severe mental illness through text—A feasibility study. *Australasian Psychiatry*, *28*(5), 548–551. https://doi.org/10.1177/1039856220917073.

Göransson, C., Wengström, Y., Ziegert, K., Langius-Eklöf, A., & Blomberg, K. (2020). Self-care ability and sense of security among older persons when using an app as a tool for support. *Scandinavian Journal of Caring Sciences*, *34*(3), 772–781. https://doi.org/10.1111/scs.12782.

Hu, J., Amirehsani, K. A., McCoy, T. P., Wallace, D. C., Coley, S. L., & Zhan, F. (2020). Reliability and validity of the Spoken Knowledge in Low Literacy in Diabetes in measuring diabetes knowledge among Hispanics with type 2 diabetes. *The Diabetes Educator*, *46*(5), 465–474. https://doi.org/10.1177/0145721720941409.

Jenkins, G. T., Shafer, M. S., & Janich, N. (2020). Critical issues in leadership development for peer support specialists. *Community Mental Health Journal*, *56*(6), 1085–1094. https://doi.org/10.1007/s10597-020-00569-9.

Johnson, D. A., Katz, P. O., Armstrong, D., et al. (2017). The safety of appropriate use of over-the-counter proton pump inhibitors: An

S

evidence-based review and Delphi consensus. *Drugs*, *77*(5), 547–561. https://doi.org/10.1007/s40265-017-0712-6.

Kauric-Klein, Z., Peters, R. M., & Yarandi, H. N. (2017). Self-efficacy and blood pressure self-care behaviors in patients on chronic hemodialysis. *Western Journal of Nursing Research*, *39*(7), 886–905. https://doi.org/10.1177/0193945916661322.

Kes, D., & Gökdoğan, F. (2020). Reliability and validity of a Turkish version of the hypertension self-care profile. *Journal of Vascular Nursing*, *38*(3), 149–155. https://doi.org/10.1016/j.jvn.2020.05.001.

Kim, H., & Kim, K. (2017). Health-related quality-of-life and diabetes self-care activity in elderly patients with diabetes in Korea. *Journal of Community Health*, *42*(5), 998–1007. https://doi.org/10.1007/s10900-017-0347-2.

Labore, N., Mawn, B., Dixon, J., & Andemariam, B. (2017). Exploring transition to self-management within the culture of sickle cell disease. *Journal of Transcultural Nursing*, *28*(1), 70–78. https://doi.org/10.1177/1043659615609404.

Lelorain, S., Bachelet, A., Bertin, N., & Bourgoin, M. (2017). French healthcare professionals' perceived barriers to and motivation for therapeutic patient education: A qualitative study. *Nursing and Health Sciences*, *19*(3), 331–339. https://doi.org/10.1111/nhs.12350.

Lim, R. B. T., Wee, W. K., For, W. C., et al. (2020). Correlates, facilitators and barriers of physical activity among primary care patients with prediabetes in Singapore—A mixed methods approach. *BMC Public Health*, *20*(1), 1. https://doi.org/10.1186/s12889-019-7969-5.

Mackintosh, N., Agarwal, S., Adcocok, K., et al. (2020). Online resources and apps to aid self-diagnosis and help seeking in the perinatal period: A descriptive survey of women's experiences. *Midwifery*, *90*, 102803. https://doi.org/10.1016/j.midw.2020.102803.

Marzband, R., & Zakayi, A. A. (2017). A concept analysis of self-care based on Islamic sources. *International Journal of Nursing Knowledge*, *28*(3), 153–158. https://doi.org/10.1111/2047-3095.12126.

Merius, H. N., & Rohan, A. J. (2017). An integrative review of factors associated with patient attrition from community health worker programs that support diabetes self-care. *Journal of Community Health Nursing*, *34*(4), 214–228. https://doi.org/10.1080/07370016.2017.1369811.

Miano, S. J., Douglas, S. L., Hickman, R. L., DiMarco, M., Piccone, C., & Daly, B. J. (2020). Exploration of decisional control preferences in adolescents and young adults with cancer and other complex medical conditions. *Journal of Adolescent and Young Adult Oncology*, *9*(4), 464–471. https://doi.org/10.1089/jayao.2019.0135.

Morgan, H. M., Entwistle, V. A., Cribb, A., et al. (2017). We need to talk about purpose: A critical interpretive synthesis of health and social care professionals' approaches to self-management support for people with long-term conditions. *Health Expectations*, *20*(2), 243–259. https://doi.org/10.1111/hex.12453.

Murfield, J., Moyle, W., Jones, C., & O'Donovan, A. (2020). Self-compassion, health outcomes, and family carers of older adults: An integrative review. *Clinical Gerontologist*, *43*(5), 485–498. https://doi.org/10.1080/07317115.2018.1560383.

Nicoloro-Santa Barbara, J., Rosenthal, L., Auerbach, M. V., Kocis, C., Busso, C., & Lobel, M. (2017). Patient-provider communication, maternal anxiety, and self-care in pregnancy. *Social Science & Medicine*, *190*, 133–140. https://doi.org/10.1016/j.socscimed.2017.08.011.

Novak, L. L., Baum, H. B. A., Gray, M. H., et al. (2020). Everyday objects and spaces: How they afford resilience in diabetes routines. *Applied Ergonomics*, *88*, 103185. https://doi.org/10.1016/j.apergo.2020.103185.

Orellana-Rios, C. L., Radbruch, L., Kern, M., et al. (2017). Mindfulness and compassion-oriented practices at work reduce distress and enhance self-care of palliative care teams: A mixed-method evaluation of an "on the job" program. *BMC Palliative Care*, *17*(1), 3. https://doi.org/10.1186/s12904-017-0219-7.

O'Shea, E. R., Lavallee, M., Doyle, E. A., & Moss, K. (2017). Assessing palliative and end-of-life educational needs of pediatric health care professionals: Results of a statewide survey. *Journal of Hospice and Palliative Nursing*, *19*(5), 468–473. https://doi.org/10.1097/NJH.0000000000000374.

Powell, K. R., & Deroche, C. (2020). Predictors and patterns of portal use in patients with multiple chronic conditions. *Chronic Illness*, *16*(4), 275–283. https://doi.org/10.1177/1742395318803663.

Pumar-Méndez, M. J., Mujika, A., Regaira, E., et al. (2017). Stakeholders in support systems for self-care for chronic illness: The gap between expectations and reality regarding their identity, roles and relationships. *Health Expectations*, *20*(3), 434–447. https://doi.org/10.1111/hex.12471.

Rhee, H., Love, T., Harrington, D., & Walters, L. (2020). Comparing three measures of self-efficacy of asthma self-management in adolescents. *Academic Pediatrics*, *20*(7), 983–990. https://doi.org/10.1016/j.acap.2020.03.001.

Safren, S. A., Harkness, A., Lee, J. S., et al. (2020). Addressing syndemics and self-care in individuals with uncontrolled HIV: An open trial of a transdiagnostic treatment. *AIDS and Behavior*, *24*(11), 3264–3278. https://doi.org/10.1007/s10461-020-02900-7.

Salamizadeh, A., Mirzaei, T., & Ravari, A. (2017). The impact of spiritual care education on the self-efficacy of the family caregivers of elderly people with Alzheimer's disease. *International Journal of Community Based Nursing and Midwifery*, *5*(3), 231–238. PMCID: PMC5478743. PMID: 28670585.

Tawalbeh, L. I., Al Qadire, M., Ahmad, M. M., Aloush, S., Sumaqa, Y. A., & Halabi, M. (2017). Knowledge and self-care behaviors among patients with heart failure in Jordan. *Research in Nursing & Health*, *40*(4), 350–359. https://doi.org/10.1002/nur.21805.

Teppala, S., Ottenbacher, K. J., Eschbach, K., et al. (2017). Variation in functional status after hip fracture: Facility and regional influence on mobility and self-care. *Journals of Gerontology Series A: Biological Sciences and Medical Sciences*, *72*(10), 1376–1382. https://doi.org/10.1093/gerona/glw249.

Toukhsati, S. R., Jaarsma, T., Babu, A. S., Driscoll, A., & Hare, D. L. (2019). Self-care interventions that reduce hospital readmissions in Patients with heart failure; towards the identification of change agents. *Clinical Medicine Insights: Cardiology*, *13*, 1179546819856855. https://doi.org/10.1177/1179546819856855.

Wales, L., Dunford, C., & Davis, K. (2020). Following severe childhood stroke, specialised residential rehabilitation improves self-care independence but there are ongoing needs at discharge. *British Journal of Occupational Therapy*, *83*(8), 530–537. https://doi.org/10.1177/0308022619894870.

Weiss, D. J., Robertson, S., & Goebel, J. R. (2019). Pilot implementation of a low-literacy zone tool for heart failure self-management. *Journal of Hospice and Palliative Nursing*, *21*(6), 475–481. https://doi.org/10.1097/NJH.0000000000000597.

Williamson, P., & Ennals, P. (2020). Making sense of it together: Youth & families co–create sensory modulation assessment and intervention in community mental health settings to optimise daily life. *Australian Occupational Therapy Journal*, *67*(5), 458–469. https://doi.org/10.1111/1440-1630.12681.

Zou, H., Chen, Y., Fang, W., Zhang, Y., & Fan, X. (2017). Identification of factors associated with self-care behaviors using the COM-B model in patients with chronic heart failure. *European Journal of Cardiovascular Nursing*, *16*(6), 530–538. https://doi.org/10.1177/1474515117695722.

Bathing Self-Care Deficit

Domain 4 Activity/rest Class 5 Self-care

Suzanne C. Ashworth, MSN, APRN, CCRN, CCNS

NANDA-I

Definition

Inability to independently complete cleansing activities.

Defining Characteristics

Difficulty accessing bathroom; difficulty accessing water; difficulty drying body; difficulty gathering bathing supplies; difficulty regulating bath water; difficulty washing body

Related Factors

Anxiety; decreased motivation; environmental constraints; impaired physical mobility; neurobehavioral manifestations; pain; weakness

At-Risk Population

Older adults

Associated Conditions

Impaired ability to perceive body part; impaired ability to perceive spatial relationships; musculoskeletal diseases; neuromuscular diseases

NOC (Nursing Outcomes Classification)

Suggested NOC Outcomes

Self-Care: Activities of Daily Living (ADLs); Self-Care: Bathing; Self-Care: Hygiene

Example NOC Outcome with Indicators

Self-Care: ADLs as evidenced by the following indicators: Bathing/Hygiene. (Rate outcome and indicators of **Self-Care: ADLs:** 1 = severely compromised, 2 = substantially compromised, 3 = moderately compromised, 4 = mildly compromised, 5 = not compromised [see Section I].)

Client Outcomes

Client Will (Specify Time Frame)

- Remain free of body odor and maintain intact skin
- State satisfaction with ability to use adaptive devices to bathe
- Maintain independency with bathing and hygiene
- Use methods to bathe safely and effectively with minimal difficulty
- Bathe with assistance of caregiver as needed and report satisfaction and dignity maintained during bathing experience
- Bathe with assistance of caregiver as needed without exhibiting defensive (aggressive) behaviors

NIC (Nursing Interventions Classification)

Suggested NIC Intervention

Self-Care Assistance: Bathing/Hygiene

Example NIC Activities—Self-Care Assistance: Bathing/Hygiene

Determine amount and type of assistance needed; Consider the culture of the client when promoting self-care activities; Provide assistance until client is fully able to assume self-care

S

Nursing Interventions and *Rationales*

- • Ask clients about their bathing preferences, which can increase client privacy and satisfaction. EBN: *A qualitative study analyzed client perceptions and experiences regarding bathing methods (n = 16). Daily washing was a necessity to maintain skin integrity and overall feelings of "wellness." Showering was the preferred method to maintain hygiene (Veje et al, 2018).*
- ✱ Adjust room temperature above 20°C (68°F) and avoid hot water bathing, especially during cold seasons. EB: *Older clients may not verbalize a dependable sense of temperature. Low bathroom temperature and higher water temperature may lead to serious physiological changes and accidents (Ono et al, 2017).*
- ✱ Bathe critically ill clients or clients outside of critical care who have a central venous access device with a nonrinse chlorhexidine-impregnated wipe or chlorhexidine solution with rinsing. EB: *Bathing with chlorhexidine gluconate reduces the risk of hospital-acquired bloodstream infections (Musuuza et al, 2019).*
- ✱ Avoid using a bath basin for bathing to avoid client exposure to multidrug-resistant pathogens from contaminated bath basins or hospital water supply. EB: *In a 44-month study by Marchaim et al (2012), hospital bath basins (n = 1103) were found 62.2% of the time to be contaminated with hospital-acquired pathogens.* EB: *An outbreak of* Pseudomonas aeruginosa *infections in a neonatal intensive care unit was attributed to contaminated water supply after 67% of environmental samples from client rooms grew* P. aeruginosa *(Bicking-Kinsey et al, 2017).*
- ✱ If a bath basin is used, use chlorhexidine gluconate solution for client bathing. EBN: *Powers et al (2012) found in a study (n = 90) that when clients are bathed with chlorhexidine gluconate the bacterial growth in the bath basin is significantly reduced.*
- ✱ Consider using a prepackaged bath for immobile clients who cannot shower. EBN: *A prospective randomized study compared soap and water with disposable packaged bathing wipes. Disposable bathing wipes caused less alterations in client skin integrity (Martin et al, 2017).* EB: *A systematic review of 33 studies found moderate- to high-quality evidence that washing without water is not inferior to traditional bed bathing techniques and should be considered for immobile clients (Groven et al, 2017).*
- • Avoid using high pressure during wiping. Monitor the client's skin and ask for feedback regarding sensation. EBN: *A quasi-experimental study examined differences in wiping pressure by nurses during bathing. Subjective data suggested that clients experienced some degree of pain during bathing (Konya et al, 2020).*
- • Consider bathing for terminally ill cancer clients who have pain and anxiety to promote comfort. EB: *The thermal effect of bathing has been found to act as an analgesic and promotes physiological and psychological relaxation (Fujimoto et al, 2017).*
- • Consider using music intervention in clients who have pain during bathing. EB: *A pilot study done in critically ill, mechanically ventilated clients found that music used during bathing significantly decreased pain intensity during bathing (Jacq et al, 2018).*
- • Use person-centered bathing approach: plan for client's comfort and bathing preferences, show respect in communications by listening, critically think to solve issues that arise, and use a gentle approach. CEB: *Focusing on the client rather than the task of bathing results in greater comfort and fewer aggressive behaviors, which are likely defensive behaviors that result from feeling threatened or anxious and increase with shower (especially) and tub bathing (Hoeffer et al, 2006).*
- ▲ Provide pain relief measures, such as ice packs, heat, and analgesics for sore joints, 45 minutes before bathing; move extremities slowly and carefully; and inform the client before movements associated with pain occur (walking; transferring to a new location; moving joints; and washing genitals, face, and between toes and under arms). Have the client wash painful areas; recognize indicators of pain and apologize for any pain caused. EB: *Pain may lead to ADL deficits such as bathing and showering (Pieber et al, 2015).*
- ▲ Use a comfortable padded shower chair with foot support or adapt a chair: pad it with towels/washcloths, cover the cold back with dry towels, and cover the arms with foam pipe insulation. CEB: *Unpadded shower chairs with large openings and no foot support contribute to pain by allowing clients to sink into the opening with their feet unsupported (Rader et al, 2006).*
- • Ensure that bathing assistance preserves client dignity through use of privacy with a traffic-free bathing area and posted privacy signs, timeliness of personal care, and encourage client participation and involvement in the delivery of care. EBN: *Clients' perceptions of being bathed are often described as being embarrassing due to being undressed in front of someone or even the opposite sex. Bed bathing has been reported to be less positive when compared to showering. Respect for privacy may lessen embarrassment and minimize client dissatisfaction (Lopes et al, 2013).*
- • For cognitively impaired clients, avoid upsetting factors associated with bathing: instead of using the terms *bath, shower,* or *wash,* use comforting words, such as *warm, relaxing,* or *massage.* Start at the client's

S

feet and bathe upward; bathe the face last after washing hands and using a clean cloth. Use a beautician/barber or wash hair at another time to avoid water dripping in the face. CEB: *Some words are associated with unpleasant bathing experiences, whereas others convey a pleasant bathing experience. Starting with the face or hair is distressing, because water drips on the face and the head becomes cold and wet (Rader et al, 2006).*

- ● Use towel bathing to bathe client in bed, a bath blanket, and warm towels to keep the client covered the entire time. Warm and moisten towels/washcloths and place in plastic bags to keep them warm. Use the towels to massage large areas (front, back) and one washcloth for facial areas and another one for genital areas. No rinsing or drying is needed, as is commonly thought for bathing. CEB: *Towel bathing is a gentle experience with less discomfort that significantly reduces aggression as well as bathing time and soap residue after showering without accumulation of pathogenic bacteria (Hoeffer et al, 2006).*
- ● For shower bathing use person-centered techniques, keep client covered with towels and cleanse under the towels, use no-rinse products, use favorite bathing items, and use a handheld shower with adjustable spray. CEB: *Covering the client is an easy means to maintain dignity, reduce embarrassment, and keep the client warm and unexposed without increasing bathing time (Rader et al, 2006).*
- ● Provide nighttime bathing or showering or a warm foot bath 1 to 2 hours before bedtime for at least 10 minutes to improve sleep. EB: *A systematic review and meta-analysis of 13 studies determined that bathing before bedtime improved sleep and shortened sleep onset latency (Haghayegh et al, 2019).*
- ▲ Request referral of client who has had a stroke to rehabilitation services. EB: *In a systematic review of 45 studies, Mehrholz et al (2018) found that electromechanical and robot-assisted arm training devices used in rehabilitation may assist in improving arm function after stroke, which is important for ADLs such as bathing.*

Geriatric

- ▲ Advocate for the use of the Bathing Without a Battle educational program for clients with dementia. EB: *In a randomized crossover diffusion study, the Bathing Without a Battle educational program that trains caregivers in methods for improving the bathing experience of clients with dementia in nursing homes was found to be effective in reducing the rate of aggressive and agitated behaviors (Gozalo et al, 2014).*
- ● Arrange the bathing environment to promote sensory comfort. Reduce noise of voices and water. Do not allow traffic into bathing room. Add fabric to absorb sound (three to four times the width of the opening for sound-absorbing folds). Play soft music. CEB: *Noise discomfort can result from high-echo tiled walls, loud voices, and running water. Traffic can compromise privacy. Absorb negative sounds, and add positive sounds through music (Ray & Fitzsimmons, 2014).* EBN: *In an observational study* (n = 53) *by Joosse (2012), sound was a predictor of agitation for those with dementia.*
- ● Design the bathing environment for comfort and safety. Use grab bars with nonslip grip and bathmats. Ensure that flooring is not slippery. EB: *Bathroom assistive devices are used to improve safety during bathing transfer. King and Novak (2017) evaluated the effectiveness of common aids. The vertical grab bar and bath mat resulted in safe bathing transfers.*
- ● Use music during shower for clients with dementia. EB: *Music may reduce agitation and improve mood to increase job satisfaction (Ray & Fitzsimmons, 2014).*
- ● Train caregivers bathing clients with dementia to avoid behaviors that can trigger assault: confrontational communication, invalidation of the resident's feelings, failure to prepare a resident for a task, initiating shower spray or touch during bathing without verbal prompts beforehand, washing the hair and face, speaking disrespectfully to the client, and hurrying the pace of the bath. CEB: *During bathing, assaults (defensive behavior) by nursing home residents with dementia are frequently triggered by caregiver actions that startle, frighten, hurt, or upset the resident. This might happen when caregivers spray water on a resident without warning or when they touch a resident's feet, axilla, or perineum, which is possibly caused by the startle reflex (Somboontanont et al, 2004).*
- ● Focus on the abilities of the client with dementia to obtain client's participation in bathing. CEB: *The use of an abilities-focused approach increases the ability of people with dementia to participate in their care (Sidani, Streiner, & Leclerc, 2012).*

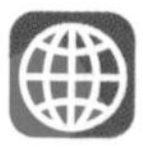

Multicultural

- ● Ask the client for input on bathing habits and cultural bathing preferences. CEB: *Bathing is a personal experience with variability in attitudes, preferences, and adaptations to disability to be considered when developing interventions for bathing (Ahluwalia et al, 2010).*

S

Home Care

- An individualized home-based caregiver training program can improve caregiver skills and competence with managing behavior issues with dementia clients during bathing. EB: *A study found that family caregivers who received a home-based training intervention were better prepared and competent to manage dementia behavior issues (Huang et al, 2013).*
- Provide home occupational therapy targeting self-bathing and environmental modifications for clients with bathing disabilities. EB: *Rehabilitation that targets improving self-care deficits with bathing improve quality of life for individuals with bathing disabilities (Zingmark et al, 2016).*
- Turn down temperature of water heater and recommend use of a water temperature-sensing shower valve to prevent scalding. EB: *Bathing at excessive water temperature can lead to shock and scalding, especially in elderly and infants. For elderly clients, water temperature of 38°C to 40°C is recommended (Wei et al, 2020).*
- Remove physical barriers in the home to maximize the client's ability to function independently and safely while bathing. EB: *A qualitative study within the randomized control trial (BATH-OUT) analyzed experiences of individuals who had received housing modifications to promote independence during bathing. Older adults with disabilities presented feeling safe, clean, and independent and had improved quality of life during bathing. This led to a greater sense of freedom due to improved functioning (Whitehead & Golding-Day, 2019).*

Client/Family Teaching and Discharge Planning

Provide client/family education regarding chlorhexidine bathing for the reduction of common hospital-acquired infections. EB: *Refusal for chlorhexidine gluconate (CHG) bathing in one study ranged from 3% to 39%. Clients expressed a low knowledge of the benefits of chlorhexidine for preventing hospital-acquired infections, and only 35% of clients reporting receiving CHG education (Caya et al, 2019).*

REFERENCES

Ahluwalia, S. C., Gill, T. M., Baker, D. I., & Fried, T. R. (2010). Perspectives of older persons on bathing and bathing disability: A qualitative study. *Journal of American Geriatric Society, 58*(3), 450–456. https://doi.org/10.1017/ice.2017.87.

Bicking-Kinsey, C., Koirala, S., Solomon, B., et al. (2017). Pseudomonas aeruginosa outbreak in a neonatal intensive care unit attributed to hospital tap water. *Infection Control and Hospital Epidemiology, 38*(7), 801–808.

Caya, T., Knoblock, M. J., Musuuza, J., Wilhelmson, E., & Safdar, N. (2019). Patient perceptions of chlorhexidine bathing: A pilot study using the health belief model. *American Journal of Infection Control, 47*(1), 18–22.

Fujimoto, S., Iwawaki, Y., Takishita, Y., et al. (2017). Effects and safety of mechanical bathing as a complementary therapy for terminal stage cancer patients from the physiological and psychological perspective: A pilot study. *Japanese Journal of Clinical Oncology, 47*(11), 1066–1072.

Gozalo, P., Prakash, S., Qato, D. M., Sloane, P. D., & Mor, V. (2014). Effect of the bathing without a battle training intervention on bathing-associated physical and verbal outcomes in nursing home residents with dementia: A randomized crossover diffusion study. *Journal of the American Geriatrics Society, 62*(5), 797–804.

Groven, F. M. V., Zwakhalen, S. M. G., Odekerken-Schröder, G., Joosten, E. J. T., & Hamers, J. P. H. (2017). How does washing without water perform compared to the traditional bed bath: A systematic review. *BMC Geriatrics, 17*(1), 31.

Haghayegh, S., Khoshnevis, S., Smolensky, M. H., Diller, K. R., & Castriotta, R. J. (2019). Before-bedtime passive body heating by warm shower or bath to improve sleep: A systematic review and meta-analysis. *Sleep Medicine Reviews, 46*, 124–135. https://doi.org/10.1016/j.smrv.2019.04.008.

Hoeffer, B., Talerico, K. A., Rasin, J., et al. (2006). Assisting cognitively impaired nursing home residents with bathing: Effects of two bathing interventions on caregiving. *Gerontologist, 46*(4), 524–532.

Huang, H. L., Kuo, L. M., Chen, Y. S., et al. (2013). A home-based training program improves caregivers' skills and dementia patients' aggressive behaviors: A randomized controlled trial. *American Journal of Geriatric Psychiatry, 21*(11), 1060–1070.

Jacq, G., Melot, K., Bezou, M., et al. (2018). Music for pain relief during bed bathing of mechanically ventilated patients: A pilot study. *PLoS One, 13*(11), e0207174.

Joosse, L. L. (2012). Do sound levels and space contribute to agitation in nursing home residents with dementia? *Research in Gerontological Nursing, 5*(3), 174–184.

King, E. C., & Novak, A. C. (2017). Effect of bathroom aids and age on balance control during bathing transfers. *American Journal of Occupation Therapy, 71*(6), 7106165030p1-7106165030p9. https://doi.org/10.5014/ajot.2017.027136.

Konya, I., Yamaguchi, S., Sugimura, N., Matsuno, C., & Yano, R. (2020). Effects of differences in wiping pressure applied by nurses during daily bed baths on skin barrier function, cleanliness, and subjective evaluations. *Japan Journal of Nursing Science, 17*(3) e12316.

Lopes, J., Nogueira-Martins, L. A., & Lbl de Barros, A. L. (2013). Bed and shower baths: Comparing the perceptions of patients with acute myocardial infarction. *Journal of Clinical Nursing, 22*(5–6), 733–740.

Marchaim, D., Taylor, A. R., Hayakawa, K., et al. (2012). Hospital bath basins are frequently contaminated with multidrug-resistant human pathogens. *American Journal of Infection Control, 40*(6), 562–564.

Martin, E. T., Haider, S., Palleschi, M., et al. (2017). Bathing hospitalized dependent patients with prepackaged disposable washcloths instead of traditional bath basins: A case-crossover study. *American Journal of Infection Control, 45*(9), 990–994.

Mehrholz, J., Pohl, M., Platz, T., Kugler, J., & Elsner, B. (2018). Electromechanical and robot-assisted arm training for improving activities of daily living, arm function, and arm muscle strength after stroke. *Cochrane Database of Systematic Reviews, 9*, CD006876. https://doi.org/10.1002/14651858.CD006876.pub5.

Musuuza, J. S., Guru, P. K., O'Horo, J. C., et al. (2019). The impact of chlorhexidine bathing on hospital-acquired bloodstream infections:

S

A systematic review and meta-analysis. *BMC Infectious Diseases, 19*(1), 416.

Ono, J., Hashiguchi, N., Sawatari, H., et al. (2017). Effect of water bath temperature on physiological parameters and subjective sensation in older people. *Geriatrics and Gerontology International, 17*(11), 2164–2170.

Pieber, K., Stamm, T. A., Hoffmann, K., & Dorner, T. E. (2015). Synergistic effect of pain and deficits in ADL towards general practitioner visits. *Family Practice, 32*(4), 426–430. https://doi.org/10.1093/fampra/cmv042. PMID:26045545.

Powers, J., Peed, J., Burns, L., & Ziemba-Davis, M. (2012). Chlorhexidine bathing and microbial contamination in patients' bath basins. *American Journal of Critical Care, 21*(5), 338–342.

Rader, J., Barrick, A. L., Hoeffer, B., et al. (2006). The bathing of older adults with dementia: Easing the unnecessarily unpleasant aspects of assisted bathing. *American Journal of Nursing, 106*(4), 40–49.

Ray, K. D., & Fitzsimmons, S. (2014). Music-assisted bathing: Making shower time easier for people with dementia. *Journal of Gerontological Nursing, 40*(2), 9–13.

Sidani, S., Streiner, D., & Leclerc, C. (2012). Evaluating the effectiveness of the abilities-focused approach to morning care of people with dementia. *International Journal of Older People Nursing, 7*(1), 37–45.

Somboontanont, W., Sloane, P. D., Floyd, F. J., Holditch-Davis, D., Hogue, C. C., & Mitchell, C. M. (2004). Assaultive behavior in Alzheimer's disease: Identifying immediate antecedents during bathing. *Journal of Gerontological Nursing, 30*(9), 22–29; quiz 55–56.

Veje, P. L., Primdahl, J., Chen, M., et al. (2018). Costs of bed baths: A scoping review. *Nursing Economics, 38*(4), 194–202.

Wei, Q., Kang, S. M., & Lee, J. H. (2020). Designing a smart bath assistive device based on measuring inner water temperature for bathing temperature monitoring. *Sensors, 20*(8), 2405. https://doi.org/10.3390/s20082405.

Whitehead, P. J., & Golding–Day, M. R. (2019). The lived experience of bathing adaptations in the homes of older adults and their caregivers (BATH-OUT): A qualitative interview study. *Health and Social Care in the Community, 27*(6), 1534–1543.

Zingmark, M., Nilsson, I., Norström, F., Sahlén, K. G., & Lindholm, L. (2016). Cost effectiveness of an intervention focused on reducing bathing disability. *European Journal of Ageing, 14*(3), 233–241.

Dressing Self-Care Deficit Domain 4 Activity/Rest Class 5 Self-Care

Suzanne C. Ashworth, MSN, APRN, CCRN, CCNS

NANDA-I

Definition

Inability to independently put on or remove clothing.

Defining Characteristics

Difficulty choosing clothing; difficulty fastening clothing; difficulty gathering clothing; difficulty maintaining appearance; difficulty picking up clothing; difficulty putting clothing on lower body; difficulty putting clothing on upper body; difficulty putting on various items of clothing; difficulty removing clothing item; difficulty using assistive device; difficulty using zipper

Related Factors

Anxiety; decreased motivation; discomfort; environmental constraints; fatigue; neurobehavioral manifestations; pain; weakness

S

Associated Conditions

Musculoskeletal impairment; neuromuscular diseases

NOC (Nursing Outcomes Classification)

Suggested NOC Outcomes

Self-Care: Activities of Daily Living (ADLs), Dressing, Hygiene

Example NOC Outcome with Indicators

Self-Care: Dressing as evidenced by the following indicators: Gets clothing from drawer and closet/Puts clothing on upper body and lower body. (Rate outcome and indicators of **Self-Care: Dressing:** 1 = severely compromised, 2 = substantially compromised, 3 = moderately compromised, 4 = mildly compromised, 5 = not compromised [see Section I].)

Client Outcomes

Client Will (Specify Time Frame)

- Dress and groom self to optimal potential
- Use assistive technology to dress and groom
- Explain and use methods to enhance strengths during dressing and grooming
- Dress and groom with assistance of caregiver as needed

NIC (Nursing Interventions Classification)

Suggested NIC Intervention

Self-Care Assistance: Dressing/Grooming

Example NIC Activities—Self-Care Assistance: Dressing/Grooming

Be available for assistance in dressing, as necessary; Reinforce efforts to dress self; Maintain privacy while the client is dressing

Nursing Interventions and *Rationales*

- ▲ Assess independence in dressing and bathing skills after rehabilitation to determine the need for follow-up care. EB: *It was found that dressing and bathing independence at rehabilitation discharge were predictors of independence at 5 years after stroke* (De Wit et al, 2014).
- ▲ Assess the motor impairment and balance of all clients after stroke. EB: *A study of 60 stroke clients demonstrated that balance reduced the ability to perform dressing activities due to the fear of falling* (Fujita et al, *2016*).
- ▲ Routinely assess functional impairment and report functional changes to the health care provider for hospitalized clients with advanced cancer. EB: *A prospective study of hospitalized cancer clients found a correlation with functional impairment and inability to perform activities of daily living (ADLs), and the study found that cancer clients had significant increase in physical and psychological symptoms and worse clinical outcomes compared to those clients without functional impairment (Lage et al, 2020).*
- ▲ Refer clients with rehabilitation needs to physical and occupational therapy for functional rehabilitation with ADLs. EB: *A prospective study of 230 stroke clients found improved ADL function with a multiprofessional rehabilitation (Langhammer et al, 2017).*
- ● For clients with spinal cord injury, encourage their self-efficacy and involve them in decision-making. EBN: *A systematic review of 6 studies* (n = 84) *showed that rehabilitation is influenced by resilience, which can be enhanced with encouragement by nurses (Kornhaber et al, 2018).*
- ● Use adaptive dressing and grooming equipment as needed (e.g., button hooks, dressing stick, elastic shoelaces, long-handled shoehorn, reacher, sock application devices, Velcro clothing and shoes, zipper pull, long-handled brushes, soap-on-a-rope, suction holders). Use of adaptive clothing and devices for dressing and grooming can improve self-care ability and promote independence.
- ● Provide client analgesics before dressing as needed, sufficient time for dressing, and assist as needed. Analgesics, adequate time, and assistance if tiring can promote independence in dressing.
- ▲ For clients who are wheelchair dependent, consider the use of functional adaptive clothing. EB: *Functional clothing for wheelchairs was newly designed and evaluated for improving ADLs. Dressing competence was improved by 24.6% and toileting was improved by 52.9%* (*Wang et al, 2014*).

Geriatric

- ▲ Gather information on the client's personal clothing style and allow the client freedom to choose from a few selected outfits. EB: *Dementia clients are more able to maintain independence when provided choices (Prizer & Zimmerman, 2018).*
- ▲ When dressing dementia clients, give short verbal instructions, provide encouragement, and provide positive reinforcement. Use gentle physical prompting when needed, never debate, and never argue. EB: *When providing simple verbal instructions and maintaining dignity, dementia clients are more able to dress themselves independently (Prizer & Zimmerman, 2018).*
- ▲ Provide training to nursing home direct care staff regarding how to assist dementia clients with dressing that maintains dignity and respect of choice. EBN: *A mixed-method study that provided online training to*

Certified Nursing Assistants (CNAs) in 10 nursing homes found that the CNAs gained additional knowledge and understanding for providing person-centered care to dementia clients (Dobbs et al, 2018).

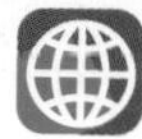

Multicultural

- Consider use of assistive technology versus personal care assistance for Native Americans. EB: *Older American Indians use more assistive technology for assistance with ADLs than the general same-age population and view the technology as allowing them to engage in activities (Reisinger & Ripat, 2014).*
- Consider cultural differences in clothing choices for Latino/Hispanic clients and respect dressing norms. EB: *Providing care for family elders is an important part of Latino/Hispanic culture. Easy-to-apply clothing, such as sweatpants, may not be deemed appropriate depending on the ethnicity (Mahoney, Coon, & Lozano, 2016).*

Home Care

- Ensure the client is dressing in a safe area. The bathroom may increase risk for falls during dressing. EB: *A systematic review of the literature for supporting ADLs of dementia clients found good evidence that the environment for dressing dementia clients should be safe and comfortable (Prizer & Zimmerman, 2018).*
- Consider home occupational therapy for elderly frail clients living at home. EB: *A systematic review and meta-analysis of home occupational therapy intervention found strong evidence that occupational therapy has a moderate improvement in ADL function (De Coninck et al, 2017).*

Client/Family Teaching and Discharge Planning

- * Include caregiver's perceptions of client rehabilitation needs after stroke. EB: *A meta-analysis of 66 studies of stroke survivors' needs as perceived by their caregivers found three areas of perceived needs that may improve outcomes by including caregivers in the rehabilitation planning (Krishnan et al, 2017).*
- Provide family caregiver training for assisting the client with dressing. EB: *A study was conducted on 36 family caregivers of dementia clients. Family training provided knowledge to assist caregivers with providing ADLs (DiZazzo-Miller et al, 2017).*

REFERENCES

De Coninck, L., Bekkering, G. E., Bouckaert, L., Declercq, A., Graff, M. J. L., & Aertgeerts, B. (2017). Home- and community-based occupational therapy improves functioning in frail older people: A systematic review. *Journal of the American Geriatrics Society*, *65*(8), 1863–1869. https://doi.org/10.1111/jgs.14889.

De Wit, L., Putman, K., Devos, H., et al. (2014). Long-term prediction of functional outcome after stroke using single items of the Barthel Index at discharge from rehabilitation centre. *Disability & Rehabilitation*, *36*(5), 353–358.

DiZazzo-Miller, R., Winston, K., Winkler, S. L., & Donovan, M. L. (2017). Family caregiver training program (FCTP): A randomized controlled trial. *American Journal of Occupational Therapy*, *71*(5), 7105190010p1–7105190010p10. https://doi.org/10.5014/ajot.2017.022459.

Dobbs, D., Hobday, J., Roker, R., Kaas, M. J., & Molinari, V. (2018). Certified nursing assistants' perspectives of the CARES® activities of daily living dementia care program. *Applied Nursing Research: ANR*, *39*, 244–248. https://doi.org/10.1016/j.apnr.2017.11.016.

Fujita, T., Sato, A., Yamamoto, Y., et al. (2016). Propensity-matched analysis of the gap between capacity and actual performance of dressing in patients with stroke. *Journal of Physical Therapy Science*, *28*(6), 1883–1887. https://doi.org/10.1589/jpts.28.1883.

Kornhaber, R., Mclean, L., Betihavas, V., & Cleary, M. (2018). Resilience and the rehabilitation of adult spinal cord injury survivors: A qualitative systematic review. *Journal of Advanced Nursing*, *74*(1), 23–33. https://doi.org/10.1111/jan.13396.

Krishnan, S., Pappadis, M. R., Weller, S. C., et al. (2017). Needs of stroke survivors as perceived by their caregivers: A scoping review. *American Journal of Physical Medicine & Rehabilitation*, *96*(7), 487–505. https://doi.org/10.1097/PHM.0000000000000717.

Lage, D. E., El-Jawahri, A., Fuh, C. X., et al. (2020). Functional impairment, symptom burden, and clinical outcomes among hospitalized patients with advanced cancer. *Journal of the National Comprehensive Cancer Network*, *18*(6), 747–754. https://doi.org/10.6004/jnccn.2019.7385.

Langhammer, B., Sunnerhagen, K. S., Lundgren-Nilsson, Å., Sällström, S., Becker, F., & Stanghelle, J. K. (2017). Factors enhancing activities of daily living after stroke in specialized rehabilitation: An observational multicenter study within the sunnaas international network. *European Journal of Physical and Rehabilitation Medicine*, *53*(5), 725–734. https://doi.org/10.23736/S1973-9087.17.04489-6.

Mahoney, D. F., Coon, D. W., & Lozano, C. (2016). Latino/hispanic alzheimer's caregivers experiencing dementia-related dressing issues: Corroboration of the preservation of self model and reactions to a "smart dresser" computer-based dressing aid. *Digital Health*, *2*, 2055207616677129. https://doi.org/10.1177/2055207616677129.

Prizer, L. P., & Zimmerman, S. (2018). Progressive support for activities of daily living for persons living with dementia. *The Gerontologist*, *58*(Suppl. 1), S74–S87. https://doi.org/10.1093/geront/gnx103.

Reisinger, K. D., & Ripat, J. D. (2014). Assistive technology provision within the Navajo nation: User and provider perceptions. *Qualitative Health Research*, *24*(11), 1501–1517. https://doi.org/10.1177/1049732314546755.

Wang, Y., Wu, D., Zhao, M., & Li, J. (2014). Evaluation on an ergonomic design of functional clothing for wheelchair users. *Applied Ergonomics*, *45*(3), 550–555. https://doi.org/10.1016/j.apergo.2013.07.010.

S

Feeding Self-Care Deficit

Domain 4 Activity/rest Class 5 Self-care

Suzanne C. Ashworth, MSN, APRN, CCRN, CCNS

NANDA-I

Definition

Inability to eat independently.

Defining Characteristics

Difficulty bringing food to mouth; difficulty chewing food; difficulty getting food onto utensils; difficulty handling utensils; difficulty manipulating food in mouth; difficulty opening containers; difficulty picking up cup; difficulty preparing food; difficulty self-feeding a complete meal; difficulty self-feeding in an acceptable manner; difficulty swallowing food; difficulty swallowing sufficient amount of food; difficulty using assistive device

Related Factors

Anxiety; decreased motivation; discomfort; environmental constraints; fatigue; neurobehavioral manifestations; pain; weakness

Associated Conditions

Musculoskeletal impairment; neuromuscular diseases

NOC (Nursing Outcomes Classification)

Suggested NOC Outcomes

Self-Care: Activities of Daily Living (ADLs), Eating

Example NOC Outcome with Indicators

Self-Care: Eating as evidenced by the following indicators: Opens containers/Uses utensils/Completes a meal. (Rate the outcome and indicators of **Self-Care: Eating:** 1 = severely compromised, 2 = substantially compromised, 3 = moderately compromised, 4 = mildly compromised, 5 = not compromised [see Section I].)

Client Outcomes

Client Will (Specify Time Frame)

- Feed self safely and effectively
- State satisfaction with ability to use adaptive devices for feeding
- Use assistance with feeding when necessary (caregiver)
- Maintain adequate nutritional intake

NIC (Nursing Interventions Classification)

Suggested NIC Intervention

Self-Care Assistance: Feeding

Example NIC Activities—Self-Care Assistance: Feeding

Provide adaptive devices to facilitate client's feeding self (e.g., long handles, handle with large circumference, or small strap-on utensils), as needed; Provide frequent cueing and close supervision as appropriate

Nursing Interventions and *Rationales*

▲ Screen for oropharyngeal dysphagia and malnutrition in elderly and high-risk hospitalized clients. EB: *A study conducted by Amaro Andrade et al (2018) aimed to determine the frequency of dysphagia risk and associated malnutrition in 909 hospitalized clients. Dysphagia prevalence was found in 10.5% and malnutrition in 13.2%. Advanced age was an associated risk factor for dysphagia.*

- ▲ The Eating Assessment Tool-10 (EAT-10) may be used to screen for dysphagia. EB: *A cross-sectional study conducted in older community members in Japan* (n = 202) *found a correlation for the presence of dysphagia when compared with the 100 mL water swallow test* (Nishida et al, 2020).
- ▲ For critical care clients who receive prolonged endotracheal intubation (>48 hours), assess swallowing using a valid tool to avoid aspiration related to dysphagia. EBN: *A prospective study conducted in four medical-surgical intensive care units* (n = 66) *tested the use of the Post Extubation Dysphagia Screening tool (PEDS). The tool was found to have a sensitivity of 81% and specificity of 69% and was determined to be reliable for assessing swallowing ability after prolonged endotracheal intubation (Johnson et al, 2018).*
- ▲ A formalized screening for dysphagia should be done in all stroke clients before any oral intake using the 3-ounce water swallow test by a trained clinician. EB: *A systematic review and meta-analysis (n = 770) found the 3-ounce water swallow test accurate and recommended for aspiration screening in poststroke clients (Chen et al, 2016b).*
- ▲ The Edinburgh Feeding Evaluation in Dementia can be used to determine the presence of behaviors that lead to feeding or eating problems in late-stage dementia clients. EBN: *The Edinburgh Feeding Evaluation in Dementia (EdFED) has been widely used in dementia clients. A recent study summarized the validity of assessment tools for dementia clients. The study determined that the EdFED continues to demonstrate high validity and inter-rater reliability (Spencer et al, 2020).*
- ▲ Assess for fatigue, sedating medications, and frailty before meals. Supervision and eating assistance may be required to avoid aspiration. EB: *In a review conducted by Cichero (2018), age >65, fatigue, hand weakness, and sedating medications were found to impair swallowing and cough reflexes.*
- ▲ Individualize the feeding process to promote interdependence, especially for younger adults who need feeding assistance. EB: *A qualitative study explored client attitudes toward feeding assistance. Younger adults had more negative feelings regarding being fed due to the loss of autonomy* (Shune, 2020).
- ▲ Consider consultation with a speech and language pathologist for clients with dysphagia for diet modifications and swallowing exercise therapy. EB: *In a study of 9 healthy older adults with dysphagia, clients had a significant improvement in swallowing ability from baseline using a high-intensity rehabilitation protocol (Balou et al, 2019).*
- ▲ Assess the ability to self-feed and communicate which clients require feeding assistance to decrease missed meals and allow for adequate nutrition. EBN: *A pilot study redesigned meal trays to include a method to communicate when assistance is needed. This resulted in an improvement of client nutritional status (Teeling et al, 2019).*
- ▲ Conduct repeat structured observations of clients at mealtime after a stroke to detect clients with eating difficulties to prevent possible social and functional consequences. EB: *A qualitative study of stroke survivors explored experiences with managing eating. Difficulties with sensory and motor function had an impact on social well-being. Clients described eating activities as being important for overall well-being and eating was a way to self-monitor recovery (Jones & Nasr, 2018).*
- ▲ Prioritize assisted feeding as important in a caregiver's assignment to allow adequate time for the client to eat. EBN: *A prospective study conducted by Chen et al (2016a) performed a before and after analysis of dementia clients' eating after implementing a Feeding Intervention Model. During the study, nurses who assisted clients allowed adequate time for clients to eat at a slow to moderate speed, ensuring consummation of the clients' meal. After implementation of the feeding intervention, clients had a significant improvement in nutritional status.*
- ▲ Consider using adaptive eating devices for clients with an upper limb motor impairment to assist with eating independently. EB: *An experimental study found significant improvements in eating and increased clients' satisfaction with introduction of an adaptive eating device (Cavalcanti et al, 2020).*
- ▲ Ensure oral care is provided to all clients using an American Dental Association–approved toothbrush and toothpaste after meals and at bedtime. Increase oral care frequency for clients who are on nothing-by-mouth (NPO) status. EBN: *Oral hygiene interventions have been shown to decrease hospital-acquired pneumonia, length of stay, and client mortality (Warren et al, 2019).*

S

Geriatric

- ▲ Assess for absent teeth and ill-fitting dentures in older clients before feeding. EB: *Tooth loss contributes to swallowing difficulties that can increase risk of aspiration in the older client. Adequate dentition is essential for effective chewing and to prevent choking* (Cichero, 2018).

▲ Establish a routine during mealtime and create a controlled stimulated environment with adequate lighting that simulates a home-like dining experience. EBN: *Promoting and maintaining eating independency is possible in nursing home residents by creating a controlled stimulated environment. Modifications to routines may trigger agitation that can affect nutritional intake (Palese et al, 2018).*

▲ Supervise the feeding of those with moderate dependency and provide physical assistance when needed. CEBN: *A feeding intervention study conducted in a nursing home with dementia clients (*n *= 30) placed emphasis on clients' autonomous eating while monitoring compliance with swallowing and chewing. The study demonstrated statistically significant improvement in food intake and independent eating compliance (Chen et al, 2016a).*

▲ When eating assistance is needed, (1) position clients in an upright position; (2) do not provide too much food at one time (approximately $^3/_4$ spoonful); and (3) offer food slowly, allowing the food to be chewed completely. For visually impaired clients, press the food to the client's lips and provide encouragement. EBN: *A prospective study of nursing home residents with dementia and dysphagia implemented a feeding intervention and found overall improvements in eating and dysphagia (Chen et al, 2016a).*

▲ Consider implementing Montessori interventions for dementia clients who have eating problems, such as playing music for sensory stimulation and employing hand-eye coordination, scooping, pouring, and squeezing activities. EB: *A systematic review of Montessori activities in dementia clients found strong evidence that eating difficulties may be improved when using Montessori interventions (Sheppard et al, 2016).*

▲ Limit activities and avoid noise and interruptions during mealtimes. EB: *A mixed-method systematic review found that interruptions can have a negative impact during mealtime (Edwards, Carrier, & Hopkinson, 2017).*

▲ Use high-calorie oral nutritional supplements for clients with advanced dementia who cannot meet their nutrition requirements by food alone. EB: *According to the European Society for Clinical Nutrition and Metabolism (ESPEN) guidelines on nutrition for dementia clients, older clients with dementia are at an increased risk for malnutrition. There is high evidence that the use of oral nutritional supplements improves nutritional status (Volkert et al, 2015).*

▲ Provide nutritional supplement drinks in a glass to older adults with cognitive impairment. EBN: *Allen, Methven, and Gosney (2014) conducted a nonblind randomized control trial that identified that the best method to provide nutritional supplement drinks to older adults with cognitive impairment is in a glass/beaker rather than using a straw in the container.*

* Provide verbal cues and encouragement during mealtimes. EBN: *A review conducted by Liu et al (2015) found good evidence that offering verbal cues and positive reinforcement leads to improved food intake.*

▲ Avoid changes or modifications to mealtime routines. EB: *Any modification or change in routine can result in agitation for nursing home residents, which can lead to decreased food intake for the individual and other residents (Palese et al, 2018).*

▲ Encourage family members to assist clients during mealtime for those who need eating assistance. EBN: *Family assistance was associated with a higher consumption of protein and energy intake for clients in a long-term care setting (Wu et al, 2020).*

▲ Play familiar soothing music during meals for clients with dementia. EB: *A systematic review by Bunn et al (2016) found evidence that music can increase food intake for dementia clients.*

▲ Provide feeding training and education programs for caregivers. EBN: *A systematic review of the literature about improving eating difficulties in older adults with dementia found good evidence that training and education programs for caregivers lead to decreased feeding difficulties (Liu et al, 2015).*

S

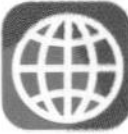

Multicultural

▲ For those with impaired hand function who use chopsticks, suggest adapted chopsticks. CEB: *In a pilot equipment study, adapted chopsticks, which can be inexpensive and easily constructed, for those with lower cervical spinal cord injury and residual gross grasp were found to convert gross grasp into 2-point pinch (Chang et al, 2006).*

▲ Use the simplified Chinese Edinburgh Feeding Evaluation in Dementia scale to measure feeding problems in people with dementia from Mainland China and other Chinese cultural groups. EBN: *Identifying client behaviors during feeding allows development of effective interventions for feeding (Liu, Watson, & Lou, 2014).*

▲ The culturally adaptive Spanish version of the Edinburgh Feeding Evaluation in Dementia Scale is valid for measuring feeding difficulties in Spanish-speaking dementia clients. EBN: *A cross-sectional study was done to determine validity of the Spanish version of the Edinburgh Feeding Assessment. The adapted version was found to be reliable (Saucedo Figueredo et al, 2018).*

Home Care

- ▲ For elderly home care clients with chronic diseases, assess nutritional status and chewing/swallowing ability. EB: *A cross-sectional study examined the nutritional status of elderly home care clients with disease burden in Germany. Chewing problems were found in 52% of the study population. More than one-third were found to have a moderate to poor appetite and a lower body mass index (Pohlhausen et al, 2016).*
- ▲ Provide multiprofessional nutritional support for home care clients by involving physical therapy, occupational therapy, and dietitians. EB: *Beck et al (2016) assessed the effect of a nutritional support team for undernourished elderly clients in a nursing home and in home care (n = 389). Improvements in quality of life, muscle strength, and oral care were found in the intervention group.*

Client/Family Teaching and Discharge Planning

- ▲ Educate family caregivers who are involved in the feeding of a family member by providing demonstration and hands-on training by a qualified trainer. EBN: *Caregivers of older adults with dementia identified the need for structured training and support. Insufficient education and lack of information were found to lead to caregiver emotional distress (Lee et al, 2019).*
- ▲ Educate family members that neither insertion of a feeding tube nor timing of its insertion affects client survival for those with advanced dementia who have eating problems. EB: *A longitudinal study of 169 clients compared hand feeding with nasogastric feeding (NGF) of bedridden dementia clients. NGF was not associated with a lower risk of pneumonia. Hospitalization and mortality were not decreased with use of NGF. Hand feeding can be considered an alternative to NGF (Chou, Tsou, & Hwang, 2020).*

REFERENCES

Allen, V. J., Methven, L., & Gosney, M. (2014). Impact of serving method on the consumption of nutritional supplement drinks: Randomized trial in older adults with cognitive impairment. *Journal of Advanced Nursing, 70*(6), 1323–1333.

Amaro Andrade, P., Araújo Dos Santos, C., Firmino, H. H., & de Oliveira Barbosa Rosa, C. (2018). The importance of dysphagia screening and nutritional assessment in hospitalized patients. *Einstein (Sao Paulo), 16*(2), eAO4189. https://doi.org/10.1590/S1679-45082018AO4189.

Balou, M., Herzberg, E. G., Kamelhar, D., & Molfenter, S. M. (2019). An intensive swallowing exercise protocol for improving swallowing physiology in older adults with radiographically confirmed dysphagia. *Clinical Interventions in Aging, 14*, 283–288. https://doi.org/10.2147/CIA.S194723.

Beck, A. M., Christensen, A. G., Hansen, B. S., Damsbo-Svendsen, S., & Møller, T. K. S. (2016). Multidisciplinary nutritional support for undernutrition in nursing home and home-care: A cluster randomized controlled trial. *Nutrition, 32*(2), 199–205. http://doi.0.1016/j.nut.2015.08.009.

Bunn, D. K., Abdelhamid, A., Copley, M., et al. (2016). Effectiveness of interventions to indirectly support food and drink intake in people with dementia: Eating and drinking well in dementia (EDWINA) systematic review. *BMC Geriatrics, 16*, 89. https://doi.org/10.1186/s12877-016-0256-8.

Cavalcanti, A., Amaral, M. F., Silva E Dutra, F., Santos, A. V. F., Licursi, L. A., & Silveira, Z. C. (2020). Adaptive eating device: Performance and satisfaction of a person with Parkinson's disease. *Canadian Journal of Occupational Therapy, 87*(3), 211–220. https://doi.org/10.1177/0008417420925995.

Chang, B. C., Huang, B. S., Chou, C. L., & Wang, S. J. (2006). A new type of chopsticks for patients with impaired hand function. *Archives of Physical Medicine & Rehabilitation, 87*(7), 1013–1015.

Chen, L. L., Li, H., Lin, R., et al. (2016a). Effects of a feeding intervention in patients with Alzheimer's disease and dysphagia. *Journal of Clinical Nursing, 25*(5–6), 699–707. https://doi.org/10.1111/jocn.13013.

Chen, P. C., Chuang, C. H., Leong, C. P., Guo, S. E., & Hsin, Y. J. (2016b). Systematic review and meta-analysis of the diagnostic accuracy of the water swallow test for screening aspiration in stroke patients. *Journal of Advanced Nursing, 72*(11), 2575–2586. https://doi.org/10.1111/jan.13013.

Chou, H. H., Tsou, M. T., & Hwang, L. C. (2020). Nasogastric tube feeding versus assisted hand feeding in-home healthcare older adults with severe dementia in taiwan: A prognosis comparison. *BMC Geriatrics, 20*(1), 60. https://doi.org/10.1186/s12877-020-1464-9.

Cichero, J. A. Y. (2018). Age-related changes to eating and swallowing impact frailty: Aspiration, choking risk, modified food texture and autonomy of choice. *Geriatrics, 3*(4), 69. https://doi.org/10.3390/geriatrics3040069.

Edwards, D., Carrier, J., & Hopkinson, J. (2017). Assistance at mealtimes in hospital settings and rehabilitation units for patients (>65years) from the perspective of patients, families and healthcare professionals: A mixed methods systematic review. *International Journal of Nursing Studies, 69*, 100–118. https://doi.org/10.1016/j.ijnurstu.2017.01.013.

Johnson, K. L., Speirs, L., Mitchell, A., et al. (2018). Validation of a postextubation dysphagia screening tool for patients after prolonged endotracheal intubation. *American Journal of Critical Care, 27*(2), 89–96. https://doi.org/10.4037/ajcc2018483.

Jones, N., & Nasr, N. (2018). The experiences of stroke survivors with managing eating 6 months post stroke. *British Journal of Occupational Therapy, 81*(2), 106–115. https://doi.org/10.1177/0308022617738487.

Lee, M., Ryoo, J. H., Campbell, C., Hollen, P. J., & Williams, I. C. (2019). Exploring the challenges of medical/nursing tasks in home care experienced by caregivers of older adults with dementia: An integrative review. *Journal of Clinical Nursing, 28*(23-24), 4177–4189. https://doi.org/10.1111/jocn.15007.

Liu, W., Galik, E., Boltz, M., Nahm, E. S., & Resnick, B. (2015). Optimizing eating performance for older adults with dementia living in long-term care: A systematic review. *Worldviews on Evidence-Based Nursing, 12*(4), 228–235. https://doi.org/10.1111/wvn.12100.

Liu, W., Watson, R., & Lou, F. L. (2014). The Edinburgh Feeding Evaluation in Dementia Scale (EdFED): Cross-cultural validation of

S

the simplified Chinese version in mainland China. *Journal of Clinical Nursing, 23*(1–2), 45–53.

Nishida, T., Yamabe, K., Ide, Y., & Honda, S. (2020). Utility of the Eating Assessment Tool-10 (EAT-10) in evaluating self-reported dysphagia associated with oral frailty in Japanese community-dwelling older people. *The Journal of Nutrition, Health & Aging, 24*(1), 3–8. https://doi.org/10.1007/s12603-019-1256-0.

Palese, A., Bressan, V., Kasa, T., Meri, M., Hayter, M., & Watson, R. (2018). Interventions maintaining eating independence in nursing home residents: A multicentre qualitative study. *BMC Geriatrics, 18*(1), 27. https://doi.org/10.1186/s12877-018-0985-y.

Pohlhausen, S., Uhlig, K., Kiesswetter, E., et al. (2016). Energy and protein intake, anthropometrics, and disease burden in elderly home-care receivers—A cross-sectional study in Germany (ErnSIPP Study). *The Journal of Nutrition, Health & Aging, 20*(3), 361–368. https://doi.org/10.1007/s12603-015-0586-9.

Saucedo Figueredo, M. C., Morilla Herrera, J. C., San Alberto Giraldos, M., et al. (2018). Validation of the Spanish version of the Edinburgh Feeding Evaluation in Dementia Scale for older people with dementia. *PLoS One, 13*(2), e0192690.

Sheppard, C. L., McArthur, C., & Hitzig, S. L. (2016). A systematic review of Montessori-based activities for persons with dementia. *Journal of the American Medical Directors Association, 17*(2), 117–122. https://doi.org/10.1016/j.jamda.2015.10.006.

Shune, S. E. (2020). An altered eating experience: Attitudes toward feeding assistance among younger and older adults. *Rehabilitation Nursing, 45*(2), 97–105. https://doi.org/10.1097/rnj.0000000000000147.

Spencer, J. C., Damanik, R., Ho, M. H., et al. (2020). Review of food intake difficulty assessment tools for people with dementia. *Western Journal of Nursing Research*. https://doi.org/10.1177/0193945920979668. [Online ahead of print].

Teeling, S. P., Coetzee, H., Phillips, M., McKiernan, M., Ní ShÉ, É., & Igoe, A. (2019). Reducing risk of development or exacerbation of nutritional deficits by optimizing patient access to mealtime assistance. *International Journal for Quality in Health Care, 31*(Suppl. 1), 6–13. https://doi.org/10.1093/intqhc/mzz060.

Volkert, D., Chourdakis, M., Faxen-Irving, G., et al. (2015). ESPEN guidelines on nutrition in dementia. *Clinical Nutrition, 34*(6), 1052–1073. https://doi.org/10.1016/j.clnu.2015.09.004.

Warren, C., Medei, M. K., Wood, B., & Schutte, D. (2019). A nurse-driven oral care protocol to reduce hospital-acquired pneumonia. *American Journal of Nursing, 119*(2), 44–51. https://doi.org/10.1097/01.NAJ.0000553204.21342.01.

Wu, S. A., Morrison-Koechl, J., Slaughter, S. E., et al. (2020). Family member eating assistance and food intake in long-term care: A secondary data analysis of the M3 study. *Journal of Advanced Nursing, 76*(11), 2933–2944. https://doi.org/10.1111/jan.14480.

Toileting Self-Care Deficit Domain 4 Activity/rest Class 5 Self-care

Suzanne C. Ashworth, MSN, APRN, CCRN, CCNS

NANDA-I

Definition

Inability to independently perform tasks associated with bowel and bladder elimination.

Defining Characteristics

Difficulty completing toilet hygiene; difficulty flushing toilet; difficulty manipulating clothing for toileting; difficulty reaching toilet; difficulty rising from toilet; difficulty sitting on toilet

Related Factors

Anxiety; decreased motivation; environmental constraints; fatigue; impaired physical mobility; impaired transfer ability; neurobehavioral manifestation; pain; weakness

Associated Conditions

Musculoskeletal impairment; neuromuscular diseases

NOC (Nursing Outcomes Classification)

Suggested NOC Outcomes

Self-Care: Activities of Daily Living (ADLs), Toileting

Example NOC Outcome with Indicators

Self-Care: Toileting as evidenced by the following indicators: Responds to full bladder and urge to have a bowel movement in a timely manner/Gets to toilet between urge and passage of urine/Between urge and evacuation of stool. (Rate the outcome and indicators of **Self-Care: Toileting:** 1 = severely compromised, 2 = substantially compromised, 3 = moderately compromised, 4 = mildly compromised, 5 = not compromised [see Section I].)

S

Client Outcomes

Client Will (Specify Time Frame)

- Remain free of incontinence and impaction with no urine or stool on skin
- State satisfaction with ability to use adaptive devices for toileting
- Explain and demonstrate use of methods to be safe and independent in toileting

NIC (Nursing Interventions Classification)

Suggested NIC Interventions

Environmental Management; Self-Care Assistance: Toileting

Example NIC Activities—Self-Care Assistance: Toileting

Assist client to toilet/commode/bedpan/fracture pan/urinal at specified intervals; Institute a toileting schedule, as appropriate

Nursing Interventions and *Rationales*

- ✱ Assess clients for fall risk using established and valid fall risk assessment tools and implement fall prevention interventions for those at risk for falling. **EBN:** *A retrospective study of 409 fall incidents within a hospital setting found that 34% of all falls were related to toileting and 44% of falls occurred at night; in 80% of nighttime falls, clients mobilized without calling for assistance as recommended (Rose et al, 2020).*
- ✱ Implement purposeful hourly or 2-hourly rounding that targets toileting needs of the client. **EBN:** *A quality improvement project conducted on a medical-surgical unit implemented a purposeful rounding protocol that address the four Ps (pain, position, potty, possessions) to decrease the number of client falls. The project led to a 41% increase in toileting and a 50% decrease in client falls (Daniels, 2016).*
- ● Perform a bladder scan for postvoid residual in neurological clients who are at high risk for neurogenic bladder and urinary retention. **EBN:** *A study conducted on poststroke clients found 53% of clients to have postvoid residuals >100 mL (Smith & Schneider, 2020).*
- ✱ Use disposable underpads versus reusable washable underpads for hospitalized adult clients with urine or fecal incontinence. **EBN:** *A study conducted in four medical-surgical units (n = 462) found that disposable pads reduced the rate of hospital-acquired pressure injuries (Francis et al, 2017).*
- ● In the acute care setting, use absorbent pads left open under the client for fecal and urine incontinence. **EB:** *Incontinence absorbent pads that are occlusive around the client create a warm environment and increase the risk for incontinent-associated dermatitis (Thayer, Rozenboom, & Baranoski, 2016).*
- ● Consider use of external urinary collection devices and avoid use of an indwelling urinary catheter for the purpose of incontinence. **EBN:** *Introduction of a female external urinary collection device reduced rates of catheter-associated urinary tract infection in a community hospital setting (Eckert et al, 2020).*
- ● Perform intermittent straight catheterization for clients who are unable to empty their bladder and have urinary retention. **EB:** *A retrospective study conducted in a trauma population demonstrated statistically significant improvements in rate of urinary tract infections after implementation of an intermittent straight catheterization protocol (Kelley et al, 2017).*
- ● Ensure a timely planned evacuation of bowel for spinal cord injury clients by implementing a low-fiber diet and digital stimulation. **EB:** *Spinal cord injury clients have increased morbidity due to symptoms of neurogenic bowel. Understanding physiology and working collaboratively with the client can improve quality of life (Stoffel et al, 2018).*
- ● Assess bowel symptoms and self-management strategies of clients who have had sphincter-saving surgery. Develop client-specific interventions to continue to support and meet client needs. **EBN:** *In a quantitative descriptive study of self-care strategies used by clients who had sphincter-saving surgery and bowel symptoms (n = 143), the strategy of proximity and knowing the location of a toilet at all times was used most by those with more bowel symptoms (Landers et al, 2014).*
- ● Consider use of a female urinal for female cancer clients who are receiving palliative care. **EBN:** *A qualitative study using a female urinal prototype was found to be easier to use compared to a bedpan, was more comfortable, and provided more dignity (Farrington et al, 2016).*
- ▲ Before use of a bedpan, discuss its use with clients. **EBN:** *A study conducted on women in labor with epidural analgesic, nurse education, and training regarding bedpan use increased nurse comfort and client ability to use a bedpan, decreasing the need for urinary catheters (McLain, 2019).*

S

* Promote use of assistive toileting equipment when needed for toileting transfer assistance. EB: *A study of 193 older people living at home found a greater sense of independence and improved quality of life when using bathroom assistive products (De-Rosende-Celeiro et al, 2019).*
* Avoid prolonged time sitting on a toilet, commode, or bedpan to reduce pressure-related skin injury risk. Use padded toilet cushions if needed. EB: *Lustig et al (2018) confirmed that prolonged time on a toilet seat leads to potential pressure injury. This risk was reduced with specialized cushions.*
* Consider use of toilet alarm systems for clients who are at risk for falling and not cognitively impaired. EBN: *The use of a toilet alarm was studied in two community-based hospitals; clients rated higher privacy, greater toileting independence, and less fear of falling (Jones et al, 2021).*
• Close toilet lid before flushing toilet and teach client to do so. EB: *A study conducted in hospital bathrooms that measured potential infectious aerosols after toilet flushing during client care found a significant increase of bioaerosol after flushing, which can lead to environmental contamination (Knowlton et al, 2018).*

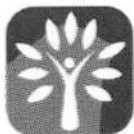

Geriatric

• Assess residents without dementia for risk factors associated with toileting disability (such as rating health as fair or poor; living in a residence with four or less residents or that is for-profit; incontinence; physical, visual, or hearing impairment; and need for ADL or transferring assistance to guide prevention interventions). EBN: *In a cross-sectional analysis of adults 65 years or older without dementia in residential care facilities (n = 2395), 15% were found to have toileting disability that was associated with rating health as fair or poor; living in a residence with four or fewer residents or that is for-profit; incontinence; physical, visual, or hearing impairment; and need for ADL or transferring assistance (Talley et al, 2014).*
• Promote a toileting pattern using timed voiding and verbal prompts to develop habits and promote continence in dementia clients. EB: *Clients with memory impairment may forget how to ask for help with toileting or how to use the toilet. Developing a toileting schedule may help maintain continence (Payne, 2020).*
• Assess the client's functional ability to manipulate clothing for toileting, and if necessary, modify clothing with Velcro fasteners, elastic waists, drop-front underwear, or slacks. EB: *For clients with impaired dexterity or weakness, wearing shirts or pants with Velcro attachments can be easier to remove and promote independence during toileting (Mlinac & Feng, 2016).*
• Consider an exercise training of routine walking and pelvic floor exercises for frail incontinent women. EBN: *A randomized control trial of 42 women with urinary incontinence found improvement of symptoms after a 12-week therapy program that combined lifestyle, behavioral, and physical therapy (Talley et al, 2017).*

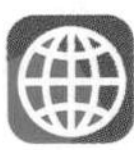

Multicultural

• Remove barriers to toileting, support client's cultural beliefs, and protect dignity during continence care. EB: *A concept analysis literature search defined the key attributes of dignity for continence care in a long-term care setting as privacy, respect, autonomy, empathy, trust, and communication (Ostaszkiewicz et al, 2020).*

S

Home Care

▲ Instruct client/family member or caregiver to develop a bladder diary to obtain a better understanding of incontinent patterns. EB: *Bladder diaries should be used for a minimum of 3 days for the initial assessment of incontinence or overactive bladder (National Institute for Health and Care Excellence [NICE], 2019).*
▲ Involve the client's caregiver in developing a written plan for managing incontinence in dementia clients. EB: *Providing optimal support of caregivers through use of planning can help avoid long-term conditions associated due to stress (Robinson, 2018).*
▲ Consider consultation with occupational therapy to evaluate home bathroom design, to evaluate assistive device needs, and to provide training for proper body mechanics for home caregivers. EB: *Improving safety and avoiding musculoskeletal injuries of caregivers is necessary. Caregivers often identify toileting assistance as a difficult activity (King et al, 2019).*
• Consider the use of technology-assisted toilets with perineal washing ability. EB: *A pilot study of stroke rehabilitation clients found effective cleaning and improved psychosocial outcomes (Yachin et al, 2017).*

Client/Family Teaching and Discharge Planning

- Instruct clients with mixed (stress and urge) urinary incontinence to perform pelvic floor exercises for at least 3 months and increase walking to build muscle strength. EBN: *A 12-week study of behavioral incontinence treatments found 50% improvement in urine leakage and toileting abilities (Talley et al, 2017).*
- Instruct female clients not to use sanitary pads for urinary incontinence. *Sanitary pads are not manufactured for absorbing urine and do not protect the skin (Payne, 2020).*
- Explain to family and caregivers of clients with dementia that toilet self-care activities decrease when self-awareness is lost. EB: *An observational study of toileting self-care in older adults with dementia revealed that toilet activities are affected and decline when self-awareness is lost (composed of theory of mind, self-evaluation, and self-consciousness) (Uchimoto et al, 2013).*

* Educate male clients who perform self-straight catheterization on use of the coude tip catheter to avoid difficulties with insertion. EBN: *With proper training and education, use of the Tiemann (coude) tip catheter can benefit clients by preventing failed catheterization (Rew, Lake, & Brownlee-Moore, 2018).*

REFERENCES

Daniels, J. F. (2016). Purposeful and timely nursing rounds: A best practice implementation project. *JBI Database of Systematic Reviews and Implementation Reports*, *14*(1), 248–267. https://doi.org/10.11124/jbisrir-2016-2537.

De-Rosende-Celeiro, I., Torres, G., Seoane-Bouzas, M., & Ávila, A. (2019). Exploring the use of assistive products to promote functional independence in self-care activities in the bathroom. *PLoS One*, *14*(4), e0215002. https://doi.org/10.1371/journal.pone.0215002.

Eckert, L., Mattia, L., Patel, S., Okumura, R., Reynolds, P., & Stuiver, I. (2020). Reducing the risk of indwelling catheter-associated urinary tract infection in female patients by implementing an alternative female external urinary collection device: A quality improvement project. *The Journal of Wound, Ostomy and Continence Nursing*, *47*(1), 50–53. https://doi.org/10.1097/WON.0000000000000601.

Farrington, N., Hill, T., Fader, M., & Richardson, A. (2016). Supporting women with toileting in palliative care: Use of the female urinal for bladder management. *International Journal of Palliative Nursing*, *22*(11), 524–533. https://doi.org/10.12968/ijpn.2016.22.11.524.

Francis, K., Pang, S. M., Cohen, B., Salter, H., & Homel, P. (2017). Disposable versus reusable absorbent underpads for prevention of hospital-acquired incontinence-associated dermatitis and pressure injuries. *The Journal of Wound, Ostomy and Continence Nursing*, *44*(4), 374–379.

Jones, L., Hessler, K., Winter, B., & Kupzyk, K. (2021). Use of toilet alarms in inpatient settings. *Nursing*, *51*(1), 65–69. https://doi.org/10.1097/01.NURSE.0000724412.70826.46.

Kelley, K., Johnson, T., Burgess, J., Novosel, T. J., Weireter, L., & Collins, J. N. (2017). Effect of implementation of intermittent straight catheter protocol on rate of urinary tract infections in a trauma population. *The American Surgeon*, *83*(7), 747–749.

King, E. C., Boscart, V. M., Weiss, B. M., Dutta, T., Callaghan, J. P., & Fernie, G. R. (2019). Assisting frail seniors with toileting in a home bathroom: Approaches used by home care providers. *Journal of Applied Gerontology*, *38*(5), 717–749. https://doi.org/10.1177/0733464817702477.

Knowlton, S. D., Boles, C. L., Perencevich, E. N., Diekema, D. J., Nonnenmann, M. W., & CDC Epicenters Program. (2018). Bioaerosol concentrations generated from toilet flushing in a hospital-based patient care setting. *Antimicrobial Resistance and Infection Control*, *7*, 16. https://doi.org/10.1186/s13756-018-0301-9.

Landers, M., McCarthy, G., Livingstone, V., & Savage, E. (2014). Patients' bowel symptom experiences and self-care strategies following sphincter-saving surgery for rectal cancer. *Journal of Clinical Nursing*, *23*(15–16), 2343–2354.

Lustig, M., Levy, A., Kopplin, K., Ovadia-Blechman, Z., & Gefen, A. (2018). Beware of the toilet: The risk for a deep tissue injury during toilet sitting. *Journal of Tissue Viability*, *27*(1), 23–31. https://doi.org/10.1016/j.jtv.2017.04.005.

McLain, S. K. (2019). A project to increase nurses' comfort in offering bedpans to women laboring with epidural analgesia. *Nursing for Women's Health*, *23*(3), 200–216. https://doi.org/10.1016/j.nwh.2019.04.001.

Mlinac, M. E., & Feng, M. C. (2016). Assessment of activities of daily living, self-care, and independence. *Archives of Clinical Neuropsychology*, *31*(6), 506–516. https://doi.org/10.1093/arclin/acw049.

National Institute for Health and Care Excellence (NICE). (2019). NICE guidance—Urinary incontinence and pelvic organ prolapse in women: Management. *BJU International*, *123*(5), 777–803. https://doi.org/10.1111/bju.14763.

Ostaszkiewicz, J., Dickson-Swift, V., Hutchinson, A., & Wagg, A. (2020). A concept analysis of dignity-protective continence care for care dependent older people in long-term care settings. *BMC Geriatrics*, *20*(1), 266. https://doi.org/10.1186/s12877-020-01673-x.

Payne, D. (2020). Managing incontinence in people with dementia. *British Journal of Community Nursing*, *25*(9), 430–436. https://doi.org/10.12968/bjcn.2020.25.9.430.

Rew, M., Lake, H., & Brownlee-Moore, K. (2018). The use of Tiemann tip catheters for male intermittent self-catheterisation. *British Journal of Nursing*, *27*(9), S18–S25. https://doi.org/10.12968/bjon.2018.27.9.S18.

Robinson, G. (2018). *Supporting the carers of people with dementia*. Nursing Standard. https://doi.org/10.7748/ns.2019.e11239. [Online ahead of print].

Rose, G., Decalf, V., Everaert, K., & Bower, W. F. (2020). Toileting-related falls at night in hospitalised patients: The role of nocturia. *Australasian Journal on Ageing*, *39*(1), e70–e76. https://doi.org/10.1111/ajag.12696.

Smith, C. E., & Schneider, M. A. (2020). Assessing postvoid residual to identify risk for urinary complications post stroke. *Journal of Neuroscience Nursing*, *52*(5), 219–223. https://doi.org/10.1097/JNN.

Stoffel, J. T., Van der Aa, F., Wittmann, D., Yande, S., & Elliott, S. (2018). Neurogenic bowel management for the adult spinal cord injury patient. *World Journal of Urology*, *36*(10), 1587–1592. https://doi.org/10.1007/s00345-018-2388-2.

Talley, K. M. C., Wyman, J. F., Bronas, U., Olson-Kellogg, B. J., & McCarthy, T. C. (2017). Defeating urinary incontinence with exercise training: Results of a pilot study in frail older women. *Journal of the American Geriatrics Society*, *65*(6), 1321–1327. https://doi.org/10.1111/jgs.14798.

Talley, K. M. C., Wyman, J. F., Bronas, U. G., Olson-Kellogg, B. J., McCarthy, T. C., & Zhao, H. (2014). Factors associated with toileting disability in older adults without dementia living in residential care facilities. *Nursing Research*, *63*(2), 94–104.

S

Thayer, D. M., Rozenboom, B., & Baranoski, S. (2016). "Top down" injuries: Prevention and management of moisture-associated skin damage (MASD), medical adhesive-related skin injury (MARSI), and skin tears. In D. B. Doughty, & L. L. McNichol (Eds.), *Wound, Ostomy and Continence Nurses Society core curriculum: Wound management* (pp. 281–312). Philadelphia: Wolters Kluwer.

Uchimoto, K., Yokoi, T., Yamashita, T., & Okamura, H. (2013). Investigation of toilet activities in elderly patients with dementia from the viewpoint of motivation and self-awareness. *American Journal of Alzheimer's Disease and Other Dementias*, *28*(5), 459–468.

Yachnin, D., Gharib, G., Jutai, J., & Finestone, H. (2017). Technology-assisted toilets: Improving independence and hygiene in stroke rehabilitation. *Journal of Rehabilitation and Assistive Technologies Engineering*, *4*, 2055668317725686. https://doi.org/10.1177/2055668317725686.

Readiness for Enhanced Self-Concept

Domain 6 Self-perception Class 1 Self-concept

Marina Martinez-Kratz, RN, MS, CNE

NANDA-I

Definition

A pattern of perceptions or ideas about the self, which can be strengthened.

Defining Characteristics

Expresses desire to enhance acceptance of limitations; expresses desire to enhance acceptance of strengths; expresses desire to enhance body image satisfaction; expresses desire to enhance confidence in abilities; expresses desire to enhance congruence between actions and words; expresses desire to enhance role performance; expresses desire to enhance satisfaction with personal identity; expresses desire to enhance satisfaction with sense of worth; expresses desire to enhance self-esteem

NOC (Nursing Outcomes Classification)

Suggested NOC Outcomes

Self-Esteem; Personal Well-Being; Psychosocial Adjustment Life Change

Example NOC Outcome with Indicators

Self-Esteem as evidenced by the following indicators: Verbalizations of self-acceptance/Open communication/Confidence level/Description of pride in self. (Rate the outcome and indicators of **Self-Esteem:** 1 = never positive, 2 = rarely positive, 3 = sometimes positive, 4 = often positive, 5 = consistently positive [see Section I].)

Client Outcomes

Client Will (Specify Time Frame)

- State willingness to enhance self-concept
- State satisfaction with thoughts about self, sense of worthiness, role performance, body image, and personal identity
- Demonstrate actions that are congruent with expressed feelings and thoughts
- State confidence in abilities
- Accept strengths and limitations

NIC (Nursing Interventions Classification)

Suggested NIC Intervention

Self-Esteem Enhancement

Example NIC Activities—Self-Esteem Enhancement

Encourage client to identify strengths; Assist client in setting realistic goals to achieve higher self-esteem

S

Nursing Interventions and *Rationales*

- Encourage client to express feelings through songwriting. EB: *Study findings suggested that people who find songwriting has strong meaning for them might be more likely to start accepting their emotions and as a result experience decreases in anxiety and depression (Baker et al, 2016).*
- Refer to nutritional and exercise programs to support weight loss. EB: *Study findings suggested that weight-loss treatments emphasize changes in self-perception (Annesi & Porter, 2015).*
- Offer client complementary and alternative medicine (CAM) interventions such as acupressure, aromatherapy, compress, and massage. EBN: *A study reviewed the development of a complex nursing intervention including CAM for breast and gynecological cancer clients during chemotherapy to improve quality of life (Klafke et al, 2016).*
- Support homeless individuals to identify and endorse a positive self-concept. EB: *A study found that assumption of positive identity meanings, even a stigmatized identity such as being a homeless person, may provide support for a more general sense of self-esteem (Parker et al, 2016).*
- Support unemployed individuals to cope with identity threats and support individual identity growth. EB: *Research shows that to cope with self-definition threats, mature-aged workers protect and restructure their self-definitions with alternative goals of either remaining in paid employment or opting out from it (Kira & Klehe, 2016).*
- Support establishing community-based partnerships to address health needs. EBN: *To prevent suicide and substance abuse, a community-based participatory research approach was used to obtain community input, which led to the development of a strengths-based intervention incorporating the Gathering of Native Americans curriculum (Holliday et al, 2018).*
- For clients with a history of trauma, offer a mindfulness-based intervention of hatha yoga. EB: *A qualitative study explored the experiences of women with posttraumatic stress disorder (PTSD) who participated in a 10-week Trauma Sensitive Yoga (TSY) class. It was found that they specifically perceived changes in symptoms and feelings of gratitude and compassion, relatedness, acceptance, centeredness, and empowerment (West et al, 2017).*

Pediatric

- Facilitate healthy relationships with teachers, coaches, and other supportive adults in the adolescents' lives. EB: *Research found that the presence of supportive teachers and coaches in an adolescent's social network is associated with healthier self-concept and decreased substance use (Dudovitz et al, 2017).*
- Provide parents with information designed to promote body satisfaction, healthy eating, and weight management in early childhood. EB: *Research evaluated Confident Body, Confident Child (CBCC), which is an intervention for parents of 2- to 6-year-old children, and found significant increases in parents' intentions to use positive behaviors and knowledge of child body image and healthy eating patterns (Hart et al, 2016).*
- Promote the adoption of a recovery identity through online interactions and support groups for individuals with eating disorders. EB: *A study found that an eating disorder identity is seen as problematic and most interventions are targeted at changing an individual's self-concept. The study suggested that interventions could instead focus on identity resources to support a transition to a recovery identity (McNamara & Parsons, 2016).*
- Provide activities to bolster physical self-concept. EB: *A meta-analytic review found that physical activity interventions increased positive self-concept in adolescents (Spruit et al, 2016).*
- ▲ Provide overweight adolescents access to group-based weight control interventions. EB: *A 12-week group-based exergaming intervention was associated with positive effects on overweight and obese adolescent girls' television viewing, self-efficacy, and intrinsic motivation (Staiano et al, 2017).*
- Provide an alternative school-based program for pregnant and parenting adolescents. EB: *Despite Title IX legislation mandating equal educational opportunities for pregnant and parenting teens, only 50% of adolescent parents graduate high school. A study found themes of struggle, support, hope, perseverance, and transformation in a cohort of young mothers' descriptions of finishing high school (Watson & Vogel, 2017).*

Geriatric

- Encourage clients to consider online support programs when they are in a caregiving situation. EBN: *Research found that participation in a Web-based family support network provided a venue to share experiences, to be informed, and to gain insights into care issues. Participation reinforced the caregiver's sense of competence, helped them meet caregiving demands, and allowed them to identify the positive aspects of their situation (Andersson et al, 2017).*

- Encourage activity and a strength, mobility, balance, and endurance training program. EB: *Older participants in a fitness training trial demonstrated beneficial effects on muscular strength, functionality, and confidence* (*Schreier et al, 2016*).
- Support meaning and purpose in the lives of older adults through a focus on everyday well-being and facilitation of personally treasured activities. EBN: *An exploratory study found four key experiences that promote meaning and purpose in life: (1) physical and mental well-being, (2) belonging and recognition, (3) personally treasured activities, and (4) spiritual closeness and connectedness* (*Drageset et al, 2017*).
- Use an approach that reduces the emphasis put on ageist self-concept attributions when working with older clients. EB: *Ageism includes cognitive, behavioral, and emotional manifestations. Ageism tends to reinforce social inequalities because it is more pronounced toward older women, poor people, or those with dementia* (*Ayalon & Tesch-Römer, 2017*).

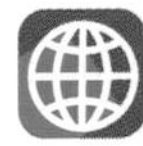

Multicultural

- Refer to the care plans Disturbed **Body Image,** Readiness for Enhanced **Coping,** Chronic Low **Self-Esteem,** and Readiness for Enhanced **Spiritual** Well-Being.

Home Care

- Previously discussed interventions may be used in the home care setting.

REFERENCES

Andersson, S., Erlingsson, C., Magnusson, L., & Hanson, E. (2017). The experiences of working carers of older people regarding access to a web-based family care support network offered by a municipality. *Scandinavian Journal of Caring Sciences*, *31*(3), 487–496. https://doi.org/10.1111/scs.12361.

Annesi, J. J., & Porter, K. J. (2015). Reciprocal effects of exercise and nutrition treatment-Induced weight loss with improved body image and physical self-concept. *Behavioral Medicine*, *41*(1), 18–24. http://doi.org/10.1080/08964289.2013.856284.

Ayalon, L., & Tesch-Römer, C. (2017). Taking a closer look at ageism: Self- and other-directed ageist attitudes and discrimination. *European Journal of Ageing*, *14*(1), 1–4. http://doi.org/10.1007/s10433-016-0409-9.

Baker, F., Rickard, N., Tamplin, J., & Roddy, C. (2016). Mechanisms of change in self-concept and well-being following songwriting interventions for people in the early phase of neurorehabilitation [abstract]. *Nordic Journal of Music Therapy*, *25*(Suppl. 1), 10–11. https://doi.org/10.1080/08098131.2016.11783620.

Drageset, J., Haugan, G., & Tranvåg, O. (2017). Crucial aspects promoting meaning and purpose in life: Perceptions of nursing home residents. *BMC Geriatrics*, *17*(1), 254. https://doi.org/10.1186/s12877-017-0650-x.

Dudovitz, R. N., Chung, P. J., & Wong, M. D. (2017). Teachers and coaches in adolescent social networks are associated with healthier self-concept and decreased substance use. *Journal of School Health*, *87*(1), 12–20. https://doi.org/10.1111/josh.12462.

Hart, L. M., Damiano, S. R., & Paxton, S. J. (2016). Confident body, confident child: A randomized controlled trial evaluation of a parenting resource for promoting healthy body image and eating patterns in 2- to 6-year old children. *International Journal of Eating Disorders*, *49*(5), 458–472. https://doi.org/10.1002/eat.22494.

Holliday, C. E., Wynne, M., Katz, J., Ford, C., & Barbosa-Leiker, C. (2018). A CBPR approach to finding community strengths and challenges to prevent youth suicide and substance abuse. *Journal of Transcultural Nursing*, *29*(1), 64–73. http://doi.org/10.1177/1043659616679234.

Kira, M., & Klehe, U. C. (2016). Self-definition threats and potential for growth among mature-aged job-loss victims. *Human Resource Management Review*, *26*(3), 242–259. http://doi.org/10.1016/j.hrmr.2016.03.001.

Klafke, N., Mahler, C., von Hagens, C., Blaser, G., Bentner, M., & Joos, S. (2016). Developing and implementing a complex Complementary and Alternative (CAM) nursing intervention for breast and gynecologic cancer patients undergoing chemotherapy—Report from the CONGO (complementary nursing in gynecologic oncology) study. *Supportive Care in Cancer*, *24*(5), 2341–2350. http://doi.org/10.1007/s00520-015-3038-5.

McNamara, N., & Parsons, H. (2016). "Everyone here wants everyone else to get better": The role of social identity in eating disorder recovery. *British Journal of Social Psychology*, *55*(4), 662–680. https://doi.org/10.1111/bjso.12161.

Parker, J., Reitzes, D. C., & Ruel, E. E. (2016). Preserving and protecting well-being among homeless men. *Sociological Perspectives*, *59*(1), 201–218. http://doi.org/10.1177/0731121415591096.

Schreier, M. M., Bauer, U., Osterbrink, J., Niebauer, J., Iglseder, B., & Reiss, J. (2016). Fitness training for the old and frail. Effectiveness and impact on daily life coping and self-care abilities. *Zeitschrift für Gerontologie und Geriatrie*, *49*(2), 107–114. http://doi.org/10.1007/s00391-015-0966-0.

Spruit, A., Assink, M., van Vugt, E., van der Put, C., & Stams, G. J. (2016). The effects of physical activity interventions on psychosocial outcomes in adolescents: A meta-analytic review. *Clinical Psychology Review*, *45*, 56–71. http://doi.org/10.1016/j.cpr.2016.03.006.

Staiano, A. E., Beyl, R. A., Hsia, D. S., Katzmarzyk, P. T., & Newton, R. L., Jr. (2017). Twelve weeks of dance exergaming in overweight and obese adolescent girls: Transfer effects on physical activity, screen time, and self-efficacy. *Journal of Sport and Health Science*, *6*(1), 4–10. https://doi.org/10.1016/j.jshs.2016.11.005.

Watson, L. L., & Vogel, L. R. (2017). Educational resiliency in teen mothers. *Cogent Education*, *4*(1), 1–22. http://doi.org/10.1080/2331186X.2016.1276009.

West, J., Liang, B., & Spinazzola, J. (2017). Trauma sensitive yoga as a complementary treatment for posttraumatic stress disorder: A qualitative descriptive analysis. *International Journal of Stress Management*, *24*(2), 173–195. https://doi.org/10.1037/str0000040.

S

Chronic Low Self-Esteem

Domain 6 Self-perception Class 2 Self-esteem

Marina Martinez-Kratz, MS, RN, CNE

NANDA-I

Definition

Long-standing negative perception of self-worth, self-acceptance, self-respect, competence, and attitude toward self.

Defining Characteristics

Dependent on others' opinions; depressive symptoms; excessive guilt; excessive seeking of reassurance; expresses loneliness; hopelessness; insomnia; loneliness; nonassertive behavior; overly conforming behaviors; reduced eye contact; rejects positive feedback; reports repeated failures; rumination; self-negating verbalizations; shame; suicidal ideation; underestimates ability to deal with situation

Related Factors

Decreased mindful acceptance; difficulty managing finances; disturbed body image; fatigue; fear of rejection; impaired religiosity; inadequate affection received; inadequate attachment behavior; inadequate family cohesiveness; inadequate group membership; inadequate respect from others; inadequate sense of belonging; inadequate social support; ineffective communication skills; insufficient approval from others; low self efficacy; maladaptive grieving; negative resignation; repeated negative reinforcement; spiritual incongruence; stigmatization; stressors; values incongruent with cultural norms

At-Risk Population

Economically disadvantaged individuals; individuals experiencing repeated failure; individuals exposed to traumatic situation; individuals with difficult developmental transition; individuals with history of being abandoned; individuals with history of being abused; individuals with history of being neglected; individuals with history of loss

Associated Conditions

Depression; functional impairment; mental disorders; physical illness

NOC (Nursing Outcomes Classification)

Suggested NOC Outcome

Self-Esteem

Example NOC Outcome with Indicators

Demonstrates improved **Self-Esteem** as evidenced by the following indicators: Verbalizations of acceptance of self and limitations/Open communication. (Rate the outcome and indicators of **Self-Esteem:** 1 = never positive, 2 = rarely positive, 3 = sometimes positive, 4 = often positive, 5 = consistently positive [see Section I].)

Client Outcomes

Client Will (Specify Time Frame)

- Demonstrate improved ability to interact with others (e.g., maintains eye contact, engages in conversation, expresses thoughts/feelings)
- Verbalize increased self-acceptance through positive self-statements about self
- Identify personal strengths, accomplishments, and values
- Identify and work on small, achievable goals
- Improve independent decision-making and problem-solving skills

S

NIC (Nursing Interventions Classification)

Suggested NIC Intervention

Self-Esteem Enhancement

Example NIC Activities—Self-Esteem Enhancement

Encourage client to identify strengths; Assist in setting realistic goals to achieve higher self-esteem

Nursing Interventions and *Rationales*

- Assess existing strengths and coping abilities, and provide opportunities for their expression and recognition. EB: *Study results found that cancer clients had lower self-esteem, and upper-level cognitive functions and problem-focused coping were worse compared with healthy controls (Inci et al, 2020).*
- Assess the client's self-esteem using valid and established tools such as the Rosenberg Self-Esteem Scale. CEB: *The use of valid and established measures of self-esteem will facilitate the identification of appropriate nursing interventions that strengthen self-esteem (Rosenberg, 1965).*
- Assess the client for addictive use of social media. EB: *Results from a study demonstrated that lower age, being a woman, not being in a relationship, being a student, lower education, lower income, lower self-esteem, and narcissism were associated with higher scores on the Bergen Social Media Addiction Scale (BSMAS) (Andreasson et al, 2017).*
- Reinforce the personal strengths and positive self-perceptions that a client identifies. EB: *A study found that self-esteem mediates the relationship between hope and life satisfaction (Du et al, 2015).*
- Encourage self-affirmations by reflecting on values and strengths, in response to daily threats. EB: *A study found that engaging in spontaneous self-affirmation was related to greater happiness, hopefulness, optimism, subjective health, personal health efficacy, and less anger and sadness (Emanuel et al, 2018).*
- Identify client's negative self-assessments. EB: *Body image was found to have significant effects on both self-esteem and depression (You et al, 2017).*
- Assess individuals with low self-esteem for nonsuicidal self-injury (NSSI). EB: *A systemic review indicated a significant negative relationship between self-esteem and NSSI (Forrester et al, 2017).*
- Assess individuals with low self-esteem for symptoms of depression. EB: *Self-esteem is related to depressive symptoms and interpersonal problems. Improvement of self-esteem during psychotherapy correlates with improvements of symptoms and interpersonal problems (Dinger et al, 2017).*
- Encourage realistic and achievable goal setting and resources and identify impediments to achievement. EB: *A combined decision support and goal-setting intervention improved diet quality, diabetes-related self-efficacy, and empowerment and reduced diabetes-related distress and depressive symptoms (Swoboda et al, 2017).*
- Assist client in challenging negative perceptions of self and performance. EB: *A study found that more often than not, self-critical thoughts were viewed as facts and would rarely be seen as distorted or biased (Kolubinski et al, 2016).*
- Encourage the client's usual religious or spiritual practices. EB: *Research supports a positive association between religious involvement and self-esteem (Schieman et al, 2017).*
- Promote maintaining a level of functioning in the community and a sense of community feeling. EB: *Research found that the community feeling is positively connected with self-esteem and psychological well-being (Kałużna-Wielobób, 2017).*

Pediatric

- Assess children/adolescents with chronic illness for evidence of reduced self-esteem and make needed referrals. EB: *A review of literature found that effective management of chronic skin conditions has been shown to increase pediatric clients' self-esteem (Vivar & Kruse, 2017).*
- Encourage parents to use active listening to foster respectful relationships with children and adolescents. EB: *A study found that self-esteem had a mediating effect on parenting practices and satisfaction with the life of the adolescent (Pérez-Fuentes et al, 2019).*
- Monitor young adolescents during the transition to middle school for changes in self-concept. EB: *A study of adolescents found that middle school transition was associated with a lower self-concept (Onetti, Fernández-García, & Castillo-Rodríguez, 2019).*

S

- Encourage mothers of premature infants to use skin-to-skin care for at least 30 minutes/day. EBN: *A study found that skin-to-skin care showed significantly positive effects on stabilizing infant physiological functions such as respiration rate, increasing maternal–infant attachment, and reducing maternal stress (Cho et al, 2016).*
- Implement interventions that promote and maintain positive peer relations for adolescent clients. EB: *A large German study found positive associations between academic achievement, perceived peer acceptance, and self-esteem (Tetzner, Becker, Maaz, 2017).*
- Encourage attendance at social support groups. EB: *A study found that lesbian, gay, bisexual, transgender, and queer (LGBTQ) youth who attended a Hatch group-level intervention that consisted of unstructured social time, consciousness-raising (education), and a youth-led peer support group had higher levels of self-esteem (Wilkerson et al, 2017).*
- Encourage parents to praise children in ways that are not overly positive or inflated. EB: *A study found that parents' inflated praise predicted lower self-esteem in children (Brummelman et al, 2017).*
- Provide parents with information designed to promote body satisfaction, healthy eating, and weight management in early childhood. EB: *Research evaluated Confident Body, Confident Child (CBCC), which is an intervention for parents of 2- to 6-year-old children, and found significant increases in parents' intentions to use positive behaviors and knowledge of child body image and healthy eating patterns (Hart et al, 2016).*
- Assess children/adolescents that express a body image of self-perceived underweight, self-perceived overweight, and/or frustration with appearance for evidence of bullying. EB: *Research indicated that self-perceived underweight, self-perceived overweight, and frustration with appearance were positively associated with being bullied (Lin et al, 2018).*
- ▲ Provide bully prevention programs and include information on cyberbullying. EB: *A moderate and statistically significant relationship exists between low self-esteem and experiences with cyberbullying (Lin et al, 2018).*

Geriatric

- Support client in identifying and adapting to functional changes. EBN: *A study outlined the importance of enquiring about feelings of uselessness, which is linked to both psychological and physical health status, especially in older people who need help in daily activities (Curzio et al, 2017).*
- Implement reminiscence therapy. EBN: *Research suggests that a reminiscence program could increase self-esteem of hospitalized elders with chronic disease (Trerin, Naka, & Nukaew, 2017).*
- Encourage older adult clients to participate in flexibility, toning, and balance exercise. EB: *Older participants in a fitness training trial demonstrated beneficial effects on muscular strength, functionality, and confidence (Schreier et al, 2016).*
- Encourage regular physical activity with prerecorded workouts. EB: *Research found that a DVD-delivered exercise intervention for older adults was associated with improved and maintained levels of self-esteem (Awick et al, 2017).*
- Encourage participation in intergenerational social activities. EB: *Older adults reported that their participation in the "Time After Time" intergenerational program enhanced their confidence, self-esteem, and social skills; contributed to their emotional and overall health and well-being; and enabled them to learn about others and feel connected to their community (Teater, 2016).*
- Encourage activities in which a client can volunteer to support/help others. EB: *Research indicates that participation in volunteering mitigates the negative effects of older adults' low self-esteem on their sense of belonging and life satisfaction (Russell et al, 2019).*
- Encourage home and community gardening activities. EB: *Research found that older adult participation in gardening activities enhanced self-esteem (Scott, Masser, & Pachana, 2020).*

S

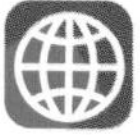

Multicultural

- Assess for the influence of cultural beliefs, norms, and values on the client's sense of self-esteem. EB: *A study of Latino youth suggested that specific cultural orientations were associated with increased global self-worth and increased levels of acculturation risk factors were associated with decreased global self-worth (Kapke et al, 2017).*
- Assess individuals with low self-esteem for symptoms of depression. EB: *Research found that low self-esteem and high depressive symptoms are more closely associated among blacks than whites (Assari, 2017).*
- Validate the client's feelings regarding ethnic or racial identity. EB: *A study found high ethnic identity to be protective against perceived stress (Espinosa et al, 2018).*

Home Care

- Assess a client's immediate support system/family for relationship patterns and content of communication. EB: *A study supported the beneficial effects of perceived family support on mental and physical health after surgery (Cardoso-Moreno & Tomás-Aragones, 2017).*
- ▲ Refer to continuous support and help from medical social services to assist the family in care of the client and support the caregiver's well-being. EB: *A study found that caregiving stress showed a significant positive correlation with depression and with economic and psychological stress, and it showed a significant negative correlation with self-esteem (Kim, 2017).*
- ▲ If a client is involved in counseling or self-help groups, monitor and encourage attendance. Help the client identify the value of group participation after each group encounter. Discussion about group participation clarifies and reinforces group feedback and support.

Client/Family Teaching and Discharge Planning

- Encourage clients to consider online support programs when they are in a caregiving situation. EBN: *Research found that participation in a Web-based family support network provided a venue to share experiences, to be informed, and to gain insights into care issues. Participation reinforced caregivers' sense of competence, helped them meet caregiving demands, and allowed them to identify the positive aspects of their situation (Andersson et al, 2017).*
- ▲ Refer to community agencies for psychotherapeutic counseling. EB: *Self-esteem is related to depressive symptoms and interpersonal problems. Improvement of self-esteem during psychotherapy correlates with improvements of symptoms and interpersonal problems (Dinger et al, 2017).*

REFERENCES

Andersson, S., Erlingsson, C., Magnusson, L., & Hanson, E. (2017). The experiences of working carers of older people regarding access to a web-based family care support network offered by a municipality. *Scandinavian Journal of Caring Sciences*, *31*(3), 487–496. https://doi.org/10.1111/scs.12361.

Andreasson, C. S., Pallesen, S., & Griffiths, M. D. (2017). The relationship between addictive use of social media, narcissism, and self-esteem: Findings from a large national survey. *Addictive Behaviors*, *64*, 287–293. http://doi.org/10.1016/j.addbeh.2016.03.006.

Assari, S. (2017). Association between self-esteem and depressive symptoms is stronger among black than white older adults. *Journal of Racial and Ethnic Health Disparities*, *4*(4), 687–695. http://doi.org/10.1007/s40615-016-0272-6.

Awick, E. A., Ehlers, D., Fanning, J., et al. (2017). Effects of a home-based DVD-delivered physical activity program on self-esteem in older adults: Results from a randomized controlled trial. *Psychosomatic Medicine*, *79*(1), 71–80. https://doi.org/10.1097/PSY.0000000000000358.

Brummelman, E., Nelemans, S. A., Thomaes, S., & Orobio de Castro, B. (2017). When parents' praise inflates, children's self-esteem deflates. *Child Development*, *88*(6), 1799–1809. https://doi.10.1111/cdev.12936.

Cardoso-Moreno, M. J., & Tomás-Aragones, L. (2017). The influence of perceived family support on post surgery recovery. *Psychology Health & Medicine*, *22*(1), 121–128. https://doi.org/10.1080/13548506.2016.1153680.

Cho, E. S., Kim, S. J., Kwon, M. S., et al. (2016). The effects of kangaroo care in the neonatal intensive care unit on the physiological functions of preterm infants, maternal–infant attachment, and maternal stress. *Journal of Pediatric Nursing: Nursing Care of Children and Families*, *31*(4), 430–438. https://doi.org/10.1016/j.pedn.2016.02.007.

Curzio, O., Bernacca, E., Bianchi, B., & Rossi, G. (2017). Feelings of uselessness and 3-year mortality in an Italian community older people: The role of the functional status. *Psychogeriatrics*, *17*(5), 300–309. https://doi.org/10.1111/psyg.12238.

Dinger, U., Ehrenthal, J. C., Nikendei, C., & Schauenburg, H. (2017). Change in self-esteem predicts depressive symptoms at follow-up after intensive multimodal psychotherapy for major depression. *Clinical Psychology & Psychotherapy*, *24*(5), 1040–1046. http://doi.org/10.1002/cpp.2067.

Du, H., Bernardo, A. B. I., & Yeung, S. S. (2015). Locus-of-hope and life satisfaction: The mediating roles of personal self-esteem and relational self-esteem. *Personality and Individual Differences*, *83*, 228–233. http://doi.org/10.1016/j.paid.2015.04.026.

Emanuel, A. S., Howell, J. L., Taber, J. M., Ferrer, R. A., Klein, W. M., & Harris, P. R. (2018). Spontaneous self-affirmation is associated with psychological well-being: Evidence from a US national adult survey sample. *Journal of Health Psychology*, *23*(1), 95–102. http://doi.org/10.1177/1359105316643595.

Espinosa, A., Tikhonov, A., Ellman, L. M., Kern, D. M., Lui, F., & Anglin, D. (2018). Ethnic identity and perceived stress among ethnically diverse immigrants. *Journal of Immigrant and Minority Health*, *20*(1), 155–163. http://doi.org/10.1007/s10903-016-0494-z.

Forrester, R. L., Slater, H., Jomar, K., Mitzman, S., & Taylor, P. J. (2017). Self-esteem and non-suicidal self-injury in adulthood: A systematic review. *Journal of Affective Disorders*, *221*, 172–183. https://doi.org/10.1016/j.jad.2017.06.027.

Hart, L. M., Damiano, S. R., & Paxton, S. J. (2016). Confident body, confident child: A randomized controlled trial evaluation of a parenting resource for promoting healthy body image and eating patterns in 2- to 6-year old children. *International Journal of Eating Disorders*, *49*(5), 458–472. https://doi.org/10.1002/eat.22494.

Inci, H., Inci, F., Ersoy, S., Karatas, F., & Adahan, D. (2020). Self-esteem, metacognition, and coping strategies in cancer patients: A case–control study. *Journal of Cancer Research and Therapeutics*. [Online ahead of print]. https://doi.org/10.4103/jcrt.JCRT_618_19.

Kałużna-Wielobób, A. (2017). The community feeling versus anxiety, self-esteem and well-being—introductory research. *Polish Psychological Bulletin*, *48*(2), 167–174. https://doi.org/10.1515/ppb-2017-0020.

Kapke, T. L., Gerdes, A. C., & Lawton, K. E. (2017). Global self-worth in Latino youth: The role of acculturation and acculturation risk factors. *Child and Youth Care Forum*, *46*(3), 307–333. http://doi.org/10.1007/s10566-016-9374-x.

S

Kim, D. (2017). Relationships between caregiving stress, depression, and self-esteem in family caregivers of adults with a disability. *Occupational Therapy International, 2017*, 1686143. http://doi.org/10.1155/2017/1686143.

Kolubinski, D. C., Nikčević, A. V., Lawrence, J. A., & Spada, M. M. (2016). The role of metacognition in self-critical rumination: An investigation in individuals presenting with low self-esteem. *Journal of Rational-Emotive and Cognitive-Behavior Therapy*, *34*(1), 73–85. http://doi.org/10.1007/s10942-015-0230-y.

Lin, Y. C., Latner, J. D., Fung, X. C. C., & Lin, C. Y. (2018). Poor health and experiences of being bullied in adolescents: Self-perceived overweight and frustration with appearance matter. *Obesity*, *26*(2), 397–404. https://doi.org/10.1002/oby.22041.

Onetti, W., Fernández-García, J. C., & Castillo-Rodríguez, A. (2019). Transition to middle school: Self-concept changes. *PLoS One*, *14*(2), e0212640. https://doi.org/10.1371/journal.pone.0212640.

Pérez-Fuentes, M. C., Molero Jurado, M. M., Gázquez Linares, J. J., Oropesa Ruiz, N. F., Simón Márquez, M. M., & Saracostti, M. (2019). Parenting practices, life satisfaction, and the role of self-esteem in adolescents. *International Journal of Environmental Research and Public Health*, *16*(20), 4045. https://doi.org/10.3390/ijerph16204045.

Rosenberg, M. (1965). *Society and adolescent self-image*. Princeton, NJ: Princeton University Press.

Russell, A. R., Nyame-Mensah, A., de Wit, A., & Handy, F. (2019). Volunteering and wellbeing among ageing adults: A longitudinal analysis. *Voluntas*, *30*, 115–128. https://doi.org/10.1007/s11266-018-0041-8.

Schieman, S., Bierman, A., Upenieks, L., & Ellison, C. G. (2017). Love thy self? How belief in a supportive God shapes self-esteem. *Review of Religious Research*, *59*(3), 293–318. http://doi.org/10.1007/s13644-017-0292-7.

Schreier, M. M., Bauer, U., Osterbrink, J., Niebauer, J., Iglseder, B., & Reiss, J. (2016). Fitness training for the old and frail. Effectiveness and impact on daily life coping and self-care abilities. *Zeitschrift für Gerontologie und Geriatrie*, *49*(2), 107–114. http://doi.org/10.1007/s00391-015-0966-0.

Scott, T. L., Masser, B. M., & Pachana, N. A. (2020). Positive aging benefits of home and community gardening activities: Older adults report enhanced self-esteem, productive endeavours, social engagement and exercise. *SAGE Open Medicine*, *8*, 2050312120901732. https://doi.org/10.1177/2050312120901732.

Swoboda, C. M., Miller, C. K., & Wills, C. E. (2017). Impact of a goal setting and decision support telephone coaching intervention on diet, psychosocial, and decision outcomes among people with type 2 diabetes. *Patient Education and Counseling*, *100*(7), 1367–1373. http://doi.org.proxy.lib.umich.edu/10.1016/j.pec.2017.02.007.

Teater, B. (2016). Intergenerational programs to promote active aging: The experiences and perspectives of older adults. *Activities, Adaptation & Aging*, *40*(1), 1–19. http://doi.org.proxy.lib.umich.edu/10.1080/01924788.2016.1127041.

Tetzner, J., Becker, M., & Maaz, K. (2017). Development in multiple areas of life in adolescence: Interrelations between academic achievement, perceived peer acceptance, and self-esteem. *International Journal of Behavioral Development*, *41*(6), 704–713. https://doi.org/10.1177/0165025416664432.

Trerin, S., Naka, K., & Nukaew, O. (2017). The effect of reminiscence program on self-esteem in hospitalized elders with chronic diseases. *Songklanagarind Journal of Nursing*, *37*(2), 106–117.

Vivar, K. L., & Kruse, L. (2017). The impact of pediatric skin disease on self-esteem. *International Journal of Women's Dermatology*, *4*(1), 27–31. https://doi.org/10.1016/j.ijwd.2017.11.002.

Wilkerson, J. M., Schick, V. R., Romijnders, K. A., Bauldry, J., & Butame, S. A. (2017). Social support, depression, self-esteem, and coping among LGBTQ adolescents participating in Hatch Youth. *Health Promotion Practice*, *18*(3), 358–365. http://doi/10.1177/152483991665446.

You, S., Shin, K., & Kim, A. Y. (2017). Body image, self-esteem, and depression in Korean adolescents. *Child Indicators Research*, *10*(1), 231–245. http://doi.org/10.1007/s12187-016-9385-z.

Situational Low Self-Esteem

Domain 6 Self-perception Class 2 Self-esteem

Marina Martinez-Kratz, MS, RN, CNE

NANDA-I

S

Definition

Change from positive to negative perception of self-worth, self-acceptance, self-respect, competence, and attitude toward self in response to a current situation.

Defining Characteristics

Depressive symptoms; expresses loneliness; helplessness; indecisive behavior; insomnia; loneliness; nonassertive behavior; purposelessness; rumination; self-negating verbalizations; underestimates ability to deal with situation

Related Factors

Behavior incongruent with values; decrease in environmental control; decreased mindful acceptance; difficulty accepting alteration in social role; difficulty managing finances; disturbed body image; fatigue; fear of rejection; impaired religiosity inadequate attachment behavior; inadequate family cohesiveness; inadequate respect from others; inadequate social support; ineffective communication skills; low self efficacy; maladaptive perfectionism; negative resignation; powerlessness; stigmatization; stressors; unrealistic self-expectations; values incongruent with cultural norms

At-Risk Population

Individuals experiencing a change in living environment; individuals experiencing alteration in body image; individuals experiencing alteration in economic status; individuals experiencing alteration in role function; individuals experiencing death of a significant other; individuals experiencing divorce; individuals experiencing new additions to the family; individuals experiencing repeated failure; individuals experiencing unplanned pregnancy; individuals with difficult developmental transition; individuals with history of being abandoned; individuals with history of being abused; individuals with history of being neglected; individuals with history of loss; individuals with history of rejection

Associated Conditions

Depression; functional impairment; mental disorders; physical illness

NOC (Nursing Outcomes Classification)

Refer to Chronic Low **Self-Esteem** for suggested NOC outcomes.

Client Outcomes

Client Will (Specify Time Frame)

- State effect of life events on feelings about self
- State personal strengths
- Acknowledge presence of guilt and not blame self if an action was related to another person's appraisal
- Seek help when necessary
- Demonstrate self-perceptions are accurate given physical capabilities
- Demonstrate separation of self-perceptions from societal stigmas

NIC (Nursing Interventions Classification)

Refer to Chronic Low **Self-Esteem** for suggested NIC interventions.

Nursing Interventions and *Rationales*

- ▲ Assess the client for signs and symptoms of depression and potential for suicide and/or violence. If present, immediately notify the appropriate personnel of symptoms. EB: *Research supported the vulnerability model of low self-esteem and depression with findings that indicated that individuals with high self-esteem have a lower risk for developing depression (Orth et al, 2016).* See care plans for Risk for Other-Directed **Violence** and Risk for **Suicidal Behavior.**
- Assess the client's environmental and everyday stressors, including evidence of abusive relationships. EB: *Research showed that dysfunctional forms of self-esteem were significantly associated with the number of negative events reported and an increased risk of developing stress-related symptoms* (Alessandri et al, 2017).
- Assess the client's self-esteem using valid and established tools such as the Rosenberg Self-Esteem Scale. CEB: *The use of valid and established measures of self-esteem will facilitate the identification of appropriate nursing interventions that strengthen self-esteem* (Rosenberg, 1965).
- Encourage expressions of gratitude through a gratitude journal or kind acts. EB: *Research shows that gratitude is significantly and positively associated with several domains of life satisfaction and overall life satisfaction in both the United States and Japan (Robustelli & Whisman, 2018).*
- Use a cognitive approach such as problem-solving education (PSE) to assist in the identification of problems and situational factors that contribute to problems and offer options for resolution. EB: *A study found that supplementing drug abuse treatment with PSE reduced relapse rates and enhanced self-efficacy and self-esteem among clients (Habibi et al, 2016).*
- Mutually identify strengths, resources, and previously effective coping strategies. EB: *A study showed that a behavioral intervention focusing on the individual's strengths showed a reduction of psychological distress and improvement of self-esteem, optimism, and quality of life compared with the control group (Victor, Teismann, & Willutzki, 2017).*
- Encourage self-affirmations by reflecting on values and strengths, in response to daily threats. EB: *A study found that engaging in spontaneous self-affirmation was related to greater happiness, hopefulness, optimism, subjective health, personal health efficacy, and less anger and sadness (Emanuel et al, 2018).*
- Accept client's own pace in working through grief or crisis situations. EB: *Rigid adherence to stage or timeline models of grief models is too simplistic and limited; they fail to represent the complex emotions and processes of grief and grieving (Stroebe et al, 2017).*

S

- Encourage the client to accept their own defenses, feelings, and urges in dealing with the crisis. EB: *Acceptance and commitment therapy (ACT) is an intervention that enhances well-being and reduces distress (Wersebe et al, 2018).*
- Teach the client mindfulness techniques to cope more effectively with strong emotional responses. EB: *A study found that mindfulness was significantly and positively related to high self-esteem (Park & Dhandra, 2017).*
- Encourage objective appraisal of self and life events and challenge negative or perfectionist expectations of self. EB: *Self-critical perfectionism has been reliably associated with poor goal progress (Moore et al, 2018).*
- Acknowledge the presence of societal stigma. Teach management tools. EBN: *Stigma toward mental illness affects both self-esteem and recovery and treatment adherence (Vass et al, 2017).*
- Validate the effect of negative past experiences on self-esteem and work on corrective measures. EB: *Negative life events influence current self-esteem (Tetzner et al, 2016).*

Pediatric, Geriatric, and Multicultural

- See care plan for Chronic Low **Self-Esteem.**

Home Care

- Establish an emergency plan and contract with the client for its use. Having an emergency plan is reassuring to the client. Establishing a contract validates the worth of the client and provides a caring link between the client and society.
- Access supplies that support a client's success at independent living.
- See care plan for Chronic Low **Self-Esteem.**

Client/Family Teaching and Discharge Planning

- Previously discussed interventions may be used in the home care setting.
- ▲ Refer to appropriate community resources or crisis intervention centers.
- ▲ Refer to resources for handicap and/or disability services.
- See care plan for Chronic Low **Self-Esteem.**

REFERENCES

Alessandri, G., Perinelli, E., De Longis, E., Rosa, V., Theodorou, A., & Borgogni, L. (2017). The costly burden of an inauthentic self: Insecure self-esteem predisposes to emotional exhaustion by increasing reactivity to negative events. *Anxiety, Stress & Coping*, *30*(6), 630–646. https://doi.org/10.1080/10615806.2016.1262357.

Emanuel, A. S., Howell, J. L., Taber, J. M., Ferrer, R. A., Klein, W. M., & Harris, P. R. (2018). Spontaneous self-affirmation is associated with psychological well-being: Evidence from a US national adult survey sample. *Journal of Health Psychology*, *23*(1), 95–102. http://doi.org/10.1177/1359105316643595.

Habibi, R., Nasrabadi, A. N., Hamedan, M. S., & Moqadam, A. S. (2016). The effects of family-centered problem-solving education on relapse rate, self efficacy and self esteem among substance abusers. *International Journal of High Risk Behaviors & Addiction*, *5*(1), e24421. http://doi.org/10.5812/ijhrba.24421.

Moore, E., Holding, A. C., Hope, N. H., et al. (2018). Perfectionism and the pursuit of personal goals: A self-determination theory analysis. *Motivation and Emotion*, *42*(1), 37–49. http://doi.org/10.1007/s11031-017-9654-2.

Orth, U., Robins, R. W., Meier, L. L., & Conger, R. D. (2016). Refining the vulnerability model of low self-esteem and depression: Disentangling the effects of genuine self-esteem and narcissism. *Journal of Personality and Social Psychology*, *110*(1), 133–149. https://doi.org/10.1037/pspp0000038.

Park, H. J., & Dhandra, T. K. (2017). The effect of trait emotional intelligence on the relationship between dispositional mindfulness and self-esteem. *Mindfulness*, *8*, 1206–1211. https://doi.org/10.1007/s12671-017-0693-2.

Robustelli, B. L., & Whisman, M. A. (2018). Gratitude and life satisfaction in the United States and Japan. *Journal of Happiness Studies*, *19*(1), 41–55. https://doi.org/10.1007/s10902-016-9802-5.

Rosenberg, M. (1965). *Society and adolescent self-image*. Princeton, NJ: Princeton University Press.

Stroebe, M., Schut, H., & Boerner, K. (2017). Cautioning health-care professionals: Bereaved persons are misguided through the stages of grief. *Omega*, *74*(4), 455–473. http://doi.org/10.1177/0030222817691870.

Tetzner, J., Becker, M., & Baumert, J. (2016). Still doing fine? The interplay of negative life events and self-esteem during young adulthood. *European Journal of Personality*, *30*(4), 358–373. https://doi.org/10.1002/per.2066.

Vass, V., Sitko, K., West, S., & Bentall, R. P. (2017). How stigma gets under the skin: The role of stigma, self-stigma and self-esteem in subjective recovery from psychosis. *Psychosis*, *9*(3), 235–244. https://doi.org/10.1080/17522439.2017.1300184.

Victor, P., Teismann, T., & Willutzki, U. (2017). A pilot evaluation of a strengths-based CBT intervention module with college students. *Behavioural and Cognitive Psychotherapy*, *45*(4), 427–431. https://doi.org/10.1017/S1352465816000552.

Wersebe, H., Lieb, R., Meyer, A. H., Hofer, P., & Gloster, A. T. (2018). The link between stress, well-being, and psychological flexibility during an acceptance and commitment therapy self-help intervention. *International Journal of Clinical and Health Psychology*, *18*(1), 60–68. http://doi.org/10.1016/j.ijchp.2017.09.002.

Risk for Chronic Low Self-Esteem

Domain 6 Self-perception Class 2 Self-esteem

Marina Martinez-Kratz, MS, RN, CNE

NANDA-I

Definition

Susceptible to long-standing negative perception of self-worth, self-acceptance, self-respect, competence, and attitude toward self, which may compromise health.

Risk Factors

Decreased mindful acceptance; difficulty managing finances; disturbed body image; fatigue; fear of rejection; impaired religiosity; inadequate affection received; inadequate attachment behavior; inadequate family cohesiveness; inadequate group membership; inadequate respect from others; inadequate sense of belonging; inadequate social support; ineffective communication skills; insufficient approval from others; low self efficacy; maladaptive grieving; negative resignation; repeated negative reinforcement; spiritual incongruence; stigmatization; stressors; values incongruent with cultural norms

At-Risk Population

Economically disadvantaged individuals; individuals experiencing repeated failure; individuals exposed to traumatic situation; individuals with difficult developmental transition; individuals with history of being abandoned; individuals with history of being abused; individuals with history of being neglected; individuals with history of loss

Associated Conditions

Depression; functional impairment; mental disorders; physical illness

NOC, NIC, Client Outcomes, Nursing Interventions and *Rationales,* and References

Refer to care plan for Chronic Low **Self-Esteem.**

Risk for Situational Low Self-Esteem

Domain 6 Self-perception Class 2 Self-esteem

Marina Martinez-Kratz, MS, RN, CNE

NANDA-I

Definition

Susceptible to change from positive to negative perception of self-worth, self-acceptance, self-respect, competence, and attitude toward self in response to a current situation, which may compromise health.

Risk Factors

Behavior incongruent with values; decrease in environmental control; decreased mindful acceptance; difficulty accepting alteration in social role; difficulty managing finances; disturbed body image; fatigue; fear of rejection; impaired religiosity; inadequate attachment behavior; inadequate family cohesiveness; inadequate respect from others; inadequate social support; individuals experiencing repeated failure; ineffective communication skills; low self efficacy; maladaptive perfectionism; negative resignation; powerlessness; stigmatization; stressors; unrealistic self-expectations; values incongruent with cultural norms

At-Risk Population

Individuals experiencing a change in living environment; individuals experiencing alteration in body image; individuals experiencing alteration in economic status; individuals experiencing alteration in role function; individuals experiencing death of a significant other; individuals experiencing divorce; individuals experiencing new additions to the family; individuals experiencing unplanned pregnancy; individuals with difficult developmental transition; individuals with history of being abandoned; individuals with history of being abused; individuals with history of being neglected; individuals with history of loss; individuals with history of rejection

Associated Conditions

Depression; functional impairment; mental disorders; physical illness

NOC (Nursing Outcomes Classification)

See Chronic Low **Self-Esteem** for suggested NOC outcomes

Client Outcomes

Client Will (Specify Time Frame)

- State accurate self-appraisal
- Demonstrate the ability to self-validate
- Demonstrate the ability to make decisions independent of primary peer group
- Express effects of media on self-appraisal
- Express influence of substances on self-esteem
- Identify strengths and healthy coping skills
- State life events and change as influencing self-esteem

NIC (Nursing Interventions Classification)

See Chronic Low **Self-Esteem** for suggested NIC interventions

Nursing Interventions and *Rationales*

- Assist client to challenge negative perceptions of self and performance. EB: *A study found that more often than not, self-critical thoughts were viewed as facts and would rarely be seen as distorted or biased (Kolubinski et al, 2016).*
- Assess the client's self-esteem using valid and established tools such as the Rosenberg Self-Esteem Scale. CEB: *The use of valid and established measures of self-esteem will facilitate the identification of appropriate nursing interventions that strengthen self-esteem (Rosenberg, 1965).*
- Encourage client to maintain highest level of community functioning. EB: *Research found that the community feeling is positively connected with self-esteem and psychological well-being (Kałużna-Wielobób, 2017).*
- Encourage self-affirmations by reflecting on values and strengths, in response to daily threats. EB: *A study found that engaging in spontaneous self-affirmation was related to greater happiness, hopefulness, optimism, subjective health, and personal health efficacy and less anger and sadness (Emanuel et al, 2018).*
- Encourage realistic and achievable goal setting and resources and identify impediments to achievement. EB: *A combined decision support and goal-setting intervention improved diet quality, diabetes-related self-efficacy, and empowerment and reduced diabetes-related distress and depressive symptoms (Swoboda et al, 2017).*
- ▲ Assess the client for symptoms of depression and anxiety. Refer to specialist as needed. Prompt and effective treatment can prevent exacerbation of symptoms or safety risks. EB: *Research supported the vulnerability model of low self-esteem and depression with findings that indicated that individuals with high self-esteem have a lower risk for developing depression (Orth et al, 2016).*
- See care plans for Disturbed personal Identity, Situational Low **Self-Esteem,** and Chronic Low **Self-Esteem.**

S

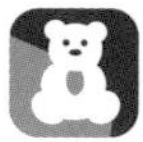

Pediatric

- Assess children/adolescents who are either a victim or an offender of cyberbullying for low self-esteem. EB: *A moderate and statistically significant relationship exists between low self-esteem and experiences with cyberbullying (Lin et al, 2018).*
- Encourage attendance at social support groups. EB: *A study found that lesbian, gay, bisexual, transgender, and queer (LGBTQ) youth who attended a Hatch group-level intervention that consisted of unstructured social time, consciousness-raising (education), and a youth-led peer support group had higher levels of self-esteem (Wilkerson et al, 2017).*
- ▲ Encourage a combination of extracurricular activity for adolescents in a safe, supportive, and empowering environment. EB: *Research suggested that enabling relations within the family, school, peer, and community are factors related to youth self-satisfaction (Simon, 2020).*

Geriatric

- Support humor as a coping mechanism. EB: *This paper identified that humor has a positive effect on all of these issues with an increasing sense of well-being and life satisfaction for the elder (Lurie & Monahan, 2015).*
- Support client in identifying and adapting to functional changes. EBN: *A study outlined the importance of enquiring about feelings of uselessness, which is linked to both psychological and physical health status, especially in older people who need help in daily activities (Curzio et al, 2017).*
- Encourage participation in intergenerational social activities. EB: *Older adults reported that their participation in the "Time After Time" intergenerational program enhanced their confidence, self-esteem, and social skills; contributed to their emotional and overall health and well-being; and enabled them to learn about others and feel connected to their community (Teater, 2016).*
- Support meaning and purpose in the lives of older adults through a focus on everyday well-being and facilitation of personally treasured activities. EBN: *An exploratory study found four key experiences that promote meaning and purpose in life: (1) physical and mental well-being, (2) belonging and recognition, (3) personally treasured activities, and (4) spiritual closeness and connectedness (Drageset et al, 2017).*
- Use an approach that reduces the emphasis put on ageist self-concept attributions when working with older clients. EB: *Ageism includes cognitive, behavioral, and emotional manifestations. Ageism tends to reinforce social inequalities because it is more pronounced toward older women, poor people, or those with dementia (Ayalon et al, 2017).*
- See care plans for Situational Low **Self-Esteem** and Chronic Low **Self-Esteem.**

Home Care

- Previously discussed interventions may be used in the home care setting.
- See care plans for Situational Low **Self-Esteem** and Chronic Low **Self-Esteem.**

Client/Family Teaching and Discharge Planning

▲ Refer the client to community agencies that offer support and environmental resources. Make referrals as needed.

- See care plans for Situational Low **Self-Esteem** and Chronic Low **Self-Esteem.**

REFERENCES

Ayalon, L., & Tesch-Römer, C. (2017). Taking a closer look at ageism: Self- and other-directed ageist attitudes and discrimination. *European Journal of Ageing, 14*(1), 1–4. https://doi.org/10.1007/s10433-016-0409-9.

Curzio, O., Bernacca, E., Bianchi, B., & Rossi, G. (2017). Feelings of uselessness and 3-year mortality in an Italian community older people: The role of the functional status. *Psychogeriatrics, 17*(5), 300–309. https://doi.org/10.1111/psyg.12238.

Drageset, J., Haugan, G., & Tranvåg, O. (2017). Crucial aspects promoting meaning and purpose in life: Perceptions of nursing home residents. *BMC Geriatrics, 17*(1), 254. https://doi.org/10.1186/s12877-017-0650-x.

Emanuel, A. S., Howell, J. L., Taber, J. M., Ferrer, R. A., Klein, W. M., & Harris, P. R. (2018). Spontaneous self-affirmation is associated with psychological well-being: Evidence from a US national adult survey sample. *Journal of Health Psychology, 23*(1), 95–102. http://doi.org.proxy.lib.umich.edu/10.1177/1359105316643595.

Kałużna-Wielobób, A. (2017). The community feeling versus anxiety, self-esteem and well-being—introductory research. *Polish Psychological Bulletin, 48*(2), 167–174. https://doi.org10.1515/ppb-2017-0020.

Kolubinski, D. C., Nikčević, A. V., Lawrence, J. A., & Spada, M. M. (2016). The role of metacognition in self-critical rumination: An investigation in individuals presenting with low self-esteem. *Journal of Rational-Emotive and Cognitive-Behavior Therapy, 34*(1), 73–85. https://doi.org/10.1007/s10942-015-0230-y.

Lin, Y. C., Latner, J. D., Fung, X. C. C., & Lin, C. Y. (2018). Poor health and experiences of being bullied in adolescents: Self-perceived overweight and frustration with appearance matter. *Obesity, 26*(2), 397–404. https://doi.org/10.1002/oby.22041.

Lurie, A., & Monahan, K. (2015). Humor, aging, and life review: Survival through the use of humor. *Social Work in Mental Health, 13*(1), 82–91. https://doi.org/10.1080/15332985.2014.884519.

Orth, U., Robins, R. W., Meier, L. L., & Conger, R. D. (2016). Refining the vulnerability model of low self-esteem and depression: Disentangling the effects of genuine self-esteem and narcissism. *Journal of Personality and Social Psychology, 110*(1), 133–149. https://doi.org/10.1037/pspp0000038.

Rosenberg, M. (1965). *Society and adolescent self-image.* Princeton, NJ: Princeton University Press.

Simon, P. (2020). Enabling relations as determinants of self-satisfaction in the youth: The path from self-satisfaction to prosocial behaviors as explained by strength of inner self. *Current Psychology, 39*, 656–664. https://doi.org/10.1007/s12144-018-9791-0.

Swoboda, C. M., Miller, C. K., & Wills, C. E. (2017). Impact of a goal setting and decision support telephone coaching intervention on diet, psychosocial, and decision outcomes among people with type 2 diabetes. *Patient Education and Counseling, 100*(7), 1367–1373. https://doi.org/10.1016/j.pec.2017.02.007.

Teater, B. (2016). Intergenerational programs to promote active aging: The experiences and perspectives of older adults. *Activities, Adaptation & Aging, 40*(1), 1–19. https://doi.org/10.1080/01924788.2016.1127041.

Wilkerson, J. M., Schick, V. R., Romijnders, K. A., Bauldry, J., & Butame, S. A. (2017). Social support, depression, self-esteem, and coping among LGBTQ adolescents participating in Hatch Youth. *Health Promotion Practice, 18*(3), 358–365. https://doi.org/10.1177/152483991665446.

S

Risk for Self-Mutilation Domain 11 Safety/protection Class 3 Violence

Marina Martinez-Kratz, MS, RN, CNE

NANDA-I

Definition

Susceptible to deliberate self-injurious behavior causing tissue damage with the intent of causing nonfatal injury to attain relief of tension.

Risk Factors

Absence of family confidant; altered body image; dissociation; disturbed interpersonal relations; eating disorder; excessive emotional disturbance; feeling threatened with loss of significant interpersonal relations; impaired self-esteem; inability to express tension verbally; ineffective communication between parent and adolescent; ineffective coping strategies; irresistible urge for self-directed violence; irresistible urge to cut self; labile behavior; loss of control over problem-solving situation; low self-esteem; mounting tension that is intolerable; negative feelings; pattern of inability to plan solutions; pattern of inability to see long-term consequences; perfectionism; requires rapid stress reduction; social isolation; substance misuse; use of manipulation to obtain nurturing interpersonal relations with others

At-Risk Population

Adolescents; battered children; incarcerated individuals; individuals experiencing family divorce; individuals experiencing family substance misuse; individuals experiencing loss of significant interpersonal relations; individuals experiencing sexual identity crisis; individuals living in nontraditional setting; individuals whose peers self-mutilate; individuals with family history of self-destructive behavior; individuals with history of childhood abuse; individuals with history of childhood illness; individuals with history of childhood surgery; individuals with history of self-directed violence; individuals witnessing violence between parental figures

Associated Conditions

Autism; borderline personality disorder; character disorder; depersonalization; developmental disabilities; psychotic disorders

NIC, NOC, Client Outcomes, Nursing Interventions and *Rationales*, Client/Family Teaching, and References

Refer to care plan for **Self-Mutilation.**

Self-Mutilation Domain 11 Safety/protection Class 3 Violence

Marina Martinez-Kratz, MS, RN, CNE

S

NANDA-I

Definition

Deliberate self-injurious behavior causing tissue damage with the intent of causing nonfatal injury to attain relief of tension.

Defining Characteristics

Abrading skin; biting; constricting a body part; cuts on body; hitting; ingested harmful substance; inhaled harmful substance; insertion of object into body orifice; picking at wound; scratches on body; self-inflicted burn; severing of a body part

Related Factors

Absence of family confidant; altered body image; dissociation; disturbed interpersonal relations; eating disorder; excessive emotional disturbance; feeling threatened with loss of significant interpersonal relations;

impaired self-esteem; inability to express tension verbally; ineffective communication between parent and adolescent; ineffective coping strategies; irresistible urge for self-directed violence; irresistible urge to cut self; labile behavior; loss of control over problem-solving situation; low self-esteem; mounting tension that is intolerable; negative feelings; pattern of inability to plan solutions; pattern of inability to see long term consequences; perfectionism; requires rapid stress reduction; social isolation; substance misuse; use of manipulation to obtain nurturing interpersonal relations with others

At-Risk Population

Adolescents; battered children; incarcerated individuals; individuals experiencing family divorce; individuals experiencing family substance misuse; individuals experiencing loss of significant interpersonal relations; individuals experiencing sexual identity crisis; individuals living in nontraditional setting; individuals whose peers self-mutilate; individuals with family history of self-destructive behavior; individuals with history of childhood abuse; individuals with history of childhood illness; individuals with history of childhood surgery; individuals with history of self-directed violence; individuals witnessing violence between parental figures

Associated Conditions

Autism; borderline personality disorder; character disorder; depersonalization; developmental disabilities; psychotic disorders

NOC (Nursing Outcomes Classification)

Suggested NOC Outcomes

Self-Control; Distorted Thought Self-Control; Impulse Self-Control; Mood Equilibrium; Risk Detection; Self-Mutilation Restraint

Example NOC Outcome with Indicators

Self-Mutilation Restraint as evidenced by the following indicators: Refrains from gathering means for self-injury/Obtains assistance as needed/Upholds contract not to harm self/Maintains self-control without supervision/Refrains from injuring self. (Rate the outcome and indicators of **Self-Mutilation Restraint:** 1 = never demonstrated, 2 = rarely demonstrated, 3 = sometimes demonstrated, 4 = often demonstrated, 5 = consistently demonstrated [see Section I].)

Client Outcomes

Client Will (Specify Time Frame)

- Have injuries treated
- Refrain from further self-injury
- State appropriate ways to cope with increased psychological or physiological tension
- Express feelings
- Seek help when having urges to self-mutilate
- Maintain self-control without supervision
- Use appropriate community agencies when caregivers are unable to attend to emotional needs

S

NIC (Nursing Interventions Classification)

Suggested NIC Interventions

Active Listening; Anger Control Assistance; Behavior Management: Self-Harm; Calming Technique; Environmental Management: Safety; Limit Setting; Mood Management; Mutual Goal Setting; Risk Identification; Self-Responsibility Facilitation

Example NIC Activities—Behavior Management: Self-Harm

Anticipate trigger situations that may prompt self-harm and intervene to prevent it; Teach client and reinforce effective coping behaviors and appropriate expression of feelings

Nursing Interventions and *Rationales*

- Before implementing interventions for nonsuicidal self-injury (NSSI), nurses should examine their own knowledge base and emotional responses to incidents of self-harm. EBN: *A study of mental health and emergency department nurses' perceptions about NSSI found that nurses from both groups had an accurate understanding of NSSI and positive attitudes about clients who self-injure. Confidence was higher among mental health nurses, and greater knowledge of NSSI was correlated with increased confidence, positive attitudes, and empathy (Ngune et al, 2021).*
- Assess clients with a diagnosis of borderline personality disorder or an eating disorder for NSSI. EB: *A systematic literature review found comorbidity with borderline personality disorder and eating disorders (Cipriano, Cella, & Cotrufo, 2017).*
- Assess veterans seeking treatment for posttraumatic stress disorder (PTSD) for NSSI behaviors. EB: *A study found that veterans who reported engaging in NSSI in the past year reported increased levels of PTSD and depressive symptoms (Calhoun et al, 2017).*
- A nonjudgmental approach to clients is critical. EBN: *A qualitative study of nurses' experiences caring for clients who self-harmed indicated the need for acceptance of the client (Moola, 2017).*
- Consider using a measure of self-harm risk that is available for clients: EBN: *A systematic review of multiple instruments rated most of their support as Grade B. The Suicide Attempt Self-Injury Interview (SASII) was reviewed as Level 3, although its length was noted as an issue (Li, 2017).*
- ▲ Provide medical treatment for injuries. Use aseptic technique when caring for wounds. Care for the wounds in a matter-of-fact manner. EB: *Clinical guidelines for the treatment of NSSI wounds indicate that the first steps in care are to examine for the depth and size of the wound, evaluate for possible contamination, and determine tetanus vaccination status. Wounds should also be evaluated for potential surgical consultation (Plener et al, 2018).*
- Assess for risk of suicide or other self-damaging behaviors. EB: *A study found that NSSI emerged as a robust predictor of recent suicide attempts and the strength of the relationship did not change in the presence of protective factors (Muehlenkamp & Brausch, 2019). Refer to the care plan for Risk for Suicidal Behavior.*
- Assess for the presence of hallucinations. Ask specific questions: "Do you hear voices that other people do not hear?" "Are they telling you to hurt yourself?" EB: *Command hallucinations occurring with schizophrenia or brief psychotic episodes may direct the client to hurt himself or herself or others. A systematic review found an association between psychosis and risk for self-injurious thoughts and behaviors (Hielscher et al, 2018).*
- Monitor the client's behavior closely, using engagement and support as elements of safety checks while avoiding intrusive overstimulation. EBN: *When lack of control exists, client safety is an important issue, and close observation is essential. Clients may feel overstimulated by intrusive close observation, resulting in agitation (Moola, 2017).*
- Focus on understanding the function that self-harm serves for the client and on managing the client's distress. EB: *Self-harm is a form of distress management. A qualitative study of mental health staff interventions and efficacy suggested that individualized care plans highlighting management of distress and identification of obstacles to interventions are more effective. If clients are unable to self-harm, prevention can lead to power struggles and the use of more harmful methods by the client (Thomas & Haslam, 2017).*
- Establish trust, listen to client, convey safety, and assist in developing positive goals for the future. EB: *Therapeutic alliance is the nature of the relationship between the client and the nurse. A systematic review of therapeutic alliance and treatment outcome found that therapeutic alliance has a positive impact on treatment outcomes among individuals engaging in or at risk for aggressive behaviors (Fahlgren, Berman, & McCloskey, 2020).*
- ▲ Refer for Treatment for Self-Injurious Behaviors (T-SIB) therapy. EB: *T-SIB is an intervention that consists of nine 1-hour-long individual weekly sessions designed to decrease the frequency of NSSI behaviors and urges. Research found decreased NSSI frequency in the T-SIB group using intent-to-treat analyses (Andover et al, 2017).*

Pediatric

- Assess children and adolescents placed in psychiatric settings for NSSI. EBN: *A study of 126 mostly nursing staff found that a minority of staff reported having formal NSSI training, and a third of respondents indicated that they did not typically assess for NSSI at all. Despite a substantial percentage of the respondents self-reporting comfort and confidence with assessing and treating NSSI, fewer than 10% demonstrated accurate skill (Pluhar et al, 2019).*

S

- ● Assess adolescents with a diagnosis of borderline personality disorder or an eating disorder for NSSI. EB: *A systematic literature review found that NSSI is most common among adolescents and young adults, with the age of onset between 12 and 14 years. The review also found comorbidity with borderline personality disorder and eating disorders (Cipriano, Cella, & Cotrufo, 2017).*
- ● Assess children and adolescents for experiences of bullying or rejection by peers. EB: *Study results indicate that being involved in bullying (as bullies, victims, or bully-victims) increases the likelihood of engagement in NSSI. Being rejected by peers increased the probability of using NSSI, for both victims and bully-victims (Esposito, Bacchini, & Affuso, 2019).*
- ● Ask adolescent clients directly if they use social media to post communication about or share images of wounds related to self-injury. EB: *Pictures that directly depicted wounds on Instagram were investigated. Researchers concluded that pictures of NSSI wounds are frequently posted on Instagram and social reinforcement might play a role in the posting of NSSI pictures (Brown et al, 2018).*
- ▲ Refer adolescents who self-harm to cognitive behavioral therapy (CBT) treatments. EB: *A study comparing the efficacies of a brief cognitive behavioral psychotherapy manual, the Cutting Down Programme (CDP), and treatment as usual (TAU) in the treatment of adolescent NSSI found that CDP was equally effective and achieved faster recovery compared with a significantly more intensive TAU (Kaess et al, 2020).*
- ▲ Refer self-injuring students for psychological or psychiatric treatment. Treatment includes starting therapy and medications, increasing coping skills, facilitating decision-making, encouraging positive relationships, and fostering self-esteem. EB: *Although the repeat rate of self-harm is around 21%, clients may have a very low treatment follow-up rate. Access to care must be a consideration (Hunter et al, 2018).*

Home Care and Client/Family Teaching and Discharge Planning

- ● Provide family teaching about NSSI and treatments. EBN: *Interviews of parents of adolescents with NSSI found that parents lack knowledge about NSSI and its treatment and experience emotional distress (Fu et al, 2020).*
- ▲ Refer family and client to outpatient family-focused cognitive behavioral treatment (F-CBT). EB: *A randomized trial found that F-CBT was associated with reductions in suicidality, depression, and NSSI (Esposito-Smythers et al, 2019).*
- ▲ Refer family and client to dialectical behavior therapy (DBT). EB: *A pilot study found that parents who received a DBT-based brief intervention reported reductions in parent self-reported depressive symptoms, emotion dysregulation, caregiver strain, psychiatric symptom distress, and interpersonal sensitivity from baseline to 6-month follow-up. Youth in the study also showed decreases in total self-harm from baseline to 6-month follow-up (Berk et al, 2020).*

REFERENCES

Andover, M. S., Schatten, H. T., Morris, B. W., Holman, C. S., & Miller, I. W. (2017). An intervention for nonsuicidal self-injury in young adults: A pilot randomized controlled trial. *Journal of Consulting and Clinical Psychology*, *85*(6), 620–631. https://doi.org/10.1037/ccp0000206.

Berk, M. S., Rathus, J., Kessler, M., et al. (2020). Pilot test of a DBT-based parenting intervention for parents of youth with recent self-harm. *Cognitive and Behavioral Practice*. [Online ahead of print]. https://doi.org/10.1016/j.cbpra.2020.10.001.

Brown, R. C., Fischer, T., Goldwich, A. D., Keller, F., Young, R., & Plener, P. L. (2018). #cutting: Non-suicidal self-injury (NSSI) on Instagram. *Psychological Medicine*, *48*(2), 337–346. https://doi.org/10.1017/S0033291717001751.

Calhoun, P. S., Van Voorhees, E. E., Elbogen, E. B., et al. (2017). Nonsuicidal self-injury and interpersonal violence in U.S. veterans seeking help for posttraumatic stress disorder. *Psychiatry Research*, *247*, 250–256. https://doi.org/10.1016/j.psychres.2016.11.032.

Cipriano, A., Cella, S., & Cotrufo, P. (2017). Nonsuicidal self-injury: A systematic review. *Frontiers in Psychology*, *8*, 1946. https://doi.org/10.3389/fpsyg.2017.01946.

Esposito, C., Bacchini, D., & Affuso, G. (2019). Adolescent non-suicidal self-injury and its relationships with school bullying and peer rejection. *Psychiatry Research*, *274*, 1–6. https://doi.org/10.1016/j.psychres.2019.02.018.

Esposito-Smythers, C., Wolff, J. C., Liu, R. T., et al. (2019). Family-focused cognitive behavioral treatment for depressed adolescents in suicidal crisis with co-occurring risk factors: A randomized trial. *Journal of Child Psychology and Psychiatry*, *60*(10), 1133–1141. https://doi.org/10.1111/jcpp.13095.

Fahlgren, M. K., Berman, M. E., & McCloskey, M. S. (2020). The role of therapeutic alliance in therapy for adults with problematic aggression and associated disorders. *Clinical Psychology & Psychotherapy*, *27*(6), 858–886. https://doi.org/10.1002/cpp.2475.

Fu, X., Yang, J., Liao, X., et al. (2020). Parents' attitudes toward and experience of non-suicidal self-injury in adolescents: A qualitative study. *Frontiers in Psychiatry*, *11*, 651. https//doi.org/10.3389/fpsyt.2020.00651.

Hielscher, E., DeVylder, J., Saha, S., Connell, M., & Scott, J. G. (2018). Why are psychotic experiences associated with self-injurious thoughts and behaviours? A systematic review and critical appraisal of potential confounding and mediating factors. *Psychological Medicine*, *48*(9), 1410–1426. https://doi.org10.1017/S0033291717002677.

Hunter, J., Maunder, R., Kurdyak, P., Wilton, A. S., Gruneir, A., & Vigod, S. (2018). Mental health follow-up after deliberate self-harm and risk for repeat self-harm and death. *Psychiatry Research*, *259*, 333–339. https://doi.org/10.1016/j.psychres.2017.09.029.

Kaess, M., Edinger, A., Fischer-Waldschmidt, G., Parzer, P., Brunner, R., & Resch, F. (2020). Effectiveness of a brief psychotherapeutic

S

intervention compared with treatment as usual for adolescent nonsuicidal self-injury: A single-centre, randomised controlled trial. *European Child & Adolescent Psychiatry*, *29*(6), 881–891. https://doi.org/10.1007/s00787-019-01399-1.

Li, Y. (2017). Evidence summary. Self-harm (adults): Validated measurement instruments. *JBI@Ovid: The Joanna Briggs Institute EBP Database*, JBI7927.

Moola, S. (2017). Evidence summary. Self-harm (inpatient mental health ward): Assessment, prevention, and treatment. *JBI@Ovid: The Joanna Briggs Institute EBP Database*, JBI18050.

Muehlenkamp, J. J., & Brausch, A. M. (2019). Protective factors do not moderate risk for past-year suicide attempts conferred by recent NSSI. *Journal of Affective Disorders*, *245*, 321–324. https://doi.org/10.1016/j.jad.2018.11.013.

Ngune, I., Hasking, P., McGough, S., Wynaden, D., Janerka, C., & Rees, C. (2021). Perceptions of knowledge, attitude and skills about non-suicidal self-injury: A survey of emergency and mental health nurses. *International Journal of Mental Health Nursing*, *30*(3), 635–642. https://doi.org/10.1111/inm.12825.

Plener, P. L., Kaess, M., Schmahl, C., Pollak, S., Fegert, J. M., & Brown, R. C. (2018). Nonsuicidal self-injury in adolescents. *Deutsches Arzteblatt International*, *115*(3), 23–30. https://doi.org/10.3238/arztebl.2018.0023.

Pluhar, E., Freizinger, M., Nikolov, R., & Burton, E. (2019). Pediatric nonsuicidal self-injury: A call to action for inpatient staff training. *Journal of Psychiatric Practice*, *25*(5), 395–401. https://doi.org/10.1097/PRA.0000000000000417.

Thomas, J. B., & Haslam, C. O. (2017). How people who self-harm negotiate the inpatient environment: The mental healthcare workers perspective. *Journal of Psychiatric and Mental Health Nursing*, *24*(7), 480–490. https://doi.org/10.1111/jpm.12384.

Self-Neglect Domain 4 Activity/rest Class 5 Self-care

Mary Rose Day, DN, MA, PGDip PHN, BSc, RPHN, RM, RGN and Susanne W. Gibbons, PhD, C-ANP/GNP

NANDA-I

Definition

A constellation of culturally framed behaviors involving one or more self-care activities in which there is a failure to maintain a socially accepted standard of health and well-being (Gibbons, Lauder, & Ludwick, 2006).

Defining Characteristics

Inadequate environmental hygiene; inadequate personal hygiene; nonadherence to health activity

Related Factors

Fear of institutionalization; impaired executive function; inability to maintain control; lifestyle choice; neurobehavioral manifestations; stressors; substance misuse

Associated Conditions

Capgras syndrome; frontal lobe dysfunction; functional impairment; learning disability; malingering; mental disorders; psychotic disorders

NOC (Nursing Outcomes Classification)

S

Suggested NOC Outcomes

Cognitive Function; Executive Function; Depression; Alcohol and Other Substance Use; Activities of Daily Living (ADLs), Instrumental Activities of Daily Living (IADLs); Safety; Nutritional Status; Social Support; Medication Safety Assessment

Examples of NOC Outcome with Indicators

Self-Neglect Status as evidenced by the following indicators: Maintains personal cleanliness and health/ Recognizes safety needs in the home. (Rate outcome and indicators of **Self-Neglect Status:** 1 = severely compromised, 2 = substantially compromised, 3 = moderately compromised, 4 = mildly compromised, 5 = not compromised [see Section I].)

Client Outcomes

Client Will (Specify Time Frame)

- Reveal improvement in cognition (e.g., if reversible and treatable)
- Show improvement in mental health problems (e.g., depression)

- Show improvement in chronic medical problems
- Demonstrate improvement in functional status (e.g., basic and IADLs)
- Demonstrate adherence to health activities (e.g., medications and medical appointments)
- Exhibit improved personal hygiene
- Exhibit improved environmental hygiene
- Have fewer hospitalizations and emergency room visits
- Increase safety of client
- Increase safety of community in which client lives
- Agree to necessary personal and environmental changes that eliminate risk/endangerment to self or others (e.g., neighbors)
- Improve social networks and social engagement
- Identify eligibility for public services and other benefits

Note: Because self-neglect is present along a continuum of severity and includes an array of behavioral and environmental issues, a change in a client's status must occur in such a way that it balances obligation for protection and respects individual rights (e.g., autonomy and self-determination) while ensuring individual health and well-being. This is accomplished through a client–provider partnership that keeps the door open, even though the client may initially decline help. Building a relationship with the client will improve trust and assist in developing an individually tailored care plan to address problems contributing to self-neglect. *Multiprofessional* collaboration and teamwork, and in some instances assistance of next of kin and/or adult protective services (APS) may be needed (e.g., a state agency or local social services program).

NIC (Nursing Interventions Classification)

Suggested NIC Interventions

Self-Neglect; Self-Care Assistance: Activities of Daily Living; Support System Enhancement

Example NIC Activities—Self-Care Assistance: Instrumental Activities of Daily Living

Determine individual's need for assistance with IADLs (e.g., shopping, cooking, housekeeping, laundry, use of transportation, managing money, managing medications, use of communication, and use of time)

Nursing Interventions and *Rationales*

- Monitor individuals with acute or chronic mental and physical illness for defining characteristics for self-neglect. EBN: *Holistic assessment includes medical and social history, cognitive status, state of mental health, well-being, physical function, social networks, medication, alcohol use, and observation of factors that limit persons' coping and self-care ability and threaten their personal safety and health (Mulcahy, Leahy-Warren, & Day, 2018; Touza & Prado, 2019).*
- Assist individuals with complex mental and physical health issues to adopt positive health behaviors so that they may maintain their health status in the community. EB: *Consequences of self-neglect can include suicidal ideation and mental health concerns (Dong, Xu, & Ding, 2017), and greater severity of self-neglect was associated with an increased 30-day hospital readmission rate (Dong & Simon, 2015).*
- Assist individuals with reconnecting with family, friends, communities, and other social networks available. EBN: *Poorer neighborhood cohesion (people do not share the same values, absent community spirit, poorer relationships, and people are unwilling to trust or help each other) (Hei & Dong, 2017), neighborhood disorder (e.g., visible signs of neglect, physical disorganization and dangerous conditions, high crime rates) (Hei & Dong, 2018), and social isolation are risk factors for self-neglect (Day, McCarthy, & Fitzpatrick, 2018; Mulcahy, Leahy-Warren, & Day, 2018).*
- Assist individuals whose self-care is failing with managing their medication regimen. EB: *Individuals who exhibit self-neglect may have difficulty managing medications because of complex medication regimens, and low adherence is significant among older adults who self-neglect (Alpert, 2014; Abada et al, 2019).*
- Assist persons with self-care deficits caused by impairments in activities of daily living (ADLs) or instrumental ADLs (IADLs). EB: *Individuals with self-care deficits may have difficulty with ADLs and IADLs because greater self-neglect severity has been associated with lower levels of physical function among older adults (Hildebrand, Taylor, & Bradway, 2014).*

S

- Assess persons with failing self-care for changes in cognitive function (e.g., dementia or delirium). EB: *Individuals with failing self-care may have changes in cognition. Decline in executive function has been associated with risk of reported and confirmed elder self-neglect, and decline in global cognitive function has been associated with risk of greater self-neglect severity (Mackay, 2017; Mills & Naik, 2018).*
- ▲ Refer persons with failing self-care to appropriate specialists (e.g., psychologist, psychiatrist, social worker) and therapists (e.g., physical therapy, occupational therapy). EBN/EB: *Individuals with self-care deficits may need assistance from other health professionals using an multiprofessional team approach, open communication, and collaboration (Braye, Orr, & Preston-Shoot, 2014; Burnett et al, 2014).*
- ▲ Responding to clients with self-neglect requires that plan of care be person centered and outcome focused and clarify how real and potential risks will be addressed, by whom, and within what timeframe. Professional judgment and complexity of cases and situations can present an exceptionally fine line in making decisions and judgments. EBN/EB: *Building relationships with the person, knowing the person's narrative/story, legal literacy, finding creative interventions, and effective multiagency working are key (Day, McCarthy, & Fitzpatrick, 2018).*
- Use behavioral modification as appropriate (describing all options and consequences of refusing care or treatment) to bring about client changes that lead to improvement in personal hygiene, environmental hygiene, and adherence to medical regimen. EB: *Person-centered interventions that take account of the circumstances, historical and current wishes and feelings of the client, the client's preferred options, and (if possible) negotiated approaches to offering support can offer better outcomes (Braye, Orr, & Preston-Shoot, 2014; Preston-Shoot, 2019).*
- Monitor persons with substance abuse disorders (i.e., drugs, alcohol, smoking) and depression for adequate health and safety. EBN/EB: *Because mental health and substance use disorders can go unrecognized and untreated in this population, identified self-neglecting clients should be screened as appropriate (Alpert et al, 2014; Hansen et al, 2016; Yu et al, 2019).*
- ▲ Refer persons with failing self-care who are significantly impaired cognitively (e.g., executive function, dementia) or functionally and/or who are suspected victims of abuse to APS. EB/CEB: *Self-neglect has been associated with mistreatment in older adults, especially those who live alone (Pavlou & Lachs, 2008).*

Geriatric

- ▲ Assess client's socioeconomic status and refer for appropriate support. EBN/EB: *Providers are advised to assess available financial and other resources to help older adults and their families obtain essential goods and services (Zhao et al, 2017; Mulcahy, Leahy-Warren, & Day, 2018).*
- ▲ Refer persons demonstrating a significant decline in self-care abilities (e.g., posing a threat to themselves or to their community) for formal evaluation of capacity and executive function. EB: *Current evidence highlights the importance of understanding the nuances of decision-making capacity and mental capacity to help clients who are self-neglecting. Tensions between autonomy and beneficence complicate decisional capacity (Day, Leahy-Warren, & McCarthy, 2016; Niforatos, Rutecki, & Yates, 2018).*

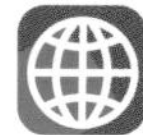

Multicultural

- Deliver health care that is sensitive to the culture and philosophy of individuals whose self-care appears inadequate. EBN: *Providers must be careful not to prematurely judge clients' health choices or living arrangements because personal values and beliefs that might appear as self-neglect do not necessarily indicate self-neglect. However, when client behavior poses a risk to self and/or others, providers have an ethical obligation to intervene (Braye, Orr, & Preston-Shoot, 2017; Braye, Orr, & Preston-Shoot, 2014; Wu et al, 2020).*

REFERENCES

Abada, S., Clark, L. E., Sinha, A. K., et al. (2019). Medication regimen complexity and low adherence in older community-dwelling adults with substantiated self-neglect. *Journal of Applied Gerontology*, *38*(6), 866–883.

Alpert, P. T. (2014). Alcohol abuse in older adults: An invisible population. *Home Health Care Management & Practice*, *26*(4), 269–272.

Braye, S., Orr, D., & Preston-Shoot, M. (2014). *Self-neglect policy and practice: Building an evidence base for adult social care.* [Project report]. London: Social Care Institute for Excellence.

Braye, S., Orr, D., & Preston-Shoot, M. (2017). Autonomy and protection in self-neglect work: The ethical complexity of decision-making. *Ethics and Social Welfare*, *11*(4), 320–335.

Burnett, J., Dyer, C. B., Halphen, J. M., et al. (2014). Four subtypes of self-neglect in older adults: Results of a latent class analysis. *Journal of the American Geriatrics Society*, *62*(6), 1127–1132. doi:10.1111/jgs.12832.

Day, M. R., Leahy-Warren, P., & McCarthy, G. (2016). Self-neglect: Ethical considerations. *Annual Review of Nursing Research*, *34*(1), 89–107.

Day, M. R., McCarthy, G., & Fitzpatrick, J. J. (2018). *Self-neglect in older adults: Global, evidence-based resource for nurses and other healthcare providers*. New York: Springer.
Dong, X., & Simon, M. A. (2015). Elder self-neglect is associated with an increased rate of 30-day hospital readmission: Findings from the Chicago Health and Aging Project. *Gerontology*, *61*(1), 41–50. doi:10.1093/gerona/glw229.
Dong, X., Xu, Y., & Ding, D. (2017). Elder self-neglect and suicidal ideation in an U.S. Chinese aging population: Findings from the PINE study. *The Journals of Gerontology: Series A, Biological Sciences and Medical Sciences*, *72*(Suppl. 1), S76–S81.
Gibbons, S., Lauder, W., & Ludwick, R. (2006). Self-neglect: A proposed new NANDA diagnosis. *International Journal of Nursing Terminologies and Classifications*, *17*(1), 10–18.
Hansen, M. C., Flores, D. V., Coverdale, J., & Burnett, J. (2016). Correlates of depression in self-neglecting older adults: A cross-sectional study examining the role of alcohol abuse and pain in increasing vulnerability. *Journal of Elder Abuse & Neglect*, *28*(1), 41–56.
Hei, A., & Dong, X. (2017). Association between neighborhood cohesion and self-neglect in Chinese-American older adults. *Journal of the American Geriatrics Society*, *65*(12), 2720–2726.
Hei, A., & Dong, X. (2018). Neighborhood disorder is associated with greater risk for self-neglect among Chinese American older adults: Findings from PINE study. *Gerontology and Geriatric Medicine*, *4*, 2333721418778185. doi:10.1177/2333721418778185.
Hildebrand, C., Taylor, M., & Bradway, C. (2014). Elder self-neglect: The failure of coping because of cognitive and functional impairments. *Journal of the American Association of Nurse Practitioners*, *26*(8), 452–462.
Mackay, K. (2017). Choosing to live with harm? A presentation of two case studies to explore the perspective of those who experienced adult safeguarding interventions. *Ethics and Social Welfare*, *11*(1), 33–46.
Mills, W. L., & Naik, A. D. (2018). Making and executing decisions for safe and independent living (MED-SAIL): A screening tool for community-dwelling older adults. In M. R. Day, G. McCarthy, & J. J. Fitzpatrick (Eds.), *Self-neglect in older adults: A global, evidence-based resource for nurses and other healthcare providers* (pp. 303–314). New York: Springer.
Mulcahy, H., Leahy-Warren, P., & Day, M. R. (2018). Health and social care professionals' perspectives of self-neglect. In M. R. Day, G. McCarthy, & J. J. Fitzpatrick (Eds.), *Self-neglect in older adults: A global, evidence-based resource for nurses and other healthcare providers* (pp. 163–174). New York: Springer.
Niforatos, J. D., Rutecki, G. W., & Yates, F. D. (2018). Decisional capacity and suspected self-neglect in a geriatric patient. *Ethics and Medicine*, *34*(3) 147–131.
Pavlou, M. P., & Lachs, M. S. (2008). Self-neglect in older adults: A primer for physicians. *Journal of General Internal Medicine*, *23*(11), 1841–1846.
Preston-Shoot, M. (2019). Self-neglect and safeguarding adult reviews: Towards a model of understanding facilitators and barriers to best practice. *Journal of Adult Protection*, *21*(4), 219–234. https://doi.org/10.1108/JAP-02-2019-0008.
Touza, C., & Prado, C. (2019). Detecting self-neglect: A comparative study of indicators and risk factors in a Spanish population. *Gerontology and Geriatric Medicine*, *5*, 2333721418823605.
Wu, M., Peng, C., Chen, Y., et al. (2020). Nurses' perceptions of factors influencing elder self-neglect: A qualitative study. *Asian Nursing Research*, *14*(3), 137–143.
Yu, M., Gu, L., Jiao, W., Xia, H., & Wang, W. (2019). Predictors of self-neglect among community-dwelling older adults living alone in China. *Geriatric Nursing*, *40*(5), 457–462. https://doi.org/10.1016/j.gerinurse.2019.02.002.
Zhao, Y., Hu, C., Feng, F., et al. (2017). Associations of self-neglect with quality of life in older people in rural China: A cross-sectional study. *International Psychogeriatrics*, *29*(6), 1015–1026.

Sexual Dysfunction Domain 8 Sexuality Class 2 Sexual function

Laura King, DNP, RN, MSN, CNE

NANDA-I

Definition

A state in which an individual experiences a change in sexual function during the sexual response phases of desire, arousal, and/or orgasm, which is viewed as unsatisfying, unrewarding, or inadequate.

Defining Characteristics

Altered interest in others; altered self-interest; altered sexual activity; altered sexual excitation; altered sexual role; altered sexual satisfaction; decreased sexual desire; perceived sexual limitation; seeks confirmation of desirability; undesired alteration in sexual function

Related Factors

Inaccurate information about sexual function; inadequate knowledge about sexual function; inadequate role models; insufficient privacy; perceived vulnerability; unaddressed abuse; value conflict

At-Risk Population

Individuals without a significant other

Associated Conditions

Altered body function; altered body structure

S

NOC (Nursing Outcomes Classification)

Suggested NOC Outcomes

Abuse Recovery: Sexual; Knowledge: Sexual Functioning, Physical Aging; Psychosocial Adjustment: Life Change; Risk Control: Sexually Transmitted Diseases (STDs); Sexual Functioning; Sexual Identity

Example NOC Outcome with Indicators

Sexual Functioning as evidenced by the following indicators: Expresses comfort with sexual expression/Expresses comfort with body/Expresses sexual interest. (Rate the outcome and indicators of **Sexual Functioning:** 1 = never demonstrated, 2 = rarely demonstrated, 3 = sometimes demonstrated, 4 = often demonstrated, 5 = consistently demonstrated [see Section I].)

Client Outcomes

Client Will (Specify Time Frame)

- Identify individual cause of sexual dysfunction
- Identify stressors that contribute to dysfunction
- Discuss alternative, satisfying, and acceptable sexual practices for self and partner
- Identify the degree of sexual interest by the client and partner
- Adapt sexual technique as needed to cope with sexual problems
- Discuss with partner concerns about body image and sex role

NIC (Nursing Interventions Classification)

Suggested NIC Interventions

Sexual Counseling; Teaching: Sexuality

Example NIC Activities—Sexual Counseling

Provide privacy and ensure confidentiality; Discuss necessary modifications in sexual activity, as appropriate; Provide referral/consultation with other members of the health care team, as appropriate

Nursing Interventions and *Rationales*

S

- ● Gather the client's sexual history, noting normal patterns of functioning and the client's vocabulary, and encouraging clients to ask questions or discuss sexual problems experienced. EBN: *A large majority of men experiencing erectile dysfunction desire for providers to initiate the subject of sexual health (Burbage-Vieth, 2020).* EB: *Sexuality is considered to be a normal component of being healthy, and as such, assessing the client's sexual history patterns along with sexual experience provides a reference base in which to evaluate potential problems (Mernone et al, 2019).* EB: *In a large cross-sectional study of men, the prevalence of erectile dysfunction (ED) increased for those with comorbidities such as hypertension, diabetes mellitus, depression, or benign prostatic hypertrophy (BPH) (Mulhall et al, 2016).*
- ● Gather a sexual history for transgender clients, including their view and importance of sexuality and the presence of coexisting sexual dysfunctions such as low desire, inability to achieve orgasm, disturbance in body image, or experiencing pain with sexual intercourse. EB: *Evaluation of the client's history is important to understand sexual dysfunction. Creating a supportive, open, and nonjudgmental environment promotes communication when evaluating the client's history to better understand the transgender client's risk for sexual dysfunction (Holmberg et al, 2019).*
- ▲ Assess duration and risk factors for sexual dysfunction and explore potential causes such as medications, medical problems, aging process, or psychosocial issues. EBN: *In a descriptive, cross-sectional survey assessing client risk factors, the number of medications taken, smoking, depression, history of stroke, and those clients taking angiotensin-converting enzyme inhibitors and statin drugs reported reduced sexual activity (Dusenbury et al, 2020).* EB: *Transgender clients undergoing medical transition may experience decreased sexual desire related to hormone therapy or psychopharmacological drugs, pain from surgical procedures, inability to achieve orgasm, or a disturbance in body image (Holmberg et al, 2019).* EBN: *In a population-based sample comparing those with a cardiac condition to those without a cardiac condition, those with*

coronary artery disease, angina, and myocardial infarction reported significantly less sexual activity, as did those who smoked, had a weight problem, had lung problems, had depression, had shortness of breath or chest pain with exertion, or took certain medications. This illustrated that multiple factors affect sexual activity and may contribute to sexual dysfunction (Steinke et al, 2018).

▲ Assess for history of sexual abuse. EB: *Clients reporting a history of childhood sexual abuse experienced higher levels of sexual dysfunction and the development of posttraumatic stress disorder (PTSD) symptoms compared with those who report no experience of abuse. It is important to identify the history of abuse and to identify symptoms of PTSD (Gerwitz-Meydan & Lahav, 2020).* EB: *Men who were forced to have sex by a woman had greater risks such as higher number of lifetime partners and greater alcohol and drug use, compared with non-victimized men, putting them at increased risk of sexually transmitted infections (Cook et al, 2016).*

▲ Assess and provide treatment for sexual dysfunction, involving the person's partner in the process, and evaluating pharmacological and nonpharmacological interventions. EB: *Results of a systematic review of men and women found that dehydroepiandrosterone (DHEA) improved sexual interest, pain, arousal, lubrication, orgasm, and frequency of sexual activity, particularly for women and those with sexual dysfunction, whereas some men had improved erectile function, but others did not (Peixoto et al, 2017).* EBN: *Treatment of ED in men should involve the sexual partner and can include a variety of treatment options, including lifestyle modifications, the use of various oral medications such as phosphodiesterase type 5 (PDE5) inhibitors, sildenafil citrate, Tadalafil, and/or the use of vacuum erection devices or penile implants to help the client achieve sexual satisfaction (Schreiber, 2019).* EB: *Sexual dysfunction as a result of cancer in female clients has been shown to be improved with the use of pelvic floor exercises, as well as vaginal lubricants or moisturizers, including those with dehydroepiandrosterone (DHEA). Cognitive behavioral therapy, couples therapy, and participation in sexual health programs have also demonstrated improved sexual function (Valpey, Kucherer, & Nguyen, 2019).*

• Assess risk factors for sexual dysfunction, especially with varying sexual partners. EB: *In substance-dependent men who were polydrug users, having occasional sexual partners resulted in 14 times the risk of ED compared with married men, illustrating the importance of a complete sexual history and evaluation of risks for sexual dysfunction (Clemente et al, 2017).*

• Observe for stress and anxiety as possible causes of dysfunction. EBN: *Low levels of sexual desire in women have been attributed to increased levels of stress and anxiety (Dahlen, 2019).* EB: *In women, fibromyalgia significantly affected sexual function, and the severity and duration of fibromyalgia, the duration of the sexual partnership, and severity of anxiety significantly increased the degree of sexual dysfunction (Hayta & Mert, 2017).* EB: *The most prevalent reasons identified by women unable to achieve orgasm were stress and anxiety; therefore, managing high levels of both is often an important objective in sexual therapy (Rowland et al, 2018).*

▲ Assess for depression as a possible cause of sexual dysfunction and institute appropriate treatment. EBN: *In women who had given birth in the prior 12 months, 24% reported postnatal depression, which was significantly associated with sexual dysfunction, not initiating partnered sexual activity, and relationship dissatisfaction, illustrating the importance of assessment and early intervention for both depression and sexual dysfunction (Khajehei & Doherty, 2017).* EB: *A large matched control study found that depression rates in the transgender population have been documented to be higher than that of the general population (Whitcomb et al, 2018).* EB: *Studies consistently identify depression in women as a factor in experiencing sexual dysfunction (Basson & Gilks, 2018).*

S

• Observe for grief-related loss (e.g., amputation, mastectomy, ostomy) because a change in body image often precedes sexual dysfunction. See care plan for Disturbed **Body** Image. EBN: *In men after lower anterior resection for rectal cancer, ED occurred in 97% compared with 76% in those undergoing colectomy, with worse overall sexual function for those with lower anterior resection, particularly for those with a stoma. This illustrates the importance of discussing sexual function and loss in those diagnosed with rectal cancer (Shieh et al, 2016).* EB: *Women are highly affected by body image concerns related to surgical loss of breast, as well as stomas from gastrointestinal and colorectal cancers. Perceived alterations in body image can lead to decreased sexual activity and function (Valpey, Kucherer, & Nguyen, 2019).*

▲ Explore physical causes of sexual dysfunction such as diabetes, cardiovascular disease, arthritis, or BPH. EBN: *Men and women with cardiovascular disease experience sexual difficulties more often than those without the disease (Gök & Korkmoz, 2018).*

▲ Consider that ED may indicate the presence of cardiovascular disease, and screening and referral of men is recommended. EB: *ED has been related to diseases such as diabetes and cardiovascular disease, indicating that it is a cardiovascular disease predictor (Hernández-Cerda et al, 2020).*

- Certain chronic diseases such as cancer often have significant effects on sexual function, and both the disease process and treatment can contribute to sexual dysfunction. **EBN:** *Although women after gynecological cancer were sexually active, 54% had impaired sexual satisfaction and experienced problems such as vaginal dryness and discomfort with vaginal penetration during sexual activity (Sekse et al, 2017).* **EB:** *For individuals with chronic diseases such as cardiovascular disease, diabetes mellitus, renal failure, asthma, and hypertension, disease symptoms and side effects lead to changes in sexuality and affect overall perceptions of health (Sabanciogullari et al, 2016).*
- Consider that neurological diseases can affect sexual function directly, with secondary effects caused by disability related to the illness and social and emotional effects. **EB:** *Studies estimate the prevalence of clients with multiple sclerosis experiencing sexual dysfunction to be 40% to 80% in women and 50% to 90% in men related to paresthesia, sensory numbness, loss of libido, decreased lubrication, and erectile dysfunction (Domingo et al, 2018).*
- Explore behavioral or other causes of sexual dysfunction, such as smoking, dietary factors, or obesity. **EB:** *A meta-analysis from 89 studies found that smoking and alcohol intake increase the risk for ED in men, whereas participation in physical activity and consuming a healthy diet lower the risk for both ED and female sexual dysfunction (Allen & Walter, 2018).*

▲ Consider medications as a cause of sexual dysfunction. **EBN:** *Evaluating all cardiac medications used by clients for potential sexual side effects is important in identifying potential causes of sexual dysfunction (Dusenbury et al, 2020).* **EB:** *The use of psychotropic drugs is known to increase the risk for sexual dysfunction in women (Leveque et al, 2020).*

▲ Refer to appropriate medical providers for consideration of medication for premature ejaculation, ED, or orgasmic problems. **EB:** *Premature ejaculation is the most commonly diagnosed sexual dysfunction and is best treated with a combination of behavioral techniques and pharmacotherapy, including selective serotonin reuptake inhibitors, tricyclic antidepressants, or PDE5 inhibitors (Pereira-Lourenço et al, 2019).* **EB:** *Treatment response for the ED drug sildenafil was better than placebo in men with no comorbidity and for those with cardiovascular disease/hypertension only, diabetes only, or depression only, regardless of age (Goldstein et al, 2017).*

- Refer to the care plan Ineffective **Sexuality** Pattern for additional interventions.

Geriatric

▲ Carefully assess the sexuality needs and sexual dysfunction of older adults and refer for counseling if needed. **EBN:** *Treatment approaches for ED in older adults include behavioral and lifestyle changes (e.g., smoking cessation, healthy diet, physical activity, limiting alcohol intake), pelvic floor muscle exercises, PDE5 inhibitors, psychotherapy, and assistive devices (Marchese, 2017).*

- Teach about normal changes that occur with aging that may be perceived as sexual dysfunction, such as reduction in vaginal lubrication and reduction in duration and resolution of orgasm for women; for men these changes include increased time required for erection and for subsequent erections, erection without ejaculation, less firm erection, and decreased volume of seminal fluid. **EBN:** *Sexual dysfunction may decrease the quality of life for the older adult and lack of knowledge of normal physiological changes may lead to that dysfunction; health care professionals must be comfortable in discussing issues related to sexual intimacy and providing information related to normal physiological changes as they relate to aging and sexual function (March, 2018).*
- If prescribed, instruct clients with chronic pain to take pain medication before sexual activity. **EB:** Clients experiencing vulvodynia may experience a decrease in pain during intercourse with the use of antiinflammatory medications and lidocaine on a short-term basis (*Goldstein et al, 2016*).
- See care plan for Ineffective **Sexuality** Pattern.

S

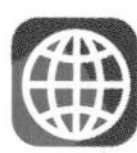

Multicultural

✱ Evaluate culturally influenced risk factors for sexual function and dysfunction. **EBN:** *Bisexual women had greater sexual coercion, more lifetime partners, physical and sexual violence, traded sex for resources, and posttraumatic stress disorder symptoms, illustrating the importance of history-taking, screening protocols, and counseling, taking into account race, ethnicity, gender, class, and sexual identity (Alexander et al, 2016).*

- Validate client feelings and emotions regarding the changes in sexual behavior by letting the client know that the nurse heard and understands what was said, promoting the nurse–client relationship. **EB:** *Culturally sensitive approaches with older adults include discussing sexual function and dysfunction regardless of culture, sexual orientation, age, gender, or marital status, and inquiring about culture in a nonjudgmental way (Atallah, 2016).*

Home Care

- Previously discussed interventions may be adapted for home care use.
- ▲ Identify specific sources of concern about sexual dysfunction and provide reassurance and instruction on appropriate expectations as indicated. EB: *Although women with breast cancer have concerns regarding sexual health, many may not feel comfortable voicing those concerns; therefore, it is important for health care professionals to facilitate communications regarding sexual function with clients (Reese et al, 2019).*
- ▲ Confirm that physical reasons for dysfunction have been addressed, and refer for therapy and/or support groups if appropriate. EB: *Most individuals with sexual problems would benefit from both pharmacological and psychological treatment, including sexual counseling and therapy (Almås, 2016).*
- See care plan for Ineffective **Sexuality** Pattern.

Client/Family Teaching and Discharge Planning

- Provide accurate information for clients regarding interventions for sexual dysfunction. EB: *To address sexual problems in those with cancer, psychosexual counseling should be offered to both men and women. Women may benefit from pelvic floor physiotherapy, hormonal therapy for vasomotor symptoms (if safe), and vaginal lubricants, whereas men might be offered PDE5 inhibitors, vacuum erectile devices, and intracavernosal injection (Barbera et al, 2017).*
- Include the partner/family in discharge instructions because partner concerns are often overlooked regarding sexual issues. EB: *Women as cervical cancer survivors wanted both information and practical advice in dealing with sexual dysfunction; physical functioning, sexual distress, relationship satisfaction, and partner perspectives should be assessed, with interventions tailored to the particular needs of the couple (Vermeer et al, 2016).*
- Teach the client and partner about condom use, for those at risk. EB: *In couples, feelings of commitment to the sexual partner resulted in reduced perceived sexual risk, illustrating that interventions for couples should include discussion of sexual risk, prevention of HIV risk (including condom use), and monogamy agreements before condoms are discontinued (Agnew et al, 2017).*
- ▲ Refer to appropriate community resources, such as a clinical specialist, family counselor, or cardiac rehabilitation, including the partner if appropriate; for complex issues, a referral to a sex counselor, urologist, gynecologist, or other specialist may be needed. EB: *Young adult clients diagnosed with cancer have many questions regarding sexual function and prefer to have those questions addressed by professionals, as well as being directed to reliable online resources (Martins et al, 2018).* EB: *Men and their partners need comprehensive information before and after treatment for prostate cancer, including support groups to help clients and partners gain education and support (Albaugh et al, 2017).*
- ▲ Refer for medical advice when ED lasts longer than 2 months or is recurring. EB: *Erectile dysfunction is a common condition in males and can be managed through a variety of treatments; therefore, it is important for providers to carefully assess at-risk clients (Irwin, 2019).*
- Teach the following interventions to decrease the likelihood of ED: limit or avoid the use of alcohol, stop smoking, exercise regularly, reduce stress, get enough sleep, deal with anxiety or depression, and see a health care provider for regular checkups and medical screening tests. EB: *In a study of nondiabetic men with cardiovascular risk factors, those with ED were more likely to be smokers and sedentary and consumed more alcohol, whereas those consuming more nuts and vegetables had less ED, illustrating the importance of counseling regarding lifestyle and its effect on ED (Ramírez et al, 2016).*
- See care plan for Ineffective **Sexuality** Pattern.

S

REFERENCES

Agnew, C. R., Harvey, S. M., VanderDrift, L. E., & Warren, J. (2017). Relational underpinnings of condom use: Findings from the project on partner dynamics. *Health Psychology*, *36*(7), 713–720. https://doi:10.1037/hea0000488.

Albaugh, J. A., Sufrin, N., Lapin, B. R., Petkewicz, J., & Tenfelde, S. (2017). Life after prostate cancer treatment: A mixed methods study of the experiences of men with sexual dysfunction and their partners. *BMC Urology*, *17*(1), 45. https://doi:10.1186/s12894-017-0231-5.

Alexander, K. A., Volpe, E. M., Abboud, S., & Campbell, J. C. (2016). Reproductive coercion, sexual risk behaviours and mental health symptoms among young low-income behaviourally bisexual women: Implications for nursing practice. *Journal of Clinical Nursing*, *25*(23–24), 3533–3544. https://doi.org/10.1111/jocn.13238Allen.

Allen, M. S., & Walter, E. E. (2018). Health-related lifestyle factors and sexual dysfunction: A meta-analysis of population-based research. *The Journal of Sexual Medicine*, *15*(4), 458–475. https://doi:10.1016/j.jsxm.2018.02.008.

Almås, E. (2016). Psychological treatment of sexual problems. Thematic analysis of guidelines and recommendations, based on a systematic literature review 2001–2010. *Sexual and Relationship Therapy*, *31*(1), 54–69. https://doi:10.1080/14681994.2015.1086739.

Atallah, S. (2016). Cultural aspects of sexual function and dysfunction in the geriatric population. *Topics in Geriatric Rehabilitation*, *32*(3), 156–166. https://doi:10.1097/TGR.0000000000000105.

Barbera, L., Zwaal, C., Elterman, D., et al. (2017). Interventions to address sexual problems in people with cancer. *Current Oncology*, *24*(3), 192–200. https://doi.org/10.3747/co.24.3583.

Basson, R., & Gilks, T. (2018). Women's sexual dysfunction associated with psychiatric disorders and their treatment. *Women's Health, 14*, 1745506518762664. https://doi:10.1177/1745506518762664.

Burbage-Vieth, J. (2020). Improving provider comfort with the assessment of erectile dysfunction in the clinic setting. *Urologic Nursing, 40*(4), 163–173.

Clemente, J., Diehl, A., Oliveira Henrique Santana, P. R., Jerônimo da Silva, C., Pillon, S. C., & de Jesus Mari, J. (2017). Erectile dysfunction symptoms in polydrug dependents seeking treatment. *Substance Abuse & Misuse, 52*(12), 1565–1574. https://doi:10.1080/10826084.2017.1290114.

Cook, M. C., Morisky, D. E., Williams, J. K., Ford, C. L., & Gee, G. C. (2016). Sexual risk behaviors and substance use among men sexually victimized by women. *American Journal of Public Health, 106*(7), 1263–1269. https://doi:10.2105/AJPH.2016.303136.

Dahlen, H. (2019). Female sexual dysfunction: Assessment and treatment. *Urologic Nursing, 39*(1), 39–46.

Domingo, S., Kinzy, T., Thompson, N., Gales, S., Stone, L., & Sullivan, A. (2018). Factors associated with sexual dysfunction in individuals with multiple sclerosis: Implications for assessment and treatment. *International Journal of MS Care, 20*(4), 191–197. https://doi: 10.7224/1537-2073.2017-059.

Dusenbury, W., Hill, T. J., Mosack, V., & Steinke, E. E. (2020). Risk factors, depression, and drugs influencing sexual activity in individuals with and without stroke. *Rehabilitation Nursing, 45*(1), 23–29. https:doi:10.1097/RNJ.0000000000000145.

Gewirtz-Meydan, A., & Lahav, Y. (2020). Sexual dysfunction and distress among childhood sexual abuse survivors: The role of post-traumatic stress disorder. *Journal of Sexual Medicine, 17*(11), 2267–2278. https://doi:10.1016/j.jsxm.2020.07.016.

Gök, F., & Korkmaz, F. D. (2018). Sexual counseling provided by cardiovascular nurses: Attitudes, beliefs, perceived barriers, and proposed solutions. *Journal of Cardiovascular Nursing, 33*(6), E24–E30. https://doi:10.1097/JCN.0000000000000535.

Goldstein, A. T., Pukall, C. F., Brown, C., Bergeron, S., Stein, A., & Kellogg-Spadt, S. (2016). Vulvodynia: Assessment and treatment. *The Journal of Sexual Medicine, 13*(4), 572–590. https://doi:10.1016/j.jsxm.2016.01.020.

Goldstein, I., Stecher, V., & Carlsson, M. (2017). Treatment response to sildenafil in men with erectile dysfunction relative to concomitant comorbidities and age. *International Journal of Clinical Practice, 71*(3–4), e12939. https://doi:10.1111/ijcp.12939.

Hayta, E., & Mert, D. G. (2017). Potential risk factors increasing the severity of sexual dysfunction in women with fibromyalgia. *Sexuality and Disability, 35*(2), 147–155. https://doi:10.1007/s11195-016-9472-6.

Hernández-Cerda, J., Bertomeu-González, V., Zuazola, P., & Cordero, A. (2020). Understanding erectile dysfunction in hypertensive patients: The need for good patient management. *Vascular Health and Risk Management, 16*, 231–239. https://doi.org/10.2147/VHRM.S223331.

Holmberg, M., Arver, S., & Dhejne, C. (2019). Supporting sexuality and improving sexual function in transgender persons. *Nature Reviews Urology, 16*(2), 121–139. https://doi.org/10.1038/s41585-018-0108-8.

Irwin, G. M. (2019). Erectile dysfunction. *Primary Care, 46*(2), 249–255. https://doi:10.1016/j.pop.2019.02.006.

Khajehei, M., & Doherty, M. (2017). Exploring postnatal depression, sexual dysfunction and relationship dissatisfaction in Australian women. *British Journal of Midwifery, 25*(3), 162–172. https://doi:10.12968/bjom.2017.25.3.162.

Leveque, E., Samarron, H., & Shaw, J. (2020). Not into sex: Women's experiences of treatment emergent sexual dysfunction. *Journal of Women and Social Work, 35*(3), 413–433. https://doi.org/10.1177/0886109919878275.

March, A. L. (2018). Sexuality and intimacy in the older adult woman. *Nursing Clinics of North America, 53*(2), 279–287. https://doi.org/10.1016/j.cnur.2018.01.005.

Marchese, K. (2017). An overview of erectile dysfunction in the elderly population. *Urologic Nursing, 37*(3), 157–170. https://doi:10.7257/1053-816X.2017.37.3.157.

Martins, A., Taylor, R. M., Lobel, B., et al. (2018). Sex, body image, and relationships: A BRIGHTLIGHT workshop on information and support needs of adolescents and young adults. *Journal of Adolescent and Young Adult Oncology, 7*(5), 572–578. https://doi:10.1089/jayao.2018.0025.

Mernone, L., Fiacco, S., & Ehlert, U. (2019). Psychobiological factors of sexual functioning in aging women—Findings from the women 40+ healthy aging study. *Frontiers in Psychology, 10*, 546. doi:10.3389/fpsyg.2019.00546.

Mulhall, J. P., Luo, X., Zou, K. H., Stecher, V., & Galaznik, A. (2016). Relationship between age and erectile dysfunction diagnosis or treatment using real-world observational data in the USA. *International Journal of Clinical Practice, 70*(12), 1012–1018. https://doi:10.1111/ijcp.12908.

Peixoto, C., Carrilho, C. G., Barros, J. A., et al. (2017). The effects of dehydroepiandrosterone one sexual function: A systematic review. *Climacteric, 20*(2), 129–137. https://doi.org/10.1080/13697137.2017.1279141.

Pereira-Lourenço, M., Vieira E Brito, D., & Pereira, B. J. (2019). Premature ejaculation: From physiology to treatment. *Journal of Family and Reproductive Health, 13*(3), 120–131. https://www.ncbi.nlm.nih.gov/pmc/articles/PMC7072026/.

Ramírez, R., Pedro-Botet, J., García, M., et al. (2016). Erectile dysfunction and cardiovascular risk factors in a Mediterranean diet cohort. *Internal Medicine Journal, 46*(1), 52–56. https://doi:10.1111/imj.12937.

Reese, J. B., Sorice, K., Lepore, S. J., Daly, M. B., Tulsky, J. A., & Beach, M. C. (2019). Patient-clinician communication about sexual health in breast cancer: A mixed method analysis of clinic dialogue. *Patient Education and Counseling, 102*(3), 436–442. https://doi:10.1016/j.pec.2018.10.003.

Rowland, D. L., Cempel, L. M., & Tempel, A. R. (2018). Women's attributions regarding why they have difficulty reaching orgasm. *Journal of Sex & Marital Therapy, 44*(5), 475–484. https://doi:10.1080/0092623X.2017.1408046.

Sabanciogullari, S., Tuncay, F. O., & Avci, D. (2016). The relationship between satisfaction and perceived health and sexuality in individuals diagnosed with a physical illness. *Sexuality and Disability, 34*(4), 389–402. https://doi.org/10.1007/s11195-016-9456-6.

Schreiber, M. L. (2019). Erectile dysfunction. *Medsurg Nursing, 28*(5), 327–330.

Sekse, R. J., Hufthammer, K. O., & Vika, M. E. (2017). Sexual activity and functioning in women treated for gynaecological cancers. *Journal of Clinical Nursing, 26*(3–4), 400–410. https://doi:10.1111/jocn.13407.

Shieh, S. I., Lin, Y. H., Huang, C. Y., et al. (2016). Sexual dysfunction in males following low anterior resection. *Journal of Clinical Nursing, 25*(15–16), 2348–2356. https://doi:10.1111/jocn.13172.

Steinke, E. E., Mosack, V., & Hill, T. J. (2018). The influence of comorbidities, risk factors, and medications on sexual activity in individuals aged 40 to 59 years with and without cardiac conditions: US National Health and Nutrition Examination Survey, 2011–2012. *Journal of Cardiovascular Nursing, 33*(2), 118–125. https://doi:10.1097/JCN.0000000000000433.

Valpey, R., Kucherer, S., & Nguyen, J. (2019). Sexual dysfunction in female cancer survivors: A narrative review. *General Hospital Psychiatry, 60*, 141–147. https://doi.org/10.1016/j.genhosppsych.2019.04.003.

Vermeer, W. M., Bakker, R. M., Kenter, G. G., Stiggelbout, A. M., & ter Kuile, M. M. (2016). Cervical cancer survivors' and partners' experiences with sexual dysfunction and psychosexual support. *Supportive Care in Cancer, 24*(4), 1679–1687. https://doi:10.1007/s00520-015-2925-0.

Whitcomb, G. L., Bouman, W. P., Claes, L., Brewing, N., Crawford, J. R., & Arcelus, J. (2018). Levels of depression in transgender people and its predictors: Results of a large matched control study with transgender people accessing clinical services. *Journal of Affective Disorders, 235*, 308–315. https://doi.org/10.1016/j.jad.2018.02.051.

Ineffective Sexuality Pattern Domain 8 Sexuality Class 2 Sexual function

Laura King, DNP, RN, MSN, CNE

NANDA-I

Definition

Expressions of concern regarding own sexuality.

Defining Characteristics

Altered sexual activity; altered sexual behavior; altered sexual partner relations; altered sexual role; difficulty with sexual activity; difficulty with sexual behavior; value conflict

Related Factors

Conflict about sexual orientation; conflict about variant preference; fear of pregnancy; fear of sexually transmitted infection; impaired sexual partner relations; inadequate alternative sexual strategies; inadequate role models; insufficient privacy

At-Risk Population

Individuals without a significant other

NOC (Nursing Outcomes Classification)

Suggested NOC Outcomes

Abuse Recovery: Sexual; Body Image; Child Development: Middle Childhood/Adolescence; Client Satisfaction: Teaching; Knowledge: Pregnancy and Postpartum Sexual Functioning; Knowledge: Sexual Functioning; Psychosocial Adjustment: Life Change; Risk Control: Sexually Transmitted Diseases (STDs); Risk Control: Unintended Pregnancy; Role Performance; Self-Esteem; Sexual Functioning; Sexual Identity

Example NOC Outcome with Indicators

Risk Control: Sexually Transmitted Diseases (STDs) as evidenced by the following indicators: Acknowledges personal risk factors for STD/Uses strategies to prevent STD transmission. (Rate the outcome and indicators of **Risk Control: Sexually Transmitted Diseases (STDs):** 1 = never demonstrated, 2 = rarely demonstrated, 3 = sometimes demonstrated, 4 = often demonstrated, 5 = consistently demonstrated [see Section I].)

Client Outcomes

Client Will (Specify Time Frame)

- State knowledge of difficulties, limitations, or changes in sexual behaviors or activities
- State knowledge of sexual anatomy and functioning
- State acceptance of altered body structure or functioning
- Describe acceptable alternative sexual practices
- Identify importance of discussing sexual issues with significant other
- Describe practice of safe sex with regard to pregnancy and avoidance of sexually transmitted infections (STIs)

NIC (Nursing Interventions Classification)

Suggested NIC Interventions

Abuse Protection Support: Child; Abuse Protection Support: Domestic Partner; Abuse Protection Support: Elder; Abuse Protection Support: Religious; Behavior Management: Sexual; Sexual Counseling; Teaching: Safe Sex; Teaching: Sexuality

Example NIC Activities—Sexual Counseling

Provide privacy and ensure confidentiality; Provide information about sexual functioning, as appropriate

Nursing Interventions and *Rationales*

- After establishing rapport or therapeutic relationship, give the client permission to discuss issues dealing with sexuality, for example, "Have you been or are you concerned about functioning sexually because of your health status?" **EBN:** *Nurses can use the PLISSIT (permission, limited information, specific suggestions, referral to intensive therapy) model to initiate communication regarding sexual concerns with clients (Kautz & Van Horn, 2017).* **EB:** *Use of the PLISSIT model has been shown to elicit information that can be used to help improve sexual function in women with multiple sclerosis (MS) (Khakbazan et al, 2016).*
- Use assessment questions and standardized instruments to assess sexual problems, where possible. **EB:** *Use of standardized scales and validated instruments to obtain information regarding current levels of sexual activity can assist in the evaluation for sexual dysfunction (Hatzichristou et al, 2016).*
- ▲ Assess any risks associated with sexual activity, particularly coronary risks. **EBN:** *For men and women, cardiac conditions including coronary heart disease, angina, and a history of myocardial infarction, along with risk factors such as smoking and obesity, and other comorbidities, symptoms, and medications can negatively affect sexual activity (Steinke et al, 2018).*
- Assess knowledge about sexual functioning and return to sexual activity after experiencing a health problem with both clients and partners. **EB:** *A population-based study found an association between coronary heart disease and reduction in sexual activity (Steptoe et al, 2016).*
- Encourage the client to discuss concerns with his or her partner. **EB:** *A systematic review of articles found that, in men with traumatic spinal cord injuries, providing information regarding the importance of communication of sexual concerns between partners, and offering resources to facilitate that communication, was beneficial for improving overall sexual health (Aikman et al, 2018).*
- Explore attitudes about sexual intimacy and changes in sexuality patterns. **EBN:** *After breast cancer, women had reduced sexual desire, frequency, and satisfaction, with no association between sexual performance and body image (Dorneles de Morais et al, 2016).* **EB:** *A cross-sectional study found that assessing attitudes and sexual patterns of individuals diagnosed with a chronic disease enabled health care professionals to recognize sexual dysfunction, which resulted in the planning of interventions to improve the quality of life and life satisfaction (Sabanciogullari et al, 2016).*
- Assess psychosocial function such as anxiety, fear, depression, and low self-esteem. **EBN:** *In a population-based study, men who had sex with men had greater depressive symptoms compared with those with partners of the opposite sex (Scott, Lasiuk, & Norris, 2016).* **EB:** *Mental health illness is a major risk factor for sexual dysfunction in women (Basson & Gilks, 2018).*
- Discuss alternative sexual expressions for altered body functioning or structure, including closeness and sexual and nonsexual touching as other forms of expression. **EBN:** *Women with fibromyalgia experienced pain with sexual activity, postcoital stiffness, anxiety about sex, and altered body image, although maintaining an active sex life was important; therefore discussion of sexual concerns, individual symptoms, and psychoemotional needs can assist in developing approaches for sexual activity, such as changes in position or alternatives to sexual intercourse when symptom burden is high (Matarín Jiménez et al, 2017).***EB:** *Alternative expressions of intimacy may play an important role in facilitating intimate relationships in women with gynecological cancers, and providing information on these alternatives can help to increase sexual health (Lee et al, 2020).*
- Assess the client's sexual orientation and usual pattern of sexual activities, and discuss prevention of illnesses for which the client may be at increased risk (e.g., anorectal cancer), asking specific questions about sexual orientation, for example, "Do you have sexual relationships with men, women, or both?" Assess use of safer sex practices (e.g., condom use); the frequency of anal intercourse; number of sexual partners in the last year; last HIV screening/results; and use of medications, alcohol, and illicit drugs. **EBN:** *Transgender women had low levels of HIV risk perception and knowledge about HIV risk and transmission, illustrating the importance of assessing transgender women's sexual health care needs and educating regarding risks (De Santis et al, 2017).*
- Specific guidelines for sexual activity for clients who have had total hip arthroplasty (THA) include the following: sexual activity can be generally resumed 1 to 2 months after surgery, and positioning to avoid hip dislocation, for example, a supine position ("missionary") at maximum abduction in extension, or the man and woman standing, with the woman's legs slightly bent and the man approaching the woman from behind (Issa et al, 2017). **EB:** *In a systematic review of THA and sexual activity, 76% of individuals identified hip arthritis as contributing to sexual problems, whereas post-THA, 44% reported improvement in sexual satisfaction, 27% reported increased intercourse frequency, and most returned to sexual activity at 4 months post-THA. Health care professionals and surgeons should discuss return to sexual activity after THA, including the best positions postsurgery (Harmsen et al, 2017).*

S

- Specific guidelines for those who have had a myocardial infarction (MI) include the following: sexual activity can generally be resumed 1 week after MI unless complications are experienced, such as arrhythmias or cardiac arrest, if the client does not have cardiac symptoms during mild to moderate physical activity; begin with activities that require less exertion, such as fondling or kissing, building confidence in tolerance for sexual activity before sexual intercourse; engage in sexual activity in familiar surroundings with the usual partner; have a comfortable room temperature, and be well rested to minimize cardiac stress; avoid heavy meals or alcohol for 2 to 3 hours before sexual activity; and choose a position of comfort to minimize stress of the cardiac client (Steinke et al, 2016). EB: *A healthy sexual life is important for all humans and it is essential for health care providers to provide clients who have experienced MI information on safely resuming sexual activity, as well as addressing client concerns in order to improve their quality of life (Farhan et al, 2020).*
- Specific guidelines include that those who have had complete coronary revascularization, in addition to those mentioned with MI, including those with successful percutaneous cardiovascular revascularization without complication, can resume sex within a few days, and those who have had standard coronary artery bypass grafting or noncoronary open heart surgery may resume sex in 6 to 8 weeks. Incisional pain with sexual activity can be managed by premedicating with a mild pain reliever, and reassurance should be provided to the partner that sexual activity will not harm the sternum as long as direct pressure is avoided (Jelavić et al, 2018). EB: *Women, particularly those with large breasts, may report more issues related to pain in the breast, chest numbness, and difficulty healing; therefore encourage these women to choose a position of comfort, support with pillows, and take a pain reliever such as acetaminophen before sexual activity (Steinke et al, 2016).*
- Specific guidelines for those with an implantable cardioverter defibrillator (ICD) include returning to sexual activity is generally safe after ICD implantation if moderate physical activity does not precipitate arrhythmias; avoid strain on the incision at the implant site; assure the client and partner that fears about being shocked during sexual activity are normal; if the ICD discharges with sexual activity, the client should stop, rest, and later notify the health care provider that the device fired so that a determination can be made if this was an appropriate shock or not; and report any dyspnea, chest pain, or dizziness with sexual activity (Steinke et al, 2016). EB: *Although most clients with ICD reported the ability to engage in sexual activity (64.6%), 51% chose to avoid sexual activity, citing reasons such as fear of shock, fear of increased heart rate, and no desire, illustrating the importance of evaluating and discussing both psychological and physical aspects of return to sexual activity (Streur et al, 2020).*
- Specific guidelines for those with chronic lung disease include planning for sexual activity when energy level is highest; use of controlled breathing techniques; avoiding physical exertion before sexual activity; using positions that minimize shortness of breath, such as a semireclining position; engaging in sexual activity when medications are at peak effectiveness; use of an oxygen cannula, if prescribed, to provide oxygen before, during, or after sex; and use of continuous positive airway pressure (CPAP) therapy, if prescribed (Steinke et al, 2016). EB: *In a systematic review of sexual dysfunction and obstructive sleep apnea in men, CPAP improved daytime sleepiness and erectile and orgasmic dysfunction, although sildenafil was superior to CPAP in improving erectile dysfunction; intervention studies for women were not available (Steinke et al, 2016).*
- Specific guidelines for those with MS include treatment of symptoms with prescribed medications, assessing changes in body image, and supportive therapies to assist with a more satisfying sexual experience, including treatment of neuropathic pain, sexual positions that are most supportive, discussing changes in sensation and stimulation with the partner, use of stretching exercise for tight muscles before sexual activity, and avoiding a distended bowel or bladder that may cause discomfort. EB: *Women with MS attending a 12-week sexual therapy program significantly improved sexual desire, arousal, lubrication, orgasm, satisfaction, overall quality of life, energy, cognitive function, and social function; designing targeted educational and sexual interventions is important to improve sexual and overall quality of life (Zamani et al, 2017).*
- Refer to the care plan **Sexual** Dysfunction for additional interventions.

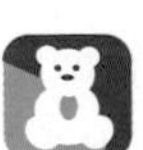

Pediatric

- Initiate discussions regarding sexual health, attitudes, and knowledge about sexual behavior and sexual abstinence, providing information that is age appropriate and accurate regarding sexual activity and risky sexual behaviors. EBN: *Lack of information regarding sexual health contributes to vulnerability and adolescents acknowledge the need for accurate information to decrease risky sexual behaviors (Grigsby, 2018).* EB: *Focus groups conducted in black churches with senior pastors, youth ministers, parents of youth, and youth ages 13 to 19 years, on the topic of youth sexual and reproductive health, resulted in the themes of engaging stakeholders, the authenticity of the curriculum, making the curriculum relevant to youth, discussion of relationships, and adaptation, providing an example that implementing sexual health programs in new settings can be successful in reaching youth and the community (Weeks et al, 2016).*

- Provide age-appropriate information for adolescents regarding HIV/AIDS and sexual behavior, and discuss STIs, particularly human papillomavirus, including the risks of perinatal transmission and methods to reduce risks among adolescents with HIV. EB: *Communication between African American fathers and their sons is an important factor in decreasing sexual risk behaviors and HIV risk (Harris et al, 2019).*
- Provide age-appropriate information regarding potential for sexual abuse. EBN: *A structured teaching program on prevention of sexual abuse with high school students resulted in improved knowledge of prevention strategies, illustrating the importance of education and directly addressing this sensitive issue (Fulgen, 2017).*

Geriatric

- Carefully assess the sexuality needs of the older client and refer for counseling as needed. EB: *Positive affect and life satisfaction was associated with increased sexual behavior in community-dwelling older men and women, regardless of depressive symptoms, physical health, and chronic diseases, whereas unpartnered adults' life satisfaction was linked with more physical tenderness and less sexual behavior, demonstrating the importance of sexual assessment of all older adults and in promoting psychological and sexual well-being (Freak-Poli et al, 2017a).*
- ▲ Explore possible changes in sexuality related to health status, menopause, medications, and sexual risk, and make appropriate referrals. EB: *Although two-thirds of older adults had experienced some sexual problems, most were not distressed by it, reporting positive sexual well-being, with positive sexual self-esteem and attitudes toward sex, high sexual satisfaction and interest, and frequently engaging in sexual activity, illustrating that although some older adults may experience challenges regarding sexual activity, many report positive sexual health (Santos-Iglesias et al, 2016).* EB: *Sexual risk-taking was prevalent among older adults, with 49% reporting engaging in vaginal sex and 43% engaging in oral sex without a condom in the prior 6 months, although 65.5% of the sample believed they were not susceptible to STIs, revealing the need for assessment, education, and intervention related to sexual risk (Syme, Cohn, & Barnack-Tavlaris, 2017).*
- Allow the client to verbalize feelings regarding loss of sexual partner, and acknowledge problems such as disapproving children, lack of available partner for women, and environmental variables that make forming new relationships difficult. EB: *Health status, frequency of sexual activity, and importance of sexual behavior were important predictors of quality of life, and these findings were independent of the presence of a spouse/partner, illustrating the importance of health care providers evaluating sexual activity as a component of quality of life with all clients (Granville & Pregler, 2018).*
- ▲ Provide a milieu that allows for discussion of sexual issues and a higher level of sexual satisfaction, including allowing couples to room together and the provision of privacy. EBN: *Sexual expression and consent should be openly addressed in long-term care settings, and results from a qualitative study of directors of long-term care facilities revealed the common themes of addressing the issue, making environmental changes, identifying staff expertise, providing education and training, assessing sexuality initially and recurrently, establishing policies and procedures for sexual expression management, developing assessment tools, and clarifying legal issues. These are all important areas that staff in long-term care facilities can use to improve the sexual health of their residents (Syme et al, 2016).*
- See care plan for **Sexual** Dysfunction.

S

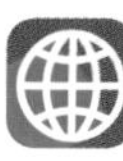

Multicultural

- ✱ Assess for the influence of cultural beliefs, norms, and values on client's perceptions of sexual behavior. EBN: *Among Hispanic men who had sex with men, parental knowledge and rejection of their sexual orientation contributed to greater depressive symptoms and no effect on safer sex behaviors, although acculturation (Americanism) may have had a protective role. These findings emphasized the importance of educating and supporting both the individual and family, including assessing mental health (Mitrani et al, 2017).*

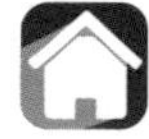

Home Care

- Previously discussed interventions may be adapted for home care use. Also see care plan for **Sexual** Dysfunction.
- Help the client and significant other identify a place and time in the home and daily living for privacy in sharing sexual or relationship activity, and, if necessary, help the client communicate the need for privacy to family members. EB: *In community-dwelling older adults, most reported experiencing physical tenderness and about half engaged in sexual activity, with sexual activity more likely in those of younger age, those*

with greater social support, those with healthier behaviors, and those with better psychological and physical health, illustrating the importance of maintaining sexual quality of life regardless of setting, not assuming that the older person is not interested in sexual pleasure, and having health care professionals proactively address sexuality and sexual health (Freak-Poli et al, 2017b).

- Confirm that physical reasons for dysfunction have been addressed, and provide support for coping behaviors, including participation in support groups or therapy if appropriate. **EB:** *A pilot study using a psychoeducational group intervention in women with MS and spinal cord injury resulted in improved sexual functioning, particularly for sexual desire and arousal, demonstrating the importance of supportive interventions to improve sexual functioning (Hocaloski et al, 2016).*

Client/Family Teaching and Discharge Planning

▲ Refer to appropriate community agencies (e.g., certified sex counselor, Reach to Recovery, Ostomy Association, American Association of Sex Educators, Counselors, and Therapists). **EB:** *Sexuality concerns should be addressed with all clients for whom sexual function might be impaired (Morton, 2017).*

▲ Sexuality education is important to all populations, whether hearing or deaf, sighted or blind, disabled or not disabled; discuss contraceptive choices as appropriate, safer sexual practices, and refer to a health professional (e.g., gynecologist, urologist, nurse practitioner). **EB:** *Sexuality education of older adults is often overlooked, and they may have inaccurate perceptions regarding sexual risk behaviors and STIs (Syme et al, 2017).*

REFERENCES

Aikman, K., Oliffe, J. L., Kelly, M. T., & McCuaig, F. (2018). Sexual health in men with traumatic spinal cord injuries: A review and recommendations for primary health-care providers. *American Journal of Men's Health*, *12*(6), 2044–2054. https://doi:10.1177/1557988318790883.

Basson, R., & Gilks, T. (2018). Women's sexual dysfunction associated with psychiatric disorders and their treatment. *Women's Health*, *14*, 1745506518762664. https:doi:10.1177/1745506518762664.

De Santis, J. P., Hauglum, S. D., Deleon, D. A., Provencio-Vasquez, E., & Rodriguez, A. E. (2017). HIV risk perception, HIV knowledge, and sexual risk behaviors among transgender women in South Florida. *Public Health Nursing*, *34*(3), 210–218. https://doi.org/10.1111/phn.12309.

Dorneles de Morais, F., Freitas-Junior, R., Macedo Sousa Rahal, R., & Maciel Reis Gonzaga, C. (2016). Sociodemographic and clinical factors affecting body image, sexual function and sexual satisfaction in women with breast cancer. *Journal of Clinical Nursing*, *25*(11–12), 1557–1565. https://doi.org/10.1111/jocn.13125.

Farhan, R., Yousuf, R., Hussain, S. N. F., et al. (2020). Sexual knowledge in post-myocardial patients: A cross sectional study. *Cureus*, *12*(6), e8480. https://doi:10.7759/cureus.8480.

Freak-Poli, R., De Castro Lima, G., Direk, N., et al. (2017a). Happiness, rather than depression, is associated with sexual behaviour in partnered older adults. *Age and Ageing*, *46*(1), 101–107. https://doi:10.1093/ageing/afw168.

Freak-Poli, R., Kirkman, M., De Castro Lima, G., Direk, N., Franco, O. H., & Tiemeier, H. (2017b). Sexual activity and physical tenderness in older adults: Cross-sectional prevalence and associated characteristics. *The Journal of Sexual Medicine*, *14*(7), 918–927. https://doi:10.1016/j.jsxm.2017.05.010.

Fulgen, F. (2017). Effectiveness of structured teaching programme on knowledge of high school children regarding prevention of sexual abuse. *International Journal of Nursing Education*, *9*(2), 61–65. https://doi:10.5958/0974-9357.2017.00037.X.

Granville, L., & Pregler, J. (2018). Women's sexual health and aging. *Journal of the American Geriatrics Society*, *66*(3), 595–601. https://doi.org/10.1111/jgs.15198.

Grigsby, S. R. (2018). Giving our daughters what we never received: African American mothers discussing sexual health with their preadolescent daughters. *The Journal of School Nursing*, *34*(2), 128–138. https://doi:10.1177/1059840517707241.

Harmsen, R. T. E., Nicolai, M. P. J., Den Oudsten, B. L., et al. (2017). Patient sexual function and hip replacement surgery: A survey of surgeon attitudes. *International Orthopaedics*, *41*, 2433–2445. https://doi:10.1007/s00264-017-3473-7.

Harris, A. L., Fantasia, H. C., & Castle, C. E. (2019). Father 2 son: The impact of African American father-son sexual communication on African American adolescent sons' sexual behaviors. *American Journal of Men's Health*, *13*(1), 1557988318804725. https://doi.org/10.1177/1557988318804725.

Hatzichristou, D., Kirana, P. S., Banner, L., et al. (2016). Diagnosing sexual dysfunction in men and women: Sexual history taking and the role of symptom scales and questionnaires. *Journal of Sexual Medicine*, *13*(8), 1166–1182. https://doi:10.1016/j.jsxm.2016.05.017.

Hocaloski, S., Elliott, S., Brotto, L. A., Breckon, E. N., & McBride, K. (2016). A mindfulness psychoeducational group intervention targeting sexual adjustment for women with multiple sclerosis and spinal cord injury: A pilot study. *Sexuality and Disability*, *34*(2), 183–198. https://doi:10.1007/s11195-016-9426z.

Issa, K., Pierce, T. P., Brothers, A., Festa, A., Scillia, A. J., & Mont, M. A. (2017). Sexual activity after total hip arthroplasty: A systematic review of outcomes. *Journal of Arthroplasty*, *32*(1), 336–340. https://doi:10.1016/j.arth.2016.07.052.

Jelavić, M. M., Krstačić, G., Perenčević, A., & Pintarić, H. (2018). Sexual activity in patients with cardiac disease. *Acta Clinical Croatica*, *57*(1), 141–148. https://doi:10.20471/acc.2018.57.01.18.

Kautz, D. D., & Van Horn, E. R. (2017). Sex and intimacy after stroke. *Rehabilitation Nursing*, *42*(6), 333–340. https://doi.org/10.1002/rnj.296.

Khakbazan, Z., Daneshfar, F., Behboodi-Moghadam, Z., Nabavi, S. M., Ghasemzadeh, S., & Mehran, A. (2016). The effectiveness of the Permission, Limited Information, Specific Suggestions, Intensive Therapy (PLISSIT) model based sexual counseling on the sexual function of women with multiple sclerosis who are sexually active. *Multiple Sclerosis and Related Disorders*, *8*, 113–119. https://doi:10.1016/j.msard.2016.05.007.

Lee, J. T., Kuo, H. Y., Huang, K. G., Lin, J. R., & Chen, M. L. (2020). Diversity of sexual activity and correlates among women with gynecological cancer. *Gynecologic Oncology*, *159*(2), 503–508. https://doi.org/10.1016/j.ygyno.2020.08.005.

Matarín Jiménez, T. M., Fernández-Sola, C., Hernández-Padilla, J. M., Correa Casado, M., Antequera Raynal, L. H., & Granero-Molina, J.

S

(2017). Perceptions about the sexuality of women with fibromyalgia syndrome: A phenomenological study. *Journal of Advanced Nursing, 73*(7), 1646–1656. https://doi:10.1111/jan.13262.

Mitrani, V. B., De Santis, J. P., McCabe, B. E., Deleon, D. A., Gattamorta, R. M., & Leblanc, N. M. (2017). The impact of parenteral reaction to sexual orientation on depressive symptoms and sexual risk behavior among Hispanic men who have sex with men. *Archives of Psychiatric Nursing, 31*(4), 352–358. https://doi:10.1016/j.apnu.2017.04.004.

Morton, L. (2017). Sexuality in the older adult. *Primary Care, 44*(3), 429–438. https://doi:10.1016/j.pop.2017.04.004.

Sabanciogullari, S., Tuncay, F. O., & Avci, D. (2016). The relationship between life satisfaction and perceived health and sexuality in individuals diagnosed with a physical illness. *Sexuality and Disability, 34*, 389–402. https://doi.org/10.1007/s11195-016-9456-6.

Santos-Iglesias, P., Byers, E. S., & Moglia, R. (2016). Sexual well-being of older men and women. *Canadian Journal of Human Sexuality, 25*(2), 86–98. https://doi:10.3138/cjhs.252-A4.

Scott, R. L., Lasiuk, G., & Norris, C. (2016). The relationship between sexual orientation and depression in a national population sample. *Journal of Clinical Nursing, 25*(23–24), 3522–3532. https://doi:10.1111/jocn.13286.

Steinke, E. E., Johansen, P. P., Fridlund, B., & Broström, A. (2016). Determinants of sexual dysfunction and interventions for patients with obstructive sleep apnoea: A systematic review. *International Journal of Clinical Practice, 70*(1), 5–19. https://doi:10.1111/ijcp.12751.

Steinke, E. E., Mosack, V., & Hill, T. J. (2018). The influence of comorbidities, risk factors, and medications on sexual activity in individuals aged 40-59 years with and without cardiac conditions: US national health and nutrition examination survey, 2011 to 2012. *Journal of Cardiovascular Nursing, 33*(2), 18–125. https://doi:10.1097/JCN.0000000000000433.

Steptoe, A., Jackson, S. E., & Wardle, J. (2016). Sexual activity and concerns in people with coronary heart disease from a population-based study. *Heart, 102*(14), 1095–1099. https//doi:10.1136/heartjnl-2015-308993.

Streur, M. M., Rosman, L. A., Sears, S. F., Steinke, E. E., Thompson, E. A., & Dougherty, C. M. (2020). Patient and partner sexual concerns during the first year after an implantable cardioverter defibrillator: A secondary analysis of the P+P randomized clinical trial. *Journal of Sexual Medicine, 17*(5), 892–902. https://doi.org/10.1016/j.jsxm.2020.01.028.

Syme, M. L., Cohn, T. J., & Barnack-Tavlaris, J. (2017). A comparison of actual and perceived sexual risk among older adults. *The Journal of Sex Research, 54*(2), 149–160. https://doi:10.1080/00224499.2015.1124379.

Syme, M. L., Lichtenberg, P., & Moye, J. (2016). Recommendations for sexual expression management in long-term care: A qualitative needs assessment. *Journal of Advanced Nursing, 72*(10), 2457–2467. https://doi:10.1111/jan.13005.

Weeks, F. H., Powell, T. W., Illangasekare, S., Rice, E., Wilson, J., Hickman, D., et al. (2016). Bringing evidence-based sexual health programs to adolescents in black churches: Applying knowledge from systematic adaptation frameworks. *Health Education & Behavior, 43*(6), 699–704. https://doi.org/10.1177/1090198116633459.

Zamani, M., Tavoli, A., Khasti, B. Y., Sedighimornani, N., & Zafar, M. (2017). Sexual therapy for women with multiple sclerosis and its impact on quality of life. *Iranian Journal of Psychiatry, 12*(1), 56–65.

Risk for Shock **Domain 11 Safety/protection Class 2 Physical injury**

Nicole Huntley, MS, RN, APN, ACCNS-AG

NANDA-I

Definition

Susceptible to an inadequate blood flow to tissues that may lead to cellular dysfunction, which may compromise health.

S

Risk Factors

Bleeding; deficient fluid volume; factors identified by standardized, validated screening tool; hyperthermia; hypothermia; hypoxemia; hypoxia; inadequate knowledge of bleeding management strategies; inadequate knowledge of infection management strategies; inadequate knowledge of modifiable factors; ineffective medication self-management; nonhemorrhagic fluid losses; smoking; unstable blood pressure

At-Risk Population

Individuals admitted to the emergency care unit; individuals at extremes of age; individuals with history of myocardial infarction

Associated Conditions

Artificial respiration; burns; chemotherapy; diabetes mellitus; embolism; heart diseases; hypersensitivity; immunosuppression; infections; lactate levels ≥2 mmol/L; liver diseases; medical devices; neoplasms; nervous system diseases; pancreatitis; radiotherapy; sepsis; sequential organ failure assessment (SOFA) score ≥3; simplified acute physiology score (SAPS III >70); spinal cord injuries; surgical procedures; systemic inflammatory response syndrome (SIRS); trauma

NOC (Nursing Outcomes Classification)

Suggested NOC Outcomes

Cardiac Pump Effectiveness; Fluid Balance; Infection Severity; Respiratory Status: Gas Exchange; Neurological Status: Autonomic; Tissue Perfusion: Cellular

Example NOC Outcome with Indicators

Neurological Status: Autonomic as evidenced by the following indicators: Apical heart rate/Systolic blood pressure/Urinary elimination pattern/Thermoregulation. (Rate the outcome and indicators of **Neurological Status: Autonomic:** 1 = severely compromised, 2 = substantially compromised, 3 = moderately compromised, 4 = mildly compromised, 5 = not compromised [see Section I].)

Client Outcomes

Client Will (Specify Time Frame)

- Discuss precautions to prevent complications of disease
- Maintain adherence to agreed-on medication regimens
- Maintain adequate hydration
- Monitor for infection signs and symptoms
- Maintain a mean arterial pressure (MAP) above 65 mm Hg
- Maintain a heart rate between 60 and 100 with a normal rhythm
- Maintain urine output greater than 0.5 mL/kg/hr
- Maintain warm, dry skin

NIC (Nursing Intervention Classification)

Suggested NIC Interventions

Admission Care; Allergy Management; Cardiac Care; Cerebral Perfusion Promotion; Electrolyte Monitoring; Fever Treatment; Fluid Management; Hemodynamic Regulation; Infection Precaution; Medication Management; Oxygen Therapy; Postanesthesia Care; Risk Identification; Shock Prevention; Teaching: Disease Process; Temperature Regulation; Vital Signs Monitoring

Example NIC Activities—Shock Prevention

Monitor circulatory status; Monitor for signs of inadequate tissue oxygenation; Administer oxygen and/or mechanical ventilation, as appropriate; Instruct client and/or family on precipitating factors of shock

Nursing Interventions and *Rationales*

- Review data pertaining to client risk status including age, primary diseases, immunosuppression, antibiotic use, and presence of hemodynamic alterations such as tachycardia, tachypnea, and decrease in blood pressure (BP). EB: *Many clients who develop shock have underlying circumstances that predispose them to shock states, as evidenced by hypotension and inadequate organ perfusion (Kleinpell, Schorr, & Balk, 2016; Balentine, 2019).*
- Review client's medical and surgical history, noting conditions that place the client at higher risk for shock, including trauma, myocardial infarction, pulmonary embolism, head injury, dehydration, infection, endocrine problems, certain medications, and pregnancy. EB: *Certain clinical conditions place clients at higher risk for shock, which requires prompt identification and treatment to improve morbidity and mortality outcomes (American Heart Association [AHA], 2016; Singer et al, 2016; Balentine, 2019).*
- Complete a full nursing physical examination. *A full nursing physical examination is crucial in identifying all factors that might place that client at risk for the development of shock, such as hypoperfusion of internal organs (manifesting as decreased urinary output and shortness of breath or laboratory values such as creatinine, coagulation measures, and adrenal insufficiency) and tissue hypoperfusion (manifesting as cool, clammy, mottled skin and diminished pulses).* EB: *The use of extremity skin temperatures alone as a predictor of decreased cardiac output (CO) cannot be validated or supported because of a lack of consensus in the literature (Hiemstra et al, 2017). However, the presence of skin mottling, especially over the knees, ears, and fingers, suggests tissue hypoperfusion states often seen in shock (Contou & de Prost, 2016; Neviere, 2021).*

- Monitor circulatory status (e.g., BP, MAP, skin color, skin temperature, heart sounds, heart rate and rhythm, presence and quality of peripheral pulses, pulse oximetry, and end-tidal carbon dioxide monitoring [$EtCO_2$]). Anticipate additional studies that will evaluate dynamic changes in cardiac tissue such as ultrasonography. **EB:** *The initial phase of shock is characterized by decreased CO and tissue perfusion, which results in immediate compensatory changes evidenced by a drop in BP, increased heart rate, and shunting of blood away from the periphery, resulting in pale, cooler, damp skin, and mottling with reduced peripheral pulses. Trending changes in contractile function can further guide treatment (Contou & de Prost, 2016; Kleinpell, Schorr, & Balk, 2016; Simmons & Ventetuolo, 2017).*
- Maintain intravenous (IV) access and provide isotonic IV fluids such as 0.9% normal saline or Ringer's lactate as ordered; these fluids are commonly used in the prevention and treatment of shock. **EB:** *Restrictive fluid resuscitation and permissive hypotension (achievement of systolic pressure around 90 mm Hg, or MAP around 65 mm Hg) may have an advantage over standard higher volume fluid resuscitation regarding overall and early intraoperative survival benefit in trauma clients experiencing shock (Carrick et al, 2016; Marik & Weinmann 2019).* **EB:** *Septic shock hypoperfusion should be initially managed with a 30 mL/kg bolus of crystalloid fluid for clients who have no underlying comorbidities (e.g., congestive heart failure or chronic renal conditions) (Rhodes et al, 2017).* There is evidence to support administering full fluid volumes to chronic organ dysfunction clients such as heart failure and liver failure. **EB:** *Sepsis mortality rates were found to be decreased in the presence of full intervention bundle application (Chang et al, 2014; Prasad et al, 2017).*
- Monitor for inadequate tissue oxygenation (e.g., apprehension, increased anxiety, altered mental status, agitation, oliguria, cool/mottled periphery) and determinants of tissue oxygen delivery (e.g., Pao_2, SpO_2, $ScvO_2/SvO_2$, MAP, hemoglobin levels, lactate levels, CO). **EB:** *Assessment of tissue oxygen delivery and oxygenation patterns provides data to assess trends in client's status and evaluates treatment responses (Standl et al, 2018; Scheeren & Ramsay, 2019). Changes in client's mental status are highly sensitive to changes in perfusion and oxygenation (Singer, 2016).* **EB:** *Invasive monitoring has not been shown to improve overall mortality. Many clinicians are using noninvasive monitoring even for hemodynamically unstable clients, including the use of bedside ultrasonography and infrared spectroscopy (Seymour & Rosengart, 2015; Rhodes et al, 2017).* **EB:** *Reduction in mortality was observed with interventions aimed at lactate-guided resuscitation (Rhodes et al, 2017).*
- ▲ Maintain vital signs (BP, pulse, respirations, and temperature) and pulse oximetry within normal parameters. **EB:** *Trending of vital signs using an early warning score (EWS) is a quick, cost-effective way to identify early clients at risk of deterioration and intervene in a timely manner (Albur, Hamilton, & MacGowan, 2016) and is more accurate than quick Sequential [sepsis-related] Organ Failure Assessment (qSOFA) (Churpek et al, 2017).* **EB:** *Increased heart rate (above 90 beats per minutes), hypotension (BP below 90 mm Hg systolic, or MAP < 65 mm Hg), tachypnea (greater than 20 breaths per minute), hypoxia (SpO_2 below 90%), lactate levels (above 2 mmol/L), and change in mentation are indicators of shock (Singer, 2016; Singer et al, 2016; Rhodes et al, 2017). Temperature greater than 38°C or less than 36°C with white blood cell count greater than 12,000/mm^3 or less than 4000/mm^3 plus symptoms listed earlier are indicators of SIRS (Bok, 2020; Singer et al, 2016; Rhodes et al, 2017).* **EB:** *qSOFA, which looks at altered mentation, systolic BP of 100 mm Hg or less, and respiratory rate greater than 22 breaths per minute, has been shown to identify clients who are likely to have poor outcomes (Singer, 2016; Singer et al, 2016; Churpek et al, 2017).*
- ▲ Administer oxygen immediately to maintain SpO_2 greater than 90%, and antibiotics and other medications as prescribed to any client presenting with symptoms of early shock. **EBN:** *The experienced nurse has an important role in the implementation of the Surviving Sepsis Campaign (SSC), which includes specific early goal-directed therapies that enhance client survival (Kleinpell, Schorr, & Balk, 2016).* **EB:** *Early goal-directed therapy protocols focusing on administration of oxygen, fluid resuscitation, antibiotics administered within an hour, and vasoactive medications provide early correction of risks for shock and improve survival of shock. Antibiotics as prescribed administered within 1 hour of diagnosis of a sepsis state facilitate a better rate of survival. For each hour in delayed antibiotic administration, survival decreases by 7.6% (Seymour & Rosengart, 2015; Rhodes et al, 2017).*
- ▲ Monitor trends in noninvasive hemodynamic parameters (e.g., MAP) as appropriate. **EB:** *MAP less than 60 to 65 mm Hg for any extended time period is associated with poor outcomes (Leone et al, 2015).* **EB:** *Restoring MAP to desired levels (above 65 mm Hg) facilitates adequate perfusion to organs (Singer, 2016; Rhodes et al, 2017).* **EB:** *An overarching goal of cardiovascular support is optimization of blood flow to tissues; however, there is no single optimum MAP that can be applied to all. In clients with chronic arterial hypertension, a higher MAP (75–85 mm Hg) may be preferable (Leone et al, 2015; Rhodes et al, 2017).*

Monitor hydration status including daily weights, postural BP changes, serum electrolytes (sodium, potassium, chloride, bilirubin, creatinine, and blood urea nitrogen), intake and output, and skin turgor. Consider insertion of an indwelling urinary catheter as ordered to measure hourly output for a goal of 0.5 mL/kg/hr (Kleinpell, Schorr, & Balk, 2016).

- ▲ Monitor serum lactate levels and interpret them within the context of each client. EB: *Elevations in serum lactate (above 2 mmol/L) may indicate circulatory failure and resultant tissue hypoxia from anaerobic metabolism that results in toxin accumulation, cellular inflammation, and cellular death with higher lactate levels predictive of higher mortality (Casserly et al, 2015).* EB: *Progression to septic shock may result as characterized by the onset of SIRS (Rhodes et al, 2017). Two or more of the following indicators suggest SIRS: altered temperatures; heart rates above 90 beats per minute; tachypnea or hypocarbia; and/or leukocytosis/leukopenia, which may or may not be related to infection as other causative factors exist (Rhodes et al, 2017). The degree of serum lactate elevation correlates with morbidity and mortality in sepsis; early detection facilitates early treatment and is a more accurate triage tool than vital signs (Casserly et al, 2015). Monitor blood glucose levels frequently and administer insulin as prescribed to targeted blood glucose levels of <180 mg/dL (Rhodes et al, 2017).*

Critical Care

- ▲ Prepare the client for the placement of an additional IV line, a central line, and/or a pulmonary artery catheter as prescribed. Adequate IV and central line access may be required for fluid resuscitation and medication delivery. Maintaining more than one IV access ensures rapid IV medication and fluid delivery in a crisis situation. Large amounts of fluid can be delivered more efficiently through centrally placed vascular access sites. Most vasoactive agents, especially vasopressors, should be delivered only through central lines because of risk of tissue sloughing. EB: *A Cochrane systematic review of 13 studies on 5686 clients found no difference in mortality rates or days spent in an intensive care unit (ICU) between those clients with a pulmonary artery catheter and those without (Rajaram et al, 2013).*
- ▲ Monitor trends in hemodynamic parameters (e.g., central venous pressure [CVP], CO, cardiac index [CI], systemic vascular resistance [SVR], pulmonary artery pressure [PAP], MAP) as appropriate. EB: *Hemodynamic indices will be altered depending on the underlying form of shock (hypovolemic, distributive, or cardiogenic). Dehydration will result in reduced CVP, CO, PAP, and ultimately MAP because of hypovolemia. Vasodilation as seen in distributive shock patterns (forms of third spacing as in neurogenic, anaphylactic, and septic shock states) will decrease BP and CVP (a surrogate for intravascular volume) and other hemodynamic indices. Cardiogenic shock will result in low CO and MAP with higher PAP and CVP indices caused by heart failure and subsequent congestion of the cardiopulmonary systems. Compensatory mechanisms to address reductions in CO and MAP include tachycardia and reduced urinary output (less than 0.5 mL/kg/hr). Both CO and SVR may temporarily increase with the onset of shock because of compensatory mechanisms; however, as shock progresses, both CO and SVR decline (Standl et al, 2018; Kislitsina et al, 2019).*
- ▲ Monitor electrocardiography. Myocardial ischemia can present as ST segment changes, which can be seen before a decrease in BP as a compensatory mechanism. EB: *As oxygen demands increase, tachycardia and cardiac dysrhythmias may be evident, such as ST segment changes (Goldberger & Prutkin, 2020).*
- ▲ Monitor arterial blood gases, coagulation, blood chemistries, blood glucose, cardiac enzymes, blood cultures, and hematology laboratory test results. EB: *Abnormalities can identify the cause of the perfusion deficits and identify complications related to the decreased perfusion or shock state. Cardiogenic shock may be identified by elevations in cardiac enzymes as a result of myocardial infarction in association with low MAP. Elevation/reduction in white blood cell counts may be indicative of septic shock when associated with alterations in MAP (Rhodes et al, 2017).*
- ▲ Administer vasopressor agents as prescribed. EB: *Norepinephrine is the vasopressor of choice for septic shock (Avni et al, 2015; Gamper et al, 2016; Rhodes et al, 2017). Norepinephrine should be administered through a central line.* EB: *Low-dose dopamine should not be started for renal protection (Gamper et al, 2016; Rhodes et al, 2017).*
- • If the client is in shock, refer to the following care plans: Risk for Ineffective **Renal** Perfusion, Risk for Ineffective **Gastrointestinal** Perfusion, Impaired **Gas** Exchange, and Decreased **Cardiac** Output.

Client/Family Teaching and Discharge Planning

- ▲ Teach client and family or significant others about any medications prescribed. Instruct the client to report any adverse side effects to his or her health care provider. Medication teaching includes the drug name, purpose, administration instructions (e.g., with or without food), and any side effects. EB: *Provision of such information using clear communication principles and with an understanding of what the health*

S

literacy level of the client/family/significant others may be can facilitate appropriate adherence to the therapeutic regimen (Balentine, 2019; Crane Cutilli, 2020; National Institutes of Health [NIH], 2021).

- Instruct the client and family on disease process and rationale for care. **EB:** *Tailoring interventions to the needs and education levels of the client and caregivers enhances learning and retention of material (Ha Dinh, 2016; Crane Cutilli, 2020; Marin, 2021).*
- Instruct clients and their family members on the signs and symptoms of low BP to report to their health care provider (dizziness, lightheadedness, fainting, dehydration and unusual thirst, lack of concentration, blurred vision, nausea, cold, clammy, pale skin, rapid and shallow breathing, fatigue, and depression). **EBN:** *Teach-back methods are among the most recommended techniques to verify client retention. Use of the teach-back method enhances individual and caregiver knowledge and adherence behaviors (Crane Cutilli, 2020). Early recognition and treatment of these symptoms may avoid more serious sequelae (AHA, 2016; Singer et al, 2016; Churpek et al, 2017).*
- Promote a culture of client safety and individual accountability. **EB:** *Organizations that promote a just culture of safety help to reduce or prevent errors and improve overall health care quality (Agency for Healthcare Research and Quality [AHRQ], 2019). Include health literacy strategies into all aspects of client-centered care and weave into organizational values (Crane Cutilli, 2020).*

REFERENCES

Agency for Healthcare Research and Quality (AHRQ). (2019). *Culture of safety*. PSNet [website]. Retrieved from https://psnet.ahrq.gov/primers/primer/5/safety-culture. [Accessed 29 July 2021].

Albur, M., Hamilton, F., & MacGowan, A. P. (2016). Early warning score: A dynamic marker of severity and prognosis in patients with Gram-negative bacteraemia and sepsis. *Annals of Clinical Microbiology and Antimicrobials, 15*, 23.

American Heart Association (AHA). (2016). Low blood pressure—When blood pressure is too low. Retrieved from https://www.heart.org/en/health-topics/high-blood-pressure/the-facts-about-high-blood-pressure/low-blood-pressure-when-blood-pressure-is-too-low. [Accessed 29 July 2021].

Avni, T., Lador, A., Lev, S., Leibovici, L., Paul, M., & Grossman, A. (2015). Vasopressors for the treatment of septic shock: Systematic review and meta-analysis. *PLoS One, 10*(8), e0129305.

Balentine, J. R. (2019). *Sepsis (blood infection)*. eMedicineHealth [website]. Retrieved from http://www.emedicinehealth.com/sepsis_blood_infection/article_em.htm. [Accessed 29 July 2021].

Boka, K. (2020). Systemic inflammatory response syndrome (SIRS). Medscape [website]. Retrieved from https://emedicine.medscape.com/article/168943-overview. [Accessed 29 July 2021].

Carrick, M. M., Leonard, J., Slone, D. S., Mains, C. W., & Bar-Or, D. (2016). Hypotensive resuscitation among trauma patients. *BioMed Research International, 2016*, 8901938.

Casserly, B., Phillips, G. S., Schorr, C., et al. (2015). Lactate measurements in sepsis induced tissue hypoperfusion: Results from the Surviving Sepsis Campaign database. *Critical Care Medicine, 43*(3), 567–573.

Chang, D. W., Huynh, R., Sandoval, E., Han, N., Coil, C. J., & Spellberg, B. J. (2014). Volume of fluids administered during rescusitation for severe sepsis and septic shock and the development of the acute respiratory distress syndrome. *Journal of Critical Care, 29*(6), 1011–1015. https://doi.org/10.1016/j.jcrc.2014.06.005.

Churpek, M. M., Snyder, A., Han, X., et al. (2017). Quick sepsis-related organ failure assessment, systemic inflammatory response syndrome, and early warning scores for detecting clinical deterioration in infected patients outside the intensive care unit. *American Journal of Respiratory and Critical Care Medicine, 195*(7), 906–911. https://doi.org/10.1164/rccm.201604-0854OC.

Contou, D., & de Prost, N. (2016). Skin mottling. *New England Journal of Medicine, 375*(22), 2187. https://doi.org/10.1056/NEJMicm1602055.

Crane Cutilli, C. (2020). Excellence in patient education; evidence-based education that "sticks" and improves patient outcomes. *Nursing Clinics of North America, 55*(2), 267–282. https://doi.org/10.1016/j.cnur.2020.02.007.

Gamper, G., Havel, C., Arrich, J., et al. (2016). Vasopressors for hypotensive shock. *Cochrane Database of Systematic Reviews, 2*, CD003709. https://doi.org/10.1002/14651858.CD003709.pub4.

Goldberger, A. L., & Prutkin, J. M. (2020). *Electrocardiogram in the diagnosis of myocardial ischemia and infarction*. Waltham, MA: UpToDate. F. V. UpToDate, D. M. Mirvis, & T. F. Dardas (Eds.). Retrieved from https://www.uptodate.com/contents/electrocardiogram-in-the-diagnosis-of-myocardial-ischemia-and-infarction. [Accessed 29 July 2021].

Ha Dinh, T. T., Bonner, A., Clark, R., Ramsbotham, J., & Hines, S. (2016). The effectiveness of the teach-back method on adherence and self-management in health education for people with chronic disease: A systematic review. *JBI Database of Systematic Reviews and Implementation Reports, 14*(1), 210–247. https://doi.org/10.11124/jbisrir-2016-2296.

Hiemstra, B., Eck, R. J., Keus, F., & van der Horst, I. (2017). Clinical examination for diagnosing circulatory shock. *Current Opinion in Critical Care, 23*(4), 293–301. https://doi.org/10.1097/MCC.0000000000000420.

Kislitsina, O. N., Rich, J. D., Wilcox, J. E., Pham, D. T., Churyla, A., Vorovich, E. B., et al. (2019). Shock—Classification and pathophysiological principles of therapeutics. *Current Cardiology Reviews, 15*(2), 102–113. https://doi.org/10.2174/1573403X15666181212125024.

Kleinpell, R. M., Schorr, C. A., & Balk, R. A. (2016). The new sepsis definitions: Implications for critical care practitioners. *American Journal of Critical Care, 25*(5), 457–464. https://doi.org/10.4037/ajcc2016574.

Leone, M., Asfar, P., Radermacher, P., Vincent, J. L., & Martin, C. (2015). Optimizing mean arterial pressure in septic shock: A critical reappraisal of the literature. *Critical Care, 19*(1), 101.

Marik, P. E., & Weinmann, M. (2019). Optimizing fluid therapy in shock. *Current Opinion in Critical Care, 25*(3), 246–251. https://doi.org/10.1097/MCC.0000000000000604.

Marin, T. (2021). *Evidence summary. Nursing care: Principles of nurse-led patient education*. JBI Evidence-Based Practice Database, JBI25516.

National Institutes of Health (NIH). (2021). *Clear communication: Health literacy*. Retrieved from https://www.nih.gov/institutes-nih/nih-office-director/office-communications-public-liaison/clear-communication/health-literacy. [Accessed 29 July 2021].

Neviere, R. (2021). *Sepsis syndromes in adults: Epidemiology, definitions, clinical presentation, diagnosis, and prognosis*. Waltham, MA: UpToDate. P. E. Parsons, & G. Finlay (Eds.). Retrieved from https://www.uptodate.com/contents/sepsis-syndromes-in-adults-epidemiology-definitions-clinical-presentation-diagnosis-and-prognosis. [Accessed 29 July 2021].

S

Prasad, P. A., Shea, E. R., Shiboski, S., Sullivan, M. C., Gonzales, R., & Shimabukuro, D. (2017). Relationship between a sepsis intervention bundle and in-hospital mortality among hospitalized patients: A retrospective analysis of real-world data. *Anesthesia & Analgesia*, *125*(2), 507–513. https://doi.org/10.1213/ANE.0000000000002085.

Rajaram, S., Desai, N. K., Kalra, A., et al. (2013). *Pulmonary artery catheters for adult patients in intensive care*. Cochrane Library. https://doi-org.proxy.hsl.ucdenver.edu/10.1002/14651858.CD003408.pub3. [Accessed 28 February 2013].

Rhodes, A., Evans, L. E., Alhazzani, W., et al. (2017). Surviving sepsis Campaign: International guidelines for management of sepsis and septic shock: 2016. *Intensive Care Medicine*, *43*(3), 307–377.

Scheeren, T. W. L., & Ramsay, M. A. E. (2019). New developments in hemodynamic monitoring. *Journal of Cardiothoracic and Vascular Anesthesia*, *33*(Suppl. 1), S67–S72. https://doi.org/10.1053/j_jvca.2019.03.043.

Seymour, C. W., & Rosengart, M. R. (2015). Septic shock: Advances in diagnosis and treatment. *JAMA*, *314*(7), 708–717.

Simmons, J., & Ventetuolo, C. E. (2017). Cardiopulmonary monitoring of shock. *Current Opinion in Critical Care*, *23*(3), 223–231. https://doi.org/10.1097/MCC.0000000000000407.

Singer, M. (2016). The new sepsis consensus definitions (Sepsis-3): The good, the not-so-bad, and the actually-quite-pretty. *Intensive Care Medicine*, *42*(12), 2027–2029. https://doi.org/10.1007/s00134-016-4600-4.

Singer, M., Deutschman, C. S., Seymour, C. W., et al. (2016). The Third International Consensus definitions for sepsis and septic shock (Sepsis-3). *JAMA*, *315*(8), 801–810. https://doi.org/10.1001/jama.2016.0287.

Standl, T., Annecke, T., Cascorbi, I., Heller, A. R., Sabashnikov, A., & Teske, W. (2018). The nomenclature, definition, and distinction of types of shock. *Deutsches Arzteblatt International*, *115*(45), 757–768. https://doi.org/10.3238/arztebl.2018.0757.

Impaired Sitting Domain 4 Activity/rest Class 2 Activity/exercise

Ruth A. Wittmann-Price, PhD, RN, CNS, CNE, CNEcl, CHSE, ANEF, FAAN

NANDA-I

Definition

Limitation of ability to independently and purposefully attain and/or maintain a rest position that is supported by the buttocks and thighs, in which the torso is upright.

Defining Characteristics

Difficulty adjusting position of one or both lower limbs on uneven surface; difficulty attaining postural balance; difficulty flexing or moving both hips; difficulty flexing or moving both knees; difficulty maintaining postural balance; difficulty stressing torso with body weight

Related Factors

Insufficient energy; insufficient muscle strength; malnutrition; neurobehavioral manifestations; pain; self-imposed relief posture

Associated Conditions

Impaired metabolism; mental disorders; neurological disorder; orthopedic surgery; prescribed posture; sarcopenia

NOC (Nursing Outcomes Classification)

Suggested NOC Outcomes

Activity Tolerance; Balance; Body Mechanics Performance; Body Positioning: Self-Initiated; Endurance; Tissue Perfusion: Peripheral; Self Care Status; Skeletal Function

Example NOC Outcome with Indicators

Body Mechanics Performance: as evidenced by the following indicators: Uses correct sitting posture/Uses supportive devices correctly. (Rate outcome and indicators of **Body Mechanics Performance:** 1 = never demonstrated, 2 = rarely demonstrated, 3 = sometimes demonstrated, 4 = often demonstrated, 5 = consistently demonstrated [see Section I].)

Client Outcomes

Client Will (Specify Time Frame)

- Verbalize importance of being able to sit as a method to engage in activities of daily living
- Understand somatic physiology of posture control
- Choose health care options that enhance ability to sit

S

- Engage in physical conditioning exercises to enhance sitting ability
- Understand relationship of posture and emotions
- Control pain to increase ability to sit

NIC (Nursing Interventions Classification)

Suggested NIC Interventions

Activity Therapy; Body Mechanics Promotion; Fall Prevention; Energy Management; Exercise Promotion: Strength Training; Exercise Therapy: Balance, Joint Mobility, Muscle Control; Functional Ability Enhancement; Positioning; Pressure Ulcer Prevention

Example NIC Activities—Exercise Therapy: Sitting

Assist client to use chair that facilitates sitting and prevents injury; Transfer safely from bed to chair; Encourage to sit in chair, as tolerated; Provide activities that can be completed while sitting

Nursing Interventions and *Rationales*

- Acknowledge the importance of being able to sit as a method to engage in activities of daily living. EB: *Park, Gong, and Yim (2017) investigated upper limb function, balance, gait, and quality of life in two groups of stroke clients (n = 26) before and after a sitting boxing program and found that the Stroke-Specific Quality of Life (SS-QOL) questionnaire scores were significantly improved in the boxing group, concluding that the sitting boxing program group had positive effects on upper extremity function, balance, gait, and quality of life.* EB: *Shambaugh et al (2020) studied clients (n = 121) with hamstring ruptures that were repaired and found that if the repair was done 6 weeks or more after the injury was sustained, there was greater sitting intolerance. This study suggests that hamstring ruptures should be repaired as soon as possible to promote normal sitting patterns without pain and discomfort.*
- Understand the somatic physiology of posture control. EB: *Lee et al (2017) studied trunk muscle activities in four types of seated postures—cross-legged, long, side, and W-shaped—in adults (n = 8) and found that trunk muscle activity did not significantly differ between the four types of sitting postures.* EB: *Massaad and colleagues (2020) studied adults with spinal deformities and found that their quality of life was adversely affected by poor postural sitting alignment. Poor posture affected every aspect of their activities of daily living.* EB: *Lee, Lee, and Shin (2017) studied forward head posture in seven different posture conditions in clients (n = 20), including sitting comfortably and sitting with the back straight, and found that head posture evaluation is a reliable assessment for evaluating proper sitting conditions.*
- Encourage engagement in physical conditioning exercises to enhance proper sitting ability. EB: *Molik et al (2017) investigated disabled clients playing volleyball in a sitting position and found that the vertical sitting position and degree of disability directly related to performance, but the exercise was beneficial.* EB: *Alghdir, Zafar, and Iqbal (2017) studied the effects of upright and slouch sitting postures and voluntary teeth clenching on hand grip strength (HGS) in clients (n = 100) and found that HGS was actually stronger during slouching than sitting upright and HGS had no effect on teeth clenching, indicating that sitting posture may matter when testing HGS in a physical assessment evaluation.* EB: *Chrisman et al (2020) studied college students (n = 22) using sitting and standing desks and the majority of participants preferred sitting to standing. The study informs health care providers of the need for education on standing desks to encourage positive physical activity in the college population.*
- Understand the relationship of posture and emotions. EB: *Oki et al (2017) investigated physical and psychological effects of the Shiatsu Stimulation (SS) (finger pressure) in a sitting position on clients (n = 20). The SS demonstrated significant change in all six mood states (tension-anxiety, depression-dejection, fatigue, and confusion decreased, whereas vigor elevated).* CEB: *A classic study about slumped and upright posture by Nair et al (2015) observed 74 participants and the results found that an upright sitting position during a stressful time can assist to maintain self-esteem, reduce negative mood, and promote a positive mood compared to those participants in a slumped posture.*
- Maintain pain levels below 3 to 4 on a 0-to-10 scale to increase ability to sit. EB: *Joshi et al (2017) studied neuropathy of the posterior femoral cutaneous nerve, which can cause pain while sitting, and performed magnetic resonance–guided cryoablation to successfully treat sitting pain caused by neuropathy.* EB: *Harvard Health (2020) reports that sore backsides during sitting can be relieved with stretching and exercise. Stretching and exercise can also reduce the incidence of sciatica and piriformis nerve discomfort.*

Pediatric

- Promote proper sitting ability to increase cognitive and physical functioning. **EB:** *Rethlefsen et al (2020) compared the way children (n = 104) sit (W-sitting to non–W-sitting) in relation to hip dysplasia and found no difference. The mode of sitting was not a causative factor for hip dysplasia in this observational study.* **EBN:** *Hitchcock (2017) reviewed the research regarding safe infant sleeping and addressed the fact that sitting devices are not recommended. Nurses should model recommended behaviors for safe infant sleep and teach parents about safe infant sleep throughout the hospital stay.*

Geriatric

- Promote proper sitting ability to increase cognitive and physical functioning. **EB:** *Researchers studied the effects of aging on clients' (n = 39) muscle control during transition from lying to sitting positions using myotonometry measurements of tone, stiffness, and elasticity; results suggested that increased age increases stiffness and tone and decreases the elasticity of muscles (Kocur et al, 2017).* **EBN:** *A meta-analysis was completed by Fazio et al (2020) and demonstrated that geriatric adults who are hospitalized spend 87% to 100% of the time sitting or lying in bed. The study suggests that tools be developed to assess mobility and that immobility be decreased to decrease health complications in this population.*

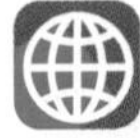

Multicultural

- Understand the importance of unimpaired sitting to different populations. **EB:** *A case study analyzed in Japan discussed the researchers' novel "hip prosthesis in the sitting posture" on a client who was an amputee and found that implanting a hip prosthesis in a sitting position enabled the client to better stand, walk, and begin balance training (Shimizu et al, 2017).* **CEB:** *Erikson et al (2011) completed a multicultural observational study about how older adults spend time in different cultures and found that there were 16 activities associated with Asian adults and one important activity among the 16 was the ability to sit and think.*

Home Care

- Encourage proper sitting posture in the home environment to promote health. **EB:** *Li et al (2017) studied clients (n = 16) in four modes of reclining wheelchairs with and without different sitting devices and found that the lumbar support with femur upward with back reclined mode provided the most significant reduction in stress load on the ischial area.* **EB:** *Arundell et al (2020) studied the amount of screen time consumed by families (n = 542). Screen time is directly related to the amount of sitting done by family members in the home. Increased screen time is inversely related to activity time needed for musculoskeletal development in children and in this study was found to affect parenting behaviors, role modeling, and the child's schooling.*

REFERENCES

Alghdir, A., Zafar, H., & Iqbal, Z. A. (2017). Effect of upright and slouch sitting postures and voluntary teeth clenching on hand grip strength in young male adults. *Journal of Back and Musculoskeletal Rehabilitation*, *30*(5), 961–965. https://doi.org.fmarion.idm.oclc.org/10.3233/BMR-150278.

Arundell, L., Parker, K., Timperio, A., Salmon, J., & Veitch, J. (2020). Home-based screen time behaviors amongst youth and their parents: Familial typologies and their modifiable correlates. *BMC Public Health*, *20*(1)1492–1492. https://doi.org/10.1186/s12889-020-09581-w.

Chrisman, M., Ye, S., Reddy, A., & Purdy, W. (2020). Assessing sitting and standing in college students using height-adjustable desks. *Health Education Journal*, *79*(6), 735–744. https://doi.org/10.1177/0017896920901837.

Erikson, G. M., Chung, J. C. C., Beng, L. H., et al. (2011). Occupations of older adults: A cross cultural description. *OTJR: Occupation, Participation and Health*, *31*(4), 182–192. https://doi.org/10.3928/15394492-20110318-01.

Fazio, S., Stocking, J., Kuhn, B., et al. (2020). How much do hospitalized adults move? A systematic review and meta-analysis. *Applied Nursing Research*, *51*, 151189. https://doi.org/10.1016/j.apnr.2019.151189.

Harvard Health. (2020). Relief for sore backsides. *Harvard Health Letter*, *45*(11), 4. Retrieved from https://www.health.harvard.edu/pain/relief-for-sore-backsides. [Accessed 29 July 2021].

Hitchcock, S. C. (2017). An update on safe infant sleep. *Nursing for Women's Health*, *21*(4), 307–311. https://doi.org/10.1016/j.nwh.2017.06.007.

Joshi, D. H., Thawait, G. V., Del Grande, F., & Fritz, J. (2017). MRI-guided cryoablation of the posterior femoral cutaneous nerve for the treatment of neuropathy-mediated sitting pain. *Skeletal Radiology*, *46*(7), 983–987. https://doi.org/10.1007/s00256-017-2617-6.

Kocur, P., Grzeskowiak, M., Wiernicka, M., Goliwas, M., Lewandowski, J., & Łochyński, D. (2017). Effects of aging on mechanical properties of sternocleidomastoid and trapezius muscles during transition from lying to sitting position—Across-sectional study. *Archives of Gerontology and Geriatrics*, *70*, 14–18. https://doi.org/10.1016/j.archger.2016.12.005.

Lee, C. H., Lee, S., & Shin, G. (2017). Reliability of forward head posture evaluation while sitting, standing, walking and running. *Human Movement Science*, *55*, 81–86. https://doi.org/10.1016/j.humov.2017.07.008.

Lee, D. G., Yu, S. J., Song, S. H., et al. (2017). Comparison of trunk electromyographic muscle activity depends on sitting postures. *Work*, *56*(3), 491–495. https://doi.org/10.3233/WOR-172515.

Li, C. T., Huang, K. Y., Kung, C. F., Chen, Y. N., Tseng, Y. T., & Tsai, K. H. (2017). Evaluation of the effect of different sitting assistive devices in reclining wheelchair on interface pressure. *BioMedical Engineering Online*, *16*(1), 108. https://doi.org/10.1186/s12938-017-0398-8.

Massaad, A., Saad, E., Rachkidi, R., et al. (2020). Sitting postural alignment and relationship with quality of life in adult spinal deformity. *Gait & Posture, 81*(Suppl. 1), 224–225. https://doi.org/10.1016/j.gaitpost.2020.08.006.

Molik, B., Morgulec-Adamowicz, N., Marzałek, J., et al. (2017). Evaluation of game performance in elite male sitting volleyball players. *Adapted Physical Activity Quarterly, 34*(2), 104–124. https://doi.org/10.1123/apaq.2015-0028.

Nair, S., Sagar, M., Sollers, J., 3rd, Consedine, N., & Broadbent, E. (2015). Do slumped and upright postures affect stress responses? A randomized trial. *Health Psychology, 34*(6), 632–641. doi:10.1037/hea0000146.

Oki, S., Ouchi, K., Watanabe, M., & Mandai, N. (2017). Physical and psychological effects of the Shiatsu Stimulation in the sitting position. *Health, 9*(8), 1264–1272. https://doi.org/10.4236/health.2017.98091.

Park, J., Gong, J., & Yim, J. (2017). Effects of a sitting boxing program on upper limb function, balance, gait, and quality of life in stroke patients. *NeuroRehabilitation, 40*(1), 77–86.

Rethlefsen, S. A., Mueske, N. M., Nazareth, A., et al. (2020). Hip dysplasia is not more common in W-sitters. *Clinical Pediatrics, 59*(12), 1074–1079. https://doi.org/10.1177/0009922820940810.

Shambaugh, B. C., Wuerz, T. H., & Miller, S. L. (2020). Does time from injury to surgery affect outcomes after surgical repair of partial and complete proximal hamstring ruptures? *Orthopaedic Journal of Sports Medicine, 8*(8), 2325967120946317. https://doi.org/10.1177/2325967120946317.

Shimizu, Y., Mutsuzaki, H., Maezawa, T., et al. (2017). Hip prosthesis in sitting posture for bilateral transfemoral amputee after burn injury: A case report. *Prosthetics and Orthotics International, 41*(5), 522–526. https://doi.org/10.1177/0309364616682384.

Impaired Skin Integrity Domain 11 Safety/protection Class 2 Physical injury

JoAnn Coar, MSN, RN-BC, A-GNP-C, CWOCN

NANDA-I

Definition

Altered epidermis and/or dermis.

Defining Characteristics

Abscess; acute pain; altered skin color; altered turgor; bleeding; blister; desquamation; disrupted skin surface; dry skin; excoriation; foreign matter piercing skin; hematoma; localized area hot to touch; macerated skin; peeling; pruritus

Related Factors

External Factors

Excessive moisture; excretions; humidity; hyperthermia; hypothermia; inadequate caregiver knowledge about maintaining tissue integrity; inadequate caregiver knowledge about protecting tissue integrity; inadequate use of chemical agent; pressure over bony prominence; psychomotor agitation; secretions; shearing forces; surface friction; use of linen with insufficient moisture wicking property

S

Internal Factors

Body mass index above normal range for age and gender; body mass index below normal range for age and gender; decreased physical activity; decreased physical mobility; edema; inadequate adherence to incontinence treatment regimen; inadequate knowledge about maintaining tissue integrity; inadequate knowledge about protecting tissue integrity; malnutrition; psychogenic factor; self mutilation; smoking; substance misuse; water-electrolyte imbalance

At-Risk Population

Individuals at extremes of age; individuals in intensive care units; individuals in long-term care facilities; individuals in palliative care settings; individuals receiving home-based care

Associated Conditions

Altered pigmentation; anemia; cardiovascular diseases; decreased level of consciousness; decreased tissue oxygenation; decreased tissue perfusion; diabetes mellitus; hormonal change; immobilization; immunodeficiency; impaired metabolism; infections; medical devices; neoplasms; peripheral neuropathy; pharmaceutical preparations; punctures; sensation disorders

NOC (Nursing Outcomes Classification)

Suggested NOC Outcomes

Tissue Integrity: Skin and Mucous Membranes; Wound Healing: Primary Intention, Secondary Intention

Example NOC Outcome with Indicators

Tissue Integrity: Skin and Mucous Membranes will be intact as evidenced by the following indicators: Skin integrity/Skin lesions not present/Tissue perfusion/Skin temperature/Skin thickness. (Rate the outcome and indicators of **Tissue Integrity: Skin and Mucous Membranes:** 1 = severely compromised, 2 = substantially compromised, 3 = moderately compromised, 4 = mildly compromised, 5 = not compromised [see Section I].)

Client Outcomes

Client Will (Specify Time Frame)

- Regain integrity of skin surface
- Report any altered sensation or pain at site of skin impairment
- Demonstrate understanding of plan to heal skin and prevent reinjury or complications
- Describe measures to protect and heal the skin and to care for any skin lesion

NIC (Nursing Interventions Classification)

Suggested NIC Interventions

Incision Site Care; Pain Management; Pressure Ulcer Care (currently referred to as Pressure Injury Care [National Pressure Ulcer Advisory Panel (NPUAP), 2016]); Pressure Ulcer Prevention (Pressure Injury Prevention [NPUAP, 2016]); Risk Identification; Skin Care: Topical Treatments; Skin Surveillance; Wound Care; Wound Irrigation

Example NIC Activities—Pressure Ulcer Care (Pressure Injury Care [NPUAP, 2016])

Monitor color of wound bed, temperature, edema, erythema, moisture, and appearance of surrounding skin; Note characteristics of any drainage

Nursing Interventions and *Rationales*

- NPUAP redefined the definition of a pressure ulcer, now referred to as pressure injuries, during the NPUAP 2016 Staging Consensus Conference. The new definitions more accurately define alterations in tissue integrity from pressure as the following: A pressure injury is localized damage to the skin and underlying soft tissue usually over a bony prominence or related to a medical or other device. The injury can present as intact skin or an open ulcer and may be painful. The injury occurs as a result of intense and/or prolonged pressure or pressure in combination with shear. The tolerance of soft tissue for pressure and shear may also be affected by microclimate, nutrition, perfusion, comorbidities, and condition of the soft tissue *(NPUAP, 2016).*
- Pressure ulcer is no longer a current clinical term; rather, pressure injury is used to describe an alteration in tissue integrity from pressure (NPUAP, 2016). Similarly, hospital-acquired pressure ulcers (HAPUs) are currently referred to as hospital-acquired pressure injuries (HAPIs).
- Assess site of skin impairment and determine cause or type of wound (e.g., acute or chronic wound, burn, dermatological lesion, pressure injury, skin tear). EB: *Identification of etiological factors, or what is causing the impairment, is the first step and requires a thorough assessment of the individual, not only the impairment. The assessment should include the medical history, current medical status, medications, and family history (Baranoski & Ayello, 2016; Murphree, 2017). Skin and tissue assessment is important in pressure injury prevention, classification, diagnosis, and treatment (NPUAP, 2016; National Pressure Injury Advisory Panel [NPIAP], European Pressure Injury Advisory Panel [EPIAP], & Pan Pacific Pressure Injury Alliance [PPPIA], 2019).*
- Use a risk assessment tool to systematically assess client risk factors for skin breakdown caused by pressure. EB: *A validated risk assessment tool such as the Norton scale or Braden scale should be used to identify*

S

clients at risk for immobility-related skin breakdown (NPIAP, EPIAP, & PPPIA, 2019). An individual identified at risk for pressure injury development or who has healed pressure injuries will need to be evaluated for pressure redistributing surfaces (Murphree, 2017). Targeting variables (e.g., age and Braden Scale Risk Category) can focus assessment on particular risk factors (e.g., pressure) and help guide the plan of prevention and care (NPIAP, EPIAP, & PPPIA, 2019).

- Determine the extent of the skin impairment caused by pressure using the revised classification system and definition for pressure injuries (NPUAP, 2016).
  - **Stage 1 Pressure Injury:** Nonblanchable erythema of intact skin. Area of localized nonblanchable erythema that may appear differently in darkly pigmented skin and changes in sensation, temperature, or firmness may precede visual changes. Color changes do not include purple or maroon discoloration, which is more likely to indicate deep tissue pressure injury (NPUAP, 2016).
  - **Stage 2 Pressure Injury:** Partial-thickness skin loss with exposed dermis. Partial-thickness skin loss with exposed dermis in which the wound bed is pink/red and moist and adipose (fat) and deeper tissues are not visible. Granulation tissue, slough, and eschar are not present. A stage 2 pressure injury may also present as an intact or ruptured blister. These injuries commonly result from adverse microclimate and shear in the skin over the pelvis and shear in the heel. This stage should not be used to describe moisture-associated skin damage (MASD) including incontinence-associated dermatitis (IAD), intertriginous dermatitis (ITD), medical adhesive–related skin injury (MARSI), or traumatic wounds (skin tears, burns, and abrasions) (NPUAP, 2016).
  - **Stage 3 Pressure Injury**: Full-thickness skin loss. Full-thickness loss of skin, in which adipose is visible and granulation tissue and epibole (rolled wound edges) are often present and undermining/tunneling may occur. Slough and/or eschar may also be visible. Fascia, muscle, tendon, ligament, cartilage, and/or bone are not exposed. The depth of tissue damage varies by anatomical location, and areas of significant adiposity can develop deep wounds. If slough or eschar obscures the extent of tissue loss, this is an unstageable pressure injury (NPUAP, 2016).
  - **Stage 4 Pressure Injury**: Full-thickness skin and tissue loss. Full-thickness skin and tissue loss with exposed or directly palpable fascia, muscle, tendon, ligament, cartilage or bone, and slough and/or eschar may be visible. Epibole, undermining, and/or tunneling often occur, and depth varies by anatomical location. If slough or eschar obscures the extent of tissue loss, this is an unstageable pressure injury (NPUAP, 2016).
  - **Deep Tissue Pressure Injury:** Persistent nonblanchable deep red, maroon, or purple discoloration. Intact or nonintact skin with localized area of persistent nonblanchable deep red, maroon, or purple discoloration or epidermal separation revealing a dark wound bed or blood-filled blister. Pain and temperature change often precede skin color changes. Discoloration may appear differently in darkly pigmented skin. This injury results from intense and/or prolonged pressure and shear forces at the bone–muscle interface. The wound may evolve rapidly to reveal the actual extent of tissue injury, or it may resolve without tissue loss. If necrotic tissue, subcutaneous tissue, granulation tissue, fascia, muscle, or other underlying structures are visible, this indicates a full-thickness pressure injury (unstageable, stage 3, or stage 4). Do not use the term deep tissue pressure injury to describe vascular, traumatic, neuropathic, or dermatological conditions (NPUAP, 2016).
  - **Unstageable Pressure Injury:** Obscured full-thickness skin and tissue loss. Full-thickness skin and tissue loss in which the extent of tissue damage within the ulcer cannot be confirmed because it is obscured by slough or eschar. If slough or eschar is removed, a stage 3 or stage 4 pressure injury will be revealed. Stable eschar (i.e., dry, adherent, intact without erythema or fluctuance) on the heel or ischemic limb should not be softened or removed (NPUAP, 2016).
  - **Mechanical Device-Related Pressure Injury:** Used to describe alterations in tissue integrity caused by pressure from mechanical devices used in the care of clients (e.g., indwelling urinary catheters, endotracheal tubes, nasogastric tubes, drains). The pressure injury typically conforms to the shape of the device (NPUAP, 2016).
  - **Mucosal Membrane Pressure Injury:** Mucosal membrane pressure injury is found on mucous membranes with a history of a medical device in use at the location of the injury. Because of the anatomy of the tissue, these ulcers cannot be staged (NPUAP, 2016).
- Inspect and monitor site of skin impairment at least once a day for color changes, erythema, edema, warmth, pain, changes in sensation, moisture, or other signs of infection. EB: *Consider assessment of temperature and subepidermal moisture as an adjunct to routine skin assessment and in darkly pigmented*

S

skin (NPIAP, EPIAP, & PPPIA, 2019). Closely assess high-risk areas such as bony prominences, skinfolds, the sacrum, and heels. Consider use of soft silicone multilayered foam protective dressings over bony prominences (NPIAP, EPIAP, & PPPIA, 2019). Systematic inspection can identify impending problems early (Baranoski & Ayello, 2016; NPIAP, EPIAP, & PPPIA, 2019).

- Monitor the client's skin care practices, noting type of soap or other cleansing agents used, temperature of water, and frequency of skin cleansing. EB: *Cleansing should not compromise the skin (Baranoski & Ayello, 2016). Keep the skin clean and hydrated. Provide prompt cleansing after episodes of incontinence, avoiding use of alkaline soaps and cleansers. Protect the skin from exposure to excessive moisture with a barrier product to reduce the risk of pressure damage (NPIAP, EPIAP & PPPIA, 2019). Products to promote healthy skin in the elderly include cleansers that are pH balanced, preferably no-rinse in soft disposable cloths, and superfatted nonalkaline soaps (Murphree, 2017).*
- Consider using physiologically compatible cleansers with each wound dressing change. EB: *Normal saline (NS) is the least cytotoxic and when delivered at a pressure of 4 to 15 PSI can safely remove wound debris (NPUAP, 2016; Cox, 2019; NPIAP, EPIAP, & PPPIA, 2019; NPUAP 2016).*
- Maintain good skin hygiene, using mild nondetergent soap, drying gently, and lubricating with lotion or emollient to reduce the risk of dermal trauma; improve circulation; and promote comfort. EB: *Avoid vigorous rubbing (NPIAP, EPIAP, & PPPIA, 2019). Provide client education on good skin hygiene practices (Doenges, Moorhouse, & Murr, 2016).*
- Urinary and fecal incontinence can cause skin breakdown. EB: *Develop and implement an individualized continence management plan. Cleanse the skin promptly after episodes of incontinence. Protect the skin from exposure to excessive moisture with a barrier product to reduce the risk of pressure damage (NPIAP, EPIAP, & PPPIA, 2019).* EB: *Chronic exposure to moisture macerates the skin, impairing its protective mechanisms and disrupting normal skin flora, which can lead to cutaneous infection (Cox, 2019).*
- For clients with limited mobility and activity, use a risk assessment tool to systematically assess immobility and activity-related risk factors. EB: *A validated risk assessment tool such as the Norton scale or Braden scale should be used to identify clients at risk for immobility-related skin breakdown (NPIAP, EPIAP, & PPPIA, 2019).* EBN: *At an organizational level, maximize workforce goals as a part of quality improvement and include evidence-based care to prevent pressure injury development. Assess the knowledge of health care professionals and provide a multifaceted education program for pressure injury prevention and treatment (NPIAP, EPIAP, & PPPIA, 2019).*
- Do not position the client on site of skin impairment. If consistent with overall client management goals, reposition the client as determined by individualized tissue tolerance and overall condition. Reposition and transfer the client with care to protect against the adverse effects of external mechanical forces such as pressure, friction, and shear. Maintain the head of the bed as flat as possible. Use a 30-degree lateral positioning (NPIAP, EPIAP, & PPPIA, 2019). EB: *Do not position an individual directly on a pressure injury. Continue to turn/reposition the individual regardless of the support surface in use. Establish turning frequency based on the characteristics of the support surface and the individual's response (NPIAP, EPIAP, & PPPIA, 2019). If the goal of care is to keep the client (e.g., a terminally ill client) comfortable, turning and repositioning may not be appropriate (NPIAP, EPIAP, & PPPIA, 2019).*
- Evaluate for use of support surfaces (specialty mattresses, beds), chair cushions, or devices as appropriate. Maintain the head of the bed at the lowest possible degree of elevation to reduce shear and friction, and use lift devices, pillows, foam wedges, and pressure-reducing devices in the bed (Brienza et al, 2016; NPIAP, EPIAP, & PPPIA, 2019).
- Implement a written treatment plan for topical treatment of the site of skin impairment. EB: *A written plan ensures consistency in care and documentation (Baranoski & Ayello, 2016).*
- Select a topical treatment that will maintain a moist wound-healing environment (stage 2) that is balanced with the need to absorb exudate. Stage 1 pressure injuries may be managed by keeping the client off of the area and using a protective dressing (Baranoski & Ayello, 2016). EBN: *Choose dressings that provide a moist environment, keep peri-wound skin dry, and control exudate and eliminate dead space (NPIAP, EPIAP, & PPPIA, 2019). Select a wound dressing based on the ability to keep the wound bed moist; need to address bacterial bioburden; nature and volume of wound exudate; condition of the tissue in the wound bed; condition of peri-wound skin; wound size, depth, and location; presence of tunneling and/or undermining; and goals and self-care abilities of the individual or caregiver (NPIAP, EPIAP, & PPPIA, 2019).*
- Avoid massaging around the site of skin impairment and over bony prominences. EB: *Research suggested that massage may lead to deep tissue trauma (NPIAP, EPIAP, & PPPIA, 2019).*

S

- Assess the client's nutritional status. Refer for a nutritional consultation and/or institute dietary supplements as necessary. EB: *Optimizing nutritional intake, including calories, fatty acids, protein, and vitamins, is needed to promote wound healing. Both the EPIAP and NPIAP (NPIAP, EPIAP, & PPPIA, 2019) endorse the application of reasonable nutritional assessment and treatment for clients at risk for and with pressure injuries.*
- Identify the client's phase of wound healing (inflammation, proliferation, or maturation) and stage of injury. EBN: *The selection of the dressing is based on the tissue in the wound bed, the condition of the skin around the wound bed, and the goals of the person with the wound. Generally, maintaining a moist wound bed is ideal when the wound bed is clean and granulating to promote healing and closure (NPIAP, EPIAP, & PPPIA, 2019). No single wound dressing is appropriate for all phases of wound healing.*

Home Care

- The interventions described previously may be adapted for home care use.
- Instruct and assist the client and caregivers in how to change dressings and maintain a clean environment. Provide written instructions and observe the client completing the dressing change before hospital discharge and in the home setting.
- Educate client and caregivers on proper nutrition, signs and symptoms of infection, and when to call the agency and/or health care provider with concerns.
- ▲ Treating wounds requires a multiprofessional approach with the frontline nurse an essential member (Cox, 2019).

Client/Family Teaching and Discharge Planning

- Teach skin and wound assessment and ways to monitor for signs and symptoms of infection, complications, and healing. Early assessment and intervention help prevent serious problems from developing. EB: *Optimize potential for healing by regularly assessing nutritional status and comorbidities and preventing contamination of wounds with regular cleansing and treatments (NPIAP, EPIAP, & PPPIA, 2019).*
- Teach the client why a topical treatment has been selected. EBN: *The type of dressing needed may change over time as the wound heals and/or deteriorates (NPIAP, EPIAP, & PPPIA, 2019).*
- If consistent with overall client management goals, teach how to reposition as client condition warrants. EB: *If the goal of care is to keep a client (e.g., terminally ill client) comfortable, turning and repositioning may not be appropriate (NPIAP, EPIAP, & PPPIA, 2019).*
- Teach the client to use pillows, foam wedges, chair cushions, and pressure-redistribution devices to prevent pressure injury (Brienza et al, 2016). EB: *Individualize the selection and periodic reevaluation of a seating support surface and associated equipment for posture and pressure redistribution with consideration of body size and configuration, the effects of posture and deformity on pressure distribution, and mobility and lifestyle needs (NPIAP, EPIAP, & PPPIA, 2019).*

S

REFERENCES

Baranoski, S., & Ayello, E. A. (Eds.). (2016). *Wound care essentials: Practice principles* (4th ed.). Philadelphia: Wolters Kluwer.

Brienza, D. M., Zulkowski, K., Sprigle, S., & Geyer, M. J. (2016). Pressure redistribution: Seating, positioning, and support surfaces. In S. Baranoski, & E. A. Ayello (Eds.), *Wound care essentials: Practice principles* (4th ed.). Philadelphia: Wolters Kluwer.

Cox, J. (2019). Wound care 101. *Nursing 2019*, *49*(10), 33–39.

Doenges, M. E., Moorhouse, M. F., & Murr, A. C. (2016). *A nurse's pocket guide: Diagnoses, prioritized interventions and rationales* (14th ed.). Philadelphia: FA Davis.

Murphree, R. W. (2017). Impairments in skin integrity. *The Nursing Clinics of North America*, *52*(3), 405–417.

National Pressure Injury Advisory Panel (NPIAP), European Pressure Injury Advisory Panel (EPIAP), & Pan Pacific Pressure Injury Alliance (PPPIA). (2019). In E. Haesler (Ed.), *Prevention and treatment of pressure ulcers: Quick reference guide*. Osborne Park, Australia: Cambridge Media

National Pressure Ulcer Advisory Panel (NPUAP). (2016). *Pressure injury stages*. Retrieved from https://npiap.com/page/PressureInjuryStages. [Accessed 29 July 2021].

Risk for Impaired Skin Integrity

Domain 11 Safety/protection Class 2 Physical injury

JoAnn Coar, MSN, RN-BC, A-GNP-C, CWOCN

NANDA-I

Definition

Susceptible to alteration in epidermis and/or dermis, which may compromise health.

Risk Factors

External Factors

Excessive moisture; excretions; humidity; hyperthermia; hypothermia; inadequate caregiver knowledge about maintaining tissue integrity; inadequate caregiver knowledge about protecting tissue integrity; inadequate use of chemical agent; pressure over bony prominence; psychomotor agitation; secretions; shearing forces; surface friction; use of linen with insufficient moisture wicking property

Internal Factors

Body mass index above normal range for age and gender; body mass index below normal range for age and gender; decreased physical activity; decreased physical mobility; edema; inadequate adherence to incontinence treatment regimen; inadequate knowledge about maintaining skin integrity; inadequate knowledge about protecting skin integrity; malnutrition; psychogenic factor; self mutilation; smoking; substance misuse; water-electrolyte imbalance

At-Risk Population

Individuals at extremes of age; individuals in intensive care units; individuals in long-term care facilities; individuals in palliative care settings; individuals receiving home-based care

Associated Conditions

Altered pigmentation; anemia; cardiovascular diseases; decreased level of consciousness; decreased tissue oxygenation; decreased tissue perfusion; diabetes mellitus; hormonal change; immobilization; immunodeficiency; impaired metabolism; infections; medical devices; neoplasms; peripheral neuropathy; pharmaceutical preparations; punctures; sensation disorders

NOC (Nursing Outcomes Classification)

Suggested NOC Outcomes

Immobility Consequences: Physiological; Tissue Integrity: Skin and Mucous Membranes

Example NOC Outcome with Indicators

Tissue Integrity: Skin and Mucous Membranes will be intact as evidenced by the following indicators: Skin intactness/Skin lesions not present/Tissue perfusion/Skin temperature. (Rate the outcome and indicators of **Tissue Integrity: Skin and Mucous Membranes:** 1 = severely compromised, 2 = substantially compromised, 3 = moderately compromised, 4 = mildly compromised, 5 = not compromised [see Section I].)

Client Outcomes

Client Will (Specify Time Frame)

- Report altered sensation or pain at risk areas as soon as noted
- Demonstrate understanding of personal risk factors for impaired skin integrity
- Verbalize a personal plan for preventing impaired skin integrity

S

NIC (Nursing Interventions Classification)

Suggested NIC Interventions

Positioning: Pressure Management; Pressure Ulcer Care (currently referred to as Pressure Injury Care [National Pressure Ulcer Advisory Panel (NPUAP), 2016]); Pressure Ulcer Prevention (Pressure Injury Prevention [NPUAP, 2016]; Skin Surveillance

Example NIC Activities—Pressure Ulcer Care

Monitor color of wound bed, temperature, edema, erythema, moisture, and appearance of surrounding skin; Note characteristics of any drainage

Nursing Interventions and *Rationales*

- The NPUAP redefined the definition of a pressure ulcer, which is now referred to as a pressure injury, during the NPUAP 2016 Staging Consensus Conference in 2016. The new definition more accurately defines alterations in tissue integrity from pressure as the following: A pressure injury is localized damage to the skin and underlying soft tissue, usually over a bony prominence or related to a medical or other device. The injury can present as intact skin or an open ulcer and may be painful. The injury occurs as a result of intense and/or prolonged pressure or pressure in combinations with shear. The tolerance of soft tissue for pressure and shear may also be affected by microclimate, nutrition, perfusion, comorbidities, and conditions of the soft tissue (NPUAP, 2016).
- Identify clients at risk for impaired skin integrity as a result of immobility, chronological age, malnutrition, incontinence, compromised perfusion, immunocompromised status, or chronic medical condition, such as diabetes mellitus, spinal cord injury, or renal failure. EB: *These client populations are known to be at high risk for impaired skin integrity (Baranoski et al, 2016). Targeting variables (e.g., age and Braden Scale Risk Category) can focus assessment on particular risk factors (e.g., pressure) and help guide the plan of prevention and care (National Pressure Injury Advisory Panel [NPIAP], European Pressure Injury Advisory Panel [EPIAP], & Pan Pacific Pressure Injury Alliance [PPPIA], 2019; NPUAP, 2016).*
- Inspect and monitor skin condition at least once a day for color or texture changes, redness, localized heat, edema or induration, pressure damage, dermatological conditions, or lesions and any incontinence-associated dermatitis. Determine whether the client is experiencing loss of sensation or pain. EB: *Systematic inspection can identify impending problems early (Baranoski et al, 2016; NPIAP, EPIAP, & PPPIA, 2019). When conducting a skin assessment in an individual with darkly pigmented skin, prioritize assessment of skin temperature, presence of edema, and change in tissue consistency in relation to surrounding tissue (NPIAP, EPIAP, & PPPIA, 2019).*
- Monitor the client's skin care practices, noting type of soap or other cleansing agents used, temperature of water, and frequency of skin cleansing. *Individualize plan according to the client's skin condition, needs, and preferences (Baranoski et al, 2016).*
- Keep skin clean and dry. Cleanse the skin gently with pH-balanced cleansers, avoiding alkaline soaps and cleansers. EB: *Avoid vigorous rubbing of skin. Consider use of skin moisturizers to hydrate skin to reduce risk of skin damage. Protect skin from exposure to excessive moisture with a barrier product to reduce the risk of pressure-related damage (NPIAP, EPIAP, & PPPIA, 2019).*
- ▲ Develop and implement an individualized continence management plan. Cleanse the skin promptly after episodes of incontinence. Use incontinence skin barriers including creams, ointments, pastes, or film-forming skin protectants as needed to protect skin and maintain intact skin (Wound, Ostomy and Continence Nurses Society–Wound Guidelines Task Force, 2017). Use highly absorbent incontinence products (NPIAP & EPIAP, 2019). EB: *Implementing an incontinence prevention plan with the use of a skin protectant or a cleanser protectant can significantly decrease skin breakdown and pressure ulcer formation (Baranoski et al, 2016; NPIAP, EPIAP, & PPPIA, 2019).*
- For clients with limited mobility, inspect and monitor condition of skin covering bony prominences. EB: *Pressure injuries usually occur over bony prominences, such as the sacrum, coccyx, trochanter, and heels, as a result of unrelieved pressure between the prominence and support surface or with shearing and friction (Baranoski et al, 2016; NPIAP, EPIAP, & PPPIA, 2019). Position individuals in the sitting position with special attention to anatomy, weight distribution, postural alignment, and support of feet (Wound, Ostomy and Continence Nurses Society–Wound Guidelines Task Force, 2017).*

S

- Implement and communicate a client-specific prevention plan. EB: *A plan of care clearly documented in the client's electronic health record will assist in ensuring consistency in care and documentation (Baranoski et al, 2016).*
- At-risk clients should be frequently repositioned. EB: *Frequency of repositioning will be influenced by variables concerning the individual's independent mobility and the support surface in use. Frequency of repositioning should be determined by the individual's tissue tolerance and medical condition (NPIAP, EPIAP, & PPPIA, 2019). Use of heel suspension devices can remove pressure from the heels and support the lower extremity of individuals who are unable to keep pressure off the heels, without placing pressure on the Achilles tendon and to the popliteal vein (Wound, Ostomy and Continence Nurses Society–Wound Guidelines Task Force, 2017; NPIAP, EPIAP, & PPPIA, 2019).*
- Evaluate for use of specialty mattresses, beds, or devices as appropriate. EB: *Select a surface that addresses the individual's need for pressure redistribution (Brienza et al, 2016; NPIAP, EPIAP, & PPPIA, 2019). Maintain the head of the bed at the lowest possible degree of elevation to reduce shear and use lift devices, pillows, foam wedges, and pressure-reducing devices in the bed. If the goal of care is to keep the client (e.g., a terminally ill client) comfortable, turning clients side to side at end of life may not be a priority or feasible. If the duration of pressure cannot be reduced, reducing the intensity may be the only option. An alternating pressure mattress with a low air loss feature is recommended (Hotaling & Black, 2018). Pressure redistributing devices are adjuncts to and not replacements for regular repositioning (Wound, Ostomy and Continence Nurses Society–Wound Guidelines Task Force, 2017).*

▲ Assess the client's nutritional status; refer for a nutritional consultation, and/or institute dietary supplements. EB: *Develop and implement an individualized nutritional care plan for individuals with or at risk for pressure injuries. Provide 1.2 to 1.5 g protein/kg body weight/day and 30 to 35 kilocalories body weight/day for individuals with pressure injuries with risk for malnutrition (NPIAP, EPIAP, & PPPIA, 2019).* EB: *Meeting nutritional needs of the client is important to prevention of skin breakdown and preventing complications of illness. Adequate nutrition is important for maintaining overall homeostasis and health (O'Hanlon et al, 2015).*

Geriatric

- Limit the number of complete baths to two or three per week, and alternate them with partial baths. Use a tepid water temperature (between 90°F [32.2°C] and 105°F [40.5°C]) for bathing or use a no-rinse alternative product. EB: *Excessive bathing, especially in hot water, depletes aging skin of moisture and increases dryness. The ability to retain moisture is decreased in aging skin because of diminished amounts of dermal proteins. One of the most common age-related changes to the skin is damage to the stratum corneum (Baranoski et al, 2016).*
- Use lotions and moisturizers to prevent skin from drying out, especially in the winter. EB: *Avoid skin care products that contain allergens such as lanolin, latex, and dyes (Baranoski et al, 2016). Use barrier products to protect aged skin from exposure to excessive moisture to reduce the risk of pressure damage (NPIAP, EPIAP, & PPPIA, 2019).*
- Increase fluid intake within cardiac and renal limits to a minimum of 1500 mL/day. EB: *Dry skin is caused by loss of fluid; increasing fluid intake hydrates the skin (Baranoski et al, 2016). Recommend that individuals with nutritional and pressure injury risks consume a minimum of 30 to 35 kcal/kg body weight per day, 1.25 to 1.5 g of protein/kg body weight per day, and 1 mL of fluid intake per kilocalorie per day, if there are no contraindications (Wound, Ostomy and Continence Nurses Society–Wound Guidelines Task Force, 2017).*
- Increase humidity in the environment, especially during the winter, by using a humidifier or placing a container of water on a warm object. Increasing the moisture in the air helps keep moisture in the skin.

Home Care

- Assess client and caregiver ability to recognize potential risk for skin breakdown. Provide resources for client/caregiver to contact health care provider with questions/concerns related to skin and incontinence care as needed. Engage family, caregivers, or legal guardian when establishing goals of care and validate their understanding of these goals. Educate the individual and his or her caregiver regarding skin changes in aging and at end of life. EB: *Early interventions can place the individual on the path to healing. Treating wounds requires a multiprofessional approach (Cox, 2019). When provided with the appropriate resources, the nurse can have a positive impact on the client's wound healing trajectory (NPIAP, EPIAP, & PPPIA, 2019).*
- See the care plan for Impaired **Skin** Integrity.

S

Client/Family Teaching and Discharge Planning

- Teach the client skin assessment and ways to monitor for impending skin breakdown. Early assessment and intervention help prevent the development of serious problems. EB: *Basic elements of a skin assessment are assessment of temperature, color, moisture, turgor, and intact skin (Baranoski et al, 2016). Seek information from the health care team to address individual pressure injury prevention and treatment needs (NPIAP, EPIAP, & PPPIA, 2019).*
- If consistent with overall client management goals, teach how to turn and reposition the client. EB: *Do not position an individual directly on a pressure injury. Continue to turn/reposition the individual even if a low air loss support surface is in use. Establish turning frequency based on the characteristics of the support surface and the individual's response (NPIAP, EPIAP, & PPPIA, 2019). If the goal of care is to keep the client (e.g., a terminally ill client) comfortable, turning and repositioning may not be appropriate (NPIAP, EPIAP, & PPPIA, 2019).*
- Teach the client and/or caregivers to use pillows, foam wedges, and pressure-reducing devices to prevent pressure injury (NPIAP, EPIAP, & PPPIA, 2019). EB: *The use of effective pressure-reducing seat cushions for older wheelchair users may significantly prevent sitting-acquired pressure injuries (Brienza et al, 2016). Pressure redistribution devices serve as adjuncts to prevention and do not replace repositioning (Wound, Ostomy and Continence Nurses Society–Wound Guidelines Task Force, 2017).*

REFERENCES

Baranoski, S., Ayello, E. A., Levine, J. M., LeBlanc, K., & Tomic-Canic, M. (2016). Skin: An essential organ. In S. Baranoski, & E. A. Ayello (Eds.), *Wound care essentials: Practice principles* (4th ed.). Philadelphia: Wolters Kluwer.

Brienza, D. M., Zulkowski, K., Sprigle, S., & Geyer, M. J. (2016). Pressure redistribution: Seating, positioning, and support surfaces. In S. Baranoski, & E. A. Ayello (Eds.), *Wound care essentials: Practice principles* (4th ed.). Philadelphia: Wolters Kluwer.

Cox, J. (2019). Wound care 101. *Nursing 2019*, *49*(10), 33–39.

Hotaling, P., & Black, J. (2018). Ten top tips: End of life pressure injuries. *Wounds International*, *9*(1), 18–21.

National. Pressure Injury Advisory Panel (NPIAP), European Pressure Injury Advisory Panel (EPIAP), & Pan Pacific Pressure Injury Alliance (PPPIA). (2019). In E. Haesler (Ed.), *Prevention and treatment of pressure ulcers: Quick reference guide*. Osborne Park, Australia: Cambridge Media.

National Pressure Ulcer Advisory Panel (NPUAP). (2016). *Pressure injury stages*. Retrieved from https://npiap.com/page/PressureInjuryStages. [Accessed July 29, 2021].

O'Hanlon, C., Dowsett, J., & Smyth, N. (2015). Nutrition assessment of the intensive care unit patient. *Topics in Clinical Nutrition*, *30*(1), 47–70.

Wound, O., & Continence Nurses Society–Wound Guidelines Task Force. (2017). WOCN 2016 guideline for prevention and management of pressure injuries (ulcers). *Journal of Wound, Ostomy and Continence Nursing*, *44*(3), 241–246. https://doi.org/10.1097/WON.0000000000000321.

Sleep Deprivation Domain 4 Activity/rest Class 1 Sleep/rest

Judith Ann Floyd, PhD, RN, FNAP, FAAN

NANDA-I

S

Definition

Prolonged periods of time without sustained natural, periodic suspension of relative consciousness that provides rest.

Defining Characteristics

Altered attention; anxiety; apathy; combativeness; confusion; decreased functional ability; drowsiness; expresses distress; fatigue; fleeting nystagmus; hallucinations; heightened sensitivity to pain; irritable mood; lethargy; prolonged reaction time; psychomotor agitation; transient paranoia; tremors

Related Factors

Age-related sleep stage shifts; average daily physical activity is less than recommended for age and gender; discomfort; environmental disturbances; environmental overstimulation; late day confusion; nonrestorative sleep-wake cycle; sleep terror; sleep walking; sustained circadian asynchrony; sustained inadequate sleep hygiene

At-Risk Population

Individuals with familial sleep paralysis

Associated Conditions

Conditions with periodic limb movement; idiopathic central nervous system hypersomnolence; narcolepsy; neurocognitive disorders; nightmares; sleep apnea; sleep-related enuresis; sleep-related painful erections; treatment regimen

NOC (Nursing Outcomes Classification)

Suggested NOC Outcomes

Rest; Sleep; Symptom Severity

Example NOC Outcome with Indicators

Sleep as evidenced by the following indicators: Hours of sleep/Sleep pattern/Sleep quality/Sleep efficiency/Feels rejuvenated after sleep/Sleeps through the night consistently. (Rate the outcome and indicators of **Sleep:** 1 = severely compromised, 2 = substantially compromised, 3 = moderately compromised, 4 = mildly compromised, 5 = not compromised [see Section I].)

Client Outcomes

Client Will (Specify Time Frame)

- Verbalize plan that provides adequate time for sleep
- Identify actions that can be taken to ensure adequate sleep time
- Awaken refreshed once adequate time is spent sleeping
- Be less sleepy during the day once adequate time is spent sleeping

NIC (Nursing Interventions Classification)

Suggested NIC Intervention

Sleep Enhancement

Example NIC Activities—Sleep Enhancement

Monitor/record client's sleep pattern and number of sleep hours; Encourage client to establish a schedule that allows age-appropriate hours of sleep with minimal environmental and personal disruptions

Nursing Interventions and *Rationales*

- Minimize care-environmental factors that may lead to sleep deprivation if they persist. See Nursing Interventions and *Rationales* for Disturbed **Sleep** Pattern.
- Address personal client factors that may lead to sleep deprivation if they persist. See Nursing Interventions and *Rationales* for **Insomnia.**
- Assess for hypersensitivity to pain in sleep-deprived clients. EB: *In a laboratory experiment using 14 healthy adults, sleep restriction protocols altered processes of pain habituation and sensitization, which may help explain why chronic pain conditions often accompany insufficient sleep (Simpson et al, 2018).* EB: *In an observational study of postoperative orthopedic surgery subjects (n = 50), a significant correlation was found between increased self-reported pain scores and decreased total sleep time (Miller et al, 2015).*
- Assess the amount of sleep obtained each night compared with the amount of sleep needed given the client's age, medical diagnoses, and personal preferences. EBN: *In an observational study (n = 141), subjects reported a large variation in how many hours of sleep they obtained in hospital as compared to home; however, the average reduction in hospital sleep duration, compared to home, was 1.8 hours (an average of 5.3 hours of sleep in hospital vs. 7.1 hours at home) (Delaney et al, 2018).*
- Assess the extent to which clients can be provided 3 to 4 consecutive hours of sleep time that is free from disturbance. CEB: *In a meta-analysis using data from 159 studies, a nurse scientist found that the deepest stages of sleep occurred during the first 3 to 4 hours of the sleep period followed by several 90- to 110-minute sleep cycles that consisted of increasingly lower percentages of deep sleep (Floyd, 2002).*
- If sleep-disrupting environmental factors that are inherent in hospitalization cannot be reduced adequately to prevent sleep deprivation, schedule specific times for rest and sleep during the day. EB: *Purposefully*

S

scheduled daytime naps may compensate in part for less sleep at night, as well as promote recovery from acute illness (Tan et al, 2019).

- If personal sleep-disrupting factors that are inherent in insomnia cannot be reduced adequately to prevent the client's sleep deprivation, consider scheduling a specific time for rest and sleep during the day. EB: *Although the number and duration of daytime naps may need to be limited if the client has difficulty initiating and maintaining nighttime sleep despite use of sleep-promoting interventions for insomnia, a purposefully scheduled nap may compensate in part for less sleep at night (Tan et al, 2019).* CEB: *Nurse scientists who conducted observational studies were the first to question the prohibition against all daytime napping by showing that carefully scheduled short naps appeared to supplement, rather than displace, nighttime sleep (Hayter, 1985; Floyd, 1995).*
- If caffeine is used by the client to alleviate daytime drowsiness, monitor amounts and time of use. CEB: *An experimental study of 12 participants found that caffeine (400 mg), even when consumed 6 hours before bedtime, had a disruptive effect on both objective and subjective sleep measures (Drake et al, 2013).*
- If naps are inadequate for preventing excessive daytime sleepiness due to sleep deprivation, consider and carefully evaluate use of unstudied, but commonly used, countermeasures for fighting drowsiness. CEB: *A descriptive study of 77 middle-aged adults identified the following unstudied strategies as possibly effective interrupters of drowsiness: (1) change physical position, (2) improve ventilation (e.g., get fresh air, turn on fan, open window), (3) reduce air temperature (e.g., turn on air conditioning, turn on fan), (4) increase auditory stimulation (e.g., play music, sing, engage in conversation, listen to debate), and (5) engage in interesting visual activity (e.g., board games, watching TV sports events, watching serial TV dramas) (Davidsson, 2012).*
- ▲ If daytime drowsiness occurs despite adequate periods of undisturbed nighttime sleep and supplemental daytime naps, consider undiagnosed sleep apnea as a possible cause. EB: *Sleep-disordered breathing affects 17% of men and 9% of women in the general population, of whom the majority are undiagnosed and untreated (Tan et al, 2019).*

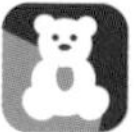

Pediatric

- Assess the amount of sleep obtained every 24 hours compared with the amount of sleep needed for the child given age, medical diagnoses, and individual differences. EB: *Caregivers of 246 hospitalized subjects ages 4 weeks to 18 years reported that subjects slept less in the hospital than at home (Erondu et al, 2019).*
- Encourage daily schedules that allow for late awakening times for adolescents. EB: *A review of evidence from 38 reports showed that delaying school start time increased sleep duration among adolescents, primarily by delaying rise times (Wheaton et al, 2016).*
- Encourage an age-appropriate nap schedule that adequately supplements the child's nighttime sleep duration. EBN: *A descriptive study of lower-income toddlers (n = 101) found that two-thirds were not getting the recommended 11 to 14 hours of sleep per 24 hours (Armstrong et al, 2019).*
- See the Pediatric section of Nursing Interventions and *Rationales* for Disturbed **Sleep** Pattern.

Geriatric

- Assess the amount of sleep obtained each night compared with the amount of sleep needed for an older adult given advancing age, medical diagnoses, and individual differences. EB: *Older adults are at risk for sleep deprivation due to normal aging-related changes in sleep architecture and the additive impact of multiple risk factors including polypharmacy, increased prevalence of symptoms such as pain and nocturia, acute disturbances such as hospitalization, and changes in social roles that normally stabilize the sleep/wake pattern (Dean et al, 2017).*
- ▲ If an older adult has daytime sleepiness despite adequate nighttime sleep, consider a referral to a sleep laboratory to rule out sleep apnea. EBN: *Nurses who studied 49 surgical subjects age 65 and older, as well as reviewed charts for an additional 52 elderly surgical subjects, found that sleep apnea was frequently undiagnosed (Qassamali et al, 2019).*
- Assess how much time the older adult spends in bed unable to sleep and their comfort with low sleep efficiency. EBN: *A meta-analysis of results from samples representing 5061 general-population adults showed a steady increase after age 50 in the amount of time in bed resting rather than sleeping, which contributed to a steady decline in sleep efficiency over the lifespan (Floyd, 2017).*
- If a client is obtaining less sleep than required for optimal daytime function, explore if daytime napping will supplement, rather than replace, nighttime sleep. CEB: *In a pretest/posttest study of 22 older adults, a consistent regimen of daily napping for 45 minutes enhanced waking function without negatively affecting nighttime sleep (Campbell et al, 2011).*
- See the Geriatric section of Nursing Interventions and Rationales for Disturbed **Sleep** Pattern and **Insomnia.**

S

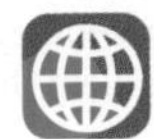

Multicultural

- Be aware of racial and ethnic disparities in sleep deprivation. **EB:** *A national survey of 444,306 American adults found that non-Hispanic black, American Indian/Alaska Native, Native Hawaiian/Pacific Islander, and multiracial populations reported a higher prevalence of sleeping less than 7 hours compared with the rest of the U.S. adult population (Liu et al, 2016).*

Home Care

- Assessments and interventions discussed previously can all be adapted for use in home care.
- ▲ If daytime drowsiness occurs despite adequate periods of undisturbed nighttime sleep and supplemental daytime naps, consider sleep apnea as a possible cause. **CEB:** *In a household survey of more than 7000 adults, unexplained excessive daytime sleepiness was identified as a predictor of undiagnosed sleep apnea (Dosman et al, 2014).*
- Teach family members about the prevalence and long-term consequences of inadequate amounts of sleep for both clients and family caregivers. **EB:** *A national survey of 444,306 American adults found that more than one-third (34.8%) were likely sleep deprived (i.e., slept less than 7 hours per night), an amount at which physiological and neurobehavioral deficits may manifest and become progressively worse under chronic conditions (Liu et al, 2016).* **CEB:** *In an integrative review of 10 studies, insufficient sleep was associated with poor attention, decreased performance, increased mortality and morbidity, and cardiovascular risk factors, including hypertension, insulin resistance, hormonal deregulation, and inflammation (Mullington et al, 2009).*
- ▲ If sleep is deprived due to insomnia, refer client to a nurse practitioner or other sleep specialist trained in cognitive behavioral therapies for insomnia (CBT-I). **EB:** *A meta-analysis of 37 comparative effectiveness studies found that chronic insomnia subjects with comorbid medical and psychiatric conditions improved their ability to initiate and maintain sleep after completion of multicomponent CBT-I programs (Wu et al, 2015).*
- Teach client/family caregivers about the need for those with medical conditions to avoid schedules and commitments that interfere with obtaining adequate amounts of sleep. **EB:** *Critical appraisal of 22 studies provided evidence that sleep disturbance was common in critically ill subjects up to 12 months after hospital discharge (Altman et al, 2017).*
- Promote adoption of behaviors that ensure adequate amounts of sleep for all family members.
- Teach family members ways to avoid chronic sleep loss.
- Advise against chronic use of caffeinated drinks to overcome daytime fatigue and drowsiness while focusing on elimination of factors that lead to chronic sleep loss. **CEB:** *In an integrative review of 26 controlled laboratory studies of adult subjects, caffeine was found helpful in the temporary management of sleepiness, but overuse and late-day use contributed to subsequent sleep disruption and caffeine habituation (Roehrs & Roth, 2008).*

REFERENCES

Altman, M. T., Knauert, M. P., & Pisani, M. A. (2017). Sleep disturbance after hospitalization and critical illness: A systematic review. *Annals of the American Thoracic Society*, *14*(9), 1457–1468. https://doi.org/10.1513/AnnalsATS.201702-148SR.

Armstrong, B., Covington, L. B., Hager, E. R., & Black, M. M. (2019). Objective sleep and physical activity using 24-hour ankle-worn accelerometry among toddlers from low-income families. *Sleep Health*, *5*(5), 459–465. https://doi.org/10.1016/j.sleh.2019.04.005 2352-7218.

Campbell, S. S., Stanchina, M. D., Schlang, J. R., & Murphy, P. J. (2011). Effects of a month-long napping regimen in older individuals. *Journal of the American Geriatric Society*, *59*(2), 224–232. https://doi.org/10.1111/j.1532-5415.2010.03264.x.

Davidsson, S. (2012). Countermeasure drowsiness by design: Using common behaviour. *Work (Reading, Mass.)*, *41*(Suppl. 1), 5062–5067. https://doi.org/10.3233/WOR-2012-0798-5062.

Dean, G. E., Weiss, C., Morris, J. L., & Chasens, E. R. (2017). Impaired sleep: A multifaceted geriatric syndrome. *Nursing Clinics of North America*, *52*(3), 387–404. http://doi.org/10.1016/j.cnur.2017.04.009.

Delaney, L. J., Currie, M. J., Huang, H. C. C., Lopez, V., & Van Haren, F. (2018). "They can rest at home": An observational study of patients' quality of sleep in an Australian hospital. *BMC Health Services Research*, *18*(1), 524. https://doi.org/10.1186/s12913-018-3201-z.

Dosman, J., Gjevre, J., Karunanayake, C., et al. (2014). Predicting sleep apnea in the clinic. *Chest*, *145*(Suppl. 3), 595A. https://doi.org/10.1378/chest.1825416.

Drake, C., Roehrs, T., Shambroom, J., & Roth, T. (2013). Caffeine effects on sleep taken 0, 3, or 6 hours before going to bed. *Journal of Clinical Sleep Medicine*, *9*(11), 1195–1200. https://doi.org/10.5664/jcsm.3170.

Erondu, A. I., Orlov, N. M., Peirce, L. B., et al. (2019). Characterizing pediatric inpatient sleep duration and disruptions. *Sleep Medicine*, *57*, 87–91. https://doi.org/10.1016/j.sleep.2019.01.030.

Floyd, J. A. (1995). Another look at napping in older adults. *Geriatric Nursing*, *16*(3), 136–138. https://doi.org/10.1016/S0197-4572(05)80047-3.

Floyd, J. A. (2002). Sleep and aging. *Nursing Clinics of North America*, *37*(4), 719–731. https://pubmed.ncbi.nlm.nih.gov/12587370/.

Floyd, J. A. (2017). Patterns of decline in sleep efficiency over the adult lifespan: Clarification via use of smoothing splines. *International Journal of Sleep Disorders*, *1*(1), 1–6. Retrieved from https://www.sciteslit.com/SleepDisorders/IJSD-ID11.pdf. [Accessed February 22, 2022].

Hayter, J. (1985). To nap or not to nap? *Geriatric Nursing*, *6*(2), 104–106. Retrieved from https://www.sciencedirect.com/science/article/abs/pii/S0197457285800100. [Accessed February 22, 2022].

Liu, Y., Wheaton, A. G., Chapman, D. P., Cunningham, T. J., Lu, H., & Croft, J. B. (2016). Prevalence of healthy sleep duration among adults United States, 2014. *MMWR: Morbidity and Mortality Weekly Report*, *65*(6), 137–141. https://doi.org/10.15585/mmwr.mm6506a1.

Miller, A., Roth, T., Roehrs, T., & Yaremchuk, K. (2015). Correlation between sleep disruption on postoperative pain. *Otolaryngology—Head and Neck Surgery*, *152*(5), 964–968. https://doi.org/10.1177/0194599815572127.

Mullington, J. M., Haack, M., Toth, M., Serrador, J. M., & Meier-Ewert, H. K. (2009). Cardiovascular, inflammatory, and metabolic consequences of sleep deprivation. *Progress in Cardiovascular Diseases*, *51*(4), 294–302. https://doi.org/10.1016/j.pcad.2008.10.003.

Qassamali, S. R., Lagoo-Deenadayalan, S., McDonald, S., Morgan, B., & Goode, V. (2019). The importance of the STOP-BANG questionnaire as a preoperative assessment tool for the elderly population. *Geriatric Nursing*, *40*(5), 536–539. https://doi.org/10.1016/j.gerinurse.2019.08.010.

Roehrs, T. A., & Roth, T. (2008). Caffeine: Sleep and daytime sleepiness. *Sleep Medicine Reviews*, *12*(2), 153–162. https://doi.org/doi:10.1016/j.smrv.2007.07.004.

Simpson, N. S., Scott-Sutherland, J., Gautam, S., Sethna, N., & Haack, M. (2018). Chronic exposure to insufficient sleep alters processes of pain habituation and sensitization. *Pain*, *159*(1), 33–41. https://doi.org/10.1097/j.pain.0000000000001053.

Tan, X., van Egmond, L., Partinen, M., Lange, T., & Benedict, C. (2019). A narrative review of interventions for improving sleep and reducing circadian disruption in medical inpatients. *Sleep Medicine*, *59*, 42–50. https://doi.org/10.1016/j.sleep.2018.08.007.

Wheaton, A. G., Chapman, D. P., & Croft, J. B. (2016). School start times, sleep, behavioral, health, and academic outcomes: A review of the literature. *Journal of School Health*, *86*(5), 363–381. https://doi.org/10.1111/josh.12388.

Wu, J. Q., Appleman, E. R., Salazar, R. D., & Ong, J. C. (2015). Cognitive behavioral therapy for insomnia co-morbid with psychiatric and medical conditions: A meta-analysis. *JAMA Internal Medicine*, *175*(9), 1461–1472. https://doi.org/10.1001/jamainternmed.2015.3006.

Readiness for Enhanced Sleep

Domain 4 Activity/rest Class 1 Sleep/rest

Judith Ann Floyd, PhD, RN, FNAP, FAAN

NANDA-I

Definition

A pattern of natural, periodic suspension of relative consciousness to provide rest and sustain a desired lifestyle, which can be strengthened.

Defining Characteristics

Expresses desire to enhance sleep-wake cycle

NOC (Nursing Outcomes Classification)

Suggested NOC Outcomes

Personal Well-Being; Rest; Sleep

Example NOC Outcome with Indicators

Sleep as evidenced by the following indicators: Hours of sleep/Sleep pattern/Sleep quality/Sleep efficiency/Feels rejuvenated after sleep/Napping appropriate for age. (Rate each indicator of **Sleep:** 1 = severely compromised, 2 = substantially compromised, 3 = moderately compromised, 4 = mildly compromised, 5 = not compromised [see Section I].)

Client Outcomes

Client Will (Specify Time Frame)

- Verbalize a current interest in what constitutes normal sleep
- Reflect on own experiences and beliefs about sleep
- Verbalize an interest in nonpharmacological approaches to sleep promotion
- Take concrete steps to establish an environment conducive to sleep initiation and maintenance

NIC (Nursing Interventions Classification)

Suggested NIC Intervention

Sleep Enhancement

Example NIC Activities—Sleep Enhancement

Assess client's sleep/activity pattern; Assist/encourage client to create an environment that facilitates sleep; Assist/encourage client to adopt personal practices that enhance sleep

Nursing Interventions and *Rationales*

- Assess client's current knowledge and beliefs about sleep need and factors affecting sleep quantity and quality. CEB: *In a descriptive study of 1707 subjects from nine primary care practices, assessment of knowledge and beliefs about sleep was identified as an essential first step in client education programs (Phillips et al, 2014).* EB: *In an observational study of 120 undergraduate students, greater maladaptive beliefs about sleep were related to greater insomnia severity, poorer sleep quality, and less sleep hygiene knowledge (Kloss et al, 2016).*
- Whenever there is a lack of knowledge or false beliefs about sleep requirements, provide information regarding sleep need and encourage clients to identify their personal sleep requirements. CEB: *In a meta-analysis (n = 180 studies), a nurse researcher found that normal-population adults averaged 7.5 to 9.0 hours of sleep per night (range of 6.5–10.0 hours) and fell asleep within 20 minutes initially and more quickly if awakened during the night; daytime was characterized by no naps or regularly scheduled brief naps, and little fatigue or sleepiness (Floyd, 2002).* EB: *In a review of research by a panel of 15 sleep experts, sleep need was found to be highly variable among adults, but 7 or more hours of sleep on a regular basis was found to promote optimal health and reduce risk of adverse health outcomes; it was unclear if averaging more than 9 hours was associated with health risk among the otherwise healthy adults (Watson et al, 2015).*
- Based on your assessment, focus on one or more of the following sleep hygiene strategies, choosing the most relevant for the client:
  - Regular scheduling of the nighttime sleep period, daytime exposure to light, exercise, napping, and mealtimes characterized by (1) exercise during the day, (2) avoidance of long periods of daytime sleep (unless a night-shift worker), (3) avoidance of large meals before bed, and (4) arising at the same time each day even if sleep was poor during the previous night. EB: *An experimental study of 173 young adults suggested that interactions among rest/activity, light/dark, sleep, and other physiological parameters (body temperature, blood pressure, and heart rate) are complex and require more study, but factors that suppress or stimulate melatonin secretion likely play a key role in circadian rhythm interactions (Gubin et al, 2017).*
  - Use of a relaxing bedtime routine that includes (1) activities that calm the mind (e.g., mindfulness or other types of meditation, listening to music, prayer) and (2) activities that relax the body (e.g., warm baths, massage, progressive muscle relaxation). EBN: *A review of evidence from nine intervention studies suggested relaxation, meditation, guided imagery, or a combination of these strategies resulted in better sleep and less fatigue in heart-failure clients (Kwekkeboom & Bratzke, 2016).*
  - Use of essential oils. EBN: *Adult rehabilitation subjects (n = 42), who were studied using a randomized crossover study design, reported better sleep quality when exposed to essential oils (Lavandula x intermedia [Lavandin Super], Citrus bergamia [bergamot], and Cananga odorata [ylang ylang]) than when exposed to a placebo oil (McConnell & Newcomb, 2019).*
  - Creation of an environment conducive to sleep, including (1) comfortable sleepwear, sleep surface, and room temperature; (2) low or masked levels of light and noise; and (3) a sleep space as free as possible from interruptions from others. EBN: *Using qualitative methods, the lived experience of client sleep in hospitals as perceived by nurses (n = 14) included several environmental factors that disturbed clients' sleep, including uncomfortable beds/mattresses/pillows, as well as light, noise, temperature, and smells (Honkavuo, 2018).*
  - Management of any sources of pain as needed before sleep. EB: *In a national survey of 1029 noninstitutionalized adults age 18 years or older, pain was associated with lower sleep quality, more sleep disruption, and greater sleep deprivation (National Sleep Foundation, 2015).* (See further Nursing Interventions and Rationales for Acute **Pain** and Chronic **Pain.**)

S

- Avoidance of late-day electronic device use. EB: *A descriptive study of 1674 adults found that participants with more screen time from TV watching and use of computers and other electronic devises reported more difficulty falling asleep and staying asleep (Vallance et al, 2015).* EB: *A representative survey of 1508 adults found that 90% of Americans used some type of electronics at least a few nights per week before bedtime and also found that adults who reported use of e-readers had reduced evening sleepiness, took longer to fall asleep, and reported reduced next-morning alertness compared with adults who read printed books at bedtime (Chang et al, 2015).*
- Monitoring of late-day intake of caffeine from all sources, including energy drinks, coffee, colas, teas, and chocolate. CEB: *In an experimental study (n = 12) researchers found that caffeine consumption (400 mg) up to 6 hours before bedtime had a disruptive effect on objectively measured and self-reported symptoms of insomnia (Drake et al, 2013).*
- Avoidance of alcoholic beverages to induce sleep. CEB: *In a descriptive study of 50 oncology outpatients, nurse researchers found that even limited alcohol use (one to two drinks) was related to shortened time to falling asleep and increased depth of sleep the first 2 hours, as well as suppressed rapid eye movement (REM) sleep, which sometimes led to REM rebound (i.e., lighter, more fragmented sleep later in the night) (Dean et al, 2010).*
- Avoidance of nicotine. CEB: *In a national survey of 6400 participants, cigarette smokers took longer to fall asleep and had shorter and lighter nighttime sleep than nonsmokers; however, acute nicotine withdrawal caused even more sleep disruption (Zhang et al, 2006).* EB: *In a survey of 498 young adults, all stimulants disturbed sleep; however, nicotine was particularly deleterious (Caviness et al, 2019).*
- Avoidance of a sedentary lifestyle. EB: *In a national survey of 1000 representative adults ages 23 to 60, excessive sitting during waking hours was associated with poor sleep quality (Buman et al, 2015).*

Geriatric

- Interventions discussed previously can all be adapted for use with geriatric clients.
- Counsel the older client regarding normal age-related sleep changes. CEB: *In a meta-analysis (n = 180 studies), a nurse researcher discovered that as adults aged, they increased time needed to fall asleep, increased the frequency and duration of waking after sleep onset, and decreased nighttime sleep amount (Floyd, 2002).* EBN: *A meta-analysis of results from samples representing 5061 general-population adults showed a steady increase after age fifty in the amount of time spent in bed with the intent to sleep, which contributed to a steady decline in sleep efficiency with aging (Floyd, 2017).*
- Elicit the older client's beliefs about sleep and correct any misconceptions, which may manifest as undue concern for some elders, but too little concern for others. CEB: *In a descriptive study comparing sleep beliefs and behaviors of 41 black and 24 white older women, the majority of women, regardless of race/ethnicity, incorrectly stated that poor sleep did not have negative effects on other health conditions (Grandner et al, 2013).*
- Review older clients' prescription medications; use of over-the-counter (OTC) medications; and use of caffeine, tobacco, and alcohol. CEB: *In a review of literature about older adults' sleep, nurse scholars found that older adults may be unaware of how their medications and commonly used psychoactive substances affect sleep (Allen et al, 2013).* EB: *A double-blind crossover study (n = 46) of adults in their fifties compared with younger adults found that caffeine interfered with initiation of deep sleep in all and that the older adults experienced even more sensitivity to caffeine intake than the younger adults (Robillard et al, 2015).*
- Assess and refer as appropriate whenever coexisting conditions may be affecting older clients' sleep. CEB: *In a review of literature about older-adult sleep, nurse scholars found that depression, sleep apnea, and restless legs syndrome are commonly missed coexisting conditions in older adults (Allen et al, 2013).*
- Expand older clients' awareness of sleep hygiene behaviors for improving sleep. EBN: *In a mixed-methods study of 18 elders, none of the study participants who used sleep hygiene practices had done so on the specific advice of a health care provider; rather, they had cobbled together some information from Internet articles and their own experience (Berkley et al, 2020).* CEB: *In a descriptive study of 195 older adults, only three strategies were heavily used by elders to address sleep concerns: ignoring the symptoms, staying in bed or resting, and praying (Sandberg et al, 2014).*
- Encourage the older client to walk and engage in other exercise outside unless contraindicated. EB: *In an evidence review of 34 research reports, exercise increased sleep efficiency and duration in healthy older adults regardless of the mode and intensity of activity, and even more so in the elderly with chronic conditions such as hypertension, obesity, diabetes, rheumatoid arthritis, or sleep disorders (Dolezal et al, 2017).*

S

Home Care

- All interventions discussed previously can be adapted for home care use.
- Assess family caregivers' readiness for enhancing sleep. EB: *A secondary analysis of quantitative data from 395 family caregivers of hospice clients found that nearly one-third experienced clinically noteworthy levels of sleep problems and/or anxiety that can interfere with sleep initiation (Washington et al, 2018).* EB: *A pretest-posttest pilot study of seven dementia clients and their family caregivers suggested that a caregiver sleep education program resulted in decreased client sleep problems and decreased caregiver depression (Tewary et al, 2018).*
- Assess the conduciveness of the home environment for promoting sleep and the resources needed to improve the sleep environment. CEB: *In an experimental study of 122 socioeconomically disadvantaged new mothers, nurse researchers found that approximately two-thirds of homes incorporated sleep hygiene recommendations consistently over 3 months (Lee & Gay, 2011).*

REFERENCES

Allen, A. M., Coon, D. W., Uriri-Glover, J., & Grando, V. (2013). Factors associated with sleep disturbance among older adults in inpatient rehabilitation facilities. *Rehabilitation Nursing, 38*(5), 221–230. https://doi.org/10.1002/rnj.88.

Berkley, A. S., Carter, P. A., Yoder, L. H., Acton, G., & Holahan, C. K. (2020). The effects of insomnia on older adults' quality of life and daily functioning: A mixed-methods study. *Geriatric Nursing, 41*(6), 832–838. https://doi.org/10.1016/j.gerinurse.2020.05.008.

Buman, M. P., Kline, C. E., Youngstedt, S. D., Phillips, B., de Mello, M. T., & Hirshkowitz, M. (2015). Sitting and television viewing: Novel risk factors for sleep disturbance and apnea risk? Results from the 2013 National Sleep Foundation Sleep in America Poll. *Chest, 147*(3), 728–734. https://doi.org/10.1378/chest.14-1187.

Caviness, C. M., Anderson, B. J., & Stein, M. D. (2019). Impact of nicotine and other stimulants on sleep in young adults. *Journal of Addictions Medicine, 13*(3), 209–214. https://doi.org/10.1097/adm.0000000000000481.

Chang, A. M., Aeschbach, D., Duffy, J. F., & Czeisler, C. A. (2015). Evening use of light-emitting eReaders negatively affects sleep, circadian timing, and next-morning alertness. *Proceedings of the National Academy of Sciences of the United States of America, 112*(4), 1232–1237. https://doi.org/10.1073/pnas.1418490112.

Dean, G. E., Finnell, D. S., Scribner, M., Wang, Y. J., Steinbrenner, L. M., & Gooneratne, N. S. (2010). Sleep in lung cancer: The role of anxiety, alcohol and tobacco. *Journal of Addictions Nursing, 21*(2-3), 130–138. https://doi.org/10.3109/10884601003777620.

Dolezal, B. A., Neufeld, E. V., Boland, D. M., Martin, J. L., & Cooper, C. B. (2017). Interrelationship between sleep and exercise: A systematic review. *Advances in Preventive Medicine, 2017*, 1364387. https://doi.org/10.1155/2017/1364387.

Drake, C., Roehrs, T., Shambroom, J., & Roth, T. (2013). Caffeine effects on sleep taken 0, 3, or 6 hours before going to bed. *Journal of Clinical Sleep Medicine, 9*(11), 1195–1200. https://doi.org/10.5664/jcsm.3170.

Floyd, J. A. (2002). Sleep and aging. *Nursing Clinics of North America, 37*(4), 719–731. Retrieved from https://pubmed.ncbi.nlm.nih.gov/12587370/. [Accessed 23 February 2022].

Floyd, J. A. (2017). Patterns of decline in sleep efficiency over the adult lifespan: Clarification via use of smoothing splines. *International Journal of Sleep Disorders, 1*(1), 1–6. Retrieved from https://www.scireslit.com/SleepDisorders/IJSD-ID11.pdf. [Accessed 23 February 2022].

Grandner, M. A., Patel, N. P., Girardin, J. L., et al. (2013). Sleep-related behaviors and beliefs associated with race/ethnicity in women. *Journal of the National Medical Association, 105*(1), 4–15. https://doi.org/doi:10.1016/s0027-9684(15)30080-8.

Gubin, D. G., Weinert, D., Rybina, S. V., et al. (2017). Activity, sleep and ambient light have a different impact on circadian blood pressure, heart rate and body temperature rhythms. *Chronobiology International, 34*(5), 632–649. https://doi.org/10.1080/07420528.2017.1288632.

Honkavuo, L. (2018). Nurses' experiences of supporting sleep in hospitals—A hermeneutical study. *International Journal of Caring Sciences, 11*(1), 4–10. Retrieved from www.internationaljournalofcaringsciences.org. [Accessed 23 February 2022].

Kloss, J. D., Nash, C. O., Walsh, C. M., Culnan, E., Horsey, S., & Sexton-Radek, K. (2016). A "Sleep 101" program for college students improves sleep hygiene knowledge and reduces maladaptive beliefs about sleep. *Behavioral Medicine, 42*(1), 48–56. https://doi.org/10.1080/08964289.2014.969186.

Kwekkeboom, K. L., & Bratzke, L. C. (2016). A systematic review of relaxation, meditation, and guided imagery strategies for symptom management in heart failure. *Journal of Cardiovascular Nursing, 31*(5), 457–468. https://doi.org/10.1097/JCN.0000000000000274.

Lee, K. A., & Gay, C. L. (2011). Can modifications to the bedroom environment improve the sleep of new parents? Two randomized controlled trials. *Research in Nursing & Health, 34*(1), 7–19.

McConnell, B., & Newcomb, P. (2019). Trial of essential oils to improve sleep for patients in cardiac rehabilitation. *Journal of Alternative and Complementary Medicine, 25*(12), 1193–1199. https://doi.org/10.1089/acm.2019.0222.

National Sleep Foundation. (2015). 2015 Sleep in America poll: Sleep and pain—Summary of findings. Retrieved from https://www.sleepfoundation.org/professionals/sleep-americar-polls/2015-sleep-and-pain. [Accessed 29 July 2021].

Phillips, S. M., Glasgow, R. E., Bello, G., et al. (2014). Frequency and prioritization of patient health risks from a structured health risk assessment. *Annuals of Family Medicine, 12*(6), 505–513. https://doi.org/10.1370/afm.1717.

Robillard, R., Bouchard, M., Cartier, A., Nicolau, L., & Carrier, J. (2015). Sleep is more sensitive to high doses of caffeine in the middle years of life. *Journal of Psychopharmacology, 29*(6), 688–697. https://doi.org/10.1177/0269881115575535.

Sandberg, J. C., Suerken, C. K., Quandt, S. A., et al. (2014). Self-reported sleep difficulties and self-care strategies among rural older adults. *Journal of Evidence-Based Complementary & Alternative Medicine, 19*(1), 36–42. https://doi.org/10.1177/2156587213510005.

Tewary, S., Cook, N., Pandya, N., & McCurry, S. M. (2018). Pilot test of a six-week group delivery caregiver training program to reduce sleep disturbances among older adults with dementia. *Dementia, 17*(2), 234–243. https://doi.org/10.1177/1471301216643191.

Vallance, J. K., Buman, M. P., Stevinson, C., & Lynch, B. M. (2015). Associations of overall sedentary time and screen time with sleep

S

outcomes. *American Journal of Health Behavior*, *39*(1), 62–67. https://doi.org/10.5993/AJHB.39.1.7.

Washington, K. T., Parker-Oliver, D., Smith, J. B., McCrae, C. S., Balchandani, S. M., & Demiris, G. (2018). Sleep problems, anxiety, and global self-rated health among hospice family caregivers. *American Journal of Hospice & Palliative Medicine*, *35*(2), 244–249. https://doi.org/10.1177/1049909117703643.

Watson, N. F., Badr, M. S., Belenky, G., et al. (2015). Recommended amount of sleep for a healthy adult: A joint consensus statement of the American Academy of Sleep Medicine and Sleep Research Society. *Sleep*, *38*(6), 843–844. https://doi.org/10.5665/sleep.4716.

Zhang, L., Samet, J., Caffo, B., & Punjabi, N. M. (2006). Cigarette smoking and nocturnal sleep architecture. *American Journal of Epidemiology*, *164*(6), 529–537. https://doi.org/10.1093/aje/kwj231.

Disturbed Sleep Pattern Domain 4 Activity/rest Class 1 Sleep/rest

Judith Ann Floyd, PhD, RN, FNAP, FAAN

NANDA-I

Definition

Time-limited awakenings due to external factors.

Defining Characteristics

Difficulty in daily functioning; difficulty initiating sleep; difficulty maintaining sleep state; expresses dissatisfaction with sleep; expresses tiredness; nonrestorative sleep-wake cycle; unintentional awakening

Related Factors

Disruption caused by sleep partner; environmental disturbances; insufficient privacy

Associated Conditions

Immobilization

NOC (Nursing Outcomes Classification)

Suggested NOC Outcomes

Personal Well-Being; Rest; Sleep

Example NOC Outcome with Indicators

Sleep as evidenced by the following indicators: Hours of sleep/Sleep pattern/Sleep quality/Sleep efficiency/Feels rejuvenated after sleep. (Rate the outcome and indicators of **Sleep:** 1 = severely compromised, 2 = substantially compromised, 3 = moderately compromised, 4 = mildly compromised, 5 = not compromised [see Section I].)

S

Client Outcomes

Client Will (Specify Time Frame)

- Verbalize plan to implement sleep promotion routines
- Maintain a regular schedule of sleep and waking
- Fall asleep without difficulty
- Remain asleep throughout the night
- Awaken naturally, feeling refreshed and is not fatigued during day

NIC (Nursing Interventions Classification)

Suggested NIC Intervention

Sleep Enhancement

Example NIC Activities—Sleep Enhancement

Determine external factors leading to sleep fragmentation; Reduce environmental disrupters of sleep

Nursing Interventions and *Rationales*

- Assess the client's sleep environment to determine its adequacy for providing undisturbed sleep. EB: *Disturbed sleep can have a detrimental impact on health and extend client recovery (Garside et al, 2018).* EBN: *Animal model studies conducted by nurse scientists suggest associations between sleep fragmentation and physical health parameters (e.g., mean arterial blood pressure and the gut microbiome/fecal metabolome), which is an association that provides insight into possible links between disrupted sleep and cardiovascular pathology (Maki et al, 2020).*
- Obtain a sleep history to identify the following: (1) the client's perception of smells, noise, and light levels in the sleep environment; (2) the client's preferred bedding; (3) client activities occurring in the sleep environment during hours of sleep, including use of handheld technology; (4) number of times the client typically awakens during the sleep period; and (5) when, during the sleep period, time is available for undisturbed sleep. EBN: *A qualitative study of hospital staff, clients, and their surrogates (n = 38) showed that many factors influenced clients' perceptions of sleep disturbances in the intensive care unit (ICU), but most environmental disturbances during hospitalization were caused by noise, light, and provision of care (Ding et al, 2017).* EBN: *Using qualitative methods, the lived experience of clients' sleep in hospitals as perceived by nurses (n = 14) included several environmental factors that disturbed clients' sleep, including uncomfortable beds, mattresses, and pillows, as well as light and noise levels, room temperatures, and smells (Honkavuo, 2018).*
- Keep environment as quiet as possible during sleep periods. EB: *A descriptive study of environmental characteristics in a 12-bed rehabilitation unit found that average noise levels were above recommended levels, and abrupt increases in noise levels were high enough to cause sleep fragmentation (Yelden et al, 2015).* EBN: *An evidence review of 51 papers showed that noise remains a persistent disruption to sleep at night in hospitals and continues to register as a concern on client satisfaction surveys (Fillary et al, 2015).*
- Consider masking hospital noise that cannot be eliminated. CEB: *In a systematic review of nine experimental studies, nurse researchers found that recorded natural sounds, music, and music videos were effective for masking noise in health care settings (Hellström et al, 2011).*
- Offer earplugs when feasible. EBN: *Results from an experimental study of subjects in intensive care (n = 50) showed that perceptions of nighttime noise decreased significantly in subjects who used earplugs (Hu et al, 2015).* EBN: *In a quasi-experimental clinical study of 135 cardiac care unit subjects, Iranian nurse researchers found that the combined use of earplugs and eye masks reduced self-reported sleep disruption (Tabas et al, 2019).*
- Dim the lights during sleep periods. CEB: *A sequential prestudy/poststudy (n = 171) found that the number of awakenings decreased when monitored lighting levels were part of a multicomponent program to decrease sleep disruption in intensive care (Patel et al, 2014).*
- Offer eye covers when lighting cannot be dimmed. EBN: *Results from an experimental study of subjects in intensive care (n = 50) showed that a combination of nonpharmacological interventions that included eye covers was useful for promoting sleep in ICU adult subjects (Hu et al, 2015).* EBN: *In a quasi-experimental clinical study of 135 cardiac care unit subjects, Iranian nurse researchers found that the combined use of earplugs and eye masks reduced self-reported sleep disruption (Tabas et al, 2019).*

✱ Be aware that use of eye covers in intubated clients may lead to sensory deprivation and anxiety. CEB: *An experimental study of eye cover use in ICU subjects (n = 18) reported less sleep fragmentation, but 72% of intubated subjects refused eye covers or removed them prematurely because of restlessness (30%), discomfort (20%), or anxiety (11%) (Simons et al, 2012).*

- Negotiate use of handheld technology whenever clients have access to electronic devices in the care setting. EB: *A representative survey of 1508 adults found that 90% of Americans used some type of electronics at least a few nights per week before bedtime and also found that adults who reported use of e-readers had reduced evening sleepiness, took longer to fall asleep, and reported reduced next-morning alertness compared with adults who read printed books at bedtime (Chang et al, 2015).*
- Consolidate essential care to provide the opportunity for uninterrupted sleep the first 3 to 4 hours of the sleep period. Follow with periods of 90 to 110 minutes between interruptions. CEB: *In a meta-analysis using data from 159 studies a nurse researcher found that the deepest stages of sleep occurred during the first 3 to 4 hours of the sleep period followed by several 90- to 110-minute sleep cycles that consisted of increasingly lower percentages of deep sleep (Floyd, 2002).*
- If the client must be disturbed during the first 3 to 4 hours of the sleep period, attempt to protect 90- to 110-minute blocks of time between awakenings. CEB: *In three studies of hospitalized subjects, nurse*

S

researchers found that the high frequency of nocturnal care interactions left subjects with no 90-minute blocks of uninterrupted time for sleep (Missildine, 2008; Missildine et al, 2010a,b). CEB: *In an experimental study that included protocols for consolidating care, the number of subject nights that contained a 3-hour window of uninterrupted sleep was increased (Patel et al, 2014).*

- When feasible, schedule newly ordered medications to avoid the need to wake the client the first few hours of the night. CEB: *A survey of sleep promotion protocols (n = 68) conducted by nurse researchers identified the need for nurses to plan ahead when initiating new medication regimens to help ensure uninterrupted sleep periods (Hofhuis et al, 2012).*
- Combine the previously mentioned interventions as feasible to create a sleep-promotion care bundle. EBN: *A qualitative study describing how experienced nurses promote sleep in hospitals* (n = 8) *identified use of a comprehensive set of cost-effective sleep-promoting measures that adapted the hospital environment for sleep and also reduced the use of sedative drugs (Salzmann-Erikson et al, 2016).* EB: *A critical appraisal of evidence from eight quantitative and qualitative studies showed that both ICU and acute ward settings affect subjects' sleep and use the same sleep-promoting strategies, including use of pharmacological aids and nonpharmacological aids (reducing noise and disturbances, eye masks, earplugs, and educational and staff behavioral changes) (Aparício & Panin, 2020).*
- Assess for medications and other stimulants that fragment sleep. Use caution when administering sleep medications. See Nursing Interventions and Rationales for **Insomnia.**

Pediatric

* ✱ Adapt interventions described above with caution because of limited empirical evidence regarding the effects of their use for pediatric clients. CEB: *A survey of 341 pediatric critical care providers worldwide found that use of earplugs, eye masks, noise reduction, and lighting optimization for sleep promotion was uncommon (Kudchadkar et al, 2014).* EBN: *During a focus-group study, nurses* (n = 30) *working on general and critical-care pediatric units identified several interrelated factors that create challenges to promoting children's sleep in hospitals and highlighted the need for formal policy and mentoring related to provision of nursing care at night in pediatric settings (Stremler et al, 2015).*
- Assess use of evening and nighttime texting and consider limiting as needed to protect sleep. EBN: *A study of 278 community-based teens found that sending and/or receiving text messages at night was significantly associated with later bedtimes, shorter time in bed, daytime tiredness, and irregular sleep habits (Garmy & Ward, 2018).*

Geriatric

- Most interventions discussed above can all be adapted for use with geriatric clients.
- Use of earplugs and eye covers with ataxic clients and clients with dementia may contribute to disorientation. CEB: *A case report and integrative review of the literature suggested that sensory deficits in subjects with dementia, which can be augmented by use of earplugs and eye covers, decrease their quality of life, increase their risk for delirium and falls, and pose a higher risk for poor outcomes (Haque et al, 2012).*

S

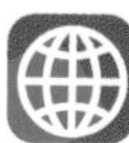

Multicultural

* ✱ Be aware that cultural sleep practices may alter the kinds of environmental sleep disruptors that require management. CEB: *As the result of an integrative review of the literature on family sleep practices, nurse scholars found that bed sharing and other aspects of the sleep environment were influenced most by ethnic factors (Jain et al, 2011).*

Home Care

- Consider the unique characteristics of each home sleep environment when addressing sleep disruption. CEB: *A longitudinal study of postpartum women* (n = 142) *showed that new mothers' sleep was disturbed 56% of the time by their infant's cries, but other environmental disrupters included (1) family, friends, and pets in the home; (2) sleeping with the television on; (3) traffic sounds; and (4) other outside noise from neighbors (Doering, 2013).*
- In addition, see the Home Care section of Nursing Interventions and Rationales for Readiness for Enhanced **Sleep.**

REFERENCES

Aparício, C., & Panin, F. (2020). Interventions to improve inpatients' sleep quality in intensive care units and acute wards: A literature review. *British Journal of Nursing, 29*(13), 770–776. https://doi.org/10.12968/bjon.2020.29.13.770.

Chang, A. M., Aeschbach, D., Duffy, J. F., & Czeisler, C. A. (2015). Evening use of light-emitting eReaders negatively affects sleep, circadian timing, and next-morning alertness. *Proceedings of the National Academy of Sciences of the United States of America, 112*(4), 1232–1237. https://doi.org/10.1073/pnas.1418490112.

Ding, Q., Redeker, N. S., Pisani, M. A., Yaggi, H. K., & Knauert, M. P. (2017). Factors influencing patients' sleep in the intensive care unit: Perceptions of patients and clinical staff. *American Journal of Critical Care, 26*(4), 278–286. https://doi.org/10.4037/ajcc2017333.

Doering, J. J. (2013). The physical and social environment of sleep in socioeconomically disadvantaged postpartum women. *Journal of Obstetric, Gynecologic, and Neonatal Nursing, 42*(1), E33–E43. https://doi.org/10.1111/j.1552-6909.2012.01421.x.

Fillary, J., Chaplin, H., Jones, G., Thompson, A., Holme, A., & Wilson, P. (2015). Noise at night in hospital general wards: A mapping of the literature. *British Journal of Nursing, 24*(10), 536–540. https://doi.org/10.12968/bjon.2015.24.10.536.

Floyd, J. A. (2002). Sleep and aging. *Nursing Clinics of North America, 37*(4), 719–731. Retrieved from https://pubmed.ncbi.nlm.nih.gov/12587370/. [Accessed 23 February 2022].

Garmy, P., & Ward, T. M. (2018). Sleep habits and nighttime texting among adolescents. *Journal of School Nursing, 34*(2), 121–127. https://doi.org/10.1177/1059840517704964.

Garside, J., Stephenson, J., Curtis, H., Morrell, M., Dearnley, C., & Astin, F. (2018). Are noise reduction interventions effective in adult ward settings? A systematic review and meta analysis. *Applied Nursing Research, 44*, 6–17. https://doi.org/10.1016/j.apnr.2018.08.004.

Haque, R., Abdelrehman, N., & Alavi, Z. (2012). "There's a monster under my bed": Hearing aids and dementia in long-term care settings. *Annals of Long-Term Care, 20*(8), 28–33. Retrieved from https://www.managedhealthcareconnect.com/articles/theres-monster-under-my-bed-hearing-aids-and-dementia-long-term-care-settings. [Accessed 23 February 2022].

Hellström, A., & Willman, A. (2011). Promoting sleep by nursing interventions in health care settings: A systematic review. *Worldviews on Evidence-Based Nursing, 8*(3), 128–142. https://doi.org/10.1111/j.1741-6787.2010.00203.x.

Hofhuis, J. G. M., Langevoort, G., Rommes, J. H., & Spronk, P. E. (2012). Sleep disturbances and sedation practices in the intensive care unit: A postal survey in The Netherlands. *Intensive and Critical Care Nursing, 28*(3), 141–149. https://doi.org/10.1016/j.iccn.2011.10.006.

Honkavuo, L. (2018). Nurses' experiences of supporting sleep in hospitals—A hermeneutical study. *International Journal of Caring Sciences, 11*(1), 4–10. Retrieved from www.internationaljournalofcaringsciences.org. [Accessed 17 October 2020].

Hu, R. F., Jiang, X. Y., Hegadoren, K. M., & Zhang, Y. H. (2015). Effects of earplugs and eye masks combined with relaxing music on sleep, melatonin and cortisol levels in ICU patients: A randomized controlled trial. *Critical Care, 19*(1), 115. https://doi.org/10.1186/s13054-015-0855-3.

Jain, S., Romack, R., & Jain, R. (2011). Bed sharing in school-age children—clinical and social implications. *Journal of Child and Adolescent Psychiatric Nursing, 24*(3), 185–189. https://doi.org/10.1111/j.1744-6171.2011.00293.x.

Kudchadkar, S. R., Yaster, M., & Punjabi, N. M. (2014). Sedation, sleep promotion, and delirium screening practices in the care of mechanically ventilated children: A wake-up call for the pediatric critical care community. *Critical Care Medicine, 42*(7), 1592–1600. https://doi.org/10.1097/CCM.0000000000000326.

Maki, K. A., Burke, L. A., Calik, M. W., et al. (2020). Sleep fragmentation increases blood pressure and is associated with alterations in the gut microbiome and fecal metabolome in rats. *Physiological Genomics, 52*(7), 280–292. https://doi.org/10.1152/physiolgenomics.00039.2020.

Missildine, K. (2008). Sleep and the sleep environment of older adults in acute care settings. *Journal of Gerontological Nursing, 34*(6), 15–21. https://doi.org/10.3928/00989134-20080601-06.

Missildine, K., Bergstrom, N., Meininger, J., Richards, K., & Foreman, M. D. (2010a). Case studies: Is the sleep of hospitalized elders related to delirium? *Medsurg Nursing, 19*(1), 39–46. Retrieved from https://pubmed.ncbi.nlm.nih.gov/20336983/. [Accessed 23 February 2022].

Missildine, K., Bergstrom, N., Meininger, J., Richards, K., & Foreman, M. D. (2010b). Sleep in hospitalized elders: A pilot study. *Geriatric Nursing, 31*(4), 263–272. https://doi.org/10.1016/j.gerinurse.2010.02.013.

Patel, J., Baldwin, J., Bunting, P., & Laha, S. (2014). The effect of a multicomponent multidisciplinary bundle of interventions on sleep and delirium in medical and surgical intensive care patients. *Anaesthesia, 69*(6), 540–549. https://doi.org/10.1111/anae.12638.

Salzmann-Erikson, M., Lagerqvist, L., & Pousette, S. (2016). Keep calm and have a good night: Nurses' strategies to promote inpatients' sleep in the hospital environment. *Scandinavian Journal of Caring Sciences, 30*(2), 356–364. https://doi.org/10.1111/scs.12255.

Simons, K. S., van den Boogaard, M., & de Jager, C. P. C. (2012). Reducing sensory input in critically ill patients: Are eye-masks a blind spot? *Critical Care, 16*(4), 439. https://doi.org/10.1186/cc11402.

Stremler, R., Adams, S., & Dryden-Palmer, K. (2015). Nurses' views of factors affecting sleep for hospitalized children and their families: A focus group study. *Research in Nursing & Health, 38*(4), 311–322. https://doi.org/10.1002/nur.21664.

Tabas, E. E., Khodadadi, F., Sarani, H., Saeedinezhad, F., & Jahantigh, M. (2019). Effect of eye masks, earplugs, and quiet time protocol on sleep quality of patients admitted to the cardiac care unit: A clinical trial study. *International Journal of Medical Surgical Nursing, 8*(3), e98762. https://doi.org/10.5812/msnj.98762.

Yelden, K., Duport, S., Kempny, A., & Playford, E. D. (2015). A rehabilitation unit at night: Environmental characteristics of patient rooms. *Disability & Rehabilitation, 37*(1), 91–96. https://doi.org/10.3109/09638288.2014.906662.

S

Impaired Social Interaction

Domain 7 Role relationship Class 3 Role performance

Marina Martinez-Kratz, MS, RN, CNE

NANDA-I

Definition

Insufficient or excessive quantity or ineffective quality of social exchange.

Defining Characteristics

Anxiety during social interaction; dysfunctional interaction with others; expresses difficulty establishing satisfactory reciprocal interpersonal relations; expresses difficulty functioning socially; expresses difficulty performing social roles; expresses discomfort in social situations; expresses dissatisfaction with social connection; family reports altered interaction; inadequate psychosocial support system; inadequate use of social status toward others; low levels of social activities; minimal interaction with others; reports unsatisfactory social engagement; unhealthy competitive focus; unwillingness to cooperate with others

Related Factors

Altered self-concept; depressive symptoms; disturbed thought processes; environmental constraints; impaired physical mobility; inadequate communication skills; inadequate knowledge about how to enhance mutuality; inadequate personal hygiene; inadequate social skills; inadequate social support; maladaptive grieving; neurobehavioral manifestations; sociocultural dissonance

At-Risk Population

Individuals without a significant other

Associated Conditions

Halitosis; mental diseases; neurodevelopmental disorders; therapeutic isolation

NOC (Nursing Outcomes Classification)

Suggested NOC Outcomes

Child Development: Middle Childhood, Adolescence; Play Participation; Role Performance; Social Interaction Skills; Social Involvement

Example NOC Outcome with Indicators

Social Involvement as evidenced by the following indicator: Interacts with close friends, neighbors, family members, and members of work groups. (Rate the outcome and indicators of **Social Involvement:** 1 = never demonstrated, 2 = rarely demonstrated, 3 = sometimes demonstrated, 4 = often demonstrated, 5 = consistently demonstrated [see Section I].)

S

Client Outcomes

Client Will (Specify Time Frame)

- Identify barriers that cause impaired social interactions
- Discuss feelings that accompany impaired and successful social interactions
- Use available opportunities to practice interactions
- Use successful social interaction behaviors
- Report increased comfort in social situations
- Communicate, state feelings of belonging, demonstrate caring and interest in others
- Report effective interactions with others

NIC (Nursing Interventions Classification)

Suggested NIC Intervention

Socialization Enhancement

Example NIC Activities—Socialization Enhancement

Encourage patience in developing relationships; Help client increase awareness of strengths and limitations in communicating with others

Nursing Interventions and *Rationales*

- Encourage the client to keep a gratitude journal. **EB:** *A study demonstrated that study participants who participated in a gratitude journal intervention experienced more positive emotions during social interactions (Drążkowski, Kaczmarek, & Kashdan, 2017).*
- Encourage dancing with Parkinson's programs for individuals with Parkinson's disease. **EB:** *Research demonstrated that dance programs provide opportunities for social interaction and nonverbal communication (Bognar et al, 2017).*
- Consider use of social cognition and interaction training (SCIT) to improve social functioning. **EB:** *Study findings suggest that individuals with serious mental illness showed improved emotion recognition skills, assertive behavior, improved relationship quality, and perceived more support from colleagues in social and professional relationships (Nienow et al, 2019).*
- Consider use of animal-assisted therapy (AAT). **EB:** *An AAT treatment group showed improvement in negative symptoms of schizophrenia such as apathy, asociality, anhedonia, and alogia (Calvo et al, 2016).*
- Encourage visually challenged clients to use text-based computer-mediated communications to facilitate social interaction. **EB:** *A study suggested that the lack of visual cues in text-based computer-mediated communications (CMCs) supported the daily social communication of visually challenged individuals (Okonji et al, 2019).*
- Provide management strategies to individuals experiencing auditory hallucinations. **EBN:** *Based on their research, Wang et al (2019) suggest that teaching people with schizophrenia to manage auditory hallucination will enhance their social interaction.*
- Refer to care plans for Risk for **Loneliness** and **Social** Isolation for additional interventions.

Pediatric

- Assess children with social impairments for experiences of bullying or victimization. **EB:** *A study found that children with autism spectrum disorder (ASD) experience more frequent bullying victimization compared to their neurotypical peers due to the increased risk of not being aware of the social situation (Forrest, Kroeger, & Stroope, 2020).*
- For adolescent clients, consider use of a peer network intervention to increase social interactions. **EB:** *Study results indicate that peer networks are effective at increasing social interactions of secondary students with ASD (Sreckovic, Hume, & Able, 2017).*
- Provide supervised interaction opportunities for children of chronically ill parents. **EBN:** *Research has identified that social isolation is a challenge for children with parents who experience chronic disabling pain (Umberger, Risko, & Covington, 2015).*
- Encourage family style dining (FSD) for preschool children to promote social interactions during mealtimes. **EB:** *A study showed that rates of interactions were increased during FSD (Lochetta, Barton, & Kaiser, 2017).*
- Use peer-mediated interaction (PMI) to increase social interactions of children on the autistic spectrum. **EB:** *A review of studies showed that PMI was an effective intervention to increase social interaction intervention for promoting social interaction between students with ASD and their peers (Watkins et al, 2015).*
- Consider Social Story with self-modeling for children with autism spectrum disorder. **EB:** *A study found that reading a Social Story with self-modeling that illustrated appropriate social behaviors improved children's initiations, responses, and affect (Youn Kang & Kim, 2020).*
- Encourage a responsive parenting style for parents of children with autism spectrum disorder. **EB:** *Structural equation models revealed that responsive parenting positively predicted prospective growth in social skills as reported by teachers (Caplan, Blacher, & Eisenhower, 2019).*

▲ Refer children with autism spectrum disorder to "Play Time/Social Time" (PT/ST) and "I Can Problem Solve" (ICPS) programs. **EB:** *A study indicated that the PT/ST program was more effective than ICPS in developing interaction skills, but both programs improved children's ability to cope with difficult social situations (Szumski et al, 2019).*

S

Geriatric

- Assess older clients for hearing loss and refer for hearing aids as needed. EB: *A study demonstrated that hearing aid fitting was associated with a subsequent improvement in older person–specific quality of life (Yamada, Švejdíková, & Kisvetrová, 2017).*
- Encourage socialization through physical activity and meaningful activities incorporated into normal daily care practices. EB: *A study showed that when activities were performed, residents of a green care farm were more engaged and had more social interaction (de Boer et al, 2017).*
- Provide live concert music for clients with dementia. EB: *A study showed that clients with mild to midstage dementia had increased levels of cooperation, interaction, and conversation after a live music concert (Shibazaki & Marshall, 2017).*
- ▲ Refer depressed clients to services for cognitive-behavioral therapy (CBT). EB: *A systematic review indicated that CBT was likely to be efficacious for depression and accompanying symptoms such as impaired social functioning in older people (Jayasekara et al, 2015).*
- Refer to care plans for **Frail** Elderly Syndrome, Risk for **Loneliness,** and **Social** Isolation for additional interventions.

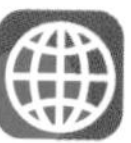

Multicultural

- Approach individuals of color with respect, warmth, and professional courtesy. EBN: *To provide person- and family-centered care, nurses must acknowledge their cultural differences, be willing to incorporate their beliefs within the health care treatment plan, and respect the values and lifeways of differing cultures (Hart & Mareno, 2014).*
- Use professional interpreters as needed. EBN: *Professional interpreters are the standard of care and will meet The Joint Commission requirements for addressing language barriers (Squires, 2018).*
- Refer to care plan for **Social** Isolation for additional interventions.

Home Care

- Previously discussed interventions may be adapted for home care use.

Client/Family Teaching and Discharge Planning

- Previously discussed interventions may be adapted for client/family teaching and discharge planning.

REFERENCES

Bognar, S., DeFaria, A. M., O'Dwyer, C., et al. (2017). More than just dancing: Experiences of people with Parkinson's disease in a therapeutic dance program. *Disability and Rehabilitation, 39*(11), 1073–1078. https://doi.org/10.1080/09638288.2016.1175037.

Calvo, P., Fortuny, J. R., Guzmán, S., et al. (2016). Animal assisted therapy (AAT) program as a useful adjunct to conventional psychosocial rehabilitation for patients with schizophrenia: Results of a small-scale randomized controlled trial. *Frontiers in Psychology, 7*, 631. https://doi.org/10.3389/fpsyg.2016.00631.

Caplan, B., Blacher, J., & Eisenhower, A. (2019). Responsive parenting and prospective social skills development in early school-aged children with autism spectrum disorder. *Journal of Autism & Developmental Disorders, 49*(8), 3203–3217. https://doi.org/10.1007/s10803-019-04039-4.

de Boer, B., Hamers, J. P. H., Zwakhalen, S. M. G., Tan, F. E. S., Beerens, H. C., & Verbeek, H. (2017). Green care farms as innovative nursing homes, promoting activities and social interaction for people with dementia. *Journal of the American Medical Directors Association, 18*(1), 40–46. https://doi.org/10.1016/j.jamda.2016.10.013.

Drążkowski, D., Kaczmarek, L. D., & Kashdan, T. B. (2017). Gratitude pays: A weekly gratitude intervention influences monetary decisions, physiological responses, and emotional experiences during a trust-related social interaction. *Personality and Individual Differences, 110*, 148–153. https://doi.org/10.1016/j.paid.2017.01.043.

Forrest, D. L., Kroeger, R. A., & Stroope, S. (2020). Autism spectrum disorder symptoms and bullying victimization among children with autism in the United States. *Journal of Autism & Developmental Disorders, 50*(2), 560–571. https://doi.org/10.1007/s10803-019-04282-9.

Hart, P. L., & Mareno, N. (2014). Cultural challenges and barriers through the voices of nurses. *Journal of Clinical Nursing, 23*(15-16), 2223–2233.

Jayasekara, R., Procter, N., Harrison, J., et al. (2015). Cognitive behavioural therapy for older adults with depression: A review. *Journal of Mental Health, 24*(3), 168–171.

Lochetta, B. M., Barton, E. E., & Kaiser, A. (2017). Using family style dining to increase social interactions in young children. *Topics in Early Childhood Special Education, 37*(1), 54–64. https://doi.org/10.1177.0271121416678078.

Nienow, T., Schulte, C., Tourville, T., Spann, D., Strom, T., & Harris, J. I. (2019). F119. Assessment of social cognition and interaction training for individuals with serious mental illness: impact on social cognitive abilities and role functioning. *Schizophrenia Bulletin, 45*(Suppl. 2), S298–S299. https://doi.org/10.1093/schbul/sbz018.531.

Okonji, P. E., Bailey, C., Lhussier, M., & Cattan, M. (2019). Adaptation to loss of visual function: implications for rehabilitation on subtle nuances of communication. *Activities, Adaptation & Aging, 43*(3), 169–185. https://doi.org/10.1080/01924788.2018.1500056.

Shibazaki, K., & Marshall, N. A. (2017). Exploring the impact of music concerts in promoting well-being in dementia care. *Aging & Mental Health, 21*(5), 468–476. https://doi.org/10.1080/13607863.2015.1114589.

S

Squires, A. (2018). Strategies for overcoming language barriers in healthcare. *Nursing Management*, *49*(4), 20–27. https://doi.org/10.1097/01.NUMA.0000531166.24481.15.

Sreckovic, M., Hume, K., & Able, H. (2017). Examining the efficacy of peer network interventions on the social interactions of high school students with autism spectrum disorder. *Journal of Autism & Developmental Disorders*, *47*(8), 2556–2574. https://doi.org/10.1007/s10803-017-3171-8.

Szumski, G., Smogorzewska, J., Grygiel, P., & Orlando, A. M. (2019). Examining the effectiveness of naturalistic social skills training in developing social skills and theory of mind in preschoolers with ASD. *Journal of Autism & Developmental Disorders*, *49*(7), 2822–2837. https://doi.org/10.1007/s10803-017-3377-9.

Umberger, W. A., Risko, J., & Covington, E. (2015). The forgotten ones: Challenges and needs of children living with disabling parental chronic pain. *Journal of Pediatric Nursing*, *30*(3), 498–507.

Wang, T. T., Beckstead, J. W., & Yang, C. Y. (2019). Social interaction skills and depressive symptoms in people diagnosed with schizophrenia: The mediating role of auditory hallucinations. *International Journal of Mental Health Nursing*, *28*(6), 1318–1327. https://doi.org/10.1111/inm.12643.

Watkins, L., O'Reilly, M., Kuhn, M., et al. (2015). A review of peer-mediated social interaction interventions for students with autism in inclusive settings. *Journal of Autism and Developmental Disorders*, *45*(4), 1070–1083. https://doi.org/10.1007/s10803-014-2264-x.

Yamada, Y., Švejdíková, B., & Kisvetrová, H. (2017). Improvement of older-person-specific QOL after hearing aid fitting and its relation to social interaction. *Journal of Communication Disorders*, *67*, 14–21. https://doi.org/10.1016/j.jcomdis.2017.05.001.

Youn Kang, V., & Kim, S. (2020). Social Stories™ with self-modeling to teach social play behaviors to Korean American children with autism. *Child & Family Behavior Therapy*, *42*(2), 73–97. https://doi.org/10.1080/07317107.2020.1738709.

Social Isolation Domain 12 Comfort Class 3 Social comfort

Marina Martinez-Kratz, MS, RN, CNE

NANDA-I

Definition

A state in which the individual lacks a sense of relatedness connected to positive, lasting, and significant interpersonal relationships.

Defining Characteristics

Expresses dissatisfaction with respect from others; expresses dissatisfaction with social connection; expresses dissatisfaction with social support; expresses loneliness; flat affect; hostility; impaired ability to meet expectations of others; low levels of social activities; minimal interaction with others; preoccupation with own thoughts; purposelessness; reduced eye contact; reports feeling different from others; reports feeling insecure in public; sad affect; seclusion imposed by others; sense of alienation; social behavior incongruent with cultural norms; social withdrawal

Related Factors

Difficulty establishing satisfactory reciprocal interpersonal relations; difficulty performing activities of daily living; difficulty sharing personal life expectations; fear of crime; fear of traffic; impaired physical mobility; inadequate psychosocial support system; inadequate social skills; inadequate social support; inadequate transportation; low self-esteem; negative perception of support system; neurobehavioral manifestations; values incongruent with cultural norms

At-Risk Population

Economically disadvantaged individuals; immigrants; individuals living alone; individuals living far from significant others; individuals moving to unfamiliar locations; individuals with history of rejection; individuals experiencing altered social role; individuals experiencing loss of significant other; individuals with history of traumatic event; individuals with ill family member; individuals with no children; institutionalized individuals; older adults; widowed individuals

Associated Conditions

Altered physical appearance; chronic disease; cognitive disorders

NOC (Nursing Outcomes Classification)

Suggested NOC Outcomes

Loneliness Severity; Mood Equilibrium; Personal Well-Being; Play Participation; Social Anxiety Level; Social Interaction Skills; Social Involvement; Social Support

Example NOC Outcome with Indicators

Social Involvement as evidenced by the following indicator: Interacts with close friends, neighbors, family members, and members of work groups. (Rate the outcome and indicators of **Social Involvement:** 1 = never demonstrated, 2 = rarely demonstrated, 3 = sometimes demonstrated, 4 = often demonstrated, 5 = consistently demonstrated [see Section I].)

Client Outcomes

Client Will (Specify Time Frame)

- Identify feelings of isolation
- Practice social and communication skills needed to interact with others
- Initiate interactions with others; set and meet goals
- Participate in activities and programs at level of ability and desire
- Describe feelings of self-worth

NIC (Nursing Interventions Classification)

Suggested NIC Intervention

Socialization Enhancement

Example NIC Activities—Socialization Enhancement

Encourage patience in developing relationships; Help client increase awareness of strengths and limitations in communicating with others

Nursing Interventions and *Rationales*

- Assess the client's feelings regarding social isolation. EBN: *Feelings that contribute to the client's perception of social isolation may include loneliness, anger, fear, despair, and sadness (Hadi & Hadi, 2017).*
- Assess individuals in quarantine or other socially isolating situations for the negative psychological effects of social isolation. EB: *Most reviewed studies reported negative psychological effects of social isolation, including post-traumatic stress symptoms, confusion, and anger. Stressors included longer quarantine duration, infection fears, frustration, boredom, inadequate supplies, inadequate information, financial loss, and stigma (Brooks et al, 2020).*
- For individuals who require quarantine, provide clear rationale for quarantine and information about protocols, and ensure sufficient supplies are provided. Tell people what is happening and why, explain how long it will continue, provide meaningful activities for them to do while in quarantine, provide clear communication, ensure basic supplies (such as food, water, and medical supplies) are available, and reinforce a sense of altruism. EB: *If quarantine is essential, research results suggest that providers should take every measure to ensure that this experience is as tolerable as possible for people (Brooks et al, 2020).*
- Provide the client with social skills training. EB: *A study concluded that social skills training can improve cognitive, affective, and behavioral interactions in clients experiencing social isolation (Nihayati et al, 2017).*
- Encourage limits on social media use. EB: *Research shows that young adults with high social media use report feeling more socially isolated than their counterparts with lower social media use (Primack et al, 2017).*
- Recommend involvement in organizations and other activities that encourage socialization. EB: *Community support and participation in activities that promote social engagement can act as protective factors to counter social isolation (Ray et al, 2019).*
- See the care plan for Risk for **Loneliness.**

S

Pediatric

- Assess for experiences of bullying and/or cyberbullying. EBN: *Bullying may manifest as social isolation or school refusal in children (Nelson et al, 2018).*
- Encourage limits on technology and social media use for children and adolescents. EB: *Research shows that young adults with high social media use report feeling more socially isolated than their counterparts with lower social media use (Primack et al, 2017).*
- Provide positive social support and assist the child to identify supportive adults in their lives. EBN: *Social isolation can be diminished when children have access to an adult who provides a secure base of emotional support (Nelson et al, 2018).*
- Promote adequate sleep time. EB: *Social isolation is a risk factor for depression and anxiety in early adolescence, but adequate sleep may act as a protective factor (Richardson et al, 2019).*
- ▲ Refer children and adolescents to mental health treatment as necessary. EB: *A randomized controlled trial found that children of substance-abusing parents showed significant improvements in social isolation after implementation of a psychoeducational preventive intervention (Bröning et al, 2019).*
- ▲ Refer parents of disabled or seriously ill children to support groups. EB: *Participation in a family-oriented support group provides community support and possible solutions to common problems in a caring and trusting environment (Mitwalli, Rabaia, & Kienzler, 2018).*

Geriatric

- The interventions described previously may be adapted for use with older clients.
- Assess for risks and experiences associated with social isolation. EB: *Research shows that approximately one-quarter of community-dwelling Americans age 65 and older are considered to be socially isolated, and a significant proportion of adults in the United States report feeling lonely (National Academies of Sciences, Engineering, and Medicine, 2020).*
- Identify social engagement activities such as volunteering, engaging in social activities, and growing spirituality that are acceptable to the client. EB: *An integrative review found that productive engagement activities are associated with improvement of social isolation in older adults (Gardiner, Geldenhuys, & Gott, 2018).*
- ▲ Refer client to pet therapy or consider pet ownership if feasible. EB: *An integrative review found that individual pet therapy reduced isolation in older adults (Gardiner, Geldenhuys, & Gott, 2018).*
- Consider telephone outreach for isolated older individuals. EB: *The Yale Geriatrics Student Interest Group implemented the Telephone Outreach in the COVID-19 Outbreak Program at three nursing homes with initial success. Nursing home residents report looking forward to their weekly phone calls and gratitude for social connectedness (van Dyck et al, 2020).*
- Consider use of technology such as computers, video conferencing, Internet, or apps to alleviate or reduce loneliness or social isolation among older adults. EB: *An integrative review found that use of these technologies reduced isolation in older adults (Gardiner, Geldenhuys, & Gott, 2018).*
- Implement fall precautions for clients experiencing social isolation. EBN: *Logistic regression models revealed that social isolation significantly predicted falls (odds ratio [OR] = 1.11; 95% confidence interval [CI] [1.05, 1.17]). The relationship remained significant after adjusting for age, gender, and education (OR = 1.08; 95% CI [1.02, 1.14]) (Pohl et al, 2018).*

S

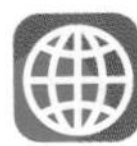

Multicultural

- The interventions described previously may be adapted for use with diverse clients.
- Assess for experiences of interpersonal and institutional racism. EB: *Experiences with overt racism and microaggressions are significantly associated with social isolation and other negative emotional responses (Ayón & Philbin, 2017).*

Home Care

- The interventions described previously may be adapted for home care use.
- Assist clients to interact and engage with neighbors when they move to a supported housing community. EB: *Clients transferring to supported housing will be placed in an unfamiliar environment that necessitates the need to develop skills to successfully adapt to their new surroundings (Kirchen & Hersch, 2015).*

Client/Family Teaching and Discharge Planning

- See the care plan for **Caregiver** Role Strain and Risk for **Loneliness.**

REFERENCES

Ayón, C., & Philbin, S. P. (2017). "Tú No Eres de Aquí": Latino children's experiences of institutional and interpersonal discrimination and microaggressions. *Social Work Research, 41*(1), 19–30. https://doi.org/10.1093/swr/svw028.

Bröning, S., Sack, P., Haevelmann, A., et al. (2019). A new preventive intervention for children of substance-abusing parents: Results of a randomized controlled trial. *Child & Family Social Work, 24*(4), 537–546. https://doi.org/10.1111/cfs.12634.

Brooks, S. K., Webster, R. K., Smith, L. E., et al. (2020). The psychological impact of quarantine and how to reduce it: Rapid review of the evidence. *The Lancet, 395*(10227), 912–920. https://doi.org/10.1016/S0140-6736(20)30460-8.

Gardiner, C., Geldenhuys, G., & Gott, M. (2018). Interventions to reduce social isolation and loneliness among older people: An integrative review. *Health and Social Care in the Community, 26*(2), 147–157. https://doi.org/10.1111/hsc.12367.

Hadi, H., & Hadi, S. (2017). Social isolation—a current reality in the corridors of our society. *Journal on Nursing, 7*(1), 29–33.

Kirchen, T. M., & Hersch, G. (2015). Understanding person and environment factors that facilitate veteran adaption to long-term care. *Physical & Occupational Therapy in Geriatrics, 33*(3), 204–219.

Mitwalli, S., Rabaia, Y., & Kienzler, H. (2018). Support groups for mothers of children with a handicap: A quantitative and qualitative study. *The Lancet, 391*(Suppl. 2), S47. https://doi.org/10.1016/S0140-6736(18)30413-6.

National Academies of Sciences, Engineering, and Medicine. (2020). *Social isolation and loneliness in older adults: Opportunities for the health care system*. Washington, DC: National Academies Press.

Nelson, H. J., Burns, S. K., Kendall, G. E., & Schonert-Reichl, K. A. (2018). The factors that influence and protect against power imbalance in covert bullying among preadolescent children at school: A thematic analysis. *The Journal of School Nursing, 34*(4), 281–291. https://doi.org/10.1177/1059840517748417.

Nihayati, H. E., Junata, A. S. P., Tristiana, R. D., & Yusuf, A. (2017). Effect of social skills training: Friendship clients of social interaction capabilities of social isolation. Proceedings of the 8th International Nursing Conference on Education, Practice and Research Development in Nursing (INC 2017). *Advances in Health Sciences Research, 3*, 143–147. https://doi.org/10.2991/inc-17.2017.37.

Pohl, J. S., Cochrane, B. B., Schepp, K. G., & Woods, N. F. (2018). Falls and social isolation of older adults in the national health and aging trends study. *Research in Gerontological Nursing, 11*(2), 61–70. https://doi.org/10.3928/19404921-20180216-02.

Primack, B. A., Shensa, A., Sidani, J. E., et al. (2017). Social media use and perceived social isolation among young adults in the U.S. *American Journal of Preventive Medicine, 53*(1), 1–8. https://doi.org/10.1016/j.amepre.2017.01.010.

Ray, M. E., Coon, J. M., Al-Jumaili, A. A., & Fullerton, M. (2019). Quantitative and qualitative factors associated with social isolation among graduate and professional health science students. *American Journal of Pharmaceutical Education, 83*(7), 6983. https://doi.org/10.5688/ajpe6983.

Richardson, C., Oar, E., Fardouly, J., et al. (2019). The moderating role of sleep in the relationship between social isolation and internalising problems in early adolescence. *Child Psychiatry and Human Development, 50*(6), 1011–1020. https://doi.org/10.1007/s10578-019-00901-9.

van Dyck, L. I., Wilkins, K. M., Ouellet, J., Ouellet, G. M., & Conroy, M. L. (2020). Combating heightened social isolation of nursing home elders: The telephone outreach in the COVID-19 outbreak program. *American Journal of Geriatric Psychiatry, 28*(9), 989–992. https://doi.org/10.1016/j.jagp.2020.05.026.

Chronic Sorrow Domain 9 Coping/stress tolerance Class 2 Coping responses

Tracy P. George, DNP, APRN-BC, CNE

NANDA-I

S

Definition

Cyclical, recurring, and potentially progressive pattern of pervasive sadness experienced (by a parent, caregiver, individual with chronic illness or disability) in response to continual loss, throughout the trajectory of an illness or disability.

Defining Characteristics

Expresses feeling that interferes with well-being; overwhelming negative feelings; sadness

Related Factors

Disability management crisis; illness management crisis; missed milestones; missed opportunities

At-Risk Population

Individuals experiencing developmental crisis; individuals experiencing loss of significant other; individuals working in caregiver role for prolonged period of time

Associated Conditions

Chronic disability; chronic disease

NOC (Nursing Outcomes Classification)

Suggested NOC Outcomes

Acceptance: Health Status; Depression Level; Depression Self-Control; Grief Resolution; Hope; Mood Equilibrium

Example NOC Outcome with Indicators

Grief Resolution with plans for a positive future as evidenced by the following indicators: Describes meaning of loss or death/Reports decreased preoccupation with loss/Reports adequate nutritional intake/Reports adequate sleep/Expresses positive expectations about the future. (Rate the outcome and indicators of **Grief Resolution:** 1 = never demonstrated, 2 = rarely demonstrated, 3 = sometimes demonstrated, 4 = often demonstrated, 5 = consistently demonstrated [see Section I].)

Client Outcomes

Client Will (Specify Time Frame)

- Express appropriate feelings of guilt, fear, anger, or sadness
- Identify problems associated with sorrow (e.g., changes in appetite, insomnia, nightmares, loss of libido, decreased energy, alteration in activity levels)
- Seek help in dealing with grief-associated problems
- Plan for the future one day at a time
- Function at normal developmental level

NIC (Nursing Interventions Classification)

Suggested NIC Interventions

Grief Work Facilitation; Grief Work Facilitation: Perinatal Death

Example NIC Activities—Grief Work Facilitation

Encourage client to verbalize memories of loss, both past and current; Assist client in identifying personal coping strategies

Nursing Interventions and *Rationales*

- Determine the client's degree of sorrow. CEB: *Use the Adapted Burke Questionnaire for the individual or caregiver, which assesses eight mood states (grief, shock, anger, disbelief, sadness, hopelessness, fear, and guilt) on a four-point scale (Whittingham et al, 2013).*
- Assess for the four discrete stages of grieving in clients with chronic disease. EB: *The four stages of grief for clients with chronic diseases can be assessed by the Acceptance of Disease and Impairments Questionnaire (Nistiandani et al, 2018).*
- Provide coping strategies for caregivers who may experience chronic sorrow. EBN: *Coping strategies for the caregivers of clients with schizophrenia may include discussing their feelings about the situation with others; reading; praying; being physically active; emotional strategies, such as crying; and cognitive strategies, such as thinking positively about the situation (Olwit et al, 2015). See care plan for* **Caregiver** Role Strain.
- Develop a trusting relationship to care for clients with chronic sorrow. EBN: *Nurses should offer compassion, empathy, consideration, and knowledge to those experiencing chronic sorrow (Glenn, 2015).*
- Provide information about support groups and counseling. EBN: *Support groups, counseling, and participating in activities are strategies that can be used with clients who are experiencing chronic sorrow (Marcella-Brienza & Mennillo, 2015).*
- Encourage use of positive coping techniques: EBN: *Encourage hobbies and physical activity for those experiencing chronic sorrow (Granek et al, 2016).*

▲ Refer the client for mental health services as needed. EB: *There may be an increase in depression among clients with chronic sorrow, so the nurse may need to refer the client for mental health care (Ghesquiere et al, 2016).*

S

▲ Refer clients for financial assistance as needed. EB: *Bereavement may be associated with financial burdens caused by the loss of income (Ghesquiere et al, 2016).*

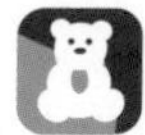

Pediatric

- Encourage the parents of children with uncommon diseases to use online resources to manage their chronic sorrow. EBN: *In a study of 16 mothers of children with a rare disease, online communication was used effectively to manage chronic sorrow (Glenn, 2015).*
- Educate parents that an increase in chronic sorrow can occur after stressful events. EB: *Worsening of the health care condition and when a child would have met developmental milestones can trigger chronic sorrow (Coughlin & Sethares, 2017).*
- Nurses should assess for chronic sorrow and discuss coping strategies for parents of children who have been in the neonatal intensive care unit (NICU). EB: *The loss an infant in the NICU can result in chronic sorrow among parents (Currie et al, 2019).*
- Educate parents that children may grieve differently than adults. EB: *Children may grieve intermittently for short periods of time in "grief puddles," certain children may grieve at each developmental stage, and some children may try to console their parents instead of going through the grieving process themselves (Gao & Slaven, 2017).*

▲ Refer grieving children to peer support groups. EB: *Peer support groups with other children who are grieving are important for children with chronic sorrow (Gao & Slaven, 2017).*

- Encourage children experiencing grief to participate in bereavement activities and camps. EB: *Hanlon et al (2018) found that family-based bereavement camps can be beneficial for parents and siblings who had experienced loss.*
- Encourage children who are grieving to participate in other forms of therapy, in addition to individual counseling and psychotherapy. EB: *Art therapy, play therapy, music therapy, and bibliotherapy are useful for children with chronic sorrow (Gao & Slaven, 2017).*
- Help the adolescent with chronic sorrow determine sources of support and refer for counseling if needed. EB: *Cognitive-behavioral therapy along with parental counseling has been useful in adolescents who experience prolonged grief (Spuij, Dekovic, & Boelen, 2015).*
- Provide family-centered care to parents of children with disabilities, and encourage parents to attend support groups. EB: *In a study of 75 children with cerebral palsy and their caregivers, Zuurmond et al (2018) found that support groups had a positive impact on the caregivers' quality of life scores, as well as their knowledge and confidence as a caregiver.*
- Encourage parents with chronic sorrow to participate in an online support group and learn coping strategies. EB: *Online bereavement support groups for parents who have lost children can be a convenient and anonymous way to obtain coping support (Elder & Burke, 2015).* EB: *Telehealth can be used to provide support groups especially in rural areas (Chang et al, 2016).*
- Parents of children with chronic illnesses may experience chronic sorrow. EB: *Six qualitative themes emerged from interviews of parents of children with chronic illnesses: surreality of diagnosis, unrealistic expectations, the battle, keeping it together, doing whatever it takes, and life goes on (Batchelor & Duke, 2019).*
- Provide information to parents who are experiencing chronic sorrow. EB: *Parents felt it was helpful when nurses provided information about the child's condition, procedures, resources, and funding sources (Coughlin & Sethares, 2017).*
- Respite care can be beneficial for parents of children with chronic illnesses. EB: *Respite care can be helpful for parents experiencing chronic sorrow who have a child with a chronic illnesses (Coughlin & Sethares, 2017).*
- Recognize that mothers who have a miscarriage or lose an infant often grieve and experience sorrow. EBN: *Providers should recognize that women who have experienced perinatal loss may have anxiety, and compassionate care should be provided (Moore & Côté-Arsenault, 2018).*

Geriatric

- Identify previous losses and assess the client for depression. EB: *The detection of depression is low in older adults; therefore, older adults should be screened for depression (Ghesquiere et al, 2018).*

- Evaluate the social support system of the older client and refer for bereavement counseling if needed. EB: *Bereavement support groups among older adults can result in improvement in grief, depression, and social support (Chow et al, 2019).*

Home Care

- In-home bereavement follow-up by nurses should be considered if available. EBN: *District nurses can be used to provide palliative care as well as bereavement visits after a loss (Johnson, 2015).*
- Assess the client for depression and refer for mental health services if appropriate. EB: *Clients experiencing bereavement are at risk for depression, so it is important to assess for depression (Ghesquierre et al, 2018).*
- Provide empathetic communication for family/caregivers. EB: *Nurses should offer compassion and empathy to those experiencing chronic sorrow (Glenn, 2015).*
- The interventions described previously may be adapted for home care use.
- See care plans for Chronic Low **Self-Esteem**, Risk for **Loneliness,** and **Hopelessness.**

REFERENCES

Batchelor, L. L., & Duke, G. (2019). Chronic sorrow in parents with chronically ill children. *Pediatric Nursing, 45*(4), 163–178. http://www.pediatricnursing.net/issues/19julaug/.

Chang, J. E., Sequeira, A., McCord, C. E., & Garney, W. R. (2016). Videoconference grief group counseling in rural Texas: Outcomes, challenges, and lessons learned. *Journal for Specialists in Group Work, 41*(2), 140–160. https://doi.org/10.1080/01933922.2016.1146376.

Chow, A. Y. M., Caserta, M., Lund, D., et al. (2019). Dual-process bereavement group intervention (DPBGI) for widowed older adults. *The Gerontologist, 59*(5), 983–994. https://doi.org/10.1093/geront/gny095.

Coughlin, M. B., & Sethares, K. A. (2017). Chronic sorrow in parents of children with a chronic illness or disability: An integrative literature review. *Journal of Pediatric Nursing, 37*, 108–116. https://doi.org/10.1016/j.pedn.2017.06.011.

Currie, E. R., Christian, B. J., Hinds, P. S., et al. (2019). Life after loss: Parent bereavement and coping experiences after infant death in the neonatal intensive care unit. *Death Studies, 43*(5), 333–342. https://doi.org/10.1080/07481187.2018.1474285.

Elder, J., & Burke, L. A. (2015). Parental grief expression in online cancer support groups. *Illness, Crises, and Loss, 23*(2), 175–190. https://doi.org/10.1177/1054137315576617.

Gao, M., & Slaven, M. (2017). Best practices in children's bereavement: A qualitative analysis of needs and services. *Journal of Pain Management, 10*(1), 119–126. Retrieved from https://search.proquest.com/openview/a2e78c7f648f69cf0c93a7d3a9b728c4/1?pq-origsite=gscholar&cbl=2034829. Accessed February 16, 2022.

Ghesquiere, A. R., Bazelais, K. N., Berman, J., Greenberg, R. L., Kaplan, D., & Bruce, M. L. (2016). Associations between recent bereavement and psychological and financial burden in homebound older adults. *Omega, 73*(4), 326–339. https://doi.org/10.1177/0030222815590709.

Ghesquiere, A. R., Pepin, R., Kinsey, J., Bartels, S. J., & Bruce, M. L. (2018). Factors associated with depression detection in a New Hampshire mental health outreach program. *Aging & Mental Health, 22*(11), 1471–1476. https://doi.org/10.1080/13607863.2017.1364346.

Glenn, A. D. (2015). Using online health communication to manage chronic sorrow: Mothers of children with rare diseases speak. *Journal of Pediatric Nursing, 30*(1), 17–24. https://doi.org/10.1016/j.pedn.2014.09.013.

Granek, L., Barrera, M., Scheinemann, K., & Bartels, U. (2016). Pediatric oncologists' coping strategies for dealing with patient death. *Journal of Psychosocial Oncology, 34*(1–2), 39–59. https://doi.org/10.1080/07347332.2015.1127306.

Hanlon, P., Guerin, S., & Kiernan, G. (2018). Reflections on the development of a therapeutic recreation-based bereavement camp for families whose child has died from serious illness. *Death Studies, 42*(9), 593–603. https://doi.org/10.1080/07481187.2017.1407012.

Johnson, A. (2015). Analysing the role played by district and community nurses in bereavement support. *British Journal of Community Nursing, 20*(6), 272–277. https://doi.org/10.12968/bjcn.2015.20.6.272.

Marcella-Brienza, S., & Mennillo, T. (2015). Back to work: Manager support of nurses with chronic sorrow. *Creative Nursing, 21*(4), 206–210. doi:10.1891/1078-4535.21.4.206.

Moore, S. E., & Côté-Arsenault, D. (2018). Navigating an uncertain journey of pregnancy after perinatal loss. *Illness, Crisis, and Loss, 26*(1), 58–74. https://doi.org/10.1177/1054137317740802.

Nistiandani, A., Juniarto, A. Z., & Dyan, N. S. (2018). The description of diabetics' acceptance stage toward diabetes mellitus' diagnoses. *Indonesian Journal of Nursing and Midwifery (Jurnal Ners dan Kebidanan Indonesia), 6*(1), 25–31. https://doi.org/10.21927/jnki.2018.6(1).25-31.

Olwit, C., Musisi, S., Leshabari, S., & Sanyu, I. (2015). Chronic sorrow: Lived experiences of caregivers of patients diagnosed with schizophrenia in Butabika Mental Hospital, Kampala, Uganda. *Archives of Psychiatric Nursing, 29*(1), 43–48. https://doi.org/10.1016/j.apnu.2014.09.007.

Spuij, M., Dekovic, M., & Boelen, P. A. (2015). An open trial of "grief-help": A cognitive-behavioural treatment for prolonged grief in children and adolescents. *Clinical Psychology & Psychotherapy, 22*(2), 185–192. https://doi.org/10.1002/cpp.1877.

Whittingham, K., Wee, D., Sanders, M. R., & Boyd, R. (2013). Sorrow, coping and resiliency: Parents of children with cerebral palsy share their experiences. *Disability & Rehabilitation, 35*(17), 1447–1452. https://doi.org/10.3109/09638288.2012.737081.

Zuurmond, M., O'Banion, D., Gladstone, M., et al. (2018). Evaluating the impact of a community-based parent training programme for children with cerebral palsy in Ghana. *PLoS One, 13*(9), e0202096. https://doi.org/10.1371/journal.pone.0202096.

S

Spiritual Distress Domain 10 Life principles Class 3 Value/belief/action congruence

Mary E. Desmond, PhD, RN, MA, MSN, AHN-BC and Barbara Baele Vinconsi, PhD, RN, FNP-BC

NANDA-I

Definition

A state of suffering related to the impaired ability to integrate meaning and purpose in life through connections with self, others, the world, or a superior being.

Defining Characteristics

Anger behaviors; crying; decreased expression of creativity; disinterested in nature; dysomnias; excessive guilt; expresses alienation; expresses anger; expresses anger toward power greater than self; expresses concern about beliefs; expresses concern about the future; expresses concern about values system; expresses concerns about family; expresses feeling abandoned by power greater than self; expresses feeling of emptiness; expresses feeling unloved; expresses feeling worthless; expresses insufficient courage; expresses loss of confidence; expresses loss of control; expresses loss of hope; expresses loss of serenity; expresses need for forgiveness; expresses regret; expresses suffering; fatigue; fear; impaired ability for introspection; inability to experience transcendence; maladaptive grieving; perceived loss of meaning in life; questions identity; questions meaning of life; questions meaning of suffering; questions own dignity; refuses to interact with others

Related Factors

Altered religious ritual; altered spiritual practice; anxiety; barrier to experiencing love; cultural conflict; depressive symptoms; difficulty accepting the aging process; inadequate environmental control; inadequate interpersonal relations; loneliness; loss of independence; low self-esteem; pain; perception of having unfinished business; self-alienation; separation from support system; social alienation; sociocultural deprivation; stressors; substance misuse

At-Risk Population

Individuals experiencing birth of a child; individuals experiencing death of a significant other; individuals experiencing infertility; individuals experiencing life transition; individuals experiencing racial conflict; individuals experiencing unexpected life event; individuals exposed to death; individuals exposed to natural disaster; individuals exposed to traumatic events; individuals receiving bad news; individuals receiving terminal care; individuals with low educational level

Associated Conditions

Chronic disease; depression; loss of body part; loss of function of a body part; treatment regimen

NOC (Nursing Outcomes Classification)

S

Suggested NOC Outcomes

Coping; Dignified Life Closure; Grief Resolution; Hope; Spiritual Health; Stress Level

Example NOC Outcome with Indicators

Spiritual Health as evidenced by the following indicators: Quality of faith, hope, meaning, and purpose in life/Connectedness with inner-self and with others to share thoughts, feelings, and beliefs. (Rate each indicator of **Spiritual Health:** 1 = severely compromised, 2 = substantially compromised, 3 = moderately compromised, 4 = mildly compromised, 5 = not compromised [see Section I].)

Client Outcomes

Client Will (Specify Time Frame)

- Express meaning and purpose in life
- Express sense of hope in the future
- Express sense of connectedness with self

- Express sense of connectedness with family/friends
- Express ability to forgive
- Express acceptance of health status
- Find meaning in relationships with others
- Find meaning in relationship with a higher power
- Find meaning in personal and health care treatment choices

NIC (Nursing Interventions Classification)

Suggested NIC Interventions

Active Listening, Forgiveness Facilitation, Grief Work Facilitation, Hope Inspiration, Humor, Music Therapy, Presence, Referral, Reminiscence Therapy, Self-Awareness Enhancement, Simple Guided Imagery, Simple Massage, Simple Relaxation Therapy, Spiritual Support, Therapeutic Touch, Touch

Example NIC Activities—Spiritual Support

Encourage use of spiritual resources if desired; Be available to listen to client's feelings

Nursing Interventions and *Rationales*

- Observe clients for cues indicating difficulties in finding meaning, purpose, or hope in life. EB: *In a correlational study of 132 participants with American Heart Association (AHA)/American College of Cardiology (ACC) classification of stage B heart failure, Mills et al (2015) found that spiritual well-being was associated with fewer depressive episodes, especially when focusing on increasing meaning and peace in clients' lives.* EB: *In a state of the science consensus report, spirituality included meaning and peace, hope, forgiveness, and gratitude (Steinhauser et al, 2017).*
- Observe seriously ill clients with poor prognosis or life-changing conditions for loss of meaning, purpose, and hope in life. EB: *A scoping review on inpatient spiritual distress with seriously ill clients and family experiences indicated that the majority of studies described clients' spiritual distress in relationship to self and others (Roze des Ordons et al, 2018).*
- Promote a sense of love, caring, and compassion in nursing encounters. EB: *Batstone et al (2020), in a systematic literature review to better understand provision of spiritual care by nurses at end of life using 11 studies (10 with palliative care nurses), found three themes: nurse value of holistic care; nurse–client relationship; and provision of nursing care that radiates warmth, love, and acceptance.*
- Be physically present and actively listen to the client. EBN: *Desmond et al (2018) developed a spiritual care for a veteran simulation and performance checklist based on a review of the literature, content validity expert review, and pilot testing with practicing nurses who care for veterans and found that spiritual care includes a caring presence and listening.* EBN: *In a cross-sectional, correlational study with (n = 554) tertiary care nurses, Mamier et al (2019) found that the top three mean scores of nurse self-reported frequency of spiritual therapeutics with clients/family were presence, listening, and spiritual assessment.*
- Assist clients to participate in their usual religious rituals or practices that support coping with cancer and its treatment. EB: *In a cross-sectional study with cancer clients in Brazil, Noronha Silva et al (2019) found that those who had negative religious/spiritual coping correlated to higher levels of spiritual distress (p <0.001) and those with positive religious coping (prayer/connection to God) had an inverse correlation to spiritual distress.*
- Help the client find a reason for living, be available for support, and promote hope. EB: *Swinton et al (2017) conducted 208 semistructured interviews with 70 dying clients, 76 family members, and 150 health care providers in an intensive care unit (ICU) to describe how spirituality was expressed during the dying process. The outcome was the development of a program to support the expressions of spirituality during the dying process (i.e., peace, connections, spiritually enhanced environments, and specific expressions of spirituality).*
- Respect the client's beliefs; avoid imposing your own spiritual beliefs on the client. Be aware of your own belief systems and accept the client's spirituality. EB: *In a state of the science consensus report, spirituality is not a monism but is holistic and infuses all aspects of being human and requires honoring individuality, promoting conversations, and capturing the breadth of experience (Steinhauser et al, 2017).*
- Monitor and promote supportive social contacts and spiritual and religious practices. EB: *In a meta-analytic review, Sherman et al (2015) found that those with greater spiritual and religious involvement have*

a greater ability to maintain satisfying social roles and relationships in individuals with cancer. EB: *In a qualitative study with cancer clients in Turkey, Cinar et al (2018) found three themes that promoted coping with cancer: hope in the future, strength from spiritual practices, and social support from family and friends.*

- Integrate and assist family in searching for meaning in the client's health care situation. EB: *A scoping review indicated that spirituality and spiritual practices can support resilience and coping with life-altering conditions, including spinal cord injury (Jones et al, 2016) and palliative care (Balboni et al, 2017).*
- Offer spiritual support to family and caregivers. EB: *In a state of the science report, clients and families who experience serious illness have spiritual needs (Balboni et al, 2017).* EB: *Borji et al (2019) found that Iranian caregivers of heart failure clients (n = 71) had significantly decreased anxiety levels (p = 0.001) 3 weeks after a spiritual care education program using pre-post methodology.*
- Screen for spiritual needs and if a need arises, offer chaplain referral. EB: *In a state of the science report, spiritual screening is an initial assessment for spiritual need, whereas chaplains provide a more in-depth assessment (Balboni et al, 2017).* EBN: *A qualitative descriptive study by Burkhart et al (2019) with nurses at a Veterans Affairs (VA) health system (n = 39) found that spiritual care actions when clients are in spiritual distress included referral to other professionals, including the chaplain for religious need, or nonreligious resources such as social worker.*
- Support mind–body interventions (e.g., meditation, guided imagery, relaxation, massage). Support outdoor activities. EB: *In a state of the science report, mind–body interventions are encouraged to promote spiritual healing (Balboni et al, 2017).*
- Encourage journaling. EB: *In a scoping review, Jones et al (2016) found use of narratives helpful in coping with spinal cord injury.* EB: *In a state of the science report, journaling was a spiritual care intervention (Balboni et al, 2017).*
- Provide privacy or a "sacred space." EB: *In a state of the science report, meditation and life review were spiritual care interventions that may require privacy (Balboni et al, 2017).*
- Integrate spiritual care in multiprofessional palliative care teams. EB: *A state of the science report indicated that multiprofessional palliative care teams incorporate a spiritual care component (Balboni et al, 2017).*
- Encourage life review at end of life, including recalling, evaluating, and integrating life experiences. EB: *A state of the science report indicated that life review enhanced a personal sense of legacy and promoted dignity when facing terminal illness (Balboni et al, 2017).*

Geriatric

- Offer opportunities to practice one's religion. EBN: *In a descriptive cross-sectional study of older adult clients admitted to a coronary care unit, Elham et al (2015) found a significant difference in the means between those who received spiritual care interventions by nurses regarding state-trait anxiety levels, but not in the control group.*

Pediatric

- Offer adolescents with cancer opportunities for reflection to express their spirituality and spiritual needs to enhance efficient coping strategies. EB: *In a single-group, quasi-experimental, pre-post study with 32 adolescents with one type of cancer in an Iranian hospital, Torabi et al (2018) found that participating in a 1:1 spiritual care program over six 45-minute sessions had a statistically significant difference between the pretest and posttest mean coping subscales (p < .001).*
- Foster spiritual activities among adolescents. EB: *Mirghafourvand et al (2016) found that in a sample of 520 Iranian adolescent girls, spiritual well-being was highly correlated with health-related quality of life (r = .60, p < .001).*

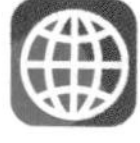

Multicultural

- Recognize the importance of spirituality and provide culturally competent spiritual care to specific populations:
  - African American. EBN: *One of four themes identified in analyzing secondary data with content analysis indicated that spirituality for African American women was a source of inner peace, joy, strength, hope, comfort, calm, coping, and other positive aspects contributing to well-being and potentially supportive of health-promoting behaviors (Conway-Phillips & Janusek, 2016).*
  - Latino/Hispanic. EB: *With diabetes having a high prevalence in the Hispanic population, Rivera-Hernandez (2016) found a positive relationship between religiosity/spirituality with diabetes care and blood sugar control in a sample of 2216 Latino/Hispanic population 50 years and older living in Mexico.*

S

- ❍ Muslim. **EBN:** *In a cross-sectional descriptive study by Akgül and Karadağ (2016), fecal ostomies were found to be a barrier to incorporating specific religious practices of salat, fasting, and pilgrimage in the lives of 150 Muslims postoperatively, providing an opportunity for nurses to assist clients in meeting their religious needs through adaptation or facilitation around this barrier.*
- ❍ Veterans of armed services. Recognize the unique spiritual needs of veterans and provide spiritual support or appropriate referrals. **EB:** *An exploratory study by Ganocy et al (2016) found an inverse relationship to suicidal ideation, posttraumatic stress disorder (PTSD), and alcohol use with existential and spiritual well-being for National Guard members who had ever been deployed overseas at least once.* **EB:** *Desmond et al (2018) developed a spiritual care for a veteran simulation and performance checklist based on a review of the literature, content validity expert review, and pilot testing with practicing nurses who care for veterans and found that spiritual care includes recognition of veteran culture environmental cues to past experiences and current veteran connections.*

Home Care

- ● All the nursing interventions described previously apply in the home setting.

REFERENCES

Akgül, B., & Karadağ, A. (2016). The effect of colostomy and ileostomy on acts of worship in the Islamic faith. *Journal of Wound, Ostomy, and Continence Nursing, 43*(4), 392–397. https://doi.org/10.1097/WON.0000000000000237.

Balboni, T. A., Fitchett, G., Handzo, G. F., et al. (2017). State of the science of spirituality and palliative care research. Part II: Screening, assessment, and interventions. *Journal of Pain and Symptom Management, 54*(3), 441–453. http://dx.doi.org/10.1016/j.j.painsymman.2017.07.029.

Batstone, E., Bailey, C., & Hallett, N. (2020). Spiritual care provision to end of life patients: A systematic literature review. *Journal of Clinical Nursing, 29*(19-20), 3609–3624. https://doi.org./10.1111/jocn.15411.

Borji, M., Mousavimoghadam, S. R., Salimi, E., Otaghi, M., & Azizi, Y. (2019). The impact of spiritual care education on anxiety in family caregivers of patients with heart failure. *Journal of Religion and Health, 58*(6), 1961–1969. https://doi.org/10.1007/s10943-018-0689-9.

Burkhart, L., Bretschneider, A., Gerc, S., & Desmond, M. E. (2019). Spiritual care in nursing practice in veteran health care. *Global Qualitative Nursing Research, 6*, 2333393619843110. https://doi.org/10.1177/2333393619843110.

Cinar, D., Yildirim, Y., Yesilbalkan, O. U., & Pamuk, A. (2018). Experiences of cancer patients: A qualitative study. *International Journal of Caring Sciences, 11*(3), 1456–1466.

Conway-Phillips, R., & Janusek, L. W. (2016). Exploring spirituality among African American women: Implications for promoting breast health behaviors. *Holistic Nursing Practice, 30*(6), 322–329. https://doi.org/10.1097/HNP.000000000173.

Desmond, M. B., Burkhart, L., Horsley, T. L., Gerc, S. C., & Bretschneider, A. (2018). Development and psychometric evaluation of a spiritual care simulation and companion performance checklist for a veteran using a standardized patient. *Clinical Simulation in Nursing, 14*, 29–44. https://doi.org/10.1016/j.ecns.2017.10.008.

Elham, H., Hazrati, M., Momennasab, M., & Sareh, K. (2015). The effect of need-based spiritual/religious intervention on spiritual well-being and anxiety of elderly people. *Holistic Nursing Practice, 29*(3), 136–143. https://doi.org/10.1097/HNP.0000000000000083.

Ganocy, S., Goto, T., Chan, P. K., et al. (2016). Association of spirituality with mental health conditions in Ohio National Guard soldiers. *Journal of Nervous and Mental Disease, 204*(7), 524–529. https://doi.org/10.1097/NMD.0000000000000519.

Jones, K., Simpson, G. K., Briggs, L., & Dorsett, P. (2016). Does spirituality facilitate adjustment and resilience among individuals and families after SCI? *Disability and Rehabilitation, 38*(10), 921–935. https://doi.org/10.3109/09638288.2015.1066884.

Mamier, I., Taylor, E. J., & Wehtje Winslow, B. (2019). Nurse spiritual care: Prevalence and correlates. *Western Journal of Nursing Research, 41*(4), 537–554. https://doi.org/10.1177/0193945918776328.

Mills, P., Wilson, K., Iqbal, N., et al. (2015). Depressive symptoms and spiritual wellbeing in asymptomatic heart failure patients. *Journal of Behavioral Medicine, 38*(3), 407–415. https://doi.org/10.1007/s10865-014-9615-0.

Mirghafourvand, M., Charandabi, S. M. A., Sharajabad, F. A., & Sanaati, F. (2016). Spiritual well-being and health-related quality of life in Iranian adolescent girls. *Community Mental Health Journal, 52*(4), 484–492. https://doi.org/10.1007/s10597-016-9988-3.

Noronha Silva, G. C., Dos Reis, D. C., Prado Simão Miranda, T., et al. (2019). Religious/spiritual coping and spiritual distress in people with cancer. *Revista Brasileira De Enfermagem, 72*(6), 1534–1540. https://10.1007/s10943-015-0150-7.

Rivera-Hernandez, M. (2016). Religiosity, social support and care associated with health in older Mexicans with diabetes. *Journal of Religion and Health, 55*(4), 1394–1410. http://dx.doi.org/10.1590/0034-7167-2018-0585.

Roze des Ordons, A. L., Sinuff, T., Stelfox, H. T., Kondejewski, J., & Sinclair, S. (2018). Spiritual distress within inpatient settings: A scoping review of patients' and families' experiences. *Journal of Pain and Symptom Management, 56*(1), 122–145. https://doi.org/10.1016/j.jpainsymman.2018.03.009.

Sherman, A. C., Merluzzi, T. V., Pustejovsky, J. E., et al. (2015). A meta-analytic review of religious or spiritual involvement and social health among cancer patients. *Cancer, 121*(21), 3779–3788. https://doi.org/10.1002/cncr.29352.

Steinhauser, K. E., Fitchett, G., Handzo, G. F., et al. (2017). State of the science of spirituality and palliative care research. Part I: Definitions, measurement, and outcomes. *Journal of Pain and Symptom Management, 54*(3), 428–440. https://doi.org/10.1016/j.jpainsymman.2017.07.028.

Swinton, M., Giacomini, M., Toledo, F., et al. (2017). Experiences and expressions of spirituality at the end of life in the intensive care unit. *American Journal of Respiratory and Critical Care in Medicine, 195*(2), 198–204. https://doi.org/10.1164/rccm.201606-1102OC.

Torabi, F., Rassouli, M., Nourian, M., et al. (2018). The effect of spiritual care on adolescents coping with cancer. *Holistic Nursing Practice, 32*(2), 149–159. https://doi.org/10.1097/HNP.0000000000000263.

S

Risk for Spiritual Distress

Domain 10 Life principles Class 3 Value/belief/action congruence

Mary Beth Flynn Makic, PhD, RN, CCNS, CCRN-K, FAAN, FNAP, FCNS

NANDA-I

Definition

Susceptible to an impaired ability to integrate meaning and purpose in life through connectedness within self, literature, nature, and/or a power greater than oneself, which may compromise health.

Risk Factors

Altered religious ritual; altered spiritual practice; anxiety; barrier to experiencing love; cultural conflict; depressive symptoms; difficulty accepting the aging process; inadequate environmental control; inadequate interpersonal relations; loneliness; loss of independence; low self-esteem; pain; perception of having unfinished business; self-alienation; separation from support system; social alienation; sociocultural deprivation; stressors; substance misuse

At-Risk Population

Individuals experiencing birth of a child; individuals experiencing death of significant other; individuals experiencing infertility; individuals experiencing life transition; individuals experiencing racial conflict; individuals experiencing unexpected life event; individuals exposed to death; individuals exposed to natural disaster; individuals exposed to traumatic events; individuals receiving bad news; individuals receiving terminal care; individuals with low educational level

Associated Conditions

Chronic disease, depression; loss of a body part; loss of function of a body part; treatment regimen

NIC, NOC, Client Outcomes, Nursing Interventions and *Rationales,* and References

Refer to care plan for **Spiritual** Distress.

Readiness for Enhanced Spiritual Well-Being

Domain 10 Life Principles Class 2 Beliefs

Mary E. Desmond, PhD, RN, MA, MSN, AHN-BC and Barbara Baele Vincensi, PhD, RN, FNP-BC

NANDA-I

Definition

S

A pattern of integrating meaning and purpose in life through connectedness with self, others, art, music, literature, nature, and/or a power greater than oneself which can be strengthened.

Defining Characteristics

Expresses desire to enhance acceptance; expresses desire to enhance capacity to self-comfort; expresses desire to enhance comfort in one's faith; expresses desire to enhance connection with nature; expresses desire to enhance connection with power greater than self; expresses desire to enhance coping; expresses desire to enhance courage; expresses desire to enhance creative energy; expresses desire to enhance forgiveness from others; expresses desire to enhance harmony in the environment; expresses desire to enhance hope; expresses desire to enhance inner peace; expresses desire to enhance interaction with significant other; expresses desire to enhance joy; expresses desire to enhance love; expresses desire to enhance love of others; expresses desire to enhance meditative practice; expresses desire to enhance mystical experiences; expresses desire to enhance oneness with nature; expresses desire to enhance oneness with power greater than self; expresses desire to enhance participation in religious practices; expresses desire to enhance peace with power greater than self; expresses desire to enhance prayerfulness; expresses desire to enhance reverence; expresses desire to enhance satisfaction with life; expresses desire to enhance self-awareness; expresses desire to enhance self-forgiveness; expresses desire to enhance sense of awe; expresses desire to enhance sense of harmony within oneself; expresses desire to enhance sense of identity; expresses desire to enhance sense of magic in the environment; expresses desire to enhance serenity; expresses desire to enhance service to others; expresses desire to enhance strength in one's faith; expresses desire to enhance surrender

NOC (Nursing Outcomes Classification)

Suggested NOC Outcomes

Personal Health Status; Coping; Dignified Life Closure; Grief Resolution; Hope; Personal Health Status; Psychosocial Adjustment: Life Change; Quality of Life; Social Involvement; Spiritual Health

Example NOC Outcome with Indicators

Hope as evidenced by the following indicators: Expresses expectation of a positive future/Faith/Optimism/Belief in self/Sense of meaning in life/Belief in others/Inner peace. (Rate each indicator of **Hope:** 1 = never demonstrated, 2 = rarely demonstrated, 3 = sometimes demonstrated, 4 = often demonstrated, 5 = constantly demonstrated [see Section I].)

Client Outcomes

Client Will (Specify Time Frame)

- Express hope
- Express sense of meaning and purpose in life
- Express peace and serenity
- Express love
- Express acceptance
- Express surrender
- Express forgiveness of self and others
- Express satisfaction with philosophy of life
- Express joy
- Express courage
- Describe being able to cope
- Describe use of spiritual practices
- Describe providing service to others
- Describe interaction with spiritual leaders, friends, and family
- Describe appreciation for art, music, literature, and nature

NIC (Nursing Interventions Classification)

Suggested NIC Interventions

Active Listening, Coping Enhancement, Counseling, Crisis Intervention, Decision-Making Support, Grief Work Facilitation, Hope Instillation, Meditation Facilitation, Mutual Goal Setting, Presence, Religious Ritual Enhancement, Imagery, Simple Relaxation Therapy, Socialization Enhancement, Spiritual Growth Facilitation, Spiritual Support, Support System Enhancement, Touch, Values Clarification

Example NIC Activities—Spiritual Support

Encourage use of spiritual resources if desired; Be available to listen to client's expression of feelings

Nursing Interventions and *Rationales*

▲ Perform a spiritual assessment that includes the client's relationship with God, meaning and purpose in life, religious affiliation, and any other significant beliefs. EBN: *In a pre/post nonrandomized interventional study, researchers Vlasblom et al (2015) found referrals to spiritual caregivers (chaplains) increased after implementing a spiritual assessment instrument by nurses at client admission, in spite of nurse hesitancy in using the tool.*

• Be present and actively listen to the client. EB: *In a state of the science report, spirituality requires observations and understanding of human experience (Steinhauser et al, 2017).* EBN: *In a cross-sectional, correlational study with (n = 554) tertiary care nurses Mamier et al (2019) found that the top three mean scores of nurse self-reported frequency of spiritual therapeutics with clients/family were presence, listening, and spiritual assessment.*

- Encourage the client to engage in other spiritual meditative or mind–body practices. **EBN:** *In a quasi-experimental interprofessional study with nursing, Sun et al (2016) discovered that religious affiliation and practices improved coping, comfort, and faith in palliative care clients.* **EB:** *In a state of the science report, mind–body interventions are encouraged to promote spiritual healing (Balboni et al, 2017).*
- Coordinate or encourage nurses to participate in spiritual care education courses and simulation. **EBN:** *Hu et al (2019), using a nonrandomized controlled trial, found that oncology nurses who received specific education on spiritual care over 12 months in China had significantly higher overall spiritual health, spiritual care competency scores, and higher individual scores ($p < 0.05$) than the control group.* **EBN:** *For use with the veteran population, Desmond et al (2018) developed a spiritual care simulation and performance checklist based on a review of the literature, content validity expert review, and pilot testing with practicing nurses who care for veterans, indicating that simulation and debriefing with a standardized client can be used to teach spiritual care ($p < .001$).*
- Perform actions to address spiritual need. **EBN:** *Burkhart et al (2019) used a qualitative descriptive method to describe spiritual care in practice with nurses in a U.S. veteran health system, finding spiritual care interventions included promoting hope through self-reflection, facilitating both religious and nonreligious spiritual practices, encouraging connection with others, and referral to other professionals.*
- Encourage clients to reflect on what is meaningful to them in life. **EBN:** *A spiritual care for a veteran simulation and performance checklist based on a review of the literature, content validity expert review, and pilot testing with practicing nurses who care for veterans found that spiritual care includes asking about/recognition of importance of veteran culture, past service, and present meaningful connection to veteran groups (Desmond et al, 2018).*
- Offer spiritual support to family and caregivers. **EB:** *In a state of the science report, clients and families who experience serious illness have spiritual needs (Balboni et al, 2017).* **EB:** *Borji et al (2019) found that Iranian caregivers of heart failure clients (n = 71) had significantly decreased anxiety levels ($p = 0.001$) 3 weeks after a spiritual care education program using pre-post methodology.*
- Offer opportunities to facilitate religious or spiritual practices, including reflection, prayer, and relaxation techniques with deep breathing and listening to scripture verses. **EB:** *In a quasi-experimental pretest-posttest with control design with clients with gynecological cancer (n = 108), Nasution et al (2020) examined the effectiveness of a spiritual intervention on coping and spiritual well-being, finding a statistically significant increase in mean score of coping ($p = 0.001$) and spiritual well-being ($p = 0.006$) in the intervention group.*
- Support spiritual practices, including meditation, guided imagery, journaling, relaxation, and involvement in art, music, or poetry. **EB:** *In a state of the science report, mind–body interventions are encouraged to promote spiritual healing (Balboni et al, 2017).*
- Encourage expressions of spirituality. **EB:** *Swinton et al (2017) conducted 208 semistructured interviews with 70 dying clients, 76 family members, and 150 health care providers in an intensive care unit (ICU) to describe how spirituality was expressed during the dying process. The outcome of these interviews was the development of the 3 Wishes Program to support the expressions of spirituality during the dying process (e.g., peace, connections, spiritually enhanced environments, and specific expressions of spirituality).*
- Encourage integration of spirituality in healthy lifestyle choices. **EBN:** *In a phenomenological study of African-Caribbean women poststroke, Moorley et al (2016) identified one of three themes, which included the use of faith, spirituality, and church, to promote choices for healthy behaviors.*

S

Geriatric

- ▲ Offer opportunities to practice one's religion. **EB:** *Moeini et al (2016), in a randomized clinical trial with 52 elderly clients with hypertension in Iran, found that the experimental group who received a religious program based on Islam had mean scores of spiritual well-being significantly higher than in the control group ($p < 0.001$) in both the religious and existential dimensions.* **EB:** *Soriano et al (2016) found, in a sample of 200 Filipino older adults living in a community and institutional setting, that regular visits with chaplains and religious practices enhanced older adults' spiritual contentment and religion and culture quality of life.*
- Encourage social relationships and connections with family for institutionalized older adults. **EB:** *Soriano et al (2016) found that the loss of familial and peer relationships on admission to a nursing home was associated with lower religion and culture quality of life and quality of life overall.*
- For those with chronic disease, encourage individual spiritual practices that promote meaning and peace. **EB:** *Mills et al (2015), in a sample of 132 men and women with asymptomatic stage B heart failure, found that spiritual well-being, particularly meaning and peace, was associated with less depression.*

- ▲ For those with terminal illness, encourage clients to attend meaning-centered psychotherapy, spiritual therapy intervention, life review, dignity therapy, yoga, meditation, and mind-body stress reduction if appropriate. EB: *Chen et al (2018), in a systematic review of 19 studies with 1548 participants, evaluated effects of spiritual care on quality of life and spiritual well-being on clients with terminal illness and found seven types of spiritual care interventions, with the majority of studies indicating that spiritual care had a potential favorable effect on global quality of life and spiritual well-being of clients.*
- During bereavement, encourage bereavement life review to promote spiritual well-being and alleviate depression. EB: *In a sample of 20 bereaved Hawaiian Americans, Ando et al (2015) found that participating in bereavement life review statistically significantly increased spiritual well-being and decreased depression.*

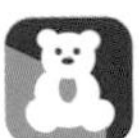

Pediatric

- Offer adolescents with cancer opportunities for reflection and storytelling to express their spirituality and spiritual needs to enhance efficient coping strategies. EB: *In a single-group, quasi-experimental, pre-post study with 32 adolescents with one type of cancer in an Iranian hospital, Torabi et al (2018) found that participating in a 1:1 spiritual care program over six 45-minute sessions had a statistically significant difference between the pretest and posttest mean coping subscales ($p < .001$).*
- Foster spiritual activities among adolescents. EB: *Mirghafourvand et al (2016) found that, in a sample of 520 Iranian adolescent girls, spiritual well-being was highly correlated with health-related quality of life ($r = .60$, $p < .001$).*

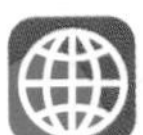

Multicultural

- Recognize the importance of spirituality and provide culturally competent spiritual care to specific populations:
  - **African American.** EBN: *One of four themes identified in analyzing secondary data with content analysis indicated that spirituality for African American women was a source of inner peace, joy, strength, hope, comfort, calm, coping, and other positive aspects contributing to well-being and potentially supportive of health-promoting behaviors (Conway-Phillips & Janusek, 2016).*
  - **Armed forces.** EB: *An exploratory study by Ganocy et al (2016) found an inverse relationship to suicidal ideation, posttraumatic stress disorder (PTSD), and alcohol use with existential and spiritual well-being for National Guard members who had ever been deployed overseas at least once.*
  - **Chinese.** EB: *Leung et al (2015) used a pretest/posttest methodology with 160 Chinese clients diagnosed with chronic disease to study the effects of a psychoeducational death preparation intervention with findings indicating that there was significant improvement in psychological, behavioral, and spiritual dimensions over time related to fear of death and preparation for death.*
  - **Homeless.** EB: *A cross-sectional mixed-methods pilot study using the Mantram Repetition Program that teaches mantram (sacred word self-selection) repetition with 29 homeless women found that 88% of the participants repeated their mantram 1 week later, with three themes emerging from the qualitative data: mantram repetition, mantram benefits, and being cared for (Weinrich et al, 2016).*
  - **Indonesian.** EBN: *In a quasi-experimental pretest-posttest with control design with a sample of 108 clients with gynecological cancer, the effectiveness of a spiritual intervention (54 each group) on coping and spiritual well-being was examined by Nasution et al (2020), finding a statistically significant increase in mean score of coping ($p = 0.001$) and spiritual well-being ($p = 0.006$) in the intervention group.*
  - **Latino/Hispanic.** EBN: *In a cross-sectional secondary analysis of a longitudinal study, Prince et al (2015) found that Hispanic stem cell transplant survivors ($n = 171$) had greater spiritual well-being and quality of life than non-Hispanic survivors, even at ≥3 years posttransplant.*
  - **Thai.** EBN: *The Thai people were found to be both religious and spiritual, using coping strategies from both areas to help manage concerns and to explain the development of kidney disease in a qualitative study by Yodchai et al (2017). Encourage both religious and spiritual coping strategies to help cope.*

Home Care

- All the nursing interventions described previously apply in the home setting.

S

REFERENCES

Ando, M., Marquez-Wong, F., Simon, G. B., Kira, H., & Becker, C. (2015). Bereavement life review improves spiritual well-being and ameliorates depression among American caregivers. *Palliative and Supportive Care, 13*(2), 319–325. https://doi.org/10.1017/S1478951514000030.

Balboni, T. A., Fitchett, G., Handzo, G. F., et al. (2017). State of the science of spirituality and palliative care research. Part II: Screening, assessment, and interventions. *Journal of Pain and Symptom Management, 54*(3), 441–453. http://dx.doi.org/10.1016/j.j.painsymman.2017.07.029.

Borji, M., Mousavimoghadam, S. R., Salimi, E., Otaghi, M., & Azizi, Y. (2019). The impact of spiritual care education on anxiety in family caregivers of patients with heart failure. *Journal of Religion and Health, 58*(6), 1961–1969. https://doi.org/10.1007/s10943-018-0689-9.

Burkhart, L., Bretschneider, A., Gerc, S., & Desmond, M. E. (2019). Spiritual care in nursing practice in veteran health care. *Global Qualitative Nursing Research, 6*, 2333393619843110. https://doi.org/10.1177/2333393619843110.

Chen, J., Lin, Y., Yan, J., Wu, Y., & Hu, R. (2018). The effects of spiritual care on quality of life and spiritual well-being among patients with terminal illness: A systematic review. *Palliative Medicine, 32*(7), 1167–1179. https://doi.org/10.1177/0269216318772267.

Conway-Phillips, R., & Janusek, L. W. (2016). Exploring spirituality among African American women: Implications for promoting breast health behaviors. *Holistic Nursing Practice, 30*(6), 322–329. https://10.1097/HNP.000000000000173.

Desmond, M. B., Burkhart, L., Horsley, T. L., Gerc, S. C., & Bretschneider, A. (2018). Development and psychometric evaluation of a spiritual care simulation and companion performance checklist for a veteran using a standardized patient. *Clinical Simulation in Nursing, 14*, 29–44. https://doi.org/10.1016/j.ecns.2017.10.008.

Ganocy, S., Goto, T., Chan, P. K., et al. (2016). Association of spirituality with mental health conditions in Ohio National Guard soldiers. *Journal of Nervous and Mental Disease, 204*(7), 524–529. https://doi.org/10.1097/NMD.000000000000519.

Hu, Y., Jiao, M., & Li, F. (2019). Effectiveness of spiritual care training to enhance spiritual health and spiritual care competency among oncology nurses. *BMC Palliative Care, 18*(1), 104. http://dx.doi.org.ezproxy.lewisu.edu/10.1186/s12904-019-0489-3.

Leung, P. Y., Wan, A. H. Y., Lui, J. Y. M., et al. (2015). The effects of a positive death education group on psycho-spiritual outcomes for Chinese with chronic illness: A quasi-experimental study. *Illness, Crises, and Loss, 23*(1), 5–19. http://dx.doi.org/10.2190/IL.23.1.b.

Mamier, I., Taylor, E. J., & Wehtje Winslow, B. (2019). Nurse spiritual care: Prevalence and correlates. *Western Journal of Nursing Research, 41*(4), 537–554. https://doi.org/10.1177/0193945918776328.

Mills, P., Wilson, K., Iqbal, N., et al. (2015). Depressive symptoms and spiritual wellbeing in asymptomatic heart failure patients. *Journal of Behavioral Medicine, 38*(3), 407–415. https://doi.org/10.1007/s10865-014-9615-0.

Mirghafourvand, M., Charandabi, S. M. A., Sharajabad, F. A., & Sanaati, F. (2016). Spiritual well-being and health-related quality of life in Iranian adolescent girls. *Community Mental Health Journal, 52*(4), 484–492. https://doi.og10.1007/s10597-016-9988-3.

Moeini, M., Sharifi, S., & Kajbaf, M. B. (2016). Effect of Islam-based religious program on spiritual wellbeing in elderly with hypertension. *Iranian Journal of Nursing and Midwifery Research, 21*(6), 566–571. https://doi.org/10.4103/1735-9066.197683.

Moorley, C. R., Cahill, S., & Corcoran, N. T. (2016). Life after stroke: Coping mechanisms among African Caribbean women. *Health and Social Care in the Community, 24*(6), 769–778.

Nasution, L. A., Afiyanti, Y., & Kurniawati, W. (2020). Effectiveness of spiritual intervention toward coping and spiritual well-being on patients with gynecological cancer. *Asia-Pacific Journal of Oncology Nursing, 7*(3), 273–279. https://doi.org/10.4103/apjon.apjon_4_20.

Prince, P., Mitchell, S. A., Wehlen, L., et al. (2015). Spiritual well-being in Hispanic and non-Hispanic survivors of alogeneic hematopoeitic stem cell transplantation. *Journal of Psychosocial Oncology, 33*(6), 635–654. https://doi.org/10.1080/07347332.2015.1082167.

Soriano, C. A. F., Sarmiento, W. D., Songco, F. J. G., Macindo, J. R. B., & Conde, A. R. (2016). Socio-demographics, spirituality, and quality of life among community-dwelling and institutionalized older adults: A structural equation model. *Archives of Gerontology and Geriatrics, 66*, 176–182. https://doi.org/10.1016/j.archger.2016.05.011.

Steinhauser, K. E., Fitchett, G., Handzo, G. F., et al. (2017). State of the science of spirituality and palliative care research. Part I: Definitions, measurement, and outcomes. *Journal of Pain and Symptom Management, 54*(3), 428–440. https://doi.org/10.1016/j.jpainsymman.2017.07.028.

Sun, V., Kim, J., Irish, T., et al. (2016). Palliative care and spiritual well-being in lung cancer patients and family caregivers. *Psycho-Oncology, 25*(12), 1448–1455. https://dx.doi.org/10.1002/pon.3987.

Swinton, M., Giacomini, M., Toledo, F., et al. (2017). Experiences and expressions of spirituality at the end of life in the intensive care unit. *American Journal of Respiratory and Critical Care in Medicine, 195*(2), 198–204. https://doi.org/10.1164/rccm.201606-1102OC.

Torabi, F., Rassouli, M., Nourian, M., Borumandnia, N., Shirinabadi Farahani, A., & Nikseresht, F. (2018). The effect of spiritual care on adolescents coping with cancer. *Holistic Nursing Practice, 32*(3), 149–159. https://doi.org/10.1097/HNP.0000000000000263.

Vlasblom, J. P., van der Steen, J. T., Walton, M. N., & Jochemsen, H. (2015). Effects of nurses' screening of spiritual needs of hospitalized patients on consultation and perceived nurses' support and patients' spiritual well-being. *Holistic Nursing Practice, 29*(6), 346–356. https://doi.org/10.1097/HNP.0000000000000111.

Weinrich, S. P., Bormann, J. E., Glaser, D., et al. (2016). Mantram repetition with homeless women: A pilot study. *Holistic Nursing Practice, 30*(6), 360–367. https://doi.org/10.1097/HNP.0000000000000138.

Yodchai, K., Dunning, T., Savage, S., & Hutchinson, A. M. (2017). The role or religion and spirituality in coping with kidney disease and haemodialysis in Thailand. *Scandinavian Journal of Caring Science, 31*(2), 359–367. https://doi.org/10.1111/scs.12355.

Impaired Standing Domain 4 Activity/rest Class 2 Activity/exercise

Tracy P. George, DNP, APRN-BC, CNE

NANDA-I

Definition

Limitation of ability to independently and purposefully attain and/or maintain the body in an upright position from feet to head.

Defining Characteristics

Difficulty adjusting position of one or both lower limbs on uneven surface; difficulty attaining postural balance; difficulty extending one or both hips; difficulty extending one or both knees; difficulty flexing one or both hips; difficulty flexing one or both knees; difficulty maintaining postural balance; difficulty moving one or both hips; difficulty moving one or both knees; difficulty stressing torso with body weight

Related Factors

Excessive emotional disturbance; insufficient energy; insufficient muscle strength; insufficient physical endurance; malnutrition; obesity; pain; self-imposed relief posture

Associated Conditions

Circulatory perfusion disorder; impaired metabolism; injury to lower extremity; neurological disorder; prescribed posture; sarcopenia; surgical procedures

NOC (Nursing Outcomes Classification)

Suggested NOC Outcomes

Activity Tolerance; Balance; Body Mechanics Performance; Body Positioning: Self-Initiated; Comfort Status: Physical; Endurance; Mobility; Risk Control: Hypotension; Skeletal Function

Example NOC Outcome with Indicators

Mobility as evidenced by the following indicators: Balance/Coordination/Body positioning performance. (Rate outcome and indicators of **Mobility:** 1 = severely compromised, 2 = substantially compromised, 3 = moderately compromised, 4 = mildly compromised, 5 = not compromised [see Section I].)

Client Outcomes

Client Will (Specify Time Frame)

- Demonstrate optimal independence and safety when standing
- Demonstrate the proper use of assistive devices
- State benefits of standing

S

NIC (Nursing Interventions Classification)

Suggested NIC Interventions

Body Mechanics Promotion

Example NIC Activities

Instruct client on structure and functional spine and optimal posture for moving and using the body

Nursing Interventions and *Rationales*

- Encourage clients to stand at intervals throughout the day. EB: *The use of standing desks reduced self-reported sedentary behaviors by 25% during a 6-month period (Resendiz et al, 2019).* EB: *Clients who engaged in standing, walking, or cycling during an 8-hour work period had lower 24-hour and postprandial blood sugars than those who sat (Crespo et al, 2016).*

- Advise clients of the physical and psychological benefits of being upright and active. EB: *In clients 1 to 3 years after suffering a stroke, depression, left hemisphere infarction, visual neglect, and difficulty with mobility and balance were associated with being less active (Kunkel et al, 2015).*
- Educate clients about the health risks of sitting. EB: *In a study of 2074 clients, sitting, for long periods of time and difficulty with standing were associated with a higher mortality rate (Olaya et al, 2018).*

Geriatric

- Advise older clients who have difficulty standing to use assistive devices. EB: *Assistive devices may allow older adults to carry out usual daily activities and participate in daily life (Freedman et al, 2017).*
- Encourage the use of trunk exercises along with walking and balance exercises in older adults. EB: *In a randomized controlled trial of 64 older adults, walking and balance exercises along with trunk strengthening exercises improved the results on the 30-second Chair Stand Test, Sitting and Rising Test, Forward Reach Test, Backward Reach Test, and Timed Up and Go Test (Shahtahmassebi et al, 2019).*
- Encourage clients who are unable to stand to consider chair exercises. EB: *In a study of 100 older adults with lower extremity osteoarthritis, the 40 adults who participated in chair yoga twice a week for 8 weeks reported less pain than the 60 participants who participated in a health education program two times per week for 8 weeks (Park et al, 2016).*
- Encourage poststroke clients to participate in rehabilitation interventions that promote standing. CEB: *In a meta-analysis using 11 studies, interventions used after strokes to improve standing were associated with faster sitting-to-standing position times and improved lateral symmetry during sitting-to-standing position changes (Pollock et al, 2014).* EB: *A study of seven participants found that a home-based intervention, Rehab@home, can be used effectively to improve the rehabilitation of balance and the movement from the sitting to standing position in clients with neurological deficits, without the presence of a physical therapist (Faria, Silva, & Campilho, 2015).*
- Mechanical sit-stand lifts can be used with clients who require assistance with transfers. EB: *Sit-stand lifts can be used with clients to prevent back and shoulder injuries among nurses (Tang et al, 2017).*
- Educate older adults who have fallen about the need for balance and muscle training of the ankle joint. EB: *In a randomized controlled trial of 26 older clients who were at risk of falling and had fallen previously, Choi and Kim (2015) found that balance and ankle muscle training resulted in improvements in the gait of older adults.*
- Educate adults older than age 80 years on the need for vitamin D. EB: *In a systematic review and meta-analysis, vitamin D deficiency was associated with a higher prevalence of orthostatic hypotension (Ometto et al, 2016).*
- Assess for risk of falls among older adults with difficulty standing. EB: *In a study among Japanese older adults, Arai et al (2020) found that the ability to stand on one leg from a 40-cm-high seat was found to predict falls in older adults, which is part of the Stand-Up Test (SUT).*
- Advise older clients who are at risk for falls to avoid doing multiple tasks at one time while standing. EB: *In a study of 243 adults ages 65 years and older, older participants' standing balance was worse than that seen in younger participants; the standing balance was worse when clients were performing a second task, which is important when considering the risk of falls (Coelho et al, 2016).*

Client/Family Teaching and Discharge Planning

- Educate clients that standing can be beneficial for their health. EB: *In a study of participants with chronic pain (n = 18) and participants without chronic pain (n = 19), Raijmakers et al (2015) found that clients with chronic pain spent more time lying and less time sitting and standing over a 1-week period.*
- Teach clients about the need to take frequent breaks when standing for long periods. EB: *Gallagher et al (2019) found that 58% (11/19) of participants who had no walking breaks when standing for 2 hours developed low back pain, compared to 26% of clients when 5-minute walking breaks were included every 25 minutes during 2-hour standing intervals.*
- Instruct clients about the use of yoga for individuals who have difficulty with standing balance. EB: *In a randomized control of obese adults with poor standing balance, participation in yoga classes three times per week was associated with improved static and dynamic standing balance (Jorrakate et al, 2015).*

REFERENCES

Arai, T., Fujita, H., Maruya, K., Morita, Y., Asahi, R., & Ishibashi, H. (2020). The one-leg portion of the Stand-Up Test predicts fall risk in aged individuals: A prospective cohort study. *Journal of Orthopaedic Science, 25*(4), 688–692. https://doi.org/10.1016/j.jos.2019.06.014.

Choi, J. H., & Kim, N. J. (2015). The effects of balance training and ankle training on the gait of elderly people who have fallen. *Journal of Physical Therapy Science, 27*(1), 139–142. https://doi.org/10.1589/jpts.27.139.

Coelho, T., Fernandes, Â., Santos, R., Paúl, C., & Fernandes, L. (2016). Quality of standing balance in community-dwelling elderly: Age-related differences in single and dual task conditions. *Archives of Gerontology and Geriatrics, 67*, 34–39. https://doi.org/10.1016/j.archger.2016.06.010.

Crespo, N. C., Mullane, S. L., Zeigler, Z. S., Buman, M. P., & Gaesser, G. A. (2016). Effects of standing and light-intensity walking and cycling on 24-h glucose. *Medicine & Science in Sports & Exercise, 48*(12), 2503–2511. https://doi.org10.1249/MSS.0000000000001062.

Faria, C., Silva, J., & Campilho, A. (2015). Rehab@home: A tool for home-based motor function rehabilitation. *Disability and Rehabilitation: Assistive Technology, 10*(1), 67–74. https://doi.org/10.3109/17483107.2013.839749.

Freedman, V. A., Kasper, J. D., & Spillman, B. C. (2017). Successful aging through successful accommodation with assistive devices. *Journals of Gerontology Series B: Psychological Sciences and Social Sciences, 72*(2), 300–309. https://doi.org/10.1093/geronb/gbw102.

Gallagher, K. M., Payne, M., Daniels, B., Caldwell, A. R., & Ganio, M. S. (2019). Walking breaks can reduce prolonged standing induced low back pain. *Human Movement Science, 66*, 31–37. https://doi.org/10.1016/j.humov.2019.03.012.

Jorrakate, C., Kongsuk, J., Pongduang, C., Sadsee, B., & Chanthorn, P. (2015). Effect of yoga training on one leg standing and functional reach tests in obese individuals with poor postural control. *Journal of Physical Therapy Science, 27*(1), 59–62. https://doi.org/10.1589/jpts.27.59.

Kunkel, D., Fitton, C., Burnett, M., & Ashburn, A. (2015). Physical inactivity post-stroke: A 3-year longitudinal study. *Disability & Rehabilitation, 37*(4), 304–310. https://doi.org/10.3109/09638288.2014.918190.

Olaya, B., Moneta, M. V., Démenech-Abella, J., et al. (2018). Mobility difficulties, physical Activity, and all-cause mortality risk in a nationally representative sample of older adults. *Journals of Gerontology Series A: Biological Sciences & Medical Sciences, 73*(9), 1272–1279. https://doi.org/10.1093/gerona/glx121.

Ometto, F., Stubbs, B., Annweiler, C., et al. (2016). Hypovitaminosis D and orthostatic hypotension: A systematic review and meta-analysis. *Journal of Hypertension, 34*(6), 1036–1043. https://doi.org/10.1097/HJH.0000000000000907.

Park, J., Newman, D., McCaffrey, R., Garrido, J. J., Riccio, M. L., & Liehr, P. (2016). The effect of chair yoga on biopsychosocial changes in English- and Spanish-speaking community-dwelling older adults with lower-extremity osteoarthritis. *Journal of Gerontological Social Work, 59*(7–8), 604–626. https://doi.org/10.1080/01634372.2016.1239234.

Pollock, A., Gray, C., Culham, E., Durward, B. R., & Langhorne, P. (2014). Interventions for improving sit-to-stand ability following stroke. *Cochrane Database of Systematic Reviews, 5*, CD007232. https://doi.org/10.1002/14651858.CD007232.pub4.

Raijmakers, B. G., Nieuwenhuizen, M. G., Beckerman, H., & de Groot, S. (2015). Differences in the course of daily activity level between persons with and without chronic pain. *American Journal of Physical Medicine & Rehabilitation, 94*(2), 101–113. https://doi.org/10.1097/PHM.0000000000000206.

Resendiz, M., Lustik, M. B., Conkright, W. R., & West, G. F. (2019). Standing desks for sedentary occupations: Assessing changes in satisfaction and health outcomes after six months of use. *Work, 63*(3), 347–353. https://doi:10.3233/WOR-192940.

Shahtahmassebi, B., Hebert, J. J., Hecimovich, M., & Fairchild, T. J. (2019). Trunk exercise training improves muscle size, strength, and function in older adults: A randomized controlled trial. *Scandinavian Journal of Medicine & Science in Sports, 29*(7), 980–991. https://doi.org/10.1111/sms.13415.

Tang, R., Poklar, M., Domke, H., Moore, S., Kapellusch, J., & Garg, A. (2017). Sit–to–stand lift: Effects of lifted height on weight borne and upper extremity strength requirements. *Research in Nursing & Health, 40*(1), 9–14. https://doi.org/10.1111/sms.13415.

Stress Overload Domain 9 Coping/stress tolerance Class 2 Coping responses

Meredith Ford, MSN, RN, CNE

S

NANDA-I

Definition

Excessive amounts and types of demands that require action.

Defining Characteristics

Difficulty with decision-making; expresses feeling pressured; expresses increased anger; expresses tension; impaired functioning; increased impatience; negative impact from stress

Related Factors

Inadequate resources; repeated stressors; stressors

NOC (Nursing Outcomes Classification)

Suggested NOC Outcomes

Anxiety Level; Caregiver Stressors; Stress Level; Health-Promoting Behavior; Knowledge: Stress Management

Example NOC Outcome with Indicators

Stress Level as evidenced by the following indicators: Increased blood pressure, restlessness, emotional outbursts, anxiety, diminished attention to detail. (Rate the outcome and indicators of **Stress Level:** 1 = severe, 2 = substantial, 3 = moderate, 4 = mild, 5 = none [see Section I].)

Client Outcomes

Client Will (Specify Time Frame)

- Review the amounts and types of stressors in daily living
- Identify stressors that can be modified or eliminated
- Mobilize social supports to facilitate lower stress levels
- Reduce stress levels through use of health promoting behaviors and other strategies

NIC (Nursing Interventions Classification)

Suggested NIC Interventions

Active Listening; Anger Control Assistance; Anxiety Reduction; Aroma Therapy; Counseling; Crisis Intervention; Emotional Support; Family Integrity Promotion; Presence; Support System Enhancement

Example NIC Activities—Support System Enhancement

Identify psychological response to situation and availability of support system; Determine adequacy of social networks; Explain to concerned others how they can help; Refer to a self-help group or Internet-based resource as appropriate; Provide services in a caring and supportive manner

Nursing Interventions and *Rationales*

- Assist client in identification of stress overload during vulnerable life events. EBN: *Research suggested that role overload, associated with high stress levels, among nurses and volunteer caregivers may negatively affect health, well-being, and job performance (Dageid et al, 2016).* EB: *When surrogates experience acute stress from participating in treatment decisions for others, it translates into posttraumatic stress disorder (PTSD), anxiety, depression, and grief in the months after the client's death (Barnato et al, 2017).* EB: *Women with breast cancer who were involved in group therapy focusing on stress reduction gained positive effects on mood and self-esteem while prolonging survival, which indirectly resulted in decreased stress (Gosain et al, 2020). Job strain has a clinically significant risk of death to men with cardiometabolic disease (Kivimäki et al, 2018).*
- Listen actively to descriptions of stressors and the stress response. EBN: *In a recent study focusing on stress and depression, these conditions are independently related to major adverse cardiovascular events (Hou et al, 2020).* EB: *Adolescents exposed to daily stress demonstrate increased risky decision-making compared with those with low stress (Uy & Galván, 2017).*
- In younger adult women, assess interpersonal stressors. EB: *A sample of 450 young adults, 62% of them being female, were at high risk for depression and anxiety related to the psychosocial effects of the COVID-19 pandemic (Kujawa et al, 2020).* CEB: *A systematic review and meta-analysis of 30 studies found that maternal exposure to the stress of domestic violence results in significantly increased risk of low birth weight and preterm birth (Shah & Shah, 2010).*
- Categorize stressors as modifiable or nonmodifiable. EB: *Strategizing on nonavoidance coping and increased socialization along with enhanced personal mastery and self-efficacy in use of problem-solving coping may minimize depression symptoms in Alzheimer's disease caregivers (Grano et al, 2017).* EBN: *Removing or minimizing some stressors, changing responses to stressors, and modifying the long-term effects of stress are all actions that can assist those with chronic illnesses and stress (Chiang et al, 2018).*
- Help clients modify or mitigate stressors identified as modifiable. EBN: *A study of 150 married working women demonstrated that role overload has a significant impact on job performance and stress (Mittal & Bhakar, 2018).* CEB: *There are numerous possible strategies to modify stressors among nurses, including team interaction and support, organizational change and enlightened leadership, and the need for a space for nurses to gather and interact (Happell et al, 2013).*

S

- Help clients distinguish among short-term, chronic, and secondary stressors. EB: *PTSD status in combination with severe trauma in Korean males who were active military in the Vietnam War had a decrease in telomere length (Kim et al, 2017).* EBN: *Social support is a critical dimension of health and health promotion and serves as a buffer in the stress response (Mette et al, 2020).*
- Provide information as needed to reduce stress responses to acute and chronic illnesses. EBN: *Nursing interventions including strategies to deal with child behavior, a focus on physical health, and planning to meet resource needs may enhance the well-being of African American grandmothers raising grandchildren (Chan et al, 2019). Proactive nursing interventions including assessment of caregiver needs for support and preparedness including early psychoeducational interventions can enhance caregiver ability to navigate the challenges associated with caring for a child with a chronic illness (Mowla et al, 2017).*
- ▲ Explore possible therapeutic approaches such as cognitive-behavioral therapy, biofeedback, neurofeedback, acupuncture, pharmacological agents, and complementary and alternative therapies. EBN: *Nonpharmacological nursing interventions, through the use of nature-based sounds played through headsets, were found to effectively decrease the stress response in mechanically ventilated clients (Rajora et al, 2019).* EB: *Those who exercised regularly were more resistant to acute stress (Bernstein & McNally, 2018). Mindfulness techniques have been suggested as an effective means of reducing stress in adolescents (Perry-Parrish et al, 2016), nursing personnel (Yang et al, 2018), and older adults (Hazlett-Stevens et al, 2019).*
- Help the client to reframe his or her perceptions of some of the stressors. EBN: *Researchers found that optimism and adaptive coping help students prevent academic burnout, positively affecting academic performance (Vizoso et al, 2019).*
- Assist the client to mobilize social supports for dealing with recent stressors. EBN: *When clients experience stronger social supports, they have less financial threat, stress, anxiety, and depression (Viseu et al, 2018).*

Pediatric

- With children, nurses should work with parents to help them reduce children's stressors. EB: *Prenatal stress and anxiety have been shown to increase stress-induced cortisol response in adolescents and adversity in early life, for example, interparental aggression and emotional maternal withdrawal (van Bodegom et al, 2017; Van Tieghem & Tottenham, 2018).*
- Help children to manage their feelings related to self-concept. CEB: *Perceived isolation as experienced in high school associated with victimization results in higher stress and longer-lasting negative psychological outcomes (Newman, Holden, & Delville, 2005).*
- Help children to deal with bullies and other sources of violence in schools and neighborhoods. EB: *Violence in schools and neighborhoods has significant effects on children's stress. A recent study of 1993 participants, ages 9 to 13 years, indicated that being bullied (victimized) was associated with increased stress, behavioral problems, and needing psychological counseling (Garaigordobil & Machimbarrena, 2019).*
- Help children to manage the complexities of chronic illnesses. EB: *Children with a chronic illness have reported moderate levels of self-management, which indicates potential problems with physical, emotional, social, and mental domains (Bravo et al, 2020).* EB: *Teenagers who had recently been diagnosed with diabetes described high levels of stress that often related to the complexities of managing the illness (Chao et al, 2016).*

S

Geriatric

- Assess for chronic stress with older adults and provide a variety of stress relief techniques. EB: *PTSD is associated with increased odds of cardiovascular, musculoskeletal, gastrointestinal, respiratory, and neurological conditions, as well as cancer, sleep disorders, and anemia (Sommer et al, 2021).*
- ▲ Encourage older adults to seek appropriate counseling. EB: *Treatment modalities for PTSD in older adults may vary depending on whether the PTSD was experienced early or late in life; however, trauma confrontation and cognitive restructuring combined with age-specific life review in cognitive-behavioral therapy may hold the most promise (Bottche et al, 2016).* CEB: *Bereavement-related major depression differs from major depression seen in other stressful life events only in relation to older age at onset. Individuals are more likely to be female; have lower levels of treatment-seeking; and have higher levels of guilt, fatigue, and loss of interest; therefore, they should not be excluded from a diagnosis of major depression (Kendler, Myers, & Zisook, 2008).*

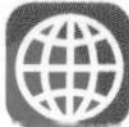

Multicultural

* ✱ Review cultural beliefs and acculturation level in relation to perceived stressors. **EBN:** *A study done to assess time-varying association of premigration and postmigration stressors in refugees' mental health indicated that there was an association between the difficulties in adjustment to life and their mental health during the resettlement period (Wu et al, 2020).* *Assess families for whether they experience high stress or low stress.* **EB:** *In a sample of 26,670 Italian fifth-grade students, first- and second-generation immigrant pupils reported being victimized more frequently than their native peers, although the incidence for second-generation pupils was lower than first generation (Alivernini et al, 2019).* **CEB:** *Stress related to racial microaggressions experienced by African Americans may have a negative cumulative effect on health outcomes (Sue et al, 2007).*

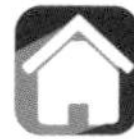

Home Care

- ● The preceding interventions may be adapted for home care use.
- ● Develop community-based programs for stress management as needed for groups with increased risk of stress overload (e.g., firefighters, policemen, military personnel, nurses). **CEB:** *Some situations have higher risks of stress overload. Stress management interventions may prevent or modify the experience of stress overload (McNulty, 2005).*
- ● Support and encourage neighborhood stability. **CEB:** *A "significant proportion of health differentials across neighborhoods is due to disparate stress levels across [Detroit] neighborhoods," and neighborhood stability was a buffer to reduce the negative effects of high stress (Boardman, 2004).*

Client/Family Teaching and Discharge Planning

- ● Diagnose the possibility of stress overload before teaching.
- ● Establish readiness for learning.
- ● Provide manageable amounts of information at the appropriate educational level.
- ● Evaluate the need for additional teaching and learning experiences.

REFERENCES

Alivernini, F., Manganelli, S., Cavicchiolo, E., & Lucidi, F. (2019). Measuring bullying and victimization among immigrant and native primary school students: Evidence from Italy. *Journal of Psychoeducational Assessment*, *37*(2), 226–238. https://doi.org/10.1177%2F0734282917732890.

Barnato, A. E., Schenker, Y., Tiver, G., et al. (2017). Storytelling in the early bereavement period to reduce emotional distress among surrogates involved in a decision to limit life support in the ICU: A pilot feasibility trial. *Critical Care Medicine*, *45*(1), 35–46. doi:10.1097/CCM.0000000000002009.

Bernstein, E. E., & McNally, R. J. (2018). Exercise as a buffer against difficulties with emotion regulation: A pathway to emotional wellbeing. *Behaviour Research and Therapy*, *109*, 29–36. https://doi.org/10.1016/j.brat.2018.07.010.

Boardman, J. D. (2004). Stress and physical health: The role of neighborhoods as mediating and moderating mechanisms. *Social Science & Medicine*, *58*(12), 2473–2483.

Bottche, M., Kuwert, P., Pietrzak, R. H., & Knaevelsrud, C. (2016). Predictors of outcome of an internet-based cognitive-behavioural therapy for post-traumatic stress disorder in older adults. *British Psychological Society*, *89*(1), 82–96.

Bravo, L., Killela, M. K., Reyes, B. L., et al. (2020). Self-management, self-efficacy, and health-related quality of life in children with chronic illness and medical complexity. *Journal of Pediatric Health Care*, *34*(4), 304–314. https://doi.org/10.1016/j.pedhc.2019.11.009.

Chan, K. L., Chen, M., Lo, K. M. C., Chen, Q., Kelley, S. J., & Ip, P. (2019). The effectiveness of interventions for grandparents raising grandchildren: A meta-analysis. *Research on Social Work Practice*, *29*(6), 607–617. https://doi.org/10.1177%2F1049731518798470.

Chao, A. M., Minges, K. E., Park, C., et al. (2016). General life and diabetes-related stressors in early adolescents with type 1 diabetes. *Journal of Pediatric Health Care*, *30*(2), 133–142. https://doi.org/10.1016/j.pedhc.2015.06.005.

Chiang, J. J., Turiano, N. A., Mroczek, D. K., & Miller, G. E. (2018). Affective reactivity to daily stress and 20-year mortality risk in adults with chronic illness: Findings from the National Study of Daily Experiences. *Health Psychology*, *37*(2), 170–178. https://doi.org/10.1037/hea0000567.

Dageid, W., Akintola, O., & Saeberg, T. (2016). Sustaining motivation among community health workers in AIDS care in Kwazulu-Natal, South Africa: Challenges and prospects. *Journal of Community Psychology*, *44*(5), 569–585. https://doi.org/10.1002/jcop.21787.

Garaigordobil, M., & Machimbarrena, J. M. (2019). Victimization and perpetration of bullying/cyberbullying: Connections with emotional and behavioral problems and childhood stress. *Psychosocial Intervention*, *28*(2), 67–73. https://doi.org/10.5093/pi2019a3.

Gosain, R., Gage-Bouchard, E., Ambrosone, C., Repasky, E., & Gandhi, S. (2020). Stress reduction strategies in breast cancer: Review of pharmacologic and non-pharmacologic based strategies. *Seminars in Immunopathology*, *42*(6), 719–734.

Grano, C., Lucidi, F., & Violani, C. (2017). The relationship between caregiving self-efficacy and depressive symptoms in family caregivers of patients with Alzheimer disease: A longitudinal study. *International Psychogeriatrics*, *29*(7), 1095–1103. https://doi.org/10.1017/S1041610217000059.

Happell, B., Dwyer, T., Reid-Searl, K., Burke, K. J., Caperchione, C. M., & Gaskin, C. J. (2013). Nurses and stress: Recognizing causes and seeking solutions. *Journal of Nursing Management*, *21*(4), 638–647. https://doi.org/10.1111/jonm.12037.

Hazlett-Stevens, H., Singer, J., & Chong, A. (2019). Mindfulness-based stress reduction and mindfulness-based cognitive therapy with older adults: A qualitative review of randomized controlled outcome

S

research. *Clinical Gerontologist*, *42*(4), 347–358. https://doi.org/10.1080/07317115.2018.1518282.

Hou, Y., Zhang, D., Zhu, J., et al. (2020). Depression and anxiety symptoms as predictors of adverse cardiovascular events in Chinese patients after percutaneous coronary intervention. *Psychology: Health & Medicine*.[Online ahead of print]. https://doi.org/10.1080/13548506.2020.1837388.

Kendler, K. S., Myers, J., & Zisook, M. (2008). Does bereavement-related major depression differ from major depression associated with other stressful life events? *American Journal of Psychiatry*, *165*(11), 1449–1455.

Kim, T. Y., Kim, S. J., Choi, J. R., et al. (2017). The effect of trauma and PTSD on telomere length: An exploratory study in people exposed to combat trauma. *Scientific Reports*, *7*(1), 4375.

Kivimäki, M., Pentti, J., Ferrie, J. E., et al. (2018). Work stress and risk of death in men and women with and without cardiometabolic disease: A multicohort study. *Lancet Diabetes & Endocrinology*, *6*(9), 705–713. https://doi.org/10.1016/S2213-8587(18)30140-2.

Kujawa, A., Green, H., Compas, B. E., Dickey, L., & Pegg, S. (2020). Exposure to COVID–19 pandemic stress: Associations with depression and anxiety in emerging adults in the United States. *Depression and Anxiety*, *37*(12), 1280–1288. https://doi.org/10.1002/da.23109.

McNulty, P. A. F. (2005). Reported stressors and health care needs of active duty Navy personnel during three phases of deployment in support of the war in Iraq. *Military Medicine*, *170*(6), 530–535.

Mette, J., Wirth, T., Nienhaus, A., Harth, V., & Mache, S. (2020). "I need to take care of myself": A qualitative study on coping strategies, support and health promotion for social workers serving refugees and homeless individuals. *Journal of Occupational Medicine and Toxicology*, *15*, 19.

Mittal, M., & Bhakar, S. S. (2018). Examining the impact of role overload on job stress, job satisfaction and job performance-A study among married working women in banking sector. *International Journal of Management Studies*, *2*(7), 1–11. http://dx.doi.org/10.18843/ijms/v5i2(7)/01.

Mowla, F., Khanjari, S., & Inanlou, M. (2017). Contribution of Benson's relaxation technique and brief psycho-educational intervention on quality of life of primary caregivers of Iranian children with chronic diseases. *Journal of Pediatric Nursing*, *35*, 65–71. https://doi.org/10.1016/j.pedn.2017.02.037.

Newman, M. J. L., Holden, G. W., & Delville, Y. (2005). Isolation and the stress of being bullied. *Journal of Adolescence*, *28*(3), 343–357.

Perry-Parrish, C., Copeland-Linder, N., Webb, L., Shields, A. H., & Sibinga, E. M. (2016). Improving self-regulation in adolescents: Current evidence for the role of mindfulness-based cognitive therapy. *Adolescent Health, Medicine and Therapeutics*, *7*, 101–108. https://dx.doi.org/10.2147%2FAHMT.S65820.

Rajora, M. A., Goyal, H., & Guleria, R. (2019). Effectiveness of Nature-based sounds on psychological stress (agitation and anxiety) in patients under mechanical ventilation support. *International Journal of Advances in Nursing Management*, *7*(3), 169–175. http://dx.doi.org/10.5958/2454-2652.2019.00041.6.

Shah, P. S., Shah, J., & Knowledge Synthesis Group on Determinants of Preterm/LBW Births. (2010). Maternal exposure to domestic violence and pregnancy and birth outcomes: A systematic review and meta-analyses. *Journal of Women's Health*, *19*(11), 2017–2031.

Sommer, J. L., Reynolds, K., El-Gabalawy, R., et al. (2021). Associations between physical health conditions and posttraumatic stress disorder according to age. *Aging & Mental Health*, *25*(2), 234–242. https://doi.org/10.1080/13607863.2019.1693969.

Sue, D. W., Capodilupo, C. M., Torino, G. C., et al. (2007). Racial microaggressions in everyday life: Implications for clinical practice. *American Psychologist*, *62*(4), 271–286.

Uy, J. P., & Galván, A. (2017). Acute stress increases risky decisions and dampens prefrontal activation among adolescent boys. *NeuroImage*, *146*, 679–689.

Van Bodegom, M., Homberg, J. R., & Henckens, M. J. A. G. (2017). Modulation of the hypothalamic-pituitary adrenal axis by early life stress exposure. *Frontiers in Cellular Neuroscience*, *11*(87), 1–33.

Van Tieghem, M. R., & Tottenham, N. (2018). Neurobiological programming of early life stress: Functional development of amygdala-prefrontal circuitry and vulnerability for stress-related psychopathology. *Current Topics in Behavioral Neurosciences*, *38*, 117–136.

Viseu, J., Leal, R., de Jesus, S. N., Pinto, P., Pechorro, P., & Greenglass, E. (2018). Relationship between economic stress factors and stress, anxiety, and depression: Moderating role of social support. *Psychiatry Research*, *268*, 102–107. https://doi.org/10.1016/j.psychres.2018.07.008.

Vizoso, C., Arias-Gundín, O., & Rodríguez, C. (2019). Exploring coping and optimism as predictors of academic burnout and performance among university students. *Educational Psychology*, *39*(6), 768–783. https://doi.org/10.1080/01443410.2018.1545996.

Wu, S., Renzaho, A. M. N., Hall, B. J., Shi, L., Ling, L., & Chen, W. (2020). Time-varying associations of pre-migration and post-migration stressors in refugees' mental health during resettlement: A longitudinal study in Australia. *Lancet Psychiatry*, *8*(1), 36–47. https://doi.org/10.1016/S2215-0366(20)30422-3.

Yang, J., Tang, S., & Zhou, W. (2018). Effect of mindfulness-based stress reduction therapy on work stress and mental health of psychiatric nurses. *Psychiatria Danubina*, *30*(2), 189–196.

Acute Substance Withdrawal Syndrome

Domain 9 Coping/stress tolerance Class 3 Neurobehavioral stress

Marina Martinez-Kratz, MS, RN, CNE

NANDA-I

Definition

Serious, multifactorial sequelae following abrupt cessation of an addictive compound.

Defining Characteristics

Acute confusion (00128); anxiety (00146); disturbed sleep pattern (00198); nausea (00134); risk for electrolyte imbalance (00195); risk for injury (00035)

Related Factors

Developed dependence to addictive substances; excessive use of an addictive substance over time; malnutrition; sudden cessation of an addictive substance

At-Risk Population

Individuals with history of withdrawal symptoms; older adults

Associated Conditions

Significant comorbidity

NOC (Nursing Outcomes Classification)

Suggested NOC Outcomes

Anxiety Level; Comfort Status; Drug Abuse Cessation Behavior; Electrolyte Balance; Seizure Severity; Substance Addiction Consequences; Substance Withdrawal Severity; Symptom Severity; Vital Signs

Example NOC Outcome with Indicators

Substance Withdrawal Severity as evidenced by the following indicators: Substance cravings/Change in vital signs/Irritability/Nausea. (Rate the outcome and indicators of **Substance Withdrawal Severity:** 1 = severe deviation from normal range, 2 = substantial deviation from normal range, 3 = moderate deviation from normal range, 4 = mild deviation from normal range, 5 = no deviation from normal range [see Section I].)

Client Outcomes

Client Will (Specify Time Frame)

- Stabilize and remain free from physical injury
- Verbalize effects of substances on body
- Maintain vital signs and laboratory values within normal range
- Verbalize importance of adequate nutrition

NIC (Nursing Interventions Classification)

Suggested NIC Interventions

Behavior Management; Drug Withdrawal; Electrolyte Monitoring; Emotional Support; Nausea Management; Seizure Precautions; Smoking Cessation Assistance; Substance Use Treatment: Alcohol Withdrawal; Substance Use Treatment: Anxiety Reduction

Example NIC Activities—Substance Use Treatment: Alcohol Withdrawal

Monitor vital signs during withdrawal, Monitor for delirium tremens, Administer medications, Provide symptom management, Implement seizure precautions

S

Nursing Interventions and *Rationales*

Alcohol-Induced Withdrawal Syndrome

- Assess for the client's pattern of alcohol use, last drink, and current blood alcohol levels. EB: *Because of ethanol's short action, withdrawal symptoms begin within 6 to 8 hours after blood alcohol levels decrease, peak at 72 hours, and are markedly reduced by days 5 through 7 (Long, Long, & Koyfman, 2017).*
- Implement seizure precautions. EB: *Clients in alcohol withdrawal are at risk for developing withdrawal seizures related to central nervous system hyperstimulation caused by loss of gamma-aminobutyric acid inhibitory effect (Long, Long, & Koyfman, 2017). The development of acute symptomatic seizures during an alcohol withdrawal episode is associated with a fourfold increase in the mortality rate that is caused by complications of severe alcohol use disorder (Jesse et al, 2017).*
- Rule out other causes of symptoms. EB: *The presence of other disease processes requires immediate treatment and stabilization (Long, Long, & Koyfman, 2017). Other assessments should include a check of blood*

gases, a review of glucose and electrolyte laboratory panels, a review of potential medication reactions, presence of infection, and other conditions.

- Monitor vital signs. **EB:** *Tachycardia and hypertension are among the broad symptoms of alcohol withdrawal (Long, Long, & Koyfman, 2017).*
- Assess for progression of withdrawal symptoms such as insomnia, anxiety, nausea/vomiting, tremulousness, headache, diaphoresis, palpitations, increased body temperature, tachycardia, and hypertension. **EB:** *These are the broad symptoms of alcohol withdrawal that can progress in intensity without treatment (Makic, 2017).*
- Monitor severity of withdrawal symptoms with the Clinical Institute Withdrawal Assessment (CIWA-Ar). **CEB:** *The CIWA-Ar is a 10-item scale for clinical quantification of the severity of the alcohol withdrawal syndrome (Sullivan et al, 1989). The CIWA-Ar scale is available at* https://umem.org/files/uploads/1104212257_CIWA-Ar.pdf.
- Evaluate the client for progression to delirium tremens (DTs). **EB:** *DTs are severe and life-threatening withdrawal symptoms that occur in 3% to 5% of clients on about the third day of withdrawal. DT symptoms have a rapid onset and include the broad alcohol withdrawal symptoms, fluctuating levels of cognition and attention, and autonomic instability. Associated risk factors are previous DTs, untreated seizures, CIWA-Ar score >15, heart rate >100, history of sustained drinking, systolic blood pressure >150 mm Hg, alcohol intake >2 days, age >30 years, recent misuse of benzodiazepines, and concurrent medical illness (Long, Long, & Koyfman, 2017).*
- Assess nutritional status for risk of malnutrition. Assess for thiamine (B_1) deficiency, which is associated with chronic alcohol abuse, folate deficiency, and vitamin D deficiency associated with a history of inadequate exposure to sunlight. Consult with health care provider as needed for supplement order. **EB:** *Alcoholism is a major cause of malnutrition in the United States. Thiamine deficiencies contribute to the development of Korsakoff's syndrome and Wernicke's encephalopathy, which are neurological complications of alcohol abuse (Dugum & McCullough, 2015). Vitamin D insufficiency is associated with cognitive impairment (Goodwill & Szoeke, 2017).*
- Address hydration needs. **EB:** *Clients in alcohol withdrawal require administration of fluids to correct dehydration (Mirijello et al, 2015; Long, Long, & Koyfman, 2017).*
- Determine hepatic and renal functioning before administration of medications. **EB:** *Hepatic or renal disease can slow the clearance of medications and lead to complications or toxicities (Long, Long, & Koyfman, 2017).*

Opioid-Induced Withdrawal Syndrome

- Assess for the client's opioid of choice, last use, and current withdrawal symptoms. **EB:** The onset of withdrawal symptoms depends on the half-life of the opioid used. Heroin withdrawal occurs 6 to 8 hours after the last use, and methadone and fentanyl withdrawal occur 1 to 3 days after the last dose *(Donroe & Tetrault, 2017).*
- Monitor severity of withdrawal symptoms with the Clinical Opiate Withdrawal Scale (COWS). **CEB:** *A standardized assessment tool is necessary for evaluating and treating opioid withdrawal. The COWS is scored numerically based on severity, with values summed to give a cumulative score. A threshold score indicates when treatment should be initiated (Wesson & Ling, 2003).*
- Nurses should wait to administer the first dose of buprenorphine to opioid-dependent clients until clients are experiencing mild to moderate opioid withdrawal symptoms. **EB:** *The American Society of Addiction Medicine (ASAM) National Practice Guidelines recommended waiting to administer the first dose of buprenorphine until clients are experiencing mild to moderate opioid withdrawal symptoms to reduce the risk of precipitated withdrawal (Kampman & Jarvis, 2015).*
- Assess and manage early opioid withdrawal symptoms (agitation, anxiety, insomnia, muscle aches, increased lacrimation, rhinorrhea, sweating, and yawning) and late opioid withdrawal symptoms (abdominal cramping, diarrhea, pupillary dilation, nausea, vomiting, and piloerection). **EBN:** *Severe withdrawal can lead to fluid and electrolyte imbalances, cardiac dysrhythmias, acute kidney injury, or rhabdomyolysis. A failure to treat could result in client injury or in clients leaving the clinical setting against medical advice (Turner et al, 2018).*
- Monitor vital signs. **EBN:** *Parameters for blood pressure should be followed especially for clients treated with clonidine or other alpha-2 agonists, which can cause hypotension (Turner et al, 2018).*
- Teach the client about the anticipated withdrawal symptoms and opioid cravings while offering support and encouragement. **EBN:** *A lack of knowledge and decreased nurse empathy and engagement are barriers to treatment (Worley, 2017).*

- ▲ Monitor laboratory reports and report to health care provider. **EBN:** *Serum electrolytes are closely evaluated for abnormalities and replaced as indicated (Turner et al, 2018).*
- ▲ Refer client for buprenorphine, methadone, or naltrexone treatment. **EB:** *Using medications for opioid withdrawal management is recommended over abrupt cessation of opioids. Abrupt cessation of opioids may lead to strong cravings, which can lead to continued use (Kampman & Jarvis, 2015). A study showed that emergency department–initiated buprenorphine was associated with increased engagement in addiction treatment and reduced illicit opioid use during the 2-month interval when buprenorphine was continued in primary care (D'Onofrio et al, 2017).*

Benzodiazepine-Induced Withdrawal Syndrome

- ● Assess for the client's last benzodiazepine use and current withdrawal symptoms. **EB:** *The onset of withdrawal symptoms occurs within 1 to 3 days of drug cessation. Common withdrawal symptoms include any of the following: autonomic instability (tachycardia, elevated blood pressure), tremulousness, diaphoresis, insomnia, anxiety, depression, psychosis (hallucinations, delusions), sensory hypersensitivity (photophobia, hyperacusis), perceptual distortions, depersonalization, agoraphobia, flulike symptoms, paresthesias, muscle stiffness, ataxia, visual disturbances, DTs, and seizures (Puening et al, 2017).*
- ● Implement seizure precautions. **EB:** *Clients withdrawing from benzodiazepines may also experience seizures on withdrawal (Puening et al, 2017).*
- ● Rule out delirium from other causes or other withdrawal syndromes. **EB:** *The symptoms of benzodiazepine withdrawal appear similar to delirium, as well as barbiturate or alcohol withdrawal (Puening et al, 2017).*
- ▲ Anticipate use of the same treatment protocols as for alcohol withdrawal and use of a long-acting benzodiazepine in tapering doses over time. **EB:** *A tapering schedule will assist with prevention of relapse (Donroe & Tetrault, 2017).*

Cocaine/Methamphetamine-Induced Withdrawal Syndrome

- ● Assess for the client's last stimulant use and current withdrawal symptoms. **EB:** *The onset of withdrawal symptoms occurs within 24 hours after abrupt discontinuation of using high amounts of amphetamine-type substances over a prolonged period of time. Common stimulant withdrawal symptoms include depressed mood with any of the following: fatigue, vivid dreams, insomnia, increased appetite, psychomotor retardation, and agitation. Cocaine withdrawal is mild and treated supportively. Methamphetamine use can result in significant psychiatric withdrawal symptoms and intense craving after abrupt cessation (Donroe & Tetrault, 2017).*

Cannabis-Induced Withdrawal Syndrome

- ● Assess for the client's last cannabis use and current withdrawal symptoms. **EB:** *The onset of withdrawal symptoms occurs within a week of cannabis cessation. Common cannabis withdrawal symptoms include any of the following: anxiety, irritability, malaise, dysphoria, decreased appetite, restlessness, and sleep disturbances (Zehra et al, 2018).*
- ● Direct nursing actions to address anxiety, irritability, sleep disturbances, and decreased appetite. **EB:** *Nursing care should target the specific symptoms of cannabis withdrawal as part of a treatment that targets cannabis use reduction and prevention of relapse (Zehra et al, 2018).*

Nicotine-Induced Withdrawal Syndrome

- ● Assess for the client's last nicotine use and current withdrawal symptoms. **EB:** *The onset of withdrawal symptoms occurs within hours of last use. Common nicotine withdrawal symptoms include craving for nicotine, irritability, anger, frustration, anxiety, difficulty concentrating, restlessness, decreased heart rate, increased appetite, weight gain, tremor, headaches, craving, delirium, and sleep disturbance (Ginige, 2016).*
- ● Rule out nicotine withdrawal as the cause of delirium in critically ill clients. **EB:** *Chronic consumption of nicotine can cause desensitization and upregulation of acetylcholine receptors. In an acute nicotine withdrawal state, the lack of sufficient nicotinic stimulation leads to acetylcholine deficiency, which is associated with delirium (Ginige, 2016).*

All Withdrawal Syndromes

- ● Obtain a drug and/or alcohol history using a tool such as the AUDIT-C or the DAST-10. **EB:** *The Audit-C is a simple 3-question screen for hazardous or harmful drinking that can stand alone or be incorporated into* *general health history questionnaires. The DAST-10 is a 10-item, yes/no self-report instrument that takes less than 8 minutes to complete* (*Mulvaney-Day et al, 2018*).

- Implement and follow institutional withdrawal protocols. EB: *A study suggested that using a protocol for treatment of critical care clients with alcohol withdrawal leads to decreased intensive care unit (ICU) length of stay and reduced ICU cost* (*Tavani et al, 2018*).
- Assess for signs of recent trauma or head injury. EB: *A study found that trauma clients who present to the hospital in a delayed fashion have unique characteristics and are more likely to suffer negative outcomes, including substance withdrawal* (*Kao et al, 2017*).
- Assess the client's level of consciousness, monitor for changes in behavior, and orient to reality as needed. EB: *Reality orientation will support the client with changes in level of consciousness or behavior and may indicate progression of withdrawal (Mirijello et al, 2015).*
- Assess vital signs and monitor for existing medical conditions and current medications. EB: *Withdrawal symptoms can be exacerbated or masked by existing medical conditions, medications, or treatments (Long, Long, & Koyfman, 2017).*
- Assess and monitor for expression of psychological distress. EB: *Withdrawal can cause or exacerbate current emotional, psychological, or mental problems (Harford et al, 2018).*
- Collect urine/serum samples for laboratory tests. EB: *Routine treatment for substance withdrawal should include serum (or breath) alcohol concentrations, complete blood count, renal function tests, electrolytes, glucose, liver enzymes, urinalysis, and urine toxicology screening* (*Mirijello et al, 2015*).
- Address craving for substances with mindfulness-based techniques. EB: *Compared with those receiving usual care, a study found that mindfulness-based addiction treatment participants reported lower anxiety, concentration difficulties, craving, and dependence, as well as higher self-efficacy for managing negative affect without smoking* (*Spears et al, 2017*).
- Respond to agitated behavior with deescalation techniques. EBN: *Research shows that staff intervention can modify processes and reduce further conflict (Berring, Pedersen, & Buus, 2016).*
- Administer as-needed (PRN) medications for agitation and symptom control as ordered. EB: *A study found that symptom-triggered treatment for alcohol withdrawal syndrome individualizes treatment, is safe, decreases treatment duration and the use of benzodiazepines, and consequently reduces health care costs* (*Soravia et al, 2018*).
- Provide a quiet room without dark shadows, noises, or other excessive stimuli. EB: *Supportive care includes controlling environmental stimuli that may increase client agitation or irritability (Mirijello et al, 2015).*
- Provide suicide precautions and 1:1 staffing for clients who are delirious or who may present a danger to themselves or others. EB: *A study showed that substance use disorders are associated with self- and other-directed violence (Harford et al, 2018).*

Client/Family Teaching and Discharge Planning

▲ After withdrawal symptoms have subsided, refer the client to substance use treatment and long-term management. EB: *Collaborative discharge planning can increase the likelihood of the client's success with substance abstinence. Referral to appropriate services can reduce discharges against medical advice and increase follow-up in postdischarge addiction treatment centers (Donroe & Tetrault, 2017).*

▲ Refer for smoking cessation services that target nicotine craving. EB: *A study found that nicotine craving may be a useful therapeutic target for increasing the effectiveness of smoking-cessation treatment (Magee, Lewis, & Winhusen, 2016).*

S

REFERENCES

Berring, L. L., Pedersen, L., & Buus, N. (2016). Coping with violence in mental health care settings: Patient and staff member perspectives on de-escalation practices. *Archives of Psychiatric Nursing*, *30*(5), 499–507. https://doi.org/10.1016/j.apnu.2016.05.005.

D'Onofrio, G., Chawarski, M. C., O'Connor, P. G., et al. (2017). Emergency department-initiated buprenorphine for opioid dependence with continuation in primary care: Outcomes during and after intervention. *Journal of General Internal Medicine*, *32*(6), 660–666. https://doi.org/10.1007/s11606-017-3993-2.

Donroe, J. H., & Tetrault, J. M. (2017). Substance use, intoxication, and withdrawal in the critical care setting. *Critical Care Clinics*, *33*(3), 543–558.

Dugum, M., & McCullough, A. (2015). Diagnosis and management of alcoholic liver disease. *Journal of Clinical Translational Hepatology*, *3*(2), 109–116.

Ginige, S. (2016). Nicotine withdrawal: An often overlooked and easily reversible cause of terminal restlessness. *European Journal of Palliative Care*, *23*(3), 128–129.

Goodwill, A. M., & Szoeke, C. (2017). A systematic review and meta-analysis of the effect of low vitamin D on cognition. *Journal of the American Geriatric Society*, *65*(10), 2161–2168. https://doi.org/10.1111/jgs.15012.

Harford, T. C., Yi, H. Y., Chen, C. M., & Grant, B. F. (2018). Substance use disorders and self- and other-directed violence among adults: Results from the national survey on drug use and health. *Journal of Affective Disorders, 225*, 365–373. https://doi.org/10.1016/j.jad.2017.08.021.

Jesse, S., Bråthen, G., Ferrara, M., et al. (2017). Alcohol withdrawal syndrome: Mechanisms, manifestations, and management. *Acta Neurologica Scandinavica, 135*(1), 4–16. https://doi.org/10.1111/ane.12671.

Kampman, K., & Jarvis, M. (2015). American Society of Addiction Medicine (ASAM) national practice guideline for the use of medications in the treatment of addiction involving opioid use. *Journal of Addiction Medicine, 9*(5), 358–367.

Kao, M. J., Nunez, H., Monaghan, S. F., et al. (2017). Trauma patients who present in a delayed fashion: A unique and challenging population. *Journal of Surgical Research, 208*, 204–210. https://doi.org/10.1016/j.jss.2016.09.037.

Long, D., Long, B., & Koyfman, A. (2017). The emergency medicine management of severe alcohol withdrawal. *American Journal of Emergency Medicine, 35*(7), 1005–1011. https://doi.org/10.1016/j.ajem.2017.02.002.

Magee, J. C., Lewis, D. F., & Winhusen, T. (2016). Evaluating nicotine craving, withdrawal, and substance use as mediators of smoking cessation in cocaine- and methamphetamine-dependent patients. *Nicotine & Tobacco Research, 18*(5), 1196–1201. https://doi.org/10.1093/ntr/ntv121.

Makic, M. B. F. (2017). Alcohol withdrawal syndrome. *Journal of PeriAnesthesia Nursing, 32*(2), 140–141. https://doi.org/10.1016/j.jopan.2017.01.007.

Mirijello, A., D'Angelo, C., Ferrulli, A., et al. (2015). Identification and management of alcohol withdrawal syndrome. *Drugs, 75*(4), 353–365. https://doi.org/10.1007/s40265-015-0358-1.

Mulvaney-Day, N., Marshall, T., Piscopo, K. D., et al. (2018). Screening for behavioral health conditions in primary care settings: A systematic review of the literature. *Journal of General Internal Medicine, 33*(3), 335–346. https://doi.org/10.1007/s11606-017-4181-0.

Puening, S. E., Wilson, W. P., & Nordstrom, K. (2017). Psychiatric emergencies for clinicians: Emergency department management of benzodiazepine withdrawal. *Journal of Emergency Medicine, 52*(1), 66–69. https://doi.org/10.1016/j.jemermed.2016.05.035.

Soravia, L. M., Wopfner, A., Pfiffner, L., Bétrisey, S., & Moggi, F. (2018). Symptom-triggered detoxification using the alcohol-withdrawal-scale reduces risks and healthcare costs. *Alcohol and Alcoholism, 53*(1), 71–77. https://doi.org/10.1093/alcalc/agx080.

Spears, C. A., Hedeker, D., Li, L., et al. (2017). Mechanisms underlying mindfulness-based addiction treatment versus cognitive behavioral therapy and usual care for smoking cessation. *Journal of Consulting and Clinical Psychology, 85*(11), 1029–1040. https://doi.org/10.1037/ccp0000229.

Sullivan, J. T., Sykora, K., Schneiderman, J., Naranjo, C. A., & Sellers, E. M. (1989). Assessment of alcohol withdrawal: The revised Clinical Institute Withdrawal Assessment for alcohol scale. *British Journal of Addiction, 84*(11), 1353–1357.

Tavani, L., Gahagen, L., Atwood, J., Shaw, D., Farraj, M., & Gajera, M. (2018). A protocol for the management of alcohol withdrawal in the intensive care unit: A pilot study. *Critical Care Medicine, 46*(1 Suppl. 1), 357. https://doi.org/10.1097/01.ccm.0000528755.55400.b6.

Turner, C. C., Fogger, S. A., & Frazier, S. L. (2018). Opioid use disorder: Challenges during acute hospitalization. *Journal for Nurse Practitioners, 14*(2), 61–67. https://doi.org/10.1016/j.nurpra.2017.12.009.

Wesson, D. R., & Ling, W. (2003). The Clinical Opiate Withdrawal Scale (COWS). *Journal of Psychoactive Drugs, 35*(2), 253–259.

Worley, J. (2017). A primer on heroin and fentanyl. *Journal of Psychosocial Nursing and Mental Health Services, 55*(6), 16–20. https://doi.org/10.3928/02793695-20170519-02.

Zehra, A., Burns, J., Liu, C. K., et al. (2018). Cannabis addiction and the brain: A review. *Journal of Neuroimmune Pharmacology, 13*(4), 438–452. https://doi.org/10.1007/s11481-018-9782-9.

Risk for Acute Substance Withdrawal Syndrome

Domain 9 Coping/stress tolerance

Class 3 Neurobehavioral stress

Marina Martinez-Kratz, MS, RN, CNE

S

NANDA-I

Definition

Susceptible to serious, multifactorial sequelae following abrupt cessation of an addictive compound, which may compromise health.

Risk Factors

Developed dependence to addictive substance; excessive use of an addictive substance over time; malnutrition; sudden cessation of an addictive substance

At-Risk Population

Individuals with history of withdrawal symptoms; older adults

Associated Conditions

Significant comorbidity

NOC (Nursing Outcomes Classification)

Suggested NOC Outcomes

Anxiety Level; Comfort Status; Drug Abuse Cessation Behavior; Electrolyte Balance; Seizure Severity; Substance Addiction Consequences; Substance Withdrawal Severity; Symptom Severity; Vital Signs

Example NOC Outcome with Indicators

Substance Withdrawal Severity as evidenced by the following indicators: Substance cravings/Change in vital signs/Irritability/Nausea. (Rate the outcome and indicators of **Substance Withdrawal Severity:** 1 = severe deviation from normal range, 2 = substantial deviation from normal range, 3 = moderate deviation from normal range, 4 = mild deviation from normal range, 5 = no deviation from normal range [see Section I].)

Client Outcomes

Client Will (Specify Time Frame)

- Stabilize and remain free from physical injury
- Verbalize effects of substances on body
- Maintain vital signs and laboratory values within normal range
- Verbalize importance of adequate nutrition

NIC (Nursing Interventions Classification)

Suggested NIC Interventions

Anxiety Reduction; Behavior Management; Electrolyte Monitoring; Emotional Support; Nausea Management; Seizure Precautions; Smoking Cessation Assistance; Substance Use Treatment: Alcohol Withdrawal; Substance Use Treatment: Drug Withdrawal

Example NIC Activities—Substance Use Treatment: Alcohol Withdrawal

Monitor vital signs during withdrawal, Monitor for delirium tremens, Administer medications, Provide symptom management, Implement seizure precautions

Nursing Interventions and *Rationales*

Risk for Alcohol-Induced Withdrawal Syndrome

- Assess for the client's pattern of alcohol use, last drink, and current blood alcohol levels. EB: *Because of ethanol's short action, withdrawal symptoms begin within 6 to 8 hours after blood alcohol levels decrease, peak at 72 hours, and are markedly reduced by days 5 through 7 (Long, Long, & Koyfman, 2017).*
- Implement seizure precautions. EB: *Clients in alcohol withdrawal are at risk for developing withdrawal seizures related to central nervous system hyperstimulation caused by loss of gamma-aminobutyric acid inhibitory effect (Long, Long, & Koyfman, 2017). The development of acute symptomatic seizures during an alcohol withdrawal episode is associated with a fourfold increase in the mortality rate caused by complications of severe alcohol use disorder (Jesse et al, 2017).*
- Rule out other causes of symptoms. EB: *The presence of other disease processes requires immediate treatment and stabilization (Long, Long, & Koyfman, 2017). Other assessments should include a check of blood gases, a review of glucose and electrolyte laboratory panels, a review of potential medication reactions, presence of infection, and other conditions.*
- Monitor vital signs. EB: *Tachycardia and hypertension are among the broad symptoms of alcohol withdrawal (Long, Long, & Koyfman, 2017).*
- Assess for progression of withdrawal symptoms such as insomnia, anxiety, nausea/vomiting, tremulousness, headache, diaphoresis, palpitations, increased body temperature, tachycardia, and hypertension. EBN: *These are the broad symptoms of alcohol withdrawal that can progress in intensity without treatment (Makic, 2017).*

S

- Monitor severity of withdrawal symptoms with the Clinical Institute Withdrawal Assessment (CIWA-Ar). CEB: *The CIWA-Ar is a 10-item scale for clinical quantification of the severity of the alcohol withdrawal syndrome (Sullivan et al, 1989; Kattimani & Bharadwaj, 2013). The CIWA-Ar scale is available at* https://umem.org/files/uploads/1104212257_CIWA-Ar.pdf.
- Evaluate the client for progression to delirium tremens (DTs). EB: *DTs are severe and life-threatening withdrawal symptoms that occur in 3% to 5% of clients on about the third day of withdrawal. DT symptoms have a rapid onset and include the broad alcohol withdrawal symptoms, fluctuating levels of cognition and attention, and autonomic instability. Associated risk factors are previous DTs, untreated seizures, CIWA-Ar score >15, heart rate >100, history of sustained drinking, systolic blood pressure >150 mm Hg, alcohol intake >2 days, age >30 years, recent misuse of benzodiazepines, and concurrent medical illness (Long, Long, & Koyfman, 2017).*
- Assess nutritional status for risk of malnutrition, thiamine (B_1) deficiency associated with chronic alcohol abuse, folate deficiency, and vitamin D deficiency–associated history of inadequate exposure to sunlight. Consult with health care provider as needed for supplement order. EB: *Alcoholism is a major cause of malnutrition in the United States. Thiamine deficiencies contribute to the development of Korsakoff's syndrome and Wernicke's encephalopathy, which are neurological complications of alcohol abuse (Dugum & McCullough, 2015). Vitamin D insufficiency is associated with cognitive impairment (Goodwill & Szoeke, 2017).*
- Address hydration needs. EB: *Clients in alcohol withdrawal require administration of fluids to correct dehydration (Mirijello et al, 2015; Long, Long, & Koyfman, 2017).*
- Determine hepatic and renal functioning before administration of medications. EB: *Hepatic or renal disease can slow the clearance of medications and lead to complications or toxicities (Long, Long, & Koyfman, 2017).*

Risk for Opioid-Induced Withdrawal Syndrome

- Assess for the client's opioid of choice, last use, and current withdrawal symptoms. EB: *The onset of withdrawal symptoms depends on the half-life of the opioid used. Heroin withdrawal occurs 6 to 8 hours after the last use, and methadone and fentanyl withdrawal occur 1 to 3 days after the last dose (Donroe & Tetrault, 2017).*
- Monitor severity of withdrawal symptoms with the Clinical Opiate Withdrawal Scale (COWS). CEB: *A standardized assessment tool is necessary for evaluating and treating opioid withdrawal. The COWS is scored numerically based on severity, with values summed to give a cumulative score. A threshold score indicates when treatment should be initiated (Wesson & Ling, 2003).*
- Assess and manage early opioid withdrawal symptoms (agitation, anxiety, insomnia, muscle aches, increased lacrimation, rhinorrhea, sweating, and yawning) and late opioid withdrawal symptoms (abdominal cramping, diarrhea, pupillary dilation, nausea, vomiting, and piloerection). EBN: *Severe withdrawal can lead to fluid and electrolyte imbalances, cardiac dysrhythmias, acute kidney injury, or rhabdomyolysis. A failure to treat could result in client injury or in clients leaving the clinical setting against medical advice (Turner et al, 2018).*
- Monitor vital signs. EBN: *Parameters for blood pressure should be followed especially for clients treated with clonidine or other alpha-2 agonists, which can cause hypotension (Turner et al, 2018).*
- Clients should be taught about risk of relapse and other safety concerns from using opioid withdrawal management as stand-alone treatment for opioid use disorder. EB: *Opioid withdrawal management on its own is not a treatment method (Kampman & Jarvis, 2015).*
- Teach the client about the anticipated withdrawal symptoms and opioid cravings, while offering support and encouragement. EBN: *A lack of knowledge and decreased nurse empathy and engagement are barriers to treatment (Worley, 2017).*

▲ Monitor laboratory reports and report to health care provider. EBN: *Serum electrolytes are closely evaluated for abnormalities and replaced as indicated (Turner et al, 2018).*

▲ Refer client for buprenorphine or methadone treatment. EB: *Using medications for opioid withdrawal management is recommended over abrupt cessation of opioids. Abrupt cessation of opioids may lead to strong cravings, which can lead to continued use (Kampman & Jarvis, 2015). A study showed that emergency department–initiated buprenorphine was associated with increased engagement in addiction treatment and reduced illicit opioid use during the 2-month interval when buprenorphine was continued in primary care (D'Onofrio et al, 2017).*

S

Risk for Benzodiazepine-Induced Withdrawal Syndrome

- Assess for the client's last benzodiazepine use and current withdrawal symptoms. EB: *The onset of withdrawal symptoms occurs within 1 to 3 days of drug cessation. Common withdrawal symptoms include any of the following: autonomic instability (tachycardia, elevated blood pressure), tremulousness, diaphoresis, insomnia, anxiety, depression, psychosis (hallucinations, delusions), sensory hypersensitivity (photophobia, hyperacusis), perceptual distortions, depersonalization, agoraphobia, flulike symptoms, paresthesia, muscle stiffness, ataxia, visual disturbances, DTs, and seizures (Puening et al, 2017).*
- Implement seizure precautions. EB: *Clients withdrawing from benzodiazepines may also experience seizures on withdrawal (Puening et al, 2017).*
- Rule out delirium from other causes or other withdrawal syndromes. EB: *The symptoms of benzodiazepine withdrawal appear similar to delirium, as well as barbiturate or alcohol withdrawal (Puening et al, 2017).*
- ▲ Anticipate use of the same treatment protocols as for alcohol withdrawal and use of a long-acting benzodiazepine in tapering doses over time. EB: *A tapering schedule will assist with prevention of relapse (Donroe & Tetrault, 2017).*

Risk for Cocaine/Methamphetamine-Induced Withdrawal Syndrome

- Assess for the client's last stimulant use and current withdrawal symptoms. EB: *The onset of withdrawal symptoms occurs within 24 hours after abrupt discontinuation of using high amounts of amphetamine-type substances over a prolonged period of time. Common stimulant withdrawal symptoms include depressed mood with any of the following: fatigue, vivid dreams, insomnia, increased appetite, psychomotor retardation, and agitation. Cocaine withdrawal is mild and treated supportively. Methamphetamine use can result in significant psychiatric withdrawal symptoms and intense craving after abrupt cessation (Donroe & Tetrault, 2017).*

Risk for Cannabis-Induced Withdrawal Syndrome

- Assess for the client's last cannabis use and current withdrawal symptoms. EB: *The onset of withdrawal symptoms occurs within a week of cannabis cessation. Common cannabis withdrawal symptoms include any of the following: anxiety, irritability, malaise, dysphoria, decreased appetite, restlessness, and sleep disturbances (Zehra et al, 2018).*
- Direct nursing actions to address anxiety, irritability, sleep disturbances, and decreased appetite. EB: *Nursing care should target the specific symptoms of cannabis withdrawal as part of a treatment that targets cannabis use reduction and prevention of relapse (Zehra et al, 2018).*

Risk for Nicotine-Induced Withdrawal Syndrome

- Assess for the client's last nicotine use and current withdrawal symptoms. EB: *The onset of withdrawal symptoms occurs within hours of last use. Common nicotine withdrawal symptoms include craving for nicotine, irritability, anger, frustration, anxiety, difficulty concentrating, restlessness, decreased heart rate, increased appetite, weight gain, tremor, headaches, craving, delirium, and sleep disturbance (Ginige, 2016).*
- Rule out nicotine withdrawal as the cause of delirium in critically ill clients. EB: *Chronic consumption of nicotine can cause desensitization and upregulation of acetylcholine receptors. In an acute nicotine withdrawal state, the lack of sufficient nicotinic stimulation leads to acetylcholine deficiency, which is associated with delirium (Ginige, 2016).*

S

All Withdrawal Syndromes

- Obtain a drug and/or alcohol history using a tool such as the AUDIT-C or the DAST-10. EB: *The Audit-C is a simple 3-question screen for hazardous or harmful drinking that can stand alone or be incorporated into general health history questionnaires. The DAST-10 is a 10-item, yes/no self-report instrument that takes less than 8 minutes to complete (Mulvaney-Day et al, 2018).*
- Implement and follow institutional withdrawal protocols. EB: *A study suggested that using a protocol for treatment of critical care clients with alcohol withdrawal leads to decreased intensive care unit (ICU) length of stay and reduced ICU cost (Tavani et al, 2018).*
- Assess for signs of recent trauma or head injury. EB: *A study found that trauma clients who present to the hospital in a delayed fashion have unique characteristics and are more likely to suffer negative outcomes, including substance withdrawal (Kao et al, 2017).*

- Assess the client's level of consciousness, monitor for changes in behavior, and orient to reality as needed. **EB:** *Reality orientation will support the client with changes in level of consciousness or behavior and may indicate progression of withdrawal (Mirijello et al, 2015).*
- Assess vital signs and monitor for existing medical conditions and current medications. **EB:** *Withdrawal symptoms can be exacerbated or masked by existing medical conditions, medications, or treatments (Long, Long, & Koyfman, 2017).*
- Assess and monitor for expression of psychological distress. **EB:** *Withdrawal can cause or exacerbate current emotional, psychological, or mental problems (Harford et al, 2018).*
- Collect urine/serum samples for laboratory tests. **EB:** *Routine treatment for substance withdrawal should include serum (or breath) alcohol concentrations, complete blood count, renal function tests, electrolytes, glucose, liver enzymes, urinalysis, and urine toxicology screening (Mirijello et al, 2015).*
- Address craving for substances with mindfulness-based techniques. **EB:** *Compared with those receiving usual care, a study found that mindfulness-based addiction treatment participants reported lower anxiety, concentration difficulties, craving, and dependence, as well as higher self-efficacy for managing negative affect without smoking (Spears et al, 2017).*
- Respond to agitated behavior with deescalation techniques. **EBN:** *Research shows that staff intervention can modify processes and reduce further conflict (Berring, Pedersen, & Buus, 2016).*
- Administer as-needed (PRN) medications for agitation and symptom control as ordered. **EB:** *A study found that symptom-triggered treatment for alcohol withdrawal syndrome individualizes treatment, is safe, decreases treatment duration and the use of benzodiazepines, and consequently reduces health care costs (Soravia et al, 2018).*
- Provide a quiet room without dark shadows, noises, or other excessive stimuli. **EB:** *Supportive care includes controlling environmental stimuli that may increase client agitation or irritability (Mirijello et al, 2015).*
- Provide suicide precautions and 1:1 staffing for clients who are delirious or who may present a danger to themselves or others. **EB:** *A study showed that substance use disorders are associated with self- and other-directed violence (Harford et al, 2018).*

Client/Family Teaching and Discharge Planning

▲ After withdrawal symptoms have subsided, refer client to substance use treatment. **EB:** *Collaborative discharge planning can increase the likelihood of the client's success of substance abstinence. Referral to appropriate services can reduce discharges against medical advice and increase follow-up in postdischarge addiction treatment centers (Donroe & Tetrault, 2017).*

▲ Refer for smoking cessation services that target nicotine craving. **EB:** *A study found that nicotine craving may be a useful therapeutic target for increasing the effectiveness of smoking-cessation treatment (Magee, Lewis, & Winhusen, 2016).*

REFERENCES

S

Berring, L. L., Pedersen, L., & Buus, N. (2016). Coping with violence in mental health care settings: Patient and staff member perspectives on de-escalation practices. *Archives of Psychiatric Nursing, 30*(5), 499–507. https://doi.org/10.1016/j.apnu.2016.05.005.

D'Onofrio, G., Chawarski, M. C., O'Connor, P. G., et al. (2017). Emergency department-initiated buprenorphine for opioid dependence with continuation in primary care: Outcomes during and after intervention. *Journal of General Internal Medicine, 32*(6), 660–666. https://doi.org /10.1007/s11606-017-3993-2.

Donroe, J. H., & Tetrault, J. M. (2017). Substance use, intoxication, and withdrawal in the critical care setting. *Critical Care Clinics, 33*(3), 543–558.

Dugum, M., & McCullough, A. (2015). Diagnosis and management of alcoholic liver disease. *Journal of Clinical Translational Hepatology, 3*(2), 109–116.

Ginige, S. (2016). Nicotine withdrawal: An often overlooked and easily reversible cause of terminal restlessness. *European Journal of Palliative Care, 23*(3), 128–129.

Goodwill, A. M., & Szoeke, C. (2017). A systematic review and meta-analysis of the effect of low vitamin D on cognition. *Journal of the American Geriatric Society, 65*(10), 2161–2168. https://doi.org/10.1111/jgs.15012.

Harford, T. C., Yi, H. Y., Chen, C. M., & Grant, B. F. (2018). Substance use disorders and self- and other-directed violence among adults: Results from the National Survey on Drug Use and Health. *Journal of Affective Disorders, 225*, 365–373. https://doi.org/10.1016/j.jad.2017.08.021.

Jesse, S., Bråthen, G., Ferrara, M., et al. (2017). Alcohol withdrawal syndrome: Mechanisms, manifestations, and management. *Acta Neurologica Scandinavica, 135*(1), 4–16. https://doi.org/0.1111/ane.12671.

Kampman, K., & Jarvis, M. (2015). American Society of Addiction Medicine (ASAM) national practice guideline for the use of medications in the treatment of addiction involving opioid use. *Journal of Addiction Medicine, 9*(5), 358–367.

Kao, M. J., Nunez, H., Monaghan, S. F., et al. (2017). Trauma patients who present in a delayed fashion: A unique and challenging population. *Journal of Surgical Research, 208*, 204–210. https://doi.org/10.1016/j.jss.2016.09.037.

Kattimani, S., & Bharadwaj, B. (2013). Clinical management of alcohol withdrawal: A systematic review. *Industrial Psychiatry Journal, 22*(2), 100–108.

Long, D., Long, B., & Koyfman, A. (2017). The emergency medicine management of severe alcohol withdrawal. *American Journal of Emergency Medicine, 35*(7), 1005–1011. https://doi.org/10.1016/j.ajem.2017.02.002.

Magee, J. C., Lewis, D. F., & Winhusen, T. (2016). Evaluating nicotine craving, withdrawal, and substance use as mediators of smoking cessation in cocaine- and methamphetamine-dependent patients. *Nicotine & Tobacco Research, 18*(5), 1196–1201. https://doi.org/10.1093/ntr/ntv121.

Makic, M. B. F. (2017). Alcohol withdrawal syndrome. *Journal of PeriAnesthesia Nursing, 32*(2), 140–141. https://doi.org/10.1016/j.jopan.2017.01.007.

Mirijello, A., D'Angelo, C., Ferrulli, A., et al. (2015). Identification and management of alcohol withdrawal syndrome. *Drugs, 75*(4), 353–365. https://doi.org/10.1007/s40265-015-0358-1.

Mulvaney-Day, N., Marshall, T., Piscopo, K. D., et al. (2018). Screening for behavioral health conditions in primary care settings: A systematic review of the literature. *Journal of General Internal Medicine, 33*(3), 335–346. https://doi.org /10.1007/s11606-017-4181-0.

Puening, S. E., Wilson, W. P., & Nordstrom, K. (2017). Psychiatric emergencies for clinicians: Emergency department management of benzodiazepine withdrawal. *Journal of Emergency Medicine, 52*(1), 66–69. https://doi.org/10.1016/j.jemermed.2016.05.035.

Soravia, L. M., Wopfner, A., Pfiffner, L., Bétrisey, S., & Moggi, F. (2018). Symptom-triggered detoxification using the alcohol-withdrawal-scale reduces risks and healthcare costs. *Alcohol and Alcoholism, 53*(1), 71–77. https://doi.org/10.1093/alcalc/agx080.

Spears, C. A., Hedeker, D., Li, L., et al. (2017). Mechanisms underlying mindfulness-based addiction treatment versus cognitive behavioral therapy and usual care for smoking cessation. *Journal of Consulting and Clinical Psychology, 85*(11), 1029–1040. https://doi.org/10.1037/ccp0000229.

Sullivan, J. T., Sykora, K., Schneiderman, J., Naranjo, C. A., & Sellers, E. M. (1989). Assessment of alcohol withdrawal: The revised clinical institute withdrawal assessment for alcohol scale. *British Journal of Addiction, 84*(11), 1353–1357.

Tavani, L., Gahagen, L., Atwood, J., Shaw, D., Farraj, M., & Gajera, M. (2018). A protocol for the management of alcohol withdrawal in the intensive care unit: A pilot study. *Critical Care Medicine, 46*(1 Suppl. 1), 357. https://doi.org/10.1097/01.ccm.0000528755.55400.b6.

Turner, C. C., Fogger, S. A., & Frazier, S. L. (2018). Opioid use disorder: Challenges during acute hospitalization. *Journal for Nurse Practitioners, 14*(2), 61–67. https://doi.org/10.1016/j.nurpra.2017.12.009.

Wesson, D. R., & Ling, W. (2003). The Clinical Opiate Withdrawal Scale (COWS). *Journal of Psychoactive Drugs, 35*(2), 253–259.

Worley, J. (2017). A primer on heroin and fentanyl. *Journal of Psychosocial Nursing and Mental Health Services, 55*(6), 16–20. https://doi.org/10.3928/02793695-20170519-02.

Zehra, A., Burns, J., Liu, C. K., et al. (2018). Cannabis addiction and the brain: A review. *Journal of Neuroimmune Pharmacology, 13*(4), 438–452. https://doi.org/10.1007/s11481-018-9782-9.

Ineffective Infant Suck-Swallow Response **Domain 2 Nutrition Class 1 Ingestion**

Margaret Quinn, DNP, CPNP, CNE

NANDA-I

Definition

Impaired ability of an infant to suck or to coordinate the suck-swallow response.

Defining Characteristics

Arrhythmia; bradycardic events; choking; circumoral cyanosis; excessive coughing; finger splaying; flaccidity; gagging; hiccups; hyperextension of extremities; impaired ability to initiate an effective suck; impaired ability to sustain an effective suck; impaired motor tone; inability to coordinate sucking, swallowing, and breathing; irritability; nasal flaring; oxygen desaturation; pallor; subcostal retraction; time-out signals; use of accessory muscles of respiration

S

Related Factors

Hypoglycemia; hypothermia; hypotonia; inappropriate positioning; unsatisfactory sucking behavior

At-Risk Population

Infants born to mothers with substance misuse; infants delivered using obstetrical forceps; infants delivered using obstetrical vacuum extraction; infants experiencing prolonged hospitalization; premature infants

Associated Conditions

Convulsive episodes; gastroesophageal reflux; high flow oxygen by nasal cannula; lacerations during delivery; low Appearance, Pulse, Grimace, Activity, & Respiration (APGAR) scores; neurological delay; neurological impairment; oral hypersensitivity; oropharyngeal deformity; prolonged enteral nutrition

NOC (Nursing Outcomes Classification)

Suggested NOC Outcomes

Bottle Feeding Establishment: Infant; Bottle Feeding Performance; Breastfeeding Establishment: Infant, Maternal; Breastfeeding: Maintenance; Hydration; Nutritional Status: Food and Fluid Intake

Example NOC Outcome with Indicators

Breastfeeding Establishment: Infant as evidenced by the following indicators: Proper alignment and latch-on/Correct suck and tongue placement/Urinations per day appropriate for age/Weight gain appropriate for age. (Rate the outcome and indicators of **Breastfeeding Establishment: Infant:** 1 = not adequate, 2 = slightly adequate, 3 = moderately adequate, 4 = substantially adequate, 5 = totally adequate [see Section I].)

Client Outcomes

Infant Will (Specify Time Frame)

- Consume adequate calories that will result in appropriate weight gain and optimal growth and development
- Have opportunities for skin-to-skin experiences
- Have opportunities for "trophic" (i.e., small volume of breast milk/formula) enteral feedings prior to full oral feedings
- Progress to stable, neurobehavioral organization (e.g., motor, state, self-regulation, attention-interaction)
- Demonstrate presence of mature oral reflexes that are necessary for safe feeding
- Progress to safe, self-regulated oral feedings
- Coordinate the suck-swallow-breathe sequence while nippling
- Display clear behavioral cues related to hunger and satiety
- Display approach/engagement cues, with minimal avoidance/disengagement cues
- Have opportunities to pace own feeding, taking breaks as needed
- Display evidence of being in the "quiet-alert" state while nippling
- Progress to and engage in mutually positive parent/caregiver–infant/child interactions during feedings

Parent/Family Will (Specify Time Frame)

- Recognize necessity of adequate calories for appropriate weight gain and optimal growth and development
- Learn to read and respond contingently to infant's behavioral cues (e.g., hunger, satiety, approach/engagement, stress/avoidance/disengagement)
- Learn strategies that promote organized infant behavior
- Learn appropriate positioning and handling techniques
- Learn effective ways to relieve stress behaviors during nippling
- Learn ways to help infant coordinate suck-swallow-breathe sequence (i.e., external pacing techniques)
- Engage in mutually positive interactions with infant during feeding
- Recognize ways to facilitate effective feedings: feed in quiet-alert state; keep length of feeding appropriate; burp; prepare/structure environment; recognize signs of sensory overload; encourage self-regulation; respect need for breaks and breathing pauses; avoid pulling and twisting nipple during pauses; allow infant to resume sucking when ready; provide oral support (cheek and/or jaw) as needed; use appropriate nipple hole size and flow rate

NIC (Nursing Interventions Classification)

Suggested NIC Interventions

Bottle Feeding; Fluid Monitoring; Kangaroo Care; Lactation Counseling; Nutritional Monitoring; Teaching: Infant Safety

Example NIC Activities—Lactation Counseling

Provide information about psychological and physiological benefits of breastfeeding; Refer to a lactation consultant

Nursing Interventions and *Rationales*

- Refer to care plans for Disorganized **Infant** Behavior, Ineffective **Breastfeeding**, Interrupted **Breastfeeding,** Insufficient **Breast Milk Production**, Ineffective Infant **Feeding** Dynamics as needed.

Mother–Baby Dyad Interventions

- Assess for any factors that may disrupt successful breastfeeding after birth. EBN: *Interventions after birth, separation of mother and baby, or excessive newborn suctioning may negatively affect the newborn transition and breastfeeding (Lau et al, 2018).*
- Provide opportunities for skin-to-skin care. EBN: *Placing a newborn skin to skin on the mother is the essential first step to promote and establish successful breastfeeding (Jefferson & Bibb, 2019).*
- Allow the stable newborn to breastfeed within the first 30 to 60 minutes after birth. EBN: *The first hour after birth is the optimal time to achieve successful breastfeeding because the sucking effort of the newborn peaks within 45 minutes of birth and declines during the next 2 hours (Jefferson & Bibb, 2019).*
- Encourage rooming-in. EBN: *Exclusive rooming-in enhances breastfeeding (Jefferson & Bibb, 2019).*
- Assess and document the effectiveness of mixed breastfeeding and bottle-feeding. EBN: *The Neonatal Eating Assessment Tool (NeoEAT—Mixed Feeding) for mixed breastfeeding and bottle-feeding is a parent-report assessment of symptoms of problematic feeding in infants who are fed by both breast and bottle. The reported reference values may be used to identify infants that require further assessment, referral, and intervention (Pados, Johnson, & Nelson, 2020).*
- Position infant in semiupright position, with head, shoulders, and hips in a straight line facing the mother with the infant's nose level with the mother's nipple. EB: *Breastfeeding improves in the semireclined position because the infant is more positionally stable and better able to coordinate sucking, swallowing, and breathing (Douglas & Keogh, 2017).*

▲ Refer to a multiprofessional team (e.g., neonatal/pediatric nutritionist, physical or occupational therapist, speech pathologist, lactation specialist) as needed. EBN: *Follow-up visits with lactation consultants, nurses, and health care providers are beneficial for breastfeeding mothers' support after delivery (Keenan-Devlin et al, 2019).*

Maternal Interventions

- Assess for any maternal issues related to breastfeeding. EBN: *A study found that breastfeeding self-efficacy was a dominant factor affecting maternal breastfeeding satisfaction. Researchers concluded that increased breastfeeding satisfaction may promote breastfeeding (Awaliyah, Rachmawati, & Rahmah, 2019).*
- Support the mother's confidence in her ability to breastfeed. EBN: *Nurses have the unique opportunity to assist with the physical initiation and maintenance of breastfeeding (Shattnawi, 2017).*
- Educate mothers to recognize and respond to their infant's cues for feeding. EB: *Hands to mouth, sucking motions, rooting, and body flexion are all common infant feeding cues. A study found that significantly more frequent feeding cues were observed at the beginning of feeding than at the end, showing that cue frequency changes with satiation (Shloim et al, 2017).*
- Assess for proper latch at the breast. EB: *Latching on is the first step for essential breastfeeding. A neonate with a correct latch will have the lips flanged, will have the tongue under the nipple and extending over the gum line, and will be sucking behind the nipple on the areola (Smith, 2016).*
- Determine the reason for the poor latch, including inverted nipples, flat nipples, ankyloglossia, small mandible, or nipple confusion, and offer alternatives to mothers for unsuccessful latch. EB: *Treatment may consist of help with positioning, nipple shell or shields, and counseling from a lactation specialist (Smith, 2016).*
- Council mothers on various feeding positions to encourage successful latch. EB: *Teaching the mother to change the newborn's position on the breast will prevent persistent pressure in one area of the nipple and areola and facilitate emptying of all quadrants of the breast (Smith, 2016).*

Infant Interventions

- Observe coordination of infant's suck, swallow, and gag reflex. EB: *Adequate coordination of sucking, swallowing, and breathing is essential for safe feeding (Geddes et al, 2017).*
- Assess for neonatal signs of inadequate milk supply/intake. EBN: *Adequate intake can be assessed by 8 to 12 feedings in 24 hours with the number of wet and stool diapers equaling the newborn's age in days and increasing each day after birth (Jefferson & Bibb, 2019).*

Premature Infants/Infants Requiring Specialty/Intensive Care

- Provide developmentally supportive neonatal intensive care for preterm infants. EB: *Early term delivery is independently associated with lower rates of breastfeeding compared to delivery after 39 weeks gestation (Keenan-Devlin et al, 2019).*
- Foster direct breastfeeding as early as possible and enable the first oral feed to be at the breast in the neonatal intensive care unit (NICU). EB: *Breast milk feeding is associated with lower neonatal morbidity in the very preterm infant (<32 weeks gestation) and breastfeeding is beneficial for maternal health (Wilson et al, 2018).*
- Before the infant is ready for oral feedings, implement gavage feedings (or other alternative) as ordered, using expressed breast milk whenever possible. EB: *The transition from gavage to oral feeding requires coordination of sucking, swallowing, and breathing and organized sleep/wake cycles in premature infants (Unal et al, 2019).*
- Provide a naturalistic environment for tube feedings (naso-orogastric, gavage, or other) that approximates a pleasurable oral feeding experience: hold infant in semiupright/flexed position; offer nonnutritive sucking; pace feedings; allow for semidemand feedings contingent with infant cues; offer rest breaks; burp, as appropriate. EBN: *Nonnutritive sucking reduces the time infants need to transition from tube to full oral feeding, and from start of oral feeding to full oral feeding. It also reduces the length of hospital stay (Foster, Psaila, & Patterson, 2016).*
- Continue to provide support for the mother discharged before the infant by encouraging skin-to-skin technique and regular breastfeeding. EBN: *The Academy of Breastfeeding Medicine recommends follow-up for ongoing support and troubleshooting (Noble et al, 2018).*

Home Care

- The previously mentioned appropriate interventions may be adapted for home care use.
- Provide breastfeeding mothers instruction on the technique of expressing milk by hand or pump. EB: *The mother should be taught how to alleviate engorgement, increase her milk supply, maintain her milk supply, and obtain milk for feeding to the infant should she and the infant be separated or if the infant is unable to feed directly from the breast (Jefferson & Bibb, 2019).*
- ▲ Provide lists of various local peer support groups and services (e.g., mother-to-mother support groups such as La Leche League; hospital/clinic-based support groups; and governmental supported groups such as Special Supplemental Nutrition Program for Women, Infants, and Children [WIC] in the United States, with phone numbers, contact names, and addresses). EB: *The Academy of Breastfeeding Medicine recommends providing a written discharge summary for the parents and primary care physician that includes detailed nutrition support recommendations, community support referrals, visiting nurse, skilled lactation consultant visits, and social services (Noble et al, 2018).*

S

Client/Family Teaching and Discharge Planning

- Before discharge, anticipation of breastfeeding problems should be assessed based on maternal and/or infant risk factors. EB: *The Academy of Breastfeeding Medicine recommends assessing the adequacy of breastfeeding and addressing any problems or potential problems (Noble et al, 2018).*
- Include mothers and appropriate others (e.g., fathers, partners, grandmothers, support persons) in teaching of anticipatory guidance for key discharge issues. EB: *The Academy of Breastfeeding Medicine recommends providing a written discharge summary for the parents and primary care physician that includes detailed nutrition support recommendations, community support referrals, visiting nurse, skilled lactation consultant visits, and social services (Noble et al, 2018).*

REFERENCES

Awaliyah, S. N., Rachmawati, I. N., & Rahmah, H. (2019). Breastfeeding self-efficacy as a dominant factor affecting maternal breastfeeding satisfaction. *BMC Nursing*, *18*(Suppl. 1), 30. https://doi.org/10.1186/s12912-019-0359-6.

Douglas, P., & Keogh, R. (2017). Gestalt breastfeeding: Helping mothers and infants optimize positional stability and intraoral breast tissue volume for effective, pain-free milk transfer. *Journal of Human Lactation*, *33*(3), 509–518. https://doi.org/10.1177/0890334417707958.

Foster, J. P., Psaila, K., & Patterson, T. (2016). Non–nutritive sucking for increasing physiologic stability and nutrition in preterm infants. *Cochrane Database of Systematic Reviews*, *10*, CD001071. https://doi.org/10.1002/14651858.CD001071.pub3.

Geddes, D. T., Chooi, K., Nancarrow, K., Hepworth, A. R., Gardner, H., & Simmer, K. (2017). Characterisation of sucking dynamics of breastfeeding preterm infants: A cross sectional study. *BMC Pregnancy and Childbirth*, *17*(1), 386. https://doi.org/10.1186/s12884-017-1574-3.

Jefferson, U. T., & Bibb, D. (2019). A breastfeeding algorithm to guide bedside health care practice for term newborns. *Nursing for Women's Health*, *23*(1), 49–58. https://doi.org/10.1016/j.nwh.2018.11.003.

Keenan-Devlin, L. S., Awosemusi, Y. F., Grobman, W., et al. (2019). Early term delivery and breastfeeding outcomes. *Maternal and Child Health Journal*, *23*(10), 1339–1347. https://doi.org/10.1007/s10995-019-02787-4.

Lau, Y., Tha, P. H., Ho–Lim, S. S. T., et al. (2018). An analysis of the effects of intrapartum factors, neonatal characteristics, and skin-to-skin contact on early breastfeeding initiation. *Maternal and Child Nutrition*, *14*(1), e12492. https://doi.org/10.1111/mcn.12492.

Noble, L. M., Okogbule-Wonodi, A. C., & Young, M. A. (2018). Academy of Breastfeeding Medicine (ABM) Clinical protocol #12: Transitioning the breastfeeding preterm infant from the neonatal intensive care unit to home, revised 2018. *Breastfeeding Medicine*, *13*(4), 230–236. https://doi.org/10.1089/bfm.2018.29090.ljn.

Pados, B. F., Johnson, J., & Nelson, M. (2020). Neonatal eating assessment tool—mixed breastfeeding and bottle-feeding. *Journal of the American Association of Nurse Practitioners*. [Online ahead of print]. https://doi.org/10.1097/JXX.0000000000000476.

Shattnawi, K. K. (2017). Healthcare professionals' attitudes and practices in supporting and promoting the breastfeeding of preterm infants in NICUs. *Advances in Neonatal Care*, *17*(5), 390–399. https://doi.org/10.1097/ANC.0000000000000421.

Shloim, N., Vereijken, C. M. J. L., Blundell, P., & Hetherington, M. M. (2017). Looking for cues—Infant communication of hunger and satiation during milk feeding. *Appetite*, *108*, 74–82. https://doi.org/10.1016/j.appet.2016.09.020.

Smith, E. (2016). If its natural, why does it hurt? Examining the reasons mom may feel pain with breastfeeding. *International Journal of Childbirth Education*, *31*(4), 40–43.

Unal, S., Demirel, N., Bas, A. Y., Arifoğlu, İ., Erol, S., & Isik, D. U. (2019). Impact of feeding interval on time to achieve full oral feeding in preterm infants: A randomized trial. *Nutrition in Clinical Practice*, *34*(5), 783–788. https://doi.org/10.1002/ncp.10244.

Wilson, E., Edstedt Bonamy, A. K., Bonet, M., et al. (2018). Room for improvement in breast milk feeding after very preterm birth in Europe: Results from the EPICE cohort. *Maternal and Child Nutrition*, *14*(1), e12485. https://doi.org/10.1111/mcn.12485.

Risk for Sudden Infant Death **Domain 11 Safety/protection Class 2 Physical injury**

Marina Martinez-Kratz, MS, RN, CNE

NANDA-I

Definition

Infant susceptible to unpredicted death.

Risk Factors

Delayed prenatal care; inadequate prenatal care; inattentive to second-hand smoke; infant < 4 months placed in sitting devices for routine sleep; infant overheating; infant overwrapping; infant placed in prone position to sleep; infant placed in side-lying position to sleep; soft sleep surface; soft, loose objects placed near infant

At-Risk Population

Boys; infants aged 2-4 months; infants exposed to alcohol in utero; infants exposed to cold climates; infants exposed to illicit drug in utero; infants fed with expressed breast milk; infants not breastfed exclusively; infants of African descent; infants whose mothers smoked during pregnancy; infants with postnatal exposure to alcohol; infants with postnatal exposure to illicit drug; low birth weight infants; Native American infants; premature infants

S

NOC (Nursing Outcomes Classification)

Suggested NOC Outcomes

Knowledge: Infant Care; Parenting Performance; Safe Home Environment; Safe Sleep Environment

Example NOC Outcome with Indicators

Knowledge: Infant Care as evidenced by the following indicators: Proper infant positioning/Age-appropriate cardiopulmonary resuscitation techniques. (Rate the outcome and indicators of **Knowledge: Infant Care:** 1 = no knowledge, 2 = limited knowledge 3 = moderate knowledge, 4 = substantial knowledge, 5 = extensive knowledge [see Section I].)

Client Outcomes

Client Will (Specify Time Frame)

- Explain appropriate measures to prevent sudden infant death syndrome (SIDS)
- Demonstrate correct techniques for positioning and blanketing the infant, protecting the infant from harm

NIC (Nursing Interventions Classification)

Suggested NIC Interventions

Infant Care; Teaching: Infant Safety 0 to 3 Months

Example NIC Activities—Teaching: Infant Safety

Instruct parent/caregiver to place infant on back to sleep and keep loose bedding, pillows, and toys out of crib; Instruct parent/caregiver to avoid holding infant while smoking or holding hot liquids

Nursing Interventions and *Rationales*

- Position the infant supine to sleep during naps and night; do not position in the prone position or side-lying position. EB: *In a research review, evidence showed that sleeping prone or in a side-lying position is associated with an increased risk of SIDS (Carlin & Moon, 2017).*
- Avoid overbundling, overheating, and swaddling the infant. The infant should not feel hot to touch. EB: *Swaddling increases the risk of SIDS twofold in infants 6 months or younger (Pease et al, 2016). Swaddling has been associated with infant death, especially when the infant has shown the ability to roll over (Carlin & Moon, 2017).*

Home Care

- Most of the interventions and client teaching information are relevant to home care.
- Evaluate home for potential safety hazards, such as inappropriate cribs, cradles, or strollers.
- Determine where and how the child sleeps, and provide instructions on safe sleeping positions and environments as needed.

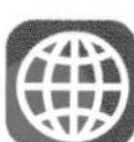

Multicultural

- Safe to Sleep recommendations should be tailored to include the mother's culture and experience, provided to all members of the family, and reviewed frequently. EB: *An ethnographic study found that African American mothers were aware of the Safe to Sleep recommendations but did not follow because of lack of comfort, feeling they are unable to comply, finding it unnecessary to comply, or finding the effort too stressful (Stifler, Matemachani, & Crane, 2020).*
- Provide teaching to African American mothers on how pacifier use reduces SIDS risk. EB: *A study of African American mothers found that many parents were unaware that pacifier use reduces SIDS risk (Joyner, Oden, & Moon, 2016).*
- Recommend to African American and Hispanic mothers the need to abstain from smoking during the prenatal period. EB: *A study found that prenatal smoking may explain a substantial portion of the disparities in birth adverse outcomes and SIDS for African American and Hispanic women (Mohlman & Levy, 2016).*

S

Client/Family Teaching and Discharge Planning

- Teach the safety guidelines for infant care in the previous interventions.
- Teach parents and caregivers the following measures for a Safe Infant Sleeping Environment recommended by the American Academy of Pediatrics (AAP) Task Force on Sudden Infant Death Syndrome (2016):
  - Place infant in supine positioning.
  - Use a firm sleep surface.
  - Room-sharing without bed-sharing.
  - Avoidance of soft bedding.
  - Avoid overheating.
  - Offer infant a pacifier.
  - Avoid smoke exposure during pregnancy and after birth.
  - Avoid alcohol and illicit drug use during pregnancy and after birth.

- ❍ Infants should be immunized in accordance with AAP and Centers for Disease Control and Prevention (CDC) recommendations.
- ❍ Do not use home cardiorespiratory monitors as a strategy to reduce the risk of SIDS.
- ❍ Breastfeeding is a protective factor.

- Provide parents of both term and preterm infants with verbal and written education about SIDS and ways to reduce the risk of SIDS before discharge to home. **EBN:** *Study results demonstrated that providing current written material along with modeling safe sleep practices in the hospital before discharge to home can help further reduce the incidence of SIDS (Dufer & Godfrey, 2017).*
- Recommend breastfeeding. **EB:** *A review identified breastfeeding as a protective factor (Carlin & Moon, 2017).*
- Teach the need to stop smoking during pregnancy and to not smoke around the infant. Do not allow the infant to be exposed to any secondhand smoke. **EB:** *Maternal smoking remains the strongest prenatal modifiable risk factor for SIDS (Friedmann et al, 2017).*

REFERENCES

American Academy of Pediatrics Task Force on Sudden Infant Death Syndrome. (2016). SIDS and other sleep-related infant deaths: Updated 2016 recommendations for a safe infant sleeping environment. *Pediatrics*, *138*(5), e20162938.

Carlin, R. F., & Moon, R. Y. (2017). Risk factors, protective factors, and current recommendations to reduce sudden infant death syndrome: A review. *JAMA Pediatrics*, *171*(2), 175–180. https://doi.org/10.1001/jamapediatrics.2016.3345.

Dufer, H., & Godfrey, K. (2017). Integration of safe sleep and sudden infant death syndrome (SIDS) education among parents of preterm infants in the Neonatal Intensive Care Unit (NICU). *Journal of Neonatal Nursing*, *23*(2), 103–108. https://doi.org/10.1016/j.jnn.2016.09.001.

Friedmann, I., Dahdouh, E. M., Kugler, P., Mimran, G., & Balayla, J. (2017). Maternal and obstetrical predictors of sudden infant death syndrome (SIDS). *Journal of Maternal-Fetal and Neonatal Medicine*, *30*(19), 2315–2323.

Joyner, B. L., Oden, R. P., & Moon, R. Y. (2016). Reasons for pacifier use and non-use in African-Americans: Does knowledge of reduced SIDS risk change parents' minds? *Journal of Immigrant and Minority Health*, *18*(2), 402–410. https://doi.org/10.1007/s10903-015-0206-0.

Mohlman, M. K., & Levy, D. T. (2016). Disparities in maternal child and health outcomes attributable to prenatal tobacco use. *Maternal and Child Health Journal*, *20*(3), 701–709. https://doi.org/10.1007/s10995-015-1870-3.

Pease, A. S., Fleming, P. J., Hauck, F. R., et al. (2016). Swaddling and the risk of sudden infant death syndrome: A meta-analysis. *Pediatrics*, *137*(6), e20153275. https://doi.org/10.1542/peds.2015-3275.

Stiffler, D., Matemachani, S. M., & Crane, L. (2020). Considerations in safe to Sleep® messaging: Learning from African–American mothers. *Journal for Specialists in Pediatric Nursing*, *25*(1), e12277. https://doi.org/10.1111/jspn.12277.

Risk for Suffocation Domain 11 Safety/protection Class 2 Physical injury

Marina Martinez-Kratz, MS, RN, CNE

NANDA-I

Definition

Susceptible to inadequate air availability for inhalation, which may compromise health.

Risk Factors

Access to empty refrigerator/freezer; eating large mouthfuls of food; excessive emotional disturbance; gas leak; inadequate knowledge of safety precautions; low-strung clothesline; pacifier around infant's neck; playing with plastic bag; propped bottle placed in infant's crib; small object in airway; smoking in bed; soft sleep surface; unattended in water; unvented fuel-burning heater; vehicle running in closed garage

Associated Conditions

Altered olfactory function; face/neck disease; face/neck injury; impaired motor functioning

NOC (Nursing Outcomes Classification)

Suggested NOC Outcomes

Knowledge: Infant Care; Parenting: Adolescent Physical Safety, Early/Middle Childhood Physical Safety, Infant/Toddler Physical Safety; Personal Safety; Risk Control; Risk Detection; Safe Home Environment; Substance Addiction Consequences

S

Example NOC Outcome with Indicators

Knowledge: Infant Care as evidenced by the following indicators: Strategies to prevent choking/ Appropriate activities for child's developmental level/First aid techniques. (Rate the outcome and indicators of **Knowledge: Infant Care:** 1 = no knowledge, 2 = limited knowledge, 3 = moderate knowledge, 4 = substantial knowledge, 5 = extensive knowledge [see Section I].)

Client Outcomes

Client Will (Specify Time Frame)

- Undertake appropriate measures to prevent suffocation
- Demonstrate correct techniques for emergency rescue maneuvers (e.g., Heimlich maneuver, rescue breathing, cardiopulmonary resuscitation [CPR]) and describe situations that require them

NIC (Nursing Interventions Classification)

Suggested NIC Interventions

Aspiration Precautions; Environmental Management: Safety; Infant Care; Positioning; Security Enhancement; Surveillance; Surveillance: Safety; Teaching: Infant Safety

Example NIC Activities—Environmental Management: Safety

Identify safety hazards in the environment (e.g., physical, biological, and chemical); Remove hazards from the environment, when possible

Nursing Interventions and *Rationales*

- Identify hospitalized clients at particular risk for suffocation, including the following:
  - Clients with altered levels of consciousness
  - Infants or young children
  - Clients with developmental delays
  - Clients with mental illness, especially schizophrenia
  - Clients who have been physically or chemically restrained
- Practice caution with physical restraints and follow all institutional policies and procedures as restraint use has been associated with mortality. EB: *A review of restraint use in nursing home clients found evidence of physical restraint–associated deaths. Neck compression was found to be the most common mechanism that resulted in asphyxia (Bellenger et al, 2018).*
- Institute safety measures such as proper positioning and feeding precautions. See the care plans for Risk for **Aspiration** and Impaired **Swallowing** for additional interventions.
- Vigilance and special protective measures are necessary for clients at greater risk for suffocation. EB: *Swallowing disorders are common in schizophrenia with associated morbidity and mortality from either acute asphyxia from airway obstruction or from aspiration and pneumonia. The death rate from acute asphyxia is significantly higher in these clients (up to 100 times greater than the general population) (Kulkarni, Kamath, & Stewart, 2017).*

S

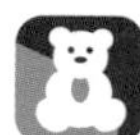

Pediatric

- Provide families with education about interventions and modifiable risk factors to prevent infant suffocation:
  - Use a firm sleep surface with a fitted sheet.
  - Do not place infants in adult beds, on couches, or in armchairs to sleep.
  - Do not overbundle the infant.
  - Avoid soft bedding and do not have loose bedding in crib with infant.
  - Use caution with infant head coverings and keep blanket end at infant chest.
  - Do not practice bed sharing or co-sleeping with infants.

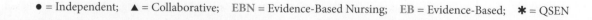

  EB: *The American Academy of Pediatrics Task Force has identified recommendations to reduce the risk of other sleep-related infant deaths such as suffocation, entrapment, and asphyxia (see care plan Risk for*

***Sudden Infant Death** for further interventions) (Moon & Task Force on Sudden Infant Death Syndrome, 2016).*

- Conduct risk factor identification, noting special circumstances in which preventive or protective measures are indicated. Note the presence of environmental hazards, including plastic bags; cribs with slats wider than 2 inches; ill-fitting crib mattresses that can allow the infant to become wedged between the mattress and crib; pillows/loose bedding in cribs; placement of crib near windows with blinds or cords; cosleeping; abandoned large appliances such as refrigerators, dishwashers, or freezers; clothing with cords or hoods that can become entangled; bibs; pacifiers on a string; necklaces in infants and children; drapery cords; and pull-toy strings. EB: *Bed sharing is associated with accidental suffocation and strangulation and sudden infant death. The risk of infant bed sharing is increased in infants who have no identified place to sleep, have health or care issues, and are breastfed. Education should support breastfeeding without bed sharing, highlight the need for safe sleep places, and address the risk factors for sleep-related deaths (Heere et al, 2017).*
- Counsel families to evaluate household furniture for safety, including large dressers, televisions, bookshelves, and appliances, which may need to be anchored to the wall to prevent the child from climbing on the furniture and it falling forward and suffocating the child. EB: *Injuries to children by falling televisions have become more frequent. Dressers and other furniture not designed for holding televisions were commonly involved. Toddlers ages 1 to 3 most frequently suffer head and neck injuries. Small children may suffer secondary brain injuries or death by mechanical asphyxia because of their small size compared with the size of the television (Cusimano & Parker, 2016).*
- Counsel families about items that are most associated with choking in children. EB: *A study found that food (hot dogs, grapes, and steak), coins, balloons, and other toys were the most common objects associated with choking in children (Duckett, Bartman, & Roten, 2020).*
- Counsel families to keep the following items away from the sight and reach of infants and toddlers: buttons, beads, jewelry, pins, nails, marbles, coins, stones, magnets, and balloons. Choose age-appropriate toys and games for children and check for any small parts that may be a choking hazard because children have the need to put everyday objects in their mouths. EB: *Reviews of foreign body injuries found that pearls, balls, coins, nuts, seeds, and toy parts were common objects ingested by children and resulted in increased morbidity and mortality (choking) (Passali et al, 2015).*
- Stress water and pool safety and stress including vigilant, uninterrupted parental supervision. EB: *A review of risk factors associated with drowning found that inadequate surveillance, inadequate availability of first responders, developmental delay, seizure disorders, lack of swimming ability, and substance misuse in adolescents were associated with an increased risk for drowning (Davey et al, 2019).*
- Underscore the necessity of not allowing children to play with or near electric garage doors and of keeping garage door openers out of the reach of young children. *Children close to the ground may not be large enough to trigger reversal mechanisms on the door and may become trapped.*
- For adolescents, watch for signs of depression that could result in suicide by suffocation. EB: *A surveillance data review of suicide in children and early adolescents found that compared with adolescents who commit suicide, in death by suicide in children, the victims were commonly male, Black, and died by hanging, strangulation, or suffocation. Children who died by suicide often experienced relationship problems with family, girlfriends, or boyfriends (Sheftall et al, 2016).*

S

Geriatric

- Monitor client during feeding for coughing or choking when eating and drinking, being unable to chew food properly, and losing food and drink from the front of the mouth. EBN: *These are common signs of dysphagia (Atkinson, 2019).*
- A swallowing assessment by a speech-language pathologist is recommended in clients with suspected or confirmed dysphagia to ensure the appropriate type and consistency of diet to mitigate choking and aspiration risk. EBN: *Safe nursing care includes a consultation with a speech-language pathologist whenever doubts arise regarding a client's ability to tolerate oral-supported nutrition in any form (Teasell et al, 2018).*
- Ensure proper positioning during and after feeding to decrease the risk of aspiration. EB: *Dysphagia in the elderly results in increased morbidity and mortality. It is important to recognize the relationship between dysphagia and aspiration pneumonia in the elderly because of the high mortality rate associated with this (Smukalla et al, 2017).*

- Recognize that older adults in depression may use hanging, strangulation, and suffocation as a means of suicide. EB: *Suicide attempts in seniors often result in death. Social isolation, poor health, frailty, loneliness, and depression are thought to be possible contributing factors. Regardless of age, suffocation, which includes hanging and strangulation, accounted for almost half of the suicides in Canada in 2012 (Skinner et al, 2016).*

Home Care

- Assess the home for potential safety hazards and refer as needed to community resources. EB: *A study found that a Mobile Safety Center's home safety educational program significantly increased home safety knowledge and spurred home safety device use (Furman et al, 2020).*
- Assist the family to develop an emergency preparedness plan for potential escape routes from the home in the event of detectors going off, fire, or other emergencies. EB: *A study of emergency preparedness found that only 24% of respondents had an Emergency Evacuation Plan (Ekenga & Ziyu, 2019).*

Client/Family Teaching and Discharge Planning

- Recommend that families who are seeking day care or in-home care for children, geriatric family members, or at-risk family members with developmental or functional disabilities inspect the environment for hazards and examine the first aid preparation and vigilance of providers. EBN: *A home accident prevention training for informal caregivers improved the knowledge, reported practices, and attitudes regarding home accident prevention among preschool children (Sabra, El-Maksoud, & El-Sayed Hegazy, 2019).*
- Ensure family members learn and practice rescue techniques, including treatment of choking and lack of breathing, as well as CPR. EB: *Family members need preparation to deal with emergency situations and should take part in the American Heart Association Basic Lifesaving Course or the American Red Cross Infant/Child CPR Course (Zackoff et al, 2020).*

REFERENCES

Atkinson, K. (2019). Neurological conditions and acute dysphagia. *British Journal of Nursing, 28*(8), 490–492. https://doi.org/10.12968/bjon.2019.28.8.490.

Bellenger, E. N., Ibrahim, J. E., Lovell, J. J., & Bugeja, L. (2018). The nature and extent of physical restraint-related deaths in nursing homes: A systematic review. *Journal of Aging and Health, 30*(7), 1042–1061. https://doi.org/10.1177/0898264317704541.

Cusimano, M. D., & Parker, N. (2016). Toppled television sets and head injuries in the pediatric population: A framework for prevention. *Journal of Neurosurgery: Pediatrics, 17*(1), 3–12. https://doi.org/10.3171/2015.2.PEDS14472.

Davey, M., Callinan, S., & Nertney, L. (2019). Identifying risk factors associated with fatal drowning accidents in the paediatric population: A review of international evidence. *Cureus, 11*(11), e6201. https://doi.org/10.7759/cureus.6201.

Duckett, S. A., Bartman, M., & Roten, R. A. (2020). *Choking.* StatPearls [Internet]. Treasure Island, FL: StatPearls Publishing. PMID:29763116.

Ekenga, C. C., & Ziyu, L. (2019). Gender and public health emergency preparedness among United States adults. *Journal of Community Health, 44*(4), 656–660. https://doi.org/10.1007/s10900-019-00638-5.

Furman, L., Strotmeyer, S., Vitale, C., et al. (2020). Evaluation of a mobile safety center's impact on pediatric home safety knowledge and device use. *Injury Epidemiology, 7*, 27. https://doi.org/10.1186/s40621-020-00254-1.

Heere, M., Moughan, B., Alfonsi, J., Rodriguez, J., & Aronoff, S. (2017). Factors associated with infant bed-sharing. *Global Pediatric Health, 4* 2333794X17690313. https://doi.org/10.1177/2333794X17690313.

Kulkarni, D. P., Kamath, V. D., & Stewart, J. T. (2017). Swallowing disorders in schizophrenia. *Dysphagia, 32*(4), 467–471. doi:10.1007/s00455-017-9802-6.

Moon, R. Y., & Task Force on Sudden Infant Death Syndrome. (2016). SIDS and other sleep-related infant deaths: Evidence base for 2016 updated recommendations for a safe infant sleeping environment. *Pediatrics, 138*(5), e20162940. https://doi.org/10.1542/peds.2016-2940.

Passali, D., Gregori, D., Lorenzoni, G., et al. (2015). Foreign body injuries in children: A review. *Acta Otorhinolaryngologica Italica, 35*(4), 265–271. PMID:26824213.

Sabra, M. T. M., El-Maksoud, M. M. A., & El-Sayed Hegazy, A. (2019). Educational program for informal caregivers about home accident prevention. *Academic Journal of Nursing & Health Education, 8*(1), 16–33.

Sheftall, A. H., Asti, L., Horowitz, L. M., et al. (2016). Suicide in elementary school-aged children and early adolescents. *Pediatrics, 138*(4), e20160436. https://doi.org/10.1542/peds.2016-0436.

Skinner, R., McFaull, S., Draca, J., et al. (2016). Suicide and self-inflicted injury hospitalizations in Canada (1979 to 2014/15). *Health Promotion and Chronic Disease Management in Canada, 36*(11), 243–251. https://doi.org/10.24095/hpcdp.36.11.02.

Smukalla, S. M., Dimitrova, I., Feintuch, J. M., & Khan, A. (2017). Dysphagia in the elderly. *Current Treatment Options in Gastroenterology, 15*(3), 382–396. doi:10.10007/s11938-017-0144-0.

Teasell, R. W., Foley, N., Martino, R., et al. (2018). *Dysphagia and aspiration following stroke.* Evidence-Based Review of Stroke Rehabilitation. Retrieved from http://www.ebrsr.com/sites/default/files/v18-SREBR-CH15-NET.pdf. [Accessed July 30, 2021].

Zackoff, M., Tegtmeyer, K., & Dewan, M. (2020). Family comes first: The importance of high-quality cardiopulmonary resuscitation training for caregivers. *Pediatric Critical Care Medicine, 21*(2), 210–211. https://doi.org/10.1097/PCC.0000000000002218.

Risk for Suicidal Behavior Domain 11 Safety/protection Class 3 Violence

Kathleen L. Patusky, PhD, MA, RN, CNS and Mamilda Robinson, DNP, APN, PMHNP-BC

NANDA-I

Definition

Susceptible to self-injurious acts associated with some intent to die.

Related Factors

Behavioral

Apathy; difficulty asking for help; difficulty coping with unsatisfactory performance; difficulty expressing feelings; ineffective chronic pain self-management; self-injurious behavior; self-negligence; stockpiling of medication; substance misuse

Psychological

Anxiety; depressive symptoms; hostility; expresses deep sadness; expresses frustration; expresses loneliness; low self-esteem; maladaptive grieving; perceived dishonor; perceived failure; reports excessive guilt; reports helplessness; reports hopelessness; reports unhappiness; suicidal ideation

Situational

Easy access to weapon; loss of independence; loss of personal autonomy

Social

Dysfunctional family processes; inadequate social support; inappropriate peer pressure; legal difficulty; social deprivation; social devaluation; social isolation; unaddressed violence by others

At-Risk Population

Adolescents; adolescents living in foster care; economically disadvantaged individuals; individuals changing a will; individuals experiencing situational crisis; individuals facing discrimination; individuals giving away possessions; individuals living alone; individuals obtaining potentially lethal materials; individuals preparing a will; individuals who frequently seek care for vague symptomatology; individuals with disciplinary problems; individuals with family history of suicide; individuals with history of suicide attempt; individuals with history of violence; individuals with sudden euphoric recovery from major depression; institutionalized individuals; men; Native American individuals; older adults

Associated Conditions

Depression; mental disorders; physical illness; terminal illness

S

NOC (Nursing Outcomes Classification)

Suggested NOC Outcomes

Depression Level; Impulse Self-Control; Loneliness Severity; Mood Equilibrium; Risk Detection; Suicide Self-Restraint

Example NOC Outcome with Indicators

Suicide Self-Restraint as evidenced by the following indicators: Expresses feelings/Refrains from attempting suicide/Verbalizes suicidal ideas/Controls impulses. (Rate the outcome and indicators of **Suicide Self-Restraint:** 1 = never demonstrated, 2 = rarely demonstrated, 3 = sometimes demonstrated, 4 = often demonstrated, 5 = consistently demonstrated [see Section I].)

Client Outcomes

Client Will (Specify Time Frame)

- Not harm self

- Maintain connectedness in relationships
- Disclose and discuss suicidal ideas and plan if present; seek help
- Express decreased anxiety and control of impulses
- Talk about feelings; express anger appropriately
- Identify a safety plan
- Identify protective factors
- Refrain from using mood-altering substances
- Obtain no access to harmful objects
- Yield access to harmful objects
- Maintain self-control without supervision

NIC (Nursing Interventions Classification)

Suggested NIC Interventions

Anxiety Reduction; Coping Enhancement; Crisis Intervention; Delusion Management; Mood Management; Substance Use Prevention; Suicide Prevention; Support System Enhancement; Surveillance

Example NIC Activities—Suicide Prevention

Determine presence and degree of suicidal risk; Encourage client to seek out care providers to talk to as urge to harm self occurs

Nursing Interventions and *Rationales*

The American Psychiatric Nurses Association (APNA, 2015) has adapted a set of essential competencies for psychiatric nurses, all of which can be useful for generalist nurses. These competencies have been incorporated in the following sections.

- Assess using suicide risk measures that are available for nurses. **EBN:** *Measures include the Nurses' Global Assessment of Suicide Risk (van Veen et al, 2015); the Center for Epidemiological Studies Depression Scale, which measures depressed mood level (Yang, Jai, & Quin, 2015); the Beck Suicide Intent Scale, which identifies a strong intent to die and may be best used in conjunction with the Karolinska Interpersonal Violence Scale (Stefansson et al, 2015); and the Suicide Assessment Checklist (Yoon, Park, & Choi, 2020).*
- Before implementing interventions in the face of suicidal behavior, nurses should examine their own emotional responses to incidents of suicide to ensure that interventions will not be based on countertransference reactions. **EBN:** *Understanding of nurses' responses to suicidal clients can facilitate suicide prevention and recovery (APNA, 2015; Morrissey & Higgins, 2019).*
- Pursue an understanding of suicide as a phenomenon at all levels of nursing practice. **EBN:** *Elements to be considered include the terminology used with suicidality and self-harm phenomena, the epidemiology of suicide, the risk of and protective influences on suicide, and the evidence-based best practices in preventing and responding to suicidality (APNA, 2015).*
- Assess for suicidal ideation when the history reveals the following: depression; substance abuse; bipolar disorder; schizophrenia; anxiety disorders, posttraumatic stress disorder, dissociative disorder, eating disorders, substance use disorders, or antisocial or other personality disorders; attempted suicide, current or past; recent stressful life events (divorce and/or separation, relocation, problems with children); recent unemployment; recent bereavement; adult or childhood physical or sexual abuse; LGBTQ+ identities, family history of suicide; and history of chronic trauma. **EBN:** *Clinicians should be alert for suicide when the previously mentioned factors are present in asymptomatic persons (American Psychiatric Association [APA], 2016).*
- Assess all medical clients and clients with chronic illnesses, traumatic injuries, or pain for their perception of health status and suicidal ideation. **EB:** *A study found that nearly all physical health conditions increased suicide risk, even after adjustment for potential confounding variables (Ahmedani et al, 2017).*
- Be alert for the following warning signs of suicide: making statements such as, "I can't go on," "Nothing matters anymore," "I wish I were dead"; becoming depressed or withdrawn; behaving recklessly; getting affairs in order and giving away valued possessions; showing a marked change in behavior, attitudes, or appearance; abusing drugs or alcohol; and suffering a major loss or life change. **EB:** *A meta-analysis found*

S

that about half of the individuals who complete suicide communicate their intentions before death (Pompili et al, 2016).

- Take suicide notes seriously and ask if a note was left in any previous suicide attempts. Consider themes of notes in determining appropriate interventions. EB: *An analysis of suicide notes by writers who died by their attempt were more likely to combine a dislike of themselves and a concern for loved ones (Synnott et al, 2018).*
- Question family members regarding the preparatory actions mentioned. EBN: *Clinicians should be alert for suicide when these factors are present in asymptomatic persons (APA, 2016).*
- Determine the presence and degree of suicidal risk. A number of questions will elicit the necessary information: "Have you been thinking about hurting or killing yourself?" "How often do you have these thoughts and how long do they last?" "Do you have a plan?" "What is it?" "Do you have access to the means to carry out that plan?" "How likely is it that you could carry out the plan?" "Are there people or things that could prevent you from hurting yourself?" "What do you see in your future a year from now?" "Five years from now?" "What do you expect would happen if you died?" "What has kept you alive up to now?" EB: *The nurse can evaluate the client's suicide risk by identifying factors associated with suicidal risk in major mood disorders (Baldessarini et al, 2019).*
- Observe, record, and report any changes in mood or behavior that may signify increasing suicide risk and document results of regular surveillance checks. EBN: *Suicidal ideation often is not continuous; it may decrease and then increase in response to negative thinking or exposure to stressors (e.g., family visits). Documentation of surveillance will alert all members of the health care team to changes in the clients' potential risk for suicide so they may be prepared to respond in the event of suicidal behavior (APNA, 2015).*
- Develop a positive therapeutic relationship with the client; do not make promises that may not be kept. Clarify with the clients that anything they share will be communicated only to other staff involved in their care. EBN: *Nurses reconnect suicidal clients with humanity by guiding the client, helping them learn how to live, and helping them connect appropriately with others. Positive support can buffer against suicide, whereas conflictual interactions can increase suicide risk (APNA, 2015).*
- Express desire to help client. Provide education about suicide and the effectiveness of intervention. Validate the client's experience of psychological pain while maintaining a safe environment for the client. EBN: *The nurse must reconcile their goal of preventing suicide with recognition of the client's goal to alleviate their psychological pain (APNA, 2015).*
- ▲ Refer for mental health counseling and possible hospitalization if evidence of suicidal intent exists, which may include evidence of preparatory actions (e.g., obtaining a weapon, making a plan, putting affairs in order, giving away prized possessions, preparing a suicide note). EBN: *Clients vary in the preparation for suicide attempts, and professional assessment is required to determine the need for hospitalization (APA, 2016).*
- Perform risk assessment for possible suicidality on admission to the hospital and thereafter during hospitalization. Alert treatment team to level of risk. EBN: *Risk assessment includes evaluating each client's risk factors, ameliorating factors, stated suicidal intent, mental status, history of physical or psychological trauma, triggers that prompt distress, tendency to minimize or exaggerate symptoms, sources of assistance, warning signs of acute risk, and history of previous suicidal or self-harm behavior (APNA, 2015).*
- Determine client's need for supervision and assign a hospitalized client to a room located near the nursing station. EBN: *Close assignment increases ease of observation and availability for a rapid response in the event of a suicide attempt (APNA, 2015).*
- Search the newly hospitalized client and the client's personal belongings for weapons or potential weapons and hoarded medications during the inpatient admission procedure, as appropriate. Remove dangerous items. EBN: *Clients who are intent on suicide may bring the means with them. Action is necessary to maintain a hazard-free environment and client safety (APNA, 2015).*
- Monitor the client during the use of potential weapons (e.g., razor, scissors) and limit access to windows and exits unless locked and shatterproof, as appropriate. EBN: *Clients with suicidal intent may take advantage of any opportunity to harm themselves (APNA, 2015).*
- Increase surveillance of a hospitalized client at times when staffing is predictably low (e.g., staff meetings, change of shift report, periods of unit disruption). EB: *A large U.S. study of hospital suicide incidence and methods found that most inpatient suicides occurred through hanging and in private areas of the hospital unit (e.g.., bathrooms, bedrooms, closets). In the data, the method for monitoring clients to ensure their safety before the suicide was poorly documented and could not be reliably determined (Williams et al, 2018).*

S

- Ensure that all oncoming staff members have adequate information to assist the client, using the acronym SBARR. **EBN:** *SBARR stands for the following: situation (current status, observations), background (relevant client history), assessment (including nurse's current risk assessment and relevant laboratory findings), recommendations (what the nurse believes is necessary going forward), and response feedback (verification of oncoming staff members' understanding) (APNA, 2015).*
- ▲ If imminent suicide is suspected or an attempt has occurred, call for assistance and do not leave the client alone. Client and staff safety will be served by assistance in the response. The client may attempt additional self-harm if left alone. **EBN:** *Staff require specialized training to respond appropriately to suicidal behaviors. A study of mental health nurses found that some participants noted the lack of competence among temporary and/or inexperienced staff led to higher demands on experienced nurses and poorer care, which may contribute to increased behavior among clients (Hagen, Knizek, & Hjelmeland, 2017).*
- Place the client in the least restrictive, safe, and monitored environment that allows for the necessary level of observation. Assess suicidal risk at least daily and more frequently as warranted. **EBN:** *Close observation of the client is necessary for safety as long as intent remains high. Suicide risk should be assessed at frequent intervals to adjust suicide precautions and limitations on the client's freedom of movement and to ensure that restrictions continue to be appropriate. Inpatient root cause analyses of suicide attempts and environmental safety checklists for units can be helpful in maintaining safety (APNA, 2015; Gøtzsche & Gøtzsche, 2017).*
- ▲ Refer for treatment and participate in the management of any mental illness or symptoms that may be contributing to the client's suicidal ideation or behavior. **EB:** *A systematic review found that individuals with a mental illness had a nearly eightfold increased risk of suicide compared with those without a mental disorder (Too et al, 2019).*
- ▲ Verify that the client has taken medications as ordered (e.g., conduct mouth checks after medication administration). **EB:** *Nurses have to prevent access to possible lethal means of harm. The client may attempt to hoard medications for a later suicide attempt (Harmer et al, 2021).*
- ▲ Maintain increased surveillance of the client whenever use of an antidepressant has been initiated or the dose increased. **EB:** *Main predictors of increased suicide risk are related to the presence of a depressive disorder and to suicidal behavior. Data suggest that depressed clients presenting at baseline with active suicidal ideation or a history of suicide attempt seem to display a poorer short-term response to antidepressants. Consequently, depressed clients with the highest risk of suicidal ideation or attempts may be poor responders to available antidepressants (Courtet, Nobile, & Lopez-Castroman, 2017).*
- Involve the client in treatment planning and self-care management of psychiatric disorders. **EB:** *A qualitative study explored experiences of treatment with clients formerly hospitalized for suicidal behaviors. The former clients reported a sense of companionship with the staff and that receiving individualized treatment and care was important for the participants (Hagen, Knizek, & Hjelmeland, 2018).*
- Explore with the client all circumstances and motivations related to the suicidality. Listen to the client's own views on his or her problems. **EBN:** *Primary reasons for suicide attempts were found to be feelings of loneliness or hopelessness and mental illness/psychological problems (APA, 2016).*
- Explore with the client reasons to live and sources of hope. **EB:** *A systematic review found that reasons to live and hope provided significant protective effects against suicide (Li, Dorstyn, & Jarmon, 2020).*
- Keep discussions oriented to the present and future. **EB:** *A factor analysis study examined factors that influence suicide resilience and found that the Positive Future factor negatively predicted suicide ideation (Clement et al, 2020).*
- ▲ Document client behavior in detail to support involuntary commitment or an overnight psychiatric observation program for an actively suicidal client. **EB:** *Failure to document suicide risk assessments, client behaviors, and interventions may lead the legal system to conclude that the documentation was not done (Sadek, 2019).*
- Use cognitive-behavioral techniques that help the client to modify thinking styles that promote depression, hopelessness, and a belief that suicide is a valid means of escaping the current situation. **EB:** *A randomized controlled trial found that Cognitive Behavioural Suicide Prevention therapy did show improvements in suicidal ideation and suicide probability (Haddock et al, 2019).*
- Engage the client in group interventions that can be useful to address recurrent suicide attempts. **EB:** *A study of a suicide-focused group therapy for veterans found that more frequent session attendance was significantly related to less suicidal ideation at 1-month measure (Johnson et al, 2019).*
- See the care plans for Risk for Self-Directed **Violence, Hopelessness,** and Risk for **Self-Mutilation.**

S

Pediatric

- The previously discussed interventions may be appropriate for pediatric clients.
- Assess specifically for bullying and cyberbullying. EBN: *A chart review of adolescents who presented to the emergency department at two Canadian hospitals found that 77% of the individuals had experienced bullying and 68.9% had suicide ideation. After controlling for age, gender, grade, psychiatric diagnosis, and abuse, a history of bullying was the most significant predictor of suicidal ideation (Alavi et al, 2017).*
- Assess for exposure to trauma and other adverse childhood experiences. EB: *A retrospective chart review of youth (n = 861) found that 52% of youth reported at least one type of trauma exposure. Emotional abuse, physical abuse, and sexual abuse/assault were found to be associated with suicidality and after controlling for other variables, children experiencing emotional abuse had a 3.2-fold increase in suicidality (Marr et al, 2021).*
- Assess for exposure to suicide of a significant other. EB: *A cross-sectional analysis of a health and well-being survey of 8500 New Zealand high school students found that students exposed to suicide attempts or completed suicide among friends and/or family members were at increased risk of reporting attempted suicide and repeated nonsuicidal self-injury (Chan et al, 2018).*
- Assess for the presence of school victimization around lesbian, gay, bisexual, and transgender (LGBT) issues and be prepared to advocate for the client. EB: *A four-stage, stepwise logistic regression for suicide attempts, suicidal ideation, and suicide planning found that anti-LGBT victimization, sexual orientation, and fear of violence at school were associated with suicidal ideation, suicide planning, and suicide attempts (Barnett et al, 2019).*
- Evaluate for the presence of self-mutilation and related risk factors. EB: *Data from self-report surveys found that nonsuicidal self-injury (NSSI) was associated with increased odds of subsequent suicide ideation and attempt. NSSI was also associated with increased risk of transitioning to a suicidal plan among those with suicidal ideation, as well as suicidal attempt among those with a plan (Kiekens et al, 2018).* Refer to care plan for Risk for **Self-Mutilation** for additional information.
- Support the implementation of school-based suicide prevention programs. *School nurses can be key to early intervention.* EB: *A randomized controlled trial including more than 11,000 students in the European Union divided the students into the following three groups: a question and refer group, a mental health awareness group, and a professional screening group. No differences between the groups showed up at 3 months. At 12 months the mental health awareness group showed significant reduction in suicide attempts and severe suicidal ideation (Wasserman et al, 2015).*

Geriatric

- Evaluate the older client's perceived mental and physical health status and financial stressors. EB: *Data from community-dwelling older adults with a current diagnosis of major depression found that perceived stress is associated with a higher risk of suicide-related ideation (Bickford et al, 2020).*
- Explore with the client perceived pressures about being a burden or being burdensome. EB: *A preliminary examination of convergent validity evidence found significant moderate correlations between the Geriatric Feelings of Burdensomeness Scale and measures of conceptually related constructs (hopelessness, suicidality, perceived burdensomeness, thwarted belongingness) (Lutz et al, 2020).*
- Conduct a thorough assessment of clients' medications. EB: *Drugs commonly used for insomnia (eszopiclone, zolpidem, and zaleplon) were associated with suicidal ideation (odds ratio [OR]=1.32 [1.14–1.54]), suicide planning (OR=1.44 [1.19–1.75]), and suicide attempts (Tubbs et al, 2021). A study of older adults found that past-year opioid misuse (adjusted odds ratio [AOR] = 1.84, 95% confidence interval [CI] = 1.07–3.19) and benzodiazepine misuse (AOR = 2.00, 95% CI = 1.01–3.94) were significantly associated with past-year suicidal ideation (Schepis, Simoni-Wastila, & McCabe, 2019).*
- When assessing suicide risk factors, note a higher degree of risk for older men and for some older adults who have lost a loved one in the previous year. EB: *A systematic review of suicide risk factors in older men found that being unmarried, single, divorced, or widowed were among the risk factors with the strongest evidence predicting suicidal behavior (Richardson, Robb, & O'Connor, 2021).*
- An older adult who shows self-destructive behaviors should be evaluated to rule out a diagnosis of dementia. EB: *A study found that clients with frontotemporal dementia had the highest prevalence of suicidal behavior (4%), with nearly 0.5% with a suicidal plan/attempt (Lai et al, 2018).*

S

▲ Refer older adults in primary care settings for integrated care management. **EB:** *A study found that geriatric client-aligned care team (GeriPACT) mental health integration is less than 50% within the Veterans Health Administration. The authors conclude that population differences between general primary care and geriatric primary care may require different care approaches and provider competencies (Moye et al, 2019).*
● Consider telephone contacts as an effective intervention for suicidal older adults. **EB:** *A systematic review of interventions to prevent suicidal behaviors and reduce suicidal ideation in older people found that telephone counseling was an effective intervention (Okolie et al, 2017).*

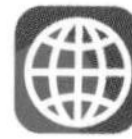

Multiculturral

● Assess for the influence of cultural beliefs, norms, and values on the client's perceptions of suicide and on the nurse's perception and approach to suicide. **EB:** *A study of multinational students found three fundamental conditions for preventing suicidal thoughts: (1) a high degree of belongingness, (2) accessibility to help-related information, and (3) healthy perceived cultural responses toward mental health (Nguyen et al, 2021).*
● Validate the individual's feelings regarding concerns about the current crisis and family functioning. **EBN:** *Validation lets the client know that the nurse has heard and understood what was said, and it promotes the nurse–client relationship (APNA, 2015).*

Home Care

● Communicate the degree of risk to family and caregivers; assess the family and caregiving situation for the ability to protect the client and to understand the client's suicidal behavior. **EB:** *A study found communication gaps between health care providers and families of individuals who had died from suicide in the month before the suicide. The authors concluded that suicide prevention strategies need strengthening of communication between these two groups (Draper et al, 2018).*
● Assess access to lethal means in the home. **EB:** *A study of lethal means assessment among emergency department (ED) clients with a positive suicide risk screen found that among 545 suicidal clients discharged home from the ED, 85% had no documentation that any provider assessed access to lethal means (Betz et al, 2018).*
● Assist the client and family to develop a suicide safety plan that includes lethal means reduction, brief problem solving and coping skills, increasing social support, and identifying emergency contacts to use during a suicide crisis. **EB:** *The Assess, Intervene and Monitor for Suicide Prevention (AIM-SP) model is a framework that recommends a safety plan that incorporates evidence-based suicide risk reduction strategies (Brodsky, Spruch-Feiner, & Stanley, 2018).*

Client/Family Teaching and Discharge Planning

● Involve the family in discharge planning (e.g., illness/medication teaching, recognition of increasing suicidal risk, client's plan for dealing with recurring suicidal thoughts, community resources). **EB:** *A qualitative study of family and friends bereaved by suicide found that family cited failures in detecting symptoms and behavioral changes, the inability of the health care provider to understand the needs of the client and their social context, and a perceived overreliance on antidepressant treatment (Leavey et al, 2017).*
● Teach cognitive-behavioral activities to the client and family, such as active problem-solving, reframing (reappraising the situation from a different perspective), or thought stopping (in response to a negative thought, picturing a large stop sign and replacing the image with a prearranged positive alternative). Teach the client to confront his or her own negative thought patterns (or cognitive distortions), such as catastrophizing (expecting the very worst), dichotomous thinking (perceiving events in only one of two opposite categories), or magnification (placing distorted emphasis on a single event). **EB:** *A randomized control trial of a cognitive-behavioral family treatment for suicide attempt prevention found that the results supported the intervention for preventing suicide attempts in adolescents presenting with recent self-harm (Asarnow et al, 2017).*
▲ Refer family members and friends to local mental health agencies and crisis intervention centers if the client has suicidal ideation or a suspicion of suicidal thoughts exists. **EBN:** *Clients at risk should receive evaluation and help (APA, 2016).*
▲ In the event of successful suicide, refer the family to a therapy group for survivors of suicide. **EB:** *A study revealed that 63% of the bereaved had elevated scores on a measure of complicated grief and that the complicated grief scores correlated moderately but positively with depression and hopelessness and negatively with subjective happiness and satisfaction with life (Bellini et al, 2018).*

S

REFERENCES

Ahmedani, B. K., Petersen, E. L., Hu, Y., et al. (2017). Major physical health conditions and risk of suicide. *American Journal of Preventive Medicine*, *53*(3), 308–315. https://doi.org/10.1016/j.amepre.2017.04.001.

Alavi, N., Reshetukha, T., Prost, E., et al. (2017). Relationship between bullying and suicidal behaviour in youth presenting to the emergency department. *Journal of the Canadian Academy of Child and Adolescent Psychiatry*, *26*(2), 70–77.

American Psychiatric Association (APA). (2016). *The American Psychiatric Association practice guidelines for the psychiatric evaluation of adults* (3rd ed.). Retrieved from http://psychiatryonline.org/guidelines.

American Psychiatric Nurses Association (APNA). (2015). *Psychiatric-mental health nurse essential competencies for assessment and management of individuals at risk for suicide*. Retrieved from http://www.apna.org/i4a/pages/index.cfm?pageid=5684. [Accessed July 30, 2021].

Asarnow, J. R., Hughes, J. L., Babeva, K. B., & Sugar, C. A. (2017). Cognitive-behavioral family treatment for suicide attempt prevention: A randomized controlled trial. *Journal of the American Academy of Child & Adolescent Psychiatry*, *56*(6), 506–514. https://doi.org/10.1016/j.jaac.2017.03.015.

Baldessarini, R., Tondo, L., Pinna, M., Nuñez, N., & Vázquez, G. H. (2019). Suicidal risk factors in major affective disorders. *British Journal of Psychiatry*, *215*(4), 621–626. https://doi.org/10.1192/bjp.2019.167.

Barnett, A. P., Molock, S. D., Nieves-Lugo, K., & Zea, M. C. (2019). Anti-LGBT victimization, fear of violence at school, and suicide risk among adolescents. *Psychology of Sexual Orientation and Gender Diversity*, *6*(1), 88–95. https://doi.org/10.1037/sgd0000309.

Bellini, S., Erbuto, D., Andriessen, K., et al. (2018). Depression, hopelessness, and complicated grief in survivors of suicide. *Frontiers in Psychology*, *9*, 198. https://doi.org/10.3389/fpsyg.2018.00198.

Betz, M. E., Kautzman, M., Segal, D. L., et al. (2018). Frequency of lethal means assessment among emergency department patients with a positive suicide risk screen. *Psychiatry Research*, *260*, 30–35. https://doi.org/10.1016/j.psychres.2017.11.038.

Bickford, D., Morin, R. T., Nelson, J. C., & Mackin, R. S. (2020). Determinants of suicide-related ideation in late life depression: Associations with perceived stress. *Clinical Gerontologist*, *43*(1), 37–45. https://doi.org/10.1080/07317115.2019.1666442.

Brodsky, B. S., Spruch-Feiner, A., & Stanley, B. (2018). The zero suicide model: Applying evidence-based suicide prevention practices to clinical care. *Frontiers in Psychiatry*, *9*, 33. https://doi.org/10.3389/fpsyt.2018.00033.

Chan, S., Denny, S., Fleming, T., Fortune, S., Peiris-John, R., & Dyson, B. (2018). Exposure to suicide behaviour and individual risk of self-harm: Findings from a nationally representative New Zealand high school survey. *Australian and New Zealand Journal of Psychiatry*, *52*(4), 349–356. https://doi.org/10.1177/0004867417710728.

Clement, D. N., Wingate, L. R., Cole, A. B., et al. (2020). The common factors of grit, hope, and optimism differentially influence suicide resilience. *International Journal of Environmental Research and Public Health*, *17*(24), 9588. https://doi.org/10.3390/ijerph17249588.

Courtet, P., Nobile, B., & Lopez-Castroman, J. (2017). Antidepressants and suicide risk: Harmful or useful? In U. Kumar (Ed.), *Handbook of suicidal behaviour* (pp. 329–347). New York: Springer. https://doi.org/10.1007/978-981-10-4816-6_18.

Draper, B., Krysinska, K., Snowdon, J., & De Leo, D. (2018). Awareness of suicide risk and communication between health care professionals and next-of-kin of suicides in the month before suicide. *Suicide and Life-Threatening Behavior*, *48*(4), 449–458. https://doi.org/10.1111/sltb.12365.

Gøtzsche, P. C., & Gøtzsche, P. K. (2017). Cognitive behavioural therapy halves the risk of repeated suicide attempts: Systematic review. *Journal of the Royal Society of Medicine*, *110*(10), 404–410. doi:10.1177/0141076817731904.

Haddock, G., Pratt, D., Gooding, P., et al. (2019). Feasibility and acceptability of suicide prevention therapy on acute psychiatric wards: Randomised controlled trial. *BJPsych Open*, *5*(1), e14. https://doi.org/10.1192/bjo.2018.85.

Hagen, J., Knizek, B. L., & Hjelmeland, H. (2017). Mental health nurses' experiences of caring for suicidal patients in psychiatric wards: An emotional endeavor. *Archives of Psychiatric Nursing*, *31*(1), 31–37. https://doi.org/10.1016/j.apnu.2016.07.018.

Hagen, J., Knizek, B. L., & Hjelmeland, H. (2018). Former suicidal inpatients' experiences of treatment and care in psychiatric wards in Norway. *International Journal of Qualitative Studies on Health and Well-Being*, *13*(1), 1461514. https://doi.org/10.1080/17482631.2018.1461514.

Harmer, B., Lee, S., Duong, T. H., & Saadabadi, A. (2021). *Suicidal ideation*. StatPearls [Internet]. Treasure Island, FL: StatPearls Publishing. https://www.ncbi.nlm.nih.gov/books/NBK565877/.

Johnson, L. L., O'Connor, S. S., Kaminer, B., et al. (2019). Evaluation of structured assessment and mediating factors of suicide-focused group therapy for Veterans recently discharged from inpatient psychiatry. *Archives of Suicide Research*, *23*(1), 15–33. https://doi.org/10.1080/13811118.2017.1402722.

Kiekens, G., Hasking, P., Boyes, M., et al. (2018). The associations between non-suicidal self-injury and first onset suicidal thoughts and behaviors. *Journal of Affective Disorders*, *239*, 171–179. https://doi.org/10.1016/j.jad.2018.06.033.

Lai, A. X., Kaup, A. R., Yaffe, K., & Byers, A. L. (2018). High occurrence of psychiatric disorders and suicidal behavior across dementia subtypes. *American Journal of Geriatric Psychiatry*, *26*(12), 1191–1201. https://doi.org/10.1016/j.jagp.2018.08.012.

Leavey, G., Mallon, S., Rondon-Sulbaran, J., Galway, K., Rosato, M., & Hughes, L. (2017). The failure of suicide prevention in primary care: Family and GP perspectives—A qualitative study. *BMC Psychiatry*, *17*(1), 369. https://doi.org/10.1186/s12888-017-1508-7.

Li, W., Dorstyn, D. S., & Jarmon, E. (2020). Identifying suicide risk among college students: A systematic review. *Death Studies*, *44*(7), 450–458. https://doi.org/10.1080/07481187.2019.1578305.

Lutz, J., Katz, E., Gallegos, J., Spalding, R., & Edelstein, B. (2020). The Geriatric Feelings of Burdensomeness Scale (GFBS). *Clinical Gerontologist*. [Online ahead of print]. https://doi.org/10.1080/07317115.2020.1838982.

Marr, M. C., Gerson, R., Lee, M., Storfer-Isser, A., Horwitz, S. M., & Havens, J. F. (2021). Trauma exposure and suicidality in a pediatric emergency psychiatric population. *Pediatric Emergency Care*. [Online ahead of print]. https://doi.org/10.1097/PEC.0000000000002391.

Morrissey, J., & Higgins, A. (2019). "Attenuating Anxieties": A grounded theory study of mental health nurses' responses to clients with suicidal behaviour. *Journal of Clinical Nursing*, *28*(5–6), 947–958. doi:10.1111/jocn.1471.

Moye, J., Harris, G., Kube, E., et al. (2019). Mental health integration in geriatric patient-aligned care teams in the Department of Veterans Affairs. *American Journal of Geriatric Psychiatry*, *27*(2), 100–108. https://doi.org/10.1016/j.jagp.2018.09.001.

Nguyen, M. H., Le, T. T., Nguyen, H. K. T., Ho, M. T., Nguyen, H. T. T., & Vuong, Q. H. (2021). Alice in suicideland: Exploring the suicidal ideation mechanism through social connectedness and help-seeking behaviors. *International Journal of Environmental Research and Public Health*, *18*(7), 3681. http://dx.doi.org/10.2139/ssrn.3776275.

Okolie, C., Dennis, M., Thomas, E. S., & John, A. (2017). A systematic review of interventions to prevent suicidal behaviors and reduce

S

suicidal ideation in older people. *International Psychogeriatrics, 29*(11), 1801–1824. https://doi.org/10.1017/S1041610217001430.

Pompili, M., Murri, M. B., Patti, S., et al. (2016). The communication of suicidal intentions: A meta-analysis. *Psychological Medicine, 46*(11), 2239–2253. https://doi.org/10.1017/S0033291716000696.

Richardson, C., Robb, K. A., & O'Connor, R. C. (2021). A systematic review of suicidal behaviour in men: A narrative synthesis of risk factors. *Social Science & Medicine, 276*, 113831. https://doi.org/10.1016/j.socscimed.2021.113831.

Sadek, J. (2019). Documentation and communication. In *A Clinician's Guide to suicide risk assessment and management* (pp. 55–58). New York: Springer. https://doi.org/10.1007/978-3-319-77773-3_6.

Schepis, T. S., Simoni–Wastila, L., & McCabe, S. E. (2019). Prescription opioid and benzodiazepine misuse is associated with suicidal ideation in older adults. *International Journal of Geriatric Psychiatry, 34*(1), 122–129. https://doi.org/10.1002/gps.4999.

Stefansson, J., Nordström, P., Runeson, B., Åsberg, M., & Jokinen, J. (2015). Combining the suicide intent scale and the Karolinska interpersonal violence scale in suicide risk assessments. *BMC Psychiatry, 15*, 226. doi:10.1186/s12888-015-0607-6.

Synnott, J., Ioannou, M., Coyne, A., & Hemingway, S. (2018). A content analysis of online suicide notes: Attempted suicide versus attempt resulting in suicide. *Suicide Life and Life Threatening Behavior, 48*(6), 767–778. https://doi.org/10.1111/sltb.12398.

Too, L. S., Spittal, M. J., Bugeja, L., Reifels, L., Butterworth, P., & Pirkis, J. (2019). The association between mental disorders and suicide: A systematic review and meta-analysis of record linkage studies. *Journal of Affective Disorders, 259*, 302–313. https://doi.org/10.1016/j.jad.2019.08.054.

Tubbs, A. S., Fernandez, F. X., Ghani, S. B., et al. (2021). Prescription medications for insomnia are associated with suicidal thoughts and behaviors in two nationally representative samples. *Journal of Clinical Sleep Medicine, 17*(5), 1025–1030. https://doi.org/10.5664/jcsm.9096.

van Veen, M., van Weeghel, I., Koekkoek, B., & Braam, A. W. (2015). Structured assessment of suicide risk in a psychiatric emergency service: Psychometric evaluation of the Nurses' Global Assessment of Suicide Risk scale (NGASR). *International Journal of Social Psychiatry, 61*(3), 287–296. https://doi.org/10.1177/0020764014543311.

Wasserman, D., Hoven, C. W., Wasserman, C., et al. (2015). School-based suicide prevention programmes: The SEYLE cluster-randomized, controlled trial. *Lancet, 385*(9977), 1536–1544. Retrieved from http://www.mdlinx.com/internal-medicine/print-preview.cfm/5874195. [Accessed February 24, 2022].

Williams, S. C., Schmaltz, S. P., Castro, G. M., & Baker, D. W. (2018). Incidence and method of suicide in hospitals in the United States. *Joint Commission Journal on Quality and Patient Safety, 44*(11), 643–650. https://doi.org/10.1016/j.jcjq.2018.08.002.

Yang, L., Jia, C. X., & Qin, P. (2015). Reliability and validity of the Center for Epidemiologic Studies Depression scale (CES-D) among suicide attempters and comparison residents in rural China. *BMC Psychiatry, 15*, 76. https://doi.org/10.1186/s12888-015-0458-1.

Yoon, S., Park, K., & Choi, K. H. (2020). The ultra brief checklist for suicidality. *Journal of Affective Disorders, 276*, 279–286. https://doi.org/10.1016/j.jad.2020.07.037.

Delayed Surgical Recovery

Domain 11 Safety/protection Class 2 Physical injury

Monica Brock, MS, RN, CCRN, CNEcl

NANDA-I

Definition

Extension of the number of postoperative days required to initiate and perform activities that maintain life, health, and well-being.

Defining Characteristics

Anorexia; difficulty in moving about; difficulty resuming employment; excessive time required for recuperation; expresses discomfort; fatigue; interrupted surgical area healing; perceived need for more time to recover; postpones resumption of work; requires assistance for self-care

Related Factors

Delirium; impaired physical mobility; increased blood glucose level; malnutrition; negative emotional response to surgical outcome; obesity; persistent nausea; persistent pain; persistent vomiting; smoking

At-Risk Population

Individuals aged ≥80 years; individuals experiencing intraoperative hypothermia; individuals requiring emergency surgery; individuals requiring perioperative blood transfusion; individuals with American Society of Anesthesiologists (ASA) Physical Status Classification score ≥3; individuals with history of myocardial infarction; individuals with low functional capacity; individuals with preoperative weight loss >5%

Associated Conditions

Anemia; diabetes mellitus; extensive surgical procedures; pharmaceutical preparations; prolonged duration of perioperative surgical wound infection; psychological disorder in postoperative period; surgical wound infection

S

NOC (Nursing Outcomes Classification)

Suggested NOC Outcomes

Endurance; Infection Severity; Mobility; Pain Control; Self-Care: Activities of Daily Living (ADLs); Surgical Recovery: Convalescence/Immediate Postoperative; Wound Healing: Primary Intention

Example NOC Outcome with Indicators

Surgical Recovery: Convalescence as evidenced by the following indicators: Extent of physiological, psychological, and role function after discharge from postanesthesia care to the final postoperative clinic visit/Vital signs/Performance of normal activities, self-care activities. (Rate the outcome and indicators of **Surgical Recovery: Convalescence:** 1 = severe deviation from normal range, 2 = substantial deviation from normal range, 3 = moderate deviation from normal range, 4 = mild deviation from normal range, 5 = no deviation from normal range [see Section I].)

Client Outcomes

Client Will (Specify Time Frame)

- Have surgical area that shows evidence of healing: no redness, induration, draining, dehiscence, or immobility
- State that appetite is regained
- State that no nausea is present
- Demonstrate ability to move about
- Demonstrate ability to complete self-care activities
- State that no fatigue is present
- State that surgical pain is controlled or relieved
- Resume employment activities/ADLs
- State no depression or anxiety related to surgical procedure

NIC (Nursing Interventions Classification)

Suggested NIC Interventions

Incision Site Care; Nutrition Management; Pain Management; Self-Care Assistance; Surgical Assistance

Example NIC Activities—Incision Site Care

Teach the client and/or the family how to care for the incision, including signs and symptoms of infection; Inspect the incision site for redness, swelling, signs of dehiscence, or evisceration

Nursing Interventions and *Rationales*

- Encourage smoking cessation before surgery. EB: *Smoking cessation restores tissue oxygenation and metabolism important to wound healing; research indicates that smoking cessation can reduce the rate of surgical site infections by more than half, as compared with active smokers (Martin et al, 2016).*
- Perform a thorough preoperative assessment of the client's health literacy level. EB: *Low health literacy, common among surgical clients, is associated with poor health outcomes (Chang et al, 2020).*
- Assess for the presence of medical conditions and treat appropriately before surgery. EB: *A chronically malnourished client may benefit from nutritional therapy before surgery (Morgensen et al, 2018). If the client is diabetic, maintain normal blood glucose levels before surgery.* EB: *High blood glucose levels slow healing and increase the risk of infection. The American Diabetes Association (ADA) recommended that blood glucose should be less than 180 mg/dL for people in the hospital or having surgery (ADA, 2019).*
- Carefully assess the client's use of herbal and dietary supplements such as feverfew, fish oil, ginkgo biloba, garlic, ginseng, ginger, valerian, kava, St. John's wort, ephedra (Ma huang or metabolite), and echinacea. It is recommended that all dietary supplements are stopped at least 1 week before major surgical or diagnostic procedures. EB: *Because herbal and dietary supplements can have unintended medical side effects as well as potential interactions with anesthetic drugs, it is important for anesthetists to be aware of their use (Levy et al, 2017).*

S

- Assess and treat for depression and anxiety in a client before surgery and postoperatively. EB: *Clients with higher levels of preoperative anxiety and depression report increased postoperative pain, nausea, and fatigue (Ghoneim & O'Hara, 2016).*
- Play music of the client's choice preoperatively, intraoperatively, and postoperatively. EBN: *Listening to self-selected music during the perioperative period can effectively reduce anxiety levels (Sibanda et al, 2019).*
- Consider using healing touch and other mind-body-spirit interventions such as stress control, therapeutic massage, and imagery. EBN: *Research indicates that use of holistic therapies in the perioperative setting can decrease pain and anesthesia complications, leading to increased client satisfaction with health care (Acar & Aygin, 2019; Guo et al, 2020).*
- Maintain perioperative normothermia. Use reflective blankets to reduce heat loss during surgery. EBN: *A randomized control trial found that reflective blankets were a more effective method of passive warming than warm blankets (Koenen et al, 2017).*
- Postoperatively, discuss vital sign parameters with the surgeon, as well as signs and symptoms that could indicate early postoperative infection. EB: *Surgical site infections are a leading cause of prolonged hospitalization, which increase cost of care and are associated with poorer client outcomes (Badia et al, 2017).*
- Use careful aseptic technique when caring for wounds. EBN: *Handwashing continues to be the most important factor in reducing health care–associated infection, but the use of an aseptic technique will further reduce the risk of infection (Berríos-Torres et al, 2017).*
- Clients should bathe before surgery. EBN: *Preoperative bathing with soap and water reduces skin colonization of microorganisms, reducing the rate of clean surgery surgical site infections by up to threefold (Maciel de Castro Franco et al, 2017; Webster & Osborne 2015).* EBN: *In an analysis of recent studies, there was no observed difference in the occurrence of surgical site infection when comparing clients undergoing preoperative bathing with soap and water or with an antiseptic agent (Maciel de Castro Franco et al, 2017).*
- Clients should be allowed to shower after surgery to maintain cleanliness, if not contraindicated because of the presence of pacemaker wires or other contraindications. EB: *In an analysis of existing studies, there was no statistically significant increase in wound infection related to early bathing. The decision to bathe the client immediately postoperatively should be specific to surgical type and site (Ljungqvist et al, 2017).*
- Optimize the client's preoperative, intraoperative, and postoperative condition to minimize client stress and retain homeostasis. EB: *Enhanced Recovery After Surgery is a multiprofessional, multimodal approach to caring for the surgical client that includes changes from overnight fasting to carbohydrate drinks 2 hours before surgery, minimally invasive approaches, management of intravenous fluids to maintain euvolemia, early removal of drains and tubes, early mobilization, and early postoperative oral intake of food and fluids. Enhanced Recovery After Surgery protocols have reduced hospital length of stay by 30% to 50% with similar reductions in complications, and have been shown to improve outcomes in nearly all major surgical specialties (Ljungqvist et al, 2017).*
- Carefully assess functional status of the client postoperatively using a fall-risk stratification tool, such as the Morse Fall Scale, to identify clients at high risk for fall. EBN: *The Morse Fall Scale has been validated in numerous studies, and it helps identify clients at high risk for falls. All clients identified as high risk should have increased monitoring and safety precautions in place (Jewell et al, 2020).*
- See care plans for **Anxiety,** Acute **Pain, Fatigue,** Risk for Perioperative **Positioning** Injury, Impaired Physical **Mobility,** and **Nausea.**

Pediatric

- Provide age-appropriate procedural information and postoperative expectations, including pain, function, and emotional care needs. EBN: *Parents and children report higher levels of satisfaction, decreased preoperative anxiety, and better surgical experiences if given the opportunity preoperatively to discuss all aspects of the surgery, including realistic postoperative expectations (Newell et al, 2020).*
- Teach imagery and encourage distraction for children for postsurgical pain relief. EBN: *Distraction decreases pain in children undergoing painful procedures (Al-Yateem et al, 2016).* EBN: *Active distraction strategies, such as use of distraction cards or viewing a kaleidoscope, resulted in significant decreases in pain and anxiety among children, as compared with passive distraction techniques (Hussein, 2015).*

Geriatric

- Clients over age 65 should undergo a comprehensive geriatric assessment before surgery. EB: *Older clients have higher rates of surgical complications and mortality than younger clients. Studies show postoperative outcomes can be improved through the use of geriatric collaborative models (Zietlow et al, 2021).*

- The condition of the client' skin should be noted and fully documented. EB: *Using an objective evaluation tool, such as the Braden scale, allows for early identification of older clients at higher risk for developing skin breakdown (Aloweni et al, 2019).*
- Routinely assess pain using a pain scale appropriate for clients with impaired cognition or inability to verbalize. EBN: *Self-report should be the first-line approach when possible, with observational assessment used as a supplementary tool, when warranted. The Pain Assessment in Advanced Dementia (PAINAD) and Pain Assessment Checklist for Seniors With Limited Ability to Communicate (PACSLAC) have been validated for reliability (Chow et al, 2016).*
- Serially evaluate the client's vital signs, including temperature. Check baseline vital signs and monitor trends. CEB: *Physiological changes of aging often result in lower baseline body temperatures and decreased heart rates, and prevent the older client from developing fever. Medications, such as blood pressure agents, may prevent the client from having an increased heart rate (Chester & Rudolph, 2011).*
- The older client should be evaluated for signs and symptoms of delirium. Ensure that hearing aids and glasses are also available as needed. EB: *The older client is at increased risk of postoperative delirium. The Confusion Assessment Method screening tool is a validated instrument widely used to screen for postoperative delirium (Hebert, 2018).* EB: *Nonpharmacological interventions for delirium include orienting to surroundings, adequate oxygen, optimizing nutrition and mobility, sleep hygiene strategies, and avoidance of restraints. Any medications known to precipitate delirium should also be avoided (Hebert, 2018).*
- Offer spiritual support. EB: *A meta-analysis found that overall religion/spirituality was associated with overall physical health, physical and functional well-being, and physical symptoms (Jim et al, 2015).*

Home Care

- The preceding interventions may be adapted for the home setting.
- Provide supportive telephone calls from nurse to client as a means of decreasing anxiety and providing the psychosocial support necessary for recovery from surgery. EBN: *A systematic review of qualitative studies found that clients report being motivated to participate in recovery but face challenges with symptoms (e.g., pain, nausea, weakness). Postoperative follow-up and phone calls provide much needed encouragement and additional assistance to facilitate recovery (Sibbern et al, 2017).*

Client/Family Teaching and Discharge Planning

- Provide discharge planning and teaching in a language that is appropriate to the client and caregiver's education and literacy level. EBN: *Do not use technical or medical jargon, and be aware that clients and caregivers may be reluctant to ask for explanation or clarification because of embarrassment and may dishonestly verbalize understanding. Allow the client to repeat their understanding of the discharge plan (Polster, 2015).*
- Create a discharge plan that includes measurable functional goals, expectations for recovery, and signs and symptoms of postoperative complications. EBN: *Client-specific discharge education equips the client with the necessary knowledge and skills to engage in their care after discharge and increases client satisfaction with the hospital experience (Kang et al, 2020).*

S

REFERENCES

Acar, K., & Aygin, D. (2019). Efficacy of guided imagery for postoperative symptoms, sleep quality, anxiety, and satisfaction regarding nursing care: A randomized controlled study. *Journal of Perianesthesia Nursing*, *34*(6), 1241–1249. https://10.1016/j.jopan.2019.05.006.

Aloweni, F., Ang, S. Y., & Fook-Chong, S. (2019). A prediction tool for hospital-acquired pressure ulcers among surgical patients: Surgical pressure ulcer risk score. *International Wound Journal*, *16*(1), 164–175. https://doi.org/10.1111/iwj.13007.

Al-Yateem, N., Brenner, M., Shorrab, A. A., & Docherty, C. (2016). Play distraction versus pharmacological treatment to reduce anxiety levels in children undergoing day surgery: A randomized controlled non-inferiority trial. *Child: Care, Health and Development*, *42*(4), 572–581. https://10.1111/cch.12343.

American Diabetes Association (ADA). (2019). Glycemic targets: Standards of Medical Care in Diabetes—2019. *Diabetes Care*, *42*(Suppl 1), S61–S70. https://10.2337/dc19-s006.

Badia, J. M., Casey, A. L., Petrosillo, N., Hudson, P. M., Mitchell, S. A., & Crosby, C. (2017). Impact of surgical site infection on healthcare costs and patient outcomes: a systematic review in six European countries. *The Journal of Hospital Infection*, *96*(1), 1–15. https://10.1016/j.jhin.2017.03.004.

Berríos-Torres, S. I., Umscheid, C. A., Bratzler, D. W., et al. (2017). Centers for Disease Control and Prevention guideline for the prevention of surgical site infection. *JAMA Surgery*, *152*(8), 784–791. https://10.1001/jamasurg.2017.0904.

Chang, M. E., Baker, S. J., Dos Santos Marques, I. C., et al. (2020). Health literacy in surgery. *Health Literacy Research and Practice*, *4*(1), e46–e65. https://doi.org/10.3928/24748307-20191121-01.

Chester, J. G., & Rudolph, J. L. (2011). Vital signs in older patients: Age-related changes. *Journal of the American Medical Directors Association*, *12*(5), 337–343. https://doi.org/10.1016/j.jamda.2010.04.009.

Chow, S., Chow, R., Lam, M., et al. (2016). Pain assessment tools for older adults with dementia in long-term care facilities: A systematic review. *Neurodegenerative Disease Management*, *6*(6), 525–538. https://doi.org/10.2217/nmt-2016-0033.

Ghoneim, M. M., & O'Hara, M. W. (2016). Depression and postoperative complications: An overview. *BMC Surgery*, *16*, 5. https://10.1186/s12893-016-0120-y.

Guo, P. P., Fan, S. L., Li, P., et al. (2020). The effectiveness of massage on peri-operative anxiety in adults: A meta-analysis of randomized controlled trials and controlled clinical trials. *Complementary Therapies in Clinical Practice*, *41*, 101240. https://10.1016/j.ctcp.2020.101240.

Hebert, C. (2018). Evidence-based practice in perianesthesia nursing: Application of the American Geriatrics Society Clinical Practice Guideline for postoperative delirium in older adults. *Journal of Perianesthesia Nursing*, *33*(3), 253–264. https://doi.org/10.1016/j.jopan.2016.02.011.

Hussein, H. A. (2015). Effect of active and passive distraction on decreasing pain associated with painful medical procedures among school aged children. *World Journal of Nursing Sciences*, *1*(2), 13–23.

Jewell, V. D., Capistran, K., Flecky, K., Qi, Y., & Fellman, S. (2020). Prediction of falls in acute care using the Morse Fall Risk Scale. *Occupational Therapy in Health Care*, *34*(4), 307–319. https://10.1080/07380577.2020.1815928.

Jim, H. S. L., Pustejovsky, J. E., Park, C. L., et al. (2015). Religion, spirituality, and physical health in cancer patients: A meta-analysis. *Cancer*, *121*(21), 3760–3768. https://doi.org/10.1002/cncr.29353.

Kang, E., Gillespie, B. M., Tobiano, G., & Chaboyer, W. (2020). General surgical patients' experience of hospital discharge education: A qualitative study. *Journal of Clinical Nursing*, *29*(1-2), e1–e10. https://doi.org/10.1111/jocn.15057.

Koenen, M., Passey, M., & Rolf, M. (2017). "Keeping them warm"—A randomized controlled trial of two passive perioperative warming methods. *Journal of Perianesthesia Nursing*, *32*(3), 188–198. https://10.1016/j.jopan.2015.09.011.

Levy, I., Attias, S., Ben-Arye, E., et al. (2017). Perioperative risks of dietary and herbal supplements. *World Journal of Surgery*, *41*(4), 927–934. https://10.1007/s00268-016-3825-2.

Ljungqvist, O., Scott, M., & Fearon, K. C. (2017). Enhanced recovery after surgery: a review. *JAMA Surgery*, *152*(3), 292–298. https://10.1001/jamasurg.2016.4952.

Maciel de Castro Franco, L., Fernandes Cota, G., Saraiva Pinto, T., & Falci Ercole, F. (2017). Preoperative bathing of the surgical site with chlorhexidine for infection prevention: Systematic review with meta-analysis. *American Journal of Infection Control*, *45*(4), 343–349. https://10.1016/j.ajic.2016.12.003.

Martin, C. T., Gao, Y., Duchman, K. R., & Pugely, A. J. (2016). The impact of current smoking and smoking cessation on short-term morbidity risk after lumbar spine surgery. *Spine*, *41*(7), 577–584. https://doi.org/10.1097/brs.0000000000001281.

Mogensen, K. M., Horkan, C. M., Purtle, S. W., Moromizato, T., Rawn, J. D., Robinson, M. K., & Christopher, K. B. (2018). Malnutrition, critical illness survivors, and postdischarge outcomes: a cohort study. *JPEN. Journal of Parenteral and Enteral Nutrition*, *42*(3), 557–565. https://doi.org/10.1177/0148607117709766.

Newell, C., Leduc-Pessah, H., Bell-Graham, L., Rasic, N., & Carter, K. (2020). Evaluating and enhancing the preparation of patients and families before pediatric surgery. *Children*, *7*(8), 90. https://doi.org/10.3390/children7080090.

Polster, D. (2015). Preventing readmissions with discharge education. *Nursing Management*, *46*(10), 30–37. https://doi.org/10.1097/01.NUMA.0000471590.62056.77.

Sibanda, A., Carnes, D., Visentin, D., & Cleary, M. (2019). A systematic review of the use of music interventions to improve outcomes for patients undergoing hip or knee surgery. *Journal of Advanced Nursing*, *75*(3), 502–516. https://10.1111/jan.13860.

Sibbern, T., Bull Sellevold, V., Steindal, S. A., Dale, C., Watt-Watson, J., & Dihle, A. (2017). Patients' experiences of enhanced recovery after surgery: A systematic review of qualitative studies. *Journal of Clinical Nursing*, *26*(9–10), 1172–1188. https://doi:10.1111/jocn.13456.

Webster, J., & Osborne, S. (2015). Preoperative bathing or showering with skin antiseptics to prevent surgical site infection. *Cochrane Database of Systematic Reviews*, *2*, CD004985. https://10.1002/14651858.cd004985.pub5.

Zietlow, K. E., Wong, S., McDonald, S. R., et al. (2021). Perioperative Optimization of Senior Health (POSH): A descriptive analysis of cancelled surgery. *World Journal of Surgery*, *45*(1), 109–115. https://doi.org/10.1007/s00268-020-05772.

S

Risk for Delayed Surgical Recovery

Domain 11 Safety/protection Class 2 Physical injury

Mary Beth Flynn Makic, PhD, RN, CCNS, CCRN-K, FAAN, FNAP, FCNS

NANDA-I

Definition

Susceptible to an extension of the number of postoperative days required to initiate and perform activities that maintain life, health, and well-being, which may compromise health.

Risk Factors

Delirium; impaired physical mobility; increased blood glucose level; malnutrition; negative emotional response to surgical outcome; obesity; persistent nausea; persistent pain; persistent vomiting; smoking

At-Risk Population

Individuals aged ≥80 years; individuals experiencing intraoperative hypothermia; individuals requiring emergency surgery; individuals requiring perioperative blood transfusion; individuals with American Society of Anesthesiologists (ASA) Physical Status classification score ≥3; individuals with history of myocardial infarction; individuals with low functional capacity; individuals with preoperative weight loss >5%

Associated Conditions

Anemia; diabetes mellitus; extensive surgical procedures; pharmaceutical preparations; prolonged duration of perioperative surgical wound infection; psychological disorder in postoperative period; surgical wound infection

NIC, NOC, Client Outcomes, Nursing Interventions and *Rationales,* Client/Family Teaching and Discharge Planning, and References

See the care plan for Delayed **Surgical** Recovery.

Impaired Swallowing **Domain 2 Nutrition Class 1 Ingestion**

Marina Martinez-Kratz, MS, RN, CNE

NANDA-I

Definition

Abnormal functioning of the swallowing mechanism associated with deficits in oral, pharyngeal, or esophageal structure or function.

Defining Characteristics

First Stage: Oral

Abnormal oral phase of swallow study; bruxism; choking prior to swallowing; choking when swallowing cold water; coughing prior to swallowing; drooling; food falls from mouth; food pushed out of mouth; gagging prior to swallowing; impaired ability to clear oral cavity; inadequate consumption during prolonged meal time; inadequate lip closure; inadequate mastication; incidence of wet hoarseness twice within 30 seconds; inefficient nippling; inefficient suck; nasal reflux; piecemeal deglutition; pooling of bolus in lateral sulci; premature entry of bolus; prolonged bolus formation; tongue action ineffective in forming bolus

Second Stage: Pharyngeal

Abnormal pharyngeal phase of swallow study; altered head position; choking; coughing; delayed swallowing; fevers of unknown etiology; food refusal; gagging sensation; gurgly voice quality; inadequate laryngeal elevation; nasal reflux; recurrent pulmonary infection; repetitive swallowing

Third Stage: Esophageal

Abnormal esophageal phase of swallow study; acidic-smelling breath; difficulty swallowing; epigastric pain; food refusal; heartburn; hematemesis; hyperextension of head; nighttime awakening; nighttime coughing; odynophagia; regurgitation; repetitive swallowing; reports "something stuck"; unexplained irritability surrounding mealtimes; volume limiting; vomiting; vomitus on pillow

Related Factors

Altered attention; behavioral feeding problem; protein-energy malnutrition; self-injurious behavior

At-Risk Population

Individuals with history of enteral nutrition; older adults; premature infants

Associated Conditions

Acquired anatomic defects; brain injuries; cerebral palsy; conditions with significant muscle hypotonia; congenital heart disease; cranial nerve involvement; developmental disabilities; esophageal achalasia; gastroesophageal reflux disease; laryngeal diseases; mechanical obstruction; nasal defect; nasopharyngeal cavity defect; neurological problems; neuromuscular diseases; oropharynx abnormality; pharmaceutical preparations; prolonged intubation; respiratory condition; tracheal defect; trauma; upper airway anomaly; vocal cord dysfunction

NOC (Nursing Outcomes Classification)

Suggested NOC Outcomes

Swallowing Status: Esophageal Phase, Oral Phase, Pharyngeal Phase

Example NOC Outcome with Indicators

Swallowing Status as evidenced by the following indicators: Delivery of bolus to hypopharynx is timed with swallow reflex/Ability to clear oral cavity/Number of swallows appropriate for bolus size and texture/Voice quality/Choking, coughing, gagging/Normal swallow effort. (Rate the outcome and indicators of **Swallowing Status:** 1 = severely compromised, 2 = substantially compromised, 3 = moderately compromised, 4 = mildly compromised, 5 = not compromised [see Section I].)

Client Outcomes

Client Will (Specify Time Frame)

- Demonstrate effective swallowing without signs of aspiration (see the section Defining Characteristics)
- Remain free from aspiration (e.g., lungs clear, temperature within normal range)

NIC (Nursing Interventions Classification)

Suggested NIC Interventions

Aspiration Precautions; Swallowing Therapy

Example NIC Activities—Swallowing Therapy

Assist client to sit in erect position (as close to 90 degrees as possible) for feeding/exercise; Instruct client not to talk during eating, if appropriate

Nursing Interventions and *Rationales*

S

- ● Assess for risk factors associated with impaired swallowing. EB: *A systematic review identified the prevalence of dysphagia as 15% of community-dwelling older adults with risk factors that included advanced age; history of clinical disease; physical frailty; and reduced ability to carry out activities of daily living (Madhaven et al, 2016).*
- ● Complete swallow screen per facility protocol. EBN: *Bedside nurse-initiated dysphagia screening with formal guidelines for the identification and management of dysphagia may have a significant effect on serious adverse outcomes such as chest infections and death (Hines, Kynoch, & Munday, 2016).*
- ▲ Do not feed clients with impaired swallowing orally until an appropriate diagnostic workup is completed. EBN: *Impaired swallow function or dysphagia places a client at greater risk for dehydration and malnutrition. Dehydration thickens secretions, increasing the risk for certain respiratory problems, and aspiration may lead to pneumonia and death (Mauk, 2017).*
- ▲ Ensure proper nutrition by consulting with a health care provider regarding alternative nutrition and hydration when oral nutrition is not safe/adequate. EBN: *A timely decision to proceed with tube feeding should be made in collaboration with the client, family (or substitute decision maker), and interprofessional team. Enteral nutrition via intravenous, nasogastric, or percutaneous endoscopic gastrostomy (PEG) tube could substantially reduce risks of aspiration and choking while providing clients with needed hydration and nutrients (Coltman, 2019).*

- ▲ Refer to a speech-language pathologist for evaluation and diagnostic evaluation of swallowing to determine swallowing problems and solutions as soon as oral and/or pharyngeal dysphagia is suspected. EBN: *Safe nursing care includes a consultation with a speech-language pathologist whenever doubts arise regarding a client's ability to tolerate oral-supported nutrition in any form (Teasell et al, 2018). Video fluoroscopic swallow study (VSS, VFSS, or MBS), or fiberoptic endoscopic examination of swallowing (FEES), should be performed on all clients considered at risk for pharyngeal dysphagia or poor airway protection based on results from the bedside swallowing assessment (McGinnis et al, 2019).*
- ▲ To manage impaired swallowing, use a multiprofessional dysphagia team composed of a speech pathologist, dietitian, nursing, health care provider, and medical staff. A comprehensive assessment from a multiprofessional dysphagia team can lead to personalized therapeutic interventions that can help the client learn to swallow safely and maintain a good nutritional status. EBN: *Elderly clients with dysphagia require a multiprofessional team working closely together to perform feeding management. Nurses have more opportunities to contact clients in clinical work, so they must learn the correct guidance of safe eating and feeding for elderly clients with dysphagia (Li et al, 2015).*
- ▲ Observe the following feeding guidelines:
  - ❍ Before giving oral feedings, determine the client's readiness to eat (e.g., alert, able to hold head erect, follow instructions, move tongue in mouth, and manage oral secretions). If one of these elements is missing, it may be advisable to withhold oral feeding and use enteral feeding for nourishment.
  - ❍ Monitor client during oral feedings and provide cueing as needed to ensure client follows swallowing guidelines/aspiration precautions recommended by speech-language pathologist or dysphagia specialist. Note: General aspiration precautions include the following: sit at 90 degrees for all oral feedings; take small bites/sips; eat at a slow rate; if client is being fed, position the feeder at eye level with the client; and no straws. However, client-specific strategies will be determined via bedside and/or instrumental swallowing evaluation performed by dysphagia specialist. EBN: *Postural changes, sensory enhancements, swallow maneuvers, or voluntary controls exerted over the swallow can improve swallow, but the use and effectiveness of these treatments will vary systematically with the client's medical diagnosis (Atkinson, 2019).*
  - ❍ Keep bolus size to 5 mL or smaller. EB: *Evidence gathered from the appraised studies generally supports the clinical hypothesis that a small bolus size (5 mL or smaller) decreases the risk of penetration or aspiration of liquids during swallowing events (Rizzo et al, 2016).*
  - ❍ During feeding, adapt environment to decrease noise and distractions. EBN: *Reducing environmental distractions will assist the client to focus on eating (Atkinson, 2019).*
  - ❍ If the client is older or has gastroesophageal reflux disease, ensure the client is kept in an upright posture for an hour after eating. EBN: *An upright position after eating is associated with decreased incidence of pneumonia in older adults (Commisso & Lim, 2019).*
- ● Monitor client during feeding for coughing or choking when eating and drinking, being unable to chew food properly, and losing food and drink from the front of the mouth. EBN: *These are common signs of dysphagia (Atkinson, 2019).*
- ● Use standardized diet and fluid descriptors such as the International Dysphagia Diet Standardisation Initiative (IDDSI) for diet and fluid modification. EB: *The IDDSI framework consists of a continuum of 8 levels (0–7), where drinks are measured from Levels 0 to 4, and foods are measured from Levels 3 to 7. The IDDSI framework provides a common terminology to describe food textures and drink thickness (Steele et al, 2018).*
- ● During meals and all oral intake, observe for wet voice, dysarthria (slurred speech), drooling, inability to cough on command, and an absent gag reflex as an indication of silent aspiration. EBN: *Silent aspiration is common in people with dysphagia (Atkinson, 2019).*
- ▲ If signs of aspiration or pneumonia are present, auscultate lung sounds after feeding. Note new onset of crackles or wheezing, or elevated temperature. EB: *Bronchial auscultation of lung sounds was shown to be specific in identifying clients at risk for aspiration (Sanivarapu & Gibson, 2021).*
- ▲ Assess for signs of malnutrition and dehydration and keep a record of food intake. EB: *A study showed that clients with diagnosed high-risk dysphagia had significantly lower scores on the geriatric nutritional risk index (Saito et al, 2018).*
- ▲ Evaluate nutritional status daily. Weigh the client weekly to help evaluate nutritional status. If the client is not adequately nourished, work with the dysphagia team to determine whether the client needs therapeutic feeding only or needs enteral feedings until the client can swallow adequately. EB: *An interprofessional approach is necessary to maintain the client's nutritional status (McGinnis et al, 2019).*

- ▲ Assist client in following dysphagia specialist's recommendations and provide open, accurate, and effective communication with dysphagia team regarding client's diet tolerance. **EB:** *Understanding and following the dysphagia specialist's recommendations is a pivotal role that nurses play in helping ensure positive dysphagia management outcomes (McGinnis et al, 2019).*
- ▲ Document and notify the provider and dysphagia team of changes in medical, nutritional, or swallowing status. **EB:** *Many negative dysphagia management outcomes can be avoided by ensuring dysphagia communication is accurate, complete, and disseminated among and between health care professionals; nurses are pivotal in this process (McGinnis et al, 2019).*
- ▲ Work with the client on swallowing exercises prescribed by the dysphagia team. **EB:** *Exercise programs can improve airway closure, the range of oral or pharyngeal structure movement during swallow, cricopharyngeal opening, and tongue strength (McGinnis et al, 2019).*
- ▲ Recognize that the client can aspirate oral feedings, even if there are no symptoms of coughing or distress. This phenomenon is called silent aspiration and is common. **EB:** *In a study of elderly long-term residents, dementia was the best predictor of silent aspiration (Sakai et al, 2016).*
- ▲ Ensure oral hygiene is maintained. **EB:** *Oral health care including toothbrushing after each meal, cleaning dentures once a day, and consistent professional oral health care reduces the incidence of aspiration pneumonia that can occur due to bacteria associated with the oral cavity (Müller, 2015).*
- ▲ For clients receiving mechanical ventilation with a tracheostomy tube or after postextubation, request a referral to a speech-language pathologist or dysphagia specialist for an instrumental swallowing evaluation before beginning oral diet. **EB:** *Objective swallowing studies and early intervention are the best ways to determine the safest oral intake and rule out silent aspiration in these clients (Alonso Rodrigues et al, 2015).*

Pediatric

- ▲ Refer children and infants who have difficulty swallowing, difficulty manipulating food, or delayed swallowing to a speech-language pathologist or dysphagia specialist for further assessment and testing. **EB:** *Assessment of dysphagia requires specialized training. Speech-language pathologists are trained to evaluate and treat pediatric dysphagia (Reynolds, 2020).*
- ▲ Consult with occupational therapy to evaluate positioning for pediatric clients related to feeding. **EB:** *Efficient oral motor movements depend on the steadiness or stability of the trunk, neck, and head (Mitchell & Paluszak, 2018).*
- ▲ For at-risk infants, consult with a feeding specialist regarding nipple selection to address sucking and swallowing coordination before bottle feeding. **EB:** *Selection of the nipple will consider the attributes of the nipple, viscosity of the fluid, and the skills and coordination of the infant (Mitchell & Paluszak, 2018).*
- ● For at-risk infants, provide external pacing by lowering the bottle to remove milk from the nipple or removing the nipple from the mouth entirely. **EB:** *External pacing is a technique in which breaks are imposed after a certain number of sucks to address suck-swallow-breathe incoordination, which may lead to apnea (Mitchell & Paluszak, 2018).*
- ● For a preterm infant, provide opportunities for patterned nonnutritive sucking (NNS) or oral stimulation. **EB:** *NNS or oral stimulation can be used to normalize responses to sensory input and to facilitate oral-motor coordination without the use of food for infants at risk for choking and aspiration (Mitchell & Paluszak, 2018).*

S

Geriatric

- ▲ Recognize that age-related changes can affect swallowing and these changes have a more pronounced effect when superimposed on neurological disease and other chronic problems. **EB:** *Age-related changes can contribute to less efficient and effective swallowing in older adults (McGinnis et al, 2019).*
- ● Assess for difficulty swallowing medications and modify medication administration as needed. **EB:** *A systematic research review suggested that approximately 14% of community-dwelling older clients have trouble swallowing medicines (Mc Gillicuddy, Crean, & Sahm, 2016).*
- ▲ Evaluate the medications the client is taking and collaborate with pharmacists and other appropriate professionals for assistance with modifications, correct dosages, and drug interactions. **EB:** *As most older adults take multiple medications, the need for enhanced knowledge in this area emphasizes the importance of interprofessional collaboration (McGinnis et al, 2019).*

Home Care

- ▲ Refer to speech therapy. Speech-language pathologists can work with clients to enhance swallowing ability and teach compensatory strategies.

Client/Family Teaching and Discharge Planning

- ▲ Teach the client and family restorative and rehabilitative techniques prescribed by the dysphagia team. EB: *Restorative and rehabilitative techniques are aimed at improving physiological swallow function (McGinnis et al, 2019).*
- • Teach the client, family, and caregivers about standardized diet and fluid descriptors such as the International Dysphagia Diet Standardisation Initiative (IDDSI) for diet and fluid modification. EB: *The IDDSI framework consists of a continuum of 8 levels (0–7), where drinks are measured from Levels 0 to 4 and foods are measured from Levels 3 to 7. The IDDSI framework provides a common terminology to describe food textures and drink thickness (Steele et al, 2018).*
- • Teach the family and caregivers how to monitor the client to prevent and detect aspiration during eating. EB: *Client's family and caregivers should be taught to monitor client during feeding for coughing or choking when eating and drinking, being unable to chew food properly, and losing food and drink from the front of the mouth as these are common signs of dysphagia (Atkinson, 2019).*

REFERENCES

Alonso Rodrigues, K., Ribeiro Machado, F., Chiari, B. M., Baccaro Rosseti, H., Lorenzon, P., & Rebelo Gonçalves, M. I. (2015). Swallowing rehabilitation of dysphagic tracheostomized patients under mechanical ventilation in intensive care units: A feasibility study. *Revista Brasiliera de Terapia Intensiva, 27*(1), 64–71. https://doi.org/10.5935/0103-507X.20150011.

Atkinson, K. (2019). Neurological conditions and acute dysphagia. *British Journal of Nursing, 28*(8), 490–492. https://doi.org/10.12968/bjon.2019.28.8.490.

Coltman, A. (2019). Implementation of a validated malnutrition screening tool in an academic medical center. Food & Nutrition Conference & Expo, 26-29 October 2019, Philadelphia, PA. *Journal of the Academy of Nutrition & Dietetics, 119*(9 Suppl. 1), A13. https://doi.org/10.1016/j.jand.2019.06.057.

Commisso, A., & Lim, F. (2019). Lifestyle modifications in adults and older adults with chronic gastroesophageal reflux disease (GERD). *Critical Care Nurse Quarterly, 42*(1), 64–74. https://doi.org/10.1097/CNQ.0000000000000239.

Hines, S., Kynoch, K., & Munday, J. (2016). Nursing interventions for identifying and managing acute dysphagia are effective for improving patient outcomes: A systematic review update. *Journal of Neuroscience Nursing, 48*(4), 215–223.

Li, M., Wang, Z., Han, W. J., Lu, S. Y., & Fang, Y. Z. (2015). Effect of feeding management on aspiration pneumonia in elderly patients with dysphagia. *Chinese Nursing Research, 2*(2-3), 40–44. https://doi.org/10.1016/j.cnre.2015.09.004.

Madhavan, A., LaGorio, L. A., Crary, M. A., Dahl, W. J., & Carnaby, G. D. (2016). Prevalence of and risk factors for dysphagia in the community dwelling elderly: A systematic review. *Journal of Nutrition, Health & Aging, 20*(8), 806–815. https://doi.org/10.1007/s12603-016-0712-3.

Mauk, K. L. (2017). *Gerontological nursing: Competencies for care* (4th ed.). Burlington, MA: Jones and Bartlett Learning.

Mc Gillicuddy, A., Crean, A. M., & Sahm, L. J. (2016). Older adults with difficulty swallowing oral medicines: A systematic review of the literature. *European Journal of Clinical Pharmacology, 72*(2), 141–151. https://doi.org/10.1007/s00228-015-1979-8.

McGinnis, C. M., Homan, K., Solomon, M., et al. (2019). Dysphagia: Interprofessional management, impact, and patient-centered care. *Nutrition in Clinical Practice, 34*(1), 80–95. https://doi.org/10.1002/ncp.10239.

Mitchell, C., & Paluszak, S. L. (2018). Adaptive feeding techniques and positioning: An occupational therapist's perspective. In J. Ongkasuwan, & E. Chiou (Eds.), *Pediatric dysphagia: Challenges and controversies* (pp. 135–146). Cham, Switzerland: Springer. https://doi.org/10.1007/978-3-319-97025-7_11.

Müller, F. (2015). Oral hygiene reduces the mortality from aspiration pneumonia in frail elders. *Journal of Dental Research, 94*(Supp. 3), 14S–16S. https://doi.org/10.1177/0022034514552494.

Reynolds, J. (2020). When a child needs an instrumental swallowing assessment: How do clinicians know when it's time to move to an instrumental assessment—And then choose the most appropriate one? *ASHA Leader, 25*(1), 40–42. https://doi.org/10.1044/leader.otp.25012020.40.

Rizzo, K., Mong, L., Helser, M., Howard, N., Katz, I., & Scarborough, D. (2016). Effects of bolus size on swallow safety: A systematic review of external evidence. *EBP Briefs, 11*(3), 1–12.

Saito, T., Hayashi, K., Nakazawa, H., Yagihashi, F., Oikawa, L. O., & Ota, T. (2018). A significant association of malnutrition with dysphagia in acute patients. *Dysphagia, 33*(2), 258–265. https://doi.org/10.1007/s00455-017-9855-6.

Sakai, K., Hirano, H., Watanabe, Y., et al. (2016). An examination of factors related to aspiration and silent aspiration in older adults requiring long-term care in rural Japan. *Journal of Oral Rehabilitation, 43*(2), 103–110. https://doi.org/10.1111/joor.12349.

Sanivarapu, R. R., & Gibson, J. (2021). *Aspiration pneumonia*. StatPearls [Internet]. Treasure Island, FL: StatPearls Publishing. Retrieved from https://www.ncbi.nlm.nih.gov/books/NBK470459/. [Accessed February 24, 2022].

Steele, C. M., Namasivayam-MacDonald, A. M., Guida, B. T., et al. (2018). Creation and initial validation of the International Dysphagia Diet Standardisation Initiative Functional Diet Scale. *Archives of Physical Medicine and Rehabilitation, 99*(5), 934–944.

Teasell, R. W., Foley, N., Martino, R., et al. (2018). *Dysphagia and aspiration following stroke.* Evidence-Based Review of Stroke Rehabilitation. Retrieved from http://www.ebrsr.com/sites/default/files/v18-SREBR-CH15-NET.pdf. [Accessed July 30, 2021].

S

Risk for Thermal Injury Domain 11 Safety/protection Class 2 Physical injury

Wendie A. Howland, MN, RN-BC, CRRN, CCM, CNLCP, LNCC

NANDA-I

Definition

Susceptible to extreme temperature damage to skin and mucous membranes, which may compromise health.

Risk Factors

Fatigue; inadequate caregiver knowledge of safety precautions; inadequate knowledge of safety precautions; inadequate protective clothing; inadequate supervision; inattentiveness; smoking; unsafe environment

At-Risk Population

Individuals exposed to environmental temperature extremes

Associated Conditions

Alcoholic intoxication; drug intoxication; neuromuscular diseases; neuropathy; treatment regimen

NOC (Nursing Outcomes Classification)

Suggested NOC Outcomes

Safe Home Environment; Parenting: Early/Middle/Adolescent; Physical Safety

Client Outcomes

Client Will (Specify Time Frame)

- Be free of thermal injury to skin or tissue
- Explain actions can take to protect self and others from thermal injury

NIC (Nursing Interventions Classification)

Suggested NIC Intervention

Environmental Management: Safety

Example NIC Activities—Environmental Management: Safety

Identify safety hazards in the environment; Modify the environment to minimize hazards and risk

Nursing Interventions and *Rationales*

- Teach the following interventions to prevent fires in the home, to handle any possible fire, and to have a readily available exit from the home:
  - Avoid plugging several appliance cords into the same electrical socket.
  - Do not use open candles or allow smoking in the home.
  - Keep a fire extinguisher within reach in case a fire should occur.
  - Install smoke alarms on every level of the home and in every sleeping area.
  - Keep furniture and other heavy objects out of the way of doors and windows.
  - Develop a fire escape plan that includes two ways out of every room and an outside meeting place. Practice the escape plan at least twice a year.
- Teach clients about home fire safety to prevent thermal injury and prevention. EB: *The National Fire Protection Association (NFPA) has teaching materials and other information for this purpose (NFPA, 2021).*
- Apply sunscreen as directed on the container when out in the sun. Also use sun-blocking clothing, and stay in the shade if possible. EB: *Sunburn is a clear indicator of overexposure to ultraviolet (UV) radiation and increases the risk of skin cancer. The estimated prevalence of sunburn in the United States is high; 34% of a survey of 31,162 U.S. adults reported one or more sunburns in the past 12 months (Guerra, Urban, & Crane, 2021).*

T

- Teach clients safety measures to prevent fires in the home in which medical oxygen is in use:
  - **Never smoke** in a home in which medical oxygen is in use. "No smoking" signs should be posted inside and outside the home. EB: *There is considerable morbidity and mortality from burns secondary to smoking while using home oxygen. Ongoing education and careful consideration of prescribing home oxygen therapy for known smokers are highly encouraged (Fields, Whitney, & Bell, 2020).*
  - Do not wear oxygen near an ignition source (e.g., open flame, gas stove, fireplace, candles, cigarettes, matches, lighters) (Fields, Whitney, & Bell, 2020). Note that petroleum jelly, lip balm, skin lotion, or the like will **not** spontaneously combust in the presence of supplemental oxygen without an ignition source (e.g., flame or spark) and are safe to use on the face and in bed in the presence of oxygen (Winslow & Jacobsen, 1998).
  - Homes with medical oxygen must have working smoke alarms that are tested monthly (Fields, Whitney, & Bell, 2020).
  - Test fire extinguishers every 3 to 6 months. Keep a fire extinguisher within reach. If a fire occurs, turn off the oxygen, leave the home, and summon the fire department (NFPA, 2021).
  - Develop a fire escape plan that includes two ways out of every room and an outside meeting place. Practice the escape plan at least twice a year (NFPA, 2021).
- Be aware that thermal injury also includes injury from cold materials and environmental conditions, including freezing injury, nonfreezing injury, and hypothermia. EB: *Frostbite causes tissue destruction similar to burns; damage may not be evident for 10 to 15 days (Basit, Wallen, & Dudley, 2021).*
- Provide adequate environmental temperatures. Older clients and others at risk for temperature dysregulation can easily become hypothermic in air-conditioned environments (e.g., a surgical suite), with inadequate clothing, inhaling cold gases, or when exposed to room temperature or chilled fluids (e.g., intravenous, gastric lavage, bowel prep, continuous renal replacement therapy [CRRT], dialysis). EB: *Inadvertent hypothermia is a common and preventable condition in surgical procedures and can predispose to infection, blood loss, pressure injury, cardiac events, and shivering that increases metabolic demands, hospital days, and costs (Conway et al, 2019).*
- Be aware that fine motor coordination decreases as a very early sign of hypothermia. Preventing progression of thermal injury is critical to client outcomes. Shivering is the body's attempt to generate heat through muscle activity; it consumes considerable metabolic energy, and is a **late** sign of hypothermia.
- Monitor temperature in vulnerable clients. Core temperature is the best measure to assess for hypothermia. If a pulmonary artery catheter is not available, use a thermometer calibrated for lower body temperature such as a distal esophageal, rectal, temporal artery, or bladder temperature probe.
- Use active warming measures to help clients maintain body temperature (e.g., warming blankets, warmed fluids, forced warm air warming devices, foil wraps, radiant warmers) as indicated. Be aware that passive devices (e.g., clothing items or blankets) do not add heat to body tissues.
- Ensure that exposed skin is protected from cold:
  - From environment, with adequate clothing
  - From cold topical applications (e.g., ice packs or circulating cold water therapy systems), with padding
- Monitor for developing cold thermal injury by checking skin color, peripheral circulation, temperature, and sensation. Be aware that fine motor coordination decreases as a very early sign of hypothermia. Shivering, the body's attempt to generate heat through muscle activity, is a late sign of hypothermia.
- Check the temperature of all equipment and other materials before allowing them to contact client skin, especially if client has increased risk factors for thermal injury.

Pediatric

- Teach the following activities to clients with young children:
  - Lock up matches and lighters out of sight and reach.
  - Never leave a hot stove unattended.
  - Do not allow small children to use the microwave until they are at least 7 or 8 years of age.
  - Keep all portable heaters out of children's reach and at least 3 feet away from anything that can burn.
  - Teach fire prevention and safety to older children.
- Install thermostatic mixer valves in a hot water system to prevent extreme hot water causing scalding burns. EB: *Scald injuries from tap water >120°F (48.9°C) are common in urban pediatric emergency department clients (Bentivigna et al, 2020; NFPA, 2021).*

T

REFERENCES

Basit, H., Wallen, T. J., & Dudley, C. (2021). *Frostbite*. StatPearls [Internet]. Treasure Island, FL: StatPearls Publishing. https://doi.org/10.1016/j.ijnurstu.2019.04.017.

Bentivegna, K., McCollum, S., Wu, R., et al. (2020). A state-wide analysis of pediatric scald burns by tap water, 2016-2018. *Burns*, *46*(8), 1805–1812.

Conway, A., Gow, J., Ralph, N., et al. (2019). Implementing a thermal care bundle for inadvertent perioperative hypothermia: A cost-effectiveness analysis. *International Journal of Nursing Studies*, *97*, 21–27.

Fields, B. E., Whitney, R. L., & Bell, J. F. (2020). Home oxygen therapy. *American Journal of Nursing*, *120*(11), 51–57. https://doi.org/10.1097/01.NAJ.0000721940.02042.99.

Guerra, K. C., Urban, K., & Crane, J. S. (2021). *Sunburn*. StatPearls [Internet]. Treasure Island, FL: StatPearls Publishing. Retrieved from https://www.ncbi.nlm.nih.gov/books/NBK534837.

National Fire Protection Association (NFPA). (2021). *Public education* [multiple resources]. Retrieved from https://www.nfpa.org/Public-Education. Accessed July 30, 2021.

Winslow, E. H., & Jacobson, A. F. (1998). Dispelling the petroleum jelly myth. *American Journal of Nursing*, *98*(11), 16RR.

Ineffective Thermoregulation

Domain 11 Safety/protection Class 6 Thermoregulation

Rosemary Timmerman, DNP, APRN, CCNS, CCRN-CSC-CMC

NANDA-I

Definition

Temperature fluctuation between hypothermia and hyperthermia.

Defining Characteristics

Cyanotic nail beds; flushed skin; hypertension; increased body temperature above normal range; increased respiratory rate; mild shivering; moderate pallor; piloerection; reduction in body temperature below normal range; seizure; skin cool to touch; skin warm to touch; slow capillary refill; tachycardia

Related Factors

Dehydration; environmental temperature fluctuations; inactivity; inappropriate clothing for environmental temperature; increased oxygen demand; vigorous activity

At-Risk Population

Individuals at extremes of weight; individuals exposed to environmental temperature extremes; individuals with inadequate supply of subcutaneous fat; individuals with increased body surface area to weight ratio

Associated Conditions

Altered metabolic rate; brain injury; condition affecting temperature regulation; decreased sweat response; impaired health status; inefficient nonshivering thermogenesis; pharmaceutical preparations; sedation; sepsis; trauma

NOC (Nursing Outcomes Classification)

T

Suggested NOC Outcomes

Thermoregulation; Thermoregulation: Newborn

Example NOC Outcome with Indicators

Thermoregulation as evidenced by the following indicators: Body temperature/Skin temperature/Skin color changes/Hydration/Reported thermal comfort. (Rate the outcome and indicators of **Thermoregulation:** 1 = severely compromised, 2 = substantially compromised, 3 = moderately compromised, 4 = mildly compromised, 5 = not compromised [see Section I].)

Client Outcomes

Client Will (Specify Time Frame)

- Maintain temperature within normal range
- Explain measures needed to maintain normal temperature

- Describe two to four symptoms of hypothermia or hyperthermia
- List two or three self-care measures to treat hypothermia or hyperthermia

NIC (Nursing Interventions Classification)

Suggested NIC Interventions

Temperature Regulation; Temperature Regulation: Inoperative

Example NIC Activities—Temperature Regulation

Institute use of a continuous core temperature-monitoring device, as appropriate; Promote adequate fluid and nutritional intake

Nursing Interventions and *Rationales*

Temperature Measurement

- Measure and record the client's temperature using a consistent method of temperature measurement every 1 to 4 hours depending on the severity of the situation or whenever a change in condition occurs (e.g., chills, change in mental status). **CEB:** *Errors in accurate temperature measurement are most often associated with instrument-related errors, choice of temperature site chosen for monitoring, and operator error (Makic et al, 2011).* **CEB:** *A consistent mode of temperature measurement for accurate trending of body temperature is important for accurate treatment decisions; if different devices are used to obtain temperature measurements, the results should not vary more than 0.3°C to 0.5°C (Makic et al, 2011).*
- Select core, near core, or peripheral temperature monitoring mode based on ability to obtain an accurate temperature from that site and clinical situation, dictating the need for mode of temperature monitoring required for clinical treatment decisions. **CEB/EB:** *Core temperature is obtained by pulmonary artery catheter and distal esophagus; near core temperature measurements include oral, bladder, rectal, tympanic membrane, and temporal artery; and peripheral measurements are obtained by skin surface measurements such as measurement in the axilla (Niven et al, 2015; Chen, 2019).*
- Caution should be taken in interpreting extreme values of temperature (less than 35°C [95°F] or greater than 39°C [102.2°F]) from a near core temperature site device. **CEB:** *Accurate oral temperature measurement requires the probe to be placed in the posterior sublingual pocket to provide a reliable near core temperature measurement (Makic et al, 2011).* **EBP:** *Research has demonstrated that the accuracy of temperature measurement from most accurate to least accurate are intravascular (pulmonary artery), distal esophageal, bladder thermistor, rectal, and oral (Niven & Laupland, 2016); axillary temperature is accurate in neonates but is not well supported in adults (Cheshire, 2016; Barbi et al, 2017).* **EB/EBN:** *Tympanic membrane and temporal artery measurements and chemical dot thermometers are least accurate and should be avoided in caring for the acutely ill adult client. Evidence is limited in testing the accuracy of temperature measurement devices outside of normal temperature ranges (Bijur, Shah, & Esses, 2016; Kiekkas et al, 2016).*
- Evaluate the significance of a decreased or increased temperature. **EB:** *Normal adult temperature is usually identified as 98.6°F (37°C), but in actuality the normal temperature fluctuates by up to 1°C; disease, injury, or pharmacological agents may cause an adaptive increase in the hypothalamic set point resulting in fever (Niven & Laupland, 2016; Chen, 2019).*

▲ Notify the health care provider of temperature according to institutional standards or written orders, or when temperature reaches 100.5°F (38.3°C) and above; use a lower threshold for immunocompromised clients who will be less likely to exhibit a fever when seriously ill (Niven & Laupland, 2016). Also notify the health care provider of the presence of a change in mental status and temperature greater than 100.5°F (38.3°C) or less than 96.8°F (36°C). **EB:** *A change in mental status may indicate the onset of septic shock (Rhodes et al, 2017).*

Fever (Pyrexia)

- Recognize that fever is characterized as a temporary elevation in internal body temperature 1°C to 2°C higher than the client's normal body temperature. **EB:** *A rise in body temperature is an innate immune response to a perceived threat and is regulated by the hypothalamus. Hyperthermia may occur when a client gains heat through either an increase in the body's heat production or is unable to effectively dissipate heat,* *and hypothermia occurs when a client loses heat or cannot generate heat (Niven & Laupland, 2016; Walter et al, 2016).*

- Recognize that fever is a normal physiological response to a perceived threat by the body, frequently in response to an infection. **EB:** *Fever is a deliberate, active thermoregulatory defense action by the body; metabolic heat accelerates the body's antibody production to defend the body and assists the body's cellular repair processes (nursing care should focus on supporting the body's normal physiological response [fever], locating the cause for the fever, and providing comfort) (Niven & Laupland, 2016; Chiappini et al, 2017).*
- ▲ Review client history, including current medical diagnosis, medications, recent procedures/interventions, recent travel, environmental exposure to infectious agents, recent blood product administration, and review of laboratory analysis for cause of ineffective thermoregulation. **EB:** *Changes in body temperature (fever) should be explored for possible problems associated with a client's health status (Barbi et al, 2017; Niven & Laupland, 2016).*
- Recognize that fever may be low grade (96.8°F–100.4°F [36°C–38°C]) in response to an inflammatory process such as infection, allergy, trauma, illness, or surgery; moderate to high-grade fever (100.4°F–104°F [38°C–40°C]) indicates a more concerted inflammatory response from a systemic infection; hyperpyrexia (40°C and higher) occurs as a result of damage of the hypothalamus, bacteremia, or an extremely overheated room (Niven & Laupland, 2016; Walter et al, 2016). **EB:** *Interventions to treat fever focus on client comfort, allowing the body to progress through the natural course of fever; exceptions may exist for the client with hyperpyrexia or when oxygen consumption threatens to exhaust metabolic reserves (Chiappini et al, 2017; Young et al, 2019).*
- ▲ Monitor and intervene to provide comfort during a fever by
  - Obtaining vital signs and accurate intake and output
  - Checking laboratory analysis trends of white blood cell counts and other markers of infection
  - Providing blankets when the client complains of being cold but removing surplus of blankets when the client is too warm
  - Encouraging fluid and nutrition
  - Limiting activity to conserve energy
  - Providing frequent oral care
  - Adjusting room temperature for client comfort

  EBN/EB: *Current evidence that examined the evidence of antipyretic therapies used to treat fever, such as administration of antipyretic medications, cooling blankets, and sponge baths, found that these therapies did not reduce the duration of illness or the mortality rate (Chiappini et al, 2017; Young et al, 2019).*

Hypothermia

- Take vital signs frequently, noting changes associated with hypothermia, such as increased blood pressure, pulse, and respirations, that then advance to decreased values as hypothermia progresses. **EB:** *Mild hypothermia activates the sympathetic nervous system, which can increase the levels of vital signs; as hypothermia progresses, the heart becomes suppressed, with decreased cardiac output, heart rate, blood pressure, and respiratory rate (Paal et al, 2016; Zafren, 2017).*
- Monitor the client for signs of hypothermia (e.g., shivering, cool skin, piloerection, pallor, slow capillary refill, cyanotic nail beds, decreased mentation, dysrhythmias) (Paal et al, 2016; Zafren, 2017).
- See the care plan for **Hypothermia** as appropriate.

Hyperthermia

- Recognize that hyperthermia is a different etiology than fever, so the cause of the elevated body temperature should be explored for definitive treatment. **EB:** *Hyperthermia is a condition in which an environmental (e.g., heat stroke), pharmacological (malignant hyperthermia), or endocrine (e.g., thyrotoxicosis) stimulus results in an increase in body temperature without a corresponding increase in the hypothalamic set point (Niven & Laupland, 2016; Lipman et al, 2019).*
- Note changes in vital signs associated with hyperthermia, such as rapid, bounding pulse; increased respiratory rate; and decreased blood pressure, accompanied by orthostatic hypotension; and signs and symptoms of dehydration (Niven & Laupland, 2016; Gaudio & Grissom, 2016). **EB:** *Consistent monitoring promotes prevention and early intervention in clients with altered cardiopulmonary status associated with hyperthermia (Gaudio & Grissom, 2016; Lipman et al, 2019).*

- Monitor the client for signs of hyperthermia (e.g., headache, nausea and vomiting, weakness, extreme fatigue, delirium, coma). EB: *Monitoring for the defining characteristics of hyperthermia allows for early intervention (Cheshire, 2016).*
- Adjust clothing to facilitate passive warming or cooling as appropriate.
- See the care plan for **Hyperthermia** as appropriate.

Pediatric

- For routine measurement of temperature, use an electronic thermometer in the axilla in infants younger than 4 weeks; for a child up to 5 years of age, use an electronic thermometer in the axilla or an infrared temporal artery thermometer. EB: *Oral and rectal routes should not be used routinely to measure the temperature of infants to children of 5 years of age (Barbi et al, 2017; National Institute for Health and Clinical Excellence [NICE], 2019). Tympanic thermometers often provide inaccurate temperature from incorrect placement in the ear canal and presence of cerumen adversely affecting temperature reading (Niven et al, 2015; Oguz et al, 2018).*
- Recognize that pediatric clients have a decreased ability to adapt to temperature extremes. Take the following actions to maintain body temperature in the infant/child:
  - Keep the head covered.
  - Use blankets to keep the client warm.
  - Keep the client covered during procedures, transport, and diagnostic testing.
  - Keep the room temperature at 72°F (22.2°C).

  EB: The combination of a relatively smaller body surface area, smaller body fluid volume, less well-developed temperature control mechanisms, and smaller amount of protective body fat limits the ability of the infant and child to maintain normal temperatures (NICE, 2019).
- Recognize that the infant and small child are both vulnerable to developing heat stroke in hot weather; ensure that they receive sufficient fluids and are protected from hot environments. EB: *Infants and young children are at risk for heat stroke for many reasons, including a decreased thermoregulatory ability in the young body and the inability to obtain their own fluids (Leon & Bouchama, 2015).*
- Antipyretic treatments typically are not indicated unless the child's temperature is higher than 38.3°C [100.4°F] and may be given to provide comfort. EB: *The use of antipyretics in febrile children should be examined in light of the therapeutic goal for treatment, which may be primarily to improve the child's discomfort; acetaminophen and ibuprofen are the only antipyretic medications recommended for pediatric clients; both agents should not be administered simultaneously because of concern for inaccurate dosing; alternating doses may be considered only if client distress is not relieved before the next dose is due (Chiappini et al, 2017; NICE, 2019).*

Geriatric

- Do not allow an older client to become chilled; keep the client covered when giving a bath and offer socks to wear in bed; be aware of factors such as room temperature (heating/air conditioning), clothing (layered/loose), and fluid intake. EB: *Older adults have a decreased ability to adapt to temperature extremes and need protection from extreme environmental temperatures; the response to cold environment is also compromised with the cutaneous vasoconstrictor response, the shivering process being less effective, decreased ability to feel cold, and medications commonly used to treat chronic age-associated diseases (Jain et al, 2018; Leyk et al, 2019).*
- Recognize that the older client may have an infection without a significant rise in body temperature. EB: *Febrile response to infection was found to be reduced with increasing age, and baseline temperatures were generally lower in older clients; therefore this blunted febrile response may lead to delayed diagnosis and treatment necessitating review of all data, including a change in temperature, rather than fever (Limpawattana et al, 2016).*
- Fever from infection in older adults does not confer a higher mortality risk; thus, fever should not be treated with antipyretic agents or other cooling methods unless the client is demonstrating limited cardiorespiratory reserves (Young et al, 2019).
- Ensure that older clients receive sufficient fluids during hot days and stay out of the sun. EB: *Older adults may have trouble walking independently to obtain fluids, have decreased thirst sensation, and have chronic illnesses that predispose them to heat stroke, which is a hyperthermic condition (Leon & Bouchama, 2015).*
- Assess the medication profile for the potential risk of drug-related altered body temperature. EB: *Anesthetics, barbiturates, salicylates, nonsteroidal antiinflammatory drugs, diuretics, antihistamines, anticholinergics,*

T

beta-blockers, and thyroid hormones have been linked to decreased body temperature (American Geriatrics Society, 2019).

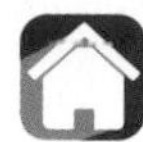

Home Care

Treating Fever

- ● Instruct client/parents on the physiological benefits of fever and provide interventions to treat fever symptoms, avoiding antipyretic agents and external cooling interventions.
- ● Ensure that client/parents know when to contact a health care provider for fever-related concerns.

Client/Family Teaching and Discharge Planning

- ● Teach the client and family the signs of fever, hypothermia, and hyperthermia and appropriate actions to take if either condition develops.
- ● Teach the client and family an age-appropriate method for taking the temperature.
- ● Teach the client to avoid alcohol and medications that depress cerebral function. **EB:** *When the client is sedated or under the influence of alcohol, mentation is depressed, which results in decreased activities to maintain an adequate body temperature (Cheshire, 2016).*

REFERENCES

American Geriatrics Society Beers Criteria® Update Expert Panel. (2019). American Geriatrics Society 2019 Updated AGS Beers Criteria® for potentially inappropriate medication Use in older adults. *Journal of the American Geriatrics Society*, *67*(4), 674–694. https://doi.org/10.1111/jgs.15767.

Barbi, E., Marzuillo, P., Neri, E., Naviglio, S., & Krauss, B. S. (2017). Fever in children: Pearls and pitfalls. *Children*, *4*(9), 81. https://doi.org/10.3390/children4090081.

Bijur, P. E., Shah, P. D., & Esses, D. (2016). Temperature measurement in the adult emergency department: Oral tympanic membrane and temporal artery temperatures versus rectal temperature. *Emergency Medicine Journal*, *33*(12), 843–847. doi:10.1136/emermed-2015-205122.

Chen, W. (2019). Thermometry and interpretation of body temperature. *Biomedical Engineering Letters*, *9*(1), 3–17. https://doi.org/10.1007/s13534-019-00102-2.

Cheshire, W. P., Jr. (2016). Thermoregulatory disorders and illness related to heat and cold stress. *Autonomic Neuroscience: Basic & Clinical*, *196*, 91–104. https://doi.org/10.1016/j.autneu.2016.01.001.

Chiappini, E., Bortone, B., Galli, L., & de Martino, M. (2017). Guidelines for the symptomatic management of fever in children: Systematic review of the literature and quality appraisal with AGREE II. *BMJ Open*, *7*(7), e015404. https://doi.org/10.1136/bmjopen-2016-015404.

Gaudio, F. G., & Grissom, C. K. (2016). Cooling methods in heat stroke. *Journal of Emergency Medicine*, *50*(4), 607–616. doi:10.1016/j.jemermed.2015.09.014.

Jain, Y., Srivatsan, R., Kollannur, A., & Zachariah, A. (2018). Heatstroke: Causes, consequences and clinical guidelines. *The National Medical Journal of India*, *31*(4), 224–227. https://doi.org/10.4103/0970-258X.258224.

Kiekkas, P., Stefanopoulos, N., Bakalis, N., Kefaliakos, A., & Karanikolas, M. (2016). Agreement of infrared temporal artery thermometry with other thermometry methods in adults: A systematic review. *Journal of Clinical Nursing*, *25*(7–8), 894–905. doi:10.1111/jocn.13117.

Leon, L. R., & Bouchama, A. (2015). Heat stroke. *Comprehensive Physiology*, *5*, 611–647. doi:10.1002/cphy.c140017.

Leyk, D., Hoitz, J., Becker, C., Glitz, K. J., Nestler, K., & Piekarski, C. (2019). Health risks and interventions in exertional heat stress. *Deutsches Arzteblatt International*, *116*(31–32), 537–544. https://doi.org/10.3238/arztebl.2019.0537.

Limpawattana, P., Phungoen, P., Mitsungnern, T., Laosuangkoon, W., & Tansangworn, N. (2016). Atypical presentations of older adults at the emergency department and associated factors. *Archives of Gerontology and Geriatrics*, *62*, 97–102. https://doi.org/10.1016/j.archger.2015.08.016.

Lipman, G. S., Gaudio, F. G., Eifling, K. P., Ellis, M. A., Otten, E. M., & Grissom, C. K. (2019). Wilderness medical Society clinical practice guidelines for the prevention and treatment of heat illness: 2019 update. *Wilderness and Environmental Medicine*, *30*(4S), S33–S46. https://doi.org/10.1016/j.wem.2018.10.004.

Makic, M. B. F., VonRueden, K. T., Rauen, C. A., & Chadwick, J. (2011). Evidence-based practice habits: Putting more sacred cows out to pasture. *Critical Care Nurse*, *31*(2), 38–62. doi:10.4037/ccn2011908.

National Institute for Health and Clinical Excellence (NICE). (2019). *Fever in under 5s: Assessment and initial management*. NICE guideline NG143. Retrieved from https://www.nice.org.uk/guidance/ng143. [Accessed 30 July 2021].

Niven, D. J., Gaudet, J. E., Laupland, K. B., Mrklas, K. J., Roberts, D. J., & Stelfox, H. T. (2015). Accuracy of peripheral thermometers for estimating temperature: A systematic review and meta-analysis. *Annals of Internal Medicine*, *163*(10), 768–777. doi:10.7326/M15-1150.

Niven, D. J., & Laupland, K. B. (2016). Pyrexia: Aetiology in the ICU. *Critical Care*, *20*(1), 247. doi:10.1186/s13054-016-1406-2.

Oguz, F., Yildiz, I., Varkal, M. A., et al. (2018). Axillary and tympanic temperature measurement in children and normal values for ages. *Pediatric Emergency Care*, *34*(3), 169–173. https://doi.org/10.1097/PEC.0000000000000693.

Paal, P., Gordon, L., Strapazzon, G., et al. (2016). Accidental hypothermia—An update. *Scandinavian Journal of Trauma, Resuscitation and Emergency Medicine*, *24*(1), 111. doi:10.1186/s13049-016-0303-7.

Rhodes, A., Evans, L., Alhazzani, W., et al. (2017). Surviving sepsis campaign: International guidelines for management of sepsis and septic shock: 2016. *Critical Care Medicine*, *45*(3), 486–552. doi:10.1097/CCM.0000000000002255.

Walter, E. J., Hanna-Jumma, S., Carraretto, M., & Forni, L. (2016). The pathophysiological basis and consequences of fever. *Critical Care*, *20*(1), 200. https://doi.org/10.1186/s13054-016-1375-5.

Young, P. J., Bellomo, R., Bernard, G. R., et al. (2019). Fever control in critically ill adults. An individual patient data meta-analysis of randomised controlled trials. *Intensive Care Medicine*, *45*(4), 468–476. https://doi.org/10.1007/s00134-019-05553-w.

Zafren, K. (2017). Out-of-hospital evaluation and treatment of accidental hypothermia. *Emergency Medicine Clinics of North America*, *35*(2), 261–279. doi:10.1016/j.emc.2017.01.003.

Risk for Ineffective Thermoregulation Domain 11 Safety/protection Class 6 Thermoregulation

Mary Beth Flynn Makic, PhD, RN, CCNS, CCRN-K, FAAN, FNAP, FCNS

NANDA-I

Definition

Susceptible to temperature fluctuation between hypothermia and hyperthermia, which may compromise health.

Risk Factors

Dehydration; environmental temperature fluctuations; inactivity; inappropriate clothing for environmental temperature; increased oxygen demand; vigorous activity

At-Risk Population

Individuals at extremes of weight; individuals exposed to environmental temperature extremes; individuals with inadequate supply of subcutaneous fat; individuals with increased body surface area to weight ratio

Associated Conditions

Altered metabolic rate; brain injuries; condition affecting temperature regulation; decreased sweat response; impaired health status; inefficient nonshivering thermogenesis; pharmaceutical preparations; sedation; sepsis; trauma

NOC, NIC, Client Outcomes, Nursing Interventions and *Rationales,* Client/Family Teaching and Discharge Planning, and References

Refer to care plans for Ineffective **Thermoregulation, Hyperthermia,** or **Hypothermia.**

Risk for Thrombosis Domain 4 Activity/rest Class 4 Cardiovascular/pulmonary responses

Dina M. Hewett, PhD, RN, NEA-BC, CCRN-A

NANDA-I

Definition

Susceptible to obstruction of a blood vessel by a thrombus that can break off and lodge in another vessel, which may compromise health.

Risk Factors

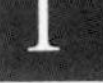

Atherogenic diet; dehydration; excessive stress; impaired physical mobility; inadequate knowledge of modifiable factors; ineffective management of preventive measures; ineffective medication self-management; obesity; sedentary lifestyle; smoking

At-Risk Population

Economically disadvantaged individuals; individuals aged ≥ 60 years; individuals with family history of thrombotic disease; individuals with history of thrombotic disease; pregnant women; women < 6 weeks postpartum

Associated Conditions

Atherosclerosis; autoimmune diseases; blood coagulation disorders; chronic inflammation; critical illness; diabetes mellitus; dyslipidemias; endovascular procedures; heart diseases; hematologic diseases; high acuity illness; hormonal therapy; hyperhomocysteinemia; infections; kidney diseases; medical devices; metabolic syndrome; neoplasms; surgical procedures; trauma; vascular diseases

NOC (Nursing Outcomes Classification)

Suggested NOC Outcomes

Tissue Perfusion: Peripheral; Tissue Perfusion: Pulmonary Risk Control: Dehydration; Hydration; Knowledge Thrombus Threat Reduction; Risk Control: Thrombus

Example NOC Outcome with Indicators

Risk Control: Thrombus as evidenced by the following indicators: Seeks current information about embolus prevention/Identifies risk factors for thrombus formation/Monitors for warning signs and symptoms of thrombus formation or embolus. (Rate outcome and indicators of **Risk Control: Thrombus:** 1 = never demonstrated, 2 = rarely demonstrated, 3 = sometimes demonstrated, 4 = often demonstrated, 5 = consistently demonstrated [see Section I].)

Client Outcomes

Client Will (Specify Time Frame)

- Not develop a thromboembolism during hospitalization
- State the relevant risk factors associated with the development of a thrombosis
- Engage in behaviors or lifestyle changes to reduce risk of developing a thrombosis

NIC (Nursing Interventions Classification)

Suggested NIC Interventions

Embolus Precautions; Embolus Care: Peripheral; Embolus Care: Pulmonary; Lower Extremity Monitoring

Example NIC Activities

Obtain a history of the client's present illness and medical history to evaluate the risk of thrombosis and implement preventative interventions

Nursing Interventions and *Rationales*

- It is estimated that 40% of clients with a deep vein thrombosis (DVT) will progress to postthrombotic syndrome (PTS); therefore, prevention of DVT is a key component. EB: *PTS is a chronic disorder characterized by pain, swelling, redness (erythema), and ulcerations. The degree will vary from client to client. Individuals with recurrent ipsilateral DVT are considered the highest risk for PTS (Kvamme & Costanzo, 2015; Lenchus et al, 2017).*
- Assess client's risk factors to develop venous thromboembolism (VTE). EB: *There are several factors that may predispose a client to VTE. According to Bruni-Fitzgerald (2015), the strongest risk factors include the following:*
  - Venous stasis as a result of dehydration, immobility, heart failure, or venous compressions from a tumor
  - Hypercoagulable states from disease, obesity, and trauma
  - Immobilization from prolonged bed rest or limb casting
  - Surgery and trauma, especially hip, pelvic, and spinal surgery and leg amputation; several burns also predispose clients to DVT
  - Pregnancy results in a hypercoagulable state placing these clients at risk; although fatal events are rare
  - Oral contraceptives and estrogen replacement may place clients at risk, which is proportional to the estrogen content; postmenopausal women on hormone replacement therapy are considered at risk
  - In malignancy cases 17% of clients with VTE have a neoplasm with the most frequent occurrence in clients with pancreatic cancer
- Use a VTE risk assessment tool to determine individual susceptibility to thrombosis. EB: *Determining a client's risk may be guided through the use of an assessment tool such as the Wells Criteria or the Caprini Risk Assessment Model. Assessment tools in the acute care setting are developed based on evidence-based research (Modi et al, 2016). The Wells Criteria was initially developed to assess an individual's risk for VTE in the*

T

outpatient setting. Recently, the Center for Evidence-Based Imaging (CEPI) scoring system was developed to more accurately predict the risk for the inpatient setting (Parks & Kohlwes, 2018).

- ▲ Implement evidence-based prevention methods, both chemical (pharmacological) and/or mechanical. EB: *The nurse must be proactive in the assessment of the client for risks for VTE and implementing prophylactic measures as prescribed (Adams, 2015).*
- ▲ Chemical thromboprophylaxis should be anticipated in the postoperative care of critically ill clients. EB: *Research has shown that chemical thromboprophylaxis, when initiated in critically ill and postoperative clients, such as anticoagulants, is not associated with clinically significant bleeding (Bartholomew, 2017). Evidence-based practice guidelines support the use of chemical and mechanical prophylaxis interventions for clients undergoing orthopedic surgery for a minimum of 14 to 35 days to reduce VTE risk (Falck-Ytter et al, 2012).*
- ● Implement mechanical prophylaxis through use of intermittent pneumatic compression (IPC) devices (Ho & Harahsheh, 2016). EB: *IPC is demonstrated to be more effective than no IPC at reducing DVT and is essential when pharmacological therapy is contraindicated because of an increased risk of bleeding (Dunn & Ramos, 2017). IPC devices reduce the risk of venous stasis by increasing the velocity of venous outflow and promoting the emptying of valvular cusps (Muñoz-Figueroa & Ojo, 2015).*
- ● Ensure proper fit and application of the device. EB: *Use a measuring tape to obtain accurate measurements and follow the manufacturer's recommendations for correct sizing. Two fingers should be easily placed between the client's leg and the sleeve. Monitor for edema and resize as needed. (Bartholomew, 2017; Link, 2018).*
- ● Implement progressive mobility and early ambulation as the client tolerates to reduce risk of VTE. EB: *Studies indicate that early mobility may reduce client deconditioning and VTE complications (Booth et al, 2016). One study conducted in a trauma critical care unit revealed a statistically significant (p = .0004) reduced rate of DVT in clients in whom early mobility and ambulation were implemented (Booth et al, 2016). A retrospective study by Cao (2021) confirmed the increased risk of DVT with prolonged bed rest. Clients with additional risk factors of age and smoking had an accumulative increased risk of developing a DVT.*
- ● Provide education to the client and family about the importance of continued use of IPC after the client is ambulatory. Ensure that IPC is reapplied after ambulation (Hanison & Corbett, 2016; Dunn & Ramos, 2017). EB: *IPC should be reapplied after the client ambulates and returns to bed to maintain prevention interventions for VTE (Bartholomew, 2017; Dunn & Ramos, 2017).*
- ● Perform a skin inspection during bathing. EB: *It is important to assess the skin with each application of the IPC and during the bath for signs of skin irritation or breakdown from the device. (Bartholomew, 2017; Dunn & Ramos, 2017).*
- ● IPC should be applied even when the client is sitting in a chair (Dunn & Ramos, 2017).
- ● Provide appropriate education or referral to a smoking cessation program. Smoking is a well-established risk factor for atherosclerotic disease that increases the client's risk for VTE (McLendon et al, 2021). CEB: *A systematic review and meta-analysis found that smoking increased the risk of VTE and the risk increased by 10.2% for every additional 10 cigarettes smoked per day or by 6.1% for every additional 10 pack-years of smoking. The study also found that smokers who were overweight had a higher risk of VTE (Cheng et al, 2013).*
- ● Obesity is an independent risk for VTE. EB: *A study found a higher incidence of VTE in clients with body mass index (BMI) ≥30 kg/m² (Peters et al, 2016). A systematic review of bariatric surgery clients found that male gender, increased BMI, smoking history, and operative procedure and time were risk factors for VTE (Bartlett, Mauck, & Daniels, 2015). Chemical and mechanical preventive interventions should be implemented to reduce the risk of VTE in the bariatric client population (Bartlett, Mauck, & Daniels, 2015).*
- ● Clients with cancer are at an increased risk of developing DVT mainly because of the release of certain chemicals from the tumor and spread of the tumor into blood vessels. Generally, bloodstream cancers such as leukemia carry the highest risk for development of DVT, followed by solid tumors of the pancreas, stomach, lungs, ovaries, uterus, bladder, and brain (Udoh, 2016).

T

Pediatric

- ● The nurse should be alert to certain diagnoses that increase the pediatric client's risk for VTE. EB: *Diagnoses associated with increased risk of VTE include mechanical ventilation, pulmonary hypertension, burns, lower extremity or pelvic fracture, spinal cord injury, surgical packing of the abdomen, sepsis, acute infection, oncological malignant growth, surgery/trauma, cardiac disease, obesity, chronic or active inflammatory disease, and immobility (Simmons, 2017).*
- ● The most frequent diagnosis associated with VTE in the pediatric population is trauma (Yen et al, 2016).

- Incidence of VTE in children is low; however, the rate of VTE in hospitalized children is much higher (Austin, Jenkins, & Hines, 2017).
- Risk factors for pediatric development of VTE include use of central venous access devices (Simmons, 2017). **EB:** *A study by Austin, Jenkins, and Hines (2017) found that pediatric clients are at risk of a catheter-associated DVT because of the size of the device and resulting damage to the fragile intima, leading to clot formation and dislodgement of the clot.*
- Neonatal and adolescent age groups are at higher risk for VTE compared with other pediatric age groups (Monagle et al, 2012). Additional studies are needed to further understand the risks and interventions for this population.

Geriatric

- The risk of VTE increases with age, increasing 90% between the ages of 15 and 80. **EB:** *Many of the risk factors for VTE are commonly seen in the older client with heart failure, chronic obstructive pulmonary disease, and malignancy. VTE is also seen in clients on bed rest and those with implantable devices such as pacemakers and hip/knee replacements (Bruni-Fitzgerald, 2015).*
- It is well established that older clients are at a greater risk of developing atrial fibrillation (Heeringa et al, 2006). **EB:** *The Framingham study indicated increasing risk of developing atrial fibrillation with increasing age (Wolf, Abbott, & Kannel, 1991). Treatment for chronic atrial fibrillation requires the use of anticoagulants to reduce the risk of an embolic event.*

Home Care

- Provide client education on the importance of continued use of compression stockings as directed. **EB:** *Ensuring the client is aware of the benefit of compression stockings reduces the risk of VTE and may facilitate compliance in wearing the compression stocking. The client may only be required to wear stockings during the day and be allowed to remove them at night (Kaur et al, 2016; Pai & Douketis, 2020).*
- Provide education to the client and/or family caregiver about the continued use of anticoagulant pharmacological therapy as directed. The client and/or family caregiver may need instruction on proper injection technique if the client is not discharged on an oral anticoagulant. **EB:** *If the client is discharged home on subcutaneous low-molecular-weight heparin or fondaparinux, the nurse needs to teach the client and/or family caregiver how to properly administer the medication by injection (Pai & Douketis, 2020; Bartholomew, 2017).*
- Clients who take the anticoagulant warfarin should have dietary education. Warfarin's effects may be decreased with a diet rich in vitamin K. **EB:** *Food containing vitamin K includes dark green leafy vegetables such as kale, Brussels sprouts, collard greens, and spinach. Avoid eating large quantities of these vegetables. Cranberry juice and alcohol should be avoided because they enhance the effects of warfarin and may lead to bleeding. (Pai & Douketis, 2020)*
- The newer anticoagulants, such as rivaroxaban, apixaban, and edoxaban, do not have the same medication–food interactions as warfarin.

REFERENCES

Adams, A. (2015). Proactivity in VTE prevention: A concept analysis. *British Journal of Nursing, 24*(1), 20–25. https://doi.org/10.12968/bjon.2015.24.1.20.

Austin, P., Jenkins, S., & Hines, A. (2017). Thromboembolic events in PICU: A descriptive study. *Pediatric Nursing, 43*(3), 132–137.

Bartholomew, J. R. (2017). Update on the management of venous thromboembolism. *Cleveland Clinic Journal of Medicine, 84*(12 Suppl. 3), 39–46. https://doi.org/10.3949/ccjm.84.s3.04.

Bartlett, M. A., Mauck, K. F., & Daniels, D. R. (2015). Prevention of venous thromboembolism in patients undergoing bariatric surgery. *Vascular Health and Risk Management, 11*, 461–477.

Booth, K., Rivet, J., Flici, R., et al. (2016). Progressive mobility protocol reduces venous thromboembolism rate in trauma intensive care patients: A quality improvement project. *Journal of Trauma Nursing, 23*(5), 284–289. https://doi.org/10.1097/JTN.0000000000000234.

Bruni-Fitzgerald, K. R. (2015). Venous thromboembolism: An overview. *Journal of Vascular Nursing, 33*(3), 95–99.

Cao, J., Li, S., Ma, Y., et al. (2021). Risk factors associated with deep venous thrombosis in patients with different bed-rest durations: A multi-institutional case-control study. *International Journal of Nursing Studies, 114*, 103825. https://doi.org/10.1016/j.ijnurstu.2020.103825.

Cheng, Y. J., Liu, H. O., Yao, F. J., et al. (2013). Current and former smoking and risk for venous thromboembolism: A systematic review and meta-analysis. *PLoS Medicine, 10*(9), e1001515. doi:10.1371/journal.pmed.1001515.

Dunn, N., & Ramos, R. (2017). Preventing venous thromboembolism: The role of nursing with intermittent pneumatic compression. *American Journal of Critical Care, 26*(2), 164–167. https://doi.org/10.4037/ajcc2017504.

Falck-Ytter, Y., Francis, C. W., Johanson, N. A., et al. (2012). Prevention of VTE in orthopedic surgery patients antithrombotic therapy and prevention of thrombosis, 9th ed: American College of Chest Physicians Evidence-Based Clinical Practice Guidelines. *Chest, 141*(Suppl. 2), e278S–e325S.

Hanison, E., & Corbett, K. (2016). Non-pharmacological interventions for the prevention of venous thromboembolism: A literature review. *Nursing Standard, 31*(8), 48–57.

Heeringa, J., van der Kuip, D. A. M., Hofman, A., et al. (2006). Prevalence, incidence and lifetime risk of atrial fibrillation: The Rotterdam study. *European Heart Journal, 27*(8), 949–953. https://doi.org/10.1093/eurheartj/ehi825.

Ho, K. M., & Harahsheh, Y. (2016). Intermittent pneumatic compression is effective in reducing proximal DVT. *Evidence-Based Nursing, 19*(2), 47.

Kaur, R., Saagi, M. K., & Choudhary, R. (2016). Evaluate the effectiveness of structured teaching program on knowledge regarding prevention and management of deep vein thrombosis (DVT) in patients among nursing staffs. *International Journal of Nursing Education, 8*(1), 127–131. https://doi.org/10.5958/0974-9357.2016.00022.2.

Kvamme, A. M., & Costanzo, C. (2015). Preventing progression of post-thrombotic syndrome for patients post-deep vein thrombosis. *Medsurg Nursing, 24*(1), 27–34.

Lenchus, J. D., Biehl, M., Cabrera, J., Gallo de Moraes, A., & Dezfulian, C. (2017). In-hospital management and follow-up treatment of venous thromboembolism: Focus on new and emerging treatments. *Journal of Intensive Care Medicine, 32*(5), 299–311. https://doi.org/10.1177/0885066616648265.

Link, T. (2018). Guideline implementation: prevention of venous thromboembolism: 1.6. *AORN Journal, 107*(6), 737–748. https://doi.org/10.1002/aorn.12146.

McLendon, K., Goyal, A., Bansal, P., & Attia, M. (2021). *Deep venous thrombosis risk factors*. StatPearls [Internet]. Treasure Island, FL: StatPearls Publishing. Retrieved from https://www.ncbi.nlm.nih.gov/books/NBK470215/. Accessed February 24, 2022.

Modi, S., Deisler, R., Gozel, K., et al. (2016). Wells criteria for DVT is a reliable clinical tool to assess the risk of deep vein thrombosis in trauma patients. *World Journal of Emergency Surgery, 11*, 24. https://doi.org/10.1186/s13017-016-007801.

Monagle, P., Chan, A., Goldenberg, N. A., Ichord, R. N., Journeycake, J. M., Nowak-Göttl, U., & Vesely, S. K. (2012). Antithrombotic therapy in neonates and children: Antithrombotic therapy and prevention of thrombosis, 9th ed. American College of Chest Physicians Evidence-Based clinical practice guidelines. *Chest, 141*(Suppl. 2), e737S–e801S. https://doi.org/10.1378/chest.11-2308.

Muñoz-Figueroa, G. P., & Ojo, O. (2015). Venous thromboembolism: Use of graduated compression stockings. *British Journal of Nursing, 24*(13), 680–685.

Pai, M., & Douketis, J. D. (2020). Patient education: Deep vein thrombosis (DVT) (beyond the basics). L. L. K. Leung, & G. Finlay (Eds.). Waltham, MA: UpToDate. Retrieved from https://www.uptodate.com/contents/deep-vein-thrombosis-dvt-beyond-the-basics. Accessed August 2, 2021.

Parks, A. L., & Kohlwes, R. J. (2018). Refining risk for deep vein thrombosis in hospitalized patients. *Journal of General Internal Medicine, 33*(1), 6. doi:10.1007/s11606-017-4194-8.

Peters, B. J., Dierkhising, R. A., & Mara, K. C. (2016). Does obesity predispose medical intensive care unit patients to venous thromboembolism despite prophylaxis? A retrospective chart review. *Critical Care Research and Practice, 2016*, 3021567. https://doi.org/10.1155/2016/3021567.

Simmons, K. (2017). Sequential compression devices in the pediatric patient population. *AORN Journal, 106*(2), 13–14. https://doi.org/10.1016/S0001-2092(17)30658-0.

Udoh, I. (2016). Understanding venous thromboembolism in patients with cancer. *Journal for Nurse Practitioners, 12*(1), 53–59.

Wolf, P. A., Abbott, R. D., & Kannel, W. B. (1991). Atrial fibrillation as an independent risk factor for stroke: The Framingham study. *Stroke, 22*(8), 983–988.

Yen, J., Van Arendonk, K. J., Streiff, M. B., et al. (2016). Risk factors for venous thromboembolism in pediatric trauma patients and validation of a novel scoring system: The risk of clots in kids with trauma score. *Pediatric Critical Care Medicine, 17*(5), 391–399. https://doi.org/10.1097/PCC.0000000000000699.

Disturbed Thought Process Domain 5 Perception/cognition Class 4 Cognition

Marina Martinez-Kratz, MS, RN, CNE

NANDA-I

Definition

Disruption in cognitive functioning that affects the mental processes involved in developing concepts and categories, reasoning, and problem solving.

Defining Characteristics

Difficulty communicating verbally; difficulty performing instrumental activities of daily living; disorganized thought sequence; expresses unreal thoughts; impaired interpretation of events; impaired judgment; inadequate emotional response to situations; limited ability to find solutions to everyday situations; limited ability to make decisions; limited ability to perform expected social roles; limited ability to plan activities; limited impulse control ability; obsessions; phobic disorders; suspicions

Related Factors

Acute confusion; anxiety; disorientation; fear; grieving; non-psychotic depressive symptoms; pain; stressors; substance misuse; unaddressed trauma

At-Risk Population

Economically disadvantaged individuals; individuals in the early postoperative period; older adults; pregnant women

Associated Conditions

Brain injuries; critical illness; hallucinations; mental disorders; neurodegenerative disorders; pharmaceutical preparations

NOC (Nursing Outcomes Classification)

Suggested NOC Outcomes

Distorted Thought Self-Control; Cognition; Cognitive Orientation

Example NOC Outcome with Indicators

Distorted Thought Self-Control as evidenced by the following indicators: Recognizes hallucinations or delusions are occurring/Refrains from attending to hallucinations or delusions/Refrains from responding to hallucinations or delusions. (Rate the outcome and indicators of **Distorted Thought Self-Control:** 1 = never demonstrated, 2 = rarely demonstrated, 3 = sometimes demonstrated, 4 = often demonstrated, 5 = consistently demonstrated [see Section I.)

Client Outcomes

Client Will (Specify Time Frame)

- Recognize and verbalize that delusions are occurring
- Verbalize reality based thoughts and ideas
- Differentiate between delusions and reality
- Refrain from acting on delusional ideation
- Remain free from injury

NIC (Nursing Interventions Classification)

Suggested NIC Intervention

Delusion Management

Example NIC Activities—Delusion Management

Establish a trusting, interpersonal relationship with client; Avoid arguing about false beliefs, state doubt matter-of-factly; Focus discussion on the underlying feelings, rather than the content of delusions

Nursing Interventions and *Rationales*

- Assess client for the presence of delusions with an established tool such as the Positive and Negative Syndrome Scale (PANSS). EB: *A systematic narrative review of terminology and assessment tools of psychosis found that the PANSS is a frequent assessment tool for individuals with psychotic disorders, individuals with nonpsychotic mental disorders, the general population, and individuals with medical conditions (Seiler et al, 2020).*
- Assess and monitor the client for suicidal ideation. EB: *A study found that suicidal ideation is extremely common in clients with persecutory delusions (Freeman et al, 2019).*
- Assess and monitor how the client copes with delusions and impaired reality testing. EB: *Coping may range from avoidance, stalking, and seeking medical care to violence, so nurses must evaluate if the cognitions will translate to action and for the potential for violence (González-Rodríguez & Seeman, 2020).*
- Assess and monitor clients for side effects associated with antipsychotic medications. EB: *A study of 679 clients with schizophrenia found that antipsychotics with high D2 receptor antagonism and illness duration were risk factors of extrapyramidal symptoms (Weng et al, 2019).*
- Use active listening to identify the meaning attributed to delusional thoughts. EB: *A qualitative study found that grandiose delusions are experienced by clients as highly meaningful. The delusions provide a sense of purpose, belonging, or self-identity or make sense of unusual or difficult events (Isham et al, 2021).*
- Respond to delusional statements with advanced empathy response techniques. Advanced empathy responses include the following:
  - Acknowledge what the person said with a "You say" statement. "You say you have microchips in your brain." Frame the question as exploratory to gain clarification.

T

- Acknowledge your understanding with a statement. "I can't see any microchips and the test results do not show microchips in your brain." State your perceptions, what you have seen, heard, or been told.
- Acknowledge how you imagine the other person feels with a perspective-taking statement such as, "I don't know what it would feel like to have microchips in my brain, but I imagine it might feel scary." Express genuine interest in the client's feelings and ask open-ended questions about their experience.
- Explore the client's feelings and methods of coping.

EB: *Lakeman (2020) states that a client's thoughts and beliefs may not be grounded in consensual reality, but the feelings associated with those thoughts and beliefs are real and require acknowledgment by professionals.*

- • Use nursing presence to provide support to clients who experience grandiose or persecutory delusions. EB: *Research indicates that people with persecutory or grandiose delusions may report distress associated with their experiences and be willing to engage in treatment (Jacobsen et al, 2019).*
- • Use asynchronous email as a method to promote engagement with clients who experience psychosis. EB: *A study found that asynchronous email support promoted engagement with online interventions for individuals with psychosis, with the potential to enable self-management of illness and improve clinical outcomes (Arnold et al, 2019).*
- • Assist the client to identify how daily stress can contribute to impaired thinking and cognitive symptoms. EB: *A study's results supported the idea that minor daily stress may play an important role in inducing a cascade of effects that may lead to psychotic experiences (Klippel et al, 2018).*
- • Provide the client with psychoeducation that includes information about their illness, treatment, disease management, problem-solving, coping skills, and how to access community mental health care services. EB: *Psychoeducation provides individuals with information so they can actively manage their illness (Morin & Franck, 2017).*
- ▲ Refer the client for cognitive behavioral therapy (CBT). EB: *A meta-analysis found that CBT was associated with a higher decrease in positive symptoms for clients with a diagnosis of schizophrenia (Bighelli et al, 2018).*
- ▲ Refer the client for metacognitive training (MCT). MCT is available in a module format, with modules that target common cognitive errors and problem-solving biases. EB: *A randomized control trial of Japanese clients diagnosed with schizophrenia found a decrease in delusions and positive symptoms and an increase in general functioning in the MCT group (Ishikawa et al, 2020).*
- ▲ Refer the client for Art Therapy group or services. EB: *Practice lessons from Art Therapy recommend encouraging reality orientation through art-based form and content, focusing on environmental understimulation and helping clients gain a sense of control to address poor reality testing symptoms (Shore & Rush, 2019).*

Geriatric

- • The previous interventions can be adapted for use with geriatric clients.

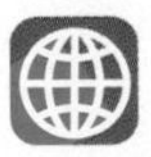

Multicultural

- • The previous interventions can be adapted for use with multicultural clients.
- • Assess for the impact of socioenvironmental risk factors, such as discrimination, on cognitions. EB: *A systematic literature review and meta-analysis found a positive association between perceived ethnic discrimination and the occurrence of psychotic symptoms and experiences (Bardol et al, 2020).*

Home Care

- • The previous interventions can be adapted for use with home care clients.

T

Client/Family Teaching and Discharge Planning

- • Assess family reactions to the client's illness. EB: *A qualitative study investigated family reactions in 14 families where one family member was experiencing a psychosis for the first time. Results indicated that some responses, such as withdrawal, guilt, fear, and stigma, led to the avoidance of seeking mental health treatment of their ill family member (Connor et al, 2016).*
- • Provide family and caregivers information about delusions. EBN: *Interviews with family caregivers found six themes: caregivers' exposure to symptoms of illness; lack of understanding about their relative's delusional beliefs; concerns about harm from their relative; efforts to conceal their relative's delusional beliefs and their consequences; fractured relationships; and learning how to cope (Onwumere, Learmonth, & Kuipers, 2016).*
- • Teach family members how to respond to delusions or expressions of impaired thinking. EBN: *The process of learning how to cope includes learning effective responses to the family member's expressions of disorganized thinking (Onwumere, Learmonth, & Kuipers, 2016).*

REFERENCES

Arnold, C., Villagonzalo, K. A., Meyer, D., et al. (2019). Predicting engagement with an online psychosocial intervention for psychosis: Exploring individual- and intervention-level predictors. *Internet Interventions, 18*, 100266. https://doi.org/10.1016/j.invent.2019.100266.

Bardol, O., Grot, S., Oh, H., et al. (2020). Perceived ethnic discrimination as a risk factor for psychotic symptoms: A systematic review and meta-analysis. *Psychological Medicine, 50*(7), 1077–1089. https://doi.org/10.1017/S003329172000094X.

Bighelli, I., Salanti, G., Huhn, M., et al. (2018). Psychological interventions to reduce positive symptoms in schizophrenia: systematic review and network meta–analysis. *World Psychiatry, 17*(3), 316–329. https://doi.org/10.1002/wps.20577.

Connor, C., Greenfield, S., Lester, H., et al. (2016). Seeking help for first-episode psychosis: a family narrative. *Early Intervention in Psychiatry, 10*(4), 334–345. https://doi.org/10.1111/eip.12177.

Freeman, D., Bold, E., Chadwick, E., et al. (2019). Suicidal ideation and behaviour in patients with persecutory delusions: Prevalence, symptom associations, and psychological correlates. *Comprehensive Psychiatry, 93*, 41–47. https://doi.org/10.1016/j.comppsych.2019.07.001.

González-Rodríguez, A., & Seeman, M. V. (2020). Addressing delusions in women and men with delusional disorder: Key points for clinical management. *International Journal of Environmental Research and Public Health, 17*(12), 4583. https://doi.org/10.3390/ijerph17124583.

Isham, L., Griffith, L., Boylan, A. M., et al. (2021). Understanding, treating, and renaming grandiose delusions: A qualitative study. *Psychology and Psychotherapy, 94*(1), 119–140. https://doi.org/10.1111/papt.12260.

Ishikawa, R., Ishigaki, T., Shimada, T., et al. (2020). The efficacy of extended metacognitive training for psychosis: A randomized controlled trial. *Schizophrenia Research, 215*, 399–407. https://doi.org/10.1016/j.schres.2019.08.006.

Jacobsen, P., McCrum, R. L., Gee, S., & Philpott, R. (2019). Clinical profiles of people with persecutory vs grandiose delusions who engage in psychological therapy during an acute inpatient admission. *Journal of Psychiatric Intensive Care, 15*(2), 67–78. https://doi.org/10.20299/jpi.2019.009.

Klippel, A., Viechtbauer, W., Reininghaus, U., et al. (2018). The cascade of stress: a network approach to explore differential dynamics in populations varying in risk for psychosis. *Schizophrenia Bulletin, 44*(2), 328–337. https://doi.org/10.1093/schbul/sbx037.

Lakeman, R. (2020). Advanced empathy: A key to supporting people experiencing psychosis or other extreme states. *Psychotherapy and Counselling Journal of Australia, 8*(1). Retrieved from https://pacja.org.au/2019/11/advanced-empathy-a-key-to-supporting-people-experiencing-psychosis-or-other-extreme-states/. Accessed February 24, 2022.

Morin, L., & Franck, N. (2017). Rehabilitation interventions to promote recovery from schizophrenia: A systematic review. *Frontiers in Psychiatry, 8*, 100. https://doi.org/10.3389/fpsyt.2017.00100.

Onwumere, J., Learmonth, S., & Kuipers, E. (2016). Caring for a relative with delusional beliefs: A qualitative exploration. *Journal of Psychiatric Mental Health Nursing, 23*(3-4), 145–155.

Seiler, N., Nguyen, T., Yung, A., & O'Donoghue, B. (2020). Terminology and assessment tools of psychosis: A systematic narrative review. *Psychiatry and Clinical Neurosciences, 74*(4), 226–246. https://doi.org/10.1111/pcn.12966.

Shore, A., & Rush, S. (2019). Finding clarity in chaos: Art therapy lessons from a psychiatric hospital. *The Arts in Psychotherapy, 66*, 101575. https://doi.org/10.1016/j.aip.2019.101575.

Weng, J., Zhang, Y., Li, H., Shen, Y., & Yu, W. (2019). Study on risk factors of extrapyramidal symptoms induced by antipsychotics and its correlation with symptoms of schizophrenia. *General Psychiatry, 32*(1), e100026. https://doi.org/10.1136/gpsych-2018-100026.

Impaired Tissue Integrity **Domain 11 Safety/protection Class 2 Physical injury**

JoAnn Coar, MSN, RN-BC, A-GNP-C, CWOCN

NANDA-I

Definition

T

Damage to the mucous membrane, cornea, integumentary system, muscular fascia, muscle, tendon, bone, cartilage, joint capsule, and/or ligament.

Defining Characteristics

Abscess; acute pain, bleeding, decreased muscle strength; decreased range of motion; difficulty bearing weight; dry eye; hematoma, impaired skin integrity; localized area hot to touch, localized deformity; localized loss of hair; localized numbness; localized swelling; muscle spasms; reports lack of balance; reports tingling sensation; stiffness; tissue exposure below the epidermis redness, tissue damage

Related Factors

External Factors

Excretions; humidity; hyperthermia; hypothermia; inadequate caregiver knowledge about maintaining tissue integrity; inadequate caregiver knowledge about protecting tissue integrity; inadequate use of chemical agent; pressure over bony prominence; psychomotor agitation; secretions; shearing forces; surface friction; use of linen with insufficient moisture wicking property

Internal Factors

Body mass index above normal range for age and gender; body mass index below normal range for age and gender; decreased blinking frequency; decreased physical activity; fluid imbalance; impaired physical mobility; impaired postural balance; inadequate adherence to incontinence treatment regimen; inadequate blood glucose level management; inadequate knowledge about maintaining tissue integrity; inadequate knowledge about restoring tissue integrity; inadequate ostomy care; malnutrition; psychogenic factor; self mutilation; smoking; substance misuse

At-Risk Population

Homeless individuals; individuals at extremes of age; individuals exposed to environmental temperature extremes; individuals exposed to high-voltage power supply; individuals participating in contact sports; individuals participating in winter sports; individuals with family history of bone fracture; individuals with history of bone fracture

Associated Conditions

Anemia; autism spectrum disorder; cardiovascular diseases; chronic neurological conditions; critical illness; decreased level of consciousness; decreased serum albumin level; decreased tissue oxygenation; decreased tissue perfusion; hemodynamic instability; immobilization; intellectual disability; medical devices; metabolic diseases; peripheral neuropathy; pharmaceutical preparations; sensation disorders; surgical procedures

NOC (Nursing Outcomes Classification)

Suggested NOC Outcomes

Tissue Integrity: Skin and Mucous Membranes; Wound Healing: Primary Intention, Secondary Intention

Example NOC Outcome with Indicators

Intact **Tissue Integrity: Skin and Mucous Membranes** as evidenced by the following indicators: Skin intactness/Skin lesions absent/Tissue perfusion/Skin temperature. (Rate the outcome and indicators of **Tissue Integrity: Skin and Mucous Membranes:** 1 = severely compromised, 2 = substantially compromised, 3 = moderately compromised, 4 = mildly compromised, 5 = not compromised [see Section I].)

Client Outcomes

Client Will (Specify Time Frame)

- Report any altered sensation or pain at site of tissue impairment
- Demonstrate understanding of plan to heal tissue and prevent reinjury
- Describe measures to protect and heal the tissue, including wound care
- Experience a wound that decreases in size and has increased granulation tissue

NIC (Nursing Interventions Classification)

Suggested NIC Interventions

Incision Site Care; Pain Management; Pressure Ulcer Care; Risk Identification; Skin Care: Topical Treatments; Skin Surveillance; Wound Care; Wound Irrigation

Example NIC Activities—Pressure Ulcer Care

Monitor color of wound bed, temperature, edema, erythema, moisture, and appearance of surrounding skin; Note characteristics of any drainage

Nursing Interventions and *Rationales*

- The National Pressure Ulcer Advisory Panel (NPUAP) redefined the definition of a pressure ulcer, which is now referred to as a pressure injury, during the NPUAP 2016 Staging Consensus Conference. The new

T

definitions more accurately define alterations in tissue integrity from pressure as follows: A pressure injury is localized damage to the skin and underlying soft tissue usually over a bony prominence or related to a medical device or another device. The injury can present as intact skin or an open ulcer and may be painful. The injury occurs as a result of intense and/or prolonged pressure or pressure in combination with shear. The tolerance of soft tissue for pressure and shear may also be affected by microclimate, nutrition, perfusion, comorbidities, and condition of the soft tissue (NPUAP, 2016).

- ● The first step is to identify etiological factors or what is causing the impairment. EB: *A thorough assessment of the individual, not only the impairment, is crucial. This includes a comprehensive medical history, current medical status, medications, and family history (Murphree, 2017). Differentiate pressure injuries from other types of wounds such as moisture-associated skin damage (MASD) (Wound, Ostomy and Continence Nurses Society–Wound Guidelines Task Force, 2017). A comprehensive assessment helps identify specific risk factors and systemic factors, which aids the clinician in a more successful wound management approach (Murphree, 2017).*
- ● Determine the size (length, width) and depth of the wound. EB: *Select a uniform, consistent method for measuring wound length, width or wound area, and depth to facilitate meaningful comparisons of wound measurements over time. A careful assessment should be performed to avoid causing injury when probing the depth of a wound bed or determining the extent of undermining or tunneling (National Pressure Injury Advisory Panel [NPIAP], European Pressure Injury Advisory Panel [EPIAP], & Pan Pacific Pressure Injury Alliance [PPPIA],* 2019).
- ▲ Classify pressure injuries (NPUAP, 2016) using national guidelines and definitions (see http://www.npuap.org/resources/educational-and-clinical-resources/npuap-pressure-injury-stages/).
  - ❍ **Pressure Injury:** A pressure injury is localized damage to the skin and underlying soft tissue usually over a bony prominence or related to a medical or another device. The injury can present as intact skin or an open ulcer and may be painful. The injury occurs as a result of intense and/or prolonged pressure or pressure in combination with shear. The tolerance of soft tissue for pressure and shear may also be affected by microclimate, nutrition, perfusion, comorbidities, and condition of the soft tissue (NPUAP, 2016).
  - ❍ **Stage 1 Pressure Injury:** Nonblanchable erythema of intact skin. Area of localized nonblanchable erythema that may appear differently in darkly pigmented skin, and changes in sensation, temperature, or firmness may precede visual changes. Color changes do not include purple or maroon discoloration, which is more likely to indicate deep tissue pressure injury (NPUAP, 2016).
  - ❍ **Stage 2 Pressure Injury:** Partial-thickness skin loss with exposed dermis. Partial-thickness skin loss with exposed dermis in which the wound bed is pink/red and moist and adipose (fat) and deeper tissues are not visible. Granulation tissue, slough, and eschar are not present. A stage 2 pressure injury may also present as an intact or ruptured blister. These injuries commonly result from adverse microclimate and shear in the skin over the pelvis and shear in the heel. This stage should not be used to describe MASD, including incontinence-associated dermatitis (IAD), intertriginous dermatitis (ITD), medical adhesive–related skin injury (MARSI), or traumatic wounds (skin tears, burns, and abrasions) (NPUAP, 2016).
  - ❍ **Stage 3 Pressure Injury:** Full-thickness skin loss. Full-thickness loss of skin, in which adipose is visible and granulation tissue and epibole (rolled wound edges) are often present, and undermining/tunneling may occur. Slough and/or eschar may also be visible. Fascia, muscle, tendon, ligament, cartilage, and/or bone are not exposed. The depth of tissue damage varies by anatomical location, and areas of significant adiposity can develop deep wounds. If slough or eschar obscures the extent of tissue loss, this is an unstageable pressure injury (NPUAP, 2016).
  - ❍ **Stage 4 Pressure Injury:** Full-thickness skin and tissue loss. Full-thickness skin and tissue loss with exposed or directly palpable fascia, muscle, tendon, ligament, cartilage, or bone and slough and/or eschar may be visible. Epibole, undermining, and/or tunneling often occur and depth varies by anatomical location. If slough or eschar obscures the extent of tissue loss, this is an unstageable pressure injury (NPUAP, 2016).
  - ❍ **Deep Tissue Pressure Injury:** Persistent nonblanchable deep red, maroon, or purple discoloration. Intact or nonintact skin with localized area of persistent nonblanchable deep red, maroon, or purple discoloration or epidermal separation revealing a dark wound bed or blood-filled blister. Pain and temperature change often precede skin color changes. Discoloration may appear differently in darkly pigmented skin. This injury results from intense and/or prolonged pressure and shear forces at the bone–muscle interface. The wound may evolve rapidly to reveal the actual extent of tissue injury, or it may resolve without tissue loss. If necrotic tissue, subcutaneous tissue, granulation tissue, fascia, muscle,

or other underlying structures are visible, this indicates a full-thickness pressure injury (unstageable, stage 3, or stage 4). Do not use deep tissue pressure injury to describe vascular, traumatic, neuropathic, or dermatological conditions (NPUAP, 2016).

- ❍ **Unstageable Pressure Injury:** Obscured full-thickness skin and tissue loss. Full-thickness skin and tissue loss in which the extent of tissue damage within the ulcer cannot be confirmed because it is obscured by slough or eschar. If slough or eschar is removed, a stage 3 or stage 4 pressure injury will be revealed. Stable eschar (i.e., dry, adherent, intact without erythema or fluctuance) on the heel or ischemic limb should not be softened or removed (NPUAP, 2016).
- ❍ **Medical Device–Related Pressure Injury:** This describes an etiology. Medical device–related pressure injuries result from the use of devices designed and applied for diagnostic or therapeutic purposes. The resultant pressure injury generally conforms to the pattern or shape of the device. The injury should be staged using the staging system (NPUAP, 2016).
- ❍ **Mucosal Membrane Pressure Injury:** Mucosal membrane pressure injury is found on mucous membranes with a history of a medical device in use at the location of the injury. Due to the anatomy of the tissue, these ulcers cannot be staged (NPUAP, 2016).

- ● Inspect and monitor the site of impaired tissue integrity at least once daily for color changes, redness, swelling, warmth, pain, or other signs of infection or per facility/agency policy. Monitor the status of the skin around the wound. Pay special attention to all high-risk areas such as bony prominences, skinfolds, sacrum, and heels. There is evidence that stage 1 pressure injuries are underdetected in individuals with darkly pigmented skin because areas of redness are not easily identified. EB: *Systematic inspection can identify impending problems early (NPIAP, EPIAP, & PPPIA, 2019).*
- ● Determine whether the client is experiencing changes in sensation or pain. EB: *An initial pain assessment, using a validated tool, should include the following four elements: a detailed pain history including the character, intensity, and duration of pressure ulcer pain; a physical examination that includes a neurological component; a psychosocial assessment; and an appropriate diagnostic workup to determine the type and cause of the pain. Select a wound dressing that requires less frequent changing, is nonadherent, and maintains a moist wound environment (NPIAP, EPIAP, & PPPIA, 2019).*
- ● Individualizing plans for bathing frequency, pH-balanced soaps, and applying moisturizing products while skin is still damp can help improve skin integrity (Murphree, 2017).
- ● Assess for incontinence and implement an individualized plan for management. EB: *Differentiate wounds caused by incontinence from other types of wounds. Cleanse the skin promptly after episodes of incontinence and use pH-balanced cleansers avoiding the use of alkaline soaps and cleansers (NPIAP, EPIAP, & PPPIA, 2019). Use incontinence skin barriers including creams, ointments, pastes, or film-forming skin protectants as needed to protect and maintain skin integrity with incontinent individuals (Wound, Ostomy and Continence Nurses Society–Wound Guidelines Task Force, 2017).*
- ● Monitor for correct placement of tubes, catheters, and other devices. Assess the skin and tissue affected by the pressure of the devices and tape used to secure these devices. EB: *Reposition the individual and/or the medical device to redistribute pressure and decrease shear forces. Reposition the individual and/or medical device to redistribute pressure and decrease shear forces. Keep skin clean and dry under medical devices. Moisture underneath a medical device can create an environment in which the skin is more vulnerable to alterations in skin integrity (NPIAP, EPIAP, & PPPIA, 2019).*
- ● Medical device–related pressure injury describes an etiology. EB: *Medical device–related pressure injuries result from the use of devices designed and applied for diagnostic or therapeutic purposes. The resultant pressure injury generally conforms to the pattern or shape of the device. The injury should be staged using the previously discussed staging system (NPUAP, 2016).*
- ● Assess frequently for correct placement of foot boards, restraints, traction, casts, or other devices, and assess skin and tissue integrity. EB: *Frequently assess for signs and symptoms of compartment syndrome (refer to the care plan for Risk for* ***Peripheral Neurovascular*** *Dysfunction). Reposition the individual and/or the medical device to redistribute pressure and decrease shear force (NPIAP, EPIAP, & PPPIA, 2019).*
- ▲ Implement and communicate a comprehensive treatment plan for the topical treatment of the skin impairment site. EB: *To improve care and outcomes for individuals with or at risk for skin impairments, evidence-based guidelines must be disseminated to ensure that health care providers are making every effort to identify individuals with or at risk for skin alterations and implement appropriate preventive and treatment interventions (Wound, Ostomy and Continence Nurses Society–Wound Guidelines Task Force, 2017).*
- ▲ Identify a plan for debridement if necrotic tissue (eschar or slough) is present and if consistent with overall client management goals (i.e., curative versus palliative care). EB: *Debride devitalized tissue within the*

T

wound bed or edge of pressure injuries (NPUAP, 2016) when appropriate to individual's condition and consistent with overall goals of care. Do not debride stable, hard, dry eschar in ischemic limbs or heels (NPIAP, EPIAP, & PPPIA, 2019).

- ● Select a topical treatment that maintains a moist, wound-healing environment and also allows absorption of exudate and filling of dead space. **EB:** *No single wound care product provides the optimal environment for healing all wounds. Choose dressings that provide a moist healing environment, keep periwound skin dry, and control exudate and eliminate dead space (NPIAP, EPIAP, & PPPIA, 2019).*
- ● Avoid positioning the client on the site of impaired tissue integrity. **EB:** *If it is consistent with overall client management goals, reposition the client based on level of tissue tolerance and overall condition, and transfer or reposition the client carefully to avoid adverse effects of external mechanical forces (pressure, friction, and shear) (NPIAP, EPIAP, & PPPIA, 2019).*
- ● Select a support surface that meets the needs of the individual based on the level of immobility/activity, size and weight, need for microclimate management, and history of pressure injuries (*NPIAP, EPIAP, & PPPIA, 2019*). **EB:** *Consider changing to a specialty support surface when an individual cannot be repositioned off of an existing pressure injury or fails to heal with current surface. Continue repositioning of individuals placed on a pressure redistribution support surface (NPIAP, EPIAP, & PPPIA, 2019).*
- ● If the goal of care is to keep the client comfortable (e.g., for a terminally ill client), repositioning may not be appropriate. **EB:** *Reposition and turn the individual, periodically, in accordance with the individual's wishes, comfort, and tolerance (NPIAP, EPIAP, & PPPIA, 2019). Maintain the head of the bed at the lowest degree of elevation possible to reduce shear and friction and use lift devices, pillows, foam wedges, and pressure-reducing devices in the bed (NPUAP, 2016; Baranoski & Ayello, 2016).*
- ▲ Assess the client's nutritional status. Refer for a nutritional consultation and/or institute dietary supplements as necessary. **EB:** *Optimizing nutritional intake, including calories, fatty acids, protein, and vitamins, is needed to promote wound healing (O'Hanlon, Dowsett, & Smyth, 2015; NPIAP, EPIAP, & PPPIA, 2019).*
- ▲ Review client nutrition plan evaluating for the intake of 1.25 to 1.5 g of protein per kilogram body weight daily, unless medically contraindicated, for adults at risk of a pressure injury or with existing pressure injuries. Offer 1 mL of fluid intake per kilocalorie per day, unless medically contraindicated (Wound, Ostomy and Continence Nurses Society–Wound Guidelines Task Force, 2017). Reassess as condition changes (*NPIAP, EPIAP, & PPPIA, 2019*).
- ▲ Develop a comprehensive plan of care that includes a thorough wound assessment, treatment interventions, support surfaces, nutritional products, adjunctive therapies, and evaluation of the outcome of care. **EB:** *Documentation of these essential elements is paramount to establishing a framework for quality care.*

Home Care

- ● Some of the interventions previously described may be adapted for home care use.
- ▲ Assess the client's current phase of wound healing (inflammation, proliferation, or maturation) and stage of injury; initiate appropriate wound management. **EB:** *A holistic assessment is required to guide correct dressing selection. Underlying pathophysiological factors need to be addressed to improve outcomes* (NPIAP, EPIAP, & PPPIA, 2019).
- ● Instruct and assist the client and caregivers in understanding how to change dressings and in the importance of maintaining a clean environment. Provide written instructions and observe them completing the dressing change.
- ▲ Initiate a consultation in a case assignment with a wound specialist or wound, ostomy, and continence nurse to establish a comprehensive plan as soon as possible. Plan case conferencing to promote optimal wound care. **EB:** *Case conferencing ensures that cases are regularly reviewed to discuss and implement the most effective wound care management to meet client needs* (NPIAP, EPIAP, & PPPIA, 2019).
- ▲ Consult with other health care disciplines to provide a thorough, comprehensive assessment. **EB:** *Consider referring to a dietitian, physical therapist, occupational therapist, and social worker/case manager as needed. Wound care management requires a multiprofessional approach with the frontline nurse as an essential member of this team (Cox, 2019).*

Client/Family Teaching and Discharge Planning

- ● Teach skin and wound assessment and ways to monitor for signs and symptoms of infection, complications, and healing. **EB:** *Early assessment and intervention help prevent serious problems from developing (Cox, 2019)*

T

- • Teach the client why a topical treatment has been selected. Explain wound bed changes that the caregiver can expect to see. Instruct on when the dressing needs to be changed. Assess pressure injuries with each wound dressing change and confirm the appropriateness of the current dressing regimen (NPIAP, EPIAP, & PPPIA, 2019). EB: *The type of wound dressing needed may change over time as the wound heals and/or deteriorates (Baranoski & Ayello, 2016; NPIAP, EPIAP, & PPPIA, 2019).*
- ▲ Teach the use of pillows, foam wedges, and pressure-reducing devices on beds and chairs to prevent pressure injury. EB: *Pressure redistributing surfaces serve as adjuncts and not replacements to regular repositioning (Wound, Ostomy and Continence Nurses Society–Wound Guidelines Task Force, 2017).*

REFERENCES

Baranoski, S., & Ayello, E. A. (Eds.). (2016). *Wound care essentials: Practice principles* (4th ed.) Philadelphia: Wolters Kluwer.

Cox, J. (2019). Wound care 101. *Nursing, 49*(10), 33–39.

Murphree, R. W. (2017). Impairments in skin integrity. *The Nursing Clinics of North America, 52*(3), 405–417.

National Pressure Injury Advisory Panel (NPIAP), European Pressure Injury Advisory Panel (EPIAP), & Pan Pacific Pressure Injury Alliance (PPPIA). (2019). In E. Haesler (Ed.), *Prevention and treatment of pressure ulcers: Quick reference guide.* Osborne Park, Australia: Cambridge Media.

National Pressure Ulcer Advisory Panel (NPUAP). (2016). *Pressure injury stages.* Retrieved from https://npiap.com/page/PressureInjuryStages. Accessed July 29, 2021.

O'Hanlon, C., Dowsett, J., & Smyth, N. (2015). Nutrition assessment of the intensive care unit patient. *Topics in Clinical Nutrition, 30*(1), 47–70.

Wound, Ostomy and Continence Nurses Society–Wound Guidelines Task Force. (2017). WOCN 2016 guideline for prevention and management of pressure injuries (ulcers). *Journal of Wound, Ostomy and Continence Nursing, 44*(3), 241–246. https://doi.org/10.1097/WON.0000000000000321

Risk for Impaired Tissue Integrity Domain 11 Safety/protection Class 2 Physical injury

Mary Beth Flynn Makic, PhD, RN, CCNS, CCRN-K, FAAN, FNAP, FCNS

NANDA-I

Definition

Susceptible to damage to the mucous membrane, cornea, integumentary system, muscular fascia, muscle, tendon, bone, cartilage, joint capsule, and/or ligament, which may compromise health.

Risk Factors

External Factors

Excretions; humidity; hyperthermia; hypothermia; inadequate caregiver knowledge about maintaining tissue integrity; inadequate caregiver knowledge about protecting tissue integrity; inadequate use of chemical agent; pressure over bony prominence; psychomotor agitation; secretions; shearing forces; surface friction; use of linen with insufficient moisture wicking property

Internal Factors

Body mass index above normal range for age and gender; body mass index below normal range for age and gender; decreased blinking frequency; decreased physical activity; fluid imbalance; impaired physical mobility; impaired postural balance; inadequate adherence to incontinence treatment regimen; inadequate blood glucose level management; inadequate knowledge about maintaining tissue integrity; inadequate knowledge about restoring tissue integrity; inadequate ostomy care; malnutrition; psychogenic factor; self mutilation; smoking; substance misuse

At-Risk Population

Homeless individuals; individuals at extremes of age; individuals exposed to environmental temperature extremes; individuals exposed to high-voltage power supply; individuals participating in contact sports; individuals participating in winter sports; individuals with family history of bone fracture; individuals with history of bone fracture

Associated Conditions

Anemia; autism spectrum disorder; cardiovascular diseases; chronic neurological conditions; critical illness; decreased level of consciousness; decreased serum albumin level; decreased tissue oxygenation; decreased tissue perfusion; hemodynamic instability; immobilization; intellectual disability; medical devices; metabolic diseases; peripheral neuropathy; pharmaceutical preparations; sensation disorders; surgical procedures

NOC, NIC, Client Outcomes, Nursing Interventions and *Rationales,* Client/Family Teaching and Discharge Planning, and References

Refer to care plan for Impaired **Tissue** Integrity.

Ineffective Peripheral Tissue Perfusion

Domain 4 Activity/rest Class 4 Cardiovascular/pulmonary responses

Susan Bonini, EdD, MSN, RN

NANDA-I

Definition

Decrease in blood circulation to the periphery, which may compromise health.

Defining Characteristics

Absence of peripheral pulses; altered motor function; altered skin characteristics; ankle-brachial index <0.90; capillary refill time >3 seconds; color does not return to lowered limb after 1 minute of leg elevation; decreased blood pressure in extremities; decreased pain-free distances during a 6-minute walk test; decreased peripheral pulses; delayed peripheral wound healing; distance in the 6-minute walk test below normal range; edema; extremity pain; femoral bruit; intermittent claudication; paresthesia; skin color pales with limb elevation

Related Factors

Excessive sodium intake; inadequate knowledge of disease process; inadequate knowledge of modifiable factors; sedentary lifestyle; smoking

Associated Conditions

Diabetes mellitus; endovascular procedure; hypertension; trauma

NOC (Nursing Outcomes Classification)

T

Suggested NOC Outcomes

Circulation Status; Fluid Balance; Hydration; Tissue Perfusion: Peripheral

Example NOC Outcome with Indicators

Demonstrates adequate **Circulation Status** as evidenced by the following indicators: Peripheral pulses strong/Peripheral pulses symmetrical/Skin color and temperature/Peripheral edema not present. (Rate the outcome and indicators of **Circulation Status:** 1 = severely compromised, 2 = substantially compromised, 3 = moderately compromised, 4 = mildly compromised, 5 = not compromised [see Section I].)

Client Outcomes

Client Will (Specify Time Frame)

- Demonstrate adequate tissue perfusion as evidenced by palpable peripheral pulses, relief of pain, increased exercise tolerance, warm and dry skin, adequate urine output, and absence of respiratory distress

- Verbalize knowledge of treatment regimen, including appropriate exercise and medications and their actions and possible side effects
- Identify changes in lifestyle needed to increase tissue perfusion

NIC (Nursing Interventions Classification)

Suggested NIC Intervention

Circulatory Care: Arterial Insufficiency

Example NIC Activities—Circulatory Care: Arterial Insufficiency

Evaluate peripheral edema and pulses; Inspect skin for arterial ulcers and tissue breakdown

Nursing Interventions and *Rationales*

▲ Assess the brachial, radial, dorsalis pedis, posterior tibial, and popliteal pulses bilaterally. If unable to palpate them, use a handheld Doppler device and notify the health care provider immediately with a decrease in pulse quality or new onset of absence of pulses along with a cold extremity. **EB:** *Audible handheld Doppler ultrasound proved to be a reliable, simple, rapid, and inexpensive bedside test of peripheral arterial disease in clients with or without diabetes (Leers, n.d.; Mitchell et al, 2019).*

● Note skin color; assess skin temperature, sensation and movement, and capillary refill.

● Assess for pain in the extremities, noting severity, quality, timing, and exacerbating and alleviating factors. Differentiate venous from arterial disease. **EB:** *When peripheral artery disease (PAD) involves the lower extremities, it produces signs and symptoms such as claudication, ischemic rest pain, skin ulceration, or gangrene (Berti-Hearn & Elliott, 2018; Berger & Davies, 2021).*

● Note skin texture and the presence of hair, ulcers, or gangrenous areas on the legs or feet. **EB:** *Nonhealing skin ulcerations and gangrene can occur in areas around the toes, boney prominences of the toes, feet, and lower legs. Chronic wounds often develop on the lower limbs as a complication of diabetes, venous insufficiency, or inadequate arterial perfusion.*

● Assess for the presence of edema in the extremities and rate severity on a four-point scale. Measure the circumference of the ankle and calf at the same time each day in the early morning (Busti, 2016).

▲ Prepare for vascular laboratory tests. **EB:** *Evaluation for PAD if signs and symptoms are present frequently involves a noninvasive vascular laboratory assessment as a next step in diagnosis (Mousa et al, 2017; Kremers et al, 2020).*

▲ Prepare for revascularization procedures. **EB:** *From 10% to 15% of clients experiencing PAD with claudication are at risk of progressing to limb ischemia. Revascularization improves claudication symptoms, minimizes tissue loss, and minimizes other lifestyle-limiting impairments (Gerhard-Herman et al, 2017).*

Arterial Insufficiency

▲ Monitor peripheral pulses. If there is new onset of loss of pulses with bluish, purple, or black areas and extreme pain, notify the health care provider immediately. *These are symptoms of arterial obstruction that can result in loss of a limb if not immediately reversed.* **EB:** *New onset of these assessment finding can result in loss of tissue, nerve damage, and loss of limb. Immediate revascularization is required to salvage the limb (Gerhard-Herman et al, 2017).*

▲ Measure ankle-brachial index (ABI) via Doppler imaging. **EB:** *Measurement of the ABI via a palpatory method offers an inexpensive, readily available alternative approach for early disease detection of PAD. Normal ABI is >0.9 (Kinlay & Gerhard-Herman, 2019; Mitchell, 2019).*

● Avoid elevating the legs above the level of the heart. With arterial insufficiency, leg elevation decreases arterial blood supply to the legs.

▲ In clients with intermittent claudication, exercise programs are recommended, such as walking or riding an exercise bicycle from 30 to 45 minutes per day, three times a week as ordered by the health care provider. **EB:** *Supervised or structured exercise programs are more effective and have been shown to improve functional status (Gerhard-Herman et al, 2017; Harding et al, 2020).*

● Keep the client warm and have the client wear clean all-cotton or all-wool socks and rounded-toe shoes or sheepskin-lined slippers when mobile. Clients with arterial insufficiency report being cold; keep extremities warm to maintain vasodilation and blood supply. Do not apply heat. Heat application can easily damage ischemic tissues.

- ▲ Pay careful attention to foot care. Refer to a podiatrist if the client has thick, overgrown nails or calluses. Ischemic feet are vulnerable to injury; meticulous foot care can prevent further injury. EB: *Symptoms or signs of PAD can be observed in up to 50% of the clients with a diabetic foot ulcer, and PAD is a risk factor for poor healing and amputation (Hinchliffe et al, 2020).*
- ● If the client has ischemic arterial ulcers, refer to the care plan for Impaired **Tissue** Integrity.
- ▲ If the client smokes, recommend the client stop smoking and offer specific smoking cessation interventions. Refer to the health care provider for medications to support nicotine withdrawal. EB: *There is a strong correlation between smoking and the risk of developing PAD. Nurses have professional responsibility to help clients stop smoking, utilizing evidence-based clinical practice guidelines (AHRQ, 2008; Gerhard-Herman et al, 2017; Hinchliffe et al, 2020).*
- ▲ If the client has diabetes, good glycemic control is recommended. EB: *Intensive cardiovascular risk management that includes good glycemic control has been shown to reduce the 5-year mortality rate in clients with PAD and diabetes (Hinchliffe et al, 2020).*
- ● Educate the client on the use and safety of antiplatelet medications. Encourage the client to wear a medical alert bracelet. EB: *Antiplatelet therapy is recommended to reduce the risk of cardiovascular ischemic events (Gerhard-Herman et al, 2017).*

Venous Insufficiency

- ● Elevate edematous legs as ordered and ensure no pressure under the knee and heels to prevent pressure ulcers. EB: *Clients who are inactive (sedentary) for long periods may have leg edema because the calf muscle pump is underused or ineffective. Elevating the ankles above the level of the heart can help relieve this type of swelling (Evans & Ratchford, 2016).*
- ▲ Apply graduated compression stockings as ordered. Ensure proper fit by measuring accurately. Remove the stockings at least twice a day, in the morning with the bath and in the evening, to assess the condition of the extremity, then reapply. Knee length is preferred rather than thigh length. EB: *Compression stockings are indicated for long-term management of chronic venous insufficiency to control edema and reduce the risk of venous ulcers (Berti-Hearn & Elliott, 2019; Youn & Lee, 2019).*
- ● Encourage the client to walk with compression stockings on and perform toe-up and point-flex exercises. Exercise helps increase venous return, builds up collateral circulation, and strengthens the calf muscles. EB: *Physical therapy modalities improve ABI, Doppler flow velocity, and blood parameters in clients with type 2 diabetes (Treat-Jacobson et al, 2019).*
- ● If the client is overweight, encourage weight loss to decrease venous disease.
- ● If the client has venous leg ulcers, encourage the client to avoid prolonged sitting, standing, and elevation of the involved leg. Encourage proper use of compression stockings. Pain may prevent compliance. EB: *Adherence to the use of compression stockings may be influenced by limited mobility, pain, appearance of stockings, discomfort with wearing, difficulty applying and wearing with shoes, and cost (Ratliff et al, 2016).*
- ▲ If the client is mostly immobile, consult with the health care provider regarding use of a calf-high intermittent pneumatic compression device for prevention of deep venous thrombosis (DVT). EB: *Below-the-knee devices have demonstrated the most efficacy, with multiple guidelines recommending usage (Ratliff et al, 2016; Berti-Hearn & Elliott, 2019).*
- ● Assess for signs of DVT, including pain, tenderness, dilated superficial veins, a palpable cord indicating a thrombosed vein, swelling in the calf and thigh, and warmth and erythema in the involved extremity. Obtain serial leg measurements of the thigh and calf circumferences. In some clients a tender venous cord can be felt in the popliteal fossa. Do not rely on Homan's sign. EB: *Screening and detection of DVT must be as accurate as possible. Consider using the Wells prediction score screening tool. It is critical to diagnose DVT because if left untreated, thrombi in the popliteal vein and above are associated with pulmonary embolism (PE) (Roberts & Lawrence, 2017).*
- ▲ Note the results of a D-dimer test and ultrasounds. EB: *Although a D-dimer test can be used during the initial workup for all clients who present to the emergency department (ED) for suspected DVT, duplex ultrasonography is a more reliable method of diagnosing DVT (Roberts & Lawrence, 2017; Berti-Hearn & Elliott, 2019).*
- ● If DVT is present, observe for symptoms of a PE. EB: *PE is a significant risk of a DVT. Signs and symptoms range from sudden onset, dyspnea, pleuritic chest pain of a sharp stabbing nature, dyspnea, palpitations, wheezing, anxiety, and cough (Roberts & Lawrence, 2017).*
- ● Educate on use and safety of anticoagulant and antiplatelet medications. EB: *DVT and PE are two manifestations of venous thromboembolism (VTE). The mainstay of therapy for DVT is anticoagulation, provided*

there is no contraindication (Roberts & Lawrence, 2017; Lip & Hull, 2021). Clients need to be aware of adverse effects of anticoagulant medications, wear a medical alert bracelet, and be aware of food–drug interactions (Berti-Hearn & Elliott, 2019).

Geriatric

- Complete a thorough lower extremity assessment, documenting the slightest change from previous assessment, and implement a plan immediately. EB: *Complete and accurate assessment is essential to guide health care providers in formulating efficacious plans of care. The prevalence of peripheral arterial disease increases with age. The elevated risk of ulcerations leading to amputation among older adults reflects not only increased rates of PAD and diabetic pathologies but also age-related changes of the vessels (Humphries et al, 2016).*
- Recognize that older adults have an increased risk for development of DVT and PE. EB: *Risk for DVT and PE increases with advanced age (age >70) and history of heart disease and/or cancer (Rali et al, 2018).*

Home Care

- The interventions previously described may be adapted for home care use.
- If arterial disease is present and the client smokes, encourage smoking cessation using motivational interviewing techniques and evidenced-based clinical practice guidelines (AHRQ, 2008; AHA, 2021; CDC, n.d.).
- Examine the feet carefully at frequent intervals for changes and new ulcerations. Encourage the client to perform regular assessment of the feet.
- ▲ Assess the client's nutritional status, paying special attention to obesity, hyperlipidemia, and malnutrition. Refer to a dietitian if appropriate.
- Monitor for development of gangrene, venous ulceration, and symptoms of cellulitis (redness, pain, and increased swelling in an extremity).

Client/Family Teaching and Discharge Planning

- Explain the importance of good foot care. Teach the client and family to wash daily with mild soap and tepid water. Teach the client and family to inspect the feet daily. Recommend that the diabetic client wear properly fitting shoes to prevent the formation of blisters and calluses. Clients with diabetes should be instructed to never walk barefoot (Berti-Hearn & Elliott, 2018).
- ▲ Teach diabetic clients that they should have a comprehensive foot examination at least annually. The examination should include sensory assessments. If good sensation is not present, refer to a footwear professional for fitting of therapeutic shoes and inserts, the cost of which may be covered by insurance and/or Medicare.
- For arterial disease, stress the importance of not smoking, following a weight loss program (if the client is obese), carefully controlling a diabetic condition, controlling hyperlipidemia, managing hypertension, maintaining intake of antiplatelet therapy, and reducing stress.
- Encourage clients to walk or engage in other forms of physical activity.
- Teach the client to avoid exposure to cold; limit exposure to brief periods if going out in cold weather and wear warm clothing.
- For venous disease, stress the importance of not smoking, and teach the importance of wearing compression stockings as ordered, elevating the legs at intervals (30 minutes, three to four times a day), weight loss if overweight, regular exercise such as walking, and watching for skin breakdown on the legs.
- Educate clients about any medications prescribed to treat their venous disease.
- Educate clients about the importance of taking prescribed medications to achieve therapeutic anticoagulation (Roberts & Lawrence, 2017).
- Teach clients to avoid crossing legs when sitting or standing for prolonged periods (Berti-Hearn & Elliott, 2019).
- Teach client to avoid long periods of sitting or standing to reduce the pooling of blood (D'Alesandro, 2016).
- Teach the client to recognize the signs and symptoms that should be reported to a health care provider (e.g., change in skin temperature, color, or sensation, or the presence of a new lesion on the foot).
- Provide clear, simple instructions about plan of care.

T

- Instruct and provide emotional support for clients undergoing hyperoxygenation treatment. **EB:** *Hyperbaric oxygen may be used as a treatment option for clients with diabetes suffering from nonhealing or delayed-healing foot ulcers (Huang et al, 2019; Longobardi et al, 2019).*

REFERENCES

Agency for Healthcare Research and Quality (AHRQ). (2008). *Treating tobacco use and dependence: 2008 update—Clinical practice guideline.* Washington, D.C.: AHRQ. Retrieved from https://www.ahrq.gov/prevention/guidelines/tobacco/clinicians/update/index.html. [Accessed August 2, 2021].

American Heart Association (AHA). (2021). *PAD toolkit for health care professionals.* Retrieved from https://www.heart.org/en/health-topics/peripheral-artery-disease/pad-toolkit. [Accessed August 2, 2021].

Berger, J. S., & Davies, M. G. (2021). Overview of lower extremity peripheral artery disease. D. L. Clement, J. F. Eidt, J. L. Mills, Sr, M. A. Creager, & K. A. Collins (Eds.). Waltham: UpToDate.

Berti-Hearn, L., & Elliott, B. (2018). A closer look at lower extremity peripheral arterial disease. *Nursing, 48*(1), 34–41.

Berti-Hearn, L., & Elliott, B. (2019). Chronic venous insufficiency: A review for nurses. *Nursing2019, 49*(12), 24–30.

Busti, A. J. (2016). *Pitting edema assessment.* Evidence-Based Medicine Consult [website]. Retrieved from https://www.ebmconsult.com/articles/pitting-edema-assessment. [Accessed August 2, 2021].

Centers for Disease Control and Prevention (CDC). (n.d.). *A practical guide to help your patients quit using tobacco.* Retrieved from https://www.cdc.gov/tobacco/basic_information/for-health-care-providers/pdfs/hcp-conversation-guide.pdf. [Accessed August 2, 2021].

D'Alesandro, M. A. (2016). Focusing on lower extremity DVT. *Nursing, 46*(4), 28–36.

Evans, N. S., & Ratchford, E. V. (2016). The swollen leg. *Vascular Medicine, 21*(6), 562–564.

Gerhard-Herman, M. D., Gornik, H. L., Barrett, C., et al. (2017). 2016 AHA/ACC guideline on the management of patients with lower extremity peripheral artery disease: Executive summary: A report of the American College of Cardiology/American Heart Association Task Force on Clinical Practice Guidelines. *Journal of the American College of Cardiology, 69*(11), 1465–1508. http://dx.doi.org/10.1016/j.jacc.2016.11.008

Harding, M. M., Kwong, J., Roberts, D., Hagler, D., & Reinisch, C. (Eds.). (2020). *Lewis's medical-surgical nursing: Assessment and management of clinical problems* (11th ed.). St. Louis: Elsevier.

Hinchliffe, R. J., Forsythe, R. O., Apelqvist, J., et al. (2020). Guidelines on diagnosis, prognosis, and management of peripheral artery disease in patients with foot ulcers and diabetes (IWGDF 2019 update). *Diabetes/Metabolism Research and Reviews, 36*(Suppl. 1),. e3276.

Huang, E., Heyboer, M., 3rd, & Savaser, D. J. (2019). Hyperbaric oxygen therapy for the management of chronic wounds: Patient selection and perspectives. *Chronic Wound Care Management and Research, 6*, 27–37.

Humphries, M. D., Brunson, A., Hedayati, N., Romano, P., & Melnkow, J. (2016). Amputation risk in patients with diabetes mellitus and peripheral artery disease using statewide data. *Annuals of Vascular Surgery, 30*, 123–131. http://doi:10.1016/j.avsg.2015.04.089.

Kinlay, S., & Gerhard-Herman, M. D. (2019). *Current status of the ABI in diagnosis, risk assessment and screening.* American College of Cardiology. Retrieved from https://www.acc.org/latest-in-cardiology/articles/2019/11/05/13/38/current-status-of-the-abi-in-diagnosis-risk-assessment-and-screening. [Accessed August 2, 2021].

Kremers, B., Wübbeke, L., Mees, B., Ten Cate, H., Spronk, H., & Ten Cate-Hoek, A. (2020). Plasma biomarkers to predict cardiovascular outcome in patients with peripheral artery disease: A systematic review and meta-analysis. *Arteriosclerosis, Thrombosis, and Vascular Biology, 40*(9), 2018–2032. https://doi.org/10.1161/ATVBAHA.120.314774.

Leers, S. A. (n.d.). Duplex ultrasound. *Society for Vascular Surgery.* Retrieved from https://vascular.org/patient-resources/vascular-tests/duplex-ultrasound. [Accessed August 2, 2021].

Lip, G. Y. H., & Hull, R. D. (2021). Overview of the treatment of lower extremity deep vein thrombosis (DVT). L. L. K. Leung, J. Mandel, & G. Finlay (Eds.). Waltham: UpToDate. Retrieved from https://www.uptodate.com/contents/overview-of-the-treatment-of-lower-extremity-deep-vein-thrombosis-dvt. [Accessed February 24, 2022].

Longobardi, P., Hoxha, K., & Bennett, M. H. (2019). Is there a role for hyperbaric oxygen therapy in the treatment of refractory wounds of rare etiology? *Diving and Hyperbaric Medicine, 49*(3), 216–224.

Mitchell, E. L. (2019). Noninvasive diagnosis of arterial disease. J. F. Eidt, J. L. Mills, & K. A. Collins (Eds.). Waltham: UpToDate. Retrieved from https://www.uptodate.com/contents/noninvasive-diagnosis-of-upper-and-lower-extremity-arterial-disease. [Accessed February 24, 2022].

Mousa, A., Morkos, R., De Wit, D., et al. (2017). Utilization of D-dimer along with clinical probability testing in determining the magnitude and location of deep venous thrombosis in a high-volume tertiary practice [abstract]. *Journal of Vascular Surgery: Venous and Lymphatic Disorders, 5*(1), 170–171.

Rali, P., Rali, M., & Sockrider, M. (2018). Pulmonary embolism part 1. *American Journal of Respiratory and Critical Care Medicine, 197*(9), P15–P16. https://doi.org/10.1164/rccm.1979P15.

Ratliff, C. R., Yates, S., McNichol, L., & Gray, M. (2016). Compression for primary prevention, treatment, and prevention of recurrence of venous leg ulcers: An evidence- and consensus-based algorithm for care across the continuum. *Journal of Wound, Ostomy, and Continence Nursing, 43*(4), 347–364.

Roberts, S. H., & Lawrence, S. M. (2017). Venous thromboembolism: updated management guidelines. *American Journal of Nursing, 117*(5), 38–47.

Treat-Jacobson, D., McDermott, M. M., Bronas, U. G., et al. (2019). Optimal exercise programs for patients with peripheral artery disease: A scientific statement from the American Heart Association. *Circulation, 139*(4), e10–e33.

Youn, Y. J., & Lee, J. (2019). Chronic venous insufficiency and varicose veins of the lower extremities. *Korean Journal of Internal Medicine, 34*(2), 269–283.

T

Risk for Ineffective Peripheral Tissue Perfusion

Domain 4 Activity/rest Class 4 Cardiovascular/pulmonary responses

Mary Beth Flynn Makic, PhD, RN, CCNS, CCRN-K, FAAN, FNAP, FCNS

NANDA-I

Definition

Susceptible to a decrease in blood circulation to the periphery, which may compromise health.

Risk Factors

Excessive sodium intake; inadequate knowledge of disease process; inadequate knowledge of modifiable factors; sedentary lifestyle; smoking

Associated Conditions

Diabetes mellitus; endovascular procedures; hypertension; trauma

NOC, NIC, Client Outcomes, Nursing Interventions and *Rationales,* Client/Family Teaching and Discharge Planning, and References

Refer to care plan for Ineffective Peripheral **Tissue Perfusion.**

Impaired Transfer Ability

Domain 4 Activity/rest Class 2 Activity/exercise

Darcy O'Banion, RN, MS, ACCNS-AG

NANDA-I

Definition

Limitation of independent movement between two nearby surfaces.

Defining Characteristics

Difficulty transferring between bed and chair; difficulty transferring between bed and standing position; difficulty transferring between car and chair; difficulty transferring between chair and floor; difficulty transferring between chair and standing position; difficulty transferring between floor and standing position; difficulty transferring between uneven levels; difficulty transferring in or out of bath tub; difficulty transferring in or out of shower stall; difficulty transferring on or off a bedside commode; difficulty transferring on or off a toilet

Related Factors

Environmental constraints; impaired postural balance; inadequate knowledge of transfer techniques; insufficient muscle strength; neurobehavioral manifestation; obesity; pain; physical deconditioning

T

Associated Conditions

Musculoskeletal impairment; neuromuscular diseases; vision disorders

NOC (Nursing Outcomes Classification)

Suggested NOC Outcomes

Balance; Body Positioning: Self-Initiated; Transfer Performance

Example NOC Outcome with Indicators

Transfer Performance as evidenced by the following indicators: Transfers from bed to chair and back/Transfers from wheelchair to toilet and back/Transfers from wheelchair to vehicle and back. (Rate the outcome and indicators of **Transfer Performance:** 1 = severely compromised, 2 = substantially compromised, 3 = moderately compromised, 4 = mildly compromised, 5 = not compromised [see Section I].)

Client Outcomes

Client Will (Specify Time Frame)

- Transfer from bed to chair and back successfully
- Transfer from chair to chair successfully
- Transfer from wheelchair to toilet and back successfully
- Transfer from wheelchair to car and back successfully

NIC (Nursing Interventions Classification)

Suggested NIC Interventions

Exercise Promotion: Strength Training; Exercise Therapy: Muscle Control

Example NIC Activities—Exercise Promotion: Strength Training

Obtain medical clearance for initiating a strength-training program, as appropriate; Assist to set realistic short- and long-term goals and to take ownership of the exercise plan

Nursing Interventions and *Rationales*

- Specify level of independence using a standardized functional scale. **EB:** *Use a nurse-driven bedside assessment tool to evaluate the client's mobility status. Regular evaluation of clients' mobility status by nurses using a standardized tool allows more awareness of the skill and equipment needed for safe client handling and mobility, reducing the risk for fall and potential injury to the nursing staff (Boynton et al, 2014; Jones et al, 2020).*
- Assess level of client ability to perform specific tasks before transfer of client. **EB:** *Valid and reliable assessment tools such as the Bedside Mobility Assessment Tool provide assessment of a client to promote safe mobility and reduce injury to staff (Boynton et al, 2014; Teeple et al, 2017; Hillrom Services, Inc., 2019).*
- Assess client's dependence, weight, strength, balance, tolerance to position change, cooperation, fatigue level, and cognition plus available equipment and staff ratio/experience to decide whether to do a manual or device-assisted transfer because devices can reduce staff injury *(American Nurses Association [ANA], 2015; Riccoboni et al, 2021).*

▲ Complications associated with immobility and resultant muscle loss begin within 48 hours of onset of injury and are greatest during the first 2 to 3 weeks (Cameron et al, 2015). Request a consultation for a physical therapist (PT) and/or occupational therapist (OT) to develop a plan of care for safe client handling and mobility. **EB:** *Progressive mobility, or mobility that starts earlier and more aggressively during a client's hospital stay, even as early as in the intensive care unit (ICU), decreases mechanical ventilation days and decreases complications such as weakness from prolonged immobilization (Arias-Fernández et al, 2018). Early exercise in the ICU improves clients' muscle strength, reduces activity limitations, and reduces restrictions in participation in activities after discharge (Tipping et al, 2017).*

▲ Obtain a consultation for a PT, OT, or orthotist to evaluate and fit clients with proper orthoses, braces, collars, and walking aids before helping them stand. **EB:** *Equipment can help increase clients' independence and decrease the level of assistance needed from caregivers (Romanoski & Swope, 2018).*

▲ Help client put on/take off collars, braces, prostheses in bed, and put on/take off antiembolism stockings and abdominal binders. If applying antiembolism stockings is prescribed to reduce the risk of DVT, apply while the client is in bed for ease of application. **EB:** *In clients with diagnosed acute DVT of the leg, compression stockings may not be routinely used to prevent postthrombotic syndrome. Postthrombotic syndrome is a complication that may occur after a DVT develops from venous insufficiency producing symptoms of pain, edema, and venous ulcers. Current guidelines recommend not routinely using compression stockings with clients who have a DVT (Kearon et al, 2016).*

▲ Collaborate with PT and OT to use algorithms to identify technological aids to handle and transfer dependent and obese clients. Use assistive mobility devices such as gait belts, lifts, and transport devices to move obese clients to avoid harm to both client and health care professional (Choi & Brings, 2015). **EB:** *Assess the client for appropriate use of assistive devices, such as powered and nonpowered stand-assist devices, mechanical lifts, stretcher-chairs, and friction-reducing devices, to prevent musculoskeletal injuries of staff and allow safe client handling (Centers for Disease Control and Prevention, National Institute for Occupational Safety and Health, 2015; Choi & Brings, 2015; Hallmark et al, 2015).*

T

- Implement and document type of transfer (e.g., slide board, pivot), weight-bearing status (non–weight-bearing, partial), equipment (walker, sling lift), and level of assistance (standby, moderate) on care plan, white board in room, and/or electronic medical record.
- Apply a gait belt with handles before transferring clients with partial weight-bearing abilities; keep the belt and client close to provider during the transfer. **EB:** *If used incorrectly, such as at arm's length, it prevents support of client and places staff at risk for back and arm injuries (Choi & Brings, 2015; Hallmark, Meachan, & Shores, 2015).*
- Help clients when wearing shoes with nonskid soles and socks/hose. Proper shoes help prevent slips/pain/pressure and improve balance. **EB:** *Suggest trying a running shoe that is comfortable and lightweight. A study found that there is inconclusive evidence that nonslip socks prevent falls as they do not adequately replace footwear and have the potential to spread infection; instead, clients should use personal footwear to prevent falls (Hartung & Lalonde, 2017).*
- Remove or swivel wheelchair armrests, leg rests, and footplates to the side, especially with squat or slide board transfers. This gives clients and nurses feet space in which to maneuver and provides fewer obstacles to trip over.
- Adjust transfer surfaces so that they are similar in height. For example, lower a hospital bed to about an inch higher than commode height. **EB:** *Similar heights between seat surfaces require less upper extremity muscular effort during transfers (Darragh et al, 2014).*
- Place wheelchair and commode at a slight angle toward the surface onto which the client will transfer. **EB:** *The two surfaces are close together yet allow room for the caregiver to adjust the client's movements during the transfer (Darragh et al, 2014).*
- Teach client to consistently lock brakes on wheelchair/commode/shower chair before transferring. **EB:** *Wheels will roll if not locked, creating risk for falls. Pneumatic wheelchair tires must be adequately inflated for brakes to lock effectively (Darragh et al, 2014; Choi & Brings, 2015).*
- Give clear, simple instructions, allow client time to process information, and let him or her do as much of the transfer as possible. **EB:** *Too much assistance by staff and family may decrease client learning, independence, self-care, and self-esteem (Choi & Brings, 2015).*

▲ Remind clients to comply with weight-bearing restrictions ordered by their health care provider. Weight-bearing may retard healing in fractured bones.

- Place client in set position before standing him or her, for example, sitting on edge of surface with bilateral weight-bearing on buttocks and hips, with knees flexed, balls of feet aligned under knees, and head in midline. **EB:** *This position prepares individuals for bearing weight and permits shifting of weight from pelvis to feet as the center of gravity changes while rising (Choi & Brings, 2015).*
- Support and stabilize client's weak knees by placing one or both of your knees next to or encircling client's knees, rather than blocking them. This allows client to flex his or her knees and lean forward to stand and transfer.
    - Squat transfer: client leans well forward, slightly raises flexed hips off the surface, pivots, and sits down on new surface.
    - Standing pivot transfer: client leans forward with hips flexed and pushes up with hands from seat surface (or arms of chair), then stands erect, pivots, and sits down on new surface.
    - Slide board transfer: client should have on pants or have a pillowcase over the board. Remove arm and leg rest from wheelchair on one side, then slightly angle chair toward new surface. Help client lean sideways, shifting his or her weight so the transfer board can be placed well under the upper thigh of the leg next to new surface. Make sure the board is safely angled across both surfaces. Help client to sit upright and place one hand on the board and the other hand on the surface. Remind and help client perform a series of pushups with arms while leaning slightly forward and lifting (not sliding) hips in small increments across the board with each pushup.

  EB: *Using different transfer techniques is necessary to facilitate clients who range from little to no weight-bearing ability (Darragh et al, 2014; Hallmark, Mechan, & Shores, 2015; Cameron et al, 2018).*
- Position walking aids appropriately so a standing client can grasp and use them once he or she is upright. **EB:** *These aids help provide support, balance, and stability to help client stand and step safely and, when used properly, can increase one's level of activity and participation (Bertrand et al, 2017).*
- Reinforce to clients who use walkers to place one hand on walker and push with opposite hand against chair arm or surface from which they are arising to stand up. Placing both hands on the walker may cause it to tip and the client to lose balance and fall.

T

- Use ceiling-mounted or bedside mechanical bariatric lifts to transfer dependent bariatric (extremely obese) clients. EB: *Lifting equipment reduces the risk of client/staff injury and is essential for clients who require a moderate/maximum assist transfer (Choi & Brings, 2015; Lee & Rempel, 2020).*
- Use bariatric devices and use available safe client handling equipment for lifting, transferring, positioning, and sliding client as an effective tool to reduce risk of injury from client handling (Choi & Brings, 2015; Lee & Lee, 2017).
- Place a mechanical lift sling in the wheelchair preventively. Place two transfer sheets or a slide board under the bariatric client. EB: *Reinforce that head should be leaning forward and that knees should be level with hips; help hold wheelchair in place as therapist directs/helps client with a scoot transfer. Client may be too fatigued to do a manual transfer back to bed after sitting, so sling/lift can be used (Choi & Brings, 2015; Lee & Lee, 2017).*
- Perform initial and subsequent fall risk assessment. Use standardized tools for fall risk assessment and interdisciplinary multifactorial interventions to reduce falls and risk of falling in hospitals. EB: *Best practice in falls reduction occurs when fall risk assessment; visual identification of individuals at high risk for falls; falls risk factor–directed interventions; and standardized multifactorial education, including visual tools for staff, families, and clients, are implemented (Low et al, 2015; Heng et al, 2020).*
- ▲ Collaborate with PT, OT, and pharmacist for individualized preventive/postfall plans; for example, scheduled toileting, balance and strength training, removal of hazards, chair alarms, call system/phone in reach, and review of medications. EB: *A systematic review of the evidence found that low-intensity exercise and incontinence care in residents in nursing homes reduced falls (Low et al, 2015; Hopkins et al, 2016).*
- Coordinate a follow-up encounter within 30 days of discharge from any inpatient facility with a licensed provider to perform a medication reconciliation, including all medications the client has been taking or receiving before the outpatient visit to provide quality care and improve quality of communication related to medications EB: *Review of medications, especially new medications added to a client plan of care, can help reduce risk for falls, changes in mentation, or mobility limitations (National Committee for Quality Assurance, 2015b).*
- Encourage an exercise component such as Tai chi, physical therapy, or another exercise for balance, gait, and strength training in group programs or at home.
- Integrate structured, progressive exercise protocols into a client's plan of care and innovative partnerships with other providers to create longer-duration interventions for clients at risk of falling. EB: *This promotes strength and aids in increasing confidence, thus reducing the risk of falling (Low et al, 2015).*
- Modify the environment for safety; recommend vision assessment and consideration for cataract removal.
- To reduce the risk of falling, assess the physical environment (e.g., poor lighting, high bed position, improper equipment). EB: *Continuous and intentional observational assessment of the environment promotes safety by reducing potential fall hazards (Low et al, 2015).*
- Recommend polypharmacy assessment with special consideration to sedatives, antidepressants, and drugs affecting the central nervous system; recommend evaluation for orthostatic hypotension and irregular heartbeats; and recommend vitamin D supplementation 800 international units/day (National Committee for Quality Assurance, 2015b).

Home Care

- ▲ Obtain referral for OT and PT to teach home exercises and balance and fall prevention and recovery. They also evaluate for potential modifications such as an entry ramp, elevated toilet seat/toilevator (raised base under toilet), tub seat or shower chair, need for shower stall with built-in seat or wheel-in shower stall without a curb/threshold, handheld flexible shower head, lever-type facets, pull-out drawers with loop handles versus cupboards, and standing lift. EB: *Interventions such as environmental modifications and assistive devices can reduce the risk of falling and promote independence by compensating for limitations in functional abilities (Putthinoi, Lersilp, & Chakpitak, 2017).*
- Develop a multifactorial/multicomponent interventions risk strategy to reduce the risk for falls that includes adaptation or modification of the home environment; withdrawal or minimization of psychoactive medications; withdrawal or minimization of other medications; management of postural hypotension; management of foot problems and footwear; and exercise, particularly balance, strength, and gait training (National Committee for Quality Assurance, 2015a).
- Assess for adequate lighting and hazards such as throw/area rugs, clutter, cords, and unfitted bedspreads. Suggest safe floor surfaces, such as use of adhesive nonslip strips in tubs, thresholds, and areas in which floor height changes; removal of wax from slippery floors; and installing low-pile carpet or nonglazed

or nonglossy tiles, wood, or linoleum coverings. Encourage relocating commonly used items to shelves/drawers in reach; applying remote controls to appliances; and optimizing furniture placement for function, maneuverability, and stability. EB: *Removing potential fall hazards and environmental barriers promotes safety and accessibility; steady furniture can be used to steady or pull oneself up if a fall occurs (Putthinoi, Lersilp, & Chakpitak, 2017; E et al, 2020; Lamb et al, 2020).*

- ● Assess clients for impairment of vision because this can result in a loss of function in activities of daily living and, consequently, result in impaired functional capacity and is an important risk factor for falls. EB: *Possible mechanisms to reduce activity restriction and improve mobility include environmental and behavioral interventions delivered by multiple types of health professionals, including OTs (E et al, 2020).*
- ● Nurses can provide further safety assessments by suggesting installing hand rails in bathrooms and by stairs, using slip-resistant floor surfaces, ensuring client's slippers and clothes fit properly, and recommending repairing or discarding broken equipment in the home (Keall et al, 2015; E et al, 2020).
- ▲ Involve social worker or case manager to educate clients about potential assistive technology, financial cost and benefits, regulations of payers, and local resources. EB: *Information helps clients understand options and cost of services in order to make informed decisions (Hamadi et al, 2018).*
- ▲ Implement approaches for home care staff and family to safely handle and transfer clients. Risk of injury is high because people often work alone, without mechanical aids or appropriate equipment such as mechanical beds and in crowded spaces, while providing care (*Hamadi et al, 2018*).
- ● For further information, refer to care plans for Impaired Physical **Mobility** and Impaired **Walking.**

Client/Family Teaching and Discharge Planning

- ● Assess for readiness to learn and use teaching modalities conducive to personal learning styles, including written instructions for home use.
- ● Supervise practice sessions in which client and family apply items such as gait belts, braces, and orthoses. Check skin once aids are removed. EB: *Repetition reinforces motor learning for safety and sound skin integrity (Low et al, 2015).*
- ● Teach and monitor client/family for consistent use of safety precautions for transfers (e.g., nonskid shoes, correctly placed equipment/chairs, locked brakes, leg rests swiveled away) and for correct performance of transfer or use of lifts/slings. *Promotes safety.*
- ● Teach client/family how to check brakes on chairs to ensure they engage and how to check tires for adequate air pressure; advise routine inspection and annual tune-up of devices. EB: *Long-term use may loosen brakes or cause them to slip; brakes work only if they make sound contact with tire or wheel. Pneumatic tires must be adequately inflated (Low et al, 2015).*
- ● Offer information on safe use of shower and commode chairs to prevent discomfort, pressure, and falls during transfer, transport, care, and hygiene.
- ● For further information, refer to the care plans for Impaired Physical **Mobility,** Impaired **Walking,** and Impaired Wheelchair **Mobility.**

REFERENCES

American Nurses Association (ANA). (2015). *Safe patient handling and mobility: Understanding the benefits of a comprehensive SPHM program*. Retrieved from https://www.nursingworld.org/~498de8/globalassets/practiceandpolicy/work-environment/health--safety/ana-sphmcover__finalapproved.pdf. [Accessed August 2, 2021].

Arias-Fernández, P., Romero-Martin, M., Gómez-Salgado, J., & Fernández-García, D. (2018). Rehabilitation and early mobilization in the critical client: Systematic review. *Journal of Physical Therapy Science, 30*(9), 1193–1201. https://doi.org/10.1589/jpts.30.1193.

Bertrand, K., Raymond, M. H., Miller, W. C., Martin Ginis, K. A., & Demers, L. (2017). Walking aids for enabling activity and participation: A systematic review. *American Journal of Physical Medicine & Rehabilitation, 96*(12), 894–903. https://doi.org/10.1097/PHM.0000000000000836.

Boynton, T., Kelly, L., & Perez, A. (2014). Implementing a mobility assessment tool for nurses. *American Nurse Today, 9*(9), 13–16.

Cameron, I. D., Dyer, S. M., Panagoda, C. E., et al. (2018). Interventions for preventing falls in older people in care facilities and hospitals. *Cochrane Database of Systematic Reviews, 9*, CD005465. doi:10.1002/14651858.CD005465.pub4.

Cameron, S., Ball, I., Cepinskas, G., et al. (2015). Early mobilization in the critical care unit: A review of adult and pediatric literature. *Journal of Critical Care, 30*(4), 664–672.

Centers for Disease Control and Prevention (CDC), National Institute for Occupational Safety and Health (NIOSH). (2015). *Safe patient handling and mobility (SPHM)*. Retrieved from http://www.cdc.gov/niosh/topics/. [Accessed August 2, 2021].

Choi, S. D., & Brings, K. (2015). Work-related musculoskeletal risks associated with nurses and nursing assistants handling overweight and obese patients: A literature review. *Work, 53*(2), 439–448.

Darragh, A. R., Shiyko, M., Margulis, H., & Campo, M. (2014). Effects of a safe patient handling and mobility program on patient self-care outcomes. *American Journal of Occupational Therapy, 68*(5), 589–596.

T

E, J. Y., Lee, T., McInally, L., et al. (2020). Environmental and behavioural interventions for reducing physical activity limitation and preventing falls in older people with visual impairment. *Cochrane Database of Systematic Reviews, 9*, CD009233. doi:10.1002/14651858.CD009233.pub3.
Hallmark, B., Mechan, P., & Shores, L. (2015). Ergonomics: Safe patient handling and mobility. *Nursing Clinics of North America, 50*(1), 153–166.
Hamadi, H., Probst, J. C., Khan, M. M., Bellinger, J., & Porter, C. (2018). Determinants of occupational injury for US home health aides reporting one or more work-related injuries. *Injury Prevention, 24*(5), 351–357.
Hartung, B., & Lalonde, M. (2017). The use of non-slip socks to prevent falls among hospitalized older adults: A literature review. *Geriatric Nursing, 38*(5), 412–416.
Heng, H., Jazayeri, D., Shaw, L., Kiegaldie, D., Hill, A. M., & Morris, M. E. (2020). Hospital falls prevention with patient education: A scoping review. *BMC Geriatrics, 20*(1), 140. https://doi.org/10.1186/s12877-020-01515-w.
Hillrom Services, Inc. (2019). *Bedside mobility assessment tool for nurses.* Retrieved from https://library.hill-rom.com/Clinical-Programs/Safe-Transfers-and-Movement-Program/Design-Your-Program/BMAT---Bedside-Mobility-Assessment-Tool-For-Nurses/. [Accessed August 2, 2021].
Hopkins, R. O., Mitchell, L., Thomsen, G. E., Schafer, M., Link, M., & Brown, S. M. (2016). Implementing a mobility program to minimize post-intensive care syndrome. *AACN Advanced Critical Care, 27*(2), 187–203.
Jones, R. A., Merkle, S., Ruvalcaba, L., Ashton, P., Bailey, C., & Lopez, M. (2020). Nurse-led mobility program: Driving a culture of early mobilization in medical-surgical nursing. *Journal of Nursing Care Quality, 35*(1), 20–26. https://doi.org/10.1097/NCQ.0000000000000404.
Keall, M. D., Pierse, N., Howden-Chapman, P., et al. (2015). Home modifications to reduce injuries from falls in the home injury prevention intervention (HIPI) study: A cluster-randomised controlled trial. *Lancet, 385*(9964), 231–238. doi:10.1016/S0140-6736(14)61006-0.
Kearon, C., Akl, E. A., Ornelas, J., et al. (2016). Antithrombotic therapy for VTE disease: CHEST guideline and expert panel report. *Chest, 149*(2), 315–352.
Lamb, S. E., Bruce, J., Hossain, A., Ji, C., Longo, R., Lall, R., & Prevention of Fall Injury Trial Study Group., et al. (2020). Screening and intervention to prevent falls and fractures in older people. *New England Journal of Medicine, 383*(19), 1848–1859. https://doi.org/10.1056/NEJMoa2001500.
Lee, S. J., & Lee, J. H. (2017). Safe patient handling behaviors and lift use among hospital nurses: A cross-sectional study. *International Journal of Nursing Studies, 74*, 53–60.
Lee, S. J., & Rempel, D. (2020). Comparison of lift use, perceptions, and musculoskeletal symptoms between ceiling lifts and floor-based lifts in patient handling. *Applied Ergonomics, 82*, 102954. https://doi.org/10.1016/j.apergo.2019.102954.
Low, L. F., Fletcher, J., Goodenough, B., et al. (2015). A systematic review of interventions to change staff care practices in order to improve resident outcomes in nursing homes. *PLoS One, 10*(11), e0140711. doi:10.1371/journal.pone.0140711.
National Committee for Quality Assurance–Health Care Accreditation Organization. (2015a). *Geriatrics: Percentage of patients aged 65 and older with a history of falls who had a plan of care for falls documented within 12 months.* National Quality Measures Clearinghouse. Retrieved from https://www.guidelinecentral.com/share/quality-measures/49449#h2_measure-domain. [Accessed November 27, 2021].
National Committee for Quality Assurance–Health Care Accreditation Organization. (2015b). *Geriatrics: Percentage of patients aged 65 and older discharged from any inpatient facility (e.g., hospital, skilled nursing facility, or rehabilitation facility) and seen within 30 days of discharge in the office by the physician, prescribing practitioner, registered nurse, or clinical pharmacist who had reconciliation of the discharge medications with the current medication list in the outpatient medical record documented.* National Quality Measures Clearinghouse. Retrieved from https://www.guidelinecentral.com/share/quality-measures/49444#h2_measure-domain. [Accessed November 27, 2021].
Putthinoi, S., Lersilp, S., & Chakpitak, N. (2017). Home features and assistive technology for the home-bound elderly in a Thai suburban community by applying the international classification of functioning, disability and health. *Journal of Aging Research*, 2865960 2017. https://doi.org/10.1155/2017/2865960.
Riccoboni, J. B., Monnet, T., Eon, A., Lacouture, P., Gazeau, J. P., & Campone, M. (2021). Biomechanical comparison between manual and motorless device assisted patient handling: Sitting to and from standing position. *Applied Ergonomics, 90*, 103284. https://doi.org/10.1016/j.apergo.2020.103284.
Romanoski, N. L., & Swope, K. (2018). Durable medical equipment that supports activities of daily living, transfers and ambulation. *Essentials of Rehabilitation Practice and Science.* Retrieved from https://now.aapmr.org/durable-medical-equipment-that-supports-activities-of-daily-living-transfers-and-ambulation/. [Accessed August 2, 2021].
Teeple, E., Collins, J. E., Shrestha, S., Dennerlein, J. T., Losina, E., & Katz, J. N. (2017). Outcomes of safe patient handling and mobilization programs: A meta-analysis. *Work, 58*(2), 173–184. doi:10.3233/WOR-172608.
Tipping, C. J., Harrold, M., Holland, A., Romero, L., Nisbet, T., & Hodgson, C. L. (2017). The effects of active mobilisation and rehabilitation in ICU on mortality and function: A systematic review. *Intensive Care Medicine, 43*(2), 171–183. https://doi.org/10.1007/s00134-016-4612-0

Risk for Physical Trauma

Domain 11 Safety/protection Class 2 Physical injury

Julianne E. Doubet, BSN, RN, EMT-B

NANDA-I

Definition

Vulnerable to accidental tissue injury (e.g., wound, burn, fracture), which may compromise health.

Risk Factors

External

Absence of call for aid device; absence of stairway gate; absence of window guard; access to weapon; bathing in very hot water; bed in high position; children riding in front seat of car; defective appliance; delay in ignition of gas appliance; dysfunctional call for aid device; electrical hazard (e.g., faulty plug, frayed wire, overloaded outlet/fuse box); exposure to corrosive product; exposure to dangerous machinery; exposure to radiation; exposure to toxic chemical; extremes of environmental temperature; flammable object (e.g., clothing, toys); gas leak; grease on stove; high-crime neighborhood; icicles hanging from roof; inadequate stair rails; inadequately stored combustible (e.g., matches, oily rags); inadequately stored corrosive (e.g., lye); insufficient lighting; insufficient protection from heat source; misuse of headgear (e.g., hard hat, motorcycle helmet); misuse of seat restraint; insufficient antislip material in bathroom; nonuse of seat restraints; obstructed passageway; playing with dangerous object; playing with explosive; pot handle facing front of stove; proximity to vehicle pathway (e.g., driveway, railroad track); slippery floor; smoking in bed; smoking near oxygen; struggling with restraints; unanchored electric wires; unsafe operation of heavy equipment (e.g., excessive speed while intoxicated with required eyewear); unsafe road; unsafe walkway; use of cracked dishware; use of throw rugs; use of unstable chair; use of unstable ladder; wearing loose clothing around open flame

Internal

Alteration in cognitive functioning; alteration in sensation (e.g., resulting from spinal cord injury, diabetes mellitus); decrease in eye–hand coordination; decrease in muscle coordination; economically disadvantaged; emotional disturbance; history of trauma (e.g., physical, psychological, sexual); impaired balance; insufficient knowledge of safety precautions; insufficient vision; weakness

NOC (Nursing Outcomes Classification)

Suggested NOC Outcomes

Risk Control; Fall Prevention Behavior

Example NOC Outcome with Indicators

Accomplishes **Risk Control** as evidenced by the following indicators: Acknowledges risk/Develops effective risk-control strategies/Follows selected risk control strategies. (Rate the outcome and indicators of **Risk Control:** 1 = never demonstrated; 2 = rarely demonstrated; 3 = sometimes demonstrated; 4 = often demonstrated; 5 = consistently demonstrated [see Section I].)

Client Outcomes

Client Will (Specify Time Frame)

- Remain free from trauma
- Explain actions that can be taken to prevent trauma

NIC (Nursing Interventions Classification)

Suggested NIC Interventions

Environmental Management: Safety; Skin Surveillance

Example NIC Activities—Environmental Management

Provide family/significant other with information about making home environment safe for client; Remove harmful objects from the environment

T

Nursing Interventions and *Rationales*

- Provide vision aids for visually impaired clients. EB: *Low-vision rehabilitation enables people to restart and/or maintain the capability of performing the tasks of daily living (Virgili et al, 2013).* EB: *Electronic low vision aids have been linked to an improvement in the visually impaired client's psychological health and welfare (Garcia et al, 2017).*
- Assist the client with ambulation. Encourage the client to use assistive devices in activities of daily living (ADLs) as needed. EB: *Studies reviewed by Edelstein (2013) have shown the advantages, if used correctly, of using time-honored assistive devices (e.g., crutches, walker).* EBN: *According to the results of a study by Ali et al (2020), assistive devices can ease the effects of diminished day-to-day capabilities, plus add support for strength and flexibility, enhance motor control, and increase sensory function.*

- Evaluate client's risk for burn injury. CEBN: *Grant (2013) stated that the very young and the elderly are at an increased risk for burn injuries compared with any other age group.* EBN: *It is apparent to Goodarzi et al (2014) in their research that there is a continuing need for further safety.* EBN: *Comparatively small burns can be a threat to the health status of elderly victims (Sheaffer, 2018).*
- Assess the client for causes of impaired cognition. EB: *Adults with intellectual disabilities are likely to have an elevated risk for traumatic injury compared with the general populace (Finlayson et al, 2014).* EBN: *The earlier that cognitive problems are recognized, the sooner the client can be referred for advanced evaluation, which will give them the opportunity to review possible reversible causes and the option to discuss their concerns (Scott & Mayo, 2018).*
- Provide assistive devices in the home. EBN: *According to Johnston et al (2014), shared conclusions between the health caregiver and the client with disabilities allows the client to choose the best assistive devices and services that are vital to achieving their goals of education, community living, and employment.* EB: *Health care professionals who assess for and advocate for assistive devices (ADs) for their clients should promote a mutual decision-making relationship with those same clients (Tuazon et al, 2019).*
- ▲ Question the client concerning his or her sense of safety. EBN: *In their study, Edwards et al (2014) stated that clients who wish to remain at home at the end of life are at increased risk for trauma caused by declining cognitive and/or physical capabilities, environmental dangers, and concerns with caregivers.* EBN: *Kenward et al (2017) advocate maintaining consistent quality care for clients so that nurses can be a factor in the decrease of clients' perceptions of being exposed and at risk.*
- ▲ Assess for a substance abuse problem and refer to appropriate resources for drug and alcohol education. EB: *According to Choi, DiNitto, and Marti (2016), older adults who abuse alcohol and/or illicit drugs should be sent to the most appropriate service that meets their needs, both for rehabilitation and for any mental health challenges that may be involved. Although drinking and driving among student drivers has declined in recent years, driving after the use of marijuana has increased; therefore, O'Malley and Johnston (2013) believed that more attention should be focused on preventing those under the influence of illicit drugs from driving.* EBN: *"Screening, Brief Intervention, and Referral to Treatment (SBIRT)" is an evidence-based intercession for those with symptoms of substance abuse (Thoele et al, 2020).*
- Review drug profile for potential side effects that may inhibit performance of ADLs. EB: *In their study of pain management in the elderly, Veal and Peterson (2015) found that older adults are at increased risk for detrimental medication side effects caused by changes in drug metabolism and due to polypharmacy that may put them at risk for drug interactions. A study by Graziano et al (2018) found that many medications taken by older clients have the potential to interact and may cause an exacerbation of symptoms and side effects.*
- See care plans for Risk for **Aspiration,** Risk for **Falls,** Impaired **Home** Maintenance, Risk for **Injury,** Risk for **Poisoning,** and Risk for **Suffocation.**

Pediatric

- Assess the client's socioeconomic status. EB: *The presently used evaluations that measure evidence of adverse childhood experiences may be insufficient to recognize the extent of adversity to which low-income urban children are exposed (Wade et al, 2014).* EBN: *As a consequence of children living with the threat of housing uncertainty, there is a good probability that they will have reduced opportunities to utilize the health care system, therefore triggering more emergency department visits and, in addition, impeded awareness of their basic physical and mental health care needs (Parry et al, 2020).*
- Never leave young children unsupervised. EB: *According to van Beelen et al (2014), the death, disability, and loss of quality of life among young children is directly related to injuries that occur in the home.* EBN: *Homes remain ripe locations for accidental mishaps, as they have numerous high-risk areas that could be lethal for children (e.g., windows, stairs, sharp objects, cleaning supplies) (Soares Silva et al, 2016).*
- Keep flammable and potentially flammable articles out of reach of young children. EB: *Infants and toddlers who scald themselves by spilling hot liquids on themselves or touching irons and hair straighteners are a main cause for concern for targeted prevention (Kemp et al, 2014).* EBN: *Hollywood and O'Neill (2014) maintained that nurses working with children in hospitals, schools, and the community can connect with parents, families, school staff, and children to offer professional advice and health and safety guidance for burn prevention.* EB: *Juškauskienė and Raškelienė (2018), in their review of studies concerning children's burns, found that the lack of supervision is a key issue in childhood thermal injuries and that the danger of injury is strongly associated with a deficiency in parental awareness.*
- Lock up harmful objects such as guns. EB: *Easy access to firearms in the home is responsible for injury to thousands of children in the United States (Barton & Kologi, 2015). There is an increased risk for childhood*

T

injury when firearms are left loaded and unlocked (Schwebel et al, 2014). EBN: *Beal (2019), in her article concerning gun safety for children, states that nurses are essential to the research and prevention of pediatric firearm injuries and deaths.* EB: *Evidenced-based firearm restriction programs are necessary to decrease firearm morbidity and mortality in youth (Ngo et al, 2019).*

Geriatric

- Assess the geriatric client's cognitive level of functioning. EB: *Patel et al (2015) agreed that the occurrence of neurocognitive disorders can be an obstacle to the capability of older adults to perform ADLs and this deficit will continue to escalate with age.* EB: *Early interventions can hold back cognitive deterioration, help maintain functional capacities, and even postpone the need for long-term care (Evans, 2018).*
- Assess for routine eye examinations. EBN: *The older client may find it difficult to adjust to vision loss and aging because of the psychological, functional, social, and health implications that play a significant role in the process (Mac Cobb, 2013).* EB: *Vision diminishes with age in every racial and ethnic group (Umfress & Brantley, 2016).*
- Perform a home safety assessment and recommend the following preventive measures: keep electrical cords out of the flow of traffic; remove small rugs or make sure they are slip resistant; increase lighting in hallways and other dark areas; place a light in the bathroom; keep towels, curtains, and other items that might catch fire away from the stove; store harmful products away from food products; provide at least one grab bar in tubs and showers; check prescribed medications for appropriate labels; store medications in original containers or in a dispenser of some type (e.g., egg carton, 7-day plastic dispenser). If the client cannot administer medications according to directions, secure someone to administer medications. Mark stove knobs with bright colors (yellow or red) and outline the borders of steps. CEBN: *As part of a person-centered, evidence-based approach, a professional case manager/care coordinator can perform a thorough assessment of the client's needs and will design and put into operation an all-inclusive care plan to meet the clinical, psychosocial, and environmental requirements of the client (Johansson & Harkey, 2014).*
- Discourage driving at night. EB: *Gruber et al (2013) suggested that there is an increasing number of older adults who continue to drive, and the population of drivers who are affected by deteriorating night vision is increasing.* EB: *Early visual assessment may expose conditions that could impair driving skills (Cummings & Fernandez, 2020).*
- Encourage the client to participate in resistance and impact exercise programs as tolerated. EB: *In their review of current evidence, Carvalho et al (2014) suggested that physical activity may not only aid in improving cognitive function in older adults but could also play a part in delaying the development of cognitive impairment in the older adult.* EBN: *Niebauer et al (2018) noted that when age-adjusted exercise was introduced into geriatric day care, significant improvement was made in the clients' muscle strength and balance.*

Client/Family Teaching and Discharge Planning

- Educate the family regarding age-appropriate child safety precautions, environmental safety precautions, and intervention in an emergency. EB: *Safety education for parents of young children is essential in the prevention of accidental injuries in and/or around the home (van Beelen et al, 2013).* EB: *In their study, Morrongiello, McArthur, and Bell (2014) found that to decrease a child's risk of harm, the child must first understand the safety issue.* EBN: *Pediatric professionals will find it necessary to evaluate, ascertain, and employ interventions to combat the high rate of unintentional injuries that occur within the pediatric population, states Welch (2017).*
- Teach the family to assess the child care provider's knowledge regarding child safety. EB: *Home safety interventions not only aid in reducing children's injuries, but they also enhance the general safety of the home (Kendrick et al, 2013).* EBN: *Safeguarding and ensuring client safety is a critical component of competent health care delivery and includes both physical and psychosocial protection (Conroy et al, 2017).*
- Educate the client and family regarding helmet use during recreation and sports activities. EB: *It has been proven repeatedly that wearing a bicycle helmet has averted or reduced the risk of serious head injuries (Basch et al, 2014).* EB: *Opinions about helmet utilization can fluctuate depending on the cyclist and also due to culturally associated dynamics; assessment of attitudes in particular areas and within distinct populations will afford an enhanced basis for designing interventions (Ledesma et al, 2019).*
- Encourage the proper use of car seats and safety belts. EB: *Himle and Wright (2014) stated that child passenger safety restraint, when used correctly, can diminish the risk of severe injury and/or death in motor vehicle crashes.* EB: *According to Sicinska and Dabrowska-Loranc (2018), vehicle safety restraints for both children and adults are the easiest and most efficient passive safety devices that will significantly reduce injuries during an accident.*

- Teach parents to restrict driving for teens. EB: *According to Taubman-Ben-Ari et al (2014), research studies have shown that parents are the most important influence on young people's driving conduct.* EB: *Findings by Naz and Scott-Parker (2017) imply that parents of teens need to be knowledgeable about the consequences of their involvement in the teen's driver's licensing process, the importance of coaching, and their own driving performance.*
- Teach parents the importance of monitoring children after school. EB: *In a study by Freisthler et al (2014), children who are not supervised appropriately, either by inattentive parents and/or caregivers, could be considered neglected.* EB: *Smith and Bradshaw (2017) note that afterschool programs are developing into strategic settings for the avoidance of problem conduct for unsupervised youth and that they also play a role in the formation of positive behavior.*
- Teach firearm safety. EB: *According to Schwebel et al (2014), firearms in the home that are loaded and unlocked are sources of increased risks for trauma.* EB: *Health care professionals must have knowledge and skills to address safe gun ownership in older adults (Pinholt et al, 2014).* EBN: *Nurses, no matter what their specialty, can influence others with their competence and concern and help solve the problem of gun safety (Kronebusch, 2020).*
- For further information, refer to care plans for Risk for **Aspiration,** Risk for **Falls,** Impaired **Home** Maintenance, Risk for **Injury,** Risk for **Poisoning,** and Risk for **Suffocation.**

REFERENCES

Ali, J. S., El-sayed Ramadan, R. M., & Aboushady, R. M. N. (2020). *Stroke rehabilitation strategies to enhance activities of daily living.* Moldova: Lambert Academic Publishing. Retrieved from researchgate.net. [Accessed November 3, 2020].

Barton, B. K., & Kologi, S. M. (2015). Why do you keep them there? A qualitative assessment of firearms storage practices. *Journal of Pediatric Nursing, 30*(2), 285–293.

Basch, C. H., Ethan, D., Rajan, S., Samayoa-Kozlowsky, S., & Basch, C. E. (2014). Helmet use among users of the Citi Bike bicycle-sharing program: A pilot study in New York City. *Journal of Community Health, 39*(3), 503–507.

Beal, J. A. (2019). Children and gun safety: a call to action for nurses. *American Journal of Maternal Child Nursing, 44*(3), 171. https://doi10.1097/NMC.0000000000000522.

Carvalho, A., Rea, I. M., Pariman, T., & Cusack, B. J. (2014). Physical activity and cognitive function in individuals over 60 years of age: A systematic review. *Clinical Interventions in Aging, 9*, 661–682.

Choi, N. G., DiNitto, D. M., & Marti, C. N. (2016). Risk factors for self-reported driving under the influence of alcohol and/or illicit drugs among older adults. *Gerontologist, 56*(2), 282–291.

Conroy, T., Feo, R., Boucaut, R., Alderman, J., & Kitson, A. (2017). Role of effective nurse-patient relationships in enhancing patient safety. *Nursing Standard, 31*(49), 53–63. https://doi:10.7798/ns.2017.e10801.

Cummings, K., & Fernandez, H. (2020). Driving. In A. Chun (Ed.), *Geriatric practice: A competency based approach to caring for older adults* (pp. 335–344). Cham, Switzerland: Springer. https://doi.org/10.1007/978-3-030-19625-7_27.

Edelstein, J. E. (2013). Assistive devices for ambulation. *Physical Medicine and Rehabilitation Clinics of North America, 29*(2), 291–303.

Edwards, S. B., Galanis, E., McGarvey, K., Prestwich, C., Ritcey, S., & Wulf, K. (2014). Safety issues at the end of life in the home setting. *Home Healthcare Nurse, 32*(7), 396–401.

Evans, S. C. (2018). Ageism and dementia. In L. Ayalon, & C. Tesch-Römer (Eds.), *Contemporary perspectives on ageism* (pp. 263–275). Cham, Switzerland: Springer. Retrieved from http://www.springer.com/series/8818. [Accessed November 3, 2020].

Finlayson, J., Jackson, A., Mantry, D., Morrison, J., & Cooper, S. A. (2014). The provision of aids and adaptations, risk assessments, and incident reporting and recording procedures in relation to injury prevention for adults with intellectual disabilities: Cohort study. *Journal of Intellectual Disability Research, 59*(6), 519–529.

Freisthler, B., Johnson-Motoyama, M., & Kepple, N. J. (2014). Inadequate child supervision: The role of alcohol outlet density, parent drinking behaviors, and social support. *Children and Youth Service Review, 43*, 75–84.

Garcia, G. A., Khoshnevis, M., Gale, J., et al. (2017). Profound vision loss impairs psychological well-being in young and middle-aged individuals. *Clinical Ophthalmology, 11*, 417–427. htpps://doi:10.2147/OPTH.S113414.

Goodarzi, M., Reisi-Dehkordi, N., Daryabeigi, R., & Zargham-Boroujeni, A. (2014). An epidemiologic study of burns: Standards of care and patients' outcomes. *Iranian Journal of Nursing and Midwifery Research, 19*(4), 385–389.

Grant, E. J. (2013). Preventing burns in the elderly: A guide for home healthcare professionals. *Home Healthcare Nurse, 31*(10), 561–575.

Graziano, O., Giovannini, S., Sganga, F., et al. (2018). Interactions between drugs and geriatric syndromes in nursing home and home care: results from Shelter and IBenC projects. *Aging and Clinical and Experimental Research, 30*(9) 1025-1021. https://doi.org/10.1007/s40520-018-0893-1.

Gruber, N., Mosimann, U. P., Müri, R. M., & Nef, T. (2013). Vision and night driving abilities of elderly drivers. *Traffic Injury Prevention, 14*(5), 477–485.

Himle, M. B., & Wright, K. A. (2014). Behavioral skills training to improve installation and use of child passenger safety restraints. *Journal of Applied Behavior Analysis, 47*(3), 549–559.

Hollywood, E., & O'Neill, T. (2014). Assessment and management of scalds and burns in children. *Nursing Children and Young People, 26*(2), 28–33.

Johansson, B., & Harkey, J. (2014). Care coordination in long-term home- and community-based care. *Home Healthcare Nurse, 32*(8), 470–475.

Johnston, P., Currie, L. M., Drynan, D., Stainton, T., & Jongbloed, L. (2014). Getting it "right": How collaborative relationships between people with disabilities and professionals can lead to acquisition of needed assistive technology. *Disability and Rehabilitation: Assistive Technology, 9*(5), 421–431.

Juškauskienė, E., & Raškelienė, V. (2018). *Parent's knowledge about burns prevention of their children* [thesis]. Kaunas, Lithuania: Lithuanian University of Health Sciences. Retrieved from https://hdl.handle.net/20.500.12512/97314. [Accessed February 28, 2022].

T

Kemp, A. M., Jones, S., Lawson, Z., & Maguire, S. A. (2014). Patterns of burns and scalds in children. *Archives of Diseases in Childhood, 99*(4), 316–321.

Kendrick, D., Mulvaney, C. A., Ye, L., Stevens, T., Mytton, J. A., & Stewart-Brown, S. (2013). Parenting interventions for the prevention of unintentional injuries in childhood. *Cochrane Database of Systematic Reviews, 3,* CD006020.

Kenward, R., Wiffin, C., & Spalek, B. (2017). Feeling unsafe in the healthcare setting: patients' perspective. *British Journal of Nursing, 26*(3), 143–149. https://doi.org/10.12968/bjon.2017.26.3.143.

Kronebusch, B. (2020). Activating nurse collective energy. *Nursing Economics; Pitman, 38*(2), 97,103. Retrieved from https://nursingeconomics.net/nec files/2020/MA20. [Accessed November 3, 2020].

Ledesma, R. D., Shinar, D., Valero-Mora, P. M., et al. (2019). Psychosocial factors associated with helmet use by adult cyclists. *Transportation Research Part F: Traffic Psychology and Behaviour, 65,* 376–388. https://doi.org/10.1016/j.trf.2019.08.003.

Mac Cobb, S. (2013). Mobility restriction and comorbidity in vision-impaired individuals living in the community. *British Journal of Community Nursing, 18*(12), 608–613.

Morrongiello, B. A., McArthur, B. A., & Bell, M. (2014). Managing children's risk of injury in the home: Does parental teaching about home safety reduce young children's hazard interactions? *Accident; Analysis and Prevention, 71,* 194–200.

Naz, S., & Scott-Parker, B. (2017). Obstacles to engaging in young driver licensing: perspectives of parents. *Accident; Analysis and Prevention, 99*(Part A), 312–320. https://doi.org/10.1016/j.aap.2016.12.006.

Ngo, Q. M., Sigel, E., Moon, A., et al. (2019). State of the science: A scoping review of primary prevention of firearm injuries among children and adolescents. *Journal of Behavioral Medicine, 42*(4), 811–829. https://doi.org/10.1007/s10865-019-00043-2.

Niebauer, J., Schreier, M. M., Bauer, U., Reiss, J., Osterbrink, J., & Iglseder, B. (2018). Combined endurance and resistance training during geriatric day care improve exercise capacity, balance and strength. *Sports Orthopaedics and Traumatology, 34*(1), 15–22. https://doi.org/10.1016/j.orthtr.2017.09.009.

O'Malley, P. M., & Johnston, L. D. (2013). Driving after drug or alcohol use by US high school seniors, 2001-2011. *American Journal of Public Health, 103*(11), 2027–2034.

Parry, Y., Willis, E., Kendall, S., Marriott, R., Sivertsen, N., & Bell, A. (2020). Meeting the needs of marginalised children: An innovative nurse practitioner led health care model at Uniting Care Wesley Bowden. *Australian Nursing and Midwifery Journal, 26*(10), 48–49. Retrieved from. https://issuu.com/australiannursingfederation/docs/anmj___2020___apr-june___issuu. [Accessed November 2, 2020].

Patel, D., Syed, Q., Messinger-Rapport, B. J., & Rader, E. (2015). Firearms in frail hands: An ADL or public health crisis. *American Journal of Alzheimer's Disease and Other Dementias, 30*(4), 337–340. pii:1533317514545867.

Pinholt, E. M., Mitchell, J. D., Butler, J. H., & Kumar, H. (2014). "Is there a gun in the home?" Assessing the risks of gun ownership in older adults. *Journal of the American Geriatrics Society, 62*(6), 1142–1146.

Schwebel, D. C., Lewis, T., Simon, T. R., et al. (2014). Prevalence and correlates of firearm ownership in the homes of fifth graders: Birmingham, AL., Houston, TX., and Los Angeles, CA. *Health Education & Behavior, 41*(3), 299–306.

Scott, J., & Mayo, A. M. (2018). Instruments for detection and screening of cognitive impairment for older adults in primary care settings: A review. *Geriatric Nursing, 39*(3), 323–329. https://doi.org/10.1016/gerinurse.2017.11.001.

Sheaffer, J. (2018). Nursing considerations in the care of elderly burn patients. In A. Rodriguez, R. D. Barraco, & R. R. Ivatury (Eds.), *Geriatric trauma and acute care surgery* (pp. 465–474). Cham, Switzerland: Springer. https://doi.org/10.1007/978-3-319-57403-5_53.

Sicinska, K., & Dabrowska-Loranc, M. (2018). Influence of social campaigns promoting use of safety belts and child restraint systems: Results of survey on road users behaviour regarding restraints. *Transport Problems, 13*(4), 77–90. https://doi:10.20858/tp.2018.13.4.8.

Smith, E. P., & Bradshaw, C. P. (2017). Promoting nurturing environments in afterschool settings. *Clinical Child and Family Psychology Review, 20*(2), 117–126. https://doi.org/10.1007/s10567-017-0239-0.

Soares Silva, E. C., Neyrian de Fátima Fernandes, M., Nascimento Sá, M. C., et al. (2016). The effect of educational intervention regarding the knowledge of mothers on prevention of accidents in childhood. *The Open Nursing Journal, 10,* 113–121. https://doi.org/10.2174/1874434601610010113.

Taubman-Ben-Ari, O., Musicant, O., Lotan, T., & Farah, H. (2014). The contribution of parents' driving behavior, family climate for road safety, and parent-targeted intervention to young male driving behavior. *Accident; Analysis and Prevention, 72,* 296–301.

Thoele, K., Draucker, C. B., & Newhouse, R. (2020). *Implementation of screening, brief intervention, and referral to treatment (SBIRT) by nurses on acute care units: A qualitative descriptive study.* Substance Abuse [Online ahead of print]. https://doi:10.1080/08897077.2020.1823549.

Tuazon, J. R., Jahan, A., & Jutai, J. W. (2019). Understanding adherence to assistive devices among older adults: A conceptual review. *Disability and Rehabilitation: Assistive Technology, 14*(5), 424–433. https://doi:10.1080/17483107.2018.1493753.

Umfress, A. C., & Brantley, M. A., Jr. (2016). Eye care disparities and health-related consequences in elderly patients with age-related eye disease. *Seminars in Ophthalmology, 31*(4), 432–438. https://doi:10.3109/08820538.2016.1154171.

van Beelen, M. E. J., Beirens, T. M. J., den Hertog, P., van Beeck, E. F., & Raat, H. (2014). Effectiveness of web-based tailored advice on parents' child safety behaviors: Randomized controlled trial. *Journal of Medical Internet Research, 16*(1), e17.

van Beelen, M. E. J., Vogel, I., Beirens, T. M. J., et al. (2013). Web-based ehealth to support counseling in routine well-child care: Pilot study of E-Health4Uth home safety. *Journal of Medical Internet Research, 2*(1) e9.

Veal, F. C., & Peterson, G. M. (2015). Pain in the frail or elderly patient: Does tapentadol have a role? *Drugs & Aging, 32*(6), 419–426.

Virgili, G., Acosta, R., Grover, L. L., Bentley, S. A., & Giacomelli, G. (2013). Reading aids for adults with low vision. *Cochrane Database of Systematic Reviews, 10,* CD003303.

Wade, R., Jr., Shea, J. A., Rubin, D., & Wood, J. (2014). Adverse childhood experiences of low-income urban youth. *Pediatrics, 134*(1), e13–e20.

Welch, M. K. (2017). *Pediatric providers knowledge on unintentional childhood injury* [dissertation]. Tucson, AZ: University of Arizona. Retrieved from http://hdl.handle.net/10150/626653. [Accessed November 2, 2020].

Unilateral Neglect Domain 5 Perception/cognition Class 1 Attention

Wendy R. Worden, MS, APRN, CNS, CRRN, CWCN

NANDA-I

Definition

Impairment in sensory and motor response, mental representation, and spatial attention of the body, and the corresponding environment, characterized by inattention to one side and overattention to the opposite side. Left-side neglect is more severe and persistent than right-side neglect.

Defining Characteristics

Altered safety behavior on neglected side; disturbed sound lateralization; failure to dress neglected side; failure to eat food from portion of plate on neglected side; failure to groom neglected side; failure to move eyes in the neglected hemisphere; failure to move head in the neglected hemisphere; failure to move limbs in the neglected hemisphere; failure to move trunk in the neglected hemisphere; failure to notice people approaching from the neglected side; hemianopsia; impaired performance on line bisection tests; impaired performance on line cancellation tests; impaired performance on target cancellation tests; left hemiplegia from cerebrovascular accident; marked deviation of the eyes to stimuli on the non-neglected side; marked deviation of the trunk to stimuli on the non-neglected side; omission of drawing on the neglected side; perseveration; representational neglect; substitution of letters to form alternative words when reading; transfer of pain sensation to the non-neglected side; unaware of positioning of neglected limb; unilateral visuospatial neglect; uses vertical half of page only when writing

Related Factors

To be developed

Associated Conditions

Brain injuries

NOC (Nursing Outcomes Classification)

Suggested NOC Outcomes

Body Image; Body Positioning: Self-Initiated; Mobility; Self-Care: Activities of Daily Living (ADLs)

Example NOC Outcome with Indicators

Mobility as evidenced by the following indicators: Balance/Coordination/Gait/Muscle movement. (Rate the outcome and indicators of **Mobility:** 1 = severely compromised, 2 = substantially compromised, 3 = moderately compromised, 4 = mildly compromised, 5 = not compromised [see Section I].)

Client Outcomes

Client Will (Specify Time Frame)

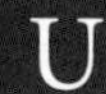
U

- Use techniques that can be used to minimize unilateral neglect (UN)
- Care for both sides of the body appropriately and keep affected side free from harm
- Return to the highest functioning level possible based on personal goals and abilities
- Remain free from injury

NIC (Nursing Interventions Classification)

Suggested NIC Intervention

Unilateral Neglect Management

Example NIC Activities—Unilateral Neglect Management

Ensure that affected extremities are properly and safely and positioned; Rearrange the environment to use the right or left visual field

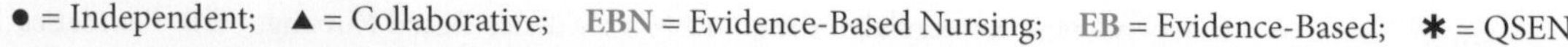

Nursing Interventions and *Rationales*

- ▲ Assess the client for signs of UN (e.g., not washing, shaving, or dressing one side of the body; sitting or lying inappropriately on affected arm or leg; failing to respond to environmental stimuli contralateral to the side of lesion; eating food on only one side of plate; reading words on one side of the page; or failing to look to one side of the body). EB: *Many tests for UN exist, but there is no consensus about which is the most valid. Joint assessments that include clinical observation, behavioral assessment, and precise testing perform better than any used individually (Azouvi, 2017; Grattan & Woodbury, 2017).* EB: *Single use of the National Institutes of Health Stroke Scale (NIHSS) led to underdiagnosis of UN in 56% of cases. In one study, 72.8% of clients had UN on admission to inpatient rehabilitation (Puig-Pijoan et al, 2018; Tarvonen-Schröder et al, 2020).*
- ▲ Collaborate with health care provider for referral to a rehabilitation team (including, but not limited to, rehabilitation clinical nurse specialist, physical medicine and rehabilitation health care provider, neuropsychologist, occupational therapist, physical therapist, and speech and language pathologist) for continued help in dealing with UN. EB: *There is some evidence that rehabilitation for unilateral spatial neglect using tools such as visual scanning and prism adaptation improves function, but their effect on disability is not clear (Gillen et al, 2015).* EB: *Challenging the client in the complexity of everyday tasks and environments can assist clients in physical and cognitive recovery (Brown & Powell, 2017).*
- ● Use the principles of rehabilitation to progressively increase the client's ability to compensate for UN by using assistive devices, feedback, and support. EB: *Studies demonstrated that recovery from UN generally resolves within 1 month of stroke, but it can still be detectable after 3 months and/or at discharge from inpatient rehabilitation (Chen et al, 2015).*
- ● Teach the client to be aware of the problem and modify behavior and environment. EB: *Awareness of the environment decreases risk of injury. There is some evidence that use of virtual environment therapy aids the client in creating some independence to perform everyday tasks such as crossing the street (Conti & Arnone, 2016).*
- ● Set up the environment so that essential activity is on the unaffected side:
  - ❍ Place the client's personal items within view and on the unaffected side.
  - ❍ Position the bed so that client is approached from the unaffected side.
  - ❍ Monitor and assist the client to achieve adequate food and fluid intake.

  Helps in focusing attention and aids in maintenance of safety.
- ● Implement fall prevention interventions as clients with right hemisphere brain damage are twice as likely to fall as those with left hemisphere damage. EB: *Clients with impaired balance, decreased mobility, depression, and reduced safety awareness after stroke have higher fall rates than the general population (Xu et al, 2018).*
- ● Position affected extremity in a safe and functional manner. EB: *A study found that poststroke musculoskeletal pain, shoulder subluxation, spasticity, and joint contracture were among the most common complications during the subacute and chronic stages (15 days to >3 months) (Paolucci et al, 2016).* EB: *One study found that in stroke survivors with visuospatial neglect or an affected left arm, use of vision as a strategy does not help compensate for impaired position sense (Herter, Scott, & Dukelow, 2019).*
- ▲ Collaborate closely with rehabilitation professionals to identify and reinforce therapies aimed at reducing neglect symptoms. EB: *Techniques such as repeated scanning, visual cuing approaches, virtual reality, limb activation strategies, prisms, mirror therapy, mental imagery, music, neck vibration, and transcranial magnetic stimulation are being used to treat UN (Winstein et al, 2016), but the evidence is limited and inconclusive on the most effective approach (Azouvi, Jacquin-Courtois, & Luauté, 2017).*

Home Care

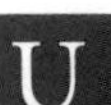

- ● Many of the previously listed interventions may be adapted for use in the home care setting.
- ● Position bed at home so that client gets out of bed on unaffected side. *Positioning the bed so that the client gets out on the unaffected side can increase safety.*

Client/Family Teaching and Discharge Planning

- ● Engage discharge planning specialists for comprehensive assessment and planning early in the client's stay. EB: *Clients with UN have longer lengths of stay and are more disabled due to functional motor and cognitive impairments (Spaccavento et al, 2017).*
- ● Encourage family participation in care to promote safety. EB: *One study found that safety issues (falls, crossing the street, driving) become problematic and related to lower levels of independence (Conti & Arnone, 2016).*

- Explain pathology and symptoms of UN to both the client and family. Family members may not understand that inattention is a complication of the neurological injury.
- Teach the client how to scan regularly to check the position of body parts and to regularly turn head from side to side for safety when ambulating, using a wheelchair, or doing self-care tasks. EB: *In one study, incorporating task-specific treatments, such as eating food from a plate and grooming, improved functional outcome and reduced neglect symptoms (Patole et al, 2015).*
- Teach caregivers to cue the client to the environment.

REFERENCES

Azouvi, P. (2017). The ecological assessment of unilateral neglect. *Annals of Physical and Rehabilitation Medicine*, *60*(3), 186–190. https://doi.org/10.1016/j.rehab.2015.12.005.

Azouvi, P., Jacquin-Courtois, S., & Luauté, J. (2017). Rehabilitation of neglect: Evidence-based medicine. *Annals of Physical and Rehabilitation Medicine*, *60*(3), 191–197. https://doi.org/10.1016/j.rehab.2016.10.006.

Brown, E. V. D., & Powell, J. M. (2017). Assessment of unilateral neglect in stroke. Simplification and structuring of test items. *British Journal of Occupational Therapy*, *80*(7), 448–452. https://doi.org/10.1177/0308022616685582.

Chen, P., Chen, C. C., Hreha, K., Goedert, K. M., & Barrett, A. M. (2015). Kessler Foundation Neglect Assessment Process uniquely measures spatial neglect during activities of daily living. *Archives of Physical Medicine and Rehabilitation*, *96*(5), 869–876.e1. https://doi.org/10.1016/j.apmr.2014.10.023.

Conti, R. P., & Arnone, J. M. (2016). Unilateral neglect: Assessment and rehabilitation. *International Journal of Neuroscience and Behavioral Science*, *4*(1), 1–10. https://doi.org/10.13189/ijnbs.2016.040101.

Gillen, G., Nilsen, D. M., Attridge, J., et al. (2015). Effectiveness of interventions to improve occupational performance of people with cognitive impairments after stroke: An evidence-based review. *American Journal of Occupational Therapy*, *69*(1), 9 6901180040p1. https://doi.org/10.5014/ajot.2015.012138.

Grattan, E. S., & Woodbury, M. L. (2017). Do neglect assessments detect neglect differently? *American Journal of Occupational Therapy*, *71*(3) 7103190050p1–7103190050p9. https://doi.org/10.5014/ajot.2017.025015.

Herter, T. M., Scott, S. H., & Dukelow, S. P. (2019). Vision does not always help stroke survivors compensate for impaired limb position sense. *Journal of NeuroEngineering and Rehabilitation*, *16*(1), 129. https://doi.org/10.1186/s12984-019-0596-7.

Paolucci, S., Iosa, M., Toni, D., et al. (2016). Prevalence and time course of post-stroke pain: A multicenter prospective hospital-based study. *Pain Medicine*, *17*(5), 924–930. https://doi.org/10.1093/pm/pnv019.

Patole, R. R., Kulkarni, V. N., Rairikar, S. A., Shyam, A. K., & Sancheti, P. (2015). Effect of task specific treatment in patients with unilateral neglect. *Indian Journal of Physiotherapy & Occupational Therapy*, *9*(1), 74–77. https://doi.org/10.5958/0973-5674.2015.00016.7.

Puig-Pijoan, A., Giralt-Steinhauer, E., Zabalza de Torres, A., et al. (2018). Under diagnosis of unilateral spatial neglect in stroke unit. *Acta Neurologica Scandinavica*, *138*(5), 441–446. https://doi.org/10.1111/ane.12998.

Spaccavento, S., Cellamare, F., Falcone, R., Loverre, A., & Nardulli, R. (2017). Effects of subtypes of neglect on functional outcome in stroke patients. *Annals of Physical and Rehabilitation Medicine*, *60*(6), 376–381. https://doi.org/10.1016/j.rehab.2017.07.245.

Tarvonen-Schröder, S., Niemi, T., & Koivisto, M. (2020). Comparison of functional recovery and outcome and discharge from subacute inpatient rehabilitation in patients with right or left stroke with and without contralateral spatial neglect. *Journal of Rehabilitation Medicine*, *52*(6), jrm00071. https://doi.org/10.2340/16501977-2698.

Winstein, C. J., Stein, J., Arena, R., et al. (2016). Guidelines for adult stroke rehabilitation and recovery: A guideline for healthcare professionals from the American Heart Association/American Stroke Association. *Stroke*, *47*(6), e98–e169. https://doi.org/10.1161/STR.0000000000000098.

Xu, T., Clemson, L., O'Loughlin, K., Lannin, N. A., Dean, C., & Koh, G. (2018). Risk factors for falls in community stroke survivors: A systematic review and meta-analysis. *Archives of Physical Medicine and Rehabilitation*, *99*(3), 563–573.e5. https://doi.org/10.1016/j.apmr.2017.06.032.

Impaired Urinary Elimination

Domain 3 Elimination and exchange Class 1 Urinary function

Kenneth J. Oja, PhD, RN

U

NANDA-I

Definition

Dysfunction in urine elimination.

Defining Characteristics

Dysuria; frequent voiding; nocturia; urinary hesitancy; urinary incontinence; urinary retention; urinary urgency

Related Factors

Alcohol consumption; altered environmental factor; caffeine consumption; environmental constraints; fecal impaction; improper toileting posture; ineffective toileting habits; insufficient privacy; involuntary sphincter relaxation; obesity; pelvic organ prolapse; smoking; use of aspartame; weakened bladder muscle; weakened supportive pelvic structure

At-Risk Population

Older adults; women

Associated Conditions

Anatomic obstruction; diabetes mellitus; sensory motor impairment; urinary tract infection

NOC (Nursing Outcomes Classification)

Suggested NOC Outcome

Urinary Elimination

Example NOC Outcome with Indicators

Urinary Elimination as evidenced by the following indicators: Urine clarity/urine odor, fluid intake, pain with urination. (Rate the outcome and indicators of **Urinary Elimination:** 1 = severely compromised 2 = substantially compromised, 3 = moderately compromised, 4 = mildly compromised, 5 = not compromised [see Section I].)

Client Outcomes

Client Will (Specify Time Frame)

- State absence of pain or excessive urgency during urination
- Demonstrate voiding frequency no more than every 2 hours

NIC (Nursing Interventions Classification)

Suggested NIC Intervention

Urinary Elimination Management

Example NIC Activities—Urinary Elimination Management

Monitor urinary elimination, including frequency, consistency, odor, volume, and color, as appropriate; Teach client signs and symptoms of urinary tract infection (UTI)

Nursing Interventions and *Rationales*

- Ask the client about urinary elimination patterns and concerns. EB: *Urinary elimination problems have many presenting signs and symptoms. Asking the client questions may help understand the subtle signs and symptoms associated with urinary elimination (Mayo Clinic, 2020).*
- Question the client regarding the following:
  - Presence of symptoms such as incontinence, dribbling, frequency, urgency, dysuria, and nocturia
  - Presence of pain in the area of the bladder
  - Pattern of urination and approximate amount
  - Possible aggravating and alleviating factors for urinary problems

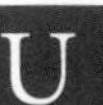

- Ask the client to keep a bladder diary/bladder log. EB: *Use of a bladder diary may provide the client with insight into their urinary patterns, afford them the opportunity to participate purposefully in their treatment plan, and assist them in identifying techniques to manage their symptoms (Dixon & Nakib, 2016).*
- For interventions on urinary incontinence, refer to the following nursing diagnosis care plans as appropriate: Stress Urinary **Incontinence,** Urge Urinary **Incontinence,** Reflex Urinary **Incontinence,** Overflow Urinary **Incontinence,** or Functional Urinary **Incontinence.**

▲ Perform a focused physical assessment including inspecting the perineal skin integrity, percussion, and palpation of the lower abdomen looking for obvious bladder distention or an enlarged kidney. EB: *A palpable kidney or bladder provides direct evidence of a dilated urinary collection system (Policastro, 2016).*

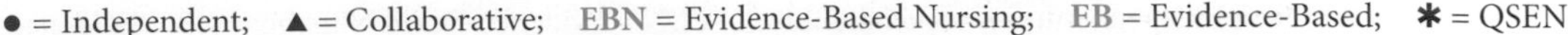

- ▲ If signs of urinary obstruction are present, refer client to a urologist. EB: *Unrelieved obstruction of urine can result in renal damage and, if severe, renal failure (Policastro, 2016). Refer to the nursing care plan for Urinary Retention if retention is present.*
- ● Check for costovertebral tenderness. EB: *Costovertebral tenderness is seen with pyelonephritis and kidney stones (Gupta & Trautner, 2015; Pietrucha-Dilanchian & Hooton, 2016).*
- ▲ Review results of urinalysis for the presence of urinary infection such as white blood cells, red blood cells, bacteria, and positive nitrites. EB: *If urinalysis results are not available, request a midstream specimen of urine (urine obtained during voiding, discarding the first and last portions) for a urinalysis (Pietrucha-Dilanchian & Hooton, 2016).*
- ▲ If blood or protein is present in the urine, recognize that both hematuria and proteinuria are serious symptoms, and the client should be referred to a urologist to receive a workup to rule out pathology.
- ● Inquire about the client's history of smoking. EB: *Bladder symptoms such as incomplete emptying, frequency, intermittency, urgency, weak stream, straining, and nocturia may be higher among clients who smoke or who have smoked in the past (Pethiyagoda & Pethiyagoda, 2016).*

Urinary Tract Infection

- ▲ Consult the provider for culture and sensitivity testing and antibiotic treatment in the individual with evidence of a symptomatic UTI. EB: *UTI is a transient, reversible condition that is usually associated with urgency or urge urinary incontinence (Nicolle & Norrby, 2016). Eradication of UTI will alleviate or reverse symptoms of suprapubic pressure and discomfort, urgency, daytime voiding frequency, and dysuria (Nicolle & Norrby, 2016).*
- ▲ Teach the client to recognize symptoms of UTI, such as dysuria that crescendos as the bladder nears complete evacuation; urgency to urinate followed by micturition of only a few drops; suprapubic aching discomfort; malaise; voiding frequency; and sudden exacerbation of urinary incontinence with or without fever, chills, and flank pain. Recognize that cloudy or malodorous urine, in the absence of other lower urinary tract symptoms, may not indicate the presence of a UTI and that asymptomatic bacteriuria in the older adult does not justify a course of antibiotics. EB: *Laboratory tests alone cannot distinguish between asymptomatic bacteriuria and infection. Thus, providers need to be cautious in prescribing antibiotics based on nonspecific findings. Recognizing asymptomatic bacteriuria decreases inappropriate administration of antibiotics in the older adult population preventing adverse drug events and polypharmacy (Cortes-Penfield, Trautner, & Jump, 2017).*
- ▲ Refer the individual with chronic lower urinary tract pain to a urologist or specialist in the management of pelvic pain. EB: *Bladder pain and storage symptoms, in the absence of an acute urinary infection, may indicate the presence of interstitial cystitis, which is a chronic condition requiring ongoing treatment (Interstitial Cystitis Association, 2019).*

Pediatric

- ● Initial management of childhood urinary incontinence: (1) thorough history and physical examination; (2) bladder diary; (3) urinalysis; (4) urinary tract ultrasound; (5) screening for behavioral problems (Maternik, Krzeminska, & Zurowska, 2015).
- ● Standard practice recommendations when caring for pediatric clients include an aggressive bowel regimen, timed voiding, and escalating urotherapy with biofeedback. Medications may be considered as a secondary measure (Arlen, 2017).
- ● Encourage children to void on a timed schedule every 2 hours, void two times with every void, drink two bottles of water during and after school, stop drinking 2 hours before bed, and void two times before bed. EBN: *Providing children with a simplified approach helps them to better understand, practice, and comply with urotherapy guidelines. With the "Rule of 2," all urotherapy guidelines are presented using the number 2 so that children can easily remember what to do (Marcella, 2019).*

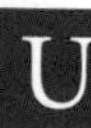

Geriatric

- ● Evidence for behavioral interventions include the following: (1) Prompted voiding is suitable for older adult clients, with or without cognitive impairment, who have a consistent caregiver; (2) prompted voiding is unsuccessful in clients who require more than one person for transfers, are not able to follow one-step commands, and a successful toileting rate of less than 66% after a 3-day prompted voiding trial; and (3) a key factor in the success of prompted voiding is caregiver education (Newman, 2019).

- Encourage older women to consume one to two servings of fresh blueberries and consider drinking at least 10 ounces of cranberry juice daily or supplement the diet with cranberry concentrate capsules as ordered. EB: *There is an ongoing debate about the effectiveness of using cranberry products to prevent UTIs (Gupta, Grigoryan, & Trautner, 2017). However, some evidence suggests that cranberry products may have a protective effect against UTIs (Foxman et al, 2015; Luis, Domingues, & Pereira, 2017).*
- ▲ Refer the older woman with recurrent UTIs to her health care provider for possible use of topical estrogen creams for treatment of atrophic vaginal mucosa from decreased hormonal stimulation, which can predispose to UTIs (Nicolle & Norrby, 2016).
- Postresidual volumes (PRVs) should be assessed in older women with overactive bladder (OAB). A volume of greater than 200 mL is significant. EB: *A history of back or pelvic injury or surgery increases the risk of greater PRV (Park & Palmer, 2015; Porritt, 2019).*
- ▲ Recognize that UTIs in older men are typically associated with prostatic hyperplasia or strictures of the urethra. Refer the client to a urologist (Nicolle & Norrby, 2016).
- Analysis of urinary elimination patterns of clients could help in clinical follow-up of elderly postoperative clients and in the selection of best nursing interventions. EB: *A study exploring NOC indictor interrater reliability showed classifications can be useful for monitoring clinical changes related to urinary elimination. High agreements for the indicators of urine odor, leukocytes, nitrates, blood, painful urination, and urinary continence were found (Ribeiro Bitencourt et al, 2016).*
- Frailty, not age, should guide urinary elimination treatment decisions. EB: *Caring for individuals with urinary incontinence and cognitive impairment needs to be tailored to the individual's abilities (Newman, 2019).*
- Managing incontinence-associated dermatitis in the geriatric population involves regular, ongoing skin assessments to identify damaged skin as well as areas for potential skin damage. EBN: *Cleanse and carefully dry the skin as soon as possible after each episode of incontinence. Use a skin product that is designed to protect against excess moisture and increased damage to the skin. Address causative factors of incontinence before using invasive approaches such as urinary catheters. Educate the client on the care and prevention of incontinence-associated dermatitis (Lumbers, 2019).*

Client/Family Teaching and Discharge Planning

- Teach the client/family methods to keep the urinary tract healthy. Refer to Client/Family Teaching in the care plan for Readiness for Enhanced **Urinary** Elimination.
- Teach the following measures to women to decrease the incidence of UTIs:
  - Urinate at appropriate intervals. Do not ignore need to void, which can result in stasis of urine.
  - Drink plenty of liquids, especially water.
  - Wipe from front to back. This helps prevent bacteria in the anal region from spreading to the vagina and urethra.
  - Wear underpants that have a cotton crotch. This allows air to circulate in the area and decreases moisture in the area, which predisposes to infection.
  - Avoid potentially irritating feminine products.

  EB: *Drinking water helps dilute the urine, allowing bacteria to be flushed from the urinary tract before an infection can begin (Nicolle & Norrby, 2016).* EB: *Using deodorant sprays, bubble baths, or other feminine products, such as douches and powders, in the genital area can irritate the urethra. There are multiple commonsense measures that can be used to decrease the incidence of UTIs (Gupta & Trautner, 2015; Mayo Clinic, 2020).*
- Teach the sexually active woman with recurrent UTIs prevention measures:
  - Void after intercourse to flush bacteria out of the urethra and bladder.
  - Use a lubricating agent as needed during intercourse to protect the vagina from trauma and decrease the incidence of vaginitis.
  - Watch for signs of vaginitis and seek treatment as needed.
  - Avoid use of diaphragms with spermicide.

  EB: *Sexually active women have the highest incidence of UTIs (Nicolle & Norrby, 2016). The vagina and periurethral area can become colonized with organisms from the intestinal flora, such as* Escherichia coli, *and increase the risk for UTIs (Gupta & Trautner, 2015; Pietrucha-Dilanchian & Hontoon, 2016).*

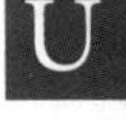

- Teach clients with spinal cord injury and neurogenic bladder dysfunction to consider adding cranberry extract tablets or cranberry juice or fruits containing D-mannose (e.g., apples, oranges, peaches, blueberries) on a daily basis and to monitor fluid intake. The client is encouraged to discuss the use of probiotics and antibiotic therapy with the provider for frequent recurrent symptomatic UTIs. **EB:** *Limited evidence suggested that clients who regularly consume cranberry extract tablets experience fewer UTIs than clients who do not routinely consume cranberry extract tablets (Foxman et al, 2015; Luis, Domingues, & Pereira, 2017). Additionally, clients with spinal cord injury and neurogenic bladder dysfunction are at higher risk for UTI, and more frequent monitoring of symptomatic infection is necessary (Brusch, 2018; Castle et al, 2018).*
- Teach all persons to recognize hematuria and to promptly seek care if this symptom occurs.

REFERENCES

Arlen, A. M. (2017). Dysfunctional voiders—Medication versus urotherapy? *Current Urology Reports, 18*(2), 14. https://doi.org/10.1007/s11934-017-0656-0.

Brusch, J. L. (2018). *Urinary tract infections in spinal cord injury*. Medscape [website]. Retrieved from https://emedicine.medscape.com/article/2040171-overview. [Accessed 3 August 2021].

Castle, A. C., Park, A., Mitchell, A. J., Bliss, D. Z., Gelfand, J. A., & De, E. J. B. (2018). Neurogenic bladder: Recurrent urinary tract infections—Beyond antibiotics. *Current Bladder Dysfunction Reports, 13*, 191–200. https://doi.org/10.1007/s11884-018-0481-4.

Cortes-Penfield, N. W., Trautner, B. W., & Jump, R. L. P. (2017). Urinary tract infection and asymptomatic bacteriuria in older adults. *Infectious Disease Clinics of North America, 31*(4), 673–688. https://doi.org/10.1016/j.idc.2017.07.002.

Dixon, C. A., & Nakib, N. A. (2016). Are bladder diaries helpful in management of overactive bladder? *Current Bladder Dysfunction Reports, 11*, 14–17. https://doi.org/10.1007/s11884-016-0343-x.

Foxman, B., Cronewett, A. E. W., Spino, C., Berger, M. B., & Morgan, D. M. (2015). Cranberry juice capsules and urinary tract infection after surgery: Results of a randomized trial. *American Journal of Obstetrics and Gynecology, 213*(2), 194.e1–194.e8. https://doi.org/10.1016/j.ajog.2015.04.003.

Gupta, K., Grigoryan, L., & Trautner, B. (2017). Urinary tract infection. *Annals of Internal Medicine, 167*(7), ITC49–ITC64. https://doi.org/10.7326/AITC201710030.

Gupta, K., & Trautner, B. (2015). Urinary tract infections, pyelonephritis, and prostatitis. In D. L. Kasper, A. S. Fauci, S. L. Hauser, D. L. Longo, J. L. Jameson, & J. Loscalzo (Eds.), *Harrison's principles of internal medicine* (19th ed.). New York: McGraw Hill Education.

Interstitial Cystitis Association. (2019). *Pain & IC*. Retrieved from https://www.ichelp.org/about-ic/symptoms-of-ic/pain-ic/. [Accessed 3 August 2021].

Luis, Â., Domingues, F., & Pereira, L. (2017). Can cranberries contribute to reduce the incidence of urinary tract infections? A systematic review with meta-analysis and trial sequential analysis of clinical trials. *Journal of Urology, 198*(3), 614–621. http://dx.doi.org/10.1016/j.juro.2017.03.078.

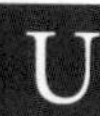

Lumbers, M. (2019). How to manage incontinence-associated dermatitis in older adults. *British Journal of Community Nursing, 24*(7), 332–337. https://doi.org/10.7257/1053-816X.2019.39.3.145.

Marcella, E. (2019). The rule of "2": Teaching a simplified approach to behavioral urotherapy. *Urologic Nursing, 39*(3), 145–146.

Maternik, M., Krzeminska, K., & Zurowska, A. (2015). The management of childhood urinary incontinence. *Pediatric Nephrology, 30*(1), 41–50. https://doi.org/10.1007/s00467-014-2791-x.

Mayo Clinic. (2020). *Urinary tract infection (UTI)*. MayoClinic.org [website]. Retrieved from https://www.mayoclinic.org/diseases-conditions/urinary-tract-infection/symptoms-causes/syc-20353447. [Accessed 3 August 2021].

Newman, D. K. (2019). Evidence-based practice guideline: Prompted voiding for individuals with urinary incontinence. *Journal of Gerontological Nursing, 45*(2), 14–26. https://doi.org/10.3928/00989134-20190111-03.

Nicolle, L. E., & Norrby, S. R. (2016). Approach to the patient with urinary tract infection. In L. Goldman, & A. Schafer (Eds.), *Goldman's Cecil medicine* (25th ed.) (pp. 1872–1876). Philadelphia: Elsevier.

Park, J., & Palmer, M. H. (2015). Factors associated with incomplete bladder emptying in older women with overactive bladder symptoms. *Journal of the American Geriatrics Society, 63*(7), 1426–1431.

Pethiyagoda, A. U. B., & Pethiyagoda, K. (2016). Impact of smoking on lower urinary tract symptoms (LUTS): Single tertiary centre experience. *International Journal of Scientific and Research Publications, 6*(5), 119–123.

Pietrucha-Dilanchian, P., & Hooton, T. M. (2016). Diagnosis, treatment and prevention of urinary tract infection. *Microbiology Spectrum, 4*(6). https://doi.org/10.1128/9781555817404.ch3.

Policastro, M. A. (2016). *Urinary obstruction*. Medscape [website]. Retrieved from http://emedicine.medscape.com/article/778456-overview. [Accessed 3 August 2021].

Porritt, K. (2019). *Post-operative urinary retention: Assessment and diagnosis*. Joanna Briggs Institute. JBI Evidence Summary. JBI21696. May 1, 2019.

Ribeiro Bitencourt, G., de Almeida Ferreira Alves, L., Ferreira Santana, R., & Venicios de Oliveira Lopes, M. (2016). Agreement between experts regarding assessment of postoperative urinary elimination nursing outcomes in elderly patients. *International Journal of Nursing Knowledge, 27*(3), 143–148.

Urinary Retention

Domain 3 Elimination and exchange Class 1 Urinary function

Kenneth J. Oja, PhD, RN

NANDA-I

Definition

Incomplete emptying of the bladder.

Defining Characteristics

Absence of urinary output; bladder distention; dysuria; increased daytime urinary frequency; minimal void volume; overflow incontinence; reports sensation of bladder fullness; reports sensation of residual urine; weak urine stream

Related Factors

Environmental constraints; fecal impaction; improper toileting posture; inadequate relaxation of pelvic floor muscles; insufficient privacy; pelvic organ prolapse; weakened bladder muscle

At-Risk Population

Puerperal women

Associated Conditions

Benign prostatic hyperplasia; diabetes mellitus; nervous system diseases; pharmaceutical preparations; urinary tract obstruction

NOC (Nursing Outcomes Classification)

Suggested NOC Outcome

Urinary Elimination

Example NOC Outcome with Indicators

Urinary Elimination as evidenced by the following indicators: Empties bladder completely/Absence of urinary leakage/Urine clarity. (Rate the outcome and indicators of **Urinary Elimination:** 1 = severely compromised, 2 = substantially compromised, 3 = moderately compromised, 4 = mildly compromised, 5 = not compromised [see Section I].)

Client Outcomes

Client Will (Specify Time Frame)

- Demonstrate consistent ability to urinate when desire to void is perceived
- Have measured urinary residual volume of less than 300 mL
- Experience correction or relief from dysuria, nocturia, postvoid dribbling, and voiding frequently
- Be free of a urinary tract infection

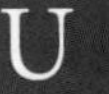

NIC (Nursing Interventions Classification)

Suggested NIC Interventions

Urinary Catheterization; Urinary Retention Care

Example NIC Activities—Urinary Retention Care

Perform a comprehensive urinary assessment focusing on incontinence (e.g., urinary output, urinary voiding pattern, cognitive function, and preexistent urinary problems); Use the power of suggestion by running water or flushing toilet

Nursing Interventions and *Rationales*

- Obtain a focused urinary history including questioning the client about episodes of acute urinary retention (UR; complete inability to void) or chronic retention (documented elevated postvoid residual volumes), as well as symptoms such as dysuria, nocturia, postvoid dribbling, and voiding frequently. **EB:** *A history of pain, changes in the amount of urine produced, difficulty urinating, blood in the urine, repeated urinary tract infections, or hypertension may be signs of urinary obstruction (Mayo Clinic, 2020).*
- Question the client concerning specific risk factors for UR:
  - ❍ Medications, including antispasmodics/parasympatholytics, alpha-adrenergic agonists, antidepressants, sedatives, narcotics, psychotropic medications, illicit drugs
  - ❍ Vaginal delivery within the past 48 hours
  - ❍ Bowel elimination patterns, history of fecal impaction, encopresis
  - ❍ Metabolic disorders such as diabetes mellitus, chronic alcoholism, and related conditions associated with polyuria and peripheral polyneuropathies
  - ❍ Spinal cord injuries
  - ❍ Ischemic stroke
  - ❍ Herpetic infection
  - ❍ Heavy-metal poisoning (lead, mercury) causing peripheral polyneuropathies
  - ❍ Advanced stage HIV infection
  - ❍ Recent surgery requiring general or spinal anesthesia
  - ❍ Recent surgical procedures
  - ❍ Recent prostatic biopsy

  EB: *UR is related to multiple factors affecting either detrusor contraction strength or urethral resistance to urinary outflow (Policastro, 2016).*
- Complete a pain assessment including pain intensity using a self-report pain tool, such as the 0 to 10 numerical pain rating scale. Also determine location, quality, onset/duration, intensity, aggravating/alleviating factors, and effects of pain on function and quality of life. **EB:** *Acute onset of obstruction with inability to void is associated with significant pain; partial obstruction causes minimal pain, which may delay diagnosis (Policastro, 2016). Symptoms of bladder distention may include difficulty urinating, a constant feeling that the bladder is full, a slow stream of urine, abdominal pain, urinary incontinence, or waking in the night to urinate (Young, 2018).*
- Perform a focused physical assessment including perineal skin integrity and inspection, percussion, and palpation of the lower abdomen, looking for obvious bladder distention or an enlarged kidney. **EB:** *A palpable kidney or bladder provides direct evidence of a dilated urinary collection system (Policastro, 2016).*
- Recognize that unrelieved obstruction of urine can result in kidney damage and, if severe, kidney failure. UR can be a medical emergency and should be reported to the primary provider as soon as possible. **EB:** *As urine backs up in the urinary tract, the pressure increases inside the ureters, which results in pressure on the nephrons, damaging the nephrons and decreasing glomerular blood flow (Policastro, 2016).*
- Review laboratory test results, including serum electrolytes, blood urea nitrogen (BUN), and creatinine, along with calcium, phosphate, magnesium, uric acid, and albumin. **EB:** *Serum electrolytes (sodium, potassium, chloride, bicarbonate, BUN, and creatinine) and calcium, phosphate, magnesium, uric acid, and albumin should be measured. Elevations of BUN and creatinine and changes in electrolytes may be caused by kidney failure secondary to obstruction (Policastro, 2016).*

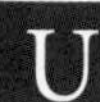

- Monitor for signs of dehydration, peripheral edema, elevated blood pressure, and heart failure. **EB:** *The kidney can develop concentrating defects associated with partial obstruction of urine flow, resulting in symptoms that indicate kidney insufficiency (Policastro, 2016).*
- Ask the client to complete a bladder diary including patterns of urine elimination, urine loss (if present), nocturia, and volume and type of fluids consumed for a period of 3 to 7 days.

▲ Consult with the health care provider concerning eliminating or altering medications suspected of producing or exacerbating UR.

- Both men and women may develop UR from obstruction of the bladder outlet and abnormalities in detrusor contractility. **EB:** *A common cause of bladder outlet obstruction (BOO) is caused by prostate/bladder neck enlargement, urethral stricture, vaginal vault prolapse, obstructing urethral sling, or impacted stool. Long-term use of medications such as alpha-agonists and tricyclic antidepressants contributes to the problem (Stoffel et al, 2016).* **EB:** *Assess for postresidual void (PVR) greater than 300 mL because it is the minimal volume at which a bladder becomes palpable (Stoffel et al, 2016).*

- In clients treated with an indwelling urethral catheter (IUC), complications such as catheter-associated urinary tract infections are common, whereas underuse of IUC may cause harmful UR. EB: *A quality improvement (QI) program aimed at staff ability to identify and manage client risk, prevention, and treatment of UR optimizes appropriate IUC use (Andersson et al, 2017).*
- Advise the male client with UR related to benign prostatic hyperplasia (BPH) to avoid risk factors associated with acute UR:
  - Avoid over-the-counter (OTC) cold remedies containing a decongestant (alpha-adrenergic agonist) or antihistamine, such as diphenhydramine, which has anticholinergic effects.
  - Avoid taking OTC dietary medications (frequently contain alpha-adrenergic agonists).
  - Discuss voiding problems with a health care provider before beginning new prescription medications.
  - After prolonged exposure to cool weather, warm the body before attempting to urinate.
  - Avoid overfilling the bladder by regular urination patterns and refrain from excessive intake of alcohol.

  EB: *Botulinum toxin injection into the bladder neck is a promising minimally invasive, tolerated, and cost-effective approach for the treatment of UR in clients with benign prostatic obstruction who are not candidates for surgery and for whom medical treatments have failed (Alam et al, 2016). These modifiable factors predispose the client to acute UR by overdistending the bladder and decreasing muscle contraction (Mayo Clinic, 2021).*
- Advise the client who is unable to void of specific strategies to manage this potential medical emergency as follows:
  - Attempt urination in complete privacy.
  - Place the feet solidly on the floor.
  - If unable to void using these strategies, take a warm sitz bath or shower and void (if possible) while still in the tub or shower.
  - Drink a warm cup of caffeinated coffee or tea to stimulate the bladder, which may promote voiding.
  - If unable to void within 6 hours or if bladder distention is producing significant pain, seek urgent or emergency care.

  EB: *Attempting urination in complete privacy and placing the feet solidly on the floor help relax the pelvic muscles and may encourage voiding. Warm water also stimulates the bladder and may produce voiding; the cooling experienced by leaving the tub or shower may again inhibit the bladder (Porritt, 2019).*
- Perform sterile (in acute care) or clean intermittent catheterization at home as ordered for clients with UR. Refer to care plan for Reflex Urinary **Incontinence** for more information about intermittent catheterization.

▲ Insert an indwelling catheter only as ordered by a health care provider. Understand the indication for the urinary catheter to be placed as part of client management. Catheter-associated urinary tract infections (CAUTIs) are among the most common health care–associated infections and result in unnecessary health care costs. A CAUTI also increases the risk of a bloodstream infection. EB: *Although certain conditions among hospitalized clients may require the use of a urinary catheter, limiting their use and decreasing the length of use are the most effective methods of reducing clients' exposure to CAUTIs (American Academy of Nursing, 2018).*

- Nurse-led and computer-based reminders are both successful in reducing how long urinary catheters remain in place (Timmons et al, 2017).
- Nurse-driven practice recommendations to reduce CAUTI risk include securing catheters; maintaining drainage bags lower than level of bladder; emptying drainage bags every 8 hours, when two-thirds full, and before any transfer; daily evaluation of catheter indication/need to promote removal; and use of bladder scanner to prevent reinsertion. EB: *Incorporating practice policies that use nurse-driven catheter practices appear to have a positive impact on the clinical predictors and prevalence of CAUTIs (Durant, 2017).*
- Current practice recommendations support aseptic catheter insertions, whereas the use of hydrophilic-coated catheters for clean intermittent catheters can reduce the rate of CAUTIs. Suprapubic catheterization is not more effective than urethral catheterization in reducing the incidence of catheter-related bacteremia. EB: *Evidence does not support routine use of antimicrobial-impregnated catheters to prevent CAUTIs (Majeed et al, 2019).*
- For the individual with UR who is not a suitable candidate for intermittent catheterization, recognize that the catheter can be a significant cause of harm to the client through development of a CAUTI or through genitourinary trauma when the catheter is pulled. EB: *An indwelling catheter provides continuous drainage of urine; however, the risks for serious urinary complications, such as chronic CAUTIs, with prolonged use*

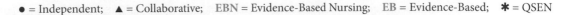

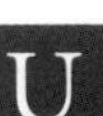

are significant (Porritt, 2019). **EB:** *One study identified that complications associated with urethral catheters can be infectious and noninfectious including UTI, pain or discomfort, trauma to the skin related to catheter securement or placement, and bladder or kidney stones (Saint et al, 2018).* **EBN:** *Indwelling urinary catheters are associated with up to 80% of hospital-acquired CAUTIs. Appropriate use of bladder ultrasonography can reduce the rate of bladder damage and the need to use catheters. Incorporating bladder ultrasonography into the client's assessment can lead to decreased use of urinary catheter and rate of CAUTIs, lower risk for spread of multiresistant gram-negative bacteria, and lower hospital costs (Guadarrama Ortega et al, 2020).*

- Advise clients with indwelling catheters that bacteria in the urine is an almost universal finding after the catheter has remained in place for more than 1 week and that only symptomatic infections warrant treatment. **EB:** *The long-term indwelling catheter is inevitably associated with bacterial colonization, with formation of biofilm on the catheter surfaces (Nicolle & Norrby, 2016).*
- Use the following strategies to reduce the risk for CAUTI whenever feasible:
  - ❍ Insert the indwelling catheter with sterile technique, only when insertion is indicated.
  - ❍ Remove the indwelling catheter as soon as possible; acute care facilities should institute a policy for regular review of the necessity of an indwelling catheter.
  - ❍ Maintain a closed drainage system whenever feasible.
  - ❍ Maintain unobstructed urine flow, avoiding kinks in the tubing and keeping the collecting bag below the level of the bladder at all times.
  - ❍ Regularly cleanse the urethral meatus with a gentle cleanser to remove apparent soiling.
  - ❍ Change the long-term catheter every 4 weeks; more frequent catheter changes should be reserved for clients who experience catheter encrustation and blockage.
- Educate staff about the risks for CAUTI development and specific strategies to reduce these risks. **EB:** *These strategies are supported by sufficient evidence to recommend routine use (Gould et al, 2019). Numerous nursing studies have demonstrated that nurse-controlled methods to decrease the length of catheterization such as chart reminders and computerized interventions lead to decreased incidences of CAUTI (Durant, 2017).*

Postoperative Urinary Retention

- UR is a common complication of surgery, anesthesia, and advancing age. If conservative measures do not help the client pass urine, the bladder needs to be drained using either an intermittent catheter or IUC, which places the client at risk for development of CAUTI (Lee et al, 2017). **EB:** *A study demonstrated decreased risk of UTI and repeat UR episodes after transurethral resection of the prostate in clients with benign prostatic hyperplasia (BPH) (Lin et al, 2018).*
- Remove the IUC at midnight in the hospitalized postoperative client to reduce the risk for acute UR.
- Perform a bladder scan before considering inserting a catheter to determine PVR volume after surgery. **EBN:** *A study in postoperative clients demonstrated a significant decrease in the number of catheterizations when ultrasonic bladder scanning was done to monitor postoperative UR (Daurat et al, 2015).* **EB:** *A retrospective cohort study of 803 clients who underwent unilateral hip or knee arthroplasty were evaluated for postoperative urinary retention (POUR). Following a nurse-led routine bladder scan protocol postoperatively found a 12.9% incidence of POUR that was treated with a nurse-led intervention and reduced recovery room time (Kort et al, 2018).*
- Spinal anesthesia is a risk factor associated with postoperative urinary retention (Bjerregaard et al, 2015).

U

Geriatric

- Aggressively assess older clients, particularly those with dribbling urinary incontinence, urinary tract infection, and related conditions, for UR. **EB:** *Older women and men may experience UR with few or no apparent symptoms; a urinary residual volume and related assessments are necessary to determine the presence of retention in this population. Providing routine skin care and scheduled voiding can reduce risks of skin breakdown and/or infections associated with urinary incontinence (Podder, 2019).* **EBN:** *A cohort study of 4061 older adults living in nursing homes found that older individuals with involuntary leakage of urine experienced a 24% increased risk of falls and 11% increase risk of mortality associated with urinary incontinence (Damián et al, 2017).*
- Assess older clients for impaction when UR is documented or suspected; monitor older male clients for retention related to BPH or prostate cancer. Prostate enlargement in older men increases the risk for acute and chronic UR.

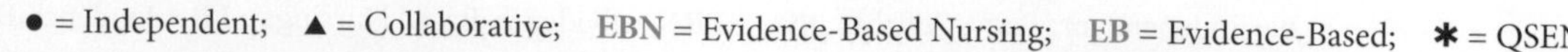

Home Care

- Encourage the client to report any inability to void.
- Maintain an up-to-date medication list; evaluate side-effect profiles for risk of UR. New medications or changes in dose may cause UR.
- ▲ Refer the client for health care provider evaluation if UR occurs. Identification of cause is important. Left untreated, UR may lead to urinary tract infection or kidney failure.

Client/Family Teaching and Discharge Planning

- Teach the client with mild to moderate obstructive symptoms to double void by urinating, resting in the bathroom for 3 to 5 minutes, and then trying again to urinate. EB: *Double voiding promotes more efficient bladder evacuation by allowing the detrusor to contract initially and then rest and contract again (Mayo Clinic, 2021).*
- Teach the client with UR and infrequent voiding to urinate by the clock. EB: *Timed or scheduled voiding may reduce UR by preventing bladder overdistention (Mayo Clinic, 2021).*
- Teach the client with an indwelling catheter to assess the tube for patency, maintain the drainage system below the level of the symphysis pubis, and routinely cleanse the bedside bag as directed.
- Teach the client with an indwelling catheter or undergoing intermittent catheterization the symptoms of a significant urinary infection, including hematuria, acute-onset incontinence, dysuria, flank pain, fever, or acute confusion.

REFERENCES

Alam, M., Zgheib, J., Dalati, M. F., & El Khoury, F. (2016). Botulinum toxin A injection in the bladder neck: A promising treatment for urinary retention. *Case Reports in Urology*, 2016, 6385276. http://dx.doi.org/10.1155/2016/6385276.

American Academy of Nursing. (2018). *Don't place or maintain an indwelling urinary catheter in a patient unless there is a specific indication to do so*. ChoosingWisely.org [website]. Retrieved from http://www.choosingwisely.org/clinician-lists/american-academy-nursing-urinary-catheters-without-specific-indication/. [Accessed August 4, 2021].

Andersson, A. C., Johansson, R. M., Elg, M., Gäre, B. A., & Christensson, L. (2017). Using quality improvement methods to implement guidelines to decrease the proportion of urinary retention in orthopaedic care. *International Archives of Nursing and Health Care*, *3*(1), 065. http://doi.org/10.23937/2469-5823/1510065.

Bjerregaard, L. S., Bogø, S., Raaschou, S., et al. (2015). Incidence of and risk factors for postoperative urinary retention in fast-track hip and knee arthroplasty. *Acta Orthopaedica*, *86*(2), 183–188.

Damián, J., Pastor-Barriuso, R., García López, F. J., & de Pedro-Cuesta, J. (2017). Urinary incontinence and mortality among older adults residing in care homes. *Journal of Advanced Nursing*, *73*(3), 688–699. https://doi.org/10.1111/jan.13170.

Daurat, A., Choquet, O., Bringuier, S., Charbit, J., Egan, M., & Capdevila, X. (2015). Diagnosis of postoperative urinary retention using a simplified ultrasound bladder measurement. *Anesthesia & Analgesia*, *120*(5), 1033–1038.

Durant, D. J. (2017). Nurse-driven protocols and the prevention of catheter-associated urinary tract infections: A systematic review. *American Journal of Infection Control*, *45*(12), 1331–1341. https://doi.org/10.1016/j.ajic.2017.07.020.

Gould, C. V., Umscheid, C. A., Agarwal, R. K., Kuntz, G., & Pegues, D. A. (2019). Guideline for prevention of catheter-associated urinary tract infections 2009. Healthcare Infection Control Practices Advisory Committee (HICPAC). Retrieved from https://www.cdc.gov/infectioncontrol/pdf/guidelines/cauti-guidelines-H.pdf. [Accessed August 4, 2021].

Guadarrama Ortega, D., Díaz Díaz, R., Aránzazu Martín Hernandez, M., Peces Hernandez, M. T., Vallejo Paredes, J., & Chuvieco Gonzalez, Y. (2020). Impact of a portable volumetric ultrasound on bladder catheterizations due to urinary retention in an internal medicine unit. *Enfermeria Global*, *19*(1), 42–62. http://dx.doi.org/10.6018/eglobal.19.1.347591.

Kort, N. P., Bemelmans, Y., Vos, R., & Schotanus, M. G. M. (2018). Low incidence of postoperative urinary retention with the use of a nurse-led bladder scan protocol after hip and knee arthroplasty: a retrospective cohort study. *European Journal of Orthopaedic Surgery & Traumatology*, *28*(2), 283–289. https://doi.org/10.1007/s00590-017-2042-5.

Lee, K. S., Koo, K. C., & Chung, B. H. (2017). Risk and management of postoperative urinary retention following spinal surgery. *International Neurology Journal*, *21*(4), 320–328. https://doi.org/10.5213/inj.1734994.497.

Lin, Y., Hou, C., Chen, T., et al. (2018). Transurethral resection of the prostate provides more favorable clinical outcomes compared with conservative medical treatment in patients with urinary retention caused by benign prostatic obstruction. *BMC Geriatrics*, *18*(1), 15. https://doi.org/10.1186/s12877-018-0709-3.

Majeed, A., Sagar, F., Latif, A., et al. (2019). Does antimicrobial coating and impregnation of urinary catheters prevent catheter-associated urinary tract infection? A review of clinical and preclinical studies. *Expert Review of Medical Devices*, *16*(9), 809–820. https://doi.org/10.1080/17434440.2019.1661774.

Mayo Clinic. (2020). *Ureteral obstruction*. MayoClinic.org [website]. Retrieved from https://www.mayoclinic.org/diseases-conditions/ureteral-obstruction/symptoms-causes/syc-20354676. [Accessed August 5, 2021].

Mayo Clinic. (2021). *Benign prostatic hyperplasia (BPH)*. MayoClinic.org [website]. Retrieved from https://www.mayoclinic.org/diseases-conditions/benign-prostatic-hyperplasia/diagnosis-treatment/drc-20370093. [Accessed August 4, 2021].

Nicolle, L. E., & Norrby, S. R. (2016). Approach to the patient with urinary tract infection. In L. Goldman, & A. Schafer (Eds.), *Goldman's cecil medicine* (25th ed.) (pp. 1872–1876). Philadelphia: Elsevier.

Podder, V. (2019). *Urinary incontinence: conservative management*. Joanna Briggs Institute. JBI Evidence Summary. JBI17400. June 5, 2019.

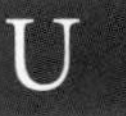

Policastro, M. A. (2016). *Urinary obstruction*. Medscape [website]. Retrieved from http://emedicine.medscape.com/article/778456-overview. [Accessed August 3, 2021].
Porritt, K. (2019). *Post-operative urinary retention: assessment and diagnosis*. Joanna Briggs Institute. JBI Evidence Summary. JBI21696. May 1, 2019.
Saint, S., Trautner, B. W., Fowler, K. E., et al. (2018). A multicenter study of patient-reported infectious and noninfectious complications associated with indwelling urethral catheters. *JAMA Internal Medicine*, *178*(8), 1078–1085. https://doi.org/10.1001/jamainternmed.2018.2417.
Stoffel, J., Lightner, D., Peterson, A., Sandhu, J., Suskind, A., & Wei, J. (2016). *AUA white paper on non-neurogenic chronic urinary retention: consensus definition, management strategies, and future opportunities*. American Urological Association. Retrieved from https://www.auanet.org/guidelines/guidelines/chronic-urinary-retention. [Accessed August 4, 2021].
Timmons, B., Vess, J., & Conner, B. (2017). Nurse-driven protocol to reduce indwelling catheter time: A health care improvement initiative. *Journal of Nursing Care Quality*, *32*(2), 104–107.
Young, B. (2018). *Enlarged bladder*. Healthline.com [website]. Retrieved from https://www.healthline.com/health/enlarged-bladder. [Accessed August 4, 2021].

Risk for Urinary Retention

Domain 3 Elimination and exchange Class 1 Urinary function

Mary Beth Flynn Makic, PhD, RN, CCNS, CCRN-K, FAAN, FNAP, FCNS

NANDA-I

Definition

Susceptible to incomplete emptying of the bladder.

Related Factors

Environmental constraints; fecal impaction; improper toileting posture; inadequate relaxation of pelvic floor muscles; insufficient privacy; pelvic organ prolapse; weakened bladder muscle

At-Risk Population

Puerperal women

Associated Conditions

Benign prostatic hyperplasia; diabetes mellitus; nervous system diseases; pharmaceutical preparations; urinary tract obstruction

NOC, NIC, Client Outcomes, Nursing Interventions and *Rationales,* Client/Family Teaching and Discharge Planning, and References

Refer to care plan for **Urinary Retention.**

Risk for Vascular Trauma

Domain 11 Safety/projection Class 2 Physical injury

Elyse Bueno, MS, ACCNS-AG, C NE-BC

NANDA-I

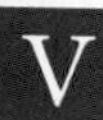

Definition

Susceptible to damage to vein and its surrounding tissues related to the presence of a catheter and/or infusion solutions, which may compromise health.

Risk Factors

Inadequate available insertion site; prolonged period of time catheter is in place

Associated Conditions

Irritating solution; rapid infusion rate

NOC (Nursing Outcomes Classification)

Suggested NOC Outcomes

Risk Control; Tissue Integrity: Skin and Mucous Membranes

Example NOC Outcome with Indicators

Accomplishes **Risk Control** as evidenced by the following indicators: Monitors environmental risk factors/Develops effective risk control strategies/Modifies lifestyle to reduce risk. (Rate the outcome and indicators of **Risk Control:** 1 = never demonstrated, 2 = rarely demonstrated, 3 = sometimes demonstrated, 4 = often demonstrated, 5 = consistently demonstrated [see Section I].)

Client Outcomes

Client Will (Specify Time Frame)

- Remain free from vascular trauma
- Remain free from signs and symptoms that indicate vascular trauma
- Remain free of signs and symptoms of vascular inflammation or infection
- Remain free from impaired tissue and/or skin
- Maintain skin integrity, tissue perfusion, usual tissue temperature, color, and pigment
- Report any altered sensation or pain
- State site is comfortable

NIC (Nursing Interventions Classification)

Suggested NIC Interventions

Intravenous Therapy; Medication Administration: Intravenous

Example NIC Activities—Intravenous Therapy

Monitor intravenous (IV) flow rate and IV site during infusion; Perform IV site care according to agency protocol

Nursing Interventions and *Rationales*

Client Preparation

- ▲ Verify objective and estimate duration of treatment. Check health care provider's order. EB: *Verify if client will remain hospitalized during the entire treatment or will go home with the device (Phillips, 2014).*
- • Assess client's clinical situation when venous infusion is indicated. EB: *Consider possible clinical conditions that cause changes in temperature, color, and sensitivity of the possible venous access site. Verify situations that alter venous return (e.g., mastectomy, stroke) (Phillips, 2014). The site of catheter insertion influences the risk of infection and phlebitis, such as preexisting catheters, anatomical deformity, and bleeding diathesis (Kaur, 2019).*
- • Assess if client is prepared for an intravenous (IV) procedure. Explain the procedure if necessary, to decrease stress. EB: *Stress may cause vasoconstriction that can interfere in the visualization of the vein and flow of the infused solution (Kaur, 2019).*
- • Provide privacy and make the client comfortable during the IV insertion. EB: *Privacy and comfort help decrease stress (Phillips, 2014).*
- • Teach the client what symptoms of possible vascular trauma he or she should be alert to and to immediately inform staff if any of these symptoms are noticed. EB: *Prompt attention to adverse changes decreases the chance of adverse effects from complications (Phillips, 2014).*

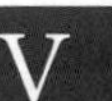

Insertion

- • Wash hands before and after touching the client, as well as when inserting, replacing, accessing, repairing, or dressing an intravascular catheter (O'Grady et al, 2011; Infusion Nurses Society [INS], 2016; Kaur, 2019).

- • Maintain aseptic technique for the insertion and care of intravascular catheters. EB: *Using an approved antiseptic solution, wearing gloves during insertion of an IV catheter, and immediately covering the insertion site with a transparent sterile semipermeable dressing are important interventions to reduce the risk of infection (Kaur, 2019).*
- • In preparation, assess the client's medical history for disease processes such as diabetes and hypertension, frequent venipuncture, variations in skin color, skin alteration, age, obesity, fluid volume deficit, and IV drug use; these factors may lead to difficult vascular visualization (INS, 2016).
- • When vascular visualization is difficult, consider the use of visible light devices that provide transillumination of the peripheral veins or ultrasonography (INS, 2016). Ultrasonography reduces the number of venipuncture attempts and procedure time.
- • Avoid areas of joint flexion or bony prominences. EB: *Movement in these sites can cause mechanical trauma in veins (INS, 2016).*
- • Avoid the use of the antecubital area, which has high failure rates, and do not use lower extremities unless necessary because of the risk of tissue damage, thrombophlebitis, and ulceration (INS, 2016).
- ▲ Avoid the dorsal hand, radial wrist, and the volar (inner) wrist, if possible. EB: *These are high-risk areas for venipuncture-related nerve injury (INS, 2016).*
- ▲ Consider topical anesthetic before IV cannula insertion to reduce pain (Kaur, 2019).
- • Choose an appropriate vascular access device (VAD) based on the types and characteristics of the devices and insertion site. Consider the following:
  - ○ Peripheral cannulae: these are short devices that are placed into a peripheral vein. They can be straight, winged, or ported and winged.
  - ○ Midline catheters or peripherally inserted central catheters (PICCs) that range from 7.5 to 20 cm.
  - ○ Central venous access devices (CVADs) are terminated in the central venous circulation and are available in a range of gauge sizes; they can be nontunneled catheters, skin-tunneled catheters, implantable injection ports, or PICCs.
  - ○ Polyurethane venous devices and silicone rubber may cause less friction and, consequently, may reduce the risk of mechanical phlebitis (Phillips, 2014).
- ▲ Choose a device with consideration of the nature, volume, and flow of prescribed solution. EBN: *Choosing the right gauge size reduces the risk of vascular trauma. Verify that the osmolarity of the solution to be infused is compatible with the available access site and device (Phillips, 2014; Loubani & Green, 2015).*
- • If possible, choose the venous access site considering the client's preference. Engaging the client in choosing the venous access site, when possible, may facilitate line patency.
- • Select the gauge of the venous device according to the duration of treatment, purpose of the procedure, and size of the vein. EB: *Emergency situations require short, large-bore cannulae. Hydration fluids and antibiotics can be delivered through much smaller cannulae (Loubani & Green, 2015). Select the smallest gauge necessary to achieve the prescribed flow rate (INS, 2016). The time of infusion of the drug, especially chemotherapy and vasoactive agents, can contribute to the occurrence of phlebitis (Loubani & Green, 2015).*
- • Verify whether the client is allergic to fixation or device material.
- • Disinfect the venipuncture site. Assess that skin is dry before puncturing to achieve maximal benefit of the disinfection agent.
- • Provide a comfortable, safe, hypoallergenic, easily removable stabilization dressing, allowing for visualization of the access site. EB: *Catheter stabilization should be used to preserve the integrity of the access device, to minimize catheter movement at the hub, and to prevent catheter migration and loss of access (INS, 2016). Some peripheral cannulae have stabilization wings (which increase the external surface area) and/or ports (which are used to administer bolus medication) incorporated into their design.*
- • Use sterile, transparent, semipermeable dressing to cover catheter site. Replace dressing with catheter change, or at a minimum every 7 days for transparent dressings *(INS, 2016)*. EB: *The use of a transparent occlusive dressing can facilitate regular monitoring by visually inspecting the VAD (Kaur, 2019). Use of gauze may be necessary if the client is diaphoretic, if the site is oozing or bleeding, or if it becomes damp; if gauze is used, it should be changed every 2 days (INS, 2016).*
- • Document insertion date, site, type of VAD, number of punctures performed, other occurrences, and measures/arrangements.
- • Always decontaminate the device before infusing medication or manipulating IV equipment. EB: *Disinfect the hub with an alcohol pad or according to hospital policy for a minimum of 15 seconds. Friction and decontamination before accessing the device port is essential in reducing contamination and/or infections (Helm et al, 2015; Kaur, 2019).*

▲ Verify the sequence of drugs to be administrated. *Vesicants should always be administered first in a sequence of drugs (Loubani & Green, 2015).*

Monitoring Infusion

- Monitor permeability and flow rate at regular intervals.
- Monitor catheter–skin junction and surrounding tissues at regular intervals, observing possible appearance of burning, pain, erythema, altered local temperature, infiltration, extravasation, edema, secretion, tenderness, or induration. Remove promptly. EB: *The infusion should be discontinued at the first sign of infiltration or extravasation, the administration set disconnected, and all fluid aspirated from the catheter with a small syringe (INS, 2016).*

▲ Replace device according to institution protocol. EBN: *Remove peripheral IV cannula if there are signs of phlebitis or infection or if the cannula is no longer functioning. There is no need to routinely change the catheter every 72 to 96 hours (Webster et al, 2010; Porritt, 2018).*

▲ Flush vascular access according to organizational policies and procedures and as recommended by the manufacturer. *A pulsating flushing technique should be used (Porritt, 2016).* EB: *VADs should be flushed after each infusion to clear the infused medication from the catheter lumen, preventing contact between incompatible medications (INS, 2016). Sodium chloride 0.9% or heparinized sodium chloride has been studied to determine optimal solution for catheter patency.* EB: *A Cochrane review found little difference in catheter patency between either solution; thus given the cost and possible client risks to heparin exposure, sodium chloride flush solution is recommended (López-Briz et al, 2014).*

- When locking a catheter, use enough fluid to fill the entire catheter and use a positive pressure technique when disconnecting the syringe (Porritt, 2016).
- Remove catheter on suspected contamination, if the client develops signs of phlebitis or infection, the catheter is malfunctioning, or when the catheter is no longer required. EB: *VADs should be removed on unresolved complication, on therapy discontinuation, or if deemed unnecessary (INS, 2016). Replace any catheter inserted under emergency conditions within 24 hours because the sterility of the procedure may have been compromised.*
- Encourage clients to report any discomfort such as pain, burning, swelling, or bleeding (Kaur, 2019).

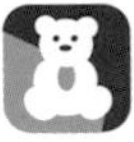

Pediatric

- The preceding interventions may be adapted for the pediatric client. EB: *Consider age, culture, development level, health literacy, and language preferences (INS, 2016).*
- Inform the client and family about the IV procedure; obtain permissions, maintain client's comfort, and perform appropriate assessment before venipuncture. Assess the client for any allergies or sensitivities to tape, antiseptics, or latex. EB: *Choose a healthy vein and appropriate site for insertion of selected device (Abolfotouh et al, 2014).*
- Consider using a two-dimensional ultrasound for venous cannulation. EBN: *Ultrasound has been shown more effective than traditional techniques and should be considered for pediatric clients (Jayasekara, 2017).* EBN: *The cephalic vein in the proximal forearm is the best initial site for ultrasound-guided catheterization when veins are not visible or palpable (Jayasekara, 2017).*
- The use of an appropriate device to obtain blood samples reduces discomfort in the pediatric client. CEB: *Accessing a pediatric client's vein successfully can be difficult, and measures to optimize the health care provider's skill are important to ensure successful venous cannulation (Goff et al, 2013).*
- Avoid areas of joint flexion or bony prominences. EB: *Cannulae inserted away from joints remain patent for longer periods of time (INS, 2016).*
- For insertion in pediatric clients, use upper extremities, lower extremities, or the scalp in neonates or young infants (O'Grady et al, 2011).

▲ Consider whether sedation or the use of local anesthetic is suitable for insertion of a catheter, taking into consideration the age of the pediatric client. EB: *The use of effective local anesthetic methods and agents before each painful dermal procedure should be discussed with the health care provider (INS, 2016; Stoltz & Manworren, 2017).*

▲ Use diversion while performing the procedure. EB: *Diversion reduces anxiety (Goff et al, 2013).*

Geriatric

- The preceding interventions may be adapted for the geriatric client.
- Consider the physical, emotional, and cognitive changes related to older adults.

- Use strict aseptic technique for venipuncture of older clients. EB: *Older adults are at an increased risk of infection because of decreased immunological function (Azar & Ballas, 2020).*

Home Care

- Some devices may remain after discharge. Provide device-specific education to the client and family members about care of the selected device.
- Help in the choice of actions that support self-care. The nurse can provide valuable information that can be used to guide decision-making to maximize the self-care abilities of clients receiving home infusion therapy.
- Select, with the client, the insertion site most compatible with the development of activities of daily living (ADLs).
- Minimize the use of continuous IV therapy whenever possible. CEBN: *Clients who received intermittent IV therapy via a saline lock were more independent regarding ability to perform self-care ADLs than those who received continuous IV therapy (O'Halloran, et al, 2008).*

REFERENCES

Abolfotouh, M. A., Salam, M., Bani-Mustafa, A., White, D., & Balkhy, H. H. (2014). Prospective study of incidence and predictors of peripheral intravenous catheter-induced complications. *Therapeutic and Clinical Risk Management*, *10*, 993–1001.

Azar, A., & Ballas, Z. K. (2020). Immune function in older adults. R. Marsh, & A.M. Feldweg, (Eds.). Waltham, MA : UpToDate. Retrieved from https://www.uptodate.com/contents/immune-function-in-older-adults?search=immune%20function%20in%20older%20adults&source=search_result&selectedTitle=1~150&usage_type=default&display_rank=1. [Accessed February 24, 2022].

Goff, D. A., Larsen, P., Brinkley, J., et al. (2013). Resource utilization and cost of inserting peripheral intravenous catheters in hospitalized children. *Hospital Pediatrics*, *3*(3), 185–191.

Helm, R. E., Klausner, J. D., Klemperer, J. D., Flint, L. M., & Huang, E. (2015). Accepted but unacceptable: Peripheral IV catheter failure. *Journal of Infusion Nursing*, *38*(3), 189–203.

Infusion Nurses Society (INS). (2016). Infusion therapy standards of practice. *Journal of Infusion Nursing*, *39*(Suppl. 1), 1–169. Retrieved from https://source.yiboshi.com/20170417/1492425631944540325.pdf. [Accessed August 4, 2021].

Jayasekara, R. (2017). *Intravenous cannulation (pediatric): Clinical information*. Joanna Briggs Institute EBP Database, JBI166.

Kaur, A. (2019). *Peripheral intravenous cannula (PIVC): Insertion*. Joanna Briggs Institute EBP Database, JBI140045.

López-Briz, E., Ruiz Garcia, V., Cabello, J. B., Bort-Marti, S., Carbonell Sanchis, R., & Burls, A. (2014). Heparin versus 0.9% sodium chloride intermittent flushing for prevention of occlusion in central venous catheters in adults. *Cochrane Database of Systematic Reviews*, *10*, CD008462.

Loubani, O. M., & Green, R. S. (2015). A systematic review of extravasation and local tissue injury from administration of vasopressors through peripheral intravenous catheters and central venous catheters. *Journal of Critical Care*, *30*(3), 653. e9–e17.

O'Grady, N. P., Alexander, M., Burns, L. A., et al. (2011). Guidelines for the prevention of intravascular catheter-related infections. *American Journal of Infection Control*, *39*(4 Suppl. 1), S1–S34. Retrieved from https://www.cdc.gov/infectioncontrol/pdf/guidelines/bsi-guidelines-H.pdf. [Accessed February 24, 2022].

O'Halloran, L., El-Masri, M. M., & Fox-Wasylyshyn, S. M. (2008). Home intravenous therapy and the ability to perform self-care activities of daily living. *Journal of Infusion Nursing*, *31*(6), 367–374.

Phillips, L. D. (2014). *Manual of IV therapeutics: Evidence-based practice for infusion therapy* (6th ed.). Philadelphia: F.A. Davis.

Porritt, K. (2016). *Intravascular therapy: Maintaining catheter lumen patency*. Joanna Briggs Institute EBP Database, JBI14448.

Porritt, K. (2018). *Peripheral intravenous cannula: Removal*. Joanna Briggs Institute EBP Database, JBI14184.

Stoltz, P., & Manworren, R. C. B. (2017). Comparison of children's venipuncture fear and pain: Randomized controlled trial of EMLA® and J-Tip® needleless injection system. *Journal of Pediatric Nursing*, *37*, 91–96.

Webster, J., Osborne, S., Rickard, C., & Hall, J. (2010). Clinically-indicated replacement versus routine replacement of peripheral venous catheters. *Cochrane Database of Systematic Reviews*, *3*, CD007798.

Impaired Spontaneous Ventilation Domain 4 Activity/rest Class 4 Cardiovascular/pulmonary responses

Debra Siela, PhD, RN, ACNS-BC, CCRN-K, CNE, RRT

NANDA-I

Definition

Inability to initiate and/or maintain independent breathing that is adequate to support life.

Defining Characteristics

Apprehensiveness; decreased arterial oxygen saturation; decreased cooperation; decreased partial pressure of oxygen; decreased tidal volume; increased accessory muscle use; increased heart rate; increased metabolic rate; increased partial pressure of carbon dioxide (PCO_2); psychomotor agitation

Related Factors

Respiratory muscle fatigue

Associated Conditions

Impaired metabolism

NOC (Nursing Outcomes Classification)

Suggested NOC Outcomes

Neurological Status: Central Motor Control; Respiratory Status: Gas Exchange, Ventilation

Example NOC Outcome with Indicators

Achieves appropriate **Respiratory Status: Ventilation** as evidenced by the following indicators: Respiratory rate/Respiratory rhythm/Depth of inspiration/Symmetrical chest expansion/Ease of breathing/ Moves sputum out of airway/Accessory muscle use not present/Adventitious breath sounds not present/ Chest retraction not present/Tidal volume/Vital capacity. (Rate the outcome and indicators of **Respiratory Status: Ventilation:** 1 = severe deviation from normal range, 2 = substantial deviation from normal range, 3 = moderate deviation from normal range, 4 = mild deviation from normal range, 5 = no deviation from normal range [see Section I].)

Client Outcomes

Client Will (Specify Time Frame)

- Maintain arterial blood gases within safe parameters
- Remain free of dyspnea or restlessness
- Effectively maintain airway
- Effectively mobilize secretions

NIC (Nursing Interventions Classification)

Suggested NIC Interventions

Artificial Airway Management; Mechanical Ventilation: Invasive; Respiratory Monitoring; Resuscitation: Neonate; Ventilation Assistance; Mechanical Ventilation Management: Noninvasive

Example NIC Activities—Mechanical Ventilation Management

Invasive

Monitor for conditions indicating a need for ventilation support (e.g., respiratory muscle fatigue, neurological dysfunction second to trauma, anesthesia, drug overdose, refractory respiratory acidosis); Consult with other health care personnel in selection of a ventilator mode

Nursing Interventions and *Rationales*

- ▲ Collaborate with the client, family, and provider regarding possible intubation and ventilation. Ask whether the client has advance directives and, if so, integrate them into the plan of care with clinical data regarding overall health and reversibility of the medical condition. EB: *Client preferences and goals of care need to be acknowledged and discussed when planning care. Advance directives protect client autonomy and help ensure that the client's wishes are respected. Many states now have Physician Orders for Life-Sustaining Treatment (POLST), Medical Orders for Life-Sustaining Treatment (MOLST), Medical Orders for Scope of Treatment (MOST), Physician Order for Scope of Treatment (POST), Do Not Resuscitate Order/Clinician Orders for Life-Sustaining Treatment (DNR/COLST), and Transportable Physician Orders for Patient Preferences (TPOPP) (House & Ogilvie, 2021). Explore the client's wishes, if possible, before requiring mechanical ventilation support.*

- ● Assess and respond to changes in the client's respiratory status. Monitor the client for dyspnea, increase in respiratory rate, use of accessory muscles, retraction of intercostal muscles, flaring of nostrils, decrease in O_2 saturation, cyanosis, and subjective complaints (Gallagher, 2017; Loscalzo, 2018).

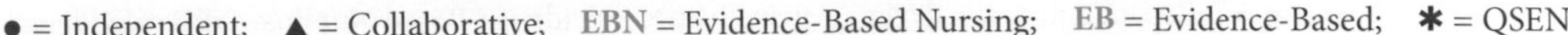

- Have the client use a numerical scale (0–10) or visual analog scale to self-report dyspnea before and after interventions. EB: *The numerical rating scale is a valid measure of dyspnea and has been found to be easiest for clients to use. Incorporating client self-report of dyspnea assists with assessment of symptom intensity, distress, progression, impact, and resolution of dyspnea (Mahler & O'Donnell, 2015; Campbell, 2017). Determine intensity, unpleasantness, or distress of dyspnea using a rating scale such as an intensity-focused modified Borg Scale, Respiratory Distress Observation Scale, or visual analog scale (Parshall et al, 2012; Campbell, 2017).*
- Assess for history of chronic respiratory disorders when administering oxygen .EB: *When managing acute respiratory failure in clients with chronic obstructive pulmonary disease (COPD), continually assess the client's oxygenation needs. Long-term administration of oxygen (>15 hours per day) has been shown to increase survival in clients with severe, resting hypoxemia (Global Initiative for Chronic Obstructive Lung Disease [GOLD], 2020).*
- ▲ Collaborate with the health care provider and respiratory therapists in determining the appropriateness of noninvasive positive pressure ventilation/noninvasive ventilation (NPPV/NIV) for the decompensated client with respiratory diseases (including COPD). Ventilatory support during an exacerbation can be provided by either noninvasive or invasive ventilation (GOLD, 2020). NIV improves respiratory acidosis and decreases respiratory rate, severity of breathlessness, incidence of ventilator-associated pneumonia (VAP), and hospital length of stay (American Association of Critical Care Nurses, 2017a; GOLD, 2020).
- ▲ Assist with implementation, client support, and monitoring if NPPV/NIV is used. EB: *In a client with exacerbation of COPD, NPPV/NIV can be as effective as intubation with use of a ventilator (GOLD, 2020). NPPV/NIV has also been found to improve outcomes in clients with acute cardiogenic pulmonary edema (Pierce, 2021; Sauls, 2021). It can also be used in acute respiratory failure causes such as asthma, pneumonia, postextubation failure, and thoracic trauma. The use of continuous positive airway pressure and bilevel positive airway pressure has been shown to improve oxygenation and decrease the rate of endotracheal intubation in clients with acute pulmonary edema (Frazier, 2017; GOLD, 2020).*
- If the client has apnea, respiratory muscle fatigue, somnolence, hypoxemia, and/or acute respiratory acidosis, prepare the client for possible intubation and mechanical ventilation. EB: *These indicators may predict the need for invasive mechanical ventilation to support the client's respiratory efforts (Gallagher, 2017). The indications for initiating invasive mechanical ventilation during a COPD exacerbation include a failure of an initial trial of NIV (Gallagher, 2017; GOLD, 2020).*
- If a client with acute respiratory failure (ARF) has a Rapid Shallow Breathing Index (RSBI) >105, endotracheal intubation is likely needed with invasive mechanical ventilation. A client with ARF with an RSBI of <105 may require only noninvasive ventilation (Karthika et al, 2016).

Ventilator Support

- ▲ Explain the endotracheal intubation and mechanical ventilation process to the client and family as appropriate, and during intubation administer sedation for client comfort according to the health care provider's orders. EB: *Explanation of the procedure decreases anxiety and reinforces information; premedication allows for a more controlled intubation with decreased incidence of insertion problems (Gallagher, 2017).*
- Secure the endotracheal tube in place using either tape or a commercially available device, auscultate bilateral breath sounds, use a CO_2 detector, and obtain a chest radiograph to confirm endotracheal tube placement. EBN: *Security of the tube is needed to prevent inadvertent extubation. Nursing studies have shown conflicting results regarding the preferable way to secure the endotracheal tube (Goodrich, 2017a).* EB: *Auscultation alone is an unreliable method for checking endotracheal tube placement. A CO_2 detector can be used to confirm tube placement in the trachea (Goodrich, 2017b); However, correct position of the endotracheal tube in the trachea (3 to 5 cm above the carina) must be confirmed by chest radiograph (Goodrich, 2017a, 2017b). Calorimetric CO_2 detectors have also been used successfully to detect inadvertent airway intubation during gastric tube placement (Goodrich, 2017a, 2017b).*
- ▲ Review ventilator settings with the health care provider and respiratory therapy to ensure support is appropriate to meet the client's minute ventilation requirements (Chacko et al, 2015). EB: *Ventilator settings should be adjusted to prevent hyperventilation or hypoventilation. A variety of new modes of ventilation are currently available that are responsive to client effort (pressure support) (Gallagher, 2017).*
- ▲ Suction as needed and hyperoxygenate according to facility policy.
- Check that monitor alarms are set appropriately at the start of each shift. EB: *This action helps ensure client safety (Gallagher, 2017).*

- Respond to ventilator alarms promptly. If unable to immediately locate the source/cause of an alarm, use a manual self-inflating resuscitation bag to ventilate the client while waiting for assistance. EB: *Common causes of a high-pressure alarm include secretions, condensation in the tubing, biting of the endotracheal tube, decreased compliance of the lungs, and compression of the tubing. Common causes of a low-pressure alarm are ventilator disconnection, leaks in the circuit, and changing compliance. Using a manual self-inflating resuscitation bag with supplemental oxygen, the nurse can provide immediate ventilation and oxygenation as needed (Gallagher, 2017; Pierce, 2021).*
- Prevent unplanned extubation by maintaining stability of endotracheal tube (Goodrich, 2017b). EB: *Prevent unplanned extubation with use of weaning protocol (Pierce, 2021).*
- Drain collected fluid from condensation out of ventilator tubing as needed. EB: *This action reduces the risk for infection by decreasing inhalation of contaminated water droplets (Gallagher, 2017).*
- Note ventilator settings of flow of inspired oxygen, peak inspiratory pressure, tidal volume, and alarm activation at intervals and when removing the client from the ventilator for any reason. EB: *Checking the settings ensures that safety measures are taken and that the client is not left on 100% oxygen after suctioning (Gallagher, 2017).*

▲ Administer analgesics and sedatives as needed to facilitate client comfort and rest. Use behavioral and sedation scales for nonverbal clients to provide a consistent way of monitoring pain and sedation levels and ensuring that therapeutic outcomes are being met. EB: *Clients receiving mechanical ventilation frequently require sedation to help attenuate the anxiety, pain, and agitation associated with this intervention. The overall goal of sedation during mechanical ventilation is to provide physiological stability, ventilator synchrony, and comfort for clients (Makic et al, 2015; Devlin et al, 2018).*

- Tools such as the Riker Sedation-Agitation Scale, the Motor Activity Assessment Scale, the Ramsey Scale, or the Richmond Agitation-Sedation Scale may be useful in monitoring levels of sedation. EB: *Each of these instruments has established reliability and validity and can be used to monitor the effect of sedative therapy (Devlin et al, 2018).*
- Alternatives to medications for decreasing anxiety should be attempted, such as music therapy with selections of the client's choice played on headphones at intervals. EBN/EB: *Music therapy has been reported to decrease anxiety and reduce heart and respiratory rate in critically ill and intubated clients (Ergin et al, 2018).*
- Analyze and respond to arterial blood gas results, end-tidal CO_2 levels, and pulse oximetry values. Ventilatory support must be closely monitored to ensure adequate oxygenation and acid-base balance. EB: *End-tidal CO_2 monitoring is best used as an adjunct to direct client observation and is used to monitor a client's ventilatory status and pulmonary blood flow (Gallagher, 2017).*
- Use an effective means of verbal and nonverbal communication with the client. Barriers to communication include endotracheal tubes, sedation, and general weakness associated with a critical illness. EB: *Basic technologies should be readily available to the client, including eyeglasses and hearing aids. A variety of communication devices are available, including electronic voice output communication aids, alphabet boards, picture boards, computers, and writing slate. Ask the client for input into their care as appropriate (Vollman et al, 2017; Pierce, 2021).*
- Move the endotracheal tube from side to side at least every 24 hours, and tape it or secure it with a commercially available device. Assess and document client's skin condition, and ensure correct tube placement at lip line (Vollman et al, 2017).
- Implement steps to prevent ventilator-associated events (VAEs), such as ventilator-associated pneumonia (VAP), including continuous removal of subglottic secretions, elevation of the head of bed to 30 to 45 degrees (Hospital Quality Institute, 2015; American Association of Critical Care Nurses, 2017a) unless medically contraindicated, change of the ventilator circuit no more than every 48 hours, and handwashing before and after contact with each client.
- The accumulation of contaminated oropharyngeal secretions above the endotracheal tube may contribute to the risk of aspiration. EB: *Use endotracheal tubes that allow for the continuous aspiration of subglottic secretions (Vollman et al, 2017; Pierce, 2021).* EB: *Subglottic secretion drainage during mechanical ventilation results in a significant reduction in VAEs, including late-onset VAP (Vollman et al, 2017). Use of continuous subglottic suctioning endotracheal tubes for intubation in clients who are predicted to require more than 48 hours likely results in decreased incidence of VAP (American Association of Critical Care Nurses, 2017a).*

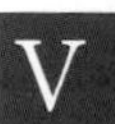

- Position the client in a semirecumbent position with the head of the bed at a 30- to 45-degree angle to decrease the aspiration of gastric, oral, and nasal secretions (Hospital Quality Institute, 2015; American Association of Critical Care Nurses, 2017a; Vollman et al, 2017).
- Consider use of kinetic therapy, using a kinetic bed that slowly moves the client with 40-degree turns. EB: *Rotational therapy may decrease the incidence of pulmonary complications in high-risk clients with increasing ventilator support requirements, at risk for VAP, and clinical indications for acute lung injury or acute respiratory distress syndrome with worsening PaO_2:FiO_2 ratio, presence of fluffy infiltrates via chest radiograph concomitant with pulmonary edema, and refractory hypoxemia* (Hanneman et al, 2015; St. Clair & MacDermott, 2017).
- Perform handwashing using both soap and water and alcohol-based solution before and after all mechanically ventilated client contact to prevent spread of infections *(Centers for Disease Control and Prevention, 2019).*
- Provide routine oral care using tooth brushing and oral rinsing with an antimicrobial agent if needed (American Association of Critical Care Nurses, 2017b, 2017b; Vollman et al, 2017). EB: *Reducing bacterial colonization of oral cavity includes interventions of daily oral assessment, deep suctioning every 4 hours, tooth brushing twice per day with a plaque reducer, and oral tissue cleaning with peroxide every 4 hours. A Cochrane review found that routine oral care that included chlorhexidine mouthwash or gel resulted in a 40% reduction in development of VAP (Zhao et al, 2020).*
- Maintain proper cuff inflation for both endotracheal tubes and cuffed tracheostomy tubes with minimal leak volume or minimal occlusion volume to decrease risk of aspiration and reduce incidence of VAP (American Association of Critical Care Nurses, 2016; Johnson, 2017).
- Reposition the client as needed. Use rotational bed or kinetic bed therapy in clients for whom side-to-side turning is contraindicated or difficult. EBN: *Changing position frequently decreases the incidence of atelectasis, pooling of secretions, and resultant VAP. Continuous, lateral rotational therapy has been shown to improve oxygenation and decrease the incidence of VAP (St. Clair & MacDermott, 2017).*
- ▲ Clients mechanically ventilated for more than 24 hours can benefit from protocolized rehabilitation directed toward early mobilization (Schmidt et al, 2017).
- Assess bilateral anterior and posterior breath sounds every 2 to 4 hours and as needed; respond to any relevant changes (Gallagher, 2017).
- Assess responsiveness to ventilator support; monitor for subjective complaints and sensation of dyspnea (Gallagher, 2017).
- ▲ Collaborate with the interdisciplinary team in treating clients with acute respiratory failure. Collaborate with the health care team to meet the client's ventilator care needs and avoid complications. EB: *A collaborative approach to caring for mechanically ventilated clients has been demonstrated to reduce length of time on the ventilator and length of stay in the intensive care unit (Devlin et al, 2018).*
- Document assessments and interventions according to policy.

Geriatric

- Recognize that critically ill older adults have a high rate of morbidity when mechanically ventilated.
- ▲ NPPV may be used during acute treatment of older clients with impaired ventilation. EB: *Current standards suggest that the use of NPPV may facilitate either not placing an older client on a mechanical ventilator or assist with preventing reintubation (Ouellette et al, 2017).*

Home Care

- ▲ Some of the interventions listed previously may be adapted for home care use. Begin discharge planning as soon as possible with the case manager or social worker to assess the need for home support systems, assistive devices, and community or home health services.
- ▲ With help from a medical social worker, assist the client and family to determine the fiscal effect of care in the home versus an extended care facility.
- Assess the home setting during the discharge process to ensure the home can safely accommodate ventilator support (e.g., adequate space and electricity).
- Have the family contact the electric company and place the client residence on a high-risk list in case of a power outage. Some home-based care requires special conditions for safe home administration.
- Assess the caregivers for commitment to supporting a ventilator-dependent client in the home.
- Be sure that the client and family or caregivers are familiar with operation of all ventilation devices, know how to suction secretions if needed, are competent in doing tracheostomy care, and know schedules for

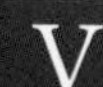

cleaning equipment. Have the designated caregiver or caregivers demonstrate care before discharge. Some home-based care involves specialized technology and requires specific skills for safe and appropriate care.

- Assess client and caregiver knowledge of the disease, client needs, and medications to be administered via ventilation-assistive devices. Avoid analgesics. Assess knowledge of how to use equipment. Teach as necessary.
- A client receiving ventilation support may not be able to articulate needs. Respiratory medications can have side effects that change the client's respiration or level of consciousness.
- Establish an emergency plan and criteria for use. Identify emergency procedures to be used until medical assistance arrives. Teach and role-play emergency care. A prepared emergency plan reassures the client and family and ensures client safety.

Client/Family Teaching and Discharge Planning

- Explain to the client the potential sensations that will be experienced, including relief of dyspnea, the feeling of lung inflations, the noise of the ventilator, and the reality of alarms. EB: *Knowledge of potential sensations and experiences before they are encountered can decrease anxiety. Administration of sedatives and/or narcotics may be needed to provide adequate oxygenation and ventilation in some clients (Baldwin & Cox, 2016; Gallagher, 2017).*
- Explain to the client and family about being unable to speak, and work out an alternative system of communication. See previously mentioned interventions (Gallagher, 2017).
- Demonstrate to the family how to perform simple procedures, such as suctioning secretions in the mouth with a tonsil-tip catheter, providing range-of-motion exercises, and reconnecting the ventilator immediately if it becomes disconnected. EB: *Families are a critical part of the client's care, may be present at the bedside for prolonged periods of time, and need information about the plan of care (Gallagher, 2017).*
- Offer both the client and family explanations of how the ventilator works and answer any questions. EB: *Having questions answered is often cited as an important need of clients and families when a client is on a ventilator (Gallagher, 2017).*

REFERENCES

American Association of Critical Care Nurses. (2016). AACN practice alert: Prevention of aspiration in adults. *Critical Care Nurse*, *36*(1), e20–e24. Retrieved from https://www.aacn.org/~/media/aacn-website/clincial-resources/practice-alerts/preventionaspirationpracticealert.pdf. [Accessed August 4, 2021].

American Association of Critical Care Nurses. (2017a). AACN Practice Alert: Prevention of ventilator-associated pneumonia in adults. *Critical Care Nurse*, *37*(3), e22–e25. Retrieved from https://www.aacn.org/~/media/aacn-website/clincial-resources/practice-alerts/preventingvapinadults2017.pdf. [Accessed August 4, 2021].

American Association of Critical Care Nurses. (2017b). AACN Practice alert: Oral care for acutely and critically ill patients. *Critical Care Nurse*, *37*(3), e19–e21. Retrieved from https://www.aacn.org/~/media/aacn-website/clincial-resources/practice-alerts/oralcarepractalert2017.pdf. [Accessed August 4, 2021].

Baldwin, J., & Cox, J. (2016). Treating dyspnea: Is oxygen therapy the best option for all patients? *Medical Clinics of North America*, *100*(5), 1123–1130. https://doi.org/10.1016/j.mcna.2016.04.018.

Campbell, M. L. (2017). Dyspnea. *Critical Care Nursing Clinics of North America*, *29*(4), 461–470. https://doi.org/10.1016/j.cnc.2017.08.006.

Centers for Disease Control and Prevention (CDC). (2019). *Hand hygiene in healthcare settings*. Retrieved from http://www.cdc.gov/handhygiene/Basics.html. [Accessed August 4, 2021].

Chacko, B., Peter, J. V., Tharyan, P., John, G., & Jeyaseelan, L. (2015). Pressure-controlled versus volume-controlled ventilation for acute respiratory failure due to acute lung injury (ALI) or acute respiratory distress syndrome (ARDS). *Cochrane Database of Systematic Reviews*, *1*, CD008807.

Devlin, J. W., Skrobik, Y., Gélinas, C., et al. (2018). Clinical practice guidelines for the prevention and management of pain, agitation/sedation, delirium, immobility, and sleep disruption in adult patients in the ICU. *Critical Care Medicine*, *46*(9), e825–e873. https://doi.org/10.1097/CCM.0000000000003299.

Ergin, E., Sagkal Midilli, T., & Baysal, E. (2018). The effect of music on dyspnea severity, anxiety, and hemodynamic parameters in patients with dyspnea. *Journal of Hospice and Palliative Nursing*, *20*(1), 81–87. https://doi.org/10.1097/NJH.0000000000000403.

Frazier, K. (2017). Weaning mechanical ventilation. In D. L. Wiegand (Ed.), *AACN procedure manual for high acuity, progressive, and critical care* (7th ed.) (pp. 277–285). Philadelphia: Elsevier.

Gallagher, J. (2017). Invasive mechanical ventilation (through an artificial airway): Volume and pressure modes. In D. L. Wiegand (Ed.), *AACN procedure manual for high acuity, progressive, and critical care* (7th ed.) (pp. 227–248). Philadelphia: Elsevier.

Global Initiative for Chronic Obstructive Lung Disease (GOLD). (2020). *Global strategy for the diagnosis, management, and prevention of chronic obstructive pulmonary disease*. Retrieved from https://goldcopd.org/wp-content/uploads/2019/12/GOLD-2020-FINAL-ver1.2-03Dec19_WMV.pdf. [Accessed August 4, 2021].

Goodrich, C. (2017a). Endotracheal intubation (assist). In D. L. Wiegand (Ed.), *AACN procedure manual for high Acuity, progressive, and critical care* (7th ed.) (pp. 23–31). Philadelphia: Elsevier.

Goodrich, C. (2017b). Endotracheal intubation (perform). In D. L. Wiegand (Ed.), *AACN procedure manual for high Acuity, progressive, and critical care* (7th ed.) (pp. 8–22). Philadelphia: Elsevier.

Hanneman, S. K., Gusick, G. M., Hamlin, S. K., et al. (2015). Manual vs automated lateral rotation to reduce preventable pulmonary complications in ventilator patients. *American Journal of Critical Care*, *24*(1), 24–32.

Hospital Quality Institute. (2015). *Eliminating ventilator-associated events (VAP) and ventilator-associated pneumonia (VAP/VAE)*. HQI Toolkit.

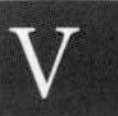

Retrieved from http://www.hqinstitute.org/hqi-toolkit/eliminating-vapvae. [Accessed August 4, 2021].
House, S. A., & Ogilvie, W. A. (2021). *Advance directives.* StatPearls [Internet]. Treasure Island, FL: StatPearls Publishing. Retrieved from https://pubmed.ncbi.nlm.nih.gov/29083680/. [Accessed February 24, 2022].
Johnson, R. (2017). Tracheostomy cuff and tube care. In D. L. Wiegand (Ed.), *AACN procedure manual for high acuity, progressive, and critical care* (7th ed.) (pp. 89–102). Philadelphia: Elsevier.
Karthika, M., Al Enezi, F. A., Pillai, L. V., & Arabi, Y. M. (2016). Rapid shallow breathing index. *Annals of Thoracic Medicine, 11*(3), 167–176. https://doi.org/10.4103/1817-1737.176876.
Loscalzo, J. (2018). Hypoxia and cyanosis. In J. L. Jameson, A. S. Fauci, D. L. Kasper, et al. (Eds.), *Harrison's principles of internal medicine* (20th ed.). New York: McGraw-Hill.
Mahler, D. A., & O'Donnell, D. E. (2015). Recent advances in dyspnea. *Chest, 147*(1), 232–241.
Makic, M. B. F., Rauen, C., Jones, K., & Fisk, A. C. (2015). Continuing to challenge practice to be evidence based. *Critical Care Nurse, 35*(2), 39–50.
Ouellette, D. R., Patel, S., Girard, T. D., et al. (2017). Liberation from mechanical ventilation in critically ill adults: An official American College of Chest Physicians/American Thoracic Society clinical practice guideline: Inspiratory pressure augmentation during spontaneous breathing trials, protocols minimizing sedation, and noninvasive ventilation immediately after extubation. *Chest, 151*(1), 166–180. https://doi.org/10.1016/j.chest.2016.10.036.
Parshall, M. B., Schwartzstein, R. M., Adams, L., et al. (2012). An official American thoracic society statement: Update on the mechanisms, assessment, and management of dyspnea. *American Journal of Respiratory and Critical Care Medicine, 185*(4), 435–452.
Pierce, L. N. B. (2021). Ventilatory assistance. In M. Sole, D. Klein, M. Moseley, et al. (Eds.), *Introduction to critical care nursing* (pp. 173–219). St. Louis: Elsevier.
Sauls, J. L. (2021). Acute respiratory failure. In M. Sole, D. Klein, M. Moseley, et al. (Eds.), *Introduction to critical care nursing* (pp. 375–403). St. Louis: Elsevier.
Schmidt, G. A., Girard, T. D., Kress, J. P., et al. (2017). Official executive summary of an American Thoracic Society/American College of Chest Physicians clinical practice guideline: Liberation from mechanical ventilation in critically ill adults. *American Journal of Respiratory and Critical Care Medicine, 195*(1), 115–119.
St. Clair, J., & MacDermott, J. (2017). Continuous lateral rotation therapy. In D. L. Wiegand (Ed.), *AACN procedure manual for critical care* (7th ed.) (pp. 111–115). Philadelphia: Elsevier.
Vollman, K., Sole, M., & Quinn, B. (2017). Endotracheal tube care and oral care practices for ventilated and non-ventilated patients. In D. L. Wiegand (Ed.), *AACN procedure manual for high acuity, progressive, and critical care* (7th ed.) (pp. 32–39). Philadelphia: Elsevier.
Zhao, T., Wu, X., Zhang, Q., Li, C., Worthington, H. V., & Hua, F. (2020). Oral hygiene care for critically ill patients to prevent ventilator-associated pneumonia. *Cochrane Database of Systematic Reviews, 12*, CD008367. doi:10.1002/14651858.CD008367.pub4.

Dysfunctional Adult Ventilatory Weaning Response

Domain 4 Activity/rest Class 4 Cardiovascular/pulmonary responses

Debra Siela, PhD, RN, ACNS-BC, CCRN-K, CNE, RRT

NANDA-I

Definition

Inability of individuals >18 years of age, who have required mechanical ventilation at least 24 hours, to successfully transition to spontaneous ventilation.

Defining Characteristics

Early Response (30 minutes)

Adventitious breath sounds; audible airway secretions; decreased blood pressure (<90 mm Hg or >20% reduction from baseline); decreased heart rate (>20% reduction from baseline); decreased oxygen saturation (<90% when fraction of inspired oxygen ratio >40%); expresses apprehensiveness; expresses distress; expresses fear of machine malfunction; expresses feeling warm; hyperfocused on activities; increased blood pressure (systolic pressure >180 mm Hg or >20% from baseline); increased in heart rate (>140 bpm or >20% from baseline); increased respiratory rate (>35 rpm or >50% over baseline); nasal flaring; panting; paradoxical abdominal breathing; perceived need for increased oxygen; psychomotor agitation; shallow breathing; uses significant respiratory accessory muscles; wide-eyed appearance

Intermediate Response (30-90 minutes)

Decreased pH (<7.32 or >0.07 reduction from baseline); diaphoresis; difficulty cooperating with instructions; hypercapnia (>50 mm Hg increase in partial pressure of carbon dioxide or >8 mm Hg increase from baseline); hypoxemia (partial pressure of oxygen 50% or oxygen >6 L/min)

Late Response (>90 minutes)

Cardiorespiratory arrest; cyanosis; fatigue; recent onset arrhythmias

Related Factors

Altered sleep-wake cycle; excessive airway secretions; ineffective cough; malnutrition

At-Risk Population

Individuals with history of failed weaning attempt; individuals with history of lung diseases; individuals with history of prolonged dependence on ventilator; individuals with history of unplanned extubation; individuals with unfavorable pre-extubation indexes; older adults

Associated Conditions

Acid-base imbalance; anemia; cardiogenic shock; decreased level of consciousness; diaphragm dysfunction acquired in the intensive care unit; endocrine system diseases; heart diseases; high acuity illness; hyperthermia; hypoxemia; infections; neuromuscular diseases; pharmaceutical preparations; water-electrolyte imbalance

NOC (Nursing Outcomes Classification)

Suggested NOC Outcomes

Respiratory Status: Gas Exchange; Ventilation

Example NOC Outcome with Indicators

Achieves appropriate **Respiratory Status: Ventilation** as evidenced by the following indicators: Respiratory rate/Respiratory rhythm/Depth of inspiration/Symmetrical chest expansion/Ease of breathing/Moves sputum out of airway/Accessory muscle use not present/Adventitious breath sounds not present/Chest retraction not present/Tidal volume/Vital capacity. (Rate the outcome and indicators of **Respiratory Status: Ventilation:** 1 = severe deviation from normal range, 2 = substantial deviation from normal range, 3 = moderate deviation from normal range, 4 = mild deviation from normal range, 5 = no deviation from normal range [see Section I].)

Client Outcomes

Client Will (Specify Time Frame)

- Wean from ventilator with adequate arterial blood gases
- Remain free of unresolved dyspnea or restlessness
- Effectively clear secretions

NIC (Nursing Interventions Classification)

Suggested NIC Interventions

Mechanical Ventilation Management: Invasive; Mechanical Ventilatory Weaning

Example NIC Activities—Mechanical Ventilatory Weaning

Monitor for optimal fluid and electrolyte status; Monitor to ensure client is free of significant infection before weaning

Nursing Interventions and *Rationales*

▲ Assess client's readiness for weaning as evidenced by the following:
- ❍ Physiological and psychological readiness. CEBN: *Assess fears and anxieties that can contribute to prolonged and repeated failure of ventilator weaning. Fear and anxiety have been found to correlate with the client's successful weaning (r = 0.77; p <.001) (Chen et al, 2011).*
- ❍ Resolution of initial medical problem that led to ventilator dependence.
- ❍ Hemodynamic stability.
- ❍ Normal hemoglobin levels.
- ❍ Absence of fever.
- ❍ Normal state of consciousness.
- ❍ Metabolic, fluid, and electrolyte balance.
- ❍ Adequate nutritional status with serum albumin levels >2.5 g/dL.

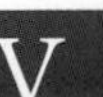

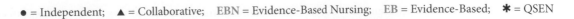

- ❍ Adequate sleep.
- ❍ Adequate pain management and minimal sedation.

EB: *The rapid shallow breathing index (RSBI) may predict weaning success (Peñuelas, Thille, & Esteban, 2015; Furqan et al, 2019; Lin et al, 2020). A spontaneous breathing trial (SBT) is often preceded by evaluation of the client's level of consciousness, physiological and hemodynamic stability, adequacy of oxygenation and ventilation, spontaneous breathing capability, and respiratory rate and pattern. Routine weaning predictor parameters include negative inspiratory force (NIF), vital capacity (VC), tidal volume (VT), respiratory rate (RR), minute ventilation (VE), and RSBI (Kacmarek, 2021; Pierce, 2021). However, applying these weaning predictors should not delay extubation decisions (Peñuelas, Thille, & Esteban, 2015; Lin et al, 2020). Decreased heart rate variability and respiratory rate variability are associated with weaning/extubation failure and should be assessed to help predict weaning outcomes (Kacmarek, 2021; Pierce, 2021). Assessment of the percent of change in diaphragm thickness (Δtdi%) between end-expiration and end-inspiration can reflect diaphragm strength. This measurement is analogous to ejection fraction of the heart (Peñuelas, Thille, & Esteban, 2015; Jansson et al, 2019). Neuromuscular weakness related to respiratory muscle strength at time of extubation was common, reinforcing the need for early ambulation while on mechanical ventilation (Ouellette et al, 2017). Predictors of extubation failure include disease severity, secretion burden, higher minute ventilation, and lower oxygenation (Kacmarek, 2021).*

- ▲ Evaluate serum electrolytes, complete blood count, and nutritional status as a measure of client readiness to wean. **EB:** *The integrative index combining serum albumin, hemoglobin, and Glasgow Coma Scale (GCS) can predict extubation outcomes better than RSBI in an adult medical intensive care unit (Wu et al, 2019).* **EB:** *Multiple SBT attempts, weak cough, and low albumin were associated with failed extubation and resulted in increased reintubation in medicalclients (Xiao & Duan, 2018).*
- ▲ Assess arterial blood gas analysis as part of weaning interventions. Monitor pulse oximetry and not correlation of pulse oximeter reading with arterial blood gas results. **EB:** *Arterial blood gases with abnormal values after an SBT may identify clients who will experience extubation failure (Keyal et al, 2020).*
- ▲ If the client has a central venous catheter, monitor changes in values during weaning as a symptom of hemodynamic stability along with changes in blood pressure and heart rate. **EB:** *An early rise in CVP after starting an SBT was associated with an increased risk of extubation failure (Dubo et al, 2019; Mallat et al, 2020).*
- ▲ Monitor respiratory parameters for weaning and extubation determination. Review and collaborate with respiratory therapists and providers to note improvements in NIF. **EB:** *An NIF threshold of ≤−25 cm H_2O was a moderate-to-good predictor for successful ventilator liberation in mechanically ventilated chronic obstructive pulmonary disease (COPD) clients with hypercapnic respiratory failure (Vahedian-Azimi et al, 2020).*
- ▲ Monitor respiratory rate and volume of independent breaths while on mechanical ventilation. Supporting independent breathing strengthens the diaphragm. **EB:** *Loss of force and reduced diaphragm muscle mass can occur from lack of use while a client is supported on mechanical ventilation (MV) (Petrof, 2018). Even brief periods of MV may result in diaphragm weakness (i.e., ventilator-induced diaphragm dysfunction [VIDD]), which may be associated with difficulty weaning from the ventilator, as well as mortality (Peñuelas et al, 2015). Critical illness–associated diaphragm weakness is consistently associated with poor outcomes, including increased intensive care unit (ICU) mortality, difficult weaning, and prolonged duration of mechanical ventilation (Dres et al, 2017).*
- ▲ Collaborate with respiratory therapy and provider tests to evaluate diaphragm strength for readiness to wean. **EB:** *Diaphragmatic excursion (DE,cm) and inspiration time ($TPIA_{dia}$cm/s) and diaphragmatic contraction speed and velocity measured by ultrasonography are good predictors of extubation success (Varón-Vega et al, 2021). A meta-analysis of 436 mechanically ventilated clients found that diaphragmatic excursion (DE) and diaphragmatic thickening fraction (DTF) showed good diagnostic performance to predict weaning success (Qian et al, 2018). Current literature suggests that diaphragmatic ultrasonography can be a useful and accurate tool to detect diaphragmatic dysfunction in critically ill clients to predict extubation success or failure, to monitor respiratory workload, and to assess atrophy in clients who are mechanically ventilated (Zambon et al, 2017).*
- ▲ Assess the presence and strength of the client's gag reflexes. **EB:** *In individuals with prolonged ventilation the presence of one or both gag reflexes could predict a reduction in extubation failure related to aspiration or excessive upper airway secretions (Houzé et al, 2020).*
- ▲ Collaborate with respiratory therapy and providers to review client readiness to wean using a standardized checklist. Checklist may be referred to as mechanical ventilator liberation protocols or spontaneous awakening trails with spontaneous breathing trials (SAT/SBT) protocols. **EB:** *Implementing an extubation checklist is associated with fewer failed extubations (Bobbs et al, 2019; Jansson et al, 2019).* **EB:** *Clients managed with ventilator liberation protocols spent fewer hours on mechanical ventilation and had earlier ICU*

discharge than did clients managed with without a protocol (Schmidt et al, 2017; Jansson et al, 2019). **EB:** *Goal-directed weaning decreased ventilator days, as well as ICU and hospital length of stay (Zhu et al, 2015). Pairing SAT and SBT interventions has been found to reduce ICU and hospital length of stay, duration of mechanical ventilation, and ventilator-associated events (Klompas et al, 2015; Rose, 2015).*

- ▲ Use evidence-based weaning and extubation protocols as appropriate. **EB:** *The American Thoracic Society recommends use of ventilator liberation protocols to manage clients who have been mechanically ventilated for over 24 hours (Schmidt et al, 2017). Protocol-directed weaning has been demonstrated to be safe and effective allowing for timely and ongoing clinical decision-making by expert nurses and health care providers (Devlin et al, 2018).* **EB:** *The use of lighter sedation resulted in less duration of mechanical ventilation, more ventilator-free days, more ICU-free days, and reduced mortality (Schmidt et al, 2017).*
- ▲ A client may require noninvasive ventilation (NIV) or bilevel positive airway pressure (BiPAP) once extubated from mechanical ventilation to reduce the risk of reintubation. **EB:** *After a spontaneous breathing trial to extubation high-risk clients receiving mechanical ventilation for more than 24 hours should be placed on NIV (Schmidt et al, 2017). Early use of NIV as a prophylactic intervention can be used to prevent reintubation for clients considered at high risk (Bajaj et al, 2015).* **EB:** *The American College of Chest Physicians and American Thoracic Society recommend inspiratory augmentation during an initial SBT, protocols minimizing sedation, and preventive NIV in relation to ventilator liberation (Ouellette et al, 2017).*
- ▲ An early mobility and walking program can promote weaning from a ventilator support as a client's overall strength and endurance improve. Collaborate with respiratory therapy and physical therapy to implement early mobility programs for clients on mechanical ventilation. **EB:** *Acutely hospitalized clients who are mechanically ventilated for greater than 24 hours require early mobilization to build endurance and support successful weaning and extubation (Peñuelas, Thille, & Esteban, 2015; Schmidt et al, 2017).* **EB:** *Early mobility and physical rehabilitation can reduce muscle weakness, mechanical ventilation duration, ICU stay, and hospital stay (Peñuelas, Thille, & Esteban, 2015; Devlin et al, 2018).* **EB:** *The American Thoracic Society/American College of Chest Physicians recommends that acutely hospitalized adults mechanically ventilated for more than 24 hours receive protocolized rehabilitation directed toward early mobilization, and be managed with a ventilator liberation protocol (Girard et al, 2017).*
- ▲ Evaluate client nutritional status as a critical element for successful weaning and ability to be successful with rehabilitation program. **EB:** *When assessing clinical outcomes of survivors of critical illness requiring prolonged mechanic ventilation (PMV), the combination of high protein and a mobility-based rehabilitation program leads to increased rates of discharge home and ventilator weaning success (Wappel et al, 2017).*
- ▲ Provide adequate nutrition to ventilated clients, using enteral feeding when possible. **EB:** *When assessing clinical outcomes of survivors of critical illness requiring PMV, the combination of high protein and a mobility-based rehabilitation program leads to increased rates of discharge home and ventilator weaning success (Wappel et al, 2017).* **EB:** *The Academy of Nutrition and Dietetics strongly recommends that people with COPD have their body weight and medical nutrition therapy be assessed and monitored by a registered dietitian nutritionist (Hanson et al, 2021).*
- • Identify reasons for previous unsuccessful weaning attempts, and include that information in development of the weaning plan. **EB:** *Pressure support reduces respiratory effort compared with T-piece. Continuous positive airway pressure of 0 cm H_2O and T-piece more accurately reflect the physiological conditions after extubation (Peñuelas, Thille, & Esteban, 2015). For difficult/prolonged weaning clients with COPD, use of a T-piece may be associated with a longer time to ventilator liberation than use of pressure support ventilation (Santos Pellegrini et al, 2018).* **EB:** *A meta-analysis of seven studies involving 634 clients suggested that proportional assist ventilation (PAV) is superior to pressure support ventilation (PSV) in terms of weaning success (Ou-Yang et al, 2020).*
- ▲ Collaborate with respiratory therapy and provide for optimal oxygen delivery plan once the client is successfully weaned from mechanical ventilation. **EB:** *Compared with the Venturi mask, high-flow nasal cannula oxygen use results in better oxygenation for the same set FiO_2 after extubation. Use of high-flow nasal cannula is associated with better comfort, fewer desaturations and interface displacements, and a lower reintubation rate (Peñuelas, Thille, & Esteban, 2015; Zhu et al, 2019). The use of high-flow nasal oxygen with NIV immediately after extubation significantly decreased the risk of reintubation compared with high-flow nasal oxygen alone (HIGH-WEAN Study Group & REVA Research Network, 2019).*
- ▲ Clients with neurological diseases may need special considerations to successfully wean from mechanical ventilation. **EB:** *Extubation failure may be avoided in clients with neurological disease by using protective ventilation, early enteral nutrition, antibiotic therapy standardization, and systematic testing extubation compared with a conventional strategy (Peñuelas, Thille, & Esteban, 2015).*

- ▲ Collaborate with an interdisciplinary team (provider, nurse, respiratory therapist, physical therapist, and dietitian) to develop a weaning plan with a timeline and goals; revise this plan throughout the weaning period. **EB:** *Decisions related to weaning trials should be made in conjunction with members of the interdisciplinary team (Devlin et al, 2018; Jansson et al, 2019; Pierce, 2021).*
- ● Assist client to identify personal strategies that result in relaxation and comfort (e.g., music, visualization, relaxation techniques, reading, television, family visits). Support implementation of these strategies. **EBN:** *Evidence supports music as an effective intervention that can lesson symptoms related to mechanical ventilation and promote effective weaning (Hetland, Lindquist, & Chlan, 2015). Music therapy increases weaning duration on daily weaning and also decreases respiratory rate and dyspnea (Hu et al, 2015; Liang et al, 2016). Clients who received a guided imagery intervention had reduced length of hospital stay (1.4 less days) and 4.88 less mechanical ventilation days compared with the comparison group (Spiva et al, 2015).*
- ● Provide a safe and comfortable environment. Orient the client to the call light button. Ensure that the call light button is readily available, and assure the client that needs will be met responsively. **CEB:** *Reduce fears and anxiety for the client by reinforcing their ability to call for assistance as needed (Chen et al, 2011).*
- ▲ Coordinate pain and sedation medications to minimize sedative effects while optimizing analgesia needs. **EB:** *Appropriate levels of analgesia and sedation are necessary for successful weaning (Devlin et al, 2018; Pierce, 2021). Daily interruption of sedation (SAT) is safe in mechanically ventilated medical ICU clients. Current practice evidence suggests that sedation should be client specific to avoid overuse of sedating agents (Klompas et al, 2015; Makic et al, 2015; Aitken et al, 2018; Devlin et al, 2018; Pierce, 2021).*
- ● Administer analgesics and sedatives as needed to facilitate client comfort and rest. Use behavioral and sedation scales for nonverbal clients to provide a consistent way of monitoring pain and sedation levels and ensuring that therapeutic outcomes are being met. **EB:** *Clients receiving mechanical ventilation frequently require sedation to help attenuate the anxiety, pain, and agitation associated with this intervention (Aitken et al, 2018; Devlin et al, 2018; Pierce, 2021).*
- ● Tools such as the Riker Sedation-Agitation Scale, the Motor Activity Assessment Scale, the Ramsey Scale, or the Richmond Agitation-Sedation Scale may be useful in monitoring levels of sedation (Devlin et al, 2018).
- ● Schedule weaning periods for the time of day when the client is most rested. Cluster care activities to promote successful weaning. Avoid other procedures during weaning: keep the environment quiet and promote restful activities between weaning periods.
- ● Promote a normal sleep-wake cycle, allowing uninterrupted periods of nighttime sleep. **EB:** *Limit visitors during weaning to close and supportive persons; ask visitors to leave if they are negatively affecting the weaning process. Communication with a client and/or the client's family is important to assess the client's typical pattern of sleep (Kacmarek, 2021; Pierce, 2021).*
- ● During weaning, monitor the client's physiological and psychological responses; acknowledge and respond to fears and subjective complaints. Validate the client's efforts during the weaning process.
- ● Involve the client and family in the weaning plan. Inform them of the weaning plan and possible client responses to the weaning process (e.g., potential feelings of dyspnea). Foster a partnership between clients and nurses in care planning for weaning.
- ● Coach the client through episodes of increased anxiety. Remain with the client or place a supportive and calm significant other in this role. Give positive reinforcement, and with permission use touch to communicate support and concern. **EB:** *It is not unusual for a client with lung disease to experience self-limiting episodes of increased shortness of breath. Supporting and coaching a client through such episodes allows weaning to continue (Baldwin & Cox, 2016; Campbell, 2017).*
- ● Terminate weaning when the client demonstrates predetermined criteria or when the following signs of weaning intolerance occur:
  - ❍ Tachypnea, dyspnea, or chest and abdominal asynchrony
  - ❍ Agitation or mental status changes
  - ❍ Decreased oxygen saturation: SaO_2 <90%
  - ❍ Increased $PaCO_2$ or end-tidal CO_2 ($EtCO_2$)
  - ❍ Change in pulse rate or blood pressure or onset of new dysrhythmias
- ▲ If the dysfunctional weaning response is severe, consider slowing weaning to brief periods. Continue to collaborate with the team to determine whether an untreated physiological cause for the dysfunctional weaning pattern remains. Consult with health care provider regarding use of noninvasive ventilation immediately after discontinuing ventilation. Consider an alternative care setting (subacute, rehabilitation facility, home) for clients with prolonged ventilator dependence as a strategy that can positively affect outcomes.

V

Geriatric

- ● Recognize that older clients may require longer periods to wean.
- ▲ NPPV may be used during acute treatment of older clients with impaired ventilation. **EB:** *Current standards suggest that the use of NPPV may facilitate either not placing an older client on a mechanical ventilator or assist with preventing reintubation (Ouellette et al, 2017).*
- ● Explore the client's wishes, if possible, before requiring mechanical ventilation support. Collaborate with the client, family, and provider regarding possible intubation and ventilation. Ask whether the client has advance directives and, if so, integrate them into the plan of care with clinical data regarding overall health and reversibility of the medical condition. **EB:** *Client preferences and goals of care need to be acknowledged and discussed when planning care. Advance directives protect client autonomy and help ensure that the client's wishes are respected. Many states now have Physician Orders for Life-Sustaining Treatment (POLST), Medical Orders for Life-Sustaining Treatment (MOLST), Medical Orders for Scope of Treatment (MOST), Physician Order for Scope of Treatment (POST), Do Not Resuscitate Order/Clinician Orders for Life-Sustaining Treatment (DNR/COLST), and Transportable Physician Orders for Patient Preferences (TPOPP) (House & Ogilvie, 2020).*

Home Care

- ● Weaning from a ventilator at home should be based on client stability and comfort of the client and caregivers under an intermittent care plan. Generally the client will be safer weaning in a hospital environment.

REFERENCES

Aitken, L. M., Bucknall, T., Kent, B., Mitchell, M., Burmeister, E., & Keogh, S. J. (2018). Protocol–directed sedation versus non–protocol–directed sedation in mechanically ventilated intensive care adults and children. *Cochrane Database of Systematic Reviews, 11*, CD009771. https://doi.org/10.1002/14651858.CD009771.pub3.

Bajaj, A., Rathor, P., Sehgal, V., & Shetty, A. (2015). Efficacy of noninvasive ventilation after planned extubation: A systematic review and meta-analysis of randomized controlled trials. *Heart & Lung, 44*(2), 150–157.

Baldwin, J., & Cox, J. (2016). Treating dyspnea: Is oxygen therapy the best option for all patients? *Medical Clinics of North America, 100*(5), 1123–1130. https://doi.org/10.1016/j.mcna.2016.04.018.

Bobbs, M., Trust, M. D., Teixeira, P., et al. (2019). Decreasing failed extubations with the implementation of an extubation checklist. *The American Journal of Surgery, 217*(6), 1072–1075. https://doi.org/10.1016/j.amjsurg.2019.02.028.

Campbell, M. L. (2017). Dyspnea. *Critical Care Nursing Clinics of North America, 29*(4), 461–470. https://doi.org/10.1016/j.cnc.2017.08.006.

Chen, Y. J., Jacobs, W. J., Quan, S. F., Figueredo, A. J., & Davis, A. H. T. (2011). Psychophysiological determinants of repeated ventilator weaning failure: An explanatory model. *American Journal of Critical Care, 20*(4), 292–302.

Devlin, J. W., Skrobik, Y., Gélinas, C., et al. (2018). Clinical practice guidelines for the prevention and management of pain, agitation/sedation, delirium, immobility, and sleep disruption in adult patients in the ICU. *Critical Care Medicine, 46*(9), e825–e873. https://doi.org/10.1097/CCM.0000000000003299.

Dres, M., Goligher, E. C., Heunks, L. M. A., & Brochard, L. J. (2017). Critical illness-associated diaphragm weakness. *Intensive Care Medicine, 43*(10), 1441–1452. https://doi.org/10.1007/s00134-017-4928-4.

Dubo, S., Valenzuela, E. D., Aquevedo, A., et al. (2019). Early rise in central venous pressure during a spontaneous breathing trial: A promising test to identify patients at high risk of weaning failure? *PLoS One, 14*(12), e0225181. https://doi.org/10.1371/journl.pone.0225181.

Furqan, A., Rai, S. A., Ali, L., & Ahmed, R. A. (2019). Comparing the predicted accuracy of pO_2/FIO_2 ratio with rapid shallow breathing index for successful spontaneous breathing trial in intensive care unit. *Pakistan Journal of Medical Sciences, 35*(6), 1605–1610. https://doi.org/10.12669/pmd.35.6.788.

Girard, T. D., Alhazzani, W., Kress, J. P., et al. (2017). An official American thoracic society/American college of chest physicians clinical practice guideline: Liberation from mechanical ventilation in critically ill adults, rehabilitation protocols, ventilator liberation protocols and cuff leak tests. *American Journal of Respiratory and Critical Care Medicine, 195*(1), 120–133. https://doi.org/10.1164/rccm.201610-2075ST.

Hanson, C., Bowser, E. K., Frankenfield, D. C., & Piemonte, T. A. (2021). Chronic obstructive pulmonary disease: A 2019 evidence analysis center evidence-based practice guideline. *Journal of the Academy of Nutrition and Dietetics, 121*(1), 139–165. e15. https://doi.org/10.1016/j.jand.2019.12.001.

Hetland, B., Lindquist, R., & Chlan, L. L. (2015). The influence of music during mechanical ventilation and weaning from mechanical ventilation: A review. *Heart & Lung, 44*(5), 416–425.

HIGH-WEAN Study Group, & REVA Research Network. (2019). Effect of postextubation high-flow nasal oxygen with noninvasive ventilation vs high-flow nasal oxygen alone on reintubation among patients at high risk of extubation failure: A randomized clinical trial. *JAMA, 322*(15), 1465–1475. https://doi.org/10.1001/jama.2019.14901.

House, S. A., & Ogilvie, W. A. (2020). Advance directives. StatPearls [Internet]. Treasure Island, FL: StatPearls Publishing. Retrieved from https://pubmed.ncbi.nlm.nih.gov/29083680/. [Accessed February 28, 2022].

Houzé, M. H., Deye, N., Mateo, J., et al. (2020). Predictors of extubation failure related to aspiration and/or excessive upper airway secretions. *Respiratory Care, 65*(4), 475–481. https://doi.org/10.4187/respcare.07025.

Hu, R. F., Jiang, X. Y., Chen, J., et al. (2015). Non-pharmacological interventions for sleep promotion in the intensive care unit. *Cochrane Database of Systematic Reviews, 10*, CD008808. https://doi.org/10.1002/14651858.CD008808.pub2.

Jansson, M. M., Syrjälä, H. P., & Ala-Kokko, T. I. (2019). Implementation of strategies to liberate patients from mechanical ventilation in a tertiary-level medical center. *American Journal of Infection Control, 47*(9), 1065–1070. https://doi.org/10.1016/j.ajic.2019.03.010.

Kacmarek, R. M. (2021). Discontinuing ventilatory support. In R. M. Kacmarek, J. K. Stoller, & A. J. Heuer (Eds.), *Egan's fundamentals of respiratory care* (12th ed.) (pp. 1184–1211). St. Louis: Elsevier.

Keyal, N. K., Amatya, R., Shrestha, G. S., Acharya, S. P., Shrestha, P. S., & Marhatta, M. N. (2020). Influence of arterial blood gas to guide extubation in intensive care unit patients after spontaneous breathing trial. *Journal of Nepal Health Research Council, 18*(1), 21–26. https://doi.org/10.33314/jnhrc.v18i1.2114.

Klompas, M., Anderson, D., Trick, W., et al. (2015). The preventability of ventilator-associated events. The CDC prevention epicenters wake up and breathe collaborative. *American Journal of Respiratory and Critical Care Medicine, 191*(3), 292–301.

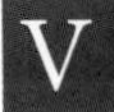

Liang, Z., Ren, D., Choi, J. Y., Happ, M. B., Hravnak, M., & Hoffman, L. A. (2016). Music interventions during daily weaning trials-A 6 day prospective randomized crossover trial. *Complementary Therapies in Medicine, 29*, 72–77.
Lin, F. C., Kuo, Y. W., Jerng, J. S., & Wu, H. D. (2020). Association of weaning preparedness with extubation outcome of mechanically ventilated patients in medical intensive care units: A retrospective analysis. *PeerJ, 8*, e8973. https://doi.org/10.7717/peerj.8973. eCollection2020.
Makic, M. B. F., Rauen, C., Jones, K., & Fisk, A. C. (2015). Continuing to challenge practice to be evidence based. *Critical Care Nurse, 35*(2), 39–50.
Mallat, J., Baghdadi, F. A., Mohammad, U., et al. (2020). Central venous-to-arterial pCO_2 difference and central venous oxygen saturation in the detection of extubation failure in critically ill patients. *Critical Care Medicine, 48*(10), 1454–1461. https://doi.org/10.1097/CCM.0000000000004446.
Ou-Yang, L. J., Chen, P. H., Jhou, H. J., Su, V. Y. F., & Lee, C. H. (2020). Proportional assist ventilation versus pressure support ventilation for weaning from mechanical ventilation in adults: A meta-analysis and trial sequential analysis. *Critical Care, 24*(1), 556. https://doi.org/10.1186/s13054-020-03251-4.
Ouellette, D. R., Patel, S., Girard, T. D., et al. (2017). Liberation from mechanical ventilation in critically ill adults: An official American College of Chest Physicians/American Thoracic Society clinical practice guideline: Inspiratory pressure augmentation during spontaneous breathing trials, protocols minimizing sedation, and noninvasive ventilation immediately after extubation. *Chest, 151*(1), 166–180. https://doi.org/10.1016/j.chest.2016.10.036.
Peñuelas, Ó., Thille, A. W., & Esteban, A. (2015). Discontinuation of ventilatory support: New solutions to old dilemmas. *Current Opinion in Critical Care, 21*(1), 74–81.
Petrof, B. J. (2018). Diaphragm weakness in the critically ill: Basic mechanisms reveal therapeutic opportunities. *Chest, 154*(6), 1395–1403. https://doi.org/10.1016/j.chest.2018.08.1028.
Pierce, L. N. B. (2021). Ventilatory assistance. In M. L. Sole, D. G. Klein, M. J. Moseley, M. B. F. Makic, & L. T. Morata (Eds.), *Introduction to critical care nursing* (8th ed.) (pp. 173–219). St. Louis: Elsevier.
Qian, Z., Yang, M., Li, L., & Chen, Y. (2018). Ultrasound assessment of diaphragmatic dysfunction as a predictor of weaning outcomes from mechanical ventilation: A systematic review and meta-analysis. *BMJ Open, 8*(9), e021189. https://doi.org/10.1136/bmjopen-2017-021189.
Rose, L. (2015). Strategies for weaning from mechanical ventilation: A state of the art review. *Intensive and Critical Care Nursing, 31*(4), 189–195.
Santos Pellegrini, J. A., Manozzo Boniatti, M., Corrêa Boniatti, V., et al. (2018). Pressure-support ventilation or T-piece spontaneous breathing trials for patients with chronic obstructive pulmonary disease—A randomized controlled trial. *PLoS One, 13*(8), e0202404. https://doi.org/10.1371/journal.pone.0202404.
Schmidt, G. A., Girard, T. D., Kress, J. P., et al. (2017). Official executive summary of an American thoracic society/American college of chest physicians clinical practice guideline: Liberation from mechanical ventilation in critically ill adults. *American Journal of Respiratory and Critical Care Medicine, 195*(1), 115–119.
Spiva, L. A., Hart, P. L., Gallagher, E., et al. (2015). The effects of guided imagery on patients being weaned from mechanical ventilation. *Evidence-Based Complementary and Alternative Medicine, 2015*, 802865. http://dx.doi.org/10.1155/2015/802865.
Vahedian-Azimi, A., Bashar, F. R., Boushra, M. N., Quinn, J. W., & Miller, A. C. (2020). Disease specific thresholds for determining extubation readiness: The optimal negative inspiratory force for chronic obstructive pulmonary disease patients. *International Journal of Critical Illness and Injury Science, 10*(2), 99–104. https://doi.org/10.4103/UCHS.IJCHS_37_20.
Varón-Vega, F., Hernández, A., López, M., et al. (2021). Usefulness of diaphragmatic ultrasound in predicting extubation success. *Medicina Intensiva, 45*(4), 226–233. https://doi.org/10.1016/j.medin.2019.10.007.
Wappel, S., Ali, O., & Verceles, A. (2017). The effects of high protein intake and mobility-based rehabilitation on ventilator weaning and discharge status in survivors of critical illness [Abstract]. *American Journal of Respiratory and Critical Care Medicine, 195*, A7575.
Wu, T. J., Shiao, J. S. C., Yu, H. L., & Lai, R. S. (2019). An integrative index for predicting extubation outcomes after successful completion of a spontaneous breathing trial in an adult medical intensive care unit. *Journal of Intensive Care Medicine, 34*(8), 640–645. https://doi.org/10.1177/0885066617706688.
Xiao, M., & Duan, J. (2018). Weaning attempts, cough strength and albumin are independent risk factors of reintubation in medical patients. *Clinical Respiratory Journal, 12*(3), 1240–1246. https://doi.org/10.1111/crj.12657.
Zambon, M., Greco, M., Bocchino, S., Cabrini, L., Beccaria, P. F., & Zangrillo, A. (2017). Assessment of diaphragmatic dysfunction in the critically ill patient with ultrasound: A systematic review. *Intensive Care Medicine, 43*(1), 29–38. https://doi.org/10.1007/s00134-016-4524-z.
Zhu, B., Li, Z., Jiang, L., et al. (2015). Effect of a quality improvement program on weaning from mechanical ventilation: A cluster randomized trial. *Intensive Care Medicine, 41*(10), 1781–1790.
Zhu, Y., Yin, H., Zhang, R., Ye, X., & Wei, J. (2019). High-flow nasal cannula oxygen therapy versus conventional oxygen therapy in patients after planned extubation: A systematic review and meta-analysis. *Critical Care, 23*(1), 180. https://doi.org/10.1186/s13054-019-2465-y.

Dysfunctional Ventilatory Weaning Response

Domain 4 Activity/rest Class 4 Cardiovascular/pulmonary responses

Mary Beth Flynn Makic, PhD, RN, CCNS, CCRN-K, FAAN, FNAP, FCNS

NANDA-I

V

Definition

Inability to adjust to lowered levels of mechanical ventilator support that interrupts and prolongs the weaning process.

Defining Characteristics

Mild

Breathing discomfort; expresses feeling warm; fatigue; fear of machine malfunction; increased focus on breathing; mildly increased respiratory rate over baseline; perceived need for increased oxygen; psychomotor agitation

Moderate

Abnormal skin color; apprehensiveness; blood pressure increased from baseline (<20 mm Hg); decreased air entry on auscultation; diaphoresis; difficulty cooperating; difficulty responding to coaching; facial expression of fear; heart rate increased from baseline (<20 beats/min); hyperfocused on activities; minimal use of respiratory accessory muscles; moderately increased respiratory rate over baseline

Severe

Adventitious breath sounds; agitation; asynchronized breathing with the ventilator; blood pressure increased from baseline (≥20 mm Hg); deterioration in arterial blood gases from baseline; gasping breaths; heart rate increased from baseline (≥20 beats/min); paradoxical abdominal breathing; profuse diaphoresis; shallow breathing; significantly increased respiratory rate above baseline; use of significant respiratory accessory muscles

Related Factors

Physiological Factors

Altered sleep-wake cycle; ineffective airway clearance; malnutrition; pain

Psychological Factors

Anxiety; decreased motivation; fear; hopelessness; inadequate knowledge of weaning process; inadequate trust in health care professional; low self-esteem; powerlessness; uncertainty about ability to wean

Situational

Environmental disturbances; inappropriate pace of weaning process; uncontrolled episodic energy demands

At-Risk Population

Individuals with history of unsuccessful weaning attempt; individuals with history of ventilator dependence >4 days

Associated Conditions

Decreased level of consciousness

NOC, NIC, Client Outcomes, Nursing Interventions and *Rationales,* Client/Family Teaching and Discharge Planning, and References

Refer to care plan for Dysfunctional Adult **Ventilatory Weaning** Response.

Risk for Other-Directed Violence

Domain 11 Safety/protection Class 3 Violence

Marina Martinez-Kratz, MS, RN, CNE

NANDA-I

Definition

Susceptible to behaviors in which an individual demonstrates that he or she can be physically, emotionally, and/or sexually harmful to others.

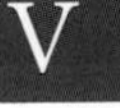

Risk Factors

Easy access to weapon; negative body language; pattern of aggressive anti-social behavior; pattern of indirect violence; pattern of other-directed violence; pattern of threatening violence; suicidal behavior

At-Risk Population

Individuals with history of childhood abuse; individuals with history of cruelty to animals; individuals with history of fire-setting; individuals with history of motor vehicle offense; individuals with history of substance misuse; individuals with history of witnessing family violence

Associated Conditions

Neurological impairment; pathological intoxication; perinatal complications; prenatal complications; psychotic disorders

NOC (Nursing Outcomes Classification)

Suggested NOC Outcomes

Abuse Cessation; Abusive Behavior Self-Restraint; Aggression Self-Restraint; Distorted Thought Self-Control; Impulse Self-Control; Risk Detection

Example NOC Outcome with Indicators

Aggression Self-Restraint as evidenced by the following indicators: Refrains from harming others/ Expresses/Vents needs and negative feelings in a nondestructive manner/Identifies when angry. (Rate the outcome and indicators of **Aggression Self-Restraint:** 1 = never demonstrated, 2 = rarely demonstrated, 3 = sometimes demonstrated, 4 = often demonstrated, 5 = consistently demonstrated [see Section I].)

Client Outcomes

Client Will (Specify Time Frame)

- Stop all forms of abuse (physical, emotional, sexual; neglect; financial exploitation)
- Display no aggressive activity
- Refrain from verbal outbursts
- Refrain from violating others' personal space
- Refrain from antisocial behaviors
- Maintain relaxed body language and decreased motor activity
- Identify factors contributing to abusive/aggressive behavior
- Demonstrate impulse control or state feelings of control
- Identify impulsive behaviors
- Identify and talk about feelings; express anger appropriately
- Displace anger to meaningful activities
- Communicate needs appropriately
- Identify responsibility to maintain control
- Express empathy for victim
- Obtain no access or yield access to harmful objects
- Use alternative coping mechanisms for stress
- Obtain and follow through with counseling

Victim (and Children if Applicable) Will (Specify Time Frame)

- Have safe plan for leaving situation or avoiding abuse
- Resolve depression or traumatic response

Parent Will (Specify Time Frame)

- Monitor social/play contacts
- Provide supervision and nurturing environment
- Intervene to prevent high-risk social behaviors

NIC (Nursing Interventions Classification)

Suggested NIC Interventions

Abuse Protection Support; Anger Control Assistance; Behavior Management; Calming Technique; Coping Enhancement; Crisis Intervention; Delusion Management; Dementia Management; Distraction; Environmental Management: Violence Prevention; Mood Management; Physical Restraint; Seclusion; Substance Use Prevention

Example NIC Activities—Environmental Management: Violence Prevention

Remove other individuals from the vicinity of a violent or potentially violent client; Provide ongoing surveillance of all client access areas to maintain client safety and therapeutically intervene as needed

Nursing Interventions and *Rationales*

- Aggressive/violent behavior may be impulsive, but more commonly it evolves in reaction to the environment (internal or external). In either case, nursing staff must go through specialized training to be prepared for a quick response. EBN: *Aggression management may include the use of physical or chemical restraints (medications), but the former should be used for brief periods only, and the latter should include monitoring for side effects. Music therapy may positively influence the environment (Fong, 2016).*
- Monitor the environment, evaluate situations that could become violent, and intervene early to deescalate the situation. Know and follow institutional policies and procedures concerning violence. Consider that family members or other staff may initiate violence in all settings. Enlist support from other staff rather than attempting to handle situations alone. EBN: *American Psychiatric Nurses Association (APNA) guidelines (2020) warn that workplace violence can occur in all settings and from a variety of sources. Nurses need to be aware and informed of department policies and procedures. Policies should be developed and training programs should be provided in proper use and application of restraints. All nursing units should develop a proactive plan for dealing with violent situations.*
- Assessment with tools that measure violence may be useful in predicting or tracking behavior and serving as outcome measures. EBN: *The Broset Violence Checklist (BVC) is an appropriate tool for acute psychiatric setting that predicts imminent threats and physical violence throughout hospitalizations (Lockertsen et al, 2021).*
- Identify clients with interpersonal hostile-dominance personality characteristics. EBN/EB: *A study found that interpersonal hostile-dominance personality characteristics were most strongly associated with aggression (Podubinski et al, 2017).*
- Assess for the presence of command hallucinations. EB: *Command hallucinations may direct the client to behave violently. Command hallucinations were identified as an independent significant risk factor associated with acute severe or fatal violence in clients with serious mental illness (Chan & Shehtman, 2019).*
- Apply verbal deescalation techniques when clients show increased irritability, hostility, or aggression. EBN: *A small quality improvement study found a clinically significant reduction in the rate of charted aggressive behavior after educating psychiatric nurses on verbal deescalation skills (Haefner, Dunn, & McFarland, 2021).*
- Apply **STAMPEDAR** as an acronym for assessing the immediate potential for violence. EB: *A review of current literature about violence against health care workers identified the following as factors and behaviors indicating the likelihood of a violent episode: staring, tone of voice, anxiety, mumbling, pacing, emotions, disease process, assertive/nonassertive behavior, and access to resources that might be used for violent behavior (STAMPEDAR) (d'Ettore et al, 2018).*
- Determine the presence and degree of homicidal or suicidal risk. EB: *Specific questions will elicit the necessary information: "Have you been thinking about harming someone?" "If yes, who?" "How often do you have these thoughts, and how long do they last?" "Do you have a plan"?" "What is it?" "Do you have access to the means to carry out that plan?" "What has kept you from hurting the person until now?" (Gunn, 2019).* Refer to the care plan for Risk for **Suicidal** Behavior.
- Establish trust, listen to client, convey safety, and assist in developing positive goals for the future. EB: *Therapeutic alliance is the nature of the relationship between the client and the nurse. A systematic review of therapeutic alliance and treatment outcome found that therapeutic alliance has a positive impact on treatment outcomes among individuals engaging in or at risk for aggressive behaviors (Fahlgren, Berman, & McCloskey, 2020).*
- Review state laws and mental health codes to determine local mandates for threat reporting by specific health care professionals. Many mental health providers are required to report harm or threats of harm to another person, referred to as the "duty to warn." EB: *Health care providers must be familiar with the law that applies to where they practice, as the jurisdictional law even in a given state can be dynamic and unpredictable (Felthous et al, 2021).*
- Place the client on the appropriate precaution monitoring and observation protocol. EBN: *A nursing study of continuous client monitoring found that the addition of a protocol designed to prevent violent and impulsive behavior significantly reduced the number of continuous monitoring hours (Ray et al, 2017).*
- Monitor the client's behavior closely, using engagement and support as elements of safety checks while avoiding intrusive overstimulation. EBN: *When lack of control exists, client safety is an important issue, and close*

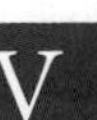

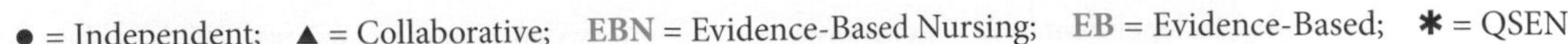

observation is essential. Clients may feel overstimulated by intrusive close observation, resulting in agitation (Moola, 2017).

- Offer information about treatment, unit rules, and procedures. EB: *A review of the literature found support for interventions targeting improvement of staff communication skills. The improvement of skills included a protocol for talking to clients who exhibited aggressive behavior, discussing treatment goals with the client shortly after admission, explaining why the ward's door was locked and the exit rules, providing a schedule of staff meetings to explain staff members' absence from the ward, and clarifying the procedure for making an appointment with the psychiatrists (D'Ettore & Pellicani, 2017).*
- Implement recovery-focused care interventions. EBN: *A study found that the following recovery-focused care interventions could be used to reduce the risk of client aggression: (1) identifying the reason for the behavior before responding; (2) being sensitive to the client's trigger for aggression; (3) focusing on the client's strengths and support, not risks; (4) being attentive to the client's needs; and (5) reconceptualizing aggression as a learning opportunity (Lim, Wynaden, & Heslop, 2019).*
- ▲ After a violent event on a unit, debriefing and support of both staff and clients should be made available. EBN: *Debriefing shortly after a violent episode may restore a sense of control and autonomy. Debriefing can reveal clients' responses to the event and provides the opportunity for staff to offer reassurance and support. The evaluation of past aggression might prevent new aggressive incidents and prevent the use of coercive measures (Vermeulen et al, 2019).*
- ▲ Initiate and promote staff attendance at aggression management training programs. EBN: *Nurses who attended 32 hours of an aggression management training course showed a significant decrease in the mean total score of perceived stress after attending the training (Masa'Deh et al, 2020).*

Pediatric

- Assess for predictors of anger that can lead to violent behavior. EBN: *A correlational study of adolescent anger predictors identified trait anger, anxiety, depression, stress, exposure to violence, and parental drinking behaviors as predictors of anger. Frequency of religious participation was associated with decreased anger (Pullen et al, 2015).*
- ▲ In the case of child abuse or neglect, refer to child protective services. EB: *Nurses are mandated reporters and required by law to report suspected abuse of minor children or vulnerable adults (Lavigne et al, 2017).*
- ▲ Refer the adolescent client to a violence prevention program. EB: *Participation in a school-based violence prevention program for youth exposed to violence in their home, school, or community found that boys and girls decreased in reactive and proactive aggression perpetration. Boys also showed a decline in teen dating violence perpetration and victimization (Reidy et al, 2017).*

Geriatric

- Assess for aggressive behavior in clients with a diagnosis of dementia or severe mental illness. EB: *In a multivariate study of residents at an assisted living facility, dementia and severe mental illness were significant risk factors for resident aggression and abuse (Gimm, Chowdhury, & Castle, 2018).*
- For clients with dementia, provide music therapy. EB: *A systematic review of interventions with aggression in adults with dementia demonstrated significant improvement with music therapy. Person-centered care, communication skills training, and dementia care matching showed reductions in aggression for up to 6 months (Lizarondo, 2016).*
- Document and record suspected elder abuse according to mandated reporter regulations. EB: *The risk for elder abuse is increased during times of social isolation. Nurses are mandated reporters and required by law to report suspected abuse of vulnerable adults (Makaroun, Bachrach, & Rosland, 2020).*

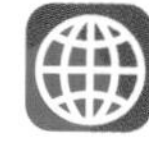

Multicultural

- Exercise caution when using violence risk instruments for populations that have not been included in the testing of the instrument. EB: *A study to address the cross-cultural disparities in the forensic risk literature found concerns with negative labeling capacity, lack of cultural contextualization, individualized focus, and absence of cultural norms and practices in violence risk instruments (Shepherd & Willis-Esqueda, 2018).*

Home Care

- Be alert to the potential for violent behavior in the home setting. Respond to verbal aggression with interventions to deescalate negative emotional states. Violence is a process that can be recognized early. Deescalation involves reducing client stressors, responding to the client with respect, acknowledging the client's feeling state, and assisting the client to regain control. If deescalation does not work, the nurse should leave the home.

- ● Assess family members or caregivers for their ability to protect the client and themselves. The safety of the client between home visits is a nursing priority. Caregivers often need assistance with recognizing or admitting fear of or danger from a loved one. **EBN:** *A qualitative study with home care staff and caregivers of clients with dementia advised that staff use a calm, compassionate approach and minimize controlling strategies such as medications or restraints in dealing with aggressive behavior. A person-centered approach was recommended (Lizarondo, 2016).*
- ● Assess access to lethal means risk factors in the home. **EB:** *A study of lethal means assessment among emergency department (ED) clients with a positive suicide risk screen found that among 545 suicidal clients discharged home from the ED, 85% had no documentation that any provider assessed access to lethal means (Betz et al, 2018).*
- ▲ For situations of suspected neglect or abuse, assist the client to develop an emergency plan with access to a cell phone. **EB:** *Client safety is a nursing priority. An emergency plan with access to a cell phone should address either immediate removal to a safe environment or identification of appropriate steps to take in the event of abuse and the securing of resources for the anticipated action (e.g., financial resources, packed bag, alternative living arrangements) (Souza Marques et al, 2020).*
- ● Encourage safe storage of firearms. **EB:** *To prevent firearm injuries, safe storage of firearms needs to be publicized and emphasized for firearm owners. Nurses can watch the following safe storage video with clients:* https://www.facs.org/quality-programs/trauma/advocacy/ipc *(Duncan et al, 2020).*

Client/Family Teaching and Discharge Planning

- ● Teach relaxation and exercise as ways to release anger and deal with stress. **EB:** *A study of the effect of progressive relaxation therapy found decreased signs and symptom of aggression among clients with risk of violent behavior (Lucya, Hadiyani, & Juniarni, 2019).*
- ● Teach cognitive-behavioral activities, such as active problem-solving, reframing (reappraising the situation from a different perspective), or thought stopping (in response to a negative thought, picture a large stop sign and replace the image with a prearranged positive alternative). Teach the client to confront his or her own negative thought patterns (or cognitive distortions), such as catastrophizing (expecting the very worst), dichotomous thinking (perceiving events in only one of two opposite categories), magnification (placing distorted emphasis on a single event), or unrealistic expectations (e.g., "should get what I want when I want it"). **EB:** *A study of the effects of Rockwood's prison-based Cognitive Behavioral Therapy/Risk–Needs–Responsivity (CBT/RNR) sex offender program found low rates of violence recidivism when compared with untreated offenders (Olver et al, 2020).*
- ▲ Refer perpetrators of violence to acceptance and commitment therapy. **EB:** *A study that examined the impact of an Acceptance and Commitment Therapy (ACT)–based program (Achieving Change Through Values-Based Behavior [ACTV]) found that fewer ACTV participants acquired any new criminal charges, domestic assault charges, or violence charges (Zarling, Bannon, & Berta, 2019).*
- ● Teach clients and families the use of appropriate community resources in emergency situations (e.g., hotline, economic resources access, community mental health agency, ED, 911 in most places in the United States, the toll-free National Domestic Violence Hotline [1-800-799-SAFE]). Virtual resources are increasing and should be made available to clients. **EB:** *The global pandemic has exacerbated the needs of clients and families experiencing violence. A survey of individuals with safety concerns found the need for increased support and economic resource access, coupled with modified safety planning and improved virtual approaches (Wood et al, 2021).*

REFERENCES

American Psychiatric Nurses Association (APNA). (2020). *Position paper: Violence prevention*. Retrieved from https://www.apna.org/i4a/pages/index.cfm?pageID=6081. [Accessed 6 August 2021].

Betz, M. E., Kautzman, M., Segal, D. L., et al. (2018). Frequency of lethal means assessment among emergency department patients with a positive suicide risk screen. *Psychiatry Research*, *260*, 30–35. https://doi.org/10.1016/j.psychres.2017.11.038.

Chan, B., & Shehtman, M. (2019). Clinical risk factors of acute severe or fatal violence among forensic mental health patients. *Psychiatry Research*, *275*, 20–26. https://doi.org/10.1016/j.psychres.2019.03.005.

D'Ettorre, G., & Pellicani, V. (2017). Workplace violence toward mental healthcare workers employed in psychiatric wards. *Safety and Health at Work*, *8*(4), 337–342. https://doi.org/10.1016/j.shaw.2017.01.004.

D'Ettorre, G., Pellicani, V., Mazzotta, M., & Vullo, A. (2018). Preventing and managing workplace violence against healthcare workers in Emergency Departments. *Acta BioMedica: Atenei Parmensis*, *89*(4-S), 28–36. https://doi.org/10.23750/abm.v89i4-S.7113.

Duncan, T. K., Weaver, J. L., Zakrison, T. L., et al. (2020). Domestic violence and safe storage of firearms in the COVID-19 era.

Annals of Surgery, 272(2), e55–e57. https://doi.org/10.1097/SLA.0000000000004088.

Fahlgren, M. K., Berman, M. E., & McCloskey, M. S. (2020). The role of therapeutic alliance in therapy for adults with problematic aggression and associated disorders. *Clinical Psychology & Psychotherapy, 27*(6), 858–886. https://doi.org/10.1002/cpp.2475.

Felthous, A. R., O'Shaughnessy, R., François-Purssell, I., Medrano, J., & Carabellese, F. (2021). The clinician's duty to warn or protect: In the United States, England, Canada, New Zealand, France and Spain. In A. R. Felthous, & H. Saß (Eds.), *The Wiley international handbook on psychopathic disorders and the law* (2nd ed.). Hoboken, NJ: John Wiley & Sons. https://doi.org/10.1002/9781119159322.ch48.

Fong, E. (2016). *Aggressive behavior management: Acute care.* Joanna Briggs Institute EBP Database. JBI@Ovid, JBI1725.

Gimm, G., Chowdhury, S., & Castle, N. (2018). Resident aggression and abuse in assisted living. *Journal of Applied Gerontology, 37*(8), 947–964. https://doi.org/10.1177/0733464816661947.

Gunn, J. C. (2019). Extended suicide, or homicide followed by suicide. *Criminal Behaviour and Mental Health, 29*(4), 239–246. https://doi.org/10.1002/cbm.2125.

Haefner, J., Dunn, I., & McFarland, M. (2021). A quality improvement project using verbal de-escalation to reduce seclusion and patient aggression in an inpatient psychiatric unit. *Issues in Mental Health Nursing, 42*(2), 138–144. https://doi.org/10.1080/01612840.2020.1789784.

Lavigne, J. L., Portwood, S. G., Warren-Findlow, J., & Brunner Huber, L. R. (2017). Pediatric inpatient nurses' perceptions of child maltreatment. *Journal of Pediatric Nursing, 34*, 17–22. https://doi.org/10.1016/j.pedn.2017.01.010.

Lim, E., Wynaden, D., & Heslop, K. (2019). Changing practice using recovery-focused care in acute mental health settings to reduce aggression: A qualitative study. *International Journal of Mental Health Nursing, 28*(1), 237–246. https://doi.org/10.1111/inm.12524.

Lizarondo, L. (2016). *Evidence summary. Aggression in the elderly with dementia: Non-pharmacological interventions.* Joanna Briggs Institute EBP Database. JBI@Ovid, JBI1527.

Lockertsen, Ø., Varvin, S., Færden, A., & Vatnar, S. K. B. (2021). Short-term risk assessments in an acute psychiatric inpatient setting: A re-examination of the brøset violence checklist using repeated measurements—Differentiating violence characteristics and gender. *Archives of Psychiatric Nursing, 35*(1), 17–26. https://doi.org/10.1016/j.apnu.2020.11.003.

Lucya, V., Hadiyani, W., & Juniarni, L. (2019). Effectiveness of progressive relaxation therapy among clients with risk of violence behavior in Indonesia. *KnE Life Sciences, 4*(13), 342–348. https://doi.org/10.18502/kls.v4i13.5264.

Makaroun, L. K., Bachrach, R. L., & Rosland, A. M. (2020). Elder abuse in the time of COVID-19-increased risks for older adults and their caregivers. *American Journal of Geriatric Psychiatry, 28*(8), 876–880. https://doi.org/10.1016/j.jagp.2020.05.017.

Masa'Deh, R., Masadeh, O., Jarrah, S., AlAzzam, M., & Alhalaiqa, F. (2020). Effect of aggression management training on perceived stress levels of nurses working in mental health care settings in Jordan. *Journal of Psychosocial Nursing and Mental Health Services, 58*(10), 32–38. https://doi.org/10.3928/02793695-20200817-03.

Moola, S. (2017). *Evidence summary. Self-harm (inpatient mental health ward): Assessment, prevention, and treatment.* The Joanna Briggs Institute EBP Database. JBI@Ovid, JBI18050.

Olver, M. E., Marshall, L. E., Marshall, W. L., & Nicholaichuk, T. P. (2020). A long-term outcome assessment of the effects on subsequent reoffense rates of a prison-based CBT/RNR sex offender treatment program with strength-based elements. *Sexual Abuse, 32*(2), 127–153. https://doi.org/10.1177/1079063218807486.

Podubinski, T., Lee, S., Hollander, Y., & Daffern, M. (2017). Patient characteristics associated with aggression in mental health units. *Psychiatry Research, 250*, 141–145. https://doi.org/10.1016/j.psychres.2017.01.078.

Pullen, L., Modrcin, M. A., McGuire, S. L., Lane, K., Kearnely, M., & Engle, S. (2015). Anger in adolescent communities: How angry are they? *Pediatric Nursing, 41*(3), 135–140.

Ray, R., Perkins, E., Roberts, P., & Fuller, L. (2017). The impact of nursing protocols on continuous special observation. *Journal of the American Psychiatric Nurses Association, 23*(1), 19–27. https://doi.org/10.1177/1078390316668993.

Reidy, D. E., Holland, K. M., Cortina, K., Ball, B., & Rosenbluth, B. (2017). Evaluation of the expect respect support group program: A violence prevention strategy for youth exposed to violence. *Preventive Medicine, 100*, 235–242. https://doi.org/10.1016/j.ypmed.2017.05.003.

Shepherd, S. M., & Willis-Esqueda, C. (2018). Indigenous perspectives on violence risk assessment: A thematic analysis. *Punishment & Society, 20*(5), 599–627. https://doi.org/10.1177/1462474517721485.

Souza Marques, E., Leite de Moraes, C., Hasselmann, M. H., Ferreira Deslandes, S., & Reichenheim, M. E. (2020). A violência contra mulheres, crianças e adolescentes em tempos de pandemia pela COVID-19: Panorama, motivações e formas de enfrentamento. *Cadernos de Saúde Pública, 36*(4), e00074420. https://doi.org/10.1590/0102-311x00074420.

Vermeulen, J. M., Doedens, P., Boyette, L. L. N. J., Spek, B., Latour, C. H. M., & de Haan, L. (2019). "But I did not touch nobody!"—patients' and nurses' perspectives and recommendations after aggression on psychiatric wards—A qualitative study. *Journal of Advanced Nursing, 75*(11), 2845–2854. https://doi.org/10.1111/jan.14107.

Wood, L., Baumler, E., Schrag, R. V., et al. (2021). "Don't know where to go for help": Safety and economic needs among violence survivors during the COVID-19 pandemic. *Journal of Family Violence* [Online ahead of print]. https://doi.org/10.1007/s10896-020-00240-7.

Zarling, A., Bannon, S., & Berta, M. (2019). Evaluation of acceptance and commitment therapy for domestic violence offenders. *Psychology of Violence, 9*(3), 257–266. https://doi.org/10.1037/vio0000097.

V

Risk for Self-Directed Violence

Domain 11 Safety/protection Class 3 Violence

Kathleen L. Patusky, PhD, MA, RN, CNS, and Mamilda Robinson, DNP, APN, PMHNP-BC

NANDA-I

Definition

Susceptible to behaviors in which an individual demonstrates that he or she can be physically, emotionally, and/or sexually harmful to self.

Risk Factors

Behavioral cues of suicidal intent; conflict about sexual orientation; conflict in interpersonal relations; employment concern; engagement in autoerotic sexual acts; inadequate personal resources; social isolation; suicidal ideation; suicidal plan; verbal cues of suicidal intent

At-Risk Population

Individuals aged 15-19 years; individuals aged ≥45 years; individuals in occupations with high suicide risk; individuals with history of multiple suicide attempts; individuals with pattern of difficulties in family background

Associated Conditions

Mental health issues; physical health issues; psychological disorder

NOC (Nursing Outcomes Classification)

Refer to care plans for Risk for **Suicide**, **Self-Mutilation,** and Risk for **Self-Mutilation.**

Client Outcomes

Client Will (Specify Time Frame)

- Stop all forms of abuse/violence to self (physical, self-injurious emotional, sexual; neglect)
- Refrain from self-deprecation
- Identify factors contributing to abusive/self-injurious behavior
- Demonstrate impulse control or state feelings of control
- Identify impulsive behaviors
- Identify precursors to impulsive actions
- Identify consequences of impulsive actions to self
- Avoid high-risk environments and situations
- Identify and talk about feelings; express anger appropriately
- Communicate needs appropriately
- Demonstrate self control
- Use alternative coping mechanisms for stress
- Obtain and follow through with counseling

Client (and Children if Applicable) Will

- Have safe plan for leaving situation
- Resolve depression or traumatic response

Parent/Caregiver Will

- Monitor social/play contacts
- Provide supervision and nurturing environment
- Intervene to prevent high-risk social behaviors

NIC (Nursing Interventions Classification)

Suggested NIC Interventions

Abuse Protection Support; Anger Control Assistance; Behavior Management; Calming Technique; Coping Enhancement; Crisis Intervention; Mood Management; Dementia Management; Distraction; Environmental Management: Violence Prevention; Physical Restraint; Seclusion; Substance Use Prevention

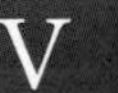

Example NIC Activities Environmental Management: Violence and Self-Harm Prevention

Remove self from the vicinity of a violent or potentially violent client; Provide ongoing surveillance of all children's access areas to maintain child's safety and therapeutically intervene as needed

Nursing Interventions and *Rationales*

- Assess with suicide-screening tools as a part of a comprehensive clinical practice. Such tools can be helpful predictors of future self-harm. **EBN:** *Clients with an increased risk for suicide were 3 to 16 times more likely to attempt suicide and 7 to 25 times more likely to engage in self-directed violence over the next 12 months (Doran et al, 2016).*
- Screen clients for adverse childhood experiences (ACEs) and refer to ACE-informed services. **EB:** *A systematic review and meta-analysis found that risk for self-directed violence was very strong for individuals with at least 4 ACEs. Screening of adult clients for a history of ACEs can help both clients and professionals understand the underlying causes of health problems and enable better-informed treatment options (Hughes et al, 2017).*
- Assess the client's use of substances such as cigarettes, alcohol, and other drugs, and suggest monitoring and/or decreasing usage. **EB:** *Research suggests that substance use correlates to the likelihood of self-harm. There is an association between daily cigarette smoking and increased self-directed violence, therefore strategies should promote smoking cessation as well as the cessation of other substance misuse with the hopes of mitigating the risk of violence (Lewis et al, 2016). "Alcohol use disorder alone and drug use disorder(s) alone were both associated with significantly increased odds of committing self-directed, other-directed, and combined aggression" (Ghossoub et al, 2019).*
- Assess parental mental health history and recommend treatment for parents who suffer from psychiatric disease. Parental history of mental illness is a risk factor for self-harming behaviors, equally for males and females. **EB:** *Research shows that the risks for offspring suicide attempt were elevated across virtually the full spectrum of parental psychiatric disease. Incidence rate ratios were the most elevated for parental diagnoses of antisocial personality disorder, cannabis misuse, and for parental suicide attempt. Parental mood disorders conferred additional modest risk increases. A history of mental illness or suicide attempt in both parents was associated with twice the risks (Mok et al, 2016).*
- Place the client on the appropriate precaution monitoring and observation protocol. **EBN:** *A nursing study of continuous client monitoring found that the addition of a protocol designed to prevent violent and impulsive behavior significantly reduced the number of continuous monitoring hours (Ray et al, 2017).*
- ▲ Refer the client to dialectical behavior therapy (DBT). **EB:** *A meta-analysis found that DBT reduced self-directed violence (d = −.324, 95% CI = −.471 to −.176), and reduced frequency of psychiatric crisis services (DeCou, Comtois, & Landes, 2019).*
- ▲ Refer the client to an emergency department for monitoring and/or surveillance. **EB:** *Clients who are prone to self-harm and self-directed violence can be closely monitored in the emergency department for safety (Zwald et al, 2020).*

Pediatric

- Assess levels of violence in the home environment, and if necessary, take steps to decrease aggression in the family. **EBN/EB:** *High levels of self-harm were reported by youth witnessing and experiencing family aggression. (Zhang et al, 2015).*
- Discuss the client's experience in school, as students who feel unconnected to school, are unhappy at school, or feel that teachers are unfair may be more likely to self-harm in the future. **EB:** *Identification of those at risk of self-harm will enable preventive measures (Kidger et al, 2015).*
- Review the client's experience online, because victims—and also, but to a lesser extent, perpetrators—of cyberbullying have a greater incidence of self-harm. **EB:** *Individuals who are cyberbullied are at a greater risk than nonvictims of both self-harm and suicidal behaviors (John et al, 2018).*
- Investigate the use of cell phone applications to address and monitor self-harming tendencies. **EB:** *BlueIce is an app developed specifically for adolescents, and the "outcome data" are "encouraging" as a means to prevent self-harm (Tingley, Greenhalgh, & Stallard, 2020).*

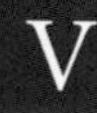

Geriatric

- Conduct a comprehensive assessment, reviewing previous mental and physical disease diagnoses. **EB:** *A study found that previous mental health diagnoses were twice as prevalent and previous physical health conditions were 20% higher in the self-harm cohort compared with the comparison cohort (Morgan et al, 2018).*
- Closely monitor medication prescribing and dosage in this population. Provide medication education and discuss alternatives to avoid potential adverse situations. **EB:** *Older clients are often prescribed antidepressants, and some correlate more closely with self-harm (Morgan et al, 2018).*

Client/Family Teaching and Discharge Planning

- Teach clients about healthy sleep patterns. EB: *Adequate education on sleep hygiene should be provided to client and family. The COVID-19 pandemic has had an impact on sleep-wake cycles, thus proper hygiene is warranted (Courtet et al, 2020).*
- Involve family members in the care of geriatric clients, whose incidents of self-harm may indicate distress that cannot easily be expressed in words. EB: *Research has shown that in individuals 80 years or older, family member's involvement and support is highly significant (Wand et al, 2018).*

REFERENCES

Courtet, P., Olié, E., Debien, C., & Vaiva, G. (2020). Keep socially (but not physically) connected and carry on: Preventing suicide in the age of COVID-19. *Journal of Clinical Psychiatry*, *81*(3). https://doi.org/10.4088/JCP.20com13370.

DeCou, C. R., Comtois, K. A., & Landes, S. J. (2019). Dialectical behavior therapy is effective for the treatment of suicidal behavior: A meta-analysis. *Behavior Therapy*, *50*(1), 60–72. https://doi.org/10.1016/j.beth.2018.03.009.

Doran, N., De Peralta, S., Depp, C., et al. (2016). The validity of a brief risk assessment tool for predicting suicidal behavior in veterans utilizing VHA mental health care. *Suicide and Life-Threatening Behavior*, *46*(4), 471–485. https://doi.org/10.1111/sltb.12229.

Ghossoub, E., Adib, S. M., Maalouf, F. T., Fuleihan, G. E. H., Tamim, H., & Nahas, Z. (2019). Association between substance use disorders and self- and other-directed aggression: An integrated model approach. *Aggressive Behavior*, *45*(6), 652–661. https://doi.org/10.1002/ab.21859.

Hughes, K., Bellis, M. A., Hardcastle, K. A., et al. (2017). The effect of multiple adverse childhood experiences on health: A systematic review and meta-analysis. *The Lancet Public Health*, *2*(8), e356–e366. https://doi.org/10.1016/S2468-2667(17)30118-4.

John, A., Glendenning, A. C., Marchant, A., et al. (2018). Self-harm, suicidal behaviours, and cyberbullying in children and young people: Systematic review. *Journal of Medical Internet Research*, *20*(4), e129. https://doi.org/10.2196/jmir.9044.

Kidger, J., Heron, J., Leon, D. A., Tilling, K., Lewis, G., & Gunnell, D. (2015). Self-reported school experience as a predictor of self-harm during adolescence: A prospective cohort study in the south west of england (ALSPAC). *Journal of Affective Disorders*, *173*, 163–169. https://doi.org/10.1016/j.jad.2014.11.003.

Lewis, A. S., Oberleitner, L. M. S., Morgan, P. T., Picciotto, M. R., & McKee, S. A. (2016). Association of cigarette smoking with interpersonal and self-directed violence in a large community-based sample. *Nicotine & Tobacco Research*, *18*(6), 1456–1462. https://doi.org/10.1093/ntr/ntv287.

Mok, P. L. H., Pedersen, C. B., Springate, D., et al. (2016). Parental psychiatric disease and risks of attempted suicide and violent criminal offending in offspring. *JAMA Psychiatry*, *73*(10), 1015–1022. https://doi.org/10.1001/jamapsychiatry.2016.1728.

Morgan, C., Webb, R. T., Carr, M. J., et al. (2018). Self-harm in a primary care cohort of older people: Incidence, clinical management, and risk of suicide and other causes of death. *The Lancet Psychiatry*, *5*(11), 905–912. https://doi.org/10.1016/s2215-0366(18)30348-1.

Ray, R., Perkins, E., Roberts, P., & Fuller, L. (2017). The impact of nursing protocols on continuous special observation. *Journal of the American Psychiatric Nurses Association*, *23*(1), 19–27. https://doi.org/10.1177/1078390316668993.

Tingley, J., Greenhalgh, I., & Stallard, P. (2020). Technology matters: BlueIce–using a smartphone app to beat adolescent self–harm. *Child and Adolescent Mental Health*, *25*(3), 192–194. https://doi.org/10.1111/camh.12397.

Wand, A. P. F., Peisah, C., Draper, B., & Brodaty, H. (2018). Why do the very old self-harm? A qualitative study. *American Journal of Geriatric Psychiatry*, *26*(8), 862–871. https://doi.org/10.1016/j.jagp.2018.03.005.

Zhang, W., Finy, M. S., Bresin, K., & Verona, E. (2015). Specific patterns of family aggression and adolescents' self- and other-directed harm: The moderating role of personality. *Journal of Family Violence*, *30*(2), 161–170. https://doi.org/10.1007/s10896-014-9662-x.

Zwald, M. L., Holland, K. M., Annor, F. B., et al. (2020). Syndromic surveillance of suicidal ideation and self-directed violence—United States, January 2017–December 2018. *MMWR. Morbidity and Mortality Weekly Report*, *69*(4), 103–108. https://doi.org/10.15585/mmwr.mm6904a3.

Impaired Walking **Domain 4 Activity/rest Class 2 Activity/exercise**

Wendie A. Howland, MN, RN-BC, CRRN, CCM, CNLCP, LNCC

NANDA-I

Definition

Limitation of independent movement within the environment on foot.

Defining Characteristics

Difficulty ambulating on decline; difficulty ambulating on incline; difficulty ambulating on uneven surface; difficulty ambulating required distance; difficulty climbing stairs; difficulty navigating curbs

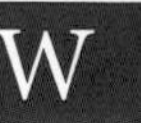

Related Factors

Altered mood; environmental constraints; fear of falling; inadequate knowledge of mobility strategies; insufficient muscle strength; insufficient physical endurance; neurobehavioral manifestations; obesity; pain; physical deconditioning

Associated Conditions

Cerebrovascular disorders; impaired postural balance; musculoskeletal impairment; neuromuscular diseases; vision disorders

NOC (Nursing Outcomes Classification)

Suggested NOC Outcomes

Ambulation, Mobility

Example NOC Outcome with Indicators

Ambulation as evidenced by the following indicators: Walks with effective gait/Walks at moderate pace/Walks up and down steps/Walks moderate distance. (Rate the outcome and indicators of **Ambulation:** 1 = severely compromised, 2 = substantially compromised, 3 = moderately compromised, 4 = mildly compromised, 5 = not compromised [see Section I].)

Client Outcomes/Goals

Client Will (Specify Time Frame)

- Demonstrate optimal independence and safety in walking
- Demonstrate the ability to direct others on how to assist with walking
- Demonstrate the ability to use and care for assistive walking devices properly and safely

NIC (Nursing Interventions Classification)

Suggested NIC Intervention

Exercise Therapy: Ambulation

Example NIC Activities—Exercise Therapy: Ambulation

Assist client to use footwear that facilitates walking and prevents injury; Encourage to sit in bed, on side of bed ("dangle"), or in chair, as tolerated

Nursing Interventions and *Rationales*

- Progressive mobilization as tolerated (gradually raising head of bed [HOB], sitting in reclined chair, standing, with assistance). Progressing mobility gradually from bed rest to increased sit-to-stand times to short-distance walking and timed testing can result in shorter admission stays and time to recovery (Snow, 2019). See also the care plan for Impaired Physical **Mobility.**
- Consider and monitor for side effects of prescribed hydration and medications; medical diagnosis, physical condition; length of immobility contributing to orthostatic hypotension; and/or if lightheadedness, dizziness, syncope, or unexplained falls occur. EB: *Orthostatic hypotension is highly prevalent in clients with a number of neurogenic and nonneurogenic conditions, associated medications, and antihypertensive drugs (Biswas, Karabin, & Turner, 2019).*
- ▲ Assess for orthostatic hypotension if systolic pressure falls 15 mm Hg or diastolic pressure falls 7 mm Hg from sitting to standing within 3 minutes. If this occurs, replace client in bed and notify prescriber. Evaluation of change in heart rate can be useful to determine if orthostatic hypotension could be neurogenic. EB: *Orthostatic hypotension increases fall risk (Biswas, Karabin & Turner, 2019).*
- Apply thromboembolic deterrent (TED) stockings and/or elastic leg wraps as prescribed; raise HOB slowly in small increments to sitting, have client move feet/legs up and down, and then stand slowly; avoid prolonged standing. Movement enhances venous return, improving cardiac output and decreasing syncope.

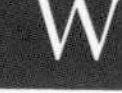

- Assess for cognitive, neuromuscular, and sensory deficits that will affect safety when walking (e.g., stroke, diabetic neuropathy, history of falls).
- ▲ Take pulse rate/rhythm, respiratory rate, and pulse oximetry before walking clients, and reassess within 5 minutes of walking, then ongoing as needed. If abnormal, have the client sit for 5 minutes, then remeasure. If still abnormal, walk clients more slowly and with more help or for a shorter time, or notify physician. If

uncontrolled diabetes/angina/arrhythmias/tachycardia (100 beats per minute or more) or resting systolic blood pressure at or above 200 mm Hg or diastolic blood pressure at or above 110 mm Hg occurs, do not initiate walking exercise. Refer to the care plan Decreased **Activity** Tolerance.

- ● Assist clients to apply orthosis, immobilizers, splints, braces, and compression stockings as prescribed before walking.
- ● Eat frequent small, low-carbohydrate meals. Low-carbohydrate meals help prevent postprandial hypotension.
- ● Reinforce correct use of prescribed mobility devices, and remind clients of weight-bearing restrictions.
- ● Emphasize the importance of wearing properly fitting, low-heeled shoes with nonskid soles and socks/hose and of seeking medical care for foot pain or problems with abnormal toenails, corns, calluses, or diabetes. Refer to podiatric consultation if indicated.
- ▲ Use a snug gait belt with handles and assistive devices while walking clients, as recommended by the physical therapist. EB: *A gait belt should be applied before and during all ambulation and functional gait activities; it should be applied securely around the waist and held firmly. Do not rely on clothing for a safe grip (Tang et al, 2018).*
- ● Walk clients frequently with an appropriate number of people; have one team member state short, simple motor instructions. EB: *Standing/weight-bearing benefits gut motility, spasticity, and respiratory/bowel/bladder function and promotes muscle stretching (Tang et al, 2018).*
- ● Cue and manually guide clients with neglect as they walk. *Prevents clients bumping into objects/people.*
- ● Document the number of helpers, level of assistance (e.g., maximum, standby), type of assistance, and devices needed in communication tools (e.g., plan of care, client room signage, verbal report).

Special Considerations: Lower Extremity Amputation

- ▲ Consult with physical therapist for best practices for postoperative mobilization for the individual case. In most cases, a prosthesis will not be fitted until wound healing occurs.
- ● Recognize that ambulation with a prosthesis is more labor-intensive than with a native limb. EB: *Allow for slower walking speed and monitor for fatigue with any person with a new or old amputation (Myers & Chauvin, 2021).*
- ● Teach clients the importance of avoiding prolonged hip and knee flexion. If contractures occur, they will affect prosthesis fit and function and ability to achieve a more normal gait. EB: *Limit amount of time the client is permitted to sit to no more than 40 minutes of each hour. Ensure that when client sits, stands, or is recumbent, the hip and knee are in extension and periodic prone lying is recommended (Myers & Chauvin, 2021).*

Geriatric

- ▲ Assess for swaying, poor balance, weakness, and fear of falling while elders stand/walk using an objective fall-risk tool if possible. If present, implement fall protection precautions and refer for physical therapy evaluation and recommendations (Thiamwong et al, 2020).
- ▲ Review medications for polypharmacy (more than five drugs) and medications that increase the risk of falls, including sedatives, antidepressants, and drugs affecting the central nervous system. EB: *Consult with pharmacist as part of polypharmacy assessment (Nguyen, Wong, & Ciummo, 2020).*
- ● Encourage tai chi, physical therapy, or another exercise for balance, gait, and strength training in group programs or at home.
- ● Recommend vision assessment and consideration for cataract removal if needed.

Home Care

- ✱ Establish a support system for emergency and contingency care (e.g., wearable medical alert alarm, Internet-connected smart speaker; notify local emergency medical services [EMS] of potential need). Impaired walking may be life-threatening during a crisis (e.g., fall, fire, orthostatic episode).
- ● Assess for and modify any barriers to walking in the home environment.
- ▲ Use a standardized tool to assess need for referral for occupational therapist (OT) or physical therapist (PT). If indicated, refer to OT/PT for home assessment and evaluation for home assessment for barriers, individualized strength, balance retraining, an exercise plan, and environmental modifications for safety (Tan et al, 2021).
- ▲ Refer to home health services for support and assistance with activities of daily living (ADLs).

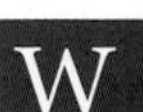

Client/Family Teaching and Discharge Planning

- • Teach clients to check ambulation devices weekly for cracks, loose nuts, or worn tips and to clean dust and dirt on tips.
- • Teach diabetics that they are at risk for foot ulcers and teach them preventive interventions. See care plan for Risk for Ineffective Peripheral **Tissue Perfusion.**
- ▲ Instruct clients at risk for osteoporosis or hip fracture to bear weight, walk, engage in resistance exercise (with appropriate adjustments for conditions), ensure good nutrition (especially adequate intake of calcium and vitamin D), drink milk, stop smoking, monitor alcohol intake, and consult a physician for appropriate medications.

REFERENCES

Biswas, D., Karabin, B., & Turner, D. (2019). Role of nurses and nurse practitioners in the recognition, diagnosis, and management of neurogenic orthostatic hypotension: A narrative review. *International Journal of General Medicine*, *12*, 173–184. https://doi.org/10.2147/IJGM.S170655.

Myers, M., & Chauvin, B. J. (2021). *Above the knee amputations.* StatPearls [Internet]. Treasure Island, FL: StatPearls Publishing. Retrieved from https://www.ncbi.nlm.nih.gov/books/NBK544350. [Accessed February 28, 2022].

Nguyen, T., Wong, E., & Ciummo, F. (2020). Polypharmacy in older adults: Practical applications alongside a patient case. *Journal for Nurse Practitioners*, *16*(3), 205–209. https://doi.org/10.1016/j.nurpra.2019.11.017.

Snow, T. M. (2019). *The use of a progressive mobility protocol to enhance patient outcomes* [dissertation]. Newark, DE: Delaware: University of Delaware, School of Nursing. https://udspace.udel.edu/handle/19716/25160.

Tan, E. S. Z., Mackenzie, L., Travassaros, K., & Yeo, M. (2021). A pilot study to investigate the feasibility of the modified Blaylock Tool for Occupational Therapy Referral (MBTOTR) for use by nurses in acute care. *Disability and Rehabilitation*, *43*(3), 414–422. https://doi.org/10.1080/09638288.2019.1624840.

Tang, R., Holland, M., Milbauer, M., et al. (2018). Biomechanical evaluations of bed-to-wheelchair transfer: Gait belt versus walking belt. *Workplace Health & Safety*, *66*(8), 384–392. https://doi.org/10.1177/2165079917749862.

Thiamwong, L., Sole, M. L., Ng, B. P., Welch, G. F., Huang, H. J., & Stout, J. R. (2020). Assessing fall risk appraisal through combined physiological and perceived fall risk measures using innovative technology. *Journal of Gerontological Nursing*, *46*(4), 41–47. https://doi.org/10.3928/00989134-20200302-01.

Wandering Domain 4 Activity/rest Class 3 Energy balance

Olga F. Jarrín, PhD, RN, Linda J. Hassler, DNP, RN, GCNS-BC, FGNLA, and Nishat S. Poppy, BSN, RN

NANDA-I

Definition

Meandering, aimless, or repetitive locomotion that exposes the individual to harm; frequently incongruent with boundaries, limits, or obstacles.

Defining Characteristics

Eloping behavior; frequent movement from place to place; fretful locomotion; haphazard locomotion; hyperactivity; locomotion interspersed with nonlocomotion; locomotion into unauthorized spaces; locomotion resulting in getting lost; locomotion that cannot be easily dissuaded; long periods of locomotion without an apparent destination; pacing; periods of locomotion interspersed with periods of nonlocomotion; persistent locomotion in search of something; scanning behavior; searching behavior; shadowing a caregiver's locomotion; trespassing

Related Factors

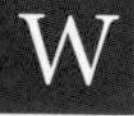

Altered sleep-wake cycle; desire to go home; environmental overstimulation; neurobehavioral manifestations; physiological state; separation from familiar environment

At-Risk Population

Individuals with premorbid behavior

Associated Conditions

Cortical atrophy; psychological disorder; sedation

NOC (Nursing Outcomes Classification)

Suggested NOC Outcomes

Safe Wandering; Safe Home Environment; Safe Health Care Environment; Surveillance: Safety; Caregiver Emotional Health; Caregiver-Client Relationship; Family Normalization: Autism Spectrum Disorder; Family Normalization: Dementia; Community Competence

Example NOC Outcome with Indicators

Safe Wandering as evidenced by the following indicators: Moves about without harming self or others/Sits for more than five minutes at a time/Paces a given route/Appears content in environment/Distracts easily/Can be redirected from unsafe activities. (Rate the outcome and indicators of **Safe Wandering:** 1 = never demonstrated, 2 = rarely demonstrated, 3 = sometimes demonstrated, 4 = often demonstrated, 5 = consistently demonstrated [see Section I].)

Client Outcomes

Client Will (Specify Time Frame)

- Remain safe and free from falls
- Maintain psychological well-being and reduce need to wander
- Reduce episodes of wandering in restricted areas/getting lost/elopement
- Maintain appropriate body weight
- Maintain physical activity and remain comfortable and free of pain

Caregiver Will (Specify Time Frame)

- Be able to explain interventions they can use to provide a safe environment for a care receiver who displays wandering behavior
- Develop strategies to reduce caregiver stress levels

NIC (Nursing Interventions Classification)

Suggested NIC Interventions

Dementia Management: Wandering; Anxiety Reduction; Area Restriction; Exercise Promotion; Environmental Management; Family Mobilization; Family Support; Normalization Promotion

Example NIC Activities—Dementia Management: Wandering

Include family members in planning, providing, and evaluating care to the extent desired; Identify usual patterns of wandering behavior; Alert neighbors and police about the person's wandering behavior; Provide a secure and safe place for wandering; Encourage physical activity during the daytime; Consider use of electronic devices (i.e., GPS tracking devices, door alarms) to locate person and monitor wandering.

Nursing Interventions and *Rationales*

- Provide safe and secure surroundings that deter and detect accidental elopements, using perimeter control devices (door alarms) or electronic tracking systems (including radiofrequency identification [RFID] tags, global positioning system [GPS] locator, smart watch, or cell phone application). EB: *Electronic tracking and tagging can provide a sense of safety for caregivers and encourage individual autonomy (Mangini & Wick, 2017).*
- Assess for physical distress or unmet needs (e.g., hunger, thirst, pain/discomfort, elimination needs). EBN: *Behavioral signs of unmet need for bowel movement or urination include anxiety, taking off/putting on clothes, restlessness, attempting to go elsewhere, scratching skin, repetitive behavior, and making strange sounds (Shih et al, 2015).*
- Assess for emotional or psychological distress, such as anxiety, fear, or feeling lost, considering the situated experience of the client. EB: *Restlessness and wandering may be understood as expressions of existential needs and feelings of anxiety, loneliness, and separation (Solomon & Lawlor, 2018).*

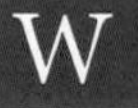

- Assess and document the pattern, rhythm, and frequency of wandering over time. EBN: *Wandering should be assessed with one or more of the following scales: the Revised Algase Wandering Scale (RAWS), or its version for community (RAWS-CV) and long-term care settings (RAWS-LTC) (Graham, 2017).*
- Obtain a psychosocial history from caregivers, including stress-coping behaviors. EBN: *A qualitative study of wandering behavior from the perspectives of older adults with mild to moderate dementia in long-term care discovered six themes: Walking as Enjoyable, Walking for Health Benefits, Walking as Purposeful, Walking as a Lifelong Habit, Walking as a Form of Socialization, and Walking to Be With Animals (Adekoya & Guse, 2019).*
- Observe the location and environmental conditions in which wandering is occurring and modify those that appear to provoke boundary transgression or unsafe wandering. EBN: *Simple environmental modifications that disguise a doorway to a potentially hazardous area may reduce entry into these spaces (MacAndrew et al, 2019).*
  - Assess the person's environment and advocate for appropriate modifications using a survey such as the Wayfinding Evidence-Based Checklist and Rating (WEBCAR) instrument (Benbow, 2013).
  - Use a full-length mirror in front of exit doors to deter elopement.
  - Use camouflage (a cloth panel, painted mural, or wall hanging) to cover doorknobs or locks (check fire safety code/policy and never obscure an emergency red EXIT sign).
  - Change the floor pattern in front of door that should not be opened to create a visual, subjective barrier (e.g., illusion of a step, black hole, or pit).
- Increase social interaction and offer structured activity and stress-reducing approaches, such as walking, exercise, music, massage, rocking chair, and activities using household methods and a prepared environment (e.g., watering plants, flower arranging, gardening, preparing meals, shining shoes, setting table, wrapping boxes, watercolor painting, sewing buttons, sorting objects, folding laundry, matching socks, stereognostic/mystery bags, doll therapy, puzzles, games, and crafts). EB: *Wandering in restricted areas was reduced 50% to 80% by the use of multimodal behavioral approaches and cognitive techniques such as problem-solving, behavioral rehearsal, and relaxation training (Nascimento Dourado & Laks, 2016).* EBN: *Low stress and mentally stimulating environments promote psychological well-being among people living with dementia in long-term care settings (Lee et al, 2017).*
- When using electronic tracking technologies, an approach emphasizing relationships, respect, and the individual needs of the person and caretaker is best suited to finding solutions that both protect and empower. EB: *Balancing the ethical principles of beneficence and respect in treating cognitively impaired persons goes beyond the necessary step of evaluating decision-making capacity to include partnering with families, caretakers, and cognitively impaired individuals who wander in a collaborative coalition of care (Yang & Kels, 2017).*
- Role model person-centered care and provide appropriate supervision, support, and education of direct-care staff. EBN: *Positive work environments for staff are associated with lower prevalence of client elopement, restlessness, and wandering behaviors compared with less positive work environments (Gu, 2015).*
- Help older adults find their rooms by placing signs with their names and portraits of themselves at a younger age next to the doorways. EB: *External memory aids in the form of signs with the person's name and portrait photograph can help people with dementia navigate their environment (Jensen & Padilla, 2017).*
- Provide a regularly scheduled and supervised exercise or walking program, particularly if wandering occurs excessively during the night or at times that are dangerous. EBN: *A structured physical activity program resulted in a statistically significant reduction in agitation and eloping behavior for individuals living with dementia in care homes (Traynor et al, 2018).*
- Refer to the care plan for **Caregiver** Role Strain. For clients with dementia, also see care plan for Chronic **Confusion.**

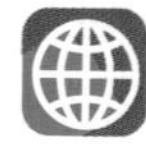

Multicultural

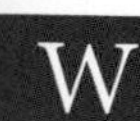

W

- Assess preferences for use of social services and family caregiver availability and willingness to provide care. EB: *A qualitative study in North Carolina found that service providers assumed that Latino families did not want to use government services and that they preferred to care for their elders; however, Latino participants expressed the need to work and not depend on family members for caregiving and financial support (Larson et al, 2017).*

Client/Family Teaching and Discharge Planning

- Teach caregivers about missing person resources such AMBER and Silver Alert public safety systems, MedicAlert Safe Return/Safely Home, Project Lifesaver, and related resources from the Alzheimer's

Association and National Autism Association; for example, the Autism Wandering Awareness Alerts Response and Education (AWAARE) Collaboration's Big Red Safety Box and Digital Toolkits for Caregivers (available in English and Spanish), First Responders, and Teachers. EB: *Similar to the AMBER alert emergency response system for missing children, the Silver alert system has been enacted in some but not all states (Gergerich & Davis, 2017).*

Home Care

- The previously mentioned interventions may be adapted for home care use.
- Help the caregiver set up a plan to reduce and manage wandering behavior, including a plan of action to use if the client elopes or is missing:
  - Assist the family to set up a plan of exercise for the client, including safe walking within appropriate geographic boundaries. EB: *Welfare concerns arise when freedom to walk outdoors is restricted; however, the risk of getting lost or injured must be minimized (Bantry White & Montgomery, 2016).*
  - Assess the home environment for modifications that will protect the client and prevent elopement. EB: *Monitoring and tracking devices are available to notify the caregiver of the client's movements, including door and bed alarms, and GPS locators worn as a necklace, bracelet/watch, shoe tag, and for clients with a cell phone can be supplemented with privacy setting for location sharing (Gu, 2015).*
  - Refer to supportive community and social services, such as an Area Office on Aging, the Alzheimer's Association, National Autism Association, home health care (psychiatric/geriatric nurse, occupational therapist, medical social worker), and companion or respite care to assist with the impact of caregiving for the wandering client.
  - Provide information about therapy dog/assistance dog resources. EB: *Therapy dogs provide a calming presence and may be trained to assist with safe walking and boundaries or to keep children with autism or adults with dementia from straying by circling them and barking to alert family members (O'Haire, 2017).*

REFERENCES

Adekoya, A. A., & Guse, L. (2019). Wandering behavior from the perspective of older adults with mild to moderate dementia in long-term care. *Research in Gerontological Nursing, 12*(5), 239–247. https://doi.org/10.3928/19404921-20190522-01.

Bantry White, E., & Montgomery, P. (2016). Supporting people with dementia to walkabout safely outdoors: Development of a structured model of assessment. *Health and Social Care in the Community, 24*(4), 473–484. https:// doi.org/10.1111/hsc.12226.

Benbow, W. (2013). Evidence-based checklist for wayfinding design in dementia care facilities. *Canadian Nursing Home, 24*(1), 4–10. Retrieved from http://wabenbow.com/wp-content/uploads/2014/02/Wayfinding-Compressed.pdf. [Accessed August 5, 2021].

Gergerich, E., & Davis, L. (2017). Silver alerts: A notification system for communities with missing adults. *Journal of Gerontological Social Work, 60*(3), 232–244. https://doi.org/10.1080/01634372.2017.1293757.

Graham, M. E. (2017). From wandering to wayfaring: Reconsidering movement in people with dementia in long-term care. *Dementia (London), 16*(6), 732–749. https://doi.org/10.1177/1471301215614572.

Gu, L. (2015). Nursing interventions in managing wandering behavior in patients with dementia: A literature review. *Archives of Psychiatric Nursing, 29*(6), 454–457. https//doi.org/10.1016/j.apnu.2015.06.003.

Jensen, L., & Padilla, R. (2017). Effectiveness of environment-based interventions that address behavior, perception, and falls in people with Alzheimer's disease and related major neurocognitive disorders: A systematic review. *American Journal of Occupational Therapy, 71*(5), 7105180030p1–7105180030p10. https://doi.org/10.5014/ajot.2017.027409.

Larson, K., Mathews, H. F., Torres, E., & Lea, C. S. (2017). Responding to health and social needs of aging Latinos in new-growth communities: A qualitative study. *BMC Health Services Research, 17*(1), 601. https://doi.org/10.1186/s12913-017-2551-2.

Lee, K. H., Boltz, M., Lee, H., & Algase, D. L. (2017). Is an engaging or soothing environment associated with the psychological well-being of people with dementia in long-term care? *Journal of Nursing Scholarship, 49*(2), 135–142. https://doi.org/10.1111/jnu.12263.

MacAndrew, M., Brooks, D., & Beattie, E. (2019). Nonpharmacological interventions for managing wandering in the community: A narrative review of the evidence base. *Health and Social Care in the Community, 27*(2), 306–319. https://doi.org/10.1111/hsc.12590.

Mangini, L., & Wick, J. Y. (2017). Wandering: Unearthing new tracking devices. *The Consultant Pharmacist, 32*(6), 324–335. https://doi.org/10.4140/TCP.n.2017.324.

Nascimento Dourado, M. C., & Laks, J. (2016). Psychological interventions for neuropsychiatric disturbances in mild and moderate Alzheimer's disease: Current evidences and future directions. *Current Alzheimer Research, 13*(10), 1100–1111. https://doi.org/10.2174/1567205013666160728143123.

O'Haire, M. (2017). Research on animal-assisted intervention and autism spectrum disorder, 2012-2015. *Applied Developmental Science, 21*(3), 200–216. https://doi.org/10.1080/10888691.2016.1243988.

Shih, Y. H., Wang, C. J., Sue, E. P., & Wang, J. J. (2015). Behavioral characteristics of bowel movement and urination needs in patients with dementia in Taiwan. *Journal of Gerontological Nursing, 41*(6), 22–29, quiz 30-31. https://doi.org/10.3928/00989134-20150414-01.

Solomon, O., & Lawlor, M. C. (2018). Beyond V40.31: Narrative phenomenology of wandering in autism and dementia. *Culture, Medicine and Psychiatry, 42*(2), 206–243. https://doi.org/10.1007/s11013-017-9562-7.

Traynor, V., Veerhuis, N., Johnson, K., Hazelton, J., & Gopalan, S. (2018). Evaluating the effects of a physical activity on agitation and wandering (PAWW) experienced by individuals living with a dementia in care homes. *Journal of Research in Nursing, 23*(2–3), 125–138. https://doi.org/10.1177/1744987118756479.

Yang, Y. T., & Kels, C. G. (2017). Ethical considerations in electronic monitoring of the cognitively impaired. *Journal of the American Board of Family Medicine, 30*(2), 258–263. https://doi.org/10.3122/jabfm.2017.02.160219.

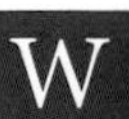

Index

A

Entries followed by *b, t,* or *f* indicate boxes, tables, or figures, respectively. **Boldface** entries indicate care plan titles. Page numbers in *italics* indicate care plan locations.